GET CONNECTED

To Content Updates, Study Tools, and More!

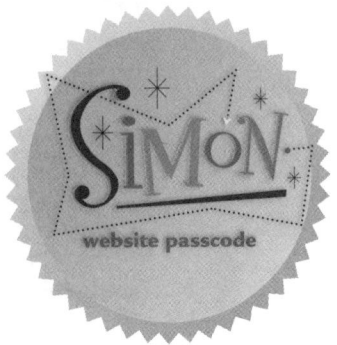

Meet SIMON

Saunders **I**nformation **M**anagement **O**nline **N**etwork

Congratulations! You now have access to SIMON for *Respiratory Care: Principles & Practice*, by Dean R. Hess, Neil R. MacIntyre, Shelley C. Mishoe, William F. Galvin, Alexander B. Adams, and Allan B. Saposnick!

Your free online website companion

sign on at:

http://www.harcourthealth.com/SIMON/Hess/

A website just for you as you learn the basics of respiratory care with *Respiratory Care: Principles & Practice*.

what you'll receive:

Whether you're a student, an instructor, or a respiratory therapist, you'll find information just for you. Things like:
● Content Updates ● Links to Related Publications
● WebLinks ● Author Information ● Frequently Asked Questions . . .
and more

plus:

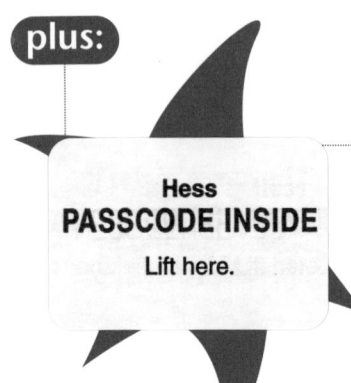

Hess
PASSCODE INSIDE
Lift here.

WebLinks

Use this passcode to access hundreds of active websites keyed specifically to the content of this book. The WebLinks are continually updated, with new ones added as they develop. **Peel only the top layer from the sticker on this page and register with the listed passcode.**

W.B. SAUNDERS COMPANY

Respiratory Care

Principles & Practice

Respiratory Care

Principles & Practice

Dean R. Hess, PhD, RRT, FAARC

Assistant Director of Respiratory Care
Massachusetts General Hospital
Assistant Professor of Anesthesia
Harvard Medical School
Boston, Massachusetts

Neil R. MacIntyre, MD, FAARC

Professor of Medicine
Respiratory Care Services
Duke University Medical Center
Durham, North Carolina

Shelley C. Mishoe, PhD, RRT, FAARC

Professor, Respiratory Therapy and
  Graduate Studies
Associate Dean, School of Allied Health
  Sciences
Medical College of Georgia
Augusta, Georgia

William F. Galvin, MSEd, RRT, CPFT

Assistant Professor, School of Allied
  Health Professions
Program Director, Respiratory Care
  Program
Administrative and Teaching Faculty,
  TIPS Program
Gwynedd Mercy College
Gwynedd Valley, Pennsylvania

Alexander B. Adams, MPH, RRT, FAARC

Senior Research Associate
Pulmonary Research
Regions Hospital
Saint Paul, Minnesota

Allan B. Saposnick, MS, RRT

Regional Director of Clinical Services
Health Care Solutions, Inc.
Sharon Hill, Pennsylvania

with 67 contributing authors and more than 800 illustrations

W.B. SAUNDERS COMPANY

A Harcourt Health Sciences Company
Philadelphia   London   New York   St. Louis   Sydney   Toronto

W.B. SAUNDERS COMPANY
A Harcourt Health Sciences Company

The Curtis Center
Independence Square West
Philadelphia, Pennsylvania 19106

Library of Congress Cataloging in Publication Data

Respiratory care: principles & practice / Dean R. Hess ... [et al.].

   p. cm.

   Includes bibliographical references and index.

   ISBN 0–7216–8077–1 (alk. paper)

   1. Respiratory therapy. I. Hess, Dean.

   RC735.I5 .R4755 2001

   616.2'0046--dc21   2001042921

Acquisitions Editor: Karen Fabiano
Developmental Editor: Mindy Copeland
Editorial Assistant: Ellen Wurm
Project Manager: Linda McKinley
Production Editor: Kristin Hebberd
Designer: Julia Ramirez
Cover Design: Julia Ramirez
Cover Illustration: Nadine Sokol

RESPIRATORY CARE: PRINCIPLES & PRACTICE   ISBN: 0–7216–8077–1

Printed in the United States of America

Last digit is print number: 9   8   7   6   5   4   3   2   1

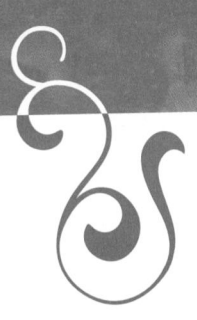

Contributors

Bekele Afessa, MD
Assistant Professor of Medicine
Mayo Medical Schools, Clinics and Foundation
Critical Care Services
Saint Mary's Hospital
Rochester Methodist Hospital
Rochester, Minnesota

Dennis H. Auckley, MD
Assistant Professor of Medicine
Case Western Reserve University
Medical Director, Sleep Disorders Program
Division of Pulmonary, Critical Care, and Sleep
    Medicine
MetroHealth Medical Center
Cleveland, Ohio

Thomas A. Barnes, EdD, RRT, FAARC
Professor of Cardiopulmonary Sciences
Director, Respiratory Therapy and Cardiovascular
    Technology Programs
Northeastern University
Boston, Massachusetts

Rajesh Bhagat, MBBS
Division of Pulmonary and Critical Care Medicine
Duke University Medical Center
Durham, North Carolina

Susan Blonshine, BS, RRT, RPFT, FAARC
Technical Director, Pediatric Pulmonary Function
    Laboratory
Michigan State University
East Lansing, Michigan;
Director
TechEd Consultants
Mason, Michigan

Richard D. Branson, BA, RRT, FAARC
Associate Professor of Surgery
University of Cincinnati
University Hospital
Cincinnati, Ohio

Pamela L. Bortner, MBA, RRT
Clinical Specialist/Case Manager
Department of Respiratory Care
The Toledo Hospital
Toledo, Ohio

Paul W. Burrowes, MD, FRCPC
Assistant Clinical Professor
University of Calgary
Deputy Director, Department of Diagnostic Imaging
Foothills Medical Centre
Calgary, Alberta, Canada

Robert S. Campbell, AS, RRT, FAARC
Instructor of Clinical Surgery
University of Cincinnati
Cincinnati, Ohio

Charles Carroll, EdD, RRT
Associate Vice President
Academic Affairs
Daytona Beach Community College
Daytona Beach, Florida

Christopher Carter, MD
Fellow in Pulmonary and Critical Care Medicine
University of Minnesota
Minneapolis, Minnesota

Robert L. Chatburn, BS, RRT, FAARC
Associate Professor of Pediatrics
Case Western Reserve University
Director of Respiratory Care
University Hospitals of Cleveland
Cleveland, Ohio

Francis C. Cordova, MD
Assistant Professor of Medicine
Temple University School of Medicine
Temple Lung Center
Philadelphia, Pennsylvania

Gerard J. Criner, MD
Professor of Medicine
Director, Pulmonary and Critical Care Medicine
Temple University
Philadelphia, Pennsylvania

Philip S. Crooke, PhD
Professor of Mathematics
Professor of Education
Vanderbilt University
Nashville, Tennessee

David A. Desautels, MPA, RRT, CHT
Consultant
Gainesville, Florida

Scott H. Donaldson, MD
Assistant Professor of Medicine
Division of Pulmonary and Critical Care Medicine
University of North Carolina
Chapel Hill, North Carolina

Thomas G. DiSalvo, MD, MPH
Assistant Professor of Medicine
Harvard Medical School
Massachusetts General Hospital
Boston, Massachusetts

Patricia English, MS, RRT
Senior Respiratory Therapist
ECMO Coordinator
Massachusetts General Hospital
Boston, Massachusetts

Bruce E. Estrem, BA, RRT
Perinatal/Pediatric Specialist
Adjuvant Faculty
The College of St. Catherine
Minneapolis, Minnesota;
Education Coordinator
Pediatric Home Service
Saint Paul, Minnesota

Michael A. Farrell, MB, FFRRCSI
Assistant Professor of Radiology
Mayo Clinic
Rochester, Minnesota

James B. Fink, MS, RRT, FAARC
Research Associate
Division of Pulmonary and Critical Care
Loyola University Chicago Stritch School of Medicine
Maywood, Illinois;
Fellow, Respiratory Science
Aerogen, Inc.
Sunnyvale, California

Michael Duane Frye, MD
Assistant Professor of Medicine
Medical University of South Carolina
Chief, Pulmonary Section
Ralph H. Johnson Veterans Hospital
Charleston, South Carolina

George W. Gaebler, MSEd, RRT
Cardiovascular Service Line Administrator
Administrative Director for Pulmonary Services
Upstate Medical University
University Hospital
Syracuse, New York

Andrew J. Ghio, MD
Assistant Consulting Professor of Medicine
Division of Pulmonary and Critical Care Medicine
Duke University Medical Center
Durham, North Carolina

Gul Gursel, MD
Associate Professor
Division of Respiratory Medicine
Consultant in Intensive Care Unit
Gazi University School of Medicine
Ankara, Turkey

Carl F. Haas, MLS, RRT, FAARC
Educational Coordinator
University Hospital Respiratory Care
Critical Care Support Services
University of Michigan Health System
Ann Arbor, Michigan

John E. Heffner, MD
Professor of Medicine
Associate Dean
Medical University of South Carolina
Charleston, South Carolina

Kathleen M. Hernlen, MBA, RRT
Instructor, School of Allied Health Sciences
Medical College of Georgia
Augusta, Georgia

John Hotchkiss
Assistant Professor of Medicine
University of Minnesota
Minneapolis, Minnesota;
Member, Biomathematics Study Group
Vanderbilt University
Nashville, Tennessee

Yuh-Chin T. Huang, MD
Adjunct Assistant Professor
Duke University Medical Center
Durham, North Carolina

David W. Hudgel, MD
Head, Section of Sleep Medicine
Pulmonary Division
Henry Ford Health System
Detroit, Michigan;
Professor of Medicine
Case Western Reserve University
Cleveland, Ohio

James M. Hurst, MD
Professor of Surgery
Vice-Chairman
Clinical Department of Surgery
University of Cincinnati Medical Center
Cincinnati, Ohio

For Susan, Terri, and Lauren.

DH

To my wife, Suzanne, and my children, Catherine, Neil, Douglas, Charles, Elizabeth, and Stephen.

NM

With love to my husband, Ken, and our sons, Wesley and Jeffrey, for all the weekends that I worked on this project rather than spent time with them. My family's understanding and encouragement make my work possible and my life meaningful.

SCM

To my students, perhaps my greatest teachers. To Gwynedd, for the supportive environment that nourished this endeavor. To the "big rocks" in my life—Denise, Ryan, Tim, and Connor— who endure my frequent absences and nurture my passions.

BG

I thank my wife, Debra, and my son, Zachary, for their patience during the preparation of this text. I also want to express my gratitude to the hundreds of respiratory therapists who have supported and encouraged me over the years.

AA

To Susan for your love, dedication, understanding, and help every day of our 35 years together.
To Nealla and Debra for making me a very proud father.

AS

Garry W. Kauffman, MPA, CHE, RRT
Columbia, Pennsylvania

Joseph B. Khoury, MD
Medical Director
Sleep Center
Centra Health
Lynchburg, Virginia

Atul Malhotra, MD, FRCPC
Instructor in Medicine
Pulmonary and Critical Care Unit
Massachusetts General Hospital and Harvard Medical
    School
Boston, Massachusetts

Steven C. Mason, BS, RRT
Senior Respiratory Therapist
Perinatal/Pediatric Specialist
Massachusetts General Hospital
Boston, Massachusetts

James R. Mault, MD
Assistant Professor
Division of Cardiothoracic Surgery
University of Colorado Health Sciences Center
Denver, Colorado

Robert A. May, MD, RRT
Department of Anesthesiology
Medical Director, Department of Respiratory Care
The Toledo Hospital
Medical Director, Respiratory Care Program
University of Toledo
Toledo, Ohio

Andrew McKibben, MD
Associate Director of Critical Care Medicine & ICU
The Miriam Hospital
Assistant Professor of Surgery and Medicine
Brown University School of Medicine
Providence, Rhode Island

Benjamin D. Medoff, MD
Instructor in Medicine
Harvard Medical School
Pulmonary and Critical Care Unit
Massachusetts General Hospital
Boston, Massachusetts

Timothy R. Myers, BS, RRT
Clinical Studies Coordinator
Case Western Reserve University
Administrative Manager, Pediatric Respiratory Care
Rainbow Babies and Children's Hospital
Cleveland, Ohio

Margaret J. Neff, MD, MSc
Senior Fellow/Acting Instructor
Division of Pulmonary and Critical Care
University of Washington
Harborview Medical Center
Seattle, Washington

Scott M. Palmer, MD, MHS
Associate in Medicine
Medical Director
Lung Transplant Program
Duke University Medical Center
Durham, North Carolina

Sanjay A. Patel, MD
Fellow, Division of Pulmonary, Allergy, and Critical Care
    Medicine
University of Pittsburgh Medical Center
Pittsburgh, Pennsylvania

Edward F. Patz, Jr., MD
Professor of Radiology
Duke University Medical Center
Durham, North Carolina

Rodney A. Radtke, MD
Duke University Medical Center
Durham, North Carolina

James E. Ramage, Jr., MD
Clinical Associate Professor of Medicine
Mercer University School of Medicine
Macon, Georgia;
Chairman, Division of Pulmonary Medicine
Memorial Health University Medical Center
Savannah, Georgia

Carl E. Ravin, MD
Professor and Chairman
Department of Radiology
Duke University Medical Center
Durham, North Carolina

Peggi Robart, MEd, RRT
Clinical Educator
MEDi-RENTS Respiratory Home Care
Boston, Massachusetts

Ray Ritz, BA, RRT, FAARC
Clinical Manager of Respiratory Care
Beth Israel Deaconess Medical Center
Boston, Massachusetts

Sharona Sachs, MD
Assistant Professor
State University of New York at Stony Brook School
    of Medicine
Director, Medical Step-Down Unit
Program Director, Lung Cancer Evaluation Center
Stony Brook University Hospital
Stony Brook, New York

Evelyn H. Schlenker, PhD
Professor
Division of Basic Biomedical Sciences
University of South Dakota School of Medicine
Vermillion, South Dakota

David R. Schwartz, MD
Attending Physician
Pulmonary and Critical Care Division
New York University
New York, New York

Frank C. Sciurba, MD
Associate Professor of Medicine
Division of Pulmonary, Allergy, and Critical Care
    Medicine
Director, Emphysema Research Center
University of Pittsburgh Medical Center
Pittsburgh, Pennsylvania

Robert L. Sheridan, MD
Associate Professor of Surgery
Harvard Medical School
Director of Trauma/Critical and Burn Care
Massachusetts General Hospital
Assistant Chief of Service
Shriners Hospital for Children
Boston, Massachusetts

Mark Simmons, MSEd, RPFT, RRT
Director, School of Respiratory Care
York College of Pennsylvania
York Hospital
York, Pennsylvania

Priscilla Simmons, EdD, RN, CS
Assistant Professor
School of Nursing
Penn State University
Hershey, Pennsylvania

Randy S. Smith, MPH, RD, LDN
Clinical Dietitian
Duke University Medical Center
Durham, North Carolina

Christine Solberg, PharmD, BCPS
Director of Pharmacy Programs
Blue Cross and Blue Shield of Minnesota
Prime Therapeutics
Eagan, Minnesota

Kenneth P. Steinberg, MD
Associate Professor of Medicine
University of Washington School of Medicine
Medical Director, Medical and Respiratory Intensive
    Care Unit
Harborview Medical Center
Seattle, Washington

Mary K. Stone, RRT
Senior Respiratory Care Practitioner
Regions Hospital
Saint Paul, Minnesota

Victor F. Tapson, MD
Associate Professor of Medicine
Division of Pulmonary and Critical Care Medicine
Duke University Medical Center
Durham, North Carolina

Andrew Wang, MD
Assistant Professor of Medicine
Duke University Medical Center
Durham, North Carolina

Bethany Weaver, DO
Senior Fellow Trainee, Infectious Diseases
University of Washington, Department of Medicine
Harborview Medical Center
Seattle, Washington

Robert R. Weilacher, BS, RRT
Chief Executive Officer
Convalescent Aids
Palestine, Texas

James R. Yankaskas, MD
Professor of Medicine
Pulmonary and Critical Care Medicine
The University of North Carolina
Medical Director, Medical and Respiratory Intensive
    Care Units
University of North Carolina Hospitals
Chapel Hill, North Carolina

Foreword

"παντα ρει: All Things Change"
(Attributed to the Greek philosopher, Heraclitus, ca. 540-480 BC)

While the oft-quoted statement by Heraclitus on change as a constant in our world may not have created an enduring philosophy, it is well applied to health care delivery in the twentieth century in this country. Perhaps no profession of health care better exemplifies the constancy of change than respiratory therapy. The first edition of *Respiratory Care: Principles & Practice,* not only reflects such change, but it in fact also embodies that change.

The birth of respiratory therapy as a formal profession dates to 1947. However, the reality of respiratory *care* can be traced to developments in the physical and biologic sciences. In fact, it is not without merit to say that Harvey's understanding of the circulation formed a necessary if not sufficient basis for the management of cardiopulmonary disease. Certainly an immediate scientific precursor of respiratory care is the identification of oxygen by Priestley and Lavoisier in 1774 and 1775 and the therapeutic application of this life-supporting gas after World War I. The pace of change that brings respiratory therapy to its current state was fostered by a coincidence of several factors after World War II: (1) dissemination of medical techniques learned in war, (2) continual development of technology and techniques in combination with healthy funding of medical research, and (3) a generous system of payment to use the technology and procedures for medical care in the United States. In particular, the payment for health care, together with postwar scientific research, formed a synergism resulting in an explosion of medical capability. The profession of respiratory therapy was a manifestation of part of the development of medical care, and even in its beginnings reached beyond treatment and support of pulmonary disease alone to support cardiac, trauma, and other types of patients.

Many of the techniques described in Part IV of this text (Respiratory Therapeutics) and Part V (Respiratory Disease Management) resulted from these factors and constituted the core of our expertise as respiratory care professionals from the late 1940s until the 1980s. Having personally participated in respiratory care for 30 years, I have seen the ongoing development of the profession, paralleling that in the other areas of medical care. From a limited selection of two or three bronchodilators, such as epinephrine, isoproterenol, and isoetharine at the beginning of the 1970s, we have pro-

gressed to a veritable menu of isomer-specific agents, short-acting agents, as well as slow but long-acting and quick but long-acting β-agonists. Neonatal ventilation today far surpasses our early attempts in the mid-1970s to support newborns weighing less than 1000 g.

The inevitability of change was manifested again in the 1980s and more intensely in the 1990s as a concern for the ever-increasing cost of health care and in calls for increased accountability to document "quality, access, or effectiveness of care" (Mishoe and Hernlen, Chapter 3). The therapist of today must not only be an expert in the technology and procedures of patient care, but in a cost-contained environment must also be able to evaluate the need for care and assess the effective outcome of the care. This role demands far more than mere technical competency from the respiratory care practitioner. The ability to analyze a situation, synthesize an interpretation, and decide on appropriate actions are now essential skills.

The development in respiratory care is no longer merely a proliferation of drugs, procedures, and equipment, but also a change in mind-set and the way in which we practice caregiving. Now we must be able to decide whether care is needed, administer the care competently, and determine whether the care provided is in fact efficacious. Respiratory therapists must be able to think critically and solve problems. Other traits, not emphasized in the early decades of the profession, that have become valuable as changes have occurred in the U.S. medical system and in American society include the interpersonal skills necessary to work with a variety of people and specialties and the ability to effectively communicate one's knowledge to persons about their disease and care. In the complex and changing setting of twenty-first century medical care in the United States, communication and the ability to work well with others is absolutely essential.

The continual evolution in respiratory care practice is reflected in several parts of this text. Part I offers a more thorough presentation than is usually provided regarding professionalism, decision making, patient education, understanding and interpretation of the professional literature, medical economics, and information management. This information is necessary to prepare practitioners for today and hopefully for the future. With the role of the respiratory therapist as a thinking, assessing caregiver, the information contained in Part III on assessment forms the basis for the development and evaluation of respiratory care. Even in Part V, which discusses disease management, the pathophysiology is complemented and infused with assessment, decision making, critical thinking, and application of the therapeutic modalities available and described in Part IV.

Dean Hess, Neil MacIntyre, Shelley Mishoe, William Galvin, Alex Adams, and Allan Saposnick, all highly respected leaders in our profession, have assembled a text that not only reflects the change occurring in respiratory

care but also, perhaps more importantly, offers a tool to facilitate such changes. Those of us who practice and teach respiratory care are indebted to them and to all of the contributing authors for their dedication and expertise.

"You cannot step twice into the same river, for fresh waters are continually flowing on." (Heraclitus, Fragment 91,12)

Joseph L. Rau, PhD, RRT, FAARC
Cardiopulmonary Care Sciences
Georgia State University
Atlanta, Georgia

Quotations of Heraclitus: From Copleston F. A History of philosophy: Greece & Rome. Vol. I. Part I. Chapter 5. Garden City, NY: Image Books; 1960.

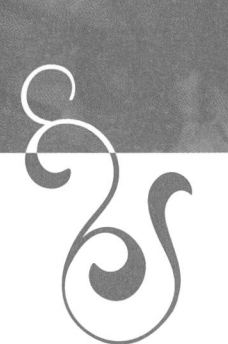

Preface

Why should we develop a new comprehensive textbook of respiratory care? First, the respiratory care profession has evolved considerably over the past 20 years. This book reflects current practice, both technically and professionally. Second, respiratory therapists are increasingly expected to function as consultants, an expectation that requires critical thinking skills, the ability to develop care plans, strong communication skills, patient education, and clinical leadership. For these reasons we have designed *Respiratory Care: Principles & Practice,* and the previously stated therapist roles are developed throughout. Our intent is for this to be the most comprehensive, up-to-date, readable, and student-friendly textbook of respiratory care available.

The book is a fresh synthesis of respiratory care and considers the professional tenets needed for respiratory care practice in the twenty-first century. We believe that it is a road map for the evolving role of the respiratory therapist. Part I covers the professional role of the respiratory therapist, including issues related to ethics, communication, decision making, patient education, reimbursement, documentation, and interpretation of the literature. Part II is a comprehensive review of the applied basic sciences as they relate to the practice of respiratory care. Part III covers all aspects of assessment of the patient with respiratory disease—an increasingly important aspect of the expanding role of the respiratory therapist. Part IV covers all the techniques and procedures included in the expanding armamentarium of the respiratory therapist. Part V focuses on management of the variety of diseases encountered by the respiratory therapist. Relevant aspects of the clinical practice guidelines of the American Association for Respiratory Care are included throughout the text.

Care of the adult, child, and newborn is addressed, as is respiratory care across the continuum of care.

We sought the best contributing authors to write these chapters. Many of them are not only experts in their assigned topics but also have extensive teaching experience. We encouraged all contributors to present a new synthesis of existing material infused with new ideas and perspectives. The result is a comprehensive yet refreshing coverage of the material that forms the basis for respiratory care practice. The contributor team consists of both respiratory therapists and physicians, underscoring the close working relationships between these clinicians in everyday practice. The entire book was edited in detail by the editor team to facilitate consistency in writing style.

I am indebted to many persons who helped realize this book. I am most grateful to my co-editors, who shared my vision and worked hard to make this project a success. I also thank all the contributing chapter authors for bringing new insights and up-to-date information to the text. I cannot thank enough the entire Harcourt Health Sciences team for their efforts in making this book a reality. In particular, Mindy Copeland and Kristin Hebberd worked unselfishly to bring this project to fruition. Mindy and Kristin brought a level of devotion and professional expertise to this project that went far beyond usual expectations.

So we present to you the fruits of our efforts. This editor team is committed to the evolution of respiratory care practice, and we all hope that this book contributes to the expanding role of the respiratory therapist as an essential member of the health care team.

Dean R. Hess

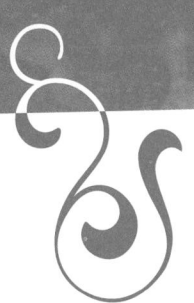

Contents

Respiratory Care

Principles & Practice

PART I

The Respiratory Care Profession

History of the Respiratory Care Profession

Robert R. Weilacher

CHAPTER OUTLINE

Significant Historic, Scientific, and Technologic Advances
Establishing Credibility
Licensure
Educational Considerations
Accreditation

National and State Credentialing
Professional Publications
Funding and Philanthropy
Medical Direction

OBJECTIVES

1. Explain the significant developments leading to the current practice of respiratory care in North America.
2. Describe the way in which professional societies affect the evolution of a profession.
3. Identify the various historical names of the professional associations for respiratory care.
4. Describe the roles of credentialing, medical directorships, professional publications, and funding in the evolution and growth of the respiratory care profession.
5. Explain the educational opportunities and considerations in respiratory care.
6. Describe the educational program accreditation throughout the history of respiratory care.
7. Discuss national and state credentialing of respiratory care professionals.
8. Describe the way in which the professional association for respiratory care meets its educational purposes.
9. Identify key individuals in the origins of respiratory care as a distinct health care profession.
10. Discuss the unique contributions of the respiratory care professional from a historical perspective.

KEY TERMS

American Association of Inhalation Therapists (AAIT)
American Association for Respiratory Care (AARC)
American Registry of Inhalation Therapists (ARIT)
American Respiratory Care Foundation (ARCF)

Certified Pulmonary Function Technologist (CPFT)
Certified Respiratory Therapist (CRT)
Clinical Simulation Examination (CSE)
Committee on Accreditation for Respiratory Care (CoARC)
Criterion-Referenced Validation Studies
Inhalation Therapy Association (ITA)

Medical Direction
National Board for Respiratory Care (NBRC)
Perinatal/Pediatric Respiratory Care Specialist
Registered Pulmonary Function Technologist (RPFT)
Registered Respiratory Therapist (RRT)

Although all of medical history influences the present and future of respiratory care, those events primarily since 1943 are particularly of interest. This chapter focuses on those events, as well as the North American model of practice of respiratory care, which varies considerably from practice elsewhere in the world.[1]

Contemporary respiratory care was established as a discrete health care discipline shortly after World War II (WWII). Unlike other medical professions, no single event describes the definitive moment of the profession's birth.

In the twentieth century, advances in medical science and technology shifted from Europe to North America.

The two world wars that decimated Europe and to a lesser degree, the Far East, left North America relatively unscathed. By the midpoint of the century the United States and Canada, with stable economies, viable technologic infrastructures, and abundant resources, were positioned to serve as the major socioeconomic support for a large part of the world. This dominance explains in part the unique character of the North American model.

Significant Historic, Scientific, and Technologic Advances

Historic, scientific, and technologic advances before 1943 that paved the way for the birth of respiratory care are beyond the scope of this book. However, some such advances, along with other notable events from more recent years, are summarized briefly in Table 1-1.[2,3]

TABLE 1-1

Historic Moments in the Evolution of Respiratory Therapy

Year	Event
1628	Blood circulation described (William Harvey)
1774	Oxygen "discovered" (Joseph Priestley)
1775	Oxygen described and named (Antoine-Laurent Lavoisier)
1800	Pneumatic Institute established in Bristol, England (Thomas Beddoes and James Watts)
1864	Full-body "iron lung" invented (Alfred F. Jones)
1886	Oxyhemoglobin dissociation curve constructed (Christian Bohr)
1895	Fractional distillation of liquid air performed (Karl von Linde)
1904	Process of oxygen and carbon dioxide transport described (Niels Bohr, Karl A. Hasselbalch, August Krogh)
1917	Logarithmic hydrogen ion activity (pH) described (Karl A. Hasselbalch)
1920	Oxygen therapy for individuals gassed in World War I described (John Barcroft)
1922	Modern therapeutic use of oxygen described (Alvin L. Barach)
1926	Oxygen tent developed (Alvin L. Barach)
1946	Inhalational Therapy Association (ITA) organized
1947	Inhalational Therapy Association incorporated; IPPB use described (Hurley L. Motley and colleagues)
1948	ITA name changed to Inhalation Therapy Association (vote on December 26, 1947)
1953	American College of Chest Physicians (ACCP) named official sponsor of ITA
1954	ITA name changed to American Association of Inhalation Therapists (AAIT); Medical Advisory Board formed
1955	First AAIT annual meeting held; first AAIT affiliate society formed: Illinois (Alpha) Chapter
1956	*Inhalation Therapy,* now *Respiratory Care,* established
1958	AAIT Code of Ethics adopted
1963	Board of Schools of Inhalation Therapy Technicians formed
1964	Canadian Society of Inhalation Therapy Technicians chartered by Canadian secretary of state
1966	AAIT House of Delegates formed; AAIT Editorial Board created
1967	AAIT name changed to American Association for Inhalation Therapy; MA-1 electronic adult ventilator marketed (V. Ray Bennett Corp., Kansas City, Kan.)
1969	Technician certification program begun; AAIT made member in National Health Council
1970	American Respiratory Care Foundation (American Association for Inhalation Therapy Foundation) incorporated; Joint Review Committee for Inhalation Therapy Education formed
1971	*Inhalation Therapy* journal renamed *Respiratory Care*
1972	AAIT executive offices opened in Dallas; AAIT now sponsored by American Thoracic Society
1973	AAIT name changed to American Association for Respiratory Therapy (AART)
1974	Conference on the Scientific Basis of Respiratory Therapy held; American Registry of Inhalation Therapists (ARIT) reorganized as National Board for Respiratory Therapy; AART specialty membership section formed
1976	AART Services Corporation formed; now restructured as Daedalus Enterprises, Inc.
1978	*AARTimes* monthly publication introduced
1982	First National Respiratory Therapy Week celebrated (November, 7 through 13, 1982)
1984	AART name changed to American Association for Respiratory Care (AARC)
1996	AARC Research Program established to sponsor research studies
1997	AARC now sponsored by National Association for Medical Direction of Respiratory Care (NAMDRC)
1998	Committee on Accreditation for Respiratory Care formed
1999	49 Clinical Practice Guidelines posted on AARC website
2000	*Respiratory Care* accepted into *Index Medicus*

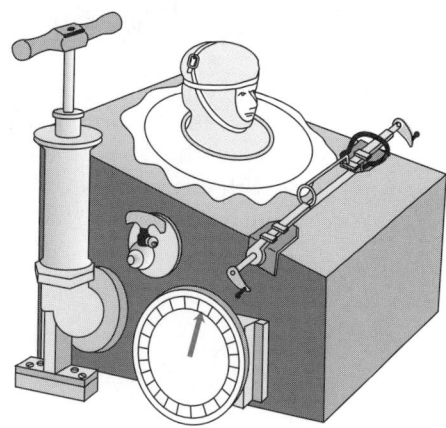
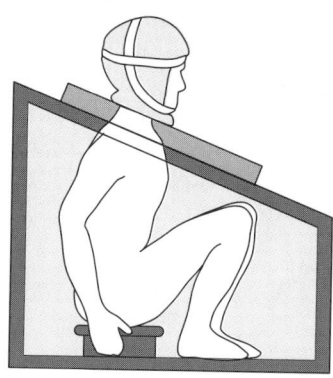

Figure 1-1 Alfred F. Jones' body-enclosing iron lung. (Modified from Emerson JH: The evolution of iron lungs. Cambridge, Mass: [private publication]; 1978.)

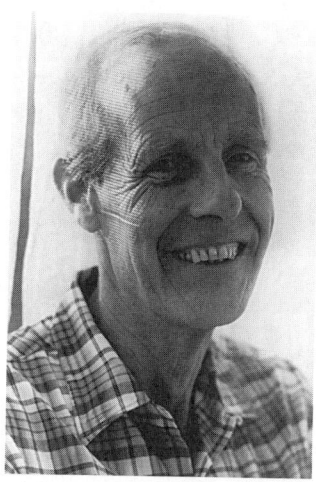

Figure 1-2 John Haven Emerson introduced the Emerson Respirator, which made mechanical ventilation practical because of its design, simplicity, and electric motor. (Courtesy J.H. Emerson Company, Cambridge, Mass.)

One of the most significant technologic advances was in response to the poliomyelitis epidemic in the 1930s. Poliomyelitis patients suffered from impaired or destroyed breathing capabilities and required mechanical ventilation. Such treatment was performed primarily through the use of negative-pressure tank ventilators later nicknamed "iron lungs."

Several physicians and scientists experimented with negative pressure, but Alfred F. Jones developed one of the first full-body iron lungs in 1864 (Figure 1-1). This device evolved into the Emerson respirator, developed by John Haven Emerson (Figure 1-2). With the increasing availability of electricity in urban areas, the Emerson respirator supplied a simply designed electric motor that hospitals could afford to answer the demand for respirators caused by the poliomyelitis epidemic.[4]

Another important advance came in 1895 with Karl von Linde's fractional distillation of liquefied air, which resulted in large quantities of relatively inexpensive oxygen, essentially a byproduct of nitrogen production. The efficacy of oxygen therapy was not clearly established, however, until the 1920s, spurred in part by John Barcroft's classification of anoxia (hypoxia) and description of his treatment modalities.[5,6] By the close of WWII, oxygen administration was available in virtually every hospital in the United States.

The world wars contributed significantly to the transition from oxygen therapy to inhalation therapy. WWII itself brought about three fundamental advances—(1) antibiotics, (2) demand breathing valves for combat pilots, and (3) nonrebreathing valves and masks for aviators.[7] Antibiotics reduced mortality associated with overwhelming infections and, in so doing, also greatly expanded thoracic surgical opportunities.[7]

ℛespiratory Recap

Leading Diseases in 1900
Heart failure
Shock
Pneumonia and pleurisy
Angina pectoris
Cerebrovascular disorders

The new therapies, such as antibiotics, vaccines, and insulin, coupled with war-proven technology in the civilian marketplace, placed growing demands on the health care community. A 1995 report noted that in 1900 the leading diseases were heart failure, shock, pneumonia and pleurisy, angina pectoris, and cerebrovascular disorders, all conditions necessitating respiratory care treatments.[7]

Oxygen demand valves, used by WWII combat aviators flying above 5000 meters, found a practical application in medicine by 1947.[8] These valves were marketed as intermittent positive pressure breathing (IPPB) devices with side-arm nebulizers. These early breathing devices were powered by large cylinders of compressed gas and could deliver bland aerosols, antibiotics, mucolytic agents, and bronchodilators. At the same time, the turning and ambulating of postsurgical patients to prevent pneumonia and other complications was gaining increased attention and importance. This growth and development marked the next phase in the history of respiratory care, gradually expanding the duties of oxygen technicians.

The availability of the famous B-L-B nonrebreathing mask used by WWII aviators that allowed for a simple, practical way to deliver a controlled percentage of oxygen further metamorphosed the respiratory therapist from an oxygen technician.[9] The inventors wrote the following in their patent application:

It is well known that a provision of inhalation apparatus which will be economical in the use of oxygen and which at the same time permits the administration of 100 per cent oxygen will open up a whole new field of oxygen therapy of great value in certain classes of cases…

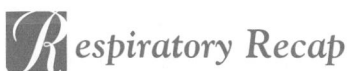 *espiratory Recap*

Origins of Inhalation Therapists

The first step in the metamorphosis of the respiratory therapist from an oxygen technician was the availability of the famous B-L-B nonrebreathing mask used by WW II aviators. In less than a decade the better-trained, more respected inhalation therapist replaced the oxygen technician.

Another contributing factor to the transition of inhalation therapy was the brief monograph, "Manual of Oxygen Therapy Techniques," written by Albert H. Andrews (Figure 1-3) in 1943. Andrews was a noted otolaryngologist from Chicago. He proposed that inhalation therapy departments should operate under the medical direction of an influential staff physician. The departmental architecture suggested in this monograph was copied across North America, contributing significantly to the beginnings of the profession.[10]

Edward R. Levine, a pioneer in pulmonary medicine, recounted the evolution of technology-driven respiratory care in his memoirs. As a young attending physician, Levine tried to involve resident physicians in his earliest efforts in caring for pulmonary patients, especially postsurgical ones. As he expressed it "…the results were uneven in quality." He wrote that nurses were somewhat better trained than physicians in bedside care but that they simply did not have the time to handle all the pulmonary patients.[11] Levine in turn organized an early inhalation ther-

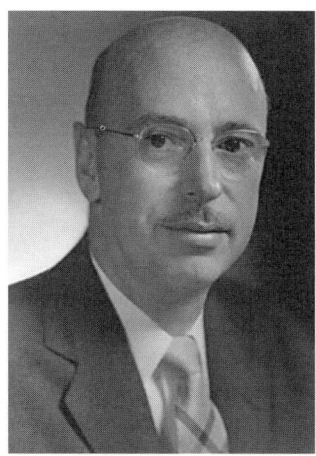

Figure 1-3 Albert H. Andrews, a noted otolaryngologist from Chicago, described the purpose and structure of the hospital-based oxygen service in 1943. (Courtesy American College of Chest Physicians, Chicago.)

apy program as part of a department of chest diseases he started in Chicago's Michael Reese Hospital in 1943. On-the-job trained (OJT) technicians were employed to manage the bedside care of postsurgical patients.

During the mid-1940s the oxygen therapy devices were heavy, bulky, and unwieldy, characteristics that created a significant problem. Hospital gas supply systems were multi-yoked, high-pressure cylinders. Consequently, strong men working in central supply or orderly departments were pressed into service to ensure that oxygen therapy was available on demand. These generally unappreciated oxygen orderlies, or oxygen technicians, were the direct ancestors of the modern respiratory therapist.

In less than a decade the somewhat more respected, better-trained inhalation therapist replaced the oxygen technician. The cause for this change was the realization that IPPB technology permitted practitioners to change various components of ventilation at will. The inhalation therapist could modify the administered pressure and the fraction (percent) of inspired oxygen, FIO_2, thus altering the inspiratory phase of ventilation.

In the following two decades a remarkable variety of mechanical respirators and ventilators became commercially available. The abundance of machines is testimony to the inventive skills of the engineers and their collaborating clinical practitioners. The marketing and distribution of the MA-1 adult ventilator (Bennett Respiration Products, Santa Monica, Calif.) in 1967 was an exciting advance.[12] This ventilator represented a class of simple, electrically driven devices capable of ventilating acutely ill individuals over a prolonged period with reasonable expectations that they would survive. These machines introduced complex electronic microprocessing, circuit boards, relays, photoelectric controls, potentiometers, and system monitoring cards.

Another newly applied technology, arterial blood gas (ABG) analysis, permitted the rapid and accurate measure-

$\mathcal{R}$*espiratory Recap*

Origins of Respiratory Care

Advances in medical science and technology shifting to North America
Manufacture of oxygen and oxygen therapy
Polio epidemic and the "iron lung"
Prevalence of cardiopulmonary diseases
Anesthesia and increased thoracic surgeries
World War II technology: antibiotics, demand breathing valves, and nonrebreathing masks
MA-1 and other electrical ventilators
Continual advances in technology and computers

ment of pH, P_{CO_2}, and P_{O_2}, allowing for the quantification of mechanical ventilation. Taken together, these were enormous advances that furthered fairly sophisticated control of respiration. *Respiratory* therapy now was being provided in contrast to the more primitive *inhalation* therapy.

Fortunately, the unending pressure of technologic development continues. This continuum of change has forged the present era, in which respiration must be considered in its three components—ventilation, diffusion, and perfusion—not simply as external respiration.

Establishing Credibility

Students in Chicago-area schools of nurse anesthesia, along with OJT inhalation therapy technicians from Michael Reese and Alexian Brothers hospitals, formed the nuclear group that organized the **Inhalation Therapy Association (ITA)** on July 13, 1946, at the University of Chicago Hospital.[12]

By early 1947, budgetary needs related to medical sponsorship, development of credentials, and national educational endeavors dictated a more formal organizational structure. On March 7, articles of incorporation were filed with the Illinois secretary of state to form the ITA. On April 5, 1947, the ITA was chartered, and the following purposes were stated in the articles of incorporation:

- To promote higher standards in methods and the professional advancement of members of the association
- To create mutual understanding and cooperation among the technician, physician, and all others working in the interest of individual or public health
- To advance the knowledge of inhalation therapy through institutes, lectures, and other means under the sponsorship of doctors of the Society of Anesthesia (currently the American Society of Anesthesiologists [ASA])

The incorporates of the ITA were George A. Kneeland, Richard E. Goss, Vincent T. McCue, Brother Roland Maher (who served as its first president), and Brother

Silverius Case. Professionally, Kneeland was a registered pharmacist; Maher and Case were nurse-anesthetists; McCue was an inhalation therapy department manager; and Goss was a manufacturer of vinyl oxygen tent canopies. The 59 members included nine physicians, a pharmacist, an attorney, seven nurse-anesthetists, and eight registered nurses.

$\mathcal{R}$*espiratory Recap*

Formation of the Professional Association

On March 7, 1947, the Articles of Incorporation were filed with the Illinois secretary of state to form the professional respiratory therapy association, originally named the *Inhalation Therapy Association (ITA)*, which is now the *American Association for Respiratory Care (AARC)*.

The Tri-State Hospital Assembly, comprising the state hospital associations of Illinois, Indiana, and Michigan, provided an early forum for the educational and political expression of the new organization. The assembly was important for its positive name recognition and as a venue to promote the specialty within the hospital community.

Without significant support the ITA struggled during the first years of its existence. Two notable events in the mid-1950s helped the ITA overcome its perception as a mere regional association. First, the name was changed to the more global **American Association of Inhalation Therapists (AAIT).** Second, under the presidency of Sister Mary Borromea, OSF, CRNA, (Figure 1-4; OSF, Order of Saint Francis; CRNA, certified registered nurse anesthetist) and with the encouragement of the physician directors, a multiclient public relations firm, Carrière and Jobson, Inc. was hired to manage the business affairs of the AAIT.[13] In May 1955, Albert Carrière, a principal in the firm, was named the AAIT executive director.[14] Carrière

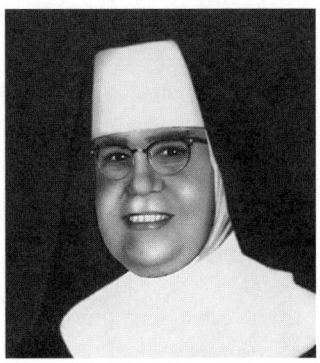

Figure 1-4   Sister Mary Borromea, OSF, CRNA, (deceased) was the fourth president of the Inhalation Therapy Association (1955-1956). During her terms of office the first paid executive director was hired; the first annual convention was held; and the *Respiratory Care* journal first was published. *OSF,* Order of Saint Francis; *CRNA,* certified registered nurse anesthetist. (Courtesy American Association for Respiratory Care, Dallas.)

directed the business operations of the AAIT for the next 12 years.

By 1967 the perception was that the AAIT's executive director held the association in virtual financial thrall. Although many of his organizational colleagues saw Carrière as a financial savior, Easton R. Smith, 1967 AAIT president, vigorously challenged that notion. He forced the executive director to resign in late 1967, effectively ushering in the present organizational strategy of financial control by the members.[15]

By the 1970s, nearly all the organization's infrastructure, as well as that of the profession, was in place, as follows:

- Practitioner roles and functions were defined.[16]
- The House of Delegates was functioning.
- Education essentials were established.
- Practitioner credentials received national recognition.
- Association member growth was clearly evident.

The profession, however, had never examined the efficacy of the modes of therapy it was using. This extraordinarily important activity was essentially left to others. Modes of respiratory therapy were based primarily on clinical impressions, not rigorous clinical studies.

A Conference on the Scientific Basis of Respiratory Therapy, supported jointly by the then-National Heart and Lung Institute (NHLI) and the American Thoracic Society (ATS), was convened in May 1974 at Temple University Conference Center at Sugarloaf in Philadelphia. Prominent scientists nationwide reviewed the efficacy of oxygen therapy, aerosol therapy, physical therapy, and IPPB therapy.

The proceedings of that conference were published in December 1974,[17] engendering considerable angst on the part of respiratory therapists. IPPB therapy, the major clinical task, was scrutinized with discouraging implications. The studies of Barach,[18] Cournand,[19] and especially Motley,[20] published as early as 1947, had served as the underpinning for the unparalleled use and misuse of IPPB therapy for more than a quarter century. The initial fears of the respiratory therapists after the proceedings proved unfounded simply because the pathologic processes that had been treated previously with IPPB still needed to be treated. Other modes of therapy with better efficacy replaced the pervasive use of IPPB.

Just as important, if not more so, is that the organization, currently known as the **American Association for Respiratory Care (AARC),** has successfully used the Sugarloaf Conference example as a template for scientific examination of every form of clinical respiratory therapy since 1974 (Table 1-2).

*T*ABLE 1-2

AARC Conference Proceedings Published in Respiratory Care

Year	Topic	Publication
1982	Complications of Respiratory Therapy	Vol 27:4
1983	The Management of Acute Respiratory Failure	Vol 28:5
1984	Perioperative Respiratory Care	Vol 29:5-6
1985	Monitoring of Critically Ill Patients	Vol 30:6-7
1986	Neonatal Respiratory Care	Vol 31:6-7
1987	Mechanical Ventilation	Vol 32:6-7
1988	PEEP	Vol 33:6-7
1989	Pulmonary Function Testing	Vol 34:6-7
1990	Noninvasive Monitoring in Respiratory Care	Vol 35:6-7
1991	Respiratory Care of Infants and Children	Vol 36:6-7
1991	Consensus Conference I: Aerosol Delivery	Vol 36:9
1992	Emergency Respiratory Care	Vol 37:6-7
1992	Consensus Conference II: The Essentials of Mechanical Ventilators	Vol 37:9
1993	Oxygenation in the Critically Ill Patient	Vol 38:6-7
1994	Controversies in Home Respiratory Care	Vol 39:4-5
1995	Resuscitation in Acute Care Hospitals	Vol 40:4-5
1995	Consensus Conference III: Assessing Innovation on Mechanical Ventilatory Support	Vol 40:9
1996	Mechanical Ventilation: Ventilatory Techniques, Pharmacology, and Patient Management Strategies	Vol 41:4-5
1997	Emerging Health Care Delivery Models and Respiratory Care	Vol 42:1
1997	Consensus Conference IV: Noninvasive Positive Pressure Ventilation	Vol 42:4
1998	Sleep-Disordered Breathing	Vol 43:4-5
1999	Inhaled Nitric Oxide	Vol 44:2-3
1999	Artificial Airways	Vol 44:6-7
2000	Oxygen Therapy	Vol 45:1-2
2000	Palliative Respiratory Care	Vol 45:11-12
2001	Tracheal Gas Insufflation	Vol 46:2
2001	Evidence-Based Respiratory Care	Vol 46:11-12

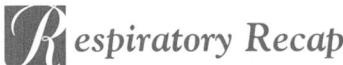

espiratory Recap

> ### Implications of the Sugarloaf Conference
>
> A conference on the scientific basis for respiratory care was convened at the Sugarloaf conference center in Philadelphia in 1974.
> Prominent scientists from around the nation met at Sugarloaf to review the efficacy of oxygen therapy, aerosol therapy, physical therapy, and IPPB.
> The Sugarloaf Conference was supported jointly by the then-National Heart and Lung Institute (NHLI) and the American Thoracic Society (ATS).
> The proceedings from Sugarloaf were published in 1974.
> The organization now known as the AARC has successfully used the Sugarloaf Conference example as a template for scientific examination of nearly every form of clinical respiratory therapy.

Licensure

As late as 1970, AAIT then-president Robert A. Dittmar recalled that, in the context of public health issues, licensure was considered a substandard solution to subvert the national Registry credentialing programs.[21] Then, in 1971 the U.S. Department of Health, Education, and Welfare (DHEW) imposed a voluntary 2-year moratorium on additional state licensing. In the spirit of cooperative citizenship the organization enthusiastically supported the moratorium.[22] Furthermore, physician mentors of that era were against any form of licensure on the part of the affiliated organizations chartered by the AARC.[23]

A significant organizational milestone was reached in 1980. AARC president at the time, Sam P. Giordano, using persuasive arguments, challenged the conventional wisdom that state licensure was not in the best interests of respiratory therapists—an official position held by the AARC for more than 20 years. After the spring meeting of the board of directors in 1980, Giordano wrote the following[24]:

> … the Board decided that the association needs to develop a plan to assist the chartered affiliates in their efforts to pursue meaningful, nonrestrictive licensure. A national organization is limited in what it can do on a state level by virtue of the fact that there is a great deal of inconsistency in how the legislative process works from state to state. However, it has been felt that the association can play a key role in educating and informing the membership on the common steps that must be taken to assure a successful licensure effort on the state level.

With this public announcement, the AARC launched one of the most ambitious, sustained, and successful undertakings in its history. Giordano appointed Jeri E. Eiserman to the post of licensure coordinator, in which she served as the chief architect of this massive undertaking. Eiserman's zealous pursuit of state licensure in 1980 carried over to her own AARC presidency in 1986. As she characterized her administration, she stated the following[25]:

> I attended 40 plus state society meetings as AARC president. Nearly everywhere I went one of the speeches that I gave addressed the critical nature of state licensure. Too, I did everything I could to marshal the AARC's resources to help states that were willing to pursue licensure. Our model credentialing act was one such resource, one that supported a whole compendium of like materials.

espiratory Recap

> ### Establishing Professional Credibility
>
> Forming a professional organization
> Developing the organization
> Examining modes of therapy to promote highest levels of practice
> Facilitating state licensure

Clearly the first purpose enunciated in the 1947 incorporation document, although still in continual evolution, has been faithfully met. The association continues to promote increasingly high standards of practice and the professional advancement of its constituents. By mid-1999, respiratory therapists were licensed in 39 states, the District of Columbia, and Puerto Rico. Four states have certification laws, and one state has a registration law.[26]

Educational Considerations

Education is the fundamental reason for the existence of the AARC and has been since its organizational inception. A key purpose listed in the Articles of Incorporation of the newly chartered ITA was, "To advance the knowledge of Inhalation Therapy through institutes, lectures, and other means…" Modern amplification of that purpose is codified in the AARC bylaws that read in part as follows[27]:

> The Association is formed to: a.) Encourage, develop, and provide educational programs for those persons interested in respiratory therapy and diagnostics…

In other words the AARC actively promotes the sequential functions of higher education—research, archiving, and dissemination of knowledge.

The original ITA purpose emphasized that the institutes, lectures, and so forth were to be "…given under the sponsorship of doctors of the Society of Anesthesia." The practical design of such sponsorship was the hope that these educational endeavors would find credibility and immediate legitimacy in the broad medical community.

The AARC was formally recognized by the medical community as the preeminent organization for respiratory care education in the United States in 1954.[28] Presently the AARC supports two related constituency groups—the education specialty section and the education committee—along with sponsorship of the **Committee on Accreditation for Respiratory Care (CoARC).** Furthermore, the AARC is prepared to act as an ombudsman in matters of education for those individuals and agencies not formally allied with it.

The centerpiece of the organization's educational thrust is the annual convention and exhibition. In 1955, only 83 people met at the first convention in Chicago. Currently, approximately 7000 conventioneers gather annually. Attendees participate in programs approved for more than 20 contact hours of continuing respiratory care education (CRCE) units. Additionally, this convention is a vehicle used to expose original research by respiratory therapists and others to the scrutiny of the medical community.

The AARC's continuing education program enjoys nearly universal recognition in the United States. The point accreditation system, designed and developed in 1968, has matured into the CRCE program. CRCE units are recognized by nearly all states requiring continuing education for license maintenance and retention.

In 1972, researchers at Providence Hospital in Seattle and Parkland Memorial Hospital in Dallas independently approached the AARC Program Committee asking to present their findings at the convention. The committee quickly developed the scientific paper competition portion of the program. This segment of the convention was overwhelmingly successful. The competition was eventually restructured, and in 1973 it debuted as the enormously popular Open Forum segment.

The AARC started an education forum in 1966, bringing together a handful of respiratory care educators to discuss issues of common interest. This forum slowly evolved into the popular meeting, the Summer Forum.

Accreditation

The roots of formal accreditation of respiratory care educational programs trace back to 1950. That year the New York Academy of Medicine's Committee on Public Health Relations published a widely circulated report, "Standard of Effective Administration of Inhalation Therapy,"[29] outlining a need for trained technical personnel in the care of both medical and surgical pulmonary patients.

In collaboration with the New York State Society of Anesthesiologists, the Medical Society of the State of New York formed a Special Joint Committee on Inhalation Therapy (SJCIT) in 1954.[30] One of its objectives was "…to establish the essentials of acceptable schools of inhalation therapy (not to include administration of anesthetic agents)…" By April 1956 this committee had finished its task, reporting the completed "essentials."[31] Within 2 months the House of Delegates of the American Medical Association (AMA) adopted the resolution in-

troduced by the Medical Society of the State of New York, with the delegates stating the following[32]:

> Resolved, that the Council on Medical Education and Hospitals is hereby requested to endorse such or similar "Essentials" and to stimulate the creation of schools of inhalation in various parts of these United States of America.

A report entitled "Essentials for an Approved School of Inhalation Therapy Technicians" was adopted by sponsors (AAIT, AMA, American College of Chest Physicians [ACCP], and ASA) at a conference in 1957. The validity of these essentials was tested during a subsequent 3-year trial, with the AMA Council on Medical Education and Hospitals recommending final adoption to the AMA's House of Delegates, which granted formal approval in December 1962.[33]

The first official meeting of the Board of Schools of Inhalation Therapy Technicians was held at the AMA's Chicago headquarters in 1963.[34] At that time the board was deemed officially functional. The Joint Review Committee for Inhalation Therapy Education (JRCITE), later renamed the *Joint Review Committee for Respiratory Therapy Education (JRCRTE,* which was later known as the *Joint Review Committee for Respiratory Care Education [JRCRCE]),* came into being in January 1970 as a Minnesota corporation under the guidance of the highly respected physician and aviation physiologist, H. Frederic Helmholz, Jr.[35] (Figure 1-5).

A maturing and increasingly assertive AARC leadership was poised to overcome perceived barriers to professional identity, self-determination, and responsibility. A core issue was the lack of therapist-physician parity on the Board of Schools. The prevailing sense among respiratory therapists was that issues concerning the profession, including education, were not adequately represented by the therapists, those individuals making up the profession. Consequently, the physicians could and did present a

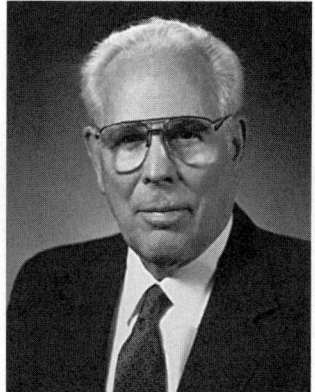

Figure 1-5   H. Frederic Helmholz, Jr., a highly respected physician and aviation physiologist, guided the formation of the Joint Review Committee for Inhalation Therapy Education (JRCITE) on January 9, 1970, as a Minnesota corporation. The JRCITE was later renamed the *Joint Review Committee for Respiratory Care Education (JRCRCE).*

united front in the deliberations of the boards they controlled at the time—Board of Schools, Registry Board, and AAIT Medical Advisory Board. Over time the respiratory therapist's role in determining the direction of the profession grew. The JRCITE's corporate articles and bylaws addressed the therapists' points of contention.

By early 1993, relations between the JRCRTE and the AARC were strained again, perhaps exacerbated by the AARC's effort to map out an educational direction for respiratory therapists into the next century.[36] In 1994 the AARC immediately sponsored a newly formed Respiratory Care Accreditation Board (RCAB). From these events arose a new structure for accreditation of respiratory care training programs. In 1998 this responsibility was transferred from the JRCRTE and RCAB to CoARC.

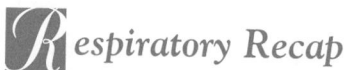

*R*espiratory Recap

Educational Considerations

Professional organization role in education
Development of accreditation standards
Formation of accreditation bodies

National and State Credentialing

A core responsibility of the accreditation process is quality assurance. That is, accredited educational programs generally prepare their graduates to pass appropriate examinations at the level to which they were trained and earn appropriate credentials.

At the dawn of the new millennium, the **American Registry of Inhalation Therapists (ARIT),** which later became the **National Board for Respiratory Care (NBRC),** had conferred nearly a quarter million credentials on health care professionals worldwide.[37] These credentials are **registered respiratory therapist (RRT), certified respiratory therapist (CRT), registered pulmonary function technologist (RPFT), certified pulmonary function technologist (CPFT),** and **perinatal/pediatric respiratory care specialist.**

The sources of these credentials are inextricably tied to those early actions and circumstances that ultimately resulted in the formation of the AARC and CoARC.[30,31] The ITA Articles of Incorporation contain the impetus for the NBRC: "To grant certificates of qualification to such as have successfully completed the prescribed requirements. To establish a central registry for members of the Association."

James E. Peo, AARC president in 1958, described the administrative mechanics of qualifying for listing in the "central registry," that is, for ITA membership, as follows[38]:

It was the custom at the time that after having completed a series of lectures given by the doctors, we would take a written examination covering the topics which the doctors had lec-

tured on. Everyone received an attendance certificate. If we passed the test, we would receive the Registry certificate.

These early experiences in examining and credentialing met with limited acceptance in the medical community. The association, however, persisted, and by mid-1960 Carrière was able to report the following[39]:

The final revisions in the Registered By-Laws (sic) have been duplicated by our attorney and sent to members of the Advisory Board. ... we are awaiting final approval by the American Society of Anesthesiologists, whose committee on Inhalation Therapy is meeting during the first week in October.

The Registry Board organized quickly, offering a two-part pilot examination in November 1960 in Minneapolis. The written and oral examinations were administered and proctored by physicians because no registered therapists yet existed to participate. To take the exam, the candidate must be an active member in good standing of the AAIT.[40] In May 1961, 12 candidates taking the examination were designated *registered inhalation therapists,* along with 23 others who took the exam that month in Chicago[41] (Figure 1-6). Written and oral examinations were conducted until 1979, when **clinical simulation examinations (CSEs)** replaced the oral forms.

During its first decade the NBRC credentialed only 1594 practitioners,[3] whereas in that same period the AARC's membership rolls grew from 750 to 5147 members, representing about 33% of all active practitioners. Increasingly apparent was that the profession was becoming conspicuous in the health care field because of its inordinately low number of credentialed practitioners—about 10%.

To rectify the situation the AARC in 1969 launched a new credentials effort. Then-President John Julius succinctly described as follows the opening of what became an organizational success story[42]:

Louise Hemmel, the (AARC) secretary, outlined for me what should be done to recognize people who weren't registered, but represented the majority of workers in the field.

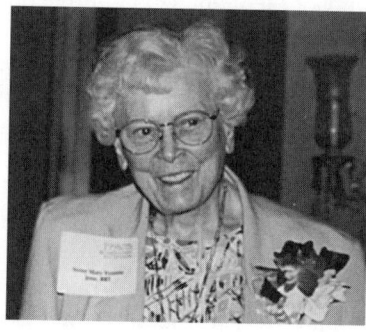

Figure 1-6   Sister Mary Yvonne Jenn, a registered respiratory therapist shown here in 1998, was the first registered therapist in North America. She was the first registrar of the American Registry of Inhalation Therapists (ARIT), now the National Board for Respiratory Care (NBRC). (Courtesy NBRC, Lenexa, Kan.)

Basically, her proposal was the Technician Certification Program.

The technician certification program proved enormously successful. During the 5 years that the AARC managed it, more than 10,000 practitioners were recognized as certified respiratory therapy technicians (CRTTs), now known as *CRTs*.

By 1972, having developed a viable, proven credential, AARC President James A. Liverett, Jr. made plans to hand the certification process over to the NBRC, as follows[43]:

I carried the message of our thinking to Kansas City where the NBRC met in 1972. I responded to the Board's invitation to address them on this topic. I must say that the trustees were a bit skeptical about this proposal. They didn't appear to be too sure about our motives in giving this program to them. All I could do was (to) openly discuss the logic of my reasoning—that credentialing should be with credentialing—planting seeds that flourished in 1974, when ARIT, Inc. and the AART Technician Certification Board merged to form the National Board for Respiratory Therapy.

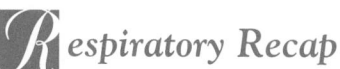

espiratory Recap

Origins of Professional Credentialing
Formation of American Registry of Inhalation Therapists (ARIT) Evolution of National Board for Respiratory Care (NBRC) Validation of examinations Incorporation of the national credentialing examinations for state licensure

The NBRC enjoys unconditional membership in the National Commission for Health Certifying Agencies (NCHCA) because the NBRC is now a leader among health certification agencies. The validity of its examinations rests on a national job analysis conducted every 5 years. **Criterion-referenced validation studies** are conducted on each examination before it is given for the first time.[3] In addition, use of the federally trademarked NBRC fulfills the vision of those individuals who founded the profession in the 1940s.

Professional Publications

Historically, the first regularly appearing publication of the profession was the *Inhalation Therapy Association Bulletin* (Figure 1-7). This quarterly periodical appeared between 1950 and mid-1954, after which a series of newsletter-type publications were distributed, essentially focusing on association news.

Medical periodicals such as the *Journal of the American Medical Association (JAMA)* and the *New England Journal of Medicine (NEJM)* exert a significant social impact. They

are highly regarded by the lay public and frequently quoted in the popular media. Stimulated by the presence of these powerful journals and other models, such as *Chest, Anesthesiology,* and the *American Review of Respiratory Disease,* the respiratory care profession sought to emulate them. By 1956, sufficient resources had been amassed to launch and sustain a quarterly journal.

Respiratory Care is a monthly science journal established as the quarterly publication, *Inhalation Therapy,* under the editorship of longtime educator James F. Whitacre (Figure 1-8). *Respiratory Care* is published currently for the AARC by Daedalus Enterprises, Inc., and its contents include editorials; original, previously unpublished contributions; case reports; guidelines, recommendations, and statements; reviews of books, films, tapes, and software; classic reprints; and more. The section devoted to guidelines, recommendations, and statements reflects the historical influence of the AARC on the scientific basis for clinical practice (Box 1-1). The material appearing in *Respiratory Care,* especially the special proceedings and consensus conferences, is tremendously valuable to the entire field of pulmonary medicine.

In 1969 William F. Miller (Figure 1-9), a pulmonary physiologist from Dallas, and his colleague, Dr. William W. Waring from New Orleans, along with publications Editor-in-Chief and RRT Allan Saposnick of Philadelphia, led a movement to restructure the contents of the journal. They set in motion the administrative actions that resulted in *Inhalation Therapy/Respiratory Care* becoming a science journal; its contents were to be free of all political influences that could be exerted by its owner, the association.[44]

In early 1981 Dr. John B. Downs, a member of the *Respiratory Care* editorial board, suggested that a special symposium be planned, held, and published in the journal. "Complications of respiratory therapy" was recommended as an appropriate theme for the symposium, held in San Francisco in 1981 as a joint venture of the AARC and the ACCP. Editor Philip Kittredge wrote the following in his foreword[45]:

The result is that this is probably the single most important issue so far in *Respiratory Care's* first 27 years. As a body of knowledge about the complications of respiratory therapy, gathered in one place, this material stands unique. Every article is pertinent and of value. Some of the topics have not been reviewed before at all. Some of these reviews will now stand as *the* authoritative sources in the literature.

In the year 2000, after 44 years of continuous publication, *Respiratory Care* was accepted in *Index Medicus,* the principle bibliographic database of the National Library of Medicine and its online counterpart, MEDLINE.

The introductory issue of another association publication, *AARC Times,* then titled *AARTimes,* appeared in July 1977. Then-AART President Thomas A. Barnes described the publication as a new service to the profession, reporting that the editorial thrust of the magazine would

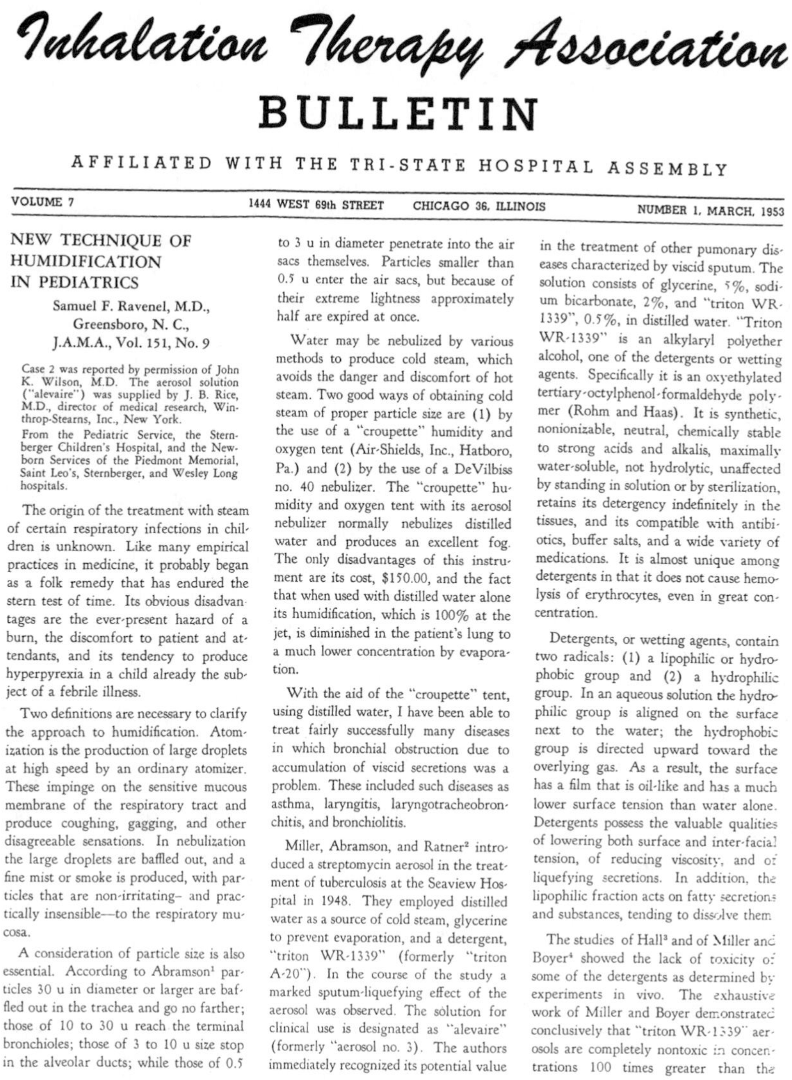

Inhalation Therapy Association
BULLETIN

AFFILIATED WITH THE TRI-STATE HOSPITAL ASSEMBLY

| VOLUME 7 | 1444 WEST 69th STREET | CHICAGO 36, ILLINOIS | NUMBER 1, MARCH, 1953 |

NEW TECHNIQUE OF HUMIDIFICATION IN PEDIATRICS

Samuel F. Ravenel, M.D.,
Greensboro, N. C.,
J.A.M.A., Vol. 151, No. 9

Case 2 was reported by permission of John K. Wilson, M.D. The aerosol solution ("alevaire") was supplied by J. B. Rice, M.D., director of medical research, Winthrop-Stearns, Inc., New York.
From the Pediatric Service, the Sternberger Children's Hospital, and the Newborn Services of the Piedmont Memorial, Saint Leo's, Sternberger, and Wesley Long hospitals.

The origin of the treatment with steam of certain respiratory infections in children is unknown. Like many empirical practices in medicine, it probably began as a folk remedy that has endured the stern test of time. Its obvious disadvantages are the ever-present hazard of a burn, the discomfort to patient and attendants, and its tendency to produce hyperpyrexia in a child already the subject of a febrile illness.

Two definitions are necessary to clarify the approach to humidification. Atomization is the production of large droplets at high speed by an ordinary atomizer. These impinge on the sensitive mucous membrane of the respiratory tract and produce coughing, gagging, and other disagreeable sensations. In nebulization the large droplets are baffled out, and a fine mist or smoke is produced, with particles that are non-irritating– and practically insensible—to the respiratory mucosa.

A consideration of particle size is also essential. According to Abramson[1] particles 30 u in diameter or larger are baffled out in the trachea and go no farther; those of 10 to 30 u reach the terminal bronchioles; those of 3 to 10 u size stop in the alveolar ducts; while those of 0.5

to 3 u in diameter penetrate into the air sacs themselves. Particles smaller than 0.5 u enter the air sacs, but because of their extreme lightness approximately half are expired at once.

Water may be nebulized by various methods to produce cold steam, which avoids the danger and discomfort of hot steam. Two good ways of obtaining cold steam of proper particle size are (1) by the use of a "croupette" humidity and oxygen tent (Air-Shields, Inc., Hatboro, Pa.) and (2) by the use of a DeVilbiss no. 40 nebulizer. The "croupette" humidity and oxygen tent with its aerosol nebulizer normally nebulizes distilled water and produces an excellent fog. The only disadvantages of this instrument are its cost, $150.00, and the fact that when used with distilled water alone its humidification, which is 100% at the jet, is diminished in the patient's lung to a much lower concentration by evaporation.

With the aid of the "croupette" tent, using distilled water, I have been able to treat fairly successfully many diseases in which bronchial obstruction due to accumulation of viscid secretions was a problem. These included such diseases as asthma, laryngitis, laryngotracheobronchitis, and bronchiolitis.

Miller, Abramson, and Ratner[2] introduced a streptomycin aerosol in the treatment of tuberculosis at the Seaview Hospital in 1948. They employed distilled water as a source of cold steam, glycerine to prevent evaporation, and a detergent, "triton WR-1339" (formerly "triton A-20"). In the course of the study a marked sputum-liquefying effect of the aerosol was observed. The solution for clinical use is designated as "alevaire" (formerly "aerosol no. 3). The authors immediately recognized its potential value

in the treatment of other pumonary diseases characterized by viscid sputum. The solution consists of glycerine, 5%, sodium bicarbonate, 2%, and "triton WR-1339", 0.5%, in distilled water. "Triton WR-1339" is an alkylaryl polyether alcohol, one of the detergents or wetting agents. Specifically it is an oxyethylated tertiary-octylphenol-formaldehyde polymer (Rohm and Haas). It is synthetic, nonionizable, neutral, chemically stable to strong acids and alkalis, maximally water-soluble, not hydrolytic, unaffected by standing in solution or by sterilization, retains its detergency indefinitely in the tissues, and is compatible with antibiotics, buffer salts, and a wide variety of medications. It is almost unique among detergents in that it does not cause hemolysis of erythrocytes, even in great concentration.

Detergents, or wetting agents, contain two radicals: (1) a lipophilic or hydrophobic group and (2) a hydrophilic group. In an aqueous solution the hydrophilic group is aligned on the surface next to the water; the hydrophobic group is directed upward toward the overlying gas. As a result, the surface has a film that is oil-like and has a much lower surface tension than water alone. Detergents possess the valuable qualities of lowering both surface and inter-facial tension, of reducing viscosity, and of liquefying secretions. In addition, the lipophilic fraction acts on fatty secretions and substances, tending to dissolve them.

The studies of Hall[3] and of Miller and Boyer[4] showed the lack of toxicity of some of the detergents as determined by experiments in vivo. The exhaustive work of Miller and Boyer demonstrated conclusively that "triton WR-1339" aerosols are completely nontoxic in concentrations 100 times greater than the

Figure 1-7   *Inhalation Therapy Association Bulletin,* volume 7, number 1, 1953. Historically, the bulletin was the first regularly appearing publication of the profession, published quarterly between 1950 and mid-1954.

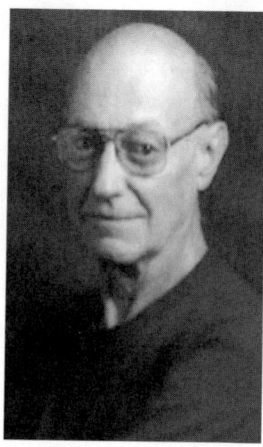

Figure 1-8   James F. Whitacre, a registered respiratory therapist, was among the first group of registered therapists in the United States. During his long career, he served on the boards of the American Association for Respiratory Care (AARC), the National Board of Respiratory Care (NBRC), and the Joint Review Committee for Respiratory Therapy Education (JRCRTE).

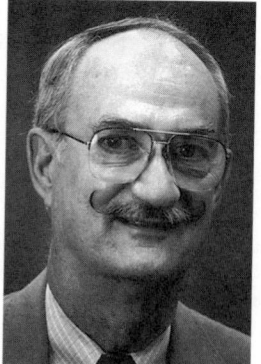

Figure 1-9   William F. Miller, a pulmonary physiologist from Dallas, led a movement to restructure the contents of the respiratory journal. They set in motion the administrative actions that resulted in *Inhalation Therapy/Respiratory Care* becoming a peer-reviewed science journal. (Courtesy of AARC.)

Box 1-1

AARC Clinical Practice Guidelines (CPGs)

Spirometry, 1996 Update (CPG 1)
Oxygen Therapy in Acute Care Hospital (CPG 2)
Nasotracheal Suctioning (CPG 3)
Patient-Ventilator System Checks (CPG 4)
Directed Cough (CPG 5)
In-Vitro pH and Blood Gas Analysis and Hemoximetry (CPG 6)
Use of Positive Airway Pressure Adjuncts to Bronchial Hygiene Therapy (CPG 7)
Sampling for Arterial Blood Gas Analysis (CPG 8)
Endotracheal Suctioning of Mechanically Ventilated Adults and Children with Artificial Airways (CPG 9)
Incentive Spirometry (CPG 10)
Postural Drainage Therapy (CPG 11)
Bronchial Provocation (CPG 12)
Selection of Aerosol Delivery Device (CPG 13)
Pulse Oximetry (CPG 14)
Single-Breath Carbon Monoxide Diffusing Capacity, 1999 Update (CPG 15)
Oxygen Therapy in the Home or Extended Care Facility (CPG 16)
Exercise Testing for Evaluation of Hypoxemia and/or Desaturation (CPG 17)
Humidification during Mechanical Ventilation (CPG 18)
Transport of the Mechanically Ventilated Patient (CPG 19)
Resuscitation in Acute Care Hospitals (CPG 20)
Bland Aerosol Administration (CPG 21)
Fiberoptic Bronchoscopy Assisting (CPG 22)
Intermittent Positive Pressure Breathing (IPPB) (CPG 23)
Application of CPAP to Neonates Via Nasal Prongs or Nasopharyngeal Tube (CPG 24)
Delivery of Aerosols to the Upper Airway (CPG 25)
Neonatal Time-Triggered, Pressure-Limited, Time-Cycled Mechanical Ventilation (CPG 26)
Static Lung Volumes (CPG 27)

Surfactant Replacement Therapy (CPG 28)
Ventilator Circuit Changes (CPG 29)
Metabolic Measurement Using Indirect Calorimetry during Mechanical Ventilation (CPG 30)
Transcutaneous Blood Gas Monitoring for Neonatal and Pediatric Patients (CPG 31)
Body Plethysmography (CPG 32)
Capillary Blood Gas Sampling for Neonatal and Pediatric Patients (CPG 33)
Defibrillation during Resuscitation (CPG 34)
Infant/Toddler Pulmonary Function Tests (CPG 35)
Management of Airway Emergencies (CPG 36)
Assessing Response to Bronchodilator Therapy at Point of Care (CPG 37)
Discharge Planning for the Respiratory Care Patient (CPG 38)
Long-Term Invasive Mechanical Ventilation in the Home (CPG 39)
Capnography/Capnometry during Mechanical Ventilation (CPG 40)
Selection of an Aerosol Delivery Device for Neonatal and Pediatric Patients (CPG 41)
Polysomnography (CPG 42)
Selection of an Oxygen Delivery Device for Neonatal and Pediatric Patients (CPG 43)
Selection of a Device for Delivery of Aerosol to the Lung Parenchyma (CPG 44)
Training the Health-Care Professional for the Role of Patient and Caregiver Educator (CPG 45)
Providing Patient and Caregiver Training (CPG 46)
Removal of the Endotracheal Tube (CPG 47)
Suctioning of the Patient in the Home (CPG 48)
Selection of Device, Administration of Bronchodilator, and Evaluation of Response to Therapy in Mechanically Ventilated Patients (CPG 49)

AARC, American Association for Respiratory Care; CPAP, continuous positive airway pressure.

include "...articles dealing with management, education, and clinical practice ... and with the activities of the Association."[46]

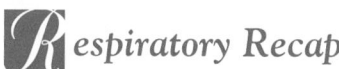

espiratory Recap

Professional Publications

Early publication efforts (*Inhalation Therapy Association Bulletin, Inhalation Therapy* journal)
Respiratory Care as a "science" journal
AARC Times, reflecting the "art" of the profession

This magazine, published monthly by Daedalus Enterprises, Inc. for the AARC, may be considered a true historical archive. The annual financial reports of the organ-

ization are printed, as are reports of the activities of the board of directors, the House of Delegates, and so forth. It is an accurate mirror of those issues with which respiratory therapists in the United States are most concerned.

Funding and Philanthropy

In 1968 the Parker B. Francis Foundation (PBFF), a private foundation formed by the Puritan-Bennett Corporation, offered a $50,000 grant to the association for the development of new multilevel training media for hospital inservice programs and formal educational programs. The grant was to be disbursed in five annual installments of $10,000.[47]

AARC then-president Robert A. Dittmar accepted the grant in 1969, contingent on the formation of a tax-exempt organization under specific provisions of the Internal Revenue Service (IRS) code.[21] The **American Respiratory Care Foundation (ARCF)** was incorporated in

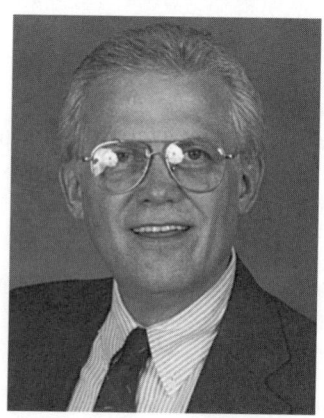

Figure 1-10   Philip R. Cooper, a registered respiratory therapist, was elected the American Respiratory Care Foundation's (ARCF's) first president in 1971, a position he held for 3 years. Cooper was named president emeritus of the ARCF in 1975. In 1994 he became a lifetime AARC member and, because of his contributions to the formation of the ARCF, was elected the only member of the AARC Presidents Council not to have served as a president of the association.

July 1970 as a California not-for-profit corporation. It was known then as the *American Association for Inhalation Therapy Foundation (AAITF)*. By the time the IRS issued a declaration of status in mid-1971 and the first $10,000 was received, more than 3 years of work and other resources had been expended.

The organizational meeting of the foundation convened in May 1971. Philip R. Cooper, an RRT, was elected as the foundation's first president (Figure 1-10). The early years were spent developing the administrative infrastructure of the ARCF with a focus on fund-raising. At the end of the first year of operations, the foundation had obligations of nearly $9000, of which only $3700 was covered because of severely restricted funds. In 1972 the situation was alleviated somewhat when the AARC presented the foundation with a nonrestricted check for nearly $2200 for administrative purposes, which covered trustee expenses for the first year's operation. Concurrently, responsibility for administration of the Mead-Johnson Fellowship Funds was transferred to the foundation from the AARC's research and education fund committee. Shortly thereafter, restricted contributions

Respiratory Recap

History of Funding Organizations
Role of Parker B. Francis Foundation
Organization of the American Respiratory Care Foundation and its continued funding role

from the 3M Company, RCI, Bard-Parker, Arbrook, Inc., and Travenol Laboratories followed.

In November 1971 the first solicitation for grant money came from the University of Alabama, Birmingham; its respiratory therapy program had a project under way, already partially funded by the DHEW. Additionally, the Pediatric Pulmonary Center, New Mexico Regional Medical Program, appealed to the ARTF for cosponsorship of its program for children and young adults.

The achievements of the ARCF over the intervening decades are remarkable. The trustees currently administer more than $20,000 annually in awards, education and literary recognition, fellowships, and grants (Box 1-2). They have made other tangible contributions to the profession through financial support of the AARC's consensus and special proceedings conferences, for instance. The ARCF recognizes achievements through its awards programs and promotes scholarly investigation through sponsored conferences and research grants. Students, educators, managers, and clinicians benefit directly and indirectly by the work recognized and funded through the ARCF.

Medical Direction

Albert Andrews wrote the following in the 1947 edition of his book:

> The physician at the head of the service, and the head should be a physician, should have a deep interest in respiration and in the application of oxygen and inhalation therapy. His specialty, if he has one, is not of first importance. Because of the 24 hour nature of this therapy ... it is believed by some that the physician should be employed full time by the hospital.[10]

His idea for **medical direction** finds contemporary expression in the AARC's highly visible and active Board of Medical Advisors (BOMA) and the National Association for Medical Direction of Respiratory Care (NAMDRC), a corporate sponsor of the AARC. A unique characteristic of the respiratory care profession is the close, interpersonal relationship between respiratory therapists and their medical directors, the ongoing legacy of Andrews' recommendation.

When the association first was formed, a tiny body of physicians held tremendous power. Known simply as the organization *medical directors* from 1947 through 1953, they ratified or vetoed every decision made by the board of directors. This core of highly motivated, caring physicians, including Andrews and Levine, used the prestige of their positions in the medical community to ensure the viability of the fledgling society, the ITA. The ITA, thus the AARC, may have foundered without the guidance of these physicians.

A case in point, Levine, the only physician to have served as president of the AARC, was elected to office in 1952. That year the American College of Hospital Ad-

Box 1-2

1999 ARCF Award Programs

General Awards
Dr. Charles H. Hudson Award for Cardiopulmonary Public Health
Forrest M. Bird Achievement Award
Invacare Award for Excellence in Home Respiratory Care

Education Recognition Awards
Jimmy A. Young Memorial Education Recognition Award
Morton B. Duggan, Jr., Memorial Education Award
NBRC/AMP Robert M. Lawrence, MD, Education Recognition Award
NBRC/AMP William W. Burgin, Jr., MD, Education Recognition Award
William F. Miller, MD, Postgraduate Education Recognition Award

Literary Awards
Dr. Allen DeVilbiss Literary Award
Radiometer Awards for Best Features in Science Journal Respiratory Care

Research Fellowships
Glaxo Wellcome Care Management Fellowship for Asthma Education
Monaghan/Trudell Fellowship for Aerosol Technique Development
Respironics Fellowship in Mechanical Ventilation
Respironics Fellowship in Non-Invasive Respiratory Care

Research Grants
Jerome M. Sullivan Research Fund (awarded periodically)
NBRC/AMP H. Frederic Helmholz, Jr., MD, Educational Research Fund
Parker B. Francis Respiratory Research Grant (awarded periodically)

ARCF, *American Respiratory Care Foundation;* NBRC/AMP, *National Board for Respiratory Care/Applied Measurement Professionals.*

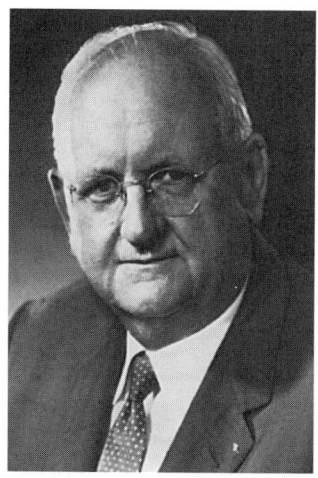

Figure 1-11   Paul M. Wood, an honored anesthesiologist and historian, was a member of the Special Joint Committee on Inhalation Therapy (SJCIT), formed in 1955. (Courtesy Wood Library-Museum, Park Ridge, Ill.)

ministrators (ACHA) was about to adopt a recommendation that "...no inhalation therapy department will be permitted in any hospital, and banned in the future."[11] He volunteered to use his medical credentials to convince the ACHA that such a resolution would destroy a significant development in emerging modern patient care.

The medical directors became the Medical Advisory Board in 1954 and the Board of Medical Advisors in 1963. The board was doubled in 1958, seating three representatives each from the ACCP and the ASA.

Dr. Paul M. Wood (Figure 1-11) also played a key role in the society's survival. Wood was an honored anesthesiologist, an historian, and a member of the SJCIT, formed in 1954.[30] Wood's subcommittee on certification reported "...that a registry of technicians ...was desirable." His sub-

committee further recommended "...that a national association of inhalation therapists ... formulate the processing, registration, and maintain the registry."[31] The personal stature he brought to this report captured the attention of the entire medical community. Then, 4 years later with little debate the ARIT was born in the format generally described by Wood.

The SJCIT operated until early 1969, when it was dissolved by legal expert and ASA president Dr. Carl E. Wasmuth.[48] Many felt the organization had become a sub rosa committee that had outlived its original purpose—to firmly establish inhalation therapy as a separate health specialty. It was a pivotal point in organized respiratory care, particularly with respect to physician-therapist relations. Subtly, allied physicians became mentors rather than remaining simply directors, and therapists became physician-extenders.

Perhaps the most worthy legacy handed down from the physicians of that era was the understanding that to share information is a professional imperative best done through publications. This understanding continues to propel both the art and science of respiratory care.

In 1978 NAMDRC was formed, originally chartered in January 1979 as a Nebraska corporation. It became an official sponsor of the AARC in 1997. Historically, the

ℛespiratory Recap

Medical Direction
Medical director idea advanced by Andrews
Shift from director to medical advisor
Early medical directors/advisors

core interest of this group has been to offer support to those who provide clinical leadership and management in pulmonary care. NAMDRC assists physicians over a broad range of pulmonary services, including critical care, hyperbaric oxygen therapy, pulmonary rehabilitation, pulmonary medicine, pulmonary physiology assessment, respiratory home care, and sleep disorders.

𝒦EY 𝒫OINTS

- Respiratory care emerged as a discrete discipline in North American health care shortly after WWII.
- In the mid-1900s a human resources vacuum was developing in the bedside care of pulmonary patients, and available technology generally required strong young men for its application.
- The formation of the ITA facilitated the development of the profession. The ITA's original corporate purposes have served as an accurate guideline on organizational structure, education, credentials, and medical direction.
- Nearly all the structure of what is now the AARC was in place by the early 1970s.
- The accreditation of respiratory therapy schools evolved into the present-day CoARC.
- The NBRC provides credentialing for respiratory therapists.
- Supported by the efforts of the AARC since 1980, respiratory therapists are licensed in most states.
- *Respiratory Care* is the scientific journal of the AARC, and the *AARC Times* is its monthly publication.
- The ARCF is the philanthropic organization for respiratory care.
- Medical direction has been an important aspect of respiratory care throughout its history.

References

1. Sullivan JM, Miyagawa T. Global respiratory care: a case of common interests, not common credentials [editorial]. Respir Care 1999;44(1):22-23.
2. Masferrer R, Dolan GK, Ward JJ. History of the respiratory care profession. In: Burton GG, Hodgkin JE, Ward JJ. Respiratory care: a guide to clinical practice. 3rd ed. Philadelphia: JB Lippincott; 1991. pp. 3-17.
3. Smith GA, editor. Respiratory care: evolution of a profession. Lenexa, Kan: Applied Measurement Professionals; 1989.
4. The evolution of irons lungs. Cambridge, Mass: JH Emerson; 1978.
5. Sackner MA. A history of oxygen usage in chronic obstructive pulmonary disease. Am Rev Respir Dis 1974;110(6 Part 2):25.
6. Barcroft J, Hunt GH, Dufton D. The treatment of chronic cases of gas poisoning by continuous oxygen administration in chambers. Quart J Med 1919-1920;13:179-200.
7. Ad-hoc literature committee. Evolution & utilization of respiratory services. Dallas: American Association for Respiratory Care; 1995.
8. Boothby WM, Lovelace WR, Bulbulian AH, inventors, assignees. Apparatus for delivering and permitting normal breathing of mixtures of gases. US patent 2,241,535. 1941 May 13.
9. Motley HL, Werko L, Cournand A, et al. Observations on the clinical use of intermittent positive pressure. J Aviat Med 1947;18:417.
10. Andrews AH Jr. Manual of oxygen therapy techniques. Chicago: Year-Book; 1947.
11. Levine ER. Unpublished memoirs in possession of author. Aug 10, 1993 [date written].
12. Etheredge SL. Summary of activities, ITA [report]. Committee on Scientific Education. Chicago: Inhalation Therapy Association; 1951.
13. Gilbert DE. Interview by author. Orlando, Fla; Aug 1, 1994.
14. Minutes. American Association of Inhalation Therapists board of directors. Chicago; 1955 May 4.
15. Smith ER. Interview by author. Orlando Fla; Aug 1, 1994.
16. American Association for Respiratory Care. Delineation of roles and functions of respiratory therapy personnel. Final report for Division of Allied Health Manpower, Bureau of Health Manpower Education, National Institutes of Health, Department of Health, Education & Welfare (US); Dallas: The Association; 1973 July 31.
17. Proceedings on the scientific basis of respiratory therapy. Am Rev Respir Dis 1974;110(6 Part 2):1-204.
18. Barach AL. The physiology of pressure breathing. J Aviat Med 1947;18:73.
19. Cournand A, Motley HL, Werklo L, et al. Physiological studies of the effects of intermittent positive pressure on cardiac output in man. Am J Physiol 1948;152:162.
20. Motley HL, Tomashefski JF. Treatment of chronic pulmonary disease with intermittent positive pressure breathing. Arch Indust Hyg Occup Med 1952;5:1.
21. Dittmar RA. Interview by author. Kettering, Ohio; July 2, 1993.
22. American Association of Inhalation Therapists board of directors. State licensure of inhalation therapy practice. Respir Care 1971;16(5):249-250.
23. Joint ad hoc committee, American College of Chest Physicians, American Society of Anesthesiologists, American Thoracic Society. Licensure for allied health workers in respiratory therapy. Respir Care 1971;16(5):255.
24. Giordano SP. Executive column. AARTimes 1980;4(6):19.
25. Eiserman JE. Interview by author. Nashville, Tenn; Dec 13, 1993.
26. Eicher J. State overview. AARC Times 1999;23(4):8.
27. AARC bylaws. Art II. Sec 1.
28. Collins VJ. Inhalation therapy education and training programs. JAMA 1969;207:329.
29. Committee on Public Relations, NY Academy of Medicine. Standards of effective administration of inhalation therapy. JAMA 1950;144:23-34.
30. Collins VJ. Report of the special joint committee on inhalation therapy. NY State J Med 1955;55:1028.
31. Standards for inhalation therapy (sec 96). NY State J Med 1956;56:1319.
32. Inhalation therapy schools. ASA Newsl 1956;20:4.
33. Collins VJ. Inhalation therapy education and training programs. JAMA 1969;207:330.

34. Taylor AN. Letter from AMA representative to Bernard Kew, AAIT president. Oct 8, 1963 [author's possession].

35. Kracum VD. Chronology of events related to the establishment of the Joint Review Committee for Inhalation Therapy Education. Undated report.

36. American Association for Respiratory Care. Year 2001: delineating the educational direction for the future of respiratory care practitioners; 1993 Oct 15-17; Dallas.

37. National Board for Respiratory Care. 1998 active credentialed practitioners. Lenexa, Kan; The Board; 1996. p. xiii.

38. Peo JE. In: Weilacher RR. Presidential reflections. Palestine, Texas; In press 2001. pp. 24-25.

39. Carrière A. Registry report. AAIT Newsletter 1960(Autumn):1.

40. Announcement. Inhalation therapy. 1960;5(6):14-15.

41. ARIT announcements. May 1961.

42. Julius JJ. Interview by author. Nashville, Tenn; Dec 12, 1993.

43. Liverett JA Jr. Interview by author. New Orleans; July 30, 1994.

44. Schoenbachler MA Jr. Interview by author. Jackson, Tenn; June 17, 1993.

45. Kittredge P. Complications of respiratory therapy [foreword, special issue]. Respir Care 1982;27(4):399.

46. Barnes TA. Letter from the president. AARTimes 1977;1(1):5.

47. Cooper PR. Extrapolation of interview by author. Louisville, Ky; July 3, 1993.

48. Wasmuth CE. Letter to Mark T. Bowers, AAIT executive secretary. Feb 10, 1969 [author's possession].

CHAPTER 2

Professional Organizations

George W. Gaebler

CHAPTER **OUTLINE**

OBJECTIVES

1. Describe the organization of the AARC.
2. Describe the roles of the NBRC and CoARC.
3. Describe the way in which medical professional organizations contribute to the respiratory care profession.
4. Discuss the accreditation, credentialing and medical direction aspects of the respiratory care profession.
5. Identify the primary medical sponsors of the respiratory care profession.
6. Discuss the physician organizations that contribute to the art and science of the respiratory care profession.
7. Identify the role that each professional must play in the future growth of the respiratory care profession.

*K*EY TERMS

AARC Times	Committee on Accreditation for	National Board for Respiratory Care
Accreditation	Respiratory Care (CoARC)	(NBRC)
American Association for Respiratory	Credentialing	President's Council
Care (AARC)	Credentials	*Respiratory Care*
Board of Directors (BOD)	House of Delegates (HOD)	Specialty Sections
Board of Medical Advisors	Licensure	
(BOMA)	National Association for Medical Direc-	
Certification	tion of Respiratory Care (NAMDRC)	

This chapter describes the role of professional organizations in the respiratory care profession, identifying each organization and discussing its importance to the profession's principles and practice (Table 2-1). The primary professional organization for respiratory care is the **American Association for Respiratory Care (AARC).** The AARC and related organizations contribute to the scientific basis, governance, stature, and growth of respiratory care. Nearly all the organizations described in this chapter have been involved with the respiratory care profession since its inception, either in the current form or via a former name or function. Respiratory care would not be as valued a member of the health care team without the contributions of such organizations.

American Association for Respiratory Care

The AARC is the national association that represents the respiratory care profession to communities of interest. A profession is described by its advancing science, technology, and practice; continuing education; active participation of its members; credentials; leadership; research; and innovation. The AARC was organized in 1946 as the Inhalation Therapy Association (ITA). As the profession progressed, the name changed and the organization evolved into the professional entity it is today.

The art and science of respiratory care are supported by the journals of the AARC, which include *Respiratory Care,* **AARC Times,** *Education Annual, Sub Acute Care Today,* and others published by specialty sections. The editorial board for the AARC's scientific journal, **Respiratory Care,** comprises researchers who are also respiratory therapists or physicians. The AARC has various standing and special committees to support the profession.

The funding for operations of the AARC is derived from member dues, advertising, and revenues from educa-

tional programs and conventions throughout the year. The AARC has an average membership of 32,000, with approximately 24,000 active members and 53 life members as of 2000; it also offers student, associate, and honorary memberships. The AARC has consistently provided some of the highest member benefits found in the health professions while maintaining nearly the lowest dues of all national health care organizations. The AARC has nine specialty sections that support major subsets of therapists, including management, education, perinatal/pediatrics, adult critical care, home care, subacute care, transport, diagnostics, and continuing care and rehabilitation. Many AARC members belong to different specialty sections based both on their work activities and on their personal interests.

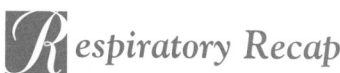

Respiratory Recap

Description of a Profession
Advancing science and technology
Evolving practice, scope, credentialing, and accreditation
Advanced degrees and continuing education
Active participation by members
Leadership, research, and innovation

Currently, the profession is undergoing a major transition. The AARC and its many allied organizations are implementing planned organizational and functional changes. For example, during the last few years, the profession has seen the emergence of the Respiratory Care Accreditation Board (RCAB), the dissolution of the Joint Review Committee for Respiratory Therapy Education (JRCRTE), and the merging of these **accreditation** groups into the Committee on Accreditation for Respiratory Care (CoARC). Changes in the profession reflect the changes in health care, science, technology, education, and communications. Consequently, the AARC has critically examined its structure, organization, and operations; relationships to its members; current practices; communities of interest; and larger societal changes.

AARC in 1999

The AARC comprises several governance and advisory bodies, including the board of directors (BOD), House of Delegates (HOD), Board of Medical Advisors (BOMA), and executive office, located in Dallas.[1,2] The AARC underwent major restructuring, passing substantial bylaws changes, during the fall 1998 meetings. The BOD enacted transition policies and timelines during 1999, with input from the HOD, BOMA and executive office. The structure for the AARC during 1999 is described relative to the changes in governance. A new structure is in process, resulting from election and bylaws changes in

TABLE 2-1

Common Acronyms in Respiratory Care

Acronym	Organization
AARC	American Association for Respiratory Care
BOMA	Board of Medical Advisors
BOD	(AARC) board of directors
CoARC	Committee on Accreditation for Respiratory Care
HOD	(AARC) House of Delegates
NBRC	National Board for Respiratory Care
NAMDRC	National Association for Medical Direction of Respiratory Care
ACCP	American College of Chest Physicians
ATS	American Thoracic Society
ALA	American Lung Association
ASA	American Society of Anesthesiologists
SCCM	Society of Critical Care Medicine

2000, with the help of a special committee known as the *transition committee*.

Board of Directors

The AARC **board of directors (BOD)** is composed of an executive committee, consisting of the president, president-elect, immediate past president, vice president, treasurer, secretary, immediate past speaker of the HOD, and chairperson of BOMA.[1,2] In general the AARC term for offices is 1 year, with the president-elect serving 3 years as president-elect, president, and past president, respectively. In addition, eight at-large members of the BOD have staggered 4-year terms, with two new BOD members elected annually by the active and life members of the AARC. The immediate past speaker of the HOD and current chairperson of BOMA serve 1-year terms as members of the BOD.[1-4]

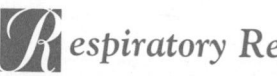

Board of Directors Responsibilities

The board of directors (BOD) is the governing body of the American Association for Respiratory Care (AARC), with fiduciary responsibility for the professional organization and its members.

The current executive director of the AARC serves as an advisor to the BOD, reporting to the current AARC president. In addition, the incoming AARC president appoints a parliamentarian to the BOD to help with procedure for BOD activities before, during, and between board meetings. The BOD meets three times per year, usually during March, directly after the AARC Summer Forum, and directly preceding the AARC International Congress in the fall. The BOD and HOD meet simultaneously during the summer and fall meetings, facilitating communications, costs, and actions required by bylaws that govern some activities of the budget, nominations, and joint members of various BOD and HOD committees.

House of Delegates

The **House of Delegates (HOD)** is a representative body for the chartered affiliates societies to contribute to the growth, existence, governance, and future of the respiratory care profession. The general membership can bring wishes and concerns to the national organization through local representatives in the HOD. The

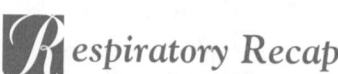

House of Delegates

Each chartered affiliate of the HOD elects active members of the AARC (from their respective affiliates) to represent the membership of the professional association.

HOD further serves as a communication bridge, reporting activities, data, information, and needs to the AARC chartered affiliates and members. Its structure, organization, and function are similar to the United States Congress. The HOD is an advisor to the BOD helps govern the AARC through approval of bylaws, budgets, nominations, and audits and through consideration of resolutions and motions forwarded to the BOD for consideration.[3-5]

Any AARC member may bring issues to the respective state delegations, which in turn broach the issue in a resolution or motion for consideration by the entire HOD. The current HOD meets semiannually in the summer, directly after the AARC Summer Forum, and directly preceding the AARC Annual Meeting in the fall.[6-8] The HOD is composed of two elected members from each chartered affiliate. Currently, 50 delegations represent 48 states, one two-state delegation comprises Vermont and New Hampshire, one state-and-district combination is composed of Maryland and the District of Columbia, and the territory of Puerto Rico has its own delegation. The HOD elects officers, including the speaker-elect, speaker, immediate past speaker, treasurer, and secretary. The speaker appoints the parliamentarian for a 1-year term. As with the BOD, HOD officers also serve 1-year terms, with the exception of the 3-year term as speaker-elect, speaker and past speaker.

Board of Medical Advisors

The **Board of Medical Advisors (BOMA)** consists of four AARC-sponsoring professional medical societies that provide significant input to the art and science of the profession of respiratory care. The current societies include the American Society of Anesthesiologists (ASA), the American College of Chest Physicians (ACCP), the American Thoracic Society (ATS), and the Society of Critical Care Medicine (SCCM). BOMA consists of four members nominated from each society who serve staggered terms. BOMA provides medical guidance in the art and science of respiratory care through service to the AARC, and the board's chairperson is designated in a rotation so that each society has a representative serve as chair.

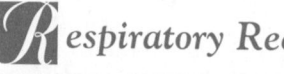

Board of Medical Advisors

The BOMA comprises the following four medical societies:
American Society of Anesthesiologists (ASA)
American College of Chest Physicians (ACCP)
American Thoracic Society (ATS)
Society for Critical Care Medicine (SCCM)

Specialty Sections

AARC **specialty sections** consist of members with special interests in specific areas of respiratory practice. Like AARC membership, specialty section membership is voluntary, but members of a section must pay special dues over and above their annual AARC dues. The current membership in the specialty sections ranges from approximately 450 to 1900 members. Each section has a chairperson, a chair-elect, and various committee chairpersons and committee members and publishes a newsletter approximately six times per year, with a circulation to the section's members. Many AARC professionals are members of multiple specialty sections.

The specialty sections usually meet during the Summer Forum and the International Respiratory Care Congress in the fall. The sections may introduce recommendations directly to the BOD through their liaison, and the board takes action on such reports during meetings. The AARC vice president serves as the liaison between the specialty sections and the BOD. In response to the fast pace of health care policy and practice changes, the sections will likely play a broadened role in governing the AARC.

Respiratory Recap

AARC Specialty Sections	
Management	Home care
Education	Diagnostics
Adult acute care	Continuing care and
Perinatal/pediatrics	rehabilitation
Subacute	Transport

Executive Office The executive office is composed of those individuals employed on behalf of the AARC. Unlike the BOD, HOD, and BOMA, which are composed of professional volunteers who meet membership requirements and work on behalf of the profession, members of the executive office are hired to focus on the daily activities of the AARC.

The AARC executive office has an executive director who reports to the president of the AARC. In addition, associate executive directors and many staff members support the membership, journal, and educational functions of the AARC. The AARC has an in-depth webpage (http://www.aarc.org), at which users can access membership and respiratory care information, special articles, and announcements and AARC members can visit a special members-only section for specific information and services.

AARC in 2000 and Beyond

In response to pressures and fast-paced changes in health care, the AARC's BOD, HOD, and BOMA have initiated changes in governance to improve the organization's responsiveness to its members. Before the most recent changes in 1998, the AARC had more than 60 committees of various types that transacted business for the organization.[1-4] Professional associations generally have no

more than 12 to 15 committees for business transactions. The reporting mechanisms of the AARC crossed lines and created confusion, duplication, gaps, and delays in importance activities.

Therefore efforts focused on ways to streamline and improve the AARC. A new organizational structure was proposed, modified, and approved in the 1998-99 year, creating a streamlined governance that includes the specialty sections and the HOD more directly than the past structure. The changes place more of the day-to-day work responsibilities on the AARC executive office, which has actually performed many of these official duties for years. For example, the AARC controller performs most of the treasurer's duties; this sort of real separation of elected officer and employee duties, for the AARC and the profession, is the primary basis of the changes outlined in the following sections.

Board of Directors The BOD has officers who include a president-elect, president, immediate past president, two vice presidents, and a secretary/treasurer. The immediate past speaker of the HOD, chairperson of BOMA, and chairperson of the President's Council are ex-officio members of the BOD, who nominate officer candidates directly for the election process, thereby decreasing the potential loss of highly qualified candidates each year when they lose an election.

The current number of standing committees are seven—bylaws, elections, executive, finance, judicial, program, and strategic planning. This structure significantly streamlines the committee structure and helps unravel some of the previously overlapping lines of authority. In addition, the combination of the treasurer and secretary reflects the reality that the AARC executive office provides much of the support for these functions, with a controller for financial activities and an administrative assistant who records and distributes the minutes of all BOD meetings.

Respiratory Recap

AARC Standing Committees	
Bylaws	Judicial
Elections	Program
Executive	Strategic Planning
Finance	

At-large directors, equal in number to the specialty sections that exceed 1000 active members, replace the past director structure. The system of specialty section chairpersons continues, with each chairperson serving a dual role as BOD director. The HOD nominates directly the complimentary at-large directors for the election process. The significance of the section chairpersons is magnified by their inclusion as BOD directors (provided that section that more than 1000 members), which allows growth of the AARC through potential inclusion of new associations and specialties that relate to the profession.

House of Delegates

The HOD includes delegations composed of one to three members at the discretion of the chartered affiliate. Some affiliates may elect to restructure themselves, which may yield the current two-delegate structure or use combinations that may include the president-elect, president, or past president to form some or all the delegation. The HOD officer structure also may change as the house moves through changes associated with the overall changes in AARC governance, and certain committee structures and reporting mechanisms will change for similar reasons. Most of the formulations for HOD structural change will take place beyond the year 2000.

President's Council

The **President's Council** formed in the 1971-72 year, consisting of past presidents of the AARC, has been an advisory body in the past. With the new structure the President's Council will play a greater role, with the chairperson being an ex-officio member of the BOD. This council has significant experience and wisdom gained through its members' experiences as elected officials of the AARC. The change should prove an invaluable resource for the BOD as it deliberates the profession's most pressing issues.[6,7]

National Board for Respiratory Care

The **National Board for Respiratory Care (NBRC)** is a voluntary health-certifying board founded in 1960 for the evaluation of professional competence of respiratory therapists.[8] The organization first was named the *American Registry of Inhalation Therapists (ARIT)* to reflect the designation of the profession at that time. The primary purpose of the NBRC and its board of trustees is to provide high-quality voluntary credentialing examinations for respiratory care and pulmonary function technology.

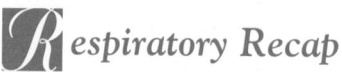

*R*espiratory Recap

National Board for Respiratory Care
The NBRC is the national credentialing body for respiratory care professionals.

The NBRC has established standards for the **credentialing** of practitioners who work under medical direction, publishes a newsletter called *NBRC Horizons* and a directory of credentialed individuals, supports the ethical and educational standards of respiratory care, and cooperates with accrediting agencies to support respiratory care education. To date the NBRC has issued more than 220,000 professional **credentials** to more than 140,000 individuals and currently tests nearly 30,000 candidates annually. The NBRC has established itself as a credible credentialing organization; its respiratory therapy examinations are used as the standard for **licensure** or **certification** in the current 42 states that regulate the profession. The national offices of the NBRC have been in Greater Kansas City since 1974 (with the offices in Lenexa, Kan.), when the ARIT and the technician certification board of the AARC merged to form a single, independent credentialing organization.

The NBRC is accredited by the National Commission for Certifying Agencies (NCCA) and is a member of the National Organization for Competency Assurance (NOCA). The NBRC is sponsored by the AARC, ACCP, ASA, ATS, and the National Society for Pulmonary Technology (NSPT). Each such sponsoring organization appoints members who serve on the 31-member NBRC board of trustees. The three physician groups and the NSPT appoint five members each, and the AARC appoints 10 members; a public member then is added.

The NBRC uses periodic assessments of the practice of respiratory care and pulmonary laboratory technology through direct profiles of current practice provided by active practitioners. The board's credentialing examinations are consistent with the federal government's Uniform Guidelines on Employee Selection Procedures and the American Psychological Association's standards for job-relatedness, validity, and criterion-referenced passing points. This continuous quality improvement has established the NBRC as a valid provider of quality credentialing examinations consistent with leading measurement standards and techniques. The clinical simulation examination was one of the first credentialing examinations of its kind in the United States. All credentialing examinations are developed, prepared, and administered through Applied Measurement Professionals, Inc., a wholly owned subsidiary of the NBRC. As of the year 2000, all NBRC examinations are administered by computer.

Examinations

All NBRC examinations have a common education requirement that includes graduation from a program recognized by CoARC or its predecessor, the JRCRTE, or accredited by the Commission on Accreditation of Allied Health Education Programs (CAAHEP). In addition, all exam candidates must be 18 years of age or older. Table 2-2 provides an overview of the different professional credentials.

All NBRC examinations are graded with a minimum pass level preestablished by the examination committee. Canadian registered respiratory therapists (RRTs) may be admitted as candidates for the certification examination (certified respiratory therapists [CRTs]) and seek reciprocity for their credential in the United States by successful

TABLE 2-2

NBRC *Respiratory Care Credentials*

Credential	Initials
Registered respiratory therapist	RRT
Certified respiratory therapist	CRT
Registered pulmonary function technologist	RPFT
Certified pulmonary function technologist	CPFT
Perinatal/pediatric respiratory care specialist	None

NBRC, *National Board for Respiratory Care.*

completion of the clinical simulation section of the registry examination. All NBRC credentialing examinations have specific admittance criteria for applicants, which may be reviewed through applications available from the NBRC and most employers of respiratory care personnel.

Certified Respiratory Therapist
The certification examination is the entry-level credential for practice in respiratory care. This credential was changed in July 1999 to a certified respiratory therapist (CRT) designation, coinciding with the introduction of a new exam based on revised test matrices. Candidates for the CRT exam must be graduates of an entry-level approved program. The graduate respiratory therapist must attempt and successfully complete the CRT exam before attempting any portion of the registry exam. Competence exhibited through successful completion of the CRT exam is the primary credential used for licensure by most state licensure boards.

Registered Respiratory Therapist
The RRT examination contains two parts that may be taken on the same day or at separate times. The RRT credentialing examinations include the written registry exam with a multiple-choice question format and the clinical simulation exam, which presents layered clinical problems that can be solved successfully in many ways. On the written registry examination the graduate therapist demonstrates a sufficient factual database of information, whereas the clinical simulation examination focuses on the graduate's ability to sufficiently process and assess patient data into clinical practice components. Candidates for the RRT exam must possess the CRT credential and have satisfied the other degree or semester-hour requirements.

Certified Pulmonary Function Technologist
The certified pulmonary function technologist (CPFT) examination is an entry-level certification exam for pulmonary function technologists. It is designed to validate a core competency in pulmonary function testing, data analysis, equipment, and instrumentation. Candidates must have a certificate from an approved program as stated previously; another way to attain eligibility is graduation and a certificate from a pulmonary function technology educational program approved by the NSPT.

Registered Pulmonary Function Technologist
The registered pulmonary function technologist (RPFT) examination is for advanced practice credentialing in pulmonary function technology. The areas of core competency are the same as for the CPFT exam—but at a higher level of practice. Candidates must meet the common eligibility requirements previously stated and must possess the CPFT credential.

Perinatal/Pediatric Respiratory Care Specialist
The perinatal/pediatric specialty certification examination recognizes advanced practice in perinatal, neonatal, and pediatric respiratory care. The successful candidate must demonstrate advanced practice knowledge desirable by employers seeking to hire individuals to perform primary duties. The exam validates competency in core areas of clinical data, equipment, and therapeutic procedures. Candidates must meet the common eligibility requirements stated previously and hold either the RRT or the CRT credential, plus 1 year of clinical experience in perinatal/pediatric respiratory care after attaining NBRC certification.

Committee on Accreditation for Respiratory Care

The **Committee on Accreditation for Respiratory Care (CoARC)** is located in Euless, Texas, and was founded in 1995 as the successor to the JRCRTE and RCAB. The initial composition of CoARC included board members from each organization, with sponsorship from the AARC, ACCP, ASA, ATS, the Association of Schools of Allied Health Professions, and the National Network of Health Career Programs in Two-Year Colleges. The CAAHEP is the overarching accreditation organization that validates CoARC through a requirement that CoARC meet similar standards of excellence required for all allied health education programs. CoARC reports accreditation findings and is scrutinized by CAAHEP, which makes all final accreditation decisions.

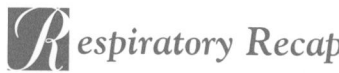

*R**espiratory Recap***

Committee on Accreditation for Respiratory Care

CoARC, as the committee is known, is the national accreditation body for respiratory care education programs.

Accreditation is voluntary, but failure to submit to the accreditation process may be construed as a program's failure to meet the standards and expectations set forth for all allied health education programs. Furthermore, the NBRC requires graduation from an accredited educational program for eligibility for its credentialing examinations.

More information about CoARC may be found via the Internet at http://www.coarc.com.

Accreditation Process

Respiratory care educational programs prepare for the critical CoARC on-site survey visit by following the committee's manual of policies and procedures detailing the expectations for accreditation of a program. The expectations, background knowledge, skills, and sensitivities of site-visit team members also are published in the accreditation manual as an objective guide as to what the CoARC team expects.

The standards by which CoARC measures programs include sponsorship, outcome orientation, resources, student disclosure, instructional planning, and program evaluation. Each critical area has objective standards of expectation established through careful scrutiny of successful high-quality programs. The manuals, policies, procedures, and written information provided by the prospective program for the accreditation decision process are confidential. The confidentiality requirement protects the hard work of each program's educators in their preparation for accreditation. CoARC uses periodic written reviews, reports, and evaluations with an on-site visit by a team of accreditation experts to determine the worthiness of an applicant program for accreditation.

The on-site review process ensures that policies and procedures submitted before an on-site visit reflect the reality of the educational experience at any prospective school. In addition, the accreditation and review process provides a measurable benchmark to which all such programs can be compared. The on-site evaluation team is composed of two individuals, usually one physician and one respiratory therapist, both of whom have completed a site-visitor-training program. The assignment process for site-visit teams allows CoARC to ensure that any on-site visit team members do not have any potential or real conflicts of interest that might be construed to decrease their objectivity.

CoARC publishes on-site team behavioral expectations so that the heads of any program in the review process are aware of the expectations of on-site accreditation visitors. The policies and procedures create a formal matrix that guides the on-site team in its objective consideration of the quality of a prospective program. The accreditation process allows outsiders, prospective students, and government educational oversight groups an objective measure of a program's accomplishments and the quality of respiratory care education. The on-site survey team provides its written findings to the referee for the program's accreditation process, and a final written report is provided to the program, along with the accreditation decision and a candid and analytic report of CoARC findings. The prospective program then provides written evaluation feedback about the on-site survey team, which provides CoARC with information about the objectivity,

knowledge, and demeanor of its on-site team members. CoARC submits written recommendations to CAAHEP regarding initial accreditation and reaccreditation of educational programs every 5 to 10 years.

National Association for Medical Direction of Respiratory Care

The **National Association for Medical Direction of Respiratory Care (NAMDRC)** has existed for more than two decades with the main goal of furthering the role that respiratory care medical direction plays in the achievement of high-quality respiratory care. NAMDRC national offices are located in Chevy Chase, Maryland. In addition, NAMDRC provides an established physician constituency with common professional respiratory care interests and practice. Currently, NAMDRC's members that comprise the medical directors at more than 2000 hospitals. Medical direction of respiratory care departments has been described in many states and through the Joint Commission for Accreditation of Healthcare Organizations (JCAHO) as most appropriate for those physicians with special training and background in respiratory disease and management. Therefore NAMDRC members provide respiratory care medical direction consistent with guidelines prescribed by most oversight agencies.

Most frequently, medical direction for respiratory care has stemmed from pulmonary medicine physicians, followed by practicing anesthesiologists, and a small percentage in other medical specialties. NAMDRC seeks to provide support across a full range of pulmonary care related services, including respiratory care, critical care, pulmonary rehabilitation, pulmonary physiology assessment, respiratory home health care services, hyperbaric oxygen therapy, and sleep disorders.

The NAMDRC reputation has a proven track record of response to its membership and maintains a highly respected profile with regulating agencies and legislators. More extensive information about NAMDRC may be obtained though its publications or the Internet at http://www.namdrc.org.

Publications

NAMDRC prints several publications that include *The Washington Watchline, The Presidential Update, The Clinical and Management Quarterly Newsletter, Understanding Oxygen Therapy,* and *The Medical Director's Handbook. The Washington Watchline* is a monthly publication that keeps NAMDRC membership current on legislative and reimbursement issues associated with pulmonary care. NAMDRC also publishes and distributes position and policy statements in *The Medical Director's Handbook.* Examples of pertinent position statements for respiratory care include "The Delivery of Hospital Respiratory Care and Duties" and "Responsibilities of the

Medical Director of Respiratory Care Services and Pulmonary Function Laboratories."

In many cases, related organizations use these position statements when justification for certain issues requires a respected physician perspective. The AARC may use the position statement entitled "The Delivery of Hospital Respiratory Care" as a basis for the promotion of the respiratory therapist as the best provider of high-quality respiratory care. Evident from the following descriptions of related organizations is that cardiopulmonary care involves closely interacting communities of interest. The related professional organization may have members in multiple roles, such as NAMDRC or BOMA members or representatives of a sponsoring organization.

American College of Chest Physicians

The ACCP provides resources for the improvement of cardiopulmonary health and critical care worldwide. Its primary mission is to promote prevention and treatment of diseases of the chest through leadership, education, research, and communication through publication of *Chest—the Cardiopulmonary and Critical Care Journal*, creation and approval of clinical practice guidelines and consensus statements, government relations' activities, membership, and philanthropy via the Chest Foundation. The ACCP, established 65 years ago, is located in Chicago. Up-to-date information about conferences, new initiatives, and current publications for ACCP is available at http://www.chestnet.org.

Membership

Membership includes more than 15,000 physicians and other professionals in this unique multidisciplinary society dedicated to the advancement of research, teaching, and clinical practice of cardiopulmonary medicine, surgery, and critical care. The designation *FCCP* indicates recognition as a specialist in the field. Allied health professionals who spend at least 50% of their time engaged in clinical work related to cardiopulmonary medicine, surgery, or critical care are eligible for ACCP membership as allied members. The ACCP also grants the FCCP designation to nonphysicians, specialists, and scientists with distinguished accomplishments in cardiopulmonary research, teaching, and clinical practice.

Educational Offerings

The ACCP offers and sponsors a large array of educational materials through meetings, video, audiotapes, CD-ROMS (compact disk–read-only memory), hands-on workshops, and online self-study. The ACCP is accredited for physician continuing medical education, holding large seminars and meetings and cosponsoring educational meetings with professional organizations,

such as the AARC. The Health and Science Policy Committee of the ACCP is a leading resource for the assessment of the science and development of clinical policy in cardiopulmonary medicine and critical care. Its mission is to oversee and monitor significant clinical developments in the scientific and clinical development of cardiopulmonary health and critical care, to transfer research findings to clinical practice, and to provide scientific conferences where research initiatives are discussed and ideas are formulated for future research activities.

Relationship with Respiratory Care

The ACCP is a sponsor of the AARC, NBRC, and CoARC through monetary support and provision of board members for the aforementioned organizations. The ACCP provides leadership for the AARC by naming ACCP members to BOMA.

American Thoracic Society

The ATS was founded in 1905 as an international professional and scientific society focusing on respiratory and critical care medicine. Currently the society has about 12,500 members, 75% of whom reside in the United States. The primary mission of ATS is the prevention and treatment of respiratory disease and the decrease in morbidity and mortality for respiratory disease through research, education, and patient care.

The ATS has a long history of cooperation and advocacy through the American Lung Association (ALA), for which the ATS serves as the medical section. This relationship formed early when a group of physicians from the American Sanitorium Association interested in tuberculosis formed the American Trudeau Society in 1938, which became the ATS in 1960. Early activities in treatment and prevention of tuberculosis formed the mission as it stands today. In the past decade, ATS has become more active in critical care medicine and in the prevention, control, and treatment of diseases such as pneumonia, tuberculosis, and human immunodeficiency virus (HIV) infection. Recently the ALA and ATS have severed their organizational ties. More information may be obtained through the Internet at http://www.thoracic.org.

Primary Missions

Research The ATS promotes research through discovery of new knowledge related to respiratory and critical care medicine in health and disease, assistance to the ALA in peer review, interaction with agencies and organizations that fund new research, and creation of new research funds through philanthropic organizations.

Education Educational initiatives at ATS promote the dissemination of new scientific information, encourage high standards for training and education, encourage research and clinical practice, facilitate rapid transfer of new scientific information to practice, and synthesize new information for the public through the ALA. The ATS publishes the *American Journal of Respiratory and Critical Care Medicine* (AJRCCM) and the *American Journal of Respiratory Cell and Molecular Biology* (AJRCMB), two highly respected journals used by pulmonary and critical care practitioners worldwide.

Patient Care   Patient care initiatives include promotion of the highest standards for quality in health care, establishment of partnerships between pulmonary and critical care medicine, and evaluation of the relationship between cost and quality in the delivery of health care.

Advocacy   The ATS encourages growth in programs and methods that provide high-quality care. In addition, the ATS advises and promotes cooperation by and between governmental and nongovernmental agencies for matters with common interests. For example, the ATS sponsors the AARC, which includes direction activities in BOMA, NBRC, CoARC, and AARC.

American Society of Anesthesiologists

The ASA is an educational, research, and scientific association of physicians organized in 1905 to raise and maintain the standards of anesthesiology and improve patient care. Contact with respiratory care usually involves postsurgical care but most prominently in the area of critical care. The anesthesiologist maintains analgesia and life functions during the surgical procedures in the operating suite. Postoperatively the anesthesiologist maintains contact with the patient's care to ensure a comfortable and stable recovery after surgery.

Members of ASA must be doctors of medicine or osteopathy who are licensed practitioners and have successfully completed a training program approved by the Accreditation Council for Graduate Medical Education (ACGME) or the American Osteopathic Association (AOA). Currently more than 34,000 practitioners are ASA members. The ASA is currently located in Park Ridge, Illinois, a suburb of Chicago. More information is available on the Internet at http://www.asahq.org.

Relationship with Respiratory Care

ASA is currently a sponsoring member of the AARC, NBRC, and CoARC. Through monetary support, clinical expertise, provision of members to BOMA for AARC and other support mechanisms similar to other physician organizations, the ASA contributes to the practice and science of respiratory care. The ASA supports AARC activities and professional issues, developing position state-

ments and clinical practice guidelines to denote the need for respiratory therapy personnel in all areas of clinical practice. The anesthesiologist is the perioperative physician who provides medical care to the patient throughout his or her surgical experience. True to this definition the anesthesiologist may order preoperative testing, including arterial blood gases and pulmonary function studies, to determine the current health status of the patient. In addition, the anesthesiologist may order respiratory care procedures to help promote a higher level of lung function in preparation for surgery. Since 1970 the number of deaths attributed to anesthesia have dropped from 1 in 10,000 to 1 in 250,000.

Mission

The ASA supports the world's largest educational program for anesthesiology practice and science. The annual meeting of ASA, with over 18,000 participants, provides up-to-date research, scientific, and educational continuing education to its members. The ASA sponsors the self-education and evaluation (SEE) program and publishes its own monthly peer-reviewed journal, *Anesthesiology*, which contains most current research findings.

A current initiative of the ASA is public education and government representatives on the hazards of secondhand smoke, especially as it relates to children. The association alerts the public about outcomes related to secondhand smoke, such as preponderance to development of asthma and its role in complications when children have surgery. A copy of the public-education alert for secondhand smoke issues related to children and other pertinent issues related to anesthesia care may be found on the ASA website.

Governmental Affairs

The ASA's Office of Governmental Affairs (OGA) located in Washington, D.C., monitors legislative activities at the state and federal levels to ensure the continuance of high-quality care in all areas of health care for which federal, state, and local governments promulgate regulations. Examples include Medicare and Medicaid. ASA works closely with others groups, such as the AMA and AARC, with which clinical practice issues of regulation may influence anesthesiology and respiratory care.

Governance

The ASA governance structure is similar to that of the AARC in that the ASA has a House of Delegates distributed by geographic region that meets at the ASA annual meeting, where the officers, past presidents, editor in chief of *Anesthesiology*, chairs of sections for education and residency all contribute to the practice, governance, and direction of anesthesiology.

Society of Critical Care Medicine

The SCCM, formed in 1970, is the youngest organization related to the practice of respiratory care. The SCCM was formed to further a multidisciplinary and multiprofessional approach to the care of the critically ill patient. Currently the society boasts more than 9000 members. SCCM membership is evidence of its multiprofessional approach; members include intensivists, nurses, respiratory therapists, pharmacists, pharmacologists, scientists, researchers, bioengineers, critical care industry executives, and other interested allied health professionals. Even the intensivist group is composed of varied physician specialties, such as pediatrics, internal medicine, pulmonary medicine, anesthesia, and surgery.

The SCCM is unique in its multidisciplinary approach to critical care medicine. The use of a multidisciplinary approach to research and patient care promotes a continuum of care, which begins at the moment of injury or illness and proceeds through full recovery. Critical care may be practiced at the site of an accident or in the perioperative setting. However, most activity involving respiratory care practice occurs in the emergency care and intensive care areas. More information may be found through the Internet at http://www.sccm.org.

Journals and Publications

SCCM publishes *Critical Care Medicine*, a monthly journal dedicated to the science and treatment of critically ill patients. More than 15,000 patient care providers receive these journals annually to augment their knowledge and expertise in critical care specialty practice.

Relationship with Respiratory Care

As a multidisciplinary organization, SCCM is engaged in respiratory care in ways similar to previously described medical groups and professional organizations. SCCM is directly involved in the AARC through BOMA and as a BOD member during its rotation as BOMA chair. SCCM sponsors AARC, NBRC, and CoARC, providing a valuable multiprofessional perspective to advances in care and regulatory issues affecting respiratory care.

Key Points

- Many organizations sponsor and support the profession of respiratory care.
- Certain organizations have very specific and limited missions, whereas others are more diverse in purpose and mission.
- The goals of each supporting organization ultimately improve the scope, practice, education, credentials, quality, and professional growth of respiratory care.
- The AARC provides various forms of education and educational opportunities through meetings, publications, grants, awards, fellowships, activities, and services for its members to facilitate continued growth of the profession.
- Although some supporting organizations are restricted to physician membership, many are not, providing numerous opportunities for participation by respiratory therapists.
- The AARC and related professional organizations enhance the entire respiratory care profession, with far-reaching effects beyond each organization's membership.
- Membership in the AARC should not only be desired, but also considered an integral part of a respiratory care professional's identity.

References

1. American Association for Respiratory Care. AARC bylaws. Dallas: The Association; 1996.
2. American Association for Respiratory Care. AARC bylaws. Dallas: The Association; 1998. AARC House of Delegates rules. Dallas: The Association; 1996.
3. American Association for Respiratory Care. AARC House of Delegates rules. Dallas: The Association; 1997.
4. American Association for Respiratory Care. AARC House of Delegates rules. Dallas: The Association; 1998.
5. American Association for Respiratory Care. AARC House of Delegates rules. Dallas: The Association; 1999.
6. American Association for Respiratory Care. AARC House of Delegates historical overview. Dallas: The Association; 1997.
7. American Association for Respiratory Care. AARC House of Delegates historical overview. Dallas: The Association; 1999.
8. National Board for Respiratory Care. NBRC general information brochure. Lenexa, Kan: The Board; 1999.

CHAPTER 3

Health Care Trends and Evolving Roles of Respiratory Care Professionals

Shelley C. Mishoe
Kathleen M. Hernlen

CHAPTER OUTLINE

Health Care Trends
Economic
Demographic
Epidemiologic
Sociologic
Technologic
Educational
Health Care Reform
Traditional Roles of Respiratory Therapists
History of Traditional Roles
Traditional Services Provided
Emergence of Nontraditional Roles

Nontraditional Roles for Respiratory Therapists
Diagnostics
Home Health
Subacute Care
Disease Prevention and Wellness Management
Case Management
Physician Extender
Industry
Research and Technical Writing

OBJECTIVES

1. Describe the economic, demographic, epidemiologic, sociologic, technologic, and educational forces affecting health care trends in the United States.
2. Discuss the historical and traditional role of the respiratory care therapist.
3. Describe how current trends in the U.S. health care delivery system influence the future of health care and respiratory care.
4. Elaborate on the emergence of nontraditional roles for respiratory care professionals.
5. Describe the role of respiratory care professionals in home health, diagnostics, subacute care, wellness and disease prevention, case management, industry, and research.
6. Discuss the role of respiratory therapists as physician extenders.
7. Explain how the respiratory therapy profession must continue to evolve within a continuously changing health care delivery system.

KEY TERMS

Case manager
Diagnostics
Diagnosis-Related Group (DRG)
Fee-for-service
Home health

Managed care
Medicaid
Medicare
Physician extender
Prospective payment

Provider
Pulmonary rehabilitation
Subacute care
Wellness programs

This chapter familiarizes students and respiratory therapists alike with the current and projected trends in health care, including the various forces affecting the health care delivery system in the United States. Its primary purpose is to elaborate traditional and emerging roles for respiratory therapists, presenting numerous possibilities and strategies for their work across the continuum of patient care and addressing the career opportunities in industry, education, management, research, and other venues. Respiratory therapists will continue to play a major role in health care, as well as an important role in the changes with health care delivery. With continuing education, experience, credentials, and documented value, respiratory therapists can continue to assume leadership roles in the constantly evolving health care system.

Health Care Trends

Between World War II (WWII) and the late 1970s the institutional and professional organizations that made up the U.S. health care system remained stable. For the most part, doctors and nurses delivered health care through small, local, and nonprofit organizations. Eventually, other specialists, including respiratory therapists, emerged and thrived. An unrestricted insurance system based on fees for service paid for a level of health care that was unsurpassed. Health care costs continued to escalate at an accelerating rate, however, without sufficient documentation of improvements in quality, access, or effectiveness of care. Consequently, during the 1990s the United States witnessed unprecedented change in health care.

The 1990s was one of the most dynamic decades ever faced by the nation's health professionals. "As disruptive as this period has been, however, it may only have been the prelude."[1] Despite dramatic changes the rate of health care reform continues to accelerate to further improve health care in this country. The health care system will continue to change as it attempts to deliver the highest-quality and most resource-responsible care. Thus health professionals, including respiratory therapists, must continually reconsider ways in which to best add value to the delivery of health services.[1]

Health care reform has centered around four main issues—(1) decreasing costs, (2) improving quality, (3) evaluating effectiveness using measurable outcomes, and (4) improving resource allocation, including access to health care. The ultimate goal is to improve the way health care resources are used so that more people receive better health care at the least possible cost. Obviously, differing opinions exist as to how the United States can achieve this objective and its related goals. Policymakers, government, insurers, providers, scholars, administrators, educators, special interest groups, and the lay public are voicing their opinions on ways to improve health care. In general, all parties agree that many forces shape health care, with economic considerations often receiving the greatest attention.

Numerous factors in both the private and public sectors influenced the change in emphasis from hospitals to other health care settings. Private-sector forces include managed care and the emergence of health care as a major social issue. In addition, public-sector policy and regulation changes to the Medicaid and Medicare systems have had tremendous impacts on the delivery of health care. The traditional delivery system, with the acute care hospital providing the majority of the care, has been replaced with a system that has broadened the continuum of care. This system, although still in the process of defining itself, has seen the emergence and importance of subacute care facilities, home health agencies and disease prevention/wellness programs. In the future, patients may spend more time in nontraditional areas of care, as opposed to the traditional hospital setting. The following sections briefly describe the economic, demographic, epidemiologic, sociologic, technologic, and educational forces affecting health care and health care reform in the United States.

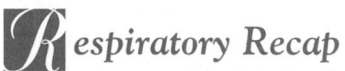

espiratory Recap

Major Health Care Reform Issues
Decrease in costs of health care
Improvement in quality of health care
Evaluation of its effectiveness through outcomes
Improvements in access and resource allocation

Economic

With the inception of **Medicare** and **Medicaid** in the 1960s, health care flourished in the United States. The reimbursement policies allowed consumers to choose their own **providers** in a **fee-for-service** agreement, in which an individual or insurance carrier paid the health care providers when services were rendered based on retrospective payment. (That is, the payment occurred after the service was provided.) Consequently, the use and costs of health care dramatically and suddenly increased in the United States. The fee-for-service system contained few limitations or constraints, and retrospective payment greatly affected inflation, with health care costs consuming continually greater amounts of the gross domestic product. Medicare is now the nation's largest payer for health services, covering approximately 37 million beneficiaries.[2]

Innovation and technologic advances flourished under the fee-for-service system. Health care providers, including physicians and nurses, became increasingly specialized. The respiratory care profession emerged in the 1940s and grew considerably during this time. Eventually, health care in the United States became the envy of other nations.[1] However, quality health care came at a price. As the century neared its end, U.S. health care had become the most expensive in the world. Powerful public and private efforts emerged in the century's last two decades to significantly alter the delivery and financing of health care.

The health care system has come under demands from public and private payers who are no longer willing to financially support a system with such high inflationary costs. Such demands have fueled the managed care industry and created lengthy debates on national health care reform. Because of the increased costs of health care, employers have decreased the amount of money they are willing to spend for employee health benefits. Consequently, insurers are finding ways to offer the same services at lower costs. Predicting how this $1.1 trillion health service industry will look in the 21st century is impossible.[1]

Managed care evolved to place constant pressure on health care providers to restrain health care costs and control use. Managed care requires doctors, nurses, and ancillary service providers to reorganize their work and reallocate duties. Managed care can be defined best as "structures and interventions to control the price, volume, delivery site and intensity of health services provided, the goal of which is to maximize the value of health benefits and the coordination of health care management for the covered population."[3]

With managed care came prospective-payment systems to replace fee-for-service agreements. Managed care companies, such as health maintenance organizations (HMOs) and preferred provider organizations (PPOs), provide enrollees with medical and hospital care in exchange for a preestablished fee. The goal is to ensure that the patient receives adequate care in the appropriate health care setting. Utilization reviews determine and assess requirements for continued stays in each health care setting. When a patient no longer meets the acuity level required, the patient is transferred to a less-costly setting. With managed care the hospital receives a set fee per diagnosis on each patient covered. If health care providers can provide care for less cost than this set fee, they profit; conversely, if the cost of care exceeds the set fee, the health care provider takes a loss. This type of reimbursement is **prospective payment.**

Prospective-payment systems (PPSs) have become increasingly popular as a replacement for the more traditional, fee-for-service agreements. With PPS, health care professionals provide the care they feel is appropriate and, as previously mentioned, can profit from lower-cost care. The fee with PPS is often based on the diagnosis, examples being the federal government's Medicare systems **diagnosis-related groups (DRGs)** or a payment per day of hospitalization (per diem). However, payment can be based on a fixed amount of reimbursement per patient, per year, in a specific geographic area. Fixed payment is also referred to as *capitated payment.* In any such system the health care provider has an incentive to carefully scrutinize the delivery of services and minimize inappropriate or excessive use.

Managed care is becoming increasingly popular among Medicare and Medicaid beneficiaries. Recent data from the Health Care Financing Administration (HCFA) indicate that almost 4 million Medicare beneficiaries and more than 11 million Medicaid recipients participate in managed care programs.[4] This increasing use of managed care among Medicare and Medicaid patients, along with the reductions in payments for respiratory services in home health and subacute care, has contributed to the current changes currently in health care delivery. Doubts about the ability of managed care to provide savings and expand coverage are reinforced by Medicare's experience with managed care. Data show that Medicare loses money on each patient who leaves traditional Medicare for a managed care plan.[5] Although many in the industry assume that a change in the premium formula for Medicare managed care plans will fix this problem,[6] the hoped-for savings in the turning of Medicare into a managed care system are not guaranteed.

During the mid-1960s and into the 1970s, for-profit corporations became a powerful new influence on the way hospitals and physician practices operated. With these changes come both rewards and liabilities for society. Today the U.S. health care system is in constant state of almost revolutionary flux. The system is becoming more efficient in its use of resources, but it has disenfranchised more than 43 million people who do not have health insurance—public or private.[1]

Demographic

Although public- and private-sector changes have been responsible for many of the changes in health care delivery, perhaps the factor that will have the most impact in the future is the changing demographic makeup of the United States. Significant changes continue to occur in the age, ethnicity, economic status, and geographic distribution of the U.S. population—changes that have direct influence on the health care system through alterations in the diseases and population groups seeking services. Population growth and changing demographics contribute to the increased use of health care and its associated costs.

The number of individuals continues to grow, as does the advancing age of those using health care services. The U.S. population is expected to continue to grow until the year 2038, when it should peak. In addition, the population is aging and living longer. By 2010 the estimated life expectancy will be 77.9 years.[7] By 2050, projections state that the number of individuals older than 65 years will be 69 million, representing more than 30% of the population;[8] the over-85 population is the fastest-growing segment of society. Society refers to this change in demographics as the "graying of America." Expectations are that the number of individuals needing respiratory care will increase with the aging demographics. Caring for the these elderly patients will place additional burdens on the U.S. health care system, requiring further innovation in the use of health care resources.

Age-Specific Angle

The over-85 years population is the fastest growing segment of American society.

Ethnicity is also changing and influencing health care needs. Birthrates and immigration rates determine the ethnicity of the U.S. population. Hispanics, African-Americans, and other ethnic groups continue to represent greater percentages of the U.S. demographics. Consequently, health care services directed at specific ethnic groups are increasingly needed to improve access and quality of care without adversely affecting costs.

In addition, demographic imbalances in health care between urban and rural communities exist. Despite a surplus of physicians and other health professionals, certain rural communities do not have a single physician and have only limited access to health care. Rural and inner-city America remains removed from the rich resource base that hospitals and other health care providers offer.[9] Consequently, health care reform is focused on ways to improve access and quality of health care to rural, inner-city, and ethnic groups, as well as the aging population.

Epidemiologic

Another reason for the development and expansion of outpatient and subacute care is the number and types of patients, especially those with chronic problems and lifestyle-related illnesses. Cigarette smoking is an important health risk, contributing to an increased incidence of cancer, heart disease, and chronic obstructive pulmonary disease (COPD). The percentage of current cigarette smokers who smoke a pack or more per day has remained relatively constant in the United States and averages about 25% of the adult population.[10] COPD is the fourth-leading cause of death, killing more than 100,000 people annually, and pneumonia is the sixth-leading cause of death, killing 80,000 annually.[11] According to the National Heart, Lung and Blood Institute, in 1998 the annual cost to the nation for COPD was $26 billion, including $13.6 billion in direct health care costs.[12] The number of Americans diagnosed with asthma increased to more than 14.8 million in 1995.[13] The prevalence of diseases such as asthma, chronic bronchitis, pneumonia, and congestive heart failure, especially among the elderly, will remain a challenge for respiratory care therapists in the twenty-first century.

Sociologic

Sociologic factors affect the way individuals and society think, feel, and act about all aspects of life, including health and health care delivery. To the individual, access to high-quality health care is a priority. However, access is determined by the individual's economic status, which usually involves education and that individual's value to society. Putting aside the problems of racial and ethnic discrimination, minority Americans are at higher risk of living in poverty, being uninsured, and having poorer health-status indicators.[1]

Health care in the United States, with its success in biomedical science, has made enormous advances in confronting the challenges presented by specific diseases. However, recognition is growing that other challenges to health care are equally important. Many factors have converged to create demand for a more integrated approach to care, one that takes into account the multiple factors that interact to promote health or cause illness. Increasingly, sociologic variables are shifting, with growing recognition that health care requires individual responsibility for one's own health, as well as collective responsibility for the health of the population at large.

The focus of health care can no longer be on specific illnesses for individual patients. The construct of illness places the organ system or pathophysiologic state at the center of what it means to be healthy or sick. Emerging societal constructs of health focus on the patient's experience, including the psychologic, sociologic, and spiritual variables as well as biologic. This deepened perspective on health and illness will shape future care. In the face of a growing chronic-disease burden and the aging of the population, such a perspective promotes a deeper and more humane approach to care, encouraging practitioners to help individuals—even those for whom a cure is not possible or those who may be dying—become as wholly functional as possible.[9] No longer are patients referred to in terms of their disease or their status as patients; the current ideology realizes that health care involves real people.

Increasingly, patient satisfaction, wellness, and quality of life are important determinants of health and outcomes of effective health care. The respiratory therapist should incorporate outcomes to evaluate the biopsychosocial determinants of health. Students and respiratory therapists should think of their work in terms of whole people and broader society, not strictly in terms of diseases, treatments, and individual patients.

Technologic

The scientific knowledge base is estimated to double every 22 months.[14] Although it is hard to imagine, advances in medical technology over the next decade will make our current health care practices seem primitive. Technologic influences on health care include drugs, devices, medical, and surgical procedures, as well as the support systems and organizations that deliver care. The advances in telemedicine, telecommunications, and information technology alone are mind-boggling. Could anyone have anticipated that electronic signatures and faxed medical histories would become common practice? Did anyone expect that bar-coding would eliminate much of the previous data-entry needs or that palm computers and cell phones would become commonplace? This textbook reviews some of the most common strategies for information technology, ventilation management, and numerous other aspects of respiratory care; however, because of the time involved in the production of a textbook of this size, how many additions and changes will occur in technology before the book is even in print?!

Technologic advances such as vaccinations, organ transplants, and mechanical ventilation have greatly contributed to health. For the most part, the evolution of the respiratory care profession is intricately and inextricably tied to technology. However, just as technology has contributed to the growth of the profession, changing technologies will create new health professionals and realign others. The traditional lines of distinction among health care providers will continue to change as new skills are needed and acquired.

The year 2000 heralded the mapping of the human genome. This discovery alone has profound and dramatic implications for health care. Specifically in respiratory care are implications for new screening and treatment strategies for chronic cardiopulmonary diseases, such as cystic fibrosis, asthma, and emphysema and infectious diseases, such as tuberculosis and human immunodeficiency virus (HIV). Other implications related to health and illnesses are deep and wide. Technologic influences on health care include advances in diagnostics, therapeutics, drug delivery, gene therapies, organ transplants, laser surgeries, biosensors, and implants. Computer technology and automated systems continue to flourish with ever-increasing applications for information systems, artificial intelligence, and robotics.

In respiratory care, advances in technology have influenced the way in which patients are managed (for example, those with acute respiratory distress syndrome [ARDS] or asthma). Advances in technology have contributed to improvements in ventilators and ventilator graphics, taking the guesswork out of many strategies for oxygenation and ventilation of the most difficult patients. Improvements in drug-delivery devices have altered the uses and recommendations for aerosol therapies. Increasingly, students, faculty, and practicing respiratory therapists must continually consult reference materials because what they learned only a few months previously may have been modified, influencing what such professionals do and say. Technologic advances and continued applications have enormous educational implications, requiring advanced and continued training so that health care professionals can safely and effectively use the latest devices and methods.

Technology also indirectly influences educational needs because of its effects on the sociologic determinants of health and health care. For example, patients increasingly use the Internet as a source of medical information. Consequently, many patients no longer see the physician or other health care provider as the expert. These changes have most likely contributed to the growth of alternative, complementary, and Eastern approaches to health care because consumers now have increased access to global information. In addition, technologic advances have influenced a growing number of health care professionals who provide patient education via computer, including the Internet. Technologic advances will continue to flourish in the 21st century, with dramatic implications and consequences on the numerous determinants of health and health care.

Educational

As society continues to refine and redefine its understanding of health and health care, several questions arise. How can health care practitioners reform their approach to patient care to correspond with these new and evolving health care trends? How can professional education programs train health practitioners who approach patient care by addressing the complex processes in health and illness, including their interconnectedness? How can educational programs address values and beliefs related to patient care? How can the regulatory systems for health professional practice be reinvented to remove barriers while continuing to ensure the highest level of practice from professionals? How can accreditation of educational programs and licensing of health care professional be improved to ensure safety but remove artificial constraints? Health care professions and the public and private sectors continue to grapple with these and numerous additional questions into the 21st century.

Current literature consistently points to the need for reforms in education to prepare health care professionals who have the skills and traits required under current and future health care delivery systems.[15-18] These changes include managed care, seamless care, patient-focused care, and numerous new models and settings to deliver health care. The impact of prospective payment has changed the way providers must plan, manage, and think about health care.[19-21] As a result the roles, skills, and traits expected from health care professionals, including respiratory therapists, also have changed. Practitioners of every discipline are learning or must learn how to cope with managed care systems.

No longer sufficient is the health care personnel who know discreet pockets of knowledge or who have specific clinical skills. Pressure is increasing to train health care practitioners with professional competence exceeding technical training or clinical skills. At the same time, pressure is mounting for allied health professionals with additional technical skills so that clinicians are multiskilled and multicompetent.[14-17] The pressure to change old models, paradigms, and traditions of practice are not unique to respiratory care or allied health but are experienced across health care professions, including nursing and medicine. Employers, educators, and patients of respiratory care professionals argue that practitioners should not only have medical knowledge and technical skills but also professional competencies and characteristics to work in the dynamic health care system. Technical knowledge alone does not equal professional competence.[22]

The National Consensus Conference on Respiratory Care Education identified and ranked the 41 most important areas that will be included in the scope of practice for the respiratory therapist of the future.[23] (See Box 3-1 for specific descriptions of the types of training today's respiratory therapist needs.) This proposed scope of practice coincides with similar studies and reports, including the Pew Commission,[1,9,18,19] the report of the National Commission on Allied Health (NCAH),[16] and the National Health Care Skills Standards Project.[15] According to the NCAH report, curricular content must emphasize rural and urban health, aging, maternal and child health, and minority health in new ways that should result in measurable improvements in quality of care.[16] Community-based health care, patient and family education, and care at alternative sites are additional content areas that must be incorporated.[9]

Many in the industry argue that the current education systems are preparing practitioners for yesterday, not for today, much less for the future.[1,19] Box 3-1 lists 21 competencies that the Pew Commission recommends for the preparation of allied health professionals for the twenty-first century.[1] The respiratory care profession can continue to thrive if it proactively and realistically modifies its curricula to meet the educational needs of preparing respiratory therapists for the current health care markets.[24] The future of allied health professions will be determined in part by the ability of each profession to prepare the type and number of graduates needed for health care today and into the future.

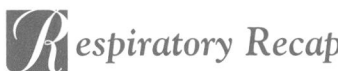

Respiratory Recap

Changes Increasing the Need for Respiratory Therapy

Aging American population
Increased life expectancy
Increased incidence of chronic pulmonary diseases
Steady rate of cigarette smokers and other lifestyle-related risk factors
Technologic advances
Increased focus on health promotion, wellness, and disease management
More well-informed public with greater access to medical information
Increased need for patient education related to changes with managed care

Health Care Reform

The previous sections described the various factors influencing health care reform in this country and some of the changes. The beginning discussion detailed the numerous problems with the U.S. health care system and the way in which health care delivery has undergone and continues rapid and perpetual change. However, this chapter would be incomplete if it failed to mention some of the problems with health care reform.

The nation's preoccupation with the transformation of the health care delivery system to managed care has tended to obscure the importance of a number of other, simultaneous trends,[5] including the declining ability of health care providers to deliver uncompensated care; the declining proportion of individuals with private insurance;

Box 3-1

Allied Health Competencies for the Twenty-First Century

1. Embrace a personal ethic of social responsibility and service.
2. Exhibit ethical behavior in all professional activities.
3. Provide evidence-based, clinically competent care.
4. Incorporate the multiple determinants of health in clinical care.
5. Apply knowledge of the new sciences.
6. Demonstrate critical thinking, reflection, and problem-solving skills.
7. Understand the role of primary care.
8. Rigorously practice preventive health care.
9. Integrate population-based care and services into practice.
10. Improve access to health care for those individuals with unmet health needs.
11. Practice relationship-centered care with individuals and families.
12. Provide culturally sensitive care to a diverse society.
13. Partner with communities in health care decisions.
14. Use communication and information technology effectively and appropriately.
15. Work in interdisciplinary teams.
16. Ensure care that balances individual, professional, system, and societal needs.
17. Practice leadership.
18. Take responsibility for quality of care and health outcomes at all levels.
19. Contribute to continuous improvement of the health care system.
20. Advocate public policy that promotes and protects the health of the public.
21. Continue to learn and help others learn.

From O'Neil EH and the Pew Health Professions Commission. Recreating health professional practice for a new century. San Francisco: The Commission; 1998.

despite a robust economy, the continued growth in the total number of uninsured people; an expected increase in the rate of inflation in health care costs; and budget reductions in Medicare and Medicaid.[5] Some of these trends, such as the decline in uncompensated care, result directly from widespread managed care; the limitations of managed care insurance as it has evolved and the false expectations imposed on it have contributed to many problems in health care today. The failure of reform to effectively address the multifaceted problems of the U.S. health care system continues to be a national concern. Respiratory therapists are increasingly involved in contributing to the improvements in health care as they face growing challenges not only as health care providers but also as health care consumers.

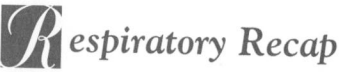

espiratory Recap

Health Care Reform Issues
More individuals than ever before are without access to the health care system.
Health care providers have a declining ability to provide uncompensated care.
Patients must frequently change providers based on insurance criteria.
Professionals, patients, and policy makers are experiencing growing dissatisfaction with the health care delivery system.
Managed care does not necessarily reduce the costs of health care, as intended.
The health care system continues to struggle to reduce costs and improve quality.

Traditional Roles of Respiratory Therapists

History of Traditional Roles

Respiratory therapy has a long and interesting history that lead to its evolution as a health profession. Therapists can trace their roots to the modern use of oxygen at the turn of the twentieth century. During the first two decades of the century, devices such as oxygen tents, nasal catheters, and oxygen masks were developed and used in clinical settings. Modern uses of oxygen created a need for knowledgeable individuals who could administer the gas; thus the field of respiratory therapy was born. Today the government recognizes respiratory therapy as a health profession according to the definition under the Public Health Service Act, title VII, section 701.[24]

In the 1940s a group of physicians and "oxygen technicians" in Chicago began meeting to discuss oxygen therapy. These discussions lead to the creation of the Inhalation Therapy Association (ITA) in 1946 (see Chapter 1). Over the next few years the number of members grew, and

in 1954 the group was renamed the *American Association of Inhalation Therapists (AAIT)*.

The 1970s saw even more advancements in the field of respiratory therapy as air/oxygen blenders, pulse oximetry, oxygen concentrators, portable liquid oxygen systems, and intermittent mandatory ventilation (IMV) were developed and incorporated into clinical practice. In 1978 the National Board for Respiratory Care (NBRC) developed an entry-level concept setting the standards for entry into the field. In 1979 the NBRC administered the first clinical simulation examination for advanced practitioners, replacing the previously used oral exam.

As technology continued to improve in the 1980s and 1990s, advancements in the profession included the development and use of pressure control ventilation, continuous flow ventilation, extracorporeal membrane oxygenation (ECMO), and home care ventilators. The profession saw tremendous growth, especially among specialty fields. The certified pulmonary function exam first was administered in 1984, followed in 1987 with the advanced pulmonary function exam and in 1991 with the first perinatal pediatric exam.

The development of respiratory care emphasized the importance of respiratory care provision by trained, qualified individuals in the hospital setting. Educational programs and respiratory care departments evolved and expanded. Eventually, respiratory therapists assumed roles as managers and educators. As new trends in health care emerged, respiratory therapists quickly responded to best meet patient's needs and establish the new profession. This adaptability has been an asset in recent years as health care continues to change rapidly. The profession began to require personnel with advanced technical training and experience in clinical decision making and critical thinking.[22-24] Respiratory therapy departments capital-

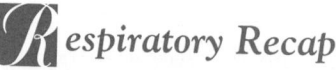

espiratory Recap

Evolution of Respiratory Therapy
Respiratory therapy can trace its roots to oxygen therapy in the early twentieth century.
A professional organization was established in 1946 as the Inhalational Therapy Association (ITA), renamed the *American Association of Inhalation Therapists (AAIT)* in 1956.
The first certification exam for inhalation therapy was administered in 1969.
Entry-level standards were established for the profession in 1978.
Protocol-based care began in the early 1980s.
Respiratory therapy was recognized as a profession by the government in the 1990s.
Respiratory therapy continues to evolve into the twenty-first century.

ized on the therapists' skills in clinical decision-making by implementing protocol-based care.[3]

Traditional Services Provided

Since its birth the primary or traditional setting for the delivery of respiratory therapy was in the hospital. Typically a centralized respiratory therapy department provided a variety of respiratory services, usually divided into two major areas—general patient care and critical care. The categories of services provided by respiratory care professionals included (1) oxygen therapy, (2) other respiratory therapies, (3) physiologic monitoring, (4) ventilation, and (5) specialized skills.

Oxygen therapy involved routine oxygen administration, transport, and hyperbaric oxygen administration. Other respiratory therapies included jet nebulizers, metered dose inhalers (MDIs), intermittent positive pressure breathing (IPPB), and chest physical therapy (CPT). Physiologic monitoring encompassed techniques and procedures such as arterial blood gas sampling and interpretation, pulmonary function testing (PFT), pulse oximetry, and capnography. Ventilator management included adult, pediatric, infant, and noninvasive ventilation. Specialized skills, such as transports, cardiopulmonary resuscitation (CPR), and airway care were also part of respiratory therapy's scope of practice. Respiratory therapists delivered many of these services in both general care and critical care; others, such as ventilator management, were delivered only in the context of critical care. Formal programs trained respiratory therapy students to work in hospitals, providing acute care in the treatment of cardiopulmonary disease.

During the past decade in particular, the traditional role and related career expectations have dramatically changed, coinciding with the changes in health care delivery. Today, educational program and continuing education programs must prepare respiratory therapists to work in nontraditional roles across numerous health care settings in addition to acute care in hospitals. Table 3-1 highlights the traditional roles of respiratory therapists.

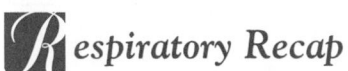
espiratory Recap

Traditional Respiratory Therapy Services
Centralized respiratory therapy departments emerged.
Both general care and critical care were available.
Care was provided primarily in hospitals
Services provided by respiratory therapists included oxygen therapy, medication delivery, airway clearance, physiologic monitoring, ventilator management, and specialized skills.

Emergence of Nontraditional Roles

In the past few years the traditional delivery system, with the acute care hospital providing the majority of the health care,

TABLE 3-1

Traditional Respiratory Care Services Provided by Respiratory Therapy Departments

Service	% Providing Service in 1992
Oxygen therapy	100
Mechanical ventilation	96
Chest physiotherapy	96
Bland aerosol therapy	81
IPPB therapy	93
Intermittent mask CPAP	63
Incentive spirometry	96
Aerosol bronchodilator therapy	100
MDI bronchodilatory therapy	82
MDI steroid therapy	66
Pulse oximetry	98
Blood gas analysis	83
Pulmonary function testing	96
Pulmonary rehabilitation	43
Home care and/or DME	32

From Cullen DL, Sullivan JM, Bartel RE et al. Year 2001: delineating the educational direction for the future respiratory care practitioner. Proceedings of a national consensus conference on respiratory care education. Dallas: American Association for Respiratory Care; 1992.
IPPB, Intermittent positive pressure breathing; CPAP, continuous positive airway pressure; MDI, metered dose inhaler; DME, durable medical equipment.

has been replaced with a system that has broadened the continuum of care. This system has already seen the emergence and importance of subacute care facilities, home health agencies, and prevention/wellness programs, and in the future, patients may spend more time in nontraditional areas of care. Private- and public-sector factors are precipitating these changes.

The changes in reimbursement strategies, the increase in managed care, and the aging population challenged hospitals to develop ways to decrease costs. Hospitals underwent restructuring and reorganization in the 1990s. A recent survey of American Association for Respiratory Care (AARC) found that 67% of its members worked in organizations that have restructured in the past 5 years.[3] Recent changes include decreasing the levels of management, labor substitution, decentralization of respiratory care departments, patient-focused care, and alternative or contract employees.

Many respiratory care departments in the United States have undergone some form of decentralization. With total decentralization, hospitals no longer assign respiratory therapists to a respiratory care department but instead assign respiratory therapists to a nursing unit, where the practitioners report directly to nursing supervisors.[3,25] Other hospitals have adopted a partially decentralized structure in which some of the respiratory duties or personnel have decentralized, whereas other duties, usually the more technically advanced, are provided by a core respiratory therapy department.

The use of protocols have emerged with labor substitution for a variety of services in the traditional setting. With protocols, respiratory therapists have been able to expand their skills by providing assessments and choosing treatment plans for patients. On the other hand, nurses or other health care personnel have begun to assume selected respiratory therapist duties in some settings. Considerable concern exists as to the competencies of these alternative personnel, even for basic, technical skills. Studies have shown that respiratory therapists demonstrate better technique in the delivery of respiratory procedures than do other providers.[3,26,27] Hospitals using respiratory therapists and protocol-directed care have significantly less overuse of respiratory therapy treatments.[28] Patient assessment and education cannot be overlooked, even during routine aspects of care.

The cost of caring for patients is greater in the acute care setting due to the number of fixed costs, such as staff members and equipment. Therefore cost-containment concerns have lead to the development of lower-cost, postacute care delivery sources, such as home health, subacute care, and outpatient programs. The estimated cost of caring for a patient in a hospital (nonintensive care) ranges from $300 to $800 per day, with the cost of intensive care ranging from $800 to $2000 per day.[29] Alternatively, the cost of subacute care ranges from $600 to $700 per day.[29]

According to the American Healthcare Association, during the 1990s the number of subacute care beds increased dramatically. At the end of the decade the United States had between 35,000 and 45,000 subacute care beds.[30] The National Subacute Care Association predicts that within 5 years, subacute care will account for 40% of all Medicare expenditures.[31]

To adapt to changes in the health care system, respiratory therapists have had to change as well. Many therapists have capitalized on this new way of thinking because they have the necessary skills needed to thrive under managed care. Respiratory therapists have strong, specialized backgrounds in the diagnosis, treatment, and prevention of cardiopulmonary diseases, which constitute a large portion of the high cost of chronic diseases currently challenging managed care companies. Respiratory therapists have strong assessment skills and the ability to create treatment plans that can lower the cost of caring for patients. Therapists also are experts on respiratory equipment, products, and medications. Because of their knowledge of cardiopulmonary diseases, respiratory therapists make excellent patient educators and can use their assessment, communication, and critical-thinking skills in prevention and wellness programs, such as those for pulmonary rehabilitation and asthma management. As cardiopulmonary specialists, respiratory therapists may represent the best alternative for patient education to facilitate improved adherence to treatment plans.

Respiratory therapists have been using these strong clinical backgrounds and assessment skills to create new careers in nontraditional settings. Although 80% of all therapists work in hospitals, recent studies conclude that many job opportunities in the coming years will be in nontraditional settings.[3] To make this transition more complete, therapists must add to their existing skills, proving their cost-effectiveness, adapting to new practice settings, and dealing with the chronic aspects of disease management, not just the acute phase. They must be willing to take on new responsibilities and be open to risks,[3] advancing their skills in communication and patient education and their knowledge of managed care and reimbursement.

Respiratory therapists have always been valued for their clinical expertise, knowledge, and management of respiratory diseases; however, working in nontraditional roles requires different skills. What may be of importance in an acute care setting, may not be as important to a respiratory therapist working in a subacute care or a home health setting. The professional and personal skills usually change from environment to environment, requiring adaptability, flexibility, problem-solving skills, and continuing education. Respiratory therapists must be able to provide effective care and document their worth in this competitive health care system.

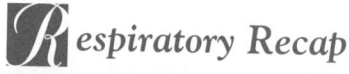

Respiratory Recap

Qualifications of Respiratory Therapists for New Health Care Roles
Strong clinical backgrounds in the diagnosis, treatment, and prevention of cardiopulmonary disease
Technologic skills (computer skills)
Patient assessment skills and the ability to create effective treatment plans
Patient education abilities, valuable because self-care teaching is increasingly important in today's health care environment
Ability to train as new technologies and practices emerge
Adaption of education and credentialing related to scopes of practice and needs

Nontraditional Roles for Respiratory Therapists

The development of nontraditional arenas for health care has offered new, challenging opportunities. Respiratory therapists have taken advantage of this enlarged continuum of care to create new niches for themselves, expanding their clinical skills into areas such as cardiopulmonary diagnostic testing and polysomnography. Emerging nontraditional therapist roles include home health, diagnostics, subacute care, wellness and disease management, and case management. In addition, respiratory therapists also work in industry, in research, sales, technical development, and medical writing. Roles in education and management continue to be available, although the duties and

Box 3-2
Evolving Scope of Practice for Respiratory Therapy

Mechanical ventilation management/life support systems
Invasive and noninvasive cardiodiagnostics and cardiopulmonary monitoring/cardiac monitoring/arterial line/indwelling catheter
Traditional basic therapies (oxygen therapy, aerosol therapy, humidity therapy, incentive spirometry, for example)
Management
Pulmonary function testing
Treatment assessment/outcome assessment
Home care
CPR/resuscitation
Respiratory care of neonatal and pediatric patients
Arterial blood gases
Rehabilitation/cardiopulmonary rehabilitation
Patient/family education
Protocols
Health promotion/disease prevention
Smoking cessation/nicotine intervention
Hyperbaric oxygenation
ECMO/other life-support techniques
Management
Discharge planning
Sleep studies

Research
Medication administration
Stress/exercise testing
Alternative-site care delivery
Bronchoscopy
Infection control
Electrolyte analysis
Geriatrics
Quality/performance assessment
Case management
EEG/neurodiagnostics
Computerization/information management
Transport/trauma in-flight specialist
Metabolics
ACLS/NRP/PALS
Mechanical cardiac support
Ethics
Teaching/team management with other health professions
Patient-focused care
Technology assessment
Charting and record keeping

From Cullen DL, Sullivan JM, Bartel RE et al. Year 2001: delineating the educational direction for the future respiratory care practitioner. Proceedings of a national consensus conference on respiratory care education. Dallas: American Association for Respiratory Care; 1992.
CPR, Cardiopulmonary resuscitation; ECMO, extracorporeal membrane oxygenation; EEG, electroencephalogram; ACLS/NRP/PALS, advanced cardiac life support/neonatal resuscitation program/pediatric advanced life support.

responsibilities also have changed. Since its inception, the respiratory therapy profession has benefited from strong relationships with physicians. Consequently, therapists have become physician extenders—a role that continues to evolve, although reimbursement constraints may limit its potential outside traditional, acute care settings.

Box 3-2 lists some nontraditional roles of respiratory therapists. In addition, the following sections elaborate the nontraditional roles for respiratory therapists across the health care industry.

Diagnostics

Respiratory therapists have intense education and training in **diagnostics** to include comprehensive aspects of (1) blood gas analysis; (2) nutritional, cardiac, pulmonary, exercise, and sleep assessments; (3) chest radiology; (4) bronchoscopy; (5) PFT; and, (6) hemodynamics and gas exchange monitoring. Chapters 19 through 30 provide detailed discussion on the important role of respiratory therapists in the assessment of patients with respiratory impairment. The following sections highlight some nontraditional roles in diagnostics, with a focus on cardiopulmonary diagnostics and polysomnography.

Cardiopulmonary Diagnostics   One area the AARC has identified as an opportunity for respiratory therapy ex-

pansion is cardiopulmonary diagnostics.[32] Use of technology for diagnostics has dramatically increased within hospitals and alternative health care sites; PFT, blood gas analysis, and cardiac testing are already a part of the scope of care of respiratory therapists in many acute care settings. However, the growing trend is to perform these tests in outpatient settings or by independent, contract services. Many subacute care facilities do not have laboratories on site but contract with outside laboratories for these services. Respiratory therapists have clinical backgrounds in cardiopulmonary diseases, which make them ideal candidates to work in cardiopulmonary diagnostic laboratories.

Many therapists have seized this opportunity by establishing their own laboratories. Therapists have created companies that offer laboratory services such as pulmonary function and sleep study testing and have contracted with managed care companies to provide services for clients enrolled in managed care programs. Other respiratory therapists have focused on providing diagnostic testing in industrial settings. Federal law requires employers to provide safe workplaces, and tests required by the Occupational Safety and Health Administration (OSHA) include fit testing for respirators, asbestosis testing, and audiometric testing for noise levels.

Skills and Rewards   Respiratory therapists working in diagnostic testing require outstanding technical abilities. They should enjoy working with and maintaining equipment; possess strong computer skills, especially with hardware, software, and telecommunication processes; and be familiar with the various organizations that accredit laboratories, as well as the related governmental regulations. Those respiratory therapists who serve industries should be familiar with OSHA standards and testing requirements and may need to complete additional continuing education courses to meet OSHA compliance levels.

Respiratory therapists involved in diagnostics enjoy providing a needed service to patients concentrating on the diagnostic aspect of disease. As opportunities for new ventures expand, some respiratory therapists have even opened their own businesses, combining their creativity and business savvy.

Respiratory Recap

> **Opportunities and Rewards of Cardiopulmonary Diagnostics**
>
> Expansion of the scope of practice
> Satisfaction of helping with the diagnosis of disease and treatment planning
> Opportunities to use clinical, computer, creative, and business skills
> Expanded markets with potential to establish new business ventures
> Opportunities for consult and contract work

Polysomnography   During the last two decades polysomnography has witnessed tremendous growth as the public and medical professionals have become more aware of the importance of sleep and the consequences of sleep deprivation. Centers that perform special testing have gained stature in the diagnosing and treatment of sleep-related diseases. Sleep studies include two main tests—the polysomnography and multiple sleep latency test (MSLT). Testing facilitates the diagnosis of sleep disorders such as narcolepsy, sleep apnea, and restless leg syndrome.

Sleep testing requires the use of various types of equipment to monitor body movement. Typical sleep studies involve placement of electrodes on the scalp to monitor brain activity for sleep staging with the electroencephalogram (EEG), electrodes to monitor eye movement, electrodes to monitor limb movement with the electromyogram (EMG), belts or strain gauzes to monitor abdominal and chest wall movement, and nasal and oral airflow transmistors to monitor apnea. In addition, pulse oximeters monitor oxygen saturation levels and electrocardiogram (ECG) electrodes monitor cardiac rate/rhythms. Many hospitals have developed their own sleep laboratories, but because of the expensive equipment and specialized personnel needs, other hospitals have contracted with independent sleep laboratories. The majority of sleep tests are performed in the outpatient setting, and many laboratories now perform sleep studies in the patient's home.

Skills and Rewards   Respiratory therapists interested in polysomnography should be skilled in performing and evaluating diagnostic procedures, specifically sleep studies, and be able to operate a variety of equipment. These therapists also must work night shifts and should enjoy quiet environments. Many patients feel ill at ease with the prospect of someone watching them sleep. The polysomnographer should possess strong people skills and must be able to put patients at ease to ensure both patient comfort and test validity. The testing procedure itself is intimidating to patients because it involves the application of electrodes and monitors to the body.

Many respiratory therapists have the basic background needed to begin working in sleep laboratories but require additional training in the equipment and procedures related to such testing. A variety of educational programs for additional education in polysomnography are available, ranging from 2-year programs to 1- to 2-week courses on sleep-related subjects. Advancement in the field requires further education in the scoring of sleep studies, which involves interpretation of data after the test is completed. Many sleep laboratories employ polysomnographers who provide scoring services only and do not perform the actual sleep testing, allowing some polysomnographers to work during the day. The Board of Registered Polysomnographic Technologists offers an examination to assess the competence of individuals performing polysomnography; those who successfully complete the test earn the credential *registered polysomnographic technologist (RPSGT)*. Examination candidates must complete 18 months experience in polysomnography, or 12 months of experience if they possess credentials in a health-related field.

Probably the biggest reward for polysomnographers is the ability to correctly diagnose sleep disorders and participate in the development and implementation of effective care plans. Effective treatment of sleep disorders, such as sleep apnea syndrome, has a tremendous impact on patients' quality of life, making the work self-satisfying.

Respiratory Recap

> **Opportunities and Rewards of Polysomnography**
>
> Possession of basic background needed to begin working in sleep laboratories
> Credentialing examination by Board of Registered Polysomnographic Technologists to assess competence of individuals performing polysomnography
> Further education to score sleep studies
> Opportunity to work independently in sleep centers and patients' homes
> Ability to assist with diagnosis and development of effective care plans
> Self-satisfaction of dramatically improving patients' quality of life

Home Health

Home health has been defined as "the provision of services and equipment to the patient in the home for the purpose of restoring and maintaining his or her maximal level of comfort, function and health."[33] At the turn of the twentieth century, primarily doctors and nurses provided the majority of health care in the home. Due to the advancement of medical knowledge and technology, this practice soon became impossible and hospitals became the choice site for health care provision. During the past century, most patients recovered from illnesses in acute care hospitals. Patients did not return to their homes until they were able to care for themselves. Recently, however, this thinking has changed, and the financial incentives realized by managed care companies, coupled with the desire of more patients to recover in their homes, has resulted in the increasing use of home health.

Today, health care professionals can provide home health services to patients with acute illnesses or exacerbations of chronic illnesses, as well as those with long-term disabilities who do not require hospitalization. Home health services fall into five different categories—home health agencies, hospice care, home medical equipment, home infusion therapy, and homemaker services/private-duty nursing.

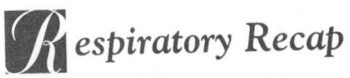

Types of Home Health Services
Home health agencies Hospice care Home medical equipment Home infusion therapy Homemaker/private-duty nursing

Skills and Rewards   A typical day in home care may take the respiratory therapist from the most expensive subdivision to a government housing project, and from the cleanest home to the most unkempt. Therefore the respiratory therapist must be adaptable and ready to work in any environment with a variety of people. Being able to relate to the patient in a nonjudgmental manner helps build the therapist-patient relationship. For example, many patients have difficulty adjusting to the permanence of the oxygen equipment or the need for lifelong medication use.

Respiratory therapists may not truly appreciate the reality of chronic cardiopulmonary disease until they work in home care. One of the biggest rewards may be the ability to offer suggestions to deal with potential problems, such as the need to plan patient outings in advance to ensure an adequate supply of oxygen. Patients may decide not to wear their oxygen equipment or not to take their medications because they feel better or have begun to deny that they have problems. Respiratory therapists must

be able to persuasively educate such patients about the consequences of their choices.

Therapists in the home care setting also need a strong knowledge of reimbursement policies and case management. Physicians may order prescriptions or treatments for patients, thinking that they are using the most cost-effective means when often less-costly alternatives exist. For example, an MDI may be the most cost-effective method of delivering bronchodilator therapy in the hospital, but not in the home. In some states, Medicare may not pay for the MDI but may pay for the unit-dose albuterol via mobilization. Therefore the role of the respiratory therapist is critical in reducing the cost of care for both the health care provider and the patient.

Despite the concerns about reimbursement, home health therapists find many aspects of their jobs rewarding. Many respiratory therapists enjoy the flexibility of setting their own schedules and consider the job less stressful than acute care work, which involves dealings with frequent emergencies. Home health respiratory therapists enjoy personal interaction and build stronger relationships with patients and their families. Being able to follow a patient for a significant amount of time is another reward. The chance to educate patients about specific diseases, equipment, and ways to improve quality of life is one of the most rewarding aspects of home health.

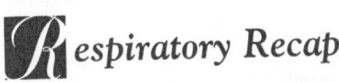

Opportunities and Rewards of Home Health
Ability to work in various environments Chance to educate patients and family members dealing with chronic cardiopulmonary diseases Opportunity to gain continued knowledge of reimbursement policies Cost-effective nature in comparison to acute care Recognition of the value of respiratory therapists in home health, including reimbursement for services Possibility for increased opportunity if respiratory therapy is included in reimbursement for skilled visits

Subacute Care

As hospitals look for ways to decrease the number of patient days per stay, postacute care has gained popularity. **Subacute care** attributes its growth to the Medicare prospective-payment system. Managed care sets limits to the amount of money provided to hospitals for patient care and uses strict review criteria to ensure that patients meet the requirements for acute care. Although still in the process of defining itself, subacute care has become a feasible alternative to patients who no longer require acute care, often serving as an intermediary between the acute care hospital and the patient's return home. The prevalence of managed care has shown a trend toward the increased use of subacute care as more patients are discharged from acute care hospitals more quickly. If the trend continues, the number of long-term acute care facilities (LTACs) and rehabilitation hospitals will increase, providing more opportunities for respiratory therapists.

Some confusion has persisted in health care delivery as to which criteria require subacute care. Medicare reimbursement policies further complicate the confusion. The American Subacute Care Association defines subacute care as follows:

> Subacute patients are sufficiently stabilized to no longer require acute care services, but are too complex for treatments in a traditional nursing center. Subacute care centers and programs typically treat patients who present with rehabilitation and/or medically complex needs and require physiological monitoring.[34]

All subacute care facilities require respiratory care services, the degree of which is determined by the type of facility and acuity of the patient. The Joint Commission on Accreditation of Healthcare Organizations (JCAHO) has specifically identified respiratory care as a necessary component for accreditation of subacute care.[3,34]

Subacute care is experiencing rapid growth due to several factors, primarily including managed care and Medicare reimbursement policies and the aging population. In 1994, subacute care was a $1 billion industry;[3,34] during 2001, subacute services accounted for 40% of Medicare expenditures, with revenues of approximately $20 billion. Subacute facilities have 20% more revenue from managed care than do nursing homes and 14% more revenue from managed care than do rehabilitation centers.[3]

As mentioned previously, the type and amount of services provided by respiratory therapists in subacute care varies, depending on the setting and patient acuity. In most cases, if ventilator management is offered, respiratory therapists are available 24 hours a day. If ventilator management is not a component of care, respiratory therapists may be available daily. Therapists working in hospitals have become more specialized in recent years, whereas those working in subacute care facilities have become more generalized in the services they provide. Ironically, however, administrative supervisors of subacute care facilities value respiratory therapists for their respiratory specialization.

Services provided may be complex and often are similar to duties performed by hospital therapists; they include assessment, treatment, care planning, airway care, monitoring, diagnostics, and other traditional therapies. Because respiratory therapists are experts in subacute care, they provide more of the airway care, such as tracheostomy care and suctioning, in subacute care facilities than in traditional settings. The patients in subacute care are generally medically stable and do not require extensive diagnostic workups. For this reason the emphasis in such settings is less on diagnostic procedures and more on assessment and monitoring. Subacute care involves less therapist-physician interaction, and respiratory therapists usually use protocols for oxygenation, ventilator management, and other therapies.

The interdisciplinary team—nurses, physical therapists, occupational therapists, speech pathologists, and other specialists depending on the patients' needs—is essential for effective subacute care delivery. Two critical members of the interdisciplinary team for subacute care are the patient and the patient's family, both of who play vitally important roles in the planning and implementation of care plans. Therapists' close work relationships with other disciplines helps ensure that patients receive the necessary information to help them achieve their treatment goals.

Types Different types of subacute care facilities currently include LTACs, skilled nursing facilities (SNFs), specialty hospitals, rehabilitation hospitals, and respiratory units within acute care hospitals. The HCFA defines the types of postacute care settings by the following criteria: nursing hours per day, rehabilitation requirements, length of stays, and cost within a particular institution.

LTACs are licensed hospitals that are exempt from the Medicare prospective-payment system as long as they maintain an average patient length of stay greater than 25 days. Patients usually stay between 10 and 60 days. Long-term hospitals receive payment from Medicare on a reasonable-cost basis and usually specialize in patients with pulmonary or medically complex problems. Such patients no longer require extensive diagnostic workups but do need additional therapy and nursing support. If the LTAC has patients on ventilators, respiratory therapy is available 24 hours per day.

SNFs are identified beds certified by the HCFA to participate in the Medicare program and serve its long-term care benefits. One way to differentiate SNFs from LTACs is in the number and amount of services provided; SNFs generally provide fewer services than LTACs. SNFs offer an average of 2 to 3 nursing hours per day and occupational therapy, physical therapy, and respiratory therapy as needed. The length of stay for patients averages 60-plus days, with an average cost of $100 to $150 per day. SNFs may be free standing or hospital based, but as a rule the cost of care is higher in a hospital-based SNF.

Many hospitals have created their own SNFs to deal with patients who require long-term ventilation or have medically complex problems. These units were among the first subacute care programs in the country.[3] SNFs have

ℛespiratory Recap

Differentiating SNFs and LTACs

LTACs are licensed hospitals.
LTACs are exempt from the Medicare prospective-payment system as long as they maintain an average patient length of stay greater than 25 days.
SNFs are identified beds certified by the HCFA to participate in the Medicare program for its long-term care benefits.
SNFs may be free standing or hospital based.

been proven to be cost effective in many cases. For instance, Shawnee Mission Medical Center in Kansas implemented a SNF with respiratory therapists providing services and demonstrated improved health care outcomes. The LOS for pneumonia patients decreased from 8 days to 4 days, which decreased the costs of caring for pneumonia patients by 50%.[35] The American Health Care Association sponsored a study that concluded that Medicare could save at least $142 million per year if clinically stable ventilator-dependent patients were treated in SNFs instead of acute care facilities.[3]

The AARC commissioned a study to determine the cost effectiveness of respiratory therapists providing services to patients with respiratory diagnoses in SNFs.[36] This study compared outcomes and costs between patients who received respiratory services from respiratory therapists with those who received services from nonrespiratory personnel. The analysis revealed that Medicare beneficiaries treated by respiratory therapists had better outcomes and lower costs that those with nonrespiratory providers.[36] Patients treated by respiratory therapists stayed 3.6 days less, with a projected annual cost savings of $97.9 million to Medicare in 1996.[36] Approximately 31% more beneficiaries treated by a nonrespiratory therapist during an initial SNF visit required subsequent services in a hospital emergency room or outpatient setting; Medicare spent 23% more to treat these patients.[36] In addition, Medicare beneficiaries treated by respiratory therapists had a 42% lower mortality rate at their next encounter with the Medicare system, compared with a similar group who received respiratory care from nonrespiratory therapist caregivers.

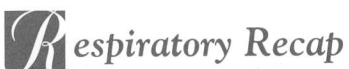 *espiratory Recap*

SNF Patients Treated by Respiratory Therapists
Patients had a 3.6-day shorter length of stay. Patient mortality was reduced by 42%. Medicare saved $97.9 million.

From Muse and associates, for American Association for Respiratory Care: A comparison of Medicare nursing home residents who receive services from a respiratory therapist with those who did not. Executive Summary. 1999. p. 1. [http://www.aarc.org/professional_resources/muse].

Skills and Rewards   Although many of the same skills used in subacute care settings are the same as those used by respiratory therapists in traditional hospital settings, some important differences exist. Respiratory therapists who work in subacute settings have less physician interaction, so they must be self-directed, able to use protocols and reimbursement criteria, willing and able to make decisions, and able to implement treatment plans for their patients. They must be aware of costs and reimbursement requirements so that the care they provide is covered by insurance and possess strong clinical, disease management,

critical-thinking, and problem-solving skills, plus experience working with protocols and care plans before working in subacute care.

Subacute care respiratory therapists find more of an educational component in their jobs. Therefore they must possess excellent communication and teaching skills. Subacute care places an emphasis on interdisciplinary care planning and teamwork; in addition to working independently, the respiratory therapist also must function as an interdisciplinary team member. A good knowledge of the skills and services provided by other allied health professionals is essential, as is a cooperative nature. A strong background in the development and implementation of care plans, outcomes assessment, and discharge planning also are needed.

The rewards of working in subacute care differ from the intrinsic motivators involved in acute care. Many patients in subacute settings have long-term or chronic illnesses. The ability to wean a patient who has been ventilated for weeks or sometimes months from mechanical ventilation is just one of the rewards. Other respiratory therapists enjoy being involved and spending more time with patients, finding satisfaction from improving a patient's quality of life. Some therapists enjoy the less-hurried, one-on-one contact with their patients. Many respiratory therapists who work in subacute care enjoy the opportunities they have to get to know not only the patients, but patients' family members as well to help them see the patient as a whole person. Other respiratory therapists enjoy the opportunity to be self-directed by using protocols; therapists are able to assess their patients and implement the care they deem necessary. The opportunity to work closely with other disciplines also appeals to many therapists who work in subacute care.

espiratory Recap

Opportunities and Rewards of Subacute Care
Necessity of respiratory care for accreditation of subacute care facilities
Subacute services accounting for 40% of Medicare expenditures
Opportunities and rewards from working with interdisciplinary teams
Ability to develop and use protocols and care plans to provide and evaluate care
Rewards from focusing on the whole person for holistic care
Addressing of the emotional and physical impacts of chronic disease
Improvement in the quality of life of patients with chronic disease

Disease Prevention and Wellness Management

As society's construct of health and health care changes, an unprecedented focus is placed on wellness, as opposed to the previous preoccupation with illness. Discussion of the current economic climate regarding disease prevention, disease management, and wellness programs is interspersed and elaborated throughout this textbook. The following sections provide overviews of the increasingly important role respiratory therapists play in disease prevention and wellness.

Pulmonary Rehabilitation   With greater emphasis on education and disease prevention to control costs, many hospitals have developed **pulmonary rehabilitation** centers and wellness programs for chronic diseases. Pulmonary rehabilitation, although not a new concept in respiratory care, has gained importance in recent years. The National Institutes of Health (NIH) defines pulmonary rehabilitation as "a multidimensional continuum of services directed to persons with pulmonary disease and their families, usually by an interdisciplinary team of specialists, with the goal of achieving and maintaining the individual's maximum level of independence and functioning in the community."[37]

The goals of pulmonary rehabilitation involve helping patients increase their activity through exercise training and education. Pulmonary rehabilitation programs usually are divided into three phases. Phase I is the pretesting portion of the program in which the patient performs tests, such as pulmonary function studies, stress tests, and the 6- to 12-minute walking test. Patients usually complete questionnaires, which assess their nutritional, psychologic, lifestyle, and vocational needs. Phase II includes education and exercise. Educational topics include lung anatomy, breathing and pulmonary hygiene techniques, nutritional guidelines, medications, equipment, and the importance of exercise conditioning; exercise is introduced during Phase II. Respiratory therapists monitor patients for oxygen saturation levels, breathing techniques, pulse, rhythm rates, and blood pressure while the patients perform exercise, which may be as simple as walking or riding a stationary bike. As the patient progresses through the program, the workload is gradually increased. Phase III includes follow-up care and long-term maintenance.

Age-Specific Angle

Respiratory therapists working in pulmonary rehabilitation should have strong backgrounds in geriatrics.

Skills and Rewards   A good understanding of cardiopulmonary physiology and pathophysiology is important for work in pulmonary rehabilitation. Understanding PFTs is essential, as is the practical ability to perform and use the PFTs. Therapists in this field need strong interpersonal and communication skills and the ability to motivate people. In addition, they should have strong backgrounds in geriatrics but be able to work with individuals of all ages as needed.

Respiratory therapists who work in pulmonary rehabilitation and wellness programs enjoy building positive relationships with their patients and those patients' families. They often get to know the patients as individuals much better than do traditional therapists. In many cases they become the primary source of health education for patients and their families, so a strong bond may become established. Making a difference in their patients' quality of life is a major reward for therapists working in pulmonary rehabilitation.

Respiratory Recap

Opportunities and Rewards of Pulmonary Rehabilitation

Way to control costs for patients suffering from chronic lung disease

Duties that include assessment, education, exercise training, and long-term maintenance

Use of multidisciplinary approach for evaluation, education, and care

Focus on the psychosocial and quality-of-life aspects of chronic pulmonary diseases

Wellness Programs   Managed care has emphasized the provision of education and programs not only for ill individuals but also for those who are healthy, to maintain their good health. This approach attempts to decrease the long-term costs to provide health care services because healthy people require less health care.

To help ensure that the healthy remain healthy, hospitals and managed care companies have established **wellness programs,** which include classes that educate consumers in ways to maintain and even improve quality of life. Wellness programs cover topics such as the benefits of diet, good sleep habits, relaxation techniques, routine exercise, diagnostic screenings, and the psychosocial aspects of health. The emphasis is placed on disease prevention and the establishment and maintenance of healthy life habits. Because paying for health care has become a stressor, wellness programs can and should focus on access and reimbursement issues related to acute and chronic care.

Managed care companies also offer wellness programs to their enrollees to keep hospital readmissions low. By reducing hospital admissions, managed care companies benefit financially while improving the health of their clients. Many managed care companies now employ respiratory therapists as disease managers or case managers, realizing that therapists can provide expert education to clients with asthma, COPD, and other pulmonary diseases. Instead of waiting for an acute episode, this approach addresses the chronic aspect of the disease by providing the patient with an individual treatment plan and an expert to help guide further care. Disease specialists develop treatment plans in conjunction with physicians for enrollees. They monitor the enrollee's progress, either by telephone or during home visits, evaluate the enrollee's progress, and offer moral support and expert education.

Entrepreneurial respiratory therapists have welcomed these opportunities and challenges, working either for managed care companies or starting their own businesses to market educational programs to managed care companies or physicians. Many physicians do not have the time or up-to-date information to provide for their patients' education. Respiratory therapists have been able to meet this need.

Skills and Rewards   Respiratory therapists who work in pulmonary rehabilitation or wellness programs require well-developed educational skills. They must have strong backgrounds in the lifestyle changes that promote good health, as well as the pathophysiology and treatment of pulmonary diseases.

These therapists strive to motivate individuals to make positive, healthy lifestyle changes. An added benefit is that in the process the respiratory therapists themselves may become healthier. Therapists can provide hope and encouragement to individuals who have seen their lives change with chronic illnesses. Many rehabilitation therapists enjoy the work because the patients are committed to learning and benefiting from the program; the patients are not there because of acute care needs but because they want to learn how to stay healthy by preventing or managing disease. Helping individuals achieve and maintain the highest possible quality of physical, emotional, and social life is a primary reward of wellness programs.

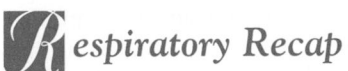 *espiratory Recap*

Opportunities and Rewards of Wellness Programs
Opportunity work with healthy individuals and focus on disease prevention
Focus on a healthier lifestyle for therapists themselves
With managed care, greater demand for therapists in pulmonary rehabilitation and wellness programs
Entrepreneurial opportunities
Financial rewards for managed care companies employing therapists
Opportunity to help individuals achieve the highest possible quality of physical, emotional, and social life

Case Management

Case management has become an essential component of all health care professions and includes two entities related to respiratory care. The first is the incorporation of case management into the daily activities of respiratory therapists. The second is ability of respiratory therapists to act as **case managers** for patients.

Many hospitals, insurance companies, HMOs, and PPOs use respiratory therapists as case mangers to remain cost effective. Respiratory therapists are qualified to be-

come case managers because of their experience in patient assessment, patient education, care planning, implementation, monitoring, and evaluation of the course of therapy.[38] The number of therapists working as case managers has increased, especially in dealing with patients with chronic pulmonary diseases. These diseases are often difficult to supervise under managed care, and respiratory therapists are experts in dealing with patients with chronic pulmonary problems because of their knowledge and management of the disease, equipment, and services needed for treatment.

A recent study by the AARC found that within the past 5 years, respiratory therapists have added case management to their duties as a routine part of their daily work;[3] for 24% of respondents, case management has become a routine part of daily activities. These numbers will grow with a continued emphasis on cost reduction for cardiopulmonary care. Consequently, hospitals have incorporated disease management programs into the services provided by respiratory therapy departments.

Respiratory therapists also have used case management in the development and implementation of protocol-based care. Hospitals have seen the benefits of using protocols in the reduction of length of stay and in the costs savings incurred in the treatment of patients with pulmonary diseases.[3] Hospital-based case mangers have varied job duties; they must work closely with insurance companies to ensure that the patient still meets requirements for acute care, perform daily clinical reviews, coordinate discharge planning, and function almost as social workers with patients and their families. They also may be involved in disease prevention because one of their goals is to decrease hospital readmissions. HMOs that employ respiratory therapists as case mangers tend to use them for education and provision of clinical services.[3]

In spite of these benefits, nursing homes and home health organizations surprisingly are four times more likely to use respiratory therapists as case mangers than are hospitals.[3] Case managers also review hospital daily censuses to identify hospitalized case management patients and interface with the hospital-based case manager. Together the two case managers work to coordinate discharge planning. The managed care case manager must confirm patient eligibility and authorize all referrals for home health and equipment.

Physicians also employ respiratory therapists as case managers in their offices. Physicians who participate in managed care plans often have their patient outcomes monitored by the managed care companies. Managed care companies also evaluate price, patient satisfaction, access to physicians, quality improvement processes, use of clinical guidelines, and patient outcomes. Morbidity and mortality are the most common outcomes, but others include complications, functionality, patient satisfaction, and quality of life. If a company's outcomes are inappropriate, that organization could be in jeopardy of losing managed care contracts, prompting some physicians to hire respiratory therapists. Therapists help physicians decide which pulmonary tests may be beneficial for which patient and educate patients on topics such as disease processes and medication delivery.[3]

Skills and Rewards   A respiratory therapist's entry into case management requires a bachelor's degree and an RRT credential. In addition, the therapist should have a strong clinical background, knowledge of the diagnosis and treatment of pulmonary diseases, and outstanding patient assessment skills, as well as effective social, organizational, and communication skills. To foster communication and understanding, the therapist must be able to balance the needs of the patient and family with the needs of the managed care company, often meeting with family members for daily updates. The therapist becomes the liaison among the family members, physician, and managed care company.

In addition, respiratory therapists should have strong knowledge of reimbursement and health plan benefits, patient care settings, support services, and current legislation. They also serve as the intermediary between the insurance company and the physician, so effective communication in this regard is necessary. Respiratory therapists must be able to work independently and prioritize their duties.

Therapists also must be able to deal with many different health care disciplines and see the patient as a whole and not just as a patient with respiratory illness. Case management entails social work, discharge planning, and disease management, so the therapist must be ready to wear different hats and juggle many aspects of the job simultaneously.

Rewards of case management include helping patients improve their quality of life through effective education and use of health care services. Patients often develop strong relationships with their case managers, which can help them make life changes because they have the therapist to motive them. Another reward involves coordination of the total care of the patient instead of only the cardiopulmonary component.[3] Most importantly, case managers find rewards

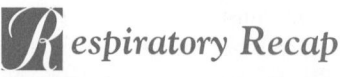espiratory *Recap*

Opportunities and Rewards of Case Management
Cost effectiveness to providers
Coordination of total care of patient, not solely cardiopulmonary aspects
Opportunity to develop long-term relationships with patients and their families
Liaison role between the patient and health care industry
Directly contribution to control of health care costs
Promotion of fiscal responsibility and appropriate allocation of finite health care resources
Assistance to consumers in the complex health care delivery system

in helping individuals and society effectively and responsibly use the expensive and finite health care resources.

Physician Extender

Respiratory therapists often have functioned as **physician extenders** in acute care and traditional hospital settings. The role of respiratory therapists is evolving from task performer to collaborative decision maker and physician extender. Other chapters and sections of this textbook address this topic in detail. Another avenue recently opened to respiratory therapists is as a physician extender in nontraditional settings, including physician offices. Managed care emphasizes treatment of the patient before acute situations occur—and the best place is the physician's office. To meet the goals of decreasing emergency room visits and hospital admissions, physicians have employed respiratory therapists, who have the necessary clinical backgrounds and expertise, to provide the services their patients need.[24]

Respiratory therapists working in physician offices perform many of the same duties they do in acute care settings, but they also may be able to advance their clinical and patient care skills. In particular, working in physician offices provides more opportunity for primary care, rather than acute or critical care. In addition to patient assessment and clinical duties, physician extenders spend a large portion of their time educating patients about disease, treatment techniques, and medications. They have more time to spend with the patients than the physicians do and often follow up with patients, becoming an important liaison between the patient and physician. In addition, they may help arrange home care services and negotiate with HMOs and insurance companies for provision and certification of care.

Skills and Rewards   Respiratory therapists who work as physician extenders in primary care should have excellent clinical skills, with several years experience in acute care. They should possess strong educational skills and the ability to teach at all levels because much of their time involves educating patients and their families. Although physician extenders work under the authority of a physician, they enjoy a large degree of autonomy and can assume a variety of duties and responsibilities that overlap with other health care professionals.

Licensure laws are nonrestrictive in most states, which means that scopes of practice for providing health care services are not restricted to any single health care profession. Therefore a respiratory therapist working as a physician extender can assume a scope of practice, including medical technology, radiologic services, nursing, and physician-assistant responsibilities under the direction and authority of the physician(s). Adequately trained personnel from a number of disciplines can provide health care in physician offices and other practice sites, depending on the state laws regulating physicians, nurses, and other health care personnel.

Therapists seeking work as physician extenders should feel comfortable working independently. They need good organizational skills to function in a busy medical practice. Above all, they need high levels of professionalism because they function as the doctors' extension. These therapists can expand not only their skills but their profession as well. Many such therapists enjoy a greater or positive impact on the lives of patients as one of the best rewards of the job. Although the work may be similar to that in an acute care setting, one of the benefits of being a physician extender is the chance to spend more time with patients.

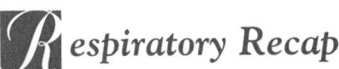 espiratory Recap

---

> **Opportunities and Rewards of the Physician Extender**
>
> Opportunity to advance skills through provision of clinical services traditional therapists do not provide
> Time to educate patients about their diseases, treatment techniques, and medications
> Reimbursement to physician offices for primary care and education provided by respiratory therapists
> Ability to make a greater or positive impact on the lives of patients

Industry

Many respiratory therapists have made the transition in recent years from staff therapists to therapists employed in industry. Corporations and companies who relied on respiratory therapists in minor roles in the past are now using their skills more than ever before. Jobs in industry include technologic design, consulting, product development, marketing, and sales. Management, education, research, and medical writing are also components of industry-related jobs. As the technology advances in respiratory therapy, companies realize that therapists should be involved in the planning, design, and marketing of respiratory equipment. Although these fields are just beginning to realize the greater importance and potential that respiratory therapists can make to their industries, they offer hope for the future growth of the profession.

Industries such as pharmaceuticals and biotechnical corporations hire respiratory therapists to aid in product design\development, market development, marketing, education, research, technical writing, and sales. These companies realize the benefits of involving therapists, with their strong backgrounds in health care, anatomy, physiology, and cardiopulmonary disease management, in the market analysis of new or existing products. Because marketing positions often involve sales and such positions involve territories that often cover several hundred miles, across several states, these jobs often provide opportunities for domestic or international travel.

Therapists can assess the market by communicating with physicians, researchers, and respiratory therapists in geographic areas. They also educate physicians and research scientists about the company's current products and provide the most updated research outcomes and studies. By interacting with the medical community, they help determine the research necessary for a product and recruit research participants. Consultants often coordinate educational programs or present lectures. In return, other respiratory therapists and health care professionals share their outcomes, clinical studies, and the need for future products with the industry consultant.

When an industry establishes a need in health care, respiratory therapists work with engineers to design the product. As a team, they must not only design a product that meets the users' needs but also address regulatory issues, such as Food and Drug Administration (FDA) guidelines. Once the FDA approves a product, therapists often help their companies market it and provide the needed clinical expertise to the sales force, many of whom may be respiratory therapists themselves. In many cases, therapists are important members of the sales force, providing the technical education about the product needed to sell and market it. Furthermore, respiratory therapists may be involved in contract negotiations with distributors and purchasing groups.

Skills and Rewards   Respiratory therapists who work in industry need strong backgrounds in the basic sciences, with an emphasis on anatomy, physiology, physics, and math. Industry consultants must know the geographic area they cover in terms of the experts in their field and require extensive knowledge of research methodologies, past and current research performed on the product, and proposed research needs. Consultants enjoy autonomy in their work, so they must be self-directed and motivated, with strong organizational and prioritization skills.

Therapists working in industry need not only self-direction but also well-developed time-management skills and a knowledge of the different environments posed by industry. The hours are usually long and unpredictable, with traveling often required. Although they often have no patient contact, they still need strong clinical backgrounds and the ability to turn their clinical background knowledge into visions of the future.

Respiratory therapists involved in the design and development of technology find examining patient care from

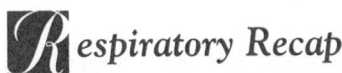 espiratory Recap

---

> **Opportunities and Rewards of Industry**
>
> Ability to view patient care from a different angle to improve health care
> Assistance with the identification, development, marketing, and sales of new products that improve respiratory care and health
> Directly contribution to growth of the profession and other therapists' professional development
> Opportunity to travel and network
> Rewarding use of creative talents in innovative ways

a different angle rewarding and enjoy being able to make a difference in the lives of patients and fellow respiratory therapists. These therapists have the prospect of ensuring the products used are best for the patient and directly contribute to advances within the profession.

Research and Technical Writing

Most of the research reported today by respiratory therapists results from questions that therapists have encountered in day-to-day practice. All respiratory therapists should be interested in research because it validates the care they provide and promotes the growth of the profession.

Therapists interested in conducting research should start small, often beginning with their daily activities concerning the outcomes or the cost effectiveness of therapies, for example. They should choose research in an area in which they have some clinical expertise. The opportunities for performing research are greater in colleges, universities, and large hospitals associated with educational institutes, but research can and has been performed at all levels of care. Today, managed care has influenced the demand for outcomes research and evidence-based medicine, often funding studies to promote cost-containment strategies.

Before undergoing a research project the novice researcher should find a mentor, someone who has experience in conducting and presenting research. Research mentors should be experienced and familiar with research techniques and publication criteria. Even seasoned researchers, such as clinicians, benefit from interaction with those who can provide constructive feedback, questions, insights, suggestions, and ideas. Experienced researchers often suggest that new researchers begin with an abstract presentation because it takes less time and effort; abstracts may be case reports, device evaluations, or original studies. Another research option is to write critical reviews and\or clinical papers for submission to peer-reviewed journals.

Most research conducted at this level does not require funding. If funding is needed, several sources are available. Often, industries provide funding for limited or preliminary projects or sometimes, for projects with larger scope and budgets. Researchers should negotiate a contract before the project starts so that the corporation cannot withdraw funding if it is disappointed with the preliminary results. Other organizations, such as the AARC, the American Respiratory Care Foundation (ARCF), and the American Lung Association (ALA), offer competitive grants and monetary awards to promote research.

A tremendous need exists for research demonstrating the effectiveness of respiratory care and the value of respiratory therapists in all aspects of the health care industry. Outcomes research to provide objective evidence of the value of respiratory therapists and the care they provide is the best way to ensure the continued growth of the profession.

Skills and Rewards Many respiratory therapists feel the need to earn advanced degrees to enter into research, but it is not always the case. However, a background in statistics is encouraged. Research in all aspects of respiratory therapy is needed, the main requirement being a background in the area of respiratory therapy in which the researcher is pursuing. Research is time consuming, usually requiring many months for conduction, data collection, analysis, and publication. Respiratory therapists interested in research must be willing to make a time commitment because research often means working during free time.

Therapists interested in conducting research must be self-motivated to sustain and persevere throughout all phases of a study. Although some therapists work full time on research, most are doing so either in conjunction with their full-time jobs or as independent endeavors. Researchers also should be able to withstand criticism and rejection because all research undergoes extensive peer review that often engenders criticism before it is published. Many articles are rejected or require several rewrites before publication. Researchers must be skilled writers because their work must be published in peer-reviewed journals.

However, respiratory therapists can work in yet another avenue of research as medical writers, without being required to research original studies. Therapists have extensive backgrounds in cardiopulmonary anatomy and pathophysiology, making them ideal candidates for medical writing. Medical writers may write for journal articles, research articles, and textbooks, to name a few. They not only write information but also assist authors in their writing, serve as editors, or create and edit tables and graphs and present statistical information.

Medical writers are needed to write and edit information presented at professional conferences or symposiums, such as pamphlets, brochures, slides, and handouts. Medical writers also help companies obtain FDA approval for drugs. Before the FDA approves a drug, extensive documentation must be presented. Medical writers complete the application, which requires extensive writing skills. Managed care has created new opportunities for medical writers to educate patients, create clinical pathways and document outcomes measured by research.

$\mathcal{R}$ espiratory Recap

Opportunities and Rewards of Research and Technical Writing

Ability to demonstrate effectiveness of care and value of respiratory therapists

Contribution to the growth and development of the profession, giving researchers a personal and professional sense of achievement

Variety of writing venues, including journal articles, research articles, and textbooks

New opportunities for researchers and medical writers to educate patients, create clinical pathways, and document outcomes measured by research

Increased focus in managed care on research about costs and outcomes of health care

Respiratory therapists interested in medical writing must demonstrate strong backgrounds in English and its rules, with a master's degree the preferred credential. Medical writers also must be able to work alone and demonstrate computer proficiency. Respiratory therapists interested in medical writing should contact the American Medical Writers Association, which offers certification programs and education.

KEY POINTS

- Numerous economic, demographic, epidemiologic, sociologic, technologic, and educational forces are affecting health care and its reform in the United States.
- Health care costs continue to escalate at an accelerating rate, without sufficient documentation of improvements in quality, access, or effectiveness of care. Consequently, the 1990s has witnessed unprecedented change in U.S. health care.
- Managed care, including HMOs and PPOs, evolved to place constant pressure on health care providers to restrain health care costs and control use.
- Health care reform has centered around four main issues—(1) decreasing costs, (2) improving quality, (3) evaluating effectiveness with measurable outcomes, and (4) improving resource allocation, including access to health care.
- The ultimate goal of health care reform is to improve the way health care resources are used in such a way that more individuals receive better health care at the least possible cost.
- Health care trends include the declining ability of health care providers to deliver uncompensated care, the declining proportion of individuals with private insurance, the continued growth in the total number of uninsured individuals, the continued increase in the rate of inflation in health care costs, and the budget reductions in Medicare and Medicaid.
- The respiratory care profession can continue to thrive only if those in the profession proactively and realistically modify the curricula to meet the educational needs required to prepare respiratory therapists for the current health care markets.
- Current health care markets include nontraditional roles and new opportunities for respiratory therapists in diagnostics, home care, subacute care, disease management and wellness promotion, case management, industry, research, and medical writing.
- The role of the respiratory therapist as a physician extender is expanding in acute care, physician practices, and nontraditional health care settings.
- With continuing education, experience, credentials, professionalism, and documented value, respiratory therapists will continue to play a major role in health care, as well as an important role in the changes with health care delivery.

References

1. O'Neil EH and the Pew Health Professions Commission. Recreating health professional practice for a new century. San Francisco, Calif: The Commission; 1998.
2. Health Care Financing Administration (US). Office of the Actuary. 1996.
3. American Association for Respiratory Care. Lewin Group Report: respiratory care practitioners in an evolving health care environment. Dallas: The Association; 1999.
4. Health Care Financing Administration (US). Office of Managed Care. 1996.
5. Smith BM. Trends in health care coverage and financing and their implications for policy [editorial]. N Eng J Med 1997; 337(14):1000-1003.
6. Brown R, Bergeron JW, Clement DG, et al. The Medicare risk program for HMOs—final summary report on findings from the evaluation. Washington, DC: Mathematica Policy Research, 1993.
7. Department of Commerce Bureau of Census (US). Statistical abstract of the U.S. 11th ed. Washington, DC: The Department; 1991.
8. General Accounting Office (US): Long-term care—projected needs of baby boom generation. GAO/HRD. Vol 91:86. Washington, DC: The Office; 1991.
9. Tresolini CP and the Pew-Fetzer Task Force. Health professions education and relationship-centered care. San Francisco: The Commission; 1994.
10. Weiss S. Epidemiology of cardio-respiratory disease for the year 2020. Year 2001: delineating the educational direction for the future respiratory care practitioner. Proceedings of a national consensus conference on respiratory care education. Dallas: American Association for Respiratory Care; 1992.
11. Centers for Disease Control. National Center for Health Statistics. Chronic obstructive pulmonary disease. http://www.cdc/nchs/fstats/copd.htm. Hyattsville, Md: The Center; 2000.
12. American Lung Association, Epidemiology and Statistics Unit. Trends in chronic bronchitis and emphysema: morbidity and mortality. www.lungusa.org/data/copd/copd1.pdf: The Association; 2000.
13. Centers for Disease Control. National Center for Health Statistics. Asthma. http//www.cdc/nchs/fstats/asthma.htm. Hyattsville, Md: The Center; 2000.
14. Paavola FG. Future trends affecting health care service and practice. Proceedings of a national consensus conference on respiratory care education. Dallas: American Association for Respiratory Care; 1992.
15. National Health Care Skill Standards Project. Quality and excellence: national health care skill standards. San Francisco: Far West Laboratory for Educational Research and Development; 1995.
16. Department of Health and Human Services (US). Report of the National Commission on Allied Health. Rockville, Md.: Government Printing Office (US); 1995.
17. Larson PF, Osterweis M, Rubin ER, editors. Health workforce issues for the 21st century. Washington, DC: Association of Academic Health Centers; 1994.
18. Pew Health Professions Commission. Critical challenges: revitalizing the health professions for the twenty-first century. San Francisco: UCSF Center for the Health Professions; 1995.
19. Reforming health care workforce regulation: policy considerations for the 21st century. San Francisco: Pew Health Professions Commission; 1995.
20. Dougherty CJ. Back to reform: values, markets, and the health care systems. New York: Oxford University Press; 1996.

21. Calkins D, Fernandopulle RJ, Marino BS, editors. Health care policy. Cambridge: Blackwell Science; 1995.

22. Mishoe SC. Critical thinking, educational preparation and development of respiratory care practitioners. Distinguished Papers Monograph 1993;1:29-43.

23. Cullen DL, Sullivan JM, Bartel RE, et al. Year 2001: Delineating the educational direction for the future respiratory care practitioner. Proceedings of a national consensus conference on respiratory care education. Dallas: American Association for Respiratory Care; 1992.

24. Mishoe SC, MacIntyre NR: Expanding professional roles for respiratory care practitioners. Respir Care 1997; 2:17.

25. Scott F: The downside of downsizing. Adv Respir Care Pract 1996;2:45-46.

26. Hanania NA, Wittman R, Keston S, et al. Medical personnel's knowledge and ability to use inhaling devices. Chest 1994;105:111-116.

27. Guidyt GG, Brown WD, Stogner SW, et al. Incorrect use of metered dose inhalers by medical personnel. Chest 1992;101:31-33.

28. Kollef MH, Shapiro SD, Clinkscale D, et al. The effects of respiratory therapist-initiated treatment protocols on patient outcomes and resource utilization. Chest 2000;17:467-475.

29. Walton J. Understanding the costs of healthcare with specific attention to respiratory care. Respir Care 1997;42:54-70.

30. American Health Care Association. Consumer information: subacute care. www.ahca.org/info/subacute.htm. Washington, DC: The Association; 2000.

31. National Subacute Care Association. General information: subacute care and the industry. www.nsca.net/info/index.htm. Washington, DC: The Association.

32. American Association for Respiratory Care. Clinical Practice Guidelines. www.aarc.org. Dallas: The Association; 2001.

33. Council of Scientific Affairs. Home care in the 1990s. JAMA 1990;263:1241-1244.

34. Cornish K. Subacute care offers opportunities for respiratory therapists. AARC Times 1995;19:22-27.

35. Bunch D. Muse study shows respiratory therapists' positive impact. AARC Times 1999;23:20-27.

36. Muse and associates. A comparison of Medicare nursing home residents who receive services from a respiratory therapist with those who did not. Executive Summary 1999. pp. 1-3. [http:www.aarc.org/professional_resources/muse].

37. Ries AL, Carlin BW, Carrieri-Kohlman V, et al: Pulmonary rehabilitation: joint ACCP/AACVPR evidence-based guidelines. Chest 1997;112:1363-1396.

38. Heiden D. Charting a new course. RT J Respir Care Pract 1996;9:46-48.

CHAPTER 4

Critical Thinking and Problem-Based Learning in Respiratory Care

Shelley C. Mishoe

CHAPTER **OUTLINE**

Essential Skills for Critical Thinking in Practice
  Prioritization
  Anticipation
  Troubleshooting
  Communication
  Negotiation
  Decision Making
  Reflection
Abilities and Characteristics of Critical Thinkers
Teaching Critical Thinking
  Traditional Teaching Methods
  Role of Faculty in a Traditional Curriculum
  Role of Students in a Traditional Curriculum
  Evaluation of Students in a Traditional Curriculum

Problem-Based Learning
  Rationale
  Definition
  Implementation
  Goals
  Role of Facilitator
  Challenges for Students
  Evaluation of Students
Curriculum Changes to Facilitate Critical Thinking
Evaluation of Critical Thinking

OBJECTIVES

1. Develop a personal definition of critical thinking.
2. List, define, and give examples of the essential skills for critical thinking in respiratory care practice.
3. Describe abilities and characteristics of critical thinkers.
4. Describe Problem-Based Learning (PBL).
5. Compare traditional teaching methods and PBL for the teaching of critical thinking.
6. Explain why self-directed and lifelong learning is essential for respiratory therapists.
7. Discuss ways to facilitate critical thinking in respiratory care practice.

*K*EY TERMS

Affective Characteristics	Decision Making	Problem Solving
Analytic Paradigm	Fallacies	Reasoning
Anticipation	Logical Reasoning	Reflection
Communication	Negotiation	Troubleshooting
Critical Thinker	Prioritization	
Critical Thinking	Problem-Based Learning	

Respiratory therapists often hear from their managers, supervisors, and even peers that they must become **critical thinkers** or that they should develop **critical-thinking** skills. Therapists may read journal articles that highlight the significance of critical thinking and wonder about its job-related importance and personal significance. Licensing and accreditation agencies stress the importance of critical thinking in respiratory care. Patients may ask practical questions that challenge respiratory therapists to question some conventional practices. For all medical professionals, information processing and decision making are at the core of clinical practice. Therefore respiratory care students and practitioners must become better thinkers, with the critical thinking skills and traits to be effective in practice.

The respiratory care profession has placed considerable emphasis on the need to train practitioners who can gather information and make appropriate clinical decisions using critical thinking. This emphasis is particularly evident in the National Board for Respiratory Care (NBRC) credentialing examinations for advanced respiratory therapists (registered respiratory therapists [RRTs]) and through the outcome-oriented essentials for respiratory therapy educational programs accredited by the Committee for Accreditation of Respiratory Care (CoARC). The current clinical simulation examinations from the NBRC are recognized by experts in critical thinking theory, assessment, and research as examples of commercially available, domain-specific critical-thinking assessment tools.[1]

Additional emphasis on the importance of critical thinking in respiratory care is further evident in an examination of the AARC Delphi Study,[2] the 1991 report by the AARC board of directors (BOD) on the respiratory therapist of 2001[3] and the proceedings of the AARC Education Consensus Conference.[4] Clearly, it is important to examine how successful respiratory therapy has been under existing programs designed for professional preparation and continuing education in the development of respiratory therapists with critical-thinking skills for the present and future.

To be an effective practitioner and a vital, functioning member of today's health care team, respiratory therapists need more than just a knowledge base. Because of the dynamic and expanding medical knowledge, the average health care professional cannot hope to survive and advance in the workplace by relying solely on information gained in school. Health care professionals must possess the ability to think independently, adapt to changes in practice, and continuously learn new approaches to patient care. Mastering the thinking and reasoning skills necessary to process both old and new knowledge is the most important task for today's respiratory therapist. Therapists must be critical thinkers who are self-directed and lifelong learners if they wish to maintain their vital role in health care today and into the future.

Critical thinking merges principles of **logical reasoning, problem solving,** and reflection.[5] Judgment, **decision making,** scientific reasoning, and lifelong learning are highly related and often used synonymously to mean *critical thinking*. In recent years the term *critical thinking* has become widely and loosely used and misused. Almost all individuals who refer to critical thinking have their own unique interpretations, often based on personal agendas, purposes, beliefs, biases, and perspectives. Complex thinking involves various intellectual activities that encompass creative and critical aspects. The creative aspect of thinking allows for the origin of ideas and alternatives, whereas the critical aspect enables the testing and evaluation of the product of creative thinking. One leading critical thinking expert and researcher cautions that one should not put too much emphasis on any particular definition because each has its limitations.[6] Table 4-1 lists common definitions of critical thinking, but after reading this chapter, readers should derive a personal definition

*T*ABLE 4-1

Common Definitions of Critical Thinking

Definition	Source
Political awareness and personal development[a]	Brookfield, 1987
Cognitive problem solving[b]	Dressel and Mayhew, 1954
Thinking in order to believe or act[c]	Ennis, 1962
Logical reasoning[d]	Hallet, 1984
Rational and purposeful attempt to use thought to move toward a future goal[e]	Halpern, 1989
Discipline-specific knowledge, skills and attitudes to solve real problems[f]	McPeck, 1990
Logical reasoning, problem solving and reflection[g]	Mishoe, 1995
An understanding of and an ability to formulate, analyze, and assess the elements of thought[h]	Paul, 1993

[a]Brookfield SD. *Developing critical thinkers.* San Francisco: Jossey-Bass; 1987.
[b]Dressel P, Mayhew LB. *General education: explorations in evaluation. Final report of the Cooperative Study of Evaluation in General Education.* Washington, DC: American Council on Education; 1954.
[c]Ennis R. *A concept of critical thinking.* Harv Educ Rev 1962;32(1):81-111.
[d]Hallet GL. *Logic for the labyrinth: a guide to critical thinking.* Washington, DC: University Press of America; 1984.
[e]Halpern DF. *Thought and knowledge: an introduction to critical thinking.* 2nd ed. Hillside, NJ: Erlbaum; 1989.
[f]McPeck JE. *Teaching critical thinking: dialogue and didactic.* New York: Routledge; 1990.
[g]Mishoe SC. *Critical thinking in respiratory care practice.* Dissertation Abstracts International; 1995;55(10):3066A (University Microfilms No. 9507227).
[h]Paul RW. *Critical thinking: what every person needs to survive in a rapidly changing world.* Rohnert Park, Calif: Center for Critical Thinking and Moral Critique; 1993.

unique to a clinical setting and applicable to a number of situations that might possibly be encountered in respiratory care practice.

Essential Skills for Critical Thinking in Practice

Critical thinking may involve numerous thoughts and activities, and each activity usually has many steps. The size and complexity of the events or situations that trigger critical thinking may determine the direction and extent of the activities involved. The majority of research on critical thinking has been conducted within academic settings involving college students. Therefore, that critical thinking is most often associated with intellectual abilities is not surprising. However, focusing on cognitive or intellectual abilities does not fully grasp the ways practitioners think and act in professional practice. Furthermore, the extent to which critical thinking in an academic setting transfers to actual professional practice is unclear. Although the intellectual and cognitive aspects of critical thinking are essential, it also contains a practical or everyday aspect.

What is known about critical thinking in health care comes primarily from the studies conducted in medicine and nursing. However, one study of critical thinking in respiratory care describes the actual critical thinking skills and traits important to respiratory care practice, including **prioritization, anticipation, troubleshooting, communication, negotiation,** decision making, and **reflection.**[7-9] The following section describes the skills of critical-thinking processes that are essential in respiratory care practice. Figure 4-1 illustrates the interrelationship among these various skills.

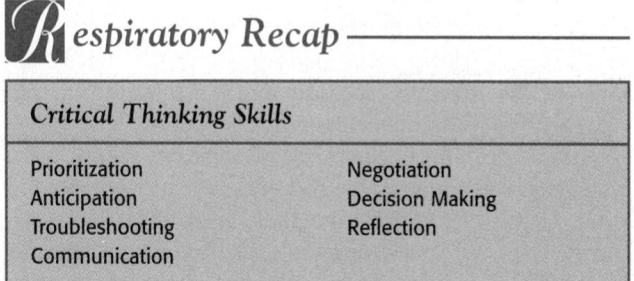

Respiratory Recap

Critical Thinking Skills	
Prioritization	Negotiation
Anticipation	Decision Making
Troubleshooting	Reflection
Communication	

Prioritization

Prioritization is the ability to arrange work according to the importance of the task. Prioritizing may be defined as "organized think" and "rapid think."[7-9] The work that is already scheduled or "expected" requires organized think, whereas the "unexpected" or emergency work requires rapid think. In clinical areas, respiratory therapists perform many scheduled, routine tasks but must also respond to emergency situations. Both types of work often cause conflicting demands and require respiratory therapists to quickly judge the importance of various tasks and situations. After the therapist makes the initial judgment, the order of the tasks must be adjusted to accommodate the highest priority.

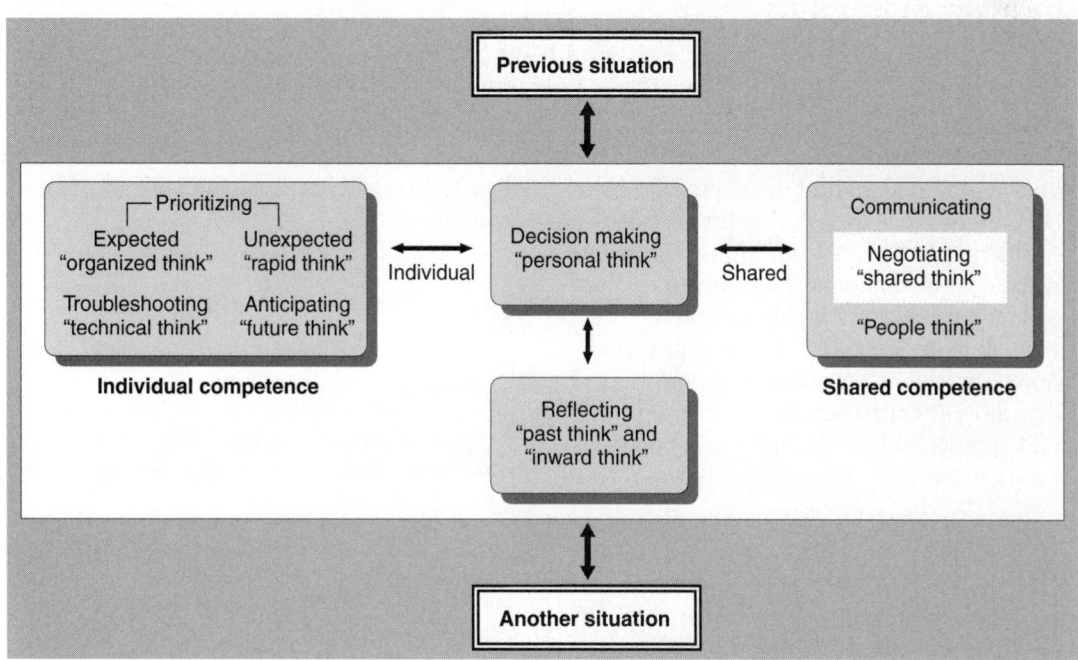

Figure 4-1 The interrelationship of skills for critical thinking in practice. (From Mishoe SC, Martin S. Critical thinking in the laboratory. The Learning Laboratorian Series 1994;6(4):1-63.)

ℛespiratory Recap

> ### Prioritization
>
> Prioritization is "organized think" and "rapid think."

In a busy intensive care unit (ICU), for example, a respiratory therapist may be drawing an arterial blood gas on a patient receiving mechanical ventilation. At the same time, a patient in a nearby bed may suddenly go into respiratory arrest, requiring immediate intubation. The respiratory therapist must quickly seek help from another health care professional who can either intubate the other patient or complete the arterial blood gas sampling so that the therapist can provide optimal patient care. Additional work lasting as long as 1 hour or more may be required for the resuscitation and stabilization of the patient. At the same time the respiratory therapists' pager may indicate that emergency assessment and treatment are needed for the patient with a severe asthma attack in the emergency department (ED). A few minutes later the radiology department may call to say that another patient's computed tomography (CT) scan is complete and the patient can be transported back to the ICU. During this time multiple trauma patients from a car accident also may arrive in the ED. This respiratory therapist must quickly prioritize responsibilities and tasks so that all these patients receive optimal care and must communicate quickly and effectively with others, including nurses, physicians, and fellow respiratory therapists, to assist or to be aware of any delays in patient care. Patients' lives may depend on the therapist's ability to prioritize work efficiently and effectively.

Anticipation

Anticipation involves the ability to think ahead and envision possible problems. Anticipation is "future think"[7-9] and pertains to the continuous and total approach to the resolution of a situation, including the ability to "see the big picture." Anticipation differs from prioritization because the emphasis in anticipation is the ability to respond quickly to a problem or prevent a problem entirely.

However, both skills are interrelated. The ability to anticipate influences the therapist's ability to prioritize and vice versa. Respiratory therapists are better able to prioritize and respond appropriately to problems or routine aspects of their work when they also anticipate what might

ℛespiratory Recap

> ### Anticipation
>
> Anticipation is "future think."

happen as a result of their actions or decisions. On the other hand, the ability to prioritize allows therapists to use their time more effectively to prevent problems.

Respiratory therapists anticipate when they modify patient care or change respiratory care; expect a new patient or face a new situation; plan ahead for equipment needs and actions; prepare what they intend to discuss with physicians; and notice subtle changes in their patients that might indicate problems. Anticipation in respiratory care practice involves the therapist's ability to continuously and holistically assess the patients, data, technology, and situation to prevent problems and develop early solutions. This skill requires global, or gestalt, thinking to grasp the whole situation and effectively formulate plans and solutions to prevent problems from occurring in respiratory care practice. Respiratory therapy students can develop their anticipation skills by working through "what-if" questions, especially during clinical rotations.

Troubleshooting

Respiratory care is a highly technical health care profession. At the same time, it is a profession that requires significant interaction with patients and other health care providers. Respiratory therapists are intimately involved in numerous aspects of patient care diagnostics, therapeutics, and education. Therefore respiratory care can be described as a health care profession that is "high tech" and also "high touch." The technical aspects of respiratory care require the critical-thinking skill of troubleshooting.

Troubleshooting of equipment involves the ability to locate, correct, and process technical problems; it is "technical think."[7-9] Respiratory therapists should be able to introduce new equipment and methodology, modify and adapt new technology for particular needs and situations, and identify and/or correct equipment malfunctions or breakdowns. Logical thinking and problem solving are integral components of troubleshooting. Therapists can obtain help in this process from manufacturers' manuals, online technical assistance, and colleagues familiar with the equipment.

ℛespiratory Recap

> ### Troubleshooting
>
> Troubleshooting is "technical think."

Troubleshooting may range from simple (ensuring a machine is turned on) to complex (the appearance of error message after proper corrective steps have been taken). Nurses and physicians may not realize that a laboratory result such as an arterial blood gas has been delayed due to a machine error. Respiratory therapists are expected to properly maintain and use their equipment for therapy and diagnostics. Proper maintenance and quality controls (part of anticipation) can help prevent equipment malfunction.

Developing troubleshooting skills is an important part of respiratory therapy training. However, students should not rely on their instructors; they must gain independent skills to comprehend and use resources for technologic troubleshooting. For example, students should be encouraged to use instruction manuals and computer help menus to solve technologic problems whenever possible, rather than relying on the instructor to solve equipment problems that occur during laboratories or clinical rotations.

Communication

The reflective dimension of critical thinking includes the communicative aspect that guides beliefs, decisions, and actions within a social context. Critical thinking in practice is very much dependent on communication with others as a primary means to give and receive information necessary for patient care. Communication is "people think."[7-9]

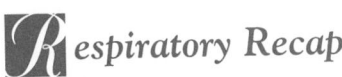

Communication
Communication is "people think."

Although cognitive skills are important, information gathering in practice does not involve merely the selection of data from a list of possibilities as presented on a clinical simulation exam. Respiratory therapists must be able to communicate effectively to gather the appropriate information to interpret, analyze, evaluate, infer, judge, or explain. If a therapist cannot communicate effectively, he or she is unable to think critically during a given situation in clinical practice. Although a therapist may possess developed cognitive skills to critically analyze data, critical thinking in practice is not likely to occur unless that therapist can access and share information with others. Effective communication depends on working relationships. Therefore not surprising is that critical thinking in actual respiratory care practice not only involves communication

but is also affected by personal traits.[8] The personal traits or dispositions that facilitate critical thinking in practice are discussed in more detail later in this chapter.

Respiratory therapists must be able to share information with other members of the health care team. For example, if they cannot properly communicate test results or other data and their meanings to physicians and nurses, patient care may be limited or even jeopardized. Respiratory therapists may obtain abnormal or conflicting laboratory results and need to speak with a physician or nurse to inquire as to the patient's clinical condition or diagnosis. If therapists cannot communicate competently, they cannot think critically in actual practice. The goal in communication is to obtain more information or to give others information. If insufficient information is due to a lack of communication, the respiratory therapist may not be able to interpret, analyze, evaluate, infer, judge, or explain. For example, a respiratory therapist may be able to critically analyze laboratory data or troubleshoot technical errors, but if that individual cannot communicate, he or she cannot perform critical thinking in actual practice because prompt access to needed information is missing. This situation is similar to an individual who tries to work a puzzle without all the pieces.

Communication in respiratory care practice is practitioner specific and situation specific.[7,8] Communication style, duration, and frequency vary greatly depending on the key players involved, including the therapists, patients, nurses, physicians, and others. Communication is essential to educate patients and their families, reassure or explain care to patients, function as part of the broader health care team, and mentor respiratory therapy students and other new clinicians.

Negotiation

Critical thinking in practice also requires the ability to negotiate patient care, including medical orders and responsibilities. Negotiation is the initiation of discussion to influence others. It is an umbrella term that can include teamwork, use of influence, making of recommendations for patient care, accepting of verbal orders, and contacting of physicians to discuss a patient. Practitioners must negotiate for what they believe is best for a given situation in practice. Negotiation also is involved in patient care during interaction with patients and their families to achieve patient compliance with care plans.

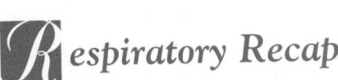

Rationale for Effective Communication
Respiratory therapists must be able to communicate effectively to gather the appropriate information needed to interpret, analyze, evaluate, infer, judge, or explain. If a respiratory therapist cannot communicate effectively, he or she is unable to think critically during a given situation in clinical practice.

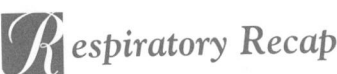

Negotiation
Negotiation is "shared think."

Negotiation does not necessarily mean conflict, confrontation, or difficulty. It takes into account the diversity of roles and opinions in the real world and the ways professionals learn to interact to maximize their efforts for better patient-care outcomes. Negotiation is "shared think."[7-9]

Negotiating patient care responsibilities and medical orders is essential for critical thinking in clinical practice to collectively solve problems. If respiratory therapists cannot negotiate, then their patients have only limited access to their professional expertise, including their cognitive critical-thinking skills. Respiratory therapists must be skilled negotiators to participate in decision making and influence patient-care medical orders regarding the management of respiratory care.

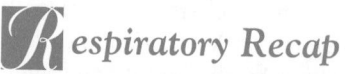

Respiratory Recap

Negotiation Versus Conflict

Negotiation does not necessarily mean conflict. *Negotiation* is an umbrella term that can include teamwork, use of influence, making of recommendations, and discussion of verbal orders.

An intimate relationship exists between communication and negotiation. Although negotiation requires communication skills, all communication is not negotiation. With negotiation the intent is to impart information and ask questions to influence others' decisions and actions. Cognitive performance on a clinical simulation exam requires the respiratory therapists to make the right clinical decision after assessing appropriate data. However, in actual practice the therapists must negotiate power through the medical order to do what they believe is right or best for the patient under specific circumstances. To negotiate effectively, respiratory therapists need good communication skills and the ability to make judgments.[7-9] They also must be able to explain how they came to their conclusions and suggestions. Successful negotiators in respiratory care practice often phrase their suggestions as questions or make indirect implications and inferences as to possible alternative actions.[8] The ability to effectively communicate enhances the therapists' opportunities to negotiate patient-care decisions, which are ultimately controlled by the medical order. Only through negotiation can respiratory therapists expand their opportunities to improve patient care based on their unique expertise.

Respiratory Recap

Rationale for Negotiation Skills

Respiratory therapists must be skilled negotiators to participate in decision making and influence patient-care medical orders for respiratory care.
If the therapist cannot negotiate, the patient has only limited access to that therapist's expertise.

The criteria for negotiation in respiratory care practice include the extent to which a particular solution is evident, the need to clarify medical orders or obtain assistance, the particular physician or physician service, the seriousness of the patient's problem, whether a cardiopulmonary problem is present, the therapist's feelings at the time, and the therapist's confidence in the ability to influence medical orders or patient care decisions.[8] Physicians have final authority regarding the medical orders and patient-care decisions. Respiratory therapists should understand that they have a responsibility to make appropriate recommendations regarding respiratory care but should also realize their limitations.

Physician support, teamwork, critical thinking, and professionalism are essential for effective respiratory care practice.[10,11] Negotiation is an important aspect of professional practice and critical thinking, so practitioners should not shy from the realization that they must learn how to negotiate. Students and novices in respiratory care can develop their communication and negotiation skills through direct observation and interaction with effective models in clinical practice.

Decision Making

Decision making is the ability to reach a conclusion; it is "personal think."[7-9] Respiratory therapists often have the opportunity to participate in clinical judgments or decision making and certainly have the ability to make decisions about their own work flow, work patterns, and work space by practicing three of the previously described aspects of critical thinking—prioritization, anticipation, and troubleshooting.

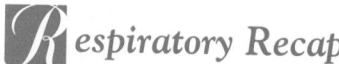

Respiratory Recap

Decision Making

Decision making is "personal think."

Decision making is one of many critical-thinking skills evident in clinical practice. The terms *reasoning, problem solving, decision making,* and *critical thinking* are closely related, and the skills and tasks they involve overlap.[12] Some authors have claimed that "making a decision is the end point of using critical thinking and scientific reasoning in problem resolution."[13] This view is acceptable if critical thinking is conceived solely as cognitive activity. However, clinical practice also involves emotive, practical, and social aspects of critical thinking. Consequently, critical thinking can be described in terms of skills, abilities, and traits in addition to and as a result of cognitive skills.

The development of cognitive skills can enhance the clinical reasoning needed for effective decision making. **Reasoning** involves the review of evidence against and in favor of a position. Inaccurate decision making can result when conflicting evidence is discounted, disconfirming evidence is ignored, and biases determine explanations. Studies of decision making in medicine demonstrate that physicians who are inaccurate with medical diagnoses tend to discount evidence that contradicts a favored hypothesis.[14]

Physicians who make accurate medical assessments pay attention to information that contradicts and supports a diagnosis. Furthermore, practitioners should be able to recognize and avoid **fallacies,** or errors or mistakes in thinking. For example, the degree to which an individual values an outcome can be confused with the probability that it will occur.[15] Avoiding formal and informal fallacies can enhance clinical reasoning and decision making in clinical practice. When respiratory therapists seek input from other health care professionals, it can sometimes result in conflicting evidence, recognition of biases, and multiple alternatives. Expert respiratory therapists should be able to appreciate multiple perspectives and be willing to reconsider their positions when presented with conflicting alternatives in practice. These traits contribute to improved clinical reasoning and decision making because the therapists can avoid fallacies and improve their reasoning abilities.

Research suggests that cognitive skills can be enhanced, resulting in improved decision making, by increases in content and procedural knowledge and clear-thinking skills. All clinicians can benefit from improved judgmental processes using scientific reasoning and clear-thinking skills because individuals often have difficulty integrating diverse sources of information as required in clinical decision making. Furthermore, that experts may make the same mistakes as novices when confronting unfamiliar problem areas suggests the need for cognitive skills and metacognitive strategies. Respiratory therapists must be able to provide reasons when sharing in patient-care decision making and negotiating medical orders with physicians. Therefore improved cognitive skills can facilitate critical thinking in practice but alone are insufficient for these purposes. To be effective in practice, respiratory therapists also must have practical skills and be able to communicate and negotiate effectively; they must reflect on their decisions, beliefs, and actions to further develop critical-thinking skills and traits.

Decision making and the role of the respiratory therapist as a consultant is discussed further in Chapter 7, which provides specific examples and further elaboration on the topic's importance.

Reflection

Reflection is the ability to "think about thinking" so as to explore assumptions, opinions, biases, and decisions. Reflection may be considered introspective, or "inward think."[7-9] If retrospective thinking is considered part of reflection, then reflection becomes "past think."[7-9] Respiratory therapists may reflect on their work, patients, decisions, and profession. Reflection helps them learn from previous mistakes and problems; handle the pain of errors

in judgment; and gain satisfaction from their work, as well as contribution to health care and their profession.

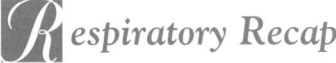

Reflection
Reflection is "inward think" and "past think."

Reflection changes as respiratory therapists grow in their careers and assume different roles and responsibilities.[8] Generally speaking, as therapists become more experienced and make less errors, they begin to reflect more on the wider context of their profession and health care. One of the most profound outcomes of reflection is the realization of the multiple perspectives of circumstances, the gray areas of decision making, and the many levels of interpretation. In other words, usually more than one correct translation of reality exists. Therefore reflection helps therapists develop the disposition of critical thinkers that is important for the implementation of critical thinking in actual practice.

Abilities and Characteristics of Critical Thinkers

Researchers and faculty members have explored various ways in which the relationships among thinking skills, disposition to think, and discipline content. Not only do critical thinkers have certain abilities, but they also demonstrate distinct characteristics. No matter which definition of critical thinking is used, certain common attributes emerge that help to distinguish the critical from the uncritical thinker. The critical thinker has an acquired ability to examine, command, and perfect the elements of thought.[6] This thinker also understands and can formulate, analyze, and assess the elements of thought as shown in Box 4-1. The uncritical thinker, however, usually is perceived as unclear, imprecise, vague, shallow, illogical, unreflective, superficial, inconsistent, inaccurate, or trivial.[6,16]

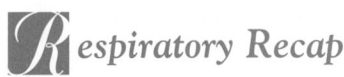

Critical Thinkers
Critical thinkers are inquisitive, alert, well informed, open-minded, honest, flexible, and reasoned.

Critical thinkers also demonstrate common affective qualities, also called *characteristics* or *dispositions*.[1,17] The critical thinker is characterized as someone who has a general approach to living that includes inquisitiveness, a

Box 4-1

Core Cognitive Critical Thinking Skills

1. Interpretation
    Categorization
    Decoding of significance
    Clarification of meaning
2. Analysis
    Examination of ideas
    Identification of arguments
    Analysis of arguments
3. Evaluation
    Assessment of claims
    Assessment of arguments
4. Inference
    Querying of evidence
    Conjecture of alternatives

concern to be well-informed, alertness to opportunities to use critical thinking, trust in the process of reasoning inquiry, self-confidence in one's own ability to reason, open-mindedness, flexibility, understanding of the opinions of others, fair-mindedness, honesty, prudence in suspension of judgment, and willingness to reconsider.

In the health professions a study of expert respiratory therapists revealed the following traits related to critical thinking in practice: (1) willingness to reconsider, (2) appreciation of multiple perspectives, (3) willingness to challenge another regardless of the power structures, (4) understanding of how other therapists' behavior affects them and their profession, (5) responsibility for their own learning and understanding, and (6) openness to continuing change in their personal and professional lives.[8] These traits were evident in a sample of expert respiratory therapists nominated by their peers and supervisors as examples of critical thinkers. This sample of therapists displayed **affective characteristics** of critical thinkers as described in the literature. No matter the profession, a broad listing of characteristics seems to indicate that differing degrees of critical thinking exist and that all adults possess some of the attributes, qualities, and abilities of critical thinkers.[16,18] Respiratory therapists are challenged not only to foster the development of their own critical thinking skills but also to develop the dispositions of the critical thinker in their personal and professional lives.

Teaching Critical Thinking

Teaching critical thinking should be fundamental to the educational experiences of every respiratory therapist because it is a skill used daily in respiratory care. Critical-thinking education may occur in a variety of settings; however, only in recent years has critical thinking been recognized "officially" and been included as part of a formal curriculum program. New graduates may have had some training in critical thinking; on the other hand, some students may have

heard the term *critical thinking* but have had no opportunities to apply and practice the skill. All adults possess some critical-thinking abilities, but a well-designed educational program can help enhance them. The setting may be a technical school or college, undergraduate or graduate program, in-service or continuing education. Faculty members share the responsibility for developing students' thinking skills and cultivating the dispositions to use them.

In respiratory care education, textbooks can be outdated before they are published because the profession undergoes rapid and perpetual change. Traditional curricula have emphasized factual knowledge and rote skills, not thinking and reasoning skills. In the real world the ability to handle situations effectively and safely is more important than the ability to state facts. Practitioners emerge from educational programs and are not realistically prepared to handle the day-to-day problems encountered across the many settings where respiratory care is practiced today. The goals of respiratory care education must change so that students are not taught *what* to think but instead *how* to think.

Respiratory Recap

Traditional Teaching

With traditional teaching the instructor retains control over students' learning by using learning objectives and lectures to convey scientific knowledge derived from research, task analysis, and expert opinion.

Traditional Teaching Methods

Most educational programs were designed to convey scientific and medical knowledge, derived from research, through the accomplishment of specific, set learning objectives. This traditional method of teaching is often called the **analytic paradigm.**

Respiratory Recap

Student Roles in Traditional Teaching

Traditional education places students in passive roles, with an emphasis on teaching versus learning.

With the analytic paradigm the traditional instructor retains control over the learning process—from setting objectives to determining evaluations. Students remain in largely passive roles and are assumed to remain receptive to new information. Educational experiences are highly structured, the dominant instructional strategy is the lecture method, and course work is usually organized according to competency- and/or performance-centered categories based on research, expert opinion, and task analysis.

Role of Faculty in a Traditional Curriculum

Faculty members in traditional settings assume the major responsibility for determining the content, sequence, pace, emphasis, and evaluation of students' learning. Traditional education places more emphasis on faculty teaching rather than on student learning. Some faculty members may rely too heavily on textbook sources and lecture notes as primary resources even though the information may be dated or unnecessarily biased. Controversial aspects of practice usually are not discussed beyond the instructor's mention that the topic is *controversial* or *under investigation*. Some instructors in fact may discourage questions from students or even refuse to answer questions because they find it distracting to the lecture. In some cases, instructors may not enjoy being put on the spot and having to formulate responses to questions they have not anticipated.

The traditional approach perpetuates the assumption that usually *one* correct answer exists and that the teacher is the expert who has all the answers. Of course, in actual practice multiple approaches usually exist to patient care, as do numerous possibilities to address the best course for each patient. Today, that any *one* individual has all the answers to the clinical problems that occur is rare. Lectures do not provide students with much role modeling and experience with the skills and traits needed for professional practice. In health care today the team approach is emphasized and required so that patients can benefit from the collective expertise of specialists in medicine and the other health care disciplines. The traditional role of faculty members has been one of expert rather than role model, colleague, and team member.

Role of Students in a Traditional Curriculum

Students have become accustomed to passive roles during lectures. In traditional education the students' role is to listen to lectures, take notes, use the learning objectives and materials required by the teacher, and memorize facts to regurgitate on tests. Students have been rewarded with passing grades even when they actually understand little about the subject. Generally, students taught by the lecture method cannot apply their knowledge to solve problems or make decisions, and not surprisingly these students learn little of the classroom teaching and cannot apply any knowledge to the clinical setting. Students have been trained by the analytic model to surrender their own responsibility for learning to the so-called expert teacher. Consequently, they cannot grasp their discipline as a whole and do not fully understand their role in professional practice.

Traditional teaching does not expect students to research topics of interest or review areas of weakness independently. Furthermore, students do not bring up topics for discussion, such as related clinical cases or relevant knowledge from previous classes. The traditional method does not allow for much deviation from the lesson plan; therefore the students' role has been to rely on the teacher to set the learning pace, direction, content, and goals.

Evaluation of Students in a Traditional Curriculum

Students have been rewarded for their efforts in lecture courses by demonstrating their ability to recall factual knowledge on course examinations. Little attention has been placed on the development and assessment of students' reasoning, problem-solving, communication, and other professional skills and attitudes. Traditional teaching and evaluation mechanisms have rewarded students who can recall large amounts of scientific information, without adequate evaluation of their professional development, and have perpetuated the notion that a "right answer" can always be found and that good grades on course exams are sufficient for professional practice. Assuming that because the student knows information, that student will perform well in professional practice is a tremendous leap; yet surprisingly, that assumption is what often happens with a traditional curriculum.

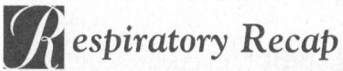 *espiratory Recap*

Evaluation in Traditional Teaching

Traditional evaluation methods give students the false impression that one "right" answer usually exists and equates knowledge of facts with intelligence.

Traditional teaching approaches also may incorporate laboratory and clinical experiences to coincide with lecture-based courses in which students have more active roles. However, even in such situations the learning environment is highly structured, with emphasis often placed on the acquisition of respiratory therapy content and psychomotor skills. Insufficient attention is given to the development and evaluation of students' reasoning, decision-making, and communication skills, all of which are important in practice.

The practicing health care professional must be able to seek information and answers to patient problems using a variety of resources and have the skills to effectively solve clinical problems, adapt to change, and interact with other clinicians, patients, and their families. Respiratory therapists need the experience and skills to seek information and alternatives to solve work-related problems in the real world. Passively listening to lectures does not contribute to a student's abilities to critically read, write, speak, or think. Therefore traditional approaches to teaching do not adequately prepare health care professionals to acquire the skills required in clinical practice. Consequently, newer approaches are needed to foster the necessary critical-thinking skills and characteristics.

Problem-Based Learning

Rationale

After examination of critical-thinking definitions, the characteristics of critical thinkers, and traditional teaching methods, what becomes obvious is that a different model must be used to train competent respiratory therapists. Continued educational reform in respiratory care is necessary for the development of practitioners who possess the necessary critical-thinking skills and traits. The heavy reliance on lectures is a grossly inappropriate means for development of students' critical thinking abilities.

ℛespiratory Recap ——————

Problem-Based Learning

Problem-based learning (PBL) uses student-centered, self-directed, small-group discussions whereby students, with faculty facilitators, solve clinical problems similar to those they may encounter in respiratory care practice.

Problem-based learning (PBL) is one teaching and learning model designed to facilitate critical thinking. Over the past few decades, many schools of medicine have adopted PBL as a teaching-learning method specifically designed to facilitate students' critical-thinking and clinical decision-making abilities. The problem-based curriculum in medicine is built on research into the problem-solving skills of physicians and principles of educational psychology.[19] PBL also has been advocated as a useful way to educate allied health practitioners for the future and has been used in clinical psychology, nursing, occupational therapy, physical therapy, respiratory therapy, and physician assistant programs.[5,20] In addition, PBL has been applied to other disciplines, including business, education, biology, chemistry, physics, general education, architecture, and calculus.[21]

Definition

PBL is student centered rather than teacher centered and allows for individualized instruction. The PBL approach assumes that students are self-directed learners and permits them to have some influence over the direction, speed, and depth of their instruction. The instructional setting for PBL is usually a small group (6 to 10 students) with a faculty tutor. A skilled facilitator may be able to handle a larger group discussion; however, as the number of students in a group increases, the ability for equal participation can be jeopardized. Equal participation of students promotes self-directed learning and enhances stu-

dents' abilities to develop their reasoning and communication skills. Therefore small groups are recommended.

Implementation

During PBL courses, students are given a clinical problem that gradually unfolds over multiple group sessions. Each session may last from 2 to 4 hours, depending on the clinical problem, learning issues, size of the group and students' abilities. One group member is the reader who reads aloud the clinical problem. The group may decide to read one line at a time, one paragraph at a time, or one page at a time. Another member is the scribe and records the group discussions on a blackboard, overhead projector, computer with projection, or newsprint so that all members can see the notes. The scribe creates five columns to record information from that information the group members know, need to know, hypothesize, need to learn, and recommend, as shown in Figure 4-2. The medical model for PBL uses three or four columns. However, an additional column for respiratory therapy recommendations is recommended (see Figure 4-2). The recommendations column helps prepare students for the NBRC examinations, especially the clinical simulations, because graduates are expected to make and evaluate respiratory care recommendations throughout each simulation. Furthermore, the professional role of respiratory therapists requires clinicians who are prepared to make recommendations and provide input and feedback for the acute and chronic management of cardiopulmonary disease.[10]

ℛespiratory Recap ——————

Describing the Clinical Problem

1. Knowledge base
2. Knowledge to be gathered
3. Hypothesis
4. Recommendations
5. Learning issues

With each problem, students evaluate what they know, need to know, and hypothesize. Based on group discussions, they make recommendations for respiratory care and collectively determines their learning issues. The last column is used to record learning issues, which students decide when the group members realize they need to review or investigate a topic further to fully understand the clinical problem. The learning issues are essentially the

	Biologic	Clinical	Psychosocial	
What do we know?	What do we need to know?	What do we hypothesize?	What do we recommend?	What topics will we research? (learning issues)

Figure 4-2   Format to record group problem-based learning discussions.

subject areas and questions that require further research. Available research resources include textbooks, journal articles, indexes, dictionaries, medical experts on and off campus, the Internet, and the faculty.

At the end of each group discussion, group members negotiate who will research each learning issue and report back to the group at the next session. When the group reconvenes, each member presents learning issues and provides handouts and information for the group to present solutions. Students must indicate the sources of their information so that the group can evaluate the accuracy, validity, and relevance of the information. Group interaction and discussion are vital to the success of this approach. Therefore facilitator and peer evaluations of each student's group performance are recommended.

Goals

PBL enables students to direct their own learning by using a variety of resources to manage and solve work-related problems that are similar to the realistic problems they will encounter in professional practice. Students are encouraged to discuss and evaluate the biologic, clinical, and psychosocial issues related to the clinical problem. Biologic issues include application of knowledge from the basic sciences that explain physiology and pathophysiology. Clinical issues include the various aspects in the prevention, diagnosis, treatment, and long-term management of disease. Psychosocial issues include patient understanding, education, compliance, and self-management, as well as societal factors such as cost and access, which influence health care. Emphasis is placed on the development of skills such as analysis, synthesis, and hypothesis generation for the successful completion, assessment, and evaluation of the learning sequence. PBL also gives students experience discussing and evaluating the numerous issues involved in the diagnosis and management of acute and chronic cardiopulmonary disease.

The PBL approach requires students to draw on their abilities to work collaboratively with others, manage time and resources, and develop the skills and characteristics of criti-

cal thinking. Most importantly the students have the opportunity to interact with faculty mentors who serve as role models for critical-thinking skills, perhaps one of the best strategies for the development of critical-thinking ability.[5,16]

Role of Facilitator

PBL facilitators are guides and coaches, not lecturers or resources. PBL emphasizes learning versus teaching. Although each facilitator has a personal style, the individual's principal role is to promote student-centered learning and critical thinking within the group. Facilitators pose nondirective questions at appropriate times to encourage analytic thought and aid in the group process. The facilitator also helps handle conflict within a group, promotes professional debate on controversial issues, provides feedback on individual and group performance, and provides direction to facilitate group learning.

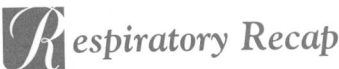

espiratory Recap

> ### Role of Facilitator in PBL
>
> The PBL facilitator guides students, providing direction to the group and feedback on individual and group performance, promoting professional debate, and helping resolve group conflict.

Challenges for Students

The students' major challenge with PBL is to learn to rely on their own abilities to understand, discover, and apply knowledge and skills applicable to the real world. A major obstacle from the students' perspective is the degree to which they have been taught to rely on the so-called expert. Students are naturally curious and eager to solve problems. However, traditional learning methods have stifled the natural tendencies for learners to ask questions and seek additional information. PBL shifts the role from "passive student" to "active learner." Students have come to rely on the role of the "expert" who will tell them what they need to know. Unfortunately, the traditional approach has placed too much emphasis on knowing facts and not enough on solving problems. Thus PBL works best when faculty members shift from teachers to mentors and students shift from mere listeners to their primary role as learners. Students may initially be reluctant to assume so

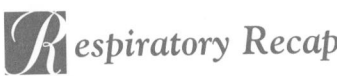

espiratory Recap

> ### Student Role in PBL
>
> PBL shifts the role of respiratory therapy students from *passive* listener to *active* learner.

espiratory Recap

> ### Goals for PBL
>
> | |
> |---|---|
> | Acquire a well-retained body of knowledge available for retrieval and later use in the clinical setting | Develop skills and attitudes of a critical thinker and lifelong learner |
> | Develop the ability to use knowledge effectively in the evaluation and care of patient health problems | Gain experience discussing and evaluating the biologic, clinical, and psychosocial issues associated with cardiopulmonary disease and respiratory care practice |

much responsibility for their learning, including the research and preparedness for class discussions. However, every student has a responsibility to come prepared to participate fully to develop the needed skills and traits.

Some students are naturally reserved or quiet and therefore hesitant to join group discussions, a quality that is counterproductive in PBL. The different experiences, knowledge, perceptions, and viewpoints within the group applied in active discussions make PBL a powerful learning method.[22] Speaking up in a group is the only way a student can test ideas, a hallmark of critical thinking. Students who do not express their own thoughts and understanding miss the opportunity to test the accuracy and validity of their ideas. Group participation is an opportunity to learn ways to communicate, negotiate, and reflect on ideas, beliefs, and actions. Quietness in a group discussion also can be misinterpreted as ignorance. Each student must participate so that the faculty tutor and group members can assess how well that individual understands the group discussions and how much the students has learned.

Evaluation of Students

The evaluation methods for PBL should include an assessment of students' abilities to summarize issues clearly; offer information from diverse sources; use information from previous cases, including clinical experiences; and reconsider hypotheses and decisions. PBL assessment techniques can include oral and written examinations, course assignments or projects, research papers related to the problems or clinical cases, concept map development, clinical simulations (computerized or written text), group discussion, group interaction, and peer evaluation. Discussion questions relevant to the cases are particularly useful to assess students' grasp of the content, as well as their problem-solving abilities. PBL evaluations also should provide feedback on questioning skills, communication skills, learning issues, peer teaching and presentations, and critical-thinking skills.

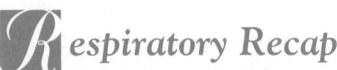espiratory *Recap*

Role of Group Participation

Group participation provides students the opportunity to learn to communicate, negotiate, and reflect on ideas, beliefs, and actions. Speaking up in a group discussion is the primary way the student can test the validity and accuracy of individual ideas, the hallmark of critical thinking.

Peer evaluation is an important aspect of PBL and should be incorporated into the course, laboratory, or clinical grade. Peers should have the opportunity to evaluate their classmates' presentation of learning issues, incorporation of resources, preparedness for group discussion, and participation in group discussion. Peer evaluation should address both the quantity and quality of each group member's participation. Forms can be used to obtain peer scores and comments, which should be incorporated into each student's evaluation for grading purposes. Grading of specific assignments can be determined by an overall score or pass/fail. Course grades also can be assigned by a numeric or letter grade or some form of pass/fail.

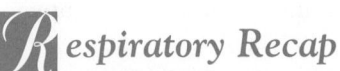espiratory *Recap*

Role of Peer Evaluation

Peers should have the opportunity to evaluate their classmates' presentation of learning issues, incorporation of resources, preparedness for group discussion, and quantity and quality of group participation.

Teaching or facilitating critical thinking requires innovative teaching approaches, dynamic learning experiences, and creative evaluation strategies. A variety of methods should be incorporated to include PBL, discussion, debate, case studies, puzzles, games, logic analyses, troubleshooting, observations, journal writing, case presentations, paper writing, group projects, research studies, clinical apprenticeships, and clinical simulations using computers, videotape, and videodiscs.[5]

Curriculum Changes to Facilitate Critical Thinking

Most respiratory care curricula are overburdened already with professional courses; as a result, present curricula cannot accommodate new courses. Neither can educators rely on general technical school or college curricula to meet the learning needs of critical thinkers. Courses already a part of the traditional curriculum, such as introductory, management, education, and ethics courses, can easily accommodate the teaching of critical thinking through changes in teaching methods that incorporate critical-thinking strategies. Teaching critical-thinking skills also can be taught through the inclusion of PBL in traditionally "hard-science" courses.

Evaluation of Critical Thinking

Because no overall consensus exists on the definition of critical thinking and the skill's process may depend on the individual and circumstances, the measurement of critical thinking is a very controversial topic. Many authors note that a disposition toward critical thinking is a key issue; however, measuring for this ability is extremely difficult in almost any testing format, particularly multiple choice. Furthermore, the tendency to think critically is affected by circumstantial or contextual variables that cannot be accounted for by most standardized tests. The organizational climate can either promote or limit opportunities for critical thinking in the workplace. Critical thinking in respiratory care practice is facilitated when a supportive medical director, strong department leadership, a progressive climate, and specific role delineations are in place.[8,10,23]

Currently, more than 12 critical-thinking assessment tests are commercially available. Some tests focus on general critical-thinking skills or cognitive ability, whereas others concentrate on critical reading or writing. A few instruments can assess dispositional traits of a critical thinker. However, no test is currently available to measure all the macroabilities or affective characteristics of a critical thinker. Each test has its own unique strengths and weaknesses.[18]

Most aspects of professional and continuing education, including evaluation mechanisms such as examinations, require professionals to make individual decisions. The ways that professionals earn formal degrees and obtain credentials generally involve individual competencies. However, shared decision making and shared cognition, which require communication and negotiation are characteristic features of critical thinking in practice. The collective management and treatment of patients by a variety of professionals, including respiratory therapists, is a common practice. Shared competence involves decision making, communication, and negotiation. Therefore an evaluation mechanism should assess respiratory therapy students in each of these areas, not solely in declarative knowledge or individual analysis and evaluation.

A panel of 46 scholars, educators and leading figures in critical-thinking theory, assessment, and research produced a consensus list of cognitive critical-thinking skills and subskills. This list of critical thinking skills, as shown in Box 4-1, may be helpful in that it provides a platform for the establishment of minimal educational goals and standards for incorporation and evaluation of critical-thinking skills within respiratory therapy education. In addition, educational goals should focus on development of the critical-thinking skills and traits important to respiratory care practice, which are described in this chapter.

Use of a variety of evaluation methods to assess respiratory therapy students' cognitive, psychomotor, and affective abilities is important in any educational program. Equally important for any such program is the assessment respiratory therapists' critical-thinking skills and traits to include logical reasoning, problem solving, reflection, and the disposition of a critical thinker.

KEY POINTS

- Fostering critical thinking has become an important issue for respiratory therapists and all medical professionals. Although many respiratory therapists may regularly practice one or more critical-thinking skills, the capacity to improve critical thinking may be enhanced through awareness and education.
- The development of a personal definition of critical thinking based on terms already proposed by experts in the field may be a helpful exercise for any individual interested in increasing critical-thinking capacity.
- All respiratory therapists who aspire to career advancement need to expand the capacity to perform critical thinking by developing related skills, dispositions, and a conducive work context.
- The essential skills for critical thinking in practice include prioritization, anticipation, troubleshooting, communication, negotiation, decision making, and reflection. These skills may be used alone or in combination and adapted or modified for clinical applications.
- In addition to practicing critical-thinking skills, critical thinkers exhibit certain characteristics. Although an extensive list has been compiled by experts, desirable attributes for respiratory therapists include problem solving, common sense, initiative, judgment, critical evaluation, objectivity, decision making, motivation, inquisitiveness, and lifelong learning.
- A problem-based learning (PBL) approach can help teach students to think critically. In the PBL curriculum, students are active learners who confront questions, problems, and situations by using critical-thinking skills and dispositions. Teaching is based on total patient and workplace circumstances and the gathering, assessment, analysis, synthesis, and evaluation of all available information to resolve problems. Faculty members act as facilitators, tutors, and role models. Teaching is performed not by lecture but through interactive techniques incorporating discussion, simulation, role play, debate, case study, games, and puzzles.
- Critical-thinking education can come in many forms: formal degree programs, science/technical/medical courses, management or education courses, practical experiences, continuing education, or in-service settings.
- Critical-thinking skills can be measured through commercially available tests or tests developed specifically to measure one skill or situation. Many concerns and controversies surround the assessment of critical thinking, but those individuals who administer critical-thinking tests must be aware of the strengths and limitations of the tests and the relationship of questions to workplace and personal skills. Consideration also must be given to question format, scoring, test length, cost, and timing.
- The emphasis placed on critical thinking in respiratory care practice will continue to increase, and skills, dispositions, education, and measurement will remain topics for discussion and debate.

References

1. Facione PA. Critical thinking: a statement of expert consensus for purposes of educational assessment and instruction. ERIC Document Reproduction Service No. ED 315 423; 1990.
2. O'Daniel CO, Cullen DL, Douce FH, et al. The future educational needs of respiratory care practitioners: a Delphi study. Respir Care 1992;37(1):65-78.
3. Dunne P. Shaping a vision of the future respiratory care practitioner. AARC Times 1992;16(4):28-30.
4. Cullen DL, Sullivan JM, Bartel RE, et al. Year 2001: delineating the educational direction for the future respiratory care practitioner. Proceedings of a national consensus conference on respiratory care education. Dallas: American Association for Respiratory Care; 1992.
5. Mishoe SC. Critical thinking, educational preparation and development of respiratory care practitioners. Distinguished Papers Monograph 1993;1(2):29-43.
6. Paul RW. Critical thinking: what every person needs to survive in a rapidly changing world. Rohnert Park, Calif: Center for Critical Thinking and Moral Critique; 1993.
7. Mishoe SC, Courtenay B. Critical thinking in respiratory care practice. Proceedings of the 35th Annual Adult Education Research Conference. Knoxville: University of Tennessee, 1994. pp. 276-281.
8. Mishoe SC. Critical thinking in respiratory care practice. Dissertation Abstracts International, 55(10):3066A. University Microfilms No. 9507227; 1995.
9. Mishoe SC. Critical thinking in respiratory care practice [abstract]. Respir Care 1996;41(10):958.
10. Mishoe SC, MacIntyre NR. Expanding professional roles for respiratory care practitioners. Respir Care 1997;42(1):71-91.
11. Giordano SP. Conference summary: emerging health care delivery models and respiratory care. Respir Care 1997;42(1):14-17.
12. Gambrill E. Critical thinking in clinical practice. San Francisco: Jossey-Bass; 1990.
13. Bandman EL, Bandman B. Critical thinking in nursing. Norwalk, Conn: Appleton & Lange; 1988.
14. Elstein AS, Shulman LS, Sprafka SA, et al. Medical problem-solving: an analysis of clinical reasoning. Cambridge, Mass: Harvard University Press; 1978.
15. Elstein AS. Cognitive processes in clinical inference and decision making. In: Turk DC, Salovey P, editors. Reasoning, inference and judgment in clinical psychology. New York: Free Press; 1988.
16. Brookfield SD. Developing critical thinkers. San Francisco: Jossey-Bass; 1987.
17. Facione PA, Facione NC. The California Critical Thinking Disposition Inventory (CCTDI) and CCTDI test manual. Millbrae, Calif: California Academic Press; 1992.
18. Mishoe SC, Martin S. Critical thinking in the laboratory. The Learning Laboratorian Series 1994;6(4):1-63.
19. Barrows HS. How to design a problem-based curriculum for the preclinical years. New York: Springer Verlag; 1985.
20. Bruhn JG. Problem-based learning: an approach toward reforming allied health education. J Allied Health 1992;21(3):161-173.
21. Wilkerson L, Gijselaers W, editors. Bringing problem-based learning to higher education: theory and practice. New directions for teaching and learning. No. 68. San Francisco: Jossey-Bass; 1996.
22. Barrows HS. What your tutor may never tell you: a guide for medical students in problem-based learning. Springfield, Ill: Southern Illinois University School of Medicine; 1997.
23. Mishoe SC. The effects of institutional context on critical thinking in the workplace. Proceedings of the 36th Annual Adult Education Research Conference. Edmonton, Alberta: University of Alberta; 1995. pp. 221-228.

CHAPTER 5

Ethics of Health Care Delivery

Kathleen M. Hernlen
Charles Carroll

CHAPTER OUTLINE

OBJECTIVES

1. Define ethics.
2. Describe methods by which an ethical orientation is formed.
3. Distinguish between ethical and legal behavior.
4. Describe an ethical dilemma.
5. State the role of ethics in the delivery of effective respiratory care.
6. Define common ethical theories.
7. Define seven contemporary ethical principles.
8. Describe the way the analysis method is used to solve ethical dilemmas.
9. Describe three common ethical dilemmas associated with the delivery of respiratory care.
10. Describe key components of the American Association for Respiratory Care's statement of ethics and professional conduct.
11. Discuss the role of ethics committees.
12. Discuss the Patient's Bill of Rights.
13. Discuss the way technology has increased the incidence of confidentiality violations.
14. Discuss the way managed care has affected the basic ethical principles.

KEY TERMS

AARC Code of Ethics	Ethics	Personal Belief System
Advance Directive	Fidelity	Personal Value System
Analysis Method	Informed Consent	Surrogate
Autonomy	Justice	Teleological Theory
Beneficence	Moral Philosophy	Veracity
Confidentiality	Nonmaleficence	
Deontological Theory	Patient's Bill of Rights	

How can respiratory therapists continue to provide quality patient care while staffs are undergoing reduction? How can therapists maintain patient confidentiality in the information age? What role do respiratory therapists play in assisting families with the difficult decision to use life support equipment or agree to "do not resuscitate" orders for their loved ones? These are examples of ethical questions confronting members of the profession every day. Ethical discussions and decisions are never easy. With ethical questions in particular, answers are rarely black or white and often lie within gray zones. Ethical decisions depend on the specific values systems and decisions of the individuals involved.

Although discussions about medical **ethics** have increased in recent years, the topic is not a new one. Medical ethics has been discussed since the days of ancient Greece. The Hippocratic oath, which was established in the fourth century BC, outlines ethical guidelines and behaviors for physicians, who vow "to keep their patients from harm and injustice."[1] Other provisions address the provision of confidentiality for patients and the role of the physician. The issues have transcended time, but each society must continually establish and define its code of ethics for health care.

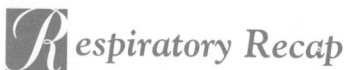 *Respiratory Recap*

Ethics
Ethical principles have long been a part of medical practice, dating back to the time of Hippocrates.
Ethics determine the ways societies and individuals make decisions regarding right or wrong.
Ethics is a decision-making process.

Definition of Ethics

The study of ethics is not the determination of right or wrong answers but the study of the ways in which individuals make judgments regarding right or wrong; ethics is the study of the decision-making process one takes in determining right from wrong. No individual is born knowing what is right or wrong. Ethics are based in part on the values individuals develop as they mature, values shaped by

religious convictions, family, political beliefs, education, life experiences, and culture. Other theories have proposed that values are shaped by gender and social and economic standards.

Foundation of Ethical Thinking

Personal Belief System

As individuals experience life and are educated in the morals and mores of our society, they develop a set of personal beliefs. These beliefs are not necessarily "right" or "wrong" and are certainly not objective. Yet they are deeply ingrained in individuals' thoughts and decision-making processes.

Attitudinal Orientation

Attitudinal orientation is the outward expression of an individual's **personal belief system.** It is what a person says and how that person behaves and is based on what the individual believes. Attitudes have a large effect on behavior, which is most evident when individuals are confronted with ethical dilemmas.

Personal Value System

The **personal value system** is formed when the decision is made to continue to believe and express a conviction even when a person or event challenges it. For example, having a particular belief about the death penalty is easy, as is ex-

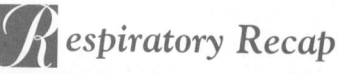 *Respiratory Recap*

Value Systems
Personal beliefs include the mores and morals of our society.
Attitudinal orientation is the outward expression of a personal belief system.
The personal value system is formed when beliefs becomes convictions.
An individual's moral philosophy can be viewed as a behavioral code.

pression of that belief when no opposition exists. However, maintaining this belief when opposition is expressed becomes more difficult. When an individual is willing to maintain a belief in the face of opposition, that belief becomes a conviction. When the individual integrates convictions into a personal value system, maintaining them in the face of opposition, they become personal principles. This progression is an important step in the formation of an individual's ethical orientation because personal principles influence that individual's ethical orientation and decision making.

Moral Philosophy

An individual's **moral philosophy** can be viewed as a behavioral code. Morals define what individuals will or will not do in a given situation, and moral philosophy is based on the individual's previously adopted personal principles. Ethics can be viewed as a work in progress, and ethical principles often reflect society. As a society evolves and changes, so do its ethical beliefs; two timely examples include abortion and the death penalty. Changes in the way society views these issue are reflected in newer laws governing these practices.

Ethical Versus Legal Behavior

Ethical Orientation

A discussion of ethical behavior is difficult without at least an allusion to legal behavior. Legal behavior in this sense simply means abiding by the law. Sometimes the line between the ethical and the legal is fine; sometimes that line disappears and the behaviors merge; other times the gap between the two widens. Although a given behavior can be described as both ethical and legal, it often has the same foundation. Ethical and legal behaviors differ primarily in the individual freedom allowed for decision making. For example, an individual may be free to adhere to a given ethical code but required to abide by the legal code under the threat of punishment by law.

Legal Standards

Ideally, behavior would always be both ethical and legal. In reality, however, that standard is not always met. Several reasons exist for the discrepancy between the legal and the ethical, the primary reason being that neither ethical behavior nor legal requirements are static standards. Ethical and legal standards of behavior change as society grows and changes.

Abortion is a classic example in recent history that demonstrates the way major societal issues influence both ethical and legal standards. Before 1973, when the Supreme Court's *Roe v. Wade* decision was handed down, abortion was clearly illegal. Needless to say, the Supreme Court did not decide in a vacuum on that day to legalize abortion. In-

stead, the argument had grown over the previous decades that all abortions should not be illegal. It may not have been stated as such, but this view marked a gradual change in society's ethical orientation. Although not every American citizen agreed that abortion should be legalized, at the time of the Supreme Court decision society's ethical orientation had shifted significantly so that the Court's interpretation was inevitable. Some legal scholars might argue that the Court simply interpreted the Constitution and the ruling had nothing to do with society's ethical orientation. However, constitutional interpretation is usually related to society's ethical orientation. Take, for example, the Supreme Court's decisions on the death penalty and slavery. The range of legal decisions handed down by courts, whether deemed positive or negative, reflect society's orientation at those times.

A major ethical and legal shift in the area of death and dying is pending. The "right to die" appears to have gained a growing acceptance from an ethical standpoint. Customary in these kinds of shifts is for legal standards to lag behind ethical development. For example, Jack Kevorkian, a Michigan pathologist, was recently found legally responsible for the death of one of his patients. Close examination of the opinions surrounding his work reveals a subtle shift from a view that his work is ethically wrong to one of a right to die. This shift in ethical viewpoints in the United States toward euthanasia is primarily evident in the nonscientific literature.[2] Discussion is under way in at least one state, California, to introduce legislation to legalize physician-assisted suicide.

The preceding discussion on legal standards and ethical orientation may appear unrelated to ethics for the respiratory therapist. However, it is important in helping respiratory therapists to understand the dynamics of ethical dilemmas. Ethical dilemmas are not static issues that remain constant but change as society changes. Thus the most important point for the therapist to learn is how to deal with ethical dilemmas in situational settings.

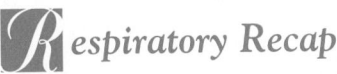espiratory *Recap*

Ethical Versus Legal Behavior
Legal behavior simply means abiding by the law.
Legal and ethical behaviors are not static.
Ideally, behavior would always be both ethical and legal.
A major pending shift in ethical and legal behavior is in death and dying.

The respiratory therapist may encounter many ethical dilemmas, ranging from dramatic life support and end-of-life issues to the basic staffing and level of care issues prevalent in today's managed care environment. In fact, most dilemmas the average therapist faces are the less dramatic ones. However, that these dilemmas are less dramatic does not make them less important.

Ethical Theories

Two main theories are used to describe the decision-making process an individual undertakes in deriving an ethical conclusion to a dilemma. Teleological and deontological theories guide ethical decision making. In addition to these two major ethical theories, the analysis method is used, which combines teleological and deontological theory, recognizing that most ethical decisions require systematic analysis.

Teleological Theory

Teleological theory is based on consequences. The right or wrong of an action is based on the outcomes or consequences of predicted outcomes. The most common type of consequential theory is known as *utilitarianism*, in which an individual chooses the act that brings about the best outcome. To determine the best outcome the individual must follow a system of steps, during which the problem first is described, all solutions then are listed, and the solutions finally are compared with the good each can provide. The correct answer is the most useful solution and becomes the *best* outcome. For example, enough money is available for either a heart transplant for one patient or vaccines for hundreds of infants. Using the teleological theory, the consequences of helping hundreds would be better than helping one patient. Therefore the best outcome would be to use the money to buy the vaccines.

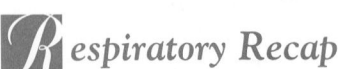

espiratory Recap

Teleological Theory
Teleological theory is consequential theory, based on consequences. The most common type of consequential theory is known as utilitarianism. Utilitarianism looks for the best outcome.

Deontological Theory

Deontological theory is based on duty and states that an act is either right or wrong based on its intrinsic character rather than on its consequences. Although teleological theory is concerned with doing the best thing, it tries to

espiratory Recap

Deontological Theory
Deontological theory is an ethical theory based on duty. An act is either right or wrong based on its intrinsic character (duty), rather than on its consequences. The philosophical works of Immanuel Kant, as well as many religions, identify with this theory.

do the right thing. The philosophical works of Immanuel Kant, as well as many religions, identify with this theory.

The steps involved in the deontological theory are much more complicated than those in teleological theory and are outlined in Figure 5-1.

Analysis Method

One other theory used in ethics is the **analysis method,** which combines key components from teleological and deontological theories. It recognizes that in the final analysis, most ethical decisions are made by a systematic analytic process devised by the individual.[3]

The analysis method has become increasingly popular in the 1980s and 1990s. Most ethical dilemmas are solved with analysis method, which combines the best of the ethical theories, as judged by an individual's ethical orientation, with critical-thinking and problem-solving skills. The actual process varies but includes the following steps:

1. Identification of the problem
2. Clarification of the problem
3. Formulation of possible solutions
4. Testing of possible solutions against consequences, feasibility, sense of right and wrong, with each individual free to place a different emphasis on each test
5. Selection and application of a solution

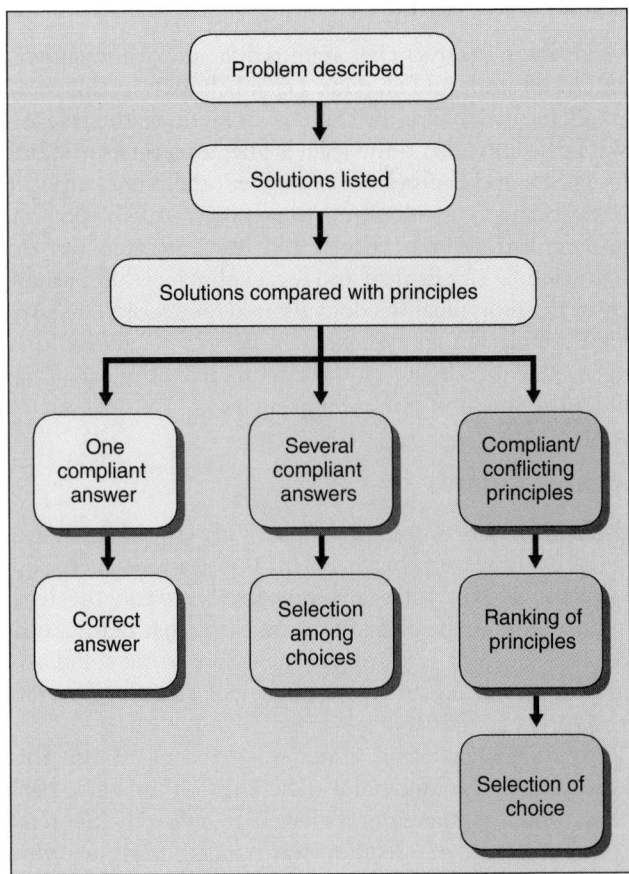

Figure 5-1 Deontological theory for reasoning.

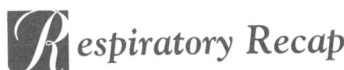espiratory Recap

Analysis Method
The analysis method combines key components from teleological and deontological theories. Health professionals resolve most ethical dilemmas using the analysis method.

Ethical Principles

Using ethical theories, society has developed several principles or standards of behavior to help determine right or wrong actions. These principles change over time as societies change. Seven important ethical principles considered important in contemporary medicine are (1) beneficence, (2) nonmaleficence, (3) veracity, (4) autonomy, (5) confidentiality, (6) justice, and (7) role fidelity.

Beneficence

Beneficence means *charity* or *mercy*. This principle imposes on the practitioner the responsibility to seek good for the patient under all circumstances. The health care professional should do only what will benefit the patient.

Health care workers enter their professions with the genuine desire to help patients and receive intrinsic rewards by helping and caring for those who need their expertise. Beneficence has long played a role in the delivery of health care. Hippocrates wrote, "I will apply dietetic measures for the benefit of the sick according to my ability and judgment."[1] This desire to provide care to benefit patients has been a continuing principle. Health care and professional organizations recognize the need for continued education to foster growth and competence in health care.

However, determining what is good is a difficulty encountered with beneficence. If beneficence means the seeking of good for the patient, who should decide what is good? Should the patient make the determination or the health care worker? Just as individuals have different values, so will patients have different opinions as to what will benefit them the most.

Beneficence is becoming increasingly more difficult to determine in today's advanced technologic world. For example, the technology now exists to prolong lives that would have been lost just two decades ago. At the same time remains the question of whether this technology should be used to save every life. An individual with terminal cancer could be kept alive for months on life support. Should technology be used in this case? Would it benefit the patient? Is it good for the patient? Is it good for the family?

Nonmaleficence

Nonmaleficence is the principle that requires therapists to avoid or refrain from harm. It is often viewed as the opposite of beneficence. This principle is outlined in the Hippocratic oath with the words "I will keep them from harm and injustice."[1] Violations of this principle are the basis for most lawsuits.

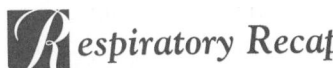espiratory Recap

Nonmaleficence
Nonmaleficence is the principle that requires practitioners to avoid or refrain from harm. The principle of double effects occurs when the benefit (or beneficence) of a treatment is accompanied by undesirable side effects that could case harm.

As with beneficence, nonmaleficence can be seen as a double-edged sword. Often the benefits or beneficence of a treatment is accompanied by undesirable side effects that could cause harm, known as the *principle of double effects*. A common example of this dilemma is the use of narcotics to relieve pain. Although use of narcotics may relieve a patient's pain (beneficence), the patient also may suffer respiratory depression (nonmaleficence).

Practitioners can use the following guiding elements to deal with the principle of double effects[4]:

1. The action taken must be good or at least morally neutral.
2. The good must not follow as a consequence of the secondary harmful effects.
3. The harm must never be intended but tolerated as casually connected with the good intended.
4. The good must outweigh the harm.

Veracity

Veracity means *truth*. This principle implies that the practitioner should tell the patient the truth at all times and is based on the belief that health care is best served in a relationship of trust in which the practitioner and the patient are both bound by truth.

Veracity has not always been the norm in medical practice. A few decades ago, doctors made decisions about

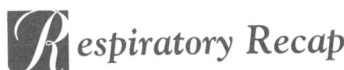espiratory Recap

Beneficence
Beneficence imposes the responsibility to seek good for the patient under all circumstances. Determining what is good can be difficult. Beneficence is becoming increasingly more difficult to determine in today's advanced technologic world.

what their patients should or should not be told about their conditions. In a 1961 study 90% of the 219 physicians surveyed stated that they would not disclose a diagnosis of cancer to a patient,[5] believing that the patient would not be able to handle the news or would give up. Then 20 years later, 264 physicians were surveyed, with 97% stating that they would disclose a diagnosis of cancer.[5] Research also demonstrates that patient attitudes concerning veracity have changed in recent years. Patients are more knowledgeable about medical treatments and more active in the decision-making process involving their health care. They expect that health care providers to be truthful with them.

Truth in medicine serves several purposes. By telling patients the truth concerning their medical conditions, an important trust is formed between the public and the medical community. Without this trust, many patients would not seek medical attention or make informed decisions about their conditions. However, the absence of veracity can result in legal action. Before undergoing procedures or participating in research studies, health professionals must give patients adequate information about the procedure or research. Patients must have an opportunity to ask questions and understand the risks involved.

ℛespiratory Recap

> ### Veracity
>
> This principle states that the practitioner should tell the patient the truth at all times.
> Benevolent deception is the view that the practitioner can lie to a patient for that patient's own good.
> Veracity has not always been the norm in medical practice.

Although the medical community realizes the importance of veracity, it also recognizes that in certain instances a physician's not telling the patient the truth is equally important. Benevolent deception is the view that the physician can withhold information from a patient for that patient's own good. For instance, telling the patient the truth can result in psychological or physiological harm in certain situations; other times patients may not wish to know everything about their medical conditions. Some patients do not want to know all the possible side effects or risks involved in a procedure and may rely on the principle that ignorance is bliss.

Asian cultures, for example, do not regard the truth as we know it to be as important as it is in the American culture. Family members with this type of cultural background may ask that information such as terminal conditions be kept from the patient. This situation requires patience, tact, and respect for cultural differences, and the health care professional must work closely with the family to establish the best course for the patient.

Autonomy

Autonomy is the right and the ability to govern one's self. In medical terms, it allows patients to make decisions about the medical treatment they will receive and decide which treatments they do not wish to receive. In the past, physicians took a more paternalistic role in the delivery of care, making the treatment choices for their patients, and were questioned rarely. Patients viewed doctors as the experts who would take care of them.

With recent advancements in medical science and telecommunications, patients have become more aware of treatment options and more vocal about making decisions regarding their health. The Patient's Bill of Rights and informed consent are the results of this changing view of autonomy.

Patient's Bill of Rights   The American Hospital Association established the **Patient's Bill of Rights** in 1975. It outlines the rights and responsibilities patients have regarding their medical care (Box 5-1). Provision four of the Bill of Rights states that the patient has the right to refuse treatment to the extent permitted by law and to be informed of the medical consequences of his or her action.[6]

Informed Consent   **Informed consent** includes disclosure, understanding, voluntarism, competence, and permission. Before undergoing or refusing treatments, a patient must be provided with all of this information. The Patient's Bill of Rights has a provision dealing specifically with informed consent, in which patient has the right to receive information necessary to give consent. The patient also has the right to know about significant medical alternatives and the names of the individuals responsible for the treatment and/or procedure.[6]

Refusal of Treatment   The patient must obtain certain criteria to refuse treatment, including an understanding of the nature of the condition and the consequences of various options. The patient also must have the mental capacity, or competency, to process the information required to make these decisions, which must be within the law.

Advance Directives   If the patient is deemed incompetent, several things could happen regarding treatment. In

ℛespiratory Recap

> ### Autonomy
>
> Autonomy is the ability and right to govern oneself.
> The Patient's Bill of Rights outlines the rights and responsibilities of patients regarding their medical care.
> For a patient to refuse treatment that individual must understand the nature of the condition and the consequences of various options.
> Advance directives, living wills, and medical power of attorney specify which treatments patients desire.

Box 5-1

A Patient's Bill of Rights

Introduction

Effective health care requires collaboration between patients and physicians and other health care professionals. Open and honest communication, respect for personal and professional values, and sensitivity to differences are integral to optimal patient care. As the setting for the provision of health services, hospitals must provide a foundation for understanding and respecting the rights and responsibilities of patients, their families, physicians, and other caregivers. Hospitals must ensure a health care ethic that respects the role of patients in decision making about treatment choices and other aspects of their care. Hospitals must be sensitive to cultural, racial, linguistic, religious, age, gender, and other differences as well as the needs of persons with disabilities.

The American Hospital Association presents *A Patient's Bill of Rights* with the expectation that it will contribute to more effective patient care and be supported by the hospital on behalf of the institution, its medical staff, employees, and patients. The American Hospital Association encourages health care institutions to tailor this bill of rights to their patient community by translating and/or simplifying the language of this bill of rights as may be necessary to ensure that patients and their families understand their rights and responsibilities.

Bill of Rights*

1. The patient has the right to considerate and respectful care.
2. The patient has the right to and is encouraged to obtain from physicians and other direct caregivers relevant, current, and understandable information concerning diagnosis, treatment, and prognosis.

   Except in emergencies when the patient lacks decision-making capacity and the need for treatment is urgent, the patient is entitled to the opportunity to discuss and request information related to the specific procedures and/or treatments, the risks involved, the possible length of recuperation, and the medically reasonable alternatives and their accompanying risks and benefits.

   Patients have the right to know the identity of physicians, nurses, and others involved in their care, as well as when those involved are students, residents, or other trainees. The patient also has the right to know the immediate and long-term financial implications of treatment choices, insofar as they are known.
3. The patient has the right to make decisions about the plan of care prior to and during the course of treatment and to refuse a recommended treatment or plan of care to the extent permitted by law and hospital policy and to be informed of the medical consequences of this action. In case of such refusal, the patient is entitled to other appropriate care and services that the hospital provides or transfer to another hospital. The hospital should notify patients of any policy that might affect patient choice within the institution.
4. The patient has the right to have an advance directive (such as a living will, health care proxy, or durable power of attorney for health care) concerning treatment or designating a surrogate decision maker with the expectation that the hospital will honor the intent of that directive to the extent permitted by law and hospital policy.

   Health care institutions must advise patients of their rights under state law and hospital policy to make informed medical choices, ask if the patient has an advance directive, and include that information in patient records. The patient has the right to timely information about hospital policy that may limit its ability to implement fully a legally valid advance directive.
5. The patient has the right to every consideration of privacy. Case discussion, consultation, examination, and treatment should be conducted so as to protect each patient's privacy.
6. The patient has the right to expect that all communications and records pertaining to his/her care will be treated as confidential by the hospital, except in cases such as suspected abuse and public health hazards when reporting is permitted or required by law. The patient has the right to expect that the hospital will emphasize the confidentiality of this information when it releases it to any other parties entitled to review information in these records.
7. The patient has the right to review the records pertaining to his/her medical care and to have the information explained or interpreted as necessary, except when restricted by law.
8. The patient has the right to expect that, within its capacity and policies, a hospital will make reasonable response to the request of a patient for appropriate and medically indicated care and services. The hospital must provide evaluation, service, and/or referral as indicated by the urgency of the case. When medically appropriate and legally permissible, or when a patient has so requested, a patient may be transferred to another facility. The institution to which the patient is to be transferred must first have accepted the patient for transfer. The patient must also have the benefit of complete information and explanation concerning the need for risks, benefits, and alternatives to such a transfer.
9. The patient has the right to ask and be informed of the existence of business relationships among the hospital, educational institutions, other health care providers, or payers that may influence the patient's treatment and care.
10. The patient has the right to consent to or decline to participate in proposed research studies or human experimentation affecting care and treatment or requiring direct patient involvement, and to have those studies fully explained prior to consent. A patient who declines to participate in research or experimentation is entitled to the most effective care that the hospital can otherwise provide.
11. The patient has the right to expect reasonable continuity of care when appropriate and to be informed by physicians and other caregivers of available and realistic patient care options when hospital care is no longer appropriate.
12. The patient has the right to be informed of hospital policies and practices that relate to patient care, treatment, and responsibilities. The patient has the right to be informed of available resources for resolving disputes, grievances, and conflicts, such as ethics committees, patient representatives, or other mechanisms available in the institution. The patient has the right to be informed of the hospital's charges for services and available payment methods.

Courtesy American Hospital Association. A patient's bill of rights. Chicago: The Association; 1992.

These rights can be exercised on the patient's behalf by a designated surrogate or proxy decision maker if the patient lacks decision making capacity, is legally incompetent, or is a minor.

Continued

Box 5-1

A Patient's Bill of Rights—cont'd

The collaborative nature of health care requires that patients, or their families/surrogates, participate in their care. The effectiveness of care and patient satisfaction with the course of treatment depend, in part, on the patient fulfilling certain responsibilities. Patients are responsible for providing information about past illnesses, hospitalizations, medications, and other matters related to health status. To participate effectively in decision making, patients must be encouraged to take responsibility for requesting additional information or clarification about their health status or treatment when they do not fully understand information and instructions. Patients are also responsible for ensuring that the health care institution has a copy of their written advance directive if they have one. Patients are responsible for informing their physicians and other caregivers if they anticipate problems in following prescribed treatment.

Patients should also be aware of the hospital's obligation to be reasonably efficient and equitable in providing care to other patients and the community. The hospital's rules and regulations are designed to help the hospital meet this obligation. Patients and their families are responsible for making reasonable accommodations to the needs of the hospital, other patients, medical staff, and hospital employees. Patients are responsible for providing necessary information for insurance claims and for working with the hospital to make payment arrangements, when necessary.

A person's health depends on much more than health care services. Patients are responsible for recognizing the impact of their life style on their personal health.

Conclusion

Hospitals have many functions to perform, including the enhancement of health status, health promotion, and the prevention and treatment of injury and disease; the immediate and ongoing care and rehabilitation of patients; the education of health professionals, patients, and the community; and research. All these activities must be conducted with an overriding concern for the values and dignity of patients.

Courtesy American Hospital Association. A patient's bill of rights. Chicago: The Association; 1992.

many cases a **surrogate** is designated to make decisions for that patient. Many individuals have made provisions for this scenario by obtaining legal documents, such as advance directives, living wills, and medical power of attorney. These documents specify what treatments they want or do not want. They also specify whom they name as a surrogate to make decisions in the event that they are unable to make them.

Advance directives grew from efforts by the courts and government to resolve ethical dilemmas. In 1990 the U.S. Supreme Court, in an attempt to determine whether a patient has a right to refuse medical treatment, handed down a decision in *Missouri v. Cruzan* recognizing a competent patient's right to refuse medical treatment.[7] Although the decision clarified the rights of competent patients, it raised many questions about informed consent, which is based on the ethical principle of autonomy. An opposing ethical principle no longer considered valid is the principle of paternalism, which stems from the word *parent* and assumes that an individual with more knowledge, in this case the health care professional, is more capable of making decisions for the patient.

As a result of the Court's decision and the autonomy-paternalism conflict related to informed consent, Congress passed the Patient Self-Determination Act, effective December 1991.[8] The act requires health care facilities receiving Medicaid or Medicare reimbursement to inform patients of their right to refuse treatment and of the availability of advance directives. Because these facilities depend financially on Medicaid and Medicare reimbursement, all states immediately passed statutes recognizing advance directives.

Confidentiality

Confidentiality ensures that the information entrusted to health care professionals in the line of duty is not revealed to others except when necessary to carry out their duties. This principle has a long past and is included in the Hippocratic Oath, which states: "What I may see or hear in the course of treatment … I will keep to myself holding such things shameful to be spoken aloud."[1] The principle of confidentiality remains one of the most cherished medical ethical principles, and the Patient's Bill of Rights guarantees confidentiality by stating that "the patient has the right to expect that all communication and records pertaining to his care should be treated as confidential."[6]

Need   Maintaining confidentiality is important because it contributes to necessary trust in the practice of medicine. Patients often reveal personal or embarrassing information

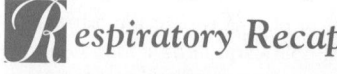

espiratory Recap

Confidentiality

Confidentiality ensures that the information entrusted to health care professionals in the line of duty is not revealed to others except when necessary to carry out such duties.

Maintaining confidentiality is important because it contributes to the trust patients need in the medical community.

Confidentiality has become more difficult to maintain due to technologic advances.

in the course of receiving medical treatment. If this information is not guarded, they lose this trust and may not provide health care professionals with the information they need to be properly diagnosed and treated. Many laws have been passed to protect patient confidentiality, including the Privacy Act of 1974, the Conditions of Participation for Hospitals in Medicare and Medicaid Programs, the Conditions of Participation for Long Term Care Facilities, and the Uniform Health Care Information Act.

Violations of Confidentiality

Confidentiality is the most violated of the ethical principles. As the medical system has expanded in recent years, so has the number of individuals with access to medical records. Estimations are that more than 75 individuals see a medical chart during a patient's hospital stay.[9] Confidentiality has become more difficult to maintain due to technologic advances;[10] although fax machines, cellular phones, and computers have made health care jobs easier, they also have helped decrease patient confidentiality. For example, patient records have been faxed accidentally to restaurants, and conversations have been overheard easily over cellular phones.

Computers offer even faster and more dangerous access to medical records. Databases can be accumulated containing information gathered legitimately by businesses. For example, drug companies may enter prescription purchases into a billing database; if an insurance company obtains these records, they could screen potential clients for high-risk conditions and deny them coverage.

Breaking Confidentiality

Although respect for confidentiality is an important tenet, at times health care professionals must break confidentiality. In such situations the practitioner must balance the need to protect others from foreseeable harm with the need to protect confidentiality. For example, if a patient threatens to harm someone, the health care worker has a responsibility to warn the individual potentially in danger.

An example of this is the case of *Tarasoff v. Regents of the University of California*.[11,12] In this case a psychologist had reason to believe that one of his patients would kill a woman whose name was Tatiana Tarasoff. The psychologist had the campus police arrest his patient, but the police later released the man when he assured them he would not contact Tarasoff. Neither the campus police nor the psychologist warned Tarasoff of the potential danger to her, and the man in question later killed Tarasoff. The woman's family brought a lawsuit against the University of California, resulting in an important decision in which the courts ruled that health care providers have a duty to warn individuals of foreseeable danger.

Breaking confidentiality is often necessary when the public's welfare may be jeopardized. Many states have laws requiring certain diseases, such as tuberculosis or sexually transmitted diseases, to be reported to public health agencies so that others who might have been exposed to the disease are informed and can receive the necessary treat-

ment. Most states have laws requiring health care workers who suspect child or elder abuse to file confidential reports. In such cases a concern exists for the public's welfare, so confidentiality may be violated.

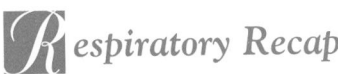 *espiratory Recap*

Confidentiality
When confidentiality is broken, one must balance the need to protect others from foreseeable harm with the need to protect confidentiality. Confidentiality may be broken when a concern exists for the public's welfare.

Justice

Justice is the principle that deals with fairness and equity in the distribution of scarce resources, such as time, services, equipment, and money. Although this concept may seem simple, in reality it is one of the most difficult principles to implement, creating numerous questions. For example, which criteria should be used to decide who receives life-saving organ transplants? Should a person's lifestyle (for instance, smoking or drinking) be considered?

Theories

How should limited health care resources be distributed? Several theories deal with this question, with the egalitarian theory stating that all individuals should have equal access to goods and services. However, this theory does not always translate into reality. For instance, health care available in rural areas of the country is not the same as availability in metropolitan areas.

Other theories approach the question from different angles. The utilitarian theory of justice states that the distribution of resources should be such that it achieves the greatest good for the greatest number of individuals. The libertarian theory emphasizes the personal rights to society and economic liberty. Another theory is the maximin view of justice. Using this theory the individual maximizes the minimum, even if doing so does not maximize the total amount of good done. In other words the individual needing the resources is helped the most, even if others are not helped. Another way to look at this theory is that the maximum amount of health care goes to a minimum number of patients (that is, the most critical).

With health care resources stretched these days, decisions about who gets the resources are never easy decisions. This question has created discussions from Congress to homes nationwide. The distribution of health care can be seen in changes in payment structures for Medicare and insurance companies, which have influenced the country's health care system. The distribution of justice affects all levels of health care and remains one of the most common ethical principles facing health care professionals today.

Respiratory Recap

> ### Justice
>
> Justice is the principle that deals with fairness and equity in the distribution of scarce resources, such as time, services, equipment, and money.
>
> The egalitarian theory of justice states that all individuals should have equal access to goods and services.
>
> The utilitarian theory of justice states that the distribution of resources should be such that it achieves the greatest good for the greatest number of individuals.
>
> The maximin theory of justice states that the individual most needing the resources is helped, even if others are not helped.

Managed Care and Justice   The implementation of managed care has changed the distribution of medical resources. Managed care uses a variety of techniques that influence the clinical behavior of health care providers and patients. These techniques, including that utilization restraints and preapproved criteria, often integrate the payment and delivery of heath care and are used with the overall goal of cost efficiency.

To keep costs down, managed care reduces resources such as time spent with patients, medications, tests, and treatments and offers incentives to physicians who are cost effective. Many physicians receive bonuses if they stay within the guidelines of the managed care provider. Those who are not cost efficient may be penalized with reduced income or receive peer pressure from superiors to become more cost efficient.

The distribution of health care resources often is debated, but managed care has added new fuel to the fire, as efforts to contain the rising cost of health care compete with its fair distribution. Companies and policies, instead of health care professionals, often dictate the decisions as to how resources are distributed. As managed care continues to expand, health care professionals will continue to face more ethical dilemmas, particularly those dealing with justice.

Respiratory Recap

> ### Managed Care and Justice
>
> Managed care uses techniques that influence the clinical behavior of health care providers and patients.
>
> To meet efficiency goals, managed care companies offer incentives to physicians who control costs.
>
> As managed care grows, so will the ethical dilemmas associated with justice.

Role Fidelity

Fidelity to Patients   **Fidelity** implies an obligation or faithfulness to duty. Each member of the health care team has a role with specific tasks and responsibilities or a scope of practice, which is usually set by tradition and/or the state legislature that regulates health care practice. Each practitioner has a duty to practice within this role (role fidelity). Keeping within the scope of practice is considered in the best interests of the patient. The American Association for Respiratory Care (AARC) has made this preference clear in its statement on ethics, as shown in Box 5-2. Respiratory care practitioners shall perform only those procedures or functions in which they are individually competent and that are within the scope of accepted and responsible practice. The nature of this role is one in which a relationship is established between the health care provider and the patient and in which the patient expects truth and the loyalty of the provider. Patients place trust in their providers to perform their duties to the best of their abilities and refrain from duties not in their expertise.

Fidelity to Colleagues   Role fidelity exists among colleagues, with an obligation of loyalty to co-workers and the profession. At times this loyalty may interfere with loyalty to the patient, and loyalty to colleagues does have exceptions. For example, most professional organizations have ethical codes that require members to report incompetent or dishonest practices or impaired colleagues. In such cases, loyalty to the patient would outweigh loyalty to colleagues. The AARC states in its position statement that the respiratory care practitioner "shall refuse to conceal illegal, unethical or incompetent acts of others."

Conflicts with Fidelity   Role fidelity creates a number of problems. In many cases, roles that once were clearly established by tradition are now changing. Managed care and a desire for cost efficiency have created overlapping jobs. Various professionals now perform tasks that were once assigned to one particular profession, creating conflicts with role fidelity.

Other practices, such as joint ventures and referrals, have added to the fidelity question. Joint ventures involve physicians who have investments in health care services to which they may refer their patients (for example, a physician who owns a radiology center and refers all of his patients to that facility for radiographs). Referrals also create problems with role fidelity. For instance, a therapist refers or recommends a home health company or equipment company to a patient and then collects a finder's fee from that company. To deal with this problem the AARC issued a statement regarding the ethical performance of therapists and prohibiting this type of conduct. In some states, self-referral and finder's fees are illegal, resulting in legal violations in addition to ethical misconduct.

Box 5-2

AARC Statement of Ethics and Professional Conduct

In the conduct of professional activities the respiratory care practitioner shall be bound by certain ethical and professional principles and demonstrate the following:

1. Demonstrate behavior that reflects integrity, supports objectivity, and fosters trust in the profession and its professionals
2. Actively maintain and continually improve their professional competence and represent it accurately
3. Perform only those procedures or functions in which they are individually competent and that are within the scope of accepted and responsible practice
4. Respect and protect the legal and personal rights of patients they treat, including the right to informed consent and refusal of treatment
5. Divulge no confidential information regarding any patient or family unless disclosure is required for responsible performance of duty or is required by law

6. Provide care without discrimination on any basis, with respect for the rights and dignity of all individuals
7. Promote disease prevention and wellness
8. Refuse to participate in illegal or unethical acts and refuse to conceal illegal, unethical, or incompetent acts of others
9. Follow sound scientific procedures and ethical principles in research
10. Comply with state or federal laws governing and related to their practice
11. Avoid any form of conduct that creates a conflict of interest and follow the principles of ethical business behavior
12. Promote the positive evolution of the profession and health care in general through improvement of the access, efficacy, and cost of patient care
13. Refrain from indiscriminate and unnecessary use of resources, both economic and natural, in practice

AARC, *American Association for Respiratory Care.*

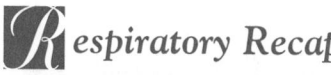 **espiratory Recap**

Role Fidelity
Fidelity implies an obligation or faithfulness to duty. Each practitioner has a duty to practice within this role. Problems with role fidelity occur more often today because of changes in traditional roles, managed care, joint ventures, and referrals.

Role of Professional Organizations in Ethics

Need for Professional Ethics

Professional medical organizations recognize the need for guidelines in helping their members maintain high ethical standards. The respiratory care profession, although still new compared with other professions, has established a code of ethics for its members. New professions must es-

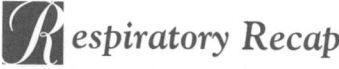 **espiratory Recap**

Professional Organizations' Role in Ethics
Professional medical organizations recognize the need for guidelines in helping their members maintain high ethical standards. The AARC code tends to the legal and professional growth needs of the profession.

tablish themselves as entities that embraces guidelines and standards and are willing to set direction and provide some degree of self-governance for their members. Along the same lines, new professionals must establish themselves as responsible practitioners who adhere to guidelines and standards. Important characteristics of a professional include the abilities to operate with integrity and demonstrate self-governance and direction.

AARC Code of Ethics

The **AARC Code of Ethics** and professional conduct has evolved through several revisions over the life of the respiratory therapy profession. In its present form (see Table 5-2), it closely resembles the ethical theories and principles discussed in this chapter and embraces the major legal concerns that all professionals face today in the performance of their professional duties. The following discussion analyzes each of the code's discrete components:

- Item 1: Demonstrate behavior that reflects integrity, supports objectivity, and fosters trust in the profession and its professionals

Item 1 of the statement addresses the need for integrity, objectivity, trust, and role fidelity for respiratory care professionals. These traits can be incorporated into the principle of veracity, or truth. By fostering integrity, health care practitioners demonstrate that in performing their duties, they adhere to unimpaired standards of care that are free of flaws. Fidelity is upheld as long as practitioners work within their professional competence.

A common trait is that all professionals adhere to a community standard of care. Community in this case may refer to both the profession and a physical community, as in a state or region of the country. Adherence to a community standard of care can be extremely important when practitioners are required to defend themselves in legal actions. Objectivity in the delivery of care ensures that the practitioner does not discriminate on any basis—ethnicity, gender, or type of disease. The objective practitioner simply delivers the best care possible to whoever needs it. Public trust in the professional is essential both to establish and maintain professional status and to maximize adherence to the service and directions of the professional.

- Item 2: Actively maintain and continually improve their professional competence and represent it accurately
- Item 3: Perform only those procedures or functions in which they are individually competent and that are within the scope of accepted and responsible practice

Items 2 and 3 reflect the need for research and continuing education, along with the requirement for professionals to self-govern themselves by acknowledging their own limitations. These items also address fidelity in reflecting the need for continuing education because the therapist's scope of practice will grow. Therapists must continue to enhance their education by learning about new procedures, treatments, and equipment. With continual learning beneficence and nonmaleficence are served; therapists will be better able to treat their patients and provide them with the best care while avoiding unnecessary therapy or harm.

- Item 4: Respect and protect the legal and personal rights of patients they treat, including the right to informed consent and refusal of treatment

Item 4 of the AARC statement emphasizes the need for informed consent, which relates to autonomy, the patient's right to decide care. This item respects the patient's right to make decisions regarding care, including the right to refuse treatments.

- Item 5: Divulge no confidential information regarding any patient or family unless disclosure is required for responsible performance of duty or is required by law

Item 5 refers to one of the oldest and best-established ethical principles, confidentiality, a mainstay of health care delivery. The respiratory therapist has a duty to uphold the confidentiality of information shared in the course of treatment unless the information is required to perform the job or disclosure is required by law.

- Item 6: Provide care without discrimination on any basis, with respect for the rights and dignity of all individuals

Item 6 refers to the principles of justice and autonomy. The distribution of health care resources should be provided without discrimination. At the same time, respiratory therapists must respect the autonomy and dignity of the patient.

- Item 7: Promote disease prevention and wellness

Item 7 supports the principles of role fidelity, justice, beneficence, and nonmaleficence. Role fidelity is addressed by the need for respiratory therapists to educate the public about disease prevention and wellness. Because therapists are the allied health experts, their involvement in the cardiopulmonary aspect of health is vital. By educating individuals about disease prevention and wellness, the public may become healthier, thus lowering the demand for respiratory resources. Justice can be served by provision of these services to those who need them. Through education, practitioners can provide good to their patients and prevent harm, serving beneficence and nonmaleficence.

- Item 8: Refuse to participate in illegal or unethical acts and refuse to conceal illegal, unethical, or incompetent acts of others
- Item 11: Avoid any form of conduct that creates a conflict of interest and follow the principles of ethical business behavior

Items 8 and 11 discuss the importance of fidelity and veracity. With fidelity, patients expect loyalty from their therapists, a trait evident in competent, ethical respiratory therapists. Therapists also have a duty to the profession to identify members of the profession who are not maintaining competency and ethical behavior, thus enforcing nonmaleficence.

In addition, sound research includes veracity. Research subjects must be informed of the risks of any research and have the opportunity to ask questions and receive truthful answers. Individuals have the right to refuse to participate in research studies without any adverse effects or discontinuance of their health care.

- Item 9: Follow sound scientific research procedures and ethical principles in research
- Item 10: Comply with state or federal laws governing and related to their practice

Items 9 and 10 again deal with fidelity. State and federal laws dictate the scope of practice, and respiratory therapists should be familiar with these laws, particularly state laws that usually define the scope of care. Item 9 also addresses the need for ethical research, which has lead to many breakthrough discoveries and enhanced beneficence. Ethical standards must be maintained so that patients can bene-fit from research, not be harmed by it.

- Item 12: Promote the positive evolution of the pro-fession and health care in general through improve-ment of the access, efficacy, and cost of patient care
- Item 13: Refrain from indiscriminate and unneces-sary use of resources, both economic and natural, in practice

Items 12 and 13 deal with justice. The current distri-bution of resources in the United States is imperfect and unequal. To deal with this problem the AARC has stated that every respiratory therapist has a duty to try to improve the principle of justice. Respira-tory therapists should be aware of the distribution of health care resources and constantly seek measures to improve their delivery and access. They should be conscious of the cost of the care provided and seek cost-efficient, effective ways to deliver care.

Ethics Committees

In 1991 the Joint Commission on Accreditation of Health-care Organizations (JCAHO) adopted guidelines requiring each accredited organization to establish a mechanism to consider ethical issues in patient care and education for health care practitioners. Most facilities responded by es-tablishing ethics committees, the composition, duties, and activities of which vary widely from institution to institu-tion. A typical committee is composed of approximately 12 members ranging from medical staff, administration, and various service departments. A member of the clergy also may serve on the ethics committee, along with a medical ethicist, often an ethics professor or researcher.

Committees may develop policies and procedures, sponsor educational activities, and serve as clearing-houses for the distribution of information on ethical is-sues. The committee may consider specific ethical dilem-mas, but when ethics committees become involved in patient care, their only goal is to issue a recommendation. Little research has been done on the effectiveness of ethics committees, which are currently required for JCAHO accreditation.

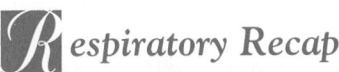*espiratory Recap* ―――――

Ethics Committees
Ethics committees were formed to consider ethical issues in patient care and education for the health care practitioner. Committees may develop policies and procedures, sponsor educational activities and serve as clearinghouses for the distribution of information on ethical issues.

Adherence to ethical standards decreases the likelihood that a facility will encounter accountability problems, im-proves patient outcomes, and assures patients that they can trust their health care system. Given the current state of health care accountability, more important than ever is that health care providers, including respiratory therapists, take every precaution possible to ensure that the services they provide meet the highest ethical standards.

CASE STUDIES

Case One
Double-Edged Sword

Casey is a respiratory therapist working in a regional burn center. One of her patients has second-degree burns on his lower extremities and is in considerable pain. He is crying and thrashing about in his bed, begging Casey "please give me something for the pain!" Casey is concerned that the patient will pull out his intravenous (IV) tube and hurt himself if he doesn't stop thrashing. The intern on call or-ders more morphine, but Casey is concerned that the ad-ditional morphine could depress the patient's respiratory drive. Should the additional morphine be given?

Using the guiding principles presented in this chapter, delivery of the narcotic would be beneficial for the patient because it would relieve his pain and keep the patient from dislodging his intravenous catheter. The narcotic is admin-istered for a good purpose, the relief of pain, and the unde-sirable side effect of respiratory depression is not intended. In this particular case, pain relief outweighs the possibility of respiratory depression and the patient should be care-fully monitored for any potential undesirable side effects.

Case Two
To Intubate or Not to Intubate

Mrs. Ray is 68 years old and has a history of chronic ob-structive pulmonary disease (COPD), congestive heart failure (CHF), and renal disease. She has been admitted to the hospital numerous times in the past 3 years, and the respiratory therapy staff members know her well. On pre-vious admissions, she stated to several respiratory therapy staff members that she never wanted to be intubated or placed on mechanical ventilation.

Mrs. Ray's current admission is for pneumonia. The res-piratory therapist assigned to give Mrs. Ray her nebulizer treatments receives a stat page; on arrival in the patient's room, the therapist finds Mrs. Ray's daughter and physi-cian in a discussion outside. Mrs. Ray is unresponsive and in impending respiratory failure. The physician explains that the antibiotics have not had time to treat Mrs. Ray's pneumonia and that without mechanical ventilation, the woman will suffer respiratory failure and die.

The physician says that they must decide whether to intubate Mrs. Ray. The daughter insists, "I want everything done for my mother! Put her on the breathing machine!" The physician agrees with the daughter and asks the respiratory therapist to intubate and ventilate the woman per the respiratory care protocol. The therapist informs the physician of Mrs. Ray's previous requests regarding intubation and mechanical ventilation, but the physician angrily states, "Mrs. Ray doesn't have an advance directive. It is the daughter's decision to make. We can treat the pneumonia and then probably extubate her."

Should Mrs. Ray be intubated and placed on mechanical ventilation? Which ethical principles are involved? What decision-making processes are the respiratory therapist and physician each using to make their judgments?

This case involves several ethical principles, including autonomy, beneficence, and nonmaleficence. The respiratory therapist, knowing that Mrs. Ray previously requested *not* to be intubated or placed on mechanical ventilation, may think that Mrs. Ray's autonomy is being compromised with intubation. Although the patient did not formally put her wishes in writing, she made her wishes well known to the respiratory staff members. Whether the patient fully understood the nature of her condition and the consequences of this decision are not known. These two criteria are required for a patient to make an autonomous decision to refuse therapy. If she understood that her medical condition could at some point in time require intubation with mechanical ventilation and that refusing this therapy could result in her death, then she made a conscious decision invoking her autonomy. She had the right to make this decision for herself.

The physician's decision to intubate could be based on the principle of beneficence, which involves the performance of procedures and treatments to benefit the patient. The assumption may be made that Mrs. Ray did not inform the physician of her past decision to refuse intubation and mechanical ventilation. The physician believes the pneumonia can be treated and that Mrs. Ray will be extubated. By performing these procedures, the physician thinks that in the long run, the patient will benefit and that beneficence must be upheld in this matter. From this viewpoint, not treating Mrs. Ray would result in nonmaleficence or harm.

The physician is guided by a consequential, or teleological, theory and is basing the decision to intubate on the possible consequences or outcomes of the actions. If the patient is not placed on mechanical ventilation, the physician believes she will die. If she is placed on mechanical ventilation and treated for her pneumonia, the physician believes that recovery and subsequent extubation are likely. According to the physician's beliefs the consequences or likely outcomes of this situation should direct the decision making. Based on this reasoning the physician has sufficient reason to intubate.

The respiratory therapist is guided by the principle of duty, or deontology, in the decision to inform the doctor of Mrs. Ray's wishes. The therapist believes in a duty to the patient to abide by previously stated wishes and that the patient's autonomous decision should be upheld, despite her daughter's wishes. Because the therapist appears to have known Mrs. Ray and has discussed intubation with her in the past, the respiratory therapist may be aware of possible psychologic or financial impacts on Mrs. Ray if her autonomy is not upheld. By refusing to uphold the patient's autonomous decision regarding life support, the therapist may believe that the principle of nonmaleficence is being violated and that intubating her against the patient's wishes would harm her.

This situation is not uncommon in today's medical practice. The absence of advanced directives and poor communication among family members and attending physicians often leads to ethical dilemmas in which all parties involved in the patient's care must balance the beneficence of an action with its nonmaleficence.

Case Three
Nosy Therapists

Bill and Lisa are respiratory therapists working in a hospital. They have discovered that they can uncover personal information about their co-workers by using the hospital computer. They already have learned that two of their co-workers are living together and that one of these individuals has a history of psychologic problems. In addition, they have discovered that the husband of another co-worker, Ann, recently tested positive for human immunodeficiency virus (HIV) and are concerned that Ann, who frequently draws arterial blood gases on patients, may be HIV positive and could be a risk to the patients. They wonder whether they should inform their boss.

In this case, two employees have learned to use the computer for some dangerous snooping. In the process they not only have most likely violated hospital policy regarding computer access but also violated patient confidentiality. They have learned that one of their co-workers has been exposed to HIV, are concerned about patient risk, and are making some assumptions regarding that co-worker, including the assumption that their boss does not know about her husband's positive HIV test. This may not be the case. They also are assuming that Ann has tested HIV positive, which may not be true. Furthermore, none of these matters involves them because they are not supervisors, and neither has a right or need to know the information in question.

From a deontological viewpoint, Bill and Lisa could argue they should inform their boss of their discovery. They believe that patients are at risk for harm and that they have a duty to protect their patients. Informing their supervisor could protect Ann's patients from potential harm.

A teleological view of this scenario involves listing of all of the consequences. Bill and Lisa believe that if they do not tell their boss, Ann could be placing her patients at risk. They could tell their boss but would most likely have to admit how they gained this information, which would place them both at risk for punishment. Bill and Lisa would have to decide which consequence would have the best outcome.

Case Four
You Can Tell Mom

A patient has been admitted to the hospital with an acute myocardial infarction (MI). The respiratory therapist on duty receives a phone call from his mother, who works with the patient's wife. His mother asks the therapist to ensure that the physicians are telling the patient's wife the full story.

In this case the respiratory therapist would violate patient confidentiality if he provided his mother with this information. He has a duty to respect the confidentiality of the patient by not revealing anything about the case to his mother. Although his mother's intentions may be good, they do not justify a breach of confidentiality. The therapist should inform his mother why he is not able to give her the information.

Case Five
Should You Tell?

Mr. Hart is 60 years old and has suffered a MI. Due to a prior MI and CHF, he has a poor prognosis. The patient does not want his wife of 42 years to know about his poor prognosis because he is afraid she cannot handle the news and wants to spare her emotional pain. The respiratory therapist has been working with Mr. Hart for several days and has established a good rapport with both the patient and his wife. While walking down the hallway the therapist runs into a tearful Mrs. Hart, who says, "I know something is wrong with my husband. What's happening to him? Please tell me!" How should the respiratory therapist respond?

In this case the patient has made his wishes known. He does not want his wife to know about his poor prognosis. The therapist has no reason to suspect foreseeable harm to Mrs. Hart, and divulging of the information is not in the public's best welfare. In addition, the therapist does not need to reveal the information to perform the duties of a therapist. Although the respiratory therapist may not agree or understand Mr. Hart's request, the patient's confidentiality should be respected and the therapist should not divulge the information to Mrs. Hart. The respiratory therapist should offer reassurance, saying something such as, "We are doing everything possible to respect Mr. Hart's wishes and help him overcome his heart attack."

Case Six
Who Gets the Therapy?

John is a respiratory therapy supervisor at a large metropolitan hospital. When he arrives to start his shift, the departing supervisor notifies him that two members on his shift have called in sick for the night and that replacements for both are unavailable. The hospital is extremely busy that night, with each staff member already taking a full load of patients, and performance of all of the respiratory therapy procedures needed is impossible. John must decide how to distribute the available resources.

Policy states that patients who are either in the intensive care units (ICUs) or on mechanical ventilation receive priority over those receiving general floor therapy. John knows that several ventilator patients are stable and have not been weaned in several weeks. However, several asthmatic patients cannot afford to be without therapy. He also knows that the nurses in the ICU are educated in respiratory therapy procedures and in a better position to help with treatments than the nurses in the general nursing units.

He could decide that all patients will receive one less treatment during this shift. For instance, a patient who was scheduled to receive three jet nebulizer treatments would receive only two treatments. He also could decide that several patients will not receive any therapy so that the others who need their treatments the most will receive therapy as ordered. Furthermore, he could assign all the procedures and allow his staff members to decide who receives the therapy. What should John do?

In making his decision, John may choose to look at issues from several viewpoints. If he decides to reduce the therapy received by all patients he would be taking an egalitarian position. This theory states all individuals should have equal access to goods and services. In this case, he could argue that all patients would be treated fairly in that they all would receive reduced services.

John may choose to assume a maximin position of justice. This theory states that justice would be served if the therapists maximized the minimum. In other words, John and the staff would provide therapy to those who need it most. John would not deliver therapy to some patients but instead would concentrate his resources on those with the greatest need.

A respiratory care policy addresses the way in which care should be delivered during a shortage of staff members, stating that respiratory care should be prioritized to treat patients in the ICU first. However, John does not think this policy fairly distributes the resources. If John were to approach the problem with a utilitarian theory, he would look at the consequences of all the possible alternatives and decide on the choice that maximizes the total amount of good done, regardless of who benefits. Because John believes the patients with asthma have the greatest need for respiratory care, he could utilize the utilitarian theory to support his decision to perform the treatments on the asthmatic patients instead of the stable, ventilated ICU patients. According to John's values the asthmatic patients would receive the greatest good from the treatments and thus would receive therapy.

By making a decision in opposition to hospital policy, John places his values above those of the hospital. By violating policy as a supervisor, he sets a poor example for his staff members. Failure to follow policies can result in detrimental actions not only to the individual disregarding the policy but also to the hospital. The hospital could face legal action if policies are not followed and patients suffer ill consequences. John will have to deal with any consequences that occur as a result of his actions. If he believes the policy is incorrect, he should address this issue with his superiors.

Case Seven
A Couple of Beers

After a busy evening shift, respiratory therapist Tony is glad when Sam arrives to relieve him. While giving his report, Tony smells alcohol on Sam's breath and notices that Sam's speech is slurred. Tony knows that Sam had mentioned he was going to watch the football game at a bar with some friends before coming in to work the night shift. Tony suspects that Sam might have had some alcohol and might not be in shape to work. He decides to question him about his suspicion. Sam admits, "I had a couple of beers. It's no big deal." Tony asks him whether he is competent to do his job, and Sam replies, "Be a friend. Don't make so much out of this. Don't worry; I can do my job." Tony is not convinced but is unsure what to do. He doesn't want to jeopardize his friendship with Sam, but he is concerned that Sam could harm a patient. What should Tony do?

Tony is torn between fidelity to his patients and fidelity to his co-worker. He can allow his colleague to maintain his autonomy and do nothing. However, Tony is not convinced his colleague has the capacity to make that decision because he believes Sam is impaired by alcohol.

Tony believes that his patients could be at risk if Sam is allowed to care for them. Following this line of thinking, he believes that fidelity to his patients and nonmaleficence take precedence. The respiratory therapy code of ethics also states he has a duty to the profession to report incompetence among fellow members. Thus Tony would do best to report the incident to his supervisor immediately so that managerial decisions about staffing for the shift can be made.

𝒦EY 𝒫OINTS

- Ethics is the study of the ways individuals and societies make judgments regarding right and wrong.
- Many factors affect decisions about right and wrong, including culture, religion, morals, and societal mores.
- Seven important ethical principles help guide health care—beneficence, nonmaleficence, veracity, autonomy, confidentiality, justice, and role fidelity.
- Beneficence is the principle that imposes on the health care practitioner the responsibility to seek good for the patient.
- Nonmaleficence is the principle in which the health care practitioner refrains from harming the patient.
- Veracity requires the health care practitioner to tell the patient the truth.
- Confidentiality ensures that information revealed to the health care practitioner is not revealed to others except when necessary to perform duties or when silence may result in harm to an individual or the public.
- Justice deals with the fair and equitable distribution of health care resources.
- Role fidelity refers to one's faithfulness to duty.
- Professional organizations such as the AARC recognize the need to establish guidelines for professional ethical behavior.
- The AARC Code of Ethics describes the ethical behaviors for respiratory therapists that guide professional practice.
- Hospitals have established ethics committees to deal with ethical issues in patient care and educate health care professionals.
- Each respiratory therapist has a duty and responsibility to provide quality health care guided by legal and ethical principles.

References

1. Hippocrates. The Oath. In: Jones WHS, translator. Hippocrates (the Loeb Classic Library). vol. 1. Cambridge, Mass: Harvard University Press; 1923. pp. 299-301.
2. Evans RW. The physician-assisted-killing fallacy. Life Adv 1999 May/June;13(6).
3. Carrol C. Ethical theories and methods. In: Carrol C. Legal issues and ethical dilemmas in respiratory care. Philadelphia: FA Davis; 1996. pp. 68-74.
4. Edge RS, Groves JR. Basic principles of healthcare ethics—a guide for clinical practice. Albany, NY: Delmar; 1994. p. 38.
5. Hebert PC, Hoffmaster B, Glass KC, et al. Bioethics for clinicians: truth telling. CMAJ 1997;156:225-228.
6. American Hospital Association. Patient's Bill of Rights. Chicago: The Association; 1975.
7. *Cruzan v. Director Missouri Dept. of Health.* US Supreme Court. 88-1503; 1990.
8. Logue B. Rights: death control and the elderly in America. New York: Macmillan; 1993.
9. Edge RS, Groves JR. Basic principles of healthcare ethics—a guide for clinical practice. Albany, NY: Delmar; 1994.
10. Dodek DY, Dodek A. From Hippocrates to facsimile: protecting patient confidentiality is more difficult and more important than ever. CMAJ 1997;156:847-852.
11. *Tarasoff v. Regents of the University of California.* 529 P2d 553,118 Cal Rpt 129; 1974.
12. *Tarasoff v. Regents of the University of California.* Reargued 17 Cal 3d 425,551 P2d 334,131 Cal Rptr 333; 1976.

CHAPTER 6

Communication Skills

William F. Galvin

CHAPTER OUTLINE

Miscommunication: the Case for Effective Communication Skills
Miscommunication #1: Watch the Borders!
Miscommunication #2: Orson Welles' War of the Worlds
Miscommunication #3: Put this Blood Gas on Ice!
Miscommunication #4: Know Bronchodilators!
Basic Concepts of Communication
Commonly Used Expressions
Levels of Communication
Principles and Assumptions
Multidimensional Communication
Transactional Communication
Process of Communication
Communication Defined
Factors Affecting Communication
Environmental Factors
Emotional/Sensory Factors

Verbal Expressions
Nonverbal Cues
Intrapersonal Factors
Physical Appearance and Status
Barriers to Effective Communication
Basic Goals and Purpose of Communication
Four Major Goals
Conveying Believability
Effective Communication
Skills of the Sender
Skills of the Receiver
Bridges to the Relationship
Questioning Techniques
Examples Used in Respiratory Care

OBJECTIVES

1. Identify common miscommunication problems.
2. Identify and explain the basic concepts of communication, including commonly used expressions, levels of communication, principles and assumptions, and a working definition.
3. List and explain the factors that affect communication, including environmental factors, emotional/sensory factors, verbal expressions, nonverbal cues, intrapersonal factors, and physical appearance and status.
4. Identify barriers to communication.
5. State the true purpose and four major subgoals of communication.
6. Explain the importance of conveying believability.
7. Identify and explain skills of the sender.
8. Identify and explain skills of the receiver.
9. List and discuss the characteristics and qualities of a nurturing relationship.
10. Identify and explain questioning strategies and techniques.
11. Illustrate the effective use of questioning strategies and techniques in the practice of respiratory care.

KEY TERMS

Channel	Confrontation	Encoding
Clarification	Decoding	Facilitation
Closed-Ended Questions	Dialogue	Feedback
Communication	Emotional Filters	Grapevine
Compound Questions	Empathy	Jargon
Confidentiality	Empowerment	Kinesics

Continued

Leading Questions	Nonverbal Communication	Proxemics
Medium	Nonverbal Cues	Transactional
Message	Open-Ended Questions	Verbal Expressions
Mindset	Paralinguistics	"White Lab Jacket" Phenomenon
Mutuality	Personal Space	

Communication is a complex and dynamic process at the heart of all human interaction. It is universally applicable and has been identified as one of the most formidable problems individuals face in any encounter. The importance of its effectiveness cannot be overstated, underestimated, or trivialized; communication is clearly one of the most vital of the basic life skills. If communication is not mastered and used effectively, it can result in misunderstanding, disagreement, and conflict.

The urgent and critical nature of health care renders it markedly more vulnerable to the devastating consequences and repercussions of poor communication. Respiratory therapists use communication skills in health care assessment, disease management, and multidisciplinary collaboration. Communication has been identified an as essential component of future respiratory care curriculum.[1] Little doubt remains as to its central role in the practice of respiratory care.

The intention of this chapter is to enhance and strengthen the interpersonal communication among the respiratory therapist and the physician, nurse, allied health professional, patient, and family member. Practical and everyday examples of miscommunication are provided, along with a wide array of definitions and perspectives, and an extensive list of factors affecting communication is discussed. The major goals and the purpose of communication are highlighted, along with the importance of the conveyance of believability. This chapter addresses the skills of the sender and receiver and provides an overview of questioning strategies and techniques, concluding with examples of the ways these communication strategies and techniques apply to respiratory care practice.

Miscommunication: the Case for Effective Communication Skills

One way to make the case for effective communication skills is to provide examples of communication blunders. Some rather amusing yet pointed examples illustrate the serious nature and magnitude of the problem. These are general in nature and also specific to respiratory care, highlighting some specific pitfalls to communication.

Miscommunication #1: Watch the Borders!

A story is circulating through the federal government regarding the famous and feared former director of the Fed-

eral Bureau of Investigation (FBI), J. Edgar Hoover. Its authenticity and origin are mysterious and sketchy, but its **message** is quite powerful. According to the story, Hoover asked his secretary to type an important memo to all his high-level, worldwide regional directors. The content of the memo is insignificant, but after the memo was typed and returned to Hoover, he wrote on the bottom of the memo the words *Watch the borders!* The memo then was copied and circulated to all the recipients. The directors read and interpreted the memo to mean that they were to increase security and surveillance at their respective regional borders. However, later determined was that what Hoover meant with the words *Watch the borders!* was that his secretary reduce the size of the memo's page borders.

Whether real or contrived, this story does bring home a message. The communication pitfalls were misinterpretation and a lack of rapport between Hoover and his secretary. Hoover was not addressing the borders of the countries but rather the borders of the memo, identifying the margins surrounding the sheet of paper. He was concerned that the margins of the text were either too narrow or too broad, but his ruthlessness, short temper, and feared personality prevented his secretary from seeking **clarification** to prevent the ensuing calamity. The consequence could have resulted in a costly outlay of additional funds to satisfy personnel expenses for what was thought to be a need for more security and surveillance at the borders of these countries.

Miscommunication #2: Orson Welles' "War of the Worlds"

Perhaps one of the most popular radio broadcasts was the 1938 version of the "War of the Worlds." The talented actor Orson Welles narrated a spell-binding and convincing broadcast over national radio on Halloween Eve, telling a story of the United States being invaded by Martians. The session began with a disclosure that the story was purely fictitious and merely done as a form of entertainment. The listeners were captivated because Welles told the story with considerable conviction and a tremendous sense of reality. The audience was terrified, and the results were nearly catastrophic. As the story goes a number of listeners from a small New Jersey community were so convinced of its authenticity that they fetched their guns and passed through the streets looking to confront what they believed were invaders from Mars. What was the problem?

This story represents a classic example of an incomplete message and how incomplete facts can have potentially serious consequences. Simply stated the audience did not hear those opening remarks about the story being fiction. However, the power of the speaker and the circumstances surrounding the broadcast (Halloween Eve) were so convincing that the listening audience actually believed it to be true. So convincing was the broadcast that some listeners were prepared to go to battle. The message is a simple one; be certain that you hear and/or observe the entire message and monitor your emotions before jumping to conclusions.

Miscommunication #3: Put this Blood Gas on Ice!

A new respiratory therapy student was attending to his first-ever cardiac arrest. He was all eyes and ears and eager to help. During the resuscitation the senior therapist drew an arterial blood gas and asked that it be sent to the lab immediately. The sample was handed back to the new student, and with it, directions to immediately put it on ice and take it to the stat laboratory. The student went down the corridor to the ice machine, secured a cup of ice, took the cap off the syringe, and instilled the blood into the cup before he ran it down to the laboratory. What is the problem?

Besides the young student being placed in a totally inappropriate situation, gross assumptions were made that commonly used medical **jargon** was understood by this novice, inexperienced, aspiring practitioner. Although any seasoned therapist would have understood the instructions, the new student's placement in this situation is grossly unfair and unacceptable. The student obviously was unfamiliar with medical language, and although willing and eager to help and make a good impression, he was asked to perform a task without proper education, supervision, and training. The case may appear extreme and even amusing, but it nonetheless makes the point about assumptions regarding the understanding of commonly used medical expressions.

Miscommunication #4: Know Bronchodilators!

A respiratory therapy student just starting out in the program visited the office of her program director to complain about the fairness of her first respiratory pharmacology examination. The director initially was reluctant to listen because previous experience had taught him that many students make unfair accusations about the difficulty and validity of exams. However, being somewhat familiar with the student's mild manner and studious work ethic, he decided to engage her in further discussion.

The student stated that during the course of the exam review session the faculty member indicated the students should "know bronchodilators." The student stated that she had studied for hours and hours thereafter. She arrived early for the morning of the exam, feeling confident and well prepared, and progressed through the exam, at one point noting five or six questions on Bronkosol, albuterol, and other bronchodilating agents. Believing these to be normal pharmacology questions, the director nodded affirmatively. However, with this nodding the student became distraught and even enraged. She began to raise her voice in displeasure and said, "But that's not fair; we were told that bronchodilators would not be on the exam." The director appeared perplexed and said, "Clearly you have to agree that questions on bronchodilators are obviously appropriate for an exam in respiratory pharmacology." The student then responded, "But he said *no bronchodilators!*" The director then realized that the student was interpreting the statement to mean *no* instead of *know*.

Although the story is alarming, it also reflects a significant finding within schools—an increase in the cultural diversity of the student body. The message is that the obvious cannot be assumed, and virtually all communications occurring with students from different cultures requires care, diligence, and attention to detail. Continual efforts must be made to enhance students' understanding of language and cultural norms.

Some of the previously discussed miscommunication stories are amusing, but they nonetheless reflect serious flaws and problems in the transmittal and receipt of messages. At issue is that medicine leaves little margin for error. The medical literature is replete with examples in which a misplaced decimal point hurriedly transcribed by a health care practitioner has resulted in the death of a patient. Other patients have had the wrong limbs amputated; angry managers have been frustrated by staff members who seemingly disregard their directives; and patients can appear noncompliant with treatment regimes designed and developed by health care professionals to meet their specific needs. At the heart of these issues is a complex process that entails considerable complication. An appreciation of the concepts involved in communication can help the health care professional alleviate the complexity.

Basic Concepts of Communication

Commonly Used Expressions

Communication can be expressed in a variety of ways. In a social context as a form of small talk, or "chit-chat," it follows a pattern of social amenities in which prescribed rules, ceremonies, or customs are observed. When a therapist says *hello* to a colleague or patient, it is a simple greeting that abides by a socially acceptable custom. Often this small talk encompasses mundane topics and simply wastes time, tests reactions, avoids involvement, or serves as a bridge to more significant conversation.[2] When friends and colleagues exchange information informally and spontaneously, it is sometimes called the **grapevine** and often viewed as gossip, rumors, half-truths, and even distorted or inaccurate information but nonetheless a normal growth of organizational life and a fulfillment of the desire to be "in the know."[3] Communication also can be expressed in the form of a **dialogue,** which involves purposeful, reciprocal, and close or intimate expression between participants.[2] Dialogue is particularly significant and valuable in health care settings, in which meaningful communication must occur between therapist and patient or therapist and health care professional.

Levels of Communication

Communication exists on five different levels,[4-6] which are summarized in Table 6-1 and discussed briefly in the following section.

Level-five communication (cliché conversation) is considered the lowest level of human interaction and is characterized by meaningless statements and clichés. No genuine human sharing takes place at this superficial level. For example, you pass a casual friend and say, "Hi. How are you?" At this point you expect the response, "I'm fine. How are you?" Nothing meaningful occurs, but each party abides by expected social niceties. However, if the acquaintance responded by saying, "I feel terrible. I have a bad cold, the kids are sick, and my wife is angry with me," that individual is trying to enter into a higher level of communication. Such a detailed response is generally frowned on because the expectation is a simple "I'm fine." As the initiator of the message, you can either express concern and encourage further dialogue or simply say "Oh! That's too bad" while looking down at your watch and hurriedly walk away. In choosing the latter, you are essentially communicating, "I don't want to hear your problems. I was just trying to be friendly." Your intention was to engage in a level-five communication.

Level-four communication (fact reporting) is still a relatively shallow form of interaction in which neutral topics are discussed and small talk ensues. It entails such issues as the news, the weather, or sports scores. Neither party shares anything personal, and the interaction remains impersonal, safe, and noncontroversial. An example of level-four communication is a situation in which you are waiting outside the conference room for a lecture to begin, you see a familiar medical student, and you say "Hi! How are you?" The student may respond, "Fine, thanks" (a level-five communication), after which a silence ensues as you both continue to wait for the conference door to open. If you choose to enter level-four communication, you say, "What a beautiful day outside." Although still shallow and without risk, this conversation is more engaging and entails a higher level of communication. The medical student has the option of engaging you in level four or providing a short response that essentially says, "I don't want to talk to you" in which he chooses to stay at level five.

If a person enters into a level-three interaction (personal ideas or judgments), that individual begins to share personal ideas, opinions, or judgments. The information is usually guarded and closely monitored; in fact if the listener indicates disapproval, boredom, or confusion, the sender may become anxious or hesitate to continue. In level three, the participants take more risk and engage in self-disclosure to begin to build a relationship, which also requires some degree of trust and time to develop. A level-three exchange requires both parties to participate. If you begin expressing your views while the other person either remains silent or evades the issue, you may be in a level three while the other person is still at a level four. At this point you may want to end the conversation or move back up to level four. Level-three communications, for example, can occur between you and a fellow therapist when you are both willing to share personal views on controversial health-related issues, such as termination of life support.

If the relationship continues, you can enter into a level-two communication (feelings and emotions), in which more self-disclosure ensues and both parties begin to share the more personal and emotional aspects of their lives. The second level of communication is characterized by individuals who have spent a considerable amount of time together; shared their innermost thoughts, fears, joys and emotions; developed a solid foundation of trust; and enjoy true friendship.

The last and highest level of communication is level one (peak communication), which is limited to a select few and generally restricted to married partners, family

TABLE 6-1

Five Levels of Communication

Level	Type	Characteristics
Five	Cliché conversation	No genuine sharing; shallow; simple; superficial; explanation of shallow answers
Four	Fact reporting	Some sharing; neutral topics; no personal information; safe, nonconfrontational topics
Three	Personal ideas and judgments	Beginning of self-disclosure; some risk; guarded and closely monitored; usually reserved for co-workers and social friends
Two	Feelings and emotions	Used within atmosphere of trust and mutual respect; reserved for very close friends and family members
One	Peak communication	Highest level; intimate; reserved for select few (marriage partner, immediate family member, extremely close and intimate friend)

Data from Purtilo R. Health professional and patient interaction, 4th ed. Philadelphia: WB Saunders; 1990.

members, and intimate friends. This level of communication is characterized by significant sharing, **empathy,** and the mastery of a deep relationship.

Although the five levels of communication do not apply universally to all health care encounters, they have been addressed in the literature and have value in therapeutic relationships.[5] In any therapeutic relationship the respiratory therapist must go beyond levels four and five to establish a rapport, encourage the patient to "open up," and gain trust and cooperation. Attaining these levels can be especially tricky during the interview and physical assessment process because the therapist must maintain a professional demeanor but not be too distant or impersonal to impede the flow of valuable health-related information. Equally important is the therapist's need to avoid displaying any inappropriate emotion (level two). When faced with a hostile or emotionally-charged encounter, the therapist should stick to the facts and not succumb to useless name-calling or derisive discourse. Finally, development and maintenance of a good rapport among other members of the health care team can be invaluable in the creation of a congenial, productive, and satisfying work climate. The important point is to develop and maintain relationships built on honesty, trust, and respect.

Principles and Assumptions

Box 6-1 provides a comprehensive list of the underlying principles of communication.[6] These principles and the assumptions that follow are used to develop a working definition that to be used throughout the text.

Multidimensional Communication

Communication has a content dimension and a relationship dimension,[7] meaning that any encounter entails the words, language, and information (content dimension), as well as the perceived relationship of one communicant to another (relationship dimension), which involves attitudes, feelings, and emotions. For example, the therapist says to the patient, "Please take this treatment." Those words represent the content dimension and are fairly straightforward, whereas the relationship dimension refers to how the two "get along" or how they perceive their association. Is the relationship one of support, care, concern, compassion, and mutual respect? Or is it strained, distant, hierarchical, directive, contemptuous, or disrespectful?

Other authors[6,8,9] have alluded to this issue similarly by identifying communication as having a cognitive dimension (thoughts) and an affective dimension (emotions). Figure 6-1 represents a graphic view of this phenomenon in which the cognitive dimension (thoughts) is represented by the head and the affective dimension (feelings or emotions) by the heart. Both the relationship dimension and the affective dimension are critical for successful communication. An amicable relationships built on honesty and trust goes a long way in a patient adhering to suggested treatment regimens, a subordinate following directives, or peers cooperating and collaborating as a team.

Transactional Communication

To say the communication is **transactional** simply means that each party is both a sender and a receiver. A reciprocal relationship, a "give and take," exists in which each alternates between these two roles. When senders speak, they also receive messages from the listener; likewise, the listener does more than simply receive a message but also sends a message. This constant sending and receiving takes the form of feedback and can be done verbally or nonverbally, a transactional relationship is represented graphically in Figure 6-2.

$\mathcal{B}$OX 6-1

Principles of Communication

Each communication situation is unique.
The key to successful communication is feedback.
Face-to-face communication is most effective.
Distractions can garble the message.
The more people involved, the more complex communication becomes.
Every message contains both information and emotion.
Words are symbols used to express thoughts and are always open to interpretation.
Selective perception can distort the message.
People communicate according to their expectations of a situation.
If a person does not trust you, that person will not understand you.

Data from Dellinger S, Deane B. Communicating effectively: a complete guide for better managing. Radnor, Pa: Chilton Book; 1980.

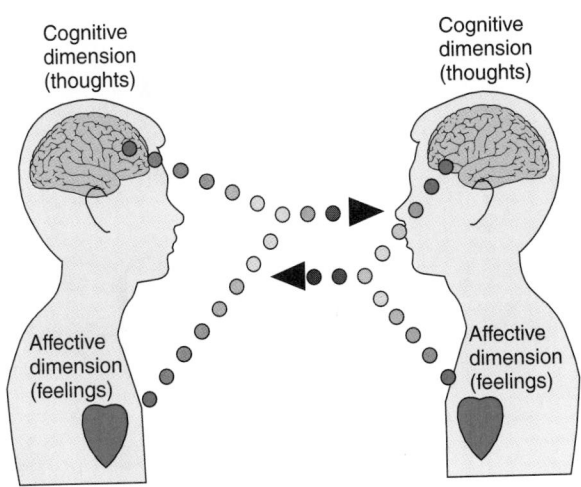

Figure 6-1   Cognitive and affective dimensions of communication. (Modified from Balzer-Riley JW. Communication in nursing. 4th ed. St Louis: Mosby; 2000.)

Process of Communication

Virtually every source used to research this topic explains communication as a process[7-13] that involves separate and distinct components that are essential for successful communication. One such reference expresses this process as consisting of seven components, which are graphically represented in Figure 6-3 and expressed in the following statement: "The *sender* transmits the *message*, which is *encoded* and sent through the *channel* for *decoding* by the *receiver* who then sends *feedback*."[13]

The sender, or source, is the person or group initiating the interaction. The sender can be a single individual serving as a manager and attempting to direct a depart-

ment; a patient educator communicating valuable advice or guidance to a patient or family member; a clinician or diagnostician attempting to collaborate with a physician, nurse, or fellow health care practitioner; or an institution or organization communicating its mission or philosophy. The message consists of the information, facts, data, ideas, thoughts, feelings, or attitude conveyed. It is the content to be communicated. The message is encoded in the form of words, symbols, actions, pictures, numbers, or gestures and transmitted through a **channel,** or **medium,** which can be verbal or nonverbal and involves the senses. Messages can be transmitted through sound (speaking and listening), sight (seeing), touch (feeling), smell, and taste. **Decoding** is similar to **encoding** and entails interpretation of the words, symbols, actions, pictures, numbers, or gestures back into the thought, feeling, or attitude.

The receiver is the recipient of the sender's message or the person or group for which the communication was intended. The receiver can be a student learning an important concept or principle; an employee receiving direction from a superior regarding workload; or a patient or family member receiving information, education, or training regarding treatment. **Feedback** is the final component in the process and occurs when the receiver and sender verify their perception of the message. The receiver encodes a return message either verbally or nonverbally through gestures.

A breakdown in the communication process can occur at a number of points along the path (see Figure 6-3). Any therapeutic message should adhere to the 5 C's of communication—complete, clear, concise, courteous, and cohesive.[14]

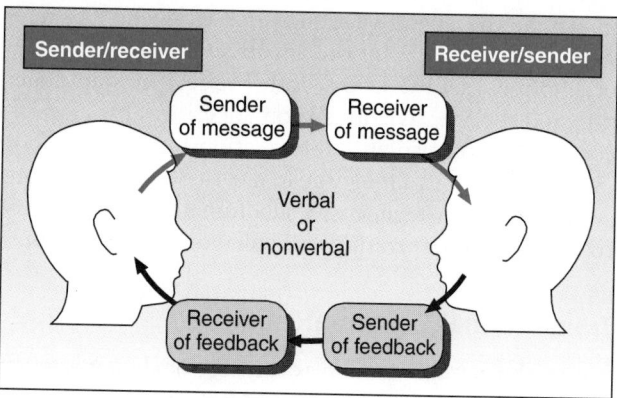

Figure 6-2   Transactional dimension of communication. (Modified from Schuster PM. Communication: the key to the therapeutic relationship. Philadelphia: FA Davis; 2000.)

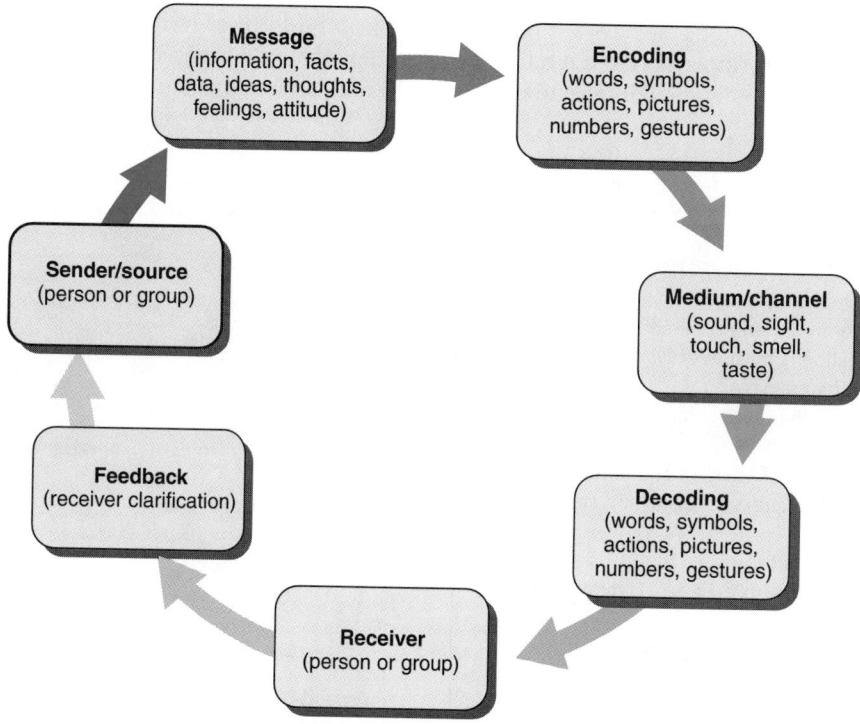

Figure 6-3   The communication process.

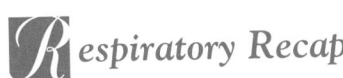

Respiratory Recap

Five C's of Communication
Complete
Clear
Concise
Courteous
Cohesive

With regard to the channel, the therapist must be aware of the extensive and increasing use of electronic media. Memos, letters, directives, bulletin boards, and other written formats are being replaced by voice mail, e-mail, and other electronic vehicles that offer real and significant advantages in speed and cost. When using such media, the wise therapist follows the KISS acronym (*keep it short and simple*). However, the most important point is to pick and choose the medium most appropriate for the circumstances and situation at hand. *Short* and *simple* do not apply to every type of interaction. Therapists must recognize the importance of face-to-face communication, in which verbal and **nonverbal communication** can help clarify meaning and nurture relationships.

Communication Defined

Communication has been defined as the sending and the receipt of a message[8] and in terms of encoding and decoding, in which information in the form of words, symbols, actions, pictures, numbers, and gestures are transformed into ideas and feelings.[2] Communication is clearly an interactive process[10] that uses a set of common rules.[7] It is continuous, dynamic, and transactional.[7] Communication can be written, verbal, or nonverbal and can even be therapeutic in that it may involve an exchange that culminates in a person's being helped to overcome stress, anxiety, fear, or other emotional experiences. Therapeutic communication also expresses support, provides information and feedback, corrects distortions, and restores hope.[9]

Although all these issues are important considerations in any understanding of the complexity of communication, any working definition must incorporate a common understanding between sender and receiver. With this view in mind, this text refers to effective communication as having a "shared meaning" between sender and receiver.[7] Posting a memo on the department bulletin board is not communication, nor is the common practice of e-mailing information to every person on the institution's mailing list. The obvious problem in both such cases is that the sender receives no assurance that the intended recipient actually read the memo or received the e-mail.

The classroom and the patient-teaching setting represent other situations in which communication problems can occur. Teachers often use written examinations and clinical competency assessments to ensure this "shared meaning," and patient education uses simple questioning techniques and return demonstration. Teachers often use a lecture or presentation to communicate a theory or principle to their students (or patients) and provide demonstration and observation in clinical situations to communicate the proper performance of a procedure. In reality, subject matter understanding and clinical competency mastery are ensured only through return demonstration. Students and patients must be able to convince the teacher of the existence of a shared meaning between the information that was taught and the knowledge that was learned. In summary, communication is not effective unless and until both the sender and the receiver share the same meaning.

Factors Affecting Communication

Why do managers complain about their subordinates not following through with directives, teachers are frustrated with their students' inability to recall information recently covered in class, or practitioners are disturbed with their patients' inability to perform a repeatedly-taught procedure? Why was a message sent not received? The answer is complex and tied to a multitude of factors.[8,11,12,15] The major categories of factors affecting communication are listed in Box 6-2 and illustrated in Figure 6-4.

Environmental Factors

Environmental factors can include physical surroundings (such as lighting, noise, temperature, and climate), a sense of formality, a lack of warmth, little privacy, unfamiliarity with the surroundings, feelings of urgency and stress, loss of personal freedom, excessive constraints, uncomfortable distance or spacing between people, overcrowding, and uncomfortable or obstructed seating arrangements.

When patients are treated in a hospital, clinic, or extended care facility, they are not in familiar surroundings. Intensive care units are busy, noisy, and crowded places, and the medical personnel working in them are absorbed in the urgency of their jobs and may uncon-

Box 6-2

Major Categories of Factors Affecting Communication

Environmental factors
Emotional/sensory factors
Verbal expressions
Nonverbal cues
Intrapersonal factors
Physical appearance and status

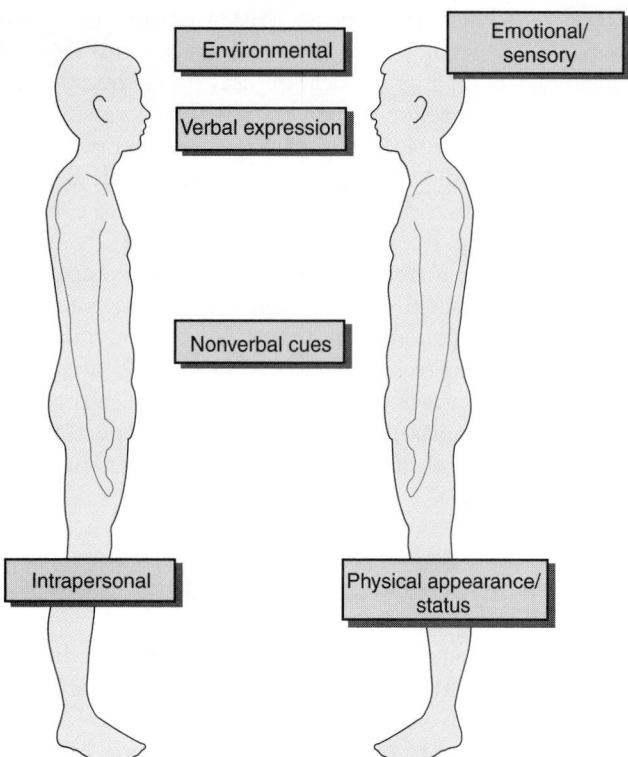

Figure 6-4 Factors influencing interpersonal communication. (Modified from Balzer-Riley JW. Communication in nursing. 4th ed. St Louis: Mosby; 2000.)

sciously be abrupt and impatient. Couple these facts with the formality of stark white lab jackets and a person could clearly feel a degree of "coolness" in the environment. The sense of urgency is exacerbated by the continuous sound of monitors and alarms and near-steady beams of bright fluorescent lights. Moving to a less critical area of the hospital is not likely to abate this feeling because hospital wards and clinics often feature lack of privacy, lack of freedom, and a significant degree of constraint.

ℛespiratory Recap

Environmental Factors Affecting Communication	
Lighting	Familiarity
Noise	Feelings of constraint
Temperature	Physical distance between
Climate	people
Formality	Mood
Warmth	Architecture
Privacy	Furniture arrangement

Privacy issues stem from cloth curtains that serve as the only barrier between the patient and visitors. History and physical assessments are performed and per-

sonal and intimate questions asked with merely a single drawn curtain separating the patient from others in the room. The meager size of the room does not allow for many personal possessions, and intravenous lines and electrocardiogram (ECG) leads limit patients' mobility and anchor them to the bed. In addition, space and distance can impede communication and threaten the comfort and openness of the conversation. Space and distance are particularly important because the therapist must avoid violations of **personal space** and the consequence of serious communications impairment. Personal space is considered within 1½ to 4 feet of an individual, and reactions to these boundaries vary according to the individual's culture and background. The four major space or distance zones are identified in Table 6-2 and illustrated in Figure 6-5.[5] A therapist who invades a patient's personal space should expect to see crossed legs, folded arms, little eye contact, and obvious movement from the sender. The offending therapist critically must discern the invasion of space and take appropriate measures to correct the situation, including moving slowly away, talking calmly, and exhibiting genuine concern, care, and compassion.

These environmental factors are not limited to just the patient. Students attempting to listen to lectures in overcrowded classrooms or engage in meaningful interaction during medical rounds are equally subject to communication problems. Distractions from their peers, uncomfortable seating, and obstructed views of the blackboard and audiovisuals all can impair reception of important information and impede effective communication.

Managers and supervisors attempting to interview new employees or conduct performance appraisals are also subject to environmental obstacles. The ringing of a telephone or the constant interruption of drop-in visitors seeking guidance and advice can wreak havoc on an interview session between a manager and a potential employee. The physical location and layout of administrative areas should be such that these obstacles and interruptions are minimized or prevented. Additionally, uncomfortable seating and the arrangement of furniture can serve as barriers between managers and subordinates and interfere with open and meaningful dialogue.

That environmental issues are significant in setting the stage for effective interaction should be apparent. Respiratory therapists and managers must be astute in identifying such factors and adept in correcting or optimizing them to enhance the relationships among subordinates, peers, and patients.

Emotional/Sensory Factors

A second major category affecting communication is emotional or sensory factors, which can consist of fear, stress, anxiety, pain, as well as limited or compromised mental acuity, sight, hearing, or speech. The health care environment involves considerable stress and anxiety, and patients, stu-

TABLE 6-2

Major Space/Distance Zones

Zone	Number of Feet	Characteristic Findings
Public space	12-25	Lecture halls or presentation areas; no physical contact; little eye contact
Social space	4-12	Typical business and work settings; more formal business and social occasions
Personal space	1½-4	Generally an arm's length; personal conversation with close friends; one-on-one patient education activities
Intimate space	within 1½	Limited to more intimate relationships in which health care measures or procedures are performed to comfort patient

Data from Purtilo R. Health professional and patient interaction. 4th ed. Philadelphia: WB Saunders; 1990.

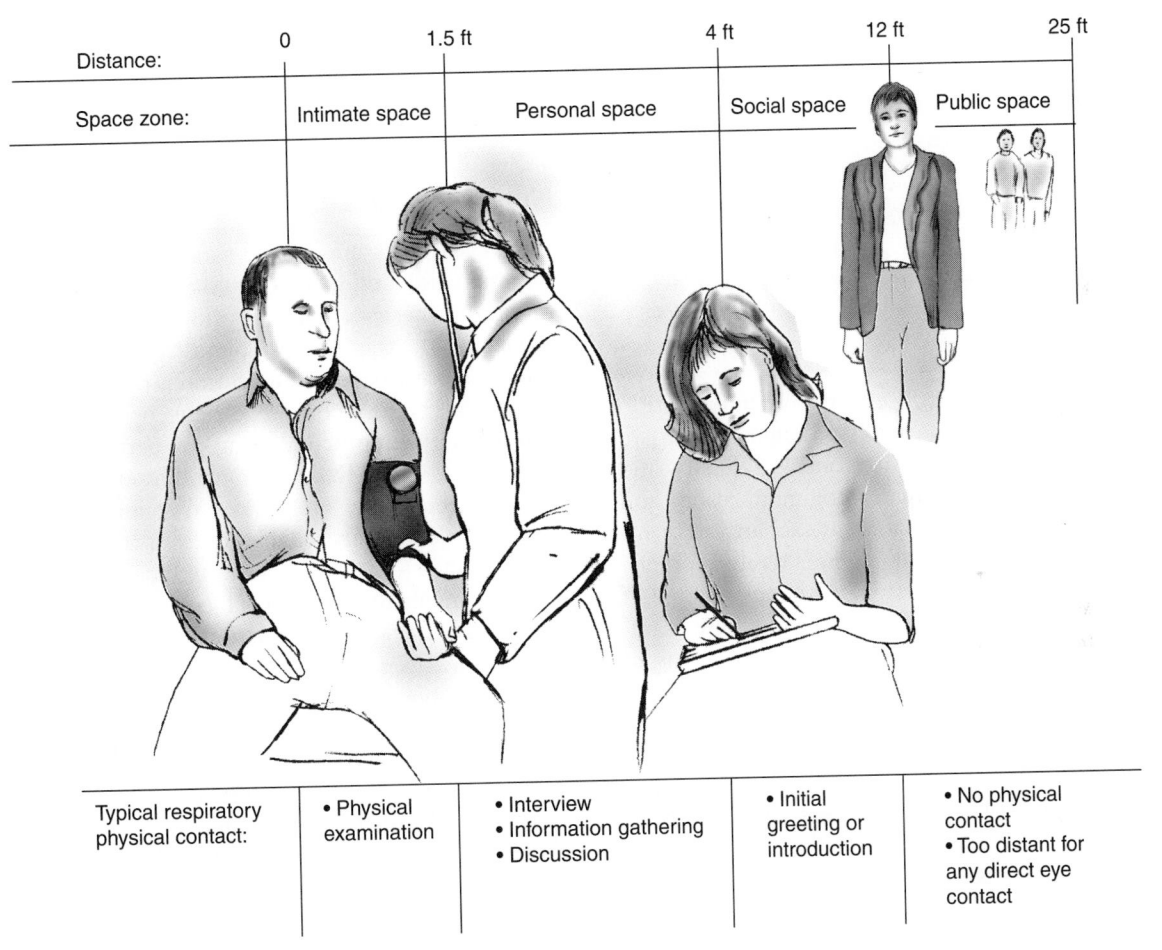

Figure 6-5   Social, personal, and intimate spaces of the patient requiring health care. (Modified from Wilkins RL, Krider SJ, Sheldon RL. Clinical assessment in respiratory care. 4th ed. St Louis: Mosby; 2000.)

dents, practitioners, and other health care providers can exhibit these emotions because of loss of control, frustration, low self-esteem, or feelings of inadequacy. Patients often demonstrate fear for their own well-being or that of their family members. A patient suspecting lung cancer may be so distraught with the thought of imminent death and the inability to care for loved ones that the ability to communicate can be significantly impaired.

The stress and tension of heavy treatment loads also can significantly affect the therapist's ability to effectively inter-

act with the patient. Wanting to do a good job and knowing that many others require treatment raises tensions, anxiety, and frustration in the mind of the conscientious therapist. Students are not immune to such feelings either and are under considerable pressure to satisfy classroom assignments and demonstrate clinical competency. In addition, pain can distract conversation. Significant degrees of physical pain and the numbing effects of medications may make communication less than optimal. Therapists attempting to instruct postoperative patients in the correct use of their incentive spirometer must be mindful and sensitive to incisional pain, which can interfere with the reception of instructions. Other patients may be seriously impaired or limited in hearing, speaking, or thinking. Respiratory therapists must be vigilant in recognizing these obstacles and prepared to adapt their behavior to ensure effective communication. Sensory communication issues, whether in patient care or the classroom, can be overcome when the sender uses multiple senses in sending messages. Multiple-sense learning may entail pictures (visual) and explanations with words (auditory). Box 6-3 represents the relative percent of remembering and learning from the use of various senses.

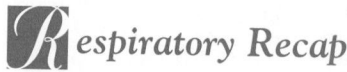

espiratory Recap

Sensory/Emotional Factors Affecting Communication	
Fear	Pain
Stress	Compromised mental acuity,
Anxiety	sight, hearing, or speech

Verbal Expressions

A third major category affecting effective communication is verbal expression, which involves language, jargon, choice of words or questions, voice tone and quality, and feedback. Language is the basis of communication, and words are the tools or symbols for the exchange. For instance, highly technical medical jargon is rarely appropriate for patient/therapist interaction. Although the use of medical jargon has the potential to increase patient confidence and credibility,[5] the loss of information and missed opportunity to build a rapport far outweigh such a suggestion. In addition to medical terms, such as *stat*, *prn*, and *NPO*, administrative terminology also must be explained. The student or young graduate may be unfamiliar with jargon, such as *FTE*, *HMO*, or *DRG*, because such issues are not always taught in school.

Additionally, verbal expression also entails the rate and volume of the spoken word. A depressed patient generally speaks slowly at a low pitch and tolerates longer periods of silence. Aggressive individuals generally speak loud and

rapidly, enunciate precisely, often interrupt, and may ridicule, tease, joke, and even insult.[2] Care must be exercised to avoid this latter style of communicating. Verbal expression also involves feedback, an important tool to ensure understanding and build rapport. For example, vague responses or squinting gestures with the eyes may indicates uncertainty, which the therapist must note and follow up with additional communication.

espiratory Recap

Verbal Expressions that Affect Communication	
Language	Voice tone and quality
Jargon	Feedback
Choice of words or questions	

Nonverbal Cues

Nonverbal cues are defined as a form of communication without words and includes messages created through body motion **(kinesics)**, the use and interpretation of space **(proxemics)**, the use of sounds **(paralinguistics)**, and touch.[7] Nonverbal communication is powerful but learned. Individuals are not born with these cues but develop them through modeling or imitating the actions or gestures of parents and peers. Recognizing and interpreting such messages can be tricky, but nonverbal communication is considered an extremely reliable index of the real meaning of what is being said or communicated[2] because a person generally is unable to exert as much conscious control over this aspect of behavior. Body positions or posture can send particular messages. An instructor at the front of the classroom with hands on the hips may be sending a nonverbal message—"Knock it off and pay attention!"—just as the hand under the chin represents thinking or mulling over.

Facial expressions are perhaps the most prominent nonverbal cue. Figure 6-6 is a graphic depiction of a variety of facial expressions and the corresponding emotion each

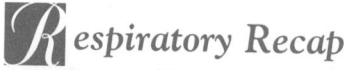

espiratory Recap

Nonverbal Cues that Affect Communication	
Body Motion (Kinesics)	**Sounds (Paralinguistics)**
Gestures	Giggling/laughing/
Position/posture	belittling
Facial expression	*Ah*'s and *um*'s
Eye movement	Knuckle cracking
Smile	Silence
Use and Interpretation	**Touch**
of Space (Proxemics)	Handshake
Distance zones (personal	Squeeze/sharp pinch
space)	Gentle touch

$\mathcal{B}$OX 6-3

Learning and Remembering

We Learn	We Remember
1% through taste	10% of what we read
1.5% through touch	20% of what we hear
3.5% through smell	30% of what we see
11% through hearing	50% of what we see and hear
83% through sight	80% of what we say
	90% of what we say and do

represents.[7] Masking or hiding one's true thoughts or feelings is difficult because facial expressions are thought to be a stronger representation of inner thoughts than are words. A smile is a universal sign of friendship and goes a long way to open the door to communication. Eye contact is another nonverbal cue, whether a wink, gaze, or movement of the eyebrow.

A patient who raises the head and eyebrows to the side when the therapist enters the room to administer a metered dose inhaler (MDI), may indicate discontent with the treatment. Words for such emotions may sound like: "Oh no, not another one of them!" An appropriate reaction by the therapist might be to engage the patient in a dialogue to accurately interpret the meaning of such gestures. The therapist must never create hostility or conflict but rather identify the reason for the sentiment, which may be as simple as the patient desiring to spend that particular moment with a visiting friend. Suggesting a return in 10 to 15 minutes may help win that patient's cooperation. Another finding regarding the eyes is that dilation conveys excitement or pleasure, whereas constriction generally reflects unpleasantness. In the United States, good eye contact is extremely important and considered to reflect a positive self concept.[2] In contrast to this finding, some Eastern cultures consider eye contact disrespectful.

Sound is another nonverbal cue—giggling, laughing, cracking knuckles, *ah*'s and *um*'s, or even silence. Although knuckle cracking can be irritating, silence or giggling when a person enters a room can create discomfort. Walking into a room and having a few colleagues instantaneously stop talking may make a person feel the colleagues are hiding something or talking behind their co-worker's back. Touching—a gentle squeeze, a firm handshake, or a sharp pinch—is another form of nonverbal expression. Slapping a person on the back is demeaning and insulting, except of course in sports in which such practice is common and considered a means to motivate or acknowledge a job well done. In medicine, touching must be done judiciously and when done appropriately can be an effective and powerful way to convey closeness, empathy, concern, care, trust, and comfort. Lightly touching the shoulder of a patient and saying, "I'm here to help you, Mrs. Jones" goes a long way in demonstrating care and compassion and enhancing the relationship. Nonverbal communication should never be taken lightly because it may be *the* thing that gets the obstinate patient to take a treatment or the staff member to stay and work that overtime shift. Being genuine and using nonverbal cues appropriately helps enhance the respiratory therapist's effectiveness; not only important is what the therapist says but also how the therapist says it.

Intrapersonal Factors

Intrapersonal factors are factors *within* the individual that affect communication. They make up the person's constitution and thus indirectly influence medical choices and decisions, but are not necessarily heard or seen. Although present in both the sender and the receiver, this discussion focuses primarily on these factors as they pertain to the patient. The specific intrapersonal factors are developmental stage, language mastery, previous experiences, attitudes, values, cultural heritage, religious beliefs, convictions, preoccupations, feelings, interest, and relative state of health.

Generally speaking, a person's developmental stage entails cognitive abilities and psychosocial development, for example the ability to think and comprehend, reading level, attention span, maturity, and independence. The developmental stage of the very young requires them to receive assistance from family members. The elderly also may need assistance because their mental acuity diminishes over time. However, 20% of American adults are illiterate and another 34% are functionally illiterate.[16] Couple this fact with the average reading level of the adult population in the United States, the eighth-grade level,[16] and whether patients understand what is being communicated at all seems questionable. Language mastery is another concern because many patients do not use English as their primary language, a cultural diversity issue that is becoming significant, with 1990 consensus data indicating that more than 21% of the U.S. population is minority. In addition, the belief system of these diverse groups can be considerably different. Western cultures are largely biomedical in health care beliefs, whereas Eastern cultures may adhere to magic, religion, or natural healing.[16] Eastern cultures are generally male dominated in hierarchy, have a strong family structure, and demonstrate considerable respect for their elderly. Communication between the therapist and such culturally diverse groups regarding terminating the ventilator of an elderly parent or a decision to use institutional care versus home care for an ailing family member is significantly affected by these values and beliefs. Interacting

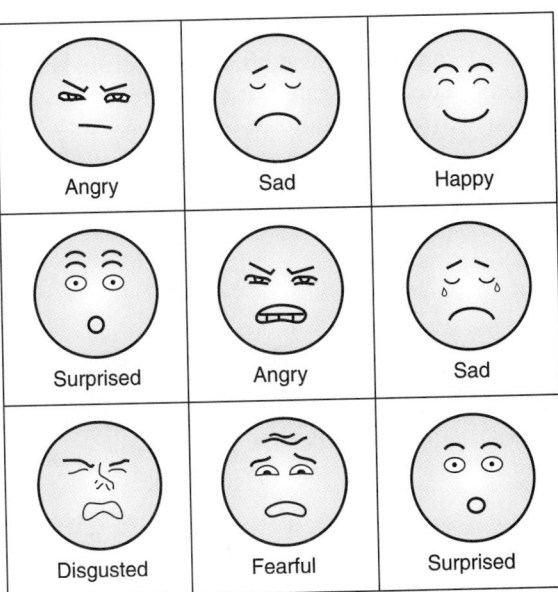

Figure 6-6 Common facial expressions and corresponding emotional meanings for each. (Modified from Harrison RP. Beyond words: an introduction to nonverbal communication. Englewood Cliffs, NJ: Prentice Hall; 1974. p. 120.)

with patients from different cultures can be challenging because eye contact, words such as *no* and *yes*, and touch can all have different meanings. Table 6-3 provides some guidelines to help therapists in cultural interactions.[16]

Additionally, a person's attitude regarding a previous unpleasant experience, such as a 5-hour wait in the hospital emergency room, could leave that person with a bad feeling and impair future communication. Other patients may simply be too physically ill to focus on any communication. Preoccupation with family matters or with the gravity of an illness also can wreak havoc on any communication encounter.

ℛespiratory Recap

Intrapersonal Factors Affecting Communication	
Developmental stage	Religious beliefs and
Language mastery	convictions
Previous experiences	Preoccupations
Attitudes/values	Feelings and interests
Cultural heritage	Relative state of health

Consider the following example. You (the therapist) enter the room of a 42-year-old man to teach him the proper use of his MDI. Minutes before, his attending physician gave him the bad news that his wife has cancer. What are the chances you can engage him in any meaningful patient education? The answer is obvious; the patient no doubt will be preoccupied with the dreadful news. Respiratory therapists must be mindful of both the magnitude and the impact that these interpersonal factors can have on communication.

Physical Appearance and Status

Physical appearance and status involve age, gender, race, body size and shape, body movements, posture, dress, hair, body adornments, body smell, role, position, organizational status and influence, and professionalism.

Communication should always be age-appropriate. In general the elderly require slower, more deliberate communication with written materials enlarged and presented in bold print. Children are usually strong auditory communicators but respond more favorably to less formal, more casual interactions; they are more comfortable with technology and thrive on media that entail pictures, games, and simulations. With regard to gender, many patients are shy and uncomfortable in dealing with members of the opposite sex. A considerable amount of sensitivity should be exercised whenever communication and interaction occurs across genders. Although blatantly inaccurate, many patients, especially the elderly, perceive that men are physicians and women are nurses.

With regard to body size and shape, many individuals perceive that large physical size conveys dominance, power, authority, and control. Posture and body movement also factor into communication because acting stern, distant, and holding the body rigid can send a message of being unapproachable. Posture and body movement also can convey openness and receptiveness, such as freely walking around the room, arm extension, or sitting back in a chair with the hands behind the head. Dress is an especially important point because people generally judge others based on attire. If a therapist were to enter a patient's room in soiled scrubs, old, oil-stained sneakers, and 2 or 3 days of facial hair growth, that therapist would not likely make a positive impression. On the other hand, if the therapist were attired in a shirt and tie and a heavily starched white lab jacket with the name embroidered over the front pocket, that therapist may well receive immediate attention and credibility. Fair or not, patients and other health care professionals do respond more favorably to a positive professional appearance. Therapists are advised to remain well groomed with minimal body adornments. Long nails, heavily-scented perfume, and large, ornate jewelry are not considered in good taste and or likely to set a professional tone.

𝒯ABLE 6-3

Guidelines to Facilitate Communication with Culturally Diverse Patients

Cultural Group	Guidelines
Asian Americans	Nonverbal communication important; no eye contact; no touching; possible hesitancy to verbalize feelings or ask questions
Chinese Americans	Shame and embarrassment commonly accompany inability to perform task; important to avoid touching the head
Japanese Americans	Important to avoid use of word *no* by asking open-ended questions; conflict avoidance common
Vietnamese Americans	*Yes* indicating respect but not always agreement; common avoidance of negative answers, which are considered disrespectful or confrontational; upward palm considered an insult
Native Americans	Important to avoid eye contact and pointing; possible answer of *yes* to please; sensitivity to nurses' note taking
African Americans	Possible language variations, with some words meaning opposite (for example, *bad* meaning *good*); use of great deal of nonverbal communication with verbal communication; eye contact usually acceptable
Hispanic Americans	Touch being dominant means of expression used more by women than men; smiling and hand-shaking part of established trust; self-disclosure difficult

Modified from Boyd M, Graham B, Gleit C, et al. Health teaching in nursing practice: a professional model. 3rd ed. Stamford, Conn: Appleton & Lange; 1998. p. 176.

Regarding role, position, and organizational status and influence, physicians and upper level health care administrators are considered to live at a higher socioeconomic level than the general population. This higher level or status can be problematic and intimidating to patients and subordinates, who may curtail or refrain from any purposeful communication. Both of these groups must be especially sensitive and make concerted efforts to remove this barrier. A related issue is the **white lab jacket phenomenon,** which essentially means that a white lab jacket generally creates an aura of instant credibility, acceptance, recognition, and stature that affords the wearer the opportunity to ask intimate questions and perform physical assessments. Departmental managers and supervisors also benefit from their elevated positions in the hierarchy of the institution, a situation fraught with advantages and disadvantages. For instance, some department members operate under a "we versus they" mentality in which they view the goals of the institution as inharmonious with their own. Within such a climate exists strained relationships and communication difficulties. Physical appearance and status have a significant bearing on communication.

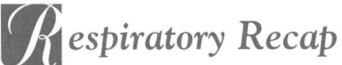espiratory Recap

Physical Appearance and Status Factors Affecting Communication	
Age, gender, and race	Body adornments
Body size and shape	Body smell
Body movements and posture	Role/position
Dress	Organizational status and influence
Hair	Professionalism

Barriers to Effective Communication

Box 6-4 is a general list of approaches and techniques that interfere with helpful communication between therapists and patients, family members, subordinates, and peers.[2] The choice of words should always be carefully considered. Abstract words, slang, and medical jargon create confusion and misunderstanding, and the separation of emotional feelings also is important. Anger, anxiety, and frustration are apparent in an individual's nonverbal communication and impair the interaction. Inappropriate facts, unrelated information, glib statements, and clichés such as, "you'll be OK" are irrelevant and may be annoying to the recipient. Being too opinionated, giving advice, and expressing unnecessary approval or undue disapproval can curtail the exchange, as can probing, requiring explanations, and belittling the person's feelings. Being defensive, interrupting the person, and interpreting behavior are also destructive tendencies. Efforts should always be directed toward relationship enhancement and satisfaction of the purpose of the communication.

Basic Goals and Purpose of Communication

Four Major Goals

In the definition of communication, the phrase *shared meaning* is highlighted and stressed. Although the transmission of a message from one person to another that is mutually understood is a vital function of the communication process, it does not stop there. The real purpose of mutual understanding is to influence the other to change.[8] The sender attempts to persuade the receiver to respond to the sender's request. Request from senders may be for (1) understanding, (2) action, (3) information, or (4) comfort.[8] Requests can be either direct or indirect. For example, you enter the room of a patient with documented asthma that physiologically requires an aerosolized bronchodilator.

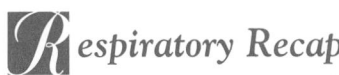espiratory Recap

Sender's Expectations from Receiver	
Understanding	Information
Action	Comfort

ℬOX 6-4
Barriers to Communication

Using the wrong words
Conveying feelings of anxiety, anger, strangeness, denial, isolation, lack of control, or lack of physical health
Failing to realize that the person's reluctance to make a message clear can prevent therapeutic communication
Making inappropriate use of facts, introducing unrelated information, offering premature explanation or counseling, choosing the wrong time, saying something important when the person is upset or not feeling well and thus unable to hear what is really said
Making glib statements or offering false reassurance
Using clichés, stereotyping responses, trite expressions, and empty verbalisms
Being too strongly opinionated
Expressing unnecessary approval
Expressing undue disapproval
Giving advice; stating personal experiences, opinions, or value judgments; giving pep talks; telling another what should be done
Asking probing, persistent, pointed, or "yes-no" questions
Requiring explanations, demanding proof, challenging or asking why
Belittling the person's feelings
Responding only literally
Interpreting the person's behavior or confronting that person
Interrupting or abruptly changing the subject
Defending or protecting someone or something

Data from Murray RB, Zentner JP. Nursing concepts for health promotion. 3rd ed. Englewood Cliffs, NJ: Prentice-Hall; 1985.

You observe him tachypneic and gasping for air, and he asks you, "When did I receive my last treatment?" His direct request is for *information* about when he had his last treatment. His indirect request is for *understanding and action*; he wants another treatment. You give him the treatment, and he is *comforted*.[8]

Conveying Believability

As noted previously the real goal in communication is to influence the other person to affect change,[8] perhaps most obvious when the respiratory therapist communicates with a physician to have an order changed or when a respiratory manager must convince his staff of the benefits of a new protocol or when the therapist must convince an asthmatic of the value of monitoring peak flows. Being able to speak convincingly and persuasively is a valuable skill because where there is no belief, there can be no action.[17] The question then becomes: How can a person convey believability in communication? The answer lies in the consistency or inconsistency of the message and more specifically with the harmony between the three V's—the verbal, vocal, and visual elements of the message.

According to Dr. Albert Mehrabian's landmark publications[18,19] on nonverbal communication, the verbal component represents a mere 7% of the communication, the vocal 38%, and the visual a hefty 55%. In other words, appearance and body language (visual) account for 55% of the way in which a message is interpreted, tone of voice (vocal) accounts for 38% of the message, and the actual spoken words (verbal) have the least importance, representing a meager 7%.[10] The implication is that 93% of the way communication is interpreted deals with the nonverbal, or the delivery of the message, whereas 7% deals with the content. Furthermore, Mehrabian's research indicates that when the message is inconsistent, the receiver is more inclined to believe the visual and vocal rather than the verbal.[17]

For example, if a therapist asks the physician to change an order from q2h to qid and in his nonverbal communication reflects uncertainty and quivering in his posture and gestures, hesitation, and an abundance of qualifiers (*ah*'s and *um*'s) in his voice, the physician may interpret these cues to mean that the therapist may not know what to do or at least that he is uncertain of his recommendation and thus may refuse to modify treatment. Although therapists undoubtedly must know the science of respira-

tory care, equally important is that they can communicate with conviction, confidence, and believability. Remember the old saying: Actions speak louder than words.

Effective Communication

From the concepts and definitions provided thus far, communication is obviously not a science. It is not governed by a strict set of scientific laws or theories. It is an art that entails skills that can be learned, developed, and with appropriate practice, mastered. Mastery of effective communication skills is a primary goal of this chapter. Box 6-5 provides some general methods for effective communication,[2] but specific communication skills related to both the sender and the receiver are identified and discussed in the following sections.

Skills of the Sender

To be an effective sender the therapist should be aware of six simple measures that can enhance this aspect of the communication. The acronym *SENDER* can help recall the six measures—(1) set the stage, (2) enunciate clearly, (3) notify the receiver of the importance, (4) demand feedback, (5) eliminate the unnecessary, and (6) receiver-orient the message.[6]

Setting the stage simply means that before commencing, the sender should decide what information is desired and

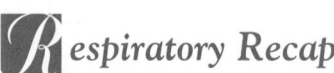spiratory Recap

Three V's of Communication
Verbal represents 7% of communication.
Vocal represents 38% of communication.
Visual represents 55% of communication.

ℬOX 6-5

Methods for Effective Therapeutic Communication

Use thoughtful silence to encourage the person to talk.
Be accepting.
Help the person strengthen self-identification in relation to others.
Suggest collaboration and a cooperative relationship.
Use open-ended, generalized, leading questions.
State related questions.
Place events in time sequence.
State perceptions about the person.
Encourage descriptions of behavior or observation.
Restate or repeat the main idea.
Reflect by paraphrasing feelings, questions, ideas, and key words.
Verbalize the implied.
Attempt to translate feelings into words.
Clarify.
Reintroduce reality.
Offer information.
Seek consensual validation.
Encourage the person's evaluation of the situation.
Encourage formulation of a plan of action.
Summarize.

Data from Murray RB, Zentner JP. Nursing concepts for health promotion. 3rd ed. Englewood Cliffs, NJ: Prentice-Hall; 1985.

decide on a time and an appropriate setting for the interaction. For example, if the occasion is a patient education session, the intention is to assess learning needs, provide instruction, and evaluate understanding and performance. The choice of time and setting should entail a time free of interruptions and distractions in a quiet, comfortable room furnished with appropriate resources (for example, blackboard, audiovisual aids, written materials). Such an environment may be the patient's room or a designated conference area. The same would hold true for a new employee interview, a staff performance appraisal, or a student clinical competency assessment.

Respiratory Recap

Skills of the Sender

Set the stage.
Enunciate clearly.
Notify the receiver of the importance of the message.
Demand feedback.
Eliminate the unnecessary.
Receiver-orient the message.

The second measure is to enunciate clearly. Frequently the therapist is under considerable pressure and has limited time at the patient's bedside. Avoiding fast-talk and garbled, inaudible, or inarticulate speech is particularly important. This issue is especially problematic for the elderly, who may need the added time to absorb and process the information. Equally important is that the therapist not speak too softly and try to energize the delivery.

A third measure is to notify the receiver of the importance of the communication. For example, before a patient education session the wise therapist would inform the patient of the imminent hospital discharge and stress that the patient must self-administer the MDI thereafter. This statement is a strong motivating factor for the patient to learn the procedure, and the therapist is more likely to gain that patient's attention and cooperation. Additionally, the therapist may indicate the length of the exchange and keep the patient informed about the time throughout the process. Finally, a summary of the key points of the exchange may help highlight important considerations.

Soliciting feedback also facilitates communication. Again with the patient education session example, the therapist may open the dialogue with a general statement inviting the patient to stop the instruction at any point with a question or concern. Periodic queries about whether the patient understands can help. Requiring a return demonstration from patients is an extremely effective way to obtain assurance of mastery and secure feedback.

The fifth measure is to eliminate the unnecessary. Research has found that most people use 30% more words than necessary.[6] The therapist should be as clear and concise as possible and when in doubt, say it and wait for feedback. Further information can always be provided as needed. The previously discussed acronym KISS is appropriate—Keep It Short and Simple.

Finally, the speaker should orient the message for the receiver. The sender's focus should not be *me* but *we*. This focus helps instill an attitude of collaboration rather than one of superiority and authority. Whenever possible, information should be *shared* rather than *told*.

Skills of the Receiver

At one time or another every person has walked away from a conversation only to say, "I have no idea what was just said." The volume and tone of the sender were more than adequate, so the message was heard. The problem was not hearing, but listening. Hearing is a physical act that acknowledges sound, whereas listening is an intellectual and emotional act that includes understanding and requires active involvement. With this information in mind, the following section addresses the five skills of the active listener—(1) listen to the content, (2) listen to the intent, (3) assess the sender's nonverbal communication, (4) monitor nonverbal communication and **emotional filters,** and (5) listen without judgment and with empathy.[20]

Respiratory Recap

Skills of the Receiver

Listen to the content.
Listen to the intent.
Assess the sender's nonverbal communication.
Monitor personal nonverbal communication and emotional filters.
Listen without judgment and with empathy.

Listening to the content means giving full attention to the speaker. A listener should eliminate internal and external distractions and if needed be prepared to take notes and physically move closer to the sender. A listener should not prepare responses while the sender is communicating but stop talking and simply listen.

Listening to the intent is a challenging skill. It means attempting to hear the whole message, not just what is implied. The intent includes the content, the nonverbal cues, the sender's background and biases, and any other factors that affect the issue at hand. For example, a patient says, "I'm not taking my treatment today because my brother told me not to. I started to shake last night when he was here, and he said that it could be due to the medication." The therapist in this case must not prematurely turn off the conversation. A busy and harried therapist may hear only the first part of the communication and prematurely pass judgment that the patient is trying to stop treatment. Listening to the intent means listening to *why* the patient says something rather than just *what* is being said. The listener may need to paraphrase or seek clarification to the sender's intention but should not use emotions to interpret the intent.

The third skill is the ability to assess the sender's nonverbal communication, which involves body language and tone of voice and represents more than 90% of the message. Nonverbal elements also represent the *how* rather than the *what*, and are considered a true reflection of the sender's innermost thoughts. When incongruity exists between what is seen and heard (the nonverbal) versus what is reflected in the verbal, the nonverbal is almost always the correct interpretation. Astute therapists note such inconsistency and seek clarification. For example, a respiratory manager asks for a volunteer to work an overtime shift, and a staff member responds, "Sure, I'll do it." The nonverbal interpretation is the more critical component of the message because the staff member may be genuine or may raise the eyes and head (a visual indicator of sarcasm) and emphasize the word *sure* (a vocal inflection signifying, "no way!").

Skillful listeners monitor their own nonverbal cues and control their emotional filters, meaning simply that just as the sender sends nonverbal messages, so does the receiver. The receiver's messages may be supportive and encouraging, such as, "Yea, I follow you; go on" or just the opposite, such as, "Yea, right (*sarcasm*); no way that could be true." Nonverbal signs of disapproval or rejection should not be used to discourage communication; the listener must maintain neutrality so as to hear the whole message. With emotional filters, both the sender and the receiver have a particular **mindset** developed over years, consisting of personal biases, experiences, and expectations. Each person has these deep-seated feelings and beliefs and should control them. A mindset may sound like this: "Nursing is a feminine job, and homosexuals are effeminate males; therefore a male nurse is a homosexual." Although this statement is obviously ridiculous, it does reflect the fact that a person's mindset stems from the particular culture in which that individual was raised. The listener should check emotional filters and not allow them to interfere with listening to the whole message.

Empathetic listening simply means the return of feedback that reflects care about the receiver and the importance of that individual's message. Being nonjudgmental means being open-minded and not entering a situation with mind already decided. In essence, the listener reflects on the whole message and at the same time says, "I am here for you."

Bridges to the Relationship

The respiratory therapist must understand the importance of exhibiting qualities and characteristics compatible with effective therapeutic relationships. Six qualities or characteristics are considered essential to nurture the relationship: care, empowerment, trust, empathy, mutuality, and confidentiality.[21]

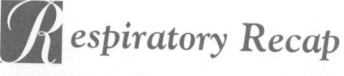

Respiratory Recap

Qualities or Characteristics of a Nurturing Relationship	
Care	Empathy
Empowerment	Mutuality
Trust	Confidentiality

Caring is an intentional human action characterized by commitment and a sufficient level of knowledge and skill to allow the therapist to support the needs of the patient.[22] It entails offering a presence, attending, affiliating, and empowering.[23] **Empowerment** involves the provision of the proper tools, resources, and environment to build, develop, and increase the ability and effectiveness of others to set and reach goals for individual and social ends.[24] Trust is present when individuals feel that they can rely on others. Building trust requires that communication is descriptive rather than evaluative, problem oriented rather than control oriented, spontaneous rather than strategic, empathetic rather than neutral, equal rather than superior, and provisional rather than certain.[7] Empathy describes individuals mutually imagining themselves in the shoes of others and then verbally conveying that understanding.[8] **Mutuality** simply means that the therapist and patient agree on the health problems and the means to resolve them.[21] Finally, **confidentiality** involves an assurance on the part of both parties that the other will not divulge private information. The sole purpose of confidentiality is to protect the patient from unauthorized disclosures. All six qualities are essential ingredients for any successful therapist/patient interaction, and their value in the nurturing of a relationship is best represented by the following saying: Patients don't care how much you know, until they know how much you care.

Questioning Techniques

Questioning techniques in respiratory care can be used between the therapist and superiors, subordinates, professional colleagues, peers, or patients during physical assessments, patient interviews, employee appraisals, student clinical assessments, or progressive discipline sessions, to name a few instances. Regardless of the purpose or motive, questioning techniques are a powerful way to obtain information, clarify uncertainties, facilitate learning, and resolve conflicts. Some of the more important questioning strategies and techniques used by the respiratory therapist include closed-ended questions, open-ended questions, clarification, leading questions, compound questions, facilitation, confrontation, silence, and support or reassurance.[2,7,9,25]

Closed-ended questions help obtain specific information, yield a limited number of possible answers, and generally can be answered with a simple *yes* or *no*. Although they are valuable in certain focused questioning sessions, they have limited value during the initial patient interview or assessment. Examples include "Have you ever had TB?" or "How many puffs of your inhaler do you use every day?"

ℛespiratory Recap

Questioning Strategies and Techniques	
Closed-ended questions	Facilitation
Open-ended questions	Confrontation
Clarification	Silence
Leading questions	Support and reassurance
Compound questions	

Open-ended questions are considered the most valuable form of questioning during the initial patient assessment. They yield the broadest amount of information and allow for more freedom of response. They generally involve short probes followed by periods of silence in which the interviewee is permitted more in-depth and personal responses. They almost always begin with the words *what, why,* or *how.* Examples include "What brings you to the hospital?" or "Tell me about your SOB."

A clarifying question attempts to correct ambiguity and clear up the meaning of confusing responses. Patients may be asked to elaborate on an ambiguous or uncertain issue. Examples include "What do you mean by the statement that you have a cold?" or "What exactly do you mean by SOB?"

Leading questions are those phrased so that a predetermined or expected response is inevitable. Such questions reflect the bias of the interviewer and should not be asked because they can produce useless, unreliable, or inaccurate responses. Examples include "You've never smoked, have you?" or "You're feeling better today, aren't you?"

Compound questions ask more than one question at a time and do not allow adequate time for each answer. They are confusing and generally result in a response to the last part of the question only. Examples include "Tell me about yourself. How old are you? Are you married? What do you do for a living?" or "Have you ever had, TB, HIV, asbestos exposure, used drugs, or smoked cigarettes?" The interviewee is likely to answer the very last part of the question, which garners the interviewer little information about the other issues.

Facilitation is actually a technique whereby words, postures, or actions encourage more detail. Facilitation is a skill that must be performed with sincerity and genuineness, with examples including "Please go on. . ." or "uh huh." Nonverbal actions that display sincerity, genuine interest, and attentiveness can include sitting forward or touching the patient.

Confrontation can be very tricky because the therapist, for example, would not want to close off communication and yet needs to be honest and bring a patient's behavior or emotional state to that individual's conscious awareness. Examples include "You said your breathing was fine, yet I noticed your rate was quite high and your breathing is labored." or "You said you are not angry, yet I observed you raising your voice and clinching your fist."

Silence allows time for reflection and is an effective way for the patient to organize thoughts and feelings. Although silence takes many forms,[2] the interviewer must learn to deal with the difficulty of prolonged periods of utter stillness. Significant delays in speech are naturally difficult between two people. Because health care is an area foreign and mysterious to the patient, that person may simply need time to process and think through the information.

Finally, support and reassurance are valuable techniques in questioning. When the therapist expresses sensitivity and sincere understanding regarding the patient's reactions, that is demonstrating support. The most important aspect of this technique is to be genuine and sincere. Even with sincerity and genuineness, the therapist is still likely to receive a curt rebuttal stating, "You have no idea what I am going through." As difficult as this response may be, a continued display of warmth, hope, dignity, empathy, and reassurance is recommended. The hope should not be false hope but should be directed at having the patient come to some degree of acceptance and peace of mind. Feelings of sympathy are feelings of sorrow *for* someone, whereas empathy describes feelings of sorrow *with* a person, meaning that the empathizer too has had similar experiences.

Examples Used in Respiratory Care

Patient Interview   You are a respiratory therapist (RT) working in a pulmonary rehabilitation department and have been asked to provide support and assistance to Mr. Saunders, a 59-year-old white man referred to you by his physician for pulmonary rehabilitation. He was recently diagnosed with chronic obstructive pulmonary disease (COPD). Your initial interview[25] with him follows:

RT: Hello, Mr. Saunders. My name is John Doe. I am a respiratory therapist and am working with your lung doctor, Dr. Smith. Before performing a physical exam, I'd like to ask you a few questions.
Patient: [nods and acknowledges the introductory remarks]

Question Session #1

RT: I have your records and know some of your medical history. However, could you tell me in your own words why you are here?
Patient: Sometimes I have a lot of trouble breathing.

Question Session #2

RT: Trouble breathing?
Patient: Yes. When I walk up the steps to the bathroom, I can't seem to catch my breath. It scares me.

Question Session #3

RT: You seem worried about this?
Patient: Well, yes. My dad died from lung disease, and he was only 61. [starts to cry]

Question Session #4

RT: [hands box of tissues to patient]

Question Session #5

Patient: Thanks. My dad was a great guy, and I think of him all the time.
RT: I'm sorry to hear of your loss. I lost my dad 4 years ago. Although relationships between people can sometimes be different, I *think* I can understand how you must feel. This must have been a very difficult moment for you.

Question Session #6

Patient: Ever since my dad died, I've taken care of my mom and frankly I'm worried about her as well. I don't want her to worry about my illness.
RT: How do you feel about your illness?

Question Session #7

Patient: I am scared to death. I don't know much about my disease and whether I will be able to take care of both of us.
RT: I'm glad you were able to tell me this. It is natural for you to feel this way.
I am here to help you. I will teach you how best to cope with your COPD.

Question Session #8

Patient: Thanks. I am glad I came.
RT: Can you tell me a little more about your COPD? Does your shortness of breath occur when you go up flights of steps or just a few steps?

Question Session #9

Patient: Flights of steps
RT: Can you tell me approximately how many steps?

Question Session #10

Patient: Approximately 12
RT: I noted in your records that you produce about a cup of sputum every day. Can you tell me whether it is thick and discolored? Explain it in your own words.
Discussion   The questioning techniques used in the previous scenario are as follows:

Question Session #	Question Technique, Strategy, and Discussion
1	Open-ended questioning: This is a very appropriate use of the open-ended questioning technique, allowing the patient to express his own feelings in his own words.
2	Facilitation: By repeating the patient's statement, the therapist helps the patient better express his condition.
3	Confrontation: The therapist picks up on an emotional feeling and confronts the patient in a non-threatening manner.
4	Silence: The therapist allows the patient to regain exposure and sympathetically addresses his emotional need.
5	Support: The therapist genuinely expresses both sympathy and empathy. The relationship appears to strengthen through this interaction.
6	Open-ended question: The therapist continues to focus on the emotional needs of the family and bring out the patient's feelings about his condition.
7	Support and reassurance: The therapist strengthens the bond by approving the openness of the relationship and provides hope, indicating that specific intervention is available to address the condition.
8	Closed-ended question: The therapist tries to obtain some specific information regarding how far the patient can move before the onset of his shortness of breath.
9	Clarifying question: The therapist asks the patient to clarify his ambiguous response.
10	Elaboration: The therapist picked up on statements in the patient's record and asked him to provide more detail.

New Hire   You are the director of the respiratory care department for a 400-bed tertiary care facility. You have an 8 AM interview with a new graduate from the local community college program for a full-time staff position on your 3 to 11 PM shift. Your candidate, Mary Jones, arrives promptly, and you greet her in the human resources conference room. Your employment interview with her follows:

Question Session #1

Director: Hello and welcome to University Hospital. Should I call you Ms. Jones, or would you prefer something else?
Candidate: Mary would be just fine. [appears nervous]

Question Session #2

Director: Well, welcome Mary. My name is Jeff Johnson, and you can call me Jeff. [pleasant smile] I am the director of respiratory care services, and I will be doing the initial interview with you this morning.
Candidate: [nods and smiles but still appears nervous]

Question Session #3

Director: I see that you are a graduate of the respiratory care program at Gwynedd Mercy College. We've had a number of their graduates and have been very pleased with their performance. It's a very good program.
Candidate: Yes, I graduated just this past month. I'm glad you have been pleased.

Question Session #4

Director: Mary, tell me a little about yourself.
Candidate: Well, as you know I graduated from Gwynedd Mercy this past May. I am single, live at home with my parents, did well in school, and am a hard worker.

Question Session #5

Director: Why would you like to work at University Hospital?
Candidate: University is only 4 miles from my home, and I've heard very good things about the hospital.

Question Session #6

Director: What have you heard?
Candidate: Well, I grew up in the area, and my family came here whenever we needed to be hospitalized. But more importantly, I know it is a large teaching hospital and that you have an active open-heart surgery program and a wide array of cardiorespiratory services.

Question Session #7

Director: Open-heart program? *[followed by pause]*
Candidate: I have an interest in working in critical care medicine. I enjoy this kind of environment and believe it will help me with my registry. I want to go as far as I can in the profession.

Question Session #8

Director: You are a member of the AARC, aren't you? *[voice inflection at end]*
Candidate: Well, yes. *[a slight hesitancy in voice]* I ah, I ah, *[stammering a bit]* think it's very important for one to be involved in their profession. I joined as a student and have every intention of maintaining membership. *[genuine and sincere tone of voice]*

Question Session #9

Director: I'm glad to hear you feel that way. *[more mild and affirming tone of voice]* You said you want to work in critical care medicine. Have you worked with Servos, Bears, and 7200s?
Candidate: Yes, I worked with the 7200 all through my clinical rotations.

Question Session #10

Director: I'm sorry. I confused you. What about *[waits for response]* the Servo *[again, waits for response]*
Candidate: Yes, I did work with the Servo while rotating through my clinicals. We also were exposed to the Servo in the laboratory.

Question Session #11

Director: Is there anything else you would like to share with me?
Candidate: I would really like to work at University. It is close to my home, and I could be available for call-outs. I feel I could fit in well with the staff. I believe my program prepared me for this kind of opportunity. And I want to provide quality patient care. I really care about my patients and will make a commitment to the institution.

Discussion   The questioning techniques used in the previous scenario are as follows:

Question Session #	Question Technique, Strategy, and Discussion
1	Closed-ended questioning/clarification: The director poses a focused question that allows only a limited response, setting the stage for the candidate to determine the degree of formality.
2	Support/clarification: The director recognizes the candidate's nervousness and tries to build rapport while clarifying the purpose of the meeting.
3	Reassurance: The director continues to use the first 2 to 3 minutes to build rapport and provide reassurance, attempting to decrease the candidate's anxiety so that she will be more comfortable and "open up" to express her true self. *[appears to be successful]*
4	Open-ended question: The director allows the candidate considerable freedom to provide information she feels is important.
5	Open-ended questioning: Once again the director tries to get the candidate to express herself to identify her motivation for wanting to work at University Hospital.
6	Clarification: The director probes to see what specifically she means by the statement, her depth of understanding.
7	Facilitation/silence: The director seeks elaboration on what this candidate sees as an "open-heart program." His comment is followed by a pause and silence, which the candidate immediately fills with elaboration.
8	Leading question: Although the director tries to identify this candidate's degree of commitment to the profession, this question is not effective. Her qualifying statement substantiates her claim in a convincing way. However, had she stopped after the word *yes,* the director would have doubts. More importantly, he makes the candidate feel defensive and runs the risk of not getting to really know her.
9	Compound question: This question is not well structured because the candidate answered only the last part, a common response to such questions. An open-ended question, such as "Which ventilators have you worked with?" would be better.
10	Clarification/closed-ended question: Recognizing his error and the confusion created, the director repeats his questions one at a time. He receives the feedback he was originally seeking.
11	Open-ended question: The director demonstrates an excellent use open-ended questioning, effectively allowing his candidate to "open up" and share her innermost feelings.

KEY POINTS

- Miscommunication can include misinterpretation of the message, incomplete messages, inappropriate use of medical terminology/expressions, and cultural influences in language.
- Communication involves accepted social customs and amenities, as well as more formal dialogue.
- Communication has a content dimension (language and information) and a relationship dimension (perceived relationship between communicants).
- Communication has a cognitive dimension (thoughts) and an affective dimension (feelings and emotions).
- Communication involves a reciprocal transaction in which each communicant alternates between the roles of sender and receiver.
- Communication is simply defined as a "shared meaning."
- Environmental factors, emotional/sensory factors, verbal expressions, nonverbal cues, internal/interpersonal factors, and physical appearance and status all affect communication.
- The degree of believability of the message is a result of congruence among the verbal, vocal, and visual components of the message.
- The vocal and visual components make up 93% of the communication.
- Effectiveness in any communication requires sending skills and receiving skills.
- Care, empowerment, trust, empathy, mutuality, and confidence are important ingredients to nurture any relationship.
- Effective questioning strategies and techniques include the appropriate use of open-ended questions, closed-ended questions, clarification, facilitation, confrontation, silence, support, and reassurance.

References

1. Cullen DL, Sullivan JM, Bartel RE, et al. Delineating the educational direction for the future respiratory care practitioner. Proceedings of a National Consensus Conference on Respiratory Care Education. Dallas: American Association for Respiratory Care; 1992.
2. Murray RB, Zentner JP. Nursing concepts for health promotion. 3rd ed. Englewood Cliffs, NJ: Prentice-Hall; 1985.
3. Haimann T. Supervisory management for health care organizations. 3rd ed. St Louis: The Catholic Health Association of the United States; 1984.
4. Powell JSJ. Why am I afraid to tell you who I am? Chicago: Argus Communications; 1969.
5. Purtilo R. Health professional and patient interaction. 4th ed. Philadelphia: WB Saunders; 1990.
6. Dellinger S, Deane B. Communicating effectively: a complete guide for better managing. Radnor, Pa: Chilton Book; 1980.
7. Northouse LL, Northouse PG. Health communication: strategies for health professionals. 3rd ed. Stamford, Conn: Appleton & Lange; 1998.
8. Balzer-Riley JW. Communication in nursing. 4th ed. St Louis: Mosby; 2000.
9. Van Servellen G. Communication skills for the health care professional: concepts and techniques. Gaithersburg, Md: Aspen; 1997.
10. Schuster PM. Communication: the key to the therapeutic relationship. Philadelphia: FA Davis; 2000.
11. Scanlon CL, Wilkins RL, Stoller JK. Egan's fundamentals of respiratory care. St Louis: Mosby; 1999.
12. Burton GG, Hodgkin JE, Ward JJ. Respiratory care: a guide to clinical practice. Philadelphia: Lippincott Williams & Wilkins; 1997.
13. Fink JB, Fink AK. The respiratory therapist as manager. Chicago: Year Book; 1986.
14. Wilkes M, Crosswait CB. Professional development: the dynamics of success. Orlando, Fla: Harcourt Brace Javanovich; 1991.
15. Wilkins RL, Krider SJ, Sheldon RL. Clinical assessment in respiratory care. 4th ed. St Louis: Mosby; 2000.
16. Boyd M, Graham B, Gleit C, et al. Health teaching in nursing practice: a professional model. 3rd ed. Stamford, Conn: Appleton & Lange; 1998.
17. Decker B. The art of communicating: achieving interpersonal impact in business. Los Altos, Calif: Crisp Publications; 1988.
18. Mehrabian A, Williams M. Nonverbal communication of perceived and intended persuasiveness. J Pers Social Psych 1969;13:37.
19. Mehrabian A. Silent messages. Belmont, Calif: Wadsworth; 1971.
20. Dugger J. Listen up: hear what's really being said. West Des Moines, Iowa: American Media Publishing; 1995.
21. Arnold E, Boggs K. Interpersonal relationships: professional communication skills for nurses. 2nd ed. Philadelphia: WB Saunders; 1995.
22. Clarke J. A view of the phenomenon of caring in nursing practice. J Adv Nurs 1992;17:1283-1290.
23. Clayton G. Connecting: a catalyst for caring. In: Chin P, editor. Anthology of caring. New York: NLN Press; 1991.
24. Hawks J. Empowerment in nursing education: concept analysis and application to philosophy, learning and instruction. J Adv Nurs 1992;17:609-618.
25. Ballweg R, Stolberg S, Sullivan EM. Physician assistant: a guide to clinical practice. Philadelphia: WB Saunders; 1994.

Recommended Reading

Axtell RE. Gestures: the do's and taboos of body language around the world. New York: John Wiley & Sons; 1998.

Bone D. The business of listening: a practical guide to effective listening. Los Altos, Calif: Crisp Publications; 1988.

Mehrabian A. Nonverbal communication. Chicago: Aldine-Atherton; 1972.

Mindell P. A woman's guide to the language of success: communicating with confidence and power. Englewood Cliffs, NJ: Prentice Hall; 1995.

Tamparo CD, Lindh WQ. Therapeutic communications for allied health professions. Albany, NY: Delmar; 1992.

CHAPTER 7

Decision Making and the Role of the Consultant

Shelley C. Mishoe

CHAPTER OUTLINE

OBJECTIVES

1. Describe the evolving role of respiratory therapists as decision makers and consultants.
2. Describe clinical practice guidelines, respiratory care protocols, and critical pathways and discuss the design, implementation, and evaluation of each.
3. Discuss the advantages and limitations of guidelines, protocols, and pathways.
4. Describe outcomes evaluation, the types of outcomes, and why their evaluation is necessary to assess the effectiveness of respiratory care.
5. Define variance and the ways used to track and assess different types.
6. Describe evidence-based medicine and its relation to respiratory care.
7. Describe internal consulting and its ability to improve organizational effectiveness.
8. Elaborate on the roles and skills of internal consultants within health care organizations.
9. Make the case that respiratory therapists can function as technical consultants and process consultants using guidelines, protocols, pathways, and evidence-based medicine to improve the effectiveness of respiratory care.

KEY TERMS

Algorithm	Evidence-Based Medicine (EBM)	Respiratory Care Protocol
Benchmarking	Managed Care	Therapist-Driven Protocol (TDP)
Clinical Practice Guideline (CPG)	Multidisciplinary	Variance Tracking
Critical Pathway (CP)	Outcomes Evaluation	

The primary purpose of this chapter is to elaborate on the emerging role of respiratory therapists as decision makers and consultants who can contribute to improved patient care through the effective use of clinical practice guidelines, respiratory care protocols, and critical pathways. This discussion presents possibilities and strategies for res-

piratory care professionals to understand, develop, use, and evaluate clinical practice guidelines, pathways, and protocols. The ultimate goal is that understanding and implementation of protocols, guidelines, and pathways will continue to improve the therapeutic value and cost effectiveness of respiratory care.

The discussion begins with the role of internal consultants, including the benefits, required skills, and ethical considerations, and makes the case for respiratory therapists as consultants, with documentation of successful use of protocols to improve the allocation and effectiveness of respiratory care. Respiratory therapists can play an important role in health care through continued contributions to effective practice, and through work with physicians and other health care professionals to make appropriate health care decisions.

Evolving Role of Respiratory Therapists as Decision Makers and Consultants

The drive to provide health care with greater access and less cost has precipitated many changes in health care delivery. Prospective-payment programs have changed the way providers plan, manage, and think about health care, in turn changing the roles, skills, and traits expected from all health care professionals. Practitioners of every discipline are learning ways to cope with **managed care** systems. Consequently, an unprecedented need exists to facilitate, support, and enhance the role of respiratory therapists as decision makers and consultants.[1]

No longer considered sufficient are health care personnel who know only discrete pockets of knowledge or who have specific clinical skills. The need for health care practitioners who have professional competence exceeding technical training or clinical skills is increasing. The pressures to change old models, paradigms, and traditions of practice are not unique to respiratory care or allied health but are experienced across health care professions, including nursing and medicine.

Employers, educators, and patients would probably agree that respiratory therapists must have not only medical knowledge and technical skills but also professional competencies and characteristics. Technical knowledge alone does not equal professional competence. Historically, respiratory care practitioners used technical knowledge as inhalation therapists in the 1940s, providing treatments requiring special equipment, such as oxygen tanks, aerosol generators, and positive pressure ventilators. The obvious advantages to these practitioners included equipment expertise and technical skills, and the therapists were vital to nurses, a role which defined most respiratory care departments early on as functional parts of nursing departments.

Eventually, separate and distinct respiratory therapy departments developed to support the growing demand for respiratory care. The traditional therapist was task oriented, performing procedures and therapies ordered by physicians under a fee-for-service system. With the former method of retrospective payment, physicians and respiratory therapists had little incentive to systematically evaluate or demonstrate the effectiveness of respiratory care. No one questioned the traditional model of health care, even when it resulted in misallocation and overuse of services.[2] Health care based much of its clinical practices and respiratory care on individual judgments through anecdotal data.

Since the 1980s, health care providers have widely acknowledged that respiratory therapy is over-ordered in hospitals and that a reduction in procedures does not adversely affect health care outcomes.[3] By the early 1990s a pattern of misallocation in respiratory care was being described, indicating that some patients received respiratory therapy that was not indicated, whereas such therapy was not ordered for other, truly needy patients.[4] Reasons such services were often misallocated included insufficient respiratory care knowledge on the part of the prescribers and the continuously variable respiratory needs of patients whose physicians may be unavailable to make changes in the medical orders.[5]

As respiratory care grew and matured, advanced respiratory therapists who achieved the registered respiratory therapist (RRT) credential became experts capable of using protocols to interface complex technology and abnormal patient physiology. By the mid to late 1990s, protocol-based respiratory care was being used to improve the effectiveness of respiratory care for hospitalized patients, including infection control practices to minimize ventilator-acquired pneumonia,[6,7] chest physiotherapy,[8] clinical use of arterial blood gases,[9] oxygen therapy,[10] inhaled bronchodilator administration,[11-13] and weaning of mechanical ventilation.[14,15] Many such protocols were designed for implementation by respiratory therapists to reduce medical care costs, unburden physicians from tasks that can be performed by respiratory therapists, and improve patient outcomes.[16] Protocols or practice guidelines have become an important means to standardize medical practices.

Increasingly complex technology and concerns about the costs of health care have placed respiratory therapists in positions in which they can be consultants and decision makers as well as technical experts who can perform tasks and care for patients. In addition, therapists are involved in delivering and evaluating patient education to improve quality of life through better patient adherence to treatment plans.

Clinical studies have demonstrated the ability of respiratory therapists to prescribe and perform standardized respiratory care for hospitalized patients.[3,10,13-21] A randomized controlled trial comparing respiratory therapist-directed respiratory care to physician-directed respiratory care found that the former demonstrated better agreement with the care plan and lower costs, without any adverse events.[20] Other studies report the positive impression of medical house staff members regarding the impact of a respiratory therapy consult service.[22]

Respiratory therapy continues to function under medical direction, but this direction is best achieved in the form of guidelines, pathways, or protocols that incorporate independent assessment, judgment, and decision making. Examples include ventilator adjustments and weaning without specific physician orders; emergency airway management, including endotracheal intubation; upper airway endoscopies for evaluation of tube function; adjustments of aerosol therapies; and placement of invasive devices, such as arterial lines or central venous lines.[1] In these roles the respiratory therapist is a health care professional who functions as a physician extender and might be more properly compared to a physician assistant.

In this advanced professional role, centralized respiratory care departments are critically important because equipment management, skill documentation, continuing education, and credentialing all require a high level of expertise. Respiratory therapists must continue to align themselves with supportive medical directors, physicians, and physician groups who value their expertise and help in providing improved patient care, including patient education. Therapists must be committed to making their jobs true professions through education, technical expertise, professional skills, protocol expertise, and effective clinical practice. Physicians, administrators, and heath care payers must recognize the cost effectiveness of health care provided by competent respiratory therapists. Incorporation of protocol-based care, outcomes assessment, and evidence-based health care will continue to facilitate the role of professional respiratory therapists as decision makers and consultants.

Guidelines, Protocols, and Pathways

Clinical guidelines, respiratory care protocols, and critical pathways have emerged as ways to standardize care, improve efficiency, reduce costs, and document the effectiveness of health care. *Clinical practice guidelines, critical pathways, therapist-directed protocols, respiratory care protocols,* and *case management* may be relatively unfamiliar terms to students and some staff respiratory therapists; these concepts are discussed in the following sections.

Clinical Practice Guidelines

Clinical practice guidelines (CPGs) are statements to assist clinicians with appropriate health care for specific clinical circumstances.[23] CPGs are developed by professional associations and related clinical groups to address the appropriateness of health care with specific indications for tests, procedures, and treatments through systematic use of the best available evidence. In other words, CPGs describe the "how to" for specific disciplines to treat certain conditions, diseases, or modalities. CPGs evolved in part because of the differences evident in patient outcomes, hospital length of stay (LOS), and cost of care, which led to concerns among third party payers and governmental agencies. The American Association for Respiratory Care (AARC) has taken a leadership role not only for the respiratory care profession but also among other allied health organizations to develop CPGs to improve the appropriateness of respiratory practice.

The AARC initiated the formal development of CPGs for respiratory care in 1990 to address the variability in clinical practice among hospitals and geographic regions.[24] The first five CPGs were published in 1991 in the journal *Respiratory Care*.

By 1999, nearly 50 CPGs were published in the journal. AARC members, invited experts, and many peer reviewers update CPGs and write, develop, and implement new guidelines. CPGs are clinical indicators for continuous quality improvement (CQI) and support the enhanced role of the respiratory care practitioner.[25] In addition, CPGs have helped to establish respiratory care protocols. CPGs should provide the basis for appropriate respiratory care while maintaining flexibility to individualize care for specific patients. Many departments and health care organizations have incorporated the AARC's CPGs into departmental policy and procedure manuals.

Development   CPGs are practical documents that address specific respiratory care modalities to help standardize care and improve the quality of care. (For an overview of the design project for CPGs, refer to editorials published in *Respiratory Care*.[26,27]) All CPGs listed in *Respiratory Care* follow the same consistent format designed to answer similar questions (Table 7-1).

Members of working groups develop a CPG after thoroughly reviewing the literature, surveying current practice, and considering the expertise of the group members. The working group makes multiple revisions and edits,

*T*ABLE 7-1

Format Used to Develop CPGs

Item	Description
Procedure	Common names by which it is known
Description	Definition of procedure in context of guideline
Setting	Places in which procedure can be appropriately performed
Indications	Recognized objectives for the procedure
Contraindications	Relative and absolute conditions in which the procedure is unsafe
Hazards/complications	Specific items associated with the procedure
Limitations	Boundaries of which the practitioner should be aware
Need	Determination that a procedure is indicated
Outcomes	Benefits (or lack thereof) derived from the procedure
Resources	Equipment or personnel required to perform the procedure
Monitoring	Related specific issues
Frequency	Statements related to how often the procedure is performed
Infection control	Related specific issues
References	Studies to support recommendations

From Hess D. The AARC clinical practice guidelines. Respir Care 1991; 36:1398-1401.
CPG, Clinical practice guideline.

and when all the members are satisfied with the draft CPG, a steering committee reviews and distributes the guideline for peer review by respiratory therapists, physicians, and others in the field. The working group carefully considers all comments provided reviewers and the steering committee, and after the completion of this process, *Respiratory Care* publishes the CPG and widely distributes it as a reprint.[27]

Advantages   Institutions can benefit from the evaluation, adoption, and use CPGs for several reasons. CPGs are excellent tools for incorporation into respiratory care protocols that are specific to institutions because they define and justify clinical practice. Respiratory care departments have incorporated CPGs into their consult services and respiratory care protocol programs.[17-20,28,29] CPGs can help therapists meet the physicians' expectations, providing a basis for therapist-physician interactions. On the other hand, CPGs are used to guide physicians to meet the expectations of respiratory therapists. Therefore CPGs provide a common frame of reference to help improve the consistency and appropriateness of care. In addition, the CPG, accepted as a standard of care, can help respiratory care departments develop triage systems so that clinicians can most appropriately allocate patient care and can serve as a guide for education and research.[28]

Limitations   CPGs are usually brief, generic, and nonspecific. Consequently they are used to establish protocols and pathways. Health care organizations can tailor CPGs to meet the needs of their specific organization and health care practices. A major limitation of CPGs is that often insufficient evidence exists to support current practices. Best available evidence is used to establish CPGs, and this evidence sometimes amounts to nothing more than the consensus of experts. This major limitation of CPGs documents the need for specific outcomes research to establish the effectiveness of conventional therapies.

The role of CPGs in respiratory care has not been studied, but in some professions (for example, anesthesiology) the adaptation of CPGs has resulted in lower malpractice premiums[30] and significant cost savings.[31] The AARC's

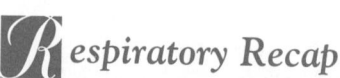
Respiratory Recap

Clinical Practice Guidelines
Specify indications for tests, procedures, and treatments to provide appropriate care
Specify treatment plans, protocols, and algorithms for patient care
Describe "how-to" in brief, generic, nonspecific language
Were developed by the profession, whose practitioners use them to treat patients
Are voluntary and evolve as the profession changes

CPGs have facilitated and promoted the development of therapist-directed protocols while also noting areas in which research is needed to gain evidence to support respiratory care practices.

Respiratory Care Protocols

The literature first described **respiratory care protocols** in 1981.[19] Since then these protocols have emerged as an integral part of many services provided by respiratory therapists. Clinicians also refer to respiratory care protocols as **therapist-driven protocols (TDPs)**, *patient-driven protocols (PDPs)*, or simply *protocols*. Respiratory care protocols are patient care plans initiated and implemented by credentialed respiratory therapists. They provide flexibility because clinicians can modify them according to the needs of the patient.

Development   One of the main purposes of respiratory care protocols is to standardize decision making. Respiratory therapists and physicians develop respiratory care protocols, which the medical staff and hospital administration must approve before implementation. Each protocol has a title, purpose or objective, description of the type of patient it is intended for (for example, geriatric), indications and contraindications, projected outcomes, and guidelines regarding appropriate times to reduce or discontinue therapy. With protocols the therapist can initiate, adjust, discontinue, and restart respiratory care procedures once the physician prescribes the protocol.

Respiratory care protocols can take several forms, such as narratives, worksheets, or **algorithms** and may be patient specific, diagnosis specific, or symptom specific. Patient-specific protocols are generic, usually patient assessment protocols, developed according to a particular patient's needs. Diagnosis-specific protocols are part of a patient's critical path of care (for example, cystic fibrosis or asthma care). Symptom-specific protocols follow a patient with a particular problem, such as wheezing, chest pain or atelectasis. Using CPGs typically generates respiratory care protocols. CPGs in respiratory care then provide profession-oriented procedures to incorporate into the institution-oriented protocol.

Once a physician orders the protocol, the respiratory therapist has the legitimate authority to evaluate, initiate care, and adjust, discontinue, or restart respiratory care procedures on a shift-by-shift, or hour-to-hour basis. For protocols to be successful in any facility, each respiratory therapist must have a strong knowledge base of cardiopulmonary care disorders and competence in the actual assessment process, which includes gathering of clinical data, formulation of a correct assessment, and appropriate treatment. Assessment and communication skills are extremely important because more time is spent with the patient for assessment and treatment, communicating with other professionals, and documenting what is done and observed.[32]

Advantages Many reasons exist why health care institutions should implement respiratory care protocols. One major advantage is that protocols are institution-specific guidelines for clinical decision making within specific clinical settings; they take into consideration the competencies of their staff members, the needs of their patients, and numerous other contextual variables that influence health care. Many advantages of such protocols have been documented, such as improvements in the allocation of respiratory care services, improvements in triage of care, objective criteria for initiation of respiratory care, discontinuation of therapy after it is no longer necessary, decreased cost of care without adverse effects, and improvements in patient care outcomes.[10-20]

Other advantages resulting from the implementation of respiratory care protocols include recruitment of better therapists because of the challenging work environment and increased job satisfaction.[32] Cost containment is a major asset for managers whose departments use protocols because patients are getting the most appropriate care, and therefore the total charges against the diagnostic-related groups (DRGs) are low. For instance, if a patient is very ill, a protocol order can achieve continuous therapy with assessment, followed by a decrease to every 2 hours, then every 4 hours, and finally twice a day as the patient's condition improves. Tremendous cost savings can be realized when respiratory therapists can decrease unnecessary therapy. Health care organizations should regularly update their protocols as respiratory care and organizational needs change to reflect the latest in technology or research. Regular updates should be part of the protocol process, ensuring little or no deleterious effects on the overall program. The AARC website (www.aarc.org) has a link to a homepage with guidelines used to prepare respiratory care protocols.

Limitations Respiratory care protocols do not have any inherent disadvantages, but successful use requires a dedicated effort by the institution. Protocols must be regularly updated to optimize clinical applicability, and they must not interfere with clinicians' abilities to alter practices based on clinical judgments. In addition, sufficient numbers of competent staff members are required to effectively use the protocols[16,33,34] Staff member competency and compliance may be important barriers for effective implementation of protocol-based care. In fact, success of protocol-based care and increased decision making by respiratory therapists may depend on several environmental factors and the organizational culture.[16,35,36]

Once a conducive organizational culture and a comprehensive system for the development, use, and evaluation of respiratory care protocols are established at an institution, the responsibility for successful implementation resides with each individual respiratory therapist. Successful implementation of protocol-based care requires competent respiratory therapists with excellent communications skills. The consultant role of respiratory therapists does not evolve simply because a protocol is implemented; suc-

cessful development and implementation depends on a partnership with physicians who have grown to respect the therapists at the bedside and have confidence in their skills, behaviors, and potential.[1,2]

A potential limitation in the protocol implementation can occur if respiratory therapists view the protocol from a task-oriented perspective rather than a decision-making perspective. Strict adherence to protocol instructions without critical thinking applied to the specific circumstance does little to promote either the protocol or the respiratory care profession. Protocol-based care is intended to standardize decision making and care without replacing the importance of clinical judgment.

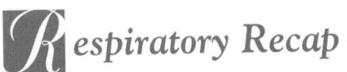

*R*espiratory Recap

> ### *Respiratory Care Protocols*
>
> Are institution-specific patient care plans, not standing orders
> Are approved by the medical staff members and hospital administrators before implementation
> Have a title, purpose or objective, description of type patients for which they are intended, indications and contraindications, projected outcomes, guidelines with appropriate times to reduce or discontinue therapy
> Provide guidelines and criteria about when to initiate the care plan
> Provide guideline for appropriate situations in which to reduce or discontinue therapy

Critical Pathways

A **critical pathway (CP)** describes a probable sequence of events during a patient's course of health care, outlining all the tests, procedures, treatments, and teaching services that patients may undergo during an LOS.[37] Many other terms are used to describe CPs, including *critical paths, clinical algorithms, care maps, care paths, collaborative plans of care, multidisciplinary action plans (MAPs), pathways, practice plans and anticipated recovery paths,* and *clinical paths* to name several. CPs define the optimal sequence or timing of the key interventions performed by each discipline involved in patient care for a particular diagnosis, procedure, or symptom.[38] Another interpretation of CP is the sequence of events in a process that takes the greatest length of time.[8] CPs in health care evolved from nursing as a blend of traditional nursing care plans, a need to provide care within the structured framework of a hospital setting, and a means to establish a standard of care for all patients.[10]

Some institutions are reluctant to use the term *critical pathway* because of the implications it may have for the patients hearing those words associated with their care. Patients and their families might mistakenly think that their condition is critical and requires some special pathway or type of health care. Some health care providers dislike the term *pathway* because it implies that one best way exists to deliver care and that any other approach is substandard. Regardless of the terms used, much of the documented success comes from the use of CPs in acute care settings. Clinicians can use CPs in any setting, and currently many health care organizations are developing CPs to meet the needs of patients across the continuum of health care.

$\mathcal{R}$espiratory Recap

Common Names for Critical Pathways	
Care plans	Practice plans
Clinical algorithms	Anticipated recovery paths
Critical paths	Care maps
Collaborative plans of care	Multidisciplinary action plans

Development   CPs originated in the construction and manufacturing industries, originally developed as tools to identify and manage rate-limiting steps in production processes.[39] CPs have maximized the efficiency of production, given multiple contractors and limited resources. All activities to be accomplished during a production process are identified and timed, with techniques such as the critical path method (CPM), program evaluation review technique (PERT), and Gantt charts. Activities then are organized in sequence according to their individual projected times of completion. By definition a *critical path* is the key sequence of events that drives the timeline of the overall project by projecting the maximum amount of time it will take to complete each process. The goal is to optimize the sequence and timing of each event to improve effectiveness and efficiency.

In health care a CP is an optimal sequencing and timing of interventions by physicians, nurses, and other disciplines for a particular diagnosis or procedure, designed to minimize delays and resource use and maximize quality of care.[38] Of all the diagnostic, therapeutic, social, and organizational interventions to be accomplished during an episode of care, the critical path is the sequence of milestone events that will have the greatest impact on clinical outcomes, LOS, and resource consumption. Initially, nurses in hospitals developed CPs for nursing care alone. Eventually multidisciplinary teams began to develop pathways to encompass all aspects of care for hospitalized patients.[40] A basic assumption behind pathway development is the "80/20 rule," meaning that 80% of patients follow a predictable path 100% of the time and an additional 20% stray from that pathway, a portion of which deviate far from the original pathway.[37]

The health professionals who use CPs should develop them. The most effective CP team includes a wide range of professions in a **multidisciplinary** task force offering a variety of views that include meetings, documents, and pathway review. Respiratory therapists are increasingly involved in the development, implementation, and evaluation of CPs. Chances are that committee members' views during implementation of CPs will mirror the views of the other staff members who are not part of the task force.

CPs are available in the literature for specific diagnoses or procedures,[41] and some agencies and professional organizations, such as the AARC, provide CPs for a fee. Although purchase of a set of CPs for implementation may seem simple, this approach does not provide a vehicle for the health care practitioners to learn about the pathways. In addition, the hasty adoption of CPs developed elsewhere does not allow organizations the time they may need to work through problems. Although the internal development of CPs is a time-consuming, complex process, it is also beneficial to the institution.

In working together to institutionalize CPs, team members gain valuable insight into their own unique contributions to patient care and a greater understanding of the roles of other health care providers. A physician or nurse customarily serves as chairperson of the group, composed of representatives from hospital administration, quality management, pharmacy, and all appropriate ancillary support services. A respiratory therapist may be responsible for developing a CP on ventilator weaning or prolonged mechanical ventilation. This developmental process can help to diminish the perception of the "cookbook approach" to care.

Time at the beginning of the process should be spent in the securing of "buy-in" within the institution. If the leadership buys in to the pathway, then the next step is to obtain such support from the staff members. To get all staff members committed to a CP is possibly the greatest challenge in any setting. Practitioner input in development and implementation also is important because the buy-in and success of the CP program increase. Achieving buy-in requires a chance for the staff to express concerns and a forum to resolve them. Like any change, staff members, including nurses, physicians, therapists, dietitians, and others, are bound to disagree about certain issues. A carefully chosen team can help ensure success in development, implementation, and evaluation of CPs.

Advantages   CPs have become an important component of case management, which organizes health care around milestone events as activities supporting the accomplishment of these events. Case management is known as the collaborative process during which the options and services required to meet an individual's health needs are assessed, planned, implemented, coordinated, monitored, and evaluated.[37] Case management uses CPs to guide communication and use of available health care resources to promote quality, cost-effective outcomes.

CPs are most likely advocated in health care today because they provide a multidisciplinary framework for the coordination and provision of health care. Consequently, health care organizations usually realize immediate, short-term benefits. These organizations frequently use CPs as a part of the CQI plan. CQI monitoring and evaluation of the appropriateness of patient care is a difficult task in a large hospital in terms of effective use of time and resources. Therefore CPs outline daily triggers that can be used to help identify potential and actual variations in the health response to a planned intervention [42] These triggers visually remind the care provider that any abnormal occurrence can have a negative impact on outcomes.

For example, a patient with cystic fibrosis may develop audible wheezing 2 days after admittance for a gastrointestinal blockage. This event is a trigger to the care providers that an unexpected event has occurred. The wheezing noted by the respiratory therapist varies from the planned course of care over time on the CP. Another example is the presence of atelectasis on the chest radiograph of a patient who underwent abdominal surgery 3 days earlier to repair an aortic aneurysm. Atelectasis triggers a variance that requires immediate attention. Practitioners can use triggers to help them respond to changes in the clinical course of the illness. An added benefit is that this model provides a means for providers to promote and document their excellence and remain competitive.

Limitations   With economic and consumer pressures on the health care industry directed at outcomes management, institution may try to hastily adopt CPs as an easy solution. Any organization's superficial approach to CPs is a mistake because such pathways require sufficient thought, preparation, and communication. CPs can promote a change in philosophy for many institutions and thus should not be undertaken lightly because of the potential impact on the organizational culture. Without a firm commitment from the leadership, CPs cannot fulfill their intended purpose—to reduce cost and LOS in the short term while improving quality and patient satisfaction in the long term.

Health care organizations may direct their professionals to incorporate CPs with little or no instruction and guidance. Outside hospitals, very few health care settings have offered continuing education activities relating to CP development and implementation. Like other promising medical innovations, CPs sometimes are used before controlled clinical trials have evaluated their effectiveness. Therefore one cannot generalize that all CPs are cost effective and cost efficient for the overall operation health care institutions over an extended time period because the data is inconclusive.

CPGs, respiratory care protocols, and CPs overlap significantly, but all three tools are appropriate for use in certain situations and at certain times. For example, an organization may develop a respiratory care protocol by using a specific CPG and may at the same time incorporate the respiratory care protocol into a CP for a specific disease or condition. In the literature, respiratory care protocols are straightforward in their description and use. However, use of CPs and CPGs present unique challenges because CPGs are written for general application, whereas

CPs are written for each specific institution, along with that facility's available resources and organization.

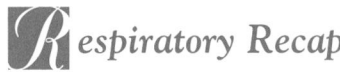

espiratory Recap

Critical Pathways
Focus on the efficiency and effectiveness of treatment decisions
Represent the completion of the protocol or guideline that results in the accomplishment of critical pathway events
Describe "when to" via specific time lines for the accomplishment of events
Are affected by any delays or complications in treatment plans
Are multidisciplinary in their development and implementation
Use practitioners' discipline-specific and professional skills from the outset of patient care
Become part of the medical record in most instances

In an era of increasing competition in health care, clinicians develop CPs to reduce costs and maintain or even improve the quality of care. Health care organizations develop CPs primarily for high-volume procedures or hospital diagnoses to provide the ideal sequence and timing of staff member actions with optimal efficiency. Despite the rapid dissemination of CPs in hospitals throughout the United States, many uncertainties remain about their development, implementation, and evaluation.[43]

Outcomes Evaluation and Evidence

Whether using CPGs, respiratory care protocols, CPs, or a combination, each organization must evaluate the outcomes, which include those related to patient care, the institution, and the care provider. Clinical outcomes are used in several ways, including but not limited to benchmarking, compliance with regulatory agencies, patient compliance, patient education, marketing, clinical operations management, and research. Health care outcomes have the potential to change practice over time. Until the use of CPs and respiratory care protocols, researchers did not scientifically evaluate the relationship between the provision of care in a certain way and the achievement of certain outcomes. The following discussion can help respiratory therapists and students understand **outcomes evaluation** and evidence-based medicine, which encompass CPGs, respiratory care protocols, and CPs.

Patient Outcomes

Morbidity and mortality rates are the most common indicators of patient outcomes, but others include complications, patient satisfaction, and improved quality of life. Increased longevity, improved functionality, and emotional health are additional examples of desirable patient outcomes. Self-care, behaviors that promote health, a positive outlook, and decreased stress can indicate improved quality of life. Questions to ask to determine which patient outcomes should be measured include the following:

1. Is the patient better off because of this treatment?
2. Is the quality of life improved or maintained, or has it declined?
3. Can the patient self-manage the disease and demonstrate health-promoting behaviors?

Patient satisfaction is gaining importance, especially with third-party payers. Health care organizations are paying more attention than ever before to patient satisfaction because of its effects on public relations and marketing in an increasingly competitive health care industry.

Institutional Outcomes

Cost and quality of care are the most common institutional outcomes, or those related to the health care facility. LOS correlates directly with the cost of health care. To decrease institutional costs, health care organizations strive for the shortest possible LOS that does not produce adverse affects. Therefore LOS is the number one variable to manipulate to preserve revenue in a health care institution. Some studies show that institutions incur the majority of health care costs within the first few days of a patient's stay.

Quantifying quality of care is much more difficult than quantifying an objective variable such as LOS. Patient understanding of the treatment plan might be used to assess quality of health care, specifically patient education. In this example, documentation of what the patient learned as opposed to the content of the education is most important. For example, patient education on a CP for asthma may include the need to assess understanding regarding indications, use of bronchodilators, and a step-up approach to exacerbations. The institutional outcome may be that the patient understands when to contact a physician as a criterion for hospital discharge. The office then follows up after discharge to document whether the patient notified the physician's office before the next emergency department visit. The evaluation of progress on the pathway or protocols can verify an institutional outcome.

Care Provider Outcomes

Studies have shown that positive care provider outcomes lead to better patient outcomes. In a study of nine critical care units, improvement in the patient outcomes for reduced mortality (risk-adjusted mortality) were reported in units with provider characteristics that included a patient-centered focus, strong leadership evidenced by shared visions, supportive visible leaders, a collaborative approach to problem solving by all members of the health care team, and effective communication.[37] Care provider outcomes include greater autonomy in clinical practice, participation

in decision-making, increased satisfaction with the care delivered, and reduced staff member turnover rates. As leaders, managers work to provide institutional climates that promote teamwork and effective problem solving to achieve improved patient outcomes. Innovative health care organizations look for these attributes while recruiting new graduates and experienced professionals alike.

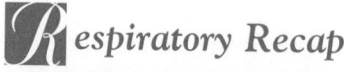 **espiratory Recap**

Types of Outcomes
Patient outcomes—patient satisfaction, functionality, quality of life
Institution outcomes—length of stay, morbidity, complications, costs of care
Provider outcomes—low staff member turnover, role in decision making, greater autonomy in clinical practice, job satisfaction

Variance Tracking

One definition of a variance is the difference between patient care and outcomes described in the pathway, protocol, or guideline and what actually happened. Simply stated, variance is the difference between the expectations and the actual findings. Good patient, institutional, or provider outcomes are expected, for instance. Variance describes any deviation from those achievement goals in health care outcomes and reflects patient or caregiver issues that can affect patient outcomes.[44] A variance occurs when a patient does not progress as anticipated or when an expected outcome is not achieved[45] and can alert health care providers to the need for action, and of equal importance, can serve as a database for CQI. Categories of variances include patient or family variance, caregiver or clinician variance, hospital or system variance, and community variances.

The guideline, pathway, or protocol helps the health care team reduce variation as part of the general improvement process.[45] For example, the achievement of an outcome earlier than expected provides clues for more cost-effective care. Timely recognition and addressing of any deviations with a CQI format is the most important step to achieve success of CPGs, CPs, or protocols and to ensure the delivery of quality patient care. As stated previously, protocols can be developed from CPGs by incorporation of an explicit review process to measure outcomes, including variances. **Variance tracking** therefore is essential to transform CPGs into protocols and pathways. Variances monitoring is a key part of the respiratory care protocol and CP processes. CQI, CPGs, CPs, and respiratory care protocols work well together, fulfilling the desired integration of an effective health care organization.

Many useful formats exist for the collection and analysis of variance. The literature provides a variety of examples of practical ways to collect data on variances but much less information on ways to analyze variances and outliers in health care. Collection of variance data tend to fall into four categories—notations written directly on the CP or respiratory care protocol document itself, retrospective chart review, the use of a separate variance data collection sheet, and the use of computerized systems. Generally, clinicians, researchers, and administrators use statistical methods to evaluate quantitative, numeric data and use qualitative methods to analyze nonnumeric data, such as variance description.

After identification of the outliers, variance analysis explains the clinical reason or reasons for the deviations. Cause-and-effect relationships can be established among medical conditions, treatment variables, and resource utilization within the given pathway or protocol. Armed with this information, health care providers and administrators can compare data from current care plans with standard performance indicators, making necessary changes to ensure maximal patient benefit. Ideally the health care providers alter the treatment approach in real time to prevent over-use or under-use of resources.

Variances also are analyzed to compare statistics relating to the effectiveness of different medical treatment plans among health care providers.[37] This peer comparison, or **benchmarking,** is a foundation for the standardization of health care delivery and the maximization of its benefits. The term *benchmarking* is a general one applied to all efforts to determine not the average use of a particular diagnosis but the most medically appropriate use per diagnosis.[37]

Variance tacking requires timely intervention to achieve desired outcomes. Ideally the designs of the variance tracking catch deviations while they occur to help individual patients. If health care providers do not track variances in a timely manner, outcome measurements do not help that particular patient but instead only future patients as problems are followed over time. Disadvantages

of tracking variances sometimes result from the audit process. Clinicians may be hesitant to implement changes in processes, even when necessary to individualize care, because the changes show up as a variance.[34] After the data are collected, analysis and reporting follow.

Case managers typically develop and implement a quality improvement process for any recurrent variances noted under CPs. By keeping track of variance data, administrators are able to document the effectiveness of provided care while reducing complications and LOS. The National Institutes of Health (NIH) and Agency for Health Care Policy and Research (AHCPR), as well as other organizations, including the AARC, have called for and funded proposals to study patient outcomes. Published outcome data do not promote any particular strategy to provide the most effective health care with the best outcomes.

Evidence-Based Medicine

The discussion thus far has described the ways organizations use outcomes to evaluate the effectiveness of health care at their specific institutions through CPGs, CPs, and protocols. Today, **evidence-based medicine (EBM),** also known as *evidence-based health care (EBH),* is used to express what is known about health care based on scientific evidence and outcomes data. The explosion of medical information and its increased accessibility has assisted the development of EBM, which requires specific criteria that include the thorough analysis of rigorous scientific data to support approaches to health care. EBM systematically and rigorously evaluates outcomes research with use of methods to increase the generalization of findings. EBM is the "conscientious, explicit and judicious use of current best evidence in making decisions about the care of individual patients."[46] EBH is a broader application of EBM across health care disciplines and may be described as a comprehensive approach to the systematic documentation of achievable health care outcomes across the disciplines.[48,49]

In EBM, research is the methodic collection of studies that meet strict quality criteria. All or portions of these studies then can be merged, distilled, and interpreted (meta-analysis). The "discoveries" in EBM are reviews and practice guidelines developed from this conservative evaluation of the effect and effectiveness of care. For example, the Cochrane Collaboration is an international research initiative established to produce, maintain, and disseminate reviews of evidence. The Cochrane Library, launched in 1995 to provide evidence needed in health care decision making, currently maintains four databases, including controlled trials, review methodologies, systematic reviews of the effects of care, and critical assessments of effectiveness.[47,49] The Cochrane Library regularly updates its databases, which are designed to make available the evidence needed to make informed health care decisions. A bimonthly publication, *Evidence-Based Medicine,* reports on recent reviews and commentaries from EBM.

℞espiratory Recap ———————

Variance Tracking

Purpose: To track differences between expectations and occurrences

Methods: Written notations on the CP or protocol, retrospective chart review, variance data collection sheets, and computerized systems

Results: Establishes cause-and-effect relationships among medical condition, treatment variables, and resource use within the given pathway or protocol; guides the CQI process

Pitfalls: Possible inhibition of individual judgments that can cause variances

Current state: NIH, AHCPR, and AARC funding promotion of outcomes research to gain additional evidence to guide clinical practice

Respiratory therapists and all health care providers should understand and apply a hierarchy for the levels of evidence when evaluating research regarding an intervention or therapy. EBM categorizes the research evidence into three levels based on the design of the study. Level-one evidence comes from a multisite, randomized clinical trial or several single-site, randomized control trials. Level-two evidence is derived from a variety of quasiexperimental studies, whereas level-three evidence includes correlational or descriptive studies. Examining the levels of evidence does not provide indications of the quality of a study or the overall strength of the body of evidence. However, examination of the levels of evidence is a useful means to address the effectiveness of a study design to establish cause and effect. The Cochrane Library and other EBM databases provide guidance for health professionals in the evaluation of the levels of evidence and quality of that evidence. Respiratory therapists can be valuable consultants and members of their organizations by using EBM to develop, implement, and evaluate CPGs, respiratory care protocols, CPs, and health care for individual patients. Figure 7-1 illustrates examples of pathways of research-based practice for health professionals, whereas

Box 7-1 provides guidelines for the appraisal of evidence from research-based CPGs.

Although a need for EBM has always existed, public health agencies, health maintenance organizations (HMOs), and cost-conscious hospitals have accelerated the need for and its

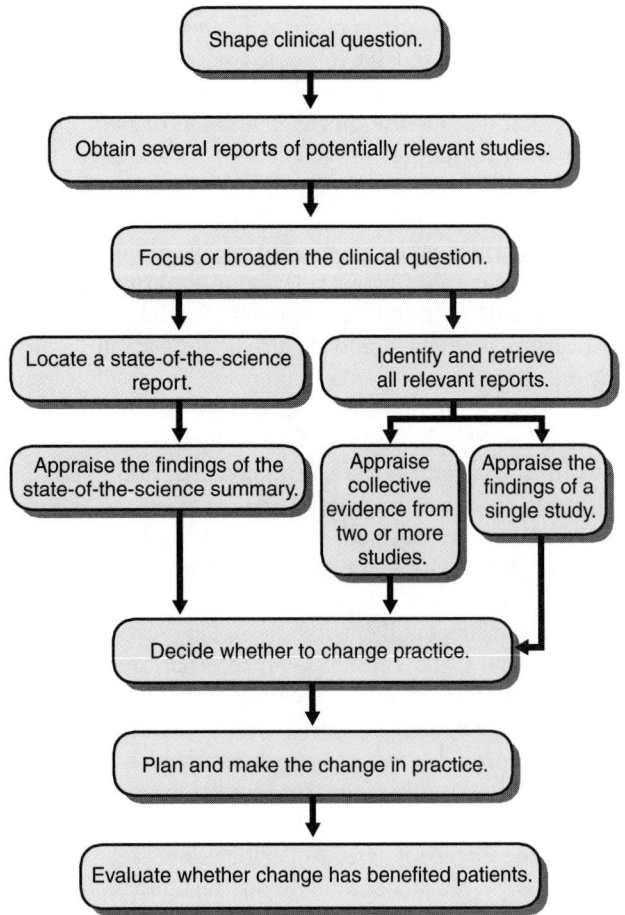

Figure 7-1   Possible pathways for research-based practice. (Modified from Brown SJ. Knowledge for health care practice: a guide to using research evidence. Philadelphia: WB Saunders; 1999.)

Box 7-1

Appraisal of Evidence from Research-Based Practice Guidelines

Citation
Cite the guideline to be appraised.

Synopsis
What does the guideline address?
For which population of patients is the guideline intended?
What are the key decision points addressed by the guideline?
What outcomes does the guideline address?
Describe the process used to develop the guideline.

Credibility Profile
Are the guidelines based on a comprehensive meta-analysis or integrative research review?
  Is the scientific basis for each recommendation provided?
  Are all key decision points addressed?
  At each decision point, was the full range of actions evaluated?
Does the discussion of the way the panel reached decisions convince us that all evidence was considered impartially?
Are the guidelines current?
Was the panel that developed the guideline composed of people with the necessary skills, expertise, and backgrounds?
Are the recommendations credible?
Yes_____ No ____

Applicability Profile
Does the guideline address a problem, decision, or situation seen in our practice?
Would we use all or part of the guideline? If part, please specify which.
Are the recommended courses of action acceptable and feasible to us and our patients?
To follow the guideline, what do we have to do differently?
Do we have the resources, skills, and equipment to implement this guideline accurately and safely?
Should we adopt this guideline in its entirety?
Yes____ No ____
Should we adopt parts of it?
Yes____ No ____

Additional Considerations
What will we have to do to implement the change?
How will we know whether our patients are benefiting from our use of the guideline?

Modified from Brown SJ. Knowledge for health care practice: a guide to using research evidence. Philadelphia: WB Saunders; 1999. p. 241.

development. Respiratory care students and instructors should use EBH to articulate the logic behind certain clinical practices and evaluate CPGs, CPs, and respiratory care protocols. Therapists should understand and use EBM in their practice to expand their effectiveness in health care, providing additional opportunities for decision making and consulting within health care settings. One caveat is to remember that EBM is not cookbook medicine nor does it strictly focus on cost-cutting health care strategies. EBM and evidenced-based practice provide a consistent framework to evaluate current health care and the methods used to improve effectiveness, without ignoring individual patient needs.

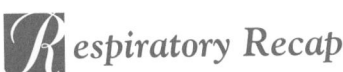

Respiratory Recap

Levels of Evidence
Level one: evidence from a multisite randomized, controlled study or several single-site controlled trials *Level two:* evidence from a variety of quasiexperimental studies *Level three:* evidence including correlational or descriptive studies

Examining levels of evidence provides no indication as to a study's quality or the overall strength of the body of evidence.

Consultation Skills for Health Care Professionals

Previous sections of this chapter have discussed the evolving role of respiratory therapists as decision makers, with an expanding consultation role through using and evaluating respiratory care protocols, CPGs, and CPs. The following sections elaborate the value, qualifications, and roles of internal consultants in health care today.

Internal Consulting

Health care comprises labor-intensive organizations filled with individuals with high-technology experience who depend on working together and consulting with one another. Internal consulting defines an effective helping relationship that leads to effective outcomes.[50] The more effective the internal consulting skills of the health care professionals, the more effective the health care organization will be. The Joint Commission on Accreditation of Healthcare Organizations (JCAHO) specifies accreditation standards that support teamwork and look to the organization to improve quality of care. Improving organizational effectiveness depends on the achievement of the highest productivity of the departments and individuals involved because these individuals account for the largest portion of any health care organization's operating budget.

Internal consultants within health care organizations include direct patient caregivers, support groups that assist care teams, and the administration. Support group consultants include departments such as human resources, education, marketing, planning, environmental services, public relations, and business. Direct patient caregivers include physicians, nurses, respiratory therapists, social workers, physical therapists, and many others.

Internal Consulting and Organizational Effectiveness

Internal consulting does not happen in a vacuum but occurs within the culture of an organization to improve its effectiveness and efficiency. When an individual within an organization works as a consultant, that person is able to think beyond the needs and functions of individual departments and assist others across the organization. Training and facilitating various members of a health care organization to become internal consultants can improve an organization's ability to deliver cost-effective health care because (1) technical skills combined with internal consulting skills can lead to effective problem identification and resolution and (2) effective problem identification and resolution lead to increased organizational effectiveness.[50]

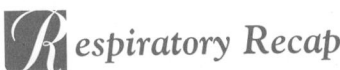

Respiratory Recap

Internal Consulting
Internal consultants can be direct patient caregivers, support personnel, or administrators. Effective health care providers possess technical expertise in addition to professional expertise, including consulting skills and traits. Internal consultants can be technical experts or process experts. Technical skills combined with consultation skills improve problem identification and resolution. Problem resolution contributes to improved organizational effectiveness. Consulting improves the effectiveness and use of human resources.

The stages of internal consulting include (1) precontracting, (2) contracting, (3) data collection, (4) data analysis, (5) presentation, (6) action planning, (7) evaluation, and (8) termination. Effective internal consultants must devote attention to each stage.

Roles and Skills of Internal Consultants

Technical skills alone are insufficient in health care today. Today's professionals need interpersonal skills that go beyond their technical expertise. The emphasis in the past has been to hire individuals with excellent technical skills, but today, respiratory therapists and other health care providers must be able to work with others in interdepartmental teams and negotiate differences. Internal consultants possess exceptional communication abilities and must be able to (1) determine the needs of the client, often another department but also possibly the patient or other health professional, (2) identify their role in relation to that department or service, (3) agree on the necessary steps for a desired outcome, (4) perform those steps, and (5) evaluate the results.

The health care professional as consultant can have multiple roles, from directive to nondirective, including advocate, information specialist, trainer and educator, joint problem solver, identifier of alternatives and linker to resources, fact finder, and process consultant. In addition, the range of consulting skills includes technical expertise and process facilitation. The approach to consulting varies, depending on whether the consultant focuses on task orientation or process orientation. However, the basic approach to consulting includes (1) problem verification, (2) problem solving, (3) feedback, (4) research, (5) involvement, (6) formation of client relationship, and (7) systems approach. Although the problem-solving process can be described in many ways, Table 7-2 outlines the basic, generic components.

Today's respiratory therapist should possess all the skills of internal consulting, as well as a comprehensive understanding of current health care. Consequently, the entire first section of this textbook is devoted to the development of professional skills, attributes, and organizational variables that facilitate the professional role in respiratory care. The case examples at the end of this chapter illustrate ways respiratory therapists can use their technical and professional expertise to enhance organizational effectiveness as internal consultants.

Respiratory Therapists as Consultants

This chapter makes the case that health care and organizational effectiveness can improve if competent respiratory therapists increase their role as decision makers. The word *competent* must include expanded responsibility and accountability to accompany the expanded role. Numerous medical directors and physician organizations support respiratory therapists at their institutions, as well as the profession in general. Position statements and letters of support from physician organizations such as the American College of Chest Physicians (ACCP), American Society of Anesthesiologists (ASA), and the California Thoracic Society (CTS) state the important role respiratory therapists play in health care.[48]

In addition, the ACCP has issued a position statement supporting the use of respiratory care protocols.[1] Physicians have published editorials, conference summaries, and original studies supporting respiratory therapists as physician extenders and practitioners of protocol-based care.[1,5,10,13-16,20,22,28,34,35] Some physicians have argued that implementation of respiratory therapy protocols would interfere with the respiratory care training of medical staff, particularly residents, fellows, and house officers. However, evidence suggests that the use of respiratory care protocols does not interfere with house staff members' knowledge of respiratory care and may actually contribute to increased knowledge of respiratory care ordering.[16,22,51,52]

Support from national professional associations and physicians at the local level and within work settings can facilitate an expanded role for respiratory therapists. Several medical directors and many physicians are involved in state and national professional associations for respiratory care, including the National Association for Medical Direction of Respiratory Care (NAMDRC), which recently issued a statement of support for respiratory care practitioners as the nonphysician caregivers best qualified to render respiratory services.[1] Many physicians also have supported state licensure of respiratory therapists and have helped their state licensure bills gain legislative approval.

Expanded roles for respiratory therapists call for continued reforms in the ways in which therapists are educated, managed, and used. Therapists who want to be vital health care professionals functioning as cost-effective health care consultants must embrace responsibility and accountability in current health care systems and demonstrate competent and effective professional practice. Responsibility and accountability lie with each individual

*T*ABLE 7-2

Problem-Solving Process

Component	Description
Awareness of problem	Recognition that something is amiss and that gap exists between what should happen and what is happening
Identification of problem	Determination and description of the exact nature of problem, which often underlies presenting problem
Selection of criteria for solutions	Specification of solution, requiring extensive communication, thinking, and work
Formulation of alternatives	Description of alternative resolutions and their criteria
Selection of strategy	Decision about which alternative will most likely achieve desired goal
Specification of action plan	Development of plan describing exact way to implement strategy
Implementation of action plan	Performance of predetermined plan
Monitoring and evaluation	Time of review to determine whether plan corrected problem and reflect on strategy, action plan, and implementation to gain further insight into its appropriateness

practitioner, as well as with physicians, educators, managers, medical directors, leaders, and researchers.

Respiratory therapists must do a better job with professional education, continuing education, and use of human resources to compete for additional duties and responsibilities as health care professionals. They also must achieve the appropriate institutional and regulatory support to make possible expanded professional roles for advanced-level therapists. To this end, more and better data are needed to document the cost effectiveness of protocol-based care, CPs, and CPGs in the delivery of quality respiratory care.

CASE STUDIES

Case One
The Crossroads: Are Respiratory Therapists Paid for What They Know or What They Do?

Jason Jeffries is the respiratory care manager at a 400-bed teaching hospital within the state university educational system. He has been working in respiratory care for almost 20 years, with more than 6 years of experience in his current position. Recently the board of regents formed an independent corporation with a board of directors to manage the hospital. Consequently, the hospital and educational portions of the state university are now separate entities. Although the state government still owns the teaching hospital, it authorized the board of directors with decision-making power to help implement managed care.

Mr. Jeffries understands that the major goals of the new organization are to decrease costs of care without jeopardizing patient safety or necessary respiratory services. He must present a plan to the senior administration on ways he intends to decrease the costs of providing respiratory care services. The current department uses time/motion studies, cost minimization strategies, consortium purchasing, and flex time to enhance productivity and limit costs. The policy and procedure manual incorporates CPGs, but the respiratory therapy department has not been involved in CPs or protocols. The staff provides respiratory care services within the hospital and outpatient clinics. How should he approach this problem, and what recommendations could he make?

Mr. Jeffries should consider several strategies, including (1) decreasing staff size, (2) increasing efficiency of staff, (3) improving allocation of services, and (4) documenting successful outcomes. As a manager, his major consideration is to think about the organization and whether the respiratory therapists are paid for what they know or what they do. Mr. Jeffries must document and then communicate to the senior administration the existing strategies that demonstrate his staff members' cost effectiveness. If he finds that his hospital has been paying respiratory therapy staff primarily for what they do, then he must actively

address this major limitation. Mr. Jeffries must critically examine how he can influence his own staff members, his physician supporters, and senior administrators to pay respiratory therapists for what they know.

Mr. Jeffries can decrease staff size by shifting technical tasks to lesser skilled employees. Technical multitasking is a broader use of the traditional task-oriented practitioner. At the present, this type of respiratory care practitioner performs basic services, such as oxygen administration, aerosol administration, and a number of other tasks linked to specific physician orders. Little or no assessment is required, and decision making is usually limited to very specific items, such as device selection and fine-tuning of therapy. These individuals often possess good procedural skills and technical knowledge, the latter of which is what makes these practitioners valuable to hospitals. On the other hand, because assessment and decision making are not major parts of the job, these individuals are often conceptually grouped by administrators with other task-oriented hospital workers, such as electrocardiogram (ECG) technologists, radiologic technologists, phlebotomists, and the like. This grouping is the force behind the creation of a broader, so-called multiskilled practitioner who can function under nurse supervision on a patient care floor. This type and level of clinician competes with the licensed practical nurse for job assignments, job recognition, and wages within health care organizations.

The role of the professional respiratory therapist implies the need for assessment and judgment. Indeed a professional is sometimes referred to as "one whose opinion matters."[1] This advanced professional career track still operates under medical direction, but the direction takes the form of guidelines or protocols that incorporate independent assessment, judgment, and decision making. In these roles the advanced respiratory care practitioner is a professional who actually functions as physician extender, comparable to a physician assistant. Mr. Jeffries must document that the respiratory care provided in his facility is truly necessary and is discontinued when the objectives are met.

Mr. Jeffries must maximize the involvement of his staff members in the creation of the new organizational climate through CP teams and other organizational committees. At the same time, he should ally himself with physicians who can help the department develop, implement, and evaluate respiratory care protocols. He should provide current evidence on ways in which protocol-based care can improve allocation of resources, patient objectives, and economic objectives without jeopardizing educational training of medical students, house staff members, and other health care professionals.

Another strategy is to find less expensive sites to provide respiratory care—alternatives to acute care settings. This hospital should transfer patients to subacute care, home care, rehabilitation, and long-term care facilities that are either affiliated with or components of the teaching hospital.

Mr. Jeffries also must develop and implement a plan to attract and retain qualified respiratory therapists who can truly function in this expanded, professional role. Otherwise, implementation of these cost-effective strategies is impossible. The department manager must develop a system documenting continuing education, credentials, performance reviews, peer reviews, and each employee's contributions to institutional and patient outcomes.

The strategies must incorporate both short- and long-term action plans and strategies to evaluate success. In the interim, Mr. Jeffries and his staff must behave competently and professionally at all times. Peer pressure and effective communication are essential for the department to pull together for the benefit of every staff member. Members who either cannot or will not adjust to the changing organization are detriments; Mr. Jeffries must nurture, mentor, and promote qualified staff members. Incompetent staffs are a liability for the department and its future potential. Therefore accountability and consequences are fundamental components for success.

Case Two
Where's Respiratory?!

Tracey is a respiratory therapist with more than 15 years of experience. She has worked in numerous acute care settings, including coronary care, neonatal intensive care, and medical intensive care units. She is an expert in airway management and mechanical ventilation and has been a member of several CP teams. Co-workers respect her because of her professionalism and interpersonal skills. Yesterday, her department manager presented her with a proposal to develop a long-term acute care (LTAC) facility on the eighth floor of the existing hospital. Her department head explained that her experience and competency makes her the ideal person to work with nursing and administration to develop, implement, and eventually manage the LTAC. How should Tracey deal with this opportunity?

First, Tracey must recognize that this opportunity is both for the department and for her own professional growth. She also should recognize that her manager sees her leadership abilities and is guiding her toward a management-related position that will allow her to retain "hands-on" patient care. Second, she must realize that the nature of the work will be much different than work in acute care. Not only will she have more management responsibilities, but the clinical work also relies heavily on a team approach. The types of patients and their needs will often be different, which is why the facility has a need for subacute care. Third, Tracey should discuss with the manager how this opportunity will affect her work hours, work commitments, wages, and fringe benefits. She should address all these issues professionally and effectively with her department head. Neither Tracey nor her manager should make assumptions about their agreement; each aspect should be negotiated until her job description and position are clearly described.

Tracey must research to find out as much as possible about subacute care. For example, she needs to know that LTACs are a form of subacute care, which is growing as hospitals look for ways to decrease the number of patient

days per stay. Subacute care attributes its growth to the Medicare prospective-payment system (PPS), initiated between 1982 and 1986. Managed care limits the amount of money provided to hospitals for patient care and uses strict review criteria to ensure that patients meet the requirements for acute care. Although still defining itself, subacute care has become a feasible alternative to patients who no longer require acute care and often serves as an intermediary between the acute care hospital and the patient's return home.

LTACs are licensed hospitals exempt from the Medicare PPS as long as they keep their average patient LOS greater than 25 days. Long-term hospitals receive payment from Medicare on a reasonable-cost basis. LTAC hospitals usually specialize in patients with pulmonary or other medically complex problems who no longer require extensive diagnostic workups but need additional therapy and nursing support. Nursing hours generally are provided 5 to 7 hours per day, and occupational, physical, and respiratory therapies are provided daily. If the LTAC has patients on ventilators, it offers respiratory therapy 24 hours per day, 7 days per week. Patients usually stay an average of 10 and 60 days, and the cost of care per day is hundreds of dollars less than acute care.

Calls for respiratory assistance should be exceedingly frequent across the continuum of care. Like anyone who has worked in respiratory therapy for any time, Tracey has heard loud, frantic calls asking, "Where is respiratory?!" In an emergency situation, especially one involving the airway, these calls are particularly commonplace, even though the nurses, physicians, and other clinicians know the names of individual respiratory therapists. In such situations the person calling for a respiratory therapist most likely wants to leave no doubt about the expertise needed and the urgency of the request. Just as respiratory therapists have become a vital component of acute care, their expertise has become increasingly important in alternative sites.

Case Three
Convince Me: Why Should Respiratory Therapists Be Internal Consultants?

You are the department manager at the local community hospital, which includes acute care, subacute care, home care, and rehabilitation services. The respiratory therapy staff members have good rapport with the pulmonologists, allergists, sleep specialists, and emergency department physicians, but the neurologists and cardiologists are less supportive and rely more on the nursing staff members. How can you convince your administration, physicians, nurses, and other health care professionals that respiratory therapists should function as internal consultants to improve organizational effectiveness and the costs of respiratory care delivery? Where will you start, and why? The following is one approach, but you are encouraged to make up your own mind and develop a strategy that you believe is worth pursuing.

As the manager, you must convince senior management that the respiratory therapists have technical and process expertise to offer the patient at the bedside, in the laboratory, in the home, and across the continuum of care. You may want to start with your physician allies to help gain additional alliances. Physicians who trust your ability to deliver what you promise and have confidence in your staff members must buy into the concept. Only after obtaining this buy-in should you approach administration.

You can elaborate and document your respiratory therapists' education, expertise, and credentials. Furthermore, you should convince upper administration that the respiratory therapy staff members are an untapped resource to improve organizational effectiveness because they have not been part of CP teams or protocol-based care. In addition, stress that the respiratory therapist is the nonphysician expert in cardiorespiratory care, with training in cardiopulmonary physiology, pathophysiology, assessment, invasive and noninvasive monitoring, treatment, education, and research. Elaborate on your knowledge that because health care is changing and moving to different/alternative care sites, so should the roles of all health care providers change. Delineate additional strategies in which physicians can use respiratory therapists as physician extenders through more protocol-based care.

Increasingly, respiratory therapists are trained to use technology to obtain data that can enhance decision making to improve ventilation of the difficult patient (for example, one with acute respiratory distress syndrome [ARDS]) or assist with the patient who is difficult to wean from mechanical ventilation. In addition, the respiratory therapist's role as educator is a good way to expand the consultant role—from inservice education to other disciplines (advanced cardiac life support [ACLS] course provided to new critical care nurses), community outreach (in areas of pulmonary rehabilitation, smoking cessation, asthma education), and institutional public relations. As the manager, you must explain ways the respiratory therapist's role extend into alternative care sites—airway management in the long-term care site or which oxygen device/delivery system is best in the home care environment.

You must elaborate that respiratory therapists know how the technology works and how it can be best used. Therapists also know anatomy, physiology, and patient assessment and how to apply procedures, monitoring, and treatments to reverse pathophysiology. Finally, therapists have the patient education expertise to design and implement age-specific education and assessment to improve patient adherence and outcomes. The literature offers many examples, as well as research, documentation of the problems with patient adherence to treatment plans, and the importance of effective patient education. Respiratory therapists can work with the organization to develop, implement, and evaluate strategies to improve patient education to patient and institutional outcomes.

Key Points

- CPGs, respiratory care protocols, and CPs have emerged to standardize care, improve efficiency, reduce costs, and document the effectiveness of health care.
- Clinical guidelines, protocols, and pathways have contributed to the increased need and use for the decision-making abilities of respiratory therapists.
- Protocol-based respiratory care has been used to improve the effectiveness of respiratory care for hospitalized patients, including its use in infection-control practices to minimize ventilator-acquired pneumonia, chest physiotherapy, the clinical use of arterial blood gases, oxygen therapy, inhaled bronchodilator administration, and weaning of mechanical ventilation.
- Many protocols were designed for implementation by respiratory therapists to reduce medical care costs, unburden physicians from tasks that can be performed by respiratory therapists, and improve patient outcomes.
- Misallocation of respiratory care services occurs for many reasons, including insufficient knowledge of respiratory care by those who prescribe the care and the continuously variable respiratory needs of patients whose physicians may be unavailable to make changes in the medical orders.
- Position statements and letters of support from physician organizations such as the ACCP, ASA, and ATS, state the important role respiratory therapists play in health care.

- Physicians have published position statements, editorials, conference summaries, and original studies supporting protocol-based care by respiratory therapists and respiratory therapists as physician extenders.
- Internal consulting defines an effective helping relationship that leads to effective outcomes. The more effective the internal consulting skills of the health care professionals, the more effective will be the health care organization.
- Internal consultants can be direct patient caregivers, support personnel, or administrators.
- Internal consultants can be technical experts or process experts. Technical skills combined with consultation skills improve problem identification and resolution, contributing to improved organizational effectiveness.
- Respiratory therapists have the education, opportunity, and potential to play an increasing role as internal consultants to improve the delivery of respiratory care and the organizational effectiveness of the health care organizations for which they work.
- Respiratory therapists can play an important role in health care through continued contributions to effective practice, working with physicians and other health care professionals to make appropriate health care decisions.

References

1. Mishoe SC, MacIntyre NR. Expanding professional roles for respiratory care practitioners. Respir Care 1997;42:71-91.

2. Hess DR. Professionalism, respiratory care practice, and physician acceptance of a respiratory consult service. Respir Care 1998;42:546-548.

3. Zibrak JD, Rossetti P, Wood E. Effects in reduction of respiratory therapy on patient outcome. N Engl J Med 1986;315:292-295.

4. Kester L, Stoller JK. Ordering respiratory care services for hospitalized patients: practices of overuse and under-use. Cleve Clin J Med 1992;59:581-585.

5. Stoller JK. The rationale for therapist-driven protocols. Respir Care Clin N Am 1996;2:1-14.

6. Kelleghan SI, Salemi C, Padilla S, et al. An effective continuous quality improvement approach to the prevention of ventilator-associated pneumonia. Am J Infect Control 1993;21:322-330.

7. Joiner GA, Salisbury D, Bollin GE. Utilizing quality assurance as a tool for reducing the risk of nosocomial ventilator-associated pneumonia. Am J Med Qual 1996;11:100-103.

8. Alexander E, Weingarten S, Mohsenifar Z. Clinical strategies to reduce utilization of chest physiotherapy without compromising patient care. Chest 1996;110:430-432.

9. Pilon CS, Leathley M, London R, et al. Practice guidelines for arterial blood gas measurement in the intensive care decreases numbers and increases appropriateness of tests. Crit Care Med 1997;25:1308-1313.

10. Konschak MP, Binder A, Binder RE. Oxygen therapy utilization in a community hospital: use of a protocol to improve oxygen administration and preserve resources. Respir Care 1999;44:506-511.

11. Goldberg R, Chan L, Haley P, et al. Critical pathway for the emergency management of acute asthma: effect on resource utilization. Ann Emerg Med 1998;31:562-567.

12. Ford RM, Phillips-Clar JE, Burns DM. Implementing therapist-driven protocols. Respir Care Clin N Am 1996;2:51-76.

13. Lierl MB, Pettinichi S, Sebastian KD, et al. Trial of a therapist-directed protocol for weaning bronchodilator therapy in children with status asthmaticus. Respir Care 1999;44:497-505.

14. Wood G, MacLeod B, Moffatt S. Weaning from mechanical ventilation: physician-directed versus a respiratory-therapist-directed protocol. Respir Care 1995;40:219-224.

15. Kollef MH, Shapiro SD, Silver P, et al. A randomized-controlled trial of protocol-directed versus physician-directed weaning from mechanical ventilation. Crit Care Med 1997;25:567-574.

16. Kollef MH. Therapist-directed protocols: their time has come. Respir Care 1999;44:495.

17. Shrake KL, Scaggs JE, England KR, et al. Benefits associated with a respiratory care assessment-treatment program: results of a pilot study. Respir Care 1994;39:715-724.

18. Walton JR, Shapiro BA, Harrison CH. Review of a bronchial hygiene evaluation program. Respir Care 1983;29:174-179.

19. Nielson-Tietsort J, Poole B, Creagh CE, et al. Respiratory care protocol: an approach to in-hospital respiratory therapy. Respir Care 1981;26:420-436.

20. Stoller JK, Haney D, Burkhart J, et al. Physician-ordered respiratory care vs physician-ordered use of a respiratory therapy consult service: early experience at the Cleveland Clinic Foundation. Respir Care 1993;38:1143-1154.

21. Torrington KG, Henderson CI. Perioperative respiratory therapy (PORT): a program of perioperative risk assessment and individualized postoperative care. Chest 1988;93:946-951.

22. Stoller JK, Michnicki I. Medical house staff impressions regarding the impact of a respiratory therapy consult service. Respir Care 1998;43:549-551.

23. Hess D. Clinical practice guidelines—valuable resources. NBRC Horizons Nov/Dec 1997;23:1,6.

24. Hess D. The AARC clinical practice guidelines. Respir Care 1991;36:1398-1401.

25. Brougher P. CPGs 1994: Where are we? Where have we been? Where are we going? Respir Care 1994;39:1146-1148.

26. Hess D. The AARC clinical practice guidelines. Respir Care 1991;36:1398-1401.

27. Hess D. Clinical practice guidelines: why, whence, and whither? Respir Care 1995;40:1264-1267.

28. Komara JJ Jr, Stoller JK. The impact of a postoperative oxygen therapy protocol on use of pulse oximetry and oxygen therapy. Respir Care 1995;40:1125-1129.

29. Orens DK. A manager's perspective on respiratory therapy consult services. Respir Care 1993;38:884-886.

30. McGinn P. Practice standards leading to premium reductions. AMA News Dec 1998;2:1,28.

31. Thompson RS, Kirz HL, Gold RA. Changes in physician behavior and cost savings associated with organizational recommendations on the use of routine chest x-rays and multichannel blood tests. Prev Med 1983;2:385-396.

32. Weber K, Milligan S. Conference summary: therapist-driven protocols: the state of the art. Respir Care 1994;39:746-756.

33. Thorens JB, Kaelin RM, Jolliet P, et al. Influence of the quality of nursing on the duration of weaning from mechanical ventilation in patients with chronic obstructive pulmonary disease. Crit Care Med 1995;23:1807-1815.

34. Ely EW, Bennett PA, Bowton DL, et al. Large scale implementation of a respiratory therapist-driven protocol for ventilator weaning. Am J Respir Crit Care Med 1999;159:439-446.

35. Clemmer TP, Spuhler VJ. Developing and gaining acceptance for patient care protocols. New Horiz 1998;6:12-19.

36. Mishoe SC. The effects of institutional context on critical thinking in the workplace. Proceedings of the 36th Annual Adult Education Research Conference. Edmonton, Alberta: University of Alberta; 1995; pp. 221-228.

37. Dykes PC, Wheeler K, editors. Planning, implementing and evaluating critical pathways: a guide for the 21st century. New York: Springer; 1997.

38. Coffey R, Richard J, Remmert C, et al. An introduction to critical paths. Qual Manag Health Care 1992;1:45-54.

39. Pearson SD, Goulart-Fisher D, Lee T. Critical pathways as a strategy for improving care: problems and potentials. Ann Intern Med 1995;123:941-948.

40. Hoffman PA. Critical path method. J Qual Improve June 1993:235-246.

41. Ignatavicius DD, Hausaman KA. Clinical pathways for collaborative practice. Philadelphia: WB Saunders; 1995.

42. Birdsall C, Sperry S. Clinical paths in medical-surgical practice. St Louis: Mosby; 1997.

43. Berger JT, Rosner F. The ethics of practice guidelines. Arch Intern Med 1996;156:2051-2056.

44. Schriefer J. Managing critical pathway variances. Qual Manag Health Care 1995;3:30-42.

45. Aronson B, Maljanian R. Critical path education: necessary components and effective strategies. J Cont Ed Nurs 1996;27:215-219.

46. Sackett DL, Rosenberg WMC, Gray MJA, et al. Evidence-based medicine: what it is and what it isn't. BMJ 1996;312:71-72.

47. Brown SJ. Knowledge for health care practice: a guide to using research evidence. Philadelphia: WB Saunders; 1999.

48. Sackett DL, Richardson WS, Rosenberg W, et al. Evidence-based medicine: how to practice and teach EBM. 2nd ed. New York: Churchill Livingstone; 2000.

49. Jones A. Second International Cochrane Colloquium—official annual meeting of the Cochrane Collaboration: a conference report. Respir Care 1995;40:171-174.

50. Ulschak FL, SnowAntle SM. Consultation skills for health care professionals: how to be an effective consultant within your organization. San Francisco: Jossey-Bass; 1990.

51. Stoller JK, Thaggard I, Piquette CA, et al. The impact of a respiratory therapy consult service on house officers knowledge of respiratory care ordering. Respir Care 2000;45:945-952.

52. Kollef MH. Medical trainee experience versus optimizing clinical outcomes: achieving the best of both. Respir Care 2000;45:938-939.

CHAPTER 8

Patient Education

William F. Galvin

OBJECTIVES

1. State the rationale for patient education in the practice of respiratory care.
2. Define patient education and related terms using several sources.
3. List the goals of patient education from the patient's perspective and that of the provider (respiratory therapy educator).
4. Identify the four major components of the patient education process.
5. Assess the learning needs of a patient.
6. Identify the factors that can adversely affect learner readiness.
7. Discuss the planning phase of the patient education process, specifically the development of goals and objectives, use of learning domains, content development, and evaluation.
8. Identify and explain the appropriate use of various teaching strategies in patient education.
9. Identify and discuss the nine basic principles of adult learning.
10. Discuss the evaluation phase of the patient education process, namely evaluation as a process and evaluation of individual learning.

KEY TERMS

Affective	Documentation	Patient Education Process
Assessment	Evaluation	PRECEDE-PROCEED Model
Audiovisual Aids	Guided Discussion	Prevention
Behavioral Contracting	Health Belief Model	Psychomotor
Behavior Modification	Health Promotion	Programmed Instruction
Client Education	Illness/Wellness Continuum	Self-Instructional
Clinical Practice Guidelines	Implementation	Teaching Moment
Cognitive	Locus of Control	Wellness
Consumer Education	Motivation	
Disease Prevention	Patient Education	

Patient education plays an important role in the delivery of health care. The goal of this chapter is to better prepare respiratory therapists to assist patients and caregivers in assuming an effective role in prevention, care, rehabilitation, and health promotion. The focus of the chapter is the increasing importance of self-care and the need to help patients develop the ability to care for themselves. Today's patients must be knowledgeable and self-sufficient; therefore health care providers must effectively transfer to them the necessary knowledge, skills, and attitudes.

The following sections provide an overview of all aspects of patient education. The areas addressed include definitions of patient education terminology; an explanation of the purpose, goals, objectives, and rationale for patient education; and a detailed discussion of the four major components of the **patient education process.** Emphasis is placed on assessment of a patient's needs and planning for instruction, identification and removal of barriers to teaching and learning, and acquisition of an understanding of the basic principles of adult learning.

Making the Case for Patient Education

Self-Management and Self-Empowerment

The traditional view of health care was rather paternalistic; the health care provider was considered the expert and the only one capable of determining the care and management of the patient. This provider, usually a physician, was considered to know what was best for patients, was solely responsible for making decisions, and did not share information with or involve patients in their own care or treatment except as recipients. Simply stated, the patient was outside the health care system and was not involved in the process. Patients were controlled by the experts, by the system.

Although much of the practice of medicine clearly is the responsibility of the health care expert, more contemporary thinking supports the idea that there are many stakeholders in the provision of health care. Perhaps the most crucial stakeholders are the patients themselves. Patients must be educated and equipped to assume greater control over their health and well-being. They must assume control rather than allow themselves to be controlled by others.

Forces Affecting the Patient Education Movement

Enabling patients to assume greater responsibility for their health care is a theme that has taken on increasing importance over the years. Patient education programs are the fastest growing component of the health care system. In 1970 about 50 hospitals in the United States had patient education programs; now almost all health care institutions engage in some form of patient education activity.[1] This increasing emphasis has been driven by economic, social, demographic, regulatory and legal, philosophic, and practical considerations (Box 8-1).

The current system clearly is driven by economic incentives to curtail costs and reduce a health care budget that is spiraling out of control. Health care expenditures have exceeded $1 trillion. More and more, costs and risk are being shifted to the consumer and from employers, insurers, and providers.

Demographic factors dictate that an increasing number of people, namely those of the baby boom generation, are approaching their retirement years, developing chronic, debilitating diseases that create significant health care needs. This places considerable economic tension on a health care delivery system that is already strained. The care and treatment of this elderly population will come from a variety of sources, among them informal caregivers, assisted living providers, and unskilled health care extenders. These new providers will require a more sophisticated understanding of the conditions and diseases affecting the elderly population.

From legislative and social perspectives, more emphasis is being placed on consumer education. The public is becoming better informed and is demanding more information about

---

Box 8-1

Rationale for Patient Education in Respiratory Care

Economic Incentive
Reimbursement requirements are shifting to an emphasis on more patient involvement and patient accountability.

Social Incentive
The consumer education movement and a well-informed public have demanded such education.

Demographic Incentive
With the "graying of America," the number of people requiring health care has risen, and the use of informal caregivers (families and friends) has increased.

Regulatory and Legal Incentives
Patient education is a requirement of the Joint Commission on Accreditation of Healthcare Organizations.

Philosophic Incentive
The wellness model of health care has become more popular compared with the traditional health care model, and self-management of one's own health has become an important issue.

Practical Incentives
Patients prefer to care for themselves, and it is more sensible and facile for them to participate in their own care.

the consequences of unhealthy lifestyle behaviors. Regulatory agencies, such as the Joint Commission on Accreditation of Healthcare Organizations (JCAHO), have established policies and requirements for patient education and have withheld accreditation for serious neglect of such programs.

Philosophically and practically, **disease prevention** and **health promotion** appear to be logical, cost-effective ways to curtail health care costs. Adoption of a disease prevention–health promotion philosophy helps instill in patients some degree of responsibility for and ownership of their health and **wellness.** Assuming individual responsibility for and having a greater degree of involvement in one's own health care is simply good medicine. Likewise, increasing the number of well-informed patients and caregivers goes a long way toward improving the efficiency and effectiveness of health care in the United States. With these points in mind, it seems only logical that effective patient education should be considered an integral component of the health care system.

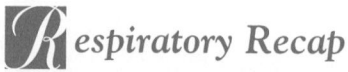
espiratory Recap

Roles of Respiratory Therapists in Patient Education	
Bedside clinician	Patient advocate
Diagnostician	Care coordinator
Technical expert	Counselor
Trouble-shooter	Patient educator

Role of the Respiratory Therapist

Bedside clinician, astute diagnostician, resourceful technical expert, and trouble-shooter are the well-established roles of the respiratory therapist. The more contemporary view includes the roles of patient advocate, care coordinator, counselor, and patient educator.

The role of patient educator has been often deemphasized, frequently misunderstood, seldom appreciated, and not uncommonly absent from the array of duties and responsibilities of today's respiratory therapist. However, as discussed previously, patient education is assuming new prominence and will be of paramount importance in future health care practice. Health care providers with sophisticated teaching skills and a savvy ability to assess patients' educational needs will be held in high esteem. Equally important will be the ability to develop educational goals, communicate accurately and effectively, and ensure that patients have an understanding of their disease and comply with treatment.

Respiratory therapists are considered the nonphysician experts in cardiorespiratory care. Their continual presence at the patient's bedside enables them to assume greater responsibility for effective patient education. Respiratory therapists must recognize that patient education is not a game of show-and-tell. It requires three important attributes: (1) savvy, sophisticated skills and knowledge of the

teaching and learning process; (2) an understanding of motivational theory and what makes people "tick"; and (3) an appreciation of the principles of adult learning. Respiratory therapists must develop a greater appreciation for the significant role they play in the patient education movement.

Definition of Terms

Client Education, Consumer Education, and Patient Education

Patient education is more than the provision of information about a disease or condition.[2] It also is more than simple identification of common signs and symptoms and explanations of therapeutic interventions. Patient education is a process[2] with succinct, discrete steps that must be followed to engage the patient effectively in the important function of self-management. Before embarking on this process, this discussion focuses on terminology, clarifies discrepancies, and provides working definitions of the key components of patient education.

A number of terms frequently are associated with patient education. Two particularly important ones are client education and consumer education. **Client education** has been defined as the use of the educational process for individuals who are partners in the health education effort.[3] Inherent in this definition is the notion that the teacher and learner work together to identify the issues to be taught and the manner in which the teaching is to be carried out. The term implies that the learner has some degree of autonomy and is self-directed.

The term **consumer education** is closely related to client education but differs in that it involves a person or a group of people who are independent decision makers; they identify the health learning need and initiate the learning process. The teacher facilitates the learning process.[3]

Patient education has been defined in a number of ways, and authors emphasize or highlight different components of their definitions. For example, one author defines it as the use of the educational process to aid individuals, their families, and other significant persons when they be-

espiratory Recap

Definitions Used in Patient Education
Client education: the use of the educational process to aid individuals who are partners in the health education effort
Consumer education: the use of the educational process by a person or a group of people who are independent decision makers
Patient education: the use of the educational process to aid individuals, their families, and other significant persons when they become dependent on the health care system for diagnosis, treatment, or rehabilitation

come dependent on the health care system for diagnosis, treatment, or rehabilitation.[3]

The three terms can be distinguished on the basis of the amount of teaching assistance learners require to make behavioral changes. As shown in Figure 8-1, consumers are highly independent and capable of exercising considerable self-responsibility, whereas patients are more dependent and require more teaching assistance; clients fall somewhere in between.

In both consumer and client education the health care provider or professional serves as a facilitator, assists in decision making, acts as a resource person, and gives encouragement and support to ideas the individual already has. In patient education the learner is highly dependent on the health care provider or professional and frequently has little if any knowledge of the content to be learned. In such situations the health care provider or professional may well need to direct the teaching process almost entirely.

Illness/Wellness Continuum

Another view of patient education is the **illness/wellness continuum** proposed by Travis and Ryan.[4] In this model, health is viewed both from a medical perspective and from a wellness perspective (Figure 8-2).

The left side of the continuum represents the medical model of health; it starts at the neutral point, the center of the continuum. The neutral point represents the absence of any physical disease, and at this point the individual is considered healthy. On moving to the left the individual is exposed to certain risks, which become signs and symptoms. If left untreated, they lead to disability and eventually premature death.

The entire continuum reflects a wellness model of health. It signifies that health is more than the absence of disease; rather, it is a state of high-level wellness over which the individual has considerable control. The person can choose to follow a lifestyle that incorporates health promotion and disease prevention principles and measures. The individual who adopts the wellness model would become knowledgeable about healthy lifestyle practices, would be sufficiently motivated to incorporate such practices into the daily routine, would use **behavior modification** techniques as needed, and ultimately would enjoy a higher level of wellness and well-being.

An example from respiratory disease may help clarify the importance of this continuum. The traditional view of health holds that the absence of disease exists at the neutral point. A man who begins smoking has moved to the left and incurred a risk factor for chronic obstructive pulmonary disease (COPD). Continued use of cigarettes could lead to increased production of mucus and shortness of breath (that is, the signs and symptoms of the disease—another move to the left). Continued and unabated use of cigarettes could lead to the man's inability to walk up a single flight of stairs, at which point he becomes a "pulmonary cripple," a disability, which is yet another move left. Progression of this process ultimately leads to premature death. Rather than living to age 72, the normal life expectancy of men in the United States, this man may die at age 60.

In contrast to this scenario, let's say the individual as a boy or young man is taught that smoking is harmful to his health. If he accepts this and is motivated to ban smoking from his lifestyle, along with following other healthy practices, he will attain a state of well-being and ultimately

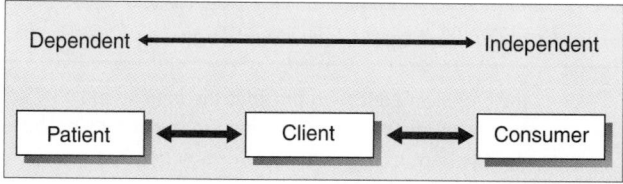

Figure 8-1 Level of learner dependency. (From Boyd MD, Graham B, Gleit C, et al. Health teaching in nursing practice: a professional model. 3rd ed. Stamford, Conn: Appleton & Lange; 1998.)

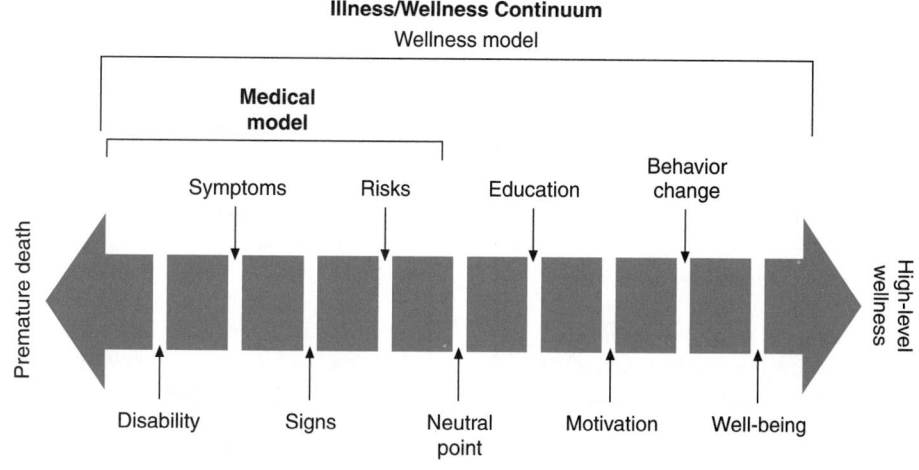

Figure 8-2 Illness/wellness continuum. (Modified from Travis JW, Ryan RS. The wellness workbook. Berkeley, Calif: Ten Speed Press; 1988. Illness/Wellness Continuum, copyright 1986, John W. Travis, MD.)

high-level wellness. Furthermore, he can benefit even after several years of smoking. If he is exposed to this teaching and accepts it, he may be motivated to eliminate this unhealthy behavior, and favorably influence his health. The critical step in the wellness model is education.

Respiratory Recap

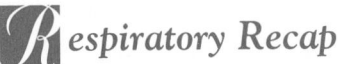

Wellness and Education
The critical step in the wellness model is education.

That patients be educated about their condition and about the ill effects of unhealthy lifestyle behaviors is vital. Effective patient education can go a long way toward effectively engaging the patient in self-management, fostering a healthy lifestyle, and addressing health concerns.

Clinical Practice Guidelines

The American Association for Respiratory Care (AARC) defines patient education through **clinical practice guidelines** (CPG 8-1 and CPG 8-2).[5,6] According to these guidelines, patient and caregiver training is a process initiated by the health care provider to help patients or caregivers acquire knowledge and skills that will help them understand the patient's medical condition and participate in its management. This training process should occur with every encounter.[5]

Teaching and Learning Aspects of Patient Education

Although patient education can be defined in numerous ways, it always entails teaching. Teaching, whether done formally or informally, is a process that facilitates learning. Learning is the process of acquiring new knowledge, skills, and attitudes, which are synthesized to bring about a change in an individual's behavior.[7] This change in behavior ultimately results in patients living longer and more productively.

CPG 8-1

Training the Health Care Professional for the Role of Patient and Caregiver Educator

- The process of training the health care professional as a patient or caregiver educator involves addressing and ensuring adequate knowledge, skills, and attitude mastery to allow both the development of patient rapport and effective teaching.
- The ultimate goal of the process is to provide patients and caregivers with an education that equips them with the knowledge, skills, and attitudes to better understand the patient's condition and participate more fully in health care.

Modified from AARC. Clinical practice guideline: training the health care professional for the role of patient and caregiver educator. Respir Care 1996;41:654-657.
CPG, Clinical practice guideline; AARC, American Association for Respiratory Care.

Respiratory Recap

Learning
Teaching facilitates learning. The foundation for learning is behavior change.

Unfortunately, too often health care providers think that "teaching" a patient or family member means telling them about the diagnosis and what can be done about it. Certainly, explaining the facts about a diagnosis is important, but it is not likely by itself to produce a change in the patient's behavior. Furthermore, this type of teaching generally is done hurriedly and at the convenience of the provider, not that of the patient or family members. Often little regard is shown for privacy or comprehension of the subject matter. The provider receives no assurance that learning has occurred.

Patient education should be viewed as a process, an orderly, sequential process, whether done in the formal setting of a classroom or in an informal manner at the bedside. Health care educators must rid themselves of the notion that

CPG 8-2

Providing Patient and Caregiver Training

- Patient and caregiver education provides the patient and family with the means of participating in the patient's health care management to the extent possible, depending on physical condition and awareness.
- The training process should occur with every encounter between the health care provider and the patient.
- The goal of the health care provider should be to elicit a positive change in the patient's or caregiver's behavior through the use of verbal, written, and visual communication in the affective, cognitive, and psychomotor domains. The coordinated efforts of health care providers should improve the patient's understanding of health-related needs, therapy, and the importance of adherence to the medical regimen and of candid communication with caregivers. These efforts should allow for better disease management through cooperation and creation of a partnership.
- Another goal of the health care educator is to provide the patient and family with the means to reap the economic benefits of improved use of the health care system.

Modified from AARC. Clinical practice guideline: providing patient and caregiver training. Respir Care 1996;41:658-663.
CPG, Clinical practice guideline; AARC, American Association for Respiratory Care.

simply informing patients of their disease and the appropriate therapeutic interventions is effective patient education. Effective patient education can occur only when learning has occurred, resulting in a change in the patient's behavior. For learning to occur, teaching must entail a logical set of steps.

Indications and Goals in Patient Education

Goals of the Patient and Provider

Although the indications for patient education are rather obvious and clear-cut, the goals should be considered from two distinct perspectives—those of the patient or informal caregiver and those of the health care professional. The caregiver usually is a person who plays a crucial role in the patient's life; this often is a family member or significant other, although the caregiver may not be legally related to the patient.[5] Important to note is that in most cases caregivers are not health care professionals; they usually are lay people who are genuinely interested in the patient's health and well-being but who do not have a sophisticated understanding of the patient's disease or condition. The health care professional, on the other hand, does have an extensive knowledge of the particular health condition and has established some degree of competence in providing health care. The goals of these participants are different.

The goals of the patient and caregiver are to (1) obtain accurate information about the condition, (2) develop the ability to make appropriate health decisions, (3) learn skills and attitudes that foster self-care and appropriate use of health services, and (4) alleviate anxiety and increase satisfaction with health matters and health care.[7]

The goals of the health care provider or professional are to (1) provide more effective and efficient health care, (2) improve patient compliance, (3) increase the patient's satisfaction with health care, (4) obtain informed consent when necessary, and (5) meet professional practice requirements.[7]

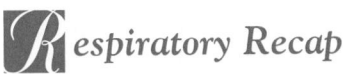

Goals of the Patient or Informal Caregiver

To obtain accurate information about the patient's condition
To develop the ability to make appropriate health decisions
To learn skills and attitudes that foster self-care and appropriate use of health services
To alleviate anxiety and increase satisfaction in health matters and health care

These two sets of goals work together toward the ultimate goal of the patient education process, that is, to equip the patient and caregiver with the knowledge, skills, and attitudes to better understand the patient's condition and to more fully participate in health care.[6] Teaching therefore is intended to foster change in the patient's adaptation to illness; it is a planned activity that is individualized to the learner's abilities, needs, resources, and support systems.[8]

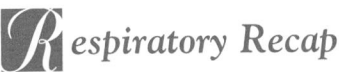

Goals of the Health Care Provider

To provide more effective and efficient health care
To improve the patient's compliance with the therapeutic regimen
To increase the patient's satisfaction with health care
To obtain informed consent when necessary
To fulfill professional practice requirements

Process of Patient Education

Most resource materials on patient education describe it as a process. The parts vary somewhat, but most sources noted four major components—assessment, planning, implementation, and evaluation. The acronym "A PIE" can be used as a mnemonic to better recall these four elements.

Overview: 'A PIE'

Assessment is the process of collecting information to help plan and implement teaching activities. The health care provider must assess both the need for patient education and the readiness of the patient, or learner, to benefit from it. Assessment requires extensive collection of data, including information about (1) the learner's readiness and ability to learn, (2) the learner's current knowledge of the subject, (3) what the learner wants to know about subject, (4) any incorrect information or misconceptions the learner may have, and (5) the educational needs of both the learner and the family.[8]

Planning is the next step in the process and involves construction of an individualized patient education program. Planning involves identification of goals, development of objectives, addressing of the learning domains, and creation, development, and refining of the information to be covered.

Implementation is the third major component. It is the actual process of teaching and requires the use of a variety of teaching methods and tools.

Evaluation, the last of the four major components, enables the teacher to determine whether learning has occurred. It basically is a feedback loop set up by the method of evaluation developed during the planning stage.

Box 8-2 presents a more detailed outline of the four components and specific steps involved in each.

The way in which the process is used varies from practitioner to practitioner, and seldom does an orderly, sequential flow come about. In their zeal to jump in and get started, respiratory therapy educators often skip from one component to another. More often than not the assessment component is overlooked, and the educator consequently becomes frustrated and discouraged when

BOX 8-2

Major Components of the Patient Education Process

Assessment
    Assess the need for patient education
    Assess the readiness of the learner for patient education.

Planning
    Establish goals and objectives.
    Determine use of learning domains (cognitive, psychomotor, and affective).
    Select content.

Implementation
    Choose teaching methods.
    Establish types of learning.

Ensure therapeutic use of time.
Determine learning needs of staff members.

Evaluation
    Evaluate patient education process.
    Evaluate individual learning.
        Written tests
        Teaching checklist
        Oral questioning
        Observational checklist
        Documentation
        Interdisciplinary patient education/family education record

Respiratory Recap

Major Components of the Patient Education Process	
Assessment	Implementation
Planning	Evaluation

obstacles to learning are uncovered later in the process. Gross errors in the practice of patient education occur with some regularity. One author noted that such errors probably are made in the following order: omission of assessment of the patient's need to learn, followed by omission of a particular step (for example, assessment of readiness, setting of goals, or systematic evaluation of learning).[1] The actual implementation component rarely is omitted.

Completion of each component is critical to successful and effective patient education. The respiratory care educator should resist the temptation to take immediate action without proper assessment, planning, and evaluation and should be vigilant in thoroughly addressing each step.

Assessment

No reputable physician would prescribe a therapeutic intervention before performing a thorough diagnostic evaluation. Equally important is that the respiratory therapy educator assesses the patient's educational needs before launching into a detailed and elaborate discussion of the disease and its treatment. Assessment, the first component of the patient education process, addresses two distinct issues—the need for patient education and the patient's readiness to learn.

Assessment of the need for patient education is directed at identification of the specific content to be covered in the teaching process. Need identification can be complicated because the educator must distinguish between a real educational need and a "felt" need, something the person or persons concerned regard as necessary. A real educational need refers to a lack of specific knowledge, skills, and attitudes that the patient needs to attain a more desirable condition.[7] A real educational need is one that can be met by means of a learning experience. In other words the patient must have a deficit in understanding, performance, or feelings about the health condition, testing, procedures, treatment, or prognosis. The assessment process addresses these issues, and the information derived helps in the planning and development of the lesson plan and learning objectives.

Assessment can be accomplished through direct questioning of the patient, consultation with family members, collaboration with other health care professionals, and review of medical records and patient information sources. Conferring directly with the patient or a family member is a technique that should not be taken lightly because many variables influence the communication process.

The educator must assess the deficits in the patient's understanding of the disease and its manifestations, progression, and resolution, a process best done systematically with some type of standardized document. Box 8-3 presents a list of questions that could be used in the patient assessment process. The list is fairly extensive, yet additional questioning may be necessary and appropriate, depending on the patient's disease or condition.

A standardized document also could be used to assess the educator's capabilities and limitations. The sample rating form for a patient education session shown in Figure 8-3 identifies some critical points used to evaluate the respiratory therapist as a patient educator. Parts one, five, and six list some of the key factors to be addressed during the opening interview and the use of appropriate counseling techniques. Parts two, three, and four focus on the educator's assessment of the patient's awareness and understanding of the medical condition.

Box 8-3

Common Assessment Questions

1. Do you understand the symptomatology?
2. How did you first respond to the symptomatology?
3. Why do you think these symptoms have occurred?
4. Are you aware of any previous illness or conditions?
5. Are you aware of any family history or previous illnesses?
6. Are you aware of the correlation among symptoms and various laboratory, radiographic, and diagnostic tests?
7. What is your psychologic state with regard to this condition?
8. How do you typically respond to exacerbations of this condition?
9. How has your illness affected family and friends?
10. Have you been provided with previous education about this condition? If so, by whom?
11. Have you responded to suggestions and recommended treatments?
12. What are your social habits?
13. Do you smoke?
14. Do you drink alcohol? If so, how much? How often?
15. Has your condition affected your employment?
16. Can you read and write?
17. What is your highest level of education?
18. Do you understand the illness and its treatment?
19. Is English the primary language spoken in your home?
20. Are your beliefs or practices affected by any particular cultural influences?
21. Do you have adequate medical coverage?

If the patient is too young or is unable to answer any or all of these questions, the caregiver may provide the answers.

Directions: Rate the patient educator's performance in each of the following areas. Using the scale below, place the appropriate number in the space next to each item. Comments and suggestions should be noted to allow for improvement where necessary.

Weak <- -> Outstanding

| 1 | 2 | 3 | 4 | 5 | 6 | 7 | 8 | 9 | 10 |

1. Opening of the interview
   - Ability to put the patient at ease
   - Use of social amenities
   - Use of eye contact
   - Professional demeanor
   - Layout of plan
2. Discussion of disease
   - Assessment of what patient wants
   - Assessment of patient's attitudes/feelings
   - Reporting of laboratory findings
   - Explanation of pathophysiology
   - Use of vocabulary appropriate to patient
   - Correctness of information
   - Assessment of patient's final understanding
3. Treatment
   - Presentation of complete plan
   - Presentation of treatment goals
   - Explanation of side effects/complications
   - Treatment individualized to patient
   - Assessment of patient compliance
   - Correctness of information
   - Assessment of patient's final understanding
4. Assessment of patient's understanding of disease and condition
   - Assessment of patient's overall understanding of disease and treatment
   - Assessment of patient's attitudes
   - Time allowed for questions
   - Flexibility in presentation

5. Appropriate use of counseling techniques
   - Attempts to clarify patient's statement
   - Reassurance and empathy
   - Appropriate use of silence
   - Appropriate vocabulary
   - Use of open-ended questions
   - Facilitation of behavior
   - Use of notes
   - Use of educational aids
   - Flexibility
   - Good use of probes
   - Good transitions
   - Appropriate pacing
   - Good use of summaries
   - Overall physical appearance
   - Nonverbal language
   - Appropriate use of patient's background
   - Clarification of the next step for patient
   - Request for questions
6. Overall effectiveness of patient counseling
   - Rapport building
   - Discussion of disease
   - Treatment program
   - Assessment of patient's understanding of disease and treatment
   - Use of counseling techniques
7. Comments and suggestions for improvement:

Figure 8-3   Sample rating form for patient education session. (From Muma RD, Lyons BA, Newman T, et al. Patient education: a practical approach. Stamford, Conn: Appleton & Lange; 1996.)

In discussing the issues on this checklist with the patient, the educator essentially is covering the presenting signs and symptoms; the patient's health history; the physical assessment; laboratory, radiographic, and diagnostic tests; evidence of any previous patient education; evidence of compliance or noncompliance; and the patient's sociocultural and economic status. This checklist is quite useful to assess the performance of the respiratory therapy patient educator, but more detailed evaluation points could be added.

Any program, survey, checklist, or questionnaire that helps the respiratory therapy educator perform a thorough assessment is a valuable tool; omitting this first and crucial step can be catastrophic. A thorough assessment prevents backpedaling during the implementation phase, contributes to the development of an effective action plan, and aids the effort to have patients assume responsibility for their care.

Readiness to Learn   Assessing the patient's readiness to learn can be a bit tricky. Some patients may mask their denial of the need for education and training or their unwillingness to accept it. Other patients may be willing but physically or mentally incapable of learning. The educator's time limitations may compound these problems. Factors that can adversely affect learner readiness are lack of awareness of the diagnosis, previous knowledge and experience of the disease, intellectual ability, motivational level, physical condition, psychologic state, and lack of a perceived need to learn.[2] Other experts have identified similar problems of the learner, including lack of readiness, physical obstacles, emotional obstacles, language barriers, and lack of motivation.[8]

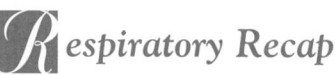

Respiratory Recap

Factors that Adversely Affect Learner Readiness
Lack of awareness of the diagnosis
Previous knowledge and experience of the disease
Intellectual ability
Motivational level
Physical condition
Psychologic state
Lack of a perceived need to learn

Patients must always be assessed to determine what they know about their condition. Health care educators should not assume that patients understand the nature of their disease. For example, patients with COPD often simply say that they have something wrong with their lungs. They may or may not fully understand the source and extent of their condition. A wise health care educator always starts with an open-ended question that allows patients to state what they know about the illness. Such a question might be, "What have you been told about your illness?"

The educator also should question patients closely about any previous knowledge or experience with the illness or condition. The educator might ask, "Did any family members have a similar problem? What do you remember about their experiences? Were they able to work? Were they hospitalized frequently? Were they severely debilitated?" These factors are likely to have influenced the way the patient views the condition and the way in which he or she deals with it.

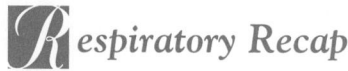

Respiratory Recap

Common Problems of the Learner
Lack of readiness
Physical obstacles
Emotional obstacles
Language barriers
Lack of motivation

The respiratory therapy educator also should take into account the patient's intellectual level, which affects the ability to comprehend the illness and determines the teaching approach. A plumber with COPD who needs frequent suctioning might be more responsive if the situation is compared to the clogging of a pipe with the resultant drainage problem and obstruction of water flow. Asking a family member to breathe through a straw for a minute or so can be quite effective in having that person live the experience of severe bronchoconstriction. Most people do not understand the complicated jargon used to describe medical conditions; therefore the teaching approach must match the patient's intellectual level.

Locus of Control   Educators also should determine whether patients are interested in changing any undesirable behaviors associated with their condition. Are they motivated to learn the best ways to deal with the condition? If so, what provides that **motivation?** For patients who want to quit smoking, is it because they want to prolong life, save money, see their grandchildren, or increase their physical activities (or all of those)? Is their motivation internal or external? Do they feel they have control over their actions, or do they believe they are helpless creatures of society? These questions get at the issue of **locus of control** and reflect whether patients are willing to assume responsibility for their actions.

Many people are of the mindset that their condition is the result of fate or happenstance. They believe that they are literally at the mercy of others, of the environment, of the system. These people have an external locus of control.

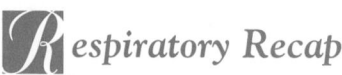

Respiratory Recap

Health Belief Model of Intrinsic Motivation
Disease prevention and action-taking depend on a person's perception of the following factors:
The person's level of susceptibility to the condition
The severity of the consequences of developing the condition
The possible benefits of the health action in preventing or reducing susceptibility
Barriers or costs related to starting or continuing the proposed behavior

They may make little effort to watch their salt intake, for example, because they believe that there is nothing they can do about the condition or that they can indulge in an unhealthy practice and simply take the magic pill. They may not have an interest in preventing the problem or practicing healthy lifestyle behaviors. These individuals simply do not take ownership of their conditions, and they feel that they can do little to influence it. Individuals with an internal locus of control believe they can direct their destiny; they therefore are more likely to assume responsibility for their actions and comply with recommended treatments and interventions. This concept obviously is centered on the notion of self-care, and a number of health models deal with the issue.

Health Models   One of the more frequently cited theories of intrinsic motivation is the **health belief model.** This model proposes that **prevention** of disease and action-taking depends on a person's perception of four issues: the person's level of susceptibility to the condition, the severity of the consequences of developing the condition, the possible benefits of the health action in preventing or reducing susceptibility, and the barriers or costs related to starting or continuing the proposed behavior.[3]

An equally popular health model that deals more with planning and focuses on extrinsic motivation is the **PRECEDE-PROCEED model.**[9] The acronym *PRECEDE* stands for predisposing, reinforcing, and enabling constructs in educational/environmental diagnosis and evaluation. *PROCEED* stands for policy, regulatory, and organizational constructs in educational and environmental development. This model, which is widely used in health promotion, focuses on factors external to the individual that shape health care behavior.

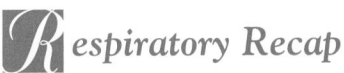

espiratory Recap

PRECEDE-PROCEED Model	
PRECEDE	**PROCEED**
• **P**redisposing	• **P**olicy
• **R**einforcing	• **R**egulatory
• **E**nabling	• **O**rganizational
• **C**onstructs	• **C**onstructs
• **E**ducational/environmental	• **E**ducational
• **D**iagnosis	• **E**nvironmental
• **E**valuation	• **D**evelopment

A person's physical or psychologic state also can have a major bearing on readiness to learn. Many patients are simply too sick to engage in any meaningful patient education or training. The respiratory therapy educator may have every good intention to inform, train, and educate, but patients may be too ill to absorb what is being said. They may be in pain, groggy from sedation, or just too weak or too tired. The educator must be adept at recognizing such situations and postpone intervention to a more appropriate time.

A mix of emotions also is likely to be a factor. Such feelings could include anxiety, fear, anger, or depression, or all of these. With such a patient state of mind, attempts to teach may be met with rejection or hostility. The respiratory therapy educator must be astute at recognizing a need to learn. If the patient is unreceptive to the need to learn, any attempt to educate will fail. Simply stated, the patient must want to learn.

In short, readiness to learn depends on three major factors: an aroused interest or motivation, relevant preparatory training, and physiologic maturity.[10] Respiratory therapy educators must not only be experts on the subject matter, they also must be able to "read" the patient effectively and follow the subtle cues provided to ensure that the patient learns.

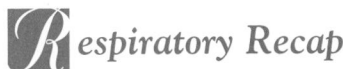

espiratory Recap

Assessment of Readiness to Learn
An aroused interest or motivation Relevant preparatory training Physiologic maturity

Planning

After assessing the need for patient education and determining the individual's readiness to learn, the respiratory therapy educator can move on to planning, the second phase of the patient education process. Planning involves establishment of goals or learning outcomes and crafting of more specific learning objectives. It also requires an understanding and appropriate use of learning domains, the development of content and subject matter, and preliminary design and development of evaluation strategies. Although evaluation is the final major step in the patient education process, its framework should be developed earlier. The planning phase is an appropriate starting point for this step, and soliciting feedback from the patient and family members during the planning phase ensures harmony among all parties.

Goals   Goals are general statements of the expected outcomes of the teaching and learning process. The expected learning outcomes are tied to the real educational need identified during the assessment phase. The goal statement must center on the learner. Each learning goal should be tailor-made for the individual patient. Also important is that the patient and family members participate in the process of goal establishment. This collaboration promotes cooperation and "buying in" from all parties and is more likely to produce the desired change in behavior

TABLE 8-1

ABCD's of Objective Development

Acronym Letter	Word	Definition	Meaning
A	Audience	The "who"	Patient, family member, or informal caregiver
B	Behavior	The "what"	Action to be achieved
C	Condition	The "givens"	Any condition that must be present or met for the objective to be completed correctly (possibly also entailing timelines)
D	Degree	How well/by when	Degree to which the action or task must be done

Modified from Boyd M, Graham B, Gleit C, et al. Teaching in nursing practice: a professional model. 3rd ed. Stamford, Conn: Appleton & Lange; 1998.

BOX 8-4

Example of a Goal

> The goal of the National Asthma Education and Prevention Program is to prepare guidelines for the diagnosis and management of asthma.

From Department of Health and Human Services (US), National Institutes of Health (NIH), National Heart, Lung, and Blood Institute. Practical guide for the diagnosis and management of asthma. NIH Pub No 97-4053. Bethesda, Md: The Institutes; October 1997.

that drives the patient education activity. Goals give direction to the teaching and learning process. Box 8-4 presents an example of a goal.

Objectives   Objectives are stated more specifically than goals and allow for fine-tuning; they are smaller steps along the path to goal achievement.

'SMART' Objectives   A good objective can be characterized as "SMART": **s**pecific, **m**easurable, **a**ttainable, **r**elevant, and having **t**imelines.

General statements, such as "I will lose weight," are far too vague and should be avoided. Much better is the specification of an actual value, such as "I will lose 10 pounds."

Measurability is important because it allows the educator to determine whether the objective has been reached, and attainability ensures that the objective is reasonable and possible. Losing 30 pounds in one week is hardly likely, let alone healthy or desirable.

Relevancy simply means that the objective must relate to the goal. For example, losing weight and quitting smoking are two separate behaviors, even though a person may

gain weight after quitting smoking. These are distinct behaviors and should be approached separately.

Timelines are an important part of an objective because they establish closure or an end point to the process.

ABCD's of Objectives   In addition to characteristics, a well-written objective has elements. These elements can be expressed as the ABCD's of objective development (Table 8-1).[3]

A stands for audience and should reflect the "who" in the objective. The audience is the patient, the family member, or the informal caregiver. *B* is the behavior and signifies the "what," or the action to be achieved. An action word (for example, *list, explain, apply, perform,* or *express*) is the hallmark of this part of the objective. C stands for condition, which means any specific condition that must be present or met to complete the objective correctly. This part of the objective might be stated with phrases such as *after gathering the appropriate equipment, after viewing the tape,* or *from the handouts provided.* Conditions also could involve timelines in a phrase *at the end of the teaching session* or *by the end of the semester.* D stands for degree of performance or accuracy. It states how well the action or task is to be done, with phrases such as *with 100% accuracy, as specified in the policy and procedure manual,* or *identify at least three indications.* Table 8-2 presents an example of an objective segmented according to the four elements listed.

Learning Domains   The respiratory therapy educator must be familiar with the three learning domains: **cognitive, psychomotor,** and **affective.**

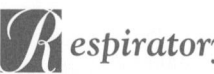 espiratory Recap

The Three Learning Domains
Cognitive = Knowing
Psychomotor = Doing
Affective = Feeling

The cognitive domain involves *knowing*, the psychomotor domain involves *doing*, and the affective domain involves *feeling*. When planning an individualized patient education program, the educator must consider us-

$\mathcal{R}$ espiratory Recap

'SMART' Objectives
Specific
Measurable
Attainable
Relevant
Timeline

TABLE 8-2

Use of the ABCD's of Objective Development

A Who	B What	C Under What Condition	D How Well/By When
John Doe	Will administer the medication in his metered dose inhaler (MDI)	After correctly assembling the device	By following all steps identified in the patient education packet; taking the medication twice daily

Modified from Boyd M, Graham B, Gleit C, et al. Teaching in nursing practice: a professional model. 3rd ed. Stamford, Conn: Appleton & Lange; 1998.

ing learning objectives from each of these three domains to obtain the desired learning outcome. For example, an asthma education program clearly entails the use of all three domains. In teaching the patient about the signs, symptoms, pathophysiology, mechanism of action of medications, and adverse effects of the asthmatic condition, the respiratory therapy educator might best establish objectives that fall into the cognitive domain, because this is largely information that the patient must *know.*

When teaching the use of a metered dose inhaler (MDI), the educator is using the psychomotor domain and therefore should develop objectives that engage the patient in the actual performance of the maneuver; the patient must *do.*

Finally, when a family member is asked to show compassion, patience, or understanding for what the patient is experiencing, that person is exhibiting an affective quality, expressing *feelings.* Many patient educators are somewhat uncomfortable in dealing with the affective domain because it focuses on values, attitudes, and emotions. Although such issues are difficult to discuss, the key to writing affective objectives is to focus on measurable behaviors. For example, the educator can observe a person placing a hand on the patient's shoulder in an attempt to console and comfort; such a display represents affective behavior and is clearly measurable.

Content and Subject Matter

Obviously, content and subject matter vary according to the topic. A vast amount of material is available on almost every cardiorespiratory condition. The respiratory therapy educator should focus on the goals and objectives already determined and develop the specific content from these points. Programs such as "Open Airways,"[11] which was developed by the American Lung Association, and "Guidelines for the Diagnosis and Management of Asthma,"[12] written by a panel of experts under the guidance of the National Institutes of Health, are excellent models used to plan and identify the detailed content of a patient education program.

Implementation

The third phase of the patient education process is implementation. In this phase, respiratory therapy educators can "roll up their sleeves" and get down to the business of

putting the teaching plan into action. However, as mentioned previously, the educator should not jump in too quickly; simply providing an explanation of the disease and its treatment does not constitute effective patient education or ensure understanding and compliance. Various teaching and learning strategies should be considered, and sending the message does not ensure reception, let alone understanding or adherence to the treatment plan.

Implementation of a teaching plan requires a dynamic, interactive encounter between the respiratory therapy educator and the patient, family member, or caregiver. Numerous techniques can be used. Some of the more popular ones are the lecture, the modified lecture or guided discussion, the demonstration, use of printed materials, case studies or simulations, role playing, problem solving, self-instructional materials or programmed instruction, drills, and behavioral contracting. Combining techniques could have a synergistic effect that can enhance the learning process.

Respiratory Recap

Teaching Strategies for Patient Education

Lecture	Problem solving
Modified lecture (guided discussion)	Self-instructional materials and programmed instruction
Demonstration	
Printed materials	Drills
Case studies or simulations	Behavioral contracting
Role playing	

Teaching Techniques

Lecture Perhaps the single most popular teaching method is the lecture, which is also referred to as simply "talking to" or "talking at" the patient. The advantages of such an approach are that (1) a considerable amount of material can be presented at one time, (2) the presentation time can be controlled to the minute, (3) many instructors can be used, (4) topics can be specialized, (5) additional questions and discussion can be elicited, and (6) a certain degree of spontaneity and instantaneous modification of the subject matter can occur. Disadvantages include (1) the potential for passivity on the part of the audience or recipient, (2) the need for preparation on the part of the presenter, (3) the need to avoid a lengthy, preachy approach that can result in boredom and resentment, and (4) the risk that the patient simply will not use the information provided. The respiratory therapy educator must be astute in identifying problems and modifying this approach to better engage the patient in the learning process.

Demonstration   Another popular approach is the demonstration. Demonstrations allow the patient both to see and to hear the necessary information. More important, demonstrations allow the patient to engage in more active learning. Information can be provided simultaneously, and discussion and questioning can be enhanced.

Demonstrations can be more time consuming and resource dependent than lectures. They should follow a planned sequence, and dividing the tasks into smaller components generally results in a more successful encounter.

Of considerable importance is the return demonstration, which requires the learner to repeat for the instructor predetermined steps essential to the proper performance of the procedure in question. Demonstration should be followed by practice and skill refinement. Frequent repetition of the procedure, coupled with remediation and feedback, leads to a higher degree of competency.

Printed Materials   The use of printed materials—in the form of books, pamphlets, brochures, or handouts—is an especially effective teaching strategy. The use of such materials is especially valuable when the respiratory therapy educator has a limited amount of time. Printed materials can address a wide variety of topics and at a variety of reading levels. They also can serve as reinforcement for other teaching strategies. The limitations of printed materials lie in the reading level and ability of the patient and in the expense, lack of social contact and interaction between the educator and patient, and need to evaluate the huge amount of material available.

Case Studies, Role Playing, and Problem Solving   Although they are used less often, case studies, role playing, and problem solving all have a place in patient edu-

cation. They generally are effective in urging patients to think critically about problems and situations that could arise because of their condition. These techniques are inexpensive, usually take little time to implement, and require direct interaction with others. **Self-instructional** materials and **programmed instruction** allow patients to learn at their own pace, are helpful in clarifying complex issues, and require little time on the part of the instructor. Many provide direct feedback and reinforcement of critical material. Their limitations are that they require a motivated, disciplined patient; can be boring; may require resources; and are extremely impersonal.

Drills   Drills are valuable in that they are a quick way to learn sequences of a required skill or procedure, allow for repetition and reinforcement of tasks, and generally break down the specific elements of a task into separate elements. The disadvantages are that they require a high degree of patient cooperation and may require the continual presence of additional resources and equipment.

Behavioral Contracting   **Behavioral contracting** is a highly accountable technique. It can create a higher level of responsibility and call on the patient's integrity and autonomy. It has an added advantage of identifying expectations up front and creating a strong alliance between patient and instructor. However, some patients might refuse to use this technique or may be reluctant to assume responsibility for behavior change.

Aligning Teaching Strategies and Learning Domains

The respiratory therapy educator should make an effort to identify the teaching strategies that might be more effective for a particular learning domain. For example, if the educator is attempting to teach a cognitive objective, the compatible teaching strategies would be the lecture, **guided discussion, audiovisual aids,** and printed materials, or a combination of these techniques. Table 8-3 matches the learning domain of the objective with teaching methodologies.[7]

Common Problems of the Provider   Like patients, educators face obstacles in the teaching and learning process (Box 8-5). One of the more important problems, inadequate assessment, can arise for a number of reasons. It may be as simple as a burning desire on the part of ed-

*T*ABLE 8-3

Choosing a Teaching Method

Learning Domain	Teaching Method of Choice
Cognitive	Lecture
	Guided discussion
	Audiovisual aids
	Printed materials
Psychomotor	Demonstration
	Drills
	Instructional guide
Affective	Group discussion
	Role playing
	Case study or simulation

Modified from Chatham MAH, Knapp BL. Patient education handbook. Bowie, Md: Robert J Brady; 1982.

*B*OX 8-5

Common Problems of the Provider

Inadequate assessment
Cost limitations
Inadequate support
Time limitations
Environmental limitations
Sociocultural differences between teacher and learner
Inadequate evaluation

Modified from Bopp A, Lubkin I. Chronic illness: impact and interventions. 2nd ed. Boston: Jones & Bartlett; 1990.

ucators to jump in and get started without acquainting themselves with patient or family conditions. Clinicians often assume that they know what is best for the patient and what needs to be taught. They fail to individualize the teaching program and center it on the specific needs of the patient. They may overlook social or environmental issues, such as a broken family or cramped living conditions in the home. They may use poor communication skills or poor observational techniques and miss important information. The value of a thorough, complete assessment can not be overstated. Vigilance in this first step is essential and goes a long way toward prevention of later problems.

Another problem cited by respiratory therapy educators is the financial limitations imposed by the institution, a form of inadequate support. A number of health care administrators and decision makers consider patient education a nonessential or at least less essential health care service. However, the JCAHO and the consumer movement do not concur. Managed care organizations are demanding better patient outcomes. Patient education has been cited as a means to increase patient compliance and to reduce costs, the length of the hospital stay, and the need for more expensive acute care. The JCAHO has developed standards that require patient education in all health care institutions; most institutions designate a department to ensure that the requirements are met. These mandates and the emergence of a savvier health care consumer likely will change the perception of patient education in the future and promote more widespread acceptance.

Environmental limitations, sociocultural differences, and inadequate evaluation are related to the educator's ability to function successfully as a teacher. Environmental limitations involve issues such as privacy, room temperature, lighting, noise, and distractions. Privacy can be dealt with if the educator shows sensitivity and awareness. Patients are not likely to share their innermost thoughts without some degree of privacy, confidence, and confidentiality. Sociocultural differences also must be recognized and require a caring, nonjudgmental demeanor on the part of the educator. Inadequate evaluation is always a concern because patient educators must be astute enough in their observations to note nonverbal and verbal cues that indicate the patient does not understand or accept the material.

Perhaps the most frequently cited problem of patient educators is the serious time limitation imposed by the high treatment load expected of health care providers. This is a recurrent theme and a product of the times. Health care administrators are constantly reminding their workforce of the need to "do more with less." Direct patient care will always win out over education, but greater appreciation is needed for the value of effective patient teaching. A strong argument can be made that effective patient education is cost effective because a well-informed, motivated patient places fewer demands on the health care system, especially with emergency room visits. Ultimately, patient education can curtail the use of health care services and reduce health care costs.

Levels of Patient Education   When the respiratory therapy educator is faced with the problem of time limitations, the teaching plan can be modified according to the three levels of education (Table 8-4).[13]

Level 1 education is used in cases in which the educator is informed that the patient is leaving in 2 hours and must be educated about the condition. In such cases the teaching method is limited to literature in the form of a well-written fact sheet. This fact sheet must be written in language comfortable for the patient, and the educator must read it in advance so as to circle or highlight key points and address questions before the patient is discharged.

Level 2 education is used when the educator has a few days to accomplish the teaching plan. It involves literature and reinforcement of the written material by some other means, such as a videotape. Educators should preview such material so that they or other members of the health care team can highlight key points and follow up with a discussion of the material.

Level 3 education is used when the educator has considerable time for the program. This optimal situation allows for the incorporation of all four major components of the patient education process. Level 3 education includes a counseling role and is more likely to result in a successful intervention.

Principles of Adult Learning   The basic principles of adult learning are important elements of any patient

TABLE 8-4

Levels of Patient Education

Level	Time Constraints	Teaching Method
1	Only a few hours available before patient is discharged	Provide literature, fact sheets, and teaching guides and discuss with patient to the extent possible
2	A few days available for teaching	Provide literature and reinforce with an instructional videotape
3	A considerable amount of time available for teaching	Use four-step process (assess, plan, implement, and evaluate) Use counseling skills (active listening, coaching, clarifying, summarizing)

Modified from Winthrop E. Patient teaching tips. St Louis: Mosby; 1995.

teaching program. Numerous courses, books, and articles have been written on this topic, but a useful and meaningful delineation has been provided by Kroehnert,[14] who uses the mnemonic "RAMP-2-FAME" to represent nine critical principles of adult learning.

R stands for recency, which means that the principles or concepts taught last are most likely to be remembered best. This stems from human beings' tendency to remember material that was addressed most recently. The implication for respiratory therapy educators is that they should plant important information in the patient's mind before leaving the room. Keeping sessions short and summarizing often helps the patient remember essential information.

*R*espiratory Recap

Principles of Adult Learning: RAMP-2-FAME
R = Recency
A = Appropriateness
M = Motivation
P = Primacy
2 = 2-Way communication
F = Feedback
A = Active learning
M = Multiple-sense learning
E = Exercise

The second letter in the mnemonic, *A*, stands for appropriateness and signifies that learners engage in the learning process only if the material presented has meaning and relevance for their needs. Explaining the biochemistry of leukotriene inhibitors in the discussion of medication for the treatment of airway obstruction would be inappropriate and futile. Equally inappropriate would be a discussion of detailed respiratory anatomy, such as the pores of Kohn. A more appropriate discussion would be to explain the inflammatory reaction as being similar to a sunburn or to describe bronchoconstriction as similar to breathing through a narrow straw. Such everyday examples have more meaning and more relevance. They are more likely to be received favorably.

The *M* stands for motivation. Patients must be moved to take action; they must want to learn. Imparting a sense of urgency or a strong need to learn the subject matter can create this motivation. For example, a parent whose child recently experienced a serious asthmatic attack while playing soccer would be greatly motivated to learn the correct use of the child's MDI. Patient educators must find the motivating factors and push those buttons to get the point across and engage the patient or family member in patient education.

The fourth letter, *P*, stands for primacy, meaning that the information the patient learns first is usually learned best. Primacy gets at the issue of first impressions and the need to deliver the most important information first. More often than not, the respiratory therapy educator has a receptive audience at the first meeting with the patient because the patient is curious about what the educator has to say. This is a golden opportunity for educators to put their best foot forward and make their case.

The numeral *2* in the mnemonic signifies the need for two-way communication. The conversation should be *with*, not *at* the patient. Interaction should be encouraged.

The *F* stands for feedback, which should be given both to the patient and to the educator. People simply need to know how they are doing. Feedback provides the opportunity for both parties to validate their roles and their understanding of the interaction.

The second *A* stands for active learning, which entails participation in the learning process. This point is extremely important because patient passivity progresses to boredom, loss of concentration, and ultimately, very little learning.

The second *M* stands for multiple-sense learning, one of the most important points. Whenever another sense is brought into the learning process, the amount of material that will be remembered has been suggested to double. People learn in different ways, and educators should use as many different techniques as possible. Although explaining a procedure to patients may be effective, showing them a picture and letting them touch or handle the equipment adds considerable value to the learning experience; it clearly results in a heightened sense of understanding and ultimately subject mastery.

The last letter, *E*, is exercise and refers to the value of the educator's repeating the new information over and over to better ensure retention. The repetition of the time's tables in elementary school is a classic example of the power of repetition. The more often patients repeat the material, the more likely they are to remember it.

In addition to these adult learning principles, respiratory therapy educators should become knowledgeable about the unique learning needs of children and older adults. Table 8-5 presents a list of some age-specific considerations.

The 'Teaching Moment' The respiratory therapy educator must take advantage of the **teaching moment,** or any opportunity to impart meaningful information to a captive audience. Such an opportunity likely will occur only after a certain degree of trust, comfort, and mutual respect has been established between patient and educator. It behooves the respiratory therapy educator to establish this relationship as soon as possible and be prepared to take advantage of the teaching moments.

Evaluation

Evaluation, the last major component of the patient education process, involves measurement and documentation of the results of the interventions. It is the culmination of

TABLE 8-5

Age-Related Considerations in Patient Teaching

Patient's Age	Teaching Considerations
Infant or toddler	Involvement of parents (key players) is important.
	Parents should be present to alleviate separation anxiety.
	Educator must establish a relationship with patient and caregiver (trust).
	Story reading, pictures, and puppets are useful tools.
	Terminology should be kept simple (concrete, nonthreatening).
	Familiar surroundings are comforting.
	Session should be kept short (2 to 5 minutes).
	Teaching session should be held close to the occurrence of the event.
	Activity should be incorporated into learning.
Preschool	Child may participate in planning.
	If possible, a choice between two options should be allowed.
	A group size of five to eight is best.
	Physical and visual stimuli are better than verbal stimuli.
	Neutral, concrete, and action-oriented words should be used whenever possible.
	A safe, secure environment for learning should be created.
	Sessions should be kept short (15 minutes or less) and slow paced; the focus should be present oriented.
	Tangible rewards work well and should be given immediately.
School age	Participation in activities is important.
	Repetition and summarizing are useful methods.
	This age group is responsive to modeling and to peer-group and mass-media influence.
	Decision making is based on simple scientific knowledge of cause and effect.
	Groups of friends of the same age are important.
	Safety and security are less important than with preschoolers.
	Sessions can be longer (15 to 30 minutes).
	Careful listening is important.
	This age group can be assisted to move from the concrete (how) to the abstract (why).
	These children often have misconceptions that may need clarification.
	Time is needed to clarify, validate, and expand the child's knowledge.
	Privacy is important.
	Praise is very effective.
Adolescent	Cognitive abilities allow for greater participation in learning and planning.
	Patient can begin to process future health implications.
	Written information is more meaningful and useful.
	Privacy is also important.
	Learning can be enhanced by use of group methods.
	Issues may need to be clarified.
	Reinforcement through recognition is a valuable motivator.
Adult	Independence in self-care and decision making should be promoted.
	Actions may be influenced by experience, economics, sociocultural factors, and values.
	Learning needs should be determined.
	Readiness to learn should be recognized.
	Relevancy should be maintained.
	Connecting to patient's knowledge and experience is important.
	Analogies can be used for complex ideas.
	Patient should be involved in planning and decision making.
Older adult	Distinct, large configurations should be used in visual aids.
	Good lighting and high-contrast colors are helpful.
	Educator should speak clearly, adjusting the rate and loudness as necessary.
	Short learning sessions involving a small amount of material work best.
	Adequate response time should be allowed.
	Repetition aids learning.
	Goals should be mutually established and reachable.
	New learning should be integrated with previously established information.
	Patient should be encouraged to participate in planning and decision making.
	Family involvement should be encouraged.

Modified from Boyd M, Graham B, Gleit C, et al. Health teaching in nursing practice: a professional model. 3rd ed. Stamford, Conn: Appleton & Lange; 1998.

all the effort that has been expended throughout the patient-educator interaction. The evaluation component can be divided into two subcategories—process evaluation and evaluation of learning.

Process Evaluation   Process evaluation is a continuous reassessment of the effectiveness of all components of the teaching-learning interaction. Respiratory therapy educators must constantly ask themselves, "Did I gather all the information needed during the assessment phase? Did I achieve my goals and objectives? Was my decision to use a demonstration technique the right one? Did I use appropriate language?" and "Did I progress too quickly?"

Evaluation of Learning   Evaluation of learning requires the respiratory therapy educator to take a step back and look at each component of the teaching-learning interaction individually, with a view to corrective intervention and remediation. It often requires educators to ask themselves, "What did the patient learn?" or "How can I enhance teaching or learning?"

Evaluation of the patient's learning involves measurement of the learner's achievement, a task easily performed through rephrasing of the learning objectives as a series of oral questions or as questions on a written test, teaching checklist, or observational checklist that the patient completes. This evaluation must be as objective as possible, and judgments must be determined against an accepted standard. Figure 8-4 is an example of a teaching checklist used to evaluate a patient's use of an inhaler.[12]

Documentation   Documentation of the patient education process is crucial and serves a number of purposes, including (1) cataloguing the respiratory therapist's involvement in teaching; (2) demonstrating a systematic, planned approach to teaching; (3) serving as a means of communication among health care professionals; (4) satisfying legal and regulatory requirements; (5) reflecting patients' levels of understanding or misunderstanding of the subject matter, and (6) providing patients the opportunity to express their responses to the intervention.[3]

Figure 8-4   Example of a teaching checklist for use of an inhaler. (From Department of Health and Human Services (US), National Institutes of Health (NIH), National Heart, Lung, and Blood Institute. Practical guide for the diagnosis and management of asthma. NIH Pub No 97-4051. Bethesda, Md: The Institutes; July 1997.)

1. ___ Remove the cap and hold the inhaler upright.
2. ___ Shake the inhaler.
3. ___ Tilt your head back slightly and breathe out slowly.
4. ___ Position the inhaler (either with mouth opened and inhaler 1 to 2 inches away or directly in the mouth using spacer/holding chamber).
5. ___ Press down on the inhaler to release medication as you start to breathe in slowly.
6. ___ Breathe in slowly (3 to 5 seconds).
7. ___ Hold your breath for 10 seconds to allow the medicine to reach deep into your lungs.
8. ___ Repeat puff as directed. Waiting 1 minute between puffs may permit a second puff to penetrate your lungs better.
9. ___ Spacers/holding chambers are useful for all patients. They are particularly recommended for young children and older adults and for use with inhaled corticosteroids.

Interdisciplinary Patient Education/Family Education Record

Patient's name: _____

Date: _____ Time of intervention: _____

Subject matter/content addressed: _____
_____
_____
_____

Method of instruction: _____
_____
_____
_____
_____

Response of learner/results of learning: _____
_____
_____
_____
_____

Initials/signature of health care provider: _____

Figure 8-5   Sample of an interdisciplinary patient education/family education record.

Documentation can take many forms. Some institutions use electronic documentation, whereas others use such techniques as anecdotal chart entries, checklists, and standardized forms. An informal survey of a variety of institutions showed that almost all believed that documentation of patient education should be included as part of the patient's permanent record and that such documentation should be interdisciplinary. The following five key components were identified:

1. Date and time of the intervention
2. Initials of the health care provider
3. Subject matter or content addressed
4. Method of instruction
5. Response of the learner or the results of the learning

Figure 8-5 shows a sample interdisciplinary patient education/family education record that includes some of the points identified previously.

For ease of charting, some institutions used a coded checklist. For example, under method of instruction, the educator would check off *E* for explanation, *D* for demonstration, *P* for printed materials, or *V* for video. Under response of the learner, *1* might stand for communicates understanding, *2* for return demonstration provided, *3* for requires reinforcement, *4* for referral indicated, or *5* for refused interaction. Almost all methods of documentation included a section for educator comments, and some had a more elaborate section for factors noted at the initial assessment, such as barriers to learning and the patient's motivational level and learning preferences.

Above all, respiratory therapy educators must be mindful of the need to constantly update and refine their teaching skills. Observation of colleagues, formal training through academic and professional courses and programs, and practice can help the patient educator attain this goal and become a more effective teacher.

Key Points

- Patient education plays an increasingly important role in health care delivery.
- Regulatory, social, demographic, economic, and philosophic practical incentives drive patient education.
- The health care system must better prepare the patient and informal caregiver to engage in preventive, maintenance, and restorative health care measures.
- Respiratory therapists must be aware of the highly dependent nature of patients.
- The goals and indications of patient education focus on the creation of behavior change.
- Patient education is a detailed, sequential process.
- Assessment is the first step; it involves determination of the patient's learning needs and readiness to learn.
- The planning phase involves development of goals and well-written objectives and addressing of the three learning domains.
- The implementation phase involves actual teaching, which requires a variety of strategies and techniques.
- Common barriers to learning include lack of readiness, physical and emotional obstacles, language barriers, and lack of motivation.
- The nine principles of adult learning produce the mnemonic RAMP-2-FAME: recency, appropriateness, motivation, primacy, two-way communication, feedback, active learning, multiple-sense learning, and exercise.
- Evaluation, the last phase in patient education, should be a continual process encompassing evaluation of the entire teaching process and of the effectiveness of the patient's learning.
- Respiratory therapy educators should always be alert to take advantage of the "teaching moment."

References

1. Redman BK. The practice of patient education. 8th ed. St Louis: Mosby; 1997.
2. DuBrey SR, Jean R. Promoting wellness in nursing practice: a step-by-step approach in patient education. St Louis: Mosby; 1982.
3. Boyd M, Graham B, Gleit C, et al. Health teaching in nursing practice: a professional model. 3rd ed. Stamford, Conn: Appleton & Lange; 1998.
4. Travis J, Ryan RS. Wellness workbook. 2nd ed. Berkeley, Calif: Ten Speed Press; 1988.
5. American Association for Respiratory Care. Clinical practice guideline: providing patient and caregiver training. Respir Care 1996;41:658-663.
6. American Association for Respiratory Care. Clinical practice guideline: training the health-care professional for the role of patient and caregiver educator. Respir Care 1996;41:654-657.
7. Chatham MAH, Knapp BL. Patient education handbook. Bowie, Md: Robert J Brady; 1982.
8. Lubkin IM. Chronic illness: impact and interventions. Boston: Jones & Bartlett; 1990.
9. McKenzie J, Smeltzer J. Planning, implementing and evaluating health promotion programs: a primer. 2nd ed. Boston: Allyn & Bacon; 1997.
10. Babcock D, Mary M. Client education: theory and practice, St Louis: Mosby; 1994.
11. National Heart, Lung, and Blood Institute. Open airways: asthma self-management program. National Institutes of Health Pub No 84-2365. Bethesda, Md: The Institute; 1984.
12. National Asthma Education and Prevention Program. Expert panel report 2: guidelines for the diagnosis and management of asthma. National Institutes of Health Pub No 97-4051. Bethesda, Md: The Program; 1997.
13. Winthrop E. Patient teaching tips. St Louis: Mosby; 1995.
14. Kroehnert G. Basic training for trainers: a handbook for trainers. 2nd ed. New York: McGraw-Hill; 1995.

Recommended Reading

American Association for Respiratory Care. Year 2001: delineating the educational direction for the future respiratory care practitioner. Proceedings of a National Consensus Conference on Respiratory Care Education; 1992 Oct 2-4; Dallas.

Canobbio M. Handbook of patient education. St Louis: Mosby; 1996.

Ferri F. Ferri's patient teaching guides. St Louis: Mosby; 1999.

Katz J. Back to basics: providing effective patient education. Am J Nurs 1997;5:33-36.

Redman BK. Measurement tools in patient education. New York: Springer; 1998.

Smith C. Patient education: nursing partnership with other professionals. Philadelphia: WB Saunders; 1987.

CHAPTER 9

Documentation and Medical Information Management

Susan Blonshine

CHAPTER OUTLINE

Forms Committee
Verbal Orders
Medical Record Authentication
Patient Confidentiality Issues
Elements of a Patient Medical Record
Electronic Charts
  Computer-Based Patient Record
  Electronic Signature
Appropriate Handling of Patient Information
  Information Security
  National Research Council Report
  Facsimile Reports
  Telemedical Records
  Retention of Medical Records
  Destruction of Patient Health Information
Ethical, Economic, and Legal Issues

OBJECTIVES

1. Describe the purpose of a forms committee.
2. Describe situations in which verbal orders are acceptable.
3. Define *medical record authentication*.
4. List medical record entries that require authentication.
5. List elements of a patient medical record.
6. Describe the different forms of medical records.
7. Describe the three criteria for a computer-based patient record, as envisioned by the Institute of Medicine.
8. Define the limitations and requirements for electronic signatures.
9. List five principles necessary for a comprehensive confidentiality system.
10. Describe the respiratory therapist's responsibilities in maintaining patient confidentiality.
11. Describe information security.
12. List three types of controls used in information security.
13. Describe several methods used to protect electronic health care information.
14. Describe guidelines for use of facsimile reports.
15. List information challenges related to telemedical records.
16. List the steps to follow in the destruction of patient health information.
17. Describe the components of an occurrence management system.

KEY TERMS

Authentication	Durable Power of Attorney	Medical Record
Clinical Repository	Electronic Signature	ORYX
Computer-Based Patient Record (CPR)	HEDIS	Power of Attorney
Confidential	Incident Report	Telemedical Record
Cryptography	Information Management	
Documentation System	Information Security	

*T*ABLE 9-1

Acronyms Related to Medical Information

Acronym	Meaning
ASTM	The American Society for Testing and Materials
AHIMA	American Health Information Management Association
CPR	Computer-based patient record
CPRI	Computer-Based Patient Record Institute
HCFA	Health Care Financing Administration
HEDIS	Health Plan Employer Data and Information Set
HIPAA	Health Insurance Portability and Accountability Act
IOM	Institute of Medicine
JCAHO	Joint Commission on Accreditation of Healthcare Organizations
NCQA	National Committee for Quality Assurance
OIG	Office of the Inspector General
ORYX	Name of JCAHO's initiative to integrate performance measures into accreditation process; Webster's dictionary definition—a kind of gazelle
OSHA	Occupational Safety and Health Administration

The **documentation system** and management of information is the backbone of a quality health care delivery system. Health **information management** requires the understanding and use of both paper records and electronic records. In either case the fundamental question remains as to the best means to efficiently capture the information. The paper record (form) and the computer screen are tools used to access and control information processing within a health care system; both control the information system by demanding and standardizing action, issuing instructions, standardizing vocabularies, fixing responsibilities, and improving communication. Paper and computer records both can be effective means to control quality and data accuracy in an information system. The emphasis on health care outcomes requires improved documentation of patient care, and studies have estimated that 40% to 50% of a clinician's time is spent writing notes in patient records.[1,2,3]

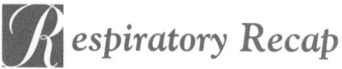*espiratory Recap*

Rationale for Effective Communications
Respiratory therapists must develop skills to document, manage, and access patient information to be effective clinicians.

Respiratory therapists must develop the necessary skills to document, manage, and access patient information if they are to be effective clinicians. Therapists also must remain informed about the various medical, ethical, legal, and financial issues involved in the documentation and use of medical information. Serious mismanagement and even patient harm can result from careless or insufficient documentation of medical information. Denial of reimbursement for services, penalties, and lawsuits can occur when patient records are mismanaged.

Table 9-1 contains a list of acronyms and abbreviations related to medical information documentation and management as used in this chapter.

Forms Committee

The forms committee in any health care system develops, reviews, and controls all methods used to capture and record patient information, methods commonly referred to as *information capture tools*. Specific elements are included for the design of both paper forms and computer forms. Although issues related to paper forms may be applied to computer-view design, the computer view features a number of unique issues. Several organizations have developed standards to automate patient information, and each forms committee within the health care system should review and use these external standards for automation when appropriate. Table 9-2 lists the current standards.

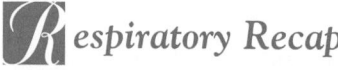*espiratory Recap*

Forms Committee
The forms committee develops, reviews, and controls all methods used to capture and record patient information within a health care delivery system.

Verbal Orders

The Joint Commission on Accreditation of Healthcare Organizations (JCAHO) specifies standards for all medical orders. Verbal orders may be accepted by authorized individuals and transcribed by qualified personnel identified by title or category in the medical staff rules and regulations.[4] Respiratory therapists are generally identified as qualified medical personnel capable of accepting verbal orders but require authorization by medical staff members to accept verbal orders per JCAHO standards. Respiratory therapy students, however, are not qualified to accept verbal orders and therefore must be properly identified and supervised during their clinical experiences.

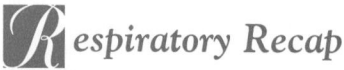*espiratory Recap*

Students and Verbal Orders
Respiratory therapy students are not qualified to accept verbal orders. Therefore proper student identification and supervision is vital.

TABLE 9-2

Standards for Automation of Patient Information

Standard of Group	Purpose or Intent of Standard or Guideline
E1384 standard guide for content and structure for the computer-based patient record National Committee on Vital and Health Statistics on Core Health Data Elements Data elements for emergency department systems (DEEDS) Health level seven (HL7)	This standard, developed by ASTM subcommittee E31.19 on vocabulary for computer-based patient records content and structure, was the first standard for the computer-based patient record to focus on identification of content vocabulary. It has five major purposes. The committee has completed the first iteration of a process to identify a set of core health data elements on persons and encounters or events that can serve multiple purposes and would benefit from standardization. This data set recommends specifications for many of the observations, actions, instructions, and conclusions entered into emergency department records. The role of HL7 is to develop standards to facilitate the electronic interchange of information on admissions, discharges, and transfers within medical institutions; financial transactions within institutions; orders; scheduling; and nursing management within institutions.

ASTM, *American Society for Testing and Materials.*

Patient name and identification number

Date

Perform lung volumes and airway resistance today 4 hours after MDI administration with albuterol.

v.o. T. Smith, MD
Mary Jane Jones RRT, RPFT
5-25-99 10:12 AM

Figure 9-1   Example of a transcribed verbal order.

Each health care system has specific policies and procedures governing who may accept verbal orders, their scope of practice, and the procedure used to document the order in the **medical record.** Physician-directed orders drive the course of care for all patients. All medical orders, whether written or verbally accepted, must be recorded accurately to ensure patient safety and accurate care.

Qualified individuals must strictly follow the institution's procedure for recording of verbal orders. Respiratory therapists providing any clinical care of patients should understand and review the institution's procedures for acceptance and recording of verbal orders. Figure 9-1 provides an example of a transcribed verbal order.

Medical Record Authentication

Accrediting organizations, Medicare conditions of participation, state laws, and other bodies specify requirements for medical records. The health care delivery system must comply with various requirements to maintain accreditation, meet legal standards, and receive reimbursement. The level of authentication of each entry in a medical record varies, depending on the regulatory agency. For example, JCAHO does not require physician signatures on all verbal orders. As of July 1996 for hospital accreditation programs,

JCAHO requires each verbal order be dated and identified by the names of all the individuals who gave the order, received the order, and implemented the order. When required by state or federal law and regulation, verbal orders are authenticated within a specified period. For those health care delivery systems in which authentication of the verbal order is required, the process of verification that the order is complete, accurate, and final occurs within a preestablished time frame. For example, in a hospital all verbal orders are authenticated within 24 hours of their writing.

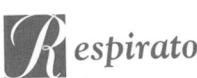 *espiratory Recap*

Requirements for Medical Records

Health care delivery systems must comply with various requirements for medical records to maintain accreditation, meet legal standards, and obtain reimbursement.

Medical record entries generally require some level of **authentication,** which is the process used to verify that an entry is complete, accurate, and final. Every medical record entry must be dated, with its author identified, and when necessary, authenticated, and the authors must authenti-

espiratory Recap

Authentication

Authentication is the process used to verify that an entry in a medical record is complete, accurate, and final. Authentication must be ensured for history and physical exams, operative reports, consultations, and discharge summaries.

cate those entries required by hospital policy. Authentication must be ensured at least for history and physical examinations, operative reports, consultations, and discharge summaries. Behavioral health entries have additional requirements. Authentication requirements also vary among ambulatory care, long-term health, and home health settings. All health care providers must be familiar with requirements for verbal orders and medical record entries for each organization.

As health care delivery systems change and ambulatory care increases, the requirements for medical records will continue to change. Respiratory therapists working in alternative settings, such as managed care organizations, may specify other requirements through quality initiatives. One example is the National Committee for Quality Assurance (NCQA), which accredits managed care plans. The NCQA evaluates how well a health care plan manages all parts of its delivery system, including physicians, hospitals, other providers, and administrative services. The NCQA standards for ambulatory records require provider identification and dating on each medical record entry but not authentication. The requirements for medical record entries may be vastly different based on the setting, and each therapist should review the policies and procedures for each clinical site or setting.

Each health care organization must develop policies and procedures to address authentication requirements and acceptable methods to authenticate medical record entries. Respiratory therapists must be aware of the content of the policies and procedures to maintain compliance, whereas respiratory students must be instructed on their role working with staff to ensure authentication and use of medical records. Documentation of care and authentication of records during students' clinical training must be supervised by qualified personnel in accordance with institutional policy. A lack of compliance with medical record authentication standards may adversely affect patient care, reimbursement, and accreditation of the specific health care system.

Patient Confidentiality Issues

All health care systems must develop policies and procedures to protect patient confidentiality, just as all medical personnel must ensure such confidentiality in all aspects of their work by following policies and procedures. Employees must be familiar with their system's information security plan, which outlines steps governing those who can access

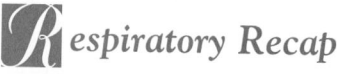
espiratory Recap

Confidentiality
All health care systems must ensure patient confidentiality. Respiratory therapy students and clinicians should carefully follow policies and procedures to protect patient confidentiality.

medical information, the content or type of information each employee is allowed to access, information that can be released to other internal or external individuals, ways in which information can be released, individuals who can release information, and those to whom information can be released. The protection of an individual's medical records has become a political issue as well.

Health care delivery systems must have policies that address internal and external release of patient information. New employees are required to sign confidentiality statement pledges before they have access to **confidential** information. Patient information should be shared only with employees who need to know, such as practitioners, and employees who are directly involved in the care. Federal and various state laws require patient confidentiality. Any health care provider may be fired or risk legal action if a breach in confidentiality occurs. When faced with making a quick decision about confidentiality, the provider must always consider the patient's need first.

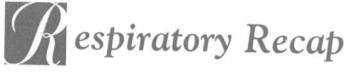
espiratory Recap

Protecting Patient Confidentiality
To protect patient confidentiality and prevent firing or lawsuits, medical personnel should not discuss patients in hallways, cafeterias, elevators, and public places.

In addition, practitioners should refrain from discussing patients in the hallways, cafeterias, and elevators. Such discussions outside the care setting is unprofessional behavior because of the risk for serious breaches in patient confidentiality. Public pressures also have forced politicians to consider legislative action for privacy protection. As legislation is passed to ensure patient confidentiality, so are standards established to ensure compliance with the law. In a 1997 speech, Secretary of Health and Human Services Donna E. Shalala listed the following five principles necessary for comprehensive confidentiality purposes[5]:

1. Establishment of boundaries so that disclosure of health care information is limited to health care purposes only
2. Security measures so that individuals are assured of the safety of their health care information
3. Consumer control so that citizens have the right to access their health records, know who is looking at them, determine their accuracy, and change incorrect information
4. Accountability standards that hold individuals and not just organizations accountable for confidentiality violations
5. Public responsibility that creates a balance among individual rights, the need to support national health priorities, and enforcement

Table 9-3 identifies several confidentiality risks and proposed controls.

TABLE 9-3
Confidentiality Risks and Controls

Technology	Risks	Controls
Copiers	• Originals are left in the copier feeder or on the copier glass, where someone who should not see the information may find it. • Imperfect copies are discarded in the nearest trash can. • Repair personnel discover confidential information while clearing paper jams.	• Implement an awareness training program. • Provide secure disposal container near machine. • Insert confidentiality clauses in repair contracts.
Facsimile (fax) machines	• A fax is sent to the wrong location. • A fax is sent to an unauthorized person. • Fax machines are shared by departments with different information needs. • Confidential faxes (incoming or outgoing) are left on the tray or table. • The fax machine is located in an area where information can be seen by unauthorized persons. • Extra copies from transmission failures are discarded in open trash containers.	• Verify fax numbers. • Verify recipients' authority to receive confidential information. • Provide separate machines for departments with differing needs. • Place fax machine in secure location.
Telephones	• Conversations are overheard. • Confidential information is given to unauthorized persons. • An unauthorized person gains access to a voice-response system.	• Implement an awareness training program. • Limit information that can be distributed. • Control access to voice-response systems.
Printers	• Machines are shared by departments with differing information needs. • Locations allow visitors to see information. • Extra or imperfect copies are discarded in open containers. • Print jobs are directed to the wrong location. • Printers require repair work.	• Provide separate printers based on need. • Locate printers in a secure area. • Provide secure disposal containers nearby. • From print menu, verify location of printers used. • Include confidentiality agreements in repair contracts.
Cordless and cellular phones	• Conversations are overheard, particularly when these devices are used in public places. • Scanning equipment can allow eavesdropping on conversations.	• Implement an awareness training program. • Refrain from discussing confidential information. • Use cordless phones that encrypt the transmitted signal.
Voice pagers	• Confidential messages received on pagers can be overheard.	• Implement an awareness training program. • Prohibit transmission of confidential messages via voice pagers. • Increase awareness about voice-mail systems that forward to pagers.
E-mail	• Confidential messages are sent or forwarded to wrong person. • Messages are sent via the Internet, resulting in disclosure of patient information. • Messages are stored on backup media and viewed by unauthorized persons.	• Establish policies for use of e-mail. • Implement an awareness training program.
Voice mail	• Confidential messages are left on the wrong mail box or answering machine. • Messages are played on speaker phones or answering machines.	• Implement an awareness training program. • Develop policies for use with confidential information.
PC displays	• Displays are located where visitors and others can see them. • Displays of confidential information are left unattended.	• Locate displays where screens cannot be seen by unauthorized persons. • Implement an automatic timeout to a blank screen.

Modified from Miller DW. In: Confidence, current technology: confidentiality risks and controls. Chicago: American Health Information Management Association; July/Aug 1998.

Continued

*T*ABLE 9-3

Confidentiality Risks and Controls—cont'd

Technology	Risks	Controls
Telemedicine	• Patient may be seen in a video used with another patient. • Video and image links are sent to the wrong location. • Videotapes or sessions are not properly protected.	• Provide private facilities. • Use system controls to protect the system and files.
Dictation and transcription systems	• Physician is overheard while dictating. • Poor management of passwords allows unauthorized access. • Transcription service and report files are inadequately controlled. • Transcription is performed in insecure locations, such as the home, where unauthorized persons may see confidential information.	• Implement an awareness training program. • Provide security controls on transcription systems. • Include confidentiality clauses in contracts.
Handheld PC	• Computer is lost or stolen. • Display information is viewed by unauthorized users.	• Implement an awareness training program. • Use encryption to protect information stored in portable devices.
PC modems	• Modems installed on personal computers for dial-out may permit unauthorized dial-in.	• Implement an awareness training program. • Use encryption to protect information stored in portable devices.
Internet	• Unencrypted patient information is transmitted, resulting in unauthorized disclosure. • Unauthorized access to the organization's system is gained via the Internet.	• Prohibit transmission of patient-identifiable information via the Internet. • Implement encryption. • Install firewalls between the Internet and the organization's system.

Modified from Miller DW. In: Confidence, current technology: confidentiality risks and controls. Chicago: American Health Information Management Association; July/Aug 1998.

The release of patient information should always ensure confidentiality as the first premise. Patients must authorize the release of their health information in most situations. The medical records department should be able to answer queries about whether a signed release is necessary. If the patient is unable to authorize release of information, other guidelines apply. For example, in the event of death the executor of the patient's estate or an individual appointed by the probate court may authorize the release; next of kin may be consulted if an executor or probate appointee does not exist. A guardian or next of kin may authorize release of information for patients who are mentally incapacitated. An agent named in a directive, such as **power of attorney,** is authorized to serve for a patient; this power or a direct agent is often named when a patient is critically ill and cannot make decisions. For example, a spouse designated with power of attorney would make medical decisions until the patient's condition improves to a level at which that person can make competent decisions.

Many states provide for a medical power of attorney specific to situations in which a person is unable to make medical decisions and allow for the designation of a specific individual to make decisions for the patient. A document known as a **durable power of attorney** for health

care names an individual or agent who can make decisions specifically related to health care for another individual. Releasing only specific medical information that is requested and authorized, and no more, is a good practice. Hospital departments generally involved with the release of medical information include medical records, risk management, quality management, and utilization management. These departments may coexist or be organized under a health information management division. Corporate offices or headquarters may serve as the institutional authority for an entire health care network within a state, regional, national, or international network.

Elements of a Patient Medical Record

Every health care delivery system must have a model for each patient's medical record. Common clinical data included in the medical record include documentation of patient assessment, problem identification, care plans, treatments, and outcomes. The paper record continues to be the most common form of a medical record and is typically composed of discharge summaries, progress notes, physician orders, laboratory results, and flow sheets. With

TABLE 9-4

Components of a Patient Medical Record

Component	Examples
Progress notes	Notes of daily assessment and progress by physician or other members of the health care team
Physician orders	All medical orders written by physician or recorded as verbal orders by authorized individual
Discharge summary	Summary of patient condition on discharge, postdischarge instructions, and care plan
Flow sheets/graphic sheets	Input and output records, daily graph of vital signs, mechanical ventilation records, and therapy records
Laboratory reports	Clinical laboratory reports and pulmonary function laboratory reports
Pharmacy reports	Medication log
Photographs	Photographs from specific procedures, such as ultrasound or bronchoscopy
Videotapes	Videotapes from procedures, such as sleep studies or bronchoscopy
Radiology reports	X-rays, scans, and images
Monitoring strips	Electrocardiogram strips
Admissions sheet	Demographics, pertinent patient information, admitting diagnosis, and physician
History and physical	Body system review by physician and all pertinent history information
Consultation sheet	Review, impressions, and recommendations of patient by specialists consulted
Consent forms	Forms signed by patient or representative for special procedures, such as surgery or bronchoscopy
Surgical records	Recording of all events occurring immediately before, during, and after surgery
Audio recordings	Tapes of special procedures, such as sleep studies, including home studies to record snoring

technologic progression the medical record has gained additional media, which may include online reports, photographs, videotapes, films, and audio recordings.

Although online computer data may be available, a hard copy (paper) is still required on the chart as part of the complete medical record. A monitoring strip, such as an electrocardiogram, is one example of the type of paper (hard) copies found in the medical record. Photographs from medical procedures, such as a bronchoscopy, also are placed in the medical record. Videotapes, audio recordings, radiographs, and other types of media are considered a part of the medical record. Table 9-4 includes examples of elements of the medical record and types of media that may be considered part of such record. Each facility must design, document, and implement a thorough process to bring together all the patient health information into a complete medical record.

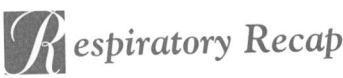

Respiratory Recap

> **Medical Records**
>
> Data in medical records includes patient assessment, problem identification, care plans, treatments, and outcomes.
> Paper records include discharge summaries, orders, laboratory results, and flow sheets.
> Media records include photographs, films, videotapes, and audio recordings.

The transition from paper records that document episodes of care to electronic records that document longitudinal care is a critical component in the building of a health care information infrastructure. In many of the current health care delivery systems, paper records are generated each time a patient visits any system site. Typically the paper records are not easily shared between sites, often creating the need for duplication and making viewing of the patient's complete health status more difficult. The transition to electronic records allows for the maintenance of each episode of care in a central medical record repository from patient birth to death.

Electronic Charts

Computer-Based Patient Record

The Institute of Medicine (IOM) released a report in 1991 outlining the vision for a **computer-based patient record (CPR)** and also recommended the establishment of a Computer-Based Patient Record Institute (CPRI). In 1997 a revised report confirmed the previous findings and requirements, envisioning a CPR with multimedia capabilities; high-resolution images; sounds, such as auscultation; full-motion video; and elaborate coding schemes. The IOM proposes that the expected results would include access, quality, security, flexibility, connectivity, efficiency, links to other databases, and decision support tools.

The CPRI describes the CPR as electronically maintained information about an individual's lifetime health status and health care. Box 9-1 outlines the three threshold criteria that the IOM envisions for a CPR. Currently, most health care systems continue to rely on the paper record as the development of the CPR continues meeting the challenge of the three threshold criteria.

*B*ox 9-1

CPRI Threshold Criteria for a CPR System

A CPR system should meet the following three criteria:
1. The CPR system must acquire, store, transmit, and retrieve data, information, and knowledge from multiple sources.
2. The CPR system must possess information-processing tools that provide added value to support decisions about patient management.
3. Caregivers must consult the CPR system as their primary source of information for patient care.

CPR, Computer-based patient record; CPRI, Computer-Based Patient Record Institute.

Although many vendors have tried to meet the challenge, the vision of the CPR has not yet been fully realized. The IOM has identified several barriers contributing to this delayed development, including the (1) lack of consensus on content, (2) complex characteristics of CPR technology, (3) high cost of systems, (4) unpredictable user behavior, (5) lack of adequate networks for data transmission, (6) insufficient leadership to resolve the issues, (7) lack of training for CPR developers, and (8) various legal and social issues. In response to the barriers and delays in development of the CPR, a government project emerged to develop a CPR from off-the-shelf products for use by all government agencies, a project known as G-CPR.

The primary advantages of the CPR are the clinical data repositories, each of which combines data from multiple entry points and visits into a single storage location. For example, you visit your physician today for the first time, after visiting the emergency department. With a **clinical repository,** your physician can review all the information from the emergency department visit online and add information from today's visit. You visit the same health care delivery system 3 years later, and all your previous entries are available for review in the repository, where additional data also can be added. A single data storage location increases a facility's and a physician's effectiveness in collecting data to deliver longitudinal care without duplication.

Another advantage of the CPR is its ability to store multimedia records under a single unique identifier. Currently, most systems are limited to supplying data for direct patient care events. Advancements are moving delivery systems toward the integration of clinical and financial information into a single system. As all the medical information moves into a single data source, the vision of a comprehensive medical record will be achieved.

The health care information systems of the future and the management of the medical record will continue to improve. Future changes will respond to regulatory and accrediting bodies as outlined in the JCAHO's **ORYX** (the initiative to integrate performance measures into the accreditation process) requirements, NCQA's HEDIS (Health Plan Employer Data and Information Set) re-

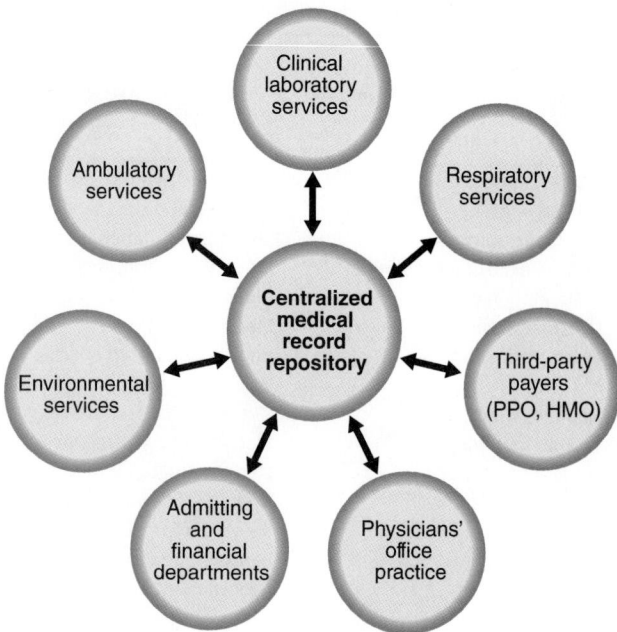

Figure 9-2   An integrated information system. All delivery sites and departments across the continuum of care can access and retrieve data from the central repository based on their security level.

quirements, and the revision of Medicare conditions of participation. JCAHO's future strategies affecting the ways health care organizations earn accreditation will incorporate ORYX requirements, which place a much greater emphasis on performance as measured against external norms. JCAHO officially describes a performance measure as a quantitative tool (rate, ratio, index, and percentage) that provides an indication of an organization's performance in relation to a specified process or outcome. Both health plans and purchasers will influence the changes in health information management through data collection systems such as **HEDIS,** which is a set of standardized measures developed by the NCQA allowing purchasers to compare health plans.

CPR systems are the tools that supply data and provide robust rules engines to use clinical guidelines, protocols, and pathways. The electronic medical record is the "central nervous system" of future health care delivery systems. Figure 9-2 illustrates an integrated information system.

Electronic Signature

According to the 1998 Comprehensive Accreditation Manual for Hospitals, **electronic signatures** are acceptable to JCAHO. The Joint Commission outlines specific requirements for the use of rubber-stamp and electronic signatures, including (1) that the practitioner must sign a statement that he or she alone will use it and (2) that no one will use the stamp or electronic signature authorized for someone else. JCAHO accepts electronic signatures in ambulatory care, long term care, and mental health. An additional JCAHO requirement allows the

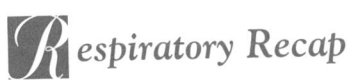

author to review the document online before signing it electronically.

In a CPR the health care practitioners may sign the record in several different ways, generally with a unique code or password that verifies the individual creating the entry and creates an individual "signature" on the record. The American Society of Testing and Materials (ASTM) has developed guidelines for the use of electronic signatures based on accountability, data integrity, and nonrepudiation. The record of the electronic signature is ultimately stored on magnetic, optical, or some other computer storage media.

Medicare also has developed several standards for the use of electronic signatures in hospitals as outlined in the Medicare conditions of participation. Medicare requires the organization's governing body to approve the use of electronic signatures; according to the conditions of participation the use of electronic signatures outside the hospital setting varies. Public law 104-191, the Health Insurance Portability and Accountability Act (HIPAA), mandates that the secretary of Health and Human Services and the secretary of Commerce shall adopt standards specifying procedures for the electronic transmission and authentication of signatures. The notice of a proposed ruling (Public Law 104-191) on electronic signatures was published in August 1998. State laws and regulations on authentication of electronic signatures and medical records vary widely, but the American Health Information Management Association (AHIMA) can provide guidance as the regulations continue to change.

Appropriate Handling of Patient Information

Information Security

Information security describes the protection of the integrity, availability, and confidentiality of computer-based information and the resources used to enter, store, process, and communicate information. A major focus of information security is to prevent unauthorized individuals from accessing, creating, or modifying information, but no system used today has absolute security. An acceptable level of security must be based on the threats to the system and the confidential information they contain. The security

measures must be cost effective and appropriate for the level of risk. Checks and balances should be developed in the system to limit the impact of a single user. For example, program changes created by one employee should have a method for verification by another employee. Another example involves the termination of employees; if a disgruntled employee leaves the health care system, security should be assigned at a level that prevents the employee from intentionally creating errors in the system. Terminated employees should be deleted from the system immediately. Users' access should be limited to the information and functions that employees need to perform their jobs.

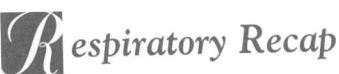

Three types of controls are used in information security—management controls, operational controls, and technical controls. Management controls focus on the management of the information security program and risk within the organization and include security policies that incorporate all applicable laws and regulations that also are designed to meet the health care organization's needs. Operational controls include contingency planning, user awareness and training, physical and environmental protections, computer support and operations, and handling of security breaches. Technical controls include user identification and authentication, access control, audit trails, and cryptography. Authentication is a method to validate the identity of the user or other system authorized to access the health care information. Authentication usually is verified with a user password prompted after log-in, but studies over the past few years have shown that this step is inadequate for authentication. Access control determines the content of information that may be entered or viewed based on the user's identification, and an audit trail identifies each log-in into the system. **Cryptography** is a process that writes the information in a code. Each of these controls is executed by the information system.

Threats to information security include, but are not limited to physical problems, disgruntled employees, malicious codes, hackers, theft, errors, omissions, and browsing. Each employee has a unique password not shared with other employees. To decrease risks, a system is usually in place to change the password at defined intervals. When an employee is terminated or retires, the identification should be immediately inactivated. Security also can be improved through deactivation of identification for individuals on prolonged leaves, such as with disability. The organization should maintain an audit trail to verify compliance with these security measures.

National Research Council Report

The National Research Council released a report in 1997 on protecting electronic health care information. The committee charged with developing this report provided recommendations in five areas, including (1) improvements in privacy and security practices, (2) creation of an industry-wide security infrastructure, (3) addressing of systemic concerns related to privacy and security, (4) development of patient identifiers, and (5) meeting of future technologic needs.

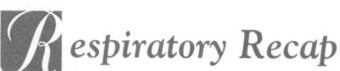 *espiratory Recap*

Recommendations for Health Care Information

The National Research Council identified five priority areas of recommendations for the use of electronic healthcare information, protection of patient rights, and assurance of confidentiality, as follows:
1. Improvements in privacy and security practices
2. Creation of an industry-wide security infrastructure
3. Addressing of systemic concerns related to privacy and security
4. Development of patient identifiers
5. Meeting of future technologic needs

Each health care organization should develop a set of technical and organizational policies, practices, and procedures to protect patient-identifiable health care information. The committee recommends that organizations adopt technical practices and procedures to include individual authentication of users, access controls, audit trails, physical security and disaster recovery, protection of remote access points, protection of external electronic communications, software discipline, and system assessment. The committee also recommends that organizations establish security and confidentiality issues and form committees, identify information security officers, establish education and training programs, develop sanctions for confidentiality and security policy violations, improve authorization forms, and permit patient access to audit logs. Recommendations for the future include the implementation of strong authentication, development of enterprise-wide authentication, use of access validation tools or software, implementation of expanded audit trails, and use of technologies for electronic authentication of electronic records.

A primary concern in the privacy and confidentiality debate concerns the use of a universal patient identifier. The committee did not recommend the use of the Social Security number (SSN) or any other number because the privacy concerns related to such numbers are subjects of fierce debate. The threats to privacy will continue to increase as the technology becomes more sophisticated, and the committee

recommends that the government take steps to improve information security technologies for health care applications.

Respiratory therapists are faced with day-to-day issues regarding patient confidentiality. The National Research Council report provides guidance on the basic principles of confidentiality for use as a reference. Clinicians, however, may be required to serve on teams to develop systems to meet the requirements of this report.

Facsimile Reports

Facsimile (fax) machines, popular tools in health care communications, open another avenue for the loss of patient confidentiality. AHIMA recommends that health information be transmitted by fax only when the original record or mail-delivered copies cannot meet the needs of immediate patient care. Before patient information is released, a properly completed and signed authorization is required, and according to AHIMA, authorizations via fax are acceptable. The fax cover page should include a confidentiality notice indicating the confidential nature of the information and limits on its use. In addition, the person sending the fax should ensure that the document will reach its intended destination.

Most regulatory and accreditation requirements do not specifically address the acceptability of health information transmission via fax. State law may restrict the transmission of certain types of health information, such as that related to acquired immunodeficiency syndrome (AIDS), human immunodeficiency virus (HIV) infection, or psychiatric care. The Bureau of Policy Development of the Health Care Financing Administration (HCFA) did address the transmission of physician orders in 1990[6] and found that the use of a fax is permissible but that fax copies may fade and require photocopying. Health care facilities are advised to take extra precautions to ensure that they retain a legible copy of the physician order with the medical record for the required period of time. Faxed orders may possibly decrease errors associated with verbal orders and thus contribute to improved care. More than 50% of states have adopted the Federal Rules of Evidence,[6] and several others have adopted the Uniform Photographic Copies of Business and Public Records Act.[6] Each of these organizations allows for the submission of record reproductions without the need to account for the original record.

Because of regulatory variances, the policies and procedures related to the receipt of a physician order via fax

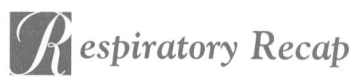 *espiratory Recap*

Policies for Facsimile Orders

Respiratory therapy students may not be qualified to accept physician orders via facsimile.
The health care system's policies and procedures should always be reviewed for information regarding facsimile transmissions.

should always be reviewed. Some regions of the country treat a faxed order in the same manner as a verbal order, but respiratory therapists and other medical personnel must remember that students are not qualified to receive even verbal orders.

Telemedical Records

In late 1998, 72 identified telemedicine programs in the United States used interactive video technology or live, real-time teleconsultations.[7] The continued growth of telemedicine raises multiple issues related to documentation, privacy, confidentiality, and legal issues. The responsible party for creating, storing, and maintaining the **telemedical record** is the first step. Coding, billing, and reimbursement of these services present additional challenges to health care professionals.

Retention of Medical Records

Each health care delivery system should develop guidelines for medical record retention, including a schedule for the length of retention. The guidelines should address the type of information to be kept, the time period the information should be kept, and the storage medium in which such information should be retained. The retention schedule must meet the needs of the patients, physicians, and researchers while complying with legal, regulatory, and accreditation requirements. The Medicare conditions of participation for hospitals require medical records and radiology service films, scans, and images to be kept for at least 5 years. The conditions of participation for other care sites vary, and respiratory therapists should be aware of the requirements for the health care delivery site at which they work. The Occupational Safety and Health Administration (OSHA) requires retention of employee medical records for the period of employment plus 30 years. States also have specific retention requirements.

Destruction of Patient Health Information

Health care facilities are unable to maintain individual patient health information indefinitely, which requires the development and implementation of retention and destruction policies and procedures. Destruction of patient information should be carried out in accordance with fed-

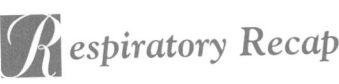

Respiratory Recap

Employee Conduct and Medical Records

The standards of conduct for each employee clearly delineate the policies of the health care delivery system regarding fraud, waste, abuse, and adherence to all statutes, regulations, and other program requirements governing federal, state, and private health benefit plans.

---

eral and state laws according to the written retention and destruction policy. Records involved in an open investigation, audit, or litigation should not be destroyed. Those records able to be destroyed, however, should be documented with the date of destruction, method of destruction, description of the disposed record series, inclusive dates covered, a statement that the records were destroyed in the normal course of business, and signatures of the individuals supervising and witnessing the destruction.

Ethical, Economic, and Legal Issues

All health care providers should be familiar with the organization's ethics statement or codes of conduct. The Office of the Inspector General (OIG) requires each health care system to develop a code of conduct available to maintain compliance with Medicare rules. The standards of conduct for each employee clearly delineate the policies of the health care delivery system regarding fraud, waste, abuse, and adherence to all statutes, regulations, and other program requirements governing federal, state, and private health benefit plans. These standards should be made available to all employees and translated, interpreted, or put into Braille as needed, with regular updates made as the policies and regulations are modified. All new employees should be asked to sign a statement certifying that they have received, read, and understood the standards of conduct. All employee certifications should be retained in a personnel file.

Each health care delivery system must maintain an occurrence management program encompassing methods to capture and analyze information about systematic problems. The program is generally linked to the risk management department, which provides management with reports that include systematic problems presenting legal or financial risk to the organization. Each department or service has a process for detecting, documenting, classifying, and correcting the problems identified.

An **incident report** is an example of an occurrence report that may be filed for an untoward happening. For example, an incident report should be completed when a patient receives an incorrect medication or when a patient accidentally falls when getting out of bed. The individual who observes or discovers the incident should begin the documentation process. An occurrence report may include specifics, such as patient name, identification number, date, time, description of the incident, immediate action taken, and the signature of the reporting employee and additional individuals involved in the incident. A supervisor should always be notified when an untoward incident is observed, and the written reporting procedure should address how and to whom incident reports should be routed. The process includes an evaluation of the incident and follow-up action. Some state laws protect incident reports from discovery in litigation and address the state's protection of the report if it is qualified or limited in any way. Access to patient-identifiable incident report information is limited to designated individuals.

𝒦EY 𝒫OINTS

- Every health care professional, including students and practicing respiratory therapists, must understand and practice within the confines of regulations and accreditation requirements, a large number of which apply to documentation and information management either directly or indirectly.
- Respiratory students and credentialed therapists alike must be familiar with all requirements related to the site where they practice. A good practice is to consult the policy and procedure manual of each practicing site and to consult an instructor. Clarification on specific issues usually can be found in the health information or risk management department.
- Patient confidentiality is a growing concern, and ensuring such confidentiality is the responsibility of every professional involved in a patient's care. Failure to comply with patient confidentiality standards may result in disciplinary actions or even dismissal.
- Technologic advances will drive many of the changes in the development, maintenance, and transfer of medical information over the next few years. The challenge of each respiratory practitioner is to understand the basic principles and to apply them in the future to improve patient care through information management.

References

1. Smith SA, Gorman CA, Murphy ME, et al. Impact of a diabetes electronic management system on the care of patients seen in a subspecialty diabetes clinic. Diabetes Care 1998;21:972-976.
2. Lusk R, Herrmann K. The computerized patient record. Otolaryngol Clin North Am 1998;31:289-300.
3. Gogola M. A joint hospital/vendor project brings CQI and point-of-care technology to home care. Comput Nurs 1995; 13:143-150.
4. Joint Commission on the Accreditation of Healthcare Organizations. Comprehensive accreditation manual for hospitals: the official guide. Oakbrook Terrace, Ill: The Commission; 1998.
5. Vincze SL. Confidentiality and compliance: political and public interests. In: Confidence. J AHIMA Nov/Dec 1997.
6. American Health Information Management Association. Practice brief: issue: facsimile transmission of health information. Chicago: The Association; 1998.
7. Grigsby B, Allen A. 4th annual telemedicine program review. Telemed Today 1997;5:30-48.

Recommended Reading

Bearden MM. Fax control: coping with the legal issues. J AHIMA 1992;63:58-64.

Detmer D, Dick R, Steen EB. The computer-based patient record: an essential technology for healthcare. rev. ed. Washington, DC: National Academy Press; 1997.

Department of Health and Human Services (US). Medicare conditions of participation proposed rules. Federal Register 62. No. 244 (Dec 1997).

CHAPTER 10

Assessing Outcomes

Garry W. Kauffman

CHAPTER OUTLINE

OBJECTIVES

1. Define *outcomes assessment* from a variety of perspectives.
2. List and discuss goals and benefits of outcomes assessment.
3. Discuss the forces driving a renewed emphasis on outcomes assessment.
4. Classify outcomes according to a variety of criteria.
5. Discuss selected outcomes assessment tools—surveys, tests, scales, and questionnaires.
6. Discuss the results of selected respiratory therapy care outcomes studies.
7. Identify the challenges and strategies for the effective use of outcomes measures.

KEY TERMS

Clinical Outcomes
Cost Outcomes
Outcomes

Outcomes Research
Qualitative Outcomes
Quality Outcomes

Quantitative Outcomes
Service Outcomes

Few issues in health care generate more interest and discussion than assessment of **outcomes.** The literature is abundant with the critical need for the health care industry to endorse the notion that health care providers and leaders can no longer afford to practice medicine without attending to the issues of quality, cost, and service important to each health care stakeholder. Such emphasis is occurring for a variety of reasons, especially the outcry to restrain the costs of health care today, which have reached and sustained double-digit inflation rates over the past several decades. Thus the quest to document the value of the care provided has assumed the focused attention of every United States citizen.

Respiratory therapists should be well versed in all aspects of outcomes assessment and measurement, even though the major focus relies heavily on costs. Compelling and undeniable evidence exists to support the notion that health care professionals of the future must justify the therapeutic, diagnostic, and rehabilitative interventions they provide. The era of health care providers serving as mere task-performers has been decisively replaced by providers who are intimately involved both with the delivery of care and with its effective management.

The role and valuation of the respiratory therapist will be determined not as much by the administration of oxygen, the delivery of aerosolized medications, the drawing of arterial blood, and the manipulation of the various mechanical ventilation controls, but on the ability to make the decisions necessary to scientifically use such interventions. The value of the respiratory therapist will be based on the knowledge of when to initiate, how to monitor and adjust, and when to discontinue oxygen therapy; which mode of delivery, medication, and dosage to deliver to relieve airway constriction; provision of both the interpretation and recommendation for therapy based on the arterial blood gas results; and the when and how to initiate, manipulate, and discontinue the mechanical ventilator.

Physician extenders, experts in cardiopulmonary medicine who know what works and why it works to improve patient care, are needed today.[1] Knowing what works and why is the business of outcomes assessment, and this chapter therefore provides the respiratory therapist with the necessary tools to use outcomes assessment from a variety of perspectives. The chapter concludes with a substantial list of recommended readings, resources, and references to help therapists understand and use outcomes assessment and measurement. This chapter reinforces the need for respiratory therapists to empower themselves to practice respiratory care at the decision-making level and provides a comprehensive review of outcomes assessment and the need for scientifically proven methodologies and tools to provide high-quality, cost-effective, and patient-focused respiratory care.

Definitions, Goals, and Benefits

Only within the last two centuries have studies of treatment effectiveness moved beyond personal observations made by individual clinicians.[2] During modern times, medicine has been based on the use of the scientific method and evidence-based practice. However, the emphasis on assessment and documentation of the efficacy and effectiveness of medical interventions has received renewed vigor within the last two decades. To fully appreciate this focus on outcomes, one must review and define the ways in which outcomes affect medical practice. Starting with the most basic definition and expanding this definition to the current times can derive a comprehensive definition of outcomes because the expanded definition captures the changing focus of the role of medical interventions and the broader societal role that health care has assumed. Although this chapter does not address the use of statistics, a basic knowledge of this area is necessary to comprehend and apply the results of **outcomes research.**

In its original focus and most basic terms the outcome of a medical intervention is simply the result of this intervention witnessed within a short time period after it is applied. Examples in respiratory care include the change in the peak flow rate after administration of an aerosolized bronchodilator, an increase in the blood oxygen level after administration of oxygen, or a change in lung compliance after application of positive end-expiratory pressure.

In each example the patient responds in an observable and measurable manner to the application of respiratory care. The response time for each intervention is within minutes to hours, and measurement of the response is limited to the individual patient receiving the medical intervention. These outcomes were the first type of measures respiratory therapists used daily to respond timely with a respiratory care modality to the specific needs of a patient.

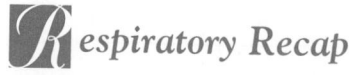
espiratory Recap

Short-Term Outcomes
Peak flow change after bronchodilator administration Increased PaO₂ after oxygen therapy Improved lung compliance with positive end-expiratory pressure (PEEP) Improved arterial blood gas (ABG) values with mechanical ventilation Decreased respiratory rate after aerosol treatment

One way to extend this immediate outcome focus is to expand the response period, observation, and measurement to include a defined episode of care rather than just the short-term response to the intervention. This definition expands the more simplistic definition of outcomes by showing that such interventions may assume a longer time frame. Thus the outcome measures are broadened through expansion of the time frame beyond the observed response to patient treatment at the bedside. Examples include (1) the percentage of patients requiring home oxygen therapy 30 days after discharge from an acute care hospital, (2) the readmission rate for patients successfully completing a pulmonary rehabilitation program versus that of a similar set of patients who did not successfully complete the program, and (3) the admission rate for pediatric patients receiving home-based respiratory care versus that of a similar set of patients who did not receive such care. These examples demonstrate the impact of outcomes research and scientific validation of interventions affecting similar patients in addition to the outcomes measures focused on the specific patient for a short-term period.

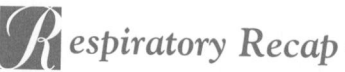
espiratory Recap

Long-Term Outcomes
Percentage of patients needing oxygen 30 days after discharge from acute care Readmission rates for patients who successfully completed pulmonary rehabilitation, compared with other similar patients Admissions rates for pediatric patients receiving home-based respiratory care

The final extension of an outcomes focus expands on the first two in terms of both the time frame and the community or societal level. This most recent extension of outcomes measures entails the most extensive and resource-intensive measurement methodology. As such, it has gained the most attention from the various perspectives within the health care delivery system, particularly in light of the increasing concern over the escalating costs of health care. Examples from respiratory care include patients' satisfaction with a pulmonary rehabilitation program and the impact of patient satisfaction on program completion, the return to work and quality of life for chronic obstructive lung disease patients, and the cost of care for ventilator-dependent patients in acute care facilities versus in subacute care facilities versus in home-based care.

 ## espiratory Recap

> **Broad Outcomes with Societal Implications**
>
> Cost comparisons of long-term mechanical ventilation in various settings, including acute care, subacute care, and home care
> Patient satisfaction with a medical intervention program, such as pulmonary rehabilitation, along with patient completion rates, return to work time, and quality of life
> Costs of care for ventilator-dependent patients in acute care facilities versus subacute care facilities
> Costs of care for disease management of children with asthma managed by respiratory therapists as compared with care provided by other health professionals

Identifying why health care professionals should understand outcomes research and application of outcomes research is important. Respiratory therapists must apply therapeutic, diagnostic, rehabilitative, and educational modalities to provide appropriate care to their patients, in both the short term and the long term. Therefore outcomes research has become an integral component of effective respiratory care, as summarized in Box 10-1. Box 10-2 outlines the goals and benefits of outcomes measurement based on the comprehensive definition discussed. These key aspects of outcomes utilization were summarized by I. K. Crombie in his definition of clinical effectiveness as ". . . doing the right thing, for the right patient, at the right time, in the right setting, by the right health care provider, using the right resources."[3]

Drivers

Many individuals and groups influence outcomes assessment in health care. These groups are called *drivers*, meaning that they set the direction of change by measuring improvement and using their influence. Medical professionals historically have been concerned with measuring

Purpose of Outcomes Research

> "Patient outcomes research provides an opportunity to improve the quality of patient care by modifying the structures and processes of care delivery. Optimal application of outcome analysis involves collaboration between the health care disciplines. The result of such an endeavor would be the identification of health care practices that lead to desired patient outcomes in the most cost-effective manner."

Jones KR. Outcomes analysis: methods and issues. Nurs Econ 1993; 11:145-152.

*B*ox 10-2

Goals and Benefits of Outcomes Measurement

> Improve service to patients and others
> Improve clinical quality
> Improve cost effectiveness of care
> Ensure appropriateness of care
> Prevent adverse effects of care
> Foster professional collaboration

the impact of care on their patients. However, this concern was contained mostly within the medical community until recent decades, during which outcomes has assumed prominence in society. With the advent of Medicare and Medicaid, health care has dramatically expanded. In addition, the nation's population has continued to age, new therapies and treatments have been developed to extend lives, and a variety of stakeholders have begun an intense scrutiny of the increasing costs of medical care. A review of those predominant forces in society can help the respiratory therapist fully comprehend the diversity of influences and appreciate the ways these factors affect their daily professional lives.

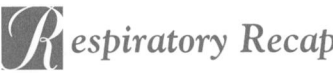 ## espiratory Recap

> **Outcomes Assessment Drivers**
>
> | | |
> |---|---|
> | Insurers | Business and industry |
> | Government | Practitioners |
> | Regulatory organizations | Consumers |
> | Provider organizations | |

Insurers

The insurance industry has witnessed a growing financial impact on its operations as the rate of inflation for health care has risen several times that of the gross domestic product over the last decades. Consequently, commercial health care insurance premiums have risen proportionately, affecting individuals, employers, and health care providers alike. This phenomenon has been at the forefront of the national movement toward managed health care. In addition to the initial focus on escalating costs, which have outstripped inflation rates, various stakeholders in health care have expanded their focus to include quality of care and access to services.

Government

The passage of the Medicare and Medicaid entitlement programs in the 1960s has culminated as one of the major drivers in the fundamental change in the way health care is delivered and reimbursed. The government has increased its use of outcomes measures to manage health care expenditures for Medicare and Medicaid patients within the constraints of the federal budget.

In 1988 the Commonwealth of Pennsylvania created the first law of its type requiring hospitals to collect and submit **clinical outcomes** data for analysis by a new agency, the Health Care Cost Containment Council.[4] This system mandated the use of a computerized acuity-adjusted system that compiles both clinical and financial information in assessing the hospital's care delivery. In March 1998, President Clinton approved the final report of a $1.8 million study by the Advisory Commission on Consumer Protection and Quality in the Health Care Industry, making more than 50 recommendations for the development of national quality improvement and performance measurement standards.[5]

Regulatory Organization

The Joint Commission on Accreditation of Healthcare Organizations (JCAHO) is the accrediting organization the federal government uses to assess whether hospitals, home care companies, and nursing homes may participate in the care of Medicare patients. As part of the accreditation process, the health care organization must demonstrate that it provides quality patient care by measuring and documenting the achievement of appropriate clinical outcomes. In its Accreditation Manual for Hospitals, the JCAHO defines patient care quality as "the degree to which patient care services increase the probability of desired outcomes, given the current state of knowledge."[6]

To improve the existing accreditation process, the JCAHO introduced the ORYX initiative, which integrates

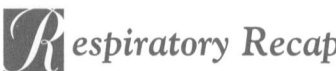

Regulatory Organization

The Joint Commission on Accreditation of Healthcare Organizations (JCAHO) is the accrediting body the federal government uses to assess whether hospitals, home care companies, and nursing homes may participate in the care of Medicare patients.

the use of outcomes and other performance measures into the accreditation process. The goal of ORYX is to establish the essential link between accreditation and the outcomes of patient/resident care through a requirement that health care organizations begin collecting, using, and transmitting performance data to the JCAHO.[7] This initiative was implemented as part of the acute care hospital accreditation process and will be expanded to other care providers.

Provider Organizations

Hospitals, home health care organizations, nursing homes, and other health care provider organizations have historically gathered outcome data focused on the specific health care event occurring in or related to each health care provider. As noted previously, as the pressure to measure the outcomes of health care interventions has increased, these organizations have broadened their measures to include cost and service outcomes in addition to quality measures. Increased pressure also exists for integration of outcomes across the continuum of health care in addition to specific outcome measures by each provider.

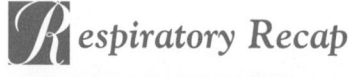

Providers that Measure Outcomes

Hospitals	Skilled nursing facilities
Nursing homes	Outpatient clinics
Home health care organizations	Other health organizations

In 1991 the Voluntary Hospitals of America, Pennsylvania (VHA/PA), began evaluating comparative outcomes data on patients admitted to its network hospitals. This information produced a rich database containing comparative measures for outcomes, including those outcomes achieved by a "best practice" hospital.[8]

Business and Industry

The increasing cost of health care also has affected the business community, particularly the maintenance of market share and profitability. This impact was noted most prominently when the chief executive officer of Chrysler Corporation announced that the cost of employee health care insurance invested in each vehicle exceeded the cost of the vehicle's steel. In short, businesses do not believe that they can be competitive in a worldwide market, given their health care costs, not to mention the government's concern over the impact of health care costs on the national deficit.[9] Within the last few years the National Committee for Quality Assurance (NCQA) developed the Health Plan Employer Data and Information Set (HEDIS), a compilation of performance measures that allow business and industry to consistently evaluate and compare managed care organizations.[10] These statistics and outcome measures are compiled as health plan "report cards" and are beginning to play a significant role as employers make decisions on the purchase of health care. One HEDIS measure directly related to respiratory care is the inpatient admission rate for asthma.

Practitioners

Within the health care delivery system, practitioners work in a variety of settings—acute care, subacute care, extended care, and home care—each of which devotes an increasing amount of resources to measuring their interventions. Clinical quality outcome measures have been part of this focus since the inception of health care delivery, but the focus has expanded to cost and service indicators and patient tracking—not only during an episode of care but also between episodes of care and throughout the patient's lifetime.

Health care practitioners are beginning to look beyond the immediate quality and cost impact of medical interventions to a broader assessment of the totality of these interventions on the long-term health status of the community. Although the cost measure appears to have reached a prominent place among outcome measures, cost containment alone (as is the case for any one outcome measure) cannot provide future security and success for providers and provider organizations. In support of this notion, many practitioners suggest that the health care system is moving from an era of cost containment into one of assessment and accountability.[11]

Consumers

Historically, consumers have played the smallest role in using outcomes to make health care decisions. However, consumers have become one of the major drivers of outcomes research and documentation of outcomes measures. In addition to cost containment, the public is actively seeking documented value for the health care premiums they pay, either directly or indirectly through employer-sponsored or employer-supported health care insurance benefits.[12] In states such as Pennsylvania consumers are provided outcomes data, reported not only by provider organizations but also by the physician of record. Most experts regard the consumer involvement in health care outcomes as only rudimentary at this point, but a consumer revolution in the near future, particularly as health care clinical and cost outcome information becomes more readily accessible, is definitely feasible.

Classification and Categorization of Outcomes

The medical literature has classification and categorization schemes for outcomes, and the following sections provide a representative sample of outcome schemes. A review of these categorizations can help students to fully understand the methodology of classification and use the information within the context of their institutions' outcomes system.

Outcomes According to Time Line

Outcomes can be categorized by time as immediate, short term, and long term. Examples from respiratory care include the following:

- *Immediate:* change in peak flow rate 30 minutes after the administration of a short-acting bronchodilator
- *Short term:* the effect of a respiratory therapist-directed ventilator weaning algorithm on the hospital length of stay (LOS) for patients undergoing coronary bypass surgery
- *Long term:* the effect of successful completion of a comprehensive pulmonary rehabilitation program on admission rates for a chronic obstructive lung disease population over 5 years

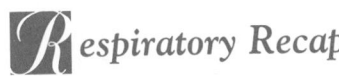

espiratory Recap

Time Line Outcomes
Immediate
Short term
Long term

Qualitative Versus Quantitative Outcomes

Classifying outcomes by qualitative or quantitative measures is a useful methodology because of its inherent simplicity. Examples of **qualitative outcomes** in respiratory care include respiratory therapist job satisfaction, patient satisfaction with a rehabilitation program, and recruitment success. Examples of **quantitative outcomes** include LOS in an acute care hospital, mortality rate, respiratory therapist turnover rates and recruitment costs, and number of missed or delayed aerosol therapy treatments.

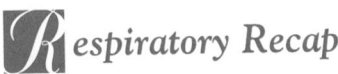

espiratory Recap

Quantitative and Qualitative Outcomes
Quantitative Outcomes Measures of health care that can be counted; *examples:* length of stay, mortality rate, and missed therapies
Qualitative Outcomes Data measures that cannot be quantified but can be analyzed to describe quality; *examples:* patient satisfaction, opinions regarding service, and patient preferences for health care options

Service, Quality, and Cost

Examples of outcome measures in respiratory care related to service include patient and family satisfaction with care provided by respiratory therapists, the time interval from an order until the performance of a sleep study, and respiratory therapist turnover rates. Examples of quality outcome measures include mortality, missed or delayed aerosol therapy treatments, and readmission rates from skilled nursing facilities for patients with pneumonia. Outcome measures categorized by cost include cost per respiratory modality, cost to recruit respiratory therapists, and cost of a pulmonary rehabilitation program in relation to readmission rates.

Continuum of Care

K. N. Lohr[13] identified a comprehensive typology of outcomes based on the continuum of care that includes mortality in the hospital or shortly after discharge, adverse events, and complications during hospitalization. Continuum of care includes a patient's inadequate recovery or complications requiring readmission, as well as any prolongation of medical problems because of the failure to assess an unrelated condition. Other aspects of continuum of care include a decline in a patient's health status because of problems or situations leading to a delay in or a denial of admission, along with a decline in a patient's quality of life that may include poorer physical, emotional, or mental function.

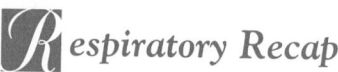

Continuum of Care
Mortality rates
Adverse events and complications
Inadequate recovery and readmission rates
Failure to assess an unrelated condition
Decline in health due to delays or denials
Decreased quality of life

Perspective

Proposed by S. T. Hegyvary[14] is a categorization of outcomes based on the perspectives of providers, consumers, and purchasers that is further categorized according to the following four areas:

1. Clinical: the patient's response to medical and nursing interventions
2. Functional: the maintenance or improvement of physical functioning
3. Financial: outcomes achieved with the most efficient use of resources
4. Perceptual: the patient's satisfaction with outcomes, care received, and providers

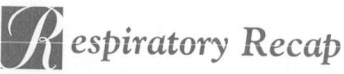

Outcomes Classified by Perspective
Providers, consumers, and purchasers can classify outcomes on perspective based on the following four areas: 1. Clinical 2. Functional 3. Financial 4. Perceptual

Measurement Instruments and Techniques

A number of methods are used to classify or categorize outcomes with the use of two different types of tools—those that measure health status and those that measure health-related quality of life, both of which include generic measures and condition-specific measures. Generic tools are comprehensive measures that assess the effects of interventions on health status, whereas condition-specific measures focus either on signs and symptoms that reflect the status of a given medical condition or on the impact of the disease or problem on the patient or group of patients.[15] Regardless of the type of tool, the use of standardized and validated tools, particularly with standardized care policies and/or protocols, provides the greatest value for clinicians (Box 10-3).[16-29]

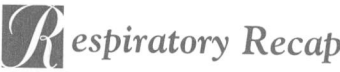

Outcomes Assessment Questions
Do patients do better? (health status) Do patients feel better? (quality of life)

Results of Outcomes Studies

This section helps reinforce the information on outcomes definitions, classification schemes, and instruments and techniques while providing practical applications used within the current health care delivery system. A review of the peer-reviewed medical literature reveals tens of thousands of research investigations dealing with the delivery of clinical medicine. In contrast to the voluminous scientific articles on clinical **quality outcomes** is the relative dearth of research seeking to evaluate service and **cost outcomes.** The scientific evaluation of service and cost outcomes has received significant interest only within the past two decades, for reasons discussed previously in this chapter. The following reviews illustrate the current state of outcomes measurement within the practice of respiratory care.

Box 10-3

Selected Outcome Tools

MOS 36-Item Short Form Health Survey[a]

A generic, health-related, quality-of-life measure used to evaluate health-related quality of life across various populations, it encompasses scores for eight domains, as well as overall physical and mental health.

About My Asthma[b]

A disease-specific questionnaire designed to assess stressors affecting the quality of life in children with asthma, the form asks children to rate the frequency with which they experience certain thoughts and feelings that can contribute to stress and decreased quality of life.

Asthma Bother Profile[c]

A self-administered questionnaire designed to measure the level of distress caused by asthma, it addresses two domains of distress in various contexts and asthma management.

Asthma Quality of Life Questionnaire—Juniper[d]

This disease-specific, health-related quality-of-life instrument was developed by E. Juniper and colleagues to identify the physical and emotional aspects of asthma.

Asthma Quality of Life Questionnaire—Marks[e]

In this self-administered questionnaire for adults covering both physical and emotional disease aspects, the respondents are asked to describe how troubling particular items have been over the past 4 weeks.

Chronic Respiratory Disease Questionnaire[f]

This interviewer-administered questionnaire measures the physical and emotional aspects of chronic respiratory disease.

Flanagan's Quality of Life Scale[g]

This self-administered questionnaire designed for patients with chronic illness addresses physical and material well-being, relationships with other people, social/community/civic activities, personal development and fulfillment, recreation, and independence.

Human Activity Profile Test[h]

Formerly the *Additive Daily Activities Profile Test (ADAPT),* this test was originally designed to measure the activity levels of individuals in rehabilitation programs for COPD but has since also been used with other patient populations. It assesses maximal activity, adjusted activity, activity age, fitness classification, activity classification, energy analysis, and dyspnea scale.

Living With Asthma Questionnaire[i]

A condition-specific, health–care-related, quality-of-life questionnaire designed to evaluate an individual's subjective experiences with asthma, including functional limitations and distress, it addresses social/leisure activity, sport, sleep, holidays, work and other activities, colds, mobility, effects on others, medication use, sexual activity, dysphoric states, and attitudes.

Perceived Control of Asthma Questionnaire[j]

This disease-specific instrument is designed to measure an individual's perceived ability to deal with asthma and its exacerbations.

Pulmonary Function Status Scale[k]

This functional status instrument is used to assess daily activities and social functioning, psychologic functioning, and sexual functioning in adult pulmonary patients.

Pulmonary Functional Status and Dyspnea Questionnaire[l]

This functional status and dyspnea questionnaire addresses functional status and dyspnea, self-care, mobility, home management, eating, recreation, and socialization in adult pulmonary patients.

Seattle Obstructive Lung Disease Questionnaire[m]

This brief, computer-scan configured, self-administered questionnaire is designed to measure the physical function, emotional function, coping skills, and treatment satisfaction of patients with COPD.

St. George's Respiratory Questionnaire[n]

This disease-specific instrument designed to measure impact on overall health, daily life, and perceived well-being was originally designed for patients with fixed and reversible airway obstruction. It addresses the frequency and severity of symptoms, activities that cause or are limited by breathlessness, and impacts regarding social functioning and psychologic disturbances that are the result of airways disease.

COPD, *Chronic obstructive pulmonary disease.*

[a]*Ware JE, Sherbourne CD. The MOS 36-Item short form health survey: conceptual framework and item selection. Med Care 1992;30:473-483.*

[b]*Mishoe SC, Baker RR, Poole S, et al. The development and evaluation of a new instrument to assess stress levels and quality of life in children with asthma. J Asthma 1998;35(7):553-563.*

[c]*Hyland ME, Ley A, Fisher DW, et al. Measurement of psychological distress in asthma and asthma management programmes. Br J Clin Psychol 1995;34:601-611.*

[d]*Juniper EF, Guyatt GH, Epstein RS, et al. Evaluation of impairment of health-related quality of life in asthma: development of a questionnaire for use in clinical trials. Thorax 1992;47:76-83.*

[e]*Marks GB, Dunn SM, Woolcock AJ, et al. An evaluation of an asthma quality of life questionnaire as a measure of change in adults with asthma. J Clin Epidemiol 1993;46:1103-1111.*

[f]*Guyatt GH, Berman LB, Townsend M, et al. A measure of quality of life for clinical trials in chronic lung disease. Thorax 1987;42:773-778.*

[g]*Flanagan JC. A research approach to improving our quality of life. Am Psychol 1978;33:138-147.*

[h]*Daughton DM, Fix AJ, Kass I, et al. Maximum oxygen consumption and the adapt quality of life search. Arch Phys Med Rehabil 1982;63:620-622.*

[i]*Hyland ME, Finnis S, Irvine SH: A scale for assessing quality of life in adult asthma sufferers. J Psychosom Res 1991;35(1):99-110.*

[j]*Katz PP, Yelin EH, Smith S, et al. Perceived control of asthma: development and validation of a questionnaire. Am J Respir Crit Care Med 1997;155:577-582.*

[k]*Weaver TE, Narsavage GL. Reliability and validity of the pulmonary impact profile scale. Am Rev Respir Dis 1989;139:A244.*

[l]*Lareau SC, Carrieri-Kohlman V, Janson-Bjerklie S, et al. Development and testing of the pulmonary functional status and dyspnea questionnaire. Heart Lung 1994;23:242-250.*

[m]*Tu SP, McDonell MB, Spertus JA, et al. A new self-administered questionnaire to monitor health-related quality of life in patients with COPD. Chest 1997;112:614-622.*

[n]*Jones PW, Quirk FH, Baveystock CM, et al. The St. George's Respiratory Questionnaire. Respir Med 1991;85:25-31.*

Asthma

"An Evaluation of Asthma Education for School Personnel Using Peak Performance USA"[30] is an investigation focusing on the role of asthma education and reinforcement as positive and prophylactic care of the asthmatic child. In particular the investigators and others believe that asthma care fails while the child is in school because of a lack of asthma training for teachers, school nurses, principals, and physical education instructors. Significant quality and cost issues exist in this type of program. Using the American Association for Respiratory Care's (AARC's) Peak Performance USA program within two school districts (one district being the control), the respiratory therapists taught asthma management to 180 school personnel. The outcomes measured included staff members' retention of learning, requests by other school districts for the program, and referral of parents to asthma management classes.

"Measuring Quality of Life in Asthma"[31] is an investigation designed to evaluate the measurement properties of an asthma quality-of-life questionnaire. The symptomatic adult asthmatics enrolled in the study were followed with physiologic metrics, documentation via the sickness impact profile, and the Rand questionnaire. The questionnaire detected changes in individuals who responded to treatment or had natural fluctuations in their asthma and differentiated them from those individuals who remained stable. The investigators noted significant longitudinal and cross-sectional correlations among asthma quality of life and other measures of both clinical asthma and generic quality of life and concluded that the questionnaire is a valid evaluative and discriminative tool with good measurement properties.

"About My Asthma"[17] (AMA) is a quality-of-life instrument designed to assess stress levels of children with asthma. The AMA established concurrent validity with the pediatric quality of life questionnaire (PAQLQ). Increased levels of stress measured by the AMA correlated with decreased quality of life measured by the PAQLQ. Children who attended a weeklong asthma camp showed decreased levels of stress associated with their asthma. The investigators concluded that the AMA is a valid and reliable instrument to measure the quantity and type of stressors experienced by children who have asthma. Asthma educational efforts should be designed for children to decrease stress levels, enhance self-management, and improve quality of life.

"Incorrect Use of Metered Dose Inhalers by Medical Personnel"[32] is the result of a test investigators designed to evaluate the didactic competency of physicians, nurses, and respiratory therapists in the proper instruction technique for use of metered dose inhalers. Of the three groups the scores indicated that respiratory therapists had a significantly higher competency than the other professionals. That no group scored 100% led the investigators to conclude that additional instruction was required for all medical personnel. This study provided outcomes data, an impetus to increase education and training. Patient response to the instructional competency of these profes-

sionals was not measured, an area for possible future investigation.

"AirLogix's Asthma Management Program Attracts HMO Attention."[33] AirLogix, founded and managed by two respiratory therapists, developed a respiratory wellness program using patient education to manage the care of asthma patients. The program has two main objectives—to empower and encourage patients to self-manage their disease and to partner with the patient, physician, case manager, and payer to achieve better financial and clinical outcomes. Given a basic cost of approximately $750 per asthma patient and approximately $1250 per chronic obstructive pulmonary disease (COPD) patient per year, the savings approach $20,000 per patient per year. In a study of 608 program members with asthma or COPD who participated in the program for between 3 and 12 months, a 73% reduction in hospitalization, a 78% reduction in hospital days, and a 73% reduction in emergency room visits were noted. For individuals with asthma the number of missed days of work dropped 55%, whereas the number of missed days of work for adults caring for children with asthma dropped 43%.

Disease Prevention

"Screening for Obstructive Sleep Apnea in Patients Presenting for Snoring Surgery"[34] was developed because of the importance of diagnosis of this high-mortality condition. Investigators performed a prospective study to evaluate whether a screening model could detect this disease in a manner comparable to polysomnographic testing. Both sensitivity and cost factors were included, and each screening model obtained 100% sensitivity, thus reducing the need for polysomnography. Additionally, the cost of these models was $35 to $80 less per patient than polysomnography.

"Get Money's Worth with Stop-Smoking Programs"[35] followed a report released by the Agency for Health Care Policy and Research revealing that smoking-cessation programs not only improve the health of the participants but also provide substantial economic savings. Investigators noted that although all types of smoking-cessation treatments are cost effective, those involving more intensive counseling and the nicotine patch proved especially beneficial. At an average cost of about $2600 per year of life saved, smoking-cessation treatment is especially cost effective in comparison with cholesterol treatment, a routine intervention that costs nearly 40 times more. Additionally, the report noted that if the interventions were provided to 75% of U.S. smokers 18 years and older, the cost to society would be $6.3 billion in the first year of implementation. As a result, society could expect to gain 1.7 million new quitters at an average savings of $3779 per quitter and $2587 per life-year saved.

Respiratory Assessment and Protocols

"The Relationship of Patient Satisfaction with Care and Clinical Outcomes"[36] is a report whose authors examined the relationship between patient satisfaction regarding quality of care, hospital care, and physician time with two ways of looking at outcomes—absolute (defined as the status at 6 months after surgery) and relative (defined as the difference between baseline and follow-up status). The authors reported that each outcome was related significantly to each satisfaction scale. However, the relative outcomes were related more strongly to satisfaction than were the absolute outcomes. Thus although outcomes and satisfaction are related, these patients' satisfaction involves more than outcomes alone. When noting their satisfaction with the care rendered, patients are more likely to focus on their present health status than consider the improvements achieved.

(The) "Establishment of a Respiratory Assessment Team Is Associated with Decreased Mortality in Patients Readmitted to the ICU."[37] The investigators of this report noted differences in mortality in intensive care unit (ICU) patient outcomes associated with improving the quality and appropriateness of respiratory care delivered to non-ICU patients on acute care floors. Specifically, they compared the outcomes between two patient groups who differed as to whether they received assessment by a respiratory therapy team and discovered that neither the overall ICU readmission rate nor those patients admitted for respiratory failure differed between the groups. However, those patients who received assessment by the respiratory assessment team had a significantly lower mortality. The investigators concluded that the respiratory assessment team enhanced the quality of patient care by identifying developing problems, which lead to a more rapid ICU readmission and thus contributed to the lower mortality rate.

"Quality of Life and Hospital Re-admission in Patients with Chronic Obstructive Pulmonary Disease"[38] involved investigators' study as to whether quality-of-life scores were capable of prospectively predicting readmission for COPD or death within 12 months of the initial admission and whether such scores predicted home nebulizer use. Increasing scientific evidence suggests that patient compliance, satisfaction, and quality of life can play a significant role in the clinical course of disease. Using several physiologic measures of disease severity and the St. George's Respiratory Questionnaire, the authors concluded that poor scores on this instrument, which measures patient distress and coping, were associated with readmission rates for COPD and use of resources (for example, nebulizers), outcomes independent of the physiologic measures of disease severity.

"Professionalism, Respiratory Care Practice, and Physician Acceptance of a Respiratory Consult Service"[39] is an editorial reviewing the results of several studies that examine the impact of respiratory care staff members performing their responsibilities and their appreciation by medical staff members. Of particular interest are misallocation of human and material resources, use of patient-focused respiratory protocols, and clinical practice guidelines. Although the studies reviewed were not done in concert, results indicate that the medical community generally views respiratory therapists as adding value, particularly when the spirits of collaboration and collegiality were

in evidence. This editorial also illustrates ways in which **service outcomes** must consider more than clinical care.

"Medical House Staff Impressions Regarding the Impact of a Respiratory Therapy Consult Service"[40] involves author evaluation of whether medical house staff members regard a respiratory therapy consult service as educationally and clinically useful. House staff members were surveyed regarding their understanding and appreciation of the respiratory consult service. The authors concluded that although staff members' knowledge of the service was excellent, they varied significantly in their recognition of the service's value. The authors suggested that more research is appropriate to determine whether these impressions about the consult service are supported by direct measure of the house staff members' knowledge of respiratory care ordering.

Challenges and Strategies for Clinicians Using Outcomes Research

Practice Variation

Two of the most serious limitations in research, especially for the practitioner working in a general care hospital, are time and financial resources. The respiratory therapist may find conducting research in a small facility difficult or even impossible because of the large number of observations required to achieve statistical relevance. Even if sufficient observations are available, the practitioner may not have the time or financial resources necessary to conduct the study.

One strategy designed to address these issues is to adopt a standard practice across multiple sites to reach the critical mass of observations within a reasonable time. The AARC's clinical practice guidelines were developed in part to address this issue of standardizing respiratory care practice and to make measurement and comparison among providers easier.

Data Collection: Timing and Source

Outcomes data are frequently collected retrospectively, often both for cost and data availability. In many instances, data collection and abstraction are tied to the organization's billing processes, which are not necessarily connected to clinical processes or decision processes affecting the real-time care of patients. The advancements witnessed most recently with computerized clinical information systems and online clinical decision support systems offer significant advantages, both in real-time data collection and in the provision of real-time feedback and interactive exchange to maximize patient care.

Patients as Data

Significant variation exists among patients based on demographics and pathophysiology as established in the literature. An aspect that has received limited attention until the last few years is the critical role of patient compliance. The "white coat hypertension" experiments documented that a white coat–attired physician's presence causes an increase in a patient's blood pressure. A more recent investigation (unpublished) regarding patient compliance with metered dose inhalers has revealed that some patients actuate the metered dose inhaler (that is, as measured by a "counter" attached to the device) while in the physician's waiting room to demonstrate to the physician compliance with the prescription. Because of this increased appreciation of the role of the patient, the respiratory therapist should begin investigations with a heightened awareness of the vital roles of the patient and family members.

Interconnection of Service, Quality, and Cost

As noted previously, the vast majority of outcomes research has focused on clinical quality. Respiratory therapists should vigorously analyze the process or program as to its potential for patient and family service and cost factors. Despite advocates' vigorous support of wellness and prevention as cost effective and clinically effective in many instances, current funding and reimbursement for such programs is insufficient. Of those programs gaining increased reimbursement are asthma prevention and smoking cessation,[39] particularly because the body of scientific evidence is growing to document their combined quality, service, and cost value.

---

*K*EY *P*OINTS

- Outcomes assessment has become increasingly popular in the past two decades, the result of numerous influences but perhaps the most critical being the compulsion to reduce health care cost and establish some degree of accountability for the services provided.
- Outcomes assessment is the witnessing of a result within a designated period after the application of a medical intervention.
- Clinical effectiveness means doing the right thing for the right patient, at the right time, in the right setting, by the right provider, with the right resources.
- Numerous forces driving the use of outcomes assessment include insurers, government, regulatory organizations, provider organizations, business and industry, practitioners, and consumers.
- Outcomes can be classified according to time line; qualitative versus quantitative; service, quality, and cost; continuum of care; and perspective.
- Many validated outcome tools are available.
- Outcomes assessment asks and then answers the following basic health care questions:
  - Does the patient do better (health status)?
  - Does the patient feel better (quality of life)?

References

1. Mishoe SC, MacIntyre NR. Expanding professional roles for respiratory care practitioners. Respir Care 1997;42(1):71-91.
2. General Accounting Office (US). Cross-design synthesis: a new strategy for medical effectiveness research. Washington, DC: The Office; 1992.
3. Crombie IK. Research in health care, design, conduct, and interpretation of health services research. West Sussex, UK: John Wiley & Sons; l996. pp. 1-20.
4. Krivenko CA, Chodroff C. The analysis of clinical outcomes: getting started in benchmarking. Joint Commission Journal on Quality Improvement 1994;20:260-266.
5. Clinton proposes standard performance measures. Healthcare Benchmarks May 1998:69-70.
6. Joint Commission on Accreditation of Healthcare Organizations. Standards. In: 1993 accreditation manual for hospitals. Oakbrook Terrace, Ill: The Commission; 1993.
7. Grachek MK. Distinguished lectures in subacute care: accreditation. Subacute Care Today May/June 1998;1:36-38.
8. Brewster AC, Karlin BG, Hyde LA, et al. Medisgroups: a clinically based approach to classifying hospital patients at admission. Inquiry 1985;22:377-387.
9. Giordano SP. Conference summary: emerging health care delivery models and respiratory care. Respir Care l997;42:15-16.
10. Sennett C. An introduction to HEDIS: the health plan employer data and information set. Hosp Phys Aug 1997:42-49.
11. Relman A. Assessment and accountability: the third revolution in health care. N Engl J Med 1988;319:1221-1222.
12. Davies AR, Doyle MA, Lansky D, et al. Outcomes assessment in clinical settings: a consensus statement on principles and best practices in project management. Joint Commission Journal on Quality Improvement 1994;20:6-16.
13. Lohr KN. Impact of Medicare prospective payment on the quality of medical care: a research agenda. Santa Monica, Calif: Rand Corporation; 1985.
14. Hegyvary ST. Issues in outcomes research. J Nurs Qual Assur 1991;5:41-44.
15. Bunch D. Using data to improve patient outcomes. AARC Times 1999;23(3):18-22.
16. Ware JE, Sherbourne CD. The MOS 36-item short form health survey: conceptual framework and item selection. Med Care 1992;30:473-483.
17. Mishoe SC, Baker RR, Poole S, et al. The development and evaluation of a new instrument to assess stress levels and quality of life in children with asthma. J Asthma 1998;35(7):553-563.
18. Hyland ME, Ley A, Fisher DW, et al. Measurement of psychological distress in asthma and asthma management programmes. Br J Clin Psychol 1995;34:601-611.
19. Juniper EF, Guyatt GH, Epstein RS, et al. Evaluation of impairment of health-related quality of life in asthma: development of a questionnaire for use in clinical trials. Thorax 1992;47:76-83.
20. Marks GB, Dunn SM, Woolcock AJ, et al. An evaluation of an asthma quality of life questionnaire as a measure of change in adults with asthma. J Clin Epidemiol 1993;46:1103-1111.
21. Guyatt GH, Berman LB, Townsend M, et al. A measure of quality of life for clinical trials in chronic lung disease. Thorax 1987;42:773-778.
22. Flanagan JC. A research approach to improving our quality of life. Am Psychol 1978;33:138-147.

23. Daughton DM, Fix AJ, Kass I, et al. Maximum oxygen consumption and the ADAPT quality of life search. Arch Phys Med Rehabil 1982;63:620-622.

24. Hyland ME, Finnis S, Irvine SH. A scale for assessing quality of life in adult asthma sufferers. J Psychosom Res 1991;35(1):99-110.

25. Katz PP, Yelin EH, Smith S, et al. Perceived control of asthma: development and validation of a questionnaire. Am J Respir Crit Care Med 1997;155:577-582.

26. Weaver TE, Narsavage GL. Reliability and validity of the pulmonary impact profile scale. Am Rev Respir Dis 1989;139:A244.

27. Lareau SC, Carrieri-Kohlman V, Janson-Bjerklie S, et al. Development and testing of the pulmonary functional status and dyspnea questionnaire. Heart Lung 1994;23:242-250.

28. Tu SP, McDonell MB, Spertus JA, et al. A new self-administered questionnaire to monitor health-related quality of life in patients with COPD. Chest 1997;112:614-622.

29. Jones PW, Quirk FH, Baveystock CM, et al. The St. George's Respiratory Questionnaire. Respir Med 1991;85:25-31.

30. Powell D. An evaluation of asthma education using Peak Performance USA. Respir Care 1998;43(10):804-810.

31. Juniper EF, Guyatt GH, Ferrie PJ, et al. Measuring quality of life in asthma. Am Rev Respir Dis 1993;147:832-838.

32. Guidry GG, Brown WD, Stogner SW, et al. Incorrect use of metered dose inhalers by medical personnel. Chest 1992;101:31-33.

33. Carr LW. AirLogix's asthma management program attracts HMO attention. Dallas Bus J 1996 (Feb 13-19):C5,11.

34. Pradhan PS, Gliklich RE, Winkleman MD, et al. Screening for obstructive sleep apnea in patients presenting for snoring surgery. Laryngoscope 1996;106:1393-1397.

35. Hasty S, editor. Get money's worth with stop-smoking programs. QI/TQM Feb 1998:19-20.

36. Kane RL, Maciejewski M, Finch M. The relationship of patient satisfaction with care and clinical outcomes. Med Care 1997;35:714-730.

37. Kirby EG, Durbin CG. Establishment of a respiratory assessment team is associated with decreased mortality in patients readmitted to the ICU. Respir Care 1996;41:903-907.

38. Osman LM, Godden DJ, Friend JAR, et al. Quality of life and hospital re-admission in patients with chronic obstructive pulmonary disease. Thorax 1997;52:67-71.

39. Hess DR. Professionalism, respiratory care practice, and physician acceptance of a respiratory consult service [editorial]. Respir Care 1998;43:546-548.

40. Stoller JK, Michnicki I. Medical house staff impressions regarding the impact of a respiratory therapy consult service. Respir Care 1998;43:549-556.

Recommended Reading

Anderson C. Measuring what works in health care. Science 1994;263:1080-1081.

Bergner M, Rothman M. Health status measures: an overview and guide for selection. Ann Rev Pub Health 1987;8:191-240.

Brewster AC, Karlin BG, Hyde LA, et al. MEDISGRPS: a clinically based approach to classifying hospital patients at admission. Inquiry 1985;22:377-387.

Charlson M, Sax F, MacKenzie C, et al. Assessing illness severity: does clinical judgment work? J Chron Dis 1986;39:439-452.

Cleary PD, McNeil BJ. Patient satisfaction as an indicator of quality care. Inquiry 1988;25:25-36.

Colditz GA, Miller JN, Mosteller F. How study design affects outcomes in comparisons of therapy. I. Medical. Stat Med 1989;8:441-454.

Daley J, Jencks S, Draper D, et al. Predicting hospital-associated mortality for Medicare patients: a method for patients with stroke, pneumonia, acute myocardial infarction, and congestive heart failure. JAMA 1988;260:3617-3624.

Detsky A, Naglie I. A clinician's guide to cost-effectiveness analysis. Ann Intern Med 1990;113:147-154.

Deyo RA. Measuring functional outcomes in therapeutic trials for chronic disease. Control Clin Trials 1984;5:223-240.

DiMatteo MR, Sherbourne CD, Hays RD, et. al. Physicians' characteristics influence patients' adherence to medical treatment: results from the medical outcomes study. Health Psychol 1993;12:93-102.

Draper D, Kahn KL, Reinisch EJ, et. al. Studying the effects of the DRG-based prospective payment system on quality of care—design, sampling, and fieldwork. JAMA 264:1956-1561.

Fisher EJ, Wennberg T, Stukel T, et al. Hospital readmission rates for cohorts of Medicare beneficiaries in Boston and New Haven. N Engl J Med 1990;331:989- 995.

Goldfield N. The hubris of health status measurement: a clarification of its role in the assessment of medical care. J Qual Health Care 1996;8:115-123.

Hansluwka HE. Measuring the health of populations, indicators and interpretations. Soc Sci Med 1985;20:1207-1224.

Hays RD, Kravitz RL, Mazl RM, et. al. The impact of patient adherence on health outcomes for patients with chronic disease in the Medical Outcomes Study. J Behav Med 1994;17:347-360.

Iezzoni LI. Risk adjustment for measuring health care outcomes. Ann Arbor, Mich: Health Administration Press; 1997.

Kaplan R, Anderson J. A general health policy model: update and applications. Health Serv Res 1988;23:203-235.

Knaus W, Draper E, Wagner D. APACHE II: a severity of disease classification system. Crit Care Med 1985;13:818-829.

Lurie N. Administrative data and outcomes research. Med Care 1990;28:867-869.

McDowell INC. Measuring health: a guide to rating scales and questionnaires. New York: Oxford University Press; 1996.

McMahon L, Billi J. Measurement of severity of illness and the Medicare prospective payment system. J Gen Intern Med 1988;3:482-490.

Miller JN, Colditz GA, Mosteller F. How study design affects outcomes in comparisons of therapy. II. Surgical. Stat Med 1989;8:455-466.

Mulrow CD, Cook DJ. Systematic reviews: synthesis of best evidence for health care decisions. Philadelphia: American College of Physicians; 1998. p. 117.

Oberle MW, Baker EL. Healthy People 2000 and community health planning. Ann Rev Pub Health 1994;15:259-275.

Pascoe G, Attkisson C. The evaluation ranking scale: a new methodology for assessing satisfaction. Eval Prog Plan 1983;6:335-347.

Patrick D, Bergner M. Measurement of health status in the 1990s. Ann Rev Pub Health 1990;11:165-183.

Petitti DB. Meta-analysis, decision analysis, and cost-effectiveness analysis: methods for quantitative synthesis in medicine. New York: Oxford University Press; 1994.

Rogers WH, Draper D, Kahn KL, et. al. Quality of care before and after implementation of the DRG-based prospective payment system: a summary of effects. JAMA 1990;264:1989-1994.

Roghmann KJ, Hengst A, Zastowny TR. Satisfaction with medical care: its measurement and relation to utilization. Med Care 1979;17:461-479.

Roos N, Black C, Frohlich N, et al. A population-based health information system. Med Care 1995;33:13-20.

Sechrest LHM. The critical importance of nonexperimental data. In: Sechrest L, Perrin E, Bunker J. Research methodology: strengthening casual interpretations of nonexperimental data. Washington, DC: Agency for Health Care Policy and Research; 1990.

Slater CH. What is outcomes research and what can it tell us? Eval Health Prof 1997;20:243-264.

Strasser S, Davis R. Measuring patient satisfaction for improved patient services. Chicago: American College of Healthcare Executives; 1991.

Tarlov A, Ware J, Greenfield S, et. al. The medical outcomes study: an application of methods for monitoring the results of medical care. JAMA 1989;262:925-930.

Thomas J, Ashcraft M. Measuring severity of illness: six severity systems and their ability to explain cost variations. Inquiry 1991;28(1):39-55.

Walker SR, Rosser RM, editors. Quality of life assessment: key issues in the 1990s. Boston: Kluwer Academic; 1993.

Wennberg JE, Roos N, Sola L, et al. Use of claims data systems to evaluate health care outcomes. JAMA 1987;257:933-936.

Websites of Interest

www.aarc.org (American Association for Respiratory Care)
www.ache.org (American College of Healthcare Executives)
www.asq.org (American Society for Quality)
www.atsqol.org (American Thoracic Society Quality of Life)
www.bayerquality.org (Bayer Quality Network)
www.hcfa.gov (Health Care Financing Administration)
www.jcaho.org (Joint Commission on Accreditation of Healthcare Organizations)
www.nahq.org (National Association for Healthcare Quality)
www.ncbi.hlm.hih.gov/PubMed (MEDLINE)
www.ncqa.org (National Committee for Quality Assurance)
www.QLMed.org (Quality of Life Assessment in Medicine)

CHAPTER 11

Health Care Reimbursement

Allan B. Saposnick
William F. Galvin

CHAPTER OUTLINE

Basic Health Care Delivery Functions
Stakeholders in Health Care Reimbursement
Respiratory Therapist's Role—Balancing Cost and Care
Forces Influencing Health Care Costs
Financing Health Care—A Brief History and Overview
  Retrospective Payment
  Prospective Payment
  Capitation
Era of Managed Care
  Health Maintenance Organizations
  Preferred Provider Organizations
  Point-of-Service Plans
  Exclusive Provider Organizations

Reimbursement Methodologies
  Fee for Service
  Cost Plus/Charge Minus
  Prospective Reimbursement
  Diagnosis-Related Groups
  Resource-Based Relative Value Scale
  Bundled Charges
  Managed Care Approaches
  Case Mix
Future of Health Care Funding
Reimbursement and the Respiratory Therapist
  Documenting Care—Charting
  Three Rights
  Demonstrating Value

OBJECTIVES

1. Explain the four major functions of the health care delivery system.
2. Explain the role of the major stakeholders in health care delivery.
3. Discuss the forces influencing health care change and costs.
4. Describe the general health care payment systems.
5. Explain the history and evolution of managed care.
6. Explain the types of managed care organizations.
7. Describe the more popular reimbursement methodologies.
8. Discuss the future of health care financing.
9. Discuss the implications of reimbursement for the respiratory therapist.

KEY TERMS

Bundled Charges
Capitation
Case Mix
Copayment
Diagnosis-Related Groups (DRGs)
Exclusive Provider Organization (EPO)
Fee-for-Service
Health Care Financing Administration (HCFA)

Health Maintenance Organization (HMO)
Indemnity Insurance Plan
Insurance
Managed Care Organizations (MCO)
Medicaid
Medicare
Minimum Data Set (MOS)
Point-of-Service Plans (POS)

Preferred Provider Organization (PPO)
Prospective Payment System (PPS)
Retrospective Payment System (RPS)
Skilled Nursing Facility (SNF)
Third-Party Payer

The way in which health care is reimbursed has a profound impact on its delivery and practice. Reimbursement and economic considerations are central issues for health care executives. In fact, some would say that the present health care system in the United States is driven almost exclusively by the dollar. Although such a statement may sound cold, greedy, impersonal, and even callous, the wise respiratory therapist must recognize the paramount importance placed on reimbursement methodologies and sources. Converting care and services into financial returns to the provider has become critical to survival, and economic pressures are not likely to change in the foreseeable future.

The problem is that respiratory therapy schools and departments have not done an especially good job in helping students and practitioners understand the critical importance of the reimbursement process and the underlying economic principles guiding the system. This chapter identifies and discusses the basic functions of health care, provides an overview of the forces driving the system, identifies and explains the role of the major stakeholders, provides a basic and simplified view of the history and various forms of reimbursement, and explains the role and function of the respiratory therapist within this system.

Basic Health Care Delivery Functions

The four major functions of the health care system in the United States are financing, insurance, delivery, and payment. Although this chapter focuses on insurance and payment, all four are discussed to set the stage for a better therapist understanding of how the system works. Table 11-1 depicts the four major functions, their roles, and the group or organization that is associated with each.

The first major function in health care delivery is *financing*, which involves the purchase of insurance and serves as the means to pay for the health care services consumed by the patient or client. Employers generally finance health care as a fringe benefit. The federal, state, and local government also can provide it.

Strictly speaking the *insurance* function entails protection of the patient, client, or consumer against catastrophic risk. Insurance also refers to the administration of the customer's benefits package and is provided by an insurance company or managed care organization (MCO) that serves as an intermediary between the purchaser and the recipient or consumer. Interestingly, providers (especially hospitals) contract directly with employers to provide health care services.

Health care *delivery*, the third major function, involves the provision of services by the physician or other health care provider to the patient or consumer. *Delivery* also can refer to the hospital, skilled nursing home, clinic, or home care company. The respiratory therapist is closely involved in this function.

Perhaps the most complex function of the system is *payment*, a major focus of this chapter that is addressed in detail in subsequent sections. The respiratory therapist must understand that payment deals specifically with reimbursement and disbursement of funds. It is an infinitely complicated process that undergoes continuous change and ceaseless revision. Payers are constantly searching for ways to optimize their profits and work the system.

The sources of these funds for disbursement are employers; the federal, state, and local governments; fraternal organizations; and MCOs. These sources take the form of premiums or entitlement payments. The insurance company is the intermediary providing payment to the provider orchestrated by way of a consumer claim. The provider or patient submits the claim to the intermediary, which settles or processes it. Payment can be made for the entire amount or a designated portion identified by the plan and addressed during contract negotiations. With managed care the patient may simply pay a small copayment, deductible, or out-of-pocket amount. More detail regarding payment is addressed under reimbursement methodologies section.

Respiratory Recap

Basic Health Care Delivery Functions	
Financing	Delivery
Insurance	Payment

The respiratory therapist should recognize that the U.S. health care system is not a well-oiled, finely tuned machine with components interconnected in such a way that

Table 11-1

Four Major Functions of Health Care

Function	Role	Affected Group or Organization
Financing	Purchase of health insurance	Private sources: employers, individuals
		Public source: federal, state, and local governments
Insurance	Protection against risk	Commercial insurance companies: Aetna US Healthcare, Met Life, Prudential, others
		Blue Cross/Blue Shield
		Quasifraternal organizations: AARP, managed care group
Delivery	Provision of services	Physicians and other health care practitioners, hospitals, alternative care sites
Payment	Determination of reimbursement methodology and disbursement of funds	Commercial insurance companies
		Blue Cross/Blue Shield
		Third-party claims processors

duplication, inconsistency, and inadequacy are prevented. Regrettably, the system is fragmented, duplicative, and disjointed, with a lack of integration among the system's four major functions. Additionally, coordination, collaboration, and integration among the major stakeholders (purchasers, insurers, payers, patients, and providers) is poor. The result is a system loosely connected, without a central oversight, brimming with confusion, and undergoing near-constant change.

Stakeholders in Health Care Reimbursement

Providing and delivering health care services involves many stakeholders. Historically, three major players existed—the patient (primary party), the provider (secondary party), and the insurer (commonly referred to as the **third-party payer**). Over the years the system has become increasingly more complicated and complex. Roles and functions of participants have expanded so that the following five significant stakeholders are involved in today's health care system (Figure 11-1):

1. Purchasers
2. Plans
3. Providers
4. Payers
5. Patient

At times the role and function of each overlaps, often clouding the lines of distinction.

Purchasers are generally employers or the federal, state, or local governments and presently subsidize much of the cost of health care. Employers are purchasers in the form of employee-benefit packages, whereas the government funds health care in the form of entitlement and shared assistance programs. Employers began providing this benefit early in the twentieth century to provide an added benefit to their employees' compensation packages. Medical coverage was viewed as a way to safeguard both the employee and the company from catastrophic health care losses. In addition, it was viewed as a way to add a benefit without having to incur a more direct expense in the form of salary increases. The federal government entered health care reimbursement by instituting Medicare and Medicaid in 1965 to assist the elderly and the poor and indigent. In recent years, purchasers have become increasingly concerned with financial risk. Their expenses have soared, and employers are interested in getting out of the business of providing benefits and the federal government preferring to exercise better control of costs.

The organization or group that provides the health care plan to the purchaser makes up the second group of stakeholders, generally the insurance company or the insurer. The insurer can be from the public or private sector and thus can be the federal government, a commercial insurance company, or a MCO. Examples of health care insurers include Blue Cross/Blue Shield, Aetna US Healthcare, and Kaiser Permanente. The health care insurer is an intermediary that negotiates and administers the health care coverage, established to take the responsibility of oversight from the employer. Health care economics grew so complex that employers simply wanted to rid themselves of the responsibility of day-to-day administration and management of such issues. The health care plan serves in this capacity; the plan is the policy, and the entity is the organization that administers the plan.

The third major stakeholder in health care delivery is the provider, which can be the hospital and all its associated health care practitioners—respiratory therapists, nurses, medical technologists, physical therapists, and others. Long-term care facilities, such as psychiatric facilities and nursing homes, and skilled nursing facilities (SNFs) are other providers, along with the medical community—primary care physicians, pulmonologists, cardiologists, surgeons, and others. Others in this category include agencies that provide home nursing care and homemaker services and companies that provide medical equipment and services to patients in their homes. Essentially any health care professional, agency, company, or service involved in the diagnosis, care, management, or treatment of the patient is considered a provider.

The provider community recently has been placed in the precarious position of being considered most responsible for increases in costs. Waste, fraud, abuse, unproductive activities, and unnecessary and inappropriate treatment and services often are cited as major factors contributing to escalating health care costs. Considerable pressure has been placed on providers to decrease costs and has included downsizing, decentralizing, restructuring, and reengineering.

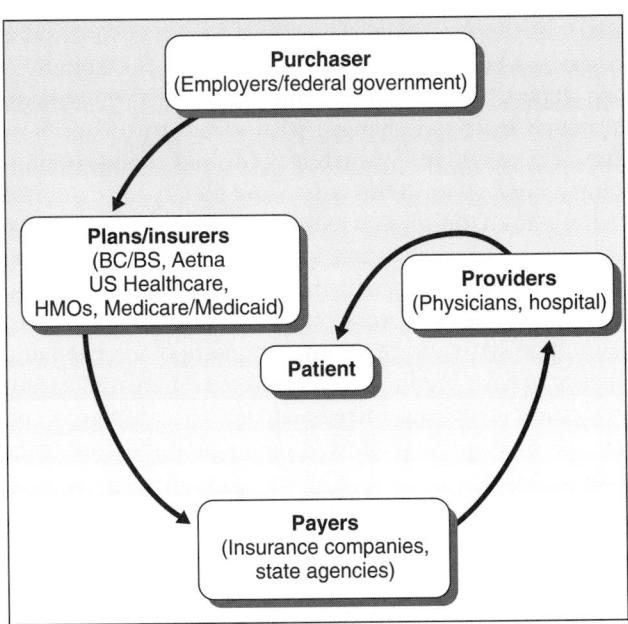

Figure 11-1   Stakeholders in health care reimbursement.

Respiratory Recap

Stakeholders in Health Care Reimbursement	
Purchasers	Payers
Plans	Patients
Providers	

The fourth stakeholder is the payer, the group or organization that processes the claim and disburses the funds. The payer can be an insurance company or a health maintenance organization (HMO) and thus the payer and the plan (or insurer) can be one and the same, the distinction being simply with regard to function. The health plan or insurer performs the insurance function, whereas the payer provides payment or disbursement. The payer holds considerable power and influence because it can accept or reject the claim and also is known as the *third-party administrator (TPA)*.

The patients are perhaps the easiest group to explain and understand. They are the consumers, the recipients of the care and services provided by the health care system. In health care delivery and specifically health care economics, patients have been a rather passive group, simply interested in receiving quality and affordable health care. Their passivity stems from their historically employer-provided health care coverage in the form of a benefit or package that can cost the employer an additional 25% to 35% of the employee's salary. However, consumer passivity is beginning to change as a result of increased consumer financial obligation. Employers are simply unable to sustain the added expense and burden of escalating health care premiums and still compete in a global economy; the escalating health care premiums are ravaging operating budgets and cutting into company profits. Consequently, employers have begun to shift some of these expenses to the employee, in the form of copayments, deductibles, out-of-pocket expenses, and curtailed health care coverage. Consumers are increasingly responsible for their health care costs today.

Currently all five stakeholders are attempting to limit their risk of exposure to financial harm. Figure 11-2 depicts a theoretic view of the amount of risk incurred by the major stakeholders during various time periods. The most

recent events in health care have exposed the provider network to considerably more risk. Employers (purchasers) simply wish to unload any risk by contracting and negotiating with the insurers (the plans/payers). Insurers are attempting to distance themselves from risk by placing more and more pressure on providers to increase productivity, cut staff members, improve patient satisfaction, eliminate inefficiency, and decrease use. Providers seem to have taken the brunt of the responsibility, with the consumer (patient) assuming the role of the silent stakeholder. Speculation is that hospitals and physicians (providers) will continue to carry the pressure and burden for change to improve the system.

At some point in the foreseeable future the consumer (patient) may be pulled into the conflict and required to participate more significantly because of the demand for them to incur additional significant financial burdens or hardships in the form of copayments, increased deductibles, or reduced services. Additionally, patients may be held more accountable for their health practices and required to participate more actively and responsibly in their own care. In some scenarios, rationing has been discussed, with a reward-and-punishment system enacted to stimulate or motivate healthy lifestyle behaviors and practices. For example, significantly reduced premiums, copayments, or deductibles can be provided to consumers who chose not to smoke or engage in healthy lifestyle behaviors that include regular exercise, annual vaccinations/immunization, and preventive health checkups.

Respiratory Therapist's Role— Balancing Cost and Care

Most respiratory therapists enter the health care profession primarily to care for patients with cardiopulmonary needs. In short, respiratory therapists' primary function is to serve as bedside clinicians and as such, the nonphysician experts in cardiorespiratory care and management. Although little has changed with regard to this primary purpose, the system in which it occurs has changed significantly. Forces within the system and society have resulted in a system that places increasing emphasis on health care costs. Respiratory therapists now compete with other health care providers for the broad array of procedures and modalities that once were considered their exclusive domain. The system is beginning to question the need and efficacy of care. Additionally, pressure is increasing to address the burgeoning increase in health care needs and costs that is outstripping what companies and consumers want to pay. Figure 11-3 provides a graphic display of the exponential growth of health care expenditures. Health care is simply becoming too costly, and cost containment is a particularly important concern to the respiratory therapist, who must learn the business of health care, develop a better understanding of the financial considerations associated with the decisions that relate to patient care,[1] and learn to strike a balance between care and costs.

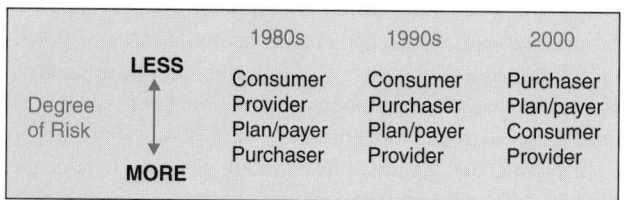

Figure 11-2 Theoretic view of risk incurred by major stakeholders in health care. (Data from Department of Health and Human Services (US), Health Care Financing Administration, Office of Information Services.)

Forces Influencing Health Care Costs

In 1996 the American Association for Respiratory Care (AARC) sponsored a conference entitled "Emerging Health Care Delivery Models and Respiratory Care" to provide the respiratory care community with critical information about the future of health care delivery and the ways it might impact respiratory care practice. A recurring theme was the emphasis placed on escalating health care costs, particularly that health care costs were surpassing general inflation at a threefold to fourfold pace during the 1970s and 1980s. Health care change in the United States is being driven by costs, quality and access, politics, and the demystification of medicine.[2] Of these four, increasing costs is clearly the principal force. But what are the reasons for escalating costs? Four broad factors have been identified—general inflation, population growth and its demographics, medical price inflation, and service intensity.[2]

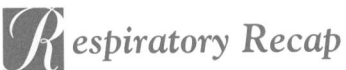espiratory Recap

Forces Driving Health Care Change	
Costs	Politics
Quality and access	Demystification of medicine

Health care consultants and industry leaders have identified service intensity as the major area of focus to effect change and curtail costs. Service intensity is influenced by technology, exemption from market forces, fragmentation, excess capacity, supplier control of demand, lack of efficacy and quality of care information, administrative costs, unnecessary care and defensive medicine, productivity costs, growth in the number of uninsured individuals, and growth in specialization.[2]

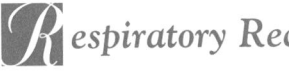espiratory Recap

Factors Influencing Growth in Health Care Costs	
General inflation	Medical price inflation
Population growth and its demographics	Service intensity

Growth in technology has added significantly to the problem because new technology is expensive, is demanded by the public and/or provider, and drives up cost. Advances in diagnostics, monitoring, and mechanical ventilation have driven the cost of such equipment to unprecedented levels. Mechanical ventilators and their accouterments—namely monitoring and graphics packages—can cost more than $30,000. Furthermore, today's health care consumer expects to benefit from advances in medicine and the latest in technology, and the system has encouraged the provider to use such advances to improve patient care, achieve higher degrees of patient satisfaction, and increase hospital revenues. In this sense, technology has been at least partially responsible for the proliferation of specialization and in some cases the performance of unnecessary or questionable procedures or services.

espiratory Recap

Factors Influencing Service Intensity	
Technology	Administrative costs
Exemption from market forces	Unnecessary care and defensive medicine
Fragmentation	Productivity costs
Excess capacity	Growth in number of uninsured
Supplier control of demand	Growth in specialization
Lack of efficacy and quality of care information	

Under a third-party insurer payment system the patient is insulated from costs, and little incentive exists for the primary party (patient) or secondary party (provider) to contain costs. In many cases, insurance is provided by either the employer or the federal, state, or local governments, and the patient does not pay at all or pays only a minimum amount in the form of a copayment or deductible. The patient has little understanding or appreciation for the value of the health care benefit. In addition, unless the insurance plan uses restraining measures, the physician (provider) is free to order diagnostic studies and therapeutic interventions with little regard to cost. The

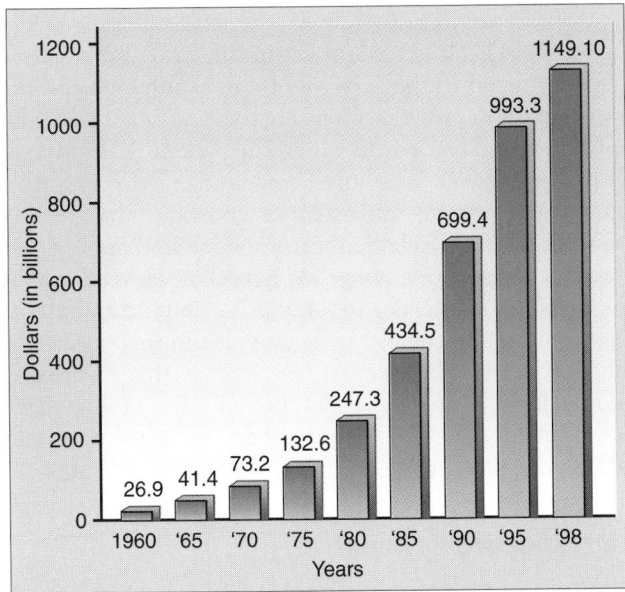

Figure 11-3 Health care expenditures for selected years. (Data from Department of Health and Human Services (US), Centers for Disease Control and Prevention, National Center for Health Statistics.)

system was created on an incentive system whereby the physician was economically rewarded for ordering more services and generating more income for that physician and the hospital. Historically the patient and provider have essentially been without the incentive to be cost conscious, with the mentality that the insurance company will cover everything. Patients and providers only recently have begun to appreciate the costs of health care services, and some of the new reimbursement methodologies are beginning to address these issues.

Traditionally the delivery and payment mechanisms have not been integrated or well coordinated; the system is fragmented. When patients are moved from one practice site to another (physician offices to acute to subacute to home care sites), services are duplicated considerably. Blood gases often are repeated, as are electrocardiograms and pulmonary function studies, resulting in excessive and unnecessary services. In addition, the system has excess capacity; in most locations, hospitals operate at 60% to 65% of capacity, relating to unproductive personnel activities, inefficiencies in practice, and increases in overhead through high-priced fixed costs spread over fewer patients. Practice variations are considerable, and only recently have the disparities in the effectiveness of care begun to be addressed. Benchmarking, practice guidelines, protocols, and best practices are giving rise to evidence-based medicine, whereby conclusive, scientific evidence drives the clinical decision-making process.

Conflict continues to exist between appropriate and necessary care and the over-ordering of unnecessary, nonessential care, often driven by defensive medicine. Physicians are still concerned about the risk of litigation and malpractice and consequently may order services of questionable value to protect their interests, resulting in waste and equally disconcerting, fraud and abuse. Fraud entails a knowing disregard for the truth and generally occurs in the form of fraudulent billing claims or fraudulent delivery but can also include a practitioner's knowingly providing unnecessary or excessive services and receiving remuneration in exchange for a referral of services. Regrettably, the home care market has been especially suspect to such concerns, especially regarding durable medical equipment. A provider referring a patient to any company with which that provider is associated or in which the provider holds a financial interest is simply inappropriate and illegal. Such practice is considered a kickback and is subject to prosecution.

The increase in the elderly population also has added significantly to medical costs inflation because the elderly consume considerably more health care services than other age groups. In fact in 1995, Medicare expenditures for the elderly averaged $5561 per beneficiary versus $3219 per capita for all Americans.[3] In addition, considerable cost is associated with the uninsured and the underinsured, with the number of uninsured growing steadily and reaching 44 million in 1998. This figure correlates to approximately 15% of the population being uninsured at any one time,[4] a significant figure that places tremendous burden on the system.

Other factors affecting costs and driving changes in health care include quality and access, politics, demystification of medicine, and disproportionate emphasis on the medical model of delivery versus the disease prevention and health promotion model. In addition to costs, the system also is concerned with quality. Providers are emphasizing such issues in the form of patient-satisfaction surveys. Competition among health care institutions demands that public perception of the institution be optimal, and health care facilities are paying close attention to the results of such surveys. In recent years the political world also has become exceedingly more involved in health care.

Little question remains that Americans are concerned about issues such as the right to health, broader access, lower costs, and measurable outcomes. Also evident is that the entire institution of medicine is being demystified. The consumer movement, patient advocacy, the proliferation of support groups, and the Internet have brought about a more intelligent and informed public that is questioning medical practices and the costs of services. Finally, the existing health care model in this country is still based on a treatment-versus-prevention model. Americans have not completely bought into the concept of practicing healthy lifestyle behaviors. For example, the Public Health Service estimates the cost per smoker for smoking-cessation interventions to be $165.61. Yet an estimated 25% of Americans continue to smoke, at an estimated expenditure of $50 billion annually.[3] A redefined focus on health promotion and disease prevention would add considerably to health care cost issues.

Financing Health Care—A Brief History and Overview

Payment for health care services in the form of reimbursement is crucial to the survival of any health care institution, facility, or provider. Gone are the days of self-pay, out-of-pocket, or direct pay in which the patient dealt directly with the provider. The more common practice entails a third party, possibly an insurance company, the government, or a MCO. Reimbursement models and methodologies are constantly evolving, and hybridization is becoming the norm. Nonetheless, an attempt to simplify and eliminate some of the complexity is provided in the sections to follow. Certain liberties are exercised in this discussion, and health care finance is addressed in terms of three general payment systems—the **retrospective payment system (RPS),** the prospective payment system, and capitation.[5]

Retrospective Payment

Traditional Health Insurance   The origins of American health insurance are rooted in the historical inability of individuals and their families to sustain the expense and resulting debt incurred by extensive medical care. Medical care, in the form of extended hospital stays or repeated house calls by the family doctor, was unaffordable to most individuals. Community hospitals and family doctors recognized that some means to finance health care was required to prevent the inevitable consequences of unpaid medical bills, personal destitution, catastrophic bankruptcy, and ultimate economic disaster for the patient, physician, and hospital. With this concern grew the concept of health **insurance,** whereby individuals pooled their limited and yet manageable amount of funds and distributed the risk of illness among a larger group. Thus grew the concepts of shared risk and shared losses.

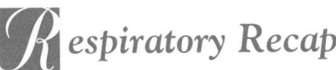

Respiratory Recap

Three General Payment Systems
Retrospective payment system (RPS)
Prospective payment system (PPS)
Capitation

The true beginning of modern private health insurance originated in 1929 when a group of teachers made a contract with Baylor Hospital in Dallas, Texas, to provide coverage against certain hospital expenses. This event was considered the birth of the first Blue Cross plan.[6] Blue Cross and Blue Shield plans, considered service plans, historically reimbursed providers for the total costs of covered benefits. This system is in contrast to the **indemnity insurance plans,** commercial in nature, that provided a benefit only if and when a medical event occurred. Indemnity plans provided payment of a fixed sum for a covered benefit.

Around this period, employers were equally concerned with the health and well being of their workers. World War II was under way, and businesses and industries, such as the railroad, steel, aluminum, and shipbuilding, needed assurance that the workforce could maintain productivity and sustain the war effort. Coupled with this desire to sustain a consistent, dependable, and healthy workforce was the desire to optimize company profits and provide additional employee incentives and rewards, the latter being especially true after the war as employers wanted to provide their employees with additional, small fringe benefits and yet avoid the costly burden of salary increases. Providing health care coverage was the perfect solution, and this benefit enhancement became a reality endorsed and sanctioned by hospitals, physicians, and employers.

Government Involvement   In 1965, the federal government entered the health care reimbursement scene with the U.S. Congress legislating and amending the Social Security Act of 1935 and establishing the Medicare (Title XVIII) and Medicaid (Title XIX) entitlement programs. **Medicare** provides health insurance for the elderly,

whereas Medicaid helps states pay for the health care of the poor and certain other groups, such as the elderly, infants and children, and the blind and other disabled. In 1973, additional legislation extended Medicare coverage to other groups, including persons with disabilities and end-stage renal disease requiring dialysis or kidney transplant. The Medicare program consisted of a Parts A and B.

Medicare Part A is considered hospital coverage, and Part B considered supplemental outpatient coverage. Part A pays the institutional provider for inpatient hospital care, care in a **skilled nursing facility (SNF),** home health services, and hospice services provided to enrolled recipients. Part A covers all inpatient hospital care, including semiprivate room, meals, regular nursing services, operating and recovery room costs, intensive care, drugs, laboratory tests, x-rays, and all other medically necessary services and supplies. However, it does not cover physician fees because it was designed solely as hospital insurance. Box 11-1 addresses the specifics of Part A as they pertain to eligibility, the benefit period, coverage, copayments, the SNF, and the hospice.

Medicare Part B is a voluntary, supplemental insurance program that covers services not provided under Part A. Part B pays for covered physician services, such as diagnostic tests, medical and surgical services, approved ambulatory services, drugs that cannot be self-administered, home health, durable medical equipment, and outpatient services. Box 11-2 addresses the specifics of Part B as they pertain to cost sharing, deductibles, and coverage of home medical and home respiratory equipment. Box 11-3 details the specific Part B coverage requirements for home respiratory equipment that the patient must meet for Medicare reimbursement.

As stated previously, **Medicaid** provides medical assistance for certain individuals and families with low incomes and resources. It is a jointly funded cooperative venture between the federal and state governments to assist states in the provision of adequate medical care to eligible needy persons. Within broad national guidelines set by the federal government, each state establishes its own eligibility standards; determines the type, amounts, duration, and scope of services; sets the rate of payment for services; and administers its own program. Thus Medicaid varies considerably from state to state.

Medicare and Medicaid have been heralded as perhaps one of the most massive and sweeping social welfare initiatives undertaken by the federal government, targeting whole segments of the population and successfully improving the health and quality of life for millions of seniors, people with disabilities, and the poor and indigent of society. Table 11-2 reflects Medicare data for selected years, and Table 11-3 represents Medicaid data for selected years.

Prospective Payment

The **prospective-payment system (PPS)** arose because of increasing pressure from employers and the federal gov-

$\mathscr{B}$OX 11-1

Medicare Part A: Financing, Eligibility, Coverage, and Benefits

Financing

Mandatory employer and employee payroll taxes are collected under Social Security—1.45% from each—paid by all working individuals, including the self-employed.

Eligibility

The benefits usually are provided automatically to persons 65 years of age or older, most people who are disabled for at least 24 months, and those who have end-stage renal disease.

Coverage

Hospital inpatient services, care in a skilled nursing facility (SNF), home health visits, and hospice care are covered.

Premiums*

No premium is required if the individual or spouse has worked for at least 10 years in Social Security/Medicare-covered employment. Other eligible individuals can purchase coverage at a monthly premium of $165 or $300 (depending on coverage status).

Deductibles/Copayments*

A cost-sharing deductible of $792 is assessed per benefit period. No copayments are required for the first 60 days of hospitaliza-

tion, with a copayment of $198 per day for days 61 through 90 and $396 per day for days 91 through 150. No copayments are assessed for skilled nursing for the first 20 days, with $99 per day for days 21 through 100. No copayments are required for home health visits, whereas small copayment are assessed for drugs through hospice care.

Benefits

The benefit period is defined as the period beginning when the beneficiary first enters the hospital and ending when the beneficiary has been out of the hospital or other facility for 60 concurrent days. Benefit periods cannot exceed 90 days of inpatient hospital care, but the number of benefit periods is unlimited. If the 90 days of inpatient hospital care are exhausted, the beneficiary can draw from a nonrenewable "lifetime reserve" of up to 60 additional days. Skilled nursing care pays up to 100 days only if it follows within 30 days of a hospitalization of 3 or more days and is certified as medically necessary. Home care through a home health agency is covered when a beneficiary is homebound and requires intermittent or part-time skilled nursing or rehabilitation care. No limits exist for time or visits for home health care. Hospice services to the terminally ill with life expectancy of 6 months or less also are covered.

Data from Department of Health and Human Services (US). Health Care Financing Administration 1999 Guide to Health Insurance for People with Medicare. Pub. No. 02110. Baltimore, Md: The Department; 1999.
Premium, deductible, and copayment information current as of March 2001. Values subject to change.

$\mathscr{B}$OX 11-2

Medicare Part B: Financing, Eligibility, Coverage, and Benefits

Financing

The voluntary program is financed by general tax revenues and requires individual premium contributions. General federal tax revenues support approximately 75% of the costs, with the remaining 25% financed through individuals choosing to enroll and pay the premiums.

Eligibility

All resident citizens over 65 years of age, even those who are not entitled to Part A services, and disabled beneficiaries entitled to Part A are eligible.

Coverage

Part B coverage is optional. Coverage of home medical equipment requires that the item be used in the home, medically useful, able to stand up to repeated use, and reasonable and necessary for the treatment of illness or injury or the improvement of function. (Equipment that satisfies this criteria is considered durable medical equipment [DME].) To be reimbursed, the supplier must have a physician's order for the items and in some cases a certificate of medical necessity (CMN).

Premiums*

Beneficiaries must pay a monthly premium of $50 per month, which in most cases is automatically deducted from the Social Security payment.

Deductibles*

An annual $100 deductible and a coinsurance payment of 20% of most allowable charges are assessed.

Benefits

Covered physician services include (excluding routine physical exams) emergency department services, outpatient surgery, diagnostic tests and laboratory services; outpatient physical, occupational, and speech therapy; outpatient mental health services; ambulance; renal dialysis; blood transfusion and blood components; medical equipment and supplies; rural health clinic services; and some limited preventive services (for example, Pap smears, mammography, and influenza shots).

Data from Department of Health and Human Services (US). Health Care Financing Administration 1999 Guide to Health Insurance for People with Medicare. Pub. No. 02110. Baltimore, Md: The Department; 1999.
Premium, deductible, and copayment information current as of March 2001. Values subject to change.

Box 11-3

Medicare Part B: Coverage of Home Respiratory Equipment

Medicare has set very specific eligibility and qualifying requirements for all durable medical equipment used in the home. That a physician prescribes a certain item is no guarantee that Medicare will pay for it. The majority of private insurers and many managed care organizations also follow the Medicare guidelines in determining eligibility and reimbursement.

Oxygen

Medicare pays a flat monthly amount for oxygen, the same whether provided from cylinders, a concentrator, or a liquid source and regardless of the liter flow. This rental fee is all-inclusive, covering the oxygen, equipment, most disposable supplies, and all services, such as delivery, maintenance, and repair.

In addition, Medicare has no required standards of service specific to providers of oxygen therapy. The supplier is not required to be accredited, perform any type of initial instruction or ongoing follow-up, or employ respiratory therapists. Suppliers who do provide these services are reimbursed at the same level as those who do not.

To qualify for home oxygen under Medicare Part B the patient must have a diagnosis of pulmonary or cardiac disease, which in the opinion of the attending physician will likely improve with the administration of oxygen. In addition, Medicare has established very specific levels of hypoxemia that the patient must demonstrate through arterial blood gases (ABGs) or pulse oximetry under specified conditions ($Pao_2 \leq 55$ mm Hg or $Sao_2 \leq 88\%$ breathing room air at rest, on exercise, or during sleep). The company providing the oxygen cannot do the testing, which must be performed by an objective third party, such as an independent laboratory, a hospital, or a physician.

Continuous Positive Airway Pressure

This intervention, more commonly known as *CPAP*, is covered if the patient has obstructive sleep apnea that has been documented during studies done in a sleep laboratory and demonstrates at least 30 episodes of apnea, each lasting a minimum of 10 seconds, during 6 to 7 hours of recorded sleep. Bilevel devices also qualify for reimbursement for treatment of obstructive sleep apnea, but only if the patient meets all of the previous criteria and CPAP has been tried without success.

Noninvasive Ventilation and Respiratory Assistive Devices

Since 1999 these devices have been covered for chronic obstructive pulmonary disease (COPD), restrictive thoracic disorders, central sleep apnea, and obstructive sleep apnea when specific qualifying awake ABGs, nocturnal oximetry, and certain other criteria are met.

Ventilators

Ventilators, either positive- or negative-pressure types, are covered if the patient has a diagnosis of neuromuscular disease, thoracic restrictive disease, or chronic respiratory failure due to COPD.

Suction Machine

A device for nasal, oral, or tracheal suctioning is covered only if the patient has difficulty raising and clearing secretions secondary to cancer or surgery of the throat, dysfunction of the swallowing muscles, unconsciousness or obtundent state, or tracheostomy.

Table 11-2

Medicare Data for Selected Years

Year	Beneficiaries (Millions)	Expenditures (Billions)
1970	20.5	$7.7
1980	28.5	$37.5
1990	34.3	$111.5
1999	39.5	$212.0

Data from Department of Health and Human Services (US), Health Care Financing Administration, Office of Information Services.

Table 11-3

Medicaid Data for Selected Years

Year	Beneficiaries (Millions)	Expenditures (Billions)
1970	17.6	$5.3
1980	21.6	$26.1
1990	25.3	$75.3
1999	41.4	$190.7

Data from Department of Health and Human Services (US), Health Care Financing Administration, Office of Information Services.

ernment to curtail spiraling health care costs. It was initiated in 1983 and involves reimbursement that establishes fixed and preestablished payment for the actual primary reason for admission. The rates are determined annually by the plan administrator, who may be the federal government (under the direction of the Health Care Financing Administration [HCFA]) and commercial insurance carriers, such as, Blue Cross or Aetna US Healthcare. The year 1983 began a multiyear phase-in of this PPS for hospital reimbursement through Medicare.

Physician reimbursement under the PPS is based on a methodology known as *resource-based relative value scale (RBRVS)*. A relative value scale is a reimbursement methodology developed by a Harvard research team that assigned values to physician services based on resource costs of providing those services.[7] The RBRVS was implemented on January 1, 1992, by HCFA as a fee schedule for physicians who participate in Medicare Part B. It is based on a national fee schedule and replaces the previous payment method outlining "usual, customary, and reasonable charges." The RBRVS assigns a relative value to each current procedural terminology (CPT) code. The relative value units are published in the *Federal Register* annually and are based on the provider's practice, malpractice, work experience, and geographic region.[8]

Capitation

Capitation is a prepaid, fixed amount negotiated in advance by the payer or plan and the provider. It involves payment for each eligible person for a particular time period regardless of the care or services provided and also is known as the *per-member, per-month (PMPM)* system, which represents or reflects the amount paid by each participating member each month enrolled in the plan. Managed care programs for primary care providers commonly use capitation, but specialists (for example, pulmonologists) are still more likely to be paid under a negotiated fee schedule.

Era of Managed Care

Managed care is actually a generic term for a payment system alternative to traditional insurance plans, such as fee-for-service or indemnity plans. The concept of managed care is considered similar to managed costs, but a distinction should be made between the techniques of care and costs management versus the organization that performs the functions. Managing care or costs may involve a variety of techniques, such as health promotion, disease prevention, wellness, disease management, patient education, and utilization control, to name a few. These are strategies or techniques and should not be confused with **managed care organizations (MCOs),** which can implement these strategies but mainly are responsible for delivering and financing health services. In other words, they are more than just the claims payers; they actively manage the delivery of the care.

A MCO is an integrated network of doctors, hospitals, and other health care providers that deliver health services to an insured population. In 1976 the United States had 174 managed care plans, with an enrollment of about 6 million individuals, or less than 3% of the population. By 1998 that number had grown to 651 plans enrolling 76.6 million individuals who represented 28.6% of the population (Table 11-4).

The four different types of MCOs are HMOs, preferred provider organizations (PPOs), exclusive provider organi-

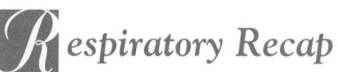

*R*espiratory Recap

Types of Managed Care
Health maintenance organization (HMO)
Preferred provider organization (PPO)
Exclusive provider organization (EPO)
Point of service (POS)

TABLE 11-4

HMO Data for Selected Years

Year	Total Number of Plans	Total Enrollees (Millions)	Population Enrolled in HMOs (%)
1976	174	6.0	2.8
1980	235	9.1	4.0
1985	478	21.0	8.9
1990	572	33.0	13.4
1995	562	50.9	19.4
1998	651	76.6	28.6

Data from Department of Health and Human Services (US), Centers for Disease Control and Prevention, National Center for Health Statistics. HMO, Health maintenance organization.

zations (EPOs), and point-of-service plans (POSs). These are discussed individually in the following sections.

Health Maintenance Organizations

Contrary to popular opinion, managed care models have been around for almost a century. The first cited example of a MCO was the Western Clinic in Tacoma, Washington, a prepaid group practice begun in 1910 to provide a broad range of medical services to lumber mill owners and their employees. These eligible individuals were provided services for a premium payment of a mere $.50 per member per month, dating PMPM's history back 90 years. A number of additional examples are cited, namely the rural workers' cooperative in Elk City, Oklahoma, the Kaiser Foundation Health Plan of Southern California, the Group Health Association of Washington, DC, the Health Insurance Plan of Greater New York, and the Group Health Cooperative of Puget Sound.

Managed care plans developed relatively slowly. However, in 1973 they received a major boost with the passage of the federal HMO Act, which reflected concern with the fee-for-service system that rewarded the system for increased volume of services. Little in the way of checks and balances were in place under this system, and the incentives were established to encourage over-use. The HMO movement is considered the brainchild of Dr. Paul Ellwood, who spearheaded the effort and is often referred to as the "father of the modern HMO movement." Because of Ellwood's expertise, President Nixon asked him to devise ways to curtail the spiraling health care costs in Medicare spending.

The **health maintenance organization (HMO)** model of health care is uniquely different from the traditional model. Rather than pay for care when the individual is ill, it provides service to maintain health, thus the term *health maintenance,* placing considerable emphasis on preventive services encouraging wellness and healthy lifestyle practices. It also provides a wide array of services for a fixed fee per month, use of which is coordinated and managed by the HMO. This type of managed care is an attempt to address the fragmentation of basic health care delivery functions alluded to previously. Under the HMO model the subscriber must secure all services from providers participating in the plan or must pay a higher amount for using a nonparticipating provider. Finally, services are provided according to established standards of quality.[3]

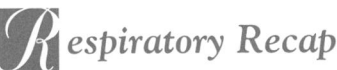

espiratory Recap

General Characteristics of an HMO
Emphasis on preventive services
Provision of a complete range of services for a fixed fee
Requirement that all care be provided by participating providers
Adherence of services to established standards of quality

HMOs have four general models—the staff model, group model, network model, and independent practice association (IPA) model. Their distinction from one another is based on the way the organization relates to its participating physicians.

The staff model entails the provision of physician services through a salaried staff of physicians employed by the HMO. The physicians in this model work exclusively for the HMO and provide care to its enrollees only. The HMO exercises considerable control over physician practice, and thus the physician's performance and practice are subject to restrictions and bonuses for curtailed costs. In the staff model the HMO is assuming the financial risk, as opposed to the physician. The staff model is considered the least popular of the four.

In the group model the HMO contracts with a multispecialty group practice. The physicians are not employees of the HMO but rather employees of the group. This model can provide more choice to the consumer when compared with the staff model, and if the practice enjoys a high degree of notoriety and respect, the HMO gains popularity and credibility with its enrollees.

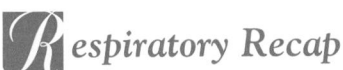

espiratory Recap

General Types of HMOs
Staff model
Group model
Network model
Independent practice association (IPA) model

The network model entails the HMO's contracting with more than one physician group and generally is more likely to occur when a large population of enrollees requires medical services. This model is more attractive to the enrollee because the number of physicians involved in the network can be quite significant, providing increased choice.

The IPA model is unique in that the association serves as an intermediary, or buffer, between the HMO and physicians, handling the logistics of arranging physician services. The responsibility for administrative issues is shifted to the IPA and not the HMO. The IPA is paid a capitated amount, reimburses the physicians based on a methodology determined by both parties, and assumes some of the risk. The IPA's degree of control over physician practices varies widely, but enrollee choice is enhanced.

Preferred Provider Organizations

Preferred provider organizations (PPOs) date back to the late 1970s. PPOs differ from traditional HMOs in that services are provided at a discounted fee-for-service basis, usually 15% to 20% below competitors or below the usual, customary, and reasonable fees. In other words, PPOs use a discounted fee-for-service system, and HMOs use capitation. Additionally, enrollees are required to use a particular group of physicians and hospitals that the PPO has preselected. Enrollees/patients are free to choose physicians or hospitals outside the system, but nonpreferred providers constitute additional charges. Thus PPOs encourage enrollees to use their preferred providers, who have agreed to abide by the PPOs guidelines. In 1998 the number of PPOs totaled 1127 in the United States.

Point-of-Service Plans

Point-of-service plans (POSs) entered the market in the late 1980s and are a hybrid of HMOs and PPOs. They represent features of both organizations, attempting to provide the tight use controls of the HMO and the ability to choose a nonparticipating provider at the point (time) at which service is received, thus the phrase *point of service*. The POS addresses the unpopular feature of limited or restricted choice that continues to plague the industry. Simply stated, a significant number of Americans insist on choosing their physician and hospital, and the POS models satisfies this need.

Exclusive Provider Organizations

Exclusive provider organizations are the most affordable of the managed care models. However, they are clearly the most restrictive. Enrollees must use the physician and hospital stipulated in the plan, completely eliminating the element of choice. The advantage is the purchaser's considerable cost savings.

The distinction among the various plans is beginning to blur, becoming less obvious. Considerable hybridization has occurred as the plans attempt to optimize their models to satisfy purchaser and consumer demands.

Reimbursement Methodologies

Reimbursement and its methodologies involve the payment for health care delivery. Intermediaries or third-party payers generally perform this function and are responsible for determining the method and amount of reimbursement, as well as the actual disbursement of funds. Examples of intermediaries are the federal government, MCOs, and insurance companies.

The methodologies for reimbursement are numerous. The four most common forms of hospital reimbursement are fee for service, per diem, diagnosis-related group (DRG), and capitation.[9] The more popular physician methodologies are fee for service and capitation. Reimbursement methodologies can involve selective contracting, national payment, utilization review, and many other techniques and strategies.

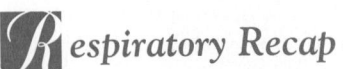
espiratory Recap

Most Common Types of Hospital Reimbursement	
Fee for service	DRG
Per diem	Capitation

Fee for Service

The **fee-for-service** option is simply a reimbursement methodology in which the provider establishes the fee for each distinct service. Billing is based on an itemized account of each service provided. For example, the pulmonologist could submit a claim for a physical examination, chest radiograph, and pulmonary function test in which each service would render a separate charge.

Initially, the insurer paid fee-for-service reimbursement after care was delivered (retrospectively) without any restrictions or limitations. However, insurers eventually adopted a "usual, customary, and reasonable" charge methodology, which limited the fee to a standard determined through regional or statewide surveys. If the provider-determined charge exceeded the usual, customary, and reasonable amount, either the patient or contracted provider was responsible for the difference. Some managed care plans, notably PPOs, adopted a discounted fee-for-service methodology. The main drawback to this method is that providers are rewarded for providing additional services, with less incentive to be cost conscious. In

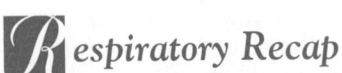
espiratory Recap

Popular Types of Physician Reimbursement
Fee for service
Capitation

fact, providers could increase their income from over-ordering unnecessary and costly services.

Cost Plus/Charge Minus

Under this methodology, rates are preestablished on a cost-plus or charge-minus basis. The cost-plus method was used by the federal government in their Medicare and Medicaid programs to establish in-patient rates for hospitals, nursing homes, and home health care. The institution was required to submit a cost report to the third-party payer detailing the total costs that facility incurred. Complicated formulas were used to determine the per-diem rate. This methodology was tied directly to costs of providing services, number of services provided, and length of stay. Historical data was essentially used to determine the amount to be paid in future years. As with the fee-for-service methodology, cost-plus also presented an incentive for providers to order costly and unnecessary services. This indiscriminate practice eventually led to the initiation of the PPS.

Prospective Reimbursement

The PPS was introduced by the federal government in 1983 under Part A of its Medicare program to curtail costs. Reimbursement was fixed at a preestablished amount in advance of the services rendered, still established annually by the HCFA. Prospective payment was applied to SNFs in 1998, and provisions were made to implement this system for hospital outpatient services and home health agencies through the balanced Budget Act of 1997.

Diagnosis-Related Groups

The **diagnosis-related group (DRG)** system, is based on patient classification of approximately 500 different groupings all entailing a predetermined amount of reimbursement. DRGs establish a rate based on bundled services for a particular diagnosis established at the time of admission. The provider receives this amount regardless of the medical care provided.

This system provides an incentive for providers to decrease overuse, misallocation, and inefficiency. Each DRG assumes that all patients with the same diagnosis require the same care and receive the same services. Differences in DRG reimbursement are provided for the following extenuating circumstances: variations in regional employee wages, location of institution, existence of residency programs, and provision of care to the indigent. Institutions located in an urban environment may require higher employee salaries, involve teaching requirements for medical training, and have a disproportionately high number of low-income patients. Such variables allow for adjustment to the fixed rates. Additionally, extensive lengths of stay and costs for extraordinary circumstances, classified as outliers, allow for higher rates.

The DRG system, based on total inpatient stay, is in direct contrast to the per-diem methodology, which is based on a daily charge. The DRG methodology is an attempt to place risk and reward solely on the hospital (provider). If the hospital provides the service for less than the predetermined DRG reimbursement rate, that facility profits. If the hospital's costs exceed the predetermined allotment, the facility incurs a loss. One concern of the DRG system is under-provision of care and services because limits on the amount of services can result in increased profits. Examples of common respiratory-related DRGs are listed in Table 11-5.

Resource-Based Relative Value Scale

The RBRVS, mentioned previously, is a new initiative to reimburse physicians according to services provided. It replaces the fee-for-service methodology and was intended to narrow the disparity in reimbursement figures between specialists and general practitioners. In reality, it merely pays for the intensity of services rendered. Pulmonologists have done fairly well under this system, whereas cardiologists have experienced a 20% to 40% reduction in gross income. The scale is based on the time, skill, and intensity of the services provided. The RBRVS, developed by the federal government under the Medicare fee schedule (MFS), is composed of more than 7000 covered services. To compute the physician's payment the relative value unit is adjusted for geographic area and then multiplied by a conversion factor, a monetary amount set annually by the federal government.

Bundled Charges

Bundled charges describe a type of packaged pricing, a form of reimbursement in which a number of related services are grouped together and provided in one fee.

TABLE 11-5

Common Respiratory-Related DRGs

DRG	Description
88	Chronic obstructive pulmonary disease
79	Pulmonary Infections and inflammations, age >17 with comorbid condition
98	Bronchitis and asthma, age 0 to 17
475	Respiratory system diagnosis with ventilator support
87	Pulmonary edema and respiratory failure
82	Respiratory neoplasms
482	Tracheostomy for face, mouth, and neck diagnosis
83	Major chest trauma with comorbid condition
78	Pulmonary embolism
462	Rehabilitation
90	Simple pneumonia and pleurisy, age >17 without comorbid condition
143	Chest pain
495	Lung transplantation

Data from DRG guidebook. Reston, Va: St. Anthony; 1995.
DRG, Diagnosis-related group.

An example of a bundled charge would be the provision of pulmonary rehabilitation. Rather than charge separately for each component, all the services falling under this service, such as education and training in pursed-lip breathing, chest physiotherapy, and pulmonary hygiene, are packaged or bundled together and a single price charged.

Managed Care Approaches

Managed care approaches consist of the HMO, PPO, POS, and EPO. The HMO plan provides or arranges for a comprehensive array of services through a defined network of providers for a monthly fee. Members are required to stay within the network of physicians, outpatient providers, and hospitals. Coverage restrictions apply to services provided outside the network, except in certain emergencies or when specific approval is provided in advance of care. The HMO receives a monthly premium in advance for each member, who then has unlimited use of most of the health plan's services as long as such services are considered medically necessary. Each member usually pays a limited fee for each physician visit, prescription, or other service stipulated in the plan, referred to as a **copayment** or *copay*.

Figure 11-4 depicts the relative level of patient choice and provider control for a variety of plans.[6] The more restrictive plans, on the righthand side of the continuum, offer fewer choices and greater restrictions, but yield lower costs. The managed care approaches are variations of a common theme all focusing on cost containment.

Case Mix

Case mix is a relatively new form of reimbursement that refers to the overall intensity of conditions requiring medical and nursing intervention. It involves extensive assessment of the patient's condition, followed by a determination of specific services or procedures considered necessary or essential to effectively manage the patient. The case mix approach is used extensively in the SNF and is driven by the **minimum data set (MDS),** which consists of a core of screening elements that are assessed for each patient admitted to the facility. These elements focus on patient care; function, health, and mental status; and treatment.

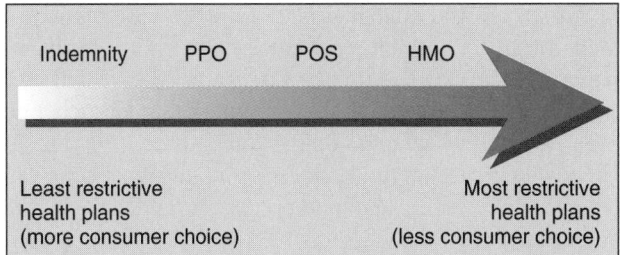

Figure 11-4 Continuum of cost control in U.S. health care.

Future of Health Care Funding

The ability to forecast the future would certainly provide considerable advantage to executives in the health care financial industry. Change appears to be the only constant in a financial market that has evolved exponentially over the past century. Interestingly enough the futurists do not anticipate any significant change in the sources of health care funding for the immediate future, meaning that the purchasers will remain relatively constant.

Research shows[4] that in 1998 approximately 168 million Americans received private health insurance from their employer or purchased it themselves, representing approximately 62% of the population. Of the remaining, 28 million were covered under Medicaid, 38 million were covered under Medicare, and 44 million had no health insurance. Employers' role as the primary provider of health care benefits for the nonelderly has dropped from approximately 69% in 1987 to approximately 64% in 1997.[4] Little question remains that employers want to absolve themselves of this role or at least limit their financial exposure. However, employer-based insurance most likely will continue to serve as the dominant source of health insurance over the next 5 to 10 years, with Medicare, Medicaid, and the uninsured continuing to represent the remaining sources.

Perhaps less predictable is the type of health care funding that will exist in the next 5 to 10 years. Employers have been successful in enticing their employees to move from the traditional indemnity plans and adopt the less expensive and more cost-effective features of the managed care programs. This movement resulted from a considerable concern for significant increases in health care premiums. Employees are concerned with out-of-pocket expenses and thus are attracted by the lower premiums, lower deductibles, and absence of co-payments. Cost sharing (sharing of the escalating costs between employer and employee) is a strong incentive for employees to join managed care programs, such as HMOs, PPOs, or POSs, and shift from indemnity, which expose them to greater risk for out-of-pocket expenses.

Reimbursement and the Respiratory Therapist

So what does the changing face of health care reimbursement mean for respiratory therapists? In short, significant reasoning supports the theory that managed care will continue to evolve and dominate the market. Under such a design, respiratory therapists must address three key points to effectively contribute to such a system—document the care they provide, ensure its appropriateness, and demonstrate value.

Documenting Care—Charting

The old adage, "if it's not charted, it wasn't done" rings especially true in a system that is attempting to reduce or curtail health care spending. Respiratory therapists must recognize that payers are looking for opportunities to deny reimbursement. Therefore therapists must document every procedure and service so that the medical coder can capture the appropriate charge and reimbursement rate.

Three Rights

Ensuring appropriateness of care can be represented by adherence to the three rights of health care delivery—provision of the right care, in the right setting, by the right provider.

Providing the right care is analogous to a balance between over-use and under-use of services. Therapists must recognize that they are rewarded for appropriate care, not for either too little or too much. Under former reimbursement methodologies, over-use of services was rewarded in that respiratory therapy departments were revenue-generators. An increase in services converted into increased revenue for the institution. In today's system, which is heavily based on capitation, DRGs, and per diems, institutions are paid on a fixed-income structure, effectively eliminating the incentives or rewards to provide additional services. In fact, too many services results in the loss of revenue for an institution.

Conversely, although underuse may at first glance appear to result in significant profit for an institution, too little health care can result in persistence of the problem and costly readmission and reentry into the system. A lack of adequate therapeutic interventions to the acutely ill asthmatic can result in a second trip to the emergency room 8 to 10 hours after a premature discharge, resulting in a more ill patient perhaps requiring more intensive and costly therapeutic interventions. The answer lies in appropriate care.

In addition to providing the right care, respiratory therapists must understand the importance of providing care in the right setting. Critical care areas represent the most expensive settings in which to provide health care services. The estimated daily charge for 1 day of admission to an intensive care unit (ICU) is approximately three to five times greater than the charge for a non-ICU ward. The number, intensity, and critical nature of services in an ICU are extremely costly and labor intensive. Respiratory therapists must recognize this fact and make every effort to assist in decision making regarding the transfer of patients to less-costly and less-intensive settings. Theoretically, the costs of care in a routine medical-surgical environment may represent per diem charges of approximately $1200. The costs of a SNF or extended care facility may result in per diems of $500. Providing care in the home could reduce costs even further, to approximately $250 per day. In addition, patients prefer the comforts and familiarity of the home to the formal and impersonal nature of the health care institution. Clearly, compelling evidence suggests that the home, when feasible, is the most desirable and the cost-effective environment for the provision of health care services. Every effort should be made to move the patient to the most appropriate care site.

Equally important is that the health care provider possess the appropriate skill, training, and education to appropriately care for the patient, satisfying professional credentialing standards and matching education and skill appropriately. A highly paid provider who routinely performs relatively low-level skills is neither economical nor cost effective. In other words a neurosurgeon should not be routinely performing phlebotomies. Nor should the nursing aid be performing chest tube insertions. These situations simply do not make good economic sense. Providers should perform services and skills appropriate to their levels of training and education. Minimizing blood gases, effectively using pharmacologic agents, and appropriately using ventilator management can earn the respiratory therapist respect and value as a member of the health care team. An experienced and knowledgeable therapist well versed in the art and science of respiratory care is indispensable in the critical care environment.

Demonstrating Value

Much has been written about the future role of the respiratory therapist, with potential roles including clinician, diagnostician, patient advocate, technical expert, consultant, counselor, and educator. Convincing and growing evidence suggests that respiratory therapists are best suited for these various roles. However, the bottom line is that therapists must demonstrate value.

Demonstrating value, central to the success of any professional, can occur clinically at the bedside, diagnostically in the pulmonary function laboratory, in consultation with the physician, nurse or other health care provider, and in counseling and education as a patient advocate and educator. Although physicians, nurses, other health care professionals, and especially patients have heralded respiratory therapists as significant contributors to quality care, therapists must continue to provide evidence through randomized controlled trials that respiratory care achieves positive outcomes. The challenge is to expand the scientific literature and document the value of the respiratory therapist in reducing costs and improving quality of care.

KEY POINTS

- The four major functions of the health care delivery system in the United States are financing, insurance, delivery, and payment.
- Managed care is an attempt to integrate and coordinate the various functions of health care and create a system that functions effectively and efficiently.
- Cost is the primary force driving health care in the United States.
- Escalating costs in health care are the result of general inflation, growth in the elderly population, a medical price index that is higher than general inflation, and unique features regarding service intensity.
- The five major players in the health care system are the patients, purchasers, plans, payers, and providers.
- The retrospective payment system uses a per-diem methodology for inpatient hospital reimbursement and a fee-for-service and "usual, customary, and reasonable" fee schedule for physician services.
- Employer-based insurance is the dominant model among most consumers, who traditionally have not been very involved or motivated to curtail costs.

- The federal government is a major player in health care reimbursement through Medicare and shared responsibility with the states through Medicaid.
- DRGs describe an attempt to curtail escalating costs with a fixed reimbursement rate based on a predetermined formula for inpatient hospital admissions.
- The RBRVS has replaced the "usual, customary and reasonable" fee payment methodology and is used to pay physicians under Medicare Part B.
- The capitated system entails a per-member, per-month payment methodology.
- The four major types of managed care are the HMO, PPO, POS, and EPO.
- The HMO emphasizes prevention, provides a complete range of services for a fixed fee, requires participants to use designated providers, and adheres to established standards of quality.
- The more popular methodologies used in health care reimbursement are fee for service, cost plus/charge minus, prospective payment, DRGs, resource-based relative value scales, bundled charges, multiple managed care approaches, and case mix.

References

1. Giordano S. Conference Summary. Respir Care 1997;42:15.
2. Fox Stoller T. What is driving change in health care delivery today? Respir Care 1997;42:20-27.
3. Singh, DA, Leiyu S. Delivering health care in America. 2nd ed. Gaithersburg, Md: Aspen; 2001.
4. Institute for the Future. Health and health care 2010: the forecast, the challenge. San Francisco: Jossey-Bass; 2000.
5. Abdelhak M, Grostick S, Hanken MA, et al. Health information: management of a strategic resource. Philadelphia: WB Saunders; 1996.
6. Williams SJ, Torrens PR. Introduction to health services. 5th ed. Albany, NY: Delmar; 1999.
7. Kimball AM, Miller EK. Making sense of managed care. vol 1. San Francisco: Jossey-Bass; 1997.
8. London A. Models of managed health care delivery in the United States. Respir Care 1997;42:30-38.
9. Kongstvedt P. Essentials of managed health care. 2nd ed. Gaithersburg, Md: Aspen; 1997.

Recommended Reading

Bashford C, Carson A. Reimbursement: what every nurse needs to know. Ohio Nurs Rev 2000(Jan):11-16.
Kongstvedt P. Essentials of managed health care. 2nd ed. Gaithersburg, Md: Aspen; 1997.
Walton J. Understanding the cost of health care with specific attention to respiratory care. Respir Care 1997;42:54-67.

CHAPTER 12

Evaluating and Accessing Medical Information

Alexander B. Adams

CHAPTER **OUTLINE**

OBJECTIVES

1. State the general sources of medical information.
2. Identify and describe the structure of a medical study.
3. Discuss differences among the types of medical studies.
4. Define the features of study design, such as randomizing, controls, crossover, blinding, matching, and inclusion and exclusion criteria.
5. Name the currently available databases and their features.
6. State the purpose of evidence-based medicine.

KEY TERMS

Animal Study	Crossover	Medical Literature
Associations	Descriptive Statistics	MEDLINE
Blinding	Entrance and Exclusion Criteria	Ovid
Case Control	Evidence-Based Medicine (EBM)	Prevalence
Case Report	Incidence	Prospective Studies
Case Series	*Index Medicus*	PubMed
CINAHL	Inferential Statistics	Randomization
Clinical Trial	Informed Consent	Retrospective Studies
Cochrane Library	Internet Grateful Med	Statistics
Cohort	Institutional Review Board (IRB)	Surveys
Controls	Matching	
Correlation and Regression Analysis	MD Consult	

Medical information continues to expand in content and complexity. Reports of new pharmaceutics, new medical devices, disease outbreaks, and patterns of disease appear daily in the popular press. Medical reporting is very much a part of increasing communication throughout the world. Everyone has a responsibility to evaluate the relevance of this information. Any health care practitioner has an ad-

ditional continuing responsibility to stay current with increasing medical information in that field.

How does one pick and choose what to read? Once read, which information should be taken as truth? For a critical care practitioner, might a newly proposed ventilator strategy reduce weaning time, reduce morbidity, be more comfortable, or simply add a feature to a ventilator?

Is a reported complication likely to occur? A responsible practitioner must be able to evaluate these types of questions. To assist in evaluating medical information, this chapter briefly outlines (1) sources of medical information, (2) reporting of studies, and (3) ways to access medical information.

Sources of Medical Information

Medical information is presented in reference texts, instructional texts, pamphlets, audiotapes, videotapes, compact discs, Internet sites, and most importantly, medical journals. Other sources are being developed for convenience and specialized instruction, but the primary sources used to obtain medical information are textbooks and journals, the focus of this chapter.

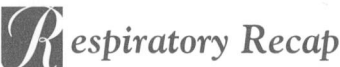

Primary Sources of Medical Information
Textbooks
Journals

Textbooks

Standard medical textbooks serve as the introduction to **medical literature** for most people. Textbooks are typically larger than journals and dedicated to specific areas of information. Generally, texts serve two important purposes—to provide instruction as part of a course of training and to serve as a reference for those interested in a specific topic or specialty. Depending on the complexity of the topic and a student's stage of training, the text can range in coverage from an entry-level requirement (anatomy and physiology) to a comprehensive volume intended to cover a course of study (such as this textbook on respiratory care).

Brief, specialized texts can be written by an individual, but course texts more often are written by a collection of contributors who have been solicited by the text's editor(s). The content of medical textbooks usually covers a topic with a certain degree of completeness. Texts are considered conservative and somewhat dated in comparison with journals. The writers are obligated to write about safe, known techniques or knowledge that is established and enduring, and the publishing process for a text takes 1 to 4 years.

Journals

The primary source for new medical information is the medical journal. Every specialty of medicine or allied health has several journals, which are published weekly, biweekly, monthly, or quarterly. However, most journals are produced monthly.

Journals often are published by professional organizations. The journal *Chest* is the publication of the American College of Chest Physicians (ACCP). *Respiratory Care* is the publication of the American Association for Respiratory Care (AARC). Membership in a professional organization often includes subscription to its journal.

Other journals are published directly by publishers and paid for by those individuals interested in a topic. For example, *Clinics in Chest Medicine* is published by and subscribed to from the publisher, W.B. Saunders Company. Journals also are published with the main purpose of distributing information about medical devices or pharmaceutics. Peer-reviewed journals meet a high standard for article acceptance. The editors of these journals accept articles only after known experts in the field (peers) have thoroughly reviewed a submitted manuscript and judge it a worthy contribution to the field. Several journals of respiratory care include *Chest*, *American Journal of Respiratory and Critical Care Medicine*, *Respiratory Care*, and *Critical Care Medicine*, all peer-reviewed journals of wide distribution.

The number of journals, articles, and authors is increasing. The number of scholarly journals has increased from 70,000 to more than 100,000 in the past 20 years.[1] Nearly 4000 journals are indexed continuously by MEDLINE,[2] the main journal database. The average number of authors per article has increased from 3.9 to 6.5 in the past 15 years.[3] How has this authorship inflation occurred? One cause for this increase involves the increasing complexity of scientific studies. Studies are larger, they take more time, and they require more resources, including people. Consultants are needed in statistics, pathology, or surveys, and they deserve authorship as well. Readers continue to be willing to pay for more journals, and editors continue to accept manuscripts.

Today, more investigators exist, and most have a noble concern for improving care and discovering new, more effective treatments. At the same time, however, is the need to publish. Those in academia hear the often-stated expression *publish or perish*. To most readers of medical literature the content and not the authorship of an article is its significance. Yet for the fraction of practitioners involved in research, authorship is important. To attain an academic appointment, gain tenure, or further one's position at a college or university, publishing is essential. A reputation as an excellent teacher may not be sufficient to maintain one's status. Therefore when research is conducted, the persons involved and those deserving authorship can be extremely important.

Certain guidelines help determine the appropriateness of authorship.[4] First, all authors must have made meaningful contributions to the study. For example, rewards for loyalty or a role in data collection do not deserve authorship. Therefore although an individual may have a great need for authorship, editors and contributors must try to enforce standards of authorship quality by limiting the number of authors to those who contributed significantly to a work. Even so, some studies are so important that the editors may accept many authors simply to publish the study. For example, a recent article reporting the discovery of a gene linked to brain, breast, and prostate cancer had 17 authors.[5]

Of seemingly minor importance but of some significance is the order of authors listed in a study.[4] Although rules about authorship order are not fixed, certain factors are related to name positioning. The first author is responsible for the work, receives credit, and is cited by other authors as the principal investigator. Authors then are positioned in decreasing order according to their amount of work and importance to the study. The last author is often the chief or head of the laboratory or section and is therefore of greater importance than the preceding authors (other than the first author).

Submission of original articles to journals for potential publication can be a major task for the investigator. The author must write up the study and receive approval from the co-authors. The article must be submitted to an appropriate journal and abide strictly to general standards of submission[6] and to the journal's specific submission criteria. Finally, the article must weave through a peer-review process. Although a study may have merit, the authors may encounter many pitfalls to its final publication, such as the back and forth of multiple revisions. The tenacity of the author and the guidance of the editor can ensure a work is printed.

A general, primary criterion for selection of certain journals or articles worth reading is to evaluate the importance of the journal in terms of readership or impact. Note, however, that individual perspectives for selecting specific journals or articles can differ. A student's perspective might be to learn and understand the discipline, whereas a clinician's perspective might be to apply or change care according to recently published studies. Still further, a researcher's perspective might be to assess current knowledge and consider other studies from the report.

A common assumption is that higher readership rates (number of subscriptions) equate with higher-quality articles of greater importance. Although this assumption is true to some extent, it is not always true, as noted by the high readership of grocery-line tabloids. On the other hand, the best work within a narrow subspecialty may have low readership. A system of status, albeit controversial, exists to evaluate the impact of a medical journal, article, or author.[7-10] Impact factors are calculated to measure how often an article or journal is referenced (cited) in other articles (Table 12-1). These numbers may seem esoteric to practitioners, but writers concerned about where an article would be best received—and acclaimed—may find them relevant.

Medical journals contain several types of articles, including editorials, reviews of topical issues, specialty columns, and original investigations. The most important of these is the original investigation report, which can report several study types. These studies are conducted to an-

TABLE 12-1

Impact Factors[*]
Journals with Highest Impact Factors in General and Respiratory Medicine

Journal Name	Impact Factor
Medicine, General, and Internal	
1. *New England Journal of Medicine*	27.77
2. *Lancet*	17.95
3. *Annals of Internal Medicine*	11.21
4. *Journal of the American Medical Association*	9.28
Respiratory System	
1. *American Journal of Respiratory and Critical Care Medicine*	4.71
2. *American Journal of Respiratory Cell Molecular Biology*	4.16
3. *Journal of Heart and Lung Transplantation*	2.65
4. *Chest*	2.34
5. *Thorax*	2.31
Emergency Medicine and Critical Care	
1. *American Journal of Respiratory and Critical Care Medicine*	4.71
2. *Critical Care Medicine*	3.64
3. *Journal of Neurotrauma*	3.09
4. *Shock*	2.38
5. *Resuscitation*	1.82

Impact factors are based on citations in the previous 2 years (articles published in those years). Therefore the factor is the average number of citations per article in the previous 2-year period.

swer a compelling question with use of the currently available resources. Knowing the type of study conducted and the ways it may answer the study question are important pieces of information. Several types of studies conducted in medical research are described in the following sections.

Study Types

Case Reports or Case Series A detailed report of an unusual, interesting case is known as a *case report* or in some instances a *case series*. **Case reports** are observational and can be reported easily. The disease described in the case may be rare, the treatment unusual, or specific instructional points outlined. Several cases reported over time constitute a **case series**. Reports of cases or case series may lead to studies that clarify the disease or its treatment.

Example: During a routine test to measure functional residual capacity (FRC) in the pulmonary function testing (PFT) laboratory, the technician discovered that the individual's helium concentration continued to decline after 7 minutes, indicating a leak in the circuitry. However, no leak could be found. On further inquiry the patient reported a history of a perforated tympanic membrane. Repeating the test with earplugs prevented the leak.[11]

Case Control Studies

Case control studies initially involve the accumulation of a number of cases, which then are matched as much as possible with those of individuals who do not have the specified condition. The matching can be to age, gender, location, or other related medical history. Both the cases and noncases (controls) then are studied for differences that may account for reasons why the cases contracted the disease. Those differences then can help researchers find the association (perhaps not the actual cause) for the case. Case control studies involve exhaustive medical record investigation.

Example: In a case control study of adult onset of wheezing, 103 adults with wheezing were compared with 217 controls. Important factors in adult wheezing included current smoking, current allergies, and a family history of allergies in all subgroups.[12] Despite the range of labeling, symptoms and risk factors for wheezing, all individuals who wheeze may share a common allergic basis.

Cohort Sudies

Cohort studies attempt to definitively answer an important question about the cause, treatment, or prevention of disease. These studies enroll large numbers of participants and follow them over time, with the researchers measuring, testing, or treating them and following up after years. Their incidence or avoidance of disease is often the outcome measure. Cohort studies take time and continual effort to track participants and maintain records.

Example: The Framingham heart study has followed many individuals in Framingham, Massachusetts, (the cohort) over decades to identify factors associated with many diseases, particularly coronary heart disease.[13,14]

Animal Studies

The use of animals for medical research is controversial, but nearly all significant advancements in medicine have been possible through **animal studies.** The study of animals is often of "models" of human disease, with limitations to the transfer of knowledge from animal studies to humans always considered.

Example: To simulate acute respiratory distress syndrome (ARDS) in animals, oleic acid is infused through the pulmonary artery to lodge in the lungs and disrupt the alveolar-capillary membrane.[15] This method has been the investigative model for the study of ARDS.

Clinical Trials

The **clinical trial** is the most important study of medical interventions. Proposed changes in care must undergo the scrutiny of clinical trials, which investigate a change in treatment or a new treatment in the clinical setting through comparison of current (or usual) therapy with the new therapy. Specific phases of an investigation of new therapy (Phases I-III) examine its safety, effectiveness, and applicability to the public. Most clinical trials are lengthy (1 to 3 years) and expensive and often investigate pharmaceutics.

Example: In a clinical trial of a lung protective strategy in ventilated ARDS patients, the use of higher positive end-expiratory pressure (PEEP) and lower tidal volume was compared with a usual setting control group. The new strategy found a decreased mortality at 28 days, a decreased incidence of barotrauma, and a higher weaning rate.[16]

Equipment Evaluations

Many instruments are used in the monitoring and diagnosis of illness. As technology improves, new instruments are compared with the "gold standard" (or not always so gold but the best available) for approval based on their supposed advantages. If measurements from the new instrument provide comparable values, or if the instrument measures "nature" more accurately or is more convenient, its use may be adopted. Although some comparisons can be made easily in the laboratory, the convincing comparisons are in the clinical settings that challenge the safety and accuracy of the instrument.

Respiratory Recap

Study Types	
Case reports or case series	Clinical trials
Case control studies	Equipment evaluations
Cohort studies	Surveys
Animal studies	

Example: A new metabolic monitor that measures dead space to tidal volume ratio was compared with the standard Douglas bag method. The comparison was favorable, with the monitor allowing further automation of the measurement.[17]

Surveys

Surveys use questionnaires, or a set of questions sometimes called the *instrument.* Their goal is to pinpoint opinions, practice patterns, or purchasing intentions.

Example: In three surveys over 10 years the number of ventilator-assisted individuals increased by 18 per year in Minnesota. In the most recent survey, noninvasive ventilation had become an important aspect of long-term ventilator care.[18]

Structure of a Medical Report

The format of a medical report is often unfamiliar to nonmedical readers. Reports of original studies currently have an *IMRAD* structure, an acronym that stands for the components of the reports—**I**ntroduction, **M**ethods, **R**esults, **A**nd **D**iscussion. More than 20 years ago authors did not necessarily adhere to this structure, but the standard format now appears in all studies. Although abstracts precede each medical report, their use and format is less standardized and continues to evolve.

Abstracts

Although not included in the *IMRAD* acronym the abstract appears before the introduction of an article. Abstracts are one-paragraph descriptions of the investigation. The growth in the use of abstracts parallels trends in society. An abstract is a brief, convenient, and efficient way to convey information about the investigation, but readers should beware of hazards in relying completely on abstracts for medical information. Abstracts do not contain the necessary details to evaluate the study critically and therefore should be used to help the reader determine whether the paper relates to topics of individual interest.

In the past an abstract was an enticement for the reader to read the article, but as they have come into common use, the length and complexity of abstracts have increased. Most abstracts now must be structured; that is, in place of a continuous narrative describing the study is a format of title, authors, institution, background/introduction, methods, results, and conclusion.

Two types of abstracts exist, and a distinction between them may not be immediately apparent.[19,20] Conference abstracts are submitted for presentation at a conference and published (without extensive peer review) to provide conference attendees with a preview of the reports to be presented. The report usually is a poster session in which the investigators display the details of their work on a poster board. Although abstract presenters are encouraged to format their complete work for full publication, only a fraction of conference abstracts become complete reports.[10]

The other type of abstract precedes the full report of an original investigation and serves as a synopsis of the study to follow. The complete study has been peer reviewed and accepted for publication, and the abstract of a full report is often circulated as the representation of the work. Today, many journals have this form of abstract online and even full-text versions of the article available to the reader during a search of the literature.

Introduction

The introduction is the background of the study and consists of several paragraphs that offer a succinct rationale for conduct of the study. Knowledge of the topic from previous investigations is outlined in this section. After reading the introduction, the reader should know clearly the reason the study was conducted and the basic question under investigation. The purpose of the study, research questions, and specific aims should be evident in the introduction, with further elaboration in the methods section.

Methods

The methods section has one primary purpose—to describe as precisely as possible what was done; it should describe the research in detail. This section is provided so that readers or other investigators can verify, repeat, or expand on the work. The type of study, its design characteristics, and its measurements are key to the understanding of its importance, validity, and reliability. Certain design characteristics are critical to the conduct of a sound study. For example, a study should be, as much as possible prospective, controlled, and double blinded.

To appraise studies critically, the reader must understand study design characteristics.[21,22] The methods section should address major decisions in sample size determination, study design, data collection, and data analysis. Prevention of researcher bias and study limitations should be apparent in the methods, and the section should support the conclusions drawn from the study. The results and conclusions are only as good as the methods used to answer the research question. Following is a list and brief description of 10 design characteristics and other study terms:

Controls: **Controls** are study participants that do not receive the new treatment but receive instead the usual treatment, a placebo, or a sham treatment. An effective treatment must beat the controls.

Matching: The controls must be similar to the treatment group in other respects in that they must be matched. This **matching** is necessary to prevent other factors from confounding (confusing) the results. For example, the controls can not enter the study more ill than the treatment group members. A beneficial treatment effect then could be due in part to a difference in precondition.

Randomization: To attempt equal matching (similar patients) between treatment group and control group members, the **randomization** method is used to assign treatment or control without the possibility of bias. This step can be done via coin flip, dice, or randomization software. Randomization is seemingly simple but potentially complex because bias can be suspected if groups are not well matched.

Blinding or masking: As much as possible the investigators and participants should remain unaware of the treatment being studied. The tendency to prefer a specific outcome (bias) is prevented through **blinding.** When both investigators and participants are blinded, the study is known as *double blinded.* When the participants are unaware of their treatment status, the study is *single blinded.* For example, in a drug study the tablets can be dispensed in coded bottles to blind the investigators and the participants.

Crossover: Ideally the treatment group and control group are the same patients, in which case age, gender, and disease state are identical. **Crossover** means that the participant is randomized to one group (treatment or control), measurements are made, and the participant then is restudied in the opposite group. If possible, the participant can be crossed over again to prevent a sequencing effect.

Entrance and exclusion criteria: To enter or be excluded from a study, clearly specified conditions must be stipulated before the study begins, known as **entrance and exclusion criteria.** In addition, conditions often are stated for withdrawal from a study. Missing data also must be explained.

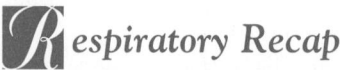

espiratory Recap

Issues in Study Design	
Controls	Prospective and retrospec-
Matching	tive qualities
Randomization	IRB and informed consent
Blinding or masking	Measurements
Crossover	Incidence and prevalence
Entrance and exclusion	
criteria	

Prospective and retrospective: **Prospective studies** are proposed and then conducted and couple with the other design features, can prevent bias. **Retrospective studies** look back at records to study what has been done. The selection of data from records has a greater potential for bias in retrospective studies than in prospective studies.

IRB and informed consent: Studies are proposed and must be approved by an **institutional review board (IRB)** before they can be conducted. The IRB assures that participants are not treated as "guinea pigs" for a new treatment. In addition, **informed consent** forms must be signed by the patient, nearest relative, or guardians to approve the participant's entry into the treatment or control group.

Measurements: The measured variables of interest in the study should have a known, acceptable degree of accuracy and variability. The measurement should have the ability to help detect (sensitivity) or excluded (specificity) a condition.

Incidence and prevalence: The **incidence** determines the frequency with which a disease or condition is contracted or diagnosed in a given time period. **Prevalence** is the number of individuals in a given population who have the disease or condition at a given time.

Results

The results of a study describe the findings or raw information obtained from its conduction. Results often are presented more clearly and efficiently in tables, graphs, or figures. The data are usually presented initially through reporting of averages (means) and variability (standard deviations [SDs]) of the study measurements. These values then are analyzed with statistical methods to allow for inference to other settings, or an answer to the question: "Why does

this study means anything elsewhere?" The strength of the study is often in the use of **statistics.** To systematically analyze the data in a meaningful way the interpretation of statistics can be quite complex, and consultation with a statistician may be necessary to help fully understand the value of a study.[23-26] Although in-depth instruction in statistics is beyond the scope of this chapter, some relevant points (termed *nuggets* and *pitfalls*) are described in the following sections.

Statistical Nuggets

Nugget #1   Consider the measurements reported by the study. Are they continuous variables, such as PaO_2 or forced expiratory volume in 1 second (FEV_1)? Are the continuous variables normally distributed (Nugget #3)? Do nominal variables exist that have a specific nature, such as dyspnea or cyanosis? Are the variables ordinal; that is, do they have an order or ranking according to an accepted scale, such as Borg scaling or APACHE scoring?

Nugget #2   Consider the purpose of the statistical analysis being reported. **Descriptive statistics,** such as mean and SD, often are used to simply present the measurements from the study. Histograms, line graphs, scatterplots, and tables present the data visually, more clearly than within the narrative of the text. Statistics are most often used to answer the questions (hypothesis) of the study and are known as **inferential statistics,** which require significance testing. A statistically significant result infers that the results can be applied to other settings (that is, beyond the study itself).

Nugget #3   Many variables are distributed in a normal distribution; that is, they are graphically characterized by a bell-shaped curve. Figure 12-1 displays a normal distribution of $PaCO_2$ values from a large number of patients. The values from a normal distribution (the $PaCO_2$ values) have an average, or mean (the peak in the center), with values distributed evenly about that mean. The dispersion of values about the mean is quantified by the SD, where ±1 SD encompasses 68% of the values, ±2 SD encompasses 95% of the values, and ±3 SD encompasses 99% of the values. The *median* is defined as the midvalue where half the values are above and half are below that median. The *mode* is the most frequent value. The mean, median, and mode are the same in a normal distribution but differ in Figure 12-2, which illustrates a set of responses to a dyspnea scoring scale. Depending on the data, a mean, median, or mode may best describe the values obtained.

Nugget #4   Whether an improvement actually has occurred with therapy, such as an improvement in FEV_1 after bronchodilator use, can be evaluated with significance testing. Before and after bronchodilator treatment, measurements can be compared to no effect (the null hypothesis; that is, nothing happening, or 0% change).

In a hypothetic study, two new bronchodilators (A and B) were tested on 10 patients by measurement of the change in FEV_1. The results of FEV_1 measurements before and after the bronchodilator administration are shown in Table 12-2. An improvement detected is considered significant if the statistical test used (a paired t-test in this

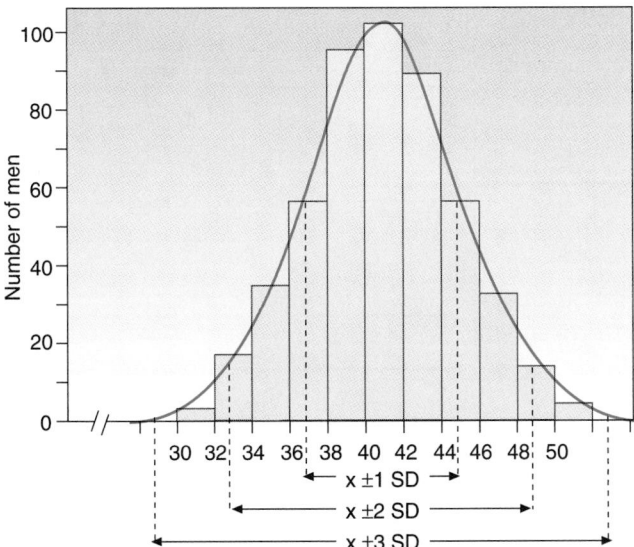

Figure 12-1   A normal distribution of $Paco_2$ values about a mean of 40 mm Hg. The values are distributed about the mean in a bell shape. The standard deviation (SD) defines the width of the bell, with ± 1 SD defining 68% of the values, ± 2 SD 95% of the values and ± 3 SD encompassing 99% of the values.

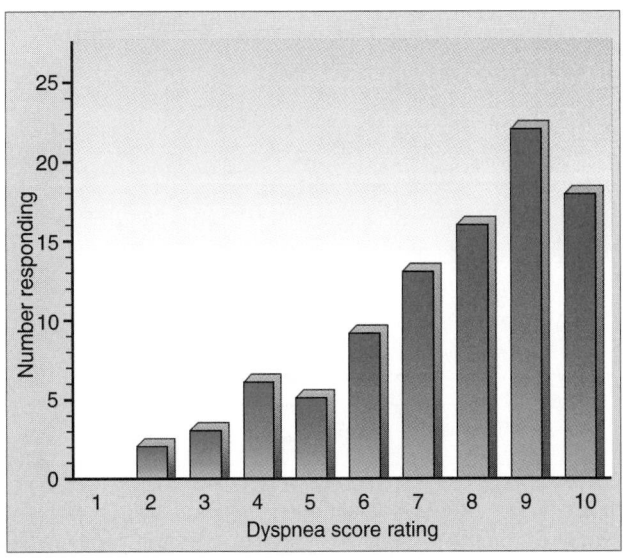

Figure 12-2   A skewed distribution in which the values have a tail. The mean, median, and mode differ, and either one may best describe the data. A dyspnea scoring scale results from a group of patients during mild exercise.

case) has a probability (p) of less than 0.05, meaning less than a 5% chance exists that the measured change is due to chance. Bronchodilator A worked in this study, demonstrated by a significant improvement in FEV_1 (p = 0.008). The use of bronchodilator B resulted in an insignificant improvement (p = 0.37), demonstrating that B did not work. The tests become more sophisticated when multiple treatments are tested on groups of patients, but the criteria for significant effects usually falls at the 5% level (that is, a less than 5% chance that the effect is due to chance).

Nugget #5   **Associations** frequently are determined to be important. As important as the relation of age to FEV_1 is the degree of association between them. Figure 12-3 demonstrates that FEV_1 is expected to decline each year by about 20 to 25 mL, which describes their association. Associations are measured by correlation and regression analysis, and their measurement and interpretation often require a statistician's assistance.

Nugget #6   Respiratory care concerns measurements and their accuracy. A new measurement instrument or method usually is compared with the current "gold standard" to assess its potential use. A Bland-Altman plot[27] often is used to display the values obtained by each method, easily illustrating the systematic differences among the measurements. The study of a new metabolic cart compared measurements with the Douglas bag collection system (referred to previously in this chapter) with a Bland-Altman plot (Figure 12-4).

Statistical Pitfalls

Although the strength of studies often relies on the statistics, acceptance of all of a study's conclusions based on statistics alone can create hazards. The interpreter must be cautious about over-interpreting

TABLE 12-2

FEV₁ Values before and after Bronchodilator Administration

Patient	Bronchodilator A		Bronchodilator B	
	Before (FEV_1)	**After** (FEV_1)	**Before** (FEV_1)	**After** (FEV_1)
1	1.65	1.82	1.65	1.70
2	2.56	3.09	2.56	2.66
3	2.11	2.27	2.11	2.13
4	3.23	3.87	3.23	3.11
5	2.99	2.90	2.99	3.04
6	3.65	4.71	3.65	3.70
7	4.55	4.88	4.55	4.50
8	2.87	2.79	2.87	2.91
9	1.95	2.88	1.95	2.24
10	3.01	3.55	3.01	2.92
Mean	2.86	3.28	2.86	2.89
SD	0.86	0.99	0.86	0.80

FEV_1, *Forced expiratory volume in 1 second;* SD, *standard deviation.*

results based on the statistics. Some problems or pitfalls with the use of statistics are described in the following sections.

Pitfall #1   Are statements or study conclusions supported by significance testing actually due to chance? A type I error is the finding of a difference when the difference is actually due to chance. A significance test with a p less than 0.05 guards against this error, but a type I error can still occur with this criterion (although less than a 5% chance if $p < 0.05$).

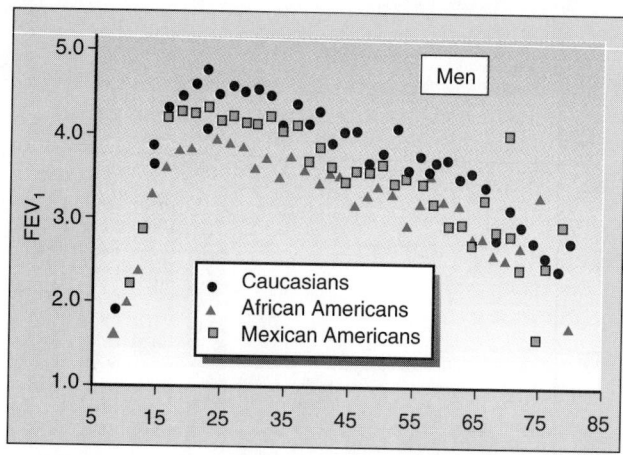

Figure 12-3   The association or regression of FEV_1 (y axis) with age (x axis) for men. (Modified from Hankinson JL, Odencrantz JR, Fedan KB. Spirometric reference values from a sample of the general U.S. population. Am J Respir Crit Care Med 1999;159: 179-187.)

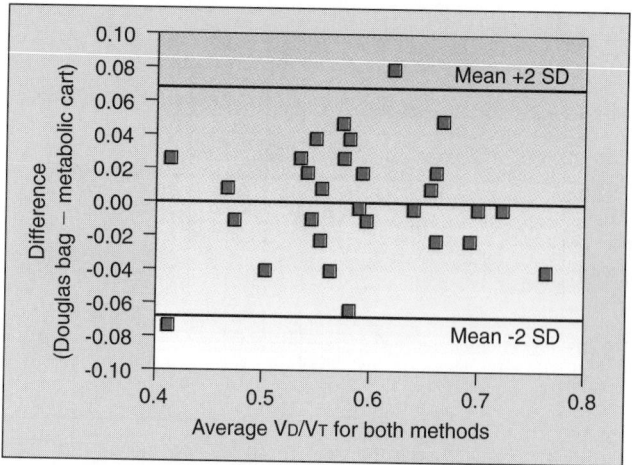

Figure 12-4   The Bland-Altman plot comparing the average of the two measurements (x axis) with the difference between them (y axis). (Modified from MacKinnon JC, Houston PL, McGuire GP. Validation of the Deltatrac metabolic cart for measurement of dead-space to tidal volume ratio. Respir Care 1997;42(7):761-764.)

Pitfall #2   The opposite of a type I error, a finding of no difference when a difference actually exists, is known as a *type II error*. What if p equals 0.06? Statistically, the conclusion is that the treatment has no effect, an assumption that may result in a type II error. If too few patients were tested, a difference may not have been detected, in which case the study may be said to be *underpowered*, (that is, not large enough to detect an actual existing difference).

Pitfall #3   Be wary of multiple comparisons. As studies become more complex, several variables often are compared to test significant effects on the outcome variable of interest. Due to the risk of the discovery of chance relationships, the significance standards must be higher for multiple comparisons, a factor that must be accounted for in the analysis.

Pitfall #4   Remember that associations do not state causality. In large studies the associations of many variables often are compared. **Correlation and regression analyses** measure these potential associations, but further conclusions must by viewed cautiously. For example, a conclusion states that the amount of crime in a city is directly related to the number of churches in the city. A reasonable person knows that churches do not cause crime; both factors are associated with city size.

The statistical findings and inferences often define the importance of a study. But ultimately the study's importance may not depend on the statistics, but on the clinical value of the findings. Although an effect measured in a study may be statistically significant, it can still be a very small effect or an unimportant effect. Therefore the reader always must judge a study's relevance in light of the author's discussion and its overall relevance to the clinician and the care of the patient.

Discussion

The discussion section of a medical report has several purposes. The authors are expected to provide their opinions about the results, and the reader expects an honest assessment of the study's importance. However, the reader must beware of an exaggeration of the study's value. The question asked by the study should be clear, and the answers in the results should support conclusions from the study. In addition, the discussion should feature a description of the study's strengths and weaknesses, and the results should be placed within the context of previous work in the area—a perspective of the current study. Speculations drawn from the study should be stated and viewed conservatively. Future work in the area should be proposed to either confirm or advance study on the topic, and a brief conclusion should summarize the study.

*R*espiratory *Recap*

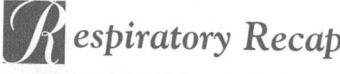

IMRAD
Abstract
Introduction
Methods
Results
And
Discussion

References

References are the citations to studies mentioned in the current report; they can occur throughout the text of a study but are usually found in the introduction and discussion. The introduction and discussion propose the study question and place the study within the context of the medical literature. Therefore these sections should be supported by the work of others. References usually are numbered in the order in which they are cited in the text. To understand more about the topic being reported, the reader should locate and read the references.

Accessing Medical Information

Medical Libraries

Medical libraries exist at medical schools, universities, and most hospitals and feature most major journals and texts. These facilities, however, are expensive to start and maintain. Ongoing subscriptions to medical journals and medical texts are expensive, and libraries are obligated to subscribe to nearly all publications and purchase the texts. To locate information the medical librarian can quickly explain the system of shelving and access to the journals and texts, the former being arranged in alphabetic order by journal name and the latter being catalogued. To direct readers or investigators to the shelves, most modern medical libraries have available computerized access to topics or authors in the journals and texts of that library.

Index Medicus

Index Medicus is a set of volumes, similar to the old encyclopedias, that systematically organizes and allows access to articles of interest. The articles from the major scientific journals are sorted and cited by author and topic. Indexed journals important to respiratory therapists include *Chest, Critical Care Medicine, Respiratory Care*, and *American Journal of Respiratory and Critical Care Medicine*. Finding articles of interest is simple; large catalogues list the columns of citations to the thousands of articles published in a specific time period. An article citation directs the researcher to locate that journal article, as the following sample citation:

Tarpy SP, Celli BR. Long-term oxygen therapy. N Engl J Med 1995;333(11):710-714.

The citation lists the authors (Tarpy SP and Celli BR), the article title (Long-term oxygen therapy), the journal in its accepted abbreviated form (New England Journal of Medicine), the year (1995) the volume and issue numbers (333 and 11, respectively), and the inclusive pages (710-714).

 espiratory Recap

Citations
Citations help to locate journal articles by listing the authors' names, article title, journal name, year, volume, issue, and inclusive page numbers.

This citation method is relatively standardized in the medical literature, and an article can be easily located in any medical library with the journal name, volume, and

page numbers. Its title alone may tell the reader whether this article is of interest. The author index of *Index Medicus* can direct readers to other articles by that author, whereas the topic index directs them to all articles on a specific topic. From the index, readers can scan the amount and nature of information on a topic. Once the reader finds an article on the topic of interest, the references can direct that individual to more information on the topic.

Searches

Accessing the medical literature by electronic searching has become greatly simplified and inexpensive over the past few years. In 1997, searches of the National Institutes of Health (NIH) database became available without charge. Searches are an automated, sophisticated type of *Index Medicus* use, with access to many other databases. Through personal computers in libraries, homes, clinics, or offices, online searches can be rapid, complete, and the cost of local access to the Internet. Entry of the topic, author, journal, or dates of interest produces a listing of the matching citations. The challenge is to zero in on the specific area of interest. The citations and their abstracts often can be viewed by the search, and an increasing number of publishers provide full-text articles from their journals online.

Increasingly, the need to browse the shelves of the medical library is being replaced by electronic access. The ability to search efficiently within databases involves the selection of key words to narrow the search. Knowledge of medical subject heading (MeSH) terms can aid searches in MEDLINE. For example, a MEDLINE search via PubMed for *emphysema* finds 14,616 citations, whereas a narrowing to *pulmonary emphysema* finds 8739 citations; *pulmonary emphysema AND oxygen therapy* finds 190 citations, and a manageable 17 citations turn up when the word *mortality* is added to the previous search.

The largest, most readily available service for access to medical literature is through the National Library of Medicine (NLM). **MEDLINE** is the premier database of the NLM, covering medicine, nursing, dentistry, veterinary medicine, the health care system, and preclinical sciences. NLM offers two free systems to search MEDLINE—**PubMed** (http://www.ncbi.nlm.nih.gov/PubMed) and **Internet Grateful Med** (http://igm.nlm.nih.gov/). Both sites allow searching of more than 11 million references and abstracts in approximately 3000 biomedical journals. PubMed has a retrieval engine that links to full-text versions of articles in more than 400 journals and features a document-retrieval service *Loansome Doc*. As a nearly immediate resource to access medical information, PubMed or Internet Grateful Med may be bookmarked on Internet browsers for ease.

NLM resources include other databases, information sources, and consensus statements. However, libraries, hospitals, research centers, and even individuals can subscribe to services that extend beyond those available from the NLM. **Ovid** Technologies provides such a service, with more than 90 databases, including MEDLINE and **CINAHL,** an acronym for Cumulative Index to Nursing and Allied

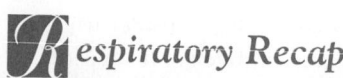

Literature Searches
Pubmed: http://www.ncbi.nlm.nih.gov/PubMed
Internet Grateful Med http://igm.nlm.nih.gov/

Health Literature, which contains the journal *Respiratory Care*. Ovid has direct full-text versions for articles in more than 300 leading medical journals and several ease-of-use features. Another site, MD Consult is designed to deliver authoritative medical information to physicians. A subscription to **MD Consult** accesses searches via MEDLINE, textbooks, practice guidelines, patient education handouts, and drug information. Therefore information services in addition to the NLM resources are direct full text (not just citations and abstracts), more extensive (CINAHL, practice guidelines . . .) and purportedly easier to use.

The explosion of medical information and its increased accessibility has assisted the development of yet another branch of medicine, **evidence-based medicine (EBM).** The research in EBM is the methodic collection of studies that meet strict quality criteria. All or portions of these studies then can be merged, distilled, and interpreted (through meta-analysis). The "discoveries" in EBM are systematic reviews developed from this conservative evaluation of the effect and effectiveness of care with various levels of evidence. Assisting this discipline is the **Cochrane Library,** a database of controlled trials, systematic reviews of the effects of care, and critical assessments of effectiveness.[28] A bimonthly publication, *Evidence-Based Medicine*, reports on recent reviews and commentaries from EBM. Although the need for EBM has always existed, public health agencies, health maintenance organizations, and cost-conscious hospitals have accelerated the need for and development of EBM.

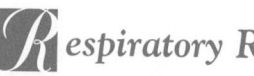

Evidence-Based Medicine and Meta-Analysis
Evidence-based medicine is the methodic collection of studies meeting strict quality criteria. A meta-analysis of these studies results in conservative reviews of the effect and effectiveness of care.

Key Points

- Medicine has a vast, expanding system for the evaluation and access of information.
- The primary sources of this information are texts and journals, with most new research being reported in journals.
- Conventions and requirements govern the conduct of studies and reporting of medical information through accepted study design methods, IMRAD, and statistical analysis.
- *Index Medicus* and computerized searches with databases such as MEDLINE allow for the rapid, efficient availability of medical information.
- Responsible practitioners will continually maintain their knowledge by reading texts and journals devoted to their areas of practice.

References

1. Hamilton DP. Publishing by-and for?-the numbers. Science 1990;250:1331-1332.
2. Stegmann J. How to evaluate journal impact factors. Nature 1997;390:550.
3. Sobal J, Ferentz KS. Abstract creep and author inflation. N Engl J Med 1990;323:488-489.
4. Huth EJ. Guidelines on authorship of medical papers. Ann Intern Med 1986;104:269-274.
5. Li J, Yen C, Liaw D, et al. PTEN, a putative protein tyrosine phosphatase gene mutated in human brain, breast, and prostate cancer. Science 1997;275:1943-1947.
6. International Committee of Medical Journal Editors. Uniform requirements for manuscripts submitted to biomedical journals. Ann Intern Med 1997;126:36-47.
7. Hansson S. Impact factor as a misleading tool in evaluation of medical journals. Lancet 1995;346:906.
8. Hecht F, Hecht BK, Sandberg AA. The journal "impact factor": a misnamed, misleading, misused measure. Cancer Genet Cytogenet 1998;104:77-81.
9. Opthof T. Sense and nonsense about the impact factor. Cardiovasc Res 1997;33:1-7.
10. Garfield E. Which medical journals have the greatest impact? Ann Intern Med 1986;105:313-320.
11. Wolf KM, Addison N. Inability to measure lung volumes in a man with congestive heart failure. Chest 1999;115:269-271.
12. Bodner CH, Ross S, Little J, et al. Risk factors for adult onset wheeze. Am J Respir Crit Care Med 1998;157:35-42.
13. Lenfant C, Friedman L, Thom T. Fifty years of death certificates: the Framingham heart study. Ann Intern Med 1998;129:1066-1067.
14. Lloyd-Jones DM, Larson MG, Beiser A, et al. Lifetime risk of developing coronary heart disease. Lancet 1999;353:89-92.
15. Shuster DP. ARDS: clinical lessons from the oleic acid model of acute lung injury. Am J Respir Crit Care Med 1994;149:245-260.

16. Amato MBP, Barbas CSV, Medeiros DM, et al. Effect of a protective-ventilation strategy on mortality in the acute respiratory distress syndrome. N Engl J Med 1998;338:347-354.

17. MacKinnon JC, Houston PL, McGuire GP. Validation of the Deltatrac metabolic cart for measurement of dead-space to tidal volume ratio. Respir Care 1997;42(7):761-764.

18. Adams AB, Shapiro RS, Marini JJ. Changing prevalence of chronically ventilator-assisted individuals in Minnesota: increases, characteristics and the use of noninvasive ventilation. Respir Care 1998;43:643-649.

19. Huth EJ. Structured abstracts for papers reporting clinical trials. Ann Intern Med 1987;106:626-627.

20. Herrmann G, Freidlander G. Fate of conference abstracts. Nature 1998;383:20.

21. MacAuley D. Critical appraisal of medical literature: an aid to rational decision making. Fam Pract 1995;12:98-103.

22. Fowkes FGR, Fulton PM. Critical appraisal of published research: introductory guidelines. BMJ 1991;302:1136-1140.

23. Yancey JM. Ten rules for reading clinical research reports. Am J Surg 1990;159:533-539.

24. Bailar JC, Mosteller F. Guidelines for statistical reporting in articles for medical journals. Ann Intern Med 1988;108:266-273.

25. Northridge ME, Levin B, Feinleib M, et al. Statistics in the journal—significance, confidence, and all that [editorial]. Am J Pub Health 1997;87:1092-1094.

26. Brown GW. Statistics and the medical journal. Am J Dis Child 1985;139:226-228.

27. Bland JM, Altman DG. Statistical methods for assessing agreement between two methods of clinical measurement. Lancet 1986;1(8476):307-310.

28. Jones A. Second International Cochrane Colloquium—official annual meeting of the Cochrane Collaboration: a conference report. Respir Care 1995;40:171-174.

PART II

Applied Sciences for Respiratory Care

CHAPTER 13

Mathematical Aspects of Respiratory Care

John R. Hotchkiss*
Philip S. Crooke
Alexander B. Adams

CHAPTER OUTLINE

OBJECTIVES

1. Describe determinant and indeterminant errors in measurements.
2. Perform calculations with the correct precedence of mathematical operations.
3. Calculate areas (rectangle, triangle) and volumes (tube, sphere).
4. Define basic algebraic relationships.
5. Define functions in terms of constants and dependent and independent variables.
6. Show that the behavior of a function can be defined by use of its limit.
7. Show that the instantaneous rate of change is a derivative.
8. Demonstrate that to integrate a function is to sum infinitely small steps.
9. Identify relationships in pulmonary mechanics as differential equations.

KEY TERMS

Algebraic Relationship	Exponent	Logarithm (log)
Algebraic	Function	Metric System
Antiderivative	Fundamental Theorem of Calculus	Numeric Integration Formula
Area	Indefinite Integral	Polynomial Functions
Constant	Independent Variable	Quadratic Functions
Definite Integral	Indeterminant Error	Rate of Change
Dependent Variable	Integral	Riemann Sum
Derivative	Integrand	Scientific notation
Determinant Error	Limit	Significant Figures
Differential Equation	Limits of Integration	Volume

Numbers are important for the monitoring and therapy of patients, and respiratory therapists must become familiar with a particular range of number types. The use of num-

bers requires an understanding of their values, respective units of measure, calculations of relationships among values, and implications about unknown values. Respiratory care places greater emphasis on mathematics than do most other health-related professions. For example, therapists must understand the mathematics of complex gas flow dy-

* John R. Hotchkiss is supported by the Scientist Development Grant of the American Heart Association.

namics, arterial blood gases (ABGs), and mechanical ventilator controls. They must have a firm basis in the principles required to use these numbers, in basic mathematical operations, and in frequently used calculations.

The body's respiratory system is governed by physical laws relating flow to pressure, resistance, and compliance. The physical characteristics of the respiratory system, together with ventilatory requirements, determine the work of breathing, airway and alveolar pressures, and minute ventilation. Mathematics is the most economical shorthand for the description of the anticipated behavior of the respiratory system to an intervention. In addition to efficiently describing the mechanical behavior of the lungs, mathematical analysis allows for the theoretic quantification and practical testing of important respiratory outcomes.

Earliest among these outcomes was the delineation of the distribution of ventilation.[1] Subsequently, extensive analyses have addressed the work of breathing, prediction of maximal expiratory flow, regional structural stresses within the lung, airway dynamics, and other clinically relevant problems.[2-6] In each case, analysis of the problem at hand was either simplified or made possible by the development of mathematical descriptions of some aspect of the respiratory system. The mathematical tools covered in this chapter form the foundation for such investigations.

Basic Mathematics

Measurements and Units

The everyday practice of respiratory therapy involves many crucial measurements. Reported values, such as pH of 7.25, O_2 at 4 L/min, FIO_2 of 0.8, compliance of 30 mL/cm H_2O, Na^+ of 135 mEq/L, high pressure limit set of 35 cm H_2O, FEV_1/FVC of 0.35, or $PaCO_2$ of 65 mm Hg have great importance. Yet the signs and symptoms of the recipient patient and the therapy being delivered carries equal importance. A therapist's understanding of these values is critical to the care of the patient and accounts for a major reason that the care rendered in intensive care units (ICUs) is considered potentially hazardous.

When a measurement is obtained and reported, several observations about the measurement must be made. The numeric magnitude of the measurement tells very little without the units. Lacking units, the quantity is deprived of an essential part of its meaning. Units must always be considered carefully because every measured quantity must be associated with the proper unit. Measured values always include an inherent degree of error in the measurement. No measurement is entirely accurate, and two types of errors can occur with any measurement.

A **determinant error** is a systematic or consistent error that occurs with each measurement. It can be fixed (a parallel shift) if the error is constant. For instance, if all PaO_2 values reported are 5 mm Hg above the actual value, that error is fixed, with a parallel shift between the measured and actual values. A determinant error also can increase with an increase in the value of the measurement (a slope shift). If the value is 5 mm Hg high at a PaO_2 of 50 mm Hg, 10 mm Hg high at a PaO_2 of 100 mm Hg, and 15 mm Hg high at a PaO_2 of 150 mm Hg, a slope shift is present. This error is systematic and varies with the magnitude of the measurement. In a plot of measured versus actual values, this type of error produces a line with a different slope than a line of identity. Determinant errors are reduced or eliminated by calibration.

An **indeterminant error** describes an inherent inaccuracy in a measurement. For example, three consecutive systolic blood pressure readings can be expected to vary a bit (for example, 138, 135, and 142 mm Hg), which might be due to the detection differences by the clinician or a slightly changing blood pressure. Indeterminant errors are common, and the clinician would reduce the reported measurement from three readings to one value by averaging the measured values and accepting the mean as the measurement value. Finally, in spite of the known errors in measurements, a measurement or its value must be weighed within its realm of clinical significance, an ability gained with training and experience.

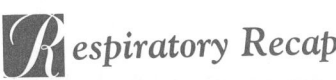 *espiratory Recap*

The metric system is the standard system of measurement in science and medicine. The standard units for length, weight, volume, temperature, and time are meter, gram, liter, degrees Celsius, and second, respectively. Divisions or multiples of these basic units (by powers of 10) are used as prefixes to indicate a workable unit for a specific measurement (Box 13-1). Commonly used units of the metric system are centimeters for length, kilograms for

Box 13-1

Metric Prefixes

Positive		Negative	
Exa	10^{18}	Deci	10^{-1}
Peta	10^{15}	Centi	10^{-2}
Tera	10^{12}	Milli	10^{-3}
Giga	10^{9}	Micro	10^{-6}
Mega	10^{6}	Nano	10^{-9}
Kilo	10^{3}	Pico	10^{-12}
Hecto	10^{2}	Femto	10^{-15}
Deco	10^{1}	Atto	10^{-18}

body weight, and milliliters for volume. Basic units in the English system are foot, pound, quart, and degrees Fahrenheit. In most cases the English system is considered obsolete in medicine. Nevertheless, because medicine involves public service and the English system sustains widespread public use, respiratory therapists must be aware of some conversions between the systems (Box 13-2).

Significant Figures and Rounding

Clarifying the precision of numbers is often necessary, especially when extremely large or small numbers are expressed. The precision of a measurement is better understood when the number of decimal places to expect is known with a defined degree of confidence. For instance, the value of PaO_2 in mm Hg is important as a whole number because the clinical variability of the measurement can be ±2 mm Hg. Therefore a PaO_2 of 63.4 mm Hg provides no more information than a value of 63 mm Hg. The number of **significant figures** in a measurement is part of the understanding of its value.

Although this rule is somewhat arbitrary, a figure is significant only if the error is less than one-half the place following the figure. Thus the number 6453 ± 40 can then be reported as 6400 or 6500 because 40 is less than one-half the hundreds place. Rounding up to 6500 would be the usual practice, rather than a truncation to 6400. With that rule a PaO_2 should be rounded to the nearest 10 or 5, but such discretion is left to the practitioner. More practically, without invoking rules, a figure is significant only to its least place of confidence. A number must not be made to seem more accurate than it is, given the limitations of the equipment, the measuring ability of the individual making the measurement, or calculations used to obtain the number. Practitioners should not be misled by extra figures; correct identification of the significant figures in a number is not as important as the acquisition of a commonsense appreciation for a number's accuracy as limited by its error. A preferable practice is to report a measurement with a percentage error, which scales with the measurement.

Rounding involves adjustment of a number to the level of confidence one has in the number's accuracy. To round is to move the number up or down in reported value to the nearest digit of confidence. If the value is to be rounded, the convention is to round up from 5, 6, 7, 8, or 9 and

down from 4, 3, 2, or 1. Rounding patient weights to the nearest kilogram would be as follows:

87.6 kg *to* 88 kg
78.4 kg *to* 78 kg
65.5 kg *to* 66 kg

Care must be taken in rounding during calculation with measured values. Rounding should be done only to the final result—not at a preliminary calculation stage.

Scientific Notation

To abbreviate numbers and make them useful in a familiar context, a common practice is to abbreviate their values with exponents. An example of a very small number is the normal concentration of hydrogen ions in blood—0.00000004 equivalents/L—whereas an example of a very large number is Avogadro's number—6,023,000,000,000,000,000,000,000 molecules/mol. Both numbers are inconvenient and difficult to compare with other values.

The practice by which large and small numbers are abbreviated as numbers with powers of ten (positive or negative) factors is called **scientific notation.** Such notation of Avogadro's number is 6.023×10^{23}, and the hydrogen ion concentration would appear as 40×10^{-9}. The superscripts, or **exponents,** of 10 (23 and −9 in this case) indicate where the decimal point should be moved to obtain the complete number. Scientific notation is the usual format used to display large or small numbers on modern calculators. For example, a calculator displays numbers in the following manner: 4.54E4 for 45,400 or 6.3342E-3 for .0063342. Laboratory results often are reported in scientific notation units to allow the values to be discussed in terms of whole numbers. For example, a statement that a red blood cell (RBC) count is 4.8 means that the RBC concentration is 4.8×10^6 cells/cm^3, or 4,800,000 cells per cubic centimeter.

Box 13-2

Common Metric–English System Conversions

Weight (Force of Gravity)	Volume
1 kilogram = 2.2 pounds	28.32 liters = 1 cubic foot
454 grams = 1 pound	29.57 mL = 1 ounce
Length	
2.54 cm = 1 inch	
1 meter = 39.37 inches	

Box 13-3

Symbols in Mathematics

Symbol	Meaning
>	Greater than
<	Less than
=	Equals
≠	Not equal to
| |	The absolute value of
Δ	Change in
∞	Infinity
. . .	Continuation of a series
*	Multiplication
≥	Greater than or equal to
≤	Less than or equal to
≈	Approximately
±	Plus or minus
≅	Approximately equal to
:	Is to
∝	Proportional to

Logarithms

An extension of the use of scientific notation is the use of **logarithms (logs),** which were originally invented to ease the difficulties of manual calculations of large or small numbers. Logs (base 10) replace a whole number and an appropriate fraction with the real number (that is, log 10 = 1, log 15 = 1.176, log 150 = 2.176). The whole-number position refers to the power of 10, and the decimals to the right refer to the actual numeric value. Tables of log values are readily available, most conveniently in modern calculators and computers. The mathematics of logs is directed by specific rules. For example, multiplication using logs actually involves the addition of the log values, whereas division involves subtraction of such values.

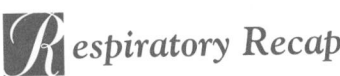 *espiratory Recap*

The common system of logs is based on powers of 10. Another log system is based on "natural" relationships, with the natural log (ln) based on the powers of e (≈2.7183). The base for this log system arises naturally to indicate growth and decay properties in science and medicine. Examples of natural logs are ln 2.7183 = 1, ln 6 = 1.7918, and ln 10 = 2.3025.

Mathematical Operations

Most mathematical operations in the clinical setting involve the basic skills of addition, subtraction, multiplication, and division. These operations are used in basic algebraic equations to many calculations performed in clinical practice. The symbols used in these operations are displayed in Box 13-3, with a precise order of precedence used to perform the calculations (Box 13-4), as follows:

1. All operations in brackets or parentheses are performed first.
2. Parentheses can be "nested." That is, if parentheses exist within parentheses, the innermost nests (parentheses) are performed first.
3. Among the mathematical operations all powers or exponents are calculated first.
4. Multiplication and division are performed next.
5. Lastly, addition and subtraction are performed.

Ratios and Proportions

Some relationships among numbers are better understood as ratios, which involve simple division. Very often a ratio

is the measurement (numerator) divided by another measurement or expected value (denominator). A common ratio is the inspiratory time to expiratory time (I:E) ratio used during mechanical ventilation. An I:E ratio of 1:2 means that the expiratory time is twice the inspiratory time. For example if the inspiratory time is 2 seconds and the I:E is 1:2, then the expiratory time is 4 seconds and the respiratory rate is 10/minute.

Some ratios are accepted as an index or indicator of disease or therapy effectiveness. Most pulmonary function test (PFT) results are comparisons of an actual measured value, such as the vital capacity, compared with a predicted value for that individual (based on age, height, and gender). Each measured parameter in a PFT usually is reported as a ratio, or a percent of the predicted value. Another ratio of interest is the portion of a tidal breath that does not participate in gas exchange, or the V_D/V_T. This fraction (ratio) is normally about 0.33 and is elevated in individuals with pulmonary disease. In these two examples the ratio has more meaning than the numerator. A proportion is similar to a ratio; it is a ratio applied to another situation (such as analogy tests). Changing the concentration of medications by dilution frequently requires the application of a proportional problem, as in Equation 13-1.

Areas and Volumes

Calculating **area** and **volume** occasionally is necessary. These calculations can be automated within the monitor or diagnostic device, but their actual calculation, or the knowledge of the mathematical algorithm used for their calculations, is useful to understand the values. The determination of areas on graphs can be completed by planimetric methods (tracing of the figure on an x-y plotting device),

Box 13-4

Examples of Precedence of Mathematical Operations

For the expression: $8 \times 2^3 - 5 + \dfrac{8}{(18 - 14)}$, the order of precedence is as follows:

1. Perform the innermost operation first, that is $18 - 14 = 4$.
2. Divide $8/4 = 2$.
3. Multiply 2^3 ($2 \times 2 \times 2 = 8$).
4. Calculate $8 \times 8 = 64$.
5. Calculate $64 - 5 + 2 = 61$.

A calculation of the alveolar gas equation when the barometric pressure $P_B = 742$ mm Hg, $F_{IO_2} = 0.80$, $Paco_2 = 54$ mm Hg, $R = 0.8$, and $P_{H_2O} = 47$ mm Hg is as follows:

1. Calculate $P_{AO_2} = F_{IO_2} \times (P_B - P_{H_2O}) - Paco_2/R$.
2. Then figure $P_{AO_2} = 0.80 \times (742 - 47) - 54/0.8$.
3. Calculate the parentheses first: $P_{AO_2} = 0.80 \times 695 - 54/0.8$.
4. Perform multiplication and division next: $P_{AO_2} = 556 - 67.5$.
5. Finally, subtract to obtain $P_{AO_2} = 488.5$ mm Hg.

EQUATION 13-1

Application of a Proportional Problem

To dilute 100 mL of a 10% solution to a 2% solution, how much diluent should be added?

$$V_1C_1 = V_2C_2$$

where:

V_1 = 100 ml
C_1 = 10%
C_2 = 2%
V_2 = Unknown

The ratio of the concentration is 2%:10% or 1:5. Applying the 1:5 ratio to the solution volumes increases the volume from 100 to 500 ml. Therefore 400 mL must be added to make a 2% solution.

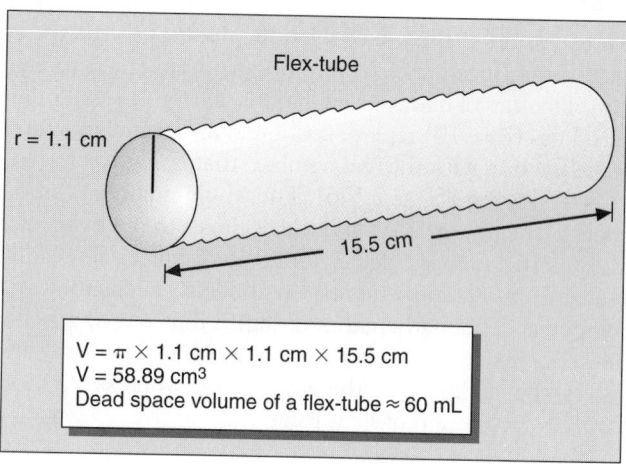

$$V = \pi \times 1.1 \text{ cm} \times 1.1 \text{ cm} \times 15.5 \text{ cm}$$
$$V = 58.89 \text{ cm}^3$$
Dead space volume of a flex-tube ≈ 60 mL

Figure 13-2   Calculation of a flex-tube volume.

BOX 13-5

Formulas for Areas

Square: l^2

Rectangle: $l \times h$

Triangle: $\frac{1}{2} \times l \times h$

Circle: $\pi \times r^2$

h, Height; r, radius; l, length.

BOX 13-6

Formulas for Volumes

Cube: l^3

Rectanguloid: $l \times h \times w$

Cylinder: $l \times \pi \times r^2$

Sphere: $\frac{4}{3} \times \pi \times r^3$

h, Height; w, width; r, radius; l, length.

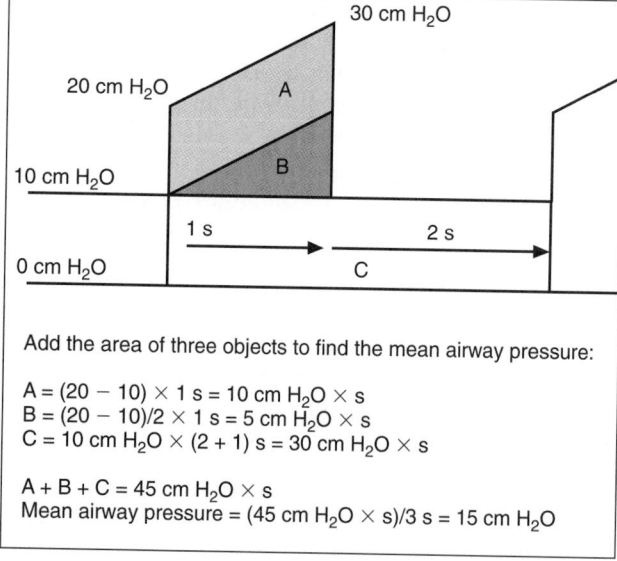

Add the area of three objects to find the mean airway pressure:

A = (20 − 10) × 1 s = 10 cm H_2O × s
B = (20 − 10)/2 × 1 s = 5 cm H_2O × s
C = 10 cm H_2O × (2 + 1) s = 30 cm H_2O × s

A + B + C = 45 cm H_2O × s
Mean airway pressure = (45 cm H_2O × s)/3 s = 15 cm H_2O

Figure 13-1   Calculation of a mean airway pressure. With an airway pressure tracing of pressure versus time, the mean airway pressure can be calculated through the addition of the pressure-time areas and division by the time.

Calculations can be made to determine the volumes of objects such as pistons, vessels, tubes, cubes, or more oddly shaped chambers, such as the lungs. These calculations can determine the capacity of an object to contain a gas. Box 13-6 provides the formulas used to determine volumes of regularly shaped objects. In a ventilator circuit, a flex-tube is often inserted between the endotracheal tube and the ventilator Y-piece, adding volume to the mechanical dead space (or rebreathable volume) of the circuitry. Figure 13-2 illustrates the calculation of the volume of a flex-tube.

Algebraic Relationships

The interrelationships among measured values are constantly being considered in the clinical setting. Some relationships are simply additive or multiplicative. Common types of **algebraic relationships** are the linear, parabolic, or exponential relationships or the more complex relationships, such as curvilinear or sigmoidal ones. A linear relationship describes a change in one value causing or corresponding to a direct effect on another value. An example of a fixed relationship is the linear comparison of the temperature scales. The conversion of Fahrenheit temperatures to the Celsius scale is linear and offset by 32 degrees. That is, every 1.8-degree change in the Fahrenheit scale changes one degree in the Celsius scale—a linear relationship. Although the relationship is defined by science, linear relationships exist throughout medicine.

Parabolic relationships are somewhat more complicated. A parabola refers to the shape formed via graphing

but the ability to complete simple calculations directly is important. Several area calculations, including triangles, rectangles, squares, and circles, are significant. Formulas used to calculate the areas of some regularly shaped figures are shown in Box 13-5; Figure 13-1 is an example of area calculation for mean airway pressure of a ventilated patient.

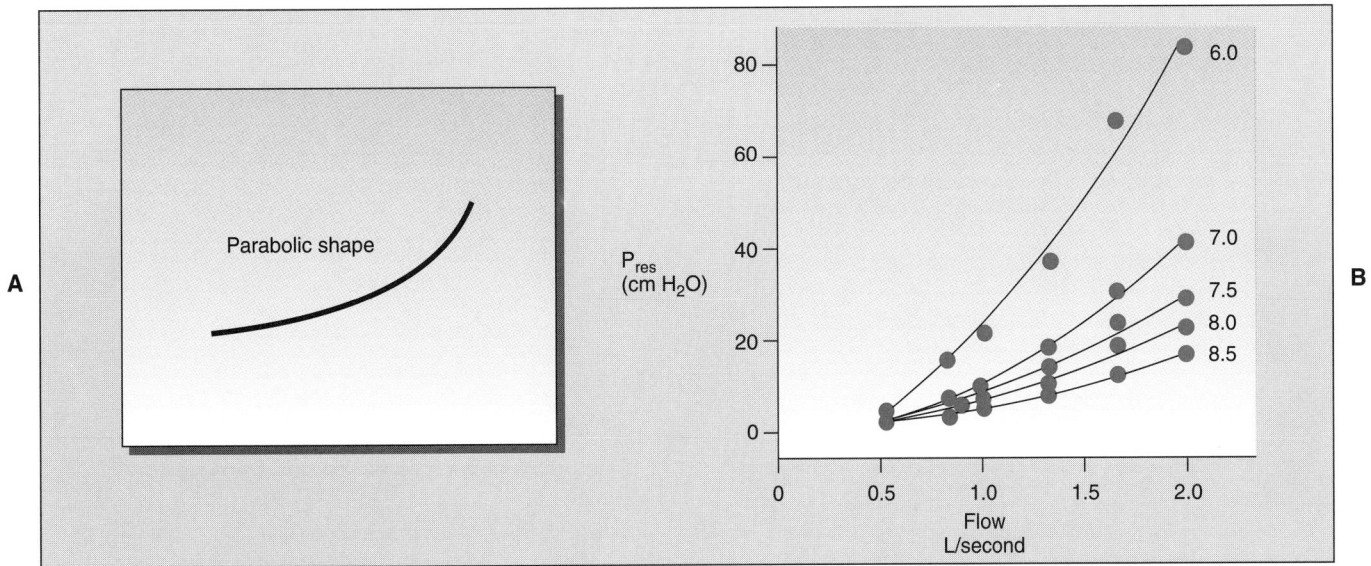

Figure 13-3   A, Parabolic curve. **B,** Example of a family of parabolic curves from a plot of the resistive pressure developed by an increase in flow through smaller endotracheal tubes. (Data from Wright PE, Marini JJ, Bernard GR. In vitro versus in vivo comparison of endotracheal tube airflow resistance. Am Rev Respir Dis 1989;140:10-16.)

of a value that is increasing in an accelerating manner (Figure 13-3). An example of this relationship is the resistive pressure generated from flow through a fixed orifice. The pressure drop between the ends of a resistive element (such as an endotracheal tube) increases with increasing flow at an increasing rate, not just a linear rate.

$\mathcal{R}$*espiratory Recap*

Algebraic Relationships	
Linear	Exponential
Parabolic	Sigmoid
Power	

In biology, where many factors can be involved, the relationships become more complicated than those established by science or based on physical principles derived from fixed objects. Accelerating growth curves for bacteria present good examples. Bacteria grown or incubated in an ideal environment multiply at an extremely rapid rate. The number of bacteria doubles in a time period called the *doubling time* or *generation time*. The generation time varies with the species of bacteria, the nutrients available, and the prevailing physical conditions (for example, temperature, moisture level, pH). The number of bacteria can be calculated (roughly) by the equation $b = B \times 2^N$, where B is the original number of bacteria, N is the number of generations (doubling periods), and b is the final number of bacteria after the incubation or total growth time. This relationship is exponential and is represented graphically in Figure 13-4. To graph this rapid growth, a specially graduated graph pa-

per, known as *logarithmic paper*, is required. The exponential growth is then a straight line on log paper. Furthermore, calculations of the number of bacteria after certain incubation periods require the mathematics of logs.

Some complex relationships involve a combination of the effects of several factors, often the case in physiology as several factors become involved in characterizing a relationship. Obvious examples of such complex relationships are the sigmoid curves that represent the oxyhemoglobin dissociation curve or the pressure-volume curve of the lung. These curves have segments with curves and line segments, generally marking the relationship as curvilinear. The oxygen-carrying capacity of the blood depends on the transient ability for oxygen molecules to bind to hemoglobin molecules, a graphically curvilinear and sigmoidal relationship. The pressure-volume relationship of the lung is shaped by the condition of alveoli or alveolar regions at different pressures. Both the dissociation curve and the pressure-volume curve are sigmoidal (Figure 13-5) and considered complex and difficult to characterize mathematically. Yet, their determinations are extremely instructive, and the curves are used to better understand physiology and patient care.

Advanced Mathematics

Functions

Practical mathematics is generally based on the quantitative description of the real world. A **function** is a rule associating two or more measurable quantities, which are called the *variables* for that function. In a mathematical function the value of one variable depends on one or more

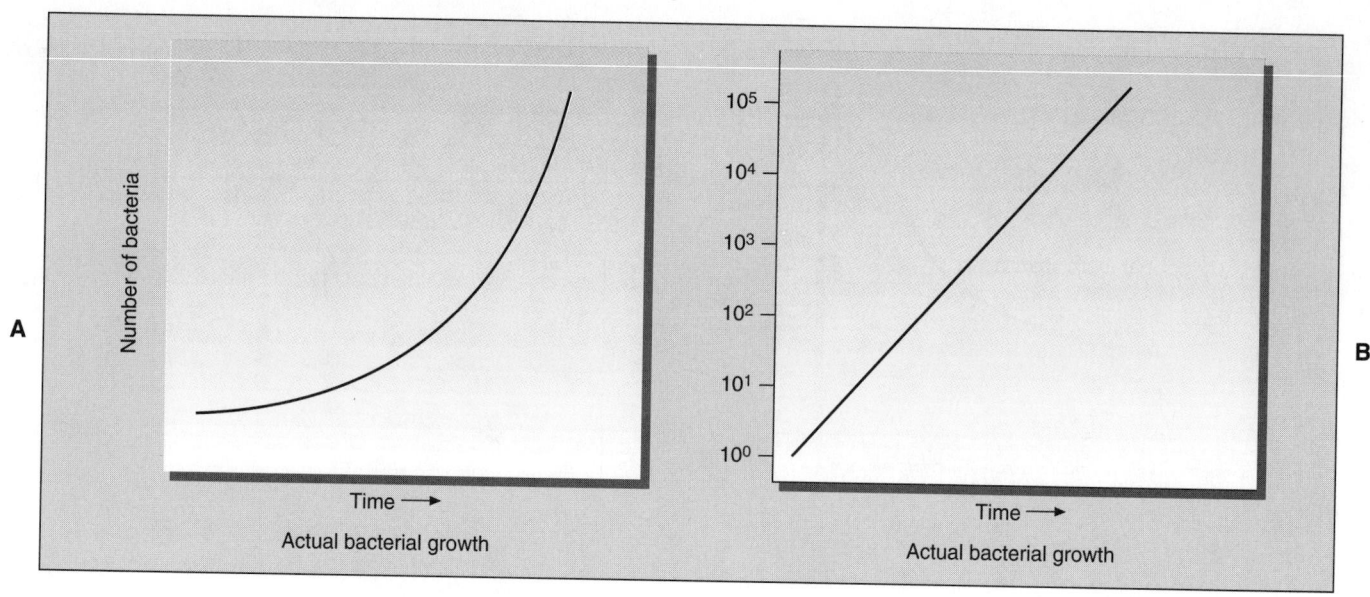

Figure 13-4   Exponential **(A)** versus logarithmic **(B)** growth of bacteria.

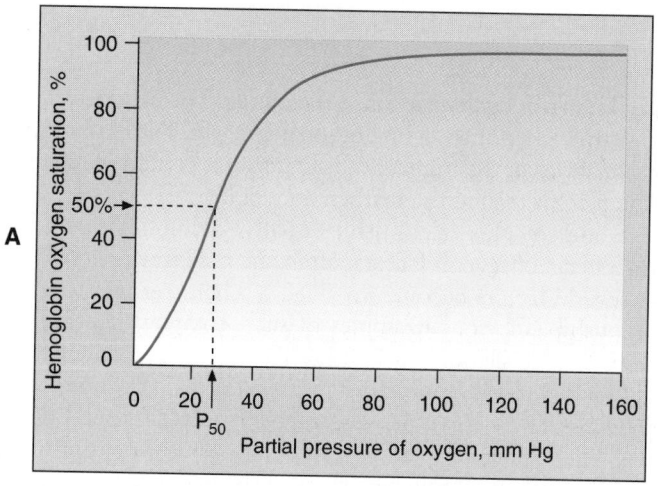

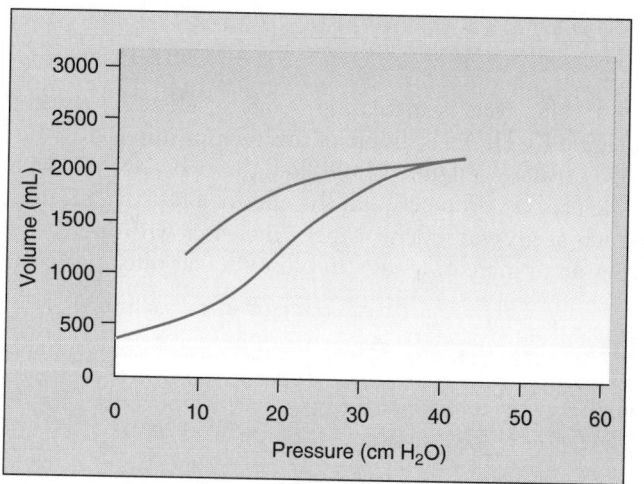

Figure 13-5   Examples of sigmoidal curves. **A,** Oxyhemoglobin dissociation curve. **B,** Pressure-volume curve of the respiratory system.

other variables (Equation 13-2). A variable with an unchanging, fixed value is called a **constant.** A function is known as **algebraic** if it can be constructed with the basic operations of algebra (addition, subtraction, multiplication, or division). Note that constants are not included in the symbol for the function, which can be linear or quadratic (Equation 13-3). Both of these functions are called **polynomial functions.** The highest power in a polynomial function is termed its *degree*. Hence, a linear function is a first-degree function, whereas a **quadratic function** is considered second degree.

Not all functions are algebraic. Commonly encountered nonalgebraic functions include the exponential, logarithmic, and trigonometric functions (Equation 13-4). Because the theoretic basis for the exponential and sine (or cosine) functions is complex, they are most practically

thought of as *rules* that generate a given *output* value for any given *input* value. The output values can be obtained from tables or calculators.

Respiratory Recap

Functions

A function is a rule associating two or more measurable quantities called *variables.*

When a function, or relationship, is set up between two variables, the **dependent variable** is said to be *defined* in terms of the **independent variable(s).** The values of the

EQUATION 13-2

Functions

An example of a function is the following gas law describing the relationship between pressure and volume for an ideal gas:

$P_1 V_1 = P_2 V_2$

The following equation helps determine the way the pressure of this gas changes as volume changes:

$$P_2 = \frac{P_1 V_1}{V_2} = F(P_1, V_1, V_2)$$

where P_2 is the dependent variable, and P_1, V_1, and V_2 are all independent variables. The value of P_2 depends on the values of P_1, V_1, and V_2.

EQUATION 13-3

Linear and Quadratic Functions

Linear Function

$$P = \frac{V}{C} = F(V)$$

where P is pressure and V is volume. This equation is a function that links pressure to volume, assuming that compliance is a constant.

Quadratic Function

$$P = R_1 \dot{Q} + R_2 \dot{Q}^2 = F(\dot{Q})$$

This equation is a function that describes the drop in pressure (P) due to a drop in flow, where R_1 and R_2 are constants and $\dot{Q}$ is flow.

EQUATION 13-4

Exponential and Trigonometric Functions

Exponential

$V = V_1 e^{kt} = F(t)$

where:

V = Volume of deflating lung
V_1 = End-inspiratory volume of deflating lung
e = Natural log
t = Time

This equation relates the volume of a passively deflating lung to its end-inspiratory volume, the natural log, and time.

Trigonometric

$\dot{Q} = k_1 \sin(k_2 t) = F(t)$

This equation gives flow ($\dot{Q}$) in terms of time (t), relating the flow a ventilator applies to the airway as a function of time during sinusoidal ventilation.

EQUATION 13-5

Limit of a Function

The limit of a function, $Y = F(x)$, as x approaches the value of interest, $x = c$, is denoted by the following equation:

$$\lim_{x \to c} F(x) = K$$

$F(x)$ is said to approach the value K as x approaches the value c. Simple techniques have been developed to find such limits. For example, $\lim_{x \to 2} (x - 2)/(x^2 - 4) = 1/4$ can be demonstrated.

independent variables and the function then assign the value for the dependent variable(s). A function may not be assigned for all values of the independent variables. However, the behavior of the function near these points may be desired, leading to the mathematical concept known as the *limit of the function*.

Limits

In relating two quantities by a function, an important change occurs. If the function is well behaved, the value of the dependent variable can be predicted as the independent variable approaches a specific point. Although this concept seems simple, for many functions the behavior of the dependent variable can become complex as the input values approach certain points. For example, what is the behavior of the function $y = (x - 2)/(x^2 - 4)$ as x approaches the point $x = 2$? Notice that the function does not make sense at $x = 2$ because division by zero is not allowed. The concept of the **limit** of a function was developed in part to address this problem (Equation 13-5). The

point to remember is that the limit of a function describes the behavior, or value, of the dependent variable as the independent variable approaches some point of interest.

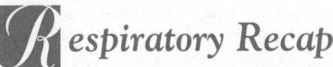 **R**espiratory Recap

Limits
A limit describes the behavior or value of the dependent variable as the independent variable approaches a point of interest.

Rate of Change

Consider a function $y = F(x)$, with x fixed at some value, for instance $x = a$. Suppose the value of the independent variable is changed to some new value, for instance $x = a + \Delta x$. The value of y then changes too. Namely, the change in the value of the function is $\Delta F = F(a + \Delta x) - F(a) = y_2 - y_1$, where $y_2 = F(a + \Delta x)$ and $y_1 = F(a)$. This difference,

EQUATION 13-6

Rate of Change of a Function

During passive ventilation the flow out of the lungs is determined by the pressure (P) within the lungs (driving pressure or alveolar pressure) and the resistance of the airway (R, assumed constant). By analogy with Ohm's law, the function of flow is as follows:

$$\dot{Q} = F(P) = \frac{P}{R}$$

where:

$\dot{Q}$ = Flow
P = Pressure
R = Resistance

The rate of change in flow when the pressure changes from one value, P_1, to another value, $P_2 = P_1 + \Delta P$ is as follows:

$$\Delta\dot{Q} = F(P_2) - F(P_1) = F(P_1 + \Delta P) - F(P_1) = \frac{P_1 + \Delta P}{R} - \frac{P_1}{R} = \frac{\Delta P}{R}$$

Hence, the change in the flow is a scaled change (by 1/R), with the change in pressure. For example, if the resistance is 40 cm H_2O/L/second and the change in pressure is $\Delta P = 5$ cm H_2O, then the rate of change in flow is $\Delta\dot{Q} = 5/40 = \frac{1}{8}$ L/second.

As another example, the driving pressure (P) during passive expiration is determined by the volume in the lung (V) and the compliance (C) of the lung (elastic recoil pressure), as follows:

$$P = F(V) = \frac{V}{C}$$

The rate of change of the pressure with a change in the lung volume, for instance, a change from a value V_1 to a value $V_2 = V_1 + \Delta V$, assuming constant compliance is as follows:

$$\Delta P = F(V_2) - F(V_1) = F(V_1 + C) - F(V_1) = \frac{V_1 + \Delta V}{C} - \frac{V_1}{C} = \frac{\Delta V}{C}$$

Again, the rate of change of the pressure is a scaled change to the change in volume.

EQUATION 13-7

Average Rate of Change

$$\bar{F} = \frac{\Delta F}{\Delta x} = \frac{F(a + \Delta x) - F(a)}{\Delta x}$$

where *F* is flow.

The average rate of change of the flow with the change in pressure is as follows:

$$\bar{\dot{Q}} = \frac{\Delta\dot{Q}}{\Delta P} = \frac{1}{R}$$

Consider Rohrer's equation for the pressure (P) as a function of flow in the quadratic equation: $P = F(flow) = R_1(\dot{Q}) + R_2(\dot{Q})^2$. Assume that $R_1 = 3$ and $R_2 = 1$. The average rate of change of the pressure if the flow changes from flow = 2 to flow = 4 is $P = (F(4) - F(2))/(4 - 2) = (28 - 10)/2 = 9$. On the other hand, a change in the flow from flow = 2 to flow = 5 is $P = (F(5) - F(2))/(5 - 2) = (40 - 10)/2 = 15$.

$\Delta F/\Delta x$, is called the **rate of change** of the function, or simply the amount of change in the dependent variable for a given change in the independent variable. The rate of change of a function is an important concept in physical systems (Equation 13-6). The average rate of change is defined as the ratio of the rate of change of a function (ΔF) to the change in the independent variable (Δx; Equation 13-7).

Derivatives

Consider the average rate of change of a function when the change of the independent variable is very small (that is, Δx close to zero). This number is called the **derivative** of F with respect to x at x = a and is denoted by the symbol F'(a) (Equation 13-8). The derivative is the instantaneous rate of change of the function at a given point (in other words a local slope). In many situations the usefulness of the derivative stems from the ease with which the rate of change of some quantity can be specified at a particular point, even if the quantity itself is changing. If the behavior of a system can be specified by a function, then the derivative of the function often can be calculated. The derivative is a measure of the instantaneous rate of change of the function to the instantaneous rate of change of its independent variable. This concept can be extended to

EQUATION 13-8

Derivatives

Consider the following limit:

$$\lim_{\Delta x \to 0} \bar{F} = \lim_{\Delta x \to 0} \frac{F(a + \Delta x) - F(a)}{\Delta x}$$

This number is called the *derivative of F* with respect to x at x = a and is denoted by the symbol F'(a). The derivative also is called the *instantaneous rate of change of the function*. Other notations also used for the derivative, as follows:

$$F'(a) = \frac{dF}{dx}\bigg|x = a = \frac{dy}{dx}\bigg|x = a = D[f](a)$$

Consider the function P = F(V) = V/C. Calculate $F'(V_0)$, where V_0 is any value for the volume of the lung. The rate of change is $\Delta P = \Delta V/C$, which implies that the average rate of change is as follows:

$$\bar{P} = \frac{\Delta P}{\Delta V} = \frac{1}{C} \to \lim_{V \to 0}\bar{P} = \lim_{V \to 0}\frac{1}{C} = \frac{1}{C}$$

Thus the derivative of P with respect to V at $V = V_0$ is 1/C. That is, $F'(V_0) = 1/C$. The derivative in this case is always the same number (1/C). However, the derivative F'(a) usually changes as (a) changes. Consider again Rohrer's equation for the pressure drop as a function of the flow: $P = F(\dot{Q}) = R_1(\dot{Q}) + R_2(\dot{Q})^2$. In this case one can show that the derivative of F at any value of the flow $\dot{Q}_0$ is $F'(\dot{Q}_0) = R_1 + 2R_2(\dot{Q}_0)$. The derivative changes as $\dot{Q}_0$ changes. For example, if $R_1 = 10$ and $R_2 = 3$, then F'(1) = 16, whereas F'(5) = 40. Hence, the instantaneous change in pressure drop is much higher at a flow of 5 than at a flow of 1.

functions that depend on more than one independent variable, but such a discussion requires considerably more mathematical structure.

A different problem arises when the equation specifying the *overall* behavior of a system is already known and the interest lies in the determination of the rate at which some variable is changing. In this case the overall behavior of the system already is known, and the process of differentiation is used to find the derivative of this function (Equation 13-9). Many rules can be used to find the derivative of a particular function. In most simple cases the derivative for a function of a particular form can simply be found in an appropriate table (Table 13-1). Differentiation has its own set of rules (for example, the derivative of the sum of two functions being the sum of the derivatives). Rules used to differentiate these equations also are available.

Integrals

Integrals are used to determine an area. In many problems the topic of interest is the addition of many small steps

EQUATION 13-9

Differentiation to Determine the Derivative of a Function

The function for the passively deflating lung is as follows:

$$V = F(t) = V_1 e^{-t/RC}$$

This function is the solution of a differential equation, a mathematical model of the way the volume of the lungs changes when they deflate. The instantaneous flow from the lung can be computed through differentiation of F with respect to t. The derivative is as follows:

$$\dot{Q} = \frac{dV}{dt} = F'(t) = \frac{V_1}{RC} e^{-t/RC}$$

Note that this new equation $\dot{Q} = G(t) = F(t)$ has the property that G(t) <0. The function G(t) gives the flow from the lung (negative flow) at any time t as a function of the initial volume of the lung and time, without the volume at the time of interest.

TABLE 13-1

Derivatives of Common Functions

Function	Derivative
F(x)	F'(x)
kx	x
kx^n	knx^{n-1}
e^{kx}	ke^{kx}
ln kx	1/x
sin kx	k cos kx
cos kx	-k sin kx

k, Constant; n, integer.

over some specified interval, such as time. For example, a respiratory therapist may wish to obtain the exhaled tidal volume of a patient. Without the use of a spirometer, such information can be obtained from the airway flow tracing. In the simplest (but nonphysiologic) case the expiratory flow remains constant from end-inhalation to end-exhalation. The exhaled volume is then the product of the flow and the expiratory time. In reality the expiratory flow declines (approaches zero exponentially) over time (Figure 13-6). The problem then becomes how to determine the exhaled volume as the expiratory flow rate varies or to determine the area under the expiratory flow curve flow (the exhaled volume).

One approach to this problem is to partition (digitize) the expiratory flow curve into a large number of small time steps, each of length Δt, as shown in Figure 13-7. The expired volume is then the sum of the areas under each step. However, the area under each step is not easily determined if flow is changing. The area of each step can be approximated under the assumption that the F(t) is essentially constant in each small interval. For example, if the flow function is defined on the interval (0,T) and this interval is partitioned into several little subintervals: $(0,t_1)$, (t_1,t_2), (t_2,t_3), . . .,(t_{n-1}, t_n) where $t_n = T$, then the assumption can be that $F(t_1) \approx F(t_2)$ on the subinterval (t_1, t_2), and so forth. In this example, $\Delta t = t_1 - 0 = t_2 - t_1 = t_3 - t_2 = . . . = T - t_{n-1}$. Then, an approximation of the exhaled volume is determined by the **Riemann sum** (Equation 13-10). If this limit can be computed, it is called the definite integral of the function F(t) over the interval (0,T) and is denoted by the following symbol:

$$V_{exhaled} = \int_0^T F(t)dt$$

In the following symbol:

$$\int_a^b f(x)dx$$

x is called the **integrand** of the definite integral, and *a* and *b* are called the **limits of integration.** The integral also can

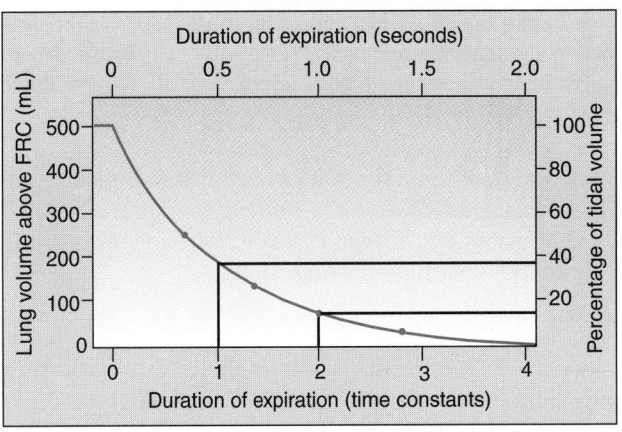

Figure 13-6   Expiratory volume decay. *FRC,* Functional residual capacity. (Modified from Marini JJ. Monitoring during mechanical ventilation. Clin Chest Med 1988;9:73-100.)

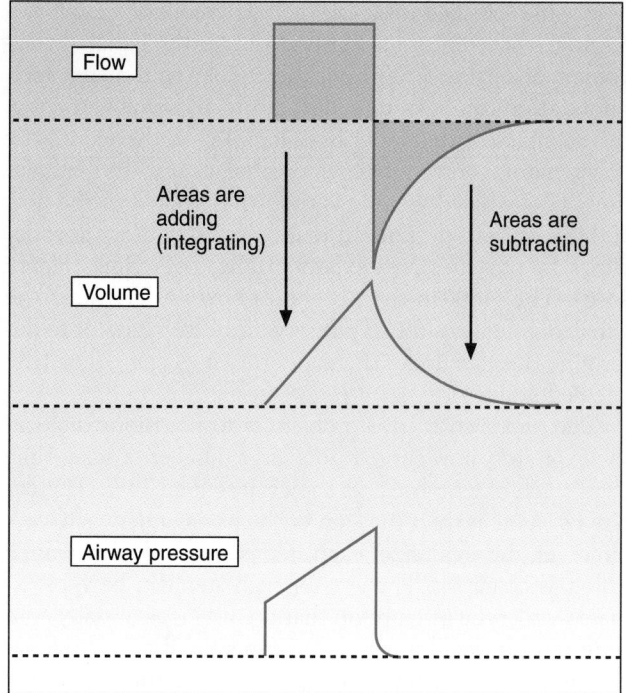

Figure 13-7   Flow/volume/pressure of a ventilated breath with integration of flow as an example of volume derivation.

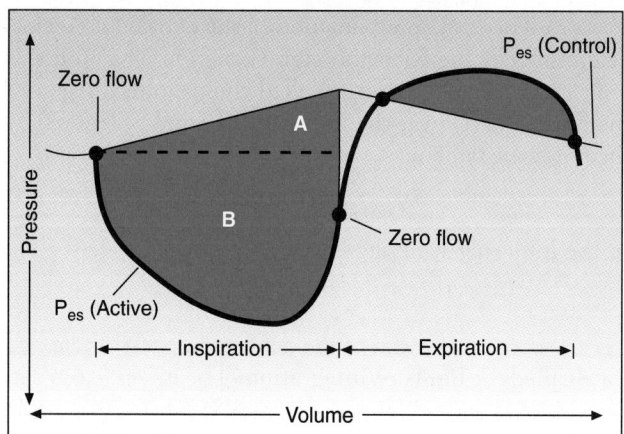

Figure 13-8   Work of breathing. The shaded area of the pressure-volume curve represents the work of breathing. Area *A* is the work done by the ventilator, and area *B* is the work done by the patient. P_{es}, Esophageal pressure. (Modified from Marini JJ. Am Rev Respir Dis 1988;138:1169-1179.)

be used to determine the work of breathing (Equation 13-11 and Figure 13-8).

Another type of integral is called the **indefinite integral,** denoted by the following symbol:

$$\int f(x)dx$$

(Note the lack of limits.) This symbol means something quite different than the **definite integral,** which produces a number. The indefinite integral gives a function:

$$\int f(x)dx = F(x)$$

EQUATION 13-10
The Riemann Sum

If the flow function is defined on the interval (0,T) and this interval is partitioned into several little subintervals: $(0,t_1)$, (t_1,t_2), $(t_2,t_3),\ldots,(t_{n-1}, t_n)$ where $t_n = T$, then the assumption could follow that $F(t_1) \approx F(t_2)$ on the subinterval (t_1, t_2), and so forth. In this instance $\Delta t = t_1 - 0 = t_2 - t_1 = t_3 - t_2 = \ldots = T - t_{n-1}$. Then, an approximation of the exhaled volume is as follows:

$$F(t_1)\Delta t + F(t_2)\Delta t + F(t_3)\Delta t + \ldots + F(t_n)\Delta t = \sum_{i=1}^{n} F(t_i)\Delta t$$

This approximation is called a *Riemann sum*. As Δt becomes smaller and smaller, this value more closely approximates the true value of the exhaled volume. In fact, if the limit is taken as Δt of 0, then, the following results:

$$V_{exhaled} = \lim_{\Delta t \to 0} \sum_{i=1}^{n} F(t_i)\Delta t$$

If this limit is computed, it is called the *definite integral* of the function F(t) over the interval [0,T], as follows:

$$V_{exhaled} = \int_0^T F(t)dt$$

EQUATION 13-11
Work of Breathing

If W_B denotes the work being done by the patient's respiratory muscles during inspiration, then the *total work* done during inspiration, 0 to T_i is as follows:

$$W_B = \int_0^{T_i} PVdt$$

and the *average work* performed by the patient's muscles is as follows:

$$W_{average} = \frac{\int_0^{T_i} PVdt}{T - 0} = \frac{1}{T}\int_0^{T_i} PVdt$$

When the definite integral of a function is known over a particular interval, then the *mean,* or *average,* value of the function (for example, work) is known over the same interval.

A property of the function F(x) is that its derivative is the integrand of the indefinite integral (Equation 13-12). Because the derivative and indefinite integral cancel each other, the indefinite integral is sometimes called the **antiderivative,** as follows:

$$\int f'(x)dx = f(x)$$

If F(x) is the antiderivative of f(x), then F(x) + C for any constant C is also an antiderivative. Hence, the following is usually written:

$$\int f(x)dx = F(x) + C$$

Many rules exist to compute antiderivatives (Box 13-7). The connection between the definite integral and the indefinite integral is called the **fundamental theorem of calculus** (Equation 13-13). In many cases, finding the antiderivative of the integrand of a definite integral is

EQUATION 13-12

Derivative of an Indefinite Integral

A property of the function F(x) is that its derivative is the integrand of the indefinite integral, as follows:

$$\frac{d}{dx}\left(\int f(x)dx\right) = \frac{dF}{dx} = f(x)$$

EQUATION 13-13

The Fundamental Theorem of Calculus

The theorem states that if the following is true:

$$\int f(x)dx = F(x) + C$$

then

$$\int_a^b f(x)dx = F(a) - F(b)$$

For example, because of the following:

$$F(x) = \int x^2 dx = \frac{1}{3}x^3 + C$$

the definite integral can be calculated, as follows:

$$\int_{-1}^{2} x^2 dx = F(2) - F(-1) = \frac{8}{3} - \frac{-1}{3} = 3$$

EQUATION 13-14

Differential Equation for Deflation of the Lungs

$$\frac{dV}{dt} = -\frac{V}{RC}$$

This differential equation states that the rate of change of lung volume during exhalation is equal to the pressure gradient driving deflation (alveolar pressure − PEEP), divided by the resistance of the airways.

PEEP, *Positive end-expiratory pressure.*

impossible, in which case the definite integral can be approximated by a Riemann sum. This simple approach, along with its more complex extensions, also is called a **numeric integration formula.** Many efficient and powerful techniques for numeric integration exist. Although numeric integration is not as convenient as exact solutions, it is powerful and can be applied to many equations that cannot be solved exactly.

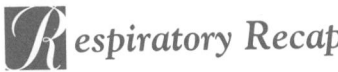

Antiderivatives

The indefinite integral, or antiderivative, is not unique. Many rules exist for the determination of antiderivatives.

BOX 13-7

Often Encountered Functions

F(x)	
K	kx + C
kx^n	$\dfrac{k}{n+1}x^{n+1} + C$
$\dfrac{k}{x}$	k ln|x| + C
k cos ax	$\dfrac{k}{a}\sin ax + C$
k sin ax	
$\int f(x)dx$	$-\dfrac{k}{a}\cos ax + C$

Differential Equations

In many cases in respiratory physiology a known equation relates the rate of change of a variable of interest to other variables, and the desired action is to predict the behavior of the system over time. The most important of these is the Equation of Motion for the lung as it is inflated from functional residual capacity (FRC) by a constant pressure (as in pressure control ventilation). In this case the rate of change of lung volume over time can be found through consideration of the pressure components of the system: $P_{applied}$, $P_{elastic}$, and $P_{resistive}$ (Figure 13-9). That is, $P_{applied} = P_{elastic} + P_{resistive}$, a conservation of pressure equation. In the case of constant pressure ventilation, $P_{applied} = P_{set}$. The pressure $P_{elastic}$ is due to the elastic recoil of the lung and expansive tension of the chest wall, whereas the resistive pressure $P_{resistive}$ is the pressure loss due to resistance. These pressures are generally modeled as shown in Equation 13-14. Many other differential equations arise in pulmonary mechanics. For example, the volume V(t) in the deflation of the lung during expiration is modeled by the differential equation in Equation 13-15. The solutions to such equations involve a vital and active area of mathematics and its application to respiratory mechanics.[7-9]

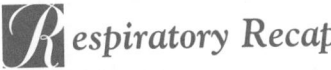

Differential Equations

Differential equations are used to define and understand static and dynamic aspects of pulmonary mechanics.

In a **differential equation,** one is interested in finding a function that satisfies a specific equation. Such a function is called the *solution* of the differential equation. For the equation of motion, the desired function can be shown to be $V(t) = Ke^{-t/RC}$, where *K* is a constant (see Equation 13-15). The constant K can be determined if the solution

EQUATION 13-15

Equation of Motion

$$P_{elastic} = \frac{V(t)}{C}$$

$$P_{resistive} = R\dot{V}(t)$$

where:

- C = Compliance
- R = Resistance are positive constants
- $V(t)$ = Volume of the lung at time t
- $P_{elastic}$ = Elastic pressure
- $P_{resistive}$ = Resistive pressure

C and R are positive constants, with $\dot{V}(t)$ being the flow at time t. Using these equations in the conservation of pressure equation, the following results:

$$P_{set} = R\dot{V}(t) + \frac{1}{C}V(t)$$

or

$$\frac{dV}{dt} = \frac{1}{R}\left(P_{set} - \frac{V}{C}\right)$$

where P_{set} is the set pressure.

This mathematical equation states that the rate of change of lung volume during inhalation is equal to the pressure gradient driving inflation (a preset pressure on the ventilator), divided by the resistance of the airways to flow. The preceding two equations are called *differential equations* for the inspiratory volume, $V(t)$. Differential equations such as these are termed *first-order differential equations* because they involve the first derivative of the variable of interest.

EQUATION 13-16

Solution for Differential Equation Describing Equation of Motion for Inhalation

$$V(t) = CP_{set} + Ke^{-t/RC}$$

where K is some constant and P_{set} is set pressure.

If an initial-condition is imposed, for instance, $V(0) = 0$, then $0 = V(0) = CP_{set} + K \rightarrow K = -CP_{set}$, which implies the following:

$$V(t) = CP_{set}(1 - e^{-t/RC})$$

has a known value at some time [for example, $V(0) = V(t)$], which implies that $V(t) = V_Te^{-t/RC}$. The condition for $V(t)$ when $V(0) = V_T$ is called an *initial condition* for the differential equation. In this example, V_T denotes the volume of the lung at which deflation starts. The solution for the Equation of Motion (see Equation 13-15) is shown in Equation 13-16. For those differential equations that cannot be solved, often functions can be found that approximate the true solutions, at least at certain points. These techniques are called *numeric methods*.

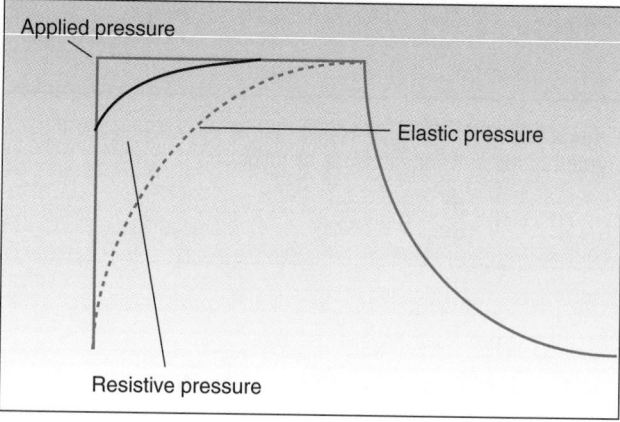

Figure 13-9 Schematic of inspiratory pressure (P) displaying $P_{applied}$, $P_{resistive}$, and $P_{elastic}$ during pressure controlled ventilation.

KEY POINTS

- A determinant error is a systematic or consistent error that occurs with each measurement, whereas an indeterminant error is an inherent inaccuracy in a measurement.
- The metric system is the standard system of measurement in science and medicine.
- A common practice is to abbreviate numbers with exponents to put them into a useful and manageable form.
- Logarithms ease the difficulties of manual calculations of large or small numbers.
- A function is a rule associating two or more measurable quantities.
- The derivative is the slope of a function (the instantaneous rate of change).
- Integrals are used to determine an area.

References

1. Otis AB, McKerrow CB, Bartlett RA, et al. Mechanical factors in the distribution of ventilation. J Appl Physiol 1955;8:427.
2. Marini JJ, Crooke PS, Truwit JD. Determinants and limits of pressure-preset ventilation: a mathematical model of pressure control ventilation. J Appl Physiol 1989;67:1081-1092.
3. Mead J, Takishima T, Leith D. Stress distribution in lungs: a model of pulmonary elasticity. J Appl Physiol 1970;28:596-608.
4. Brody AW. Mechanical compliance and resistance of the lung-thorax calculated from the flow recorded during passive expiration. Am J Physiol 1954;178:189-196.
5. Zin WA, Rossi A, Mili-Emili J. Model analysis of respiratory responses to inspiratory resistive loads. J Appl Physiol 1983;55:1565-1573.
6. Campbell D, Brown J. The electrical analog of the lung. Br J Anaesth 1963;35:684-693.

7. Crooke PS, Head JD, Marini JJ, et al. Patient-ventilator interaction: a general model for nonpassive mechanical ventilation. IMA J Math Appl Med Biol 1998;15:321-337.

8. Hotchkiss JR Jr, Crooke PS III, Marini JJ. Theoretical interactions between ventilator settings and proximal dead space ventilation during tracheal gas insufflation. Intensive Care Med 1996;22:1112-1119.

9. Hotchkiss JR Jr, Crooke PS, Adams AB, et al. Implications of a biphasic two-compartment model of constant flow ventilation for the clinical setting. J Crit Care 1994;9:114-123.

CHAPTER 14

Application of Physical Principles

Andrew McKibben

CHAPTER **OUTLINE**

OBJECTIVES

1. Identify the physical principles that are most important to respiratory physiology and respiratory care.
2. Explain the behaviors of fluids at various pressures, volumes, temperatures, and flows.
3. Describe units of measurement, molecules, and states of matter.
4. Discuss the relationships of physical principles affecting force, stress, pressure, and work.
5. Describe compliance, elastance, and resistance and their relationships to work of breathing.
6. Describe work of breathing and its assessment.
7. Describe surface tension and its relationship to lung function and work of breathing.
8. Discuss Boyle's, Charles', and Gay-Lussac's laws and the ideal gas law, explaining the way changes in pressure and temperature volume affect the behavior of gases.
9. Describe the application of physical principles for monitoring, measurement, and assessment of lung function.

KEY TERMS

Bernoulli Principle
Boyle's Law
Charles' Law
Compliance
Dalton's Law
Density
Elastance
Fick's Law

Flow
Force
Gay-Lussac's Law
Graham's Law
Gravity
Hagen-Poiseuille Equation
Hydrostatic Pressure
Ideal Gas Law

Joule
Laminar Flow
Mass
Ohm's Law
Pascal
Pressure
Resistance
Reynolds Number

Respiratory therapists must understand the physical principles important to respiratory physiology and the practice of respiratory care, such as the behavior of gases and liquids under varying conditions of pressure, temperature, and flow. Physical forces have significant effects on gas transfer, ventilation, and perfusion. Furthermore, the thorax is exposed to a wider variation of forces than other anatomic structures.

Respiratory therapy lies at a critical juncture between physical and clinical science. Therefore an understanding of the fundamental physical principles is essential to a genuine grasp of the daily practice of respiratory care. Some of the equations and relationships presented in this chapter simplify physics and physiology, but this approach provides a useful approximation of the key principles involved.

Basic Physics

Molecules and States of Matter

Molecular theory approaches physical entities and their response to physical forces by describing atoms and molecules and their interactions. Molecules are composed of atoms, the elemental unit of matter (although smaller subatomic particles have been described). A molecule may be a pure element in which all atoms are the same, or a compound of dissimilar atoms. Both elements and compounds are composed of atoms that are chemically joined (bound) by intermolecular forces that exist among the atoms in each molecule. Molecular oxygen (O_2) is composed of two atoms of an element (oxygen); carbon dioxide (CO_2) is a molecular compound made up of one carbon atom and two oxygen atoms. These chemical bonds may be covalent bonds, which are particularly strong, or weaker bonds. The intrinsic properties of atoms, as well as conditions such as pressure and temperature, determine when and in what combination atoms join to form molecules.

Molecular theory describes three states of matter—solid, liquid, and gas. The amount of kinetic energy present and interactions among molecules (based on the intrinsic properties of particular atoms or molecules) determine the ways and physical forms in which molecules interact. For example, under common conditions, water exists as a solid (ice), liquid, or gas.

A solid is a condensed structure in which intermolecular bonds determine a definite shape and volume. Solids do not move and are difficult to compress. A liquid, which is composed of molecules that move freely, has a definite volume without definite shape. Liquids have greater density than gas. Like solids, liquids are difficult to compress. The intermolecular interactions of a gas, on the other hand, are weak. A gas is compressible and completely fills an available space. Both gases and liquids are fluids; that is, substances that flow. Figure 14-1 shows a simplified model of each of the three states of matter.

$\mathcal{R}$espiratory Recap

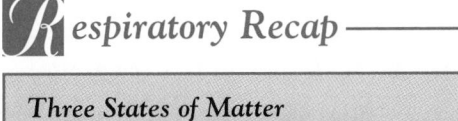

Three States of Matter
Solid
Liquid
Gas

In a mixture of gases, such as one of molecular oxygen and carbon dioxide, weak intramolecular (between molecules) interactions exist in addition to the strong chemical intermolecular bonds. Nevertheless, no chemical combination of molecular oxygen with carbon dioxide occurs. Interactions among molecules may be attractive or repulsive. In general, molecules or atoms do not attract each other unless they are quite close (that is, separated by a distance less than the diameter of the molecule or atom); in that circumstance, they repel each other.

All three states of matter have a characteristic elasticity, or reversible deformability. An ideal gas may be considered perfectly elastic. When the molecules of such a gas collide with the wall of a vessel or with each other, no energy is lost. According to kinetic theory, ideal gases demonstrate continuous movement of perfectly elastic molecules without significant intramolecular interactions. All real gases depart from this behavior, especially under extremes of pressure and temperature, when intermolecular interactions significantly affect their behavior. Nevertheless, under the conditions encountered in most aspects of respiratory care, gases may be analyzed as ideal gases.

Units of Measurement

A common system of measurement is important to establish clear, consistent communication. Unfortunately, a wide variety of units of measure have been used in respiratory physiology. The **Système International d'Unités**

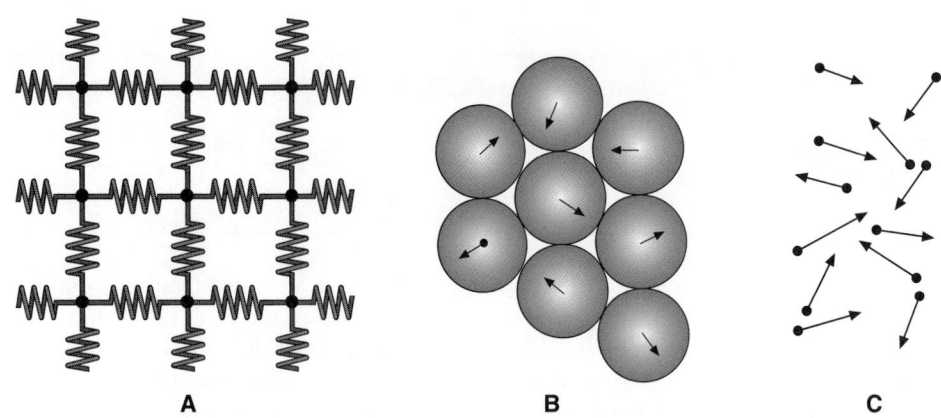

Figure 14-1　Simplified models of the three states of matter. **A,** Solid. **B,** Liquid. **C,** Gas. (Modified from Nave CR, Nave BC. Physics for the health sciences. 3rd ed. Philadelphia: WB Saunders; 1985.)

TABLE 14-1

International System (SI) Base and Derived Units

SI Base Units			SI-Derived Units			
Measurement	**Unit**	**Abbreviation**	**Measurement**	**Unit**	**Abbreviation**	**Derivation**
Length	Meter	m	Force	Newton	N	kg m s^{-2}
Mass	Kilogram	kg	Pressure	Pascal	Pa L	N m^{-2}
Time	Second	s	Work	Joule	j	N m (L kPa)
Temperature	Kelvin	°K	Frequency	Hertz	Hz	s^{-1}
Amount of substance	Mole	mol				
Luminosity (intensity)	Candela	cd				
Electrical current	Ampere	amp				

The unit of measurement kPa is commonly used in physiology because the pascal is too small in the physiologic range.

(SI system) is an international system of measurement that is widely but not universally used. SI units generally are preferred, particularly in scientific and health care settings; however, frequently both mercury and water manometers are used. Measurements expressed in centimeters of water (cm H_2O) and millimeters of mercury (mm Hg) remain in common use. Measurements in inches of water or mercury also may be used, especially in engineering environments.

In the SI system the newton (N) is the primary unit of force, and the **pascal** (Pa) (1N/m^2) is the primary unit of pressure (Table 14-1). For ease of calculation, the kilopascal (kPa) commonly is used. One standard atmosphere (at sea level) is approximately 101 kPa.

Familiarity with the symbols used in respiratory physiology is essential for a thorough understanding of terminology and clear communication. These symbols have particular meanings and may be modified by characters placed above the symbol or added as subscripts or superscripts. A dot over a symbol indicates the first-time derivative (for example,

velocity), whereas two dots indicate the second-time derivative (acceleration). For example, V indicates volume, and $\dot{V}$ is flow. A bar over a symbol indicates a mean quantity. Commonly used symbols are listed in Table 14-2.

Force, Stress, Pressure, and Work

Force is energy applied to a free body, causing it to change the magnitude or direction of its velocity. In mathematic terms, force is the product of mass and acceleration. **Mass** is the amount of a substance, independent of any applied force. The molecular weight (more properly the *molecular mass*) of a substance is the mass of 1 mole (mol) of the substance, defined as the amount of any substance containing Avogadro's number (6.023 × 10^{23}) molecules. Weight describes the acceleration of **gravity** acting on a mass (Equation 14-1). Acceleration of gravity is approximately 9.8 m/sec^2. The mass of a liquid is most easily described as **density** (ρ), or mass per unit volume. Therefore the product of density and the acceleration of gravity is also weight.

TABLE 14-2

Symbols and Modifiers Commonly Used in Respiratory Physiology

Symbol	Meaning	Modifier*	Meaning
V	Volume	I	Inspired
V_T	Tidal volume	E	Expired
$\dot{V}$	Flow	T	Total
$\dot{V}_E$	Ventilation	A	Alveolar
Q	Volume of liquid	a	Arterial
$\dot{Q}$	Blood flow, perfusion	v	Venous
C	Concentration	atm	Atmospheric
S	Saturation	rc	Rib cage
F	Fraction	cw	Chest wall
P	Pressure	pl	Pleural
T	Temperature	es	Esophageal
C	Compliance		
E	Elastance		
R	Resistance		
SG	Specific conductance		
t	Time		
f	Frequency (respiratory rate)		

*A modifier usually is expressed as a subscript or suffix.

EQUATION 14-1

Weight

$$\text{Weight} = m \times g$$
$$\text{Weight} = \rho \times g$$

where:

m = Mass
ρ = Density (mass of a liquid)
g = Acceleration of gravity

EQUATION 14-2

Pressure and Force

$$P = \frac{F}{A}$$
$$F = P \times A$$

where:

P = Pressure
F = Force
A = Area

Stress is force applied to an area. **Strain** is deformation in shape (change of intermolecular forces). A gas or liquid has no preferred shape; therefore the concept of stress is difficult to apply to fluids. **Pressure** (force per unit area) is the same concept applied to fluids (Equation 14-2). Examples include the pressure of the atmosphere (barometric pressure) compared with the pressure measured in an airway over the course of a respiratory cycle. Force is the product of pressure and area.

A gas is highly elastic, which means that physical interactions (collisions) among molecules do not result in a great loss of energy. Other fluids, such as liquids, are less elastic and demonstrate interactions among adjacent molecules that result in loss of energy. Pressure applied tangentially to a fluid generates viscosity, or shear stress. Viscosity is the force applied to the interaction among adjacent fluid molecules as the fluid slips sideways, not force applied to the fluid as a whole. Solids also have a characteristic elasticity but over a more limited range of stresses than gases or liquids. The elasticity of a solid determines the amount of *reversible* deformability and the degree of strain a particular stress generates. The strain produced may deform solid materials in their molecular bonds only; this action can alter the strength or soundness of a substance without changing its directly observed shape. A stress that bends a piece of steel or distends a lung alveolus may not change the perceptible surface, but it nevertheless affects the integrity or longevity of the structure.

A force that displaces a body does work. For gases, force can be measured as pressure and displacement as volume. Using SI units, work is expressed in newton-meters (N × m) or **joules** (J). Although not SI terms the product of liters (kilopascals) and cm H_2O often is used in respiratory physiology. Table 14-3 presents the conversion factors.

Work of breathing is the work necessary to move air (or other gas) through cycles of breathing. It can be estimated by measurement of a volume change and the associated pressure change. Positive work results in a decrease in volume or an increase in pressure. Negative work causes volume or pressure changes opposite in direction. The pressure may be measured at the airway if the person is passive (such as a relaxed patient receiving mechanical ventilation). In this case, lung volume is generated by pressure applied at the airway opening. During spontaneous breathing the pressure that generates tidal volume is pleural pressure (referenced to atmospheric pressure), which may be estimated by measurement of the esophageal pressure.

Pressure is transmitted without reduction throughout any enclosed static fluid, an observation described as *Pascal's law*. In terms of molecular theory the collisions of molecules with one another and the wall of their containing vessel generate pressure. If conditions are at equilibrium, kinetic energy and therefore pressure is constant

TABLE 14-3

Common Conversions in Units of Measurement

Measurement	Unit of Measure	Conversions*
Pressure	1 Kilopascal (kPa)	7.5 mm Hg
		10.2 cm H$_2$O
		0.00987 atm
		10^4 dyne $\times$ cm^{-2}
	1 Millimeter of mercury (mm Hg)	1 torr
		0.133 kPa
		1.36 cm H$_2$O
		1.33 $\times$ 10^3 dyne $\times$ cm^{-2}
	1 Centimeter of of water (cm H$_2$O)	0.098 kPa
		0.736 mm $\times$ Hg
		980.7 dyne $\times$ cm^{-2}
	1 Atmosphere	101.3 kPa
		760 mm Hg
		1033 cm H$_2$O
		10 m sea water
Work	1 Joule	0.239 calories
		1 L $\times$ kPa
Power	1 Watt	1 J $\times$ s^{-1}
Compliance	1 L $\times$ kPa^{-1}	0.098 L $\times$ cm H$_2$O
Resistance	1 Wood unit (mm Hg $\times$ min $\times$ L^{-1})	(dyne $\times$ s $\times$ cm^{-5})/80
		0.125 kPa $\times$ L^{-1} $\times$ s

Atmospheres (atm) and millimeters of mercury (mm Hg) are not International System (SI) units, but they are in common use. The Wood unit (mm Hg $\times$ min $\times$ L^{-1}), which is used to measure vascular resistance, also is not an SI unit.

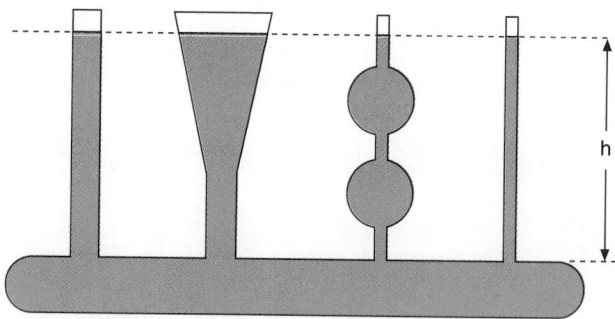

Figure 14-2 Pascal's law. Liquid pressure depends only on the height (h) of the vessel and not on the vessel's shape or the total volume of liquid. (Modified from Nave CR, Nave BC. Physics for the health sciences. 3rd ed. Philadelphia: WB Saunders; 1985.)

EQUATION 14-3

Hydrostatic Pressure

P = h $\times$ ρ $\times$ g

where:

P = Pressure
h = Height
ρ = Density
g = Acceleration of gravity

throughout the fluid, if the weight of the fluid itself is neglected. The weight of a fluid generates static fluid pressure, which varies according to the density of fluid and height, reflecting the force of gravity (Equation 14-3). This pressure is called *manometric pressure* or, in the case of water, **hydrostatic pressure.** Static fluid pressure can be observed as the pressure in a column of fluid (a manometer), such as the sphygmomanometer of a blood pressure cuff. Positive end-expiratory pressure (PEEP) can be established through attachment of the expiratory tubing of a breathing circuit to such a column. As shown in Figure 14-2, the height of the fluid and its density determine liquid pressure; pressure is not affected by the shape of the container.

Because pressure is force applied to an area, if pressure is equal throughout an enclosed fluid the force exerted at a larger area of a container must be greater than the force at a smaller area, known as the *hydraulic press principle*. Given two syringes of different diameters, the syringe with the larger diameter generates greater force than the connected syringe with the smaller diameter. Work describes the energy present in the system and must be equal throughout. Work is the product of force and distance; therefore the distance the syringe with the smaller diameter (less force)

moves is greater than the distance that the larger-diameter syringe moves. Alternatively, if equal *force* is applied simultaneously to syringes of different diameters, the greater pressure is generated in the syringe of lesser cross-sectional area.

Atmospheric (barometric) pressure is one example of static fluid pressure. Atmospheric pressure is the pressure generated at any particular altitude by the weight of atmospheric gas. Evangelista Torricelli performed some of the first investigations of atmospheric pressure at different altitudes. The *torr* ($\frac{1}{760}$ of 1 atmosphere), which is approximately equal to 1 mm Hg, or 0.13 kPa, was named in his honor and is commonly used today to measure pressure. Torricelli developed the first barometer, which measured air pressure, by placing a glass tube containing a column of mercury over a dish of mercury. This device showed changes with weather.[1] As elevation increases, atmospheric pressure decreases. The decrease in atmospheric pressure at a higher altitude can be understood as a result of a smaller column of atmospheric gas. The density of atmospheric air and the acceleration of gravity are constant, positive quantities.

Compliance and Elastance

Pressure not only is force exerted on a column of fluid or atmosphere but also a force applied to a closed, distensible unit, such as a spherical alveolus. The force required

EQUATION 14-4

Compliance and Elastance

$$\text{Compliance} = \frac{\text{Volume}}{\text{Pressure}}$$

$$\text{Elastance} = \frac{1}{\text{Compliance}}$$

$$\frac{1}{C_{rs}} = \frac{1}{C_{cw}} + \frac{1}{C_{lung}}$$

$$E_{rs} = E_{cw} = E_{lung}$$

where:

C_{rs} = Total respiratory system compliance
C_{cw} = Chest wall compliance
C_{lung} = Lung compliance
E_{rs} = Total respiratory system elastance
E_{cw} = Chest wall elastance
E_{lung} = Lung elastance

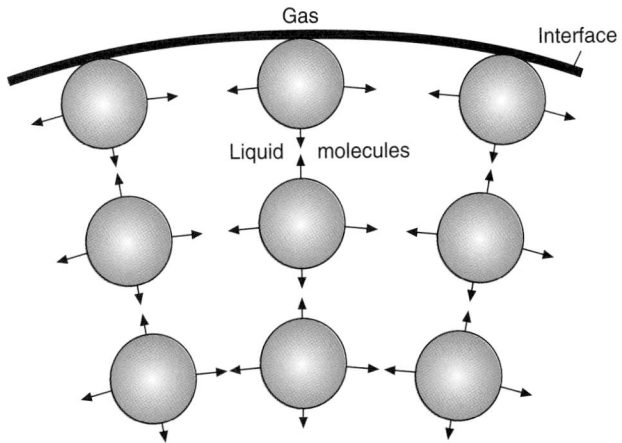

Figure 14-3   The force of surface tension in a drop of liquid. Cohesive force *(arrows)* attracts molecules inside the drop to one another. Cohesion can pull the outermost molecules inward only, creating a centrally directed force that tends to contract the liquid into a sphere. (Modified from Scanlan CL, Wilkins RL, Stoller JK. Egan's fundamentals of respiratory care. 7th ed. St Louis: Mosby; 1999.)

to distend the unit generating a particular volume may be described as **compliance,** or the stiffness of the structure (Equation 14-4). A set of compliances in series, but not in parallel, is added as reciprocals. A common arrangement of compliance in series is the compliance of the total respiratory system, composed of the two connected but independent compliances of the thorax (chest wall) and lung. **Elastance** (pressure per unit volume) is the reciprocal of compliance. Elastance in series can be added directly. Although elastance is attractive from this point of view, compliance remains the most common expression of the force characteristic of a distensible structure.

Wall Tension and Surface Tension

Although Pascal's law states that pressure is equal throughout a containing structure (neglecting fluid static pressure), wall tension varies. Laplace's law describes the tension of the wall of a sphere or cylinder (Equation 14-5). Wall tension therefore increases with radius. A structure with a larger radius has a lesser curvature per unit area; therefore the tension for the same downward component is greater. A structure such as a bubble or a lung alveolus exerts a pressure inside the bubble twice the wall tension divided by the radius. A *smaller* structure generates a *greater* pressure.

Surface tension is not the same as wall tension. The term **surface tension** describes the property of liquid that tends to reduce the surface of a liquid to a minimum, pulling the surface molecules inward. This tension is not stretch between molecules of the wall structure itself (such as in a sheet of latex) but describes the force acting at the boundary surface between two adjoining regions, such as the boundary between the liquid coating lung tissue and the adjoining air (Figure 14-3). The force generated in the

EQUATION 14-5

Laplace's Law

Sphere	Cylinder
$T = \dfrac{(P \times r)}{2}$	$T = P \times r$
$P = \dfrac{(2T)}{r}$	$P = \dfrac{T}{r}$

where:

T = Tension
P = Pressure
r = Radius

wall of a structure is a combination of wall and surface tension. Surfactant, a complex fluid that exists in the lung, reduces surface tension, thereby reducing the pressure required to expand an alveolus. Surfactant also reduces the pressure differences between alveoli of different diameters. Without surfactant, smaller alveoli would empty into

Respiratory Recap

Surface Tension and Surfactant

Surface tension tends to reduce the surface of a liquid to a minimum.
Surfactant reduces surface tension.

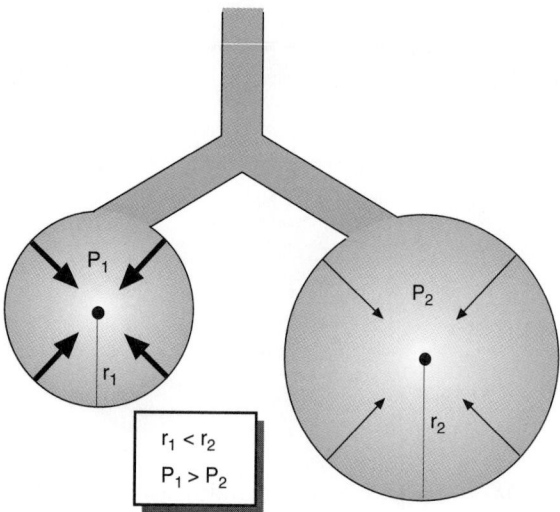

Figure 14-4 Relationship described by Laplace's law. Bubble A (left), which has the smaller radius, has the greater inward or deflating pressure and is more prone to collapse than is bubble B (right). Because the two bubbles are connected, bubble A would tend to deflate and empty into bubble B. Conversely, because of bubble A's greater surface tension, it would be harder to inflate than bubble B. (Modified from Scanlan CL, Wilkins RL, Stoller JK. Egan's fundamentals of respiratory care. 7th ed. St Louis: Mosby; 1999.)

*T*ABLE 14-4

Temperature Conversions in Kelvin, Celsius, and Fahrenheit

Degrees Kelvin (° K)	Degrees Celsius (° F)	Degrees Fahrenheit (° C)
373	100	212
363	90	194
353	80	176
343	70	158
333	60	140
323	50	122
313	40	104
310	37	98.6
303	30	86
293	20	68
283	10	50
273	0	32
263	-10	14
253	-20	-4
243	-30	-22
233	-40	-40
223	-50	-58
0	-273	-459.4

larger ones because they have greater surface tension (Figure 14-4). Surfactant is necessary for normal lung function because it reduces the work of breathing within physiologic capabilities (by reducing the surface tension) and allows alveoli of various sizes to coexist by achieving comparable surface tensions.

Temperature

Temperature describes the amount of heat, or thermal energy, present in a system. Early studies of temperature used liquid in glass tubes as thermometers. Several scales evolved, which were calibrated with the freezing and boiling points of water; these provided convenient and apparently constant points of reference (Table 14-4). The Fahrenheit scale (developed by Gabriel Fahrenheit) divided the temperature range between freezing and boiling into 180 gradations. According to this scale, pure water freezes at 32° F. The Fahrenheit scale is commonly used in the United States but not in most scientific and health care settings.

Another scale, initially referred to as *Centigrade*, was renamed *Celsius* in honor of Anders Celsius. This scale placed the freezing and boiling points of pure water 100 degrees apart. Initially the scale was the reverse of that which is familiar today, but it was later changed so that the freezing point of pure water is 0 degrees. The difference in the number of gradations between the boiling and freezing points of water accounts for the conversion factor $\frac{9}{5}$ ($\frac{180}{100}$) between the Fahrenheit and Celsius scales. A formula used for any

*E*QUATION 14-6

Celsius and Fahrenheit Temperature Conversions

Conversion from Celsius to Fahrenheit

$$\text{Fahrenheit} = 32 + \left(\text{Celsius degrees} \times \frac{9}{5}\right)$$

Conversion from Fahrenheit to Celsius

$$\text{Celsius} = (\text{Fahrenheit degrees} - 32) \times \frac{5}{9}$$

conversion between these two scales also must account for the difference in zero points (Equation 14-6).

The physical distance between degrees in either scale varies, depending on the indicator solution, because different substances, such as mercury or alcohol, expand differently. William Thompson, also known as *Lord Kelvin*, proposed an absolute scale based not on the physical ex-

*R*espiratory Recap

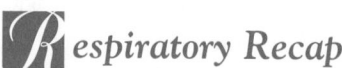

Temperature Scales
Fahrenheit (° F)
Celsius (° C)
Kelvin (absolute) (° K)

TABLE 14-5

Changes in the State of Matter

Type of Change	Conversion	Example
Exothermic Change		
Condensation (liquefaction)	Gas to liquid or solid	Steam to water
Freezing (crystallization)	Liquid to solid	Water to ice
Endothermic Change		
Sublimation	Solid to gas	Dry ice
Melting (fusion)	Solid to liquid	Ice melting
Evaporation (vaporization)	Liquid to gas	Water boiling

Substances usually condense to liquids before becoming solids.

pansion of any particular substance but on a constant change of energy per degree. In this scale, zero is called *absolute zero*, which is not reached experimentally but is considered the point at which a system reaches its minimum possible total energy. On the Kelvin scale, 273° K is equal to 0° C.

Thermodynamics and Heat Exchange

Thermodynamics describes changes in the thermal state of a system. Adding or removing energy, such as by changes in pressure, volume, or temperature, may change the state of the substance. When a change of state requires the addition of energy, the process is endothermic. An exothermic process gives off energy. Table 14-5 lists common endothermic and exothermic processes as the states of matter change among gas, liquid, and solid.

Most respiratory physiology can be understood without an allowance for thermodynamic effects. Occasionally, however, such effects are significant. Any process that occurs rapidly may not allow the flow of heat into or from the system; such a process is called *adiabatic*. If heat does not leave a system (for example, as when a volume of gas is compressed in a plethysmograph), adiabatic heating occurs. Adiabatic cooling may occur if a rapid release of pressure increases volume, such as when a gas cylinder is decompressed rapidly.

Heat exchange occurs by three processes—conduction, convection, or radiation. Conduction is the transfer of heat directly from molecule to adjacent molecule. Although metals have relatively high thermal conductivity, gases do not. Convection describes the transfer of heat caused by the motion of materials themselves rather than molecules within materials. Physical movement of a liquid or gas from an area of high heat to an area of lower heat is an example of convection. Radiation is the emission of heat energy without the movement of materials themselves.

EQUATION 14-7

Gay-Lussac's Law of Combining Volumes

$$V = k \times n$$

$$\frac{V_1}{n_1} = \frac{V_2}{n_2}$$

where:

V = Volume
k = Constant
n = Number of moles

Gas Laws

Solids and liquids follow the same basic principles but do not exhibit the perfectly elastic intermolecular behavior of an ideal gas. An ideal gas behaves precisely the same at all temperatures and pressures. In fact, real gases are not ideal under all conditions, but under the relatively low pressure and temperature conditions encountered in respiratory physiology, their behavior can be predicted well with these laws.

Gay-Lussac's law of combining volumes states that volumes of gases combine chemically in volumetric proportions that are small whole numbers (Equation 14-7). This observation confirms that under equivalent conditions, equal volumes of ideal gases contain an equal number of molecules. Under standard conditions of 0° C and barometric pressure of 1 atmosphere (1 atm), 1 mol of an ideal gas has a volume of 22.4 L.

Early in the eighteenth century, Robert Boyle performed a series of experiments in which the amount of mercury in a J-shaped tube was varied while a fixed mass of air was trapped in the closed end of the tube. Edme Mariotte independently made these observations 16 years later. This work led to a description of the direct relationship between pressure and volume in a fixed amount of gas at constant temperature, which came to be known as **Boyle's law** (or Mariotte's law), stating that pressure is directly proportional to volume (Equation 14-8). The product of pressure and volume may be expressed as a constant, *k*. Boyle's law predicts the relation of a volume of a fixed mass of gas to a pressure change. Expressed in another form, new conditions can be predicted if initial conditions and change in either pressure or volume are known, given a constant mass and temperature. Pressure changes important to respiratory physiology may include

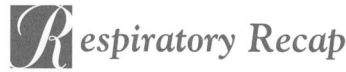

Respiratory Recap

Gas Laws	
Boyle's law	Gay-Lussac's law
Charles' law	Combined (ideal) gas law

EQUATION 14-8
Boyle's Law

$$P \times V = k$$
$$P_1 \times V_1 = P_2 \times V_2$$

where:

P = Pressure
V = Volume
k = Constant

EQUATION 14-10
Gay-Lussac's Law

$$P = k \times T$$
$$\frac{P_1}{T_1} = \frac{P_2}{T_2}$$

where:

P = Pressure
T = Absolute temperature
k = Constant

EQUATION 14-9
Charles' Law

$$V = k \times T$$
$$\frac{V_1}{T_1} = \frac{V_2}{T_2}$$

where:

V = Volume
k = Constant
T = Absolute temperature

EQUATION 14-11
Combined Gas Law

$$\frac{(P_1 \times V_1)}{T_1} = \frac{(P_2 \times V_2)}{T_2}$$

where:

P = Pressure
V = Volume
T = Absolute temperature

$$PV = nRT$$

where:

P = Pressure
V = Volume
n = Number of moles
R = Gas constant
T = Absolute temperature

changes in barometric pressure or pressure alterations during positive pressure ventilation. The same mass of gas during positive inspiratory pressure has a lower volume than during expiration, which occurs at atmospheric pressure.

Charles' law predicts the effect of temperature on a fixed amount of dry gas. At constant pressure, gas expands proportionally to changes in temperature (Equation 14-9). A constant multiplied by temperature predicts volume. This constant also may be described as a coefficient of expansion, the numeric rate of volume change in terms of temperature. Early investigators found the thermal coefficient of expansion of 37.5%, or $1/273$ per degree Celsius in the range between 0° C and 100° C. This coefficient corresponded to predicted absolute zero. Later investigation under more precise conditions did not verify this linear relationship over a greater range of temperatures. Nevertheless, at least at a qualitative level, Charles' law describes the effect of kinetic energy on volume. It remains a precise quantitative relationship over the range of conditions experienced clinically.

Because the Kelvin temperature scale is based on energy per degree and has a zero point at the point of minimum total energy, the behavior of gases is predicted with degrees Kelvin, or degrees Celsius +273 degrees. The similar proportional relationship of pressure and temperature at a constant volume and mass is described as Gay-Lussac's law (Equation 14-10).

The combined gas law mathematically combines Boyle's, Charles', and Gay-Lussac's laws. Rearranging the

terms of the combined gas law generates a set of pseudo-equations, allowing for examination of the effects of pressure, volume, or temperature on the other variables. Once again, knowledge of initial conditions and all but one new condition allows for prediction of the remaining variable (Equation 14-11). Pressure and volume are inversely related, whereas temperature is directly proportional to volume or pressure (Figure 14-5).

The term *n* in the **ideal gas law** accounts for the number of gas molecules present, allowing for comparison of gases with different molecular masses when mole terms are used. The universal gas constant, *R*, expresses the force required to move a quantity of ideal gas, or **work.** This has a value of 8.1314 joules $\times$ degrees Kelvin^{-1} $\times$ moles^{-1}. Units of joules are equivalent to the product of pressure and volume. Pressure may be expressed in millimeters of mercury or atmospheres. The constant then may be expressed as 0.08205 L $\times$ atm $\times$ K^{-1} $\times$ mol^{-1}, or 62.32 L $\times$ mm Hg $\times$ K^{-1} $\times$ mol^{-1}.

Many gases (for example, carbon dioxide, nitrous oxide, and volatile anesthetic agents) deviate from the behavior of ideal gases, even under commonly encountered conditions.[2] These nonideal gases require quantitative modifica-

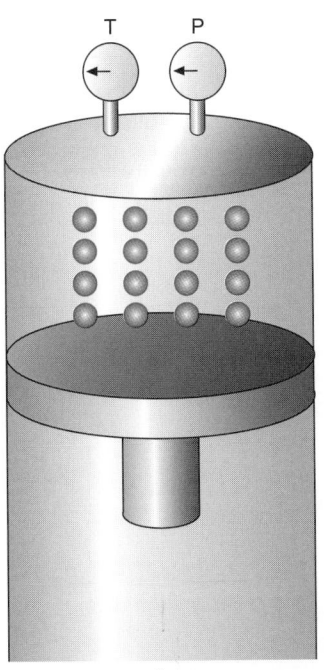 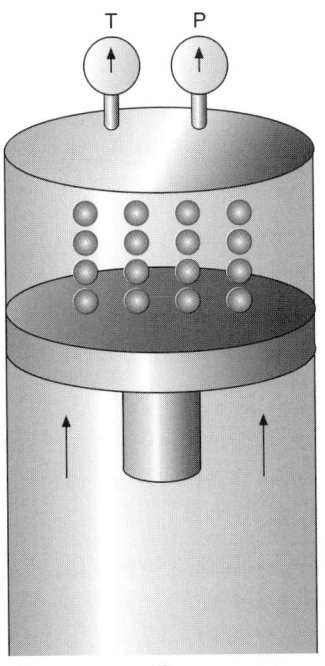 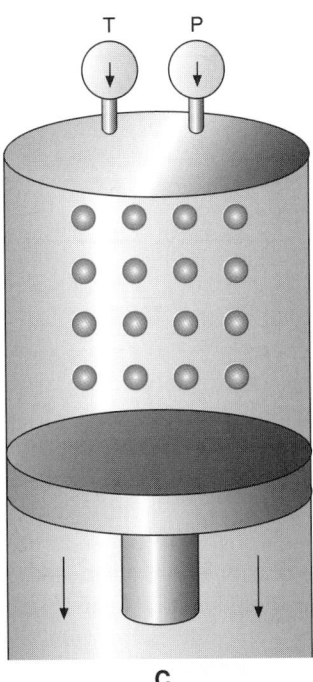

A   B   C

Figure 14-5   **A,** A mass of gas in the resting state exerts a given pressure at a given temperature in cylinder. **B,** As the piston compresses the gas, the molecules are crowded closer together, and the increased energy of molecular collisions increases both the temperature and the pressure. **C,** Conversely, as the gas expands molecular interaction diminishes, and the temperature and pressure fall. (Modified from Scanlan CL, Wilkins RL, Stoller JK. Egan's fundamentals of respiratory care. 7th ed. St Louis: Mosby; 1999.)

tions of the classic gas laws to describe their behavior. For example, under standard conditions the mole volume of carbon dioxide is 22.2 L rather than 22.4 L. Several approaches, including the Van der Waals equation, attempt to predict these changes.[2]

Gas Mixtures and Partial Pressures

Dalton's law of partial pressures describes the behavior of physical mixtures of gases and vapors. In such a mixture, each separate gas acts as predicted by the combined gas law, as if it were present alone. The partial pressure of each particular gas is proportional to the fractional concentration of that gas and equal to the product of fractional concentration and total atmospheric pressure. Oxygen accounts for 20.95% (estimated at 21%) of atmospheric air, a percentage that can be expressed as fractional oxygen content of inspired air (FIO_2) of 0.21. The pressure of any individual gas can be predicted from the total pressure in the system and the fractional concentration of a gas. At 1 atm (760 mm Hg) the pressure of inspired oxygen (PIO_2) is 159.6 (Equation 14-12). Nitrogen, which accounts for approximately 78% of air, has a partial pressure that can be calculated in a similar fashion and is 792.8 mm Hg at 1 atm. Physical combinations of gases mix uniformly. Based on kinetic theory, gases are continuously in motion regardless

EQUATION   14-12
Dalton's Law

Pressure of Oxygen at 1 Atmosphere

$PIO_2 = FIO_2 \times P_{atm}$ (Atmospheric pressure)
$PIO_2 = 0.21 \times 760$ mm Hg $= 159.6$ mm Hg

Pressure of Nitrogen at 1 Atmosphere

$PIN_2 = FIN_2 \times P_{atm}$
$PIN_2 = 0.78 \times 760 = 592.8$ mm Hg

where:

PIO_2 = Pressure of inspired oxygen
FIO_2 = Fractional oxygen content of inspired gas
P_{atm} = Atmospheric pressure
PIN_2 = Pressure of inspired nitrogen
FIN_2 = Fractional nitrogen content of inspired gas

of molecular weight and at equilibrium, are evenly distributed in any particular space. The same fractional percentages of oxygen, nitrogen, and so on are present both in Death Valley (86 m or 282 feet below sea level) and on Mount Everest (elevation 8848 m or 29,029 feet), although their partial pressures vary according to atmospheric pressure.

Box 14-1

Composition of Unconditioned Air

Nitrogen: 78.08%	Argon: 0.93%
Oxygen: 20.95%	Trace gases: 0.01%
Carbon dioxide: 0.03%	Total: 99.99%

Humidity and Water Vapor

Most gases encountered in physiologic conditions not only are combinations of various dry gases but also contain water vapor. Unconditioned air inhaled at the mouth is a combination of oxygen, nitrogen, and other gases (Box 14-1). Inhaled air is nearly completely humidified after it passes through the upper airway. Exhaled air has lower concentrations of oxygen and higher concentrations of carbon dioxide and remains humidified. The term *n* in the ideal gas law defines the number of gas molecules present. This term accounts for changes in the total number of gas molecules present, such as when water molecules are present as vapor in combination with dry gas.

Water vapor pressure represents the kinetic activity of water molecules in air. Although the words *vapor* and *gas* often are used interchangeably, reference to vapor as a gaseous substance below its critical point (that is, the temperature or pressure below which a substance can be liquefied by application of enough pressure) is more accurate. The critical point of water is approximately 374° C, or 218 atm, conditions not usually encountered. Strictly speaking, water present in the gas phase is not gaseous water, but molecular water.

Evaporation

Water is particularly important as a vapor in the physiologic conditions encountered in respiratory care. A water surface emits molecules of vapor continuously with evaporation. As vapor molecules hit the surface of a liquid, some are absorbed into the liquid with condensation. The net evaporation or condensation depends on which is greater—the rate of condensation or the rate of evaporation. Above 100° C at atmospheric pressure, water is largely a vapor. Below 0° C, it is a solid. Vapor pressure is the pressure at which water forms a gas and is approximately 760 mm Hg (1 atm) at 100° C. Under other specified conditions the mass of water existing as gas can readily be calculated or determined from standard tables (Table 14-6).

Water vapor saturation occurs when equilibrium exists between condensation and evaporation. Boiling occurs when the local vapor pressure above a liquid becomes equal to the total pressure because of heat, boiling will occur. The boiling point is the temperature at which the saturated vapor pressure is equal to atmospheric pressure. The vapor pressure in this condition is the saturation vapor pressure, which varies with temperature.

Table 14-6

Absolute Humidity and Water Vapor Pressure as a Function of Temperature (at 100% Relative Humidity)

Temperature (° C)	Absolute Humidity (mg/L)	Water Vapor Pressure (mm Hg)
0	4.8	4.6
5	6.8	6.5
10	9.4	9.2
15	12.8	12.8
20	17.3	17.5
25	23	23.8
26	24.4	25.2
27	25.7	26.7
28	27.2	28.4
29	28.7	30
30	30.3	31.8
31	32	33.7
32	33.8	35.7
33	35.6	37.7
34	37.5	39.9
35	39.6	42.2
36	41.7	44.6
37	43.9	47.1
38	46.2	49.7
39	48.5	52.4
40	51.1	55.3
41	53.7	58.4
42	56.4	61.5
43	59.3	64.8
44	62.2	68.3
45	65.3	71.9
50	82.8	92.6
55	104	118.1
60	129.7	149.5
65	160.4	187.7
70	196.9	233.8
75	240.1	289.2
80	290.7	355.3
85	349.9	433.6
90	418.5	525.9
95	497.6	634
100	588.5	759.9

Humidity can be considered the partial pressure of water (P_{H_2O}), absolute humidity, or relative humidity. A gas mixture holding all the vapor it can without droplets of liquid being formed is saturated. Absolute humidity (Equation 14-13) is the mass of water present in a volume of gas, usually measured in grams of water per cubic meter (or milligrams per liter). Humidity also can be expressed as relative humidity, or the total water content in a gas, such as air, compared with the water content of saturated air. A sample of gas having a relative humidity of 50% at 20° C has a vapor pressure of 8.75 mm Hg (0.5 × 17.5 mm Hg). At the usual body temperature of 37° C, 50% relative humidity is a water vapor pressure of 23.5 mm Hg.

EQUATION 14-13

Calculating Humidity

Absolute Humidity

Absolute humidity = $(16.42 - 0.73T) + 0.04T^2$

where *T* is temperature (Celsius)

Relative Humidity

% Relative humidity = $\left(\dfrac{\text{Absolute humidity}}{\text{Humidity capacity}}\right) \times 100\%$

Humidity Deficit

Humidity deficit = Content − Capacity at 37° C =

Content − 43.8 mg/L

Body Humidity (BH)

%BH = $\dfrac{\text{Content}}{\text{Capacity}} \times 100\%$ = $\dfrac{\text{Content}}{43.8 \text{ mg/L}} \times 100\%$

If the temperature is increased but the vapor pressure remains the same, the relative humidity is reduced. Therefore as temperature is reduced in a ventilator circuit at a distance from a heated humidifier, condensation occurs. When the molecules in a liquid gain sufficient kinetic energy, some escape from the liquid. While at a given temperature, the average kinetic energy is enough for some molecules to escape the liquid; not all molecules have the same kinetic energy. As temperature increases, more molecules gain enough kinetic energy to leave the liquid phase. Because those molecules escaping the liquid are those with more kinetic energy, evaporation is a cooling process because the remaining liquid loses kinetic energy, explaining the greater efficiency of heated humidifier systems. When a gas is not fully saturated, the water vapor content can be expressed as its relative humidity. The relative humidity of a gas is the ratio of its actual water vapor content to its saturated capacity at that temperature, expressed as a percentage. In reality relative humidity can be easily measured with a hygrometer, and it is rarely calculated using actual water vapor content.

When conditions such as pressure and temperature are constant, a vapor can be analyzed in the same manner as any gaseous substance. At 1 atm, fully humidified or saturated air at body temperature has a P_{H_2O} of 47 mm Hg. Other gases account for 760 mm Hg − 47 mm Hg, or 713 mm Hg. In clinical practice, respiratory therapists use two additional measures of humidity—percentage of body humidity (%BH) and humidity deficit. The %BH is the ratio of actual water vapor content to the water vapor capacity in a saturated gas at 37° C. The water content (absolute humidity) of fully saturated gas at body temperature is 43.8 mg/L. Therefore the capacity is fixed. A humidity deficit occurs whenever inspired gas is not fully saturated (43.8 mg/L) at body temperature, which requires the body to add the needed water to achieve full saturation. Humidity deficit is calculated through determination of the difference between the absolute content of the water vapor within an inspired gas at a given temperature and 43.8 mg/L.

As temperature, pressure, and volume change from those conditions usually encountered, compounds that exist fully in a gas may exist partly as liquid and partly as vapor. One such case involves estimation of the amount of substance in a compressed cylinder. Many gases, such as oxygen, are completely in gas form in compressed tanks. In this case the pressure in the tank directly reflects the amount of oxygen remaining. However, carbon dioxide and nitrous oxide are partly liquid at the pressure of a compressed cylinder. As the gaseous portion of the tank contents is used, more gas is formed from liquid. Therefore the pressure remains constant until all liquid is transformed into gas, when the pressure of the tank rapidly decreases. For these compounds, monitoring of the pressure in the tank is not a good reflection of the amount remaining.

Gas in Solution, Diffusion, and Osmosis

A gas present in combination with a liquid to which it does not react dissolves in a predictable manner. A portion of the gas is present in the gaseous state but dissolved in the liquid. Henry's law states that at a constant temperature, a gas dissolves in solution in proportion to its partial pressure. The solubility coefficient (mass dissolved per unit of partial pressure) for a gas decreases as temperature increases. Carbon dioxide is approximately 20 times more soluble than oxygen. The Ostwald coefficient expresses the volume of gas dissolved at the temperature and pressure conditions under which the solution occurred. The Bunsen coefficient is the volume of gas (STPD) per unit of solvent at pressure described in atmospheres. Henry's law does not predict whether a gas will combine chemically with a constituent of the fluid (such as oxygen combining with hemoglobin). Indeed, Henry's law cannot predict precisely the behavior of gas exposed to any complex fluid, such as blood.

Diffusion is the process of intermingling of molecules as a result of their random motion, reflecting kinetic energy. **Graham's law** predicts the rate of diffusion of a gas as inversely proportional to the square root of its gram molecular weight (Equation 14-14). The molecular weight determines the density of a gas. The velocity, which determines diffusion, is inversely proportional to the square root of the molecular weight of a substance, meaning that lighter gases diffuse faster than heavier gas molecules if only density is considered. However, in a liquid medium, both Graham's law and Henry's law affect the rate of diffusion of gases.

Osmosis is the movement of a solvent through a semipermeable membrane that does not permit movement of larger solute molecules. The solvent diffuses from an area of lesser concentration to one of greater concentration. **Fick's law** (Equation 14-15) describes the transfer of a solute by diffusion. The diffusion rate across a barrier is di-

TABLE 14-7

Common Sets of Conditions Affecting Gas Volume

Condition	Temperature (° C)	Atmospheres (atm)	Humidity (%)
Standard temperature and pressure, dry (STPD)	0	1 (760 mm Hg)	0
Body temperature and pressure, saturated (BTPS)	37	1	100 (47 mm Hg)
Atmospheric temperature and pressure, dry (ATPD)	Ambient (≈ 25)	Ambient	0
Atmospheric temperature and pressure, saturated (ATPS)	Ambient (≈ 25)	Ambient	100 (47 mm Hg)

EQUATION 14-14

Graham's Law (Rate of Diffusion of Gases)

$$\frac{Rate_A}{Rate_B} = \sqrt{\frac{MW_B}{MW_A}}$$

where *MW* is molecular weight

EQUATION 14-15

Fick's Law

$$V_{gas} \propto \frac{A}{T} \times D_{gas}(P_1 - P_2)$$

where:

V_{gas} = Volume of gas diffusing across a membrane
A = Surface area for diffusion
T = Thickness of the membrane
$P_1 - P_2$ = Pressure gradient
D_{gas} = Diffusibility of the gas (Solubility coefficient/Density)

$$D_{O_2} = \frac{0.023}{\sqrt{32/22.4}} = 0.0192$$

$$D_{CO_2} = \frac{0.51}{\sqrt{44/22.4}} = 0.364$$

The diffusibility of carbon dioxide (D_{CO_2}) is 19 times greater than that of oxygen (D_{O_2}).

rectly proportional to the cross-sectional area available for diffusion and the difference in concentration gradient per unit distance perpendicular to that cross-section. The concentration, in turn, is determined by Henry's law, the product of solubility and partial pressure.

Conversion of Gas Volumes

Pressure, temperature, and humidity have prominent effects on gas volume. Several sets of conditions are commonly encountered because of the way certain gases are stored (dry gas) or measured (body temperature, humidified gas). These are (1) standard temperature and pressure, dry (STPD), (2) body temperature and pressure, saturated (BTPS), (3) atmospheric temperature and pressure, dry (ATPD), and (4) atmospheric temperature and pressure, saturated (ATPS) (Table 14-7). Gas is transformed from BTPD to BTPS on inspiration, requiring calculation to determine actual volume changes after alterations caused by temperature and humidity changes. Similarly, although gas may be collected and measured under BTPS conditions, measurement of gas exchange (such as oxygen consumption) usually is reported at 1 atm and 0° C or STPD. Conversions between conditions of BTPS, STPD, and ATPD are shown in Equation 14-16. Although tables and computer programs frequently are available, the basis of these equations must be understood and some conversion factors committed to memory.

A frequently needed conversion allows computations during combination of volume measurements in STPD and BTPS. The gas constant (which is different from the universal gas constant) is used to convert between the standard temperature and pressure of 1 atm and 0° C and body temperature and pressure of 37° C and 1 atm (Equation 14-17). This conversion is especially important in the evaluation of dead space through use of carbon dioxide production and minute ventilation. Production of CO_2 usually is measured in STPD, whereas minute ventilation is directly measured in BTPS.

Respiratory Recap

Conditions Affecting Gas Volumes
STPD: **S**tandard **t**emperature and **p**ressure, **d**ry
BTPS: **B**ody **t**emperature and **p**ressure, **s**aturated
ATPD: **A**tmospheric **t**emperature and **p**ressure, **d**ry
ATPS: **A**tmospheric **t**emperature and **p**ressure, **s**aturated

Flow of Gases and Other Fluids

When fluids are put in motion, a variety of complex behaviors result. Flow is the bulk movement of a substance through space. Both liquids and gases can flow. Hydrodynamics is the study of fluids in motion. The flow of gas through tubes is a key physical phenomenon in respiratory physiology, whether in reference to the flow of air into and from the lungs or the flow of gas through a ventilator circuit. Flow is central to other areas of physiology as well, such as blood flow through vessels.

EQUATION 14-16

Gas Conversion Formulas

$$V_{BTPS} = V_{ATPS} \times \left(\frac{P_{Atm} - P_{H_2O(t)}}{P_{Atm} - P_{H_2O(37)}} \right) \times \frac{273 + 37}{273 + T}$$

$$V_{STPD} = V_{ATPD} \times \frac{P_{atm}}{P_{atm(standard)}} \times \frac{273}{273 + T}$$

$$V_{BTPS} = V_{STPD} \times \frac{P_{atm(standard)}}{P_{atm} - P_{H_2O(T)}} \times \frac{310}{273}$$

$$V_{STPD} = V_{ATPS} \frac{273}{273 + T} \times \frac{P_{atm} - P_{H_2O(t)}}{P_{atm(standard)}}$$

where:

V_{BTPS} = Volume at body temperature and pressure, saturated

V_{ATPS} = Volume at atmospheric temperature and pressure, saturated

P_{atm} = Atmospheric pressure

P_{H_2O} = Partial pressure of water

T = Temperature

V_{STPD} = Volume at standard temperature and pressure, dry

V_{ATPD} = Volume at atmospheric temperature and pressure, dry

$P_{atm(standard)}$ = Standard pressure

EQUATION 14-17

Gas Constant

$$(760 - 47) \div \left(\frac{273}{310} \times \frac{713}{760} \right) = 863$$

$$mm\ Hg - mm\ Hg \div \left(\frac{°K}{°K} \times \frac{mm\ Hg}{mm\ Hg} \right)$$

This constant is the standard partial pressure of dry gas (partial pressure of vapor pressure subtracted from standard atmospheric pressure) divided by the ratio of standard temperature and body temperature in degrees Kelvin (273 and 310 degrees, respectively) multiplied by the ratio of the partial pressure of humidified gas at body temperature to dry gas at 1 atmosphere (760 mm Hg). It is used to express moles of carbon dioxide (CO_2) production in terms of volumes measured at standard temperature and pressure, dry (STPD). As an illustration of the other conversions detailed above, units of temperature cancel.

Expressing CO_2 tension in mm Hg and CO_2 production in milliliters, the gas constant is 0.863:

$$Pa_{CO_2} = \frac{\dot{V}_{CO_2} \times 0.863}{\left(1 - \frac{V_D}{V_T} \right) \times \dot{V}_E}$$

where:

Pa_{CO_2} = Partial pressure of arterial carbon dioxide

$\dot{V}_{CO_2}$ = Carbon dioxide production

V_D = Dead space

V_T = Tidal volume

$\dot{V}_E$ = Minute ventilation

Flow is the movement of a specified volume of fluid (gas or liquid) in a particular period of time. It is also the ratio of a pressure difference and resistance. As an initial approximation, fluid can be considered as ideal (or newtonian). Such a fluid is incompressible and without internal friction, or viscosity. In fact, no gas or other fluid is truly ideal, but this analysis allows for the use of simplifying assumptions that help to illustrate key factors influencing flow. Even the behavior of highly complex fluid can be predicted with relative accuracy with such assumptions, particularly under the conditions of interest to most areas of respiratory care. In certain circumstances, such as high flow rates or frequencies, the analysis presented in this discussion may be less predictive. Some fluids rarely follow newtonian assumptions. Blood, for example, is highly complex in behavior, even under the relatively low pressure and temperature conditions commonly encountered in human physiology.

The rate, or **velocity,** of flow can be determined mathematically by differentiation of volume with respect to time. That is, the rate of volume change determines the rate of flow. A volumetric spirometer is one measuring device that uses this technique. Alternatively, volume can be calculated from integration of flow with respect to time. Devices that measure flow are capable of faster responses to changes than are devices that directly measure volume. This limitation in frequency response, or ability to faithfully reflect changes in volume over short periods,

has restricted the use of volumetric spirometers. Therefore most volume measurement devices in wide use today measure flow to calculate volume. Much of the analysis of flow and related events requires use of calculus for the most rigorous approach. This chapter uses a descriptive strategy instead.

Principle of Continuity

If any liquid flows through a rigid pipe of some arbitrary length at a constant rate, the mass of fluid entering must equal the mass leaving. This concept is the principle of continuity (Equation 14-18 and Figure 14-6). Considering geometry alone, any arbitrarily thin slice of fluid moves a particular distance in a set period. This movement of fluid over a time period is the flow velocity. The product of velocity and the diameter of the pipe defines the mass of fluid involved. If the diameter of the pipe increases for a portion of its length, the same mass of fluid per unit time must still move through it so that the mass entering the pipe equals the mass exiting. Because the diameter increases, the velocity of flow decreases. Diameter and velocity therefore are inversely related. Momentum refers to the quantity of movement. Although the flow of mass through the pipe is constant, momentum is not necessarily so. The mass flow from a garden hose may be constant, but the momentum is increased if a small-diameter nozzle is placed at the end, increasing the distance of the water spray.

Bernoulli Principle

In 1738 David Bernoulli described the properties of fluid flow through a tube, or the first law of fluid dynamics (Equation 14-19), which became known as the **Bernoulli principle.** Bernoulli explained the pressure drop when fluid passes through a constriction in a rigid tube by showing the way in which potential energy, kinetic energy, and pressure energy interact. Energy cannot be created or destroyed. Rather, energy is transformed from one form to another under normal conditions, and the sum of all energy is constant. Velocity is equivalent to the kinetic energy of a fluid, whereas the lateral forces equate to pressure energy. If a tube is held level, maintaining a constant potential energy, the sum of the kinetic energy must equal the sum of its pressure energy. Consequently, velocity and pressure have an inverse relationship. Therefore if energy is applied to increase the velocity of a fluid (that is, movement through a constriction), the energy available to exert pressure must decrease. On the other hand, if velocity decreases, lateral pressure increases.

The Bernoulli principle can be described in terms of flow through a rigid pipe. When fluid flows through a pipe with a uniform diameter, pressure progressively decreases over the tube's length. Flow results from a pressure gradient between two regions, a force acting on the fluid. Adding any pressure or gravitational force to a region of the fluid decreases the gradient and the flow. The force, or the product of mass and acceleration, generating flow then must equal the sum of the pressure and gravitational force acting on the fluid. Using the principle of continuity, velocity is inversely related to tube diameter. At a constant laminar flow and density, velocity increases as cross-sectional area decreases, and pressure must decrease as well. That is, pressure is inversely related to velocity, as shown in Equation 14-20 (Figure 14-7).

Measurement of Flow

The Bernoulli principle is not only a fundamental description of the relationships of velocity and pressure but also allows direct measurement of both. A number of devices applying this principle are used to measure flow. This measurement is not straightforward because the pressure gradient defines a *difference* in the *square* of two velocities.

The venturimeter, designed by Giovanni Venturi, is designed to prevent generation of turbulent flow in a region of reduced diameter. Ignoring any gravitational forces (minimal in low-density gases and constant in a

EQUATION 14-18
Principle of Continuity

$$\dot{V}_1 d_1 = \dot{V}_2 d_2$$

where $\dot{V}$ is flow and d is diameter.

EQUATION 14-19
First Law of Fluid Dynamics

Pressure force + Gravitational force = Mass × Acceleration

EQUATION 14-20
Bernoulli Principle

Energy at point A = Energy at point B

$$P_1 + \frac{1}{2}(mv_1^2) = P_2 + \frac{1}{2}(mv_2^2)$$

$$P_1 - P_2 = \frac{1}{2}m(v_2^2 - v_1^2)$$

where:

P = Static pressure
m = Mass
v = Velocity

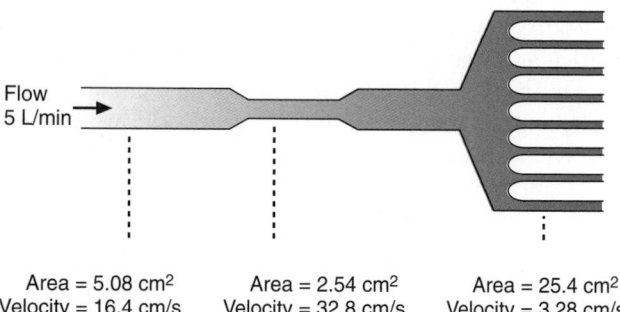

Figure 14-6   Illustration of the principle of continuity. Note that fluid velocity is related inversely to the cross-sectional area. (Modified from Nave CR, Nave BC. Physics for the health sciences. 3rd ed. Philadelphia: WB Saunders; 1985.)

Area = 5.08 cm²   Area = 2.54 cm²   Area = 25.4 cm²
Velocity = 16.4 cm/s   Velocity = 32.8 cm/s   Velocity = 3.28 cm/s

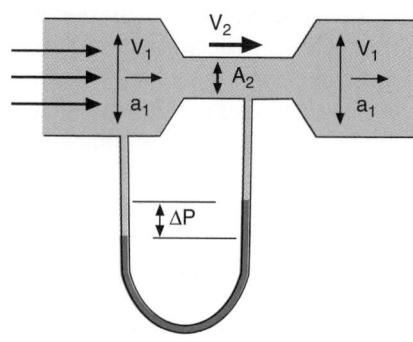

Figure 14-7   Illustration of the Bernoulli principle. A flowing fluid's lateral pressure is inversely related to its velocity.

horizontal tube), the pressure gradient across a change of diameter describes the velocity of flow. According to the principle of continuity, two known diameters allow determination of flow velocity using the pressure gradient and the ratio of the diameters (Equation 14-21). If flow occurs through constricted tubing, the pressure drop distal to the constriction can be used to entrain a second fluid to mix with the main flow (Figure 14-8). The **Venturi principle** states that pressure drop across an obstruction can be restored if the angle of divergence is less than 15 degrees. A Pitot tube (Figure 14-9) allows measurement of flow at any one point, not in a closed conduit. In this tube, dynamic pressure (measured normal to the direction of flow) and static pressure (measured at a side port) are compared (Equation 14-22). The orifice facing the flow samples the sum of dynamic and static pressure so that the pressure difference is the total subtracted from static pressure, or dynamic pressure.

With either the venturimeter or the Pitot tube, flow varies with the square root of pressure. Although these measurement devices are usable under real conditions, significant assumptions must still be acknowledged: zero viscosity and constant density and flow. Furthermore, velocity remains a squared quantity, requiring careful measurement to maximize precision. These equations and

devices do not account for energy loss, but a small amount of energy is changed to heat as frictional thermal loss.

A common thought is that air entrainment oxygen delivery masks (so-called venturi masks) operate according to this principle. This thought cannot be, however, because such masks operate by directing a flow of gas through an orifice of a mask. The system is not closed, and regions of different diameters cannot generate pressure changes. In fact, viscous gas—in this case, oxygen—explains these masks' operation. The devices use the converging funnel half of the venturi tube, increasing the velocity of flow as the same amount of gas moves through a reduced diameter. Following the Bernoulli principle, pressure does decrease as it approaches the constricted mouth of the funnel, a jet principle. This pressure gradient, however, is not maintained because the gas is at ambient pressure on exit. Air therefore cannot be entrained by a pressure differential. Rather, the higher velocity gas exiting the jet interacts with stagnant ambient air. Molecules of gas exiting the jet collide with molecules in the surrounding air. The velocity of stagnant air molecules increases as the oxygen molecules exiting the jet decrease, entraining air molecules in the forward flow of gas. These effects occur at constant pressure.[3]

Viscosity

All real fluids, both gases and liquids, have the property of **viscosity,** which adds a level of complexity for which the Bernoulli principle does not directly account. Rather, analysis using the Bernoulli principle assumes that fluids

*E*QUATION 14-21

Principle of Continuity Using a Venturimeter

$$\Delta P = \frac{(\rho \dot{V})}{2} \times \left(\frac{1 - d_1{}^2}{d_2{}^2} \right)$$

$$\Delta P = \frac{(\rho \dot{V}^2)}{2}$$

where:

ΔP = Pressure gradient
ρ = Density
$\dot{V}$ = Flow
d_1 = Diameter at point 1 in the tube
d_2 = Diameter at point 2 in the tube

*E*QUATION 14-22

Pitot Static Tube

$$\Delta P = \frac{(\rho \dot{V}^2)}{2}$$

where:

ΔP = Pressure gradient
ρ = Fluid density
$\dot{V}$ = Flow

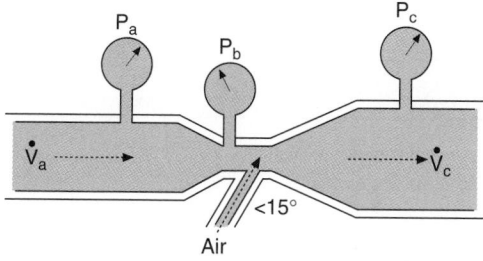

Figure 14-8   A venturi tube. The original lateral pressure at point P_a falls at the restriction (P_b). Pressure is almost completely restored distal to the restriction (P_c) if the angle of tube dilation does not exceed 15 degrees. (Modified from Scanlan CL, Wilkins RL, Stoller JK. Egan's fundamentals of respiratory care. 7th ed. St Louis: Mosby; 1999.)

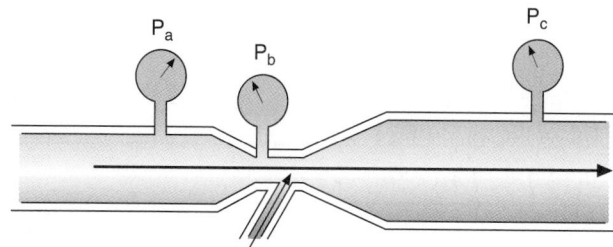

Figure 14-9   Pitot tube. Through high forward velocity and forward pressure after air entrainment, molecules of the source gas and entrained air mixture hit the sides of the tube less often. Ideally, they exert low lateral pressure so that forward pressure is maximized. (Modified from Scanlan CL, Wilkins RL, Stoller JK. Egan's fundamentals of respiratory care. 7th ed. St Louis: Mosby; 1999.)

have zero viscosity. Viscosity can be described as the internal friction of a fluid and is independent of the density of a fluid. Therefore the perception of viscosity, which may be based on experience of its density, may actually be quite different. According to concepts of kinetic theory, molecules of a liquid flowing through a pipe collide with the walls of the conduit, reducing the overall velocity of the liquid and decreasing momentum. In air, viscosity increases with temperature because the frequency of collisions between molecules is greater. Viscosity in liquids, however, is increased at lower temperatures. A viscous fluid, such as molasses or oil, demonstrates high dependence of viscosity on temperature.

Viscosity most frequently refers to dynamic, or molecular, viscosity. A fluid in motion may be viewed as a set of thin parallel layers that move past each other. Dynamic viscosity is the shear, or the stickiness, between sheets. If a constant force pushes against an upper plate while the lower one is fixed, the upper plate moves with a flow velocity. The required force to achieve a velocity depends on the area of the plate, the viscosity, and the distance between plates (Equation 14-23). Measurement of viscosity using SI units is Pa (N m^{-2}) seconds, a unit without a specific name. The poise, dyne second cm^{-2}, is a non-SI unit that remains in frequent use. Poise is approximately $^{1}/_{10}$ the SI unit.

Dynamic viscosity is similar to stress and strain in solids. Using such terms, viscosity compares shear stress to the rate of change of velocity, or shear rate. Kinematic vis-

cosity, which describes how easily a particular fluid flows, is the ratio of dynamic viscosity to the fluid density. If density is an expression of inertia, kinematic viscosity is the tendency to eliminate nonuniform motion of fluid velocity. In most clinical situations, a gas is less viscous than a liquid. Air is approximately 50 times less viscous than water. However, air is kinematically more viscous than water.

Hagen-Poiseuille Equation

If a viscous fluid is flowing without turbulence through a pipe, the fluid can be considered as composed of multiple extremely thin parallel cylinders of fluid. The layer of fluid immediately adjacent to the immobile wall of the conduit (the boundary layer) has no velocity, whereas the layer at the axis of the pipe has the maximum velocity. Its velocity is approximately twice the minimum velocity close to the wall of the conduit. The set of different flow rates present takes on a parabolic configuration. To understand the flow of a viscous fluid, analysis beyond the principle of continuity and the Bernoulli principle must be applied. If any one of the thin cylinders of fluid flowing through the pipe is considered, the force required must be the product of the pressure gradient responsible for the presence of flow and the area of the cylinder (Equation 14-24).

The product of shear stress and surface area opposes this force. Shear stress in turn is the product of viscosity and the velocity gradient. After several mathematic transfor-

Equation 14-23
Force and Viscosity

$$F = \frac{\eta \dot{V} A}{z}$$

$$\eta = \frac{Fz}{\dot{V} A}$$

where:

F = Force
η = Viscosity
$\dot{V}$ = Velocity
A = Area
z = Distance between plates

Equation 14-24
Calculating Force through a Pipe

$$F = \Delta P(2\pi r^2)$$

where:

F = Force
ΔP = Static pressure gradient
r = radius

Equation 14-25
Hagen-Poiseuille Equation

$$\dot{V} = \frac{\Delta P\, r^4}{8\eta l}$$

where:

$\dot{V}$ = Velocity
ΔP = Static pressure gradient
r = Radius
η = Viscosity
l = Length

Equation 14-26
Reynolds Number

$$Re = \frac{\text{Inertial forces}}{\text{Viscous forces}} = \frac{\nu r \rho}{\eta}$$

where:

Re = Reynolds' number
ν = Velocity
r = Radius
ρ = Density
η = Viscosity

mations the **Hagen-Poiseuille equation** can be derived (Equation 14-25). The equation calculates volume per unit time, not distance or flow velocity. Volume flow is related to the fourth power of the radius. It is directly and inversely related to the viscosity of the fluid and the length of the tube through which the fluid passes and directly related to the pressure gradient. If these variables remain constant, the pressure gradient over the length of the tubular structure in question is directly proportional to flow. Differential pressure pneumotachographs use this principle to measure flow.

The Hagen-Poiseuille equation requires **laminar flow,** which is the flow of a fluid through a straight tube as a series of concentric cylinders slide over one another (Figure 14-10). Turbulence, however, describes the circumstances in which this orderly flow is disrupted. The behavior of **turbulent flow** is quite different from that of laminar flow and much more difficult to define precisely. Instead of a parabolic distribution of velocities from the wall (slowest) through the central axis (fastest) of a conduit, flow is a jumbled mixture of velocities, more resembling a square wave of velocities. Friction has a more prominent effect (it can be ignored during laminar flow).

Reynolds number (Equation 14-26) describes factors associated with generation of laminar or turbulent flow. Reynolds number is a dimensionless number because units of measurement cancel one another when consistent units are used. The equation demonstrates that density and viscosity are independent factors affecting turbulence. Although viscosity is inversely related to Reynolds number, the fluid density, velocity, and conduit radius are directly related. On a qualitative basis,

Reynolds number describes a ratio of inertial forces to viscous forces. A fluid with significant inertia (high propensity to continue in the direction of movement) is more likely to demonstrate turbulence. A low Reynolds number (under 2000 in smooth, nonbranching pipes with a length substantially longer than the diameter) indicates laminar flow, whereas a high number (more than 3000) predicts turbulent flow.

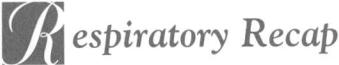

Respiratory Recap

Types of Flow
Laminar
Turbulent

In contrast to laminar flow, turbulent flow varies directly with the square of flow rate and carries a term for friction, implying greater resistance at equivalent flows. Density rather than viscosity is the prominent fluid characteristic. These differences explain the use of helium and oxygen mixtures for conditions in which the upper airways are narrowed. Although the viscosities of helium, oxygen, and air are not markedly different, helium is much less dense. Equation 14-27 describes the effects of density when flow is turbulent. Flow velocity is greater in the upper airway and trachea than in the more numerous small airways because of the principle of continuity. The total area of the smaller airways is greater; thus the velocity is less. The characteristics of turbulent flow may sometimes be used to advantage. The lack of a parabolic distribution of flow velocity implies that turbulent flow is more effective than laminar flow during purging of a tube, such as during a change of gas.

Equation 14-27
Laminar Flow and Turbulent Flow

> **Laminar Flow**
>
> $$\Delta P = \frac{8\eta l \dot{V}}{r^4}$$
>
> **Turbulent Flow**
>
> $$\Delta P = \frac{\rho l \dot{V}^2}{4\pi r^5}$$
>
> where:
>
> ΔP = Pressure gradient
> η = Viscosity
> l = Length
> r = Radius
> $\dot{V}$ = Flow
> ρ = Density

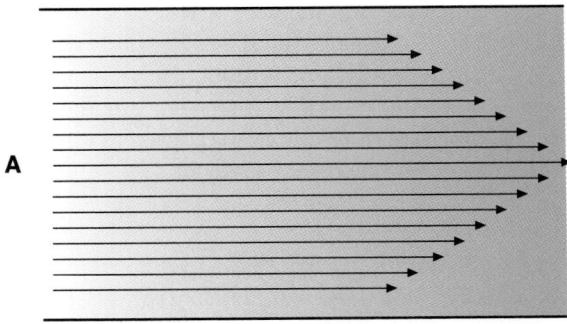

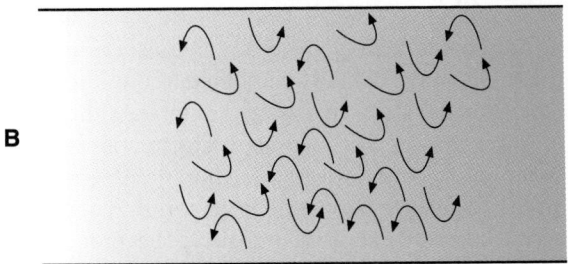

Figure 14-10   A, Laminar flow. **B,** Turbulent flow.

*E*QUATION 14-28
Ohm's Law

$$V = I \times R$$

Impedance

$$I = \frac{V}{R}$$

Resistance

$$R = \frac{V}{I}$$

where:

V = Voltage
R = Resistance
I = Impedance or amperage

Ohm's Law

Ohm's law primarily describes properties of electric systems. Similar to the Bernoulli principle, ohmic analysis assumes linear relations among a pressure, resistance, and flow term, without loss of thermal energy or turbulence. This analysis allows application of easily measured quantities, such as electrical resistance, to other circular systems of single or connected circuits in which measurement may be more technically difficult. The most general expression of Ohm's law describes the relation of voltage, resistance, and impedance (Equation 14-28).

In physiologic terms, voltage correlates with pressure and impedance with the flow rate. Thus Ohm's law gives a general expression for **resistance,** the ratio of pressure gradient to flow. This relation may be used to calculate airway resistance. Using a body plethysmography box, the subject pants or breathes with a small tidal volume. Alveolar pressure falls with inspiratory effort as a function of airway resistance. Following Boyle's law, alveolar volume increases, which is registered as an increase in pressure inside the box. Airway resistance is calculated from measurement of instantaneous airflow and pressure changes (Equation 14-29). Alternatively, airway pressures during passive inspiration can be analyzed. Many current mechanical ventilators use this method to calculate resistance. The difference in inspiratory pressure at end-inspiration and during an end-inspiratory pause determines the pressure gradient resulting from flow generated by the mechanical ventilator. This reflects the resistance of the conducting airways of the lungs and endotracheal tube.

The cardiovascular system can also be analyzed using this relationship of pressure and flow. The element of flow of most interest in the cardiovascular system is cardiac output ($\dot{Q}c$). Therefore in terms of the cardiovascular system, vascular resistance can be described as shown in Equation 14-30. By use of Ohm's law the cardiovascular system is modeled as a single circuit in which the flow out

*E*QUATION 14-29
Ohm's Law for Airway Resistance

Airway Resistance

$$R_{aw} = \frac{\Delta P_{alv}}{\dot{V}}$$

where:

R_{aw} = Airways resistance
ΔP_{alv} = Alveolar pressure
$\dot{V}$ = Flow

Resistance during Mechanical Ventilation

$$R_{aw} = \frac{PIP - P_{plat}}{\dot{V}}$$

where:

R_{aw} = Airway resistance
PIP = Peak inspiratory pressure
P_{plat} = Plateau pressure

equals the flow in, opposed by a single resistance over a particular part of the circuit. For example, systemic vascular resistance is estimated through subtraction of venous inflow pressure or right atrial (central venous) pressure from aortic pressure, usually estimated as mean arterial pressure. Similarly, pulmonary vascular resistance is estimated as the pressure difference of pulmonary artery occlusion (or wedge) pressure, an estimate of left atrial pressure, subtracted from mean pulmonary pressure. Flow is cardiac output.

Conductance (G) also is used to refer to the rate of flow generated by a pressure gradient. Conductance is the reciprocal of resistance (R) and implies the *ease* of transfer of a substance, whereas resistance implies *opposition*. These two items are logarithmically, not arithmetically, related: log R = -log G. For a constant flow the pressure gradient and conductance are hyperbolically related, whereas resistance is linearly related to the pressure gradient.

Application of Physical Principles to Measurement and Physiology

Principles of Measurement

Any measurement device converts a physical entity into a signal. Even a water column manometer converts a pressure existing somewhere in a system of interest into a column of water than can be measured. Electric or electronic transducers are commonly in use. Important considerations in the ability of measurement devices to record physical signals faithfully include linearity; the proportional output of a system without hysteresis (a difference between responses to increasing and decreasing pressure);

EQUATION 14-30
Ohm's Law for Vascular Resistance

$$\text{Vascular resistance} = \frac{\text{Pressure gradient}}{\text{Cardiac output}}$$

Systemic Vascular Resistance and Pulmonary Vascular Resistance

$$\text{SVR} = \frac{\text{MAP} - \text{CVP}}{\dot{Q}c}$$

$$\text{PVR} = \frac{\text{PAP} - \text{PCWP}}{\dot{Q}c}$$

where:

SVR = Systemic vascular resistance
MAP = Mean arterial pressure
CVP = Central venous pressure
$\dot{Q}c$ = Cardiac output
PVR = Pulmonary vascular resistance
PAP = Mean pulmonary artery pressure
PCWP = Pulmonary capillary wedge pressure

---

drift, or long-term change in the system output in response to a constant signal; and dynamic response, or distortion of the signal caused by the way the physical signal reaches the transducer.

An analog meter or gauge measures by a physical continuous scale, such as a spring (mechanical) or voltage range (electronic). Passing the signal into a suitable circuit allows simple manipulation of the signal (for example, integration or differentiation). A digital meter, on the other hand, measures the signal of interest not continuously but at regular, discrete intervals. Digital analysis permits more flexible and complicated analysis but must sample the signal at a sufficiently rapid frequency to reproduce it faithfully. According to the Nyquist sampling limit, to detect a signal of any particular periodic frequency, it must be sampled at least twice that frequency.

Noise composes the unwanted effects detected by the recording system. It may be intrinsic noise, such as oscillations occurring in a catheter system attached to a pressure manometer, or extrinsic noise, such as electrical interference occurring between a transducer and an amplifier.

Calibration refers to the process by which the output of a measurement system is adjusted to a known input. It may be passive calibration, in which the output is compared with a static input signal, such as a particular pressure, or dynamic calibration, which compares the system output with a forcing function or probe in which a varying signal is used for calibration. The latter type can be used to determine the dynamic frequency response of the recording system. Because physiologic signals frequently are periodic, a frequency response rapid enough to reflect the physiologic input is important.

To measure a periodically repeating signal, such as blood pressure or airflow, the Fourier theory can be ap-

plied. This theory allows description of a wave form by summation of a series of sinusoidal waves. A regularly repeating wave can be described by series of frequency (f, 2f, 3f . . .). These series are harmonics of the Fourier series.[4,5]

Common Flow Measurement Devices

The most straightforward method of flow measurement is direct, timed collection of volume (blood, gas). However, this method cannot be applied to a closed system. Any measurement applied must add a minimum of resistance and generate a signal that is linear over the range of expected flows. Devices used to measure the flow of some liquids include electromagnetic flowmeters, which rely on a conductor moving through a magnetic field (by use of the Faraday principle); ultrasonic flowmeters, in which frequency changes of reflected sound waves are measured (Doppler frequency shift principle); radioactivity counting devices; and direct volume measurement, in which a volume change is directly measured when outflow is occluded for a set period. All these methods have been used to determine blood flow,[6] but the underlying principles do not apply (electromagnetic, ultrasound techniques) or are impractical (plethysmography) to measure airflow.

A variety of devices are available for clinical measurement of gas flow. The rotating vane anemometer, or Wright respirometer, uses a rotating vane set in a tube with oblique slots through which air enters. This device is not linear at low flows because gas can enter the tube before the vanes rotate. The hot wire anemometer is based on the temperature dependence of electrical resistance. As gas flow cools a wire, change in resistance is detected. This device also is not linear at low flows, but electronic calculation of calibration curves can partly overcome these disadvantages. Many mechanical ventilators use a hot wire system for flow (and volume) measurement. The Wright peak flow meter uses a spring to maintain constant pressure at the mouthpiece. The peak expiratory flow alters an orifice opening that registers the amplitude of flow.

A differential pressure pneumotachograph measures airflow by detecting the reduction of pressure across a resistance, based on Hagen-Poiseuille's law. A wire grid or bundle of small tubes (introduced by Lilly and Fleisch, respectively) produces resistance, establishing laminar flow and satisfying the requirements of the Hagen-Poiseuille equation. Heating the device minimizes condensation of water vapor on the capillary tubes or screens to prevent changes in the imposed resistance.

Expiratory Flow

Expiratory flow demonstrates several physical principles important to respiratory physiology, including expiratory flow limitation and the time constant. Flow in the respiratory system, however, occurs through semicollapsible tubes. The velocity of fluid flowing through a tube is limited by the velocity of an elastic wave along its walls, gen-

Equation 14-31

Washout Function

$$y = y_0 e^{-kt} \quad or \quad y = \frac{y_0}{e^{kt}}$$

$$y = y_0 e^{-t/\tau}$$

where:

y_0 = Initial quantity in question
e = Base of natural logarithms (2.71828...)
t = Time
k = Reciprocal of the time constant, τ.

$$V = V_0 e^{-(t/RC)}$$

where:

V_0 = Initial volume
V = Volume at t
C = Compliance
R = Resistance

Equation 14-32

Equation of Motion

$$P_{aw} = P_{ex} + \dot{V} \times R_{aw} + \frac{V_T}{C}$$

where:

P_{aw} = Airway pressure
P_{ex} = End expiratory pressure
$\dot{V}$ = Flow
R_{aw} = Airway resistance
V_T = Tidal volume
C = Compliance

Equation 14-33

Conservation of Mass

$$\text{Uptake or release} = \dot{Q} \times (Ca - C\bar{v})$$

where:

$\dot{Q}$ = Blood flow
Ca = Content in arterial blood
$C\bar{v}$ = Content in mixed venous blood

Equation 14-34

Cardiac Output (Fick Principle)

$$\dot{Q}c = \frac{\dot{V}_{O_2}}{Ca_{O_2} - C\bar{v}_{O_2}}$$

where:

$\dot{Q}c$ = Cardiac output
$\dot{V}_{O_2}$ = Oxygen consumption
Ca_{O_2} = Arterial oxygen content
$C\bar{v}_{O_2}$ = Mixed venous oxygen content

erated by flow through the conduit. According to wave speed theory, flow through an airway cannot be greater than the flow at which gas velocity equals wave speed. Wave speed is the speed at which a small disturbance travels in a compliant tube filled with a fluid. When the pressure across the wall of a semicollapsible conduit is positive, the wave speed tends to be much higher than the fluid velocity. The wave speed in rigid walls is quite high and does not limit flow appreciably. When the transmural pressure falls, as during expiration, the decreased wave speed limits the fluid velocity that can be achieved. If airways are abnormally collapsible, this effect is more prominent and occurs at lower flow rates. Therefore in conditions such as emphysema, expiratory flow limitation is a prominent effect. At lower lung volumes the effects of viscosity limitation also are observed.

Passive exhalation is an example of a washout function. Other pertinent examples include the change in the partial pressure of arterial oxygen (PaO_2) or the partial pressure of arterial carbon dioxide ($PaCO_2$) after a change in the inspired oxygen concentration or minute ventilation or removal of volatile anesthetic agents from the body. In these cases the decrease in a quantity is proportional to the amount remaining (Equation 14-31). After 1 time constant, the amount remaining is $1/e$, or approximately 37% of its initial value. After 2 time constants, the amount remaining is $1/e^2$, or 13.5% of the initial value, and after 5 time constants the amount remaining is $1/e^5$, or less than 1% of the initial value.

The time constant also has some characteristics peculiar to the physical properties of passive expiration. Resistance is the ratio of pressure gradient to flow rate. Compliance is the ratio of volume to pressure. The **time constant** is the product of compliance, the force needed to distend the lungs, and resistance. Thus the tidal volume remaining in the lungs at any point during exhalation is determined by resistance and compliance (see Equation 14-31).

Equation of Motion

The Equation of Motion predicts the pressure resulting from flow through a system of tubes and a distensible (elastic) container. Although the most general form of the equation may describe the behavior or any fluid—gas or liquid—in such a system, a more particular form describes the behavior of a fluid in a system such as the lung (Equation 14-32). This equation specifies that factors such as resistance, flow, and tidal volume are not independent of the airway pressure generated. Although the equation in this form describes the behavior of the total respiratory system, the separate contributions of the thorax (chest wall and abdomen) and lung can be specified.

Conservation of Mass

Calculation of flow does not necessarily require direct measurement of volume or flow but may be based on the principle of conservation of mass. The total consumption or release of any substance is the product of the flow through an organ and the difference in arterial and venous blood content of that substance (Equation 14-33), which is the Fick principle. Measuring total oxygen consumption through measurement of inspired and expired gas and comparison of this amount with the arteriovenous oxygen difference determined by blood oxygen analysis is most often referred to as the *Fick method of calculating cardiac output* (Equation 14-34). The commonly used method to determine cardiac output clinically, the thermodilution technique, also uses the Fick principle. In that case the substance released is injection of thermal energy (cold). A thermistor at the distal end of a pulmonary artery catheter measures the speed of the dissipation of temperature to calculate cardiac output.

KEY POINTS

- Molecular theory describes physical entities and their response to physical forces by describing atoms and molecules and the interactions between them.
- Work of breathing may be estimated by measurement of volume change and the associated pressure change.
- Pascal's law describes the way in which pressure is transmitted without reduction throughout any enclosed static fluid; this law is the basis for manometric measurements.
- Laplace's law describes the tension of the wall of a sphere or cylinder (wall tension) and is useful to understand pressures in an alveolus.
- Surface tension describes the property of liquid that tends to reduce the surface of a liquid toward a minimum, pulling the surface molecules inward.
- Surfactant is necessary for normal lung function because it reduces surface tension.
- The ideal gas law states that pressure and volume are inversely related, whereas temperature is directly proportional to volume or pressure.
- Common conditions for reporting of gas volumes include STPD, BTPS, ATPD, and ATPS.
- A humidity deficit occurs whenever inspired gas is not fully saturated at body temperature.

- Graham's law predicts the rate of diffusion of a gas as inversely proportional to the gram molecular weight of the gas.
- Fick's law describes the transfer of a solute by diffusion.
- The Bernoulli principle describes the pressure drop when fluid passes through a constriction in a rigid tube.
- The Venturi principle states that a pressure drop across an obstruction can be restored, provided the angle of divergence is less than 15 degrees.
- The Hagen-Poiseuille equation states that flow is related to the *fourth* power of the radius, the *viscosity* of the fluid, the length of the tube, and the pressure gradient.
- Reynolds number is a dimensionless number used to describe laminar or turbulent flow.
- Ohm's law describes the relationship among pressure, flow, and resistance.
- Expiratory flow is an example of a washout function, in which the decrease in quantity is a function of the initial amount and time constant.
- Calculation of flow can be based on the principle of conservation of mass (Fick principle).

References

1. Astrup P, Severinghaus JW. The history of blood gases, acids, and bases. Copenhagen: Munksgaard; 1986.
2. Lumb AB. Nunn's applied respiratory physiology. 5th ed. Boston: Butterworth-Heinemann; 2000.
3. Scacci R. Air entrainment masks: jet mixing is how they work; the Bernoulli and Venturi principles are how they don't. Respir Care 1979;24:928-931.
4. Milnor RW. Hemodynamics. Baltimore: Williams & Wilkins; 1982.
5. Butler JP, Leith DE, Jackson AC. Principles of measurement: applications to pressure, volume, and flow. In: Fishman AP, Macklem PT, Mead J, editors. Handbook of physiology. Vol. II. Mechanics of breathing. Section 3. The respiratory system. Bethesda, Md: American Physiological Society; 1986.
6. Linden RJ. The measurement of blood volume: techniques in the life sciences. In: Linden RJ, editor. Cardiovascular physiology. Part 1. New York: Elsevier Scientific; 1983.

Recommended Reading

Kellogg RH. Laws of physics pertaining to gas exchange. In: Fishman AP, Farhi LE, Tenny SM, et al., editors. Handbook of physiology. Vol. IV. Gas exchange. Section 3. The respiratory system. Bethesda, Md: American Physiological Society; 1987.

Lide DR, editor. CRC handbook of chemistry and physics. 79th ed. Boca Raton, Fla: CRC Press; 1998.

Otis AB. An overview of gas exchange. In: Fishman AP, Farhi LE, Tenny SM, et al., editors. Handbook of physiology. Section 3. The respiratory system. Bethesda, Md: American Physiological Society; 1987.

Vogel S. Life in moving fluids. 2nd ed. Princeton, NJ: Princeton University Press; 1994.

CHAPTER 15

Chemistry for Respiratory Care

Carl F. Haas

CHAPTER **OUTLINE**

Basic Chemistry
  Matter
  Chemical Bonding
  Chemical Reactions
  Liquid Mixtures
Inorganic Molecules
  Water
  Oxygen and Carbon Dioxide
  Electrolytes
Organic Molecules
  Carbohydrates
  Proteins

Lipids
Nucleic Acids
Clinical Chemistry
  Fluid and Electrolyte Balance
  Acid-Base Balance
  Nutrition and Metabolism
  Carbon Dioxide Production, Oxygen Consumption,
    and Transport

OBJECTIVES

1. Describe the structure of the atom.
2. Compare ionic, covalent, and hydrogen bonds.
3. Describe synthesis, decomposition, and exchange reactions.
4. List factors that affect the solubility of solutions.
5. Compare methods used to state concentrations of solutions.
6. List colligative properties of solutions.
7. Compare organic and inorganic compounds.
8. Describe the physical and chemical properties of water, oxygen, carbon dioxide, and electrolytes.
9. Describe the chemical properties of acids, bases, buffers, and salts.
10. Discuss the biologic importance of carbohydrates, lipids, proteins, nucleic acids, vitamins, hormones, and enzymes.
11. Explain the biologic basis of fluid and electrolyte balance.
12. Discuss the biologic principles of acid-base balance.
13. Describe the energy-producing metabolic pathways.
14. Describe oxygen and carbon dioxide transport.

KEY TERMS

Acid	Boiling Point	Concentrated
Adenosine triphosphate (ATP)	Buffers	Covalent Bond
Amino Acid	Catabolism	Crenation
Anabolism	Cations	Deoxyribonucleic Acid (DNA)
Anions	Cholesterol	Dilute
Atom	Citric Acid (Krebs) Cycle	Electrons
Atomic Number	Colligative Properties	Electron Transport System
Atomic Weight	Colloid	Element
Base	Compound	Freezing Point

KEY TERMS—cont'd

Glucose	Matter	Protons
Glycolysis	Molar Solution	Ribonucleic Acid (RNA)
Hemolysis	Mole	Saturated
Henderson-Hasselbalch Equation	Neutrons	Saturated Fatty Acid
Hydrogen Bond	Nucleic Acid	Semipermeable Membrane
Hydrophilic	Osmosis	Solute
Hydrophobic	Osmotic Pressure	Solution
Hypertonic	Oxidative Phosphorylation	Solvent
Hypotonic	Peptide	Specific Heat
Ions	Percent Solution	Steroids
Ionic Bond	pH	Suspension
Isotonic	Phospholipids	Triglycerides
Isotope	Polar	Unsaturated Fatty Acid
Lipid	Precipitate	Valance Electrons
Mass Number	Proteins	Vapor Pressure

Respiratory therapists must have a basic knowledge of the principles of chemistry to better understand the functioning of the human body and to better appreciate such clinical concepts as arterial blood gas interpretation, fluid and electrolyte physiology, nutrition, and pharmacology.

Basic Chemistry

Matter

Anything that occupies space and has mass is **matter.** Matter is classified as an element or a compound. An element cannot be broken down into two or more substances; it is a pure substance. Although oxygen is a good example of an element, most living materials are not composed of pure elements but rather are a combination of elements. When two or more elements join to form a chemical combination, the result is a **compound.** Water (H_2O) is a compound because it can be broken down into the elements hydrogen (H) and oxygen (O).

The **atom** is often called the building block of the universe. It is the smallest portion of an element that retains all the properties of the element. Each atom is composed of a small, heavy, corelike nucleus with particles surrounding it at relatively great distances. The three fundamental particles that make up the atom are the proton, the electron, and the neutron. **Protons** have a positive charge (+1) and are located in the nucleus. **Neutrons** have no net charge and are also located in the nucleus. **Electrons** have a negative charge (−1) and are located outside the nucleus (Figure 15-1).

The number of protons in the nucleus defines the element and is known as the **atomic number.** Because all atoms are electrically neutral, the number of protons is the same as the number of electrons. The sum of the protons and neutrons determines the atom's **mass number.** The

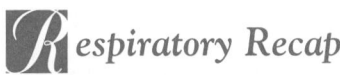

Respiratory Recap

Components of the Atom
Protons
Neutrons
Electrons

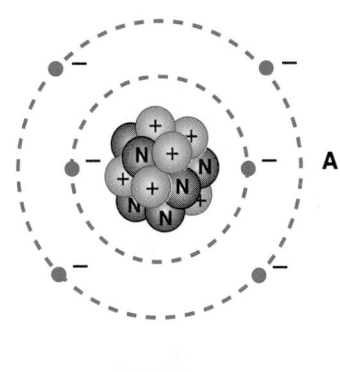

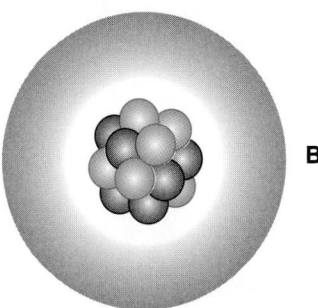

Figure 15-1   Model of the atom. **A,** The nucleus contains protons (+1 charge) and neutrons (0 charge). Electrons (−1 charge) occupy the outer regions, which are called *electron shells.* This figure represents the carbon atom, which has six protons and six neutrons in the nucleus and six electrons orbiting the nucleus. Two electrons are in the first electron shell, and the remaining four are in the outer shell. **B,** The outer shells can be thought of collectively as an *electron cloud.*

naturally occurring sodium atom has an atomic number of 11 and a mass number of 23, indicating 11 protons and electrons and 12 neutrons. The relative weight of an atom is its **atomic weight,** a term often used interchangeably with mass number. The carbon atom, which has a mass number of 12 (carbon-12), has been assigned the weight of 12 atomic mass units (amu), to which all other atoms are referenced.

Each element has a symbol that represents not only the element but also one atom of the element. The symbol "O" stands for one oxygen atom. Figure 15-2 shows the first four rows of the periodic table; it is interesting that 23 of the first 36 elements on the periodic table are found in the body. Table 15-1 lists 26 elements that are important to the functioning of the human body.

An **element** is a substance in which all the atoms have the same atomic number. Although all the nuclei of the atoms of a particular element have the same atomic number, the nuclei of a given element may not have the same mass number. **Isotopes** are atoms with nuclei that have the same number of protons (atomic number) but a different number of neutrons (mass number). Most elements have isotopes. Oxygen has three isotopes, each having eight protons and eight electrons but 8, 9, or 10 neutrons (99.8% of atmospheric oxygen is composed of oxygen-16, 0.04% is oxygen-17, and 0.16% is oxygen-18). Isotopes of the same element have the same basic chemical properties because they have the same number of electrons and protons, but they have different physical properties because they differ in the number of neutrons.

Electrons are arranged in a definite order in the atom. They occupy various principal energy levels, or shells, which can be thought of as a volume occupied by an electron cloud. Each level can hold a maximum number of electrons, which is defined by the formula $2n^2$, where n is the number of energy levels or orbits from the nucleus. The first level can hold 2 electrons, the second, 8; the third, 18, and so on.

Each energy level has sublevels, called *subshells*. As the energy level increases, so does the number of subshells. The atoms of known elements have four types of subshells, labeled *s, p, d,* and *f.* In "excited atoms," electrons may oc-

cur in subshells labeled *g, h, i,* and so on, but further detail is beyond the scope of this discussion. The number of subshells is equal to the shell (energy level) number. The first energy level has one subshell, the *s* subshell, which contains two electrons (1 pair). The second energy level has two subshells: an *s* subshell (2*s*) containing two electrons and a *p* subshell (2*p*) that has six electrons (3 pairs). The third energy level has an *s* subshell (3*s*) with two electrons, a *p* subshell (3*p*) with six electrons, and a *d* subshell (3*d*), which holds 10 electrons (5 pairs). The fourth energy level has the *s, p, d* subshells and an *f* subshell, which can hold 14 electrons (7 pairs). Electrons fill shells in an orderly manner: first the orbital 1*s*; then 2*s*; then 2*p* and 3*s*; then 3*p* and 4*s*; then 3*d*, 4*p*, and 5*s*; then 4*d*, 5*p*, and 6*s*; then 4*f*, 5*d*, 6*p*, and 7*s*; followed by 5*f*, 6*d*, and 7*p*. Overlapping of shells begins with the transition from shell 3 to shell 4.

The number of electrons in the various energy levels and a notation referred to as the *electron configuration* can represent the subshells of an element. For example, the electron configuration for the element sodium (Na, atomic number 11) is $1s^22s^22p^63s^1$. This representation indicates that the 1*s* subshell has two electrons, the 2*s* subshell has two electrons, the 2*p* subshell has six electrons, and the 3*s* (outermost) subshell has one electron. Table 15-2 shows the electron configuration for the first 20 elements.

Chemical Bonding

The outermost shell is most important to determine an element's chemical properties, because these orbitals are involved in the formation of chemical bonds and in chemical reactions. An electron dot structure, known as a *Lewis dot structure,* often is used to represent the structure of an atom. The nucleus and all the filled energy levels are represented by the element's symbol; the symbol is surrounded by dots equal to the number of electrons in the outer shell. These electrons are known as **valance electrons.** The Lewis dot structures for the first 20 elements are included in Table 15-2. The gases helium, neon, and argon, which are known as *noble gases,* have full outer shells (helium has only two electrons because it is filling

Period	IA																	0
1	1 H 1.01	IIA											IIIA	IVA	VA	VIA	VIIA	2 He 4.00
2	3 Li 6.94	4 Be 9.01											5 B 10.81	6 C 12.01	7 N 14.01	8 O 15.99	9 F 18.99	10 Ne 20.18
3	11 Na 22.99	12 Mg 24.31	IIIB	IVB	VB	VIB	VIIB	VIII	VIII	VIII	IB	IIB	13 Al 26.98	14 Si 28.09	15 P 30.97	16 S 32.06	17 Cl 35.45	18 Ar 39.95
4	19 K 39.10	20 Ca 40.08	21 Sc 44.96	22 Ti 47.88	23 V 50.94	24 Cr 51.99	25 Mn 54.94	26 Fe 55.85	27 Co 58.93	28 Ni 58.69	29 Cu 63.55	30 Zn 65.38	31 Ga 69.72	32 Ge 72.59	33 As 74.92	34 Se 78.96	35 Br 79.90	36 Kr 83.8

Figure 15-2   First 36 elements of the Periodic Table of the Elements.

only the 1s orbital, whereas the others have eight electrons). Eight electrons in the outer energy level corresponds to filled s and p orbitals, which in turn leads to great stability. This tendency to fill the s and p levels is known as the *octet rule*. Elements with the same number of valance electrons are in the same column in the periodic table. They belong to the same group or family and have similar chemical properties. Such elements tend to form similar compounds and often substitute for each other.

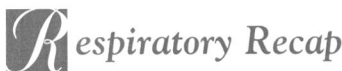

Chemical Bonds
Ionic bonds
Covalent bonds
Hydrogen bond

TABLE 15-1

Important Elements Found in the Body

Element	Symbol	Atomic Number	Percentage of Body Weight	Function or Importance
Major Elements				
Oxygen	O	8	65	Cellular respiration; a component of water and organic compounds
Carbon	C	6	18.5	Backbone of organic molecules
Hydrogen	H	1	9.5	Component of water and most organic molecules; necessary for energy transfer and respiration
Nitrogen	N	7	3.3	Component of all proteins and nucleic acids
Calcium	Ca	20	1.5	Component of bones and teeth; necessary for certain enzymes, nerve and muscle function, hormonal action, cellular motility, and blood clotting
Phosphorus	P	15	1	Main component of nucleic acids; required for bones and teeth; important in energy transfer and for phospholipids and some proteins
Potassium	K	19	0.4	Main positive intracellular ion; important in muscle and nerve function
Sulfur	S	16	0.3	Component of most proteins and some organic compounds
Sodium	Na	11	0.2	Important positive ion surrounding cells; important in muscle and nerve function and in fluid balance
Chlorine	Cl	17	0.2	Important negative ion surrounding cells
Magnesium	Mg	12	0.1	Component of many energy-transferring enzymes
Trace Elements				
Silicone	Si	14	<0.1	—
Aluminum	Al	13	<0.1	—
Iron	Fe	26	<0.1	Critical component of blood hemoglobin and many enzymes
Manganese	Mn	25	<0.1	Requirement for many enzymes
Fluorine	F	9	<0.1	Requirement for bones and teeth; inhibitor of certain enzymes
Vanadium	V	23	<0.1	Relationship to action of insulin
Chromium	Cr	24	<0.1	Relationship to action of insulin
Copper	Cu	29	<0.1	Requirement for many enzymes, for the synthesis of hemoglobin, and for normal bone formation
Boron	B	5	<0.1	—
Cobalt	Co	27	<0.1	Assistance to vitamin B_{12} in blood clot production
Zinc	Zn	30	<0.1	Requirement for many enzymes; related to action of insulin; essential for normal growth and reproduction
Selenium	Sn	34	<0.1	Close relationship to action of vitamin E
Molybdenum	Mo	42	<0.1	Key component of many enzymes
Tin	Sn	50	<0.1	—
Iodine	I	53	<0.1	Component of thyroid hormone

—, Denotes exact function unclear or unknown.

TABLE 15-2

Electron Representations of the First 20 Elements

Element	Atomic Number	Electron Configuration	Lewis Dot Structure
H	1	$1s^1$	H·
He	2	$1s^2$	He:
Li	3	$1s^2 2S^1$	Li·
Be	4	$1s^2 2s^2$	Be:
B	5	$1s^2 2s^2 2p^1$	Ḃ·
C	6	$1s^2 2s^2 2p^2$	Ċ·
N	7	$1s^2 2s^2 2p^3$	:Ṅ·
O	8	$1s^2 2s^2 2p^4$	:Ö·
F	9	$1s^2 2s^2 2p^5$	:Ḟ·
Ne	10	$1s^2 2s^2 2p^6$	:Ṅe:
Na	11	$1s^2 2s^2 2p^6 3s^1$	Na·
Mg	12	$1s^2 2s^2 2p^6 3s^2$	Mg:
Al	13	$1s^2 2s^2 2p^6 3s^2 3p^1$	Äl·
Si	14	$1s^2 2s^2 2p^6 3s^2 3p^2$	Ṡi·
P	15	$1s^2 2s^2 2p^6 3s^2 3p^3$	·Ṗ·
S	16	$1s^2 2s^2 2p^6 3s^2 3p^4$	:Ṡ·
Cl	17	$1s^2 2s^2 2p^6 3s^2 3p^5$	:Ċl·
Ar	18	$1s^2 2s^2 2p^6 3s^2 3p^6$	:Är:
K	19	$1s^2 2s^2 2p^6 3s^2 3p^6 4s^1$	K·
Ca	20	$1s^2 2s^2 2p^6 3s^2 3p^6 4s^1$	Ca:

H, *Hydrogen*; He, *helium*; Li, *lithium*; Be, *beryllium*; B, *boron*; C, *carbon*; N, *nitrogen*; O, *oxygen*; F, *fluorine*; Ne, *neon*; Na, *sodium*; Mg, *magnesium*; Al, *aluminum*; Si, *silicon*; P, *phosphorus*; S, *sulfur*; Cl, *chlorine*; Ar, *argon*; K, *potassium*; Ca, *calcium*.

EQUATION 15-1

Cations and Anions

Cations
$$Na - 1e \rightarrow Na^+$$
$$Al - 3e \rightarrow Al^{+3}$$

Anions
$$Cl + 1e \rightarrow Cl^-$$
$$S + 2e \rightarrow S^{-2}$$

EQUATION 15-2

Production of the Ionic Compound Sodium Chloride

$$Na + Cl \rightarrow Na^+ + Cl^- \rightarrow NaCl$$

positive sodium cation and a negative chloride anion are formed. The two opposite-charged ions are held together by electrostatic attraction of their opposite charges to form a sodium chloride molecule (Equation 15-2). Compounds having ionic bonds, called *ionic compounds*, share some characteristics, such as high melting and boiling points and the ability to conduct electricity in the gaseous or liquid state. Ions are very important in the chemistry of the body, especially as electrolytes and minerals.

Another type of bonding involves the sharing of one or more pairs of electrons to achieve a stable electron configuration. When each of the two bonding atoms shares one of its valence electrons, the bond is referred to as a *covalent bond*. When one of the atoms shares two of its valence electrons with another atom, the bond is called a *dative bond*. Once formed, both covalent and dative bonds produce a shared pair of electrons and therefore have identical structures. The molecular orbital theory is used to describe the sharing of electrons and the overlap of atomic orbitals. When the atomic orbital of one atom overlaps with the atomic orbital of another atom, two new molecular orbitals are formed that encompass both nuclei. Each molecular orbital can hold one spin pair of electrons, which is the property of the whole molecule, not just the atoms forming the bond. This molecular arrangement is more stable than a combination in which each nucleus retains its own electrons.

Atoms often share more than one pair of electrons. When one, two, or three pairs of electrons are shared, the covalent bonds formed are called *single* (−), *double* (=), or *triple* (≡) bonds, respectively. The carbon atom has four valence electrons that can be shared to form covalent bonds (Figure 15-3). It uses all three types of covalent bonds when bonding with another carbon atom, often with the remaining valence electrons single bonded with hydrogen atoms.

The covalent bond is particularly important in physiology because the major elements of the body (carbon, oxy-

Atoms bond in such a way that each atom participating in the chemical bond either acquires a completed outer shell and attains the configuration of the closest noble gas to satisfy the octet rule or obtains at least a spin pair of electrons in the outer shell. Stable configurations are achieved by the transfer of electrons (**ionic bond**) or by the sharing of electrons (**covalent bond**). Elements with only one, two or three valence electrons tend to give them up, thereby becoming positive ions. Positively charged ions are known as **cations.** Sodium (Na) loses its one valence electron and takes on a +1 charge (11 protons and 10 electrons); aluminum (Al) loses its three valence electrons and takes on a +3 charge (13 protons and 10 electrons) (Equation 15-1). Elements with six or seven valence electrons tend to gain electrons to reach stability. Chlorine (Cl), which has seven valence electrons, gains one electron to fill its outer shell, thereby taking on a −1 charge and becoming a negative ion. Similarly, sulfur (S) takes on two electrons to fill its outer shell and becomes an ion with a −2 charge. Negatively charged ions are also known as **anions.**

Ions of opposite charge are attracted to each other. When a sodium atom (Na) combines with a chlorine atom (Cl) to form a sodium chloride molecule (NaCl), the sodium atom loses (or donates) an electron, and the chlorine atom gains (or accepts) the electron. In the process a

Ethane (C$_2$H$_6$) single bond (sharing 2 e$^-$)

$$H-\underset{\underset{H}{|}}{\overset{\overset{H}{|}}{C}}-\underset{\underset{H}{|}}{\overset{\overset{H}{|}}{C}}-H$$

Ethylene (C$_2$H$_4$) double bond (sharing 4 e$^-$)

Acetylene (C$_2$H$_2$) triple bond (sharing 6 e$^-$)

$$H-C\equiv C-H$$

Figure 15-3   Formation of carbon-carbon single, double, and triple bonds.

EQUATION 15-3

Chemical Reactions

Synthesis Reaction

A + B	→	AB
(Reactants)	Energy	(Product)

Decomposition Reaction

AB → A + B + Energy

Exchange Reaction

AB + CD → AD + CB

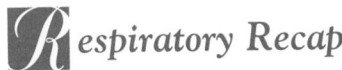
H · Lactate + NaHCO$_3$ → Na · Lactate + H$_2$CO$_3$

gen, hydrogen, and nitrogen) almost always share electrons to form bonds. Carbon, nitrogen, and oxygen form covalent bonds using atomic orbitals of the second principal energy level (elements in the second row on the periodic table). Table 15-2 shows that oxygen (atomic number 8) has six valence electrons and that the two unpaired electrons in the 2*p* subshell are available to form covalent bonds. Oxygen exists naturally as a diatomic molecule (O$_2$), which uses a double covalent bond to form. When two oxygen atoms unite to form molecular oxygen, each oxygen atom shares its two unpaired 2*p* electrons.

In addition to covalent and ionic bonds, which form molecules, a third type of bond can exist within or between biologically important molecules. The **hydrogen bond** is a weak bond and requires much less energy to break than a covalent or ionic bond. It forms as the result of unequal charge distribution on a molecule rather than from sharing or transfer of electrons. This type of molecule is called a **polar** molecule. Water is a polar molecule; although it is electrically neutral, it has a partial positive charge on the hydrogen side and a partial negative charge on the oxygen side. Hydrogen bonds weakly attach the negative (oxygen) side of one water molecule with the positive (hydrogen) side of an adjacent water molecule. This ability of water to form hydrogen bonds makes water an ideal medium for the chemistry of life. Hydrogen bonds also help maintain the three-dimensional structure of proteins and nucleic acids.

Chemical Reactions

Chemical reactions involve the formation or breaking of chemical bonds between atoms and molecules. The three basic types of chemical reactions are (1) synthesis reactions, (2) decomposition reactions, and (3) exchange reactions (Equation 15-3). Synthesis reactions combine two or more substances (reactants) to form a different, more complex substance (product). Energy is required for this reaction to occur and the new product to be formed.

Decomposition reactions break down complex substances into two or more simpler substances. During this reaction chemical bonds are broken, and energy is released. The energy can be released in the form of heat en-

ergy, or it can be captured and stored for future use. An example of a decomposition reaction is the breakdown of a complex nutrient in a cell to release energy for other cellular functions. The products of such reactions are ultimately waste products. Synthesis and decomposition reactions are opposites: synthesis forms chemical bonds and builds up, whereas decomposition undoes bonds and breaks down. Often the two opposite processes are coupled in such a way that the energy released through decomposition is used to drive a synthesis reaction.

An exchange reaction allows two reactants to exchange components and to form two new products. Exchange reactions break down two compounds and synthesize two new compounds. An example of such a reaction in the blood is the reaction of lactic acid with sodium bicarbonate to form sodium lactate and carbonic acid.

Respiratory Recap

Chemical Reactions
Synthesis reaction
Decomposition reaction
Exchange reaction

Liquid Mixtures

Most chemical reactions in the body take place in a liquid environment. Water is the primary liquid in the body, making up about 45% to 80% of the human body. Every cellular process takes place in a watery environment, and water is essential to the processes of digestion, circulation, elimination, and regulation of body temperature. Water allows substances and particles to get into a liquid form as one of three types: a solution, a suspension, or a colloid.

A **solution** is a homogeneous mixture of two or more substances, meaning that the substances mix evenly and occupy the entire volume of the solution in equal proportions. A liquid solution consists of two parts: the **solute,** which is the solid, liquid, or gaseous material being dissolved, and the

EQUATION 15-4

Calculation of Moles

$$\text{Number of moles} = \frac{\text{Number of grams}}{\text{Gram molecular weight}}$$

Example: Calculate the number of moles in 8 g of carbon. (The gram molecular weight of carbon is 12 g.):

$$\frac{8 \text{ g Carbon}}{12 \text{ g Carbon/mol}}$$

$$8 \text{ g Carbon} \frac{1 \text{ mol}}{12 \text{ g}} = 0.75 \text{ mol Carbon}$$

EQUATION 15-5

Molarity

$$\text{Molarity (M)} = \frac{\text{Number of moles (mol)}}{\text{Liter (L)}}$$

Example: Calculate the molarity of a 150 mL solution containing 10 g of NaCl.

Step 1: Determine the weight of 1 mol of NaCl.
The gram molecular weight of sodium is 23 and that of chloride is 35.

1 mol NaCl = 23 + 35 = 58 g

Step 2: Determine the number of moles of NaCl in 10 g.

$$10 \text{ g} \left(\frac{1 \text{ mol}}{58 \text{ g}} \right) = 0.172 \text{ mol}$$

Step 3: Convert 150 mL to liters.

$$150 \text{ mL} \left(\frac{1 \text{ L}}{1000 \text{ mL}} \right) = 0.15 \text{ L}$$

Step 4: Determine the molarity.

$$M = \frac{0.172 \text{ mol } H_2O}{0.15 \text{ L}} = 1.15 \text{ M}$$

EQUATION 15-6

Weight to Weight Percent Solutions

$$\text{w/w\%} = \frac{\text{Weight of solute}}{\text{Weight of solute} + \text{Weight of solvent}} \times 100$$

Example: Calculate the percent solution containing 2.5 g of sugar in 47.5 g of water. Because both the solute and solvent are expressed as weights, the weight/weight percent method is used.

$$\text{w/w\%} = \frac{2.5 \text{ g Sugar}}{2.5 \text{ g Sugar} + 47.5 \text{ g } H_2O} \times 100\% = 5\%$$

Other common solvents are alcohol, which forms the basis of medicinal tinctures, and ether, which dissolves fats and oils.

The degree to which solute particles can dissolve into a solvent is referred to as the *solubility of the solution.* A high solubility indicates that the solvent allows many solute particles to be dissolved. The following factors affect solubility:

- *The nature of the solute:* A physical characteristic of matter that determines how certain substances dissolve in a solvent.
- *The nature of the solvent:* In general, polar liquids (such as water, methyl alcohol, and ethyl alcohol) dissolve polar compounds (such as sodium chloride and potassium iodide), and nonpolar solvents (such as benzene, ether, and carbon tetrachloride) dissolve nonpolar compounds (such as oils and waxes).
- *Temperature:* Most solids become more soluble as temperature increases (that is, the solubility of solids is directly related to temperature), although sodium chloride shows little change; gases become less soluble as temperature increases (the solubility of gases is inversely related to temperature).
- *Pressure:* The solubility of a gas is directly related to pressure, although pressure has little effect on solid or liquid solutes.
- *Surface area:* Although the actual solubility is not changed, the rate of dissolution is directly related to surface area, which explains the rationale for a powder solute.
- *Agitation:* Stirring a solution brings solute particles in contact with fresh solvent more quickly, which increases the rate of dissolution but not the actual solubility.

solvent, which is the liquid material into which the solute is dissolved. Water is the most common solvent in the body.

Solutions have several common characteristics: they have a variable concentration; they are transparent; they are homogeneous; they do not settle; they may be separated by physical means; and they can pass through filter paper. When a salt crystal is dropped into a glass of water and stirred, the crystal dissolves and the solution remains clear. The same thing occurs when sugar is mixed with water. If more salt or sugar (solute) is mixed into the water (solvent), the solution becomes more concentrated but remains clear. If the solution is poured into a funnel with filter paper, the solute particles pass though, indicating that solute particles in a solution are very small. If the glass is left undisturbed for a time, the solute particles do not settle out, provided evaporation does not occur. Should the solvent evaporate, the solute particles would be left behind.

The relative concentration, or strength, of a solution is classified as dilute or concentrate. **Dilute** means that the solution contains a small amount of solute. As more solute is added, the solution becomes more **concentrated.** No specific point exists at which dilute becomes concentrated; these are relative terms, used only in a comparative sense, and they do not provide a specific quantitative meaning. The term **saturated** means that the maximum

$\mathcal{E}$QUATION 15-7

Weight to Volume Percent Solutions

$$w/v\% = \frac{\text{Grams of solute}}{100 \text{ mL of Solution}} \times 100$$

Example: What percent solution is the bronchodilator albuterol if its concentration is 2.5 mg/0.5 mL?

Step 1: Determine the number of grams in 100 mL.

$$\frac{g}{100 \text{ mL}} = \frac{2.5 \text{ mg}}{0.5 \text{ mL}} \times \frac{200}{200}$$

$$= \frac{500 \text{ mg}}{100 \text{ mL}}$$

$$= \frac{500 \text{ mg}}{100 \text{ mL}} \times \frac{1 \text{ g}}{1000 \text{ mg}}$$

$$= \frac{0.5 \text{ g}}{100 \text{ mL}}$$

Step 2: Determine the percent solution.

$$\text{Weight/volume}\% = \frac{0.5 \text{ g}}{100 \text{ mL}} \times 100\%$$

$$= 0.5\% \text{ Solution}$$

Example: How many milligrams of active drug are contained in 1 mL of a 2.25% solution of racemic epinephrine?

$$2.25\% = \frac{2.25 \text{ g}}{100 \text{ mL}}$$

$$= \frac{2250 \text{ mg}}{100 \text{ mL}}$$

$$= 22.5 \text{ mg/1 mL}$$

$\mathcal{E}$QUATION 15-8

Volume to Volume Percent Solutions

$$v/v\% = \frac{\text{Volume of solute}}{\text{Total volume of solution}} \times 100\%$$

Example: Calculate the volume of alcohol in 200 mL of beer containing 5% alcohol.

Step 1: Determine the volume of alcohol in a 5% solution.

$$5\% \text{ Alcohol} = \frac{5 \text{ mL Alcohol}}{100 \text{ mL Solution}}$$

Step 2: Determine the volume of alcohol in the 200 mL of solution.

$$\text{Volume of alcohol} = 200 \text{ mL Solution} \times \frac{5 \text{ mL Alcohol}}{100 \text{ mL Solution}} = 10 \text{ mL Alcohol}$$

---

amount of solute is dissolved for given conditions. If conditions such as temperature or pressure change, the maximum amount of solute that a given volume of solvent can dissolve also changes. An unsaturated solution contains fewer solute particles than it maximally could under normal conditions. A supersaturated solution contains more solute particles than it normally does under specific conditions. Such a solution is formed by the addition of solute as a mixture is heated, until the solution is saturated. On slow cooling, if the solution is not disturbed, excess solute remains in solution. Such a solution is very unstable, and any physical disturbance causes the excess solute to crystallize and form a solid, or **precipitate,** at the bottom of the container.

The terms related to saturation are relative and do not indicate the quantity of solute in solution. In hospitals, chemical laboratories, and industry it is important to be specific; therefore more precise terms must be used. A **molar solution** is defined as a solution that contains 1 mole (mol) of solute per liter of solution. One **mole** of a substance is equal to its gram molecular weight, which has 6.02×10^{23} atoms (Avogadro's number). Carbon-12 has an atomic weight of 12 amu, therefore the gram molecular weight of carbon-12 is 12 g. One mole of carbon-12 weighs 12 g. When 1 mole of an element combines with 1 mole

of another element, the result is 1 mole of a new molecule or substance. For example, a mole of potassium chloride (KCl) contains 1 mole of potassium (K) atoms and 1 mole of chlorine (Cl) atoms, or 6.02×10^{23} KCl molecules; KCl weighs 74.4 g (the gram molecular weight of K is 39 g and that of Cl is 35.4 g).

Given that the weight (grams) and the gram molecular weight are known, it is possible to determine the number of moles (Equation 15-4). The molarity of a solution can then be calculated (Equation 15-5). The concept of molarity is commonly used in chemistry to quantify solute in solutions.

In clinical situations, a **percent solution** is used more often. Percent concentrations usually are expressed with units of mass or volume in ratios such as weight to weight, weight to volume, and volume to volume. The weight to weight percent method (w/w%) describes the relative weight of the solute compared with the total weight of the solution (Equation 15-6). The weight to volume percent method (w/v%) is commonly used in clinical situations and in pharmacology (Equation 15-7). The volume to volume percent method (v/v%) is commonly used with liquid solutes (such as in expressions of the alcohol content of beer or wine) (Equation 15-8).

Simple ratios are sometimes used to describe the concentration of certain drugs. A ratio of 1:100 indicates

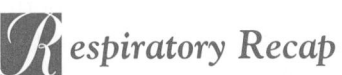

$\mathcal{R}$espiratory Recap

Methods Used to Express the Concentration of a Solution	
Molar	Ratio
Percent	mEq/L
Weight/weight	
Weight/volume	
Volume/volume	

EQUATION 15-9
Ratio Concentrations

> *Example:* How much solute (active drug) of isoproterenol is contained in 0.5 mL of a 1:200 solution?
>
> Step 1: Determine the concentration of a 1:200 solution.
>
> 1:200 = 1 g/200 mL = 1000 mg/200 mL = 5 mg/mL
>
> Step 2: Calculate the amount of solute.
>
> 0.5 mL Isoproterenol (5 mg/1 mL) = 2.5 mg Solute

EQUATION 15-10
Dilution of Stock Solutions

> $V_1 C_1 = V_2 C_2$
>
> where V_1 and V_2 are the initial and final volumes, and C_1 and C_2 are the initial and final concentrations, respectively.
>
> *Example:* Prepare 5 mL of a 10% solution, given a 20% stock solution. Given C_1 (20%), C_2 (10%), and V_2 (5 mL), solve for V_1 (x mL of stock solution).
>
> x ml stock solution × 20% = 5 mL × 10%
>
> 20x = 50
>
> x = 2.5 mL
>
> To prepare the solution, take 2.5 mL of the 20% stock solution and add 2.5 mL of water to dilute it to a final 5 mL 10% solution.

that 1 g of solute is dissolved in 100 mL of solvent (Equation 15-9). The milliequivalent per liter (mEq/L) is the unit used to describe the concentration of ions in body fluids (electrolytes). One equivalent of an ion (1 Eq) is defined as 1 mol multiplied by the value of the charge the ion carries. One Eq of sodium ion (Na^+) contains 1 mol of sodium ions, whereas 1 Eq of calcium ions (Ca^{+2}) contains $\frac{1}{2}$ mol of calcium ions. One milliequivalent (mEq) is $\frac{1}{1000}$ of an equivalent. In clinical medicine it often is necessary to prepare a weaker solution from a stronger (stock) solution. This usually is done by the addition of water or 0.9% NaCl to the stock solution (Equation 15-10).

The properties of a pure solvent are different from those of a solution. The term **colligative properties** refers to the properties of solutions that depend on the number of solute particles dissolved and not on chemical properties. Such properties include **vapor pressure, boiling point, freezing point,** and osmotic pressure. When a solute is added to a solvent, the solute dilutes the solvent and displaces some of the solvent particles at the surface of the solution. This displacement allows fewer solvent particles to escape in the form of gas particles, thereby reducing the vapor pressure of the solution. As a result of the lower vapor pressure, a higher temperature is required to raise the vapor pressure to atmospheric pressure. The solute particles in effect raise the boiling point of the solution compared to a pure solvent. For every mole of solute particles added per kilogram of water (1 kg of water has a volume of 1 L), the boiling point is raised 0.52° C. Solute particles also reduce the likelihood that water will enter the solid state and freeze, effectively reducing the freezing point of the solution. This is why salt is added to water when pasta is boiled, why salt is added to ice on sidewalks, and why antifreeze is added to radiators.

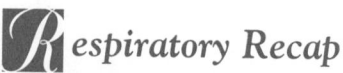

Respiratory Recap

Colligative Properties of Solutions	
Vapor pressure depression	Freezing point depression
Boiling point elevation	Osmotic pressure

Another colligative property of solutions involves osmosis. **Osmosis** is the process by which water molecules are transferred through a semipermeable membrane. A **semipermeable membrane** allows water but not other molecules to pass through it. Osmosis is very important in the maintenance of water balance between intracellular and extracellular fluid. It involves the movement of water from an area of high concentration of water to an area of low concentration in an attempt to make the concentrations equal. As an example, Figure 15-4 shows the effect of the placement of equal volumes of 20% NaCl and 40% NaCl in a U-tube container, with the two sides separated by a semipermeable membrane. Because the concentration of NaCl is higher on the right, the concentration of water must be lower on that side. Water therefore moves from an area of high water concentration (the left side) to an area of low concentration (the right side). This net movement of water results in both sides of the membrane having equal concentrations of solution, but because the membrane did not allow solute particles to pass through, the volume of fluid on the right is now much greater than on the left. The increased volume raises the height of the column of fluid, which exerts a pressure. External pressure (hydrostatic) can be applied to the right side of the column to push the higher column down and make the sides equal again. This externally applied pressure that would just stop the flow of solvent through the membrane is called the **osmotic pressure.** The osmotic pressure of pure water is always zero, whereas the osmotic pressure of a solution is directly related to the number of solute particles in solution. The greater the concentration of the solution, the greater the osmotic pressure the solution exerts.

Cells in the body can be harmed if the concentrations of solutes in the body fluids are not carefully maintained. If the concentration of water outside a red blood cell (RBC) is less than that inside the cell (that is, the osmotic pressure is higher outside the cell), water leaves the cell, causing it to shrivel, a process called **crenation.** In the reverse situation, when the water concentration is higher outside the cell (that is, the osmotic pressure is lower out-

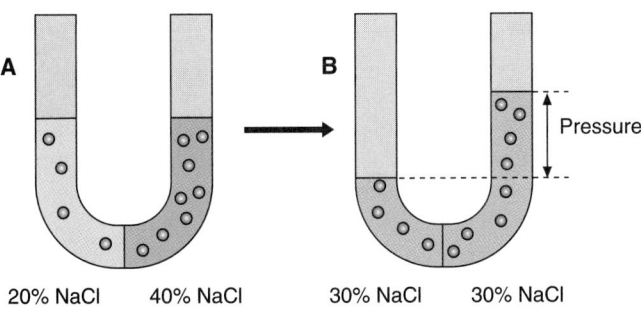

Figure 15-4 Osmotic pressure. **A,** A U-shaped tube divided by a semipermeable membrane has a 20% sodium chloride (NaCl) solution on the left side of the membrane and an equal volume of 40% NaCl solution on the right side. As time passes, water moves from the area of high solvent (water) and low solute (NaCl) concentration (left side) to the area of low solvent and high solute concentration (right side). **B,** Because the membrane allows movement only of the solvent and not of the solute, the volume on the right side increases. The difference in the height of the water columns creates back pressure, which helps stop the flow of water.

TABLE 15-3

Comparison of the Properties of Solutions, Suspensions, and Colloids

	Size	Passes through Filter Paper	Passes through Membranes	Settles	Adsorbs	Charged
Solution	<1 nm	Yes	Yes	No	No	No
Suspension	>100 nm	No	No	Yes	No	No
Colloid	1-100 nm	Yes	No	No	Yes	Yes

side the cell), water passes into the cell and may burst it, a process called **hemolysis.**

When intravenous fluids are administered, the composition of the fluid must be carefully considered. Solutions with an osmotic pressure equal to that found inside the cell are **isotonic.** A 0.9% sodium chloride solution and a 5.5% glucose solution are considered isotonic. Solutions with an osmotic pressure less than that inside the cell are considered **hypotonic.** Distilled water, tap water, and 0.45% sodium chloride are all hypotonic solutions. Solutions with an osmotic pressure greater than that inside the cell are **hypertonic.** Examples of hypertonic solutions include 5% sodium chloride and 10% glucose solutions.

A second type of liquid mixture is a **suspension.** Whereas particles in solutions consist of ions and molecules, particles in suspensions consist of large clumps of molecules. Properties of suspensions include: they consist of an insoluble substance dispersed in a liquid; they are heterogeneous; they are not clear; they settle out over time; they do not pass through filter paper; and they do not pass through membranes. Certain medications are dispensed as solutions, such as milk of magnesia. Water is often the suspending medium, although oils also can be used, as is the case with certain antibiotics. An aerosol is an example of a liquid suspended in a gas.

A third type of liquid mixture, a **colloid,** consists of tiny particles suspended in a liquid. Although similar to suspensions, they have entirely different properties. Colloids do not settle; they can pass through filter paper but not through membranes; they adsorb (hold) particles on their surface; they have electrical charges, owing to the adsorption of charged particles (ions); and they exhibit the Tyndall effect and brownian movement, which are discussed later. Table 15-3 compares the properties of colloids, solutions, and suspensions.

The particles in a colloid are larger than those in a solution (<1 nm) but smaller than those in a suspension (>100 nm); colloid particles therefore are small enough to pass though filter paper but too large to pass through a membrane. Colloids have a vast surface area because they consist of so many tiny particles. The property of adsorption is due to this tremendous surface area. Adsorption is defined as the ability to hold substances to a surface. Most colloids have selective adsorption, or the ability to adsorb only certain substances. Colloidal charcoal adsorbs large amounts of gas. Coconut charcoal selectively adsorbs poisonous gas but not ordinary gas, which is why it is used in gas masks. Colloids can selectively adsorb ions and take on an electrical charge. If a colloidal mixture consists of like charges, the particles repel each other and have minimal likelihood of coming together to form larger particles that would settle. On the other hand, if colloids of opposite charges come in contact, they attract each other and settle out. When the poison bichloride of mercury ($HgCl_2$) is swallowed, it forms a positive colloid in the stomach. Drinking egg white, a negative colloid, is the antidote. These two opposite-charged colloids neutralize each other and coagulate in the stomach. The coagulate must be pumped out of the stomach before the egg white is digested, which would expose the body to the poison again.

When a beam of light is passed thorough a colloid, the beam reflects off the colloidal particles and scatters. Such a beam passes directly though a solution without scattering because the particles are so small. This phenomenon, referred to as the *Tyndall effect,* is used as a way to distinguish between colloids and solutions. Colloids also exhibit a haphazard, irregular motion, known as *brownian movement,* which never ceases. This movement is thought to be due to constant bombardment of the colloid particles by the molecules of the suspending medium, which are in continuous, random motion. Colloidal dispersions can be **hydrophilic** (water attracting) or **hydrophobic** (water repelling). Systems in which a strong attraction exists between the colloidal particles and water (hydrophilic systems) are called *gels*. Gels, such as gelatin, are semisolid or semirigid and do not flow easily. When little attraction exists between the colloid and water (hydrophobic systems), the system is referred to as a *sol*. Such a dispersion in air is called an *aerosol* and when in water, a *hydrosol*. When a gel is heated, it turns into a sol, which returns to a gel on cooling. Protoplasm has the ability to change from gel to sol and vise versa.

Several clinical applications use the concept by which solutions and colloids are passed through membranes. Dialysis involves the separation of solute particles from colloid particles with a semipermeable membrane. Peritoneal dialysis involves bathing of the gut with a solution, after which water-soluble waste particles are allowed to pass through the semipermeable intestinal wall. Hemodialysis involves passing of blood by a semipermeable membrane, in which soluble waste products are removed and the blood cells and plasma proteins retained. Antitoxins are prepared by placement of an impure material inside a membrane suspended in running water. The soluble impurities are washed out, leaving the pure antitoxin. Low-sodium milk is produced by a similar method.

Inorganic Molecules

The compounds that make up living organisms can be divided into two broad categories: organic compounds and inorganic compounds. Organic compounds generally are composed of molecules containing carbon—carbon (C—C) or carbon—hydrogen (C—H) covalent bonds. Organic compounds usually have both types of bonds. Inorganic compounds do not have any C—C or C—H bonds, although several inorganic compounds do contain carbon. Organic compounds usually are larger and more complex than inorganic compounds. The human body contains both types of compounds. As shown in Table 15-1, the body is made up of 26 important elements. Eleven are considered major elements, and the remaining 15 are referred to as *trace elements*. More than 96% of body weight is made up of four elements: oxygen, carbon, hydrogen, and nitrogen; oxygen alone is responsible for 65% of the body's weight. The most abundant molecule in the body is water (H_2O).

Water

The importance of water in the human body is evidenced by the fact that the body can stay alive for several weeks without food but only a few days without water. Water is essential for existence. As mentioned earlier, water accounts for 45% to 80% of the total weight of the human body and is essential for proper digestion, circulation, elimination, and regulation of body temperature. Every activity in every cell in the body takes place in a watery environment.

Pure water is colorless, odorless, and tasteless. Many physical constants are based on water as a reference. The freezing point (0° C [32° F]) and the boiling point (100° C [212° F]) of water at 1 atmosphere of pressure are the standard reference points for the measurement of temperature. The calorie is defined as the amount of heat required to change the temperature of 1 g of water 1° C. The metric standard of weight, the gram, is equal to the weight of 1 mL of water at 4° C (its maximum density). The concept of specific gravity is based on water and is defined as the weight of a substance compared with the weight of an equal volume of water.

The atomic structure of water results from the combination of two covalent bonds between a single oxygen atom and two hydrogen atoms. The water molecule is not arranged in a straight line (such as HOH) but rather in a nonlinear manner, with the angle between the hydrogen atoms being approximately 105 degrees. The shared electrons between the hydrogen and oxygen are attracted to the oxygen more than the hydrogen, which results in a slight negative charge at the oxygen end of the molecule and a slight positive charge at the hydrogen end. This polar nature of water makes it such an effective solvent. As a polar solvent, water has a tendency to ionize substances in solution. This allows large compounds to be broken into smaller, more reactive particles **(ions)**, getting them ready for chemical reactions to occur.

Water also has several chemical properties worth noting (Equation 15-11). When an electric current is passed through water, it undergoes electrolysis and forms hydrogen gas (H_2) and oxygen gas (O_2). Water is extremely stable; when it boils and turns into a gas (steam), it does not decompose, even at extreme temperatures (~0.3% decomposition at 1600° C). When water reacts with a metal oxide (metals are found on the left side of the periodic table), it forms a compound known as a *base*. When water reacts with a nonmetal (nonmetals are found on the right side of the periodic table), it forms a compound known as an *acid*. When water reacts with active metals, such as sodium or potassium, a vigorous reaction occurs and hydrogen gas is formed. As already noted, water plays an important role in many bodily functions. It plays a crucial role in the transport of many essential materials in the body. For example, by dissolving oxygen and food substances in the blood, water enables these materials to enter and leave the blood capillaries in the lungs and digestive organs and eventually to enter cells in every area of the body. Water then transports waste products from the place where they are produced to the excretory organs, where they are eventually eliminated.

Water's ability to absorb and give up heat slowly gives it a major role in another unique and important bodily function—maintaining a relatively constant temperature. Chemists refer to water's ability to lose and gain large amounts of heat with little change in temperature as its high **specific heat.** Because the body has such a large water content, it can resist sudden changes in temperature. For example, it can transport the heat produced by muscle

EQUATION 15-11

Reactions of Water

Electrolysis (with the symbol ↑ indicating a gas):

$$2\ H_2O \rightarrow 2H_2\uparrow + O_2\uparrow$$
Electric current

Reaction with metal oxide to produce a base:

$$CaO + H_2O \rightarrow Ca(OH)_2$$

Calcium	Calcium
oxide	hydroxide
(metal oxide)	(base)

Reaction with nonmetals to produce an acid:

$$CO_2 + H_2O \rightarrow H_2CO_3$$

Carbon	Carbonic
dioxide	acid
(nonmetal)	(acid)

Reaction with metals:

$$2\ Na + 2\ H_2O \rightarrow 2\ NaOH + H_2\uparrow$$

EQUATION 15-12

Acid Reactions

Reactions in Water

Acids with a single ionizable hydrogen ionize into one cation and one anion:

$$HCl \rightarrow H^+ + Cl^-$$
$$HNO_3 \rightarrow H^+ + NO_2^-$$

Acids with multiple ionizable hydrogen atoms donate their protons in stages:

Stage 1: $H_2SO_4 \rightarrow H^+ + HSO_4^-$
Stage 2: $HSO_4^- \rightarrow H^+ + SO_4^{-2}$

that can be combined and represented as:

$$H_2SO_4 \rightarrow 2\ H^+ + SO_4^{-2}$$

Reactions with Metal Oxides and Hydroxides to Form Water and a Salt

$$H_2SO_4 + 2\ NaOH \rightarrow 2\ H_2O + Na_2SO_4$$

contraction during exercise to the surface of the body to be evaporated, with little change in core temperature.

Another important physical property of water is its high heat of vaporization; this refers to the fact that a significant amount of heat must be absorbed to change water from a liquid to a gas (specifically 540 calories per gram). The energy is used to break the hydrogen bonds holding adjacent water molecules together in the liquid state. When water is placed on the skin, the heat required to make it evaporate comes from the skin. In this manner the skin loses heat and is cooled. In a similar manner, the skin is cooled by the evaporation of perspiration.

Oxygen and Carbon Dioxide

Oxygen and carbon dioxide (CO_2) are inorganic substances that play an important role in cellular respiration. Oxygen is required to complete the decomposition reactions required for the release of energy from nutrients burned by the cells. CO_2 is a waste product of these same decomposition reactions and is important to acid-base homeostasis of the body. These concepts are discussed in greater detail later in the chapter.

Electrolytes

Electrolytes constitute another large group of inorganic compounds. They include acids, bases, and salts. Electrolytes are substances that break down, or dissociate, in solution to form ions. As stated earlier, positively charged ions are called *cations* and negatively charged ions are called *anions*. In solution, electrolytes are capable of carrying an electrical current.

Acids and Bases Acids and bases are common and important substances in the body. Historically, early chemists used such characteristics as taste and the ability to change

the color of certain dyes to differentiate acids and bases. Acids are sour, whereas bases are bitter; acids turn the dye litmus red, whereas bases turn it blue. Through observations such as these, it becomes clear that acids and bases are chemical opposites. Although they both dissociate in solution, they release different types of ions.

An **acid** can be defined as a compound that donates, or yields, a hydrogen ion (H^+) in an aqueous solution. Acid solutions have a sour taste. Citric acid gives a sour taste to lemons and grapefruits; acetic acid gives a sour taste to vinegar; and lactic acid makes milk taste sour. Because a hydrogen ion is the result of the hydrogen atom losing its only electron, it becomes a single proton, since it has no neutron in its nucleus. Actually, an aqueous hydrogen ion, H^+ (aq) is not a bare proton but rather a proton chemically bonded to water as H_3O^+ (aq).

According to the Brönsted-Lowry theory, an acid is the species that donates a proton in a proton transfer reaction. An acid, then, can also be thought of as a substance that donates protons. Some common acids are hydrochloric acid (HCl), sulfuric acid (H_2SO_4), nitric acid (HNO_3), carbonic acid (H_2CO_3), phosphoric acid (H_3PO_4), and acetic acid (CH_3CO_2H). Acids yield ions when placed in water (Equation 15-12). Strong acids (such as HCl,

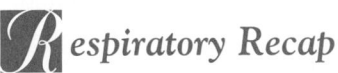

espiratory Recap

Acids and Bases
Acid: Donates hydrogen ions
Base: Accepts hydrogen ions
Buffer: Minimizes change in the hydrogen ion concentration
Salt: Produced by a reaction between an acid and a base

EQUATION 15-13

Chemical Reactions Involving Bases

> The ionization reaction of sodium hydroxide to yield OH^-:
>
> $NaOH \rightarrow Na^+ + OH^-$
>
> Reactions that accept a proton:
>
> $\underset{\text{Base}}{HCO_3^-} + \underset{\text{Proton}}{H^+} \rightarrow H_2CO_3$

EQUATION 15-14

The pH of a Solution

> $pH = -\log[H^+]$
>
> A solution with a $[H^+]$ of 10^{-7} mol/L has a pH of 7:
>
> $pH = -\log[H^+] = -\log 10^{-7} = -(-7) = 7$

EQUATION 15-15

Reactions of Buffers

> Neutralization reaction:
>
> $\underset{\text{Acid}}{HCl} + \underset{\text{Base}}{NaOH} \rightarrow \underset{\text{Salt}}{NaCl} + \underset{\text{Water}}{H_2O}$
>
> Salts in solution yield a positive and negative ion:
>
> $NaCl \rightarrow Na^+ + Cl^-$
> $K_2SO_4 \rightarrow 2 K^+ + SO_4^{-2}$

HNO_3, and H_2SO_4) almost completely ionize in solution to form H^+ ions, whereas weak acids (such as H_2CO_3) dissociate very little and therefore produce few excess H^+ ions. Acids react with metal oxides and hydroxides to form water and a salt.

An important point about water is that the water molecule dissociates continually in a reversible reaction to form hydrogen ions and hydroxide ions (OH^-) : $H_2O \leftrightarrow H^+ + OH^-$. The single unpaired valence electron makes hydrogen unstable, and by losing or donating the electron, it becomes more stable; this is why the dissociation of water occurs. Rather than share its electron with O_2, hydrogen would just as soon give up its electron to OH to maintain stability. In pure water the balance between the two ions is equal, but when an acid, such as HCl, dissociates into H^+ and Cl^-, it shifts the H^+/OH^- balance in favor of H^+ ions, increasing the acidity level.

Certain metal hydroxides are called *bases*. A **base** is a solution that yields a hydroxide ion (OH^-) in an aqueous solution. The base, or alkaline compound, shifts the H^+/OH^- balance in favor of OH^-, as shown in the ionization reaction of sodium hydroxide (Equation 15-13). A base can be thought of as the species that accepts the proton in a proton transfer reaction. With this definition the bicarbonate ion (HCO_3^-) also is a base because it can accept a proton. Basic solutions feel slippery and soapy and have a bitter, biting taste. A strong base has a high hydroxide concentration and is corrosive to tissues because of its ability to react with proteins and fats.

The concentration or strength of an acid or base is expressed by the concept of pH. The **pH** indicates the hydrogen ion concentration $[H^+]$ in a solution and is mathematically defined as the negative logarithm of the hydrogen ion concentration (Equation 15-14). A logarithm is an exponent. The logarithm (log) of 100, or 10^2, is 2, and $\log 10^{-4}$ is -4 (10^{-4} is 0.0001). Therefore a solution with a $[H^+]$ of 10^{-7} mol/L has a pH of 7. The sum of $[H^+]$ and $[HCO_3^-]$ is always 10^{-14}, therefore when the concentration of one increases, the concentration of the other must be reduced by an equal amount. The values for pH range from zero to 14. For example, a pH of zero indicates a $[H^+]$ mol/L of 10^0 mol/L (or 1 mol/L) and a $[HCO_3^-]$ of 10^{-14} mol/L. A pH of 14 indicates a $[H^+]$ of 10^{-14} mol/L and a $[HCO_3^-]$ of 10^0 mol/L. A pH of 7 indicates a neutral solution, because the concentrations of the two ions are the same,

10^{-7}. A pH above 7 indicates a base, whereas a pH below 7 indicates an acid. Because of its logarithmic relationship, a difference of 1 pH unit represents a tenfold difference in strength. This means that an acid solution with a pH of 5.5 is 10 times as strong as one with a pH of 6.5 and that a base with a pH of 9 is 10 times as strong as one with a pH of 8.

Buffers The blood has a tremendous ability to maintain a relatively narrow pH range. The normal arterial pH is 7.4 and that of venous blood is 7.37. The difference is primarily due to CO_2, which enters the venous bloodstream as a waste product of cellular metabolism. The CO_2 is carried in the blood as carbonic acid (H_2CO_3), which lowers the venous pH. At the lungs some of the carbonic acid dissociates to CO_2 and water, and the CO_2 is eliminated with the expired gas. Even though venous blood transports more than 30 L of carbonic acid each day, 1 L of venous blood has only about $\frac{1}{100,000,000}$ g more of hydrogen ions than does 1 L of arterial blood. Substances called **buffers** act as reservoirs for hydrogen ions and maintain a relative constant pH level in the blood. The specifics of buffering mechanisms are described in more detail later.

Salts When an acid and a base react, the result is a salt. When the result is a salt and water, the reaction is known as a *neutralization reaction* (Equation 15-15). Although acids (H^+) and bases (OH^-) all have an ion in common, salts do not. Salts in solution yield a positive and negative ion. Many of the major and trace minerals listed in Table 15-1 are derived from inorganic salt sources, which are common in many body fluids and specialized tissue such as bone. Often, these elements can exert a full physiologic effect only when present as an ion in solution. Some common inorganic salts are listed in Table 15-4.

TABLE 15-4

Common Inorganic Salts in the Body

Salt	Chemical Formula	Electrolyte Combination	Medicinal Use*
Sodium chloride	$NaCl$	$Na^+ + Cl^-$	Replacement therapy, irrigation, diluent
Calcium chloride	$CaCl_2$	$Ca^{+2} + 2\ Cl^-$	Reduction in blood clotting time
Sodium bicarbonate	$NaHCO_3$	$Na^+ + HCO_3^-$	Antacid, buffering agent
Potassium chloride	KCl	$K^+ + Cl^-$	Potassium replacement therapy
Sodium sulfate	Na_2SO_4	$2\ Na^+ + SO_4^{-2}$	Cathartic agent
Calcium carbonate	$CaCO_3$	$Ca^{+2} + CO_3^{-2}$	Antacid
Calcium phosphate	$Ca_3(PO_4)_2$	$3\ Ca^{+2} + 2\ PO_4^{-3}$	Replacement therapy
Magnesium sulfate	$MgSO_4$	$Mg^{+2} + SO_4^{-2}$	Cathartic agent, anticonvulsant, laxative
Potassium iodide	KI	$K^+ + I^-$	Expectorant, antitussive, mucolytic

*In addition to the physiologic use in the body.

BOX 15-1

Comparison of Organic and Inorganic Compounds

Characteristics of Most Organic Compounds	Characteristics of Most Inorganic Compounds
Complex structure	Simpler structure
Flammability	Nonflammability
Low melting point	High melting point
Low boiling point	High boiling point
Solubility in nonpolar liquids	Insolubility in nonpolar liquids
Insolubility in water	Solubility in water
Covalent bonds	Ionic bonds
Reactions usually formed between molecules	Reactions usually formed between ions
Generally many atoms	Usually relatively few atoms

Organic Molecules

Organic chemistry is the chemistry of carbon compounds. Carbon compounds have a separate category because although there are tens of thousands known inorganic compounds, there are millions of known organic compounds. Some important organic compounds in the body are carbohydrates, lipids, proteins, nucleic acids, vitamins, hormones, and enzymes. Other common materials that contain organic compounds include some drugs, wool, silk, cotton, linen, nylon, rayon, Dacron, perfumes, dyes, flavors, soaps, detergents, plastics, gasoline, and oils.

Organic compounds are different from inorganic compounds in many ways. Some of the most important differences are listed in Box 15-1. One of the unique characteristics of carbon is its ability to bond other carbon atoms to itself to form very large, complex atoms. The carbon atoms may form continuous or branched chains, creating substances known as *aliphatic compounds*. Carbon atoms also can form in the shape of a ring. If the ring is formed of all carbon atoms, the compound is called a *cyclic*, or *aromatic*, *compound*; if another element, such as nitrogen, is substituted for one of the carbon atoms in the ring, the compound is called a *heterocyclic compound*.

Because the carbon atom has four valence electrons and needs four more to reach a full shell of eight electrons, carbon can form four covalent bonds. This requirement can be satisfied by its bonding to four separate atoms by use of four single bonds; to three atoms by use of two single bonds and one double bond; or to 2 atoms by use of a triple bond and 1 single bond. This is represented in Figure 15-5. Hydrogen needs one electron to fill its outer shell and can form only one bond; oxygen forms two bonds; and nitrogen forms three bonds. With this brief overview, let us move on to the four major groups of organic substances most important in the human body: carbohydrates, lipids, proteins, and nucleic acids.

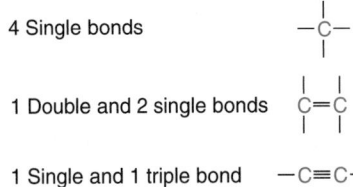

Figure 15-5 Covalent bonds formed by carbon. Each dash represents a pair of shared electrons.

Respiratory Recap

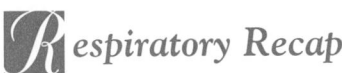

Biologically Important Organic Molecules

Carbohydrates	Vitamins
Lipids	Hormones
Proteins	Enzymes
Nucleic acids	

Carbohydrates

All carbohydrate molecules contain the elements carbon, hydrogen, and oxygen; the word *carbohydrate* literally means "carbon and water." The carbon atoms are linked to form chains of varying lengths. Sugars and starches are carbohydrates and the primary sources of chemical energy required by each cell in the body. Carbohydrates are divided into three groups based on the length of the carbon chain: monosaccharides (simple sugars), disaccharides (double sugars), and polysaccharides (complex sugars).

The basic unit of the carbohydrate molecule is the monosaccharide. **Glucose** (dextrose), the most important monosaccharide, is a six-carbon sugar with the formula $C_6H_{12}O_6$. Because it is a six-carbon molecule, it is referred to as a *hexose* (*hexa* meaning six). Glucose is present in a straight chain in the dry state but forms a cyclic compound when in solution. Glucose is the primary source of energy for the cells. Fructose and galactose are other important hexoses. Some monosaccharides consist of five-carbon atoms and are referred to as *pentoses*. Two important pentoses are ribose and deoxyribose, which are integral to the formation of the nucleic acids ribonucleic acid (RNA) and deoxyribonucleic acid (DNA).

Disaccharides and polysaccharides are composed of two or more simple sugars bonded together through a synthesis reaction that involves the removal of water. Examples of disaccharides include sucrose (table sugar from cane or beet sugar), maltose (grain sugar), and lactose (milk sugar). Each consists of two linked monosaccharides. After they are eaten, these important dietary disaccharides are broken down into monosaccharides so that the cell can use them. The combining of glucose and fructose forms sucrose.

Polysaccharides are made up of many chemically linked monosaccharides. Glycogen is the body's most important polysaccharide. It sometimes is referred to as *animal starch*. Because it has a molecular weight of several million atomic mass units, it is considered a macromolecule. When excess glucose is present in the blood, liver and muscle cells form glycogen, which can be "stored" for later use.

Proteins

Proteins are very large molecules composed of carbon, hydrogen, oxygen, and nitrogen. The molecular weight of a protein usually ranges into several million atomic mass units. The basic protein unit or building block is the **amino acid.** Proteins are composed of 20 such amino acids, and nearly all 20 are present in every protein. Of the 20, only 8 are considered essential amino acids because they cannot be produced by the body and must be included in the diet. The remaining 12 are known as *nonessential amino acids* because they can be produced from other amino acids or from simple organic molecules readily available to the body cells.

The basic structure of an amino acid consists of a carbon atom (called the α-*carbon*) to which are bonded an amino group (NH₂), a carboxyl group (COOH), a hydrogen atom, and a side chain (Figure 15-6). The side chain is a group of elements denoted by the letter R. It is the side chain that constitutes the unique and identifying characteristic of an amino acid.

To link amino acids, the OH from the carboxyl group of one amino acid and the H from the amine group of another amino acid split off to form water plus a new compound called a **peptide.** The bond between the amino acids is called a *peptide bond*. Two peptides linked together are called a *dipeptide*; three peptides linked together are called a *tripeptide*. A long chain of peptides is called a *polypeptide*, and the compound is finally considered a protein when the chain reaches about 100 amino acids or more in length.

The shape of a protein molecule determines its function. Structural proteins allow them to form essential structures of the body. Examples of such proteins are collagen, which holds most of the body tissues together, and keratin, which forms a network of waterproof fibers in the outer layer of the skin. Functional proteins are involved in the chemical processes of the body. They include some of the hormones, growth factors, cell membrane channels and receptors, and enzymes. Proteins can also bond with other organic compounds to form "mixed" molecules, such as a glycoprotein (sugar with a protein) or a lipoprotein (a lipid and a protein).

Lipids

A **lipid** is an organic biomolecule that is soluble in nonpolar organic solvents, such as ether, alcohol, or benzene. They are not soluble in water. Lipids are composed primarily of carbon, hydrogen, and oxygen, although nitrogen and phosphorus are also used. The proportion of oxygen is much lower in lipids than it is in carbohydrates. The different lipid categories include triglycerides (fats), phospholipids, steroids, and prostaglandins.

Lipids have critically important biologic functions. They provide (1) energy (they yield more energy per unit of weight than carbohydrates or proteins); (2) structure (phospholipids and cholesterol are required components of cell membranes); (3) essential nutrients in the form of vitamins (fat-soluble vitamins include vitamins A, D, E, and K); (4) protection (fat surrounds and protects organs); (5) insulation (skin fat minimizes heat loss; fatty tissue, or myelin, covers nerve cells and electrically insulates them);

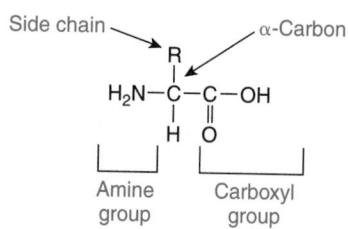

Figure 15-6 Basic structure of an amino acid.

and (6) regulation (steroid hormones such as estrogen, testosterone, and prostaglandins regulate many physiologic processes).

Triglycerides are the most abundant lipids and function as the body's most concentrated source of energy. Fats and oils are both triglycerides; fats are solid at room temperature (for example, butter and lard), and oils are liquid (such as corn or olive oil). The basic building blocks of the triglyceride are a glycerol molecule and three fatty acids. The glycerol unit is the same for all triglycerides; the specific type of fatty acid determines the identity and chemical nature of the fat.

Naturally occurring fats have long fatty acid chains, consisting of an even number of carbons, that range from 12 to 24 carbons long. A **saturated fatty acid** is one in which all available bonds of the hydrocarbon chain are filled with hydrogen atoms. The chain has all single carbon-carbon bonds. **Unsaturated fatty acids** have one or more double carbon-carbon bonds in its hydrocarbon chain because not all of the chain carbon atoms are saturated with hydrogen atoms. The degree of saturation determines the physical and chemical properties of fatty acids. Fats become more oily and liquid as the number of unsaturated double bonds increases. Double bonds cause the chain to bend or kink, thereby keeping the molecules from fitting closely together. For example, animal fats such as lard are saturated, whereas vegetable oils are not.

Phospholipids are similar to triglycerides. Instead of three fatty acids attached to a glycerol, one of the fatty acid chains is replaced by a chemical structure containing phosphorus and nitrogen. The shape of the phospholipid molecule resembles a head with two tails; the head is the phosphorus and nitrogen group, and the tails are the two fatty acids. The head is hydrophilic (attracts water), whereas the tails are hydrophobic (repel water). This unique property allows the phospholipid molecule to bridge or join two different chemical environments; for example, a water environment on one side and a lipid environment on the other. Phospholipids are a primary component of cell membranes and of pulmonary surfactant, a surface tension–reducing agent in the lungs.

Steroids are an important lipid group. They are widely distributed throughout the body and are involved in many important structural and functional roles. **Cholesterol** is a steroid lipid that combines with phospholipids in the cell membrane to help stabilize the membrane's bilayer structure. The body also uses cholesterol as a starting point for making steroid hormones such as estrogen, testosterone, and cortisol.

Prostaglandins are lipids composed of a 20-carbon unsaturated fatty acid that has a five-carbon ring. They are often referred to as *tissue hormones*. Sixteen types of prostaglandins (PGs) have been classified into nine broad categories, labeled PGA to PGI. Prostaglandins are produced by cell membranes in almost every body tissue. They are formed and released in response to specific stimuli.

Once released, they have a very local effect and are then inactivated. Prostaglandins help regulate blood pressure and the secretion of digestive juices, enhance the immune system and inflammatory response, play an important role in blood clotting, and help regulate the effects of several hormones. The use of prostaglandin and prostaglandin inhibitor drugs is gaining attention for the treatment of specific conditions ranging from relief of menstrual cramps to treatment of asthma, high blood pressure, and ulcers.

Nucleic Acids

The two principal forms of **nucleic acid** are **deoxyribonucleic acid (DNA)** and **ribonucleic acid (RNA).** The basic building block of nucleic acids are nucleotides. Just as proteins are made from chains of amino acids, nucleic acids are made from chains of nucleotides. Each nucleotide consists of a phosphate group, a five-carbon sugar, and a nitrogenous base. The sugar component in DNA is deoxyribose, whereas ribose is used in RNA. The five nitrogenous bases are uracil (U), thymine (T), cytosine (C), guanine (G), and adenosine (A). Both DNA and RNA use the bases C, G, and A; DNA also uses T, and RNA also uses U.

DNA molecules are the largest molecules in the body. They are composed of two long polynucleotide chains that run parallel to each other (Figure 15-7). The sugar-phosphate part of the molecule faces toward the outside, and its bases point inward, toward the bases of the other chain. Each base in one chain is joined to a base in the other chain by hydrogen bonds, forming a base pair. DNA base pairs always consist of A with T and G with C. The double chains coil around each other to form a double helix. The DNA molecule looks like a twisted ladder, with the rails of the ladder being the sugar-phosphate backbone of the nucleotide chain and the rungs of the ladder the base pairs connected by hydrogen bonds.

Although a DNA molecule contains only two types of base pairs (A-T and G-C), millions of them are present in each DNA molecule. It is amazing to realize that the millions of base pairs occur in the same sequence in all the millions of DNA molecules in one individual's body, but in a different sequence in the DNA of another person's body. In other words, the base pair sequence in DNA is unique to each individual.

DNA may carry the genetic information necessary for synthesis of proteins specific for a given species, but RNA acts as the machinery for this process. RNA is used to translate the genetic information stored in DNA into protein structures. RNA consists of a single strand of a polynucleotide and occurs in three basic forms: messenger RNA (mRNA), transfer RNA (tRNA), and ribosomal RNA (rRNA).

Tiny cellular particles called *ribosomes* are the sites of protein synthesis. They consist of numerous proteins and three to four rRNA molecules. In addition to providing a surface for protein synthesis, ribosomes contain enzymes

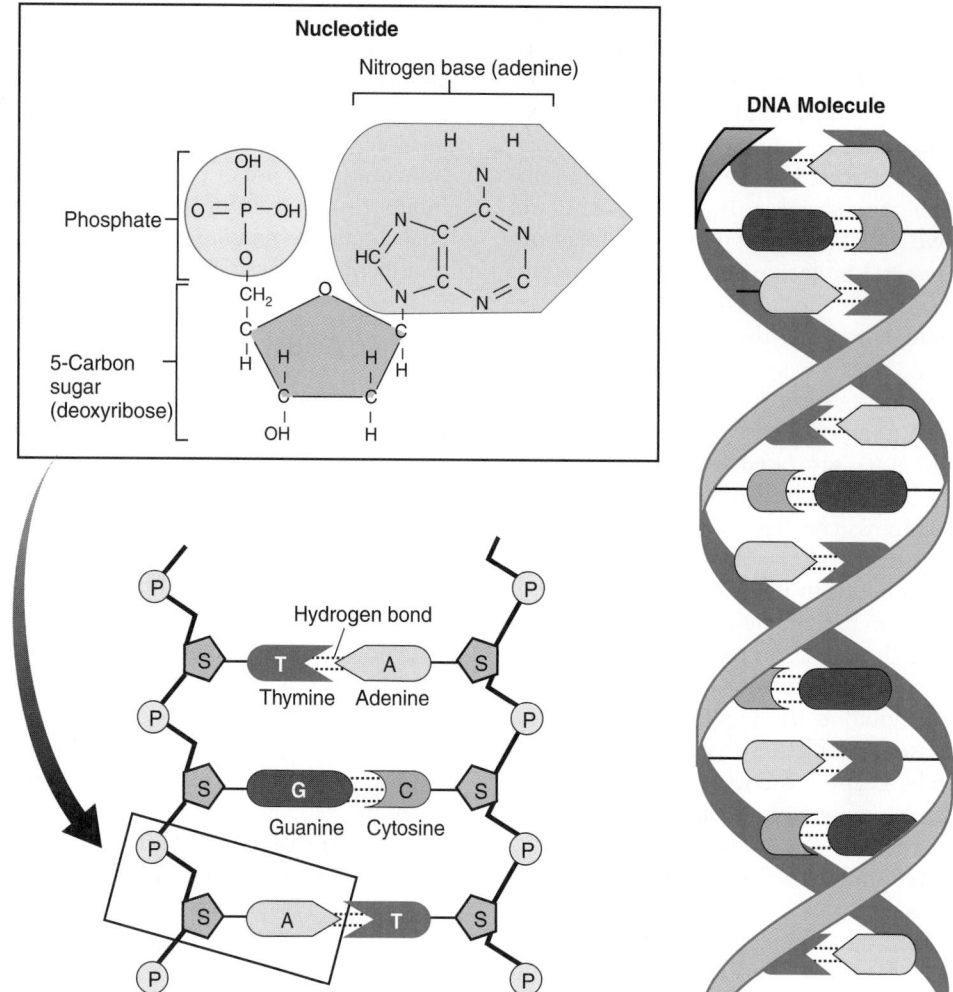

Figure 15-7   Structure of the DNA molecule.

that catalyze the process. A mRNA molecule diffuses about the cell and attaches itself to a ribosome, where it acts as a pattern for protein synthesis. A sequence of three base pairs in a mRNA molecule acts as the code for a particular amino acid. This sequence is called a *codon,* and each codon represents one of the 20 different amino acids. The attached mRNAs codons provide the sequence of amino acids for a protein that will be synthesized. A tRNA molecule then bonds to a particular amino acid and carries it to a ribosome. It attaches itself to a mRNA codon through base pairing. Once the sequence of amino acids is complete, a termination codon signals the end of the polypeptide, and the finished product, a protein, is released from the ribosome.

In addition to their role in DNA and RNA, nucleotides have other important biologic functions. Most notable is their role in the production of high-energy triphosphate, or **adenosine triphosphate (ATP),** which is the main molecule used to storage energy. Another important nucleotide group is the cyclic nucleotides, such as cyclic 3′5′-adenosine monophosphate (cAMP), which, among other

functions, is involved in relaxation of the smooth muscles of the airways (bronchodilation).

Clinical Chemistry

Fluid and Electrolyte Balance

The human body is composed primarily of water, which accounts for 45% to 80% of an individual's total body weight. The weight of a newborn infant is 75% to 80% water, that of a woman, 45% to 50%, and that of a man, 55% to 60%. These percentages vary depending on the person's age, gender, and weight. People with a higher fat content have a lower water content per kilogram of body weight. Women have relatively less total water content than men primarily because of their higher percentage of fat.

Water in the body is functionally distributed between two major areas, the intracellular compartment and the extracellular compartment. Intracellular fluid is a solvent in the cells that facilitates intracellular chemical reactions. Extracellular fluid serves the dual roles of providing a relatively constant environment for cells and transporting substances to and from the cell. Approximately 55% to 60% of the body's water is intracellular and 40% to 45% is extracellular (Figure 15-8). The extracellular fluid compartment is composed of five areas: (1) the interstitial compartment, which accounts for the fluid outside or between the cells (15% of total body water); (2) the intravascular (plasma) compartment, which accounts for the fluid in the heart and blood vessels (7.5%); (3) dense connective tissue, cartilage, and bone (15%); (4) lymph (5%); and (5) the transcellular compartment, which includes the fluid in the salivary glands, thyroid gland, gonads, mucous membranes of the respiratory and gastrointestinal tracts, kidneys, liver, pancreas, cerebrospinal fluid, joint fluid, and the fluid in the spaces of the eyes (2.5%). The interstitial and intravascular compartments are the extracellular areas most involved with fluid balance.

The normal daily water intake is 2400 to 2500 mL, which is offset by an equal amount of fluid output. Fluid is taken in primarily through daily food (~700 mL) and drink (~1500 mL), but some also comes from body metabolism (~200 mL a day). In the oxidation of food, about 14 mL of water is produced for every 100 kcal of energy released. The type of energy substrate oxidized determines the volume of water produced: 100 g of carbohydrate produces 55 g of water; 100 g of fat produces 107 g of water; and 100 g of protein produces 41 g of water.

Fluid loss occurs as a sensible loss through the kidneys as urine (~1400 mL a day) and the gastrointestinal tract as feces (~200 mL a day) or as an insensible loss through the skin as perspiration (~450 mL a day) or from the lungs as expired water vapor (~350 mL a day). The volume of insensible loss is higher with vigorous muscular exercise, with an increased respiratory rate, in a hot, dry environment, with a fever, or with severe skin burns.

The various compartments are separated by semipermeable membranes that allow certain fluids and solutes to move freely between them. The movement of water between compartments is maintained by a dynamic equilibrium among five interdependent factors: intake and output, osmotic and hydrostatic pressure, hormones, electrolyte concentration, and the cardiovascular system.

An important concept in fluid balance is that the amount of fluid taken in must equal the amount of fluid leaving the body. If this does not occur, the fluid level in the various compartments must change. The body's primary mechanism to maintain total body fluid volume is adjustment in the amount of fluid leaving the body through the volume of urine excreted. Although it is difficult for the body to control the amount a person eats or drinks, it can influence the desire to do so through thirst and hunger.

The composition of the solutions in the different compartments has a major effect on fluid balance. The principal difference in the composition of the intracellular, intravascular, and interstitial fluids is the difference in the protein and salt concentrations. As shown in Table 15-5,

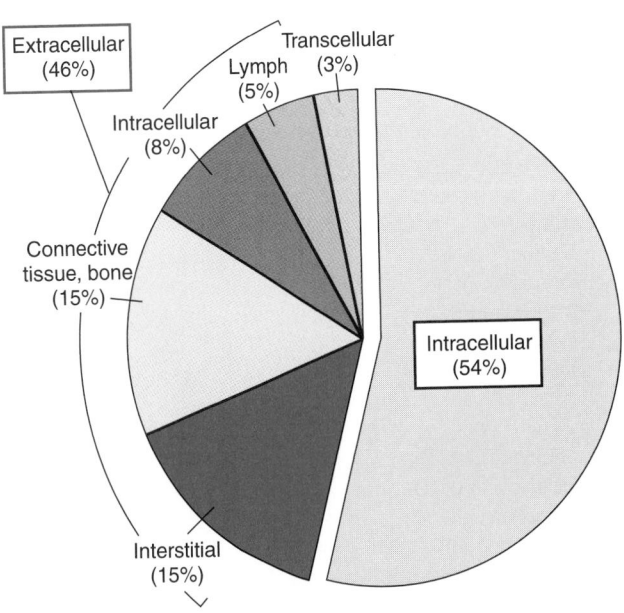

Figure 15-8   Fluid compartments of the body.

EQUATION 15-16
Calculation of mEq/L

$$mEq/L = \frac{mg/100 \text{ ml} \times 10 \times Valence}{Atomic\ weight}$$

Example: To convert 16 mg% of potassium to mEq/L, (atomic weight = 39, valence = 1):

$$mEq/L = \frac{16 \times 10 \times 1}{39} = \frac{160}{39} = 4.1$$

the electrolyte concentration of the extracellular compartments is very similar, with the major cation being sodium and the major anions being chlorine and bicarbonate. The intravascular compartment has a much higher protein concentration than the interstitial compartment, thereby generating an osmotic pressure that helps keep fluid in the vascular space and out of the interstitial space. Extracellular and intracellular fluids are more unlike chemically than they are similar. The primary intracellular cation is potassium, and the major anion is phosphate, and the protein content is highest in the cells.

The unit of measurement for electrolytes is the number of milliequivalents per liter of solution (mEq/L). Milliequivalents measure the number of ionic charges or electrovalent bonds in a solution and therefore are an accurate measure of the chemical combining power, or reactivity, of the electrolyte solution. The number of milliequivalents can be determined from the weight of the ion in 100 mL of the solution (mg%) (Equation 15-16).

TABLE 15-5

Electrolyte Concentrations of Body Fluids

Electrolyte	Intravascular Concentration (mEq/L)	Interstitial Concentration (mEq/L)	Intracellular Concentration (mEq/L)
Cations			
Sodium (Na^+)	142	145	10
Potassium (K^+)	4	4	158
Magnesium (Mg^{+2})	3	2	35
Calcium (Ca^{+2})	5	3	2
TOTAL	154	154	205
Anions			
Chloride (Cl^-)	103	115	2
Bicarbonate (HCO_3^-)	27	30	8
Phosphate (PO_4^{-2})	2	2	140
Sulfate (SO_4^{-2})	1	1	—
Protein ($Prot^-$)	16	1	55
Organic acids	5	5	—
TOTAL	154	154	205

One important mechanism used to control extracellular fluid (ECF) volume is the electrolyte concentration, specifically that of sodium. The phrase, "Where sodium goes, water soon follows," can aid in remembering this concept. When the ECF and blood volume are reduced, for example, from lack of fluid intake, the arterial blood pressure declines. This stimulates pressure receptors (baroreceptors) in the hypothalamus and thorax to stimulate the adrenal cortex to increase secretion of the hormone aldosterone. Aldosterone increases resorption of sodium in the kidney tubule, which leads to an increase in kidney tubule resorption of water and a reduction in urine volume. The reduced urine volume increases the ECF volume and steers it back toward a normal balance.

Stimulation of the hypothalamus also triggers the pituitary gland to secrete antidiuretic hormone (ADH). ADH functions to reduce the amount of water excreted by promoting resorption of water into the circulation at the renal tubules. The pituitary gland can also trigger secretion of ADH after receiving a signal from the baroreceptors in the aortic bodies that the blood pressure is low.

Two factors working together determine urine volume: the kidney glomerular filtration rate and the rate of water resorption by the renal tubules. Except under abnormal conditions, the filtration rate is fairly constant and is not a major factor in urine excretion. The rate of tubular resorption, on the other hand, fluctuates considerably. During the course of a single day, the kidneys filter 190 L of water, yet reabsorb 189 L. As already discussed, the amounts of the hormones secreted by the pituitary gland (ADH) and the adrenal cortex (aldosterone) regulate water resorption.

Another important mechanism that regulates the water and electrolyte levels in the extracellular fluid is the pres-

EQUATION 15-17

Starling's Law

Starling's law is expressed as:

$$Q_f = K_1 (P_{ch} - P_{ih}) - K_2 (P_{co} - P_{io})$$

where

Q_f = Effective filtration pressure between blood and interstitial fluid, which determines the bulk or net outward flow of fluid from the capillaries
P_{ch} = Capillary hydrostatic pressure
P_{ih} = Interstitial hydrostatic pressure
P_{co} = Capillary osmotic pressure
P_{io} = Interstitial osmotic pressure
K_1 = Capillary permeability coefficient for fluids and electrolytes
K_2 = Capillary permeability coefficient for proteins

sure gradient. According to the physical laws governing filtration and osmosis, hydrostatic pressure tends to push fluid out of its compartment, whereas osmotic pressure tends to pull water into its compartment. English physiologist Ernest Starling proposed a mechanism that controls movement across capillary membranes (Equation 15-17). Because the intravascular compartment contains a larger number of proteins than the interstitial compartment (see Table 15-5), a larger osmotic pressure is generated in the vascular space. At the arterial end of tissue capillaries, normal values for the various pressures are P_{ch}, 35 mm Hg; P_{co}, 24 mm Hg; P_{ih}, 2 mm Hg; and P_{io}, 0 mm Hg (Figure 15-9), where:

P_{ch} = Capillary hydrostatic pressure
P_{co} = Capillary osmotic pressure

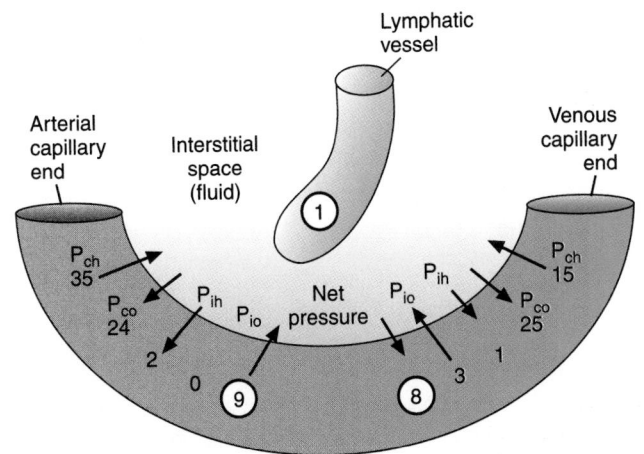

Figure 15-9 Starling's law governs the movement of fluids between the capillary and interstitial fluid compartments based on hydrostatic (capillary P_{ch} and interstitial P_{ih}) and osmotic (capillary P_{co} and interstitial P_{io}) pressure differences. (See text for details.)

P_{ih} = Interstitial hydrostatic pressure
P_{io} = Interstitial osmotic pressure

Therefore the net filtration pressure at the arterial end of the capillaries is as follows:

$$(35 - 2) - (24 - 0) = 33 - 24 = 9 \text{ mm Hg}$$

This equation means that a net pressure of 9 mm Hg tends to push fluids from the vascular space at the arterial end of the capillaries. At the venous end of the tissue capillaries, normal pressures are P_{ch}, 15 mm Hg; P_{co}, 25 mm Hg; P_{ih}, 1 mm Hg; and P_{io}, 3 mm Hg. The net filtration pressure of the venous end of the capillaries is as follows:

$$(15 - 1) - (25 - 3) = 14 - 22 = -8 \text{ mm Hg}$$

This equation means that a net pressure of 8 mm Hg tends to pull fluids in toward the vascular space at the venous end of the capillaries. As blood flows through the capillary tissue bed, the tendency is for fluid to be pushed out into the interstitial space at the arterial end (net outward pressure of 9 mm Hg) and pulled back into the capillaries from the interstitial space at the venous end (8 mm Hg). Interstitial fluid that is not pulled back into the capillaries is drained via the lymphatic system.

Of the three main body compartmental fluids, interstitial fluid varies the most. Plasma volume usually fluctuates only slightly and briefly. If an abnormally large amount of fluid shifts to the interstitial (and eventually to the intercellular) tissue space, the condition is known as *edema*. Edema can be caused by any of the factors governing the movement of fluids between the vascular and interstitial compartments, including (1) retention of electrolytes (especially sodium) in the extracellular fluid as a result of increased aldosterone secretion or after serious renal disease; (2) an increase in capillary hydrostatic pressure, as is seen in congestive heart failure caused by left ventricular failure; and (3) a decrease

in plasma proteins because of a low overall protein concentration, such as that caused by poor nutrition (reflected in a low serum albumin level) or because of increased capillary permeability, such as that caused by infection, burns, or shock. Increased capillary permeability allows protein molecules to leak out of the vascular space into the interstitial space, where they exert an osmotic pressure.

The electrolyte concentrations in the various body fluids serve important functions in addition to their role in fluid balance. Table 15-6 lists the primary functions of seven major electrolytes and important ions—sodium, potassium, calcium, chloride, bicarbonate, phosphate, and magnesium—as well as the effects on the body of abnormal levels of these components.

Acid-Base Balance

Acid-base balance is one of the crucial homeostatic mechanisms of the body. The pH at the cellular level must be maintained at a relatively constant concentration; even slight deviations can cause potentially fatal changes in metabolic activity.

Although acids and bases continuously enter the blood from absorbed foods and metabolic nutrients at the cellular level, it is the hydrogen ion concentration in the extracellular fluid that determines homeostasis of the body pH. Hydrogen ions continuously enter the body fluids in the form of carbonic acid, lactic acid, sulfuric acid, and phosphoric acid and as acidic ketone bodies.

Carbonic acid and lactic acid are metabolic products of the aerobic and anaerobic breakdown of glucose, respectively. Sulfuric acid is produced by the oxidation of sulfur-containing amino acids, and phosphoric acid accumulates after the breakdown of phosphoproteins and nucleoproteins for energy. Acidic ketone bodies, such as acetone, can be produced by the incomplete breakdown of fats.

Carbonic acid exists in an equilibrium with gaseous CO_2 and is referred to as a *volatile acid*. It is excreted in its gaseous form by the lungs. Sulfuric, lactic, and phosphoric acids are referred to as *nonvolatile*, or *fixed*, *acids*. They do not come into equilibrium with nor originate from a gaseous component. Fixed acids therefore are excreted not by the lungs but by the kidneys. The lungs eliminate most of the acid load, excreting approximately 24,000 mmol a day of CO_2 through the lungs, compared with the removal of 50 to 70 mmol a day of fixed acid by the kidneys.

After food is metabolized, the minerals that remain as byproducts are considered to be either acid or base forming, depending on whether they form an acid or a base medium when in solution. Chlorine, sulfur, and phosphorus are acid-forming elements. They are abundant in high-protein foods such as meat, fish, poultry, and eggs. Potassium, calcium, sodium, and magnesium are base-forming foods. These elements are found in fruits and vegetables. After the metabolism of these foods, the basic and acidic residues must be buffered so that the blood pH does not vary too far from the normal range.

TABLE 15-6

Primary Functions of Seven Important Ions and Effects of Abnormal Levels

Ion	Primary Functions	Normal Serum Level	Below Normal Serum Level	Above Normal Serum Level
Sodium (Na⁺)	Maintain extracellular osmotic pressure Control water retention in tissue spaces Help maintain blood pressure Maintain body's acid-base balance by means of bicarbonate buffer system Regulate irritability of nerve and muscle tissue, including the heart	136 to 145 mEq/L	**Hyponatremia** *Causes* Dilutional (water intake exceeds output) Renal failure Increased output of ADH Severe hyperglycemia Congestive heart failure Hepatic cirrhosis Third spacing of fluids (burns, pancreatitis, trauma) Diuretic excess *Clinical signs and symptoms* Cold, clammy extremities Low blood pressure Weak, rapid pulse Muscular weakness Apathy, headache, nausea, and disorientation Low specific gravity (<1.01)	**Hypernatremia** *Causes* Low water intake Excessive water loss caused by hyperventilation, excessive sweating, or fever Osmotic diuretic therapy Diabetes insipidus Diarrhea High salt intake Poor kidney excretion Hyperactivity of the adrenal cortex (Cushing's disease) Hypercalcemia, hypokalemia *Clinical signs and symptoms* Intense thirst Flushed skin, sweating Low or no urine output Dry, itchy mucous membranes Rough, dry tongue Diarrhea High urine specific gravity (>1.03)
Potassium (K⁺)	Maintain cellular osmotic pressure Maintain cellular electrical potential Maintain cell size Maintain proper heart contraction Maintain proper nerve impulse transmission	3.5 to 5.5 mEq/L	**Hypokalemia** *Causes* Inadequate intake of potassium (K⁺) ions because of starvation or malnutrition, diet deficient in potassium, or IV infusions lacking potassium Excessive loss of K⁺ ions because of use of diuretics or corticosteroids, prolonged vomiting, gastric suctioning or intestinal drainage, or diarrhea and vomiting *Clinical signs and symptoms* Lack of energy Muscular weakness Numbness of fingers and toes Cramps (especially in calf muscles) Weak pulse, reduced blood pressure ECG changes	**Hyperkalemia** *Causes* Too rapid IV infusion of potassium Renal failure Acute dehydration Sudden shift in K⁺ ions from intracellular to extracellular space because of severe burns, crush injury, or acidosis Hypoaldosteronism *Clinical signs and symptoms* Muscular weakness Listlessness Mental confusion Bradycardia, eventually cardiac arrest ECG changes

ADH, Antidiuretic hormone; ECG, electrocardiogram; IV, intravenous.

TABLE 15-6

Primary Functions of Seven Important Ions and Effects of Abnormal Levels—cont'd

Ion	Primary Functions	Normal Serum Level	Below Normal Serum Level	Above Normal Serum Level
Calcium (Ca^{+2})	Mediate neuromuscular function Mediate cellular enzyme processes	8.4 to 10.5 mg/dL	**Hypocalcemia** *Causes* Hypoparathyroidism Acute pancreatitis Septic shock Renal failure Severe trauma Vitamin D deficiency Magnesium deficiency Hypoproteinosis *Clinical signs and symptoms* Hyperactive tendon reflexes Muscular twitching and spasm Abdominal cramps ECG changes Tetany, seizures	**Hypercalcemia** *Causes* Hyperthyroidism, hyperparathyroidism Diuretic therapy Cancer with metastases to the bones Sarcoidosis Prolonged immobilization Renal failure Vitamin D intoxication *Clinical signs and symptoms* Fatigue Depression Muscle weakness Anorexia, nausea, vomiting, constipation Stupor, coma
Magnesium (Mg^{+2})	Is important for neuromuscular function Activates more enzymes than any other metal ion in the body (more than 100 metabolic reactions)	1.3 to 2.1 mEq/L	**Hypomagnesemia** *Causes* Malabsorption syndromes Condition found in hypercalcemia, hyperaldosteronism, and inappropriate secretion of ADH Diuretic therapy Nasogastric suction, diarrhea Acute pancreatitis *Clinical signs and symptoms* Severe cases (<1 mEq/L): muscle weakness (including respiratory) Tetany ECG changes Anorexia, nausea, vomiting	**Hypermagnesemia** *Causes* Hypoparathyroidism Alcoholism Dehydration Renal insufficiency *Clinical signs and symptoms* Potentiator of cardiac effect of hyperkalemia, ECG changes, and bradycardia Respiratory depression Depressed mental status
Chloride (Cl^-)	Is most prominent anion in extracellular fluid Is major component of gastric hydrochloric acid Is important in transport of oxygen and CO_2 in the blood	98 to 106 mEq/L	**Hypochloremia** *Causes* Prolonged vomiting, diarrhea Profuse sweating Diuretics Depletion of potassium ions *Clinical signs and symptoms* Vomiting Profuse sweating Diarrhea Muscle spasm	**Hyperchloremia** *Causes* Dehydration Metabolic acidosis Respiratory alkalosis *Clinical signs and symptoms* Minimal

Continued

TABLE 15-6

Primary Functions of Seven Important Ions and Effects of Abnormal Levels—cont'd

Ion	Primary Functions	Normal Serum Level	Below Normal Serum Level	Above Normal Serum Level

Bicarbonate (HCO_3^-)	Is major extracellular anion
	Is primary means of CO_2 transport
	Is important buffer in acid-base balance
		22 to 26 mEq/L	**Low Bicarbonate Level**
			Causes
			    Metabolic acidosis due to renal failure, diabetic ketoacidosis, lactic acidosis, exogenous poisons (ethanol, methanol, glycerol, salicylates), or gastrointestinal loss (diarrhea, colostomy)
			    Respiratory alkalemia
			Clinical signs and symptoms
			    Nausea, vomiting
			    Hyperpnea
			    Circulatory shock
				High Bicarbonate Level
				Causes
				    Metabolic alkalosis due to diuretic therapy, vomiting or GI drainage, or steroid administration
				    Respiratory acidemia
				Clinical signs and symptoms
				    Irritability
				    Tetany
				    Muscular weakness

Phosphate (PO_4^-)	Is primary intracellular anion
	Is important buffer in acid-base balance
	Is required for production of ATP
		2.5 to 4.5 mg/dL	**Hypophosphatemia**
			Causes
			    Hyperparathyroidism
			    Starvation
			    Uncontrolled diabetes
			    Association with hypercalcemia, respiratory alkalosis, and metabolic acidosis
			    Sepsis
			    Chronic diarrhea
			Clinical signs and symptoms
			    Possible diaphragmatic weakness during respiratory failure
			    Muscle weakness
			    Impaired cardiac contractility
				Hyperphosphatemia
				Causes
				    Tissue trauma
				    Hypoparathyroidism
				    Bowel infarction
				    Chronic renal disease and acute kidney failure
				    Association with hypocalcemia
				    Vitamin D intoxication
				    Acid-base disorders (lactic and respiratory acidosis)
				    Hypomagnesemia
				Clinical signs and symptoms
				    Tetany
				    Hypocalcemia

ATP, Adenosine triphosphate; GI, gastrointestinal.

Two major types of buffer control systems that maintain a constant pH. Chemical buffers combine immediately with any acid or alkali that enter the body. Examples are the bicarbonate and phosphate buffering systems. Physiologic buffers act as a secondary defense against major pH swings if the chemical buffers are unable to stabilize the pH. The respiratory response and the renal response are examples of physiologic buffer systems. Chemical buffers act immediately, whereas the response from the physiologic systems is delayed, occurring within 1 to 2 minutes for the respiratory system and within hours for the kidneys.

Chemical buffers consist of two kinds of substances, which are referred to as *buffer pairs*. Most of the body fluid buffer pairs consist of a weak acid and the salt of that acid (Table 15-7). The chemical buffer systems commonly are divided into two categories: the bicarbonate system, which accounts for 53% of the total blood buffering capacity, and the nonbicarbonate system, consisting of the hemoglobin, plasma proteins, and phosphate buffer pairs, which is responsible for the remaining 47% of the total blood buffering capacity.

Chemical buffers react with a strong acid or base to replace it with a relatively weak acid or base. A strong acid completely dissociates in solution, thereby forming a large number of hydrogen ions, whereas a weak acid produces fewer hydrogen ions because it does not completely dissociate. Buffer reactions replace a strong acid, which would contribute many hydrogen ions and drastically change the solution pH, with a weaker acid, which contributes fewer hydrogen ions and results in less of a pH change. As an example, consider the way the bicarbonate buffer pair handles the addition of a strong acid such

TABLE 15-7

Examples of Buffers in the Body

Type of Buffer	Total Blood Buffering Capacity (%)	Weak Acid	Salt
Bicarbonate pairs	53	H_2CO_3	$NaHCO_3$
		H_2CO_3	$KHCO_3$
Hemoglobin pairs	35	Hb	K · Hb
		HbO_2	K · HbO_2
Plasma protein pairs	7	Proteins	Na · Proteinate
Phosphate buffer pairs	5	NaH_2PO_4	Na_2HPO_4

EQUATION 15-18

Buffer Reactions

Addition of a strong acid to a buffer:

HCl	+	$NaHCO_3$	→	H_2CO_3	+	NaCl
Strong acid		Salt of weak acid		Weak acid		Salt of strong acid

Addition of a strong base to a buffer:

NaOH	+	H_2CO_3	→	$NaHCO_3$	+	H_2O
Strong base		Weak acid		Salt of weak acid		

EQUATION 15-19

Reactions Involving Carbon Dioxide in the Red Blood Cell

$$CO_2 + H_2O \rightarrow H_2CO_3$$
$$H_2CO_3 + K \cdot Hb \rightarrow KHCO_3 + H \cdot Hb$$
$$KHCO_3 \rightarrow K^+ + HCO_3^-$$

as hydrochloric acid (Equation 15-18). As a result of the buffering action of the base bicarbonate ($NaHCO_3$), the weak acid (H_2CO_3) replaces the strong acid in the reaction, thereby lowering its pH only slightly. A strong base completely dissociates, forming a large number of hydroxide ions (OH^-). Note the way the same bicarbonate buffering pair reacts to the addition of a strong base, such as sodium hydroxide. The hydrogen ion of the weak acid of the buffer pair combines with the OH^- of the strong base to form water. This reaction results in fewer OH^- ions in solution and less of a drastic rise in pH after the addition of a strong base. The buffering principles summarized here for the bicarbonate buffer pair can be applied equally to the plasma protein, hemoglobin, and phosphate buffer systems.

The bicarbonate buffer system is effective only in buffering fixed acids because one of its buffer pairs is the weak but volatile acid carbonic acid (H_2CO_3). The following changes in the blood result from buffering of fixed acids in tissue capillaries: (1) the amount of carbonic acid increases because strong acids are converted to H_2CO_3; (2) the amount of blood bicarbonate (mainly as $NaHCO_3$) decreases to become part of the H_2CO_3; (3) the blood hydrogen ion concentration increases slightly; and (4) the blood pH declines slightly.

Carbonic acid is produced by the buffering of fixed acids and from the combination of CO_2 and water. It is the most abundant acid in body fluids and is buffered by the nonbicarbonate buffer system. As a cellular waste product, CO_2 diffuses out of tissue cells into the blood plasma, where it combines with water with the help of the RBC enzyme carbonic anhydrase to form carbonic acid (Equation 15-19). Carbonic acid is buffered primarily by the potassium salt of hemoglobin inside the RBC to form $KHCO_3$. While still in the RBC, the $KHCO_3$ dissociates to potassium and bicarbonate ions, and the bicarbonate ion diffuses out of the cell. When the negative bicarbonate ion (HCO_3^-) moves out of the cell, a negative chloride ion (Cl^-) moves into the cell to maintain electrical neutrality. The process by which negative ions are exchanged,

referred to as the *chloride shift*, makes it possible for CO_2 to be buffered in the RBC and then carried as bicarbonate in the plasma to the lungs for excretion.

Chemical buffers alone cannot maintain homeostasis of the blood pH. If hydrogen ions keep entering the system, buffers prevent the pH from dropping dramatically, but they do not stop it from becoming more acidic. The physiologic buffering response systems eliminate the acids through the lungs and the kidneys.

The degree to which the blood pH changes depends on the ratio of base bicarbonate to carbonic acid buffer. A ratio of 20:1 in the extracellular fluid provides a neutral blood pH of 7.4. The relationship between the [H^+] of body fluids and the ratio of base bicarbonate to carbonic acid is mathematically expressed by the **Henderson-Hasselbalch equation.** This equation is derived from the ionization constant for carbonic acid, the acid component of the bicarbonate buffer system (Equation 15-20). The ratio of HCO_3^- to H_2CO_3 for a pH of 7.4 is 24:1.2, or 20:1. If the ratio goes up by means of an elevation in bicarbonate or a reduction in the partial

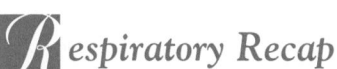

Respiratory Recap

Henderson-Hasselbalch Equation

The pH of a buffer is determined by the ratio of the concentration of base to the concentration of weak acid.

In the blood, an important base is bicarbonate, and the important acid is CO_2. Therefore the pH of the blood is determined by the ratio of bicarbonate to the partial pressure of carbon dioxide (Pco_2).

pressure of carbon dioxide (P_{CO_2},) the pH increases, or become more basic or alkaline. The opposite occurs if the ratio goes down. Either a reduction in the bicarbonate or an increase in P_{CO_2} causes the pH to decrease and become more acidic.

If all the constants are eliminated in the Henderson-Hasselbalch equation, a relationship between the kidneys and lungs is evident (Equation 15-21). The respiratory system plays a vital part in controlling body pH. Although the lungs can excrete only volatile acids (H_2CO_3), they can excrete vast amounts very quickly. Because carbonic acid is formed as the result of metabolism and from the buffering of fixed acids, the body has 500 times more of it than any other acid.

CO_2 excretion is proportional to the level of alveolar ventilation. As the level of CO_2 increases, the level of ventilation must increase to eliminate this volatile acid. The major controller of the degree of ventilation is the brain. The primary respiratory center is located in the medulla of the brain, which contains nerve cell areas that are sensitive to certain chemicals (chemoreceptors). The medullary chemoreceptors are bathed in cerebrospinal fluid (CSF) and respond directly to the pH of this fluid. As blood CO_2 rises, not only is blood pH reduced, but the

CO_2 molecules readily cross the gas permeable blood-brain barrier and act to reduce the CSF pH as well. The acidic CSF pH triggers the medullary center to cause the respirator muscles to increase the rate or depth of breathing and therefore the level of alveolar ventilation.

The nonvolatile (fixed) acids are eliminated by the kidneys in the urine through a process referred to as *acidification* of the urine. The kidney tubules help adjust the blood pH by excreting hydrogen ions or by conserving base. As stated earlier, one of the functions of the kidneys is to conserve or resorb sodium. Approximately 80% of the resorption of sodium is accomplished at the proximal tubules, where chloride is resorbed with the sodium. The remaining 20% of sodium resorption is accomplished at the distal tubules, where the sodium ion (Na^+) is exchanged for either hydrogen ions (H^+) or potassium ions (K^+).

CO_2 diffuses from the tubule capillary into the distal tubule cell, where carbonic anhydrase catalyzes it and water to form carbonic acid. The carbonic acid dissociates into hydrogen and bicarbonate ions, where the hydrogen ions diffuse into the tubular urine and displace sodium from a basic salt, such as Na_2HPO_4. The sodium ion diffuses back into the tubule cell, where it combines with the bicarbonate ion and together with the sodium bicarbonate is absorbed back into the blood. The hydrogen ions combine with $NaHPO_4^-$ ions to form the weak acid salt NaH_2PO_4 and are excreted in the urine.

Hydrogen ions also are excreted in the urine by means of another mechanism. As the amino acid glutamine moves into the tubule cell, it loses an amine group (NH_2^-), which picks up a hydrogen ion to form ammonia (NH_3). The ammonia is excreted into the tubular urine, where it combines with another hydrogen ion to form an ammonia ion (NH_4^+), which displaces sodium or some other basic ion from a salt of a fixed acid to form an ammonium salt (such as NH_4Cl). The basic ion (such as Na^+) then diffuses back into the tubule cell and combines with bicarbonate ions to form a basic salt, which then diffuses into tubular blood. The hydrogen and chloride ions excreted into the urine combine with ammonia already in the urine to form the weak acid salt NH_4Cl.

Nutrition and Metabolism

The word *metabolism* is derived from the Greek word *meta* for "change." Metabolism represents the sum of the chemical processes that convert the raw materials (nutrients) necessary to nourish living organisms into energy and the

ℰQUATION 15-20

Derivation of the Henderson-Hasselbalch Equation

$$Kc = \frac{[H^+]\,[HCO_3^-]}{[H_2CO_3]}$$

where Kc is the dissociation constant for carbonic acid. The pH is a logarithmic expression of $[H^+]$. The equation can be rearranged to become:

$$pH = pKc + \log \frac{[HCO_3^-]}{[H_2CO_3]}$$

where pKc is the negative log of the dissociation constant of carbonic acid. Normal pKc in the blood has a value of 6.1. Because of volatile carbonic acid is a transitory intermediate between CO_2 and H^+, the CO_2 is treated as the acid itself and used in the equation. The amount of H_2CO_3 can be quantified by multiplication of the dissolved partial pressure of carbon dioxide $[P_{CO_2}]$ by a factor of 0.03. The final Henderson-Hasselbalch equation then becomes:

$$pH = 6.1 + \log \frac{[HCO_3^-]}{[P_{CO_2} \times 0.03]}$$

If the normal bicarbonate level is 24 mEq/L and normal arterial P_{CO_2} is 40 mm Hg, the pH of arterial blood can be calculated as such:

$$pH = 6.1 + \log \frac{24}{40 \times 0.03}$$

$$pH = 6.1 + \log \frac{24}{1.2}$$

$$pH = 6.1 + \log 20$$
$$pH = 6.1 + 1.3$$
$$pH = 7.4$$

ℰQUATION 15-21

Application of the Henderson-Hasselbalch Equation to Illustrate the Relative Effects of the Kidneys and Lungs

$$pH \approx \frac{[HCO_3^-]}{P_{a CO_2}} \quad \begin{array}{l}\text{(Kidney controlled)}\\[4pt]\text{(Lung controlled)}\end{array}$$

chemically complex final products of the various cells. Nutrition refers to the food human beings eat, which consists of three primary types—carbohydrates, fats, and proteins—as well as essential vitamins and minerals.

Metabolism involves the processes by which these nutrients are used after they are ingested, digested, absorbed, and circulated to the cells of the body. It uses them in two ways, as an energy source to drive vital functions or as the ingredients to make complex chemical compounds. Before nutrients can be used in either way, they must be assimilated, which is the process by which the food molecules are taken into the cells, where they undergo many chemical changes. The process by which chemical energy is released from food molecules is **catabolism,** and the process by which the food molecules are used to build more complex biomolecules is **anabolism.**

Catabolism is a decomposition process involving the oxidation of nutrient molecules. It releases energy (exergonic metabolism) in two forms, as heat or as chemical energy. Heat energy helps maintain the homeostasis of body temperature, but it cannot be used as a form of energy by the cells. Chemical energy, on the other hand, can be used by the cells, but it must first be transferred to high-energy bonds of ATP molecules. These bonds break more easily than other types of chemical bonds and therefore give up their energy more readily. ATP is one of the crucial compounds of the biologic world because it supplies energy directly to the energy-using reactions of all cells in all kinds of living organisms, from one-celled plants to trillion-celled human beings. The end products of catabolism include such molecules as lactic acid, ethanol, CO_2, urea, ammonia, and water.

Anabolism is a synthesis process that assembles precursor molecules, such as amino acids, sugars, fatty acids, and nitrogenous bases, into cell macromolecules such as proteins, polysaccharides, lipids, and nucleic acids. This process requires energy (endergonic metabolism), which is supplied by the ATP generated during catabolism.

These two metabolic processes occur simultaneously in the cell in that some of the energy released and the breakdown products produced during catabolism are immediately used in the process of anabolism. The cell manages the conflicting demands of concomitant catabolism and anabolism in two ways. First, the cell maintains a tight and separate regulation of both processes through the use of literally hundreds of enzymatic reactions organized into discrete pathways. Second, the metabolic pathways are localized in different cellular compartments. For example, the enzymes responsible for fatty acid biosynthesis are found in the cytosol, whereas the fatty acid oxidation process takes place in the mitochondria.

The pathways of catabolism converge to a few end products, and the process consists of three stages (Figure 15-10). Stage 1 involves the breakdown of protein, polysaccharide, and lipid macromolecules into their respective building blocks. Proteins give up their 20 component amino acids; polysaccharides break down to carbohydrate units that are ultimately converted to glucose; and lipids

produce glycerol and fatty acids. The cells prefer glucose as their primary energy fuel and therefore catabolize most of the carbohydrates absorbed and anabolize a relatively small portion of it. Fats and proteins are catabolized only when the amount of glucose entering cells is inadequate for their energy needs.

Stage 2 converts the products from stage 1 into an even more limited set of simpler metabolic byproducts. Fatty acids break down into two-carbon units of acetyl coenzyme A (acetyl-CoA). Glucose and the glycerol from lipids generate the three-carbon α-keto acid pyruvic acid (pyruvate), which breaks down into acetyl-CoA in the presence of oxygen (aerobic metabolism) or to lactic acid when oxygen is absent (anaerobic metabolism). Amino acids give rise to pyruvate, acetyl-CoA, or intermediates fed directly into the citric acid cycle of stage 3. Stage 3 involves the combustion of the acetyl groups of acetyl-CoA by the citric acid cycle and oxidative phosphorylation to yield CO_2, water, and ATP molecules.

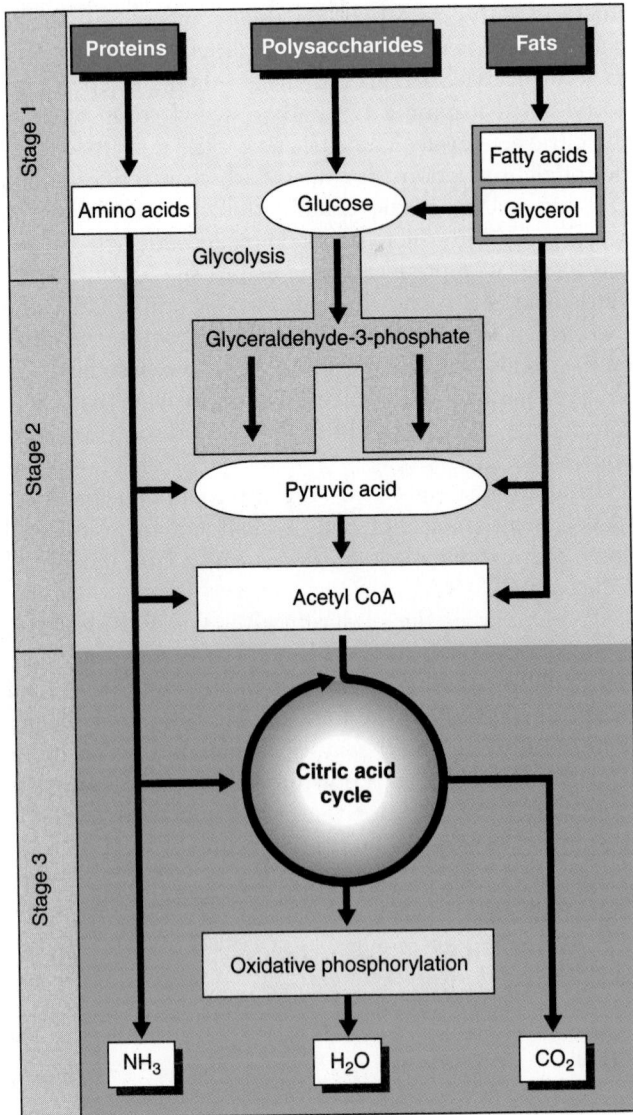

Figure 15-10   Three stages of catabolism. *CoA,* Coenzyme A.

As stated previously, carbohydrates are the primary source of energy. Glucose metabolism begins with the breakdown of a six-carbon glucose chain ($C_6H_{12}O_6$) to two three-carbon pyruvate (pyruvic acid) molecules by means of a process called **glycolysis.** Glycolysis takes place in the cytosol of the cell. It is an anaerobic process in that it does not use oxygen and as such is the only process that provides cells with energy when the oxygen supply is inadequate or even absent. Glycolysis releases about 5% of the energy stored in the glucose molecule, releasing some energy as heat and the rest as energy transferred to ATP molecules and to reduced nicotinamide adenine dinucleotide (NADH) molecules. For every glucose molecule undergoing glycolysis, a net of two ATP molecules are formed. Although only a small amount of energy is released during glycolysis, it is an essential process because it prepares glucose for the second step in catabolism, namely the citric acid cycle.

The **citric acid (Krebs) cycle** converts two pyruvic acid molecules into six CO_2 molecules and six water molecules. The citric acid cycle takes place in the presence of oxygen in the mitochondria of the cell. Before pyruvic acid molecules enter the mitochondria, they combine with coenzyme A to split off CO_2 and a pair of high-energy electrons to form acetyl-CoA. Coenzyme A then detaches from acetyl-CoA, leaving a two-carbon acetyl group to enter the citric acid cycle. The citric acid cycle consists of a series of eight reactions, the first of which is the formation of citric acid from the combination of the two-carbon acetyl group with the four-carbon oxaloacetic acid (which was formed as a product in the eighth step of the cycle). Citric acid is also known as *tricarboxylic acid (TCA)*, and the citric acid cycle therefore is also known as the *TCA cycle;* it is also known as the *Krebs cycle* because Sir Hans Krebs deciphered the cyclic nature of pyruvate oxidation, earning the 1935 Nobel Prize for his work on this metabolic pathway.

In addition to eight acids, the citric acid cycle produces CO_2, a small amount of ATP, a small amount of reduced flavin adenine dinucleotide (FAD), and a large amount of reduced NAD (NADH).

The energy produced during glycolysis and the TCA cycle is not enough to sustain life. The high-energy electrons removed during the first two processes in the form of reduced FAD and NAD enter a chain of carrier molecules that is embedded in the inner membrane of the mitochondria. This process, known as the **electron transport system,** is responsible for the production of 90% of the

ATP formed during carbohydrate catabolism. The most important fact about electron transport is that as electrons move down the carrier chain, they release small bursts of energy to pump protons between the inner and outer membranes of the mitochondria. The diffusion of the protons into the matrix in the inner compartment drives a process called **oxidative phosphorylation,** which refers to the joining of a phosphate group to adenosine diphosphate (ADP) to form ATP. At the end of the electron transport chain, oxygen serves as the final electron receptor to form water (Equation 15-22). The NAD^+—NADH system can be viewed as a shuttle that carries electrons released from catabolic substrates to the mitochondria, where they are transferred to oxygen, the ultimate electron acceptor in catabolism. In the process, the free energy is trapped in ATP molecules. The net result of oxidation of glucose is shown in Equation 15-23. Certain drugs can disrupt the coupling of electron transport and ATP synthesis. Cyanide poisoning is an example of such an uncoupler. Rather than producing ATP, the energy released in electron transport is dissipated as heat, oxygen is not consumed, and death eventually occurs.

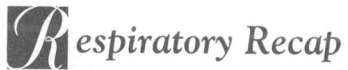

*R*espiratory Recap

Metabolic Pathways
Glycolysis
Citric acid cycle
Electron transport

Carbon Dioxide Production, Oxygen Consumption, and Transport

Respiration can be defined as the physical and chemical processes by which an organism supplies its cells and tissues with the oxygen needed for metabolism and relieves them of the CO_2 formed in energy-producing reactions. The two primary components of this process involve provision of enough oxygen to the body's respiring tissues and removal of the waste product CO_2. Each of these components has two elements: adequate alveolar ventilation via the lungs to bring oxygen into the body and to remove CO_2, and adequate transport mechanisms to carry oxygen to and CO_2 away from the tissues.

*E*QUATION 15-22

Final Reaction in Electron Transport to Generate Water from Oxygen

$$NADH + H^+ + \frac{1}{2}O_2 \rightarrow NAD^+ + H_2O$$
Reductant   Oxidant

*E*QUATION 15-23

Net Result of Oxidation of Glucose

$$Glucose + 38\ ADP + 38\ HPO_4^{-2} + O_2 \rightarrow$$
$$6\ CO_2 + 38\ ATP + 44\ H_2O$$

CO_2 is produced by the cells during the metabolism of carbohydrates, fats, and proteins. The quantity and nature of the metabolism determines the volume of CO_2 produced. When the amount of work done by the body increases, such as during exercise, the quantity of CO_2 produced increases proportionally. The metabolic rate, and therefore CO_2 production, also increases with an increase in body temperature, with severe burns, and during sepsis (bacterial infection of the blood). The nature of the substrate metabolized also determines the amount of CO_2 produced; carbohydrate metabolism produces more CO_2 than does fat or protein metabolism. Normal CO_2 production averages 200 mL/ minute but may range from 120 to 280 mL/minute.

Although CO_2 is produced at the tissue level, it is eliminated by the lungs. Some of these details were explained during the acid-base discussion, but a review is helpful to put the concepts in perspective (Figure 15-11). As CO_2 diffuses from the tissue cells into the blood, it takes one of three transport routes: (1) it can physically dissolve in solution in the plasma and exert a partial pressure (P_{CO_2}), which accounts for about 8% of CO_2 transport; (2) it can combine with carbamino groups, such as proteins (2%) or hemoglobin (10%); or (3) it can be carried as HCO_3^- (80%). Most of the CO_2 is transported as HCO_3^-, which is carried in both the plasma and RBCs. Because gases can rapidly diffuse across semipermeable membranes; therefore when CO_2 diffuses from the tissues into the plasma, it also diffuses into the RBCs. Because the enzyme carbonic anhydrase is present in the RBCs and lacking in plasma, the hydrolysis reaction forming carbonic acid (H_2CO_3) occurs 13,000 times faster in the RBCs. Almost immediately after carbonic acid is formed in the RBCs, it dissociates to HCO_3^- (which diffuses back out to the plasma) and H^+ (which combines with hemoglobin). In the tissues, chlorine ions (Cl^-) move into the RBCs as HCO_3^- leaves them (the chloride shift) to maintain electrostatic equilibrium. The opposite occurs in the lungs: as Cl^- leaves the RBCs, HCO_3^- enters it. Once in the RBCs, HCO_3^- combines with protons from hemoglobin to form carbonic acid, which dissociates to CO_2 and H_2O. The CO_2 then diffuses out to the plasma and into the alveoli, where it is exhaled.

Oxygen is taken into the body via inspired gas and enters the blood at the alveolar-capillary level. It is carried in two compartments of the blood: physically dissolved in the plasma and combined with hemoglobin. The volume of a gas that is dissolved in a liquid depends on the solubility coefficient of the gas in that particular liquid. The solubility coefficient of oxygen for blood at normal body temperature (37° C) equals 0.003 mL of O_2/dL of blood/ mm Hg pressure. This means that for each millimeter of mercury of pressure applied to blood, 0.003 mL of oxygen dissolves into 100 mL of blood. For example, a partial pressure for arterial oxygen (PaO_2) of 100 mm Hg at 37° C would indicate that 0.3 mL of oxygen is dissolved per 100 mL of blood, which is normally referred to as 0.3 vol%.

Most of the oxygen is transported combined with hemoglobin. Hemoglobin (Hb) takes up about one third of the intracellular space of the RBC and has a normal concentration of 14 to 16 g/dL of blood in men and 13 to 14 g/dL in women. In addition to carrying O_2, hemoglobin can carry CO_2 and buffer H^+ ions. When hemoglobin is chemically attached to oxygen, it is referred to as *oxyhemoglobin (HbO_2)*, and when it has not reacted with oxygen, it is called *reduced hemoglobin (HHb)*. The amount of oxygen that can attach to hemoglobin is equal to 1.34 mL of oxygen per gram of hemoglobin. The amount of oxygen carried in the blood chemically attached to hemoglobin is determined as shown in Equation 15-24. The total amount of oxygen in the arterial blood is referred to as the *arterial content of oxygen* (CaO_2) and is the sum of the oxygen dissolved in plasma and the oxygen attached to hemoglobin.

The relationship between the amount of oxygen dissolved in plasma and that combined with hemoglobin is represented by the oxyhemoglobin dissociation curve. With the partial pressure of oxygen (PO_2) on the x axis and oxygen saturation (SO_2) on the y axis, the normal curve has a sigmoidal shape (Figure 15-12) with three distinct areas. This sigmoidal shape indicates a varying affinity of hemoglobin for oxygen. At the start of the curve, a modest rise in PO_2 (PO_2 from 0 to about 20 mm Hg) results in a rather small rise in saturation (SO_2 from 0 to about 25%). The steeply sloped middle section demonstrates a high hemoglobin affinity for oxygen in that the SO_2 rises dramatically (from about 25% to about 90%) as a result in a small change in PO_2 (from about 20 to about 60 mm Hg). The flattened third section demonstrates a low hemoglobin affinity for oxygen in that large increases in PO_2 (from 90 to 150 mm Hg) are required to increase the saturation only marginally (from 90% to 100%).

Several factors can affect the overall position of the curve, shifting it to the right and downward or to the left and upward. A right downward shift corresponds to a reduced hemoglobin affinity for oxygen and can be caused by an increase in such factors as the partial pressure of carbon dioxide (P_{CO_2}), [H^+] (or a reduced pH), temperature,

EQUATION 15-24
Oxygen Content of the Blood

Oxygen Bound to Hemoglobin

Hb × So_2 × 1.34 = Volume % of O_2 attached to Hb

where So_2 is the percentage of oxygen saturation or the percentage of oxyhemoglobin. For example, given a Hb of 15 g/100 mL and a So_2 of 100% (indicating that all the available Hb is saturated with O_2, the total amount of oxygen carried on Hb is equal to 15 × 1 × 1.34 = 20.1 vol%.

Oxygen Content of Arterial Blood

Cao_2 = (0.003 × Pao_2) + (Hb) × Sao_2 × 1.34)

    Dissolved   Attached to

    in plasma   hemoglobin

or 2,3-diphosphoglycerate (2,3-DPG). For a given saturation, the P_{O_2} is higher than normal. This phenomenon normally occurs at the peripheral tissue level to allow greater unloading of oxygen from the hemoglobin, thereby making it more readily available for use by the tissues. A left and upward shift corresponds to a higher affinity of hemoglobin for oxygen, which can be caused by an decrease in P_{CO_2}, $[H^+]$ (or an increased pH), temperature, or 2,3-DPG. A left shift can also be caused by an increase in the level of abnormal hemoglobin species. Carboxyhemoglo-

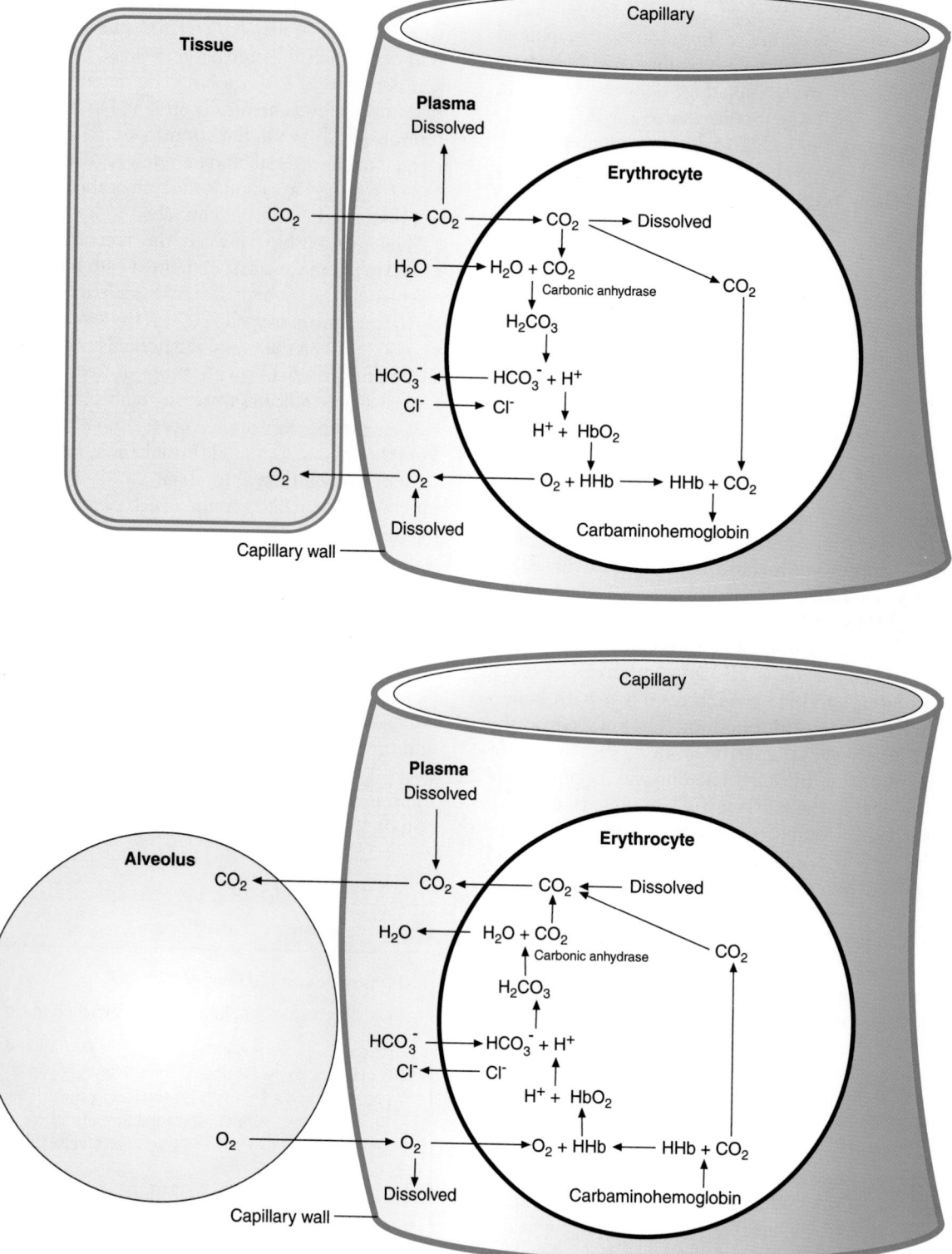

Figure 15-11   Transport of carbon dioxide (CO_2) and oxygen (O_2) at the tissue and lung levels. Note that the process of CO_2 uptake and O_2 release at the tissue level is reversed at the lung level (O_2 uptake and CO_2 release).

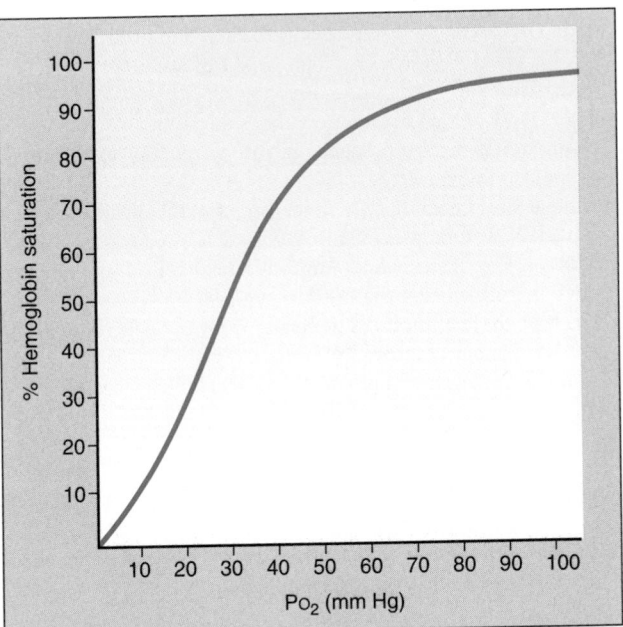

Figure 15-12 Oxyhemoglobin dissociation curve. *Po₂,* Partial pressure of oxygen.

bin (HbCO) is caused by carbon monoxide (CO) binding at the same site as O₂ because of the significantly higher affinity (200 to 250 times) hemoglobin has for CO compared with O₂. Fetal hemoglobin (HbF) is hemoglobin present until 3 to 6 months of age. Methemoglobin (Met-Hb) is caused by the administration of certain drugs, such as nitrates. A slight leftward shift in the oxyhemoglobin curve occurs normally at the lungs, making it easier for oxygen to attach itself to hemoglobin.

Hemoglobin can carry O₂ and CO₂ at the same time because they are carried at different sites on the hemoglobin molecule. The hemoglobin saturation level of O₂ and CO₂ influences the loading or unloading of the other. The affinity of hemoglobin for CO₂ is greater when it is not combined with O₂, and the influence that oxyhemoglobin has on CO₂ transport is referred to as the *Haldane effect*. As hemoglobin becomes more oxygenated at the lungs, the capacity of hemoglobin to hold CO₂ is reduced, and it is easier to unload CO₂ to be exhaled. At the tissues, where the oxyhemoglobin level is low, it is easier for CO₂ to load onto hemoglobin and be carried back to the lungs. On the other hand, the affinity of hemoglobin for O₂ is influenced by the level of CO₂ and [H⁺] and is referred to as the *Bohr effect*. This effect accounts for the normal physiologic shifting of the oxyhemoglobin dissociation curve to the right at the tissues and to the left at the lungs.

Once O₂ is taken into the body, it must be moved to the tissues. Oxygen delivery (Do_2) to the tissues is the product of the amount of O₂ in the arterial blood (arterial O₂ content, or Cao_2) and the amount of blood flowing past the tissues (cardiac output):

$$Do_2 = (Cao_2) \times (Cardiac\ output) \times 10$$

where 10 is a factor to convert the Cao_2 units of milliliters of O₂ per deciliter of blood (vol%) into milliliters of O₂ per liter of blood. Assuming normal values for hemoglobin (15 g), arterial hemoglobin oxygen saturation (Sao_2 97%), Pao_2 (100 mm Hg), and cardiac output (5 L/minute), the normal oxygen delivery or transport to the tissues is approximately 1000 mL O₂/minute.

Tissue utilization of O₂ is the final step in the oxygenation process. Oxygen is the final electron acceptor in the electron transfer chain and is necessary for maximum production of ATP molecules from glucose metabolism. Normal O₂ consumption is about 250 mL/minute, but when indexed to body weight, it is 3 to 3.5 mL O₂/kg body weight/minute.

KEY POINTS

- Atoms consist of protons, neutrons, and electrons.
- Atoms join to produce ionic, covalent, and hydrogen bonds.
- Chemical reactions involve the forming or breaking of chemical bonds.
- The degree to which solute particles dissolve into a solvent is called *solubility*.
- The concentration of a solution can be stated as moles, percent, or mEq/L.
- Colligative properties are the properties of a solution that depend on the number of dissolved solute particles.
- Living organisms are composed of organic and inorganic compounds.
- Electrolytes include acids, bases, and salts.
- Acids are hydrogen ion donors, bases are hydrogen ion acceptors, buffers minimize the change in hydrogen ion concentration, and salts are the result of reactions between acids and bases.
- Carbohydrates are monosaccharides, disaccharides, or polysaccharides.
- Proteins are composed of amino acids.
- Fats, phospholipids, steroids, and prostaglandins are lipids.
- DNA and RNA are nucleic acids.
- DNA carries the genetic information (genes) for protein synthesis.
- Fluid and electrolyte balance is normally maintained within a narrow range.
- Chemical buffers minimize changes in pH when a strong acid or a strong base is added.
- Glycolysis, the citric acid (Krebs) cycle, and electron transport are responsible for energy production in the cell.
- CO₂ is transported physically dissolved in plasma, on carbamino groups, and as bicarbonate.

Recommended Reading

Brown WH. Introduction to organic chemistry. Boston: Willard Grant Press; 1982.

Ebbing DD. General chemistry. 4th ed. Boston: Houghton Mifflin; 1993.

Grishham CM, Garrett RH. Biochemistry. 2nd ed. Fort Worth, Texas: Saunders College; 1999.

Kacmarek RM. Carbon dioxide production, carriage, and transport. In: Pierson DJ, Kacmarek RM, editors. Foundations of respiratory care. New York: Churchill Livingstone; 1992.

Kacmarek RM. Oxygen carriage, transport, and utilization. In: Pierson DJ, Kacmarek RM, editors. Foundations of respiratory care. New York: Churchill Livingstone; 1992.

Malley WJ. Clinical blood gases: application and noninvasive alternatives. Philadelphia: WB Saunders; 1990.

Ouellette RJ. Introduction to general, organic, and biological chemistry. 3rd ed. New York: Macmillan; 1992.

Pierson DJ. Overview of respiratory processes and needs. In: Pierson DJ, Kacmarek RM, editors. Foundations of respiratory care. New York: Churchill Livingstone; 1992.

Ruppel GL, Scanlon CL. Solutions, body fluids, and electrolytes. In: Scanlon CL. Egan's fundamentals of respiratory care. 6th ed. St Louis: Mosby; 1995.

Sachheim GI, Lehamn DD. Chemistry for the health sciences. 5th ed. New York: Macmillan; 1985.

Thibodeau GA, Patton KT. Anthony's textbook of anatomy and physiology. 14th ed. St Louis: Mosby; 1994.

Thibodeau GA, Patton KT. The human body in health and disease. 2nd ed. St Louis: Mosby; 1997.

Thomas G. Chemistry for pharmacy and the life sciences. Herefordshire, England: Prentice Hall; 1996.

Wojciechowski WV. Respiratory care sciences: an integrated approach. Albany, NY: Delmar; 1996.

World Book Encyclopedia of Science. Vol 3. Chicago: World Book; 1991. Chemistry Today.

CHAPTER 16

Respiratory Microbiology, Infection, and Infection Control

Christopher Carter
Mary K. Stone

CHAPTER **OUTLINE**

Basic Microbiology
   Bacteria
   Chlamydiae
   Rickettsiae
   Mycoplasmas
   Mycobacteria
   Viruses
   Fungi
   Pneumocystis carinii
   Parasites
Antibiotic Resistance
Infection Control Methods
   Cleaning, Disinfection, and Sterilization
   Equipment Surveillance
   Universal Precautions

Respiratory Infection
   Otitis and Sinusitis
   Pharyngitis, Parapharyngeal Abscess, Epiglottitis,
     Tracheitis/Tracheobronchitis (Croup)
   Bronchitis, Bronchiolitis, and Pneumonia
Nosocomial Infections Related to Respiratory Care
  Equipment
   Equipment-Related Issues
   Infection-Reducing Techniques
Diagnostic Procedures
   Sputum Induction
   Bronchoscopy
   Transtracheal Aspiration
   Nonbronchoscopic Bronchoalveolar Lavage
   Pleural Fluid Analysis
   Acceptable Specimens

OBJECTIVES

1. List the major organisms causing community-acquired, nosocomial, and ventilator-associated pneumonias.
2. Describe the routes of infection for the upper and lower respiratory tracts.
3. Describe the major risk factors associated with development of pneumonia.
4. Identify respiratory care equipment and practices that are potential sources of respiratory infection.
5. Describe techniques used to minimize nosocomial respiratory infection, including universal precautions and hand washing.
6. Define critical (sterile), semicritical (disinfected), and noncritical (clean) equipment and describe the common methods of sterilization.

KEY TERMS

Acid-Fast Bacilli (AFB)	Inoculum	Sterilization
Aerobe	Mantoux Test	Transtracheal Aspiration (TTA)
Anaerobe	Mold	Universal Precautions
Coliforms	Mycosis	Yeast
Disinfection	Normal Flora	
Enteric Bacteria	Nosocomial Pneumonia	
Gram's Stain	Purified Protein Derivative (PPD)	

Basic Microbiology

The respiratory therapist encounters upper and lower airway infections every day. The pathogens responsible for these common illnesses are diverse, representing essentially the entire spectrum of microbiology, including bacteria, viruses, and fungi (and occasionally parasites). Before discussing the clinical aspects of respiratory infection, this chapter briefly reviews the microbiology of respiratory pathogens.

Bacteria

Bacteria are single-celled organisms measuring 0.7 to 3 μm. Belonging to the kingdom Protista (Monera), they have a prokaryotic cell structure, which differs from the eukaryotic structure of plant and animal cells in several ways. As with animals and plants the bacterial genome is encoded by deoxyribonucleic acid (DNA). But unlike eukaryotes, prokaryotic DNA forms only a single, circular chromosome. Like animals and plants, bacteria use ribosomes to translate ribonucleic acid (RNA) into protein products. However these ribosomes differ from eukaryotic ribosomes in structure and size (prokaryotic ribosomes being 70S in size and eukaryotic ribosomes being 80S), a difference targeted by some antibiotics. (S is a standard measure of protein size. It is nondimensional and describes how far [relatively] the protein migrates on a gel.) Bacteria (excluding the mycobacteria) are surrounded by both a cell membrane and a rigid cell wall, which is also an antibiotic target. Eukaryotes lack a cell wall. A schematic diagram of a typical bacterium is shown in Figure 16-1.

Bacteria are free-living organisms that vary in their survival requirements. Oxygen is a variable of particular clinical importance. An **aerobe** requires oxygen for survival, an **anaerobe** requires the absence of oxygen, and a facultative anaerobe has limited oxygen tolerance. Bacteria are ubiquitous but are found preferentially in certain sites. For example, anaerobes such as *Clostridium* are found in soil, where oxygen concentrations are lower, explaining why soil-contaminated wounds are more prone to tetanus infection and gas gangrene (*C. tetani* and *C. perfringens*). *Pseudomonas aeruginosa* commonly colonizes the leaves of plants; thus live flowers are frequently banned from ventilator and burn units, where pseudomonal pneumonias and tissue infections can create difficulties. As shown in Figure 16-2, bacteria are classified and named in part based on shape (cocci, bacilli, or spirochete).

ℛespiratory Recap

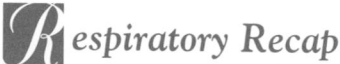

Bacterial Oxygen Requirements
Aerobe: $+O_2$
Anaerobe: $-O_2$
Facultative anaerobe: $\pm O_2$

One of the most important criteria used to classify bacteria is the ability to take up crystal violet dye, a component of **Gram's stain,** a characteristic that reflects important details about the structure of the bacterial cell wall. Diagrams of typical gram-positive and gram-negative cell walls are shown in Figure 16-3. The peptidoglycan layer of the cell wall is the structure that takes up the crystal violet. (Notice in Figure 16-3 that it is much thicker in the gram-positive cell wall.)

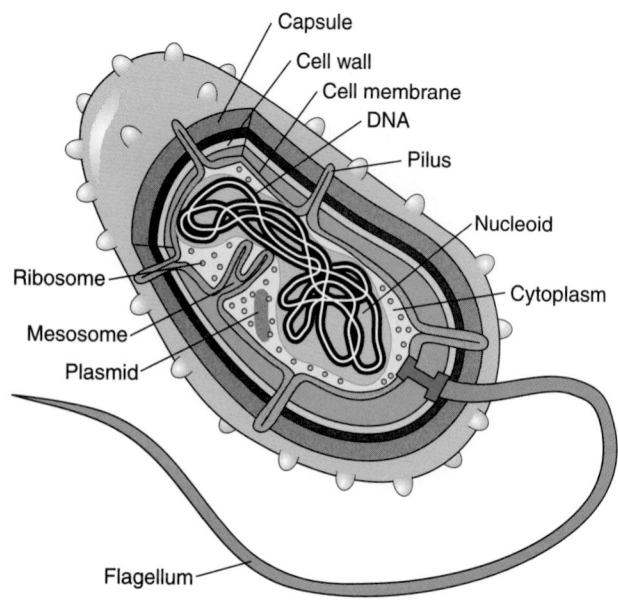

Figure 16-1   A typical bacterium.

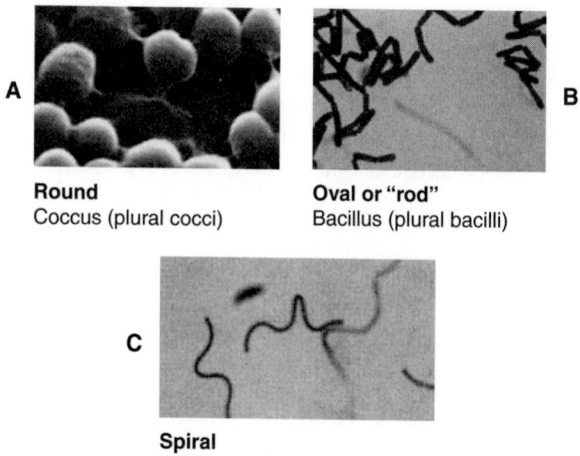

A Round
Coccus (plural cocci)

B Oval or "rod"
Bacillus (plural bacilli)

C Spiral
Spirochete (plural spirochetes)

Figure 16-2   Classifications of basic bacterial shapes. **A,** Cocci. **B,** Bacilli. **C,** Spirochetes.

Respiratory Recap

In addition, the gram-negative cell has an outer cell membrane external to the peptidoglycan cell wall. Between this outer membrane and the peptidoglycan lies the periplasmic space, which contains beta (β)-lactamases in some bacteria. These enzymes digest β-lactam antibiotics before they reach and lyse the peptidoglycan layer. The outer membrane found in gram-negative bacteria contains lipopolysaccharide (LPS, also called *endotoxin*), which contributes to the inflammatory effects of infection, such as fever and hypotension (shock). Teichoic acid may play the same role in gram-positive bacteria.

Respiratory Recap

Bacteria reproduce by binary fission, whereby each bacterium grows, makes a second copy of its own DNA, and then divides into two identical bacteria. Because this process is asexual, the ability of bacteria to vary their genetic traits is limited. However, bacteria can evolve new genetic traits through three methods—mutation, conjugation, and transduction.

Mutations, due to errors during DNA copying or damage to already completed DNA, occur regularly in all organisms. Although some mutations are repaired and most produce nonfunctional genes, an occasional fortuitous mutation occurs, producing an "improved" gene. This altered gene then is passed on as the bacterium divides, and if the new gene imparts a survival advantage, bacteria carrying it may come to predominate over normal, wild-type bacteria.

Plasmids are circular pieces of DNA that some bacteria carry in addition to the normal single chromosome. Plasmids known as *F plasmids* (fertility) encode genes that enable bacteria to mate, a process called *conjugation*, which allows for the exchange of genetic material. One or more plasmids, including the F plasmid, may be exchanged. Additionally, the F plasmid may be incorporated into the bacterial chromosome, allowing the chromosomal DNA to be transferred. Plasmid exchange is an important method in the acquisition of antibiotic resistance.

Viruses that infect bacteria, known as *bacteriophages*, may integrate a portion of the bacterial DNA into their own genetic material as they replicate. When viruses are released, they carry this DNA to newly infected bacteria. This process is known as *transduction*.

Given an environment that provides unlimited nutrients, binary fission produces rapid bacterial growth. Because the number of bacteria doubles with each division, the pattern of growth is exponential (logarithmic). The number of bacteria produced is 2^n, where *n* is the number of divisions, or generations. The time between divisions is

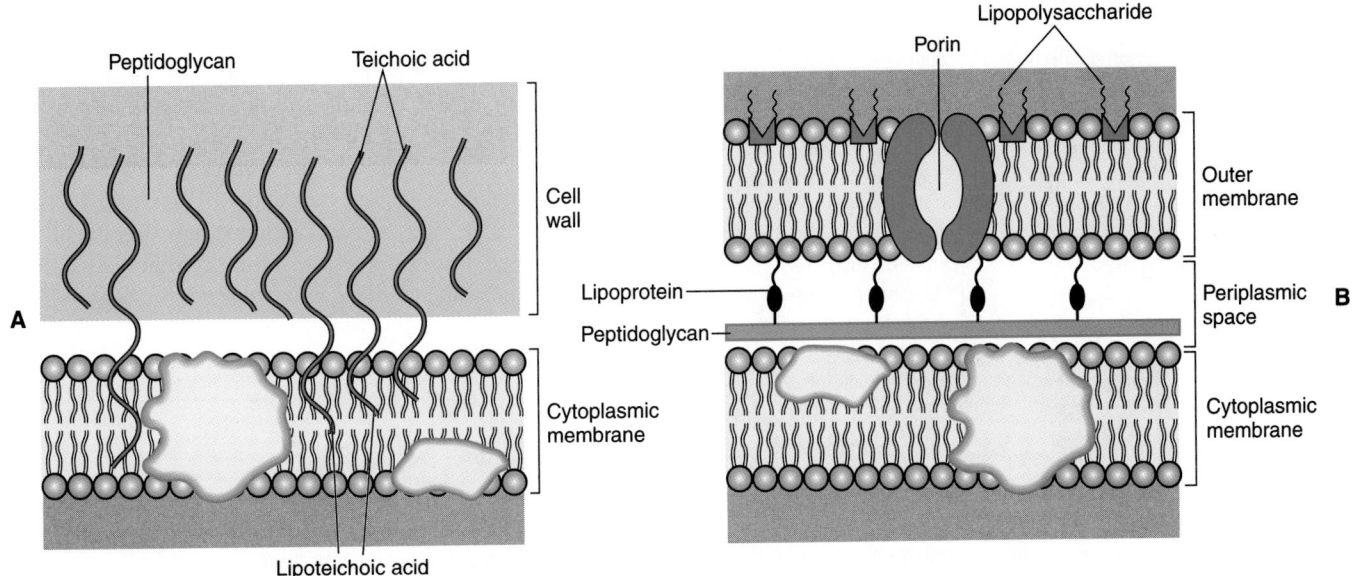

Figure 16-3   Comparative structures of gram-positive **(A)** and gram-negative **(B)** cell walls.

called the *doubling time*. Each bacterium has a characteristic doubling time under ideal conditions, ranging from 20 minutes (for *Escherichia coli*) to 24 hours (for *Mycobacterium tuberculosis*). Thus a single *E. coli* bacterium under ideal conditions can yield 2^{24}, or 16,777,216, bacteria in 8 hours. Within 24 hours the bacterial growth would fill a patient's hospital room. Fortunately, bacteria do not sustain these division rates in the infected host. Real-world growth is described in the following four phases:

- Lag phase—Initially, bacteria go through a phase of variable length, during which metabolic activities are high but division does not take place.
- Log (logarithmic) phase—Bacteria then begin to divide, growing at essentially logarithmic rates, although doubling times may be longer than under ideal conditions.
- Stationary phase—As nutrients are locally depleted and waste products accumulate, growth rate slows and the population reaches a steady state.
- Death phase—Conditions may continue to deteriorate so that bacterial counts begin to decline to low levels. This phase occurs in abscesses or as a consequence of immune system activity.

*R*espiratory Recap

Bacterial Growth
1. Lag phase   3. Stationary phase
2. Log phase   4. Death phase

*T*ABLE 16-1

Common Disease-Causing Toxins

Toxin	Producer	Effect
Toxic shock	*Staphylococcus aureus*	Causes fever, rash, shock
Diphtheria	*Corynebacterium diphtheriae*	Inhibits protein synthesis, causing cell death
Erythrogenic	*Streptococcus pyogenes*	Causes scarlet fever rash
Tetanus	*Clostridium tetani*	Inhibits release of neurotransmitter glycine, causing muscle spasm and rigidity
Botulism	*Clostridium botulinum*	Blocks release of neurotransmitter acetylcholine, causing paralysis and flaccidity
Enterotoxin	*Escherichia coli*	Stimulates adenylate cyclase, increasing fluid secretion into the gut and causing diarrhea

Bacteria cause disease through three major mechanisms—toxic formation, direct damage, and inflammatory response. In addition to the endotoxin contained in the cell walls of gram-negative bacteria, many bacteria secrete exotoxins, potent substances that cause various patterns of host tissue dysfunction. Some important examples are shown in Table 16-1. Toxic illness does not require invasion of the bacteria into tissue or even the presence of viable bacteria. Particularly in food-borne illnesses, preformed toxin may be ingested even when all bacteria have been killed during brief cooking. Cooking or sterilization must produce high enough temperatures for sufficient duration to break down toxins as well as kill bacteria.

Although some bacterial illnesses are due solely to toxins, most bacteria cause direct tissue damage by tissue invasion. Once in tissue, bacteria deplete nutrients and produce toxins that damage host tissues. More importantly, many bacteria produce substances that cause damage to adjacent tissues, facilitating bacterial spread. Examples include the collagenase and hyaluronidase produced by *Streptococcus pyogenes* bacteria, which digest components of the intercellular matrix. *Staphylococcus aureus* bacteria produce coagulase, which forms a fibrin clot around the site of infection, protecting *S. aureus* from immune attack.

The body's immune response to bacterial invasion is also a major cause of disease manifestations. Immune responses include elucidation of cytokines, which cause fever, hypotension, muscle aches, malaise, loss of appetite, confusion, and temporary liver and heart dysfunction. Immune cells also cause local tissue damage in their attempt to directly kill bacteria. This damage can manifest in pyogenic or granulomatous patterns. With the pyogenic pattern the predominant immune cells are neutrophils. Intense activity kills bacteria and host cells, producing a collection of neutrophils and dead tissue called *pus*. A cavity called an *abscess* may form where tissue has been destroyed. Because immune cells tend to travel along tissue surfaces, bacteria may survive within the center of an abscess unless it is drained. Some bacteria, of which *M. tuberculosis* is the archetype, stimulate the formation of granulomas, which are collections of macrophages arranged in a palisade, or wall, around a focus of infection. The macrophages are surrounded by T-lymphocytes, a formation that tends to "wall off" the infection, preventing its spread. Organisms then are phagocytized (ingested) by the macrophages. The interior of a granuloma may become filled with dead tissue, forming a cheesy substance that gives these granulomas the name *caseating necrotizing granulomas*.

*R*espiratory Recap

Mechanisms of Bacterial Disease
Toxin formation by bacteria
Direct local tissue damage from bacteria
Damage due to the immune response (pyogenic or granulomatous in nature)

Many areas of the body normally contain bacteria known as the **normal flora,** which do not usually cause disease at that site. However, when normal flora of one site contaminate another site, serious illness may result. Normal flora of several important sites are listed in Table 16-2. The list of bacteria that cause respiratory illness is lengthy, but just a few cause the majority of illness. Bacterial upper respiratory infections (URIs), which include pharyngitis, sinusitis, and otitis media, are caused most frequently by *Streptococcus pneumoniae* (pneumococcus), *Haemophilus influenzae* ("H. flu"), and *Moraxella catarrhalis*. All these bacteria are all found in the normal flora of the pharynx. Infection of the middle ear and sinuses probably occurs when these areas become closed off and overgrowth occurs.

The cause of lower respiratory infections varies by age and setting. Community-acquired pneumonia (CAP) originates outside a health care setting and must be distinguished from nosocomial pneumonia and ventilator-associated pneumonia (VAP). **Nosocomial pneumonia** (defined as pneumonia diagnosed more than 48 hours after hospital admission) is hospital- or nursing-home acquired, whereas VAP is a subset of nosocomial pneumonia occurring in mechanically ventilated patients. Box 16-1 lists the microorganisms responsible for each, in descending order of prevalence.

Anaerobes are not routinely cultured or reported, and their importance remains uncertain. They are thought to be a minor cause of CAP but become increasingly important in nosocomial pneumonia and VAP. Identifying the causative organisms in nosocomial pneumonia—and especially VAP—may be difficult because of the high rate of lower respiratory tract colonization. For example, the lower respiratory tracts of essentially all individuals receiving mechanical ventilation for the acute respiratory distress syndrome (ARDS), for example, are colonized with potential pathogens. Determining which microbes are pathogenic may be difficult but is important so that appropriate antimicrobial therapy may be begun. As an example, *Candida* species is frequently cultured

from endotracheal specimens in the intensive care unit (ICU) but is almost always considered a contaminant. Evaluating culture results cautiously allows for the prevention of potentially toxic antifungal therapy in these individuals.

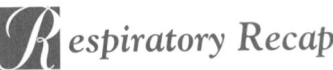 **espiratory Recap**

Pneumonia Classification
Community-acquired pneumonia (CAP) originates outside a health care setting.
Nosocomial pneumonia is acquired in a hospital or nursing home; shows symptoms more than 48 hours after admission.
Ventilator-associated pneumonia (VAP) is a subset of nosocomial pneumonia occurring in mechanically ventilated patients.

Culture is the principal method of diagnosis for bacterial infection. Somewhat increased specificity may be achieved by quantitative culture of blood, catheter tips, and bronchoscopic specimens, which involve counting of the number of colony-forming units per unit volume to distinguish contamination or colonization from active infection. After pathogens are isolated, culture allows for the determination of the bacteria's susceptibility to specific antibiotics. DNA probe, immunofluorescence, and latex agglutination methods allow for extremely rapid detection of some bacterial pathogens, including group A streptococci and *Helicobacter pylori*.

Chlamydiae

Chlamydiae are bacteria that are unable to support metabolism independently. They are therefore obligate intracellular organisms, growing only inside host cells. In the past a substantial number of pneumonias were recognized as caused by organisms that did not appear in standard culture

*T*ABLE 16-2

Normal Human Flora by Body Site

Site	Normal Flora
Pharynx and upper gastrointestinal tract	*Moraxella catarrhalis; Staphylococcus epidermidis* and *aureus;*, α-hemolytic streptococci; viridans-group streptococci; *Streptococcus pneumoniae; Peptostreptococcus, Lactobacillus,* and *Fusobacterium* species; *Actinomyces israelii; Haemophilus influenzae* and *parainfluenzae; Corynebacterium* species; *Neisseria meningitidis, Bacteroides* species and other anaerobes; and *Candida* (yeast) species
Colon	*Enterococcus* species; *E. coli; Pseudomonas, Bacteroides,* and *Clostridium* species and other gram-negatives and anaerobes; also *Candida* (yeast) species; organisms known as **coliforms** or **enteric bacteria** because of their location in the colon)
Skin	*Staphylococcus epidermidis* and *aureus;* streptococci; *Corynebacterium* species; *Clostridium perfringens; Propionibacterium acnes; Candida* (yeast) species
Lower respiratory tract	Essentially sterile; possibility of colonization when illness or structural lung disease compromise immune function

Modified from Herceg RJ, Peterson LR. Normal flora in health and disease. In: Shulman ST, Phair JP, Peterson LR, et al., editors. The biologic and clinical basis of infectious disease. 5th ed. Philadelphia: WB Saunders; 1997.

*B*OX 16-1

Etiologies of CAP, VAP, and Nosocomial Pneumonia

The microorganisms associated with each type of pneumonia are listed in descending order of prevalence.

CAP, Age Less than 60 Years
Streptococcus pneumoniae
Mycoplasma pneumoniae
Viruses
Chlamydia pneumoniae
Haemophilus influenzae
Legionella species
Staphylococcus aureus
Mycobacterium tuberculosis
Fungi (*Histoplasma, Coccidioides, Blastomyces* species)
Gram-negative bacilli, nonpseudomonal (*Klebsiella,* enteric species)

CAP, Age Greater than 60 Years
S. pneumoniae
Viruses
H. influenzae
Gram-negative bacilli, nonpseudomonal

S. aureus
Moraxella catarrhalis
Legionella species
M. tuberculosis
Fungi (*Histoplasma, Coccidioides, Blastomyces* species)

Nosocomial (Non-VAP) Pneumonia
Polymicrobial organisms
S. aureus
S. pneumoniae
Gram-negative bacilli, nonpseudomonal
Pseudomonas species

VAP
Polymicrobial organisms
S. aureus
Pseudomonas species
H. influenzae
S. pneumoniae
Gram-negative bacilli, nonpseudomonal

Modified from Lawlor DP, Emig M. Community acquired pneumonia. In: Civetta JM, editor. Critical Care. 3rd ed. Boston: Lippincott Williams & Wilkins; 1998; Niederman MS, Bass JB Jr, Campbell GD, et al. Guidelines for the initial management of adults with community-acquired pneumonia: diagnosis, assessment of severity, and initial antimicrobial therapy. Am Rev Respir Dis 1993;148:1418-1426; and Bartlett JG, Mundy LM. Community acquired pneumonia. N Engl J Med 1995;333:1618-1624.
CAP, Community-acquired pneumonia; VAP, ventilator-associated pneumonia.

techniques. These were termed *atypical pneumonias*. In addition to being culture negative the atypical pneumonias have a characteristic presentation in that they usually affect younger people, produce less leukocytosis and sputum, and tend to produce fewer crackles and other signs of consolidation on physical exam, despite significant infiltrates on x-ray films. Two important atypical pneumonias are caused by chlamydiae, the more common of which is chlamydia pneumonia, caused by *Chlamydia pneumoniae*, formerly called TWAR. This infection is spread by aerosolized secretions. The second type, psittacosis, is caused by *Chlamydia psittaci* and is classically transmitted by inhalation of the dust of dried, infected bird droppings. It is therefore not generally transmitted directly person-to-person. Chlamydiae can be grown in cell culture; characteristic inclusion bodies may be seen microscopically in infected cells. A rapid DNA probe is available for *Chlamydia trachomatis* only.

Rickettsiae

Like chlamydiae, rickettsiae are small bacteria that are obligate intracellular organisms. Rickettsiae are maintained within a mammalian reservoir (humans in the case of *Rickettsia prowazekii*). However, rickettsiae are transmitted to humans indirectly, through the bite of specific arthropods (lice, mites, fleas, or ticks) that have previously encountered the infected mammal. The agent causing

Q fever, originally named *Rickettsia burnetii* but recently renamed *Coxiella burnetii*, is an exception to this pattern; *C. burnetii* is spread by aerosol directly from cats, dogs, sheep, cattle, and goats. Aerosolization from the surface of the placenta is particularly effective, so attendance at an animal birth is a risk factor for infection.

Rickettsial diseases manifest as fever, severe headache, and influenza symptoms. Rickettsiae with important pulmonary manifestations include Q fever (*C. burnetii*), epidemic typhus (*R. prowazekii*), endemic typhus (*Rickettsia typhi*), and scrub typhus (*Rickettsia tsutsugamushi*). Cell culture is possible but not commonly used. Diagnosis is based on serology, the detection of a specific antibody response to the organism. Serology may not show positive results for up to 2 weeks after infection.

Mycoplasmas

Mycoplasmas are the smallest of bacteria, with diameters as small as 0.3 μm, similar to large viruses. Unlike viruses, chlamydiae, and most rickettsiae, however, mycoplasmas are free living, with their own independent metabolic processes; in fact they are the smallest free-living organisms. Mycoplasmas are unique among bacteria in that they are enclosed by a cell membrane only and lack a cell wall. *Mycoplasma pneumoniae* is an important respiratory pathogen, the most common cause of atypical pneumonia and among the most common causes of pneumonia in children and young adults. Diagnosis is based on serology. In addition, cold agglutinins—antibodies against red blood cells—are produced in approximately half of pneumonia cases. A cold agglutinin titer of greater than 1:128 is usually considered diagnostic for *M. pneumonia* infection.

Mycobacteria

Mycobacteria are rod-shaped bacteria, distinguished by an unusual staining pattern in response to the Ziehl-Neelson stain. Because of the presence of waxes, such as mycolic acid, the cell wall retains red carbolfuchsin stain despite rinsing with hydrochloric acid. The mycobacteria therefore are called **acid-fast bacilli (AFB).** The only other type of acid-fast bacteria is *Nocardia* species. AFB are considered neither gram-positive nor gram-negative. Tuberculous mycobacteria cause tuberculosis (TB) and include M. *tuberculosis* (MTB), *Mycobacterium bovis*, and *Mycobacterium africanum*. Nontuberculous mycobacteria include *Mycobacterium avium* complex (MAC) and M. *intracellulare*—together called *Mycobacterium avium-intracellulare* (MAI), *Mycobacterium gordonae*, *Mycobacterium kansasii*, *Mycobacterium fortuitum*, and *Mycobacterium chelonei*. Mycobacteria causing primarily nonpulmonary disease include *Mycobacterium marinum*, *Mycobacterium leprae*, M. *bovis* (used to produce bacille Calmette-Guérin [BCG] vaccine for TB), and *Mycobacterium scrofulaceum*.

Mycobacteria are obligate aerobes and most—especially MTB—are slow growing, which accounts for tuberculosis being a slowly progressive, wasting disease, often progressive over months to years. Many of the manifestations of the disease—fever and weight loss particularly—are due to the chronic granulomatous inflammatory response. Exceptions are the so-called rapidly growing mycobacteria, M. *fortuitum*, and M. *chelonei*, which produce more acute illnesses. Because of the slow growth of MTB, prolonged antimicrobial therapy of 6 to 12 months is required. Although isoniazid (INH) still is used alone for exposure without clinical illness, the widespread appearance of antibiotic-resistant and multidrug-resistant tuberculosis (MDR-TB) now requires at least two- and sometimes up to four-drug therapy for active tuberculosis.

Immunofluorescence has largely replaced actual acid-fast staining for AFB. This technique uses antibodies that bind specifically to mycobacteria and are joined to a molecule that fluoresces under ultraviolet light. The presence of fluorescence is evaluated microscopically. Like staining, this technique is limited by the very small numbers of organisms present in most cases of active disease. Therefore these techniques, although rapid, are insensitive. Additionally, neither test distinguishes MTB from other species of mycobacteria.

Mycobacterial culture remains essential to reliably detect the presence of mycobacteria, identify the species, and determine the pattern of susceptibility to antibiotics.

*T*ABLE 16-3

*Criteria for Mantoux Test Positivity**

Threshold for Positive Test	Group
5 mm	Recent TB exposure, chest x-ray suggestive of TB, or HIV-infected individuals
10 mm	Individuals with exposure risk: born in a country with high prevalence of TB, residents of nursing homes, prisons, and other institutions; and health care workers
15 mm	General population

TB, *Tuberculosis;* HIV, *human immunodeficiency virus.*
Diameter of induration at 48 to 72 hours.

The major drawback to mycobacterial culture is the slow growth rate of mycobacteria; even with newer, rapid-growth techniques, results may take longer than 1 week.

Placement of **purified protein derivative (PPD)** subcutaneously, called the **Mantoux test,** detects the presence of an immune response to mycobacteria by eliciting a delayed-type hypersensitivity response. This response manifests as induration of the injection site within 72 hours. A positive test is defined as induration of 5 to 15 mm in diameter, depending on the population group (Table 16-3), representing exposure to mycobacteria at some time in the past, but not necessarily infection. Once converted to positive PPD status, most patients remain positive indefinitely.

Some patients fail to demonstrate an immune response even after exposure and are termed *anergic*. Anergy may be assessed through placement of a control—a simultaneous subcutaneous injection of universal allergens, such as candida and mumps, that would be expected to produce a positive response in all cases. The BCG vaccine rarely produces induration greater than 15 mm into adulthood, so Mantoux tests can be useful in this population. However, the Mantoux test should not be applied to patients who have received BCG vaccine recently or to patients known to be PPD positive because a vigorous immune response may produce tissue damage at the test site.[1] A positive Mantoux test may be produced by exposure to any *Mycobacterium* species.

Viruses

With the exception of the prions, the viruses are the smallest and simplest class of pathogens. Ranging in size from 0.02 to 0.30 μm, viruses consist of genetic material, either RNA or DNA, surrounded by a protein coat called a *capsid*. Some viruses also are surrounded by a lipoprotein membrane called an *envelope*.

After gaining entry into a host, viruses attach themselves selectively to certain host cells; for example, rhinovirus infects upper airway mucosa, whereas human immunodeficiency virus (HIV) has a predilection for CD4+ lymphocytes. This specificity is imparted by different proteins embedded in the outer surface of the capsid, or (in enveloped viruses) glycoproteins embedded in the envelope. These proteins or glycoproteins bind to specific cell surface "receptors," and the virus then is taken up into the host cell and sheds its capsid or envelope to expose its genetic material, a process known as *uncoating*.

Viruses themselves are metabolically inactive, but once inside a cell they use the host cell metabolism to replicate. The mechanism of viral replication varies, depending on the type of virus, but its goal is always to produce messenger RNA (mRNA), from which viral proteins are translated by the host cell. Most positive-polarity RNA viruses simply use their genome directly as mRNA, whereas negative-polarity RNA viruses carry their own RNA-dependent RNA polymerase to transcribe their genome into positive-polarity mRNA. Some RNA viruses—the retroviruses, of which the best-known is HIV—first transcribe their RNA into DNA. Because eukaryotic cells lack the reverse transcriptase necessary for DNA production from RNA, the retroviruses must carry a copy of their own reverse transcriptase. The resulting viral DNA then is transcribed by the host cell's RNA polymerase to produce mRNA. The genome of DNA viruses is transcribed directly into mRNA by the host cell RNA polymerase.

Regardless of the mechanism used, the host cell eventually fills with newly synthesized virions—sometimes clustered together as a recognizable inclusion body—and then ruptures, releasing the viruses into the environment. Viruses cause clinical disease by the following three mechanisms:

1. Cause host cell rupture and death
2. Cause host cell dysfunction, including fusion with other cells to produce multinucleate giant cells, and sometimes malignant transformation
3. Stimulate the body's cellular host defenses against infection

Although local disease is mediated by cell dysfunction and death, the third mechanism is responsible for many systemic symptoms associated with viral infection, including fever, malaise, loss of appetite, and increased mucus production. Because a large number of virus species exist, they are usually considered in groups, with some of the more important viral respiratory pathogens listed in Table 16-4.

Viruses are grown in cell culture, where they produce recognizable cytopathic changes, a process that can take up to 2 weeks. A "rapid shell vial" culture technique is used to obtain a diagnosis of cytomegalovirus (CMV) infection within 48 hours and is frequently performed on respiratory secretions and bronchoscopy specimens. Certain viruses, especially CMV and Epstein-Barr virus (EBV), produce characteristic microscopically visible inclusion bodies in infected cells. DNA probes and enzyme-linked immunosorbent assay (ELISA) now allow for the rapid detection of influenza virus and HIV.

Fungi

Fungi differ from the other organisms in that they are eukaryotic and thus share many features with human cells. This homology makes difficult the development of antifungal therapy that is nontoxic to humans. Fungal structure does differ in the following two important ways from human cells: (1) the fungal cell membrane contains ergosterol and zymosterol instead of cholesterol; (2) fungi have a rigid cell wall composed of chitin (unlike the peptidoglycan cell wall of bacteria).

Fungi occur in two forms. **Yeasts** exist as single cells. In contrast, **molds** grow as long, multicellular forms called *hyphae*, which associate to form structures called *mycelia*. Although individual yeasts are approximately 4 μm each,

$\mathcal{T}$ABLE 16-4

Viruses Important in Human Respiratory Disease

Virus	Resulting Disease
Rhinoviruses, adenoviruses, coronaviruses	URI; "common cold"
Herpesviruses	Diverse important diseases
Herpes simplex virus (HSV)	Herpetic skin lesions; infection of the lungs and brain, causing pneumonia and encephalitis
Varicella-zoster virus (VZV)	Chickenpox and shingles, both of which may involve the lung and central nervous system
Cytomegalovirus (CMV)	Systemic infection, including pneumonia, usually in immunocompromised individuals
Epstein-Barr virus (EBV)	Infectious mononucleosis ("mono")
Retroviruses (include HIV)	Diverse respiratory manifestations resulting from HIV
Flaviviruses (include yellow fever and dengue viruses)	Yellow fever and dengue, diseases common in Central and South America
Orthomyxoviruses	Influenza
Paramyxoviruses	Measles; mumps; parainfluenza
Respiratory syncytial virus (RSV)	Bronchiolitis in infants; milder disease in children and adults
Togaviruses	Diverse illnesses, including rubella

HIV, *Human immunodeficiency virus;* URI, *upper respiratory infection.*

mycelia can be quite large, covering up to 1500 acres, and are claimed to be the world's largest organisms.[2] Some fungi are dimorphic, existing as molds in soil but forming yeasts at human body temperatures. All fungi reproduce by spore formation, which may occur either sexually or asexually, depending on the species.

With the exception of candida, which is part of the normal human flora, the natural environments of fungi include soil, bird feces, and other decaying material. Therefore they often produce disease after exposure to dust, rotting wood, or dried bird droppings. Skin infection can be caused by direct contact, as in cases of tinea pedis (athlete's foot).

Because inhalation is a significant route of fungal infection, the lung is second only to skin as the major site of fungal infection. The clinical manifestations of fungal disease, known as **mycosis**, depend somewhat on the number or organisms introduced into the lungs (the **inoculum**) and are produced by the following three mechanisms:

- *Direct tissue damage:* Most fungi form masses that destroy adjacent tissue as they grow. This is usually a minor component, but in the brain, because of the limited inflammatory response and the importance of even small mass lesions, it is the primary mechanism of disease. Another exception is the angioinvasive fungi, *Aspergillus, Mucor,* and *Rhizopus* species, which invade and destroy tissues; they have a predilection for blood vessels, destroying blood supply and causing necrosis in infected areas.
- *Inflammatory response:* More important than direct tissue damage in many cases is the damage caused by the inflammatory response, which is provoked by fungal infection. Candidal infections of the mouth and skin folds (thrush and intertrigo, respectively) are excellent examples. The painful, raw base underneath the candida plaque is caused by the granulomatous inflammatory response to the yeast.
- *Allergy:* In cases of prolonged infection or colonization, an immune response may develop. An excellent example is allergic bronchopulmonary aspergillosis (ABPA). In this condition, pulmonary colonization with aspergillus leads to chronic fevers, cough, and pulmonary infiltrates that represent a delayed-type hypersensitivity reaction (allergy), not a direct effect of the aspergillus. Because the aspergillus cannot be eradicated, treatment is with immune suppression, such as steroids.

Important fungal respiratory pathogens in normal hosts are listed in Table 16-5, whereas Table 16-6 lists mycoses known as *opportunistic* because they generally occur in response to lowered host immune activity.

Fungi may be cultured by special techniques but grow more slowly than bacteria. Diagnosis can be made either by cytology or microscopic observation after treatment with potassium hydroxide (KOH), which dissolves most tissue but leaves the chitinous fungal wall intact. Serology is often useful, but its utility is limited in endemic areas, where the majority of healthy individuals may be seropositive. Latex agglutination is frequently used as a rapid detection test for cryptococcus in cerebrospinal fluid.

Pneumocystis carinii

Little was known about *Pneumocystis carinii* before the era of acquired immunodeficiency syndrome (AIDS), and it has only recently been classified as a fungus, based on genetic studies. *P. carinii* is dimorphic, existing as trophozoites and cysts.

TABLE 16-5

Important Fungal Respiratory Pathogens in Normal Hosts

Organism	Disease	Comments
Coccidioides immitis	Coccidioidomycosis	The organism is commonly found in the arid regions of the southwest United States (for example, Arizona, central California) and the disease causes valley fever, with high fever and bilateral pneumonia, and may later form thin-walled pulmonary cavities.
Histoplasma capsulatum	Histoplasmosis	The organism is commonly found along the Mississippi and Ohio river valleys, and high inhaled *Histoplasma* inoculum may cause acute fever and pneumonia. Some patients develop disseminated infection, often causing skin lesions; in rare cases, fibrosis of the mediastinum may result. Most residents of endemic areas have had asymptomatic infection, causing elevated antibody titers, and often one or more calcified granulomas visible on chest x-ray film.
Blastomyces dermatitidis	Blastomycosis	The organism is common in the southern United States, and the disease varies from mild fever and pulmonary infiltrates to severe illness, nodular pulmonary infiltrates, and dissemination.
Paracoccidioides brasiliensis	Paracoccidioidomycosis	Occurring in Central America, this clinical disease is similar to mild coccidioidomycosis.

TABLE 16-6

Opportunistic Fungal Respiratory Pathogens

Organism	Disease	Comments
Candida albicans	Candidiasis (thrush, esophagitis, intertrigo)	Organism is commonly found in infants and the elderly and also in HIV-infected and critically ill patients. Thrush also may be precipitated by inhaled steroid deposition in the mouth. True candidal pneumonia is rare.
Aspergillus species	Aspergillosis	Disease causes otitis externa in normal hosts; may infect skin, sinuses, or lung of immunocompromised individuals; and can disseminate, with extremely high mortality. Preexisting lung cavities from tuberculosis or emphysema are particularly prone to infection, with formation of a "fungus ball" inside.
Cryptococcus neoformans	Cryptococcosis	Organism is found in kitten feces and causes pneumonia and meningitis, a feared complication of AIDS.
Mucor and *Rhizopus* species	Mucormycosis	Organism can infect the sinuses, lungs, or gut, forming a black eschar. Treatment is difficult, often requiring surgical debridement.

HIV, *Human immunodeficiency virus;* AIDS, *acquired immunodeficiency syndrome.*

P. carinii causes pneumocystis pneumonia (PCP). The organism itself is also referred to as *PCP*. Pneumocystis pneumonia was commonly found during the first decade of AIDS and remains an important complication, although its incidence has dropped since the institution of trimethoprim-sulfamethoxazole (TMP/SMX) or aerosolized pentamidine prophylactic therapy. Any immunocompromised individual is at risk for developing PCP, including patients on medium- to high-dose, long-term corticosteroids and those receiving transplants. PCP has a variable x-ray appearance but usually manifests as a diffuse pneumonia or nodular infiltrate. A hallmark of pneumocystis pneumonia is that the patient's degree of hypoxia is often greater than expected based on the chest x-ray film. A PaO_2 of less than 50 is an indication for systemic corticosteroids, which have significantly reduced mortality. Treatment is with high-dose TMP/SMX, dapsone, or intravenous (IV) pentamidine in sulfa-allergic patients.

Diagnosis is based on microscopic observation of the organisms on cytology. Bronchoalveolar lavage is the sampling method of choice and has a very high sensitivity (80%-95%) in HIV-positive patients. Yield is lower in other immunosuppressed patients.

Parasites

Parasites are important in developing areas but are rare pulmonary pathogens in the developed countries and will be discussed in this chapter only briefly. A *parasite* is defined as a plant or animal that lives with or on another, deriving benefit from the association but having a detrimental effect on the host. Essentially any pathogen can be considered a parasite by this definition, but in practical usage the term *parasite* is usually limited to protozoans and helminths. Examples of pulmonary parasitic infections include *Entamoeba histolytica* (amebiasis), *Paragonimus westermani* (paragonimiasis), and *Echinococcus multilocularis/E. granulosis* (echinococcosis: hy-

datid cysts). *Plasmodium falciparum* (malaria) may cause pulmonary manifestations in 3% to 10% of individuals.

The single-celled protozoa usually cause pulmonary disease through abscess formation or stimulation of a vigorous inflammatory response in the lungs. The multicellular helminths frequently produce focal lesions in the lungs—cysts or larvae—and usually are easily visible on chest x-ray films. Manifestations are most frequently malaise, fever, cough, and dyspnea. Chest pain may be present, and eosinophilia is a frequent occurrence.

Antibiotic Resistance

The development of widespread resistance of many bacteria to antibiotics is a growing concern worldwide and has become a major problem, especially true in environments that are constantly exposed to antibiotics, such as hospitals and especially ICUs, where resistant bacterial strains can become a dominant part of the endogenous flora (Table 16-7). Several mechanisms of antibiotic resistance exist, and Table 16-8 lists some important resistant pathogens.

Production of antibiotic-inactivating enzymes is usually encoded by a plasmid. The most important mechanism of resistance to penicillins and cephalosporins is the production of β-lactamases, which digest the β-lactam ring structure of these antibiotics. The most important mechanisms of resistance to aminoglycosides and chloramphenicol are also the production of various inactivating enzymes.

The activity of antibiotics also may be improved by modification of their targets, which usually involves a change in the chromosomal genes of the microorganism. The second-most-important mechanism of resistance to penicillins and cephalosporins is modification of the "penicillin-binding proteins" in the bacterial cell membrane to which the drugs attach. Resistance to aminoglycosides, macrolides, sulfonamides, fluoroquinolones, and rifampin is

*T*ABLE 16-7

Common Antibiotics, Mechanisms, Spectra of Activity, and Toxicities

Class	Examples	Mechanism of Action	Spectrum of Activity	Toxicity
Antibacterials				
Penicillins	Penicillin, amoxicillin, amoxicillin-clavulanate (Augmentin), piperacillin, ticarcillin	Cleave bonds contained in peptidoglycan cell wall, disrupting bacterial structural integrity	G+, G−, and anaerobic activities increasing with successive generations	Hypersensitivity, GI intolerance, hepatitis with prolonged use
Cephalosporins	Cefazolin (Ancef), cephalexin (Keflex), ceftriaxone (Rocephin), ceftazidime	Same as penicillins	Same as penicillins	Rare cytopenias
Carbapenems	Imipenem	Same as penicillins	Broad G+, G−, anaerobic coverage	Seizure, GI intolerance, occasional cytopenias
Monobactams	Aztreonam	Same as penicillins	Broad G+, G−, anaerobic coverage	Similar to penicillins
Aminoglycosides	Gentamicin, tobramycin (TOBI)	Antiribosomal: interfere with translation of proteins from mRNA by binding the bacterial ribosome 30S subunit Bacteriocidal	G−	Nephrotoxicity, ototoxicity, rare paralysis; levels requiring monitoring
Tetracyclines	Tetracycline, doxycycline, minocycline	Antiribosomal: bind the 30S subunit Bacteriocidal at high concentrations	G+, atypicals	Tooth and bone defects, phototoxicity, GI intolerance, benign intracranial hypertension, mild hepatitis
Sulfonamides	Trimethoprim/ sulfamethoxazole (TMP/SMX, Bactrim, Septra)	Blocks metabolic pathway for folate production	G+, G−, *Pneumocystis carinii*	Hypersensitivity, possible trigger of hemolysis in G6PD deficiency
Flouroquinolones	Ciprofloxacin, levofloxacin, gatifloxacin	Inhibits DNA gyrase, interfere with DNA synthesis	G−, G+, atypicals	Cartilage erosion in animals; not administered in children, except those with cystic fibrosis
Macrolides	Erythromycin, clarithromycin (Biaxin), azithromycin (Zithromax)	Antiribosomal: binds 50S subunit Bacteriostatic	G+, some G−; good atypical coverage, including *Legionella* species	GI intolerance
Others	Vancomycin	Inhibits cell wall synthesis	G+, including MRSA; *Enterococcus* species	Hypotension and rash with infusion, ototoxicity
	Metronidazole	—	Anaerobes	Ethanol intolerance, seizures, peripheral neuropathy
	Chloramphenicol	Antiribosomal: binds 50S subunit	G+, many G−, anaerobes, rickettsiae	Aplastic anemia; used only when strongly indicated
	Clindamycin	Antiribosomal: bacteriocidal at high concentrations	G+ and anaerobes	*Clostridium difficile* colitis

DNA, *Deoxyribonucleic acid;* G+, *gram-positive bacteria;* G −, *gram-negative bacteria;* GI, *gastrointestinal;* MRSA, *methicillin-resistant* Staphylococcus aureus.

Continued

*T*ABLE 16-7

Common Antibiotics, Mechanisms, Spectra of Activity, and Toxicities—cont'd

Class	Examples	Mechanism of Action	Spectrum of Activity	Toxicity
Antifungals				
Imidazoles	Fluconazole, itraconazole	Inhibita ergosterol production	*Aspergillus, Blastomyces,* and *Histoplasma* species, onychomycosis	ECG QT prolongation when given with cisapride, hepatotoxicity
Polyenes	Amphotericin B	Disrupts ergosterol-based cell membrane	All; preferred for severe infections	Fever, rigors, hypotension with infusion, nephrotoxicity, hypersensitivity, hepatotoxicity, cytopenias
Antivirals				
	Acyclovir, famciclovir, valacyclovir	Guanosine analogues incorporated into DNA, blocking further DNA synthesis; interferes with DNA synthesis	HSV, VZV, CMV	Headache, nausea
	Amantadine, rimantadine	Blocks attachment of virus and/or release of viral nucleic acid into host cell	Influenza A	Reversible neurotoxicity
	Ganciclovir	Guanine analogue incorporated into DNA, blocking further DNA synthesis; interferes with DNA synthesis	CMV	Cytopenias, impaired male fertility
	Foscarnet	Pyrophosphate analogue blocking DNA synthesis by interfering with DNA polymerase	HSV, VZV, CMV, EBV	Nephrotoxicity in most patients, electrolyte abnormalities, seizures, anemia
	Ribavirin	Unknown	RSV	Possible clogging of ventilator valves, severe bronchospasm, rash
Antituberculous				
	Rifampin	Inhibits DNA polymerase	G+, G-, MTB	Flulike syndrome, hepatotoxicity
	Isoniazid (INH)	Unknown	MTB	Hepatotoxicity, neurotoxicity, hypersensitivity
	Ethambutol (EMB)	Inhibits protein synthesis?	MTB	Optic neuritis
	Pyrazinamide (PZA)	Unknown	MTB	Hepatotoxicity, hyperuricemia
	Streptomycin	Antiribosomal: binds with 30S subunit Bacteriocidal	MTB, G-	Hypersensitivity, ototoxicity, neurotoxicity

CMV, *cytomegalovirus;* EBV, *Epstein-Barr virus;* ECG, *electrocardiographic;* HSV, *herpes simplex virus;* MTB, Mycobacterium tuberculosis; RSV, *respiratory syncytial virus;* VZV, *varicella-zoster virus.*

imparted by mutations in the bacterial ribosomes or enzymes that make up the targets of these antibiotics.

Resistance to aminoglycosides, tetracyclines, and INH results from decreased permeability of the cell wall and membrane to the antibiotic, reducing the antibiotic levels inside the bacterium. Antibiotics also may be actively transported from the bacteria by an enzymatic pump, which is usually plasmid encoded. Resistance to tetracyclines and sulfonamides also is accomplished by active transport of the antibiotic from the bacteria.

Infection Control Methods

Cleaning, Disinfection, and Sterilization

Equipment processing uses one or a combination of four modalities: (1) cleaning, (2) disinfection, (3) antisepsis, and (4) sterilization. Cleaning removes gross contamination, such as dirt and secretions, reducing the number of microorganisms and removing much of their potential growth medium. Cleaning is generally a prerequisite for

TABLE 16-8

Important Antibiotic-Resistant Respiratory Bacterial Pathogens

Bacterial Pathogen	Description
Methicillin-resistant *Staphylococcus aureus* (MRSA)	Although defined by its resistance to methicillin, MRSA is now recognized by its resistance to oxacillin in routine testing (not to be confused with *S. epidermidis*, which is always oxacillin resistant). MRSA carries a β-lactamase or has modified its penicillin-binding proteins, which usually renders it resistant to all penicillins and cephalosporins. Usual therapy is with vancomycin. MRSA is carried on skin and in the nasopharynx.
Vancomycin-resistant enterococcus (VRE)	Enterococcus is intrinsically resistant to many antibiotics, making vancomycin one of the few routinely effective antibiotics. The onset of vancomycin resistance has made this organism nearly impossible to treat. Treatment includes new agents, such as teicoplanin and Synercid (quinupristin/dalfopristin). VRE is harbored in the gastrointestinal tract.
Tuberculosis	Resistance to at least one antituberculous drug is now common worldwide, making two-, three- or even four-drug therapy mandatory.
Multidrug resistant tuberculosis (MDR-TB)	MTB resistant to two or more antituberculous drugs is termed *multidrug-resistant tuberculosis (MDR-TB)*.
Pseudomonas aeruginosa	*P. aeruginosa* is frequently resistant to antipseudomonal antibiotics and tends to develop resistance rapidly. The simultaneous use of at least two antipseudomonals is recommended.
Streptococcus pneumoniae	Resistance is moderate but increasing. First-generation penicillin and ciprofloxacin are now usually ineffective.
Haemophilus influenzae	*H. influenzae* is responsible for a large percentage of amoxicillin treatment failures for respiratory illness because resistance to amoxicillin is 80% in some areas.
Moraxella catarrhalis	Amoxicillin resistance often exceeds 80%

MTB, *Mycobacterium tuberculosis.*

the other three modalities. **Disinfection** does not remove all microorganisms but radically reduces the number of infectious organisms by killing most of those present. Spores, mycobacteria, and nonlipid viruses are the most resistant to eradication. *Antisepsis* is sometimes used synonymously with *disinfection* but usually specifically describes the use of chemical agents (antiseptics) to inhibit microbial growth. Microbes are not necessarily killed, as with disinfection, but their ability to replicate and produce toxins is impaired. Antisepsis is also used to describe disinfection of a biologic surface (for example, hand washing). **Sterilization** is the complete killing of all organisms.

In descriptions of equipment processing, equipment may be divided into three categories—critical, semicritical, and noncritical. Critical equipment, such as a chest tube, directly comes into contact with tissues and sterile areas, such as the pleural space. This equipment *must* be sterile. Semicritical equipment touches mucosal surfaces,

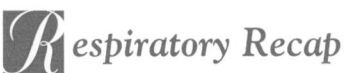

Respiratory Recap

Levels of Equipment Processing

Critical (sterile): no viable (living) organisms
Semicritical (disinfected): few organisms remaining , with spores and nonlipid viruses possibly remaining viable
Noncritical (clean): grossly appreciable organic matter ("dirt") removed

where transmission of infection is relatively easy, requiring high-level disinfection of the equipment during processing. Most respiratory care equipment is semicritical. An exception is equipment passed through an endotracheal tube, in which a protected passage to the lower airways is established, bypassing the relatively unclean upper airway. In this setting, use of sterile equipment such as suction catheters may successfully decrease the infectious load introduced to the lower airways. Noncritical equipment touches only intact skin and must be cleaned only, although disinfection is usually used.

Adequate cleaning requires four elements—water to solubilize and carry away contaminants, detergent to solubilize hydrophobic (water-insoluble) substances, mechanical agitation to dislodge contamination, and adequate duration of cleaning because time increases the amount of mechanical agitation and water used.

Most reusable respiratory care equipment is disinfected between patients. A common technique is pasteurization, which involves immersion of the equipment in water heated to below its boiling point. Respiratory care equipment is typically immersed in water at 77° C for 30 minutes.

The addition of antiseptic agents to soaps decreases bacterial activity on the skin during hand washing. Recently, waterless rub-on antiseptics have come into common use to replace hand washing. These are a blend of isopropyl alcohol and skin softeners. Although they are useful short-term measures, effective antisepsis relies on the thorough removal of organic matter first. At least occasional hand washing is necessary. In addition, wiping of surfaces with alcohol or iodine is antiseptic only; it does not kill spores.

Steam autoclaving kills microorganisms by heat-denaturing microbial proteins. Effective sterilization requires adequate heat and time, but increases in pressure or the addition of moisture enhances and hastens killing. Therefore most autoclaves use pressurized steam. Autoclaving has the advantage of being fast (typically 5 to 15 minutes plus cooling time) but damages some types of equipment.

Ethylene oxide is a dry toxic gas that sterilizes without need for heat or moisture; thus it is used to process equipment that is unable to tolerate autoclaving or immersion. Approximately 3 to 4 hours of gas exposure are required, and processed equipment usually requires ventilation for 8 to 24 hours afterward. Contact of ethylene oxide with water produces ethylene glycol (antifreeze), which may persist on the equipment as a toxic, sticky residue.

Immersion in a glutaraldehyde solution such as Cidex can disinfect equipment within 20 minutes and sterilize in 6 to 10 hours. Because glutaraldehyde is toxic, the equipment then must be rinsed and (usually) dried. Although its use is limited to immersible equipment, glutaraldehyde is convenient because the solution may be kept in a small container and reused for 14 to 30 days, without the storage issues associated with a bulky autoclave, gas sterilizer, or pasteurizer. Quaternary ammonium compounds (quats) are cationic detergents that solubilize the cell membranes of microorganisms. Their use is similar to glutaraldehyde.

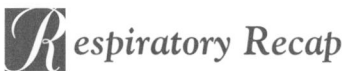espiratory Recap

Methods of Sterilization	
Autoclaving (steam)	Quats
Gas (ethylene oxide)	Irradiation
Glutaraldehyde	

Gamma (γ) irradiation is useful for equipment that does not tolerate moisture or heat; irradiation also is frequently used by manufacturers to sterilize single-use disposable items. It is not commonly used to process reusable equipment due to the expense and bulk of the equipment required.

Equipment Surveillance

Maintaining a regular program of surveillance is important to ensure that sterile and disinfected equipment is being properly processed to meet the necessary levels of cleanliness. Although indicator tapes are regularly placed in autoclaves and gas sterilizers to indicate that proper heat and gas concentrations and duration have been achieved for each run, this action does not ensure that sterilization has actually taken place. Biologic tests also are regularly run in each sterilizer. The tubes containing bacteria in growth medium are subsequently cultured to ensure complete killing. Still, this step does not guarantee that the equip-

ment itself is being sterilized. Inadequate cleaning before autoclaving, for example, may allow organisms to survive, requiring that the equipment itself be cultured periodically to verify the sterility of sterile equipment or low bacterial counts for clean equipment. One of the following three methods are typically used:

1. Aspiration: A quantity of sterile saline is drawn through the lumen of the equipment to be tested, after which the saline is cultured.
2. Plating: To culture exterior surfaces, the equipment may be rolled directly onto a culture medium, usually a Petri dish filled with agar (a plate). The culture obtained may be qualitative (measuring only the presence and type of organism) or quantitative (measuring the level of infection by counting of the number of colonies produced on the agar surface).
3. Swabbing: Irregular surfaces that are not easily rolled onto an agar plate may be rubbed with a sterile swab coated with culture medium. The swab may then be used to inoculate a plate.

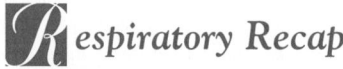espiratory Recap

Equipment Surveillance
Aspiration
Plating
Swabbing

Universal Precautions

The HIV pandemic, along with appearance of antibiotic-resistant microorganisms and increased immigration from the Third World to First World countries focused increased attention on disease transmission in the health care setting in the 1980s. A protocol was developed to minimize transmission of disease between patients and caregivers, termed **universal precautions**,[3] and gained such dramatic acceptance that adherence to it is now a major part of the day-to-day practice of respiratory care.

Universal precautions to some extent replaced a strategy of disease-specific precautions. Previously, emphasis was placed on the identification of individuals with specific diseases. Once the individual was diagnosed, specific precautions could be taken based on the known mode of transmission. Why was this approach changed?

Underlying the universal precautions are two basic ideas that reflect the changing realities mentioned at the beginning of this section. The first concept is that any person may potentially harbor any of a very large number of serious communicable diseases, including HIV, hepatitis (B, C, E, G), MDR-TB, herpes simplex virus (HSV), varicella-zoster virus (VRE), multidrug-resistant *S. aureus* (MRSA), and other yet-identified diseases. Also included are common organisms that, if transmitted to an immunocompromised individual, may be just as deadly. Given the large number of infectious diseases encountered in clinical practice, screening for all possibilities is highly impractical.

The second concept underlying universal precautions is that the presence of an infectious disease can rarely be excluded, even when an individual is specifically tested for the disease. This fact has been especially true of HIV, in which serology may be negative for 2 weeks despite very high viral loads in the blood. Therefore testing is not only impractical but also incompletely effective in the identification of transmission risks. From these two concepts sprang the central tenet of universal precautions, as follows:

Treat every person (including yourself) as if they carried a communicable disease.

Two major techniques are used to accomplish the tenet. First, "If it's wet and it isn't yours, don't touch it." Because microbes are frequently spread by contact and the majority of organisms require a moist environment to maintain viability, the use of appropriate protective barriers (gloves, boots, mask, eye protection, gown) is required when contact with any body fluid is possible. Contact with dry, intact skin does not require protective barriers. Aerosolization represents another major pathway for disease transmission. Universal use of airborne isolation procedures is less practical, but masks are worn to protect the caregiver in cases in which aerosolization of body fluids or fine particle formation is possible (such as the use of bone saws or the induction of cough for a sputum specimen). Masks also are worn to protect the patient in cases in which respiratory aerosols may transmit pathogens to an open wound, such as during dressing changes.

The second technique of universal precautions is consistent hand washing before and after patient contact, a practice designed to remove organisms that may circumvent or penetrate a protective barrier and to remove organisms that remain viable on the skin without the gross presence of body fluids. The disinfection of respiratory equipment between each patient may be viewed as an extension of this technique. Hand washing is almost certainly the most effective intervention practitioners perform to limit the spread of infectious disease. Unfortunately, numerous studies have documented generally poor compliance with regu-

lar hand washing, which can be difficult to perform regularly. This practice takes time from schedules that are already too stretched in most institutions, and sinks are sometimes inconveniently located. Despite its occasional inconvenience, the bottom line remains that hand washing is essential to the provision of good health care, and the provider is encouraged to make an ingrained habit of it.

Respiratory Infection

Otitis and Sinusitis

The nasopharynx is surrounded by several air spaces in the skull that drain into it via channels. These air spaces include the middle ear, which drains into the posterior nasopharynx via the eustachian tube, along with the frontal, sphenoid, and maxillary sinuses, which drain into the nasopharynx through ostia located above the superior turbinate and under the middle turbinate. In addition, two collections of small air cells are present in the skull—the ethmoid air cells above the nose and the mastoid cells behind the ears. Because the drainage passages to the middle ear and sinuses are vulnerable to obstruction by mucosal swelling, thick secretions, or mechanical obstruction by tubes or nasal polyps, these spaces can become essentially closed spaces, prone to infection. Anatomic differences in the child's eustachian tube predispose it to obstruction, explaining the higher incidence of otitis media in children.

The organisms that cause URIs may be acquired by inhalation of infected aerosol drops, as with *S. pneumoniae* and viruses. However, infection frequently represents an overgrowth of local flora after normal drainage of the air space is compromised, explaining why sinusitis frequently follows a viral URI that has caused mucosal edema. The most common organisms causing otitis and sinusitis therefore reflect the normal flora of the nasopharynx to a great extent. In decreasing order of frequency, they are *S. pneumoniae*, *S. aureus*, *H. influenzae*, and *M. catarrhalis*.

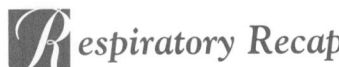*espiratory Recap*

Upper Respiratory Pathogens
Respiratory viruses
S. pneumoniae
H. influenzae
M. catarrhalis

Pharyngitis, Parapharyngeal Abscess, Epiglottitis, and Tracheitis/Tracheobronchitis (Croup)

The trachea and posterior pharynx itself are also frequent sites of infection. Overgrowth of normal flora is less commonly the culprit here because these spaces are not closed.

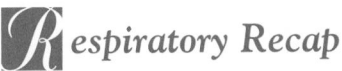*espiratory Recap*

Universal Precautions
Protect both the patient and the caregiver.
Apply precautions for every patient encounter, assuming everyone is at risk.
When body fluids (including significant aerosol) may be encountered, use appropriate barriers, including gloves, mask, eye protection, gowns, and booties.
Wash hands before and after each patient.

Infections in these regions are primarily acquired via aerosol spread. Examples include group A β-hemolytic streptococci (*S. pyogenes*) and *C. diphtheriae*. Infection of the pharynx rarely causes respiratory complications, although the thick gray peel of necrotic mucosa generated in cases of diphtheria can cause airway obstruction. Infection of the trachea can be more severe, especially in infants, in whom even minor mucosal swelling can significantly narrow the airway. Croup, the viral tracheobronchitis that causes stridor and brassy cough in infants, can produce respiratory failure in severe cases. Infection and swelling of the epiglottis (acute epiglottitis) can rapidly produce severe airway compromise in young children and represents a true emergency because acute airway obstruction may occur. If the infection spreads to the soft tissues around the pharynx and trachea (parapharyngeal abscess), local swelling can compress the airway. Alternatively, the deep tissue planes of the neck may facilitate the rapid spread of infection down into the mediastinum (Ludwig's angina).

Bronchitis, Bronchiolitis, and Pneumonia

The lung may become infected by two major routes: (1) aspiration of secretions and (2) inhalation of infected aerosols. Infection also may be carried to the lung by the bloodstream (hematogenous spread). Up to 98% of the cardiac output flows through the pulmonary capillary bed, which is the first filter encountered by organisms or objects returning to the heart from the body via the venous system of the body. Nevertheless, hematogenous infection is much less common than aspiration or inhalation.

Most lower respiratory infections are thought to originate from the person's own flora and gain access to the lung by aspiration of secretions. The usual source is via the pharynx and upper digestive tract. Organisms from the upper digestive tract find their way to the pharynx via gastroesophageal reflux, which occurs nearly universally in healthy individuals. Once organisms are present in the pharynx, they are readily aspirated into the lower respiratory tract. Up to 45% of healthy individuals aspirate small amounts of secretions (microaspiration).[4] Weakened hospital patients, spending long periods of time flat and often with nasogastric tubes traversing the pharynx, experience an even greater incidence of aspiration. Intubated, mechanically ventilated patients are believed to universally aspirate.

The aspirated organisms generally represent the normal flora, but illness and extensive exposure to antibiotics may modify it substantially, particularly evident in the increasing role of gram negatives as one moves across Table 16-2 from CAP to nosocomial pneumonia and VAP. Factors that have been shown to increase pharyngeal colonization with potentially pathogenic gram-negative bacteria are presented as follows, grouped to suggest possible mechanisms by which they operate: depressed level of consciousness (alcoholism, coma, hypotension), compromised immune function (acidosis, alcoholism, azotemia, diabetes mellitus, leukocytosis, leukopenia), anatomic alteration of the respiratory system (nasogastric or endotracheal tubes, preexisting pulmonary disease), and exposure to antibiotics. The recognized risk factors for development of nosocomial pneumonia are essentially identical, with the addition of extreme age (either young or old).

Respiratory Recap

Mechanisms of Infection	
Overgrowth of normal flora	Hematogenous spread
Aspiration of oral and gastric flora	Direct contact (rare except during instrumentation)
Aerosol inhalation	

Aerosol spread is another common route of lower respiratory infection. Coughing and sneezing project large quantities of aerosol a surprising distance, but even quiet breathing produces aerosol capable of spreading infection. In the case of fungi, large numbers of organisms may be present in the general environment. Aerosol transmission can occur in the hospital, although isolation of patients with pneumonia is not a common practice. An important exception is tuberculosis, which requires immediate respiratory (aerosol) isolation as soon as a reasonable suspicion of the disease is present.

Direct contact rarely causes pneumonia directly but is believed to be a common mode by which bacteria are spread between patients and caregivers. These bacteria often include antibiotic-resistant and unusual organisms, such as MRSA and VRE. Once spread to a new individual, these bacteria frequently reside in the nasopharynx, skin, and digestive tract, where they displace normal flora. From these locations, they infect the lower respiratory tract, providing a reason why hand washing is an effective and essential technique used to limit the spread of infectious agents in the health care setting. Direct contact does become an important mechanism of infection when instrumentation is introduced into the lower respiratory tract.

Nosocomial Infections Related to Respiratory Care Equipment

The upper and lower respiratory tracts contain an extremely large surface area—approximately 100 m^2—within a nearly ideal environment for microbes, one that is warm, humid, and dark. Several liters of air move into and from the lungs every minute, with the potential for carrying large numbers of microorganisms. Many of the patients encountered by the respiratory therapist have compromised host defenses against infection, and in the case of the mechanically ventilated patient the respiratory therapist regularly bypasses these defenses. Therefore a primary issue in respiratory care is to prevent the introduction of infection. Although the majority of nosocomial pneumonia cases arise from microaspiration, respiratory care equipment itself is a well-documented source of such infection.

Equipment-Related Issues

Ventilator Tubing During normal use, water from the ventilator humidification system condenses in the inspiratory tubing. Craven and colleagues showed that this condensate is contaminated with organisms from the patient's oropharynx.[5] The primary hazard of this contaminated condensate is inadvertent spillage into the patient's respiratory tract during tube manipulation. With normal use, contamination of the ventilator circuit is from the patient, and circuits can be used for prolonged periods without increasing the pneumonia risk.

Humidifiers and Nebulizers Approximately 30 years ago, humidifiers operated with an aerosol chamber and were implicated in cases of nosocomial pneumonia. Modern humidifiers use a wick or bubble-through system that avoids significant aerosolization, and this use has been associated with a decline in VAP rates. Nosocomial pneumonia can be a complication of small-volume nebulizer use due to contamination of medications from multidose vials[6] and *Legionella*-contaminated tap water.[7]

Respiratory Recap

Nosocomial Sources of Respiratory Infection	
Condensate in ventilator tubing	Suction catheters
Humidifiers	PFT equipment
Nebulizers	Nasotracheal and nasogastric tubes

Suction Catheters Suction catheters acquire bacterial contamination as they pass through the endotracheal tube and can deposit these bacteria in the lower airways. In-line, multiuse suction catheters become colonized over time,[8] but this colonization is likely from organisms within the patient's lower respiratory tract.

Mechanical Ventilators The 1994 Centers for Disease Control and Prevention (CDC) Guideline for Prevention of Nosocomial Pneumonia states that "the internal machinery of mechanical ventilators ... is not considered an important source of bacterial contamination of inhaled gas." Thus routine sterilization or high-level disinfection is considered unnecessary.[9]

Spirometers and Pulmonary Function Testing Equipment Pulmonary function testing (PFT) equipment, like the mechanical ventilator, is not believed to carry a high risk

of infection. However, rare cases of cross-contamination have occurred.[10,11] For this reason the use of filters between the patient and equipment has been advocated to trap aerosolized microbes.

Ventilator-Associated Pneumonia Mechanically ventilated patients are at high risk for the development of pneumonia and sinusitis. Most such cases of VAP are not attributable directly to respiratory care equipment but instead to aspiration of organisms from the patient's own flora. VAP has an incidence of 0.5% to 3.4% per day, with most patients' risk being 1% per day.[12] As shown in Box 16-1, the microbiology of VAP differs substantially from that of CAP and other nosocomial pneumonias. This difference reflects the more severe immunocompromised state of the individuals with this disease—both mechanically due to hardware in the airways and biologically due to severe underlying illness. The difference also reflects the different spectrum of bacteria that colonize ICUs.

Infection-Reducing Techniques

Reduction of Condensate within Ventilator Tubing Heated wires within the inspiratory circuit reduce, but do not eliminate, condensation. Use of a heat-moisture exchanger (HME) or artificial nose at the patient end of the ventilator circuit recycles humidity from the exhaled gas, eliminating the need for a humidifier and minimizing circuit condensation. Although one study suggested a reduction in VAP with the use of HMEs,[13] this finding has not been universal.[14-16] Regardless of the technique used, care should be taken to drain condensate and avoid spillage into the patient's airway during tubing manipulation.

Sinusitis Prevention and Surveillance The population of patients seen by respiratory therapists is particularly susceptible to the development of sinusitis. First, they are frequently debilitated, with lowered host defenses. Second, they tend to spend long periods of time in the supine position. Third, they tend to have increased amount and thickness of secretions, which plug the communicating passages to the sinuses. Finally, hardware inserted in the nares (nasal packing, nasotracheal tubes, and nasogastric tubes) can physically obstruct the orifices that drain the sinuses.

In most patients, little can be done to alter these risk factors. Orotracheal intubation does reduce the risk of sinusitis compared with nasotracheal intubation.[17] Adequate hydration of the patient and especially humidification of inspired gases thin secretions and promote drainage. Some nasal hardware may be readily moved from one nare to the other at intervals to limit the period of time that each side is obstructed. The use of a vasoconstrictor, such as oxymetazoline delivered as a nasal spray, may decrease mucosal edema and thereby maintain the patency of the drainage orifices.

Patients with respiratory illness will continue to develop sinusitis, however, and the condition remains an important cause of fever in the ICU. Because of the multiple potential sources of fever in these patients, sinusitis is frequently missed and probably resolves much later as the patient recovers and mobilizes and tubes are withdrawn. Holzapfel and colleagues[18] showed that ICU morbidity can be significantly decreased if the diagnosis of sinusitis is aggressively pursued and treated. In their study of nasotracheally intubated patients, all patients with otherwise unexplained fever underwent x-ray and/or CT scanning of the sinuses. If evidence of sinusitis was present, it was confirmed and the organism identified by needle aspiration of the sinus. All confirmed cases were treated, yielding a decrease in both VAP and mortality.

Frequency of Ventilator Circuit Changes Traditionally, regular tubing changes, as frequently as every 8 hours, were advocated for all mechanically ventilated patients to reduce the risk of VAP. Several studies have shown that less-frequent tubing changes may be superior. Lareau and colleagues[19] reported that VAP rates were reduced when tubing was changed every 24 hours instead of every 8 or 12 hours. In addition, Craven and colleagues[20] reported that an increase the interval from 24 to 48 hours did not increase inspiratory gas contamination or VAP rate. Dreyfuss and colleagues[21] reported no increase in pneumonia when ventilator circuits were left in place for the entire duration of mechanical ventilation, compared with changes every 48 hours. Similarly, Thompson[22] reported that (in a subacute care facility) the incidence of VAP was unchanged in comparison of tube changes every 7 days versus every 14 days. The optimum protocol for ventilator tubing changes is still considered uncertain, but evidence suggests that tubing-change intervals should be at 7 days,[23,24] and accumulating evidence suggests that ventilator circuits need not be changed at any regular interval.[21,25]

Frequency of HME Changes Accumulating evidence suggests that HMEs can be used for 48 to 96 hours without increasing the risk of nosocomial pneumonia.[26-32]

Frequency of Nebulizer Changes Because they produce aerosols that can carry microorganisms into the lower respiratory tract, nebulizers should be changed daily.[9] This recommendation is for both large-volume nebulizers (for example, heated aerosol, cool mist) and small-volume medication nebulizers.

Use of Sterile Water Common practice is to fill the humidification chamber with sterile water to prevent the introduction of heat-resistant organisms, such as *Legionella* species, which may contaminate the device despite its high temperatures that inactivate most common respiratory pathogens. The efficacy of this practice has not been validated but appears prudent given the demonstrated danger of *Legionella* infection from hospital tap water. Similarly, sterile water is preferred to tap water during rinsing of reusable equipment after disinfection.[33]

Use of Single-Use Versus Multiuse In-Line Suction Catheters Studies have failed to show a consistent difference between single use and in-line suction catheters in terms of pneumonia incidence.[8,34] The colonization of in-line suction catheters is likely from the patient. Evidence has shown that pneumonia rates are not increased if the in-line suction catheter is used for a prolonged time.[34]

Continuous Subglottic Suctioning Continuous suctioning of secretions pooled between the glottis and endotracheal tube balloon, through a separate port integrated into the endotracheal tube wall, may delay the onset of pneumonia in mechanically ventilated patients. Studies have demonstrated a decreased pneumonia rate with this technique.[35-37] Presumably, subglottic suctioning works by reducing the volume of secretions that are silently aspirated past the cuff of the endotracheal tube.

Use of Acid-Suppression Therapy Versus Sucralfate for Peptic Ulcer Prophylaxis Acid-suppression therapy used to treat peptic ulcer prophylaxis is currently an area of controversy. The gastric acid suppression commonly used in the ICU has been shown to increase the number of bacteria in the stomach.[38] In addition, that the increased bacteria correlate with risk of pneumonia has been demonstrated.[39,40] A suggestion has been made that through replacement of gastric acid suppressive therapy with sucralfate (which forms a protective coat over the mucosa without altering pH) the incidence of nosocomial pneumonia might be reduced. Numerous studies have addressed this question without consistent findings.

Selective Decontamination of the Digestive Tract The goal of selective decontamination of the digestive tract (SDD) is to reduce the number of gram-negative bacteria and *Candida* species from the upper digestive tract while not disturbing the anaerobic flora that helps prevent overgrowth of other organisms. This reduction is accomplished by a combination of an oral paste and an oral or tube-fed solution of polymyxin, an aminoglycoside, or fluoroquinolone, and an antifungal such as nystatin. Numerous trials of SDD have been performed, most demonstrating a reduction in the pneumonia rate. Most of the studies have contained methodologic flaws.[9] Recent controlled trials failed to show significant pneumonia reduction;[41,42] therefore the efficacy of SDD remains uncertain.

Kinetic Beds (Continuous Lateral Rotational Therapy) Immobility has been implicated as a substantial risk factor for nosocomial pneumonia, and kinetic beds, which rotate the patient from side to side, have been proposed to decrease its incidence.[43-45] Although the results of several studies have been mixed, the meta-analysis by Cook and colleagues[14] does suggest a benefit.

Diagnostic Procedures

Sputum Induction

When a patient is unable to produce sputum for analysis, the inhalation of nebulized hypertonic saline frequently yields an acceptable sample. The saline increases the tonicity of the fluid layer lining the airways, both drawing fluid into these secretions and stimulating an irritant cough response. In the patient who is able to produce sputum spontaneously, induction does not improve sensitivity. Care must be taken during sputum induction in a patient with suspected contagious illness, especially tuberculosis, to prevent transmission of the disease to the respiratory therapist.

Bronchoscopy

Fiberoptic bronchoscopy is a powerful technique that enables the collection of many sample types from the lower airways. The working channel is generally contaminated with upper airway secretions, so simple suctioned specimens yield unreliable cultures. This problem has been addressed with the protected specimen brush (PSB), also called the *protected brush catheter (PBC)*. A brush, the sterility of which is maintained within a sheath, is passed through the working channel into the bronchus. The brush is advanced from the catheter and worked back and forth to collect secretions and cells before it is withdrawn back into the protective sheath and retrieved for culture. The reported sensitivity of PSB varies from 36% to 72%, with specificity of 85% to 93%.[46-52]

Another common technique used to diagnose pneumonia, which has the ability to sample the extreme distal airways and alveoli, is bronchoalveolar lavage (BAL). The bronchoscope is positioned as far distally as possible in the airway leading to the site of interest. Aliquots of 20 to 50 mL of sterile saline, totaling up to 250 mL but usually on the order of 100 mL, are introduced via the working channel. This saline migrates distally, mixing with secretions, and each aliquot then is suctioned back and collected in a sterile trap. BAL is a sensitive technique and used to detect organisms that are not reliably isolated from sputum, including nontuberculous mycobacteria, CMV and *Pneumocystis* species, for which sensitivities may be more than 90% with near-100% specificity.[53] When used to diagnose acute nosocomial pneumonia, BAL has been reported to produce sensitivities of 63% to 82% and specificities of 85% to 96%.[51,52]

Biopsy of the lung parenchyma is useful for diagnosis of pneumonia, especially fungal and granulomatous infections, and is accomplished bronchoscopically by tearing of small pieces of tissue (approximately 1 mm) from the lung parenchyma with small grasping biopsy forceps that are placed through the working channel. For bacterial pneumonia, transbronchial biopsy (TBB) has a reported sensitivity of 57% and specificity of 100%.[54] Because the technique appears to offer little advantage over PSB and BAL and carries a much higher risk of hemorrhage and pneumothorax, TBB is not often used to diagnose acute pneumonia.

Regardless of the technique used for specimen collection, quantitative culture is superior to standard, qualitative culture techniques because of its increased ability to distinguish contaminants from true infection.

Transtracheal Aspiration

Transtracheal aspiration (TTA) is a sputum-collection technique designed to bypass the upper airway, with its potential contaminants. The method begins with a careful skin preparation of the anterior neck, followed by the insertion of a sterile needle directly into the trachea through the cricothyroid membrane. Proper position is ensured by aspiration of air from the needle, and tracheal secretions are aspirated. The obvious disadvantage of this procedure is its invasive nature, leading to a substantial number of complications, which explains why it is not commonly used in clinical practice although it remains a useful research standard.

Nonbronchoscopic Bronchoalveolar Lavage

BAL also has been described with a blind, nonbronchoscopic technique in mechanically ventilated patients. With this technique a 14-French catheter with guide wire is advanced through the endotracheal tube until resistance is felt in the distal airways of the (usually) right lower lobe, usually at a distance of 50 to 60 cm. The guide wire then is removed, and two 50-mL aliquots of sterile saline are instilled and suctioned. When compared with traditional bronchoscopic BAL (B-BAL) in the same patients, the reported sensitivities of nonbronchoscopic BAL (NB-BAL) and B-BAL were 73% and 93%, respectively; specificities were 96% and 100%, respectively.[55] Although traditional BAL is superior to NB-BAL, the nonbronchoscopic technique is useful because of its ease of performance and substantially lower cost.

Pleural Fluid Analysis

The presence of significant pleural fluid usually demands sampling and analysis of the fluid to determine its nature, unless a cause is readily apparent. Pleural fluid analysis may address two principal issues. First, the measurement of fluid characteristics, such as cell type, pH, protein, amylase, lactate dehydrogenase, and others, may provide clues to the effusion's cause. For example, demonstration of increased adenosine deaminase (ADA) in the fluid, a predominance of lymphocytes in the white blood cell (WBC) differential, and a paucity of mesothelial cells (which make up the pleural surface and are usually found in abundance) all suggest tuberculosis as a potential cause.

A second issue is frequently addressed when a pleural effusion is adjacent to an area of pneumonia. These parapneumonic effusions are at risk for becoming secondarily infected from the pneumonia, at which time they become empyemas. If organisms are cultured from the normally sterile pleural space, this technique usually identifies the cause of the pneumonia. Parapneumonic effusions also tend to be highly proteinaceous, prone to developing loculations and forming peels around the adjacent lung, permanently limiting its expansion. For this reason, parapneumonic effusions are most frequently drained completely at the time of sampling.

Acceptable Specimens

The collection of sputum specimens from which microbiologic diagnoses can be made is quite difficult, accounting for the low percentage of pneumonias identified by sputum alone (less than half). Three criteria must be met to obtain a useful sputum specimen. First, the specimen must be collected in a sterile container and handled with sterile technique. Second, the specimen must be transported to the laboratory promptly. Some respiratory pathogens are very sensitive to bacterial overgrowth, which may occur if the sputum sits. Finally, the sample must be screened to verify that it is in fact sputum from the lower respiratory tract and not saliva, which is accomplished by counting of the number of squamous epithelial cells per microscopic low power field (lpf). Because these cells originate from the oropharynx, a large number of them (>25/lpf) indicates a specimen that is unacceptably contaminated with oral secretions. Sputum with less than 25 squamous epithelial cells per lpf is considered a good specimen.

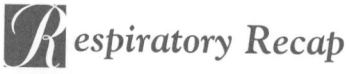

Respiratory Recap

Acceptable Sputum Specimens
Less than 25 squamous cells per low power field

KEY POINTS

- Respiratory infection is caused most frequently by bacteria, viruses, and *Mycoplasma pneumoniae*. Chlamydiae, rickettsiae, mycobacteria, and fungi also are commonly encountered.
- Bacteria are classified by three major characteristics—oxygen requirement, Gram's staining positivity versus negativity, and shape.
- Normal flora bacteria are generally present in certain areas of the body but are major causes of respiratory infection when they overgrow in the upper airway or are introduced to the normally near-sterile lower airways.
- The modes of infection and the most common respiratory pathogens vary significantly, depending on the age and setting. CAP in young patients, CAP in older patients, nosocomial pneumonia, and VAP all must be considered separately.
- Among normal adults the major pathogens of upper airway infection are *S. pneumoniae*, *H. influenzae*, and *M. catarrhalis*. The most common community-acquired lower respiratory pathogens are *S. pneumoniae*, viruses, and *H. influenzae*. *M. pneumoniae*, *C. pneumoniae*, and assorted gram-negative bacteria are also common.

- A large number of antibiotics are available to treat respiratory infection, each with toxicities that must be considered. Use of nebulized antibiotics can reduce toxicity.
- Antibiotic resistance is now a common phenomenon and has necessitated use of multiple antibiotics for some infections, such as tuberculosis and *Pseudomonas* pneumonia.
- Aspiration represents the major route of pulmonary infection, especially among hospitalized patients. However, a wide variety of respiratory care equipment has been implicated in the spread of infection.
- Several specific clinical practices have been identified that are shown to reduce the incidence of pneumonia in hospitalized, especially critically ill, patients.
- The use of universal precautions, including hand washing, has become standard practice and should be used without exception to reduce the spread of infection in the heath care setting.
- Induced sputum is frequently useful, but some infections are much more reliably diagnosed with bronchoscopy or nonbronchoscopic bronchoalveolar lavage.
- Acceptable sputum specimens must have fewer than 25 squamous epithelial cells per low-power field to distinguish them from saliva.

References

1. Hoft DF, Tennant JM. Persistence and boosting of bacille Calmette-Guerin-induced delayed-type hypersensitivity. Ann Intern Med 1999;131:32.
2. Carrier R, editor. Guinness Book of World Records. New York: Bantam Books; 1999. p. 236.
3. Garner JS. Hospital control practices advisory committee guideline for isolation precautions in hospitals. Infect Control Hosp Epidemiol 1996;17:53-80.
4. Huxley EJ, Viroslav J, Gray WR, et al. Pharyngeal aspiration in normal adults and patients with depressed consciousness. Am J Med 1973;64:564-568.

5. Craven DE, Goularte TA, Make BA. Contaminated condensate in mechanical ventilator circuits—risk factor for nosocomial pneumonia? Am Rev Respir Dis 1984;129:625-628.

6. Sanders CV, Luby JP, Johanson WG, et al. *Serratia marcescens* infections from inhaled therapy medications: nosocomial outbreak. Ann Intern Med 1970;73:315-321.

7. Mastro TD, Fields BS, Breiman RF, et al. Nosocomial Legionnaire's disease and use of medication nebulizers. J Infect Dis 1991;163:667-670.

8. Deppe SA, Kelly JW, Thoi LL, et al. Incidence of colonization, nosocomial pneumonia, and mortality in critically ill patients using a Trach Care closed-suction system versus an open-suction system: prospective, randomized study. Crit Care Med 1990;18(12):1389-1393.

9. Centers for Disease Control and Prevention. Hospital Infection Control Practices Advisory Committee Members: Guideline for Prevention of Nosocomial Pneumonia. Respir Care 1994;39:1191-1236.

10. Cunha BA, Klimek JJ, Gracewski J, et al. A common source outbreak of *Acinetobacter* pulmonary infection traced to Wright respirometers. J Postgrad Med 1980;56:169-172.

11. Gough J, Kraak WAG, Anderson EC, et al. Cross-infection by non-encapsulated *Haemophilus influenzae*. Lancet 1990;336: 159-160.

12. Fagon JY, Chastre J, Domart Y, et al. Nosocomial pneumonia in patients receiving continuous mechanical ventilation: prospective analysis of 52 episodes with use of a protected specimen brush and quantitative culture techniques. Am Rev Respir Dis 1989;139:877-884.

13. Kirton OC, DeHaven B, Morgan J, et al. A prospective, randomized comparison of an in-line heat moisture exchange filter and heated wire humidifiers: rates of ventilator-associated early-onset (community-acquired) or late-onset (hospital-acquired) pneumonia and incidence of endotracheal tube occlusion. Chest 1997;112:1055-1059.

14. Cook D, De Jonghe B, Brochard L, et al. Influence of airway management on ventilator-associated pneumonia: evidence from randomized trials. JAMA 1998;279(10):781-787.

15. Branson RD, Davis K, Brown R, et al. Comparison of three humidification techniques during mechanical ventilation: patient selection, cost, and infection considerations. Respir Care 1996;41:809-816.

16. Dreyfuss D, Kjedaini K, Gros I, et al. Mechanical ventilation with heated humidifiers or heat and moisture exchangers: effects on patient colonization and incidence of nosocomial pneumonia. Am J Respir Crit Care Med 1995;151:986-992.

17. Holzapfel L, Chevret S, Madinier G, et al. Influence of long-term oro- or nasotracheal intubation on nosocomial maxillary sinusitis and pneumonia: results of a prospective randomized clinical trial. Crit Care Med 1993;21:1132-1138.

18. Holzapfel L, Chastang C, Demingeon G, et al. A randomized study assessing the systematic search for maxillary sinusitis in nasotracheally mechanically ventilated patients: influence of nosocomial maxillary sinusitis on the occurrence of ventilator-associated pneumonia. Am J Resp Crit Care Med 1999;159: 695-701.

19. Lareau SC, Ryan KJ, Diener CF. The relationship between frequency of ventilator circuit changes and infectious hazard. Am Rev Respir Dis 1978;118:493-496.

20. Craven DE, Connolly MG, Lichtenberg DA, et al. Contamination of mechanical ventilators with tubing changes every 24 or 48 hours. N Engl J Med 1982;306:1505-1509.

21. Dreyfuss D, Djedaini K, Weber P, et al. Prospective study of nosocomial pneumonia and of patient and circuit colonization during mechanical ventilation with circuit changes every 48 hours vs. no change. Am Rev Respir Dis 1991;143:738-743.

22. Thompson RE. Incidence of ventilator-associated pneumonia (VAP) with 14-day circuit change in a subacute environment. Respir Care 1996;41:601-606.

23. Fink JB, Krasue SA, Barrett L, et al. Extending ventilator circuit change interval beyond 2 days reduces the likelihood of ventilator-associated pneumonia. Chest 1998;113:405-411.

24. Hess D, Burns E, Romagnoli D, et al. Weekly ventilator circuit changes: a strategy to reduce costs without affecting pneumonia rates. Anesthesiology 1995;82:903-911.

25. Kollef MH, Shapiro SD, Fraser VJ, et al. Mechanical ventilation with or without 7-day circuit changes: a randomized controlled trial. Ann Intern Med 1995;123:168-174.

26. Daumal F, Colpart E, Manoury B, et al. Changing heat and moisture exchangers every 48 hours does not increase the incidence of nosocomial pneumonia. Infect Control Hosp Epidemiol 1999;20:347-349.

27. Davis K, Evans SL, Campbell RS, et al. Prolonged use of heat and moisture exchangers (HME) does not affect device efficiency or incidence of nosocomial pneumonia. Crit Care Med 2000;28:1412-1418.

28. Thomachot L, Vialet R, Viguier J, et al. Efficacy of heat and moisture exchangers after changing every 48 hours rather than 24 hours. Crit Care Med 1998;26:477-481.

29. Djedaini K, Billiard M, Mier L, et al. Changing heat and moisture exchangers every 48 hours rather than 24 hours does not affect their efficacy and the incidence of nosocomial pneumonia. Am J Respir Crit Care Med 1995;152:1562-1569.

30. Thomachot L, Boisson C, Arnaud S, et al. Changing heat and moisture exchangers after 96 hours rather than after 24 hours: a clinical and microbiological evaluation. Crit Care Med 2000;28:714-720.

31. Markowicz P, Richard J, Dreyfuss D, et al. Safety, efficacy, and cost-effectiveness of mechanical ventilation with humidifying filters changed every 48 hours: a prospective, randomized study. Crit Care Med 2000;28:665-671.

32. Kollef MH, Shapiro SD, Boyd V, et al. A randomized clinical trial comparing an extended-use hygroscopic condenser humidifier with heated-water humidification in mechanically ventilated patients. Chest 1998;113:759-767.

33. Arnow PM, Chou T, Weil D, et al. Nosocomial Legionnaire's disease caused by aerosolized tap water from respiratory devices. J Infect Dis 1982;146:460-467.

34. Kollef MH, Prentice S, Shapiro SD, et al. Mechanical ventilation with or without daily changes of in-line suction catheters. Am J Respir Crit Care Med 1997;156:466-472.

35. Mahul P, Auboyer C, Jospe R, et al. Prevention of nosocomial pneumonia in intubated patients: respective role of mechanical subglottic secretions drainage and stress ulcer prophylaxis. Intensive Care Med 1992;18:20-25.

36. Valles J, Artigas A, Rello J, et al. Continuous aspiration of subglottic secretions in preventing ventilator-associated pneumonia. Ann Intern Med 1995;122:179-186.

37. Rello J, Sonora R, Jubert P, et al. Pneumonia in intubated patients: role of respiratory airway care. Am J Respir Crit Care Med 1996;154:111-115.

38. Donowitz LG, Page MC, Mileur BL, et al. Alteration of normal gastric flora in critical patients receiving antacid and cimetidine therapy. Infect Control 1986;7:23-26.

39. Atherton ST, White DJ. Stomach as a source of bacteria colonizing respiratory tract during artificial ventilation. Lancet 1978;2:968-969.

40. DuMoulin GC, Paterson DG, White JH, et al. Aspiration of gastric bacteria in antacid-treated patients: a frequent cause of postoperative colonization of the airway. Lancet 1982;2: 242-245.

41. Gastienne H, Wolff M, Destour F, et al. A controlled trial in intensive care units of selective decontamination of the digestive tract with nonabsorbable antibiotics. N Engl J Med 1992;326: 594-599.

42. Hammond JMJ, Potgieter PD, Saunders GL, et al. A double-blind study of selective decontamination in intensive care. Lancet 1992;340:5-9.

43. Fink MP, Helsmoortel CM, Stein KL, et al. The efficacy of an oscillating bed in the prevention of lower respiratory tract infection in critically ill victims of blunt trauma: a prospective study. Chest 1990;97:132-137.

44. Summer WR, Curry P, Haponik EF, et al. Continuous mechanical turning of intensive care unit patients shortens length of stay in some diagnostic-related groups. J Crit Care 1989;4:45-53.

45. Gentilello L, Thompson DA, Tonneson AS, et al. Effect of a rotating bed on the incidence of pulmonary complications in critically ill patients. Crit Care Med 1988;16:783-786.

46. Marquette CH, Copin MC, Wallet F, et al. Diagnostic tests for pneumonia in ventilated patients: prospective evaluation of diagnostic accuracy using histology as a diagnostic gold standard. Am J Respir Crit Care Med 1995;151:1878-1888.

47. Roger-Moreau I, de Bareyrac B, Ducoudre M, et al. Evaluation of bronchoalveolar lavage for the diagnosis of bacterial pneumonia in ventilated patients. Ann Biol Clin (Paris) 1992;50:587-591.

48. Papazian L, Thomas P, Garbe L, et al. Bronchoscopic or blind sampling techniques for the diagnosis of ICU-acquired pneumonia. Am J Respir Crit Care Med 1995;152:324-331.

49. Timsit JF, Misset B, Goldstein FW, et al. Reappraisal of distal diagnostic testing in the diagnosis of ICU-acquired pneumonia. Chest 1995;108:1632-1639.

50. Torres A, el Ebiary M, Padro L, et al. Validation of different techniques for the diagnosis of ventilator-associated pneumonia: comparison with immediate postmortem pulmonary biopsy. Am J Respir Crit Care Med 1994;149:324-331.

51. Sanchez-Nieto JM, Torres A, Garcia-Cordoba F, et al. Impact of invasive and noninvasive quantitative culture sampling on outcome of ventilator-associated pneumonia: a pilot study. Am J Respir Crit Care Med 1998;157:371-376.

52. Jourdain B, Joly-Guillou ML, Dombret MC, et al. Usefulness of quantitative cultures of BAL fluid for diagnosing nosocomial pneumonia. Chest 1997;111:411-418.

53. Paradis IL, Grgurich WF, Dummer JS, et al. Rapid detection of cytomegalovirus pneumonia from lung lavage cells. Am Rev Respir Dis 1988;138:697-702.

54. Rao VK, Ritter J, Kollef MH. Utility of transbronchial biopsy in patients with acute respiratory failure: a postmortem study. Chest 1998;114:549-555.

55. Pugin J, Auckenthaler R, Mili N, et al. Diagnosis of ventilator-associated pneumonia by bacteriologic analysis of bronchoscopic and nonbronchoscopic "blind" bronchoalveolar lavage fluid. Am Rev Respir Dis 1991;143:1121-1129.

CHAPTER 17

Cardiopulmonary Anatomy and Physiology

Evelyn H. Schlenker

OBJECTIVES

1. Describe the gross anatomy of the respiratory system.
2. Describe the anatomy of the upper airway.
3. Describe the anatomy of the tracheobronchial tree.
4. Discuss the relationship between the bony elements of the thorax.
5. Compare the roles of the diaphragm, accessory inspiratory muscles, and abdominal muscles.
6. Compare the pulmonary and bronchial circulations.
7. Describe the innervation of the lungs.
8. Describe the visceral pleura, parietal pleura, and pleural space.
9. Describe the anatomy of the mediastinum.
10. Describe the anatomy of the heart.
11. Describe the mucociliary apparatus.
12. Describe the smooth muscle function of the airways and the pulmonary circulation.
13. Compare macrophages and dendritic cells found within the respiratory system.
14. Compare alveolar Type I and Type II cells.
15. Describe the interstitial space within the lungs.
16. Describe the role of airways resistance and respiratory system compliance on the pressures required during the respiratory cycle.
17. Discuss factors affecting capacity and endurance of respiratory muscles.
18. Compare the distribution of ventilation and blood flow within the lungs.
19. Discuss the importance of the ventilation/perfusion ratio.
20. Describe the diffusion capacity of the lungs.

KEY TERMS

Abdominal Muscles	Atria	Compliance
Accessory Muscles	Bronchi	Conchae
Alveoli	Bronchial Circulation	Coronary Artery

Continued

The primary function of the respiratory system is to promote gas exchange, which entails movement of oxygen (O_2) into the lungs and blood and removal of carbon dioxide (CO_2), a major by-product of aerobic metabolism. Another important function of this system is acid-base regulation in conjunction with the kidneys and various body buffer systems. Because of the large volume of air moved by the lungs (12,000 to 24,000 L/day) and containing numerous pollutants and microbes, defense defines another system function.[1] Defense (prevention of clots from reaching the left side of the heart) is also a function of the pulmonary vasculature that receives the entire cardiac output of the body. Moreover, endothelial cells that line the pulmonary vasculature also produce and metabolize chemicals that affect various organ systems. For example, angiotensin-converting enzyme (ACE) found in endothelial cells converts angiotensin I to angiotensin II, a hormone affecting vasculature tone and adrenal gland function. Finally, as a consequence of air movements into and from the lungs, both heat and water are exchanged. Thus the respiratory system is involved to some extent in both temperature and water balance.[2]

Contraction of respiratory pump muscles also generates pressures within the respiratory system that consequently move air into and from the respiratory tract.[3] These pressures also affect swallowing, suckling, defecation, vomiting, and labor. Regulation of airflow patterns is important in such processes as phonation, vocalization, and musical instrument playing.[1] Moreover, the chest wall (skeletal elements and musculature) is involved in stabilization of the thoracic cavity to maintain posture and expedite locomotion. Aside from lungs, the thoracic cavity contains the heart (Figure 17-1). Both structural and functional interactions between the lungs and the heart affect venous return, cardiac output, and distribution of gas within the lung that in turn influence gas exchange and transport of O_2.

Clearly the respiratory system is involved in numerous functions. The purpose of this chapter is to describe the gross and microanatomy of the respiratory system, including the upper airways, lungs, pleural space, lymphatics, musculature of the chest wall involved in breathing, and innervation of these structures. Functionally the contributions these structures make to the generation of pressures and airflow and the diffusion of O_2 and CO_2 are described. Finally the intimate interactions between the lungs and heart are emphasized.

Gross Anatomy of the Respiratory System

In this section the gross anatomy of the upper airways and thoracic structures (Figure 17-2), including the skeletal elements, muscles, airways and lung parenchyma, is re-

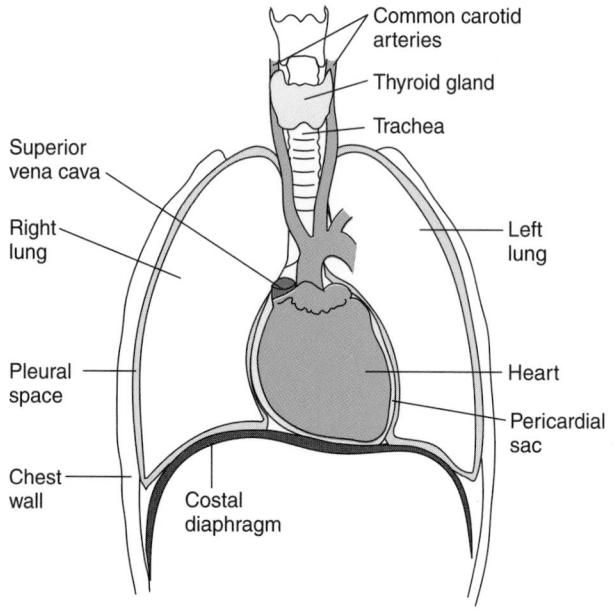

Figure 17-1   Diagram of the structures within the thoracic cavity.

$\mathcal{R}$espiratory Recap

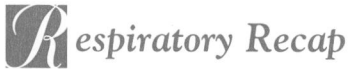

Gross Anatomy of the Respiratory System
Skeletal components
Muscles
Airways and lung parenchyma

viewed. In addition, the functional correlates of these structures associated with gas exchanged are covered.

The upper airways consist of nose, nasopharynx, oropharynx, tongue, epiglottis, laryngopharynx, and portions of the trachea situated outside the thoracic cavity.[4,5] Supporting these structures are connective tissues, muscles, bony elements, and cartilage. At rest, air flows into and from the respiratory system through the nose. Muscles that influence the patency of the nose are the transverse and alar parts of the nasalis muscles and the depressor septi. Two nasal bones form the bridge of the nose and the frontal process of the maxilla. The cavity of the nose is divided into a medial portion divided by the septum into right and left halves. The perpendicular plate of the ethmoid, the nasal cartilage, and the vomer form the septum. Three curled bony plates, or **conchae** (also known as *turbinates*), project downward from the walls of the nasal cavity, greatly enlarging the surface area of the nose, and are lined with mucous membranes containing an olfactory portion with olfactory nerve endings and a respiratory portion with goblet cells and ciliated epithelial cells. These latter cells help move mucus toward the nasopharynx. The respiratory portion is highly vascularized, which helps humidify and warm incoming air. The mucus, hairs, and tortuous turbinate structure of the nose also impede the movement of larger particles into the lungs. Innervation of the respiratory portion of the nasal epithelium is from sensory nerves from the trigeminal (V) cranial nerve. Innervation of the glands located in the nose is via the facial (VII) nerve.[6] Various reflexes associated with the nose affect sneezing, sleep behavior, and the sensation of breathlessness.[3]

The **nasopharynx** is located behind the nasal cavities, above and behind the soft palate. Air from the internal nares then enters the **oropharynx** and the larynx. Except for the soft palate, the walls of the nasopharynx are immovable and help keep this cavity patent. Tonsils or adenoids consist of lymphoid tissues and are located within its posterior wall.[7] Enlargement of these structures may impede breathing, especially during sleep.[8-10] The muscular uvula and muscles comprising the soft palate (such as the palatoglossus, palatopharyngeus, and pharyngeal constrictors) move upward and backward to prevent food and liquids from being regurgitated into the nose.[11] Constriction of these pharyngeal muscles also decreases dead space volume and stabilizes the oropharynx.[12] Inability to maintain the tone of these muscles during sleep may lead to the development of obstructive sleep apnea.[13,14]

The floor of the oral cavity consists of the tongue and the **epiglottis**.[11] Regulation of tongue movement occurs through extrinsic muscles, including the hyoglossus, genioglossus, styloglossus, and the palatoglossus. These muscles move and change the shape of the tongue.[4] The hypoglossal (XII) cranial nerve innervates both the extrinsic and intrinsic muscles. Sensory innervation of the tongue is accomplished by the glossopharyngeal (IX), lingual (V), and tympanic (VII) cranial nerves.[6]

The **larynx** (or windpipe) extends from the epiglottis to the trachea and consists of cartilage, ligaments, and muscles.[5] It is lined by a mucous membrane and bordered by the thyroid gland on its anterior surface and the esophagus on its posterior surface. Enlargement of the thyroid gland (goiter) may impinge on the upper airway, increasing air-

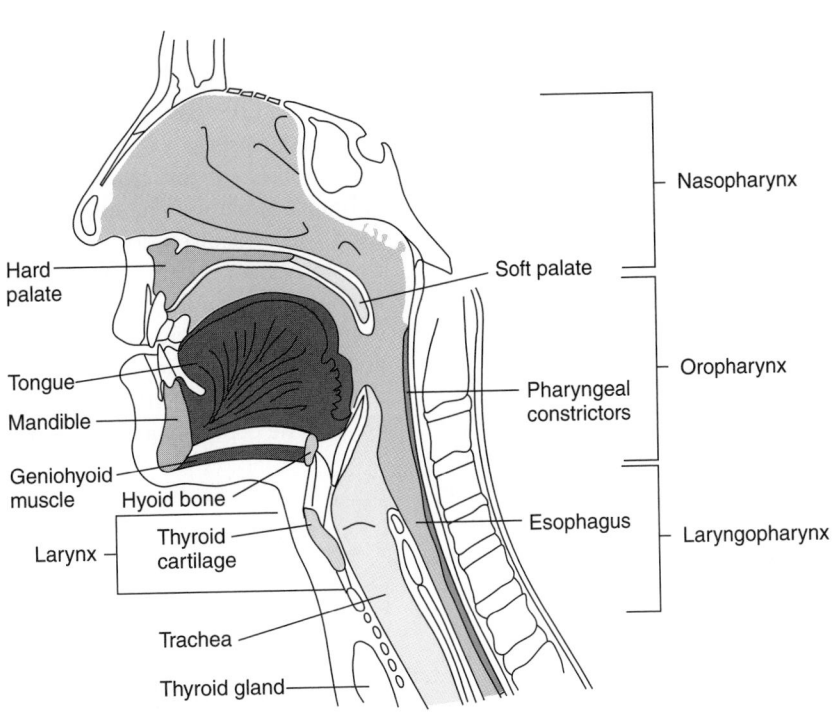

Figure 17-2 Medial section of the pharynx showing the nasopharynx, oropharynx, and laryngopharynx and associated structures.

way resistance.[10] The laryngeal cavity through which air flows consists of the vestibule, glottis, and infraglottis. Laryngeal muscles include intrinsic (cricothyroid, arytenoids, thyroarytenoids, and vocalis muscles) and extrinsic (omohyoid, sternohyoid, sternothyroid, thyrohyoid, and some suprahyoid muscles) groups.[15] These muscles are involved in the opening and closing of the glottis, swallowing, coughing, sneezing, and changes in tension on the vocal cords during phonation,[3] all of which affect airflow by affecting airway resistance. Closure of the glottis and a concomitant increase in intrathoracic pressure occur during defecation and childbirth. Both automatic (the vagus, superior laryngeal, and recurrent laryngeal nerves) and voluntary innervation from the cortex regulate their function.[6] In addition, the extrinsic muscles also may act as accessory muscles during forced inspiratory maneuvers.

The **trachea** begins at the lower border of the cricoid cartilage and measures 10 to 12 cm in length. Half the trachea is part of the neck, and the rest is located within the thoracic cavity. Approximately 15 to 20 horseshoe-shaped cartilage rings help keep the trachea open. Posteriorly the cartilage rings are bound by the tracheal muscle that is innervated by the recurrent laryngeal nerve. Changes in tension or in the position of this smooth muscle affect airway resistance and dead space volume. For example, during coughing the muscle bulges into the lumen of the trachea and increases airway resistance. The tracheal surface is covered with both ciliated and nonciliated epithelial cells, which help make up the mucociliary clearance apparatus[16] of the airways. Submucosal glands also are found on the tracheal surface.

Muscles that may be respiratory in nature are located outside the thoracic cavity, as part of the neck. They include the sternocleidomastoid and scalene muscles, the former muscle of which is innervated by the accessory (XI) nerve and the latter by the anterior primary rami of the cervical (C) nerves (C5-C8). The sternocleidomastoid muscles are known as **accessory muscles** and used during forced inspiration maneuvers. In patients with chronic obstructive lung disease, the accessory muscles become markedly hypertrophied.[3]

Anatomy of the Thorax

The thoracic structures associated with respiration include the skeletal elements that make up the bony framework of the thorax, lungs, pleura, and muscles of respiration. Within the thorax the mediastinum contains major blood vessels, the esophagus, and the heart enveloped within the pericardial sac.[4,5] Each of these structures is described and its interactions mentioned in the following sections.

Bony Thorax

The bony elements that make up the **thorax** include the sternum, ribs, thoracic vertebrae, clavicles, and scapu-

lae. These elements protect the contents of the thorax, help expand and relax the chest by the contraction of respiratory muscles to effect inspiration and expiration, and stabilize the chest wall against changes in intrapleural pressure.

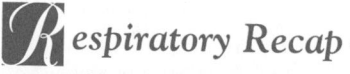

Bony Elements of the Thorax	
Sternum	Clavicles
Ribs	Scapulae
Thoracic vertebrae	

Each rib is attached to the vertebral column by two joints, the vertebrocostal and the costotransverse joint. These attachments constrain the movement of the ribs around an axis that joins these two joints. Rotation around this axis carries the upper rib forward and slightly lateral. In contrast, the lower ribs have their axis of rotation posteriorly and laterally. The costal cartilages of ribs 1 through 7 attach the anterior portions of these ribs to the manubrium and body of the sternum. Costal cartilages of ribs 8 through 10 attach to the costal cartilage of the rib above it. The 11th and 12th ribs are short, and their costal cartilages end in musculature of the anterior abdominal wall. In general, the costal cartilages confer elasticity and mobility to the ribs.

Respiratory Muscles

Chest wall muscles involved in ventilation can be divided into primary and accessory muscles. The **diaphragm** is the principal respiratory muscle and is composed of a central tendon and the costal and crural portions.[17,18] The central tendon consists of a tendinous membrane from which the muscle fibers of the crural and costal portions of the diaphragm radiate.[19] The fibers of the costal portion project from the central tendon to either the xiphoid process of the sternum or the upper margins of the six lower ribs. The fibers of the crural diaphragm project to the anterior lateral portion of the lumbar vertebrae. In the body the diaphragm assumes the shape of a dome. Contraction of the diaphragm displaces the central tendon caudally and increases the cephalocaudal dimensions of the thoracic cav-

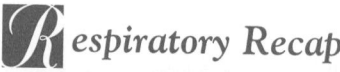

Muscles of Ventilation
Diaphragm
Accessory muscles of inhalation
Accessory muscles of exhalation

ity.[17] Moreover, the zone of apposition between the diaphragm and the rib cage decreases with increasing lung volume during inspiration.[19]

The diaphragm is a well-perfused skeletal muscle receiving major nerve supply from the cervical region via the phrenic nerve (C3-C5). Each hemidiaphragm actually receives its own innervation; thus paralysis of a hemidiaphragm is possible. The majority of muscle fibers that make up the diaphragm are oxidative (both slow and fast). Only 25% of the fiber types are fast glycolytic fibers.[18] Thus diaphragmatic muscle fibers are most useful for continuous activity. Like other skeletal muscles, however, they can fatigue and ultimately fail under conditions associated with a rapid breathing pattern or increased airway resistance.[20]

Additional muscles of inspiration include the intercostal muscles that elevate the ribs (Figure 17-3). The external intercostal muscles and the parasternal portion of the internal intercostal muscles are essentially active during inspiration.[17] The lateral portion of the internal intercostal muscles and the innermost layer (the vertebrocostal muscles) are active during expiration. The intercostal nerves that innervate these muscles are from the anterior primary rami of thoracic (T) nerves T1 through T11. Contraction of the diaphragm also increases intraabdominal pressure, facilitating nonventilatory functions, such as labor, vomiting, and defection.

Additional muscles associated with the chest wall and abdomen are involved in ventilation. These accessory muscles that affect inspiration are the pectoralis minor and major (innervated by C5-C8 and T1), serratus anterior (innervated by C5-C7), and erector spinae. These muscles help raise the ribs, push the sternum forward and upward, and straighten the concavity of the thoracic spine. **Abdominal muscles** such as the rectus abdominis, external and internal oblique muscles, and transversus abdominis muscles depress the lower ribs, increase intraabdominal pressure, and flex the thoracic spine. The more powerful muscles available for expiration result in the generation of a greater maximal expiratory than an inspiratory pressure.[21]

Lungs

Within the thoracic cavity reside the lungs, heart, esophagus, major blood vessels, and thymus. This section describes the anatomy of the lungs and their pleural coverings. Subsequently the anatomy of the mediastinal contents then is detailed.

The lungs are paired, lobed, pyramidal structures.[4] The base or inferior surface of the lung resting on the diaphragm is concave. In contrast, the mediastinal surface that faces medially is flat, with the **hilum** of the lung through which bronchi, blood vessels, nerves, and lymphatics enter and leave located centrally. Finally, the costal surface is convex, molded by the curvature of the ribs. The lung consists of right and left sides (Figure 17-4).

The larger right side contains three **lobes**—the upper, middle, and lower lobes—whereas the left lung consists of two lobes—upper and lower. The lower lobes are separated from more rostral lobes by the oblique fissure, whereas the right lung contains a second fissure, the transverse fissure. Each lobe is further subdivided into 10 bronchopulmonary **segments** that correspond to the distribution of a specific bronchus (Table 17-1). Lungs lie free in the pleural cavities except for two attachments—at their roots and at the pulmonary ligaments.

The lungs consist of two major anatomic divisions—the airways and the parenchyma.[4,5-8] The epithelial-lined airways conduct air into and from the lungs, whereas the parenchyma is involved in gas exchange with the pulmonary circulation. Starting from the trachea, two major **bronchi** distribute air into the right and left parts of the lung. The angle between the trachea and the right bronchus is less than that between the trachea and left bronchus, a difference that may facilitate the deposition of aspirates more into the right than the left lung. The bronchi are further subdivided into the segmental bronchi, large intrasegmental bronchi, and small intrasegmental bronchi. Structurally the smaller bronchi have less cartilage and more smooth muscles than larger bronchi. Even smaller branches, the bronchioles, contain no cartilage, are composed of smooth muscles, and diminish in diameter as they travel deeper into the lung. The smaller bronchioles consist of the terminal and respiratory bronchioles, with

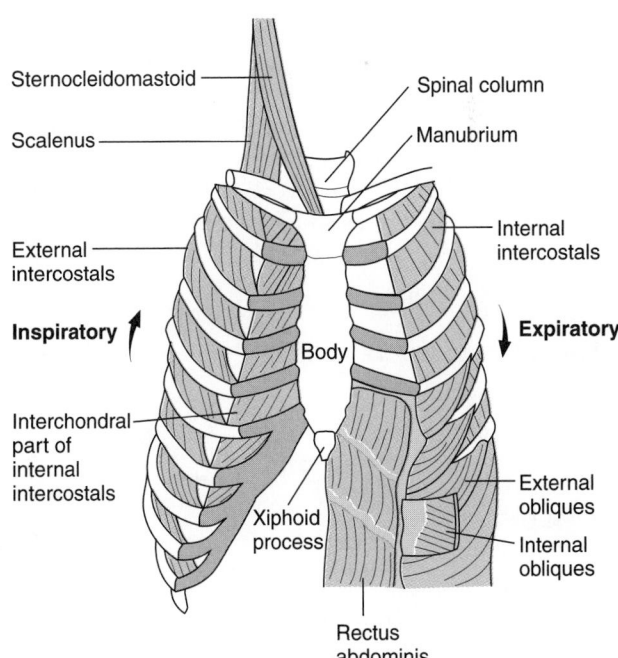

Figure 17-3 Bony components and muscles of the chest wall involved in ventilation. The red portions represent the costal cartilage and associated ribs. Arrows pointing upward represent the muscles that are active during inspiration. Arrows pointing downward denote muscles that contribute to forced expiratory maneuvers.

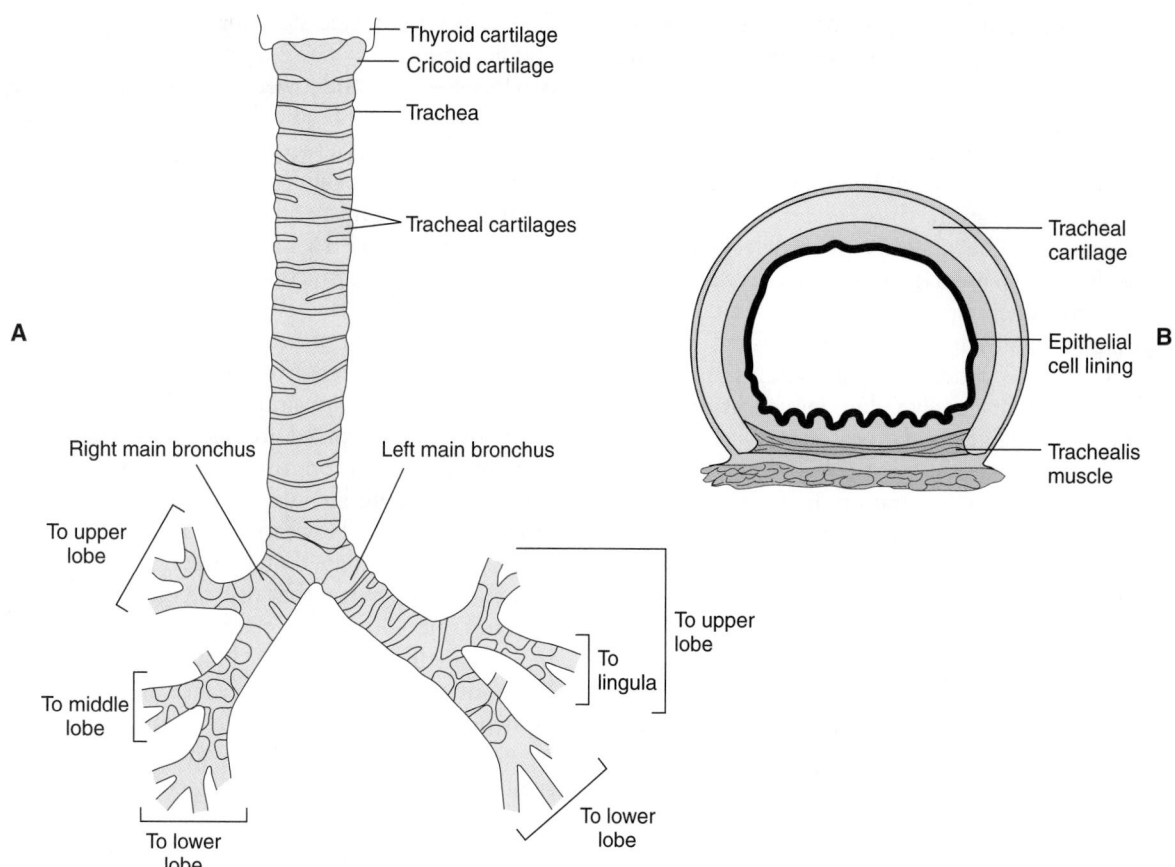

Figure 17-4 **A,** Frontal view of the trachea and major bronchi, with designations of the major lung lobes to which they conduct air. **B,** A schematic cross-sectional view of the trachea.

the latter involved in gas exchange; respiratory bronchioles also, with the alveolar sacs that contain **alveoli,** form the acinus (Figure 17-5). Distribution of gas at this level occurs via alveolar duct and **pores of Kohn** that communicate directly among alveoli. The alveoli are composed of two types of cells—Type I cells and Type II cells.[8] Their roles in gas exchange are discussed later in this chapter.

level of the alveoli and the pulmonary capillaries. Oxygenated blood travels within the venous system from venules to the pulmonary veins and finally into the left atrium. The distribution of blood flow in the lungs depends on posture (upright, prone, supine) and gravity; thus all segments of the lung do not receive a uniform amount of blood.

*R*espiratory Recap

Anatomy of the Lungs
Airways and alveoli
Lobes and segments

*R*espiratory Recap

Pulmonary Blood Flow
Pulmonary circulation
Bronchial circulation

Blood Supply to the Lungs

The lungs are well perfused.[8] **Pulmonary arteries** emanating from the right ventricle deliver deoxygenated blood to the lung and also perfuse the visceral pleura. The arteries further subdivide into arterioles and then into capillaries. Unlike the systemic vasculature the pulmonary arteries are less muscular and have a higher compliance, lower pressure, and lower resistance. Gas exchange occurs at the

The **bronchial circulation** may arise from the aorta or the intercostal arteries and supply blood to the tracheobronchial tree down to the level of the terminal bronchioles.[5] In addition, the bronchial circulation perfuses the hilar lymph nodes, visceral pleura, pulmonary arteries and veins, vagus nerve, and esophagus. Venous drainage of the bronchial circulation enters the azygos and hemiazygos veins and the pulmonary veins, bypassing the lungs. This path contributes to

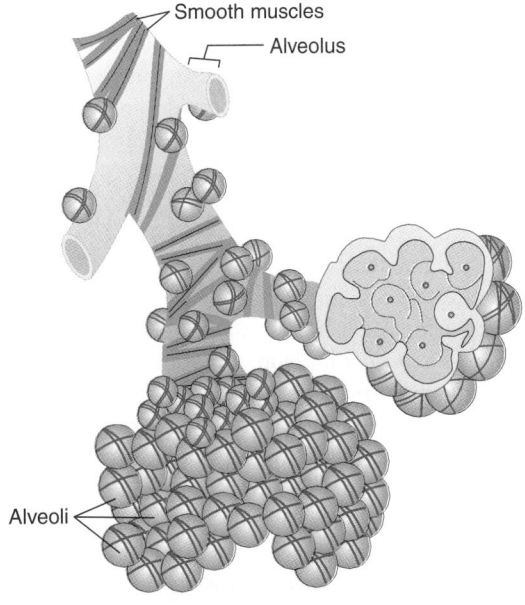

TABLE 17-1

Lobes and Segments of the Lungs

Lung	Lobe	Segments
Right	Upper	Apical
		Anterior
		Posterior
	Middle	Lateral
		Medial
	Lower	Superior
		Anterior basal
		Posterior basal
		Lateral basal
		Medial basal
Left	Upper	Apical posterior
		Anterior
		Superior lingular
		Inferior lingular
	Lower	Superior
		Anterior medial basal
		Lateral basal
		Posterior basal

Figure 17-5 The terminal bronchioles, alveolar ducts, alveolar sacs, and alveoli that make up the acinus. These intrapulmonary structures are directly associated with gas exchange.

the normal anatomic right to left shunt. Functionally the bronchial circulation is important in air-conditioning of inspired air, fluid balance in the airways, perfusion of the parietal pleura, and uptake of inspired agents.

The lungs and their covering, the **pleura,** also are well endowed with lymphatic circulation and lymph nodes.[5,7] The lymphatic system follows the veins and helps prevent the accumulation of fluid in the alveoli. Like the upper airways, the lungs are involved in defense. A component of this defense system is the bronchus-associated lymphoid tissue located at the bifurcations of bronchi.[22] This system is essential for an adequate immune response against respiratory viral infections.

Innervation of the Lungs

The nerve supply of the lung involves all this organ's components—the airways, parenchyma, and vasculature. The vagus nerves and the upper four to five thoracic sympathetic ganglia contribute fibers to the pulmonary plexus. These nerves supply the bronchi and veins. Postganglionic parasympathetic efferent fibers innervate the smooth muscles in all divisions of the airways. Although α- and β-adrenergic receptors are present on airway smooth muscles, no direct sympathetic innervation of the airways exists. Instead, human airways also are innervated by the nonadrenergic-noncholinergic nervous system that travels in parallel with the vagus nerve[23] and when stimulated, results in bronchodilation. The mediator responsible for this dilation is thought to be vasoactive intestinal polypeptide (VIP). Moreover, epinephrine released by the adrenal medulla may stimulate β-adrenergic receptors on smooth muscle cells and cause bronchodila-

tion.[24] The pulmonary vasculature contains both parasympathetic and sympathetic innervation, but vasomotor tone is influenced more by changes in the composition of alveolar gases (hypoxia and hypercapnia) than by stimulation of these nerves.

Respiratory Recap

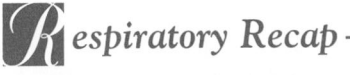

Innervation of the Lungs
Parasympathetic (cholinergic)
Sympathetic (adrenergic)
Nonadrenergic-noncholinergic

The lung contains a number of receptors associated with respiratory reflexes.[8] Axons from these receptors travel to the brain by way of the vagus nerve. For example, slowly adapting stretch receptors in the smooth muscles respond to lung inflation or increased transpulmonary pressure, causing bronchodilation, increased heart rate, and decreased peripheral systemic vascular resistance. Irritant receptors located primarily in the epithelium (the lining) of extrapulmonary airways may cause bronchoconstriction, increased ventilation, constriction of the larynx, cough, and mucous secretion. Finally, C-fibers or J-type receptors in alveolar walls, airways, and pulmonary blood vessels respond to increased interstitial congestion, chemical injury, or microemboli by initiating a rapid, shallow breathing pattern, bronchoconstriction, bradycardia, and increased mucous secretion.

Another nervous system component of the lungs are the neuroepithelial bodies found in the airways.[25] These bodies are composed of nonciliated neuroendocrine cells and contain various neuropeptides and neural markers. The function of the neuroepithelial cells is unclear, but they may be involved in chemoreception, neuropeptide production affecting bronchomotor tone, and lung remodeling.

Pleura

The lung is covered with a lining, the **visceral pleura,** whereas the chest wall is lined by the **parietal pleura** (Figure 17-6).[5,26] During quiet breathing the pleura extend beyond the lung. The visceral pleura cover the surface of the lung, extending into the fissures between the lobes. On the medial surface of the lung the visceral pleura are reflected onto the mediastinum to become part of the parietal pleura. Thus the pleura isolate the right and left lungs and the heart, which sits within its own container, the **pericardium.** The visceral pleura receive innervation from the vagus nerve and are relatively insensitive to pain. In contrast, the parietal pleura are innervated in the costal portion by the intercostal nerves and at the diaphragmatic portion by the phrenic nerve. Ciliated mesothelial cells line both pleurae.[26]

Between the two pleura is the **pleural space,** a serous cavity containing a small amount of fluid (approximately 0.3 mL/kg of body weight) that has a low protein concentration. Regulation of the fluid volume within the pleural space involves balancing of net filtration from systemic and pulmonary capillaries and drainage by lymphatic vessels located in the pleurae. The lymphatics involved in reabsorption of fluid have a relatively high capacity of approximately 700 mL per day. Distribution of pleural fluid occurs from costal to mediastinal regions. The fluid in the pleural space is vital in guaranteeing a close apposition between the lungs and the chest wall and allowing for frictionless sliding between the visceral and parietal pleurae. Both properties are necessary to couple the pump composed of the chest wall musculature and the lung for ventilation to occur. An analogy is a drop of water between two glass slides. The water allows the slides to be moved slightly, but separation of the slides is difficult. In addition, the opposition of mechanical forces between the lungs and chest wall helps ensure a negative pressure (below atmospheric pressure) within the pleural space. Intrapleural pressure first was measured through placement of a catheter within the pleural space. Intrapleural pressure is estimated today through measurement of the pressure in the middle third of the esophagus.

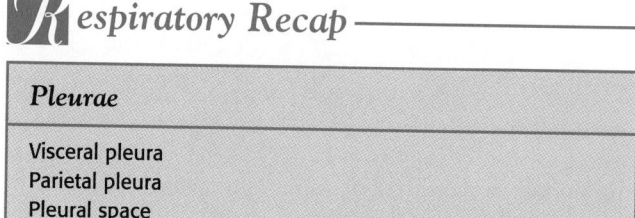

Respiratory Recap

Pleurae
Visceral pleura
Parietal pleura
Pleural space

Innervation of the visceral pleura is by the anterior and posterior pulmonary plexuses. In contrast, the intercostal nerves supply the costal and peripheral parts of the diaphragmatic parietal pleura.[4] The central portions of the diaphragmatic pleura and pleura are supplied by the phrenic nerves. Importantly, irritation of the visceral pleura does not result in pain sensation because it receives no nerves of general sensation, whereas the parietal pleura is extremely sensitive to irritations, which can result in severe pain that may be referred to the root of the neck and over the shoulder.[5]

Mediastinum

The **mediastinum** is the area between the two pleural sacs and is divided into superior and inferior (anterior, middle, and posterior) regions.[4,5] All structures within the thorax except the lungs and pleurae are located in the mediastinum. The superior mediastinum contains the thymus, great vessels associated with the heart, esophagus, trachea and thoracic duct, and numerous nerves, including the vagus and esophageal plexus. Within the other regions are located the heart (within the pericardium), main bronchi, great vessels, phrenic nerves, and portions of the thymus and esophagus.

The pericardial sac that surrounds the heart consists of the fibrous portion that protects it against sudden overfilling (Figure 17-7). The base rests on and is fused with the

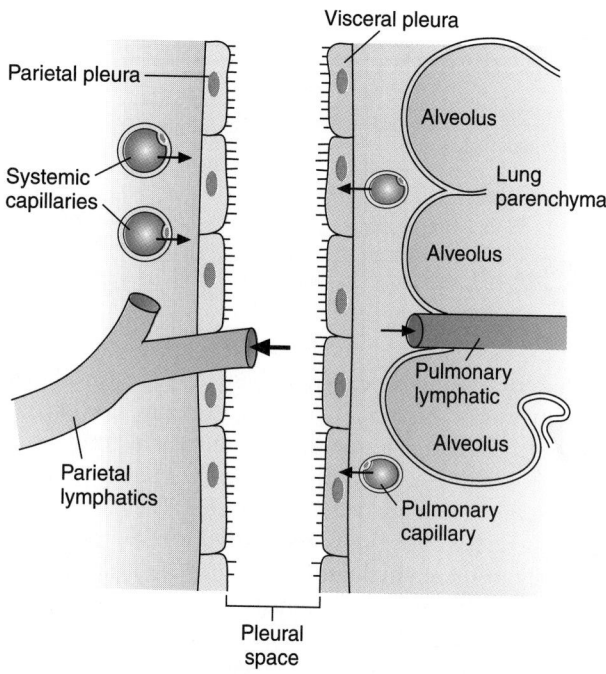

Figure 17-6 Diagram of the structures making up the pleurae and the pleural space. The pleurae are lined with mesothelial cells containing microvilli that face the pleural space. The arrows denote the direction for filtration and reabsorption of pleural fluid. Thus fluid emanates from capillaries and is predominantly reabsorbed by the lymphatics.

central tendon of the diaphragm. Anteriorly the fibrous pericardial portion is attached to the sternum by sternopericardial ligaments. The fibrous pericardium also is fused with the tunica adventitia of the great vessels entering and leaving the heart. Thus movements of the sternum, diaphragm, and heart influence movement of the pericardial sac.

The fibrous pericardium contains two layers—a parietal pericardium and a visceral pericardium. The parietal pericardium is fused to the internal portion of the fibrous surface, whereas the visceral portion covers the heart's surface. A small amount of serous fluid is contained within the potential space between the two pleurae. Like the pleural space surrounding the lung, this fluid allows the beating heart to move within the pericardial sac. Inflammation of the pericardium may increase the amount of fluid in the pericardial space, hinder the movement of the heart, and compress the pulmonary veins.

The heart is located within the pericardial sac.[5] The major function of the heart is to generate a pressure head to propel blood through the lungs and systemic circulation. In addition, movements of the heart help distribute gas within the lungs through cardiogenic oscillations. This muscular structure consists of three parts—the epicardium, myocardium, and endocardium. The epicardium, a thin membrane, lines the outside of the heart. The innermost lining of the heart is the endocardium, composed of endothelial cells. Finally, the myocardium consists of cardiac muscle. Most of cardiac muscle cells are contractile, but some make up the electrical conduction system of the heart.

Although the heart is considered a single pump, it consists of four chambers—the right and left **atria** and the right and left **ventricles.** The interventricular septum separates the two ventricles. The right side of the heart receives blood via the inferior and superior vena cavae, and the right ventricle pumps it into the pulmonary arteries. Blood returning from the pulmonary veins drains into the left atrium, into the left ventricle, and finally into the aorta, which dispenses it into the systemic circulation. Between the two right chambers is the tricuspid valve, which is held in place by chordea tendinea attached to the cardiac tissue via papillary muscles. Blood entering the pulmonary artery or leaving the pulmonary vein does so via the pulmonary (semilunar) valves. The mitral valve sits between the left atrium and ventricle. The valve regulating blood flow into the aorta is the aortic valve. These valves are imbedded into the heart matrix by fibrous rings.

The electrical conduction system of the heart consists of specialized cells.[5] Generally the major pacemaker of the heart, the sino-atrial (SA) node, is located in the right atrium. A conduction system throughout the atria coordinates propagation of electrical signals that ultimately lead to concomitant contraction of the two atrial chambers. A breaking system is located within the atrial-ventricular (AV) node. Impulses from this region travel via the bundle of His and right and left bundle branches to the Purkinje fibers, which innervate the ventricular muscles. Thus both ventricles contract simultaneously.

The blood supply to the heart or the coronary circulation arises from the ascending aorta and right and left aortic sinuses. The right **coronary artery** passes anteriorly between

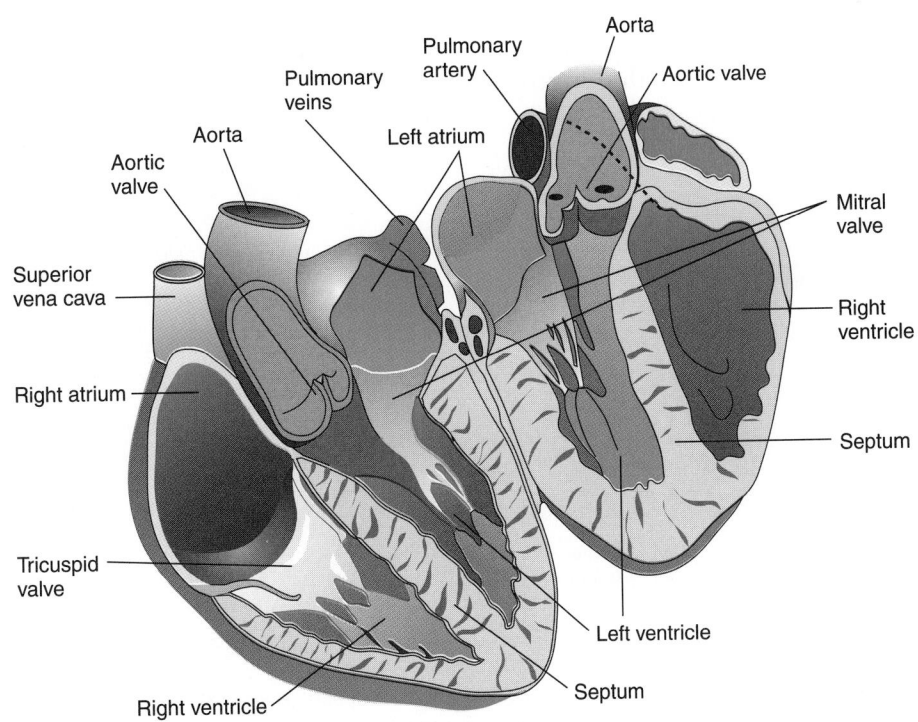

Figure 17-7   The heart and great vessels presented in a medial plane that slices the structures in half.

the pulmonary trunk on the right and the right atrium posteriorly and on the left. This artery surrounds the heart until it reaches the diaphragmatic surface, where it anastomoses with the terminal branch of the left coronary artery. Major branches of the right coronary artery include (1) the artery to the SA node, (2) the right marginal artery perfusing the inferior border of the heart and ventricular tissues, and (3) the posterior (or inferior) intraventricular artery supplying the septum, the walls of both ventricles, and the rest of the electrical conduction system of the heart.

The left coronary artery arises from the left aortic sinus and divides into the left anterior descending artery and the circumflex artery. The former supplies blood to the walls of both ventricles and the interventricular septum. A branch of the left descending artery forms the diagonal artery that supplies the wall of the left ventricular wall. The circumflex artery, a continuation of the left coronary artery, follows the surface of the heart and on the inferior portion of the heart anastomoses with the right coronary artery. Venous drainage of the heart accompanies the major branches of the coronary arteries and finally drains into the coronary sinus. This blood then returns to the right atrium posterior to the tricuspid valve and anterior to the inferior vena cava.

Innervation of the heart is via the autonomic nervous system.[6] The sympathetic efferent supply is from the upper thoracic segments of the spinal cord, through the sympathetic trunk and cardiac veins. These fibers join the cardiac plexus beneath the arch of the aorta and innervate the SA and AV nodes, the myocardium, and the coronary arteries. The efferent parasympathetic innervation is from the vagus nerves. Stimulation of the sympathetic nervous system inhibits parasympathetic outflow and increases heart rate, stroke volume, and cardiac contractility. Stimulation of the parasympathetic nervous system does the opposite. In resting individuals the amount of parasympathetic tone predominates. Afferent fibers are associated with pain sensation and sensory input for modulation of cardiac reflexes.

Microanatomy of the Respiratory System

The following sections describe the microanatomy of the respiratory system and its functional attributes. Included among these are the mucociliary clearance mechanism of the airways, airway and vascular smooth muscles, endothelial cells, alveolar cells involved in gas exchange and surfactant production, and resident cell types, such as macrophages, dendritic cells, and mast cells.

Mucociliary Clearance

Ventilation of between 12,000 and 24,000 L/day exposes the lungs to a large amount of potential damaging agents, including pollutants, viruses and bacteria, and organic agents, such as antigens. The body has developed reflex responses, such as coughing, sneezing, bronchoconstriction, altered breathing patterns, and increased mucous production, to counteract the effects of these possible damaging agents. Another important defense mechanism that uses cellular strategies is the **mucociliary apparatus** of the tracheobronchial tree (Figure 17-8).[16]

As the name implies, this complex system is found throughout the airways. In the larger airways the apparatus consists of ciliated epithelial cells, goblet cells, basal (stem) cells, and submucosal glands that contain mucous- or serous-secreting cells. The trachea contains both ciliated and nonciliated epithelial cells, and the percentage of ciliated cells increases in the bronchi. Immediately bathing the epithelial cells is a watery fluid (sol), on top of which a mucous (gel) layer sits. In the bronchioles are less-ciliated cuboidal cells and Clara cells (secretory).[27] These cells rest on a basal lamina under which fibroblasts, nerves, lymphatics, and smooth muscle cells reside.

Cilia beat at different frequencies, with the highest being in the trachea and the lowest in the small airways. One function of the mucociliary apparatus is to serve as a me-

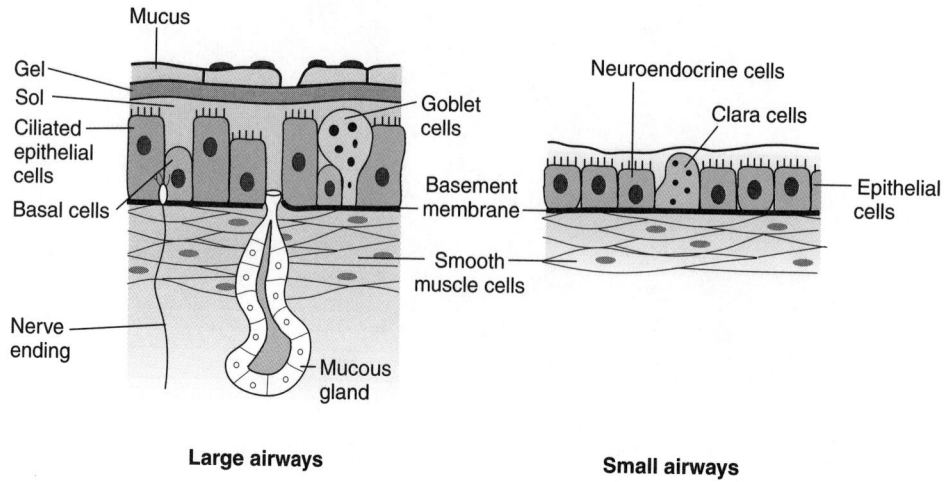

Large airways   **Small airways**

Figure 17-8   Cells that contribute to the mucociliary clearance apparatus in large and small airways. Basal cells are thought to be stem or progenitor cells that give rise to epithelial and goblet cells when the epithelium is damaged.

chanical barrier by trapping agents in the surrounding fluid and, through ciliary action, moving them to the upper airways, where the agents are either expectorated or swallowed. Secondly, the fluid itself may capture and neutralize gases and act as an antioxidant. Finally, the fluids prevent the adhesion of microorganisms to the epithelium. Fluid balance in the airways depends on the function of active transporters (for chloride and sodium) and the presence of water channels. β-Adrenergic agents such as epinephrine augment the function of these transporters and various water channels called *aquaporins*. Proper functioning of these systems is especially important in utero to help lung development and shortly after birth to remove excess lung fluid. This topic is discussed further in the section concerning Type II cells.

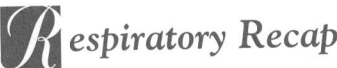

Respiratory Recap

Mucociliary Apparatus
Contains a mucous layer
Contains cilia that move mucous layer cephalad

The mucociliary apparatus is predominately innervated by the parasympathetic nervous system.[8] In addition, intraepithelial nerves and neuroendocrine bodies also have been identified near mucous cells. Surface epithelial cells and submucosal glands also contain a high number of β-adrenergic receptors. Other receptors expressed in these cells include those for VIP and substance P. Many drugs administered to patients with airway disease, such as β-adrenergic agonists and methylxanthines, enhance the function of the mucociliary apparatus. Factors that may impede its function include mechanical or chemical damage, viral infections, or disruption of fluid balance, such as during mouth or tracheal breathing (bypassing the nose). Chronic disorders such as cystic fibrosis, asthma, bronchitis, and primary ciliary dyskinesia compromise the function of the mucociliary apparatus and contribute to a higher incidence of respiratory infections in individuals with these disorders.[16]

Airway and Vascular Smooth Muscle

Both the airways and pulmonary vasculature contain large amounts of smooth muscle cells.[24,28,29] Structural and functional heterogeneity exists between and within these two smooth muscle beds. A major function of airway smooth muscles is to help regulate the distribution of gas in the lungs by altering contractility. Smooth muscles also can proliferate, hypertrophy, and transform their molecular characteristics. Changes in smooth muscle size and number also may affect airway diameter. In addition, airway smooth muscles can secrete mediators, cytokines, chemokines, and growth factors that influence airway reactivity. In turn, other cell types found in the airways, such as mast and epithelial cells, alter the function of airway smooth muscles. For example, mast cells produce histamine and leukotrienes that constrict airway smooth muscles.[30] Prostaglandin E_2 and nitric oxide (NO) produced by epithelial cells cause bronchodilation.

Smooth muscle within the pulmonary vasculature, especially the arterial bed, is much less than that found in systemic arteries.[8,29] Moreover, tone in the pulmonary vasculature is low, as are pressure and resistance. These characteristics buffer changes in blood volume between the right and left parts of the heart by recruitment and distention of blood vessels. Smooth muscles also help direct blood flow within the lung parenchyma. Thus factors that influence smooth muscle tone can influence the areas perfused and the amount of blood they receive.[29]

Chemicals that affect vascular tone are produced locally or metabolized by endothelial cells, nerves, and mast cells, or by other organs. Thus endothelial cells can produce angiotensin II, prostaglandin I_2, and endothelin (all vasoconstrictors) and degrade bradykinin. Nerve endings within the pulmonary vasculature can release acetylcholine, norepinephrine, and VIP. Finally, mast cells produce histamine and leukotrienes. Atrial natriuretic peptide, produced in the heart (and possibly the lungs), is a potent vasodilator, as is vasopressin, released by the posterior hypothalamus. Pulmonary vascular tone is potently affected by changes in surrounding gas concentrations and acid-base status. Thus hypoxia, hypercapnia, and a decrease in pH result in vasoconstriction. Hypoxia acts directly on smooth muscles cells. The functional significance of changes in alveolar gases affecting pulmonary vasomotor tone is to match alveolar ventilation and perfusion and therefore maximize gas exchange.

Mast Cells, Dendritic Cells, and Macrophages

Mast cells range from 10 to 20 μm in diameter and may be oval or more irregularly shaped. They frequently are located in the respiratory mucosal surfaces and alveolar septa. Within the lung are two types of mast cells classified according neutral protease composition (chymase and/or tryptase).[31] A major feature of mast cells is the presence of abundant granules. Mediators released from mast cell granules are one of three classes: (1) preformed, granule-associated mediators, such as histamine and serotonin, heparin, and neutral proteases; (2) membrane-derived lipid mediators or arachidonic acid metabolites, such as prostaglandins, thromboxanes, or leukotrienes; and (3) cytokines. In individuals with asthma, mast cell numbers in bronchial and alveolar cells are elevated, as are protease and histamine levels in bronchoalveolar lavage fluid. Stabilization of mast cell membranes and administration of drugs that counter the production or activity of mediators help prevent the symptoms manifested during an asthma attack.

Two cell types derived from bone marrow stem cells that reside in different parts of the lung are dendritic cells and macrophages (Figure 17-9).[32-34] A number of subtypes of each are found in specific locations within the lung. Both cell types modulate immunity within the lung, but of the two the macrophages are the most abundant and have the most varied functions.[33]

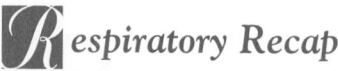

Respiratory Recap

Dendritic Cells, Macrophages, and Mast Cells
Dendrites: antigen-presenting cells Macrophages: phagocytic cells Mast cells: cells that release mediators

Dendritic cells are mobile cells with irregular shapes and long processes.[35] Normally they are found in small numbers within the airway epithelium and lung parenchyma. Their major function in the lung is as antigen-presenting cells. When exposed to antigens, dendritic cells phagocytose antigens and process them, migrate to lung-draining lymph nodes, present the antigens to T-lymphocytes, and activate them. Dendritic cells also produce adhesion molecules and cytokines and express class I and II major histocompatibility locus (HLA) molecules. If an individual is chronically exposed to inhaled irritants, the number of dendritic cells within the lung increases dramatically. Elevating the levels of inhaled or systemically administered steroids reduces the number of dendritic cells within the lung. Current studies suggest that dendritic cells actually may be derived from monocytes.

Macrophages are cells present in many locations in the lung, including the pleura, interstitium, and epithelial surface.[36] Apparently, both phenotypic and functional characteristics of macrophages from these different locations vary greatly, even if they are derived from the same stem cell line.[32] These ameboid-like cells are derived from blood monocytes or through local proliferation. The alveolar macrophages (the focus of the following discussion) have a long lifespan and are found in large numbers within the lung (about 23×10^9 cells/lung).

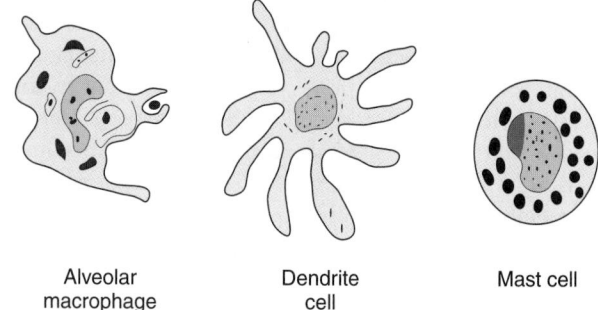

Figure 17-9 A schematic representation of an alveolar macrophage, dendritic cell, and mast cell.

These mobile cells have many functions, in large part associated with defense of the lung against inhaled agents. To conduct many of its functions, alveolar macrophages recognize and respond to signals from their environment.[33] These signals are "sensed" by receptors that recognize the Fc portion of most classes of immunoglobulin, CR1 complement receptors, and receptors for transferrin, glucocorticoids, and many cytokines, such as colony-stimulating factor, tumor necrosis factor α, interleukin 1, platelet-activating factor (PAF), several proteases and antiproteases, histamine, and leukotrienes, to mention a few. Macrophages phagocytose particulates and debris nonspecifically, or through specific ligand receptor-mediated processes. They also produce a number of secretory products, including oxidants that kill microbes, and bioactive lipids, such as thromboxanes, prostaglandins, leukotrienes, and PAF. These latter substances help recruit inflammatory cells and can modulate airway and vascular function.

Activation of macrophages in the presence of particulates or stimulation of specific receptors (such as immune complexes, cytokines, and arachidonic acid metabolites) causes changes in anatomic and functional characteristics of the alveolar macrophage. Activated macrophages are larger and exhibit pronounced membrane ruffling, an increased number of pinocytotic vesicles, increased metabolic activity, and changes in the density of surface markers. In addition, they release a number of secretory products into the lung environment.

The major function of the alveolar macrophages is to neutralize or eliminate inhaled agents that may be harmful to the lung. Phagocytosed substances and bacteria may be digested by lysosomes and the oxidant burst or removed via the epithelial surface or by the lymphatics. Macrophages also may remain in the lung. If they are chronically activated, the increased production of their metabolites actually may injure the lung. Although alveolar macrophages are expert phagocytosis machines, they are not as effective as dendritic cells for immune responses. Macrophages can, however, recruit and activate other inflammatory cells, such as neutrophils, eosinophils, and monocytes, by releasing specific mediators. Transforming growth factor β, produced by macrophages, actually acts as an immunosuppressant for both T- and B-lymphocytes. In addition, a number of macrophage-produced secretory products are involved in the maintenance and repair of the lung parenchyma by stimulating undifferentiated mesenchymal cells within the extracellular matrix. Some of these factors include platelet-derived growth factor, fibronectin, and a number of cytokines. Over-stimulation and increased macrophage numbers in individuals with acute and chronic lung diseases create a positive feedback system that can actually augment the damaging effects of released macrophage products. For example, individuals with interstitial lung disease have macrophages that increase the production of fibronectin, promoting cell adhesion and migration, differentiation, and growth.

Alveolar Cells

Just as the mucociliary apparatus consists of a number of cell types that function together, the alveolar-capillary complex is another multicellular structure involved in common functions. The alveolar-capillary complex consists of alveolar epithelial cells (Type I and Type II), a basement membrane, an interstitial space, and endothelial cells that make up pulmonary capillaries containing red blood cells (RBCs). The major function of the alveolar-capillary complex is to facilitate the diffusion of O_2 into and of CO_2 from the pulmonary capillaries. This section describes each of the cell types that makes up the alveolar-capillary complex and its function (Figure 17-10).

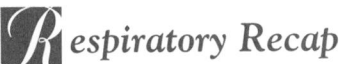

Respiratory Recap

Alveolar Cells
Type I: cover greatest surface area
Type II: produce surfactant

Type I and Type II cells make up the alveolar sacs.[8,37,38] When spread out, these cells cover a surface area equal to that of a single's tennis court. **Type I cells** are relatively large, flat, and branched squamous epithelial cells that form tight junctions. They cover a large portion (90%) of the alveolar surface and have a mean thickness of approximately 0.2 μm.[2] Because of the thinness of these cells, gases move easily across them. Terminally differentiated, Type I cells are sensitive to injury, including high levels of O_2, bacteria, bleomycin, cyclophosphamide, and particulates.[37]

The **Type II cells,** or granular pneumocytes, are cube shaped and make up only 10% of the alveolar surface.[38] They are located predominately in corners of alveolar sacs and form tight junctions with Type I cells, which helps impede the movement of excess fluid into the alveolar spaces. Type II cells exhibit a number of functions, including the production of surfactant and surfactant-associated proteins, division and differentiation into Type I cells that may have been damaged, and transport of sodium and water toward the endothelial cells and blood to help minimize fluid accumulation in the alveolar space.

Type II cells are small and functionally polarized. They contain organelles common to many cell types and laminar bodies. Distinct to this cell type, laminar bodies are organelles that contain layers of surfactant phospholipids, lysosomal enzymes, α-glucosidase, and surfactant protein A. The apical membrane of Type II cells contains short microvilli consisting of actin filaments and associated proteins. The basolateral membrane contains a high concentration of Na^+-K^+ ATPase (*ATP* being adenosine triphosphate) involved in active transport systems.

Type II cells produce, secrete, and clear surfactant.[39] This surface-active agent contains phosphatidylcholine, phospholipids, and phosphatidylglycerol, as well as surfactant-associated proteins—SP-A, SP-B, SP-C, and SP-D.[40,41] The most abundant protein is SP-A, which enhances the phagocytosis of *Staphylococcus aureus* and acts as an opsonin in the phagocytosis of herpes simplex virus (HSV) by macrophages. Similar defense roles have also been reported for SP-D. Deficiencies of SP-A and SP-D occur in children with cystic fibrosis and may contribute to the pathophysiology of this progressive lung disease.[42] Both SP-B and SP-C help adsorb tubular myelin, a form of unraveled secreted surfactant. In vivo, the major stimulus for surfactant secretion is hyperventilation. Hormonal stimuli for surfactant production include estrogen, epinephrine, thyroid hormones, and glucocorticoids. These hormones are especially important during lung development in utero. Surfactant alters the surface tension characteristics of alveoli and equalizes pressure distributions throughout the lung to prevent atelectasis, maximize gas exchange, and decrease the work of breathing. Insufficient production of normal surfactant is found in babies with infant respiratory distress syndrome and acute respiratory distress syndrome, conditions with high mortality rates.

Another major function of Type II cells is their clearance of excess alveolar fluid,[43] accomplished through active solute transport of chloride and sodium and the presence of aquaporins (water channels).[44] Agents that stimulate the production of cyclic adenosine monophosphate (cAMP), such as epinephrine, stimulate solute transport and water into the alveolar cells. In contrast, increased levels of atrial natriuretic peptide produced by the heart and lungs during heart failure actually inhibit cAMP mechanisms and increase fluid flux into the alveolar space. The nature and number of solute transporters and water

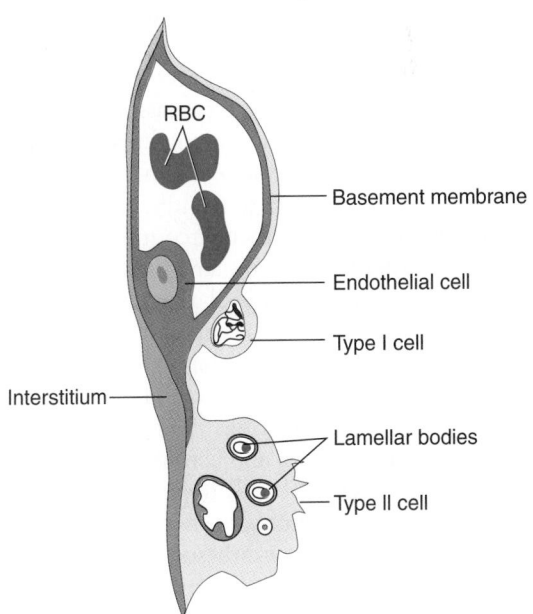

Figure 17-10 A schematic representation of the alveolar-capillary complex showing the structural relationships between Type I and Type II cells and endothelial cells that make up the pulmonary capillaries. *RBC,* Red blood cells (within the pulmonary capillary).

channels in the lung change during development. For example, around the time of birth the amount of Na^+-K^+-ATPase and amiloride-sensitive Na^+ channels, as well as the number of water channels (especially AQP-4), increase. β-Adrenergic agonists increase the function of all these transporters. However, most studies have been conducted in mammals other than humans.

Maintaining low levels of fluid within the alveolar space to decrease the distance for gas diffusion is necessary to ensure rapid and adequate gas exchange. This fact is especially important for O_2, which has a much lower diffusibility (20 times lower) in plasma membranes and fluid than does CO_2. The following six safety factors within the alveolar-capillary complex help prevent fluid invasion:

1. Tight junctions exist between alveolar cells.
2. A number of mechanisms are available for the transport of water from the alveolar spaces into the vasculature that have been reviewed previously.
3. The hydrostatic pressure within the pulmonary vasculature is very low.
4. Surfactant and its associated proteins help repel water.
5. An active defense system exists within the alveolar sacs that helps prevent injury to alveolar membranes.
6. An extensive lymphatic system exists within the lung that helps drain fluid that accumulates within the interstitial space. This system is very important.

Interstitial Space

Broadly speaking, the pulmonary interstitium is the "space" between the air space epithelial and the endothelial cells lining the vasculature.[45] The interstitium is bounded by the basement membranes that form the innermost boundary of epithelial and endothelial cells. Thus the interstitium is found in all parts of the lung and serves as mechanical support, containing various cell types associated with the maintenance of low water in the lung lumen and defense. The interstitium is a continuum that pervades the entire lung, from the visceral pleura to the hilum, where it is connected to the mediastinum. Its interconnectedness helps it maintain the interdependence among lung units. Cells within the interstitium include fibroblasts, myofibroblasts, smooth muscle cells, pericytes, lymphatic endothelial cells, and inflammatory/immune cells that include lymphocytes, mast cells, and macrophages. Structural components that form the matrix within the interstitium include collagens, elastic fibers, proteoglycans, and fibronectin.

Interstitial mesenchymal cells have numerous functions with the interstitium. Fibroblasts are highly ramified cells with long extensions that synthesize the major building blocks consisting of fibers with the lung, including collagens, proteoglycans, and fibronectin. Synthesis of these chemicals occurs during lung development in utero and postnatally, and possibly during lung injury. Fibroblasts interact with other matrix components by the presence of specific receptors, especially of the integrin family. Another important chemical produced by fibroblasts is fibroblast-pneumocyte factor (FPF). During lung development, FPF stimulates the production of cholinephosphate cytidyltransferase, the rate-limiting enzyme in phosphatidylcholine synthesis.[46] Thus fibroblasts can influence the production of surfactant.

Elastic fibers are synthesized by myofibroblasts during fetal and postnatal life.[47] Myofibroblasts are members of the fibroblast family with contractile ability. They contain actin, intermediate filaments, and microtubules and maintain parenchymal tone, affect distribution of ventilation in extremely small airways, alter interstitial compliance, and may affect capillary patency. Additional studies are needed to fully confirm these functions.

Other members of the fibroblast family are the pericytes. Within the alveolar-capillary complex, pericytes are anchored to the endothelial basement and attach directly to capillary endothelial cells. Like myofibroblasts, pericytes contain contractile filaments. The exact function of this cell type is not known but also may influence endothelial activity. Other cells found in the interstitium include smooth muscle cells and various immune/inflammatory cells that have been described previously. During the development of interstitial lung fibrosis, all these cell types increase markedly in number.

Matrix components within the interstitium contribute to the structural integrity of the lung.[45,46] These components consist of elastin and collagen fibers, fibronectin, proteoglycans, and constituents of the epithelial and endothelial basement membranes. The scaffolding that forms the alveolar walls and septa consists primarily of collagen and elastin fibers.[45,47] Collagen represents 15% to 20% of lung dry weight, and various types of collagen molecules exist within the lung. Within the matrix of alveolar septa, airways, and blood vessels, the major types of collagen are III and I, which actually copolymerize into fibrils. Type IV collagen is found within the basement membranes. Elastin fibers are composed of an amorphous elastin component and a microfibrillar component.[47] Elastin is both hydrophobic and highly insoluble. It forms a three-dimensional network that contributes to the elastic recoil characteristics of the lung matrix. Although normally the adult lung features very little elastin turnover, the presence of a large number of elastases or a deficiency of α_1-antitrypsin can lead to considerable lung remodeling and pathologic processes.

Fibronectins are large glycoproteins that form dimers and contain many receptors that allow it to interact with numerous other cell types within the interstitium.[48] These receptors include a variety of integrins and receptors that bind to fibroblasts and proteoglycans. In the normal lung, fibronectin is primarily of plasma origin, although activated macrophages can produce large amounts of it. When present in large amounts, fibronectin forms matrices involved in cell migration and development. In adult lungs, fibronectin is found within the basal lamina of alveolar capillaries, epithelial cells, and that of conducting airways, as well as in bronchoalveolar fluid. During lung injury (for example, due to infection, sarcoidosis, heavy metal exposure, or bleomycin treatment) the amount of fibronectin increases dramatically within the lung and may contribute to the development of lung fibrosis.

Another component found within the interstitium is proteoglycans, which comprise a class of complex macromolecules composed of a protein core and complex carbohydrates.[49] Proteoglycans and hyaluronic acid influence lung compliance and water balance because of their "spongelike" characteristics and location.[49] They also influence cellular events during lung development and injury. A variety of proteoglycans exist within the lung. Within the bronchioles, chondroitin sulfate proteoglycan can interact with other substances, such as link glycoproteins and hyaluronic acid, to provide a structural framework and absorb compressive forces associated with respiration.

Smaller proteoglycans are associated with collagen fibers and basement membranes within the alveolar-capillary complex, in which they may influence permeability characteristics affecting O_2 transport and form a barrier against airborne pathogens. Hyaluronic acid is a linear polysaccharide consisting of D-glucuronic acid and N-acetyl-D-glucosamine, and influences tissue viscoelasticity, or turgor. Within the lung, hyaluronic acid is found in the basolateral surfaces of the bronchiolar epithelium, the adventitia of blood vessels, the space between large blood vessels, and the respiratory pathways; normally little exists in the alveolar interstitium. During acute inflammation the amount of hyaluronic acid may increase, affecting the gas exchange characteristics of the alveolar-capillary complex.

Functional Characteristics of the Respiratory System

The proceeding sections have emphasized the structural characteristics of the lung, with some comments directed at function. The following section uses the structural components of the lung at the gross anatomic and microanatomic levels to help understand the ways they contribute to (1) the system's mechanical characteristics that influence pressure, volume changes, and production of flow rate, (2) the distribution of ventilation, and (3) gas exchange within the respiratory system.

Airflow into and from the Lungs

The major purpose of the lungs and the chest wall is to generate pressure gradients within the lung to allow air to flow into and from the lung. Before a breath is taken, no airflow exists. Thus the pressure within the lung, or the alveolar pressure, is comparable to the surrounding, or atmospheric, pressure. The atmospheric pressure can be considered a reference pressure and is designated as 0 cm H_2O. Within the pleural space the pressure is below atmospheric (for example, -5 cm H_2O) due to the opposing forces of the lung and the chest wall. When the respiratory muscles contract, especially the diaphragm during resting breathing, the pleural pressure becomes more negative, the pressure within the alveoli becomes negative, and a pressure gradient exists between the atmosphere and the alveolar compartment. Because of this pressure gradient, air flows into the lung, and a breath is taken. To allow air to flow from the lungs the pressure within the lung must become greater than the atmospheric pressure. The passive recoil of the lung and chest wall generates a positive pressure within the lung, resulting in a pressure within the lung that is greater than the reference pressure. Consequently, air flows from the lung.

Pressures within the pleural space originally were measured by introduction of a catheter attached to a pressure transducer within the pleural space.[50] This technique lead to the development of pneumothoraces (collapse of the lung). Currently a catheter with a balloon on its end is introduced into the middle third of the esophagus, and this pressure measured with a transducer used to approximate pleural pressure.[51] Airflow rate is measured with a pneumotachygraph and volume changes determined through integration of the flow signal. A pressure transducer attached to a mouthpiece measures pressure at the mouth, reflecting alveolar pressure.

Through evaluation of pleural pressure, alveolar pressure, volume changes, and airflow rate, mechanical characteristics of the respiratory system may be determined. A primary consideration is to measure the elastic recoil of the lung, chest wall, and the entire respiratory system.[51] The elastic recoil is analogous to the transmural pressure, or the pressure within a structure minus that outside the structure. For example, the alveolar pressure minus the pleural pressure determines the transmural pressure across the lung. The transmural pressure across the chest wall is determined by subtraction of the reference pressure (which is assumed to be 0 cm H_2O) from the pleural pressure. Thus the transmural pressure across the chest wall is equal to the pleural pressure. Finally, the transmural pressure across the entire respiratory system is equal to the alveolar pressure minus the reference pressure, or simply the alveolar pressure, according to the previous discussion.

Physiologically, the greater the elastic recoil of the lung, the more work is needed by the respiratory muscles to stretch the lungs—but the more rapidly and forcefully they recoil during passive expiration. This increase in elastic recoil may occur in cases of lung fibrosis, decreased surfactant production, or congestive heart disease when more fluid than normal is contained within the pulmonary vasculature or interstitium. The opposite occurs in a condition in which the lung parenchyma is damaged, such as in emphysema.[52-54] In such a situation decreased levels of elastin and collagen cause a decrease in elastic recoil of the lung. Because mechanical characteristics of the respiratory system depend on volume history (an assessment of the individual's past breathing) and lung volume, these two factors must be standardized among subjects in evaluations of elastic recoil.

Compliance and Resistance

Two mechanical parameters—compliance or elastance (the inverse of compliance) and resistance—can be calculated when the pressure-volume and flow characteristics of the respiratory system are known.[53] **Compliance** is determined through division of the change in volume divided by the corresponding change in transmural pressure. For example, at resting lung volume or functional residual capacity (FRC), the transmural pressure across the lung (alveolar minus pleural pressure) is determined to be 3 cm H_2O and the lung volume change, 0.6 L. The lung compliance would then be 0.6 L/3 cm H_2O, or 0.20 L/cm H_2O. The elastance is 5.00 cm H_2O/L. Because compliance and elastance are influenced by lung volume, another parameter is calculated, the specific compliance or specific elastance. For example, specific compliance is determined through division of compliance by lung volume.

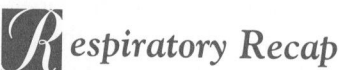

Respiratory Recap

Mechanics of Breathing

Resistance to flow through airways
Compliance of the lungs and chest wall

The previous discussion assumes that compliance or elastance was measured in a quasistatic manner. That is, a subject takes a breath and holds it briefly. Transmural pressure is determined before and after the breath is taken. Compliance also can be measured during actual breathing, called *dynamic compliance*. In a normal person the two ways to measure compliance should yield the same value. However, in areas of the lung that are not being ventilated at the same rate, dynamic compliance may be lower than static compliance. This concept is discussed further in the section on distribution of ventilation.

The static pressure volume curves for the lungs, chest wall, and respiratory system are shown in Figure 17-11. The slope of the pressure-volume curve is compliance. Note that the pressure-volume curve is sigmoidal. The compliance is low at both low and high lung volumes. The respiratory system is most compliant at a normal FRC.

Aside from evaluations of lung compliance and elastance, these characteristics also may be determined about the chest wall and the entire respiratory system. In fact, with the compliance of two components, for example, the chest wall (C_{CW}) and total respiratory system (C_T), the third (lung compliance, C_L) may be calculated with the following formula:

$$\frac{1}{C_T} = \frac{1}{C_L} + \frac{1}{C_{CW}}$$

Note also that elastance (E) then would be as follows:

$$E_T = E_L + E_{CW}$$

The **resistance** to airflow is associated primarily with the patency of the airways and relative turbulence of air-

flow. Airway resistance (R) is inversely proportional to the fourth power of the radius, as follows:

$$R \propto \frac{1}{r^4}$$

Thus physiologic factors that decrease airway radius increase resistance. Such factors include allergens that cause constriction of airway smooth muscles, edema in the airway, excess mucus production, or tumors within or impinging on airways. In cases of emphysema, airway resistance increases because the springs holding open the airways are weaker.[54] Thus during normal breathing and especially during a forced expiratory maneuver, these airways dynamically collapse.

Another factor that may increase airway resistance is turbulent flow.[8,53] As airflow rate increases, turbulence increases, as does airway resistance. Thus resistance is higher in the nose, upper airways, and larger conducting tubes (trachea and bronchi) than in the smaller airways. Resistance in the nose and larger airways is in series. Consequently, as flow rate increases during exercise, turbulence and resistance increase to the point that breathing is no longer through the nose but is initiated through the mouth. Flow in smaller airways is more laminar. Thus in the smaller airways, turbulence does not play a role in increasing resistance. Furthermore, because smaller airways are arranged in parallel, the total resistance is equal to the sum of the inverse of the individual resistances. The difference in the distribution of resistance values between the larger and smaller airways tends to "hide" increases in resistances of small airways. Specialized tests have been devised to separate the effects of increasing resistance in small versus larger airways. Moreover, an increase in small airway resistance contributes to the uneven distribution of ventilation, which directly affects gas exchange.[52]

Airway resistance is determined by division of the difference between airway opening pressure and alveolar pressure by the flow rate. In most measurements of airway resistance the resistance afforded by breathing through the nose is discounted. Also, resistance may be different during inspiration and expiration. One way to evaluate both lung volume and airway resistance is through the use of plethysmography, during which a subject sits in a closed booth, similar in size to a phone booth and the principles behind Boyle's Law (PV = k) are used to determine lung volume. Alveolar pressure also can be measured through brief occlusion of the airway. Flow rate is evaluated directly before this occlusion; thus not only resistance but also specific resistance can be measured.

Muscle Strength and Endurance

Aside from the use of volume, pleural, and alveolar pressures to evaluate pulmonary mechanics, maximum pressures generated at the mouth and the transmural pressure across the diaphragm are used to evaluate respiratory muscle strength and endurance.[17] Because respiratory muscle length is a func-

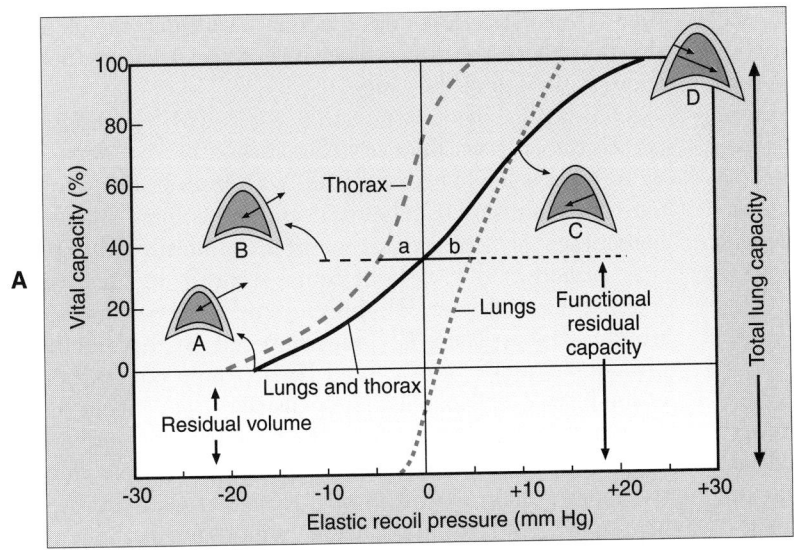

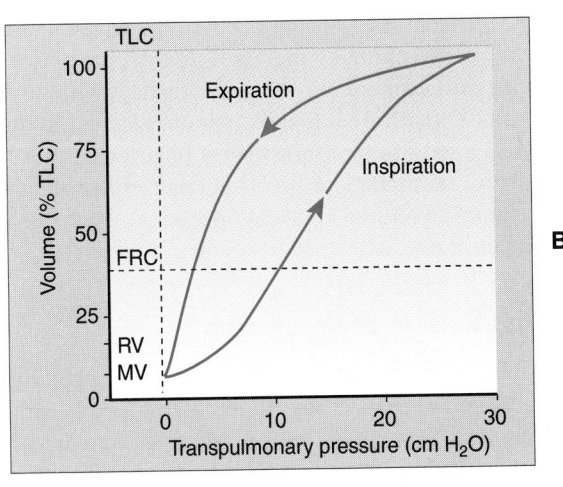

Figure 17-11 **A,** Pressure-volume curves for the lungs, chest wall, and respiratory system. Note that the respiratory system curve is the sum of those for the lungs and the chest wall and that the respiratory system compliance is greatest at functional residual capacity (FRC). **B,** Pressure-volume curve of the respiratory system. The difference between the inspiratory and expiratory curves represents hysteresis. *TLC,* Total Lung capacity; *RV,* Residual volume; *MV,* minimum volume. (**A,** Modified from Beachey W. Respiratory care anatomy and physiology. St Louis: Mosby; 1998. **B,** Modified from Berne RM, Levy MN. Physiology. 3rd ed. St Louis: Mosby; 1993.)

tion of lung volume and also affects the force that the muscle can generate, it must be considered.[17,53] The optimum length of the diaphragm occurs just below FRC. Thus maximum inspiratory (PI_{max}) and expiratory (PE_{max}) pressures may be measured at FRC. In addition PI_{max} also is measured after a subject exhales to residual volume and makes a maximal inspiratory effort to total lung capacity. Maximum expiratory pressure also is determined after a subject inhales to total lung capacity and then maximally exhales. To achieve these measurements the subject breathes through a mouthpiece connected to a tube containing a small leak and coupled to a pressure transducer. A nose clip prevents loss of pressure through the nose. Respiratory muscle strength is affected by gender, age, training, position, and underlying cardiac, pulmonary, and respiratory muscle and infectious diseases. In addition, electrolyte imbalances, acid-base disturbances, endocrine abnormalities (such as thyroid disease), and prolonged use of steroids and neuromuscular-blocking drugs may also affect maximum pressures.

*R*espiratory Recap

Strength and Endurance of the Respiratory Muscles

Maximal inspiratory pressure (PI_{max})
Maximal expiratory pressure (PE_{max})
Maximum voluntary ventilation (MVV)
Work of breathing
Oxygen cost of breathing

To more specifically evaluate diaphragmatic function, transdiaphragmatic pressure is evaluated through the introduction of two catheters containing balloons into the internal nares and then down the esophagus. One catheter-balloon system is used to evaluate pleural pressure and the other, gastric pressure just below the diaphragm. These catheters are attached to pressure transducers, and the difference in pressure (gastric-pleural pressure) is determined. During inspiration, pleural pressure becomes more negative (relative to reference pressure) and gastric or abdominal pressure becomes more positive. Thus the transdiaphragmatic pressure increases. When a subject with the catheters in place inhales at FRC against an occluded airway, the transdiaphragmatic pressure is evaluated in a standardized manner.

One way to evaluate the endurance of respiratory muscles is the measurement of maximum voluntary ventilation (MVV). This test entails measurement of ventilation when a subject is told to breathe maximally for 15 seconds. This level of ventilation is seldom reached during exercise. In a healthy individual, 75% of MVV can be sustained for 4 minutes and 60% may be sustained for 15 minutes. This latter level also is known as the *maximum sustainable ventilation.* Respiratory system endurance is influenced by respiratory muscle characteristics (size and percentage of different muscle fiber types), blood flow, and pulmonary mechanics.

The work of breathing is generally a small portion of the O_2 consumption (1% to 3%). During quiet breathing in a healthy individual, most of the work is used to overcome the elastic recoil properties of the respiratory system associated with inspiration. Only 25% of the work of breathing is needed to counter the effects of airway resistance. Increasing ventilation during exercise increases the work of breathing by increases in both the elastic and the resistive components. In individuals with lung disease, work of breathing is markedly increased and results in dyspnea, a sensation of shortness of breath that may be due in part to the inefficient breathing patterns these individuals manifest, patterns that also decrease their gas-exchange capabilities and lead to hypoxia and hypercapnia.[54]

Distribution of Ventilation

The inspired tidal volume is distributed to conducting airways and alveoli. The volume of the conducting airways does not participate in gas exchange and is called **dead space** volume. Only the alveolar volume participates in gas exchange. During disease, some alveoli may be ventilated but not perfused. These contribute to the dead space and are referred to as *alveolar dead space*. A pulmonary embolus is an example of a dead space producing disease. Dead space ventilation increases the minute ventilation required to maintain acceptable alveolar ventilation.

For optimal gas exchange, ventilation must be distributed equally throughout the lung. The distribution of ventilation may be uneven because of gravitational forces acting on the lung in the upright position. Thus a pleural pressure gradient exists from the apex (top) to the base of the lung, with the pleural pressure being lower at the apex than at the base. This difference results in a greater transpulmonary pressure at the top of the lung at FRC. Thus the alveoli at the top of the lung are more open than those at the bottom of the lung. This difference is also a function of lung volume. At total lung capacity, alveoli at both locations are equal in size, but at functional residual capacity those at the top are distended more than those at

the bottom. Therefore during normal breathing, alveoli at the bottom of the lungs receive more ventilation than those at the top of the lungs.

One way to demonstrate this fact is with the single-breath nitrogen washout test (Figure 17-12). An individual inhales a single breath of 100% O_2 from residual volume and then slowly exhales. Both lung volume and the percentage of nitrogen are constantly monitored. The first section of the washout comes from O_2 in the dead space (phases I and II). Subsequently, alveoli empty, which is called *phase III*. Superimposed on this tracing are regular oscillations caused by rhythmic contraction of the heart and thought to help distribute gas within the alveoli. Finally, nitrogen from the alveoli at the very top of the lung empties, whereas the alveoli at the bottom of the lungs remain closed, known as *phase IV*, or the *closing volume*. As ventilation becomes more unequal due to respiratory diseases, such as chronic obstructive pulmonary disease (COPD), the slope of phase III and phase IV increase.

Uneven distribution of ventilation may occur if resistance increases (for example, due to regional lung inflammation) or compliance increases or decreases (Figure 17-13).[54-56] Aside from the single-breath nitrogen washout test, measurement of static lung compliance and dynamic lung compliance at different breathing frequencies is used to demonstrate uneven distribution of ventilation. The ratio of dynamic to static compliance decreases in the face of uneven distribution because as frequency of breathing increases, lung units that have higher resistance values are no longer ventilated. Both the single-breath nitrogen washout test and the dynamic-to-static compliance measurements do not determine where in the lung the inequalities occur, just that they exist. To pinpoint where in the lung ventilation is abnormal, a subject inhales radiolabeled xenon. With a scanner, the location that contains a lower level of xenon (and thus is less ventilated) can be ascertained.[56]

Distribution of Blood Flow

Gas exchange in the lung depends not only on the distribution of ventilation but also on the distribution and amount of pulmonary blood flow, on whether ventilation and perfusion of various lung units are matched, and on the characteristics of the alveolar-capillary complex (Figure 17-14).[55,56] Hydrostatic factors and lung volume influence perfusion of the lungs in an upright individual. At the top of the lungs, alveolar pressure is greater than pulmonary vascular pressure, resulting in no blood flow (dead space), called *West Zone 1*. At the bottom of the lungs, pulmonary vascular pressure is greater than alveolar pressure called *West Zone 3*. In West Zone 2, between zones 1 and 3, blood flow is determined by the difference between pulmonary vascular pressure and alveolar pressure. Thus blood flow at the top of the lung is less than that at the bottom.

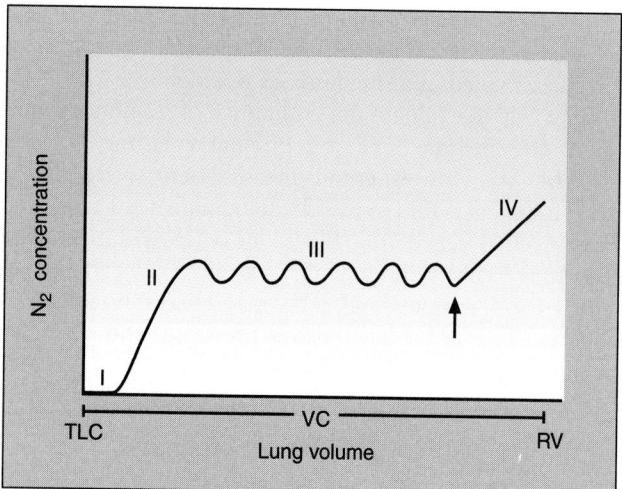

Figure 17-12 The components of the single-breath nitrogen washout test. Numbers I through IV represent different phases of the test. The arrow indicates the onset of the closing volume. *TLC,* Total lung capacity; *VC,* vital capacity; *RV,* residual volume; *N₂,* nitrogen.

The lowest resistance to blood flow in the lung is at FRC and increases at either total lung capacity or residual volume. Pulmonary vascular resistance, which influences perfusion, also is increased under conditions of hypoxia and hypercapnia. Thus perfusion of the lung is modulated by ventilation. In areas of the lung that receive less ventilation, perfusion also is decreased because the resulting hypoxia and hypercapnia contribute to the constriction of vascular smooth muscles. The major purpose of this mechanism is to match ventilation to perfusion and make gas exchange more efficient.

Ventilation/Perfusion Ratio

The **ventilation/perfusion ratio ($\dot{V}/\dot{Q}$)** ideally should be 1 to ensure the most effective gas exchange. Although a healthy individual has some heterogeneity of $\dot{V}/\dot{Q}$ ratios within the lung, most lung units have a $\dot{V}/\dot{Q}$ close to 1. With shunt (perfusion without ventilation) the $\dot{V}/\dot{Q}$ is zero. At the opposite extreme (dead space), the $\dot{V}/\dot{Q}$ is infinity. In individuals with pathologic processes of the lung the distribution of $\dot{V}/\dot{Q}$ exhibits more and more heterogeneity[54,57] and leads to increasingly poorer gas exchange. Arterial gases in these individuals indicate a greater hypoxemia and possibly hypercapnia than expected. Anatomic abnormalities, fluid in the alveolar spaces, or atelectasis (collapse of lung units) can give rise to shunts. In these situations, blood bypasses the lung and no gas exchange occurs, adding greatly to arterial hypoxemia.

ℛespiratory Recap

$\dot{V}/\dot{Q}$ Ratio	
Ideal: 1.0	Shunt: 0
Normal: 0.8	Dead space: infinity

In relationship to gas exchange the alveolar-capillary complex is thin, devoid of excess fluid either in the interstitium or in the alveolar sacs, and patent. Factors that thicken the alveolar-capillary complex (edema, fibrosis, or increased number of Type II cells), increase the distance that O_2 needs to transverse, decreasing the gas exchange for O_2 across the lung. Transport of O_2 also is influenced by the O_2 gradient. Venous partial pressure for oxygen (PO_2) is 40 mm Hg in a healthy young person at sea level, whereas alveolar PO_2 is approximately 95 mm Hg. Thus the PO_2 gradient across the lung is 55 mm Hg. As this gradient decreases, for instance, at high altitude (alveolar PO_2 being only 59 mm Hg in La Paz, Bolivia) or in the case of lung disease, less O_2 diffuses into the lung. In contrast to O_2, the high diffusibility of the lung for CO_2 necessitates only a partial pressure gradient of 5 mm Hg. Thus in individuals with lung disease, hypoxemia generally occurs before hypercapnia.

Oxygen Uptake and Diffusion Capacity

Another factor that influences gas exchange is the time that a RBC needs to transit the pulmonary capillary. In a resting individual the transit time for a RBC through the pulmonary capillary is 0.75 seconds (Figure 17-15).[18] As cardiac output increases during exercise, transit time may decrease to 0.25 seconds. In a healthy person this event may not greatly compromise O_2 diffusion, but in a person with lung disease or living at a high altitude, this decrease in time profoundly decreases O_2 diffusion across the lung and leads to further hypoxemia. Thus exercise in an individual with lung disease and without additional inhaled O_2 leads to marked dyspnea.

The number of and the biochemical characteristics of RBCs also influence gas exchange across the lung.[53] The greater the number of RBCs, the more sites for gas exchange are available. Without RBCs, which contain hemoglobin (a molecule that can carry four O_2 molecules),

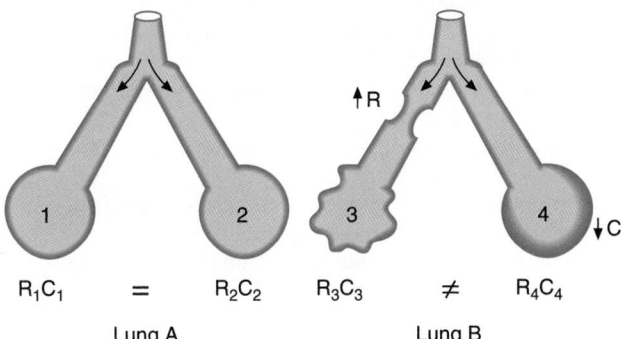

Figure 17-13   A diagrammatic representation of two lung units exhibiting equal (lung A) and unequal (lung B) resistance (*R*) and compliance (*C*) values. In lung A, airflow would be distributed equally to units 1 and 2. In lung B, distribution of airflow would be unequal due increased resistance (3) and decreased compliance (4).

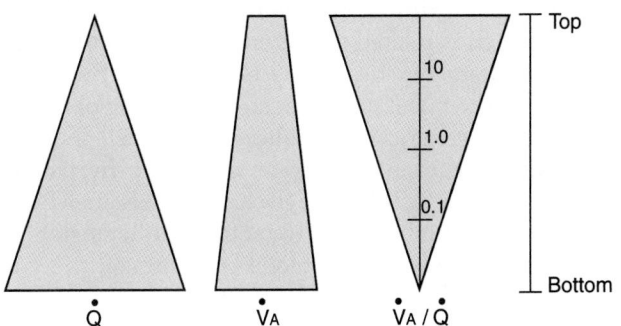

Figure 17-14   A schematic representation of the relative distribution of perfusion ($\dot{Q}$), alveolar ventilation ($\dot{V}A$), and the ratio of $\dot{V}A/\dot{Q}$ throughout the lung of an upright individual breathing at functional residual capacity. *Top* denotes alveoli and capillaries in the hilar regions of the lung, and *bottom* denotes these structures at the base of the lung.

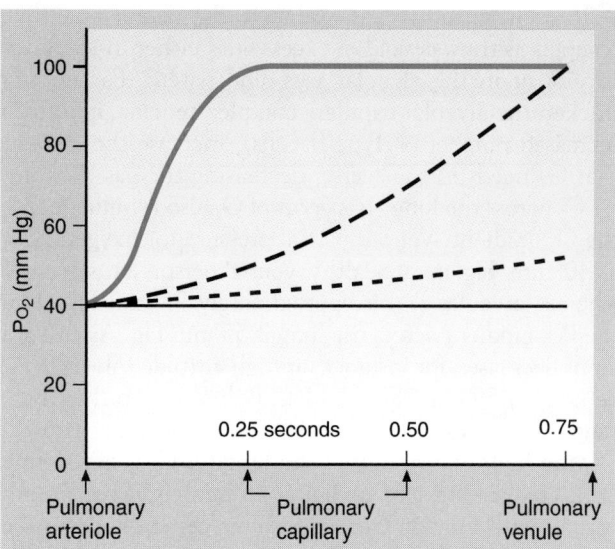

Figure 17-15 Changes in the partial pressure of oxygen (Po_2) of blood as it enters the pulmonary capillary from a pulmonary arteriole and reaches a pulmonary venule. The solid line represents increasing levels of Po_2 as blood transverses the capillary in an individual with a normal diffusion capacity. The dashed lines denote the effects of progressively poorer diffusion capabilities of individuals with lung disease on Po_2 levels in blood moving across the pulmonary capillary. At rest in a healthy individual living at sea level, the red blood cell transverses the pulmonary capillary by 0.75 seconds and picks up all the oxygen possible. This scenario is also true for the person with mild lung disease. But for the person with severe lung disease during exercise (*arrow* at 0.25 seconds), the effects of impaired diffusion capacities are magnified due to the decreased transit time.

the amount of O_2 in the blood would depend on the solubility of O_2 in plasma and the Po_2. The amount of dissolved O_2 in plasma at sea level is 0.003 mL/100 mL of blood per mm Hg of O_2. Thus arterial blood contains 0.3 mL of O_2 for every 100 mL of blood. In contrast, the amount of O_2 bound to hemoglobin is about 20 mL for 100 mL of blood. The amount of O_2 bound to hemoglobin depends on the amount of hemoglobin present, the reactivity of O_2 with hemoglobin, and the percent saturation, which is related to the arterial Po_2 and the biochemical characteristics of the hemoglobin. For example, the biochemical characteristics of hemoglobin may be altered by genetic abnormalities (sickle cell anemia), exposure to carbon monoxide or drugs, hypoxemia (which elevates 2,3-diphosoglycerate levels in RBCs), and developmental changes (fetal to adult hemoglobin). In a normal person, 5 L of blood pass through the lung per minute, and the O_2 uptake is approximately 234 mL of O_2 per minute.

Evaluation of **diffusion capacity** across the lung is done clinically with small amounts of carbon monoxide.[58] This molecule binds 210 times more tightly to hemoglobin than does O_2, is not limited by perfusion of blood through the

lung, and in nonsmokers its amount in blood is considered zero. To measure diffusion capacity with the single-breath method, a subject inhales a breathe containing 21% O_2, 0.35% carbon monoxide, and 5% helium. The subject then holds that breath for 10 seconds and exhales. Helium is used to calculate the initial fraction of carbon monoxide. At end-expiration a gas sample is collected. The diffusion capacity for carbon monoxide is determined through division of the fractional content of carbon monoxide in the alveolar samples at the beginning and end of the breath hold, which is divided by the partial pressure of carbon monoxide (Pco) left in the alveoli. The diffusion capacity of the lung for O_2 is determined by multiplication of the diffusion capacity for carbon monoxide by 1.23. This number is obtained by division of the product of the molecular weight and solubility for carbon monoxide by the same products for O_2. Some individuals may have normal lung mechanics and only a diffusion capacity abnormality that makes them breathless while exercising.

$\mathcal{K}$EY $\mathcal{P}$OINTS

- The primary function of the lungs is gas exchange.
- The upper airway consists of the nose, nasopharynx, oropharynx, laryngopharynx, and larynx.
- The lungs consist of the airways and alveoli.
- The bony thorax consists of the sternum, ribs, thoracic vertebrae, clavicles, and scapulae.
- The respiratory muscles are the diaphragm, accessory muscles of inspiration, and accessory muscles of expiration.
- The pulmonary circulation participates in gas exchange, whereas the bronchial circulation provides nutritional support for the lungs.
- The innervation of the lungs consists of cholinergic, adrenergic, and nonadrenergic-noncholinergic components.
- The visceral pleurae surround the lungs, and the parietal pleurae line the chest wall; the pleural space is between the visceral and parietal pleurae.
- The mediastinum is the area between the two pleural sacs and contains the heart, great vessels, esophagus, and thymus.
- The mucociliary apparatus clears inhaled agents from the lower respiratory tract.
- Important cells in the lower respiratory tract include mast cells, macrophages, and dendrites.
- The alveolus is composed of Type I and Type II cells.
- The interstitial space is located between the alveolar epithelia and the vascular endothelia.
- The mechanics of airflow into and from the lungs is determined by resistance and compliance.
- The $\dot{V}/\dot{Q}$ ratio is ideally 1 but can range from zero (shunt) to infinity (dead space).

References

1. Proctor DF. Form and function of the upper airways and larynx. In: Macklem PT, Mead J, editors. Mechanics of breathing. Part 1. Handbook of physiology. Section 3. The respiratory system. Bethesda, Md: American Physiological Society; 1986. pp. 63-73.

2. Irbeck D. Normal mechanisms of heat and moisture exchange in the respiratory system. Respir Care Clin N Am 1998;4:189-198.

3. Bouhuys A. Breathing: physiology, environment and lung disease. New York: Grune and Stratton; 1974.

4. Netter FH. Atlas of human anatomy. 2nd ed. East Hanover, NJ: Novartis; 1997.

5. Rogers AW. Textbook of anatomy. Edinburgh: Churchill Livingstone; 1992.

6. Wilson-Pauwels L, Akesson EJ, Stewart PA. Cranial nerves: anatomy and clinical comments. Toronto: BC Decker; 1988.

7. Sminia T. A review of the mucosal immune system: development, structure and function of the upper and lower respiratory tract. Eur Respir Rev 1996;36:136-141.

8. Murray JF. The normal lung. 2nd ed. Philadelphia: WB Saunders; 1986.

9. Dahl R, Mygind N. Mechanisms of airflow limitation in the nose and lungs. Clin Exp Allergy 1998;28(Suppl 2):17-25.

10. Glovsky MM. Upper airways involvement in bronchial asthma. Curr Opin Pulm Med 1998;4:54-58.

11. Amis TC, O'Neill N, DiSomma E, et al. Epiglottic movements during breathing in humans. J Physiol (London) 1998;512:307-314.

12. Kuna ST, Vanoye CR. Mechanical effects of pharyngeal constrictor activities on pharyngeal airway function. J Appl Physiol 1999;86:411-417.

13. Schwab RJ. Functional properties of the pharyngeal airway: properties of tissues surrounding the upper airway. Sleep 1996;19:S170-S174.

14. Kuna ST, Smickley JS, Vanoyae CR. Respiratory-related pharyngeal constrictor activity in normal human adults. Am J Respir Crit Care Med 1997;155:1991-1999.

15. van Lunteren E. Upper-airway effects on breathing. In: Crystal RG, West JB, Barnes PJ, et al., editors. The lung: scientific foundations. 2nd ed. New York: Raven Press; 1991; pp. 1631-1644.

16. Wanner A, Salath M, O'Riordan, TG. Mucociliary clearance in the airways. Am J Respir Crit Care Med 1996;154:1868-1902.

17. De Troyer A. Respiratory muscle function. In: Cherniack NS, Altose MD, Homma I, editors. Rehabilitation of the patient with respiratory disease. New York: McGraw-Hill; 1999. pp. 21-32.

18. Sahgeal V, Tetik S. Respiratory muscles—structural considerations. In: Cherniack NS, Altose MD, Homma I, editors. Rehabilitation of the patient with respiratory disease. New York: McGraw-Hill; 1999. pp. 33-51.

19. Poole DC, Sexton WL, Farkas GA, et al. Diaphragm structure and function in health and disease. Med Sci Sports Med 1997;6:738-754.

20. Stasssijin G, Lysens R, Decramer M. Peripheral and respiratory muscles in chronic heart failure. Eur Respir J 1996;9:2161-2167.

21. Pokorski M. Control of breathing. In: Cherniack NS, Altose MD, Homma I, editors. Rehabilitation of the patient with respiratory disease. New York: McGraw-Hill; 1999. pp. 69-86.

22. Bals R, Weiner DJ, Wilson JM. The innate immune system in cystic fibrosis lung disease. J Clin Invest 1999;103:303-307.

23. Widdicome JG. Autonomic regulation i-NANC/e-NANC. Am J Respir Crit Care Med 1998;158:S171-S175.

24. Reeves JT, Rubin LJ. The pulmonary circulation: snapshots of progress. Am J Respir Crit Care Med 1998;157:S101-S108.

25. Sunday ME. Neuropeptides and lung development. In: McDonald JA, editor. Lung growth and development. New York: Marcel Dekker; 1997. pp. 401-494.

26. Miserocchi G. Physiology and pathophysiology of pleural fluid turnover. Eur Respir J 1997;10:219-225.

27. Plopper G. Clara cells. In: McDonald JA, editor. Lung growth and development. New York: Marcel Dekker; 1997. pp. 181-209.

28. Stephens NL, Li W, Wang Y, et al. The contractile apparatus of airway smooth muscle: biophysics and biochemistry. Am J Respir Crit Care Med 1998;158:S80-S94.

29. Barnes PJ. Pharmacology of airway smooth muscle. Am J Respir Crit Care Med 1998;158:S123-S132.

30. Schwartz LB, Huff TF. Mast cells. In: Crystal RG, West JB, Barnes PJ, et al., editors. The lung: scientific foundations. 2nd ed. New York: Raven Press; 1991. pp. 601-616.

31. Bradding P, Okayama P, Howarth PH, et al. Heterogeneity of human mast cells based on cytokine content. J Immunol 1995;155:297-307.

32. Gjomarkaj M, Pace E, Melis M, et al. Phenotypic and functional characterization of normal rat pleural macrophages in comparison with autologous peritoneal and alveolar macrophages. Am J Respir Cell Mol Biol 1999; 20:135-142.

33. Gordon S, Hughes D. Macrophages and their origins. In: Lipcomb MF, Russell SW, editors. Lung macrophages and dendritic cells in health and disease. New York: Marcel Dekker; 1997. pp. 3-31.

34. Nicod LP. Role of antigen-presenting cells in lung immunity. Eur Respir Rev 1996;6:142-150.

35. Schneeberger EE, Takafumi S. Ontogeny and heterogeneity of lung dendritic cells. In: Lipcomb MF, Russell SW, editors. Lung macrophages and dendritic cells in health and disease. New York: Marcel Dekker; 1997. pp. 239-266.

36. Crystal RG. Alveolar macrophages. In: Crystal RG, West JB, Barnes PJ, et al., editors. The lung: scientific foundations. 2nd ed. New York: Raven Press; 1991. pp. 527-538.

37. Schneeberger EE. Alveolar Type I cells. In: Crystal RG, West JB, Barnes PJ, et al., editors. The lung: scientific foundations. 2nd ed. New York: Raven Press; 1991. pp. 229-234.

38. Mason RJ, Williams MC. Alveolar Type II cells. In: Crystal RG, West JB, Barnes PJ, et al., editors. The lung: scientific foundations. 2nd ed. New York: Raven Press; 1991. pp. 235-246.

39. Hawgood SH. Surfactant: composition, structure, and metabolism. In: Crystal RG, West JB, Barnes PJ, et al., editors. The lung: scientific foundations. 2nd ed. New York: Raven Press; 1991. pp. 247-261.

40. van Golde LMG, Batenburg JJ, Robertson B. The pulmonary surfactant system. News Physiol Sci 1994;9:13-22.

41. Korutal L, Strayer DS. SP-A as a cytokine: surfactant protein-A-regulated transcription of surfactant proteins and other genes. J Cell Physiol 1999;178:379-386.

42. Postle AD, Mander KB, Reid BM, et al. Deficient hydrophilic lung surfactant proteins A and D with normal surfactant phospholipid molecular species in cystic fibrosis. Am J Respir Cell Mol Biol 1999;20:90-98.

43. Campbell AR, Folkesson HG, Berthiaume Y, et al. Alveolar epithelial fluid clearance persists in the presence of moderate left atrial hypertension in sheep. J Appl Physiol 1999;86:139-151.

44. Yasui M, Serlachius E, Lofgrenm M, et al. Perinatal changes in expression of aquaporin-4 and other water and ion transporters in rat lung. J Physiol (London) 1997;505:1:3-11.

45. Weibel ER, Crystal RG. Structural organization of the pulmonary interstitium. In: Crystal RG, West JB, Barnes PJ, et al., editors. The lung: scientific foundations. 2nd ed. New York: Raven Press; 1991. pp. 369-380.

46. Shannon J, Deterding RR. Epithelial-mesenchymal interactions in lung development. In: McDonald JA, editor. Lung growth and development. New York: Marcel Dekker; 1997. pp. 401-494.

47. Mecham RP, Prosser IW, Fukuda Y. Elastic fibers. In: Crystal RG, West JB, Barnes PJ, et al., editors. The lung: scientific foundations. 2nd ed. New York: Raven Press; 1991. pp. 389-398.

48. Roman J, McDonald JA. Fibronectins. In: Crystal RG, West JB, Barnes PJ, et al., editors. The lung: scientific foundations. 2nd ed. New York: Raven Press; 1991. pp. 399-411.

49. Juul SE, Wight TN, Hascall VC. Proteoglycans. In: Crystal RG, West JB, Barnes PJ, et al., editors. The lung: scientific foundations. 2nd ed. New York: Raven Press; 1991. pp. 413-420.

50. Mead J, Gaensler A. Esophageal and pleural pressure in man: upright and supine. J Appl Physiol 1959;14:81-83.

51. Dawson A. Elastic recoil and compliance. In: Clausen JL, editor. Pulmonary function testing guidelines and controversies. Orlando, Fla: Grune and Stratton; 1984. pp. 193-204.

52. Macklem PT. The physiology of small airways. Am J Respir Crit Care Med 1998;157:S181-S183.

53. Staub NC. Basic respiratory physiology. New York: Churchill Livingstone; 1991.

54. Bates DV. Respiratory function in disease. Philadelphia: WB Saunders; 1989.

55. West JB, Wagner PD. Pulmonary gas exchange. Am J Respir Crit Care Med 1998;157:S82-S87.

56. West JB, Wagner PD. Ventilation-perfusion relationships. In: Crystal RG, West JB, Barnes PJ, et al., editors. The lung: scientific foundations. 2nd ed. New York: Raven Press; 1991. pp. 1289-1305.

57. Manier G, Castaing Y. Gas exchange abnormalities in pulmonary vascular and cardiac disease. Thorax 1994;49:1169-1174.

58. American Thoracic Society. Single-breath carbon dioxide monoxide diffusing capacity (transfer factor). Am J Respir Crit Care Med 1995;152:2185-2198.

CHAPTER 18

Respiratory Pharmacology

Christopher Carter
Christine Solberg

CHAPTER OUTLINE

Principles of Pharmacology
  Chemical and Physical Properties of Drugs
  Pharmacokinetics
  Pharmacodynamics
  Indications and Dosages
  Toxicity, Side Effects, and Allergic Reactions
Pharmacology of the Respiratory System
  Mediators of Inflammation
  Mediators of Bronchial Smooth Muscle Tone
  Mediators of Bronchial Secretions
  Receptor Physiology
Routes of Delivery
  Inhalation
  Intratracheal Instillation

Oral Route
Intravenous and Intramuscular Routes
Subcutaneous Route
Respiratory Drugs
  Bronchodilators
  Antiinflammatory Drugs
  Secretion Modifiers
  Surfactant Replacements
  Inhaled Antimicrobial Drugs
  Other Drugs Used in Pulmonary Medicine

OBJECTIVES

1. List the aspects of drugs described by pharmacology.
2. Describe the importance of chemical and physical properties in the activity of drugs.
3. Describe how pharmacokinetics affects the way a drug moves through the body.
4. Use pharmacodynamics to describe a drug's actions in the body.
5. Explain drug indications and dosage.
6. Define the terms *toxicity*, *side effects*, and *allergic reaction* as they apply to drug administration.
7. List mediators of bronchial smooth muscle tone and bronchial secretions.
8. Compare adrenergic, cholinergic, histaminergic, corticosteroidal, and leukotriene receptors.
9. Compare routes of drug administration.
10. Compare the three classes of bronchodilators: β-agonists, anticholinergics, and methylxanthines.
11. Compare the four classes of antiinflammatory drugs: corticosteroids, nonsteroidal antiinflammatory drugs, cromones, and leukotriene inhibitors.
12. Describe the actions of drugs that modify airway secretions.
13. Discuss the role of surfactant therapy in the treatment of neonatal respiratory distress syndrome.
14. Discuss the role of inhaled microbial therapy for patients with respiratory disease.
15. Describe the actions of the following drug groups: anticoagulants, diuretics, vasopressors, inotropic agents, vasodilators, opiates, sedatives, and neuromuscular blockers.

KEY TERMS

Agonist	Analgesic	Anticoagulant
Allergy	Antagonist	Antiemetics
α-Adrenergic	Anticholinergic	Antihistamine

Continued

KEY TERMS—cont'd

Antimicrobials	Hydrophobic	Pharmacodynamics
Antipyretic	Indication	Pharmacokinetics
Antitussive	Inflammation	Pharmacology
Anxiolytics	Inotropism	Potency
β-Adrenergic	Intramuscular (IM)	Racemic
Bronchodilator	Intravenous (IV)	Receptor
Chronotropism	Leukotrienes	Sedatives
Clearance	Lipophilic	Side Effect
Coagulant	Methylxanthines	Stereoisomer
Competitive Inhibition	Muscarinic	Subcutaneous (SC or SQ)
Contraindication	Neuromuscular Blockers	Surfactant
Corticosteroids	Nicotinic	Therapeutic Window
Cromones	Noncompetitive Inhibition	Tolerance
Diuretics	Nonsteroidal Antiinflammatory Drugs	Toxicity
Efficacy	(NSAIDs)	Vasodilator
Enteral	Opiate	Vasopressor
Half-Life	Oral (PO)	Volume of Distribution (V_d)
Hydrophilic	Parenteral	

A growing number of medicines are used to treat respiratory disease. Many of these drugs are administered directly to the lungs, because this route has the advantages of rapid onset, a large surface area over which the drug might act, and the ability to achieve high local drug concentrations with fewer or diminished systemic effects. Respiratory therapists are primarily responsible for administering and monitoring these drugs; therefore they must have a thorough understanding of the anatomy of the respiratory system and the pharmacology of respiratory drugs.

Principles of Pharmacology

Pharmacology is the science that describes the chemical entities known as *drugs* and their interactions with the body. A drug generally is defined as a chemical used to alter the body's physiology. Pharmacology describes five as-

pects of a drug: (1) its chemical and physical properties; (2) its movement into, through, and out of the body (pharmacokinetics); (3) its effect on the body (pharmacodynamics); (4) indications for its use and the dosage to be used; and (5) its possible side effects and toxicity.

Respiratory Recap

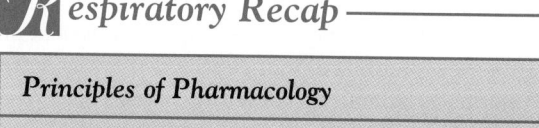

Principles of Pharmacology	
Chemical and physical properties of a drug	Pharmacodynamics
	Indications and dosage
Pharmacokinetics	Side effects and toxicity

Chemical and Physical Properties of Drugs

Stereochemistry   The molecular structure of nearly all drugs includes a stereocenter, or site where four components are joined to a common atom. A stereocenter can be assembled in one of two mirror-image forms to produce different molecules, or **stereoisomers** (Figure 18-1). Al-

Respiratory Recap

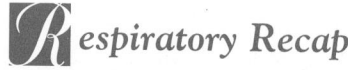

Characteristics of Stereoisomers
Two mirror-image molecules
Same constituent atoms
Not identical because of different spatial configurations
Designated R- or S-based on physical configuration and L- or D-based on the direction in which light is rotated

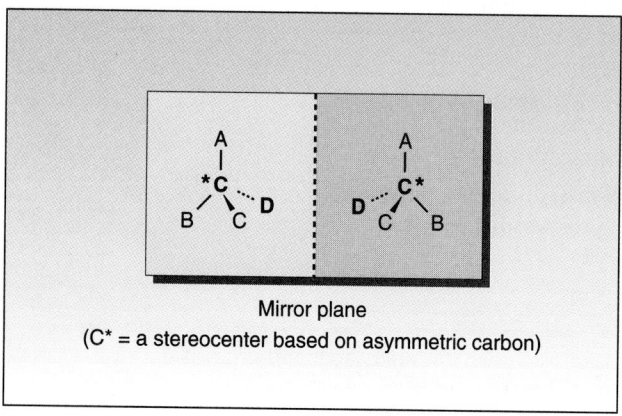

Mirror plane
(C* = a stereocenter based on asymmetric carbon)

Figure 18-1   Two complementary stereoisomers.

though their components are identical, stereoisomers (or *enantiomers*) are not the same because they are arranged differently in space.

Stereoisomers are designated right (R-, for the Latin word *rectus*) or left (S-, for the Latin word *sinister*) based on their physical configuration. They also are designated right (*D-*) or left (*L-*) according to which direction they rotate light; this designation does not necessarily correlate with the designations for the physical configuration. Substances produced biologically often are composed of only one stereoisomer, because the compounds are "assembled" in a specific way by enzymes. Chemicals produced in the laboratory usually are an equal mix of both stereoisomers, because the component atoms have an equal chance of coming together in each configuration. Because two complementary stereoisomers are called *racemates*, such a mixture is described as **racemic.** In most drugs the *L*-isomer produces the pharmacologic effect of the drug, and the *D*-isomer is inactive or may cause unwanted side effects. Through advances in technology stereoisomers can be separated, and compounds can be synthesized that contain only the active isomer. The drug levalbuterol was developed with this technology.

Electrochemistry In general, chemical substances have an overall neutral electrical charge. However, the electrical charges in the molecule may not be evenly distributed. Water, for example, carries a significant negative charge around its oxygen atom, and the two hydrogen atoms are relatively positively charged. This gives the molecule a positive "end" and a negative "end," an electrical dipole; such a molecule is described as *polar* (Figure 18-2).

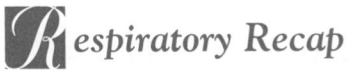

Hydrophilic and Hydrophobic

Hydrophilic: Having an affinity for water; a hydrophilic (polar) substance mixes readily with water because of its electrical polarity.
Hydrophobic: Lacking affinity for water; a hydrophobic (nonpolar) substance does not mix well with water or aqueous solutions because of its minimal electrical polarity.

Because they are highly polar, water molecules tend to aggregate strongly, the positively and negatively charged ends of adjacent molecules attracting one another. This phenomenon is responsible for water's high surface tension. Other polar molecules tend to be attracted to and mix well with water molecules; such substances are **hydrophilic,** meaning they have a strong affinity for water.

Hydrocarbons, such as oils and fats, have very little polarity because they distribute their electrical charges fairly evenly. Nonpolar compounds do not mix well with water or aqueous solutions; therefore these compounds are **hy-**

drophobic, or lacking affinity for water. However, they are **lipophilic** because they have a high affinity for fatty tissues in the body.

Another important electrochemical process is called *ionization.* Some chemical structures may acquire a positive or negative charge in certain environments. A charged molecule is called an *ion;* therefore the molecule is ionized. The overall electrical neutrality of the solution is preserved because the electrical charge is transferred from nearby molecules, which then carry the opposite charge. However, the ionized molecule becomes highly hydrophilic and is unable to cross lipid membranes unless it passes through a channel or is actively transported across. Because many drugs are weak acids or bases, the appropriate environment causes them to become ionized[1]; this prevents them from moving across the lipid cell membranes.

Pharmacokinetics

Pharmacokinetics, which literally means "drug movement," describes the way the body moves a drug through the processes of absorption, distribution, and clearance (elimination).

Absorption and Availability In most cases absorption of a drug must be ensured so that it becomes available for use by the body. For inhaled medications, however, as with intravenous drugs, absorption usually causes little concern; the mucosa provides an excellent surface for absorption of many drugs, and inhaled medications are delivered directly to the respiratory mucosa, where absorption occurs rapidly over its large surface area (approximately $100\ m^2$). Inhaled drugs are almost immediately present in the lung tissue in relatively high concentrations.

Delivery of medications to the lower airways, however, has its own problems. A substantial portion of the drug may be lost as it enters the mouth or settles in the proximal airways. Consequently, only a fraction of the medication becomes available to the lungs despite near-100% absorption. The belief is that only particles smaller than $3\ \mu m$ in diameter are carried to the distal airways. Much of the drug lost to proximal deposition eventually is absorbed systemically. In the case of albuterol, this is approximately 20% of the administered dose.[2] Therefore the availability of inhaled medications to the intended site of action tends to be somewhat low and variable despite excellent absorp-

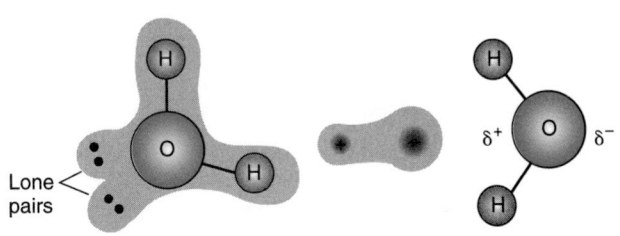

Figure 18-2 Water molecule, illustrating electrical dipole.

tion. Intravenous, intramuscular, and subcutaneous administration usually yield 100% absorption, whereas oral absorption may vary considerably for several reasons.

The rapidity of drug absorption and distribution to the target tissues also should be considered. For inhaled medications, this can be a matter of a few seconds. Intravenous medications reach their target tissues within about 1 minute. Oral medications may have quite a variable absorption rate and may even be designed to release over several hours.

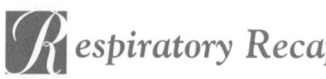espiratory Recap

---

Absorption of Inhaled Aerosols

Medications are rapidly absorbed at the respiratory mucosa, yielding high local concentrations.
Delivery to the lower airway is somewhat inefficient and variable.

Distribution Once absorbed, drugs are distributed throughout the body. However, this distribution is not uniform. In consideration of a drug's utilization in the body, it often is necessary to think of the body as a number of compartments in which the drug may exist at different concentrations and may enter and leave at different rates.

The body generally can be divided into four compartments, each accounting for a portion of the total body water (TBW), which itself makes up 50% to 60% of the body's weight. The intravascular water (plasma) makes up approximately 4% of TBW. Fluid in cells (the intracellular compartment) accounts for approximately 60% of TBW. The large amount of water surrounding the cells in body tissues (the extracellular compartment) accounts for approximately 40% of TBW. About half the extracellular compartment, approximately 20% of TBW, is located in fatty tissues and is considered separately as the lipid compartment.

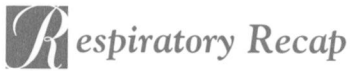espiratory Recap

---

Distribution of Body Water

Intracellular compartment (intracellular fluid): approximately 60% of total body water (TBW)
Extracellular compartment (extracellular fluid): approximately 40% TBW
Lipid compartment: accounts for half of extracellular compartment, or 20% TBW
Intravascular compartment (plasma; considered subset of extracellular compartment): 4%

Depending on its hydrophilic versus lipophilic characteristics, a drug may be taken up in the lipid compartment to varying degrees. Even in the aqueous spaces of the body,

drugs may not distribute evenly (Figure 18-3). Drugs can move across membranes between serum and extracellular and intracellular water compartments only when the drug molecules are both electrically uncharged and unbound to proteins. For example, in a relatively alkaline environment, aspirin, which is acidic, sheds its hydrogen ion (H^+), leaving a negatively charged group. Aspirin therefore becomes trapped in the alkaline space, unable to cross over lipid membranes because of its increased polarity. Uncharged aspirin from other compartments continues to cross into the alkaline space, so that the concentration in that space becomes higher than in the surrounding environment. Another example, heparin, tends to be highly bound to proteins in the serum, which keeps a disproportionate amount of the drug in the intravascular fluid space. The body also has particular spaces, notably the cerebrospinal fluid (CSF), that drugs may not effectively penetrate. Aminoglycosides are ineffective in the treatment of meningitis, for example, because they cannot cross the blood-brain barrier into the CSF. Fortunately, the respiratory system has no such spaces.

Volume of Distribution Because drug levels are measured in the plasma and both renal and hepatic elimination depend on the plasma concentration, a convenient way to

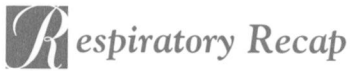espiratory Recap

---

Volume of Distribution

The volume of distribution (V_d) is the theoretical volume that a drug would occupy if it were distributed evenly at its serum concentration.
V_d is determined by the amount of drug in the body and the plasma concentration of the drug.

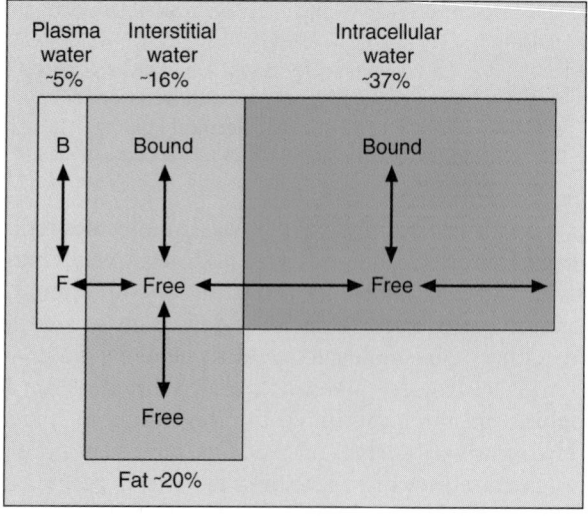

Figure 18-3 Schematic of pharmacokinetic body compartments.

describe drug distribution is to calculate the volume the drug would occupy at a uniform concentration equal to its plasma concentration; this is called the **volume of distribution (V_d)** (Equation 18-1).

Occasionally the volume of distribution is a physically real entity, but often it does not have a physical meaning. Regardless, the concept of V_d is very useful. For example, if a drug's V_d is known, the plasma concentration can be measured and the amount of drug in the body calculated. V_d also predicts the drug's elimination. Both the liver and kidneys clear drug from the plasma, which flows through

these organs in the bloodstream. Drug present outside the plasma space has no direct influence on the rate of **clearance,** but as drug is cleared from the plasma, it is replenished by drug from these other compartments, helping to maintain a consistent distribution. Elimination occurs as if the liver and kidneys were clearing a huge reservoir of plasma with a volume equal to V_d.

Clearance   Drugs may be cleared from the body by biotransformation or elimination or a combination of the two. *Biotransformation* refers to the modification of a drug's chemical structure, generally by enzymatic reactions. A large number of biotransformations are performed in the liver, many of them by a specific enzyme complex called *P-450.* This is important because drugs metabolized by the P-450 system may enhance or diminish the enzyme's activity. Therefore two such drugs may significantly alter each other's rate of clearance. Drugs that have undergone biotransformation are called *metabolites.* Some metabolites are inactive, but many retain the original drug effect and are called *active metabolites.* Other metabolites may have different effects altogether, including toxic effects.

Both metabolites and unaltered drugs can be cleared by elimination, which can be done by the kidneys, which excrete the drug in the urine, or by the liver, which excretes substances in bile to be eliminated in the stool. The most common respiratory medicine, albuterol, is cleared by the kidneys as unaltered drug.[2] The hepatic (liver) elimination rate varies with liver disease but is difficult to predict.

*E*QUATION 18-1

Volume of Distribution

$$V_d = \frac{\text{Amount of drug in the body}}{C_p}$$

where V_d is the volume of distribution of the drug in the body and C_p is the plasma concentration.

Example: A 90-kg patient is given 2 g of drug. The important values are as follows:

Patient's weight	90 kg
Total body water	50 L
Extracellular compartment	20 L
(Lipid extracellular fluid, 10 L; nonlipid extracellular fluid, 10 L)	
Plasma volume	2 L
Intracellular compartment	30 L
Total nonlipid body water	40 L

Case 1

The drug stays entirely in the blood. The measured plasma concentration is 1g/L. To find V_d, calculate the volume that the entire 2 g of drug would occupy at the plasma concentration of 1g/L, as follows:

$$\frac{2 \text{ g}}{1 \text{g/L}} = 2 \text{ L}$$

Not surprisingly, this value is the plasma volume. This result is consistent with the drug being physically distributed in the blood.

Case 2

The drug is lipophilic; over time, 90% of it goes into the lipid compartment. The portion of the drug in nonlipid body water is evenly distributed. The lipid concentration is 0.18 g/L, and the plasma concentration is 0.005 g/L. At these concentrations, 1.8 g of the drug is in body fat, as follows:

$$0.18 \text{ g/L} \times 10 \text{ L} = 1.8 \text{ g}$$

The remaining 0.2 g of drug is in nonlipid body water, as follows:

$$0.005 \text{ g/L} \times 40 \text{ L} = 0.2 \text{ g}$$

Thus the V_d is as follows:

$$\frac{2\text{g}}{0.005 \text{ g/L}} = 400 \text{ L}$$

*R*espiratory Recap

Clearance

Hepatic (liver) clearance: Clearance through the liver usually involves biotransformation, often by the P-450 enzyme system. This type of clearance is affected by liver disease and the presence of other drugs metabolized by the P-450 system.
Renal (kidney) clearance: Clearance through the kidneys involves elimination of unchanged drug or its metabolites. This type of clearance usually is proportional to creatinine clearance.

Renal (kidney) elimination generally occurs at a rate proportional to the creatinine clearance (CrCl), which indicates the amount of blood completely cleared of creatinine every minute. Creatinine is used as a marker because for the most part it is passively filtered out of the blood rather than being actively excreted or reabsorbed. Although some drugs are actively excreted into or reabsorbed from the urine, CrCl remains a good approximation of renal elimination. It can be estimated by the following formula:

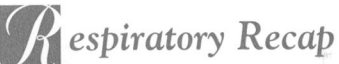

$$\text{CrCl} = \frac{(140 - \text{Age [years]}) \times \text{Weight (kg)} (\times 0.85 \text{ for women})}{72 \times \text{Serum creatinine (mg/dL)}}$$

In most cases the clearance rate increases linearly with the drug plasma concentration; this is called *first-order*, or *linear, kinetics*. However, some drugs have nonlinear clearance rates. This occurs most often when the body's clearance mechanism becomes fully occupied at submaximum drug concentrations. Although the drug level is increased, the rate of clearance cannot increase and becomes constant; this is called *zero-order*, or *saturation, kinetics*. The most important consequence of zero-order kinetics is that drug concentrations may begin to rise rapidly when doses are increased beyond the saturation point. Among the respiratory drugs, this phenomenon is most often seen with theophylline.

Half-Life   The time required for a drug's concentration to be reduced by half is called the drug **half-life** (t½). In first-order kinetics the drug concentration is cut in half after each half-life (that is, ½, ¼, ⅛, 1/16, and so on of the initial concentration). The dosing interval of a drug often is similar to its half-life, but this is not always the case, and care must be taken in the interpretation of the half-life. For example, salmeterol has a half-life of 5½ hours[2] but is administered only every 12 hours, because it can be given in doses sufficient to produce a high initial peak concentration. Thus it remains at effective concentrations even after two half-lives have elapsed. Conversely, the antiepileptic drug phenytoin has a half-life of 22 hours but is given three times a day. Because it is toxic at concentrations just over the therapeutic level (that is, it has a narrow therapeutic window), small, frequent doses are necessary to avoid toxic peak concentrations. For most respiratory medications, however, the dosing interval is on the order of one half-life. The half-life also should be considered when drug therapy is begun. When a drug is started, its concentration increases every time a dose is given (because some drug remains from previous doses) until dose-dependent clearance increases to equal the rate of administration, and the drug reaches a steady-state concentration. This process does not depend on the frequency of dosing; as long as doses are given at regular intervals, an essentially steady state is reached after four half-lives have elapsed.[1]

Pharmacodynamics

A drug's **pharmacodynamics** is its action in the body, both at a molecular level and in overall clinical effect.

Receptor Types   On reaching the target tissue, most drugs produce their effect by binding to **receptors**, either stimulating or blocking them. An agent that stimulates a receptor is called an **agonist**, and an agent that blocks a receptor is called an **antagonist**. Some agents produce ef-

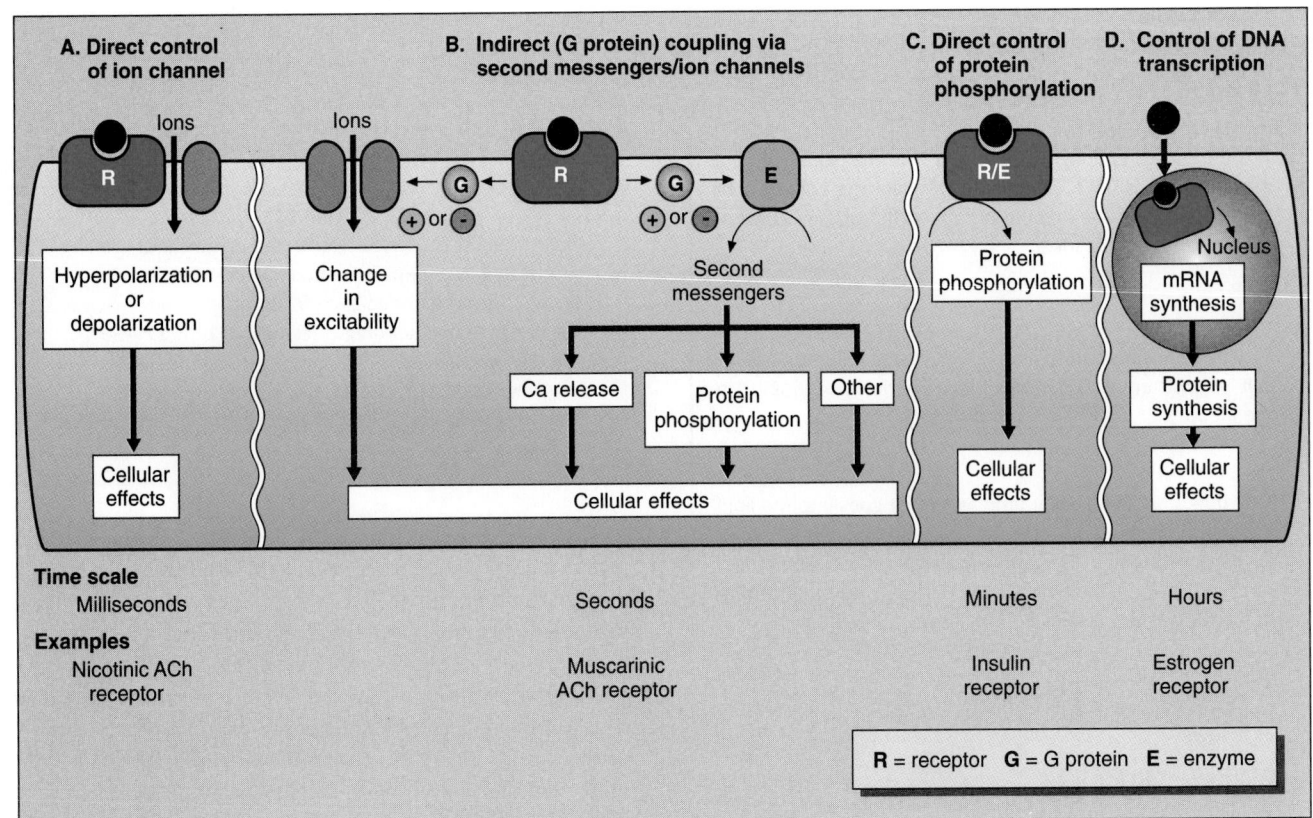

Figure 18-4   Four classes of receptor-effector linkage.

fects that fall in between, weakly stimulating a receptor while preventing it from being more strongly stimulated by other agonists. These intermediate agents are called *partial agonists*.

Most receptors fall into one of four general classes (Figure 18-4). Direct ligand-gated channel receptors are found at the cell membrane, stretching from the extracellular side to the intracellular side of the membrane; they therefore are called *transmembrane receptors*. These receptors act as passageways for specific substances into and out of the cell. A drug that binds to the transmembrane receptors opens or closes these passageways. This affects the movement of substances, often ions such as sodium and potassium, across the cell membrane. Because the drug produces this effect directly at the receptor, the mechanism is very fast.

The tyrosine-kinase–linked receptor, another transmembrane type, also uses a direct mechanism. When bound by drug at the extracellular binding domain, this receptor becomes enzymatically active at its intracellular end, acting as a tyrosine kinase. This means that it adds phosphate groups to (or *phosphorylates*) the amino acid tyrosine in proteins with which it comes into contact. Phosphorylation changes the activity of these proteins, leading to the clinical effect. The receptors for insulin and other nonsteroidal hormones are tyrosine-kinase linked.

G protein–coupled receptors are also transmembrane receptors, but they do not use a direct mechanism; rather, they act through an intermediary, the G protein (Figure 18-5). The G protein normally moves about in the cell membrane bound to a molecule of guanosine diphosphate (GDP). When it contacts a receptor that has been bound by

drug, the G protein is stimulated to exchange its GDP for a guanosine triphosphate (GTP) molecule. Effectively phosphorylated, the G protein makes its way to a separate target protein, such as an enzyme or membrane channel, that is responsible for production of the end-effect of the drug.

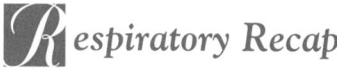

ℛespiratory Recap

> ### *Types of Drug Receptors*
>
> **Ligand-Gated Channel Receptors**
> Provide quickest mechanism by which a drug's effect is achieved
> Regulate movement of ions (such as sodium and potassium) and other molecules across membranes
>
> **Tyrosine-Kinase–Linked Receptors**
> Rapidly initiate drug's actions
> Include insulin and nonsteroidal hormone receptors
>
> **G Protein–Coupled Receptors**
> Are moderately quick at initiating drug action
> Include adrenergic, muscarinic acetylcholine, and opiate receptors
>
> **Steroid Receptors**
> Are slow in initiating drug effect
> Are located inside the cell in the cytoplasm

This indirect mechanism is somewhat slower than direct ligand-gated channel or tyrosine-kinase receptors.

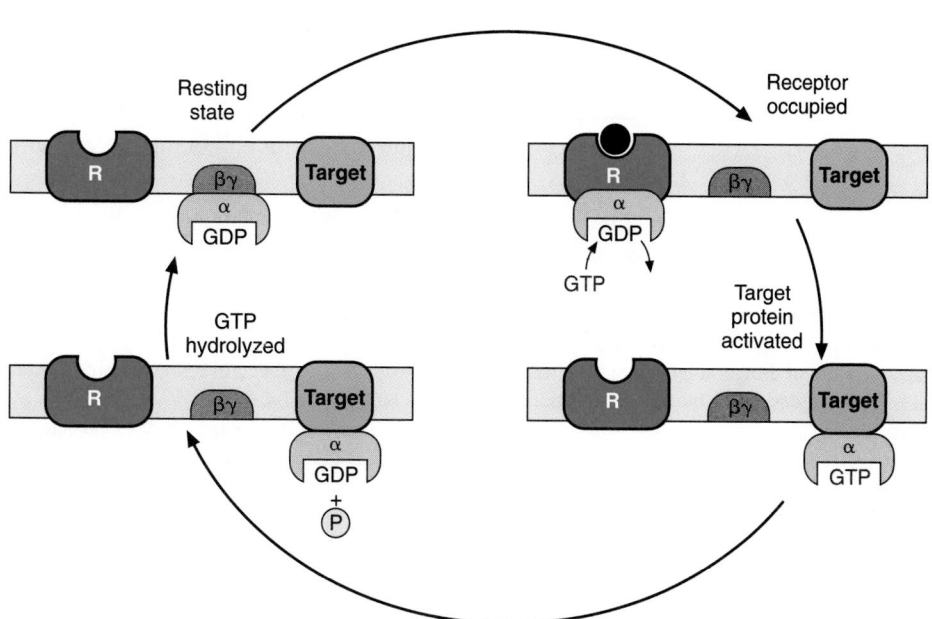

Figure 18-5   Function of the G protein-coupled receptor. Once bound by drug, the receptor causes a G protein to exchange its guanosine diphosphate (GDP) molecule for guanosine triphosphate (GTP). Thus activated, the G protein moves along the cell membrane to a target protein, which it in turn activates. In the process, GTP is cleaved to produce GDP, regenerating the starting elements. *R,* Receptor.

G protein–coupled receptors are a common feature of respiratory physiology; they include adrenergic receptors, muscarinic acetylcholine receptors, and **opiate** receptors.

Steroid receptors are not transmembrane receptors; they are located inside the cell in the cytoplasm. Because steroid molecules are lipophilic, they pass readily through the cell membrane into the cytoplasm, where they can bind their receptor. The steroid-receptor complex translocates into the nucleus, where the receptor acts directly on deoxyribonucleic acid (DNA) to modulate its transcription. In this case the end-effect of the drug does not become manifest until transcription and translation of new proteins have had time to occur, making this the slowest of the four receptor mechanisms.

Receptor Kinetics   Most drugs produce their effects by interacting with a receptor. Although this is described as binding, in almost all cases the drug is in a constant process of binding to and unbinding from its receptor, spending varying amounts of time bound and unbound depending on its affinity for the receptor. This is described in Equation 18-2.[3] For any dissociation constant (K_d), as the drug concentration increases, more receptors are bound by drug. The process of binding may compete with another substance that binds the same receptor. In such cases the agent with the smaller K_d tends to occupy more of the receptors, unless the concentration of the agent with the higher K_d is increased. This becomes important when patients are treated with both agonists and antagonists for the same receptor, such as a patient who is taking β-blockers for hypertension who is treated with the β-agonist albuterol for bronchospasm. In most cases this antagonism is called **competitive inhibition** because increasing the concentra-

tion of one of the agents forces more of that drug onto the receptors, displacing the other agent. In some cases either the agonist or the antagonist does not bind and unbind in equilibrium but rather binds irreversibly to its receptor. In such cases the interaction is called **noncompetitive inhibition** because an increase in the concentration of the other agent does not displace any of the irreversibly bound drug. The interaction of aspirin with cyclooxygenase is one example of irreversible binding. Important to note is that drugs are bound to proteins in varying degrees, and only the portion not protein bound (that is, *free drug*) is available to bind to the receptor.

The effect of a drug is not only proportional to the number of receptors that are bound, but it also depends on the effect of the drug at the receptor. For example, morphine has a purely stimulatory effect on the opiate receptor; it is a pure agonist. Nalbuphine, in contrast, is a partial agonist at the opiate receptor. Because of its molecular structure, it stimulates the receptor but induces less than full activity. Compared with a full agonist, it has a lesser effect even when the same number of receptors are occupied. This effect can be enhanced by binding of more receptors with more drug, but the maximum achievable effect, when all receptors are occupied, is always less than that produced by a pure agonist. Naloxone is a pure antagonist of the opiate receptor; it competitively displaces any agonists.

Potency Versus Efficacy   A distinction can be made between two often-confused concepts, potency and efficacy. **Potency** refers to the amount of drug necessary to achieve a given level of effect. A more potent drug produces the same effect at a lower concentration than a drug of lower potency. There may be several reasons for this. The more potent drug may be more efficiently distributed to the target tissue; it may be less protein bound; it may have a lower K_d; or it may be a more pure agonist. Alternatively, the drugs may produce their action through entirely different mechanisms, with different concentration requirements for achieving the end-effect.

ℰQUATION 18-2

Drug Binding to Receptor

$$D + R \underset{k_2}{\overset{k_1}{\rightleftharpoons}} DR$$

where *D* represents free drug, *R* is unbound receptor, *DR* is the drug-receptor complex, and k_1 and k_2 are the rates of the interconversion to and from the complexed state, respectively.[4] At any given time a proportion of the receptors is bound by drug, depending on the concentration of drug and affinity of the drug for the receptor. This affinity is described by the dissociation constant, K_d, as follows:

$$Kd = \frac{k_2}{k_1}$$

so that

$$\text{Fraction of occupied receptors} = \frac{[D]}{K_d + [D]}$$

where *[D]* is the concentration of free drug.

ℛespiratory Recap

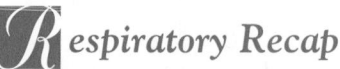

Potency and Efficacy
Potency: The ability of a drug to produce an effect at a given concentration. *Efficacy:* The maximum effect achievable by a drug.

Efficacy refers to the maximum achievable effect a drug is able to produce, regardless of concentration. A common misconception is that a more potent drug is more effective. This is not necessarily the case; for example, the opiate partial agonist buprenorphine can be compared with the opiate agonist morphine. Buprenorphine is much more potent, achieving effective analgesia with doses of 250 μg (compared with 2.5 mg for morphine), but its maximum efficacy is limited, even at the maximum dose, because of its weak agonist effect. Morphine, in contrast, has a high level of efficacy if given in sufficient doses.

Indications and Dosages

An **indication** is the condition for which a drug is given. For example, the indication for a **bronchodilator** may be asthma, chronic obstructive pulmonary disease (COPD), or nonspecific bronchospasm. When pharmaceuticals are approved by the Food and Drug Administration (FDA) in the United States, they are approved for specific indications for which they have demonstrated efficacy. Although drugs can be marketed only for their FDA-approved indications, they legitimately may be prescribed for additional indications, in what is called *off-label use*.

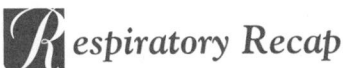 *espiratory Recap*

Indications and Contraindications
Indications: are the therapeutic applications of a drug. The two types of indications are those approved by the U.S. Food and Drug Administration (FDA) and off-label indications, which are indications other than those approved by the FDA. *Contraindications:* are conditions that preclude the use of a drug or that make its use unfavorable. The two types of contraindications are absolute contraindications, which preclude the use of the drug whenever the contraindication is present, and relative contraindications, which make the use of the drug less beneficial or more hazardous.

A **contraindication** is a condition that makes the use of a drug unfavorable, usually because of possible hazards or diminished efficacy. A contraindication may be *relative*, meaning that it makes use of the drug somewhat less favorable, or *absolute*, meaning that the drug should never be used if the contraindication is present. Absolute contraindications are uncommon in pulmonary medicine, because in many cases the possible consequences of not treating respiratory distress outweigh the possible adverse effects of a drug. Especially important contraindications are highlighted in FDA-approved drug labeling as black-box warnings.

For specific indications, dosages are established as part of the FDA approval process. As with indications, the dosages used clinically may vary. Over time new off-label uses with different dosages are established. The dosages used for the original FDA approval process also may be revised with new research and clinical findings.

Certain medications are characterized by a phenomenon called **tolerance,** which means that the dose required to achieve the same effect increases gradually over time. Important examples include the opiates and the loop diuretics.

Tolerance also may develop with intensive, long-term use of short-acting β_2-agonists because of a reduction in the number (*down-regulation*) of β_2-receptors. This phenomenon has not been demonstrated with long-acting β-agonists, other bronchodilators, or antiinflammatory drugs.

Toxicity, Side Effects, and Allergic Reactions

Toxicity and side effects are similar but not identical concepts. Strictly speaking, a **side effect** is any drug effect other than the primary intended therapeutic effect. As such it can be beneficial or harmful, although the term usually is used to denote undesirable effects. Side effects may also represent excessive therapeutic effect, such as hypotension caused by antihypertensive medications or an increased incidence of infection with the use of immunosuppressive drugs. **Toxicity** is a harmful biologic effect produced by a substance, such as liver dysfunction caused by isoniazid, an antituberculous agent. Toxicity therefore may be considered a subgroup of side effects.

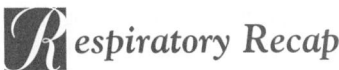 *espiratory Recap*

Toxicity, Side Effects, and Allergy
Toxicity: A harmful biologic effect (damage or disturbance of function) caused by a drug *Side effects:* Undesirable symptoms caused by a drug *Allergy:* An immune-mediated hypersensitivity reaction

Most side effects are dose related; their incidence or severity (or both) increases as the drug dose or duration of use increases. Increasing the dose gradually may reduce the incidence of side effects. The **therapeutic window** is the range of drug concentration that is bounded on the low side by the minimum effective concentration and on the high side by the onset of dose-related side effects. Some side effects, primarily toxic reactions, are idiosyncratic, meaning that they occur without any correlation to drug dose or duration of use.

The presence of side effects and toxicity must be considered whenever a drug is administered. Nearly all medications used in pulmonary medicine have potentially serious adverse effects. In addition, coexisting medical problems, such as cardiac or renal disease, may make a respiratory patient more susceptible to some adverse effects. For these reasons, it is an important responsibility of the respiratory therapist to monitor patients for adverse drug effects.

Allergy is a specific type of adverse drug reaction, defined as an immune-mediated hypersensitivity reaction. The hypersensitivity may be described as one of four types. Intermediate-type (Type I) hypersensitivity is mediated by preformed immunoglobulin E (IgE)-class antibodies to an antigen. Previous exposure to an antigen can stimulate production of specific antibodies. On reexposure, the IgE antibodies recognize the antigen and mount a response within minutes. IgE antibodies may be circulating in the serum but most often are found on the surface of mast cells, where stimulation by a specific allergen triggers activation of the mast cell. Once activated, the mast cell immediately releases granules rich in histamine and proinflammatory cytokines; this process is called *degranulation*. Primarily this histamine causes the manifestations of allergy: pruritus (itching), hives, and edema formation. The runny nose, sneezing, and itchy eyes of seasonal allergies are manifestations of edema and pruritus. More severe Type I hypersensitivity reactions that cause life-threatening systemic effects are called *anaphylactic reactions*. In anaphylaxis, massive histamine release causes small vessels throughout the body to leak, resulting in widespread edema and severe hypotension caused by loss of intravascular fluid. These effects are accompanied by intense pruritus and a severe, hivelike rash. From the respiratory perspective, the most significant complication of anaphylaxis is airway edema, which leads to stridor and possibly to airway obstruction.

Antibody-mediated (Type II) hypersensitivity occurs when non-IgE antibodies are produced that recognized specific antigens—including drugs—present on cell surfaces. These antibodies then activate the immune system, causing destruction of the presenting cell. Unlike IgE, these other antibodies do not stimulate the immediate release of histamine in great quantities. Immune complex-mediated (Type III) hypersensitivity is a common mechanism for drug allergy. In this type, non-IgE antibodies combine with antigen and activate complement (a group of inflammatory proteins), producing an inflammatory response that may remain localized or become systemic. Delayed-type hypersensitivity reactions (Type IV), such as those caused by poison ivy, usually are of less concern to the respiratory therapist.

True allergy often is confused with other unpleasant side effects, and care must be taken to establish an accurate allergy list. For example, many patients develop tachycardia when given β-agonists or agitation and insomnia when taking prednisone, and these conditions are reported as allergies. This sometimes complicates therapy when these agents are indicated.

Treatment of allergy is based on **antihistamine** therapy for the immediate effects, and antiinflammatory therapy (usually corticosteroids) for the subsequent inflammatory state. Anaphylaxis often is treated with epinephrine, which blocks the initial histamine release and to some extent vasoconstricts the peripheral vascular beds, limiting edema formation.

Pharmacology of the Respiratory System

To understand the numerous therapeutic effects that respiratory drugs have, the respiratory therapist must understand the mediators that produce physiologic changes in the lungs and the pathways by which these mediators are regulated.

Figure 18-6 shows a diagram of a medium-sized airway. The airway is lined by a pseudostratified columnar epithelium composed primarily of ciliated epithelial cells but also containing mucus-producing goblet cells. Below this lies the smooth muscle layer, which encircles the airway. Two major types of inflammatory cells, macrophages and mast cells, are present in the airways. Macrophages are more prominent in the distal airways and alveoli, where they ingest foreign material and infectious organisms. Mast cells predominate in the proximal airways, where they can be activated by a wide variety of stimuli to release histamine and other cytokines. Both macrophages and mast cells recruit other inflammatory cells, such as neutrophils and lymphocytes, from the bloodstream passing through the lungs. Numerous types of receptors are scattered throughout the epithelium and smooth muscle of the lungs (Figure 18-7); most of these are stimulated by humoral mediators that travel in the bloodstream. The cholinergic receptors, however, are stimulated by nerve fibers.

Mediators of Inflammation

Inflammation is a complex process. Acute inflammation in the airways can be divided into an early phase and a late

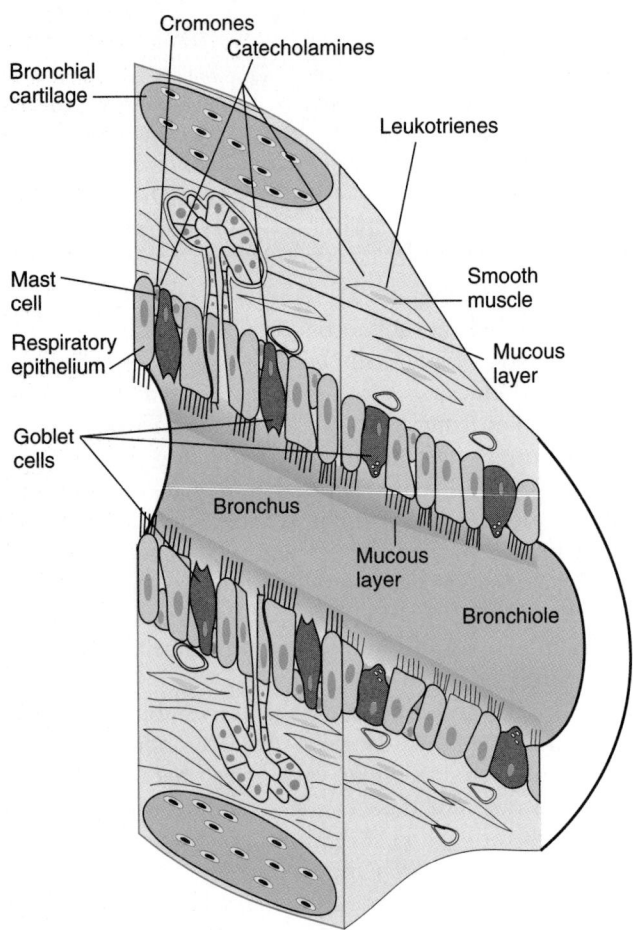

Figure 18-6   Diagram of an airway showing sites of action of different classes of drugs.

phase. The first step in the induction of inflammation is the appearance of an *antigen*, a foreign substance in the lung that stimulates an immune response. This antigen may be an allergen, such as pollen, or a component of invading infectious organisms.

As antigen enters the lung, it may encounter specific preformed IgE antibodies bound to mast cell membranes. By binding these antibodies, the antigen activates the mast cell, causing it degranulate. Mast cells may also be activated by many nonallergenic stimuli, such as cooling, drying, and mechanical trauma. Mast cell granules contain *histamine*, a powerful vasoactive molecule that causes many of the early manifestations of acute inflammation. Activated mast cells also produce proinflammatory chemicals called *cytokines*. A cytokine is a substance used by one cell to signal nearby cells. When cytokines are released into the environment, they attract and activate a number of other inflammatory cells, drawing them from the circulation into the inflamed area. In this way the inflammatory process intensifies.

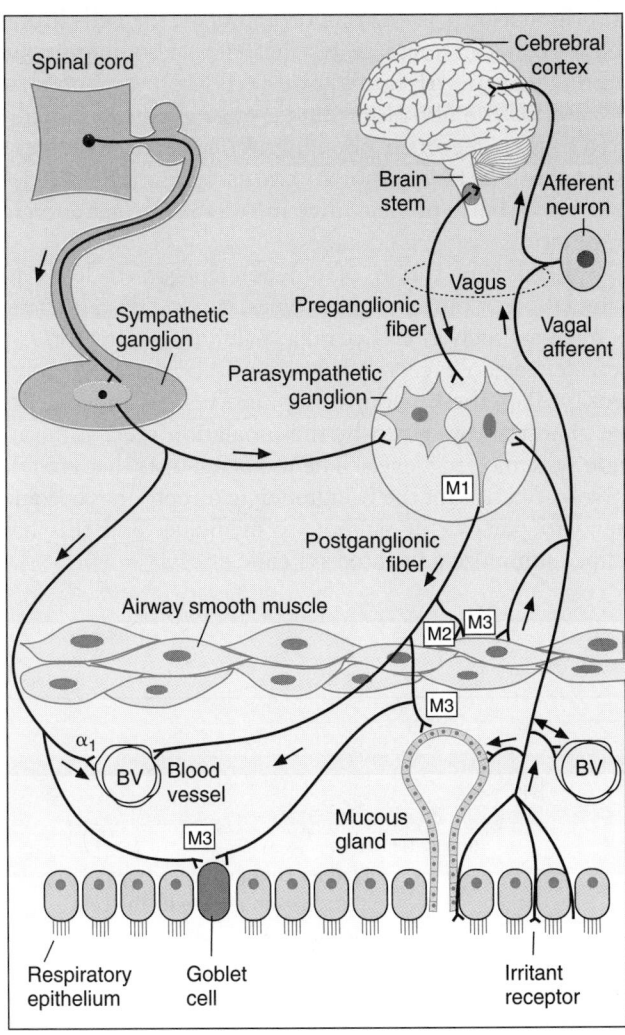

Figure 18-7   Innervation and receptor sites in the lung. *BV,* Blood vessel.

In addition to mast cells, antigen also encounters macrophages, which ingest the antigen and express pieces of it on their own surfaces. By presenting this antigen to T lymphocytes, macrophages activate the lymphocytes. Macrophages and T cells then begin to produce a number of proinflammatory cytokines, including tumor necrosis factor (TNF), interleukins, γ-interferon (γ-IFN), RANTES (which stands for *r*egulated on *a*ctivation, *n*ormal **T**-cell *e*xpressed and *s*ecreted), and three classes of molecules derived from arachidonic acid: prostaglandins, thromboxane, and **leukotrienes.**

An example of early acute inflammation is the acute asthma attack. In response to a variety of initial stimuli, including exposure to an allergen, exercise, or cold air, the airway mast cells degranulate, disgorging histamine (and other mediators), which causes bronchospasm, edema, and an increase in secretions and in mucous plugging.

All the events discussed thus far constitute the early phase of inflammation. The late phase begins as new inflammatory cells begin to arrive in the area in response to chemoattractant cytokines *(chemokines).* In asthma this occurs 12 to 24 hours after the initial attack, when symptoms can spontaneously recrudesce. The appearance of newly recruited neutrophils and their activation by cytokines in the local environment fuel the fire. After several days neutrophils begin to be outnumbered by a third inflammatory cell, the lymphocyte, which arrives on the scene. At this point, inflammation takes on a chronic appearance.

Mediators of Bronchial Smooth Muscle Tone

The smooth muscle encircling the airways is the most important determinant of airway caliber and resistance. Smooth muscle tone is regulated by the following four main types of mediators:

Adrenergic system: β$_2$-Adrenergic receptors cause smooth muscle relaxation and bronchodilation. Endogenous catecholamines produce a low level of constant stimulation, but administration of exogenous agonists produces additional bronchodilation. Conversely, β-blockers (β-receptor antagonists) are known to cause bronchospasm in susceptible patients.

Cholinergic system: Vagal nerve stimulation of M$_3$ muscarinic cholinergic receptors causes smooth muscle contraction and bronchoconstriction.

Leukotrienes: Previously known collectively as the slow-reacting substance of anaphylaxis (SRS-A), the leukotrienes LTC$_4$, LTD$_4$ and LTE$_4$ act on smooth muscle cells through their own receptor to cause tonic bronchoconstriction.

Histamine: Histamine has powerful effects on both bronchial and vascular smooth muscle, causing contraction. Unfortunately, antihistamines appear to have only mild bronchodilatory action.[4]

Mediators of Bronchial Secretions

The following four types of mediators are the primary regulators of bronchial secretions:

Adrenergic system: Although adrenergic stimulation does not directly affect secretions, it does enhance mucociliary clearance in the bronchi and fluid clearance from the alveoli and therefore may have some mitigating effect on secretions. As of now this component has not been used as a specific target of therapy.

Cholinergic system: Vagal efferents leading to the bronchial goblet cells enhance the production of mucus by means of M_3 receptors. **Anticholinergic** agents decrease both bronchial and upper airway secretions. However, the use of anticholinergics to diminish secretions is controversial because of their tendency to produce less but thicker mucus.

Histamine: Histamine increases secretions in the upper and lower airways by direct stimulation and by increasing vascular permeability, which causes airway edema.

Inflammation: Inflammation is the most common stimulus of bronchial secretions. It likely acts through direct mechanisms on the airway epithelium and by a neural feedback pathway through the vagus nerve, leading to cholinergic stimulation as described previously.

Receptor Physiology

Adrenergic Receptors   The adrenergic system mediates the "fight or flight" response. These receptors are so-named because they are sensitive to the catecholamines epinephrine (adrenaline), norepinephrine, and dopamine, which are produced by the adrenal gland. In addition to these endogenous catecholamines, many synthetic adrenergic agents have been developed. Two types of adrenergic receptors, **α-adrenergic** receptors and **β-adrenergic** receptors, were discovered in the 1950s, and their subclassifications were delineated in the late 1960s. The principal effects of each receptor subtype are listed in Table 18-1.[5]

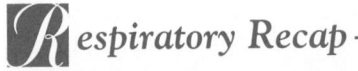

Respiratory Recap

Receptor Classes of the Respiratory System	
Adrenergic receptors	Corticosteroidal receptors
Cholinergic receptors	Leukotrienes
Histaminergic receptors	

Adrenergic receptors are G protein linked to a target enzyme called *adenylate cyclase*. This enzyme produces cyclic adenosine monophosphate (cAMP), a powerful intracellular signaling molecule that is responsible for the various effects of adrenergic stimulation. In the lungs the primary adrenergic receptor is the β_2-adrenergic receptor, which causes bronchodilation through relaxation of bronchial smooth muscle. Mast cells also have adrenergic receptors on their surfaces, which prevent them from degranulating in response to environmental stimuli. The respiratory epithelium demonstrates improved mucociliary clearance in response to adrenergic stimulation. Adrenergic receptors on the cells lining the alveoli can increase the activity of sodium-potassium adenosine triphosphatase (ATPase), a pump that helps clear the alveoli of fluid. Fewer effects are attributed to β_1-receptors in the lungs; however, this receptor is responsible for pulmonary vasoconstriction and decreased vascular permeability in response to adrenergic stimulation.

Systemic absorption of adrenergic agonists leads to stimulation of other receptor types, causing dose-limiting side effects such as tachycardia, palpitations, tremor, hyperkalemia (an excess of potassium), and possibly hypertension. For these reasons, respiratory adrenergic agents are almost always given by the inhalation route to minimize systemic drug levels. The use of agonists that are relatively selective for the β_2-adrenergic receptor has become standard practice in pulmonary medicine, and this has helped minimize unwanted systemic effects.

Table 18-1

Effects Mediated by Adrenergic Receptors

Receptor Type	Lungs	Heart and Vascular Tissues	Other
α_1	Bronchoconstriction	Vasoconstriction	Bladder contraction, glycogenolysis, potassium release by the cells
α_2	—	Vasoconstriction	Platelet aggregation
β_1	—	Increased pumping force (positive inotropism) and increased heart rate (positive chronotropism)	—
β_2	Bronchodilation, increased edema clearance	Vasodilation	Sphincter relaxation, glycogenolysis, tremor

Cholinergic Receptors Cholinergic receptors are sensitive to acetylcholine and to many exogenous cholinergic agonists. Two of these exogenous agonists, nicotine and muscarine, allowed the distinction of two types of cholinergic receptors, **nicotinic** receptors and **muscarinic** receptors. The muscarinic receptor has been subtyped into M_1, M_2, and M_3 receptors, which are all G protein linked. In the lungs M_3 receptors cause an increase in secretions and bronchoconstriction.[5] These are undesirable effects, and the use of cholinergic agonists in respiratory care is limited to nebulized methacholine, which is given to provoke bronchospasm for asthma testing. Cholinergic antagonists, or anticholinergic agents, however, are used extensively as bronchodilators and to reduce secretions.

Cholinergic receptors are unique in the lungs in that they are primarily stimulated by cholinergic nerves of the parasympathetic nervous system (with acetylcholine as the neurotransmitter) rather than by local mediators. The lungs are innervated by the vagus nerve, which carries efferent fibers (outgoing from the brain) to the smooth muscle of the airways, where this nerve causes bronchoconstriction, and to the goblet cells, which are stimulated to increase the production of mucus. The vagus nerve also carries afferent (incoming to the brain) sensory input, which may modulate the efferent activity returning to the lungs. These afferent inputs include irritant receptors in the esophagus. In this way gastroesophageal acid reflux may produce a cough reflex and bronchospasm even though the acid may not directly contact the airways.

Histaminergic Receptors Currently three subtypes of histaminergic receptor have been recognized: H_1, H_2, and H_3. The H_1 receptor is the principal receptor found in the respiratory tract; the H_2 receptor is important primarily for its effects on gastric acid secretion. The H_3 receptor, which is also found in the airway, reduces bronchoconstriction by inhibiting cholinergic and noncholinergic nerves excitatory to smooth muscle. The H_1 receptors produce their effect by increasing intracellular levels of cyclic guanosine monophosphate (cGMP), whereas H_2 receptors cause an increase in cAMP and a decrease in cGMP.

H_1 receptors are found on a number of tissues in the respiratory tract. In the mucosa of both the upper and lower airways, they stimulate the formation of secretions and cause edema by increasing vascular permeability. In the smooth muscle layer they stimulate contraction. Stimulation of H_2 receptors produces some bronchodilation, which is consistent with their reduction of cGMP, but this is not currently thought to be clinically important.

Corticosteroid Receptors In general, **corticosteroids** produce two types of effect, the glucocorticoid effect and the mineralocorticoid effect. The glucocorticoid effect is multifaceted; it reduces inflammation, increases the blood glucose level, and generally induces a catabolic state. The mineralocorticoid effect, which is active primarily at the kidneys, promotes sodium conservation. In terms of respi-

ratory medicine, steroids are used for their antiinflammatory glucocorticoid effect. Corticosteroid receptors are found throughout the lungs, but the highest concentrations are in the airway epithelial cells and bronchial vascular endothelial cells.[6]

Activation of corticosteroid receptors inhibits the production of several inflammatory mediators, including cytokines, adhesion molecules, inducible nitric oxide synthase, inducible cyclooxygenase, endothelin-1, and Neurokinin-1 (NK1)-receptors. Corticosteroids also increase the synthesis of certain antiinflammatory mediators, such as lipocortin-1, secretory leukocyte inhibitory protein, $I\kappa B$-α, interleukin-1 (IL-1), and neutral endopeptidase. Through these mechanisms corticosteroids reduce the concentrations of inflammatory mediators in the environment, thereby inhibiting the recruitment of more circulating inflammatory cells and allowing the existing inflammatory response to disperse. Important to note is that corticosteroids treat and possibly prevent the development of the later phase of inflammation, which follows the activation of mast cells and neutrophils; they have much less effect on these early phase events.

Although steroids classically act by affecting protein production at a transcriptional level, some conflicting evidence indicates that they may have more immediate effects.[7,8] They appear to exert direct antiinflammatory effects on many cells and tissues that play a role in the inflammatory process, including macrophages, eosinophils, T lymphocytes, mast cells, dendritic cells, neutrophils, endothelium, airway smooth muscle, and mucosal glands.[9] Glucocorticoids may play a role in the inhibition of microvascular leakage induced by inflammatory mediators. This theory is supported by the finding that bronchoalveolar lavage (BAL) fluid from stable asthma patients treated with inhaled corticosteroids has a lower plasma protein content. Glucocorticoids also increase the transcription of β_2-adrenergic receptors in airway smooth muscle. Theoretically this may offset the down-regulation of these receptors that occurs with prolonged β_2-agonist therapy, although in clinical settings tolerance is still observed.[10] Steroids also reduce the secretion of mucus in the airways.

Routes of Delivery

Inhalation

Most respiratory medications are delivered by the inhalation route. The advantages of this route are the rapidity of onset and the high concentrations of drug that can be achieved by direct application with far fewer systemic side effects. The primary disadvantage is the variability in the amount of drug delivered. This variability arises from several sources. For example, some patients, particularly the elderly, may have considerable difficulty actuating an inhaler and coordinating this with inhalation. A variable amount of drug is thus lost between the inhaler and the mouth. More drug is lost when large aerosol droplets are deposited on the mouth, posterior pharynx, and central airways. Only particles less than 5 μm in diameter reach the lower respiratory tract.

Intratracheal Instillation

A few medications, such as the surfactant replacers, are poured directly into the lungs via the trachea as liquids.

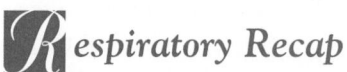

espiratory Recap

Routes of Drug Delivery	
Inhalation route	Intravenous route
Intratracheal instillation	Intramuscular route
Oral route	Subcutaneous route

Box 18-1

Drugs Commonly Used in Respiratory Therapy

Bronchodilators
Adrenergic agonists
  Nonselective
  Epinephrine
  Ephedrine
  Isoproterenol
  Short-acting β-selective
  Albuterol
  Bitolterol
  Metaproterenol
  Pirbuterol
  Terbutaline
  Long-acting β-selective
  Salmeterol
Anticholinergic agonists
  Ipratropium
Methylxanthines
  Theophylline
  Dyphylline
  Aminophylline

Antiinflammatory Drugs
Corticosteroids
  Systemic
  Prednisone
  Prednisolone
  Methylprednisolone
  Cortisone
  Hydrocortisone
  Dexamethasone
  Inhaled
  Budesonide
  Fluticasone
  Triamcinolone
  Beclomethasone
  Flunisolide
Nonsteroidal antiinflammatory drugs
Cromones
  Cromolyn sodium
  Nedocromil sodium
Leukotriene receptor blockers
  Zileuton
Leukotriene inhibitors
  Montelukast
  Zafirlukast

Surfactant Replacers
  Colfosceril palmitate
  Beractant

Secretion Modifiers
  Acetylcysteine
  Antihistamines
  Atropine
  Glycopyrrolate
  Dornase alfa

Inhaled Antimicrobials
  Tobramycin
  Ribavirin
  Pentamidine
  Colistimethate
  Amphotericin B

Coagulants and Anticoagulants
  Heparin
  Low-molecular-weight heparins
  Warfarin
  Thrombin

Opiates
  Codeine
  Morphine
  Fentanyl

Sedatives
  Benzodiazepines
  Propofol
  Phenothiazines

Vasoactive Agents
  Epoprostenol (prostacyclin)
  Nitric oxide
  Epinephrine
  Norepinephrine
  Phenylephrine
  Dobutamine
  Dopamine

Other Drugs
  Lidocaine
  Heliox

This generally is done through an endotracheal tube, and the onset of effect is rapid. Obviously, the primary disadvantage of this route is discomfort, although this is rarely a problem in practice because these medications are given to sedated, intubated patients. A secondary problem is the possibility of transiently worsening gas exchange in the lungs because of the presence of liquid in the air spaces.

Oral Route

The **oral (PO)** route is also called the **enteral** route, because it passes into the gastrointestinal system. Oral respiratory medications include prednisone and other corticosteroids, theophylline, leukotriene inhibitors, opiates, and warfarin. The advantages of the oral route are convenience and the fact that pills can be easily stored and dispensed. Because of these factors, patients generally prefer pills to inhaled medications. The disadvantages of the oral (enteral) route are the long absorption time (typically exceeding 20 minutes) and variable absorption. Many drugs are incompletely absorbed from the digestive tract; some are partly inactivated by the liver as they pass through it on the way from the digestive tract to the rest of the body (*first-pass metabolism*). Also, absorption from the digestive tract may be affected by poor digestive motility, edema of the intestine, and poor blood flow to the digestive tract. For these reasons, **antimicrobials** and other medications often are given intravenously to hospitalized patients.

Intravenous and Intramuscular Routes

Currently three **intravenous (IV)** drugs are commonly given for respiratory disease: aminophylline, methylprednisolone and other corticosteroids, and heparin. The advantages of the IV route are rapid drug delivery (within 1 minute) and essentially 100% absorption of the drug. This makes administration very predictable. Also, this route bypasses the digestive system, which otherwise would degrade drugs such as heparin.

Intramuscular (IM) administration is the injection of a bolus of drug into a muscle bed, where it is taken up into the bloodstream by the local capillary bed. It is similar to intravenous administration except that absorption generally is slower. Some IM drugs are formulated for slow release, and the muscle bed provides a convenient location to deposit these drugs.

Subcutaneous Route

Subcutaneous (SC or SQ) administration involves injection of a drug into the dermal or subdermal layer of skin, where it is taken up by the capillary bed. This is similar in most respects to intramuscular administration except that it is suitable only for very small volume drugs, such as epinephrine. Absorption generally occurs within a few minutes, nearly as quickly as with IV administration, but it can be unpredictable in patients with poor blood flow to the skin, such as patients in shock. The intravenous, intramuscular, and subcutaneous routes are the **parenteral** routes, because they bypass the gastrointestinal system.

Respiratory Drugs

Box 18-1 lists the drugs with which the respiratory therapist should be familiar, and Box 18-2 presents commonly used dosing abbreviations.

Bronchodilators

β-*Adrenergic Agonists* Adrenergic agonists (Figure 18-8) generally are the most effective class of medication for acute bronchodilation and are the most widely prescribed class of bronchodilator.[11] The archetype adrenergic agonist, epinephrine, was isolated and administered as a bronchodilator at start of the twentieth century. Unfortunately, many undesirable systemic effects, such as an increase in the heart rate and blood pressure, were observed in patients receiving it. These effects later were found to be due to stimulation of β_1-adrenergic and α-adrenergic receptors. The development of adrenergic agonists that were relatively selective for β_2-receptors greatly enhanced the clinical utility of these drugs. Although administration of exogenous epinephrine for respiratory disease was plagued by too many systemic side effects, its synthetic racemic mixture has found use in certain disorders. For example, inhaled racemic epinephrine is used for its vasoconstrictor properties in the treatment of stridor associated with laryngeal edema and croup.

The ability of another adrenergic drug, ephedrine, to produce sustained bronchodilation was questioned by several studies, but it was widely used (combined with theophylline) to treat asthma until the 1970s, when other β-agonists became available. An additional problem with ephedrine was its long-lasting stimulant effect, which often was countered by administration of barbiturates. Ephedrine was found in several over-the-counter (OTC) preparations and was commonly sold at truck stops as a central nervous system stimulant. In the 1980s all forms were removed from OTC sale because of the growing

---

Box 18-2

Dosing Abbreviations

Route	Frequency
PO: By mouth	q2h: Every 2 hours
PR: Rectally	q4d: Every 4 days
IV: Intravenously	qd: Daily
IV gtt: Intravenous drip (infusion)	qh: Hourly
	qod: Every other day
IM: Intramuscularly	bid: Twice daily
SC: Subcutaneously	tid: Three times daily
SL: Sublingual	qid: Four times daily
	prn: As needed

Epinephrine

Isoproterenol

Isoetharine

Colterol

Metaproterenol

Terbutaline

Albuterol
(R,S-isomer)

Pirbuterol

Levalbuterol
(R-isomer)

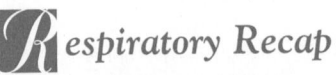

Salmeterol

Figure 18-8   Structures of adrenergic bronchodilators.

abuse of the drug for its long-lasting effect and as a starting agent in the synthesis of amphetamine. Ephedrine is now available by prescription as a component of several combination bronchodilators, including Quadrinal, Bron-

$\mathcal{R}$*espiratory Recap*

Classes of Bronchodilators
Adrenergic agonists   Anticholinergic agents
Systemic or inhaled   (cholinergic antagonists)
β₂-Selective or nonselective   Methylxanthines
Short acting or long acting

cholate, Kie, Mudrane, Marax, and Rynatuss. These are intended primarily for pediatric patients.

Isoproterenol was developed in the 1940s and was the most specific adrenergic agonist at the time because it had only β-receptor activity. Isoproterenol activates both β₁- and β₂-receptors, causing relaxation not only of tracheal and bronchial smooth muscle but also of vascular smooth muscle, resulting in a decrease in peripheral vascular resistance and blood pressure (especially diastolic). In addition, activation of β₁-receptors results in an increase in the heart rate (positive chronotropism) and contractility (positive inotropism), increasing the work of the heart and the need for oxygen. Beta₁ effects are primarily observed when isoproterenol is given intravenously, but they may occur with administration by inhalation. Tolerance to the drug's bronchodilatory effects may develop with continued use. Isoproterenol now is rarely used to treat respiratory disorders, because drugs with more specific β₂-agonist activity are available.

Selective β₂-Agonists   Modifications in the basic catecholamine structure produced agents with adrenergic activity relatively specific to β₂-receptors. This greatly reduced many of the cardiac effects seen with β₁-receptor stimulation. The modifications also changed the metabolism of the agents, resulting in longer-acting compounds. The first agents synthesized were longer acting than the natural catecholamines such as epinephrine, because they were less susceptible to breakdown by the monoamine oxidases found throughout the body. More recently, even longer acting compounds have been derived; therefore the first synthetic agents now are called *short-acting β₂-agonists*.

Short-Acting β₂-Agonists   The short-acting β₂-agonists are used therapeutically on an as-needed basis to relieve the symptoms of bronchospasm, usually in asthma and COPD. They also are used before exercise to prevent exercise-induced asthma. Some controversy exists regarding the safety of the use of short-acting β-agonists for asthma. This controversy has arisen because coincident with the increasing use of these agents has been an increase in asthma mortality worldwide. Two theories have been advanced linking the two factors. The first theory proposes that some patients and physicians use β-agonists as first-line therapy even for moderate to severe asthma, in place of antiinflammatory therapy. Although these drugs provide quick bronchodilation, this simply masks the symptoms while airway inflammation worsens. If β-agonist use is increased to compensate for asthma exacerbations, the exacerbations may be tolerated longer, and the patient may not seek care until the process is far advanced and refractory to therapy. According to the second theory, short-acting β-agonists may have proinflammatory effects in asthma that worsen the underlying pathophysiologic condition while initially controlling symptoms effectively. This has not yet been shown to be clinically significant, and short-acting β-agonists continue to be important agents for the relief of the symptoms of asthma but for not control of the disease itself.

Because the β_2 selectivity of these agents is only relative, they can still produce significant side effects from α-adrenergic and β_1-adrenergic stimulation; in fact, patients commonly notice some palpitations when taking higher doses of these drugs. For the same reason, these drugs usually are administered to adults via the inhalation route to minimize systemic drug levels.

Metaproterenol was one of the compounds created by structural changes to enhance β selectivity. It produces fewer side effects than isoproterenol because of its greater specificity for β_2-receptors, but similar side effects may still occur and are dose related. Terbutaline is structurally related to metaproterenol, but its activity is more specific to β_2-receptors. The availability of a parenteral formulation made it the drug of choice in emergency departments and in the treatment of acute bronchospasm and status asthmaticus. Currently it is less likely to be used in this manner, because inhaled β-agonist therapy has been shown to provide equivalent respiratory benefit with fewer systemic effects. The occurrence of paradoxic bronchospasm has been described but is rare. The adrenergic effects of terbutaline are not specific to the respiratory system; the drug is also used to treat premature labor by relaxing uterine smooth muscle. This is probably the most common use of terbutaline today.

Albuterol has been the mainstay of β-agonist therapy for many years and is the most commonly prescribed pulmonary medication for adults. It produces equivalent bronchodilation but has fewer side effects than the agents discussed thus far. Because it has a rapid onset, it is primarily used for symptomatic relief of bronchospasm. Inhaled doses may be scheduled or used for symptomatic relief as needed. The maximum amount recommended is 12 inhalations a day, separated by 4 hours.

Recently the R-enantiomer of albuterol was isolated and purified for use. This is the same as the levo (*L*)-enantiomer, resulting in the name levalbuterol. Laboratory studies indicate that most of the bronchodilatory effect of albuterol was found in the R-enantiomer, whereas the S-enantiomer had little effect on the airways. Levalbuterol has greater binding affinity than albuterol, which allows a smaller dose of the drug to be given. The doses of levalbuterol used clinically are approximately half those of albuterol, but laboratory studies indicate that a 0.63-mg dose of levalbuterol produces a similar change from baseline in the forced expiratory volume in 1 second (FEV_1) as a 2.5-mg dose of albuterol.

The logic in the use of the single stereoisomer is that with a smaller overall dose, the same effect is achieved with fewer side effects. Therefore fewer adverse effects from albuterol would be expected in patients receiving levalbuterol. However, in clinical trials, similar rates of tachycardia were observed. The incidences of tremor and nervousness were less in patients taking levalbuterol than

in those receiving albuterol. However, the clinical importance of this difference is unknown.

Pirbuterol is similar to albuterol in pharmacokinetics, pharmacodynamics, and use. Bitolterol is similar to albuterol in pharmacodynamics and use but has the advantage of a slightly longer duration of action. However, the popularity of this drug has suffered because of its disagreeable taste.

Long-Acting β_2-Agonists Long-acting β_2-agonists have drawn great interest because of their possible advantages in terms of slower onset of action (and therefore lower peak concentrations that cause milder side effects) and longer duration. A new class of long-acting β_2-agonists was recently developed that has a duration of effect of 12 hours. Currently only one agent from this category, salmeterol, is in clinical use in the United States. Formoterol, another long-acting β_2-agonist, is available in many other countries.

Salmeterol's long duration of action is the result of a long, lipophilic side chain that makes the molecule lipophilic. This allows the drug to embed itself in the lipophilic cell membrane, where it is maintained in proximity to the adrenergic receptors rather, than dispersing in aqueous fluids. Salmeterol's 12-hour duration of action is sufficient to maintain bronchodilation overnight, making it a good agent for the control of nighttime asthma. It is also convenient for maintenance therapy because of its twice-daily dosing schedule. If symptoms occur between doses, the number of puffs of salmeterol can be increased, or a short-acting β_2-agonist can be used as needed. However, salmeterol's onset of action is slower than that of other agents, which makes it a poor choice for controlling acute symptoms of bronchospasm.

Salmeterol generally is preferred to oral sustained-release albuterol, because it is longer acting and has fewer side effects. However, albuterol maintains its role in pediatric asthma, because salmeterol has been approved by the FDA only for patients over 12 years of age. As with all bronchodilators, salmeterol should not be used as a replacement for antiinflammatory therapy in asthma. Use of salmeterol as maintenance therapy of bronchodilator-responsive COPD is increasing.

Anticholinergics Anticholinergic compounds[12] have been inhaled as far back in time as ancient Greece. In addition to being bronchodilators, they are known to decrease respiratory and upper airway secretions. The British learned of their use for the treatment of respiratory conditions from the indigenous peoples of India and then introduced these compounds to the western world. Historically only atropine and atropine-like compounds were available, but these had many unwanted side effects, and the use of anticholinergics stagnated until ipratropium was developed in the 1980s.

Ipratropium differs from atropine in the position of the ammonium group in its structure; atropine is a tertiary ammonium compound, and ipratropium is a quaternary ammonium compound. This structure allows ipratropium to carry a positive charge, which prevents it from crossing the lipid blood-brain barrier and other cell membranes. Limiting absorption and distribution of the drug to the central nervous system (CNS) prevents most bothersome side effects, making the compound more useful therapeutically. For reasons other than decreased absorption, ipratropium does not have the secretion-drying effects common to atropine-like compounds, which mitigates concerns about thickened secretions with long-term use.[13]

Anticholinergic agents currently are indicated for the treatment of COPD but sometimes find use in difficult to control asthma. They also occasionally are used to reduce secretions. Both atropine and glycopyrrolate (Robinul) are used for this indication.

Ipratropium is the anticholinergic agent primarily used in the treatment of respiratory disorders. However, because it is poorly absorbed across the oral mucosa, it is given only by the inhalation route. The drug's half-life is 3 hours; therefore it must be dosed every 4 to 6 hours. Ipratropium is available in several formulations and in a combination metered dose inhaler (MDI) with albuterol (Combivent).

Methylxanthines

Methylxanthines are a class of pharmacologic compounds that includes caffeine (found in coffee, tea, and cola), theobromine (found in chocolate), and theophylline (found in tea). Caffeine was often used in respiratory medicine in the past, but theophylline has become the methylxanthine of choice. The water-soluble complex theophylline ethylenediamine (aminophylline) is used intravenously in the treatment of critically ill patients for whom oral therapies cannot be used. The potency of the naturally occurring methylxanthines, in decreasing order, is theophylline, caffeine, and theobromine. Theobromine is not used therapeutically.

The methylxanthines' mechanism of action is still poorly understood, but they probably act through inhibition of phosphodiesterase, thereby increasing intracellular cGMP levels. They also probably act through competitive antagonism of adenosine receptors. This is consistent with the observation that inhalation of adenosine can provoke bronchoconstriction in asthmatic individuals but has little effect in normal controls.[14] During short-term administration, the methylxanthines cause some catecholamine release, but this is not thought to contribute to their long-term effectiveness.[14]

In addition to bronchodilation, at least one of the methylxanthines, theophylline, has some antiinflammatory effect. This probably is due to inhibition of eosinophils and an increase in the antiinflammatory cytokine IL-10. Methylxanthines cause some diuresis, and they have been shown to enhance diaphragmatic contractility and mucociliary clearance; this makes them useful in the management of patients with respiratory muscle weakness, especially because these patients have difficulty with secretion clearance. Methylxanthines are most commonly

used worldwide as a CNS stimulant. Americans are estimated to take in an average of 300 mg of caffeine daily in the form of coffee and cola.

Methylxanthines have a narrow therapeutic window, meaning that toxicity is observed at levels not much higher than those used therapeutically. Consequently, careful administration and monitoring of drug levels are particularly important with these compounds. Toxicity takes the form of cardiac tachyarrhythmias and seizures. Other undesirable side effects are agitation, tremor, headache, nausea and vomiting, dizziness, and increased secretion of stomach acid.

Theophylline is one of the oldest medicinal agents used in the treatment of respiratory disorders. It was the mainstay of asthma therapy throughout the 1970s but fell out of favor with the discovery of the role of airway inflammation in asthma and the development of inhaled corticosteroids. The recent discovery of theophylline's antiinflammatory effects, along with its low cost and long duration of action, has revived interest in the compound. However, many clinicians consider theophylline a difficult drug to manage, which has tempered its use.

Theophylline has a complex pharmacokinetics. It is completely absorbed, but approximately 40% is protein bound. The drug is 90% metabolized by the liver, partly by the P-450 system. The rate of theophylline metabolism varies widely among patients, with the average half-life ranging from 4 hours in children to 10 hours in the elderly (6 hours is the quoted average half-life). In addition to the effects of age, many medications influence theophylline metabolism through their effect on P-450 activity. Smoking is an important factor affecting theophylline metabolism; active smokers may increase their clearance by 50% to 80% over baseline. Also, the metabolism of theophylline does not vary linearly with concentration. At levels above 10 μg/mL, it displays saturation kinetics.

Because of this wide variability in theophylline metabolism, complicated by a narrow therapeutic index, serum levels of theophylline should be monitored routinely. Serum concentrations of 10 to 20 μg/mL have been shown to produce satisfactory clinical effects. More recent clinical studies have demonstrated that serum concentrations of 5 μg/mL may produce therapeutic effects in most patients. Currently, the recommended therapeutic range is 5 to 15 μg/mL. This range has been lowered somewhat from the former recommendation of 10 to 20 μg/mL. Blood levels should be checked at least 48 hours after the last dosage change to allow a steady state to occur. Drug level monitoring usually is not performed with patients who are taking theophylline only once at bedtime to control nocturnal symptoms; it is assumed that the drug is largely eliminated between doses.

In clinical studies theophylline as monotherapy was not as effective as the inhaled steroid budesonide in controlling the symptoms, bronchial hyperresponsiveness, or eosinophilia of mild to moderate asthma.[15] However, adding theophylline to inhaled budesonide produced greater increases in forced vital capacity (FVC) and FEV₁ than budesonide alone. In cases of moderate asthma the addition of theophylline to low-dose budesonide achieved similar results compared with high-dose budesonide alone.[16]

The current role of theophylline in the treatment of respiratory disorders is as an alternative to inhaled corticosteroids for patients with mild persistent asthma and as an add-on therapy with inhaled corticosteroids for patients with moderate to severe asthma. In this capacity theophylline allows some reduction in the steroid dose, which may be beneficial. The sustained-release formulations have a special role (along with salmeterol) in the treatment of nocturnal asthma symptoms because the effect lasts 12 hours. Theophylline remains an alternative to oral albuterol as a bronchodilator in children too young to use an MDI. Despite its possible antiinflammatory effect, theophylline should not be used as a substitute for formal antiinflammatory therapy in any type but the mild form of asthma.

Dyphylline, a synthetic methylxanthine introduced in 1946, differs from theophylline in that it does not undergo hepatic biotransformation; in fact, 88% of the compound is excreted unchanged by the kidneys.[2] It therefore has somewhat more predictable pharmacokinetics, and the manufacturer does not recommend serum level monitoring except in patients with impaired renal function. Because dyphylline's bronchodilatory efficacy is approximately one fifth that of theophylline, dyphylline's therapeutic efficacy may be overstated.[16]

As mentioned previously, the compound aminophylline was developed by the mixture of theophylline with ethylenediamine, a water-soluble salt of theophylline. Because of its solubility, aminophylline can be administered parenterally, giving it an important niche in the armamentarium of emergency asthma treatment. Aminophylline is 86% theophylline, and its pharmacodynamics and metabolism are those of theophylline.

Antiinflammatory Drugs

Adrenocorticosteroids   Adrenocorticosteroids are endogenous hormones secreted by the adrenal cortex or synthetic analogs of these hormones. They help maintain homeostasis in many body systems and exert a variety of beneficial and detrimental effects, including formation of glucose from body proteins, retention of sodium by the kidneys, depletion of bone calcium, increase in fat production, impaired immunologic response, reduction of inflammatory response, and elevation of blood pressure. The naturally occurring corticosteroids, cortisone and hydrocortisone (cortisol), have both glucocorticoid and significant mineralocorticoid activity. This is especially evident when they are used in prolonged or high-dose courses of therapy, because sodium retention with edema and hypertension may occur. Many of the synthetic corticosteroids also have both effects, although much less mineralocorticoid activity.

The physiologic amount of hydrocortisone and cortisone produced daily by the adrenal glands in times of minimal stress is equivalent to 20 mg of hydrocortisone. Greater amounts are required during illness. The generally accepted equivalents to these amounts for the other systemically administered glucocorticoid agents are listed in Table 18-2. When exogenous steroids are given for longer than about 2 weeks in doses exceeding the body's own production, adrenal steroid production can be suppressed. Adrenal function returns when the exogenous steroids are discontinued, but this process can be protracted, requiring long tapering of steroid doses over weeks to months. For the same reason, if a patient encounters serious physical stressors while taking steroids, the exogenous dose may need to be increased to support the body's increased need. Long-term steroid administration in supraphysiologic doses also carries substantial risk of serious toxicity.

Despite these serious disadvantages, corticosteroids have powerful beneficial effects and are used in a wide variety of respiratory diseases. They are most commonly used in the treatment of asthma and COPD exacerbation, but they also are the mainstay of therapy in sarcoidosis, bronchiolitis obliterans–organizing pneumonia (BOOP), and chemical pneumonitis. They are important adjuncts in the treatment of *Pneumocystis carinii* pneumonia, Löffler's syndrome, berylliosis, and other interstitial lung diseases. Their use in acute respiratory distress syndrome (ARDS) is controversial, but they are increasingly thought to be useful in late nonresolving (defined as more than 7 days' duration) ARDS. Steroids may also be administered to mothers at risk of delivering a premature neonate to stimulate fetal surfactant production and prevent respiratory distress syndrome (RDS).

TABLE 18-2

Systemically Administered Corticosteroids and Dose Equivalents

Corticosteroid	Approximate Equivalent Dose	Relative Glucocorticoid Potency	Relative Mineralocorticoid Potency
Short Acting (Half-Life Less than 12 Hours)			
Hydrocortisone (cortisol)	20	1	1
Cortisone	25	0.8	0.8
Intermediate Acting (Half-Life 12-36 Hours)			
Methylprednisolone	4	5	0
Prednisolone	5	4	0.25
Prednisone	5	4	0.25
Triamcinolone	4	5	0
Long Acting (Half-Life Longer than 48 Hours)			
Betamethasone	0.6	25	0
Dexamethasone	0.75	25	0

Respiratory Recap

Classes of Antiinflammatory Drugs	
Corticosteroids (systemic or inhaled)	Cromones
	Leukotriene inhibitors
Nonsteroidal antiinflammatory drugs (NSAIDs)	

As the concept of asthma as a primarily inflammatory disease has developed, corticosteroids have become the mainstay of asthma treatment. The development of inhaled steroids has made sustained therapy with minimal apparent toxicity possible. Currently, continuous treatment with inhaled corticosteroids is the first-line therapy of moderate and severe asthma, with a role in mild persistent asthma as well.

Corticosteroids are also the primary treatment for exacerbations of asthma. The rise in asthma mortality coincident with the increasing use of the short-acting β_2-agonists has been partly attributed to a tendency to treat worsening asthma with bronchodilators while leaving the underlying inflammatory disease untreated. The current thinking is that the first response to worsening or poorly controlled asthma should be intensified treatment of the underlying inflammation with an increase in corticosteroids, sometimes the addition of systemic steroids. On the other hand, it is equally important to keep in mind that the effect of steroids may not manifest for several hours after administration; therefore in severe, life-threatening asthma exacerbations, there is no substitute for a short-acting bronchodilator, such as albuterol, to prevent acute respiratory failure.

Along with immediate bronchodilator therapy, systemic corticosteroids remain an important part of emergency department asthma treatment, because they can prevent the second-wave influx of proinflammatory cells to the lungs that can trigger the late-phase asthma exacerbation. There is little scientific basis for the selection of a corticosteroid dose for acute exacerbations. Intravenous methylprednisolone usually is given initially, and two common regimens (125 mg IV q12-24h and 60 mg IV q6h) have proved effective.[16] Several small studies have failed to demonstrate any added benefit to larger doses.[17-19] Current knowledge dictates that some period of increasing bronchial inflammation usually occurs in the period leading up to an asthma exacerbation. When a patient seeks treatment for a significant exacerbation, a 5- to 20-day course of oral corticosteroids often is prescribed to promote dissipation of this established inflammation. If the course of therapy is longer than 5 to 10 days, a tapering dose often is used. The initial dosage usually is 20 to 40 mg of prednisone daily.

There is continuing controversy over the role of corticosteroids in the treatment of COPD. Some degree of chronic inflammation accompanies COPD and may contribute to a decline in lung function. Inflammation may also play a role in exacerbations. However, because structural lung changes, not inflammation, are primarily responsible for the impairment in COPD, there is significant skepticism about the efficacy of steroid therapy in the treatment of the disorder. Recently, Niewoehner and colleagues[20] demonstrated significant improvement in patients with acute exacerbations of COPD who were treated with systemic corticosteroids. On the basis of current evidence, corticosteroids may be recommended at least for acute use in COPD.

Some patients with severe asthma and COPD seem to require long-term systemic corticosteroids to control the disease activity. A recent study by Rice and colleagues[21] suggests that many so-called steroid-dependent COPD patients may be able to discontinue systemic steroids with little change in their respiratory status. The same is not true of many steroid-dependent asthma patients, however, and finding a treatment plan that enables these patients to stop long-term systemic steroids is a common challenge.

Corticosteroids are also used for patients with nonresolving acute ARDS. Prolonged administration of methylprednisolone (2 mg/kg/day) for patients with nonresolving ARDS was associated with improvement in lung injury and reduced mortality in one report.[22] Although the use of steroids in late-phase (fibroproliferative) ARDS is controversial, the drugs are commonly used in this setting.

Systemic corticosteroids are notorious for their side effects and toxicity, and some patients are highly resistant to taking these drugs. The adverse effects associated with corticosteroids are indeed many and serious, but the most severe occur with long-term use. These include adrenal gland suppression, osteoporosis, cataract formation, muscle wasting and frank steroid myopathy, thinning and striae formation in the skin, and development of a cushingoid appearance (central obesity, moon facies, and a buffalo hump). Adverse effects associated with short-term use are worsened glycemic control (and possible provocation of transient diabetes mellitus), water retention, insomnia and agitation, facial flushing, appetite stimulation, stomach upset, and headache. Diabetic patients should monitor their blood sugar level carefully while undergoing therapy. Corticosteroids also cause mood changes; patients typically are slightly euphoric. However, at moderate to high doses, especially in the elderly, the drugs may cause delirium and frank mania.

Hydrocortisone is a glucocorticoid available in oral and parenteral formulations. This agent is used in the treatment of adrenal insufficiency to replace cortisol. The mineralocorticoid activity of hydrocortisone makes it less favorable for administration in respiratory conditions. However, the intravenous formulation may be administered in episodes of severe asthma or in other respiratory disorders requiring hospitalization. When the drug is used in the high doses required for these conditions for longer than 72 hours, patients should be monitored for sodium retention and resultant edema and hypertension. Dosing in these instances is largely empiric and often is based on the physician's preference.

Methylprednisolone is the glucocorticoid agent most commonly administered intravenously in severe cases of respiratory distress. It has less mineralocorticoid activity then hydrocortisone and therefore is less likely to cause edema and electrolyte abnormalities. For this reason, it may be especially preferred over hydrocortisone in patients with underlying cardiac disease and fluid retention problems.

At the time of its introduction, dexamethasone was the first and only steroid available in intravenous, oral, and inhalation formulations. Because of its availability and lack of significant mineralocorticoid activity, it was a commonly used agent in the treatment of respiratory disorders. However, there is a high level of systemic absorption from the inhalation product. The use of inhaled dexamethasone has diminished since the advent of other steroid formulations.

The steroid most often used for therapy of respiratory disease in adults is prednisone. As with dexamethasone, the drug has only minimal mineralocorticoid properties, which makes it an attractive agent especially for long-term therapy. Prednisolone, which is similar to prednisone and also has low mineralocorticoid activity, traditionally has been more commonly used in pediatric patients.

Inhaled Corticosteroids

Inhaled corticosteroids[23] were developed to reduce the side effects of systemic glucocorticoid administration and to provide direct delivery of the drug to the site of action. Although systemic absorption of inhaled corticosteroids is readily demonstrable, these levels are relatively low, and long-term use of inhaled corticosteroids is believed to be safe and relatively free of systemic side effects, including significant adrenal suppression. One exception, however, is that measurable growth suppression has been demonstrated among children using long-term inhaled corticosteroid therapy for asthma, especially large doses.[24]

Although relatively safe, the inhalation route has its own set of side effects. Deposition of steroid on the posterior pharynx and vocal cords can cause sore throat, hoarseness (which may occur in up to half of patients using inhaled steroids) and a predisposition to thrush. These complications can be largely avoided through use of a spacer to minimize proximal deposition and by rinsing of the mouth after the inhaler is used.

The success of inhaled corticosteroids has led to the development of nasal-inhaled steroids for inflammatory conditions of the nasopharynx and sinuses. These conditions include allergic rhinitis and acute and chronic sinusitis.

After dexamethasone, beclomethasone was the second inhalation product marketed in the United States. It is a medium-potency agent with a short half life. Beclomethasone dipropionate is rapidly metabolized by enzymes in the lung fluid to the active metabolite beclomethasone-17-monopropionate. It is also rapidly broken down in the gastrointestinal tract, which is why an oral preparation is not available. Beclomethasone is available as Vanceril and Beclovent for oral inhalation and Vancenase and Beconase for nasal inhalation.

Triamcinolone is a low-potency, short-acting agent. The commercial product includes a built-in spacer. Despite the drug's short duration of action, maintenance therapy may be administered twice daily if the patient tolerates it. Several new non-chlorofluorocarbon (CFC)–based triamcinolone products are in development.

Flunisolide is comparable to triamcinolone in potency. Compliance may be an issue with pediatric patients, because the commercial product is known to have a bad taste; AeroBid M includes menthol in the vehicle as a flavoring agent. Budesonide is a high-potency agent packaged in a breath-activated MDI called the *Pulmicort Turbuhaler;* this may improve drug delivery in individuals with poor coordination. Fluticasone (Flovent) is a somewhat higher potency glucocorticoid than the other available inhaled agents. As such it may have increased efficacy at recommended doses, and there is some evidence that this is the case.[25] Therefore switching an existing inhaled corticosteroid to fluticasone if asthma symptoms are poorly controlled is not uncommon. A nasal inhaler, Flonase, is also available.

Nonsteroidal Antiinflammatory Drugs

The **nonsteroidal antiinflammatory drugs (NSAIDs),** of which the archetype is acetylsalicylic acid (aspirin, or ASA), have **analgesic** (pain reducing), antiinflammatory, **antipyretic** (fever reducing), and antiplatelet (platelet aggregation reducing) properties. They exert these effects by inhibiting the enzyme cyclooxygenase in the arachidonic acid metabolism pathway, which blocks the production of the proinflammatory prostaglandins. NSAIDs are used for a wide variety of inflammatory processes, from arthritis to myocarditis, but they are not generally used for inflammatory processes of the lung such as asthma and BOOP. One reason is their lower efficacy compared with the corticosteroids. Perhaps more important, they may cause bronchospasm in sensitive individuals, which is especially undesirable when treating asthma. One important use of NSAIDs in respiratory medicine is the treatment of pleural inflammation, especially viral pleurisy. In these cases the combination of antiinflammatory effect and analgesia is convenient.

The NSAIDs are commonly used as platelet inhibitors in the treatment and prevention of acute coronary syndromes and stroke. They also are excellent antipyretics; along with acetaminophen (which is not an NSAID), they often are used to reduce fever. This effect may help alleviate respiratory distress in critically ill patients with limited respiratory reserve.

The three major adverse effects of NSAIDs are bronchospasm, gastric ulcer and hemorrhage, and inhibition of platelet function, leading to increased bruising and bleeding. For this reason, they are contraindicated in patients with aspirin-sensitive asthma and those with a history of gastrointestinal (GI) bleeding, especially the elderly. Their use in patients undergoing surgery is controversial because of an increased bleeding tendency.

The number of NSAIDs has increased dramatically; only the most common are presented here. Although the

NSAIDs share many similarities as a class, it should be noted that aspirin seems to have a greater tendency to cause bronchoconstriction than other NSAIDs and produces irreversible antagonism of cyclooxygenase. A new class of NSAIDs has been designed to selectively block the cyclooxygenase-2 (COX-2) enzyme, in contrast to the traditional NSAIDs, which block both COX-1 and COX-2 enzymes. These new drugs, called *COX-2 inhibitors*, retain antiinflammatory and analgesic effects but have less of a tendency to cause gastric ulceration.

Derived from the bark of the cinchona (willow) tree, aspirin is the original NSAID. It is also the archetype of the salicylates, a subclass of the NSAIDs. Salicylates in high doses cause a syndrome of tinnitus, decreased hearing, and nausea, known as *salicylism*, or *cinchonism*. Aspirin is unique among the NSAIDs in that it causes irreversible inhibition of cyclooxygenase; the effect is only reversed by the production of new enzyme. Because platelets lack synthetic function, the antiplatelet effect persists until new platelets are produced, or approximately 1 week. Other NSAIDs are reversible, competitive antagonists of cyclooxygenase.

Ibuprofen is the most commonly prescribed NSAID for musculoskeletal conditions, partly because it is thought to produce fewer GI side effects than aspirin. The most potent of the oral NSAIDs, indomethacin, traditionally is the favored NSAID used to treat pleural and pericardial inflammation. It also is used in neonates to stimulate closure of a patent ductus arteriosis (PDA), a cause of hypoxia in newborns. Ketorolac, one of the two NSAIDs available in parenteral form, is commonly used in emergency departments for rapid relief of pain when inflammation also is present or when narcotics are contraindicated.

Leukotriene Inhibitors: Leukotriene Receptor Antagonists and 5-Lipoxygenase Antagonists

Leukotriene inhibitors are the newest class of respiratory medications, having become available in the mid-1990s. Leukotrienes originally were described as the slow-reacting substance of anaphylaxis, a substance that produced prolonged smooth muscle contraction, including bronchospasm, and had significant proinflammatory effects. In the 1970s SRS-A was identified as the group of cysteinyl leukotrienes: leukotriene C_4 (LTC$_4$), D$_4$ (LTD$_4$) and E$_4$ (LTE$_4$). The cysteinyl leukotrienes are derived from arachidonic acid via the lipoxygenase pathway. This discovery also provides a possible mechanism for aspirin-induced asthma: as aspirin blocks the cyclooxygenase pathway, more arachidonic acid metabolism is shunted down the lipoxygenase pathway, possibly inducing bronchospasm.[26]

Several leukotriene antagonists have become available clinically. These agents have proved effective in reducing asthma activity,[27] but their clinical role is still being defined. One role in which the leukotriene antagonists are consistently efficacious is the treatment of aspirin-sensitive asthmatic patients. In asthma patients who are not aspirin sensitive, studies comparing or adding leukotriene inhibitors to corticosteroids have suggested that although the leukotriene inhibitors are not as effective in controlling asthma as the corticosteroids, they may allow reduction of the corticosteroid dose when used with them.[28,29] Treatment of allergic rhinitis and COPD are other potential uses for leukotriene inhibitors. An important advantage of the leukotriene inhibitors is the fact that they are taken orally, which may promote better patient compliance compared with MDIs.

Side effects are uncommon with leukotriene inhibitors but can include insomnia, gastric upset, aggravation of an ulcer or reflux, increased hyperactivity in some children, and difficulty with urination in elderly men with prostatic hypertrophy. The development of Churg-Strauss syndrome has been attributed to two of the leukotriene inhibitors, montelukast and pranlukast, which may represent a class effect.[30] However, that the reported cases of Churg-Strauss syndrome were caused by leukotriene receptor antagonists (LTRAs) is as yet uncertain; they may have been preexisting, masquerading as asthma and unmasked by the replacement of corticosteriods with LTRAs.[31] Overdose of these drugs can produce tachycardia and tachyarrhythmias, nausea and vomiting, CNS stimulation, headache, seizures, hyperglycemia, and hypokalemia.

Cromones

Cromones are a class of antiinflammatory drugs developed in the 1960s that appear to reduce the inflammatory response associated with asthma. The principal effect of cromones is thought to be inhibition of mast cell degranulation, or the release of granules containing histamine and other proinflammatory factors. Cromones also inhibit production of proinflammatory leukotrienes by mast cells after stimulation with antigen. In addition to their effects on mast cells, cromones appear to affect other inflammatory cell types. They alter the expression of cell surface receptors and suppress the effect of chemoattractant cytokines on neutrophils, eosinophils, and monocytes.[32]

The cromones are used as maintenance agents to prevent exacerbations of mild to moderate asthma. They are thought to be particularly useful for patients who are sensitive to environmental allergens. Cromones may be used in conjunction with, or more commonly as a replacement for, corticosteroids. Their antiinflammatory efficacy is somewhat less than that of the corticosteroids, but their side effect profile also is less severe, which makes them attractive for the milder end of the asthma spectrum.

Cromolyn is a synthetic compound derived from the naturally occurring compound khellin in 1965. Although khellin has both antiinflammatory and bronchodilation capabilities, cromolyn has only the antiinflammatory effects. Specifically, cromolyn was found to reduce antigen-induced bronchospasm in asthmatic patients and to inhibit the release of histamine and other inflammatory mediators from mast cells. Available in the United States since 1973, cromolyn's primary uses are prophylactic control both of mild, persistent asthma and of exercise-induced bronchospasm. It also is effective in the prophylaxis of early- and late-phase asthmatic reactions. Corticosteroids remain the recommended antiinflammatory agents for controlling mild, persistent asthma. However, cromolyn may be an alternative for patients who cannot tolerate or do not want to take inhaled steroids. Cromolyn may be used concomitantly with inhaled steroids. Studies have demonstrated that use of cromolyn reduces the dosage of inhaled steroids needed to control asthma symptoms.[33] Studies also have shown that individuals who use cromolyn regularly for 2 to 3 months show reduced bronchial hyperreactivity. Some patients show an improvement immediately, but for most patients it takes several weeks to achieve the maximum effect. Patients who use cromolyn to prevent exercise-induced bronchospasm should administer it at least 10 to 15 minutes but not more than 1 hour before exercising.

Nedocromil is a newer cromone approved for use in 1993. It is structurally different from cromolyn but similar in its mechanism of action and role in therapy. Clinical trials demonstrated that nedocromil improves symptoms and lung function and reduces nonspecific airway responsiveness.[34] When nedocromil and cromolyn are directly compared in trials, little clinical difference is seen between the two agents.[35] Although its half-life (3.3 hours) is slightly longer than that of cromolyn, nedocromil is also administered four times daily for best effect.

Secretion Modifiers

Abnormal volume or thickness (or both) of respiratory secretions is a hallmark of some pulmonary diseases, particularly cystic fibrosis and other forms of bronchiectasis. In fact, secretion clearance remains one of the truly challenging problems in pulmonary medicine. The anticholinergics reduce secretion volume but may thicken the secretions; antihistamines have a similar effect. These two classes of drugs have been particularly effective in the treatment of cystic fibrosis. Unfortunately, their use for other diseases, such as chronic bronchitis and pneumonia, has not produced definite benefit.

The antihistamines, which are growing in number, are commonly used to reduce the volume of secretions, especially upper airway secretions, associated with upper respiratory infections and allergies. Although they are effective in this role, they are rarely used for lower respiratory tract secretions. The most common indication for antihistamines in pulmonary medicine is the treatment of chronic cough caused by postnasal drip.

The archetype antihistamine is diphenhydramine (Benadryl), which has both H_1- and H_2-blocking activity. Its principal disadvantage is significant sedation. A new group of nonsedating antihistamines, which includes cetirizine (Zyrtec), fexofenadine (Allegra), and loratadine (Claritin), is becoming quite popular. These drugs have selective activity for the H_1 receptor.

The anticholinergics as bronchodilators were discussed with the drug ipratropium. Other anticholinergics occasionally are used to reduce secretions. This is most commonly done to facilitate procedures, although long-term use is a treatment for weakened patients who have difficulty with secretion control.

Like ipratropium, atropine has bronchodilating properties but is most commonly used for its ability to reduce the volume of secretions by blocking the muscarinic M_3 receptors. This affects primarily the aqueous (watery) portion of the secretions; consequently, secretions may thicken as their volume is reduced. Because atropine penetrates the CNS, it is associated with more of the typical anticholinergic side effects than ipratropium. Glycopyrrolate is similar to atropine in its effects and clinical use. The CNS side effects associated with glycopyrrolate are similar to but somewhat less severe than those of atropine.

N-acetyl-L-cysteine, commonly known as *acetylcysteine*, is the classic mucolytic agent, although it does not have that indication in the United States.[36] It is most commonly thought of as the antidote for acetaminophen toxicity. Acetylcysteine has been shown to reduce the viscosity of airway secretions by breaking the bonds between the sulfide compounds in the secretions. Administration of the drug may cause bronchospasm, especially in asthmatic patients; therefore a prophylactic dose of albuterol often is given first. Dornase alfa is commonly used in cystic fibrosis, but its use is often restricted by insurers because of the high cost. This drug has theoretic value in certain other patients with purulent secretions (it is not effective against mucoid secretions because they lack significant amounts of DNA), but its efficacy has not been proved in these patients other than those with cystic fibrosis.

Surfactant Replacements

Neonatal RDS, also called *hyaline membrane disease*, occurs in premature neonates who lack sufficient capacity to produce **surfactant.** Without surfactant, alveolar surface tension causes lung units to collapse, and overall compliance declines. The high mortality of this disease has been significantly reduced by a recently developed technique that allows delivery of surfactant replacers to the lungs by nebulization. Natural surfactant is a suspension of the proteins SP-A, SP-B, and SP-C in phospholipid. The phospholipid dipalmitoylphosphatidylcholine (DPPC), also called *phosphatidylcholine* and *colfosceril palmitate*, is the predominant phospholipid, comprising 70% of total surfactant by weight.

Exosurf is a protein-free product composed primarily of DPPC. Cetyl alcohol and tyloxapol are added as spreading agents, without which the DPPC is ineffective. It is instilled as a liquid directly into the endotracheal tube, which can provoke a drop in the partial pressure of arterial oxygen (PaO_2) by more than 20% in 6% to 22% of patients.[2] Reflux of Exosurf into the endotracheal tube is common but can be minimized by slow instillation. An increase in pulmonary hemorrhage has been reported in patients receiving Exosurf, from 2% to 10% in one study.

Survanta is a natural bovine (cow-derived) surfactant that has SP-B and SP-C (but not SP-A) proteins in phospholipid. The addition of the surfactant protein constituents has been shown to significantly enhance the performance of this compound relative to Exosurf.[37] Survanta also is instilled as a liquid endotracheally; the manufacturer recommends that this be done specifically with a 5 French (5 Fr) catheter during mechanical, not manual, ventilation. The patient is placed in four positions during instillation to distribute the Survanta. The adverse effects that arise during instillation are similar to those with Exosurf, except that the incidence of pulmonary hemorrhage does not appear to be significantly increased.

Infasurf (Calfactant), like Survanta, is a natural surfactant derived from bronchoalveolar lavage fluid from calves. It contains SP-B and SP-C proteins, approximately 2% by weight. Its effectiveness in the treatment of RDS has proved to be similar to that of Survanta but of longer duration (24 hours versus 6 hours).[37] It is administered as a liquid via the endotracheal tube.

Inhaled Antimicrobial Drugs

The administration of antimicrobial drugs directly into the lungs is an area of open possibilities in the treatment of respiratory infections.[38] Although it is not widely practiced, there are several specific indications for this therapy. Currently accepted applications include administration of antipseudomonal antibiotics in cystic fibrosis, pentamidine prophylaxis in patients who test positive for the human immunodeficiency virus (HIV), and administration of ribavirin for respiratory syncytial virus.

Direct administration of antibiotics to the lungs would seem to provide a valuable treatment option for lung infections, but several possible reasons explain why this route has not achieved more common use, as follows:

1. Serious bacterial respiratory infections frequently have a systemic component, mandating systemic administration of antimicrobial therapy.
2. Infections associated with consolidation or cavitation are associated with severely decreased or absent regional ventilation, preventing delivery of inhaled drug to the more severely affected areas.
3. Because of the reluctance to use this route in the treatment of infections, most studies have concentrated on "prophylactic" use of inhaled antimicrobials; therefore there remains relatively little evidence to establish efficacy and dosing protocols for treatment of established infections. Resistance has also been observed in many studies. Both contributed to dissatisfaction with this route of therapy.
4. The characterization of dose-response relationships for inhaled drugs is difficult. Doses actually delivered to the lung depend on the delivery system, the patient's breathing patterns, and the airway anatomy.

Progress is being made in response to these concerns. More reliable delivery systems and improved techniques used to measure the dose of drug delivered to the lungs are helping to identify dose responses. Improved imaging techniques are aiding the development of delivery systems capable of reaching problem areas of the lungs. Concomitant treatment of respiratory infections with systemic and local therapy has been suggested.

Ribavirin is infamous among respiratory therapists for its messiness. Exhaled aerosol tends to cause eye and mucosal irritation. Extreme care must be taken when the drug is administered to mechanically ventilated patients. Ribavirin is rather sticky and has been known to cause obstruction of the expiratory ventilatory circuit, which can be a dangerous event.[39] For these reasons, most institutions have special protocols for the delivery of ribavirin, including placement of filters in the expiratory limb of the ventilator circuit. Contact and inhalational isolation precautions must be instituted for pregnant women because ribavirin is highly teratogenic.

Colistimethate (Coly-Mycin) is a polypeptide antibiotic similar to polymyxin. This class of drugs is not commonly used because of its narrow therapeutic window and narrow spectrum of antimicrobial coverage. Colistimethate continues to be potentially useful, however, as an inhaled antibiotic for the treatment of *Pseudomonas* pneumonia.

Invasive pulmonary aspergillosis is a major cause of morbidity and mortality among immunocompromised patients, especially those who have received bone marrow transplants. Several strategies used to prevent and treat *Aspergillus* infection have been proposed. One of these is the use of nebulized amphotericin B, either in standard or liposomal form. Liposomal amphotericin B is a recently developed formulation that packages the drug in tiny lipid spheres called *liposomes*, providing some reduction in toxicity. Although administration by aerosolization has been shown to be feasible, it has not yet been demonstrated that the highly expensive liposomal preparations are required when amphotericin B is given in nebulized form.

There is some evidence that aerosolized amphotericin B (AAB) is effective for prophylaxis of pulmonary aspergillosis[40-42] with minimal toxicity.[43] Aerosolized amphotericin B also has been used to treat fungal infection, although evidence of efficacy has not yet been established.

Pseudomonas aeruginosa is a major pathogen and colonizer of patients with bronchiectasis and to a lesser extent emphysema; it has been implicated as a primary cause of lung deterioration among patients with cystic fibrosis. The treatment of *Pseudomonas* infection has been complicated by the organism's tendency to develop resistance to antimicrobial agents and by the severe systemic toxicity of most antipseudomonal drugs. These difficulties have spurred the development of inhaled aminoglycosides, such as tobramycin. Because these drugs are inhaled, systemic drug levels are relatively low, which reduces the severity of toxicity. Thus unusually high concentrations can be safely achieved in lung tissue, concentrations that may overcome bacterial resistance. The most recent aminoglycoside addition is TOBI, a tobramycin formulation that is preservative free to reduce adverse effects. As with any aminoglycoside, it is important to consider ototoxicity and nephrotoxicity. Ototoxicity, especially, appears to remain problematic with sustained use. Gentamicin, another aminoglycoside antibiotic, also is delivered in aerosolized form to treat pulmonary gram-negative infections.

Pentamidine, one of the first drugs available to treat *Pneumocystis carinii* infection, has had a major impact on mortality caused by this organism. Although pentamidine has been replaced by trimethoprim-sulfamethoxazole (TMP/SMX), it remains the second-line agent for treatment (intravenous) and prophylaxis (nebulized) of patients allergic to sulfa drugs. The mechanism of anti-*Pneumocystis* action is not known. Pentamidine has important adverse effects; infusion can cause hypotension, dyspnea, nausea and vomiting, pancreatitis, hyperglycemia, and life-threatening hypoglycemia. Inhalational therapy appears to prevent these problems. A disadvantage of nebulized pentamidine prophylaxis is a tendency for patients to be poorly protected against *P. carinii* infection in the lung apices.

Other Drugs Used in Pulmonary Medicine

Most respiratory therapists spend a great deal of their time in the intensive care unit (ICU), working with critically ill patients who have complex medication regimens. Although most of these drugs are not administered by a respiratory therapist, many are given to treat the patient's respiratory disease, and some have a significant impact on the patient's respiratory status. For this reason, a brief overview of some of these drugs follows.

Antimicrobials   The number of antibiotics in use is growing rapidly. The respiratory therapist regularly encounters a wide variety of systemically administered antibiotics and should be familiar with the general classes and most common agents.

Coagulants and Anticoagulants   Respiratory therapists rarely administer a **coagulant** or an **anticoagulant,** but the high incidence of deep venous thrombosis (DVT) and pulmonary embolism (PE) means that the therapist frequently encounters patients receiving anticoagulant drugs, sometimes as the primary therapy for the respiratory problem. These drugs are also used for a variety of coagulation disorders such as coagulopathies and atrial fibrillation. An anticoagulant blocks the formation of a new blood clot (thrombus), allowing the existing thrombus to be slowly broken down by serum thrombolytic enzymes. This is in contrast to thrombolytic drugs, such as streptokinase (SK) and tissue plasminogen activator (tPA), which occasionally are used to actively dissolve a pulmonary embolism when it is immediately life threatening. Thrombolytics are rarely administered into the airway to dissolve obstructive blood clots. The use of thrombolytics is limited by their tendency to cause serious bleeding complications.

Heparin causes anticoagulation by activating antithrombin III, a serum anticoagulant factor. Because heparin is a polymeric peptide, it must be given parenterally to avoid digestion in the stomach. It usually is given either subcutaneously twice daily to prevent DVT or by continuous intravenous infusion as a treatment for DVT or PE. Because it is highly bound to serum proteins, heparin's effect is somewhat unpredictable; dosing must be adjusted on the basis of the activated partial thromboplastin time (aPTT). For most indications, the goal aPTT is one and one half to two times normal (approximately 50 to 80 seconds).

The low-molecular-weight heparins (LMWHs) are a new class of anticoagulants produced by cleaving the heparin polymer to produce smaller polymers. The advantages of the smaller form are (1) more predictable absorption, possibly eliminating the need for monitoring and allowing intermittent subcutaneous dosing rather than continuous infusion, and (2) a theoretically improved specificity of the heparin for a preexisting clot rather than generalized anticoagulation. Although the improved clot specificity has not been shown to be clinically significant, the predictability of absorption has allowed patients with DVT and PE to be treated outside the hospital, self-administering injections twice daily without regular monitoring. The consistency of LMWH absorption recently has been questioned, and there is concern that these drugs may require monitoring of antifactor Xa levels.

Several formulations of LMWH are available, which are roughly equivalent. These include ardeparin (Normiflo), dalteparin (Fragmin), and enoxaparin (Lovenox). Differences in their molecular weights and activity are responsible for some subtle but possibly important distinctions between these products, although the clinical relevance of these distinctions has yet to be determined.

The treatment of DVT and PE requires prolonged therapy (3 to 6 months), which is most easily accomplished with the oral medication warfarin. Warfarin inhibits the vitamin K–dependent production of coagulation factors V, VII, IX, and X by the liver. Because the reduction in factor levels requires approximately 3 days, heparin or LMWH is used initially to achieve anticoagulation while warfarin takes effect. Warfarin's effect can be reversed either with additional vitamin K to overcome the metabolic inhibition or the infusion of coagulation factors with fresh-frozen plasma (FFP).

Thrombin (coagulation factor II) occasionally is administered by the respiratory therapist through a bronchoscope to help coagulate excessive airway bleeding, which may occur from bronchoscopic biopsy.

Diuretics **Diuretics** stimulate urine production and commonly are used in the ICU to promote loss of excess body water and salt. Because pulmonary edema and subsequent respiratory failure can be among the first manifestations of fluid volume overload, the respiratory therapist frequently encounters these drugs. This is especially true with patients who have congestive heart failure and those who have received large amounts of intravenous fluid in the course of resuscitation.

ℛespiratory Recap

Classes of Diuretics	
Loop diuretics	Carbonic anhydrase
Thiazides	inhibitors
Potassium-sparing diuretics	Osmotic diuretics

Five classes of diuretics, each acting on a different part of the kidney, are commonly used. The most common in the ICU are the loop diuretics: furosemide (Lasix), torsemide (Demadex), and bumetanide (Bumex). These drugs block the resorption of sodium in the ascending loop of Henle. Because water generally follows sodium passively, the kidneys excrete both more sodium and more water.

The second most common class, the thiazides, block sodium permeability of the collecting duct. Examples of this class are hydrochlorothiazide (Esidrix, Microzide, Oretic), metolazone (Zaroxolyn), chlorthalidone (Hygroton, Thalitone), and indapamide (Lozol).

The third class of diuretics is the potassium-sparing diuretics. These block sodium resorption and potassium excretion in the distal tubule; in the case of spironolactone, this is achieved through antagonism of aldosterone, the endogenous mineralocorticoid. The most common potassium-sparing diuretic is spironolactone (Aldactone); other members of the class are amiloride (Midamor) and triamterene (Dyrenium). The potassium-sparing diuretics are particularly useful in liver failure, in which they are used in an attempt to reduce ascites formation. Hyperkalemia is a possible hazard of this diuretic class, and this effect is used therapeutically to counteract the potassium wasting caused by other diuretics.

The fourth class of diuretics, the carbonic anhydrase inhibitor acetazolamide (Diamox), blocks the enzyme that interconverts bicarbonate and carbon dioxide in the proximal convoluted tubule. This prevents bicarbonate from being reabsorbed; the negative bicarbonate ion is excreted, carrying with it positive sodium ions and, in turn, water. This drug is of particular interest because it is one of the few tools available for encouraging the kidneys to excrete excess bicarbonate, thereby correcting metabolic alkalosis. However, it is rarely used to this end.

The fifth class of diuretics is the osmotic diuretics, represented by the drug mannitol. Mannitol is a highly osmotic saccharide molecule that is filtered by the kidneys and not reabsorbed. Mannitol raises the osmolarity of the urine, pulling in water, which is then excreted. This is the only class of diuretics that does not rely on sodium as a carrier of water; it therefore promotes a water diuresis more than a saline diuresis.

With the exception of acetazolamide, aggressive diuresis with any of these agents can cause a metabolic alkalosis known as *contraction alkalosis*, which is manifested by a high bicarbonate level and a low chloride level. The loop and thiazide diuretics tend to cause hypokalemia and sometimes hypomagnesemia, and potassium and magnesium are lost in the urine.

Vasopressors **Vasopressors** increase blood pressure. Each of them achieves this through a combination of vasoconstriction (causing higher flow resistance and therefore higher pressure) and increased cardiac output. Important to note is that if the heart has limited reserve, the increased resistance imposed by vasoconstriction causes cardiac output to fall.

Epinephrine is a naturally occurring catecholamine that stimulates α_1-, α_2-, β_1-, and β_2-receptors. When given parenterally as a vasopressor, it causes vasoconstriction, an increased heart rate (positive chronotropism) and increased forcefulness of cardiac contraction (positive inotropism). Like epinephrine, norepinephrine (Levophed) is a naturally occurring catecholamine. It tends to be more specific to α-receptors than epinephrine; therefore it causes more vasoconstriction with less of a side effect of tachycardia. Phenylephrine (Neo-Synephrine) is a selective α-agonist and as such acts as a powerful vasoconstrictor with little if any chronotropism or inotropism. It is becoming increasingly popular as a pressor because of its specificity.

Low-dose dopamine (Intropin) is classically described as stimulating dopaminergic receptors, which causes slight vasodilation, especially in the renal arteries. Low doses of 1 to 3 μg/kg/minute have been called *renal dose dopamine* because of the resulting increase in renal blood flow and urine output. At higher doses dopamine stimulates first β-receptors and then α-receptors. Because it has balanced β and α effects, dopamine frequently is used as a first-line pressor. However, if high levels of blood pressure support are needed, dopamine's β stimulation often causes undesirable degrees of tachycardia. Recently the concept of renal dose dopamine has become increasingly controversial. It appears that this effect is minimal and that most of the increased renal blood flow is caused by increased cardiac output as a result of β stimulation.

Inotropic Agents These drugs are not highly effective in raising blood pressure, but they improve cardiac performance, primarily through an increase in the force of cardiac contractility. Dobutamine (Dobutrex) is a relatively selective β-agonist. Its β$_1$ stimulation causes positive **inotropism** and some **chronotropism,** whereas β$_2$ stimulation causes vasodilation. The overall effect on blood pressure often is neutral but varies individually. The combination of cardiac stimulation with vasodilation (decreased resistance) can markedly increase cardiac output. Milrinone (Primacor) and amrinone (Inocor) inhibit the enzyme phosphodiesterase without significant adrenergic stimulation. Despite their differing mechanism, the effects of milrinone and amrinone are similar to those of dobutamine: positive inotropism with some vasodilation.

Vasodilators Nitroglycerin and nitroprusside are used in three settings. First, they quickly and powerfully reduce high blood pressure; second, by decreasing resistance to flow, they improve the output of a failing heart; and third, they relieve angina by reducing the workload of the heart, thereby reducing its oxygen consumption.

Nitroglycerin (Tridil, Nitrol, Nitrostat) is converted in the body to nitric oxide (NO), a powerful, naturally occurring **vasodilator** (arterial dilator) and venodilator (venous dilator). Nitroglycerin has fairly balanced vasodilation and venodilation effects; therefore it is an effective antianginal medication. Nitroprusside (Nipride) also exerts its effects through conversion to NO. Compared with nitroglycerin, nitroprusside is a more specific vasodilator with less of a venodilation effect. The metabolic products of nitroprusside include cyanide, which can reach a toxic level if nitroprusside is used at high doses for prolonged periods, especially in patients with impaired renal clearance. Cyanide causes intracellular hypoxia by blocking cellular use of oxygen in the electron transport chain. Manifestations of hypoxia such as confusion, tachycardia, anxiety, and lactic acidosis are present despite an adequate blood oxygen level.

Prostacyclin (Flolan), also known as *epoprostenol* and *PGI*$_2$, initially was used as a pulmonary vasodilator to treat idiopathic pulmonary hypertension. Infused through an implantable pump, prostacyclin effectively lowers pulmonary artery pressures, relieving strain on the right ventricle. This treatment has been demonstrated to improve function, quality of life, and life expectancy.[44]

Opiates The opiates are natural and synthetic derivatives of morphine, which is derived from the opium poppy. By stimulating mu (μ), delta (δ), and kappa (κ) opiate receptors in the brain and spinal cord, they diminish the sensation of pain. In addition to their powerful analgesic qualities, opiates are potent **sedatives,** meaning that they decrease the level of consciousness. Opiates are also excellent cough suppressants. Although as a class they are probably equivalent in their **antitussive** effect, codeine is by far the most commonly used narcotic for this indica-tion, being one of the active ingredients in the cough syrup Robitussin AC.

One of the important hazards of narcotic use is their ability to depress the central respiratory drive, resulting in hypoventilation, even apnea and death. Narcotics occasionally are used for this respiratory depressant effect to suppress the sensation of dyspnea in patients with chronic dyspnea that is unrelieved by other therapies or in patients with terminal pulmonary disease who essentially are dying of suffocation. In this role morphine and fentanyl are more commonly used. Narcotics generally are given orally or intravenously. Twice-daily formulations of morphine (MS Contin) and oxycodone (OxyContin) are available. Fentanyl is available in a once-weekly patch. Other side effects of narcotics include decreased mental status and constipation (narcotics are powerful antidiarrheal drugs). Narcotic overdose can be temporarily reversed by administration of naloxone (Narcan).

The opiates have a high addictive potential, which has severely limited their use, especially for chronic pain. This is of less concern in the terminally ill, and reticence to use narcotics to relieve pain in these patients is decreasing. It currently is believed that if opiates are used only to the extent needed to relieve active pain, addiction is uncommon.

Other Sedatives Examples of benzodiazepines include lorazepam (Ativan), diazepam (Valium), and midazolam (Versed). The benzodiazepines are called **anxiolytics** because they tend to suppress anxiety. They act as agonists at the γ-aminobutyric acid (GABA) receptors of the central nervous system. In addition to anxiolysis, benzodiazepines cause sedation and amnesia and raise the seizure threshold. Adverse effects include hypotension and oversedation. Benzodiazepines can cause respiratory depression, but their tendency to do so is much less than that of the opioids. Because of their lipophilicity and resulting large volume of distribution, even short-acting benzodiazepines can persist for long periods after repeated or continuous dosing. Benzodiazepines can be competitively reversed with flumazenil (Romazicon).

A relatively new sedative, propofol (Diprivan), can be readily identified by its opaque white color because it is packaged as a lipid emulsion. Because propofol is packaged in preservative-free lipid, bacterial contamination can occur if strict aseptic technique is not observed. Propofol has a rapid onset and short duration, even after prolonged infusion, which makes it highly desirable and can justify its relatively high cost in patients with CNS disease, because propofol allows these patients to be quickly and briefly awakened on a regular basis to asses their mental status. Major adverse effects of propofol are hypotension, bradycardia, hyperlipidemia, and respiratory depression. The use of propofol in patients who are not intubated currently is controversial. Some early events led many institutions to limit its use to intubated patients, but experience with the drug is increasing, and it is being used more often for well-supervised, spontaneously breathing patients.

Examples of phenothiazines include haloperidol (Haldol) and droperidol (Inapsine). These medications initially were used in the treatment of schizophrenia and other psychiatric diseases, but they have proved quite useful as anxiolytics and sedatives. Their primary advantage lies in the fact that they cause less hypotension than other sedatives and do not cause respiratory depression in therapeutic doses. The phenothiazines are also effective **antiemetics** (drugs that reduce nausea). Serious side effects are uncommon; the most problematic is the acute dystonic reaction, which may be treated with a centrally acting anticholinergic (other than ipratropium), such as diphenhydramine (Benadryl).

Important to note is that none of these drugs has analgesic properties; therefore they should always be used in combination with an analgesic (usually a narcotic) when a patient is exposed to painful conditions such as intubation, indwelling catheters, and trauma. This type of combination therapy generally results in synergism between the analgesic and the sedative, reducing the dose requirement of both.

Neuromuscular Blockers

Neuromuscular blockers are also known as *paralytic agents* and *muscle relaxants*. They fall into two classes, depolarizing and nondepolarizing, which have opposite molecular actions but a similar clinical result: flaccidity and paralysis of all skeletal (striated) muscles, including the diaphragm and all accessory respiratory musculature.

Striated muscle is activated by motor nerves that meet the muscle (synapse) at the motor endplate. Motor nerves are *cholinergic*, which means that they transmit their signal by releasing acetylcholine at the motor endplate. Nicotinic cholinergic receptors are present on the endplate, and when stimulated by acetylcholine, they act through direct ligand-gated channels to cause electrical depolarization of the muscular cell membranes. Depolarization causes a calcium influx to the muscle cells, leading to muscle contraction. Acetylcholine, meanwhile, is cleared from the motor endplate receptors by cholinesterase, opening the receptors to receive new signals.

A single depolarizing neuromuscular blocker, succinylcholine, has been approved in the United States. The drug binds to and stimulates nicotinic cholinergic receptors on the motor endplate; this causes muscle cell depolarization and contraction, an event observed as *fasciculations*, or brief twitches, which pass through the patient approximately 45 seconds after administration of the drug. Succinylcholine is much less susceptible than acetylcholine to cholinesterase, however, and remains bound to the receptors for approximately 10 minutes. This state of sustained depolarization renders the muscles unresponsive to any further stimuli, therefore paralyzed and flaccid.

The advantages of succinylcholine are its rapid onset and short duration. However, the drug is contraindicated in patients with a head injury, hyperkalemia, or rhabdomyolysis, because the fasciculations caused by depolarization tend to increase intracranial pressure and can cause further muscle damage, with the release of potassium into the blood.

Several nondepolarizing neuromuscular blockers are available, which differ primarily in duration of action. The earliest of these was curare, which was used on arrowheads to enhance lethality; it is used today in the form tubocurarine. This group of neuromuscular blockers also includes vecuronium, pancuronium, cisatracurium, and rocuronium. The nondepolarizing agents essentially are competitive antagonists of the nicotinic cholinergic receptors of the motor endplate. Their onset of action (~2 to 3 minutes) is slower than that of succinylcholine and gradual. They also have longer durations; the shortest-acting is rocuronium, (effective duration 15 minutes), although attempts are being made to produce an extremely short-acting agent.

The neuromuscular blockers are used primarily in three situations. They are used to facilitate intubation; by relaxing the thoracic and jaw muscles, these drugs allow the patient to be more easily bag-valve-mask ventilated and prevent biting and gagging as the endotracheal tube is inserted. They also are used during surgery, especially of the abdomen, when muscle relaxation facilitates surgical exposure. The third common use is during mechanical ventilation of tenuous patients who are poorly synchronized with the ventilator ("bucking the vent") or who have high airway pressures. Relaxation of the respiratory muscles abolishes dyssynchrony, reducing chest wall recoil and therefore airway pressure.

Paralysis clearly is a valuable aid to difficult mechanical ventilation in some cases. However, sustained neuromuscular blockade should be undertaken only with extreme caution and trepidation. Because the patient is rendered unable to participate at all in ventilation, the care team suddenly assumes full responsibility for all the patient's needs. The ventilator minute ventilation should be matched to the overall minute ventilation before paralysis, and care must be taken that the patient is fully sedated to avoid conscious paralysis, an extremely uncomfortable sensation. Neuromuscular agents, especially used in conjunction with corticosteroids, have been implicated as a cause of critical illness polyneuropathy, a profound acute weakness that occurs after severe illness.[45]

Lidocaine

Nebulized lidocaine, a topical anesthetic, is used routinely to prepare patients who are not intubated for bronchoscopy. By anesthetizing the larynx and airways, lidocaine reduces gag and cough during the procedure. For intubated patients, similar results are achieved by instilling 1% lidocaine as a liquid via the endotracheal tube. Lidocaine also has antiinflammatory properties and has been investigated for maintenance use in asthma; this use remains experimental. Lidocaine overdose produces decreased mental status and methemoglobinemia.

$\mathscr{K}$EY $\mathscr{P}$OINTS

- Pharmacology is the science that describes drugs and their interactions with the body.
- Pharmacokinetics describes how the body moves a drug through the processes of absorption, distribution, and elimination.
- Pharmacodynamics describes the drug's action on the body at a molecular level and in terms of overall clinical effect.
- Most drugs produce their effects by interacting with a receptor.
- Potency refers to the amount of drug necessary to achieve a given effect.
- Efficacy refers to the maximum achievable effect a drug is able to produce.
- An indication is the condition for which a drug is given.
- A contraindication is a condition that makes the use of a drug unfavorable.
- A side effect is any drug effect other than the primary intended therapeutic effect.
- Toxicity is a harmful biologic effect caused by a substance.
- Allergy is an immune-mediated hypersensitivity reaction.
- Smooth muscle tone is regulated by mediators.
- The primary adrenergic receptor in the lungs is the β_2 subtype.
- Cholinergic receptors are primarily stimulated by cholinergic nerves of the parasympathetic nervous system.
- Corticosteroid receptors are found throughout the lungs.

- Most respiratory medications are delivered through the inhalation route.
- The major classes of bronchodilators are adrenergic agonists, anticholinergic agents, and methylxanthines.
- The major classes of antiinflammatory drugs are corticosteroids, nonsteroidal antiinflammatory drugs (NSAIDs), cromones, and leukotriene inhibitors.
- Antihistamines are commonly used to reduce the volume of secretions, especially upper airway secretions, associated with upper respiratory infections and allergies.
- Acetylcysteine and dornase alfa are used as mucolytic agents.
- Instilled surfactant is used in the treatment of neonatal respiratory distress syndrome.
- Applications of inhaled antimicrobial drugs include antipseudomonal antibiotics in cystic fibrosis, pentamidine prophylaxis in HIV-positive patients, and ribavirin for respiratory syncytial virus.
- Diuretics stimulate urine production.
- Vasopressors are used to increase blood pressure.
- Inotropic agents are not highly effective at raising blood pressure.
- Vasodilators reduce blood pressure.
- Opiates diminish the sensation of pain and can be used as cough suppressants.
- Benzodiazepines are called *anxiolytics* because they tend to suppress anxiety.
- Neuromuscular blockers are also known as *paralytic agents* and *muscle relaxants.*

References

1. Benet LZ, Mitchell JR, Sheiner LB. Pharmacokinetics: the dynamics of drug absorption, distribution, and elimination. In: Gilman AG, editor. The pharmacological basis of therapeutics. 8th ed. New York: Pergamon Press; 1990.
2. Arky R. Physician's desk reference. 51st ed. Montvale, NJ: Medical Economics; 1999.
3. Ross EM. Pharmacodynamics: mechanisms of drug action and the relationship between drug concentration and effect. In: Gilman AG, editor. The pharmacological basis of therapeutics. 8th ed. New York; Pergamon Press; 1990.
4. American Medical Association: AMA Drug Evaluations Annual: 1992. Chicago: American Medical Association; 1992.
5. Rang HP, Dale MM. Adrenergic transmission. In: Pharmacology. 2nd ed. Edinburgh: Churchill Livingtone; 1991.
6. Adcock IM, Gilbey T, Gelder CM, et al. Glucocorticoid receptor localization in normal human lung and asthmatic lung. Am J Respir Crit Care Med 1996;154:771-782.
7. Lin RY, Pesola GR, Bakalchuk L, et al. Rapid improvement of peak flow in asthmatic patients treated with parenteral methylprednisolone in the emergency department: a randomized controlled study. Ann Emerg Med 1999;33:487-494.
8. Lin RY, Pesola GR, Westfal RE, et al. Early parenteral corticosteroid administration in acute asthma. Am J Emerg Med 1997;15:621-625.
9. Haynes RC. Adrenocorticotropic hormone; adrenocortical steroids and their synthetic analogues; inhibitors of the synthesis and actions of adrenocortical hormones. In: Gilman AG, editor. The pharmacological basis of therapeutics. 8th ed. New York: Pergamon Press; 1990.
10. Yates DH, Kharitonov SA, Barnes PJ. An inhaled glucocorticoid does not prevent loss of protection against salmeterol. Am J Respir Crit Care Med 1996;154:1603-1607.
11. Rau JL. Inhaled adrenergic bronchodilators: historical development and clinical application. Respir Care 2000;45:854-863.
12. Campbell SC. Clinical aspects of inhaled anticholinergic therapy. Respir Care 2000;45:864-867.
13. Brown JH. Atropine, scopolamine, and related antimuscarinic drugs. In: Gilman AG. The pharmacological basis of therapeutics. 8th ed. New York: Pergamon Press; 1990.
14. Rall TW. Drugs used in the treatment of asthma: the methylxanthines, cromolyn sodium, and other agents. In: Gilman AG, editor. The pharmacological basis of therapeutics. 8th ed. New York: Pergamon Press; 1990.

15. Reed CE, Offord KP, Nelson HS, et al. Aerosol beclomethasone dipropionate spray compared with theophylline as primary treatment for chronic mild to moderate asthma. The American Academy of Allergy, Asthma, and Immunology Beclomethasone Dipropionate-Theophylline Study Group. J Allergy Clin Immunol 1998;101:14-23.

16. Evans DJ, Taylor DA, Zetterstrom O, et al. A comparison of low-dose inhaled budesonide plus theophylline and high-dose inhaled budesonide for moderate asthma. N Engl J Med 1997;337:1412-1418.

17. Manser R, Reid D, Abramson M. Corticosteroids for acute severe asthma in hospitalised patients. Cochrane Database of Systematic Reviews 2000;1(2) [http://www.update-software.com/abstracts/ab001740.htm].

18. Emerman CL, Cydulka RK. A randomized comparison of 100-mg versus 500-mg dose of methylprednisolone in the treatment of acute asthma. Chest 1995;107:1559-1563.

19. Marquette CH, Stach B, Cardot E, et al. High-dose and low-dose systemic corticosteroids are equally efficient in acute severe asthma. Eur Respir J 1995;8:22-27.

20. Niewoehner DE, Erbland ML, Deupree RH, et al. Effect of systemic glucocorticoids on exacerbations of chronic obstructive pulmonary disease. Department of Veterans Affairs Cooperative Study Group. N Engl J Med 1999;340:1941-1947.

21. Rice KL, Rubins JB, Lebahn F, et al. Withdrawal of chronic systemic corticosteroids in patients with COPD: a randomized trial. Am J Respir Crit Care Med 2000;162:174-178.

22. Meduri GU, Headley AS, Golden E, et al. Effect of prolonged methylprednisolone therapy in unresolving acute respiratory distress syndrome: a randomized controlled trial. JAMA 1998;280:159-165.

23. Colice GL. Comparing inhaled corticosteroids. Respir Care 2000;45:846-853.

24. Sharek PJ, Bergman DA. The effect of inhaled steroids on the linear growth of children with asthma: a meta-analysis. Pediatrics 2000;106:E8.

25. Baraniuk J, Murray JJ, Nathan RA, et al. Fluticasone alone or in combination with salmeterol versus triamcinolone in asthma. Chest 1999;116:625-632.

26. Smith LJ. Leukotrienes in asthma: the potential therapeutic role of antileukotriene agents. Arch Intern Med 1996;156:2181-2189.

27. Israel E, Cohn J, Dube L, et al. Effect of treatment with zileuton, a 5-lipoxygenase inhibitor, in patients with asthma. JAMA 1996;275:931-936.

28. Laitinen LA, Nay IP, Binks S, et al. Comparative efficacy of zafirlukast and low-dose steroids in asthmatics on prn β_2-agonists. Eur Respir J 1997;10:4195.

29. Dahlen B, Nizankowska E, Szczeklik A, et al. Benefits from adding the 5-lipoxygenase inhibitor zileuton to conventional therapy in aspirin-intolerant asthma. Am J Respir Crit Care Med 1998;157:1187-1194.

30. Wechsler ME, Finn D, Gunawardena D, et al. Churg-Strauss syndrome in patients receiving montelukast as treatment for asthma. Chest 2000;117:708-713.

31. Stirling RG, Chung KF. Leukotriene antagonists and Churg-Strauss syndrome: the smoking gun. Thorax 1999;54:865-866.

32. Kay AB, Walsh GM, Moqbel R, et al. Disodium cromoglycate inhibits activation of human inflammatory cells in vitro. J Allergy Clin Immunol 1987;80:1-8.

33. Murphy S, Kelly HW. Cromolyn sodium: a review of mechanisms and clinical use in asthma. Drug Intelligence and Clinical Pharmacy 1987;21:22-35.

34. North American Tilade Study Group. A double-blind, multi-center-group comparative study of the efficacy and safety of nedocromil sodium in the management of asthma. Chest 1990;97:1299-1306.

35. Lal S, Dorow PD, Venho KK, et al. Nedocromil sodium is more effective than cromolyn sodium for the treatment of chronic reversible obstructive airway disease. Chest 1993;104:438-447.

36. Fuloria M, Rubin BK. Evaluating the efficacy of mucoactive aerosol therapy. Respir Care 2000;45:868-873.

37. Cummings J, Holm B, Hudak M, et al. A controlled clinical comparison of four different surfactant preparations in surfactant-deficient preterm lambs. Am Rev Respir Dis 1992;145:999-1004.

38. O'Riordan TG. Inhaled antimicrobial therapy: from cystic fibrosis to the flu. Respir Care 2000;45:836-845.

39. Hicks RA, Olson LC, Jackson MA, et al. Precipitation of ribavirin causing obstruction of a ventilation tube. Pediatr Infect Dis 1986;5:707-708.

40. Eisenberg RJ, Oatnay WH. Nebulization of amphotericin B. Am Rev Respir Dis 1971;103:289-292.

41. Riley DK, Pavia AT, Beatty PG, et al. The prophylactic use of low-dose amphotericin B in bone marrow transplant patients. Am J Med 1994;97:509-514.

42. Conneally E, Cafferkey MT, Daly PA, et al. Nebulized amphotericin B as prophylaxis against invasive aspergillosis in granulocytopenic patients. Bone Marrow Transplant 1990;5:403-406.

43. Dubois J, Bartter T, Gryn J, et al. The physiologic effects of inhaled amphotericin B. Chest 1995;108:750-753.

44. Barst TRJ, Rubin LJ, Long WA, et al. A comparison of continuous intravenous epoprostenol (prostacyclin) with conventional therapy for primary pulmonary hypertension. The Primary Pulmonary Hypertension Study Group. N Engl J Med 1996;334:296-302.

45. Larsson L, Li X, Edstrom L, et al. Acute quadriplegia and loss of muscle myosin in patients treated with nondepolarizing neuromuscular blocking agents and corticosteroids: mechanisms at the cellular and molecular levels. Crit Care Med 2000;28:34-45.

PART III

Assessment of the Patient with Respiratory Impairment

CHAPTER 19

History and Physical Examination

Priscilla Simmons

CHAPTER OUTLINE

Creating a Therapeutic Climate
Components of the Health History
    Chief Complaint
    History of Present Illness
    Occupational and Environmental History
    Geographic Exposure
    Activities of Daily Living
    Smoking History
    Cough and Sputum Production
    Family History
    Medical History
    Review of Systems
Vital Signs

Techniques of Assessment
    Inspection
    Palpation
    Percussion
    Auscultation
Physical Examination of the Lungs and Thorax
    Inspection
    Palpation
    Percussion
    Auscultation
    Signs of Respiratory Distress
Assessment of Other Body Systems
    The Heart and Blood Vessels
    The Neurologic System

OBJECTIVES

1. Discuss the factors essential in the creation of a therapeutic climate.
2. Explain three considerations of an effective health history.
3. Explain the relevance of cultural diversity in the history-taking process.
4. List the major components of a health history.
5. Identify the four major examination techniques.
6. Define common terms used in assessment of the respiratory system.
7. Explain the technique for auscultation of the chest.
8. Define terms associated with normal and abnormal breath sounds.
9. List the signs associated with respiratory distress.
10. Identify common pathologic processes of the respiratory system and pertinent physical findings that extend to other body systems.
11. Identify the significance of various chest landmarks.
12. Explain the significance of sounds heard during cardiac auscultation.
13. Explain the significance of jugular venous distention.
14. Explain common findings associated with an assessment of the neurologic system.

KEY TERMS

Auscultation	Clubbing	Hyperresonant
Barrel Chest	Crackles	Hyperventilation
Biot's Respirations	Cyanosis	Inspection
Bradypnea	Dyspnea	Jaundice
Bronchial Breath Sounds	Egophony	Kussmaul's Respirations
Bronchophony	Flail Chest	Kyphosis
Cheyne-Stokes Breathing	Hyperpnea	Lordosis

KEY TERMS—cont'd

Murmur	Pectus Excavatum	Scoliosis
Orthopnea	Percussion	Stridor
Pack Years	Platypnea	Tachypnea
Pallor	Plethora	Tactile Fremitus
Palpation	Pleural Friction Rub	Tympanic
Paradoxical Respiration	Precordium	Vesicular Breath Sounds
Paroxysmal Nocturnal Dyspnea	Resonant	Wheezes
Pectus Carinatum	Rhonchi	Whispered Pectoriloquy

This chapter provides a guide to essential assessment techniques used by the respiratory therapist. In the hospital many members of the health care team examine the patient. In the community setting, however, fewer members of the health care team assess the patient, thereby warranting a more thorough examination by the respiratory therapist. Whatever the setting, no clinician regularly uses all the available assessment techniques. In fact, some techniques are rarely used. The emphasis of this chapter is on the pathophysiology underlying common respiratory abnormalities and the typical assessment findings associated with them.

Creating a Therapeutic Climate

The patient's perception of the respiratory therapist's competence is of prime importance. When any health care provider is perceived as being uncaring, the patient may remember that attitude most vividly. Even worse, that poor image may come to characterize for the patient all the members of the profession. To ensure a therapeutic, professional relationship, competence and caring must coexist. A practitioner can communicate caring through a gentle demeanor and an unhurried, unabrupt manner. Maintaining eye contact is essential. Also appropriate is the judicious use of touch, such as patting or squeezing a patient's hand or shoulder. Respiratory therapists should dress appropriately because a professional appearance communicates respect for the patient. A patient's judgment of a health care provider often is based on physical appearance. These measures help establish rapport and a climate of professional caring, a goal in every professional relationship.

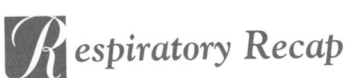

espiratory Recap

Variables Supporting a Therapeutic Climate	
Caring demeanor	Judicious use of touch
Competence	Professional image
Eye contact	

Components of the Health History

The health history provides a detailed, chronologic health record of the patient. It elicits information regarding variables affecting the patient's health status to develop an individualized plan of care. The value of the history should not be underestimated because it guides the selection of appropriate physical examination techniques and helps the respiratory therapist develop an accurate index of suspicion. Because obtaining a comprehensive history is time consuming, many health care providers primarily assess the body systems of concern. Clearly, the heart and lungs are the systems of primary interest for respiratory therapists.

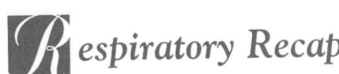

espiratory Recap

The Health History	
Chief complaint	Smoking history
History of present illness	Cough and sputum production
Occupational and environmental history	Family history
Geographic exposure	Medical history
Activities of daily living	Review of systems

Chief Complaint

The chief complaint (CC) is the problem or concern that prompted the patient to seek health care. When documenting the CC in the patient record, the examiner should use the patient's own words in quotation marks.

History of Present Illness

The history of present illness (HPI) is the chronologic, narrative account of the patient's health problem. It should describe in detail information relevant to the CC, including a description of the onset of the problem—the date the symptoms occurred and whether they developed gradually or suddenly—and the setting in which they developed. Also included is a description of the signs and symptoms associated with the problem. The mnemonic

OLD CART can help the examiner gather information accordingly, as follows:

Onset (when the problem started)

Location of pain, shortness of breath, or other symptoms

Duration of pain, shortness of breath, or other symptoms

Character, quantity, and quality of pain; shortness of breath; or other symptoms

Associated manifestations (the setting in which the pain, shortness of breath, or other symptoms developed)

Relieving factors or factors that diminish or aggravate the pain, shortness of breath, or other symptoms

Treatment (any medications or other remedies that relieve or exacerbate shortness of breath)

*R*espiratory Recap

History of Present Illness	
Onset	Associated manifestations
Location	Relieving factors
Duration	Treatment
Character	

Occupational and Environmental History

The examiner should inquire as to whether the patient is employed, retired, or laid off. Are current or past hazards at work, such as exposure to asbestos, coal dust, silica, molds, dust, or animals? Is the patient under stress at work? Is the patient satisfied with the job?

Geographic Exposure

Has the patient traveled to foreign countries? Has the patient been in military service?

Activities of Daily Living

Has the patient experienced difficulty with or change in the ability to provide self-care?

Smoking History

How long has the patient smoked cigarettes? This answer is usually expressed in **pack years** and is calculated as follows. A pack a day for 1 year is known as *one pack year*. Two packs a day for a year is *two pack years*, and so on. What is the patient's willingness to quit? The examiner should also inquire as to whether the patient smokes a pipe, cigars, or illicit drugs, such as marijuana or crack cocaine.

Cough and Sputum Production

The examiner should ask about the presence of cough and sputum. If the patient has a cough, the timing of the cough (for example, in the morning, at night, after eating) and whether sputum is produced should be noted. If sputum is produced, the examiner should determine its amount, consistency, color, and odor, as well as whether the frequency of the cough and the amount of sputum have increased recently.

Family History

Any family history of genetically transmitted disease, cancer, heart disease, tuberculosis (TB), or human immunodeficiency virus (HIV) should be noted.

Medical History

Dates of past health problems, hospitalizations, symptoms, and treatment should be noted in the history, as well as whether the problem is ongoing, resolved, or recurrent. Are immunizations current? Does the patient have any food, drug, insect, or environmental allergies?

Review of Systems

A review of the symptoms provides the opportunity for the examiner to systematically question the patient about the health of each body system. It differs from the physical examination in that the data are collected verbally. A thorough review of each system is unnecessary, but the examiner should include a detailed review of the systems affected by the present illness. If the patient answers with a negative response, a denial of that specific complaint should be noted. For example, "Patient denies pain with deep inspiration and coughing."

Vital Signs

Pulse, respirations, and blood pressure are considered *vital signs*. These are commonly measured, along with body temperature, as indicators of the patient's health status. The pulse rate and rhythm can be measured by cardiac auscultation or palpation of any artery, with the radial artery being that most commonly used for this purpose. The pulse is counted for a minimum of 15 seconds and then mathematically adjusted to the rate per minute. The normal pulse rate for adults is 60 to 100 beats per minute; the rate is more rapid for infants and children. The respiratory rate is measured by inspection of the movement of the chest for 1 minute. The normal respiratory rate for adults is 12 to 20 breaths per minute; it is more rapid for infants and children. Blood pressure is measured either with a sphygmomanometer or an indwelling arterial catheter. Normal blood pressure for adults is 120/80 mm Hg; measurements are lower for infants and children. Body temperature can be

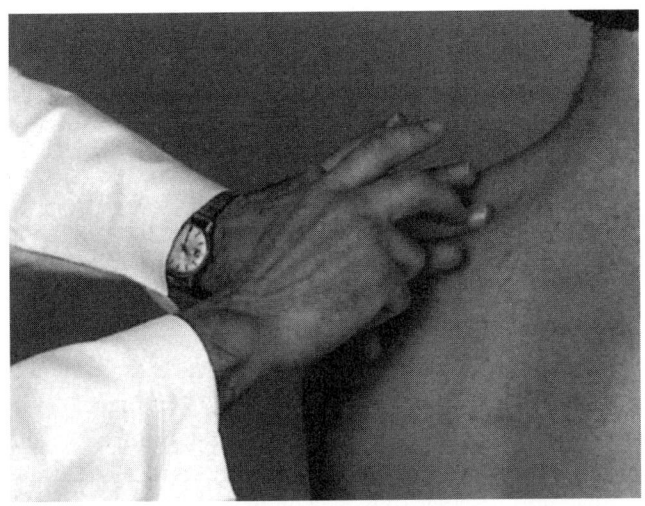

Figure 19-1 Percussion technique. (From Seidel HM, Ball JW, Dains JE, et al. Mosby's guide to physical examination. 4th ed. St Louis: Mosby; 1999.)

measured via the oral, rectal, axillary, or tympanic sites. Normal body temperature is 37° C. The term *fever* refers to a higher-than-normal body temperature (hyperthermia), whereas hypothermia is a temperature lower than normal.

Age-Specific Angle

Compared with adults, infants and children have higher respiratory rates, higher pulse rates, and lower blood pressure readings.

Techniques of Assessment

Inspection

As an examination technique, **inspection** ranges from casual observation to visual scrutiny of the patient.

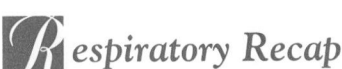espiratory Recap

Respiratory Assessment Techniques	
Inspection	Percussion
Palpation	Auscultation

Palpation

Palpation is the process whereby the examiner uses the hands to feel for body movement, lumps, masses, and skin characteristics. Palpation can be either light or deep.

Percussion

Percussion requires the examiner to place a finger firmly against a body part and strike that finger with a fingertip

from the other hand. The technique for the right-handed examiner is as follows:

1. Hyperextend the middle finger of the nondominant hand (pleximeter finger).
2. Press the distal interphalangeal joint firmly on the surface to be percussed. Avoid contact with any other part of the hand because vibrations may be dampened.
3. Hold the forearm of the other arm close to the surface, with the hand turned up at the wrist, and partially flex the middle finger (plexor).
4. Strike the pleximeter with the tip of the plexor with a quick, sharp, and relaxed wrist motion and aim at the distal interphalangeal joint (Figure 19-1). Withdraw briskly to avoid dampening the vibrations. Use one to two blows at each location.

The resulting sounds can suggest either normal underlying tissue or typical sounds associated with given abnormalities.

Five percussion tones (Table 19-1) are commonly recognized—flat, dull, resonant, hyperresonant, and tympanic. A flat percussion note is soft, high-pitched, and of short duration. It may be elicited by percussion of the thigh. A dull percussion note is of medium intensity, pitch, and duration. It is heard over the liver or a tumor. A **resonant** note is loud, low in pitch, and of long duration. It may be heard over normal lung tissue. A **hyperresonant** note is very

espiratory Recap

Percussion Notes	
Flat	Hyperresonant
Dull	Tympanic
Resonant	

*T*ABLE 19-1

Characteristics of Percussion Notes

Type of Tone	Intensity	Pitch	Duration	Quality
Flat	Soft	High	Short	Extremely dull
Dull	Medium	Medium-high	Medium	Thudlike
Resonant	Loud	Low	Long	Hollow
Hyperresonant	Very loud	Very low	Longer	Booming
Tympanic	Loud	High	Medium	Drumlike

From Seidel HM, Ball JW, Dains JE, et al. Mosby's guide to physical examination. 4th ed. St Louis: Mosby; 1999.

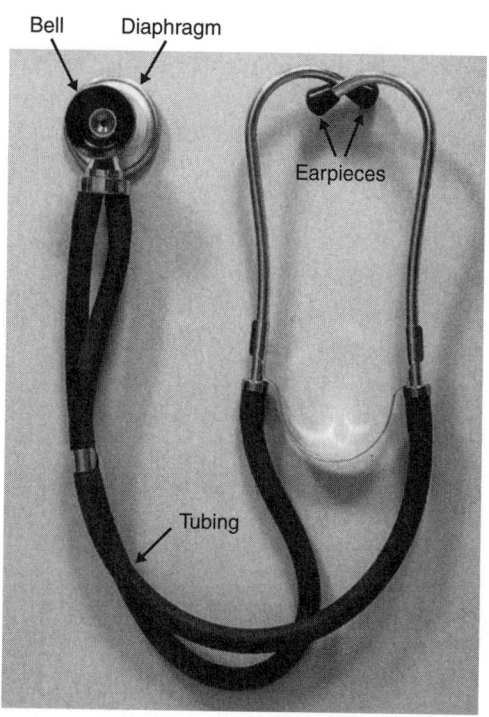

Figure 19-2 Stethoscope, illustrating the diaphragm and bell. (From Seidel HM, Ball JW, Dains JE, et al. Mosby's guide to physical examination. 4th ed. St Louis: Mosby; 1999.)

loud, lower in pitch, longer in duration, and commonly heard over an emphysematous lung. A **tympanic** note is loud and drumlike, with a high pitch. It may be heard over a gastric bubble.

Auscultation

After inspection, **auscultation** is the most commonly used physical assessment technique, particularly for assessment of the respiratory system. Auscultation involves listening to body sounds with a stethoscope placed on bare skin. The stethoscope has several important components (Figure 19-2). The diaphragm is the larger side of the stethoscope head and is made of rigid plastic. The bell is the smaller cup on the other side of the head and is covered with a plastic

or rubber ring. The bell is useful for detection of certain cardiac and vascular sounds. The diaphragm is used more frequently. Note that both adult and pediatric diaphragms and bells exist, with the latter being smaller. Some stethoscopes come with interchangeable parts. The examiner should ensure that the appropriate sizes are being used.

Quality stethoscopes have thick, heavy, and stiff tubing that conducts sound better than thinner, lighter, and more elastic tubing. An appropriate tubing length is 12 to 18 inches. Both soft and hard earpieces are available; either type is acceptable, providing the devices fit snugly and comfortably. The earpieces must point toward the nose of the examiner to project sound toward the tympanic membrane of the examiner's ears.

Physical Examination of the Lungs and Thorax

The astute examiner is thoroughly familiar with human anatomy. An in-depth knowledge of structure and function is vital to the interpretation of assessment findings in terms of underlying pathologic processes. Thoracic landmarks and the surface anatomy of the chest are illustrated in Figure 19-3.

Inspection

Observing Respirations   The examiner must be familiar with common respiratory patterns (Figure 19-4).

*R*espiratory Recap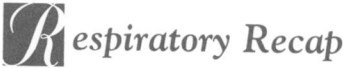

Patterns of Respiration	
Tachypnea	Orthopnea
Hyperpnea	Paroxysmal nocturnal
Kussmaul's respirations	dyspnea
Bradypnea	Cheyne-Stokes respirations
Dyspnea	Biot's respirations
Platypnea	

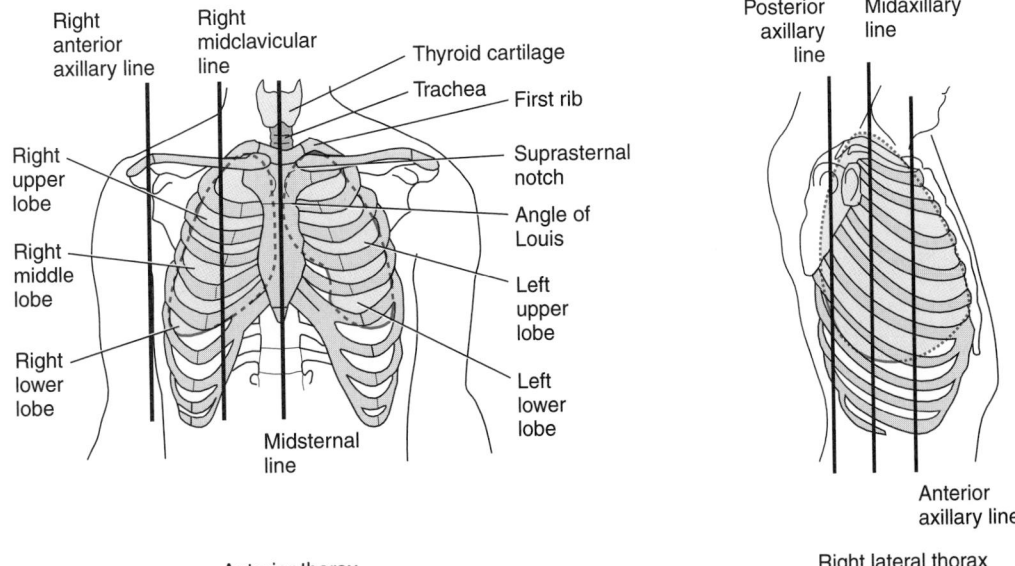

Right anterior axillary line

Right midclavicular line

Thyroid cartilage

Trachea

First rib

Right upper lobe

Suprasternal notch

Right middle lobe

Angle of Louis

Left upper lobe

Right lower lobe

Left lower lobe

Midsternal line

A

Anterior thorax

Posterior axillary line

Midaxillary line

Anterior axillary line

Right lateral thorax

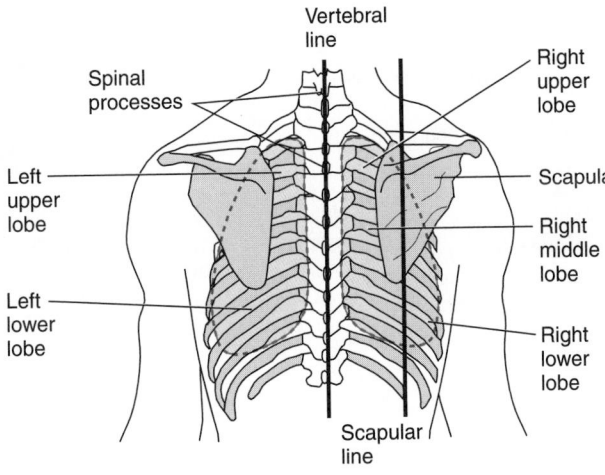

Vertebral line

Spinal processes

Right upper lobe

Left upper lobe

Scapula

Right middle lobe

Left lower lobe

Right lower lobe

Scapular line

Posterior thorax

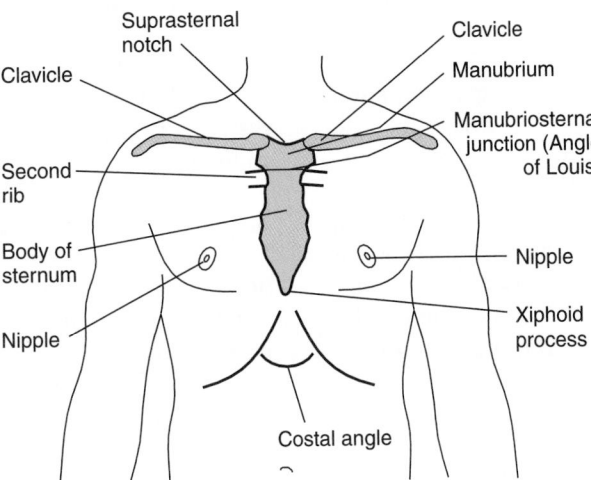

B

Suprasternal notch

Clavicle

Clavicle

Manubrium

Manubriosternal junction (Angle of Louis)

Second rib

Body of sternum

Nipple

Nipple

Xiphoid process

Nipple

Costal angle

Figure 19-3 **A,** Thoracic landmarks. **B,** Topographic landmarks of the chest.

Continued

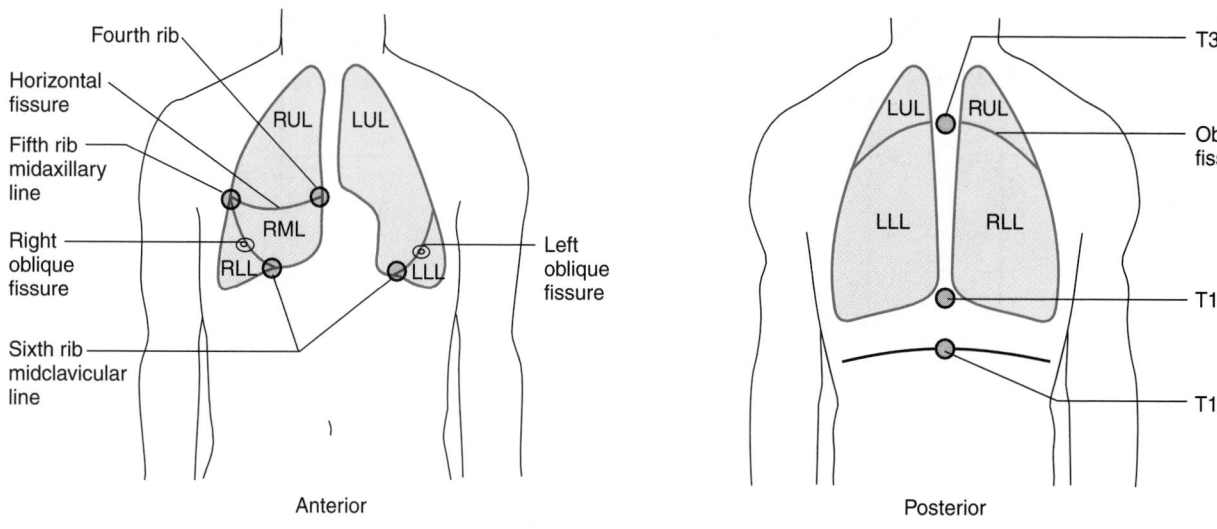

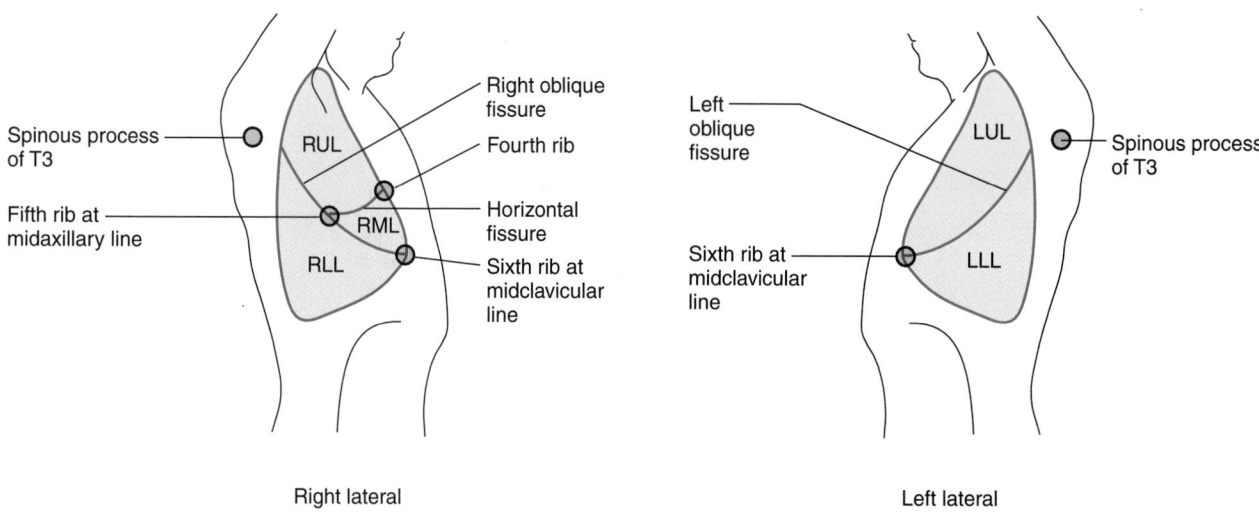

Figure 19-3—cont'd   **C,** Surface anatomy of the thorax.

Tachypnea describes a persistent rate of respiration faster than 20 breaths per minute. It may be present in individuals who are hypoxemic and those who have pain in the thoracic region. Similarly, if liver enlargement or abdominal distention compromises diaphragmatic movement, tachypnea may result. At times, however, tachypnea is merely a patient response to the realization that respirations are being observed and counted. Tachypnea also occurs in individuals with fever and in those with restrictive ventilatory defects, such as pulmonary fibrosis or pneumonectomy.

Hyperpnea describes breathing that is rapid, deep, and labored. If it results in a lowered P_{CO_2}, **hyperventilation** is the term that applies. **Kussmaul's respirations** describe hyperventilation as a compensatory mechanism for metabolic acidosis, most commonly diabetic ketoacidosis. Conversely, **bradypnea** is a rate slower than 12 breaths per minute. It may suggest neurologic impairment or acid-base disturbance but may be a normal finding in physically fit individuals.

Dyspnea is a term that simply means difficult or labored breathing, with the individual feeling short of breath. **Platypnea** refers to an individual's difficulty in breathing unless lying flat. **Orthopnea** indicates that an individual must sit or stand to breathe. Many individuals with chronic lung disease must assume an upright position to breathe well. Such individuals often find it more comfortable to sleep in a chair. **Paroxysmal nocturnal dyspnea** is characterized by sudden shortness of breath that occurs several hours after the individual lies down. It commonly suggests cardiac dysfunction in that the heart is unable to adequately pump a circulatory volume expanded by fluid reabsorbed from the legs, which became edematous during the day.

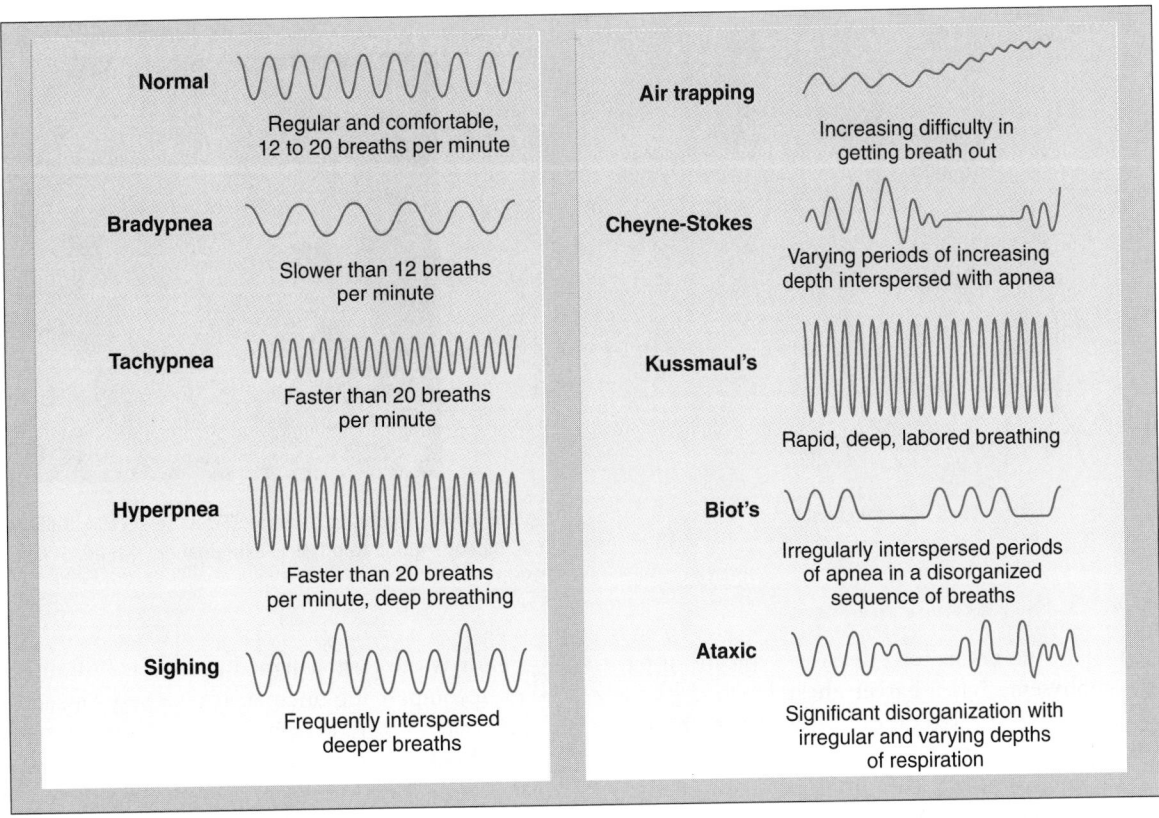

Figure 19-4   Patterns of respiration. (Modified from Seidel HM, Ball JW, Dains JE, et al. Mosby's guide to physical examination. 4th ed. St Louis: Mosby; 1999.)

Cheyne-Stokes breathing is characterized by episodes of slow, shallow breaths, which rapidly increase in depth and rate. This crescendo-decrescendo pattern is followed by periods of apnea. Such breathing may be a normal variant in young children and the elderly. Otherwise, it occurs in individuals with cerebral disease and congestive heart failure.

Biot's respirations are symptomatic of elevated intracranial pressure and meningitis. This breathing pattern is characterized by a short burst of uniform, deep respirations, followed by periods of apnea lasting 10 to 30 seconds.

Use of Accessory Muscles

Muscles of the back, neck, and abdomen are known as *accessory muscles* of respiration. Although they play a relatively minor role in normal respiration, their function becomes more prominent during exercise or respiratory distress. Use of accessory muscles implies an increased work of breathing.

Retractions suggest a barrier to inspiration, occurring anywhere along the respiratory tract. To overcome this barrier, the respiratory muscles contract more vigorously, resulting in a more negative intrapleural pressure. Retractions resemble a "sucking in" of structures, such as the intercostal spaces, suprasternal space, and subclavian spaces. In such a situation, the examiner documents that the patient "has retractions," "is retracting," or "is using accessory muscles."

Nasal Flaring and Pursed-Lip Breathing

Individuals in respiratory distress commonly exhibit nasal flaring, presumably in an attempt to decrease the resistance to airflow through the nostrils. Those with emphysema commonly use pursed lips during the expiratory phase to control expiratory flow.

Flail Chest and Paradoxical Respiration

Flail chest is a term describing the appearance of a thorax with multiple rib fractures, causing instability of the chest wall. In this situation the chest wall moves outward on expiration and inward on inspiration. This movement, which is contrary to normal chest movement, is known as **paradoxical respiration.** Flail chest with paradoxical respiration indicates a serious injury and will result in hypoxia if left untreated.

The chest and abdomen also should move in synchrony during the respiratory cycle. Paradoxical inward movement of the abdomen during the inspiratory phase indicates diaphragmatic weakness associated with paralysis. Paradoxical inward movement of the chest wall during inspiration indicates paralysis of the chest wall muscles, as may occur with high thoracic spine injury or low cervical spine injury.

Shape of the Chest

The examiner should observe the shape of the patient's chest. Abnormalities of the thorax

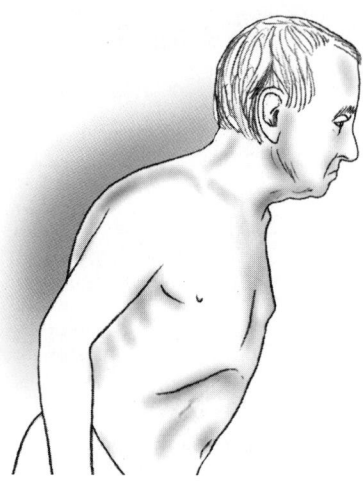

Figure 19-5   Barrel chest.

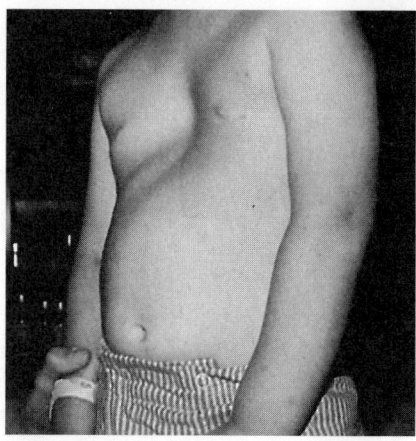

Figure 19-6   Pectus excavatum. (From Seidel HM, Ball JW, Dains JE, et al. Mosby's guide to physical examination. 4th ed. St Louis: Mosby; 1999.)

can be significant factors in lung disease. Typically, a patient with emphysema has a **barrel chest** (shaped like a barrel; Figure 19-5). The lateral diameter of the chest is normally twice the anteroposterior diameter. With a barrel-shaped chest configuration, the anteroposterior diameter is equal to the lateral diameter. Although obstructive lung disease causes this characteristic change in chest configuration, certain other abnormalities of thoracic shape result in restrictive lung disease. **Pectus excavatum,** or a funnel-shaped sternum, describes a sternum that is depressed and deviated somewhat like a funnel (Figure 19-6). Similarly, **pectus carinatum,** or a pigeon-breasted sternum, describes a chest that bows out at the sternum, similar to that of a pigeon. These abnormalities in thoracic configuration may result in lung disease as the patient ages. **Scoliosis,** for instance, causes lateral curvature of the spine, **kyphosis** causes forward curvature of the spine, and **lordosis** causes backward curvature of the spine (Figure 19-7).

The examiner also should note whether the trachea is in the midline of the neck. A tension pneumothorax causes tracheal deviation from the affected lung. Atelectasis or lung resection causes the trachea to be deviated toward the affected side.

Skin Color   The color of the patient's skin should be noted. Although several abnormalities in skin color exist, **cyanosis** is of prime significance to the respiratory therapist. When hemoglobin is poorly saturated with oxygen, the skin assumes a bluish hue, which is initially apparent in the nailbeds. Cyanosis may be present normally in the nailbeds of a person who is vasoconstricted as a result of exposure to cold temperatures. Cyanosis also may be noted in the mucous membranes of the mouth; this site is of particular use in the assessment of individuals with dark skin. Cyanosis also can appear around the mouth (circumoral). In healthy children, circumoral cyanosis is quite common, particularly when they are cold. The significance of cyanosis must be evaluated in light of other clinical findings.

Pallor is the term assigned to describe diminished skin color accompanying anemia. It also may be seen in individuals with severe peripheral vasoconstriction accompanying shock. Detecting pallor is easier in lighter-skinned individuals, but the color of darker skin also appears more pale when the individual is in shock.

ℛespiratory Recap

Skin Color Abnormalities	
Cyanosis	Plethora
Pallor	Jaundice

Plethora is the term describing the fullness of blood vessels at the skin surface. Plethora may occur with vasodilation and may be present in individuals who are hypercapnic. **Jaundice** is the yellowish skin color arising from an elevated serum bilirubin level. Any disorder resulting in bile being retained in the liver ultimately causes jaundice. Jaundice is first apparent in the sclera of the eyes.

Clubbing of Fingers   Clubbed fingers result from enlargement of the distal phalanges and develop as a compensatory mechanism when an individual has chronic hypoxia, such as with congenital heart defects or chronic lung disease. The appearance of **clubbing** is exactly as the term implies; the finger distal to the base of the nail looks like a small club (Figure 19-8). Affected fingertips appear full, fleshy, and vascular. Clubbing is associated with lung tumors, bronchiectasis, cystic fibrosis, congenital heart disease, and liver and gastrointestinal disease; it is hereditary in some cases. However, clubbing does *not* occur in conjunction with chronic obstructive pulmonary disease.

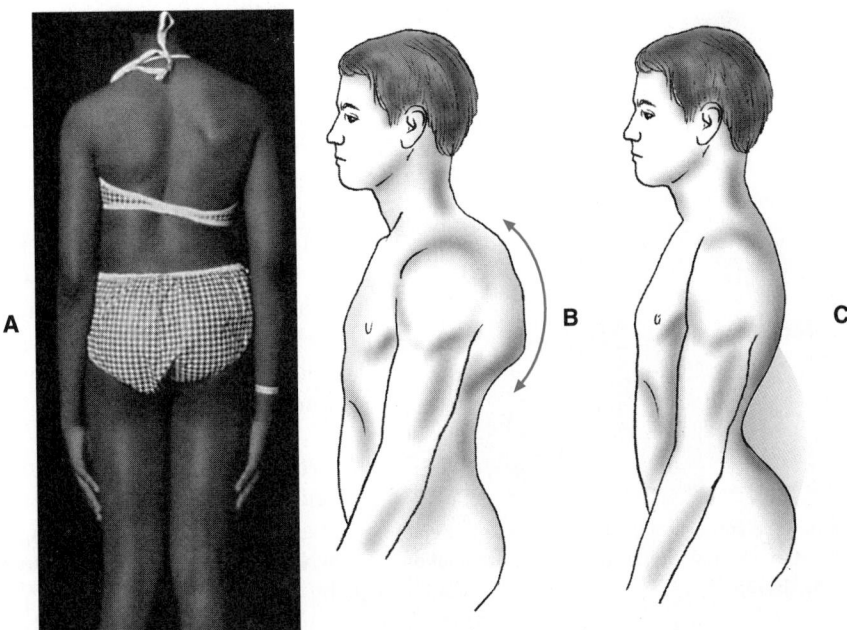

Figure 19-7   A, Scoliosis. **B,** Kyphosis. **C,** Lordosis (**A,** From Seidel HM, Ball JW, Dains JE, et al. Mosby's guide to physical examination. 4th ed. St Louis: Mosby; 1999.)

Palpation

Subcutaneous Emphysema   Subcutaneous emphysema is the presence of air in the subcutaneous tissues of the neck, chest, and face. The tissues may be painful and appear swollen. In addition, a crackling or popping sound may be auscultated when a stethoscope is placed over the tissue. An examiner also may detect subcutaneous emphysema by palpating bubbles as the finger pads are rolled over the affected areas.

Respiratory Expansion   The assessment of respiratory expansion is used primarily to determine whether the lungs are expanding symmetrically. Asymmetry of expansion may be present with a pneumothorax, atelectasis, lung resection, or main stem intubation. To perform this examination, the examiner places the thumbs along each costal margin at the back. The hands then are slid medially to raise loose skin folds between the thumbs. The patient is asked to inhale deeply, and the examiner notes the range and symmetry of respiratory expansion by observing how the skin fold spreads out.

Tactile Fremitus   **Tactile fremitus** is defined as the palpation of vibrations of the chest wall as a patient speaks. To elicit these the examiner presses the bony part of a palm at the base of the fingers against the patient's chest wall. The patient is asked to repeat the words *ninety-nine* or *one-one-one*. When the lungs are healthy, vibrations are barely palpable. When the lung tissue is consolidated, however, vibrations are increased. In the patient with large amounts of secretions in the airways, palpation of the fremitus that is produced may be possible as gas flows past the secretions.

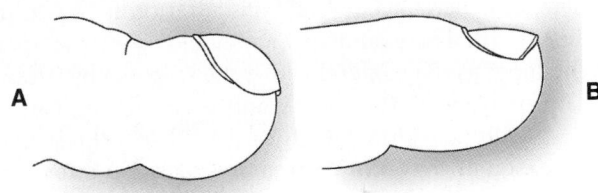

Figure 19-8   A, Clubbing of the finger. **B,** Normal digit.

Percussion

Chest percussion can be used to elicit several abnormal findings. With a pneumothorax or emphysema, the affected hemithorax produces a hyperresonant or tympanic percussion note. With consolidation, pleural effusion, or atelectasis, the percussion note is dull or flat. A useful application of percussion is to determine diaphragmatic excursion. The difference in posterior, dependent resonance between maximum inhalation and maximum exhalation represents diaphragmatic excursion (Figure 19-9). Diaphragmatic excursion is affected by emphysema, pneumothorax, pleural effusion, atelectasis, consolidation, phrenic nerve injury, and diaphragmatic weakness.

Auscultation

The stethoscope is the most frequently used instrument in respiratory assessment and yields valuable information about the status of the lungs. Because the lower lobes of the lungs are posterior in the thorax, complete ausculta-

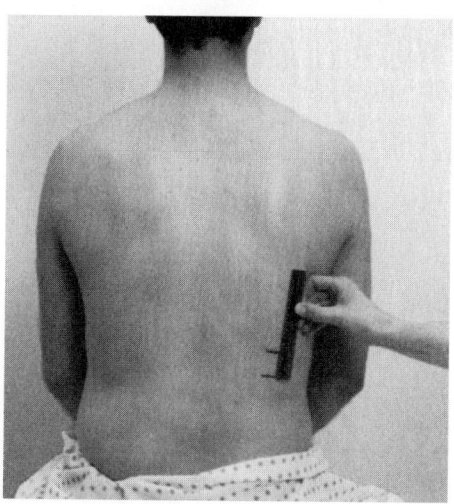

Figure 19-9 Measuring diaphragmatic excursion. (From Seidel HM, Ball JW, Dains JE, et al. Mosby's guide to physical examination. 4th ed. St. Louis: Mosby; 1999.)

tion of breath sounds through the anterior chest wall is impossible. Therefore examiners should avoid the temptation to auscultate only the anterior chest wall because of its easy accessibility. Auscultation of the posterior chest wall generally yields more useful information.

The sequence for lung field auscultation is shown in Figure 19-10. The examiner first should assess the apex of the lungs as they extend above the scapulae by listening on one side of the thorax and then moving to the corresponding area on the other side. Below the scapulae the examiner continues to move back and forth, listening to corresponding areas on both sides and comparing the sounds. Sounds generated by normal lungs differ according to location in the respiratory system (Table 19-2).

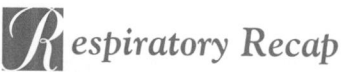

Respiratory Recap

Auscultation
Intensity of breath sounds
Presence of bronchial breath sounds
Presence of adventitious breath sounds: crackles, rhonchi, wheezes, stridor, pleural friction rubs

Intensity of Breath Sounds

Breath sounds may be reduced in individuals with a number of conditions. They can be diffusely decreased with shallow breathing or with the hyperinflation and decreased airflow that occurs with hyperinflation (for example, emphysema or acute asthma). Localized diminished breath sounds occur with airway obstruction, atelectasis, and main stem intubation. Decreased breath sounds at the lung bases are commonly associated with postoperative atelectasis.

Characteristics of Normal Breath Sounds

Bronchial breath sounds are heard over the trachea, at the manubrium anteriorly, and between the scapulae posteriorly. These breath sounds are louder and higher in pitch. Expiratory sounds are as long or slightly longer than the inspiratory component. Bronchovesicular breath sounds are heard over the junction between the bronchi and alveoli. Anteriorly, the sounds occur in the first and second interspaces between the ribs. Inspiratory and expiratory phases are equally long. **Vesicular breath sounds** are heard over the lung periphery, where the alveoli are located. These sounds are characteristically soft and low-pitched, and inspiration lasts longer than expiration.

Characteristics of Abnormal Breath Sounds

Bronchial breath sounds heard over the periphery of the lungs suggest consolidation of lung tissue. Consolidation occurs when lung tissue that is normally aerated is "made solid" by filling with fluid, mucus, pus, or cellular debris. Consequently, sounds generated by air movement through the bronchi resonate more clearly to pulmonary regions where only vesicular or bronchovesicular sounds are normally heard.

Other sounds typical of consolidation are the so-called voice sounds—bronchophony, egophony, and whispered pectoriloquy. **Bronchophony** is elicited when the examiner asks the patient to say the words *ninety-nine*. Normally, this sound is muffled, but when heard over consolidated lungs, the words are clearly audible. Similarly, **egophony** is elicited when the patient is asked to say the letter *e* and it sounds like *a* over consolidated lungs. **Whispered pectoriloquy** can be evoked when the patient is asked to whisper the numbers *1,2,* and *3*. Normally this sound is soft, but with lung consolidation, it is clearly audible.

Crackles

Crackles or rales (pronounced *rawls* although many clinicians say *rails*) are commonly heard adventitious, or abnormal, breath sounds (Figure 19-11). Crackles are discontinuous sounds usually heard at the end of inspiration; they are fine in quality and high pitched. Crackles result when the terminal airways pop open late in inspiration because fluid or secretions have accumulated. Consequently, crackles are heard most often over the lung bases.

Crackles are a common finding in individuals with congestive heart failure. In this condition, fluid accumulates in the interstitial spaces between the capillaries and alveoli. As the condition worsens, the fluid fills the alveoli. Initially the crackles are heard in the bases of the lungs. Crackles that ascend higher up the lung fields are related to an increasing degree of congestive heart failure. In cases of pneumonia, crackles are heard over the involved lobe. In some individuals who have remained supine for long periods, crackles may be auscultated in the dependent areas of the lung and will subsequently clear when the patient coughs.

Rhonchi

The definition of a *rhonchus* (singular), or **rhonchi** (plural) is subject to some debate. To a certain

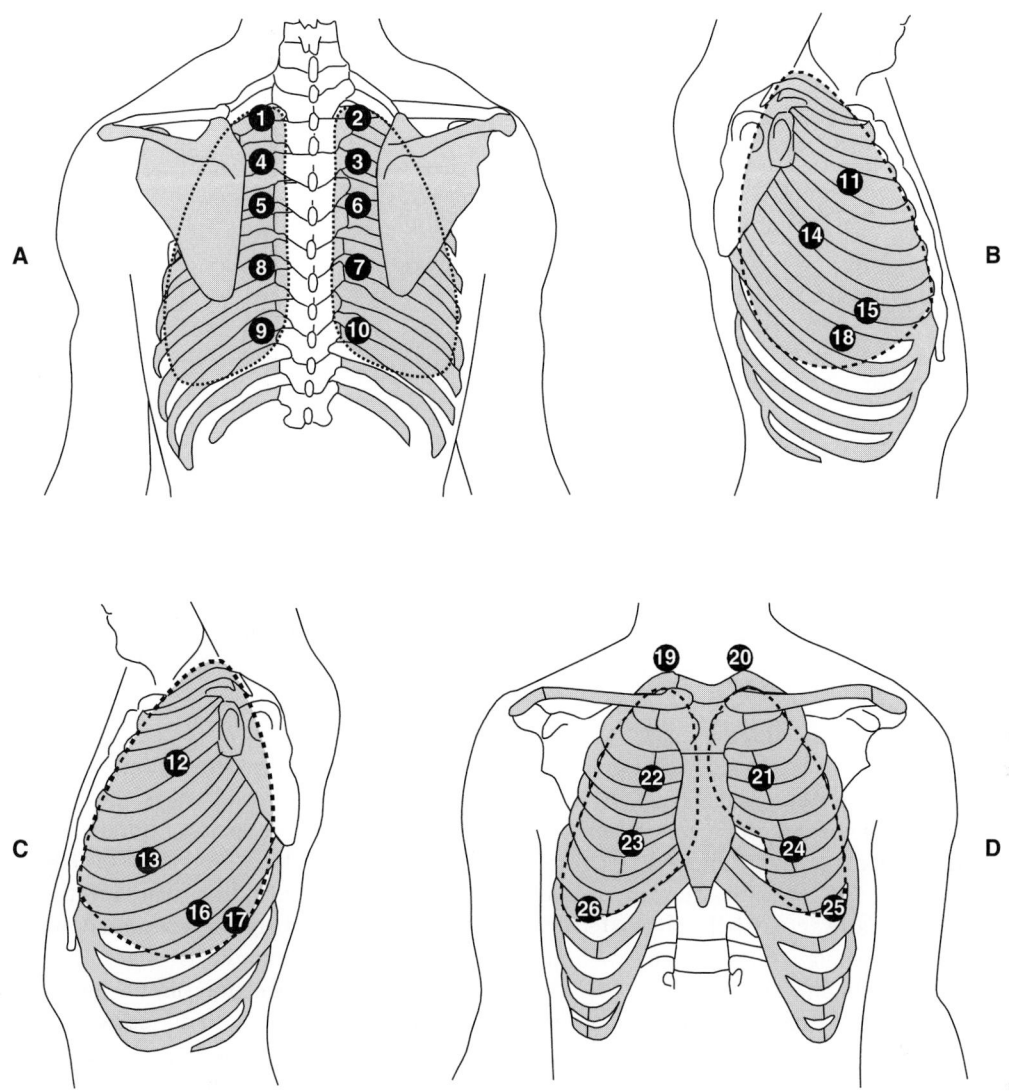

Figure 19-10   Suggested sequence for systematic percussion and auscultation of the thorax from the posterior **(A)**, right lateral **(B)**, left lateral **(C)**, and anterior **(D)** views.

TABLE 19-2

Lung Sounds Assessed by Auscultation

Sound	Characteristics	Findings
Vesicular	Heard over most of lung fields; low pitch; soft and short expirations; accentuated in thin person or child and diminished in overweight or very muscular individuals	
Bronchovesicular	Heard over main bronchus area and upper right posterior lung field; medium pitch; expiration equaling inspiration	
Bronchial/tracheal (tubular)	Heard only over trachea; high pitch; loud and long expirations, often somewhat longer than inspiration	

From Seidel HM, Ball JW, Dains JE, et al. Mosby's guide to physical examination. 4th ed. St Louis: Mosby; 1999.

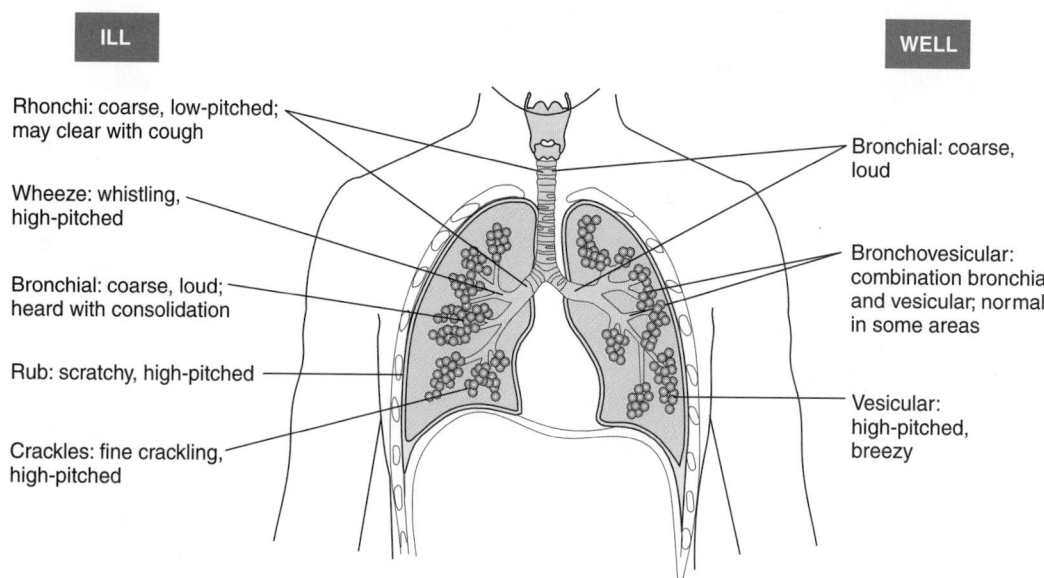

Figure 19-11   Breath sounds noted in the ill and well patient.

degree the use of the term varies among clinical practice sites. However, the American Thoracic Society (ATS) has defined *rhonchi* as being deeper, rumbling sounds that are more pronounced on expiration. These sounds are more likely to be continuous. Generally, they are caused by air passing through an airway partially obstructed by thick secretions, spasm of the airways, or presence of a tumor. Higher-pitched or sibilant rhonchi arise in the smaller bronchi, such as is the case of asthma. Lower-pitched, sonorous, or snoring rhonchi are more commonly heard in association with thick secretions in the larger airways. At times the rumbling may be palpable through the chest wall.

Wheezes   Considering that the definition of rhonchi overlaps with the generally accepted description of wheezes, there may be some confusion about terminology. During lung auscultation an examiner may detect some overlap in breath sounds. In addition, the definition of wheezes is similar to the description of sibilant rhonchi.

Wheezes may be either high or low in pitch. High-pitched wheezes are often called *sibilant* wheezes. They are musical or whistling in nature, caused by air passing through narrowed airways, such as in the bronchospasm of asthma (reactive airway disease). Most often, sibilant wheezes are heard on expiration, although they may be heard throughout the respiratory cycle. Although wheezes are most often associated with asthma, wheezes also can be present in individuals with other conditions, such as congestive heart failure and foreign body aspiration.

Stridor   **Stridor** is a crowing sound commonly caused by inflammation and edema of the larynx and trachea. It may be heard after extubation, when tracheal damage has occurred with resultant edema. Stridor is commonly associated with croup in children and frequently is accompanied by a barking cough. Usually, stridor is a nocturnal assessment finding related to the possible development of edema in the upper airway when a child is in a dependent position during sleep. Mouth-breathing related to nasal congestion often causes a thickening of secretions that further compounds the stridor. The constellation of findings includes improvement of symptoms with air humidification. Taking the child outside into the cool night air may be an effective intervention. If the child does not improve, however, the stridor must be evaluated further because of the danger of airway obstruction.

Age-Specific Angle

Stridor is associated with croup in children.

Pleural Friction Rubs   A **pleural friction rub** is a continuous grating sound such as is audible when two pieces of leather are rubbed together. Another analogy is that a friction rub sounds as though the palms of both hands are sliding against each other. This sound is produced when the visceral and parietal pleurae become inflamed and no longer glide silently against each other during the respiratory cycle. Consequently, the sound is localized and exists only over the area of pleural irritation. Pleural friction rubs may be intermittent.

TABLE 19-3

Physical Findings of Respiratory Diseases

Condition	Percussion Note	Fremitus	Breath Sounds	Adventitious Sounds
Normal	Resonant	Normal	Vesicular	None
Left heart failure	Resonant	Normal	Vesicular	Rales, occasionally wheezes
Pleural effusion	Dull or flat	Decreased	Decreased or absent	None or pleural rub
Consolidation	Dull	Increased	Bronchial	Rales, rhonchi, egophony
Bronchitis	Resonant	Normal or decreased	Prolonged exhalation	Wheezes, rales, rhonchi
Emphysema	Hyperresonant	Decreased	Decreased or absent	None
Pneumothorax	Hyperresonant	Decreased	Decreased or absent	None
Atelectasis	Dull	Decreased	Decreased or bronchial	None or rales
Asthma	Resonant or hyperresonant	Normal or decreased	Vesicular	Wheezes
Pulmonary fibrosis	Resonant	Normal	Vesicular	Rales

Modified from Chatburn RL, Lough MD. Handbook of respiratory care. 2nd ed. Chicago: Year-Book; 1990.

Pleural friction rubs may accompany a pleural effusion—the accumulation of fluid in the usually empty pleural cavity. The cause of pleural effusion includes malignant seeding of metastatic tumors onto the pleural linings. Pleural friction rubs also may be heard in individuals with infectious processes involving the pleural cavity. After thoracic surgery, residual blood in the pleural cavity eventually becomes sludge and may irritate the pleurae, resulting in a friction rub.

Signs of Respiratory Distress

Common physical findings of pulmonary diseases are shown in Table 19-3.

Assessment of Other Body Systems

The respiratory system interfaces with all other organ systems. Consequently, evaluation of the respiratory system does not occur in an assessment vacuum. The following discussion highlights assessment techniques used to monitor the heart, blood vessels, and brain.

The Heart and Blood Vessels

Location and Significance of Various Chest Landmarks

Counting Ribs   The chest wall overlying the heart is known as the **precordium.** Each heart valve is auscultated best by placement of the stethoscope in a specific location on the precordium. To do so, the cartilaginous structures, known as *interspaces*, lying between the ribs must be located, first by identification of the clavicle. (Note that the space under the clavicle does not count as an interspace.) Next, the first rib should be identified. The cartilage under the first rib is the first interspace. Counting the ribs is done by movement of the fingers down from each rib to the corresponding interspace. The second interspace is important for assessment of the semilunar valves.

The accuracy of the counting process may be verified as in the following way. The ridge of bone that is the joint between the manubrium and sternum, known as the *sternal angle* or *Angle of Louis*, must be identified. The interspace to either side immediately below the sternal angle is the second interspace. On the posterior thorax the spinous processes of the vertebrae are useful landmarks. The spinous process of the seventh cervical vertebra (C7) is identified when the patient extends the head and neck forward and down. The most prominent spinous process is C7, directly below which is the first thoracic vertebra (T1).

A thorough cardiac auscultation involves systematic movement of the stethoscope over the precordium. First, the base of the heart should be auscultated, namely the aortic and pulmonic valves. The aortic valve is assessed in the second interspace to the right of the sternal border, where it is heard best because the valve "points" in that direction (Figure 19-12). The stethoscope then is moved to the second interspace at the left sternal border, the best location for assessment of pulmonic valve function. All other assessments occur on the left side of the sternum. The tricuspid valve is heard at the fifth interspace at the left sternal border, and the mitral valve is assessed where the fifth interspace intersects the midclavicular line. The mitral valve, or apical area, is not only useful as a landmark but also provides other useful information. This relatively small left ventricular apex is the area where the left ventricle protrudes from behind the right ventricle, known as the *point of maximal impulse (PMI)*. The left ventricle taps gently against an area of the thoracic wall no more than 2 cm in diameter (Figure 19-13). Left ventricular hypertrophy may be the cause of an enlarged PMI.

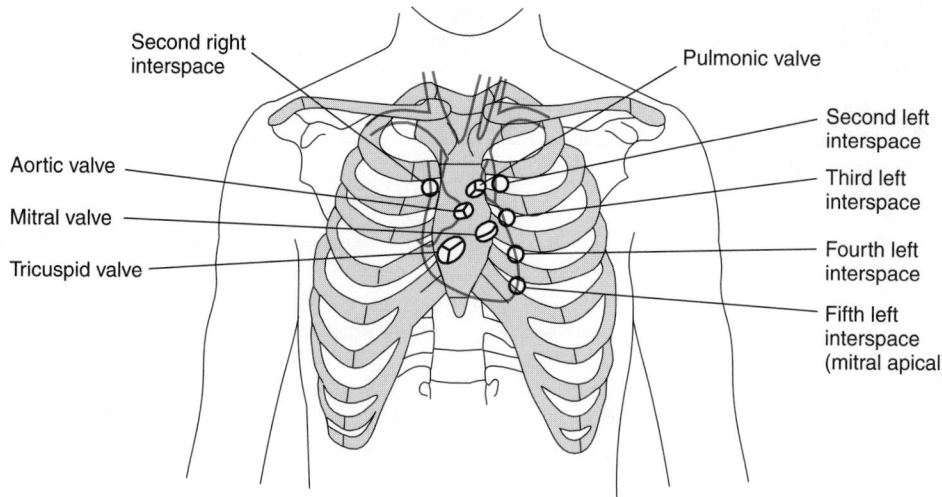

Figure 19-12   Areas for auscultation of the heart.

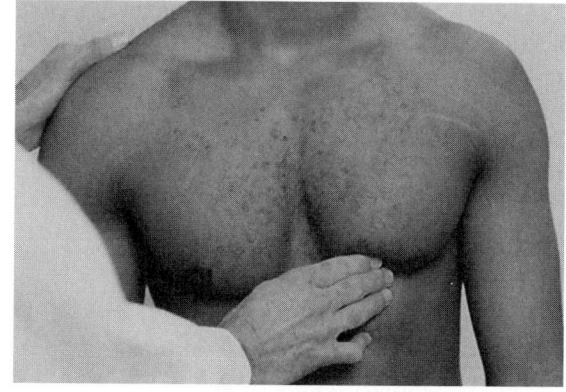

Figure 19-13   Palpation of the apical pulse. (From Seidel HM, Ball JW, Dains JE, et al. Mosby's guide to physical examination. 4th ed. St Louis: Mosby;1999.)

Cardiac Auscultation   Listening to heart sounds involves notations of rate and rhythm, extra heart sounds, and murmurs. Heart rate and rhythm should be observed first. A regular rhythm with a rate between 60 to 100 beats per minute is ideal; however, certain irregularities represent harmless variants. Conversely, other irregularities may herald serious consequences. Auscultation used to determine rate and rhythm is done with the stethoscope at the apex of the heart, a procedure commonly known as *taking an apical rate.*

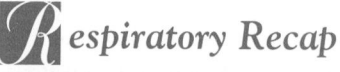 espiratory Recap

Cardiac Auscultation
Heart rate and rhythm
Extra sounds
Murmurs

S_1 and S_2   Normal heart sounds are classified as S_1 and S_2. S_1 is the first heart sound and results from closure of

the atrioventricular (mitral and tricuspid) valves. S_1 is also known as *lub*. As the ventricles eject most of their blood, ventricular pressure drops below aortic pressure, resulting in closure of the aortic and pulmonic valves, which in turn produces S_2, or the second heart sound, also known as *dub*.

A normal variant may be auscultated with the stethoscope at the second interspace along the left sternal border. In many individuals, a "split S_2" may be heard here during inspiration, a sound that occurs when pulmonic valve closure happens a few milliseconds after closure of the aortic valve. Typically, this action takes place during inspiration, as increasing intrathoracic pressure causes blood to impact the pulmonic valve with greater force.

S_3 and S_4 S_3 and S_4 are extra sounds generated by certain aberrant blood flow mechanisms. These sounds are best heard at the left fifth intercostal space at the midclavicular line, also known as the *mitral,* or *apical, area.* An S_4 immediately precedes the S_1, and the S_3 follows immediately after the S_2. These rhythms are commonly called *gallops* because of their resemblance to the sound of a horse galloping. To auscultate for either an S_3

or an S_4, the bell of a stethoscope is pressed lightly against the skin. Pressing too firmly obliterates the sounds. The S_3 and S_4 are heard best with the patient in a left–side-lying position.

An S_3 results from rapid ventricular filling. When ventricular pump failure occurs, an increased amount of residual blood remains in the heart chambers after a contraction. Consequently, the ventricles fill faster during diastole. This pumping of blood into an already partially filled ventricle causes vibrations heard as an S_3. An S_3 occurs immediately after the S_2. It resembles a split S_2 but differs in location. A split S_2 is heard in the pulmonic area, whereas the S_3 is heard at the apex.

An S_4 is a sound caused most often by a stiff ventricle, such as may be the case in hypertension or after a myocardial infarction. For an S_4 to be present, an atrial contraction must occur. Consequently, this heart sound is often known as an *atrial gallop*. An S_4 cannot exist in the presence of atrial fibrillation, a condition in which the atria do not contract. The vibrations causing an S_4 are thought to be due to atrial contraction occurring in the presence of a stiff or noncompliant ventricle. The S_4 precedes the S_1.

Murmurs

A simple description of a cardiac **murmur** is an extra sound heard in conjunction with S_1 and S_2. Several mechanisms describe the etiology of murmurs. Murmurs occur when blood regurgitates back into the chamber from which it came. Sometimes valvular dysfunction develops as a sequela to rheumatic heart disease after infection with β-hemolytic streptococci. This syndrome results in valves that are distorted in shape and calcified.

Other murmurs arise when a large volume of blood flows through a valve, such as occurs during pregnancy, anemia, or hyperthyroidism. Murmurs also result from blood flowing through a narrowed or stenotic valve. A final category of murmurs arises from congenital defects resulting in blood flow through openings not normally present.

Classification of Murmurs

Murmurs are classified as early, middle, or late systolic—that is, occurring between S_1 and S_2. Others are diastolic, coming between S_2 and the next S_1. The intensity of murmurs is graded between I and VI and is recorded in Roman numerals. A grade I murmur is very faint and may not be heard in all positions. Generally, a highly trained ear is required for detection of this sound. Murmurs that are grades II through IV increase progressively in intensity, with a grade V murmur being very loud. A grade VI murmur may be heard without the stethoscope in contact with the chest.

Murmurs differ in quality and are described as blowing, rasping, harsh, coarse, grating, whistling, or musical. In addition, they are classified according to the location at which the sound is loudest. This location corresponds to the area of the precordium where the valve in question is best auscultated, such as the fifth interspace midclavicular line or mitral area.

Murmurs and Subacute Bacterial Endocarditis

Many murmurs are classified as functional, innocent, or physiologic, meaning that they are clinically insignificant. Others are significant in that they suggest a progressive pathologic process that may eventually require surgical intervention. Some murmurs signify a defect that requires prophylaxis against subacute bacterial endocarditis (SBE), which is caused by bacteria lodging on defective valves and colonizing there. This colonization results in "vegetation" that grows on valves and interferes with efficient hemodynamics. Another danger exists if the vegetation breaks off and the resulting emboli lodge elsewhere in the body. The bacteria then reproduce in that location. *SBE prophylaxis* is the term given to antibiotic therapy administered before any invasive or surgical procedure, including dental work. Innocent or physiologic murmurs require no SBE prophylaxis; however, innocence can be determined only by echocardiogram. Diastolic murmurs—those occurring between S_1 and S_2—suggest the need for SBE prophylaxis.

Jugular Venous Distention

The inspection component of a cardiac assessment primarily involves observation of the right internal jugular vein, the vessel that reflects pressure changes better than other superficial veins. Oscillations in this vein reflect changing pressures within the right atrium. Similarly, distention of this neck vein suggests a distended right ventricle, which often suggests right ventricular failure. Distended neck veins are normal in an individual in the supine position. Furthermore, neck veins fill temporarily with any activity that raises intrathoracic pressure, such as coughing, conversing, or bearing down (the Valsalva maneuver). To assess pathologic processes, the following technique is used to determine the degree of jugular venous distention. The patient is placed in a supine position, with the head of the bed at a 45-degree angle (Figure 19-14). With a centimeter ruler, the vertical distance between the sternal angle and the highest level of jugular vein pulsation then is measured on both sides. Neck veins, which fill to a level of 2 cm or less, are considered normal. More than this level suggests increased right ventricular pressure and is associated with right-sided heart failure.

The Neurologic System

Because of the system's complexity, an assessment of the neurologic system can be daunting. This brief summary focuses on the most common neurologic abnormalities.

Level of Consciousness

When a patient experiences an alteration in the level of consciousness, because of trauma or some other hypoxic or metabolic event, the Glasgow Coma scale (Table 19-4) is commonly used. This scale uses a numeric scoring method to document eye-opening response, verbal response, and integrated motor response. Scores range from a low of 3 points, which sug-

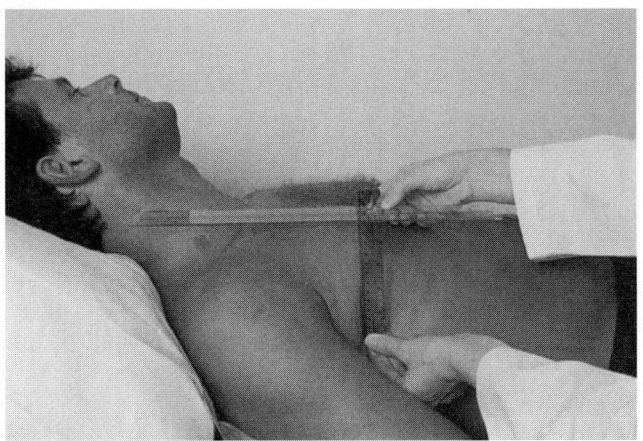

Figure 19-14 Technique used to measure jugular venous pressure. (From Seidel HM, Ball JW, Dains JE, et al. Mosby's guide to physical examination. 4th ed. St Louis: Mosby; 1999.)

TABLE 19-4
Glasgow Coma Scale

Observation	Score
Eye Opening	
Spontaneous	4
In response to voice	3
In response to pain	2
None	1
Verbal Response	
Oriented response	5
Confused response	4
Inappropriate words	3
Incomprehensible words	2
None	1
Motor Response	
Obeys commands	6
Localizes	5
Withdraws	4
Flexes (decorticate)	3
Extends (decerebrate)	2
None	1

TABLE 19-5
Ramsay Sedation Scale

Level	Response
1	Anxious, agitated, restless
2	Cooperative, oriented, tranquil
3	Responding to commands only
4	Asleep, brisk response to stimulus
5	Asleep, sluggish response to stimulus
6	Unarousable

cause sleep is itself a decreased level of consciousness, it is important to distinguish between normal sleep or a state suggesting a serious pathologic condition, such as is the case in carbon dioxide narcosis or respiratory failure. In critically ill, mechanically ventilated patients, sedation and decreased level of consciousness are often pharmacologically induced. The level of sedation in these patients is often assessed with the Ramsay Score (Table 19-5).

Posturing Patients with neurologic injury may demonstrate decerebrate or decorticate posturing (Figure 19-15). Decerebrate posturing may result from a painful stimulus of a comatose patient with a low-level brain stem compression. The patient responds with extension and internal rotation of the arms and extends the legs. Decorticate posturing results when a painful stimulus is applied to a comatose patient with a lesion in the mesencephalic region of the brain. In response to the stimulus, the patient rigidly flexes the arms at the elbows and wrists. The legs may be flexed as well.

Pupillary Dilation Pupillary dilation (Figure 19-16) can occur with cerebral edema and brain stem compression, whereas either dilation or constriction of the pupils also can be associated with the administration of some medications.

gests brain death, to a maximum of 15 points, which indicates full consciousness.

Other indications of neurologic integrity are normality and equality of strength in all extremities. Clearly, any less-than-normal finding suggests impairment and warrants full evaluation. Pupils may be evaluated for size, equality, reaction to light, and accommodation. Normal reactivity is documented as *PEARLA* or *pupils equal and reacting to light and accommodation*. However, although pupillary assessment is commonly performed, abnormalities in size and reaction are a late finding and may indicate significant brain dysfunction.

A decreasing level of consciousness is the first finding to suggest neurologic impairment. However, be-

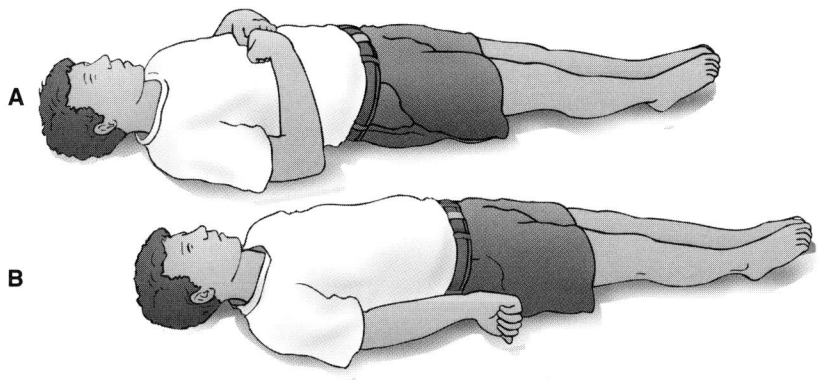

Figure 19-15   **A,** Decorticate posturing. **B,** Decerebrate posturing.

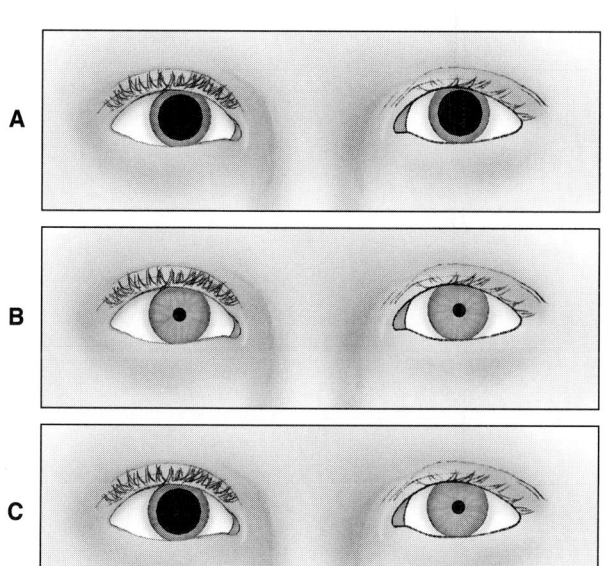

Figure 19-16   **A,** Dilated pupils. **B,** Constricted pupils. **C,** Unequal pupils. (Modified from Chatburn RL, Lough MD. Handbook of respiratory care, 2nd ed. Chicago: Year-Book; 1990.)

𝒦EY 𝒫OINTS

- The health history provides a detailed, chronologic record of the patient.
- The HPI offers a description of the onset of the problem, whether it developed suddenly, and the setting in which it developed.
- The four examination techniques commonly used are inspection, palpation, percussion, and auscultation.
- The use of accessory muscles implies an increased work of breathing.

- The assessment of respiratory expansion helps determine whether the lungs are expanding symmetrically.
- Auscultation of the chest allows assessment of diminished breath sounds, bronchial breath sounds, and adventitious breath sounds, such as crackles, rhonchi, wheezing, stridor, and pleural friction rubs.
- Listening to heart sounds involves notations of the rate and rhythm, extra heart sounds, and murmurs.
- The Glasgow Coma Score is used to assess the level of consciousness.

Recommended Reading

Barkauskas VH, Baumann LC, Stoltenberg-Allen K, et al. Health & physical assessment. 2nd ed. St Louis: Mosby; 1997.

Bickley LS, Hoekelman RA. Bates' guide to physical examination and history taking. 7th ed. Philadelphia: JB Lippincott; 1995.

Erickson B. Heart sounds and murmurs: a practical guide. 2nd ed. St Louis: Mosby; 1991.

Jarvis C. Physical examination and health assessment. 2nd ed. Philadelphia: WB Saunders; 1996.

Seidel HM, Ball JW, Dains JE, et al. Mosby's guide to physical examination. 4th ed. St Louis: Mosby; 1999.

Swartz MH. Textbook of physical diagnosis history and examination. 3rd ed. Philadelphia: WB Saunders; 1998.

Timby BK. Fundamental skills and concepts in patient care. 6th ed. Philadelphia: Lippincott; 1996.

Wilkins RL, Hodgkin JE, Lopez B. Lung sounds: a practical guide. 2nd ed. St Louis: Mosby; 1996.

Wilkins RL, Krider SJ, Sheldon RL. Clinical assessment in respiratory care. 4th ed. St Louis: Mosby; 2000.

CHAPTER 20

Blood Chemistries and Hematology

Rajesh Bhagat
Neil R. MacIntyre

CHAPTER **OUTLINE**

Serum Electrolytes
  Body Water
  Sodium
  Potassium
  Chloride
  Total Serum Carbon Dioxide
  Unmeasured Anions
  Calcium
  Magnesium
  Phosphorus
  Lactate
Serum Chemistries Associated with Renal Function
  Blood Urea Nitrogen
  Serum Creatinine

Serum Enzyme Activity
Miscellaneous Serum Chemistries
  Bilirubin
  Proteins
  Glucose
Coagulation Tests
  Prothrombin Time
  Activated Partial Thromboplastin Time
Hematology
  Hemoglobin and Hematocrit
  Platelets
  Total and Differential Leukocyte Count
Laboratory Standards and Quality Control

OBJECTIVES

1. Discuss the physiology of normal fluid and electrolyte balance.
2. List causes of abnormal electrolyte levels.
3. Discuss the effects of renal function on serum chemistry.
4. Discuss the role of serum enzymes in assessing liver and cardiac function.
5. Describe laboratory tests used to assess coagulation.
6. Discuss abnormalities of hemoglobin, platelets, and leukocytes.

KEY TERMS

Activated Partial Thromboplastin Time	Hemoglobin	Hypophosphatemia
Anion	Hypercalcemia	Intracellular Fluid
Anion Gap	Hyperchloremia	Lactate
Bilirubin	Hyperkalemia	Leukocytes
Blood Urea Nitrogen (BUN)	Hypermagnesemia	Leukocytosis
Cardiac Enzymes	Hypernatremia	Leukopenia
Cation	Hyperphosphatemia	Oncotic Pressure
Coagulation	Hypocalcemia	Platelets
Creatinine	Hypochloremia	Prothrombin Time (PT)
Extracellular Fluid	Hypokalemia	Serum Electrolytes
Glucose	Hypomagnesemia	Serum Proteins
Hematocrit	Hyponatremia	Unmeasured Anions

Circulating blood is composed of water, proteins, electrolytes, and cells. Removing only the cells from blood leaves plasma. Removing both cells and coagulation proteins leaves serum. The water component of blood can move across both tissue barriers and cell membranes, depending on hydrostatic and **oncotic pressures.** On the other hand, protein and electrolyte movements into and from blood vessels often depend on complex tissue or cell membrane pumps. Blood cells generally remain within the blood vessels except under conditions of blood vessel injury or inflammation.

Measuring the chemical and cellular properties of blood can yield considerable information about disease states. These measurements are often expressions of concentrations of a substance. Some measurements, however, measure a functional property, such as coagulation activity or osmotic pressure. This chapter covers the common measurements performed on blood samples from patients. For each measurement the discussion includes a review of the physiologic (and pathophysiologic) importance of the blood substance or property, followed by a brief review of commonly used measurement techniques. Diagnoses that should be considered in the event of an abnormal value also are reviewed.

Serum Electrolytes

Body Water

The most common **serum electrolytes** are the **cations** Na^+, K^+, Ca^{+2}, and Mg^{+2} and the **anions** HCO_3^-, PO_4^-, and SO_4^-. However, a discussion of serum electrolytes must first begin with a discussion of the body water in which these electrolytes exist. In an average person, approximately 60% of total body weight is water (Figure 20-1).

Two-thirds is in the intracellular compartment (that is, within cells) and one-third is in the extracellular compartment (that is, interstitium and blood, which make up 75% and 25%, respectively, of this compartment). The compartments are separated by cell membranes that set up active and passive forces regulating water, electrolyte, and solute movement, with resulting electrolyte concentration gradients and oncotic pressures.

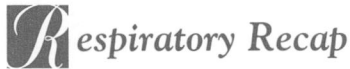
Respiratory Recap

Body Water
Approximately 60% of total body weight is water. Two thirds of body water is in the intracellular space. One third of body water is in the extracellular space.

Extracellular fluid is characterized by higher amounts of Na^+, Cl^-, and HCO_3^-, whereas **intracellular fluid** has higher amounts of K^+, Mg^{+2}, PO_4^-, and SO_4^-. These cations and anions are regulated in the compartments over a narrow normal range. Mechanical, inflammatory, and other pathologic processes frequently affect the integrity of these compartments, with consequent movement of electrolytes, proteins, and water. Moreover, a change in body or compartment level of one substance often sets off a sequence of compensatory events in the body to maintain fluid homeostasis.

Thus initial assessment of the overall water volume status is critical in any evaluation of a patient's fluid and electrolyte status. No single test precisely quantifies total body water (TBW) easily in the clinical setting. Instead, clinicians rely on history-taking and physical examination. The intent is to decide whether the patient is hypovolemic, euvolemic, or hypervolemic with respect to TBW (Box 20-1).

Sodium

The sodium cation (Na^+) is the most common electrolyte in extracellular fluid, and the normal serum values range from 135 to 145 mEq/L. Na^+ is important for a variety of cell membrane functions and in determinations of serum osmotic pressure. In the hypovolemic patient with a normal total body Na^+ content, the relationship between Na^+ and TBW allows for calculation of the free water deficit, as follows:

$$\text{Free water deficit} = TBW \times \left(1 - \frac{140}{\text{Serum } Na^+}\right)$$

$$= 0.6 \times \text{Weight (kg)} \times \left(1 - \frac{140}{\text{Serum } Na^+}\right)$$

This formula is useful in calculations of the appropriate amount of free water to be administered in water deficit

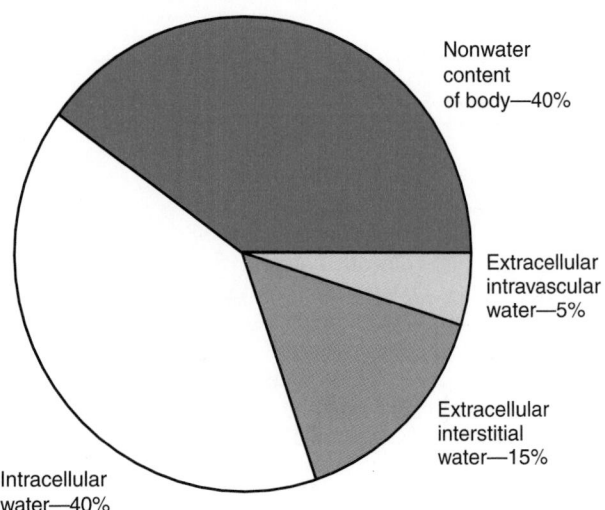

Figure 20-1   Fluid compartments in the body and the percentages of each.

states. The relationship between Na$^+$ and TBW also can be used to predict the change in serum Na$^+$ after administration of various intravenous fluids, as follows:

Change in serum Na$^+$ =

$$\frac{(\text{Infusate Na}^+ + \text{Infusate K}^+) - \text{Serum Na}^+}{\text{TBW} + 1}$$

Both low-Na$^+$ (**hyponatremia**) and high-Na$^+$ (**hypernatremia**) conditions are evident in a number of disease states and produce important clinical manifestations.

The physiologic effects of Na$^+$ depend on its concentration in extracellular water. If the serum sample has significant amounts of substances that increase the serum volume but not the water volume, the measured serum Na$^+$ will appear low even though its water concentration is normal (pseudohyponatremia). Substances that expand serum volume but not blood volume include the toxins methanol and ethylene glycol, as well as glucose, mannitol, proteins, and lipids. To assess this instance, osmolality can be measured directly and compared with an estimated value, as follows:

Estimated osmolality =

$$2\text{Na}^+ + \left(\frac{\text{BUN mg/dL}}{2.8}\right) + \left(\frac{\text{Glucose mg/dL}}{18}\right)$$

If the measured osmolality is within 20 of the estimated serum osmolality (that is, no osmolar gap), the Na$^+$ value reflects the true value and rules out the presence of unmeasured substances.

Decreased serum Na$^+$ levels are associated with water moving osmotically within cells and creating a significant shift in the relationship between intracellular and extracellular fluid compartments. This shift is associated with weakness, giddiness, lassitude, faintness, muscle cramps, anorexia, nausea, vomiting, confusion, delirium, stupor, and coma. On examination the skin turgor is low, blood pressure may be decreased, and orthostatic hypotension is usually present.

Because the relationship between Na$^+$ and fluid is so intertwined, a useful practice is to divide the causes of hyponatremia into hypovolemic, euvolemic, and hypervolemic categories, depending on the estimation of TBW by physical examination and the response of the kidney in moving Na$^+$ into the urine (Box 20-2).

Regarding hypernatremia, clinicians usually are concerned with increased Na$^+$ serum concentrations rather than increased total body sodium levels. (That is, hypervolemic hyponatremic patients have increased total body sodium levels, but their serum sodium levels are diluted because of excess water.) Hypernatremia is associated with an increased serum osmolality, and its clinical features are classically the same as those associated with water loss. The causes of hypernatremia are listed in Box 20-3.

Laboratory techniques used to estimate sodium concentration include flame atomic emission spectroscopy; ion-selective electrode (ISE) potentiometry—direct and indirect, chromogenic ionophore, and enzymatic (or enzyme activation), with ISE (either direct or indirect) being the most commonly used method. The direct ISE method has the advantage that hyperproteinemic and hyperlipidemic states do not affect the accuracy. A potential source of error is protein buildup on membrane surfaces of the measuring electrode.

Potassium

Approximately 90% of total body potassium (K$^+$) is intracellular. K$^+$ homeostasis is regulated by acid-base status, insulin, catecholamines, and aldosterone. Alkalosis and elevated insulin, catecholamine, and aldosterone levels lower serum K$^+$ through either renal excretion or intracellular potassium shifting. Acidosis and reduced insulin, catecholamine, and aldosterone levels raise serum potassium levels. K$^+$ is essential for maintenance of the electrical membrane potential; thus changes in serum K$^+$ levels affect neuromuscular activity as well as cardiac electrical impulses. Normal serum range is from 3.5 to 5.5 mEq/L.

*B*ox 20-1

Assessment Tools Used to Evaluate Total Body Water

Decreased TBW (hypovolemia) is associated with the following:

- *Symptoms:* thirst, decreased urine output, dizziness on standing up
- *Signs:* thready rapid pulse, low blood pressure, orthostatic hypotension, low skin turgor, sunken eyes, depressed fontanelle in infants, dry coated tongue; also associated with muscle tremors, rigidity, and even seizures and rarely with hallucinations, delirium, and maniac behavior; development of tachypnea and respiratory arrest before death
- *Laboratory data:* shows elevated hematocrit (if hypovolemia is not due to blood loss), sodium, and protein levels. Urine is

concentrated, and urine potassium loss (kaliuresis) is seen, associated with decreased serum potassium levels.

Increased TBW (hypervolemia) is associated with the following:

- *Symptoms:* weight gain, loss of diurnal rhythm of diuresis, pedal edema, dyspnea
- *Signs:* orthopnea, pedal edema, elevated jugular venous pressure, wheezing, ascites
- *Laboratory data:* is not characteristic but may show serum hyponatremia (dilutional) and hypoproteinemia.

TBW, Total body water.

Box 20-2

Classification of Hyponatremia

Hypovolemic Hyponatremia
Total body sodium deficit higher than TBW deficit
Renal loss (urine sodium >20 mEq/L)
Diuresis: osmotic or diuretic excess
Mineralocorticoid deficiency
Extrarenal loss (urine sodium <10 mEq/L)
Vomiting
Diarrhea
Fluid movement into the "third space"*

Euvolemic Hyponatremia
Increased TBW undetectable by clinical evaluation
Syndrome of inappropriate ADH secretion—malignancy, drugs, CNS lesions

Hypothyroidism
Immediate postoperative period (first 24 hours)
Glucocorticoid deficiency

Hypervolemic Hyponatremia
Dilutional: TBW increase greater than total body sodium
Congestive heart failure
Nephrotic syndrome
Cirrhosis
Acute and chronic renal failure

TBW, *Total body water;* ADH, *antidiuretic hormone;* CNS, *central nervous system.*
Extracellular space is sometimes grouped into three volumes. The first is plasma volume, the second is interstitial fluid volume, and the third refers to various actual or potential cavities, such as the pleural space, peritoneal space, and gut lumen.

Box 20-3

Causes of Hypernatremia

Water Loss More than Sodium Loss
Osmotic and loop diuretic
Postobstructive nephropathy
Sweating
Diarrhea and fistulas

Pure Water Loss
Diabetes insipidus: central, peripheral, and combination
Excessive sweating: exercise, fever, and hot environment

Increase in Total Body Sodium
Primary hyperaldosteronism
Cushing's syndrome
Hypertonic sodium bicarbonate administration in situations such as cardiac arrest

Serum K^+ levels below normal (Box 20-4) affect neuromuscular function, causing muscular weakness, malaise, fatigue, and myalgias. Severe K^+ depletion has been associated with paralysis and rhabdomyolysis. Life-threatening cardiac arrhythmias with electrocardiogram (ECG) changes (U waves, QT prolongation, T wave changes) are commonly associated with severe **hypokalemia.** Paraesthesias, abdominal cramps, and ileus are also common manifestations. Spuriously reduced potassium levels—pseudohypokalemia—may accompany markedly elevated white blood cell (WBC) counts, as in cases of leukemia. Prompt laboratory processing of the sample helps prevent such false-positive results.

Serum K^+ levels above normal (Box 20-5) produce hyporeflexia and muscle weakness. Paralysis can occur in cases of severe **hyperkalemia,** but death due to cardiac ar-

rhythmias usually takes place beforehand. On the ECG, peaked T waves, widened QRS, and eventually sine waves develop before the appearance of actual cardiac arrest. Falsely elevated K^+ levels may be seen when the blood sample is hemolyzed or the WBC or platelet count is unusually elevated.

Techniques used to estimate sodium and potassium levels include flame atomic emission spectroscopy, ISE (direct and indirect), chromogenic ionophore, and enzymatic (enzyme activation). ISE is most frequently used.

Chloride

Chloride (Cl^-) is the most common anion in the extracellular space. Usually, changes in serum Cl^- follow changes in serum sodium levels. Exceptions are hyperchloremic acidoses and chloride responsive, hypochloremic alkaloses. Although **hypochloremia** in experimental situations is associated with vasoconstriction and increased reactivity to norepinephrine (especially in cerebral vessels), clinically important isolated chloride changes are almost never seen. Normal Cl^- levels are 98 to 107 mmol/L in the serum and 110 to 250 mmol/L in the urine. Estimation of Cl^- is affected by other halides. Erroneously high values (**hyperchloremia**) may be found

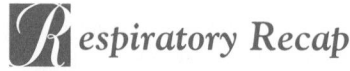

Respiratory Recap

Serum Electrolytes	
Sodium	Calcium
Potassium	Magnesium
Chloride	Phosphorus
Total carbon dioxide	Lactate
Unmeasured anions	

Causes of Hypokalemia

Increased loss of potassium
 GI losses: vomiting, especially with pyloric obstruction; villous adenoma of colon; diarrhea; non-β islet cell tumor of pancreas
 Renal losses: diuretics, such as thiazides and furosemide; renal tubular acidosis I and II; hyperaldosteronism; massive doses of penicillin G, ureteroenterostomy
Intracellular shift of potassium: insulin, testosterone, β₂ agonists, respiratory and metabolic alkalosis, hypokalemic periodic paralysis
Decreased intake: malnutrition, alcoholism, and anorexia nervosa
Miscellaneous: magnesium depletion, Bartter's syndrome, Liddle's syndrome, licorice abuse

ℬOX 20-5

Causes of Hyperkalemia

Increased intake or tissue release, especially in face of compromised renal function: tumor lysis syndrome, rhabdomyolysis, hemolysis, blood transfusion
Drugs: potassium-sparing diuretics, cyclosporin, trimethoprim, ACE inhibitors, heparin, NSAIDs
Renal causes: acute and chronic renal failure, type IV renal tubular acidosis, pseudohypoaldosteronism
Aldosterone deficiency: Addison's disease, hereditary adrenal enzyme defects

ACE, *Angiotensin-converting enzyme;* NSAIDs, *Nonsteroidal antiinflammatory drugs.*

ℬOX 20-6

Unmeasured Anions

Lactate (liver disease, tissue hypoxia)	Uremic acidosis
	Formate and lactate
Ketones (diabetic and alcoholic ketoacidosis)	Glycolate and oxalate
	Ethylene glycol
Salicylates (toxic ingestion)	Free fatty acids
PO_4^- and SO_4^-	Methyl malonate

with bromide present in the sample. Four laboratory methods are used to estimate Cl^- levels—colorimetric method (mercuric/ferric thiocyanate), coulometric titration, ISE, and enzymatic method. ISE methods are most commonly used.

Total Serum Carbon Dioxide

Serum contains carbon dioxide in the form of dissolved carbon dioxide (CO_2), carbon dioxide loosely bound to amine group of plasma proteins, bicarbonate anion (HCO_3^-), carbonate anion (CO_3^{-2}), and carbonic acid. It acts as one of the major buffering systems to control acid-base milieu of the body. The normal range is 22 to 32 mmol/L. The Henderson-Hasselbalch equation describes the relationship of dissolved CO_2, pH, and HCO_3^-, as follows:

$$pH = pK_a + \log \frac{HCO_3^-}{\alpha P_{CO_2}}$$

Methods used to estimate total serum CO_2 include gas release, pH indicator, carbon dioxide electrodes, enzymatic methods, and calculation from the acid-base estimation. Commonly used methods include the ISE or colorimetric method. Accuracy requires anaerobic handling of the sample. Most autoanalyzers permit immediate analysis of the sample. However, if the sample is left uncapped, the total CO_2 levels can decrease by 6 mmol/L/hour.

Unmeasured Anions

Anionic proteins and other substances (Box 20-6) also can exist in serum. Generally these are not measured in routine serum electrolyte determinations. However, their presence can be suspected by calculation of the **anion gap,** as follows:

$$\text{Anion gap} = ([Na^+] + [K^+]) - ([CO_2] + [CL^-])$$

If the anion gap exceeds 12 mmol/L, excessive **unmeasured anions** are likely present. Because its concentration is normally low, $[K^+]$ is often omitted from this calculation.

Calcium

Calcium (Ca^{+2}) performs multiple functions in the body. Besides being a major structural substance in bone, it plays an important role in maintaining cellular conduction in the neuromuscular system. Ca^{+2} is also an important participant or catalyst in several metabolic cascades (for example, the coagulation pathways). Ca^{+2} is mainly absorbed in the bowel and excreted in the urine. Bones serve as a major calcium reservoir. The important Ca^{+2} regulators levels are vitamin D, calcitonin, phosphate, and parathyroid hormone. In general, vitamin D and parathyroid hormone increase Ca^{+2} levels, whereas calcitonin and phosphate reduce them.

In serum, most Ca^{+2} is bound to albumin. Measured Ca^{+2} levels are thus sensitive to all the factors regulating or affecting serum protein levels (especially albumin). Because unbound (that is, ionized) calcium is what is metabolically important, measured total serum Ca^{+2} should be corrected for albumin concentration (that is, a reduction in Ca^{+2} level 0.8 mg/dL for every gram per deciliter of albumin below normal). Ionized calcium also can be measured directly. In adults, normal total serum Ca^{+2} levels are 8.6 to 10.0 mg/dL (2.15 to 2.50 mmol/L). Normal ionized Ca^{+2} levels are 4.6 to 5.3 mg/dL (1.16 to 1.32 mmol/L).

A low ionized calcium level (**hypocalcemia**) is usually due to either decreased absorption or decreased mobilization of calcium from the bones. Causes include malnutrition, parathyroid hormone activity, vitamin D abnormalities, certain drugs, and renal dysfunction (which produces hyperphosphatemia). Pancreatitis, massive blood transfu-

Causes of Hypercalcemia

Abnormal Protein Syndromes
Multiple myeloma and paraproteinemias

Increased Parathyroid Hormone or Related Peptides
Malignancy of lung or kidney

Increased Absorption
Usually vitamin D related (milk alkali syndrome), granulomatous diseases (such as tuberculosis and sarcoidosis), lymphoma

Excessive Renal Phosphate Excretion
Familial syndrome, sarcoidosis

Abnormal Bone Resorption/Formation
Prolonged bed rest, Paget's disease

Miscellaneous
Bone metastases, especially from breast and prostate cancers, drugs such as thiazides (rarely)

Causes of Hypomagnesemia

Absorption Problems
Malnutrition per se or due to alcoholism, diarrhea, intravenous alimentation, intestinal bypass surgery
Psychological problems: bulimia, laxative abuse, or aggressive weight reduction
Others: short bowel syndrome or malignancies, especially in the bowel

Excessive Loss in Urine
Use and abuse of diuretics, postobstructive diuresis, acute tubular necrosis, hypercalcemia and hereditary renal magnesium wasting

Miscellaneous
Association with hyperaldosteronism, diabetic ketoacidosis, excessive lactation
Exchange transfusions
Acute intermittent porphyria

sions, and tumor lysis syndrome can precipitate Ca^{+2} and thus reduce serum levels. Low Ca^{+2} levels frequently coexist with low magnesium levels, especially in malnourished alcoholics. Clinical features of hypocalcemia consist of perioral numbness and tingling progressing to tetany. Physical examination evidence for protein-energy malnutrition, previous parathyroidectomy, pancreatitis, and tumor lysis syndrome should increase the suspicion for reduced Ca^{+2} levels.

Increases in Ca^{+2} levels are due to multiple factors (Box 20-7). The clinical features of **hypercalcemia** include anorexia, vomiting, polyuria, mental confusion, obtundation, and death. The ECG may show a shortened QT interval.

Laboratory tests used to measure serum Ca^{+2} include atomic absorption, cresolphthalein complex formation, arsenzo III dye, and ISEs to estimate ionic calcium levels. Autoanalyzers frequently use ISEs. Atomic absorption remains the gold standard, although it is not frequently used for clinical work.

Magnesium

Magnesium (Mg^{+2}) is the other major cation in the serum (besides Ca^{+2}) that helps maintain membrane potentials at the cellular level. Mg^{+2} is also important in maintaining potassium homeostasis through regulation of cell membrane potassium channels. Only 1% to 2% of total body Mg^{+2} is present in the serum, and one third of this amount is bound to proteins. Mg^{+2} is mainly absorbed in the small bowel (mostly in the initial parts) and is excreted by the kidneys. In adults the normal serum Mg^{+2} range is 1.8 to 3.0 mg/mL (1.5 to 2.5 mEq/L).

Causes of low Mg^{+2} levels (**hypomagnesemia**) are listed in Box 20-8. Low levels often are associated with hypokalemia. Indeed, concurrent hypomagnesemia and hypokalemia makes it difficult to correct the potassium levels until the Mg^{+2} levels are corrected. Hypomagnesemia also is associated with hyponatremia, hypocalcemia, and hypophosphatemia. Low Mg^{+2} levels result in tremulousness, hyperreflexia, ataxia, convulsions, and death in extreme cases. Hypomagnesemia-induced cardiac dysrhythmias originating in the atria or the ventricles can be fatal. Hypertension in hypomagnesemic patients can be difficult to control. Hypomagnesemic dysmotility in gastrointestinal muscles is clinically manifest as dysphagia.

High Mg^{+2} levels (**hypermagnesemia**) are uncommon but can be seen in patients suffering from renal failure, especially those undergoing inappropriate dialysis or alimentation regimens. Another cause of hypermagnesemia is abuse of magnesium-based laxatives. In addition, hypermagnesemia is sometimes induced to treat eclampsia. The condition's clinical manifestations include hyporeflexia, muscle weakness, hypotension, bradycardia, coma, and death.

Laboratory methods used to estimate serum levels of Mg^{+2} include colorimetric methods using calmagite, methylthymol, or chlorophosphonazo III; ISE methods; and atomic absorption, the latter of which remains the gold standard. However, ISEs are increasingly being used to estimate serum Mg^{+2} levels.

Phosphorus

More than 80% of total body phosphorus is found in bones. Phosphate ion (PO_4^-) is a major intracellular anion participating primarily as a cofactor in intracellular meta-

Box 20-9

Causes of Hypophosphatemia

Decreased Absorption
Malnutrition, alcohol abuse, vitamin D deficiency, laxative abuse, antacid abuse

Intracellular Shift
High-energy states and parenteral nutrition with carbohydrate overload

Increased Excretion
Hyperparathyroidism, diuretics, hyperglycemia, and alcohol abuse

bolic processes. Extracellular phosphate salts function as buffers and play a role in calcium homeostasis. (That is, serum PO_4^- and Ca^{+2} exist in a reciprocal, balanced relationship.) PO_4^- is absorbed through the gastrointestinal tract (vitamin D dependent) and excreted through the kidneys (enhanced by parathyroid hormone). In adults, normal serum PO_4^- levels range between 2.7 and 4.5 mg/dL (0.87 to 1.45 mmol/L).

Low PO_4^- (**hypophosphatemia**) levels are primarily caused by decreased absorption, intracellular shifts, or increased excretion (Box 20-9). Severe stress causing glucagon and cortisol release may be responsible for the low serum PO_4^- levels seen in trauma patients. Clinical features of hypophosphatemia include decreased contractility of muscles causing cardiomyopathy, hyporeflexia, and hypoventilation. If severe, this condition can lead to rhabdomyolysis. Hypophosphatemia also can produce confusion, seizures, and coma. Chronic deficiency can cause osteomalacia.

High PO_4^- levels (**hyperphosphatemia**) are unusual but can be seen in individuals with chronic renal failure, in which the hyperphosphatemia is often overshadowed by other metabolic and electrolyte abnormalities. Other conditions producing hyperphosphatemia include hypoparathyroidism (low calcium levels also being seen), pseudohypoparathyroidism, and Paget's disease of the juvenile, which is characterized by muscle weakness and high alkaline phosphatase levels.

To estimate serum PO_4^- levels, ammonium phosphomolybdate complex levels are read directly by an ultraviolet monitor or the complex is reduced to molybdenum and its levels estimated.

Lactate

An elevated serum lactate level is an important cause of anion gap metabolic acidosis. **Lactate** is most commonly formed in ischemic cells as a consequence of anaerobic glycolysis and the use of pyruvate for generation of adenosine triphosphate (ATP). Thus it is frequently used to indicate the severity of shock and provides a rough idea of tissue perfusion, oxygen delivery, and oxygen use. For individuals in shock, increased lactic acid is associated with increased mortality. Lactic acid has the both D and L isomers. Humans normally produce L-lactic acidosis that most laboratories easily estimate. Theoretically, D-lactic acid (normally produced by ruminants and bacteria) can be elevated in certain types of individuals (for example, those with bowel abnormalities). Currently D-lactic acidosis is more of research curiosity, with rare cases involving humans. Normal values for lactate in adults are less than 2 mmol/L.

Methods used to estimate lactate levels include chemical oxidation, enzyme reactions, and enzyme electrodes. Other methods use gas chromatography and photometry. Thus enzyme electrodes have made estimation of serum lactate much simpler. Because lactate is unstable, samples should be processed immediately. Lactate increases by 0.4 mmol/L in whole blood kept at room temperature for 30 minutes (0.1 mmol/L on ice).

Serum Chemistries Associated with Renal Function

The most important tests of renal function are the quantity of urine produced and the characteristics of that urine (that is, pH, specific gravity, microscopic analysis, and culture). However, two other measurements are frequently used to assess renal function—the serum blood urea nitrogen (BUN) and creatinine levels.

Blood Urea Nitrogen

Blood urea nitrogen (BUN) levels indicate the body's ability to clear nitrogenous wastes in the form of urea in the urine. Urea (along with ammonia) is a breakdown product of amino acids. Thus it can be increased by increases in gastrointestinal protein absorption from either dietary factors or heme in the bowels (that is, gastrointestinal bleeding). Similarly, urea levels can be decreased with decreases in protein intake or liver impairment. Urea is readily filtered in the glomeruli, but approximately half of it is reabsorbed. It also is broken down into ammonia in the bowel. Levels of BUN thus reflect protein intake and metabolism, as well as glomerular and proximal tubule function in the kidney. In the adult, normal BUN values are between 7 and 21 mg/dL.

BUN is estimated from serum urea levels. Almost all the tests used estimate directly or indirectly the amount of ammonia present in the sample—calorimetric methods, indicator dye, and ISEs.

Serum Creatinine

Creatinine levels are a function of skeletal muscle breakdown. Thus the levels are directly related to muscle mass of a person. Most creatinine is filtered in the glomeruli, with very little reabsorption. A small amount also is secreted by the tubules into the urine. Thus if the individual's muscle mass is relatively stable, serum creatinine is a good indicator of glomerular filtration and, hence, renal function. Increased creatinine levels, however, also can occur in conjunction with increased muscle breakdown (for example, corticosteroids, rhabdomyolysis) or with decreased tubular excretion, as that seen with trimethoprim. Decreased creatinine levels reflect decreased muscle mass, such as those in states of malnutrition or muscle atrophy. In the adult, normal values for creatinine are 0.7 to 1.4 mg/dL.

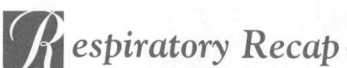espiratory Recap

Laboratory Tests Associated with Renal Function
Blood urea nitrogen Creatinine

Serum creatine level is a relatively insensitive monitor of renal function and may not increase until more than 50% of renal function has deteriorated. With complete renal shutdown, creatinine levels rise approximately 1 mg/dL/day. Creatinine levels also can be used to describe creatinine clearance (the amount of blood per minute cleared of creatinine by the kidney), a more precise measurement of renal function, as follows:

Creatinine clearance =

$$\frac{\text{Urine creatinine concentration} \times \text{24-Hour urine volume}}{\text{Plasma creatinine concentration}}$$

A simpler method used to estimate creatinine clearance is as follows:

Creatinine clearance =

$$(140 - \text{Age}) \times \frac{\text{Weight (kg)}}{72} \times \text{Serum creatinine}$$

Normal creatinine clearance is 97 to 137 mL/min (for men) and 88 to 128 mL/min (for women). Creatinine clearance decreases 6.5 mL/min/decade after 40 years of age.

Estimation of creatinine is done by spectrophotometric analysis of Jaffe's reaction, enzymatic hydrolysis of creatinine, and cation-exchange high-performance liquid chromatography.

Serum Enzyme Activity

Enzymes are chemical substances that facilitate chemical reactions. Most enzymatic reactions occur intracellularly. Nevertheless, a number of these enzymes appear in serum under physiologic conditions. In pathologic conditions, many enzymes appear in serum in increased concentrations because of either cell injury or metabolic abnormalities within the cell.

A number of serum enzymes reflect liver function but also may reflect dysfunction elsewhere. Alanine aminotransferase (ALT) is present in liver cells, and an increased serum level indicates liver cell injury. Aspartate aminotransferase (AST) is present in liver cells but also is present in cardiac, skeletal, kidney, and brain tissue. The AST:ALT ratio is normally >2. Mildly elevated AST levels (that is, <250 U/L) suggest alcoholic liver injury. Serum alkaline phosphatase (ALP) comes from either liver or bone. Elevation of liver ALP indicates intrahepatic or collecting system bile drainage abnormalities (cholestasis). Elevated γ-glutamyltransferase (GGT) serum levels also indicate cholestasis.

Lactic dehydrogenase (LDH) enzymes are a family of enzymes in which elevations can reflect liver, bone, cardiac, red blood cell (RBC), or pancreatic abnormalities. LDH assays can be fractionated to indicate the organ involved (Table 20-1).

Cardiac enzymes refer to a group of enzymes that are released from myocardial tissue and appear in the serum during myocardial injury (usually ischemia). As the understanding of cardiac ischemia has changed, so also has the use of various enzymes to estimate cardiac muscle damage. Nevertheless, cardiac enzyme abnormalities remain a standard used to diagnose cardiac ischemia, in conjunction with history and ECG changes. The initial panel of cardiac enzymes included serum lactate dehydrogenase (LDH), serum glutamic-oxaloacetic transaminase (SGOT), and creatine kinase (CK). The myocardial-specific (MB isoform) creatine kinase (CKMB) has became the standard.

CKMB levels begin rising within 4 to 8 hours of myocardial injury, with peak activity by 24 hours. CKMB levels return to baseline in 2 to 3 days. Many centers now also are measuring cardiac troponin I or T isoforms. Troponin I rises within 3 to 6 hours of an acute myocardial infarction, peaks by about 14 to 20 hours and returns to baseline in 5 to 10 days. Unfortunately, nonuniformity in the measurement of troponin has made the comparison of values from various laboratories difficult. CKMB (mass), CKMB (isoforms), troponin I, and troponin T are available in various combinations and are estimated by different methods. The situation is further complicated in the presence of renal failure and rhabdomyolysis. Rapid assays of these enzymes also are available. In the future, fatty acid-binding protein (FABP) and glycogen phosphorylase isoenzyme (BB) may prove useful.

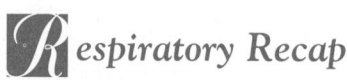espiratory Recap

Serum Enzymes
Liver enzymes Cardiac enzymes

TABLE 20-1

LDH Abnormalities

LDH Type	% of Normal	Source	Significance of Elevations
HHHH	14-26	Cardiac, RBC, kidney	Myocardial infarct, renal infarct, hemolytic anemia, megaloblastic anemia
HHHM	29-39	Cardiac, RBC, kidney	Myocadial infarct, renal infarct, hemolytic anemia, megaloblastic anemia
HHMM	20-26	Lung, lymphocytes, pancreas, spleen, platelets	Pulmonary emboli, pneumonia, cancer
HMMM	8-16	Liver	Hepatic injury
MMMM	6-16	Skeletal muscle	Skeletal muscle injury

LDH, *Lactate dehydrogenase;* RBC, *red blood cell.*

Methods used to estimate CK include electrophoresis, ion exchange chromatography, immunoinhibitors, and mass assay (specific for CKMB) with no interference by hemolysis. Normal total serum CK is 15 to 130 U/L, and CKMB is less than 6% of total CK. Potential sources of error are hemolysis, exposure of sample to daylight, and muscle mass of the patient (either too large or too small). For troponin estimation, enzyme-linked immunosorbent assay (ELISA), immunoenzyme techniques, and rapid immunochromatographic assays are available. The normal range is less than 0.1 ng/mL to 3.1 ng/mL.

Amylase and lipase are two enzymes that appear elevated as a consequence of pancreatic injury. Both may be elevated in individuals with other gastrointestinal abnormalities as well. Pancreatic disease caused by biliary tract disease usually has accompanying liver-associated abnormalities in the serum.

Miscellaneous Serum Chemistries

Bilirubin

Bilirubin is a breakdown product of hemoglobin that is metabolized in the liver. Total serum bilirubin concentration is less than 1.1 mg/dL. Approximately 80% of serum bilirubin is indirect or unconjugated. Elevation of indirect bilirubin suggests prehepatic bilirubinemia caused by increased bilirubin production (for example, hemolysis) or decreased liver uptake, as seen in Gilbert syndrome. Parenchymal liver injury and bile collecting system abnormalities (that is, posthepatic) lesions cause bile stasis (cholestasis) and lead to an increase of conjugated bilirubin levels.

Proteins

A number of **serum proteins** can be measured. Serum albumin is exclusively synthesized in the liver. Its half-life is approximately 3 weeks, and it can be used as a marker of liver synthetic function. Serum albumin also is a useful marker of nutritional status. Ferritin is an iron-binding protein that also is taken as an index of nutritional status. Serum globulins are mediators of the humoral immune system. Elevations can be seen in individuals with tumors secreting these globulins (for example, multiple myeloma) and other paraproteinemias. Low values are seen in individuals with various congenital immune deficiency states.

Glucose

Glucose metabolism is heavily influenced by a number of nutritional, liver, hormonal, and pancreatic factors. Glucagon and adrenal steroids increase glucose concentrations by promoting liver breakdown of stored glycogen. Insulin is produced by islet cells in the pancreas and is critical for the transfer of glucose into cells. Pancreatic injury or islet cell dysfunction (type 1 diabetes) impairs insulin production and results in serum hyperglycemia. If severe, this condition can produce diabetic ketoacidosis. Severe hyperglycemia also can cause a hyperosmolar state with coma. In addition, type 2 diabetes (cellular resistance to insulin) can produce hyperglycemia and deranged glucose metabolism. Insulin-secreting tumors or exogenous insulin overdoses produce hypoglycemia. Severe liver injury also can produce hypoglycemia because of a depletion or failure to metabolize liver glycogen; if severe, hypoglycemia can bring about coma and death.

Coagulation Tests

The **coagulation** system can be assessed in a number of ways (Figure 20-2). A simple and direct way to evaluate overall coagulation status is the bedside bleeding time. However, this method is time consuming and difficult to standardize. More commonly used techniques are the measurements of the prothrombin time (PT), activated partial thromboplastin time (aPTT), and platelet count.

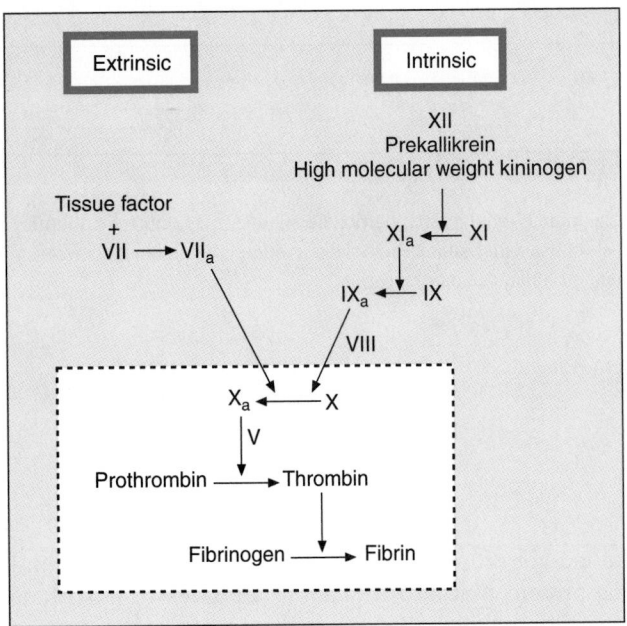

Figure 20-2 A simplified version of the role of various clotting factors in the coagulation cascade. (Modified from Goldman L, Bennett JC. Cecil textbook of medicine. 21st ed. Philadelphia: WB Saunders; 2001.)

Box 20-10

Causes of Low Hemoglobin and Hematocrit Values

Abnormal Hemoglobin
Iron in the ferric form: methemoglobinemia
Abnormalities in the polypeptide chain: hemoglobinopathies, such as thalassemias and sickle cell disease

Decreased Hemoglobin Production
Bone marrow problems: aplastic anemia, myelosuppressive drugs, idiosyncratic reaction to drugs, infiltration of bone marrow by other cells
Deficiencies: iron, vitamin B_{12} cofactors, erythropoietin
Miscellaneous: malignancy, chronic diseases, hypothyroidism, hypopituitarism

Increased Loss or Breakdown of RBCs
Fault in the RBCs: membrane defects, enzymatic deficiencies, hemoglobin disorders
Acquired causes of hemolysis: drugs, toxins, infections
Hypersplenism
Bleeding

RBC, Red blood cell.

Prothrombin Time

The **prothrombin time (PT)** is used to evaluate the extrinsic pathway and depends on the levels of factors V, VII, X, and eventually I and II (see Figure 20-2). It often is used to monitor adequate anticoagulation in patients on Coumadin, which acts on these factors. The result is usually expressed as either a time or ratio of the values with respect to normal pooled sera. To standardize oral anticoagulant therapy the PT is expressed as an international normalized ratio (INR). The goals of Coumadin therapy are to increase the INR to 2 to 3. However, in specific conditions, such as mechanical prosthetic heart valves, this ratio must be increased further.

Respiratory Recap

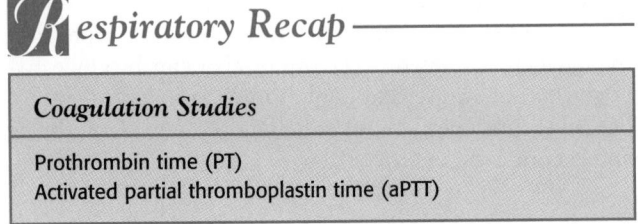

Coagulation Studies

Prothrombin time (PT)
Activated partial thromboplastin time (aPTT)

The PT can be prolonged by vitamin K deficiency and liver disease because factors II, V, VII, and X are vitamin K dependent and produced in the liver. In the presence of severe, acute liver injury, the PT may rapidly (that is, within 24 hours) become abnormal. Vitamin K absorption also is impaired in the presence of hepatocellular disease and cholestasis, contributing to the abnormal PT.

Activated Partial Thromboplastin Time

The aPTT is used to assess the intrinsic clotting pathway, especially the early stages involving factors XII, XI, IX, and VIII (see Figure 20-2). It often is used to monitor patients on heparin therapy. The goals of heparin therapy are to extend the aPTT to about twice the upper level of normal. In individuals not on anticoagulant therapy, abnormal PT or aPTT values indicate abnormalities in the coagulation system, possibly reflecting liver disorders, hematologic disorders, toxins or drugs, or disseminated intravascular coagulation (DIC) associated with a multiorgan failure syndrome. Further workup might include a number of specific clotting factor assays to identify the exact abnormality. Adding normal clotting factors to the test sample can help separate whether a coagulation abnormality is due to factor deficiency (coagulation normalizing with "mix") or a circulating anticoagulant (coagulation not normalizing with "mix").

Hematology

The complete blood count (CBC) is the most frequently ordered diagnostic test in the hospital. Under the heading of CBC is a long list of indices that vary among laboratories. Automated machines usually directly measure the hemoglobin, WBC count, RBC count, platelet count, differential **leukocyte** fractions, and RBC distribution list, as well as calculate the hematocrit, mean corpuscular volume, mean corpuscular hemoglobin, mean corpuscular hemoglobin concentration, and differential leukocyte count.

Box 20-11

Abnormalities in Platelet Function

Thrombesthenia
Abnormal platelet function with uremia
von Willebrand disease
Drugs

Thrombocytopenia (Decreased Platelet Count)
Bone marrow problems: malignancies, drugs, myelodysplasias
Increased breakdown: structural platelet defects, immune problems
Hypersplenism

Thrombocytosis (Increased Platelet Count)
Essential or idiopathic
After splenectomy
Acute blood loss
Pregnancy

Box 20-12

Causes of Leukocytosis

Physiologic
Exercise
Pregnancy
Stress: pain, psychologic, cold exposure, anesthesia, anoxia
Trauma, hemorrhage
Menstruation, pregnancy, and labor
Seizure

Pathologic
Infections: bacterial, fungal, viral, and parasitic
Leukemoid reaction due to any of the previous causes
Leukemias: uncontrolled malignant proliferation of any of the WBCs in the bone marrow

WBC, *White blood cell.*

Box 20-13

Causes of Leukopenia

Overwhelming infection, especially in the very young or very elderly
Drug actions and adverse events
Malignant involvement of the bone marrow
Collagen vascular diseases, such as lupus (infrequent cause)
Idiopathic or not–well-understood disease processes, such as myelodysplastic syndromes

Hemoglobin and Hematocrit

Hemoglobin is an iron-containing globular protein consisting of two pairs of polypeptides. Its primary function is the transport of oxygen from the lungs to the tissues. Approximately 1 g of hemoglobin binds with 1.34 mL of oxygen. Normal values for hemoglobin in the adult are 13.5 to 15.5 g/dL (for men) and 12.5 to 14.5 g/dL (for women). The **hematocrit** is the proportion of whole blood that is RBCs (the hemoglobin-carrying cell). Normal hematocrit values in the adult are 42% to 52% (for men) and 37% to 48% (for women). Causes of abnormal hemoglobin and hematocrit levels are provided in Box 20-10. High hemoglobin levels are associated with chronic hypoxia and hematologic diseases, such as polycythemia vera. High hemoglobin/hematocrit values also may be seen in individuals with dehydration and hemoconcentration.

Estimation of hemoglobin levels and types of hemoglobin is done by electrophoresis (alkaline or acid), other tests used to estimate abnormal hemoglobin (for example, solubility test for sickle cell disease), and autoanalyzers.

Platelets

Platelets are blood cells critical to clot formation after vascular injury. They are produced in the bone marrow, with normal blood concentrations ranging from 1.5 to 4.0 $\times 10^5$/mm^3. Abnormalities in platelet function are listed in Box 20-11.

Total and Differential Leukocyte Count

The primary role of WBCs is in fighting infections, and an elevated WBC count (**leukocytosis**) is often a sign of significant infection. Leukocytosis, however, also can be associated with elevated glucocorticoids (for example, stress reaction or steroid administration) and in a number of cases of hematologic malignancies (Box 20-12). A low WBC count (**leukopenia**) is invariably a bad sign in any disease process, especially in infections in which it often indicates overwhelming infection (Box 20-13). The differential percentage of various WBCs in the peripheral smear help identify the disease process. Once the percentage of different cells is known, the absolute numbers can be calculated from the total WBC counts. Normal WBC counts in adults ranges from 4000 to 11,000/mm^3.

Respiratory Recap

Hematology

Hemoglobin and hematocrit
Platelets
Leukocytes

Earlier hematology laboratories used visual counting techniques to estimate WBC concentrations. Today, most laboratories have automated instruments that use either resistance changes or flow characteristics to estimate the cell count and size of the cells. To enhance accuracy, RBCs are usually destroyed by chemicals in the blood sample before the WBC counts are performed. Currently, flow-through techniques using electrical resistance (or flow) changes, or cytometry alone or in combination with cytochemical techniques are used. The sophistication of the instrument depends on whether it provides a three-, five-, or six-part differential. Ideally the false-negative rate varies from 2% to 4%, with a false-positive rate of 8% to 15%. Falsely elevated WBC counts may be seen in individuals with undestroyed nucleated RBCs or large or aggregated platelets. Falsely low numbers may be seen in individuals with leukoagglutination; abnormal cells, such as blasts; immature granulocytes; and atypical lymphocytes. Further limitations include an inability to separate mature polymorphonuclear cells from band forms.

Autoanalyzers for CBC using spectrophotometric methods, electric impedance technique, or light-scattering phenomenon can provide reliable numbers for all the parameters in the majority of samples. Results may be compromised in the presence of hyperlipidemia, cryoproteinemia, agglutination of various cells (RBC, WBC, platelets), and abnormal shape and size of cells (for example, schistocytes and sickled cells). Atypical features are usually flagged by the machine and must be assessed by a visual review of the smear.

Laboratory Standards and Quality Control

An enormous amount of clinical information can be derived from examination of blood chemistries and hematology. Indiscriminate or routine ordering of these tests, however, should be discouraged because such practices consume unnecessary resources, cause potential harm from false-positive or false-negative results, and waste patient blood. Indeed, one of the most important causes of "ICU anemia" is blood drawing.

All hematology and blood chemistry testing procedures must be standardized to ensure optimal accuracy and precision. To this end the United States federal government in 1988 established published standards under the Clinical Laboratory Improvement Amendment (CLIA). Other organizations, such as the College of American Pathologists (CAP) and the Joint Commission on Accreditation of Healthcare Organizations (JCAHO) also have published certification standards for laboratories. All laboratories must adhere to these standards, not only to ensure quality care but also to ensure appropriate reimbursement.

As testing methodologies are made more portable, so called point-of-care devices for electrolytes, glucose, lactate, hemoglobin, and blood gases have become available. In addition to more rapid turnaround times, these devices also offer the ability to use smaller samples of blood or even return the blood to the patient after testing. However, the same quality standards mandated for central laboratories also should be applied to these devices.

Regardless of the device used, the limitations of various methods must be kept in mind. Interpretation of values requires knowledge of other medical conditions that may affect the numbers. Indeed, an appropriate first step in the assessment of an unexpected abnormality might be to simply repeat the test. Laboratory tests can provide significant information that drives clinical decision making. The clinician assessing the results should fully appreciate both the significance of the results and the potential errors that might exist.

KEY POINTS

- The most common serum electrolytes are sodium, potassium, calcium, magnesium, chloride, total carbon dioxide, and phosphorus.
- Two thirds of body water is intracellular.
- Sodium is the most common electrolyte in extracellular fluid.
- Hyponatremia and hypernatremia are associated with a number of disease states.
- Potassium is found primarily in the intracellular space.
- Changes in serum potassium concentrations affect neuromuscular activity and cardiac electrical impulses.
- Changes in serum chloride concentrations usually follow changes in serum sodium concentrations.
- Unmeasured anions are estimated through calculation of the anion gap.
- Most calcium is bound to albumin, but only ionized calcium is metabolically important.
- Magnesium plays an important role in maintaining membrane potential.
- Phosphorus is a major intracellular anion that participates in many metabolic processes.
- Increased lactate concentrations are usually due to anaerobic metabolism.
- Blood urea nitrogen and serum creatinine are used to assess renal function.
- Serum enzymes are used to assess liver and cardiac function.
- Bilirubin is a breakdown product of hemoglobin that is metabolized in the liver.
- Serum albumin is a useful marker of nutritional status.
- Hyperglycemia and hypoglycemia result from derangements in glucose metabolism.
- Prothrombin time and activated partial thromboplastin time are used to assess coagulation.
- Hematology laboratory tests include hemoglobin, hematocrit, platelets, and leukocytes.

Recommended Reading

Adrogue HJ, Madias NE. Hypernatremia. N Engl J Med 2000;342: 1493-1499.

Barth JH, Fiddy JB, Payne RB. Adjustment of serum total calcium for albumin concentration: effects of non-linearity and of regression differences between laboratories. Ann Clin Biochem 1996; 33:55-58.

Bartlett RH. Fluids and electrolytes. In: Bartlett RH, editor. Critical care physiology. Boston: Little, Brown; 1996. pp. 155-175.

Bishop ML, Duben-Engelkirk JL, Fody EP. Clinical chemistry: principles, procedures, correlations. 4th ed. Philadelphia: Lippincott Williams & Wilkins; 2000.

Dahlback B. Blood coagulation. Lancet 2000;355:1627-1632.

Dirks JL. Diagnostic blood analysis using point-of-care technology. AACN Clin Iss 1996;7:249-259.

Fulop M. Algorithms for diagnosing some electrolyte disorders. Am J Emerg Med 1998;16:76-84.

George JN. Platelets. Lancet 2000;355:1531-1539.

Gulati GL, Hyun BH. The automated CBC: a current perspective. Hematol Oncol Clin North Am 1994;8:593-601.

Harvey MA. Point-of-care laboratory testing in critical care. Am J Crit Care 1999;8:72-83.

Henderson AR. An overview and ranking of biochemical markers of cardiac disease: strengths and limitations. Clin Lab Med 1997;17:625-654.

Hood VL, Tannen RL. Mechanisms of disease: protection of acid-base balance by pH regulation of acid production. N Engl J Med 1998;339:819-826.

James JH, Luchette FA, McCarter FD, et al. Lactate is an unreliable indicator of tissue hypoxia in injury or sepsis. Lancet 1999;354: 505-508.

Jospe N, Forbes G. Fluids and electrolytes: clinical aspects. Pediatr Rev 1996;11:395-403.

Kamath PS. Clinical approach to the patient with abnormal liver test results. Mayo Clin Proc 1996;71:1089-1095.

Kaplan LA, Pesce AJ, Kaznierzak SC. Clinical chemistry: theory, analysis and correlation. 3rd ed. St Louis: Mosby; 1996.

Kellum JA. Metabolic acidosis in critically ill: lessons from physical chemistry. Kidney Int 1998;53(Suppl 66):S81-S86.

Kokko JP, Tannen RL. Fluids and electrolytes. 3rd ed. Philadelphia: WB Saunders; 1996.

Krause JR. The automated white blood cell differential: a current perspective. Hematol Oncol Clin North Am 1994;8:605-616.

Lum G. Evaluation of a laboratory critical limit (alert value) policy for hypercalcemia. Arch Pathol Lab Med 1996;120:633-636.

Mandal AK. Renal disease: hypokalemia and hyperkalemia. Med Clin North Am 1997;81:611-639.

McGee S, Abernethy WB, Simel DL. Is this patient hypovolemic? JAMA 1999;281:1022-1028.

Roberts R. Rapid MB CK subform assay and the early diagnosis of myocardial infarction. Clin Lab Med 1997;17:669-683.

Schrier RW. Renal and electrolyte disorders. 4th ed. Boston: Little, Brown; 1992.

Spital A. Diuretic induced hyponatremia. Am J Nephrol 1999;19: 447-452.

Toffaletti J. Elevations in blood lactate: overview of use in critical care. Scand J Clin Lab Invest 1996;56(Suppl 224):107-110.

Uribarri J, Oh MS, Carroll HJ. D-Lactic acidosis: a review of clinical presentation, biochemical features and pathophysiologic mechanisms. Medicine 1998;77:73-82.

Whang R, Burns JA. Clinical disorders of magnesium metabolism. Compr Ther 1997;23:168-173.

Workman ML. Magnesium and phosphorus: the neglected electrolytes. AACN Clin Iss 1992;3:655-663

CHAPTER 21

Arterial Blood Gases

Yuh-Chin T. Huang

CHAPTER OUTLINE

OBJECTIVES

1. Compare methods to measure P_{O_2}, P_{CO_2}, pH, and oxygen saturation.
2. Describe the technique used to obtain arterial blood samples by arterial puncture.
3. Describe preanalytic errors in blood gas analysis.
4. Discuss issues related to temperature correction of blood gases.
5. Describe methods of quality control and proficiency testing of blood gases.
6. Discuss the physiology of gas exchange and acid-base balance.
7. List causes of hypoxemia, hypoxia, and hypercapnia.
8. List causes of acid-base disorders.

KEY TERMS

Allen's Test	Arterial Blood Gases	Bohr Effect
Anion Gap	Bicarbonate Buffer System	Carbonic Acid

The analysis of **arterial blood gases** has become an indispensable tool in clinical practice. The primary measurements (Po_2, Pco_2, and **pH**) provide important information about oxygenation, ventilation, and acid-base status. They also guide respiratory and metabolic interventions in critically ill patients. This chapter discusses arterial blood gas measurements and the physiologic basis for the interpretation of arterial blood gas data.

History of Arterial Blood Gas Analysis

Acid-Base Balance

By the eighteenth century, normal blood was recognized as alkaline. Alkalinity was later found to be related to carbon dioxide (CO_2) content (bicarbonate) in the blood. In 1909, Lawrence J. Henderson applied the **law of mass action** to describe the relationship of bicarbonate (HCO_3^-) to dissolved CO_2 or **carbonic acid** (H_2CO_3).[1] This equation, known as the *Henderson equation*, was later transformed by Karl A. Hasselbalch into the logarithmic form known as the **Henderson-Hasselbalch equation.**[2]

Measurement of pH

Wilhelm Ostwald first measured the concentration of hydrogen ions in 1896 using a platinum electrode in solutions saturated with hydrogen gas. He discovered that the potential generated by the platinum electrode was a logarithmic function of the strength of the acid. The Ostwald platinum electrode was later modified and used by Hasselbalch in 1912 to measure blood acidity. Phyllis T. Kerridge constructed the first blood pH electrode in 1925. A thermostated blood pH apparatus was invented in 1931 but was not commercially available until the mid-1950s. Manual Sanz developed the modern ultra-micro pH electrode in the late 1950s.[3]

Measurement of Pco_2

CO_2 was discovered in 1754 by Joseph Black and later detected in exhaled air and the blood. Until the mid-1950s, Pco_2 was either derived from the CO_2-combining power, which involved the equilibration between blood and a gas with known CO_2 content, or calculated from the Henderson-Hasselbalch equation after measurement of pH with a glass electrode and CO_2 content by Van Slyke's manometric method. The polio epidemics of the 1950s, which resulted in large numbers of patients requiring ventilatory support and monitoring, led to the development of the Astrup apparatus to replace the older, more cumbersome methods.

The Astrup apparatus measured pH and Pco_2 based on the principle that the relationship between the pH and log Pco_2 of blood was linear in the clinically relevant range.[4] By measuring pH at two different Pco_2 values, a linear plot of the measured pH against log Pco_2 could be generated. The Pco_2 in the unknown sample then could be obtained by extrapolation. The deviation of the measured pH–log Pco_2 line from the normal position defines the metabolic acid-base imbalance of an individual and the concept of standard base excess.[5] The modern Pco_2 electrode was introduced by Richard Stow in 1957 and later modified by Severinghaus.[6]

Measurement of Po_2

The discovery of oxygen (O_2) is usually credited to Joseph Priestley. He termed this gas *dephlogisticated air* because it required five times as much nitric oxide saturation as ordinary air. In 1777, Antoine Lavosier changed the name to *principe acidifiant* or *principe oxygine* in the mistaken belief that all acids contained O_2. The word *oxygen* (*oxys* = acid, *gene* = to produce) became standard even before it was proved that all acids do not contain O_2. Measurement of Po_2 in the blood first was achieved in the late nineteenth century by Edward Pfluger and August Krogh, who developed a bubble method that involved equilibration of small gas bubbles with large volumes of blood followed by analysis of gas tensions in the bubble. In 1942, Francis Roughton and Per Scholander modified this method to measure carbon monoxide (CO) using a syringe with a calibrated capillary for equilibration so that only a small amount of blood was needed. This syringe method was adapted later by Richard Riley for measuring Po_2 in the blood, and it became known as the *Riley bubble method*. The Riley bubble method was widely used, primarily as a research tool to study ventilation-perfusion relationships in the lung. In 1954, Leland Clark constructed the first modern PO_2 electrode, which measured PO_2 based on the polarographic principle. Its miniaturization subsequently allowed the incorporation of the entire electrode into the modern blood gas analyzer.

Gas Exchange between the Lungs and Blood

Humphrey Davy first demonstrated the presence of both O_2 and CO_2 in blood in 1799. In 1837, Heinrich Gustav Magnus quantified the amount of O_2 and CO_2 in blood. He found that arterial blood contained more O_2, but less CO_2, than venous blood. These findings led to his hypothesis that blood gas exchange took place in the lungs while the oxidation and generation of body heat occurred elsewhere. However, the mechanism of gas exchange in the lungs was hotly debated between two schools of scientists in the eighteenth century. The Secretionists, represented by Carl Ludwig, Christian Bohr, and John Scott Haldane, believed that the lungs actively pumped the respiratory gases into the blood. The Diffusionists, led by Edward Pfluger, claimed that all exchange of respiratory gases occurred by simple diffusion. The diffusion theory eventually prevailed after a series of elegant studies by August and Marie Krogh in the early 1990s.

Hemoglobin and Oxyhemoglobin Equilibrium Curve

The discovery of **hemoglobin** is usually credited to Felix Hoppe-Seyler, who crystallized it and described its spectrum in 1862. He also found that O_2 molecules form a loose and dissociable compound with hemoglobin, which he termed *oxyhemoglobin*. Carl Gustav von Hufner reported that 1 g of crystalline hemoglobin could combine with 1.34 mL of O_2. The in vivo relationship between PO_2 and O_2 content was demonstrated first by Paul Bert in 1878. This nonlinear relationship constituted the **oxyhemoglobin equilibrium curve (OEC),** also commonly called the *oxyhemoglobin dissociation curve*. The molecular basis for the OEC was not understood until the detailed chemical structure of the hemoglobin molecule was unveiled and the conformational changes of the molecule associated with binding and release of O_2 were defined by Linus Pauling and Max Perutz in the late 1940s.

Blood Gas Analyzers

pH Electrode

Measurement of pH is based on the linear relationship between the potential differences and pH variations across a pH-sensitive glass membrane. Figure 21-1 shows the basic design of the modern pH electrode, which consists of two chemical half-cells separated by a pH-sensitive glass membrane. One half-cell has a reference electrode, usually made of mercury-mercurous chloride (calomel), and the other has a measuring electrode, usually composed of silver-silver chloride. The mercury-mercurous chloride of the reference electrode provides a constant reference voltage at a constant temperature. The silver-silver chloride measuring electrode detects the voltage difference across the glass membrane produced by two solutions with different pH levels. The measuring half-cell is embedded within a chamber containing a buffer with a pH of 6.840, which is encased in

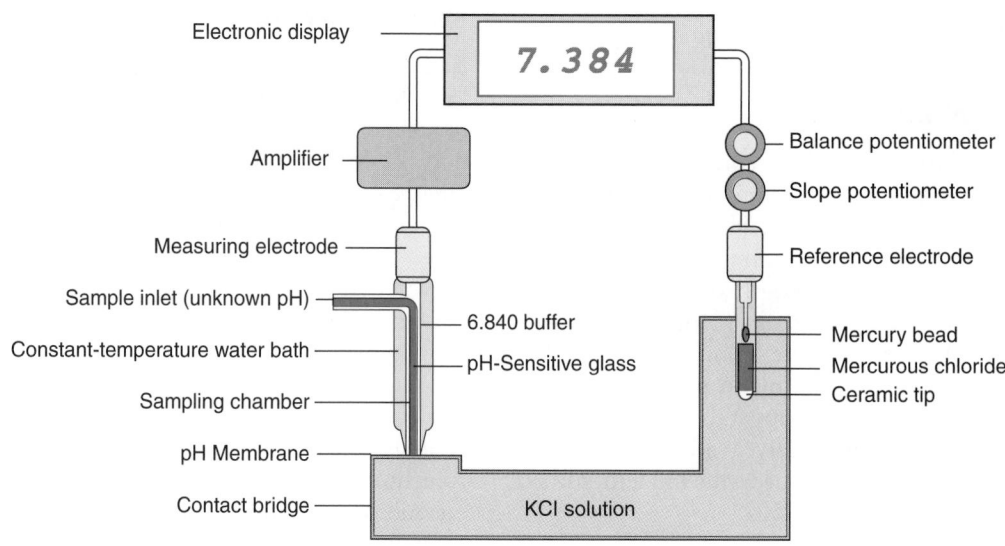

Figure 21-1   Schematic illustration of the modern pH electrode. (Modified from Shapiro BA. Clinical application of blood gases. Chicago: Year-Book; 1977.)

a constant-temperature water bath. The measuring half-cell is connected to the reference half-cell by a potassium chloride (KCl) contact bridge, which completes the electronic circuit. To prevent contamination, the KCl solution is separated from the unknown blood in the sampling chamber by a membrane. The modern pH electrode has a small sampling chamber that allows the use of aliquots of blood volume as small as 25 μL.[3] The pH electrode includes a balance potentiometer set to display 6.840 when the 6.840 buffer solution is placed in the measuring half-cell, as well as a slope potentiometer set to display 7.384 when the measuring half-cell is filled with 7.384 buffer solution. Because the potential difference is a linear function of the pH, two-point calibration (for example, pH of 6.840 and 7.384) is usually sufficient for accurate blood pH measurement. The modern pH electrode is sometimes referred to as the **Sanz electrode.**

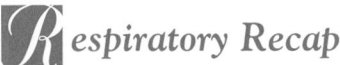

*R**espiratory Recap*

pH and Blood Gas Electrodes

A pH electrode measures the voltage difference across a glass membrane produced by two solutions of different pH.
A P_{CO_2} electrode measures pH change caused by CO_2 diffusion from the sample.
A P_{O_2} electrode uses the principles of polarography.
Oximetry uses light absorption at specific wavelengths.

P_{CO_2} Electrode

The principle of P_{CO_2} measurement is that changes of pH induced by the diffusion of CO_2 across a permeable membrane are proportional to P_{CO_2} in contact with the membrane. Thus the basic design of the P_{CO_2} electrode consists of a CO_2-permeable, but H^+-impermeable, membrane that separates the blood sample from the measuring half-cell (Figure 21-2). The measuring half-cell contains a dilute electrolyte solution (sodium bicarbonate and sodium or potassium chloride). When CO_2 in the blood sample dif-

fuses across the permeable membrane, it undergoes the following reaction:

$$CO_2 + H_2O \rightarrow H_2CO_3 \rightarrow H^+ + HCO_3^-.$$

Because H^+ concentration is directly proportional to CO_2 in contact with the membrane, pH measured by a pH electrode can be used as an indirect measure of P_{CO_2}.

The design of the P_{CO_2} electrode is slightly different from the Sanz electrode in that the pH-sensitive glass electrode is separated from the permeable membrane by nylon mesh or other spacers that allow bicarbonate solution to exist between the glass and membrane. The measuring and reference half-cells are silver-silver chloride. The entire pH electrode is bathed in electrolyte solution, which serves as the electronic bridge between the measuring and reference half-cells. The modern P_{CO_2} electrode, commonly referred to as the **Severinghaus electrode,** is a modification of the electrode developed by Stow in the early 1950s. Gas mixtures with a CO_2 concentration of 5% and 10% are commonly used to calibrate the P_{CO_2} electrode.

P_{O_2} Electrode

The P_{O_2} electrode, or **Clark electrode,** consists of a platinum cathode and silver anode immersed in a dilute, buffered potassium chloride solution (Figure 21-3). The Clark electrode measures P_{O_2} with the principle of polarography. The electric current produced by a cathode (negative electrode) in a solution is directly proportional to the availability of O_2 molecules at the cathode tip. When the O_2 molecules come in contact with the platinum cathode, they are reduced to hydroxide anion, as follows:

$$O_2 + 2H_2O + 4\ electrons \rightarrow 4\ OH^-.$$

The source of electrons comes from oxidation of the silver anode by the chloride anions attracted to the anode, forming silver chloride. Because the amount of O_2 reduced is directly proportional to the number of electrons (or current), P_{O_2} in the solution can be determined by measurement of the change in current between the anode and cathode. The modern P_{O_2} electrode system is usually covered by an O_2-permeable but electrically nonconductive membrane

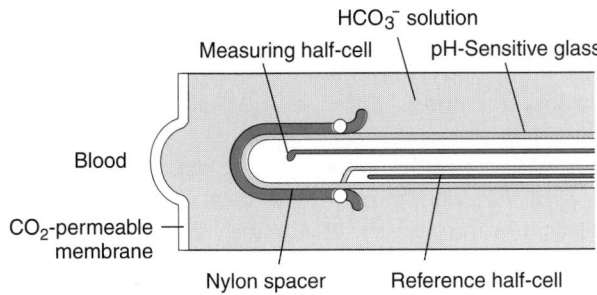

Figure 21-2 Schematic illustration of the modern P_{CO_2} electrode.

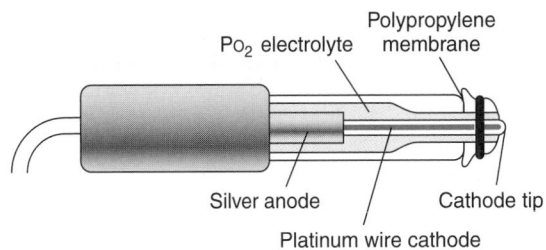

Figure 21-3 Schematic illustration of the P_{O_2} electrode. (Modified from Shapiro BA. Clinical application of blood gases. Chicago: Year-Book; 1977.)

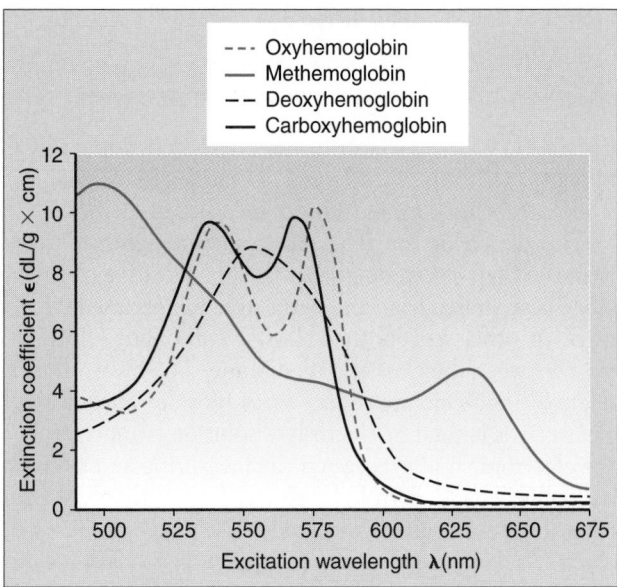

Figure 21-4   Absorption spectra for hemoglobin species.

(such as polypropylene or polyethylene), which allows slow diffusion of O_2 from the blood into the electrode while preventing degradation of the electrode by the blood.

Gas mixtures with O_2 concentrations of 0% and 12% or 20% usually are used to calibrate the electrode. For convenience and economy, the calibration gases for the P_{O_2} and P_{CO_2} electrodes usually are combined with one gas composed of 5% CO_2 and 12% or 20% O_2 balanced with nitrogen and a second gas containing 10% CO_2 and 90% nitrogen. The P_{O_2} electrode also responds to halothane, resulting in inaccurate P_{O_2} measurements in blood drawn from patients anesthetized with this drug.[7]

Oximeter

Hemoglobin content in the blood can be measured by an **oximeter,** a spectrophotometer that uses specific wavelengths in the oxyhemoglobin spectrum. The light at those wavelengths is absorbed at the vibrational frequencies of the molecule of interest (such as oxyhemoglobin) in the solution. The concentration of the molecule in the solution can be determined through quantification of the amount of light absorbed by the solution. Modern oximeters, such as the CO oximeter, can generate multiple spectra (usually four) that allow distinction among four major hemoglobin species: oxyhemoglobin, reduced hemoglobin (deoxyhemoglobin), **carboxyhemoglobin,** and **methemoglobin** (Figure 21-4).

Blood Gas Sampling

Sites of Arterial Puncture

The ideal arterial sampling site should be easily accessible, have collateral blood flow, and be relatively insensitive to pain. Based on these criteria the radial artery is the pre-

ferred site for arterial puncture and cannulation for adult patients (CPG 21-1). The brachial artery is a good alternative if the radial arteries are unavailable. Femoral artery punctures should be used only if absolutely necessary because the artery is deep under the skin and the risk of undetected postpuncture bleeding is increased. The limited collateral arterial flow makes the lower limb more susceptible to ischemia if the femoral artery is occluded by clot or hematoma. In addition, the risk of infection is higher because the femoral artery is close to the perineum.

Allen's Test

Before radial arterial puncture or cannulation is performed, the modified **Allen's test** is performed to ascertain adequate ulnar artery perfusion to the hand. This test was proposed originally in 1929 by Edgar V. Allen as a noninvasive evaluation of the patency of the arterial supply to the hand of individuals with thromboangiitis obliterans.[8] The test was later modified for use as a test of collateral circulation before arterial cannulation.[9] The patient makes a fist to force blood from the hand, and pressure is applied to compress the ulnar and radial arteries. The patient then relaxes the hand, and obstructing pressure is removed from the ulnar artery while the radial artery remains compressed. If the ulnar artery is patent, the hand should become flushed within 10 seconds, constituting a normal or positive Allen's test. If the Allen's test is abnormal, ulnar perfusion to the hand should be assumed to be poor, and the radial artery in the contralateral wrist or other alternative site should be considered for arterial blood sampling. Although the modified Allen's test has significant false-positive and false-negative rates, it remains a simple, useful screening test to assess the adequacy of ulnar collateral perfusion of the hand.

Technique for Radial Arterial Puncture

After collateral circulation has been assessed, the patient is prepared for puncture of the radial artery. A towel is rolled under the wrist, with the hand hyperextended to bring the radial artery closer to the skin surface. The radial artery is located via palpation for maximal arterial pulsation. The puncture site is cleansed with an alcohol swab, iodophor solution, or other appropriate disinfectant. The arterial puncture can be performed with either a glass syringe lubricated with a minimal amount of liquid heparin or a special, vented, preheparinized (100 to 200 IU), self-filling plastic syringe. The blood gas syringe should be fitted with a 1-inch, 22- or 23-gauge needle.

With the nondominant hand locating the maximal arterial pulsation and the dominant hand holding the syringe needle at a 45-degree angle pointing in the opposite direction of arterial flow with the needle bevel up, the skin is punctured and the needle advanced. Because the radial nerve lies laterally to the artery, care must be taken not to direct the needle toward the lateral aspect of the wrist. Once the artery is entered, a flash of arterial blood is seen

CPG 21-1

Sampling for Arterial Blood Gas Analysis

Indications

The need to evaluate the adequacy of ventilatory ($Paco_2$) acid-base (pH and $Paco_2$), and oxygenation (Pao_2 and Sao_2) status, and the oxygen-carrying capacity of blood (Pao_2, Hbo_2, Hb_{total}, and dyshemoglobins)

The need to quantitate the patient's response to therapeutic intervention, diagnostic evaluation (such as oxygen therapy or exercise testing), or both

The need to monitor severity and progression of a documented disease process

Contraindications

Negative results of a modified Allen test (collateral circulation test) are indicative of inadequate blood supply to the hand and suggest the need to select another extremity as the puncture site.

Arterial puncture should not be performed through a lesion or through or distal to a surgical shunt (such as in a dialysis patient). If evidence exists of infection or peripheral vascular disease involving the selected limb, an alternative site should be selected.

Agreement is lacking regarding the puncture sites associated with a lesser likelihood of complications. However, because of the need to monitor the femoral puncture site for an extended period, femoral punctures should not be performed outside the hospital.

A coagulopathy or medium-to-high-dose anticoagulation therapy (such as heparin or Coumadin, streptokinase, or tissue plasminogen activator [but not necessarily aspirin]) may be a relative contraindication for arterial puncture.

Hazards and Complications

Hematoma
Arteriospasm
Air or clotted-blood emboli
Anaphylaxis from local anesthetic

Introduction of contagion at sampling site and consequent infection in patient; introduction of contagion to sampler by inadvertent needle stick

Hemorrhage

Trauma to the vessel

Arterial occlusion

Vasovagal response

Pain

Assessment of Need

History and physical indicators, such as positive smoking history, recent onset of difficulty in breathing independent of activity level, or trauma

Presence of other abnormal diagnostic tests or indices, such as abnormal pulse oximetry reading, or chest x-ray film

Initiation of, administration of, or change in therapeutic modalities (for example, initiation, titration, or discontinuance of supplemental oxygen or initiation of, changes in, or discontinuance of mechanical ventilation)

Projected surgical interventions for patients at risk

Projected enrollment in a pulmonary rehabilitation program

Assessment of Test Quality

Sampling of arterial blood for any indication listed is useful for patient management only if the sampling procedure is carried out according to an established, proven protocol. The validity of test results can be voided if any of the following occur:

• The sample is contaminated by air, improper anticoagulant or inappropriate anticoagulant concentration, flush solution (if sample is drawn from an indwelling catheter), or venous blood.

• The sample clots because of improper anticoagulation of the collection device, improper mixing, or exposure to air.

• Analysis is delayed (>15 minutes for samples held at room temperature or >60 minutes for samples held at 4° C).

Modified from AARC Clinical practice guideline: sampling for arterial blood gas analysis. Respir Care 1992;37:913-917.
CPG, Clinical practice guideline.

in the needle hub. Approximately 2 to 3 mL of arterial blood is collected as the arterial pressure fills the syringe. Usually, aspiration is unnecessary.

After the desired blood volume has been obtained, the needle is withdrawn from the artery and the site compressed for at least 5 minutes. This compression decreases the possibility of hematoma formation, compartment syndromes, and ecchymosis, which may interfere with future arterial punctures. Longer compression times may be necessary for patients receiving anticoagulants (for example, heparin or Coumadin) or those with coagulation defects (for example, thrombocytopenia, chronic renal failure, or disseminated intravascular coagulation). After bleeding has stopped, an elastic bandage is applied with moderate pressure. The exposed needle should be disposed of safely in a puncture-resistant container, and air bubbles should be

expelled. Then the syringe is sealed with a cap and gently mixed for a few seconds, and the blood is analyzed immediately or placed on ice if blood gas analysis will be delayed.

Punctures of Other Arterial Sites

For brachial artery puncture the arm should be hyperextended and the hand pronated to best stabilize the artery. The brachial artery should be palpated on the medial side of the biceps tendon, 1 to 2 cm distal to the antecubital fossa. Care must be taken to not direct the puncture medially because this site is the most frequent location of the median nerve. The femoral artery is entered perpendicularly, with the patient in the supine position. The artery is best palpated and fixed just below the inguinal crease. The femoral nerve lies lateral and the femoral vein medial to the artery.

Most individuals can tolerate a single arterial puncture without local anesthesia. Sometimes a local anesthetic (such as 1% lidocaine HCl) is necessary, especially for arterial cannulation or to decrease the pain and minimize anxiety-induced changes in a patient's blood gas values. Complications associated with arterial puncture include hematoma, arteriospasm, and thrombosis, all of which may result in hand ischemia if perfusion is not restored promptly.[10] The patient's reaction to arterial puncture ranges from feelings of uneasiness to vasovagal syncope, shocklike symptoms, or convulsions.

Radial Artery Cannulation

Arterial cannulation is performed when frequent arterial blood gas measurements are required and when continuous monitoring of arterial blood pressure is necessary. Usually the radial artery is cannulated. The arterial catheter is usually placed through percutaneous puncture, although a Seldinger technique also can be used. Before insertion, the area of puncture is anesthetized with 2% lidocaine (without epinephrine, which increases the risk of arterial spasm). A 20-gauge beveled needle with a clear, plastic flash chamber is used. A straight, stiff, Teflon or polyurethane catheter with a hub at its distal end is placed over the needle. The technique for insertion of the radial artery catheter is illustrated in Figure 21-5. After insertion, the catheter is attached to a kit consisting of connective tubing, a stopcock for blood gas sampling, a transducer for blood pressure monitoring, and a continuous flush solution to prevent clotting in the catheter. The catheter is secured in place with tape or sutures.

Capillary Blood Gases

Capillary samples may be used to estimate pH and P_{CO_2} in infants or other individuals when arterial blood gas analysis is indicated but arterial access is difficult (CPG 21-2). A puncture or small incision is made with a lancet into the cutaneous layer of the skin in a highly vascular area. The site is warmed before the procedure to arterialize the blood. Blood is collected in a heparinized glass capillary tube. Capillary punctures should not be performed through previous puncture sites; through inflamed, edematous, cyanotic, or poorly perfused tissues; through areas of infection; through peripheral arteries; through the posterior curvature of the heel to avoid injuring bone; or in the fingers of neonates to avoid nerve damage. Excessive squeezing of the puncture site may result in venous or lymphatic contamination of the sample. Capillary sampling should not be performed on infants less than 24 hours old because of poor peripheral perfusion. Relative contraindications include peripheral vasoconstriction, polycythemia (caused by shorter clotting times), and hypotension. Capillary blood is handled similar to arterial blood samples; it should be free of contamination by air or blood clots and analyzed in an appropriate time frame. Extreme variability in capillary P_{O_2} values precludes the use of this technique to assess oxygenation.

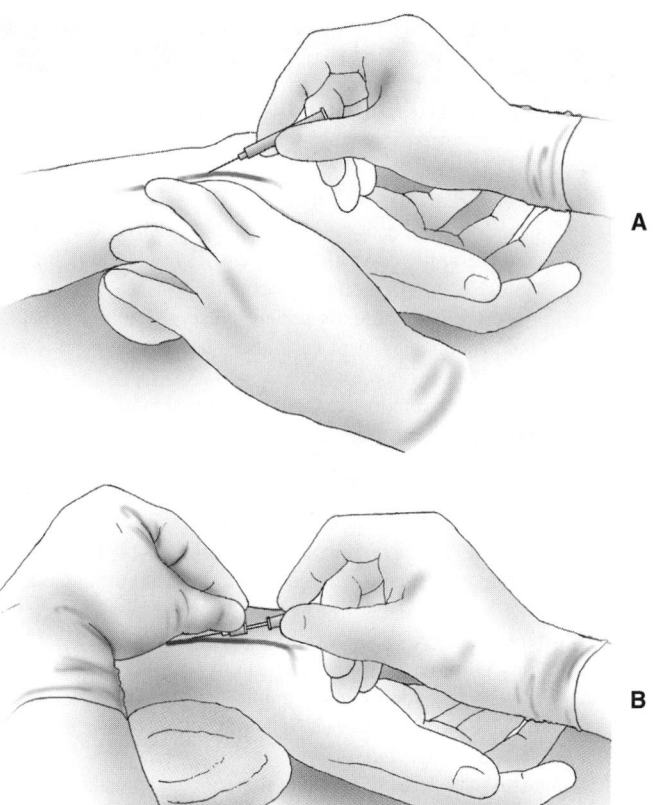

Figure 21-5   Technique of radial artery cannulation. **A,** Needle is positioned at a 30- to 45-degree angle to the plane of the skin, with the tip directly over the radial artery (bevel upward). The paths of the needle and the artery should be parallel. The needle enters the skin at an angle. Thus the insertion point should be slightly distal to the desired point for the needle to cross into the artery. With a slow, steady motion, the needle is advanced through the skin. A flash of blood indicates that the artery has been entered. **B,** Once blood is returned, the needle is lowered so that it lies much closer to the skin and then advanced 1 to 2 mm further. If blood is still flashing in the plastic chamber, the catheter can be safely advanced over the needle.

Quality Control

Sample Procurement

After the arterial blood specimen is obtained, any air bubble larger than 5% of the blood sample should be expelled. Because room air contains a P_{CO_2} of essentially zero and a P_{O_2} of approximately 150 mm Hg, air bubbles in the blood sample lower the P_{CO_2} values of the blood sample and cause the P_{O_2} to approach 150 mm Hg. The syringe must be capped immediately and placed on ice after sampling, and the technician in the blood gas laboratory must take great care to ensure that ambient air does not mix with the sample as it is introduced into the blood gas analyzer.

Because sodium heparin has a pH of approximately 7.0, too much heparin may affect the pH. In general, 0.05 to 0.1 mL of heparin per milliliter of blood does not affect the pH value and provides adequate anticoagulation.[11]

CPG 21-2

Capillary Blood Gases

Indications

Arterial blood gas analysis is indicated but arterial access is not available.

Noninvasive monitor readings are abnormal: transcutaneous values, end-tidal CO_2, pulse oximetry.

Assessment of initiation, administration, or change in therapeutic modalities (mechanical ventilation) is indicated.

A change in patient status is detected by history or physical assessment.

Monitoring the severity and progression of a documented disease process is desirable.

Contraindications

Capillary punctures should not be performed at or through the following sites: posterior curvature of the heel (because the device may puncture the bone); the heel of a patient who has begun walking and has callus development; the fingers of infants (to prevent nerve damage); previous puncture sites; inflamed, swollen, or edematous tissues; cyanotic or poorly perfused tissues; localized areas of infection; and peripheral arteries.

Capillary punctures should not be performed on patients less than 24 hours old because of poor peripheral perfusion.

Capillary punctures should not be performed when direct analysis of oxygenation is needed.

Capillary punctures should not be performed when direct analysis of arterial blood is needed.

Relative contraindications include peripheral vasoconstriction and polycythemia (caused by shorter clotting times); hypotension may be a relative contraindication.

Hazards and Complications

Infection

Introduction of contagion at sampling site and consequent infection in patient, including calcaneus osteomyelitis and cellulitis

Inadvertent puncture or incision and consequent infection in clinician's obtaining sample

Burns

Hematoma

Bone calcification

Nerve damage

Bruising

Scarring

Puncture of posterior medial aspect of heel (possibly resulting in tibial artery laceration)

Pain

Bleeding

Inappropriate patient management (possibly resulting from reliance on capillary Po_2 values)

Limitations of Method

Inadequate warming of the site before a puncture may result in capillary values that correlate poorly with arterial pH and Pco_2 values.

Undue squeezing of the puncture site may result in venous and lymphatic contamination of the sample.

A second puncture may be necessary to obtain an adequate amount of blood for analysis.

Variability in capillary Po_2 values precludes use of these samples to assess oxygenation status.

Assessment of Need

Capillary blood gas sampling is an intermittent procedure and should be performed when a documented need exists. Routine or standing orders for capillary puncture are not recommended. The following may assist the clinician in assessing the need for capillary blood gas sampling:

- History and physical assessment
- Noninvasive respiratory monitoring values: pulse oximetry, transcutaneous values, end-tidal CO_2 values
- Patient response to initiation, administration, or change in therapeutic modalities
- Lack of arterial access for blood gas sampling

Assessment of Test Quality

The validity of the test may be jeopardized if any of the following occur:

- The sample is contaminated by air.
- Clots prevent accurate analysis.
- Quantity of sample is insufficient for analysis.
- Analysis of sample is delayed (>15 minutes for samples at room temperature, or >60 minutes for samples held at 4° C).

Modified from AARC Clinical practice guideline: capillary blood gases. Respir Care 1994;1180-1183.
CPG, Clinical practice guideline.

The volume of the dead space is proportional to the size of the syringe. For example, the dead space of a 5-mL syringe with a needle is about 0.2 mL. Thus 2 to 4 mL of blood should be obtained so that it contains at least 0.05 mL heparin per 1 mL blood but no more than 0.1 mL heparin per 1 mL blood. Thus before arterial blood is obtained, the syringe should be flushed with heparin and ejected so that the volume of heparin in the syringe is kept at a minimum. The commercially available, prehep-

arinized syringes have minimized such a contamination problem because they use dry, lyophilized heparin. If electrolyte measurements are performed with the blood gas sample, lithium heparin should be used, rather than sodium heparin.

Once the arterial blood gas sample is obtained, it should be promptly transported (within 15 minutes) to the arterial blood gas laboratory for analysis. Many intensive care units (ICUs) have a vacuum tube transport system ideal for distances of 200 feet or more. A delay could lead to erroneous readings because gas diffusion through the plastic syringe wall or between a bubble and blood increases with time, especially when the blood gas tensions differ significantly from those of room air. The diffusion rate also increases with temperature (Table 21-1).

If the sample cannot be analyzed immediately, it should be placed in ice (slush or chips) to hasten cooling. Putting the sample in ice slush also slows down **oxygen consumption** by white blood cells (WBCs), which is approximately 0.1 mL of O_2 from 100 mL blood in 10 minutes at body temperature. This effect is exaggerated if the WBC count is very high (leukocyte larceny). The effect on PO_2 is more prominent if the hemoglobin saturation of the arterial blood is high. For example, if the sample is not iced, PO_2 drops to below 250 mm Hg in 1 hour if the original PO_2 is 400 mm Hg. However, if PO_2 is 50 mm Hg, the loss of 0.1 mL O_2 per 100 mL blood makes a very small change in PO_2 because the primary change occurs in the hemoglobin saturation.

Preanalytic errors are issues affecting blood gas results that occur before the sample is introduced into the blood gas analyzer. Common such errors are listed in Box 21-1.

Sample Analysis

The blood gas sample should be mixed well before the analysis. Although mixing has minimal effect on blood gases and pH, it is necessary if hemoglobin or hematocrit is to be measured by a CO oximeter. As previously mentioned, any air bubbles need to be removed before thorough mixing occurs. Blood clots also should be removed so that the blood gas analyzer does not become plugged. Expelling one or two drops of blood from the syringe tip onto a gauze pad or tissue directly before introduction into the analyzer helps ensure that clots are not present and air bubbles are not introduced.

Blood gas calibrations are required in accordance with the manufacturer's instructions, with a frequency determined by volume of use. Calibration reagents are usually standard CO_2 and O_2 gases (for example, 5% CO_2 + 20% O_2 and 10% CO_2 + 90% N_2) for PO_2 and PCO_2 sensors and phosphate buffers (for example, pH 6.840 and pH 7.384) for pH. The reagents are referenced to the National Institute of Standards and Technology (NIST). Most modern blood gas instruments perform automatic calibration at least every 30 minutes. When a blood gas sample has very high values (for example, a PO_2 value of 600 mm Hg), the operator may need to measure tonometered blood with known values at similar extreme levels to ascertain the instrument's degree of inaccuracy.

Tonometry of Blood

Because of the unique O_2-binding characteristics of hemoglobin and complex viscosity characteristics of normal fresh blood, whole blood must be carefully tonometered so that exact gas tensions can be prepared for analysis by a blood gas instrument. A **tonometry** reference method has been developed and recognized as the internationally accepted standard method. The method requires fresh blood (less than 24 hours old) from asymptomatic donors, which should be nonhemolyzed and without leukocytosis or high blood lipid levels. Gas mixtures, the composition of which have been verified by a mass spectrometer or with a CO_2 and O_2 gas analyzer, can be used to equilibrate the blood. If human blood is not available, bovine hemoglobin solutions (containing both deoxygenated and oxygenated hemoglobin) also can be used. These bovine preparations have been shown to yield data closely resembling those obtained with human blood. These solutions also can be formulated to provide precision data for the pH and electrolytes.

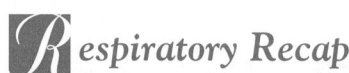
$\mathcal{R}$espiratory Recap

Calibration, Quality Control, and Proficiency Testing

Calibration adjusts the analyzer to reference standards.
Quality control analyzes materials of known values for pH, PCO_2, and PO_2.
Proficiency testing analyzes materials from an external source that have values unknown to the tester.

$\mathcal{T}$ABLE 21-1

Approximate Changes with Time and Temperature* after Sample is Drawn into Syringe

Factor	37° C	4° C
pH	0.01/10 min	0.001/10 min
PCO_2	1 mm Hg/10 min	0.1 mm Hg/10 min
PO_2	0.1 vol%/10 min	0.01 vol%/10 min

*A temperature of 37° C assumes that the blood remains at body temperature in the syringe. A temperature of 4° C assumes that the sample is properly iced immediately after being drawn.

$\mathcal{B}$OX 21-1

Common Arterial Blood Gas Preanalytic Errors

Room air contamination of sample
Heparin dilution of sample
Hyperventilation during sample collection
Long delay time between sample collection and analysis
Excessive sample metabolism (leukocyte larceny with high WBC count)
Inadequate wait time between change in inspired oxygen or ventilation and collection of blood sample

WBC, White blood cell.

Quality Control and Proficiency Testing

The quality of results is crucial for blood gas analysis. The general aspects of quality control are regulated by the federal government through the **Clinical Laboratory Improvement Amendment (CLIA).** A properly designed quality control program enables proper function of the blood gas analyzer on a routine basis. Quality control procedures for a blood gas analyzer differ from other analyses performed in the clinical laboratory environment because the patient sample is fresh, whole blood.

The optimal technique used to establish the extent of inaccuracy and imprecision of an individual blood gas analyzer is the use of whole blood tonometry with samples of fresh, anticoagulated, whole blood. However, the technical and economic advantages of whole blood tonometry must be balanced by its hazard potential and labor-intensive process. Alternatives to whole blood tonometry are commercially available, prepackaged materials such as aqueous buffer solutions, blood-based (hemoglobin containing) materials, and perfluorocarbon-oil emulsions. However, the physical and chemical properties of these controls do not match those of whole blood.

Whichever materials are chosen, the results of the quality control program should be recorded in a manner that allows the operator to easily detect changes in performance of the instrument. This detection is most commonly done with Levey-Jennings charts (Figure 21-6). CLIA requires at least two levels of control for pH, Pco_2, and Po_2 on each work shift or every 8 hours of operation. Because internal quality control programs better estimate precision than accuracy, external proficiency testing programs are used. (These programs are available from sources such as the College of American Pathologists [CAP] and the American Thoracic Society [ATS].)

Temperature Correction

Controversy exists regarding whether blood gas values should be corrected for the actual individual's body temperature in clinical practice. The argument for temperature correction (such as during hypothermia) is that blood gas values measured at 37° C may not accurately reflect the true oxygenation and acid-base status of the body. Although Po_2 changes with temperature (7% per degree Celsius), O_2 capacity, O_2 content, and hemoglobin saturation do not. Thus the Po_2 of the arterial blood in a cold extremity may be only 40 mm Hg, but the saturation value is 96%. If such a temperature-corrected value of Po_2 is reported, the Po_2 may seem dangerously low to the clinician while in fact the hypothermic patient is adequately oxygenated.

The same argument also applies to the acid-base status. Pco_2 and pH change with temperature (4% per degree Celsius for Pco_2; 0.0146 units per degree Celsius for pH), but the bicarbonate and intracellular neutrality do not. This concept is best illustrated with the example of heavy exercise (Figure 21-7).[12] Blood at the core temperature of 37° C has a pH of 7.4, which is alkaline relative to the intracellular fluid (ICF) with a pH of 6.8. Blood in the exercising muscles, which have a temperature of 41° C, has a lower pH of 7.35 and a higher Pco_2 of 48 mm Hg. Blood in the cooler skin (25° C) has a higher pH of 7.6 and a lower Pco_2 of 22 mm Hg.

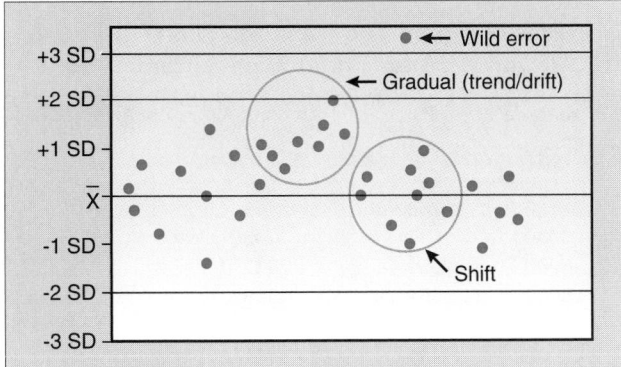

Figure 21-6 Three types of analytic errors identified on a Levey-Jennings chart: wild error (outlier), gradual error (trend, drift), and a shift to a new (in this case, lower) mean. *SD,* Standard deviation. (Modified from Branson RD, Hess DR, Chatburn RL. Respiratory care equipment. 2nd ed. Philadelphia: JB Lippincott; 1999.)

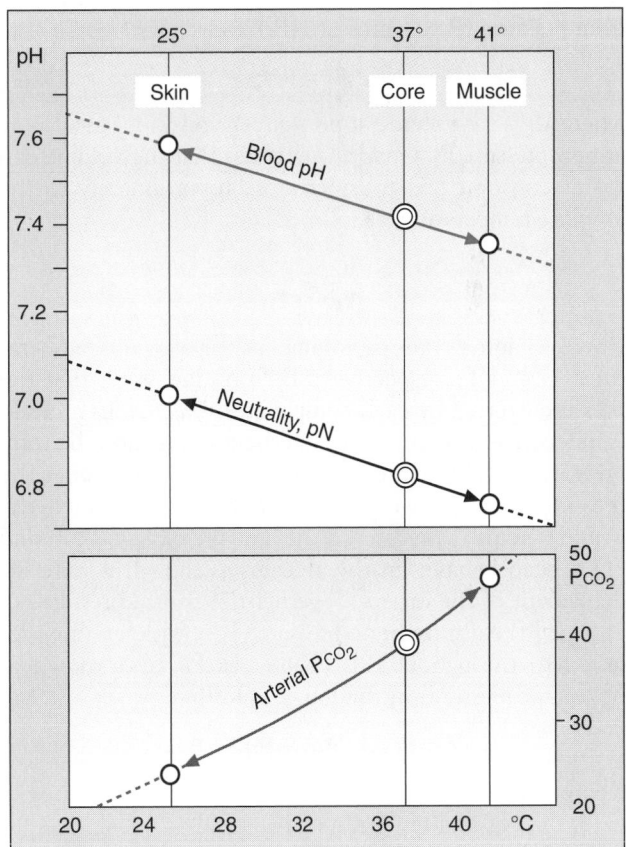

Figure 21-7 Expected changes in blood pH and Pco_2 in the arterioles of skin at 25° C and working muscle at 41° C of a healthy man with a core temperature of 37° C. (Modified from Rahn H. Body temperature and acid-base regulation. Pneumonologie 1974;151:87-94.)

Despite these striking regional variations in pH and P_{CO_2}, the CO_2 content and the relative alkalinity between blood and ICF remain constant. Thus the pH and P_{CO_2} values at 37° C reliably reflect the in vivo acid-base status of the patient. Most acid-base nomograms are valid only at 37° C,[13] and temperature correction does not improve clinical decision making. Based on these arguments, routine blood gas measurements have been recommended to be consistently reported at 37° C without correction for actual body temperature.[14,15] On rare occasions the temperature-corrected values for arterial (and alveolar) values may be more appropriate, such as for the calculation of the alveolar-arterial O_2 gradient or arterial-alveolar end-tidal CO_2 gradient in patients with abnormal temperatures. The P_{O_2} or P_{CO_2} values of the arterial blood and alveolar gas should be expressed at body temperature.

Physiology of Gas Exchange

Gas Laws

Boyle's law states that at a constant temperature, the volume of any gas (V) varies inversely with the pressure (P) to which the gas is subjected. For a perfect gas changing from pressure (P_1) to pressure (P_2), as follows:

$$P_1V_1 = P_2V_2$$

where V_1 is gas volume at pressure P_1 and V_2 is gas volume at new pressure P_2. Charles' law states that the volume of a gas at constant pressure increases proportionately to the absolute temperature, as follows:

$$\frac{V_1}{V_2} = \frac{T_1}{T_2}$$

where V_1 and V_2 are gas volumes at the absolute temperatures T_1 and T_2, respectively. Dalton's law states that the pressure exerted by each component in a gaseous mixture is independent of other gases in the mixture, and the total pressure of the mixture of gases is equal to the sum of the pressure each gas would exert if it alone occupied the whole volume. The gases in the lung are CO_2, O_2, N_2, and H_2O. Each behaves in the alveolus as though it were independent of the others. Together the partial pressures of all equal the atmospheric pressure (P_{atm}, which will be referred to throughout this chapter as P_B, also known as *barometric pressure*) in the lungs, as follows:

$$P_B = P_{CO_2} + P_{O_2} + P_{N_2} + P_{H_2O}$$

where P_{CO_2}, P_{O_2}, P_{N_2}, and P_{H_2O} are partial pressures of CO_2, O_2, N_2, and H_2O, respectively.

Partial Pressure of Gas in Ambient Air

The partial pressure of a gas in ambient air is a function of its atmospheric concentration. In dry air the partial pressure of O_2 in the inspired gas (P_{IO_2}) is equal to the following:

$$P_{IO_2} = F_{IO_2} \times P_B$$

where P_B is the atmospheric pressure and F_{IO_2} is the fractional concentration of O_2. At sea level, P_B is 760 mm Hg and F_{IO_2} is 0.21. Therefore the P_{IO_2} is 159.6 mm Hg. In moist, inspired gas fully saturated with water vapor (P_{H_2O} being 47 mm Hg at 37° C), P_{IO_2} is as follows:

$$P_{IO_2} = (P_B - P_{H_2O}) \times F_{IO_2} = (760 - 47) \times 0.21 \cong 150 \text{ mm Hg}$$

At high altitudes, where P_B is less, P_{IO_2} decreases, although the fraction of O_2 in the air remains 0.21 (Table 21-2). Alveolar P_{O_2} decreases more than the atmospheric P_{O_2} because of excreted CO_2 and the pressure of water vapor. At a temperature of 37° C the saturated water vapor pressure is 47 mm Hg, regardless of barometric pressure.

Gases dissolve in solutions depending on the solubility in that solution. Gas dissolved in solution tends to escape through the liquid surface into the gas phase. The gas also may return from the gas phase into the solution. When the partial pressure of a gas tending to come from the solution is equal to the partial pressure of the same gas tending to go back into the solution, the system is in equilibrium. The partial pressure of the gas in the solution is equal to the partial pressure of the gas in the gas phase.

Blood Gas Transport

In humans the metabolic processes of the body are supported by the integrated functions of the heart, lungs, and blood. Atmospheric O_2 brought into the air spaces of the lungs diffuses into the erythrocyte and is bound reversibly to hemoglobin. The erythrocyte travels to the tissue capillaries, where O_2 dissociates from hemoglobin and diffuses down its concentration gradient into the cells to be consumed in the mitochondria. The blood then carries CO_2

$\mathcal{T}$ABLE 21-2

Decrease of Barometric Pressure, Ambient P_{O_2} (P_{IO_2}), and Alveolar P_{O_2} at High Altitude

Altitude (Feet)	P_B (mm Hg)	Ambient P_{IO_2} (mm Hg)	Alveolar P_{O_2} (mm Hg)
0	760	159	109
3000	682	143	103
5000	630	132	92
8000	564	118	78
10,000	523	110	70
12,000	483	101	61
15,000	412	90	50
18,000	379	80	40
20,000	349	73	33
30,000	226	47	7

generated in the mitochondria to the alveolar capillaries, where it diffuses down its concentration gradient into the air spaces of the lung. CO_2 then is eliminated by ventilation. These gas-transport mechanisms use the physical processes of diffusion (between lungs and blood and between tissues and blood), chemical reactions (between O_2 or CO_2 and hemoglobin), and convection (between lungs and tissues).

Oxygen Pathway

The use of O_2 by the body occurs by a relatively simple physical pathway. This O_2 pathway begins in the atmosphere, where P_{O_2} is about 160 mm Hg, and ends at the mitochondria, where P_{O_2} is only a few millimeters of mercury (Figure 21-8). Inspired P_{O_2} decreases as soon as the ambient gas reaches conducting airways, which is caused by warming of the inhaled air and its saturation with water vapor. These processes dilute the inspired mixture of N_2 and O_2. Once the inspirate reaches the terminal respiratory units, gas exchange takes place (O_2 uptake). The blood in the pulmonary capillaries leaving the alveoli contains approximately the same P_{O_2} as the gas phase of the terminal units. The P_{O_2} in arterial blood is slightly lower because local matching of ventilation and perfusion in normal lungs is imperfect, and unoxygenated blood is added to pulmonary capillary blood from the postpulmonary shunt. O_2 then is delivered to the systemic capillaries, where it diffuses into the cells to support aerobic metabolism. The bulk of molecular O_2 (about 90%) is consumed in the mitochondria.

Oxygen Uptake

O_2 is normally taken up by the lungs' approximately 300 million alveoli, each of which is about 300 μm in diameter. The huge surface area (approximately 75 m²) and the thin septa (less than 0.5 μm thick) of the alveoli provide an extremely efficient mechanism for the human body to take up O_2 from the ambient air. With each inspiration, approximately 500 mL of air enters the lungs (tidal volume). If anatomic dead space is 150 mL and the respiratory rate is 12 breaths/min, alveolar ventilation is 4.2 L/min (350 mL × 12/min).

O_2 in the alveolar space diffuses into the pulmonary capillaries, where it binds the hemoglobin in the erythrocytes and enters the systemic circulation. Each erythrocyte traverses the pulmonary microcirculation in about 0.75 seconds (Figure 21-9). Within the first third of this brief transit time (0.25 seconds) the hemoglobin virtually becomes completely oxygenated. At the same time, CO_2 formed in the body tissues is removed from the pulmonary capillaries by ventilation. Slightly more O_2 is removed from the alveolar space than CO_2 is added, given a normal respiratory exchange ratio of 0.8. The efficiency of O_2-CO_2 exchange is determined primarily by the ventilation-perfusion ($\dot{V}_A/\dot{Q}$) relationship of the lung units. Low $\dot{V}_A/\dot{Q}$ units and right-to-left shunt ($\dot{V}_A/\dot{Q} = 0$) are associated with impaired O_2 uptake from the alveolar space, whereas high $\dot{V}_A/\dot{Q}$ units and dead space ($\dot{V}_A/\dot{Q} = $ infinity) result in inefficient elimination of CO_2 from the pulmonary arterial blood.

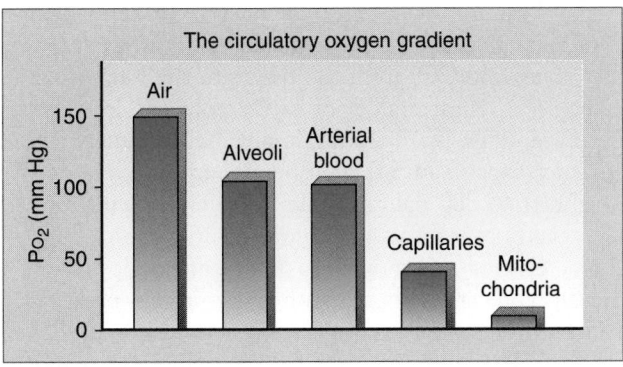

Figure 21-8 The oxygen gradient from the alveolar space to the mitochondria. Note the stepwise decrement in P_{O_2} from 100 mm Hg in the alveolar space to values of a few mm Hg at the mitochondria, where most of the oxygen is consumed. (Modified from Baum GL, Crapo JD, Celli B, et al. Textbook of pulmonary diseases. 6th ed. Philadelphia: Lippincott Williams & Wilkins; 1998.)

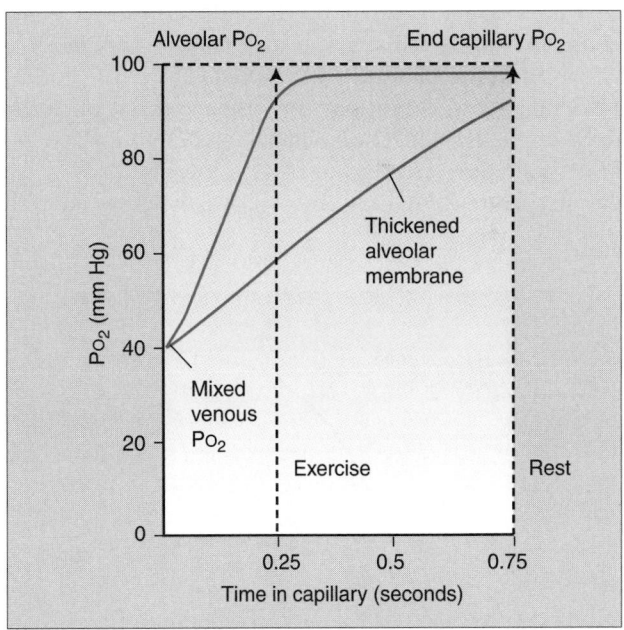

Figure 21-9 Typical time courses for the change in P_{O_2} in the pulmonary capillary. Note that it takes an average of 0.75 seconds for each erythrocyte to traverse the pulmonary microcirculation. In healthy lungs the hemoglobin becomes virtually completely oxygenated within 0.25 seconds. In abnormal lungs with significant $\dot{V}_A/\dot{Q}$ mismatch and thickened alveolar capillary membrane, the hemoglobin at end-capillary may not be fully saturated. This effect is further accentuated by exercise, which shortens the capillary transit time. (Modified from Baum GL, Crapo JD, Celli B, et al. Textbook of pulmonary diseases. 6th ed. Philadelphia: Lippincott Williams & Wilkins; 1998.)

Oxygen Transport

Once O_2 diffuses into the pulmonary capillaries, it binds rapidly to hemoglobin. The affinity of hemoglobin for O_2 increases with increasing O_2 saturation (cooperativity). The OEC has a sigmoid shape (Figure 21-10). The amount of O_2 transported in the blood to the peripheral tissues (O_2 delivery or DO_2) can be calculated by **Fick's cardiac output equation,** as follows:

$$Do_2 = 1.34 \times CO \times [Hb] \times So_2 + 0.003 \times Pao_2$$

where CO is cardiac output, [Hb] is hemoglobin concentration, So_2 is hemoglobin O_2 saturation, 1.34 is the amount of O_2 (mL) carried by 1 g of hemoglobin, and 0.003 is the solubility of O_2 in the plasma (mL/mm Hg/100 mL). In a normal adult at sea level and at rest, Do_2 is approximately 1000 mL/min (assuming hemoglobin concentration 15 g/100 mL, 100% O_2 saturation, and a cardiac output of 5 L/min). The majority of O_2 is carried by the hemoglobin (21 mL/100 mL) compared with the plasma (0.003×100, or 0.3 mL/100 mL). Without hemoglobin, a cardiac output of at least 80 L/min would be needed to support the normal resting O_2 consumption of about 250 mL/min in adult humans. In clinical practice, increases in delivery of O_2 to the peripheral tissues are most efficiently done through increases in hemoglobin concentration and cardiac output. When hemoglobin O_2 saturation is more than 90% (in other words, at the plateau of the curve), additional O_2 does not significantly enhance O_2 delivery. It simply increases the amount of O_2 dissolved in the plasma.

A number of conditions can displace the OEC to the right or the left, affecting hemoglobin O_2 saturation and thus O_2 delivery (see Figure 21-10). Increased 2,3-diglycerophosphate (2,3-DPG), acidosis, and hyperthermia shift the curve to the right and decrease hemoglobin saturation for any given PO_2. In contrast, decreased 2,3-DPG, alkalosis, and hypothermia shift the curve to the left and increase hemoglobin saturation at any given PO_2.

Oxygen Consumption

The consumption of O_2 ($\dot{V}O_2$) can be described by the Fick principle, as follows:

$$\dot{V}o_2 = \dot{Q}c \times (Cao_2 - C\bar{v}o_2)$$

where $\dot{Q}c$ is cardiac output, CaO_2 is arterial O_2 content ($1.39 \times Hb \times SaO_2$), and $C\bar{v}O_2$ is venous O_2 content ($1.34 \times Hb \times S\bar{v}O_2$). In a normal adult at rest, CaO_2 is 21 mL/dl ($1.34 \times 15 \times 100\%$) and $C\bar{v}O_2$ is 16 mL/dL ($1.34 \times 15 \times 75\%$). If the cardiac output is 5 L/min, $\dot{V}O_2$ is 250 mL/min. Thus under normal resting conditions, the tissues extract about 25% of O_2 delivered to them. The extraction of O_2 can increase under conditions such as exercise, congestive heart failure, and severe anemia, leading to a lower $C\bar{v}O_2$. The O_2 extraction can decrease in disease states (for example, sepsis), leading to a higher $C\bar{v}O_2$. Resting blood and O_2 supply of various organs are shown in Table 21-3. Brain tissue and cardiac muscle extract much more O_2 from the blood than do other organs. These two organs also are most susceptible to O_2 deprivation caused by ischemia and **hypoxia.**

The majority of O_2 (90%) used by the cell is consumed by the mitochondria. The remainder is used by other subcellular organelles. In mitochondria, molecular O_2 is reduced to water by cytochrome c oxidase after accepting electrons from the respiratory chain. High-energy phosphate compounds (such as adenosine triphosphate [ATP]) are generated by the process of oxidative phosphorylation. ATP provides most of the energy required for the biologic function of cells.

Hemoglobin

Hemoglobin is the major protein of erythrocytes, which allows humans to transport molecular O_2 from the lungs to the tissues and CO_2 from the tissues to the lungs. Human hemoglobin is a tetramer of two α-polypeptides and two β-polypeptides, each containing a heme moiety.[16] The tetramer consists of 547 amino acids and has a molecular weight of 64,800 daltons. The heme and globin interact with each other in a way that determines the O_2-binding characteristics of hemoglobin. The heme groups to which the O_2 binds are harbored within the protein parts of the molecule. Heme is the complex of chelated iron in a cyclic tetrapyrrole (porphyrin) ring. The porphyrin of hemoglobin is called *protoporphyrin IX*. The iron atom is kept in the center of the porphyrin ring between four nitrogens. The porphyrin carries side chains that maintain the heme group in the proper orientation within the protein portion of the hemoglobin molecule. The color of hemoglobin is caused by double bonds in the heme moiety; it is a bright-red color when oxygenated and a purple color when deoxygenated.

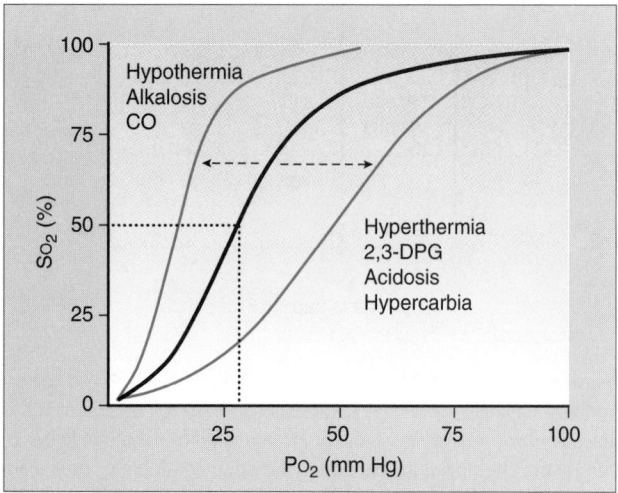

Figure 21-10 Oxyhemoglobin equilibrium (aka *dissociation*) curve of hemoglobin. The normal P_{50} value is indicated by the dashed lines. The changes in position of the curve associated with various effector molecules are indicated by the dashed arrows. (Modified from Baum GL, Crapo JD, Celli B, et al. Textbook of pulmonary diseases. 6th ed. Philadelphia: Lippincott Williams & Wilkins; 1998.)

TABLE 21-3

Oxygen Supply and Consumption of Various Organs

Organ	Blood Flow (mL/min) (% Cardiac Output)	Blood Flow (mL/100 g)	A-V Difference Volume %	O_2 Consumption (mL/min)
Heart	210 (4)	70	11.4	23.9
Brain	760 (15)	50	6.3	47.9
Kidney	1220 (24)	400	1.3	15.9
Liver	510 (10)	29	4.1	20.9
Gastrointestinal tract	715 (14)	35	4.1	29.3
Skeletal muscle	760 (15)	2.5	6.4	60.8
Skin	215 (4)	9.5	1.0	2.15
Other organs (fat, etc.)	715 (14)	—	—	—
TOTAL CARDIAC OUTPUT	5100 ml			200.9

Modified from Jain KK, Fischer B. Oxygen in physiology and medicine. Springfield, Ill: Thomas; 1989.

A standard terminology is used for the different properties of deoxyhemoglobin and oxyhemoglobin to describe the way changes in the heme structure affect the globin. Deoxyhemoglobin is said to be in the *T*, or *tense, state*, and oxyhemoglobin is said to be in the *R*, or *relaxed, state*.[17] The R state has an O_2 affinity about 150 times greater than the T state, which has a low O_2 affinity. The transition between these conformational states is induced by the shift of the heme iron when O_2 is bound or released.

Oxyhemoglobin Equilibrium Curve

The first physiologists to observe the sigmoid nature of the OEC concluded that O_2 affinity increased during progressive oxygenation. They called this phenomenon *cooperativity*. The relationship between the fractional saturation of hemoglobin with O_2 and Po_2 is the sigmoid OEC of hemoglobin (see Figure 21-10). In 1913 a simple equation was proposed by Archibald Vivian Hill to describe OEC (the Hill equation, Equation 21-1).

The sigmoid shape of the hemoglobin OEC determines the loading and unloading of O_2 under physiologic conditions. Its position often is expressed by the P_{50}, or the Po_2 at 50% hemoglobin saturation. The normal P_{50} for human hemoglobin is approximately 27 mm Hg. When the O_2 affinity increases, the OEC shifts to the left (reduced P_{50}). When the O_2 affinity decreases, the OEC shifts to the right (increased P_{50}). The actual shape and position of the OEC are influenced by many factors (Table 21-4).

The hydrogen ion concentration in erythrocytes is regulated mainly by Pco_2 (**Bohr effect**). In the pulmonary microcirculation, $[H^+]$ decreases within the red blood cells (RBCs) as CO_2 is eliminated by ventilation, and the O_2 affinity of hemoglobin increases (O_2 loading). In the peripheral capillaries the process is reversed. CO_2 produced by cellular metabolism diffuses into the RBCs, causing $[H^+]$ to rise within the cells, and the O_2 affinity of hemoglobin is decreased (O_2 unloading). The combined effect is physiologically favorable because it enhances both O_2 uptake in the lungs and O_2 release in the tissues.

The position of the OEC can be altered by organic phosphates, notably ATP and 2,3-DPG. The concentration of 2,3-DPG in RBCs is four times more plentiful than ATP because of the increased glycolytic activity.[18] An increase in 2,3-DPG facilitates release of O_2 by shifting the OEC to the right. Through this important mechanism, RBCs defend against tissue hypoxia after vigorous exercise, after ascent to high altitude, and in numerous diseases associated with reduction in O_2 availability (such as anemia, right-to-left shunt, and congestive heart failure). Low levels of 2,3-DPG in the RBCs with corresponding increases in O_2 affinity have been observed in individuals with hypophosphatemia, hexokinase deficiency, and septic shock.

Changes in temperature alter the conformation of hemoglobin and thus the position of the OEC. Hyperthermia or hypothermia increases or decreases the P_{50} by

EQUATION 21-1

Hill Equation

The Hill equation is based on the hypothetical equilibrium:

$$Hb(O_2)n \leftrightarrow Hb + nO_2$$

$$\frac{S}{1-S} = \left(\frac{Po_2}{P_{50}}\right)^n$$

where S is oxyhemoglobin saturation.

Taking the logarithms of the previous equation gives the following:

$$\log \frac{S}{1-S} = n\log Po_2 - n\log P_{50}$$

A plot of $\log [S/(1 - S)]$ versus $\log Po_2$ is called a *Hill plot*, which approximates a straight line. Its slope n at the midpoint of the binding (S = 0.5) is called the *Hill coefficient*. The value of n increases with the degree of cooperativity; the maximum value of n is equal to the number of binding sites. For hemoglobin, the value of n is about 2.7.

TABLE 21-4

Effect of Various Factors on the Affinity of Hemoglobin to Oxygen and P_{50}

Factors	Changes	O_2 Affinity	P_{50}
pH	↑ (Alkalemia)	↑	↓
	↓ (Acidemia)	↓	↑
2,3-DPG	↑	↓	↑
	↓	↑	↓
Temperature	↑	↓	↑
	↓	↑	↓
P_{CO_2}	↑	↓	↑
	↓	↑	↓
CO	↑	↑	↓
Methemoglobin	↑	↑	↓
Fetal hemoglobin	↑	↑	↓

2,3-DPG, 2,3-Diphosphoglycerate; CO, carbon monoxide.

EQUATION 21-2

Reactions whereby Methemoglobin Is Reduced

$HbF^{+3} + RedCyt\ b_5 \rightarrow HbFe^{+2} + OxCyt\ b_5$

$OxCyt\ b_5 + NADH \rightarrow RedCyt\ b_5 + NAD$ (methemoglobin reductase)

where:

HbF^{+3} = Methemoglobin

$HbFe^{+2}$ = Hemoglobin

$RedCyt\ b_5$ = Reduced cytochrome b_5

$OxyCyt\ b_5$ = Oxidized cytochrome b_5

approximately 2 mm Hg per degree Celsius. CO_2 affects the OEC through the formation of H^+ and carbamino compounds. Increases in carbamino compounds also shift the OEC to the right, similar to increases in $[H^+]$.

One of the most powerful ways to increase O_2 affinity is to bind CO to hemoglobin. CO effectively competes with O_2 for hemoglobin binding because its affinity for heme is more than 200 times that of O_2. Furthermore, when CO binds to one heme site, it increases O_2 affinity of the other binding sites and causes the leftward shift of the OEC. This latter effect on the OEC explains why the formation of 50% carboxyhemoglobin causes more severe tissue hypoxia than when various forms of anemia cause the reduction of hemoglobin concentration to half the normal concentration.

Methemoglobin is formed when the ferrous (Fe^{+2}) center of heme molecule is oxidized to the ferric state (Fe^{+3}). As this action occurs successively among the four heme groups, the O_2 affinity of the remaining unoxidized Fe atoms increases. Normal RBCs contain less the 1% methemoglobin. The methemoglobin can be reduced by serial reactions facilitated by reduced cytochrome b_5 and the enzyme cytochrome b_5 reductase (methemoglobin re-

BOX 21-2

Conditions Associated with Methemoglobinemia

Hereditary
  M hemoglobins
  Cytochrome b_5 reductase deficiency

Acquired
  Nitrites and nitrates: sodium nitrite, amyl nitrite, nitroglycerin, nitroprusside, silver nitrate, inhaled nitric oxide
  Aniline dyes: aminobenzenes, nitrobenzene
  Acetanilid and phenacetin
  Sulfonamides, sulfasalazine
  Other: lidocaine, chlorate, phenazopyridine, ferrous sulfate, quinones

ductase; Equation 21-2). The effect of methemoglobin on peripheral capillary O_2 release and the production of tissue hypoxia are qualitatively the same but quantitatively less than that produced by equal amounts of carboxyhemoglobin. Clinical conditions associated with increased methemoglobin formation are shown in Box 21-2.

Fetal hemoglobin (hemoglobin F) has higher affinity for O_2 than adult hemoglobin (hemoglobin A). The increased O_2 affinity of hemoglobin F can be attributed to the replacement of β chains in hemoglobin A by γ chains, which have decreased binding of 2,3-DPG. The high affinity of hemoglobin F to O_2 permits the fetus to extract maximal amounts of O_2 from the maternal venous blood with low O_2 content.

Genetic hemoglobin abnormalities can be associated with increases (such as Chesapeake or Yakima) or decreases (such as Seattle or Kansas) in O_2 affinity. This effect is believed to be also mediated by the altered binding of 2,3-DPG to the abnormal peptide chains.

Carbon Dioxide Dissociation Curve

The CO_2 dissociation curve of hemoglobin describes overall CO_2 transport as a function of CO_2 tension (Figure 21-11). The CO_2 content of deoxygenated blood is greater than oxygenated blood at any P_{CO_2} (**Haldane effect**). When plotted on logarithmic axes, it becomes linear.[19] The slope of the line depends on the hemoglobin concentration of blood and determines the efficiency of CO_2 exchange.[20] The logarithmic expression of the CO_2 dissociation curve also permits definition of the curve via measurement of a single experimental point and the hemoglobin concentration. The slope of the CO_2 dissociation curve is relatively steep in comparison with the O_2 equilibrium curve. Consequently, large volumes of CO_2 can be exchanged by the lungs with relatively small changes in blood P_{CO_2}. These small changes in blood P_{CO_2} minimize oscillations in blood pH, and the hydrogen ion concentration of blood at rest varies only 10% be-

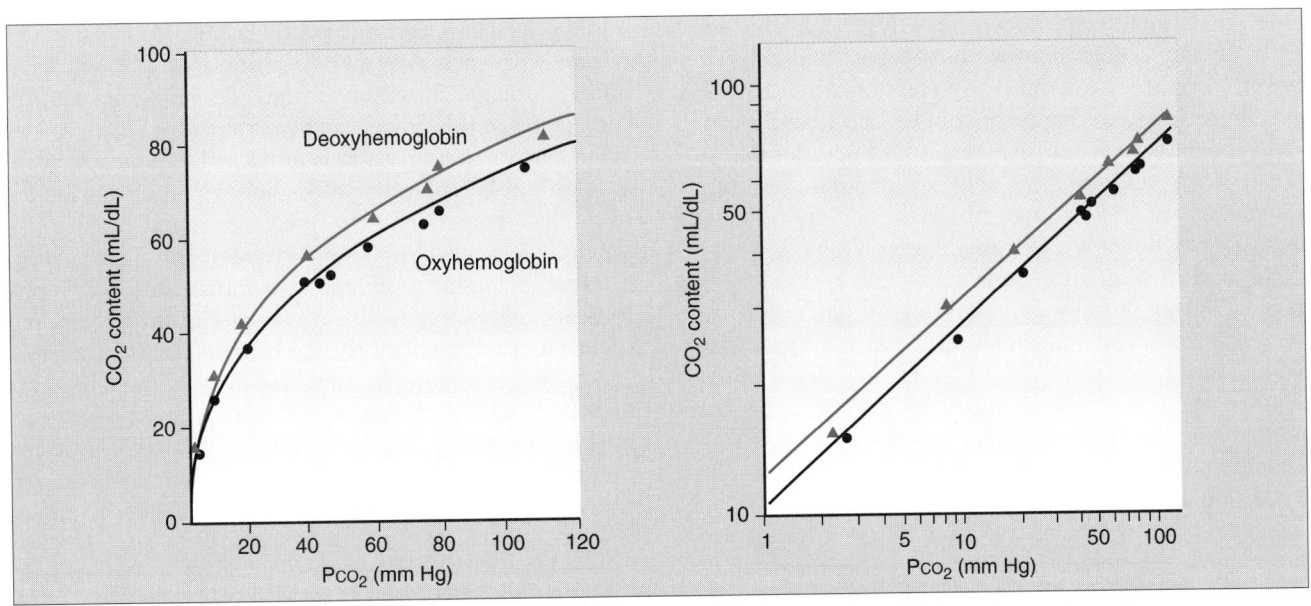

Figure 21-11   *Left,* Carbon dioxide dissociation curve of blood. *Right,* Logarithmic transformation of the curve that linearizes the relationship between CO_2 content and P_{CO_2}. (Modified from Baum GL, Crapo JD, Celli B, et al. Textbook of pulmonary diseases. 6th ed. Philadelphia: Lippincott Williams & Wilkins; 1998.)

tween arterial and mixed venous values. The steepness of the CO_2 dissociation curve also permits continued excretion of CO_2 even in the presence of significant mismatching of pulmonary ventilation and blood flow.[20,21]

Carbon Dioxide Transport

The transport pathway of CO_2 begins with the diffusion of CO_2 from tissues into the capillary blood. Most CO_2 that enters the blood passes into the RBCs, where it undergoes one of three chemical reactions: (1) it remains as dissolved CO_2; (2) it combines with the NH_2 groups of hemoglobin to form carbamino compounds; or (3) it combines with water to form H_2CO_3, which dissociates into H^+ and HCO_3^-. The remaining CO_2 is distributed in the plasma as dissolved CO_2 and carbamino compounds after reacting with NH_2 groups of plasma proteins.

Although only a small amount of bicarbonate is generated from the dissolved CO_2 in the plasma, the plasma transports more than 60% of CO_2 added to capillary blood because the chemical reactions within the RBCs provide practically all additional bicarbonate ions in the plasma. Thus the CO_2-binding capacity of the plasma is increased by the large internal buffering capacity of erythrocytes, the presence of cellular carbonic anhydrase, and the ability to exchange bicarbonate and chloride ions across the erythrocyte membrane. Although dissolved CO_2 accounts for only 5% of the CO_2 content of arterial or venous blood, it is important for CO_2 transport and exchange because the bicarbonate and carbamate pools are linked through dissolved CO_2.

Hydration of CO_2 produces carbonic acid (H_2CO_3), which is almost completely ionized to H^+ and bicarbonate

in the blood because the pK of carbonic acid (~ 3.8) is much lower than blood pH, as follows:

$$CO_2 + H_2O \rightarrow H_2CO_3 \rightarrow H^+ + HCO_3^-.$$

Hydration of CO_2 to H_2CO_3 is a slow process. In the erythrocyte this reaction is greatly facilitated by carbonic anhydrase.[21-23] The reaction occurs so quickly that the process is completed during the passage of the red cell through the peripheral capillaries. The reverse reaction, the dehydration of H_2CO_3 to CO_2, occurs in the pulmonary microcirculation and similarly requires carbonic anhydrase. Carbonic anhydrase is present within the erythrocyte in high concentrations but is virtually absent from plasma. Carbonic anhydrase also is found in the capillary endothelium of the lung[24-26] and other organs,[21,24,27] but the quantity of enzyme is small.

When carbonic anhydrase is inhibited by acetazolamide, the CO_2 that enters the blood from the tissues continues to form HCO_3^- after the blood has left the peripheral capillaries. When the blood reaches the pulmonary capillaries, the dissolved CO_2 can diffuse into alveolar gas but HCO_3^- in RBCs cannot dehydrate fast enough to maintain the P_{CO_2}. Thus the P_{CO_2} rises as blood flows through the systemic arteries, and the unloading reaction completes slowly. The overall result is a rise in tissue P_{CO_2} and **hypercapnia.**

CO_2 entering the blood from the tissues diffuses into the erythrocytes, where CO_2 is hydrated enzymatically into carbonic acid. Carbonic acid then forms bicarbonate, which is essential for blood CO_2 transport. However, the bicarbonate content of erythrocytes is low because of the rapid exchange of intracellular bicarbonate ions for extracellular chloride ions, thereby shuttling bicarbonate ions produced within the erythrocyte into the plasma (chloride shift).[28] The exchange between bicarbonate and chloride across the erythrocyte membrane is electroneutral and mediated by an anion exchange protein (AE1, or band 3 protein).[29] Some movement of water inward occurs simultaneously with the chloride shift to maintain osmotic equilibrium, resulting in a slight swelling of erythrocytes in venous blood relative to those in arterial blood.

CO_2 and hydrogen ions reversibly bind to uncharged amino groups of proteins (Equation 21-3). Under physiologic conditions, carbamic acids release H^+ and form carbamate ions, $R-NHCOO^-$. In RBCs, H^+ is buffered by hemoglobin molecules. This process is facilitated by the simultaneous loss of O_2 from capillary blood to the tissues because deoxyhemoglobin is a weaker acid and can take up additional H^+ with little change in pH.

Because both molecular CO_2 and H^+ compete for uncharged amino groups, carbamate formation is pH dependent and increases with alkalinity. Transport of CO_2 as carbamates also is influenced by P_{CO_2} and by the pK of the amino groups on the proteins. The pK values of the α-amino group of the N-termini of blood proteins lies within the physiologic range of pH.[30] Therefore these blood proteins frequently exist in the uncharged $R-NH_2$ form and are available to bind CO_2. In contrast, ε-amino groups, which are located throughout the protein chains, have a pK well above the physiologic pH range, which means that most ε-amino groups are bound to hydrogen ions and cannot bind CO_2. The concentration of carbamates in plasma is approximately 0.6 mM, and binding of CO_2 to α-amino groups accounts for 60% of this quantity. However, plasma carbamates do not participate in CO_2 exchange because the steep slope of the CO_2 dissociation curve minimizes changes in pH and P_{CO_2} between arterial and venous blood. This effect in turn minimizes changes in plasma carbamate concentrations in the lung and systemic capillaries.

The influence of O_2 on the CO_2 dissociation curve (Haldane effect) has received less attention than its converse relationship, the effect of CO_2 on the O_2 dissociation curve of blood (Bohr effect). The Bohr effect is responsible for only 2% of total O_2 exchange in the tissues, whereas the Haldane effect accounts for nearly 50% of resting CO_2 exchange.[31] O_2-dependent exchange of CO_2 occurs through the carbamate and bicarbonate pathways and is a function of pH, P_{CO_2}, and the concentration of 2,3-DPG.[32] With

EQUATION 21-3

Reactions of Carbon Dioxide and Hydrogen Ions with Uncharged Amino Acids of Proteins

$$R - NH_2 + H^+ \rightarrow R - NH_3^+$$
$$R - NH_2 + CO_2 \rightarrow R - NHCOOH$$
$$R - NHCOOH \rightarrow R - NHCOO^- + H^+$$

where R represents the protein moiety and $R - NHCOOH$ is the carbamic acid.

normal 2,3-DPG concentrations the Haldane effect increases with increasing pH, reaching its maximum value under normal acid-base conditions. The importance of the carbamates in this process increases as the pH increases because carbamate formation is promoted by the lack of H^+ and less 2,3-DPG binding at higher pH. The contribution of the bicarbonate pathway to CO_2 transport peaks in the physiologic range of pH, but it decreases at higher pH because of increasing prominence of carbamates. When protons are released from deoxyhemoglobin on O_2 binding, some are consumed by the carbamate reaction, thereby leaving fewer protons to combine with bicarbonate ion to form CO_2. CO_2 exchange would occur without a functioning Haldane effect, despite the fact that half of CO_2 excretion normally occurs by this mechanism. The cost is greater changes in arterial-venous CO_2 content, greater tissue hypercarbia, and altered acid-base status.[33]

Ventilation-Perfusion Distribution

Exchange of O_2 and CO_2 between blood in the pulmonary arterial system and alveolar gas occurs continuously in more than 100,000 terminal respiratory units of the lungs. The adequacy of function of each gas exchange unit is determined by local matching between ventilation and perfusion ($\dot{V}_A/\dot{Q}$). In general, inadequate ventilation relative to perfusion (low $\dot{V}_A/\dot{Q}$ and shunt) has the greatest effect on O_2 uptake by the lungs and thus may result in **hypoxemia**. On the other hand, excessive ventilation relative to perfusion (high $\dot{V}_A/\dot{Q}$ and dead space) has more influence on CO_2 elimination by the lungs and may cause hypercapnia in severe cases.

The effects of $\dot{V}_A/\dot{Q}$ matching on the efficiency of gas exchange in the lungs can be illustrated with the two-compartment lung model (Figure 21-12). In an ideal lung consisting of two alveolar units (A and B) with each receiving 2.0 L/min of alveolar ventilation and 2.5 L/min of blood flow, the $\dot{V}_A/\dot{Q}$ ratio is 0.8 for the individual units A and B and thus the entire lung. Assuming no barrier to diffusion of O_2 and a normal P_{O_2} in the pulmonary artery, the P_{O_2} of alveolar gas is the same as the P_{O_2} of end-capillary and arterial blood. An O_2 gradient from alveolus to capillary (alveolar-arterial P_{O_2} difference [$P(A-a)_{O_2}$]) does not exist. In a normal lung a slight degree of $\dot{V}_A/\dot{Q}$ mismatch occurs, primarily because of the greater effects of gravity on the distribution of perfusion than on ventilation (see Figure 21-12). Thus although the $\dot{V}_A/\dot{Q}$ ratio for the whole lung remains at 0.8, the $\dot{V}_A/\dot{Q}$ ratios for the two units A and B are 1.0 and 0.6, respectively, causing the mean P_{O_2} in the blood leaving the lung to decrease slightly and produces an $P(A-a)_{O_2}$ difference of 4.4 mm Hg. Uneven distribution of blood flow also may result in similar effects, especially in the upright lung.

Measurement of $\dot{V}_A/\dot{Q}$ Distribution

It has long been recognized that the lungs must contain some sort of distribution of $\dot{V}_A/\dot{Q}$ ratios. Major conceptual advances became possible with the introduction of the **multiple inert gas elimination technique (MIGET).**[34] The MIGET is based on the straightforward principles governing inert gas elimination by the lungs. When an inert gas in solution is infused into systemic veins, the proportion of gas eliminated by ventilation from a lung unit depends only on the solubility of the gas and the $\dot{V}_A/\dot{Q}$ ratio of that unit. The relationship is given by the following equation:

$$\frac{Pc'}{P\bar{v}} = \frac{\lambda}{(\lambda + \dot{V}_A/\dot{Q})}$$

where Pc' is the partial pressure of the gas in end-capillary blood and λ is the blood-gas partition coefficient. The end-capillary partial pressure divided by the mixed venous partial pressure (P$\bar{v}$) is known as the *retention*.

Experimentally a saline solution containing low concentrations of six gases of different solubility (such as sulfur hexafluoride [SF_6], ethane, cyclopropane, isoflurane, diethyl ether, and acetone) is infused slowly into a peripheral vein until a steady state is reached (about 20 minutes). Simultaneous samples of arterial and mixed venous gases and expired gas are collected and analyzed for the test gases by gas chromatography. Retention and excretion values for the inert gases are graphed against their solubility in blood (Figure 21-13, *upper panel*). With a 50-compartment model, the retention-solubility plots from the MIGET can be transformed to obtain the distribution of $\dot{V}_A/\dot{Q}$ ratios in the lung (see Figure 21-13, *lower panel*). A lung containing shunt units shows increased retention of the least-soluble gas, SF_6. Conversely, a lung having large

amounts of ventilation-to-lung units with very high $\dot{V}_A/\dot{Q}$ ratios shows increased retention of the high-solubility gases (such as ether and acetone).

Figure 21-13 shows the distribution of $\dot{V}_A/\dot{Q}$ ratios from a 22-year-old, healthy volunteer.[35] The distributions for both ventilation and blood flow (dispersion) are narrow and span only one log of $\dot{V}_A/\dot{Q}$ ratios. Essentially, no ventilation or blood flow occurs outside the range of approximately 0.3 to 3.0 on the $\dot{V}_A/\dot{Q}$ ratio scale, and no significant intrapulmonary shunt is detected. With aging the dispersion of ventilation and perfusion increases. As much as 10% of the total blood flow may go to lung units with $\dot{V}_A/\dot{Q}$ values of less than 0.1, but still no shunt is detected. The increased low-$\dot{V}_A/\dot{Q}$ regions adequately explain the decreased PaO_2 and increased alveolar-arterial O_2 difference with aging. The cause of such age-related $\dot{V}_A/\dot{Q}$ mismatch often is attributed to degenerative processes in the small airways with aging.

$\dot{V}_A/\dot{Q}$ Distributions in Lung Disease

Various abnormal patterns of $\dot{V}_A/\dot{Q}$ distributions have been demonstrated by the MIGET in diseased lungs.[36] The distribution of $\dot{V}_A/\dot{Q}$ ratios from an individual with chronic obstructive lung disease is shown in Figure 21-14. The $\dot{V}_A/\dot{Q}$ distribution is bimodal, and large amounts of ventilation go to lung units with extremely high $\dot{V}_A/\dot{Q}$ ratios (Figure 21-14, A). This $\dot{V}_A/\dot{Q}$ pattern is typically seen in individuals with predominant emphysema.[37] Presumably the high-$\dot{V}_A/\dot{Q}$ regions reflect ventilation-to-lung

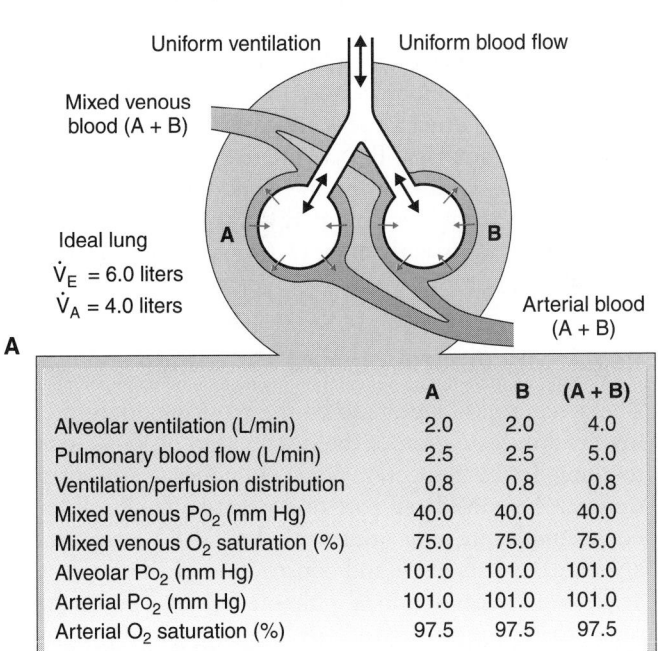

	A	B	(A + B)
Alveolar ventilation (L/min)	2.0	2.0	4.0
Pulmonary blood flow (L/min)	2.5	2.5	5.0
Ventilation/perfusion distribution	0.8	0.8	0.8
Mixed venous Po_2 (mm Hg)	40.0	40.0	40.0
Mixed venous O_2 saturation (%)	75.0	75.0	75.0
Alveolar Po_2 (mm Hg)	101.0	101.0	101.0
Arterial Po_2 (mm Hg)	101.0	101.0	101.0
Arterial O_2 saturation (%)	97.5	97.5	97.5

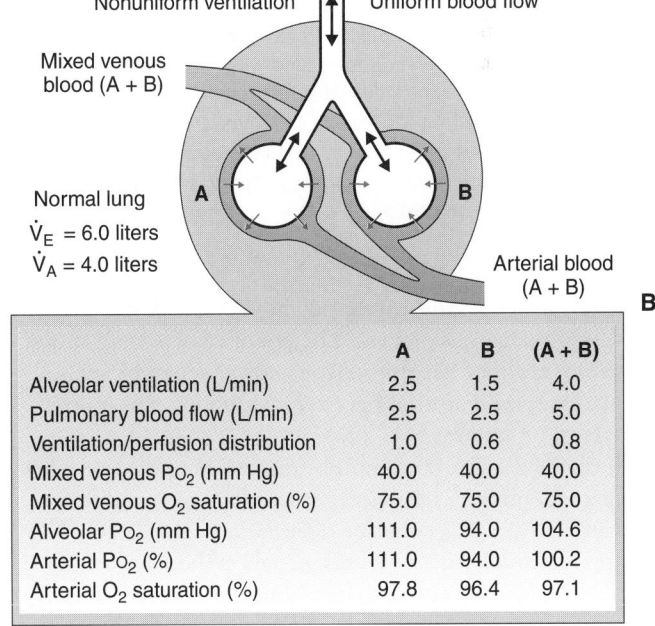

	A	B	(A + B)
Alveolar ventilation (L/min)	2.5	1.5	4.0
Pulmonary blood flow (L/min)	2.5	2.5	5.0
Ventilation/perfusion distribution	1.0	0.6	0.8
Mixed venous Po_2 (mm Hg)	40.0	40.0	40.0
Mixed venous O_2 saturation (%)	75.0	75.0	75.0
Alveolar Po_2 (mm Hg)	111.0	94.0	104.6
Arterial Po_2 (%)	111.0	94.0	100.2
Arterial O_2 saturation (%)	97.8	96.4	97.1

Figure 21-12 Ventilation/perfusion relationships of an ideal lung (**A**) and a healthy lung (**B**) are illustrated with a two-compartment model. Note that the ventilation/perfusion maldistribution is responsible for an alveolar-arterial Po_2 difference of about 4.4 mm Hg; the remainder of the normal Po_2 difference is caused by postpulmonary shunts (ignored in this illustration). (Modified from Forster RE, Dubois AB, Briscoe WA, et al, editors. The normal lung: physiological basis of pulmonary function tests. 3rd ed. Chicago: Year-Book; 1986.)

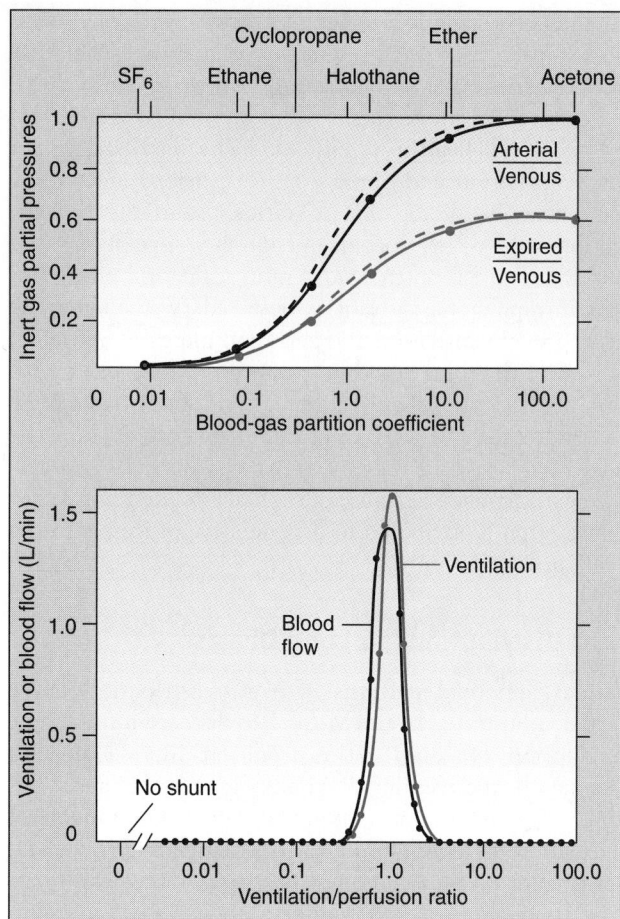

Figure 21-13 Distribution of ventilation-perfusion ratios determined by the multiple inert gas elimination technique. Data from a 22-year-old normal subject are illustrated. Upper panel features data points for inert gas retention (*upper curve*) and excretion (*lower curve*). Broken lines join the points. The two solid lines show the values of retention and excretion for a lung with no ventilation/perfusion inequality. Lower panel illustrates recovered distribution of ventilation/perfusion ratios. SF₆, sulfur hexafluoride. (Modified from Wagner PD, Laravuso R, Uhl R, et al. Continuous distributions of ventilation-perfusion ratios in normal subjects breathing air and 100% O₂. J Clin Invest 1974;54:53-68.)

units in which many capillaries have been destroyed by the emphysematous process. The presence of a small shunt (3.1%) and slight left shift of the main mode of blood flow can explain mild arterial hypoxemia found in this individual (PaO₂ 63 mm Hg).

Individuals with chronic obstructive lung disease who have predominant bronchitis generally show a different pattern of $\dot{V}A/\dot{Q}$ distribution (see Figure 21-14, *B*). The main abnormality in these individuals is the large amount of blood flow distributed to lung units with very low $\dot{V}A/\dot{Q}$ ratios between 0.003 and 0.1, which explains the more severe hypoxemia generally found in this type of individual. Presumably the low $\dot{V}A/\dot{Q}$ units in individuals with chronic bronchitis are the result of airway obstruction caused by retained secretions and mucous gland hyperplasia.

EQUATION 21-4

Fick's Law of Diffusion

$$\dot{V}_{gas} = \frac{A}{T} \times D \times (P_1 - P_2)$$

where:

V_{gas} = Amount of gas transferred
A = Surface area for diffusion
T = Thickness of the membrane
D = Diffusion constant
$(P_1 - P_2)$ = Concentration gradient across the membrane

Because the lung is too complex to determine the area and the thickness of the blood-gas barrier, the diffusion equation can be rewritten to combine the factors A, T, and D into one constant, DL, as follows:

$$V_{gas} = DL \times (P_1 - P_2)$$

Thus the diffusing capacity for a gas is given by the following equation:

$$DL = \frac{V_{gas}}{PA - Pc'}$$

where PA and Pc' are the partial pressures of the gas in alveolar space and capillary blood, respectively, and DL is the diffusing capacity of the lung.

$\dot{V}A/\dot{Q}$ Mismatch and Carbon Dioxide Retention

It is important to understand that ventilation-perfusion mismatch interferes with the efficiency of CO_2 elimination by the lung, although patients with $\dot{V}A/\dot{Q}$ mismatch often have a normal or even low PaCO₂. The reason is that the regulatory chemoreceptors increase the ventilatory drive whenever they sense a rising PaCO₂. Such patients can maintain a normal PCO₂ by increasing the total ventilation at a cost of increasing the work of breathing. However, a significant portion of this increased ventilation goes to lung units with high $\dot{V}A/\dot{Q}$ ratios that are inefficient at eliminating CO_2.

Regulatory Control of $\dot{V}A/\dot{Q}$ Matching

The alveolar PO₂ appears to be the most important factor involved in regulation of the distribution of $\dot{V}A/\dot{Q}$ within the lung. In this respect, hypoxic pulmonary vasoconstriction can be considered part of a negative feedback loop. For example, in lung units with low $\dot{V}A/\dot{Q}$ ratios, local alveolar PO₂ decreases, and constriction of the associated arterioles reduces the local pulmonary blood flow, which tends to restore the local $\dot{V}A/\dot{Q}$ ratio toward its normal value. This effect can be appreciated in people living in high altitudes, who are exposed constantly to lower ambient O₂ concentrations. High-altitude residents have better $\dot{V}A/\dot{Q}$ matching than sea-level residents, as reflected by a smaller P(A − a)O₂ difference.[38]

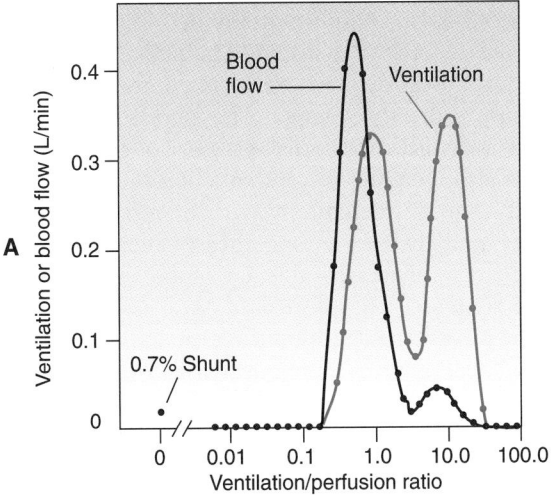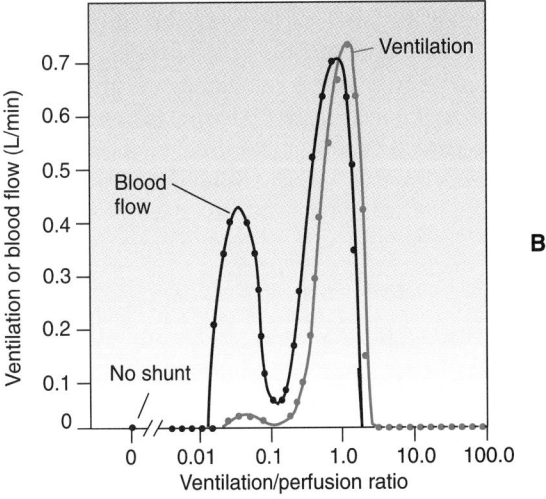

Figure 21-14 Examples of the distribution of ventilation/perfusion ratios in individuals with chronic obstructive pulmonary disease. **A,** Type A (individuals with predominantly emphysema) tend to have areas of very high $\dot{V}A/\dot{Q}$. **B,** Type B (patients with predominantly chronic bronchitis) often have areas of very low $\dot{V}A/\dot{Q}$. Shunt ($\dot{V}A/\dot{Q} = 0$) is rarely seen in either type. (Modified from Wagner PD, Dantzker D, Dueck R, et al. Ventilation-perfusion inequality in chronic obstructive pulmonary disease. J Clin Invest 1977;59:203-216.)

The intensity of hypoxic pulmonary vasoconstriction varies among different lung regions and likely depends on the smooth muscle tone in different vessels. The effectiveness of hypoxic pulmonary vasoconstriction in preserving $\dot{V}A/\dot{Q}$ ratios also depends on the type of inhomogeneity. For example, when collateral ventilation is present, the regulatory effectiveness of hypoxic vasoconstriction may be greater than if a parallel ventilatory arrangement between lung units existed.[39] More recently, a role for nitric oxide (NO) in regulating local $\dot{V}A/\dot{Q}$ matching has been suggested. The hypothesis is supported by the following observations: (1) production of NO is decreased when P_{O_2} is low; (2) NO produced endogenously by endothelial cells regulates local blood flow through its vasodilating effect; and (3) NO inhibits hypoxic pulmonary vasoconstriction. The loss of local hypoxic vasoconstriction worsens $\dot{V}A/\dot{Q}$ mismatch and hypoxemia.

Diffusion

O_2 from the ambient air is carried into the lungs by two physical processes. Bulk flow occurs in the conducting airways, and molecular diffusion is the main mechanism of gas transfer in the distal alveolar units. From the alveolar region, O_2 must diffuse across the alveolar-capillary membrane, plasma, and red cell membrane before it reacts with hemoglobin. The diffusion gradient for O_2 is the P_{O_2} difference between alveolar gas and mixed venous blood. In normal individuals this gradient is approximately 60 mm Hg. At rest the diffusion process is virtually complete within the first third (0.25 seconds) of the mean capillary transit time of 0.75 seconds (see Figure 21-9).

Diffusion of gases across the alveolar-capillary membrane behaves according to **Fick's law of diffusion** (Equation 21-4). Fick's law states that for a given gas, the amount of gas transferred across a tissue sheet is proportional to the area, diffusion constant, and difference in partial pressure. It is inversely proportional to the thickness of the barrier. The diffusing capacity includes the area, thickness, diffusion properties of the membrane, and physical properties of the gas. CO usually is the gas of choice to measure the diffusion capacity of the lung. Because the partial pressure of CO in capillary blood is very low due to its high affinity for hemoglobin (more than 200 times greater than O_2), its partial pressure in the blood generally can be neglected. In this case, diffusing capacity can be calculated as follows:

$$D_{LCO} = \frac{\dot{V}_{CO}}{P_{ACO}}$$

where D_{LCO} is the diffusing capacity of the lung for CO, $\dot{V}_{CO}$ is the amount of CO transferred across the alveolar-capillary membrane, and P_{ACO} is the partial pressure of CO in the alveolar space. The units are mL CO/min/mm Hg of alveolar partial pressure. This unit is analogous to that of conductance. Under some circumstances (such as in heavy cigarette smokers), the CO partial pressure in the blood cannot be neglected because carboxyhemoglobin in the blood is sufficiently high. In this case a correction must be made for back-diffusion of CO during the D_{LCO} calculation.

The diffusing capacity for O_2 in the lungs is higher than that for CO and can be estimated through multiplication of the diffusing capacity for CO by 1.25. However, the uptake of O_2 in the lungs is typically limited by perfusion, not diffusion, under normal conditions. Only under hypoxic conditions does diffusion begin to play some role in limiting O_2 uptake. For this reason, measurements of diffusion that use O_2 are often difficult to interpret.

Anatomically the diffusing capacity of the lung can be separated into two components: the alveolar-capillary membrane plus the erythrocyte cell membrane and the reaction with hemoglobin (Figure 21-15, A). These components can be regarded as resistances in series in the transfer of O_2. Based on this model, Roughton and Forster showed that the following relationship exists[40]:

$$\frac{1}{D_L} = \frac{1}{D_M} + \frac{1}{\theta V_C}$$

where D_M is the diffusing capacity of the membrane (which includes the alveolar-capillary membrane, the plasma, and the red cell membrane), θ is the rate of reaction of CO (or O_2) with hemoglobin, and $\dot{V}_C$ is the volume of blood in the pulmonary capillaries. In the equation, values for D_M and $\dot{V}_C$ can be obtained graphically via measurement of the diffusing capacity for CO at both high and normal alveolar PO_2 values (see Figure 21-15, B). Increasing the alveolar PO_2 reduces the value of θ for CO because CO has to compete with a higher pressure of O_2 for the hemoglobin. When the values of $1/D_L$ obtained at two different PO_2 values are plotted against $1/\theta$, as shown in Figure 21-15, the slope of the line is $1/\dot{V}_C$, whereas the intercept on the vertical axis is $1/D_M$.

The Roughton-Forster equation is useful to demonstrate the factors that influence the diffusing capacity of the lung. The diffusing capacity can be reduced if D_M is decreased (when the thickness is increased or the area is reduced). The diffusing capacity also can be reduced if θ is reduced (such as in cases of anemia or if $\dot{V}_C$ is reduced, as with pulmonary embolism).

Mathematically the term D_M is as important as $\theta\dot{V}_C$ in determination of the diffusing capacity of the lung. However, in clinical medicine the more common factor affecting the diffusing capacity is $\dot{V}_C$. Raising the pulmonary artery pressure when left atrial pressure is low can be shown to increase the D_L substantially because higher perfusion pressure recruits and distends pulmonary capillaries and thus increases $\dot{V}_C$. This effect is diminished if left atrial pressure is already elevated. The increase in D_L during exercise and with changes from the upright to the supine position also is caused by capillary dilation and recruitment, resulting in an increase in $\dot{V}_C$. The reduced diffusing capacity in many cases of lung diseases, including those characterized by increased alveolar septal thickness, also has been attributed to a decreased $\dot{V}_C$ caused by loss of pulmonary capillaries from destruction and distortion of lung parenchyma, rather than a decreased D_M.

Assessment of Gas Exchange Function

Assessment of Hypoxemia

The effectiveness of gas exchange can be assessed by several methods. The simplest approach is to measure gas tension in arterial blood. More complicated approaches rely on tracer gases and modeling of gas exchange, such as the MIGET. However, no measurement technique allows an exact description of the complex behavior of gas exchange in the lungs.

The arterial PO_2 certainly provides some information about the degree of $\dot{V}_A/\dot{Q}$ matching. The major advantage of the measurement is its simplicity. Normal values of PaO_2 decrease with age. Regression equations have been developed to predict the age-specific PaO_2 in supine and sitting positions.[41,42] Supine PaO_2 is normally lower than upright or seated PaO_2. However, these equations have relatively large standard errors of estimation. For simplicity, hypoxemia in adults usually is defined as PaO_2 of less than 80 mm Hg (Table 21-5). In general a low PaO_2 almost always indicates the presence of $\dot{V}_A/\dot{Q}$ mismatch or shunt, but a

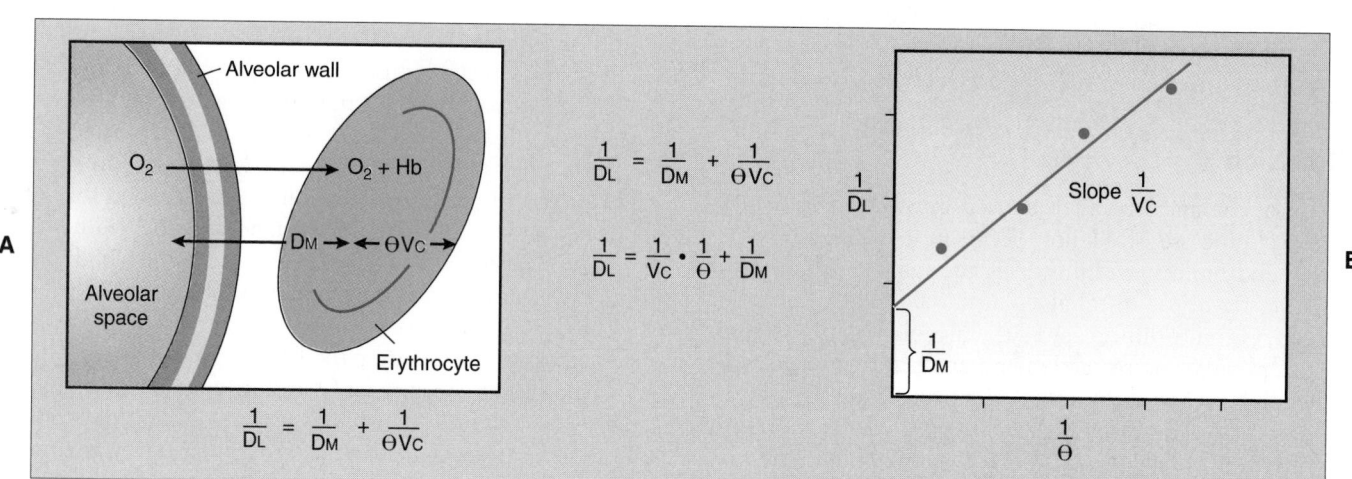

Figure 21-15 The two components of the diffusing capacity of the lung (D_L). **A,** Components attributable to the diffusion process itself and the time taken for O_2 (or CO) to react with hemoglobin. **B,** The graph solution of D_M and V_C according to the Roughton-Forster analysis. D_M and V_C are derived by plotting of $1/\theta$ against $1/D_L$. (Modified from West JB. *Textbook of respiratory medicine.* 2nd ed. Philadelphia: WB Saunders; 1994.)

normal PaO_2 (>80 mm Hg) does not necessarily imply a normal $\dot{V}A/\dot{Q}$ distribution of the lung. The alveolar-arterial PO_2 difference, $P(A - a)O_2$, is calculated as the difference between the PAO_2 and the PaO_2. PAO_2 is computed from the alveolar gas equation (Equation 21-5). The $P(A - a)O_2$ is more sensitive than the arterial PO_2 alone in the determination of $\dot{V}A/\dot{Q}$ abnormalities.

The $P(A - a)O_2$ in healthy adults breathing room air increases with age. As a general rule, the $P(A - a)O_2$ for an individual should be no more than half the chronologic age and no more than 25 mm Hg.[42] Thus the upper normal limit of $P(A - a)O_2$ for a 30-year-old person is 15 mm Hg, whereas the upper normal limit of $P(A - a)O_2$ for a 60-year-old individual is 25 mm Hg. The $P(A - a)O_2$ in normal adults is the result of the combination of mild $\dot{V}A/\dot{Q}$ mismatch and a small right-to-left shunt. Each of these mechanisms is responsible for about half the total $P(A - a)O_2$. At sea level, none of the $P(A - a)O_2$ difference in normal individuals is caused by diffusion limitation, even during heavy exercise. Diffusion dysequilibrium may contribute to increased $P(A - a)O_2$ during exercise at high altitudes.[43]

The $P(A - a)O_2$ increases with increasing alveolar PO_2.[44] In lungs with severe nonuniform $\dot{V}A/\dot{Q}$ distribution, the $P(A - a)O_2$ reaches a maximum at FIO_2 of 0.6 to 0.7 and then decreases at higher FIO_2 values (Figure 21-16). The decline in $P(A - a)O_2$ at higher FIO_2 is caused by more uniform rises in PAO_2, which overcome the nonuniform distribution of $\dot{V}A/\dot{Q}$ ratios. This nonlinear relationship between the $P(A - a)O_2$ and FIO_2 makes reference $P(A - a)O_2$ values obtained with supplemental O_2 difficult to use in critically ill patients, whose FIO_2 values vary frequently.

The PaO_2/FIO_2 ratio is a simple, bedside index of O_2 exchange when $\dot{V}A/\dot{Q}$ mismatch is the primary cause of hypoxemia. However, this ratio loses reliability when shunt becomes the major cause of hypoxemia. The PaO_2/PAO_2 ratio is another easily calculated index of oxygenation. It has similar advantages and disadvantages of the PaO_2/FIO_2 ratio. In addition, the PaO_2/PAO_2 ratio can be misleading if

$P\bar{v}O_2$ fluctuates. The PaO_2/FIO_2 ratio is affected by $PaCO_2$, but the PaO_2/PAO_2 ratio is not.

The presence of right-to-left shunt can be differentiated from low $\dot{V}A/\dot{Q}$ causes of hypoxemia through breathing of 100% O_2. While the individual breathes pure O_2, the alveolar PO_2 in different lung units differs according to differences in alveolar PCO_2. Lung units with low $\dot{V}A/\dot{Q}$ ratios increase their PO_2 values maximally with elevation of the inspired PO_2, but shunt does not. The amount of the shunt can be calculated with the following equation:

$$\frac{Qs}{QT} = \frac{Cc'O_2 - CaO_2}{Cc'O_2 - C\bar{v}O_2}$$

EQUATION 21-5

Alveolar Gas Equation

$$PAO_2 = FIO_2 (PB - PH_2O) - \frac{PACO_2}{R}$$

where:

PB = Barometric pressure
PH_2O = Water vapor pressure at body temperature (47 mm Hg at 37° C)
FIO_2 = Fractional concentration of oxygen in inspired gas
R = Respiratory exchange ratio

At room air (FIO_2 = 0.21) with an R of 0.8, the equation can be simplified as follows:

$$PAO_2 = 0.21(713) - 1.25 \times PaCO_2 = 150 - 1.25 \times PaCO_2$$

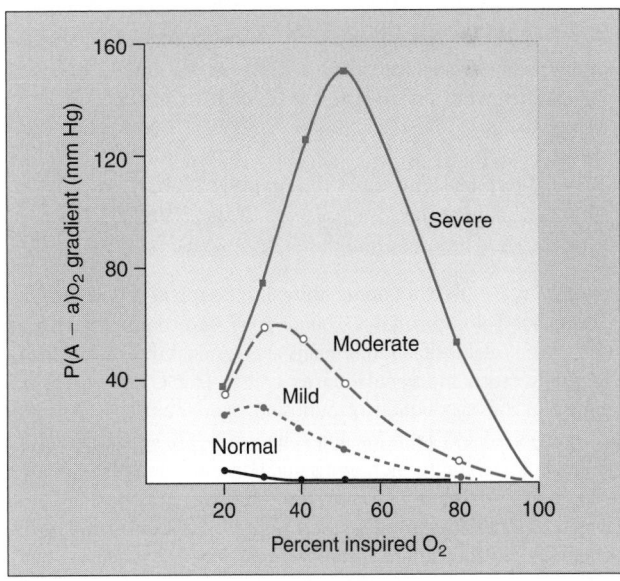

Figure 21-16 Relationship of alveolar-arterial PO_2 difference to inspired oxygen percentage under conditions of normal to severe ventilation/perfusion inequality. (Modified from Dantzker DR. Mechanisms of hypoxemia and hypercapnia. In: Bone RC, editor. Critical care: a comprehensive approach. Park Ridge, Ill: American College of Chest Physicians; 1984.)

TABLE 21-5

*Acceptable Arterial PO_2 Ranges for Adults in Supine Position**

Age (Years)	PaO_2 (mm Hg)
30	>90
40	>85
50	>80
60	>75
70	>70
80	>65
90	>60

*Values are calculated with the equation of Sorbini C, Grassi V, Solinas E. Arterial oxygen tension in relation to age in healthy subjects. Respiration 1968;25:3.

where $\dot{Q}s/\dot{Q}T$ is the shunt ($\dot{Q}s$) as a fraction of cardiac output ($\dot{Q}T$), $Cc'o_2$ is end-capillary O_2 content, Cao_2 is arterial O_2 content, and $C\bar{v}o_2$ is mixed venous O_2 content. Healthy individuals have a small shunt that amounts to 2% to 5% of the cardiac output. This shunt or venous admixture occurs because some venous blood normally drains into the pulmonary veins, left atrium, or left ventricle from bronchial and myocardial (Thebesian) circulation.

Breathing 100% O_2 increases the arterial Po_2 to greater than 600 mm Hg in normal adults. If Pao_2 only rises to 250 mm Hg during 100% O_2 breathing, the shunt is about one-fourth the cardiac output (25%). This procedure does not determine the anatomic location of a shunt, which may be intracardiac or intrapulmonary, but the calculation can help the clinician focus the differential diagnosis on causes of hypoxemia that develop predominantly by shunt mechanisms. Furthermore, because Pao_2 shows little response to

variations in Fio_2 at shunt fractions that exceed 25%, the clinician may be encouraged to reduce toxic and marginally effective concentrations of O_2. However, the shunt calculation frequently overestimates the true shunt because alveoli with very low $\dot{V}a/\dot{Q}$ ratios (<0.1) may collapse completely during O_2 breathing.

Physiologic Mechanisms of Hypoxemia

Hypoventilation decreases the Pao_2 and increases the arterial Pco_2. If $\dot{V}a/\dot{Q}$ distribution remains uniform, no alveolar-arterial difference would develop for either O_2 or CO_2. Although hypoxemia caused by hypoventilation can be corrected with supplemental O_2, the primary treatment should be directed toward support of alveolar ventilation.

$\dot{V}a/\dot{Q}$ mismatch (low $\dot{V}a/\dot{Q}$ units) is the most common cause of hypoxemia associated with lung diseases. Figure 21-17 illustrates the way $\dot{V}a/\dot{Q}$ mismatch can cause hypoxemia with a two-compartment lung model. High $\dot{V}a/\dot{Q}$ units do not cause hypoxemia directly because the blood perfusing these units is well oxygenated. Hypoxemia associated with asthma, chronic bronchitis, emphysema, pneumonia, and interstitial lung diseases is mostly caused by $\dot{V}a/\dot{Q}$ mismatch. Hypoxemia caused by $\dot{V}a/\dot{Q}$ mismatch usually responds well to supplemental O_2.

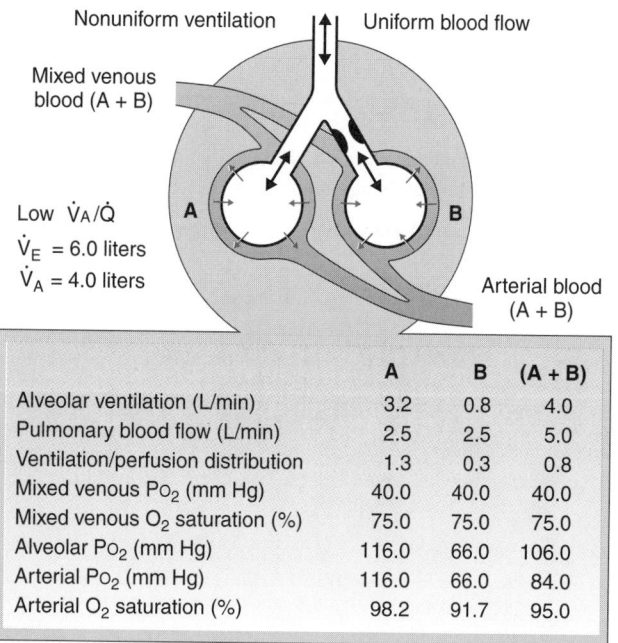

	A	B	(A + B)
Alveolar ventilation (L/min)	3.2	0.8	4.0
Pulmonary blood flow (L/min)	2.5	2.5	5.0
Ventilation/perfusion distribution	1.3	0.3	0.8
Mixed venous Po_2 (mm Hg)	40.0	40.0	40.0
Mixed venous O_2 saturation (%)	75.0	75.0	75.0
Alveolar Po_2 (mm Hg)	116.0	66.0	106.0
Arterial Po_2 (mm Hg)	116.0	66.0	84.0
Arterial O_2 saturation (%)	98.2	91.7	95.0

Figure 21-17 Effects of nonuniform distribution of ventilation with uniform blood flow on gas exchange in a two-compartment lung model. If the total ventilation remains at 4 L/min, but unit A receives 4 times as much the ventilation as unit B (3.2 L/min versus 0.8 L/min) and the distribution of perfusion is uniform (2.5 L/min for each unit), the $\dot{V}a/\dot{Q}$ ratio for unit A becomes 1.3, whereas that for unit B is 0.3. Oxygen tension and saturation must decrease in blood leaving unit B with low $\dot{V}a/\dot{Q}$; oxygen saturation must rise in blood leaving unit A with high $\dot{V}a/\dot{Q}$. Because of the sigmoid shape of the oxyhemoglobin equilibrium curve, high Po_2 in the blood leaving high-$\dot{V}a/\dot{Q}$ unit A is not sufficient to compensate for the low Po_2 contributed by low-$\dot{V}a/\dot{Q}$ unit B. The final Po_2 in the pulmonary venous blood, which is derived from blood flow-weighted average of oxygen content, decreases. The arterial blood then would have a Po_2 of 84 mm Hg instead of 100 mm Hg, as in the healthy lung. (Modified from Baum GL, Crapo JD, Celli B, et al. Textbook of pulmonary diseases. 6th ed. Philadelphia: Lippincott Williams & Wilkins; 1998.)

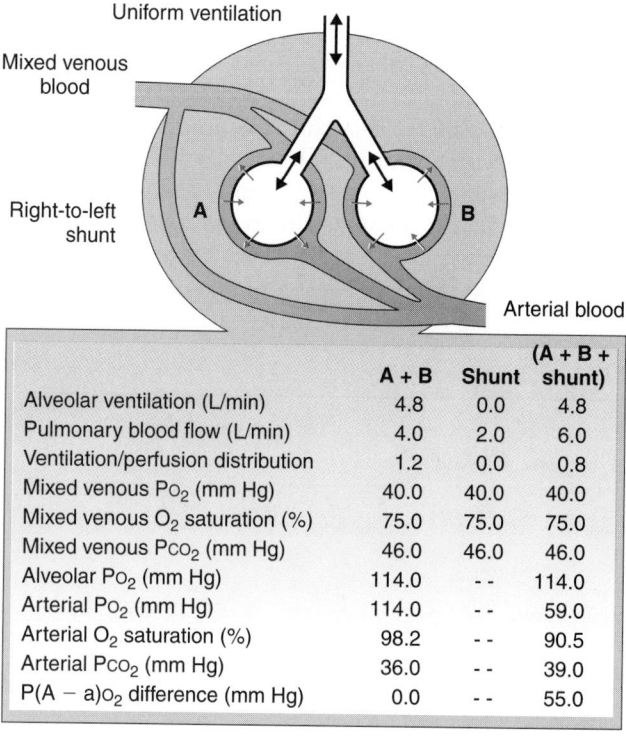

	A + B	Shunt	(A + B + shunt)
Alveolar ventilation (L/min)	4.8	0.0	4.8
Pulmonary blood flow (L/min)	4.0	2.0	6.0
Ventilation/perfusion distribution	1.2	0.0	0.8
Mixed venous Po_2 (mm Hg)	40.0	40.0	40.0
Mixed venous O_2 saturation (%)	75.0	75.0	75.0
Mixed venous Pco_2 (mm Hg)	46.0	46.0	46.0
Alveolar Po_2 (mm Hg)	114.0	- -	114.0
Arterial Po_2 (mm Hg)	114.0	- -	59.0
Arterial O_2 saturation (%)	98.2	- -	90.5
Arterial Pco_2 (mm Hg)	36.0	- -	39.0
P(A − a)o_2 difference (mm Hg)	0.0	- -	55.0

Figure 21-18 Effects of right-to-left shunt on gas exchange in a two-compartment lung model. (Modified from Baum GL, Crapo JD, Celli B, et al. Textbook of pulmonary diseases. 6th ed. Philadelphia: Lippincott Williams & Wilkins; 1998.)

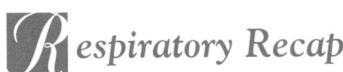

espiratory Recap

Causes of Hypoxemia
Decreased inspired oxygen (altitude)
Shunt
Ventilation/perfusion mismatch
Hypoventilation
Diffusion abnormality

The effects of a right-to-left shunt on gas exchange are shown schematically in Figure 21-18. In this example, 33% of the total blood flow (2.0 L/min) is shunt. Although gas exchange in units A and B is unimpaired, the net result from mixture of blood from these two units and the shunt pathway is a reduction of PaO_2 and the creation of the alveolar-arterial O_2 gradient. This effect on PO_2 is similar to that caused by $\dot{V}A/\dot{Q}$ mismatch. Because of the absence of ventilation in the shunt pathway, hypoxemia resulting from right-to-left shunt cannot be corrected via breathing of 100% O_2. Thus 100% O_2 breathing allows $\dot{V}A/\dot{Q}$ mismatch to be differentiated from shunt as the cause of hypoxemia. Clinical examples of right-to-left shunt include atelectasis, arteriovenous malformation caused by hereditary hemorrhagic telangiectasia (Osler-Weber-Randu disease), liver cirrhosis, and congenital heart diseases (Eisenmenger syndrome, tetralogy of Fallot).

In healthy individuals resting at sea level, O_2 equilibrates quickly between the blood and gas phases in the alveolar region of the lung, and diffusion limitation does not occur. During exercise at higher altitudes (greater than 10,000 feet), the $P(A - a)O_2$ can increase because of diffusion impairment. Such exercise-induced diffusion abnormality at high altitudes is a result of the combined effects of a lower ambient PO_2, thus decreasing the diffusion gradient, and an increase in the rate of blood flow, thus shortening the capillary transit time (see Figure 21-9). In individuals with severe lung diseases who exercise, diffusion impairment also can be an important determinant of hypoxemia because the pulmonary capillary blood volume

is decreased, further exacerbating the effect of short capillary transit time during exercise. Similar to $\dot{V}A/\dot{Q}$ mismatch, hypoxemia caused by diffusion impairment can be corrected by 100% O_2 breathing.

The O_2 content of pulmonary artery (mixed venous) blood usually has little effect on arterial PO_2 in individuals with normal lungs. In the presence of a substantial amount of either $\dot{V}A/\dot{Q}$ abnormalities, a large right-to-left shunt, or both, the O_2 content in the mixed venous blood has a considerable effect on arterial PO_2. For a given amount of $\dot{V}A/\dot{Q}$ mismatch, the lower the mixed venous O_2 content, the lower the arterial PO_2. This mechanism of hypoxemia is particularly important in critically ill individuals with serious cardiopulmonary diseases. Clearly, the response to supplemental O_2 depends on the relative contributions of $\dot{V}A/\dot{Q}$ mismatch and right-to-left shunt to hypoxemia.

Tissue Hypoxia

Complex disturbances of cellular function can be produced by hypoxia, primarily because of inadequate production of high-energy phosphate compounds such as ATP. When O_2 is insufficient, glucose is metabolized anaerobically to pyruvate and lactate. Organs that use large amounts of O_2, such as the brain and heart, are more susceptible to hypoxia. When blood PaO_2 is reduced acutely, symptoms and signs of cerebral hypoxia (such as impaired judgment, motor incoordination, or altered mental status) and cardiac hypoxia (such as myocardial ischemia or arrhythmias) tend to manifest first. When hypoxia becomes more severe and prolonged, the respiratory centers of the brain stem are affected and death usually occurs as a result of respiratory failure. Although tissue hypoxia may be associated with a variety of clinical conditions, it is generally divided into five categories (Table 21-6).

Hypoxemic hypoxia results from inadequate amount of O_2 in the blood (reduced PaO_2) caused by either lung diseases or decreased O_2 in the inspired air (such as at high altitude). Supplemental O_2 may correct tissue hypoxia by raising the PaO_2 in most cases, excepting right-to-left shunt.

Anemic hypoxia results from a reduction in the O_2-carrying capacity of hemoglobin, which may be caused by

TABLE 21-6

Mechanisms of Tissue Hypoxia

Causes of Hypoxia	Examples	Response to Oxygen
Hypoxemic	Lung diseases, high altitude	Good in most cases (except in right-left shunt)
Anemic	Severe anemia, carbon monoxide poisoning, methemoglobinemia	Generally good, depending on the arterial PO_2
Stagnant	Cardiac failure, hypovolemia, peripheral vascular diseases, cardiac arrest	Poor
Affinity	Alkalosis	Poor
Histotoxic	Cyanide poisoning	Poor

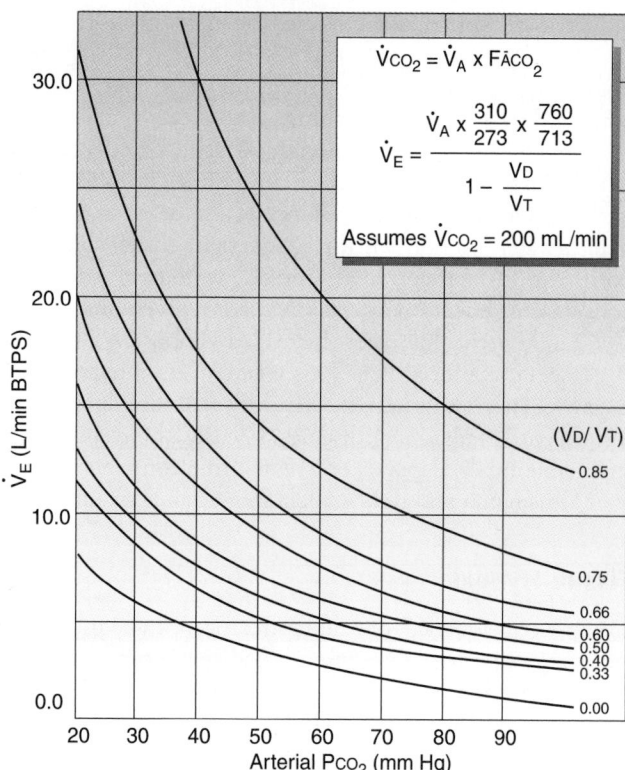

Figure 21-19 An isopleth nomogram used to estimate $\dot{V}_D/\dot{V}_T$ from minute ventilation ($\dot{V}_E$) and arterial P_{CO_2}. Assumptions and calculations are given in the box in the right upper corner. (Modified from Baum GL, Crapo JD, Celli B, et al. Textbook of pulmonary diseases. 6th ed. Philadelphia: Lippincott Williams & Wilkins; 1998.)

severe anemia, or the presence of dyshemoglobin states (such as carboxyhemoglobin or methemoglobin). In anemic individuals, PaO_2 is normal but the absolute amount of O_2 transported per unit volume of blood is diminished. Because the hemoglobin is well saturated with O_2, supplemental O_2 provides little benefit in augmenting O_2 delivery to the tissues unless the PaO_2 is raised into the hyperbaric range. CO poisoning not only decreases the O_2-binding capacity of hemoglobin but also shifts the hemoglobin dissociation curve to the left, impairing the unloading of O_2 at the peripheral tissues. O_2 is useful in CO poisoning because it displaces CO from hemoglobin and decreases the half-life of carboxyhemoglobin and CO in the tissues.

Stagnant hypoxia is a result of poor tissue perfusion, as may be seen in cases of severe cardiac failure, hypovolemic

shock, cardiac arrest, and peripheral vascular diseases. Tissue edema associated with poor perfusion increases the distance through which O_2 has to travel before it reaches the cells and contributes to localized hypoxia. Supplemental O_2 usually is not helpful unless tissue perfusion can be restored.

Affinity hypoxia occurs when hemoglobin does not adequately release O_2 to tissues because of a severe left shift of the OEC, resulting in increased affinity of the hemoglobin molecule for O_2 and decreased release of O_2 to the tissues.

Histotoxic hypoxia is an inability to use O_2 at the cellular level, as with cyanide or sulfide poisoning. These chemical poisons produce cellular hypoxia by inhibiting electron-transfer function by cytochrome oxidase so that O_2 cannot be reduced to water. Because O_2 delivered to the tissues by the blood is not used, the venous blood tends to have a high PaO_2. Supplemental O_2 has little benefit unless the underlying toxic process is reversed.

The mixed venous PO_2 ($P\bar{v}O_2$) is the PO_2 in blood of pulmonary artery. At rest, the normal $P\bar{v}O_2$ is 35 to 40 mm Hg. A value less than 35 mm Hg in a critically ill individual suggests that O_2 extraction is increased and tissues may be hypoxic. However, a normal or a higher-than-normal value does not mean that the tissues have adequate oxygenation. In cases of sepsis, blood may bypass tissues through the peripheral arterial-venous shunting. Therefore less O_2 is extracted by the tissues, leading to higher-than-normal $P\bar{v}O_2$, but tissue oxygenation is impaired. In the individual with cyanide poisoning, O_2 delivered to the tissues cannot be used because the cytochrome oxidase of the respiratory transport chain is inhibited. $P\bar{v}O_2$ increases despite severe tissue hypoxia. Thus the interpretation of $P\bar{v}O_2$ must consider the individual's clinical condition.

Physiologic Mechanisms of Hypercapnia

Physiologic dead space represents lung units with ineffective CO_2 exchange capacity. This portion of each tidal volume (V_D/V_T) can be calculated from the Bohr equation:

$$V_D/V_T = \frac{P_{ACO_2} - P\bar{E}_{CO_2}}{P_{ACO_2}}$$

where V_D is physiologic dead space, V_T is tidal volume, $P\bar{E}_{CO_2}$ is mixed expired P_{CO_2}, and P_{ACO_2} is alveolar P_{CO_2}. P_{ACO_2} is assumed to be equal to $PaCO_2$. If $PaCO_2$ is 40 mm Hg and $P\bar{E}_{CO_2}$ is 27 mm Hg, the V_D/V_T ratio is 0.33. The

*R*espiratory *Recap* ———————

Causes of Hypoxia	
Hypoxemic hypoxia	Affinity hypoxia
Anemic hypoxia	Histotoxic hypoxia
Stagnant hypoxia	

*R*espiratory *Recap* ———————

Causes of Hypercapnia
Hypoventilation
Increased dead space
Increased CO_2 production

Bohr equation requires a measurement of mixed expired gas, which is not obtained conveniently in many clinical settings. Alternatively, V_D/V_T can be estimated from the $\dot{V}_E$ and Pa_{CO_2} with an isopleth nomogram (Figure 21-19).

Physiologic dead space consists of the conducting airways (anatomic dead space) and the abnormally high $\dot{V}_A/\dot{Q}$ units in the gas exchange regions (alveolar dead space). The anatomic dead space has little CO_2 exchange. Its volume varies little in disease states but does vary moderately with V_T because airway volume increases slightly at higher lung volumes. The volume of anatomic dead space can be measured by the single-breath nitrogen washout technique.[45] However, in clinical practice, measurement of anatomic dead space usually is not necessary because its size can be predicted (anatomic dead space in mL = body weight in pounds). In patients receiving mechanical ventilation, the volume of anatomic dead space may be increased because of mechanical bronchodilation. Positive-pressure ventilation also can increase dead space because of the added ventilator tubing (mechanical dead space). An endotracheal tube or tracheostomy decreases anatomic dead space.

High $\dot{V}_A/\dot{Q}$ units or alveolar dead space participate in CO_2 exchange but less efficiently than units with normal $\dot{V}_A/\dot{Q}$. In the sitting position, V_D/V_T is about 0.3 and varies little with age. It can increase to 0.6 or more in lung disease states characterized by increased number of high $\dot{V}_A/\dot{Q}$ units, such as emphysema. During exercise, V_D/V_T normally decreases to below 0.2 primarily because of an increase in V_T.[46] In disease states, V_D/V_T may not decrease to normal levels, and in severe cases it may even increase with exercise.[47]

Although maldistribution of ventilation and perfusion usually does not cause hypercapnia, CO_2 exchange is clearly affected by severe $\dot{V}_A/\dot{Q}$ mismatch. As $\dot{V}_A/\dot{Q}$ falls, local P_{CO_2} rises, reaching the value of the mixed venous P_{CO_2} at a $\dot{V}_A/\dot{Q}$ of 0. The resulting increase in CO_2 tension is small (40 to 47 mm Hg), but CO_2 content changes considerably because of the steep slope of the CO_2 dissociation curve. In addition to the direct effect of decreased ventilation on CO_2 elimination, failure to oxygenate blood further hinders CO_2 exchange. Elimination of CO_2 retained in the blood due to low $\dot{V}_A/\dot{Q}$ usually is accomplished by alveoli with higher-than-normal $\dot{V}_A/\dot{Q}$. Because high $\dot{V}_A/\dot{Q}$ units are inefficient in CO_2 exchange, total ventilation is increased to keep the alveolar CO_2 exchange normal. The increase in ventilation occurs rapidly because of the sensitivity of central chemoreceptors to altered levels of Pa_{CO_2}.

The ventilatory work that is required for this compensation is usually small, as can be illustrated by the following extreme example. If one-half the cardiac output goes to alveoli that are no longer ventilated, the remaining alveoli would have to excrete twice the normal amount of CO_2 to prevent hypercapnia. This increased excretion can be accomplished by an increase in ventilation by 25% to 30% and maintenance of P_{CO_2} at about 30 mm Hg, which is only a small fraction of the normal ventilatory reserve. The ease of this compensation and the magnitude of normal

Box 21-3

Common Causes of Respiratory Acidosis

Associated with Alveolar Hypoventilation
Drugs: anesthetics, sedatives, hypnotics, narcotics
Neuromuscular diseases: poliomyelitis, myasthenia gravis, Guillain-Barré syndrome
Morbid obesity (pickwickian syndrome)
Severe kyphoscoliosis
Idiopathic (primary alveolar hypoventilation syndrome)

Associated with Severe Ventilation/Perfusion Mismatch
Chronic obstructive pulmonary disease
Advanced diffuse lung parenchymal diseases (such as sarcoidosis or pulmonary fibrosis)

ventilatory reserve account for the low incidence of hypercapnia in individuals with $\dot{V}_A/\dot{Q}$ mismatch. However, as the mismatch becomes greater, compensation becomes more difficult to achieve. In the previous example, if retained CO_2 was excreted in only 10% rather than 50% of the alveoli, a much higher $\dot{V}_A/\dot{Q}$ would be present in the compensating alveoli. In this circumstance a 200% increase in ventilation would be required to maintain normocapnia. Although normal ventilatory reserve is unlikely to be exceeded except in extreme $\dot{V}_A/\dot{Q}$ mismatch, the reserve may be minimal in disease. In addition, the work of breathing can be increased substantially in disease states. CO_2 produced by respiratory muscles may place an additional burden on the lungs when increments in ventilation require high levels of muscular work. Thus a decreased ventilatory reserve combined with a high work of breathing and severe $\dot{V}_A/\dot{Q}$ mismatch can lead to hypercapnia.

According to the alveolar ventilation equation, Pa_{CO_2} is inversely related to alveolar ventilation. Because alveolar ventilation is the difference between total minute ventilation and dead space ventilation, hypercapnia can be caused by a decrease in total minute ventilation or an increase in dead space. Occasionally an increase in CO_2 production (for example, caused by overfeeding) may cause hypercapnia in patients with severe $\dot{V}_A/\dot{Q}$ abnormalities and borderline ventilatory reserve. Common causes of alveolar hypoventilation are listed in Box 21-3.

Physiology of Acid-Base Balance

Henderson-Hasselbalch Equation

A discussion of acid-base problems requires a basic understanding of the chemical behavior of acids and bases in aqueous solutions. Chemical reactions proceed at a velocity proportional to the active concentrations, or activities, of the reactants (Equation 21-6). In 1909, Lawrence J. Henderson used the law of mass action to express the hydrogen ion equilibrium. Using the convention in which $[H^+]$ is ex-

EQUATION 21-6

The Henderson-Hasselbalch Equation

In a reaction that may proceed in either direction, the law of mass action may be written as follows:

$$[A] + [B] \leftrightarrow [C] + [D]$$

The reactions have rate constants for both the forward (k_1, $A + B \rightarrow C + D$) and reverse (k_2, $C + D \rightarrow A + B$) directions, which determine the concentrations of reactants until chemical equilibrium is reached, when the following occurs:

$$\frac{k_1}{k_2} = \frac{[C]\,[D]}{[A][B]}$$

The term k_1/k_2 is the equilibrium constant Ke. For an acid (HA) in solution, the equilibrium constant is known as the dissociation constant (K_a), as follows:

$$K_a = \frac{[H^+][A^-]}{[HA]}$$

K_a determines the concentration of hydrogen ion $[H^+]$. If the acid is strong, K_a is large and $[H^+]$ and $[A]$ are much higher than $[HA]$.

For carbonic acid, the following occurs:

$$[H^+] = K_a \times \frac{[CO_2]}{[HCO_3^-]}$$

where K_a is the dissociation constant for carbonic acid $[CO_2]$.

Hasselbalch rearranged Henderson's equation and applied it to the carbonic acid buffer system to obtain the following:

$$pH = pK_a + \log \frac{[HCO_3^-]}{[CO_2]}$$

When methods for the measurement of Pco_2 became available, $[CO_2]$ was replaced by Pco_2 and Henderson's equation was written as follows:

$$[H^+] = 24 \times \frac{Pco_2}{[HCO_3^-]}$$

where $[H^+]$ is in nEq/L, Pco_2 is in mm Hg, and $[HCO_3^-]$ is in mEq/L. The familiar form of the Henderson-Hasselbalch equation is as follows:

$$pH = 6.1 + \log \frac{[HCO_3^-]}{0.0301 \times Pco_2}$$

is obtained through substitution of 6.1, the pK_a of the system, and 0.0301, the solubility constant for CO_2 in plasma, into the equation. Because the Pco_2 of arterial plasma is regulated by alveolar ventilation, it is used to indicate the respiratory component of the acid-base state. The $[HCO_3^-]$ is an estimate of the nonrespiratory, or metabolic, component of the acid-base state.

pressed as pH, Hasselbalch rearranged Henderson's equation and applied it to the carbonic acid buffer system.

The Henderson-Hasselbalch equation accurately describes the equilibrium relationships among pH, Pco_2, and HCO_3^-. However, it does not describe the regulation of acid-base balance. The regulation of acid-base balance could be described by the Henderson-Hasselbalch equa-

tion only if both Pco_2 and HCO_3^- acted independently without significant influence on each other or from the other systems involved in acid-base control. This assumption is not valid because the **bicarbonate buffer system** is influenced by the independent and direct effect of Pco_2 on $[HCO_3^-]$. Thus changes in $[HCO_3^-]$ do not indicate metabolic changes alone.

This difficulty was addressed by titration studies of plasma to produce the Siggaard-Andersen nomogram (Figure 21-20), along with normalization of the Pco_2 to 40 mm Hg.[48] This approach produced the concept of base excess, the excess $[HCO_3^-]$ in arterial plasma that accounts for changes in metabolic component of acid-base disorders. However, the concept of the base excess did not hold up when applied to whole blood or plasma changes in which the acid-base adjustments were made in vivo. This issue required standardization of in vitro data to whole blood with a constant hemoglobin concentration.

The contribution of strong electrolytes, such as Na^+, K^+, and Cl^- to $[H^+]$, in the blood is another problem that has been approached conventionally through analysis of the difference between the concentrations of anions and cations. In plasma, cations predominate and exert a basic, or alkalizing, effect. The effect of strong ions other than Na^+, Cl^-, and HCO_3^- is usually expressed as the **anion gap**: $[Na^+] - ([Cl^-] + [HCO_3^-])$. The anion gap is normally 12 ± 4 mEq/L and is mostly caused by negatively charged plasma proteins, sulfate, and phosphate. The anion gap reflects the concentrations and charges of unmeasured substances; thus an increase in unmeasured anions can occur with both **metabolic acidosis** and **metabolic alkalosis.** An excessive anion gap represents additional unmeasured anions, such as lactate or ketones.

Strong Ion Difference

The working principle of the **strong ion difference (SID)** is similar to that of the anion gap, but it has the advantage of functioning as an independent variable in acid-base regulation.[49] In physiologic fluids the main strong electrolytes are Na^+, K^+, and Cl^-. These strong ions influence $[H^+]$ by the law of electrical neutrality and the dissociation of water, meaning that the net charge must be zero in any system at equilibrium. Thus in a solution of Na^+, K^+, and Cl^- in water: $[Na^+] + [K^+] + [H^+] - [Cl^-] - [OH^-] = 0$.

The effect of strong ions may be lumped into a single term that expresses the net negative or positive charge that they exert. This is the *[SID]*, which in plasma is normally: $[Na^+] + [K^+] - [Cl^-]$. Strong organic ions, such as lactate or ketones, also contribute to $[SID]$ because they may be present in high concentrations. Other strong inorganic ions are usually ignored because they are present in low concentrations. Therefore $[SID] + [H^+] - [OH^-] = 0$, where the independent variable is the $[SID]$ and the dependent variables are $[H^+]$ and $[OH^-]$. In normal plasma, $[Na^+]$ is 140 mEq/L, $[K^+]$ is 4 mEq/L, and $[Cl^-]$ is 104 mEq/L. Thus the normal $[SID]$ is approximately 40 mEq/L. Without bi-

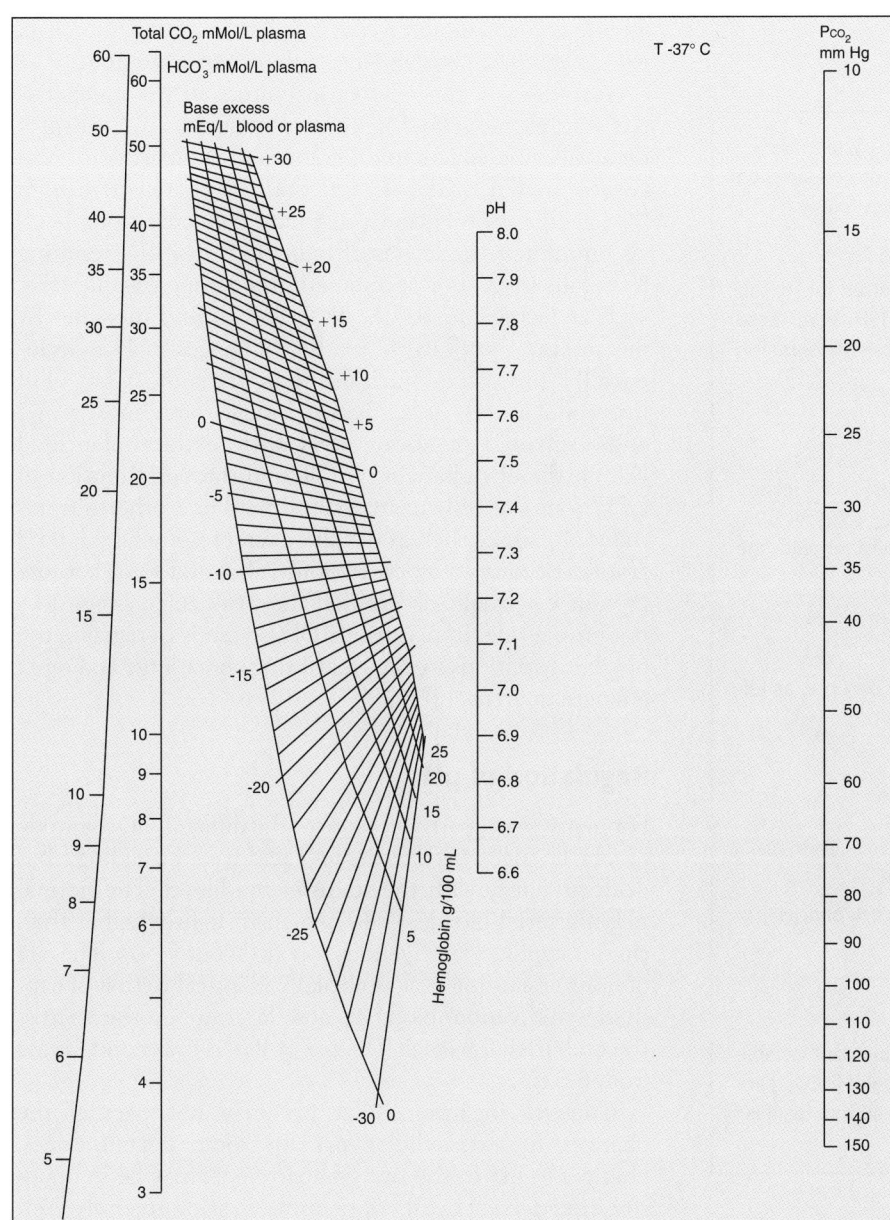

Figure 21-20 Siggaard-Andersen alignment nomogram. (1) A line is constructed between pH and P_{CO_2}; (2) actual plasma HCO_3^- is read directly at the intersection of the line; (3) base excess is hemoglobin dependent and can be read at the intersection of the constructed line and the patient's hemoglobin value; (4) standard HCO_3^- can be determined via construction of another line through the base excess-hemoglobin point and a P_{CO_2} of 40 mm Hg and by reading of the HCO_3^- scale; and (5) buffer base can be computed from the equation BB = 41.7 + (0.42 V Hb) + BE. (Modified from Mahoney JJ, Hodgkin J, Van Kessel A. Arterial blood gas analysis. In: Burton G, Hodgkin J, Ward J, editors. Respiratory care: a guide to clinical practice. Philadelphia: Lippincott; 1997.)

carbonate or other basic electrolytes in plasma, $[OH^-]$ would have to be close to 40 mEq/L, $(4 \times 10^{-2}$ Eq/L). If true, then: $[H^+] = (4.4 \times 10^{-14})/(4 \times 10^{-2})$ mEq/L = 1.1×10^{-12} Eq/L, or a pH of nearly 12. This calculation illustrates the importance of strong ions, weak acids, and the HCO_3^- buffer system in the control of $[H^+]$ in body fluids. With these systems in plasma, the $[H^+]$ is 4×10^{-8} (pH = 7.4).

Total weak acids (A_{tot}) are the buffers present in a partially dissociated state in the physiologic pH range (see Figure 21-23). These acids have dissociation constant (K_a) values between 10^{-4} and 10^{-12}. However, only those with K_a close to 4×10^{-8} (pH = 7.4) are effective buffers. These buffer systems include plasma proteins ($K_a = 3 \times 10^{-7}$), proteins and phosphates in cells ($K_a = 5.5 \times 10^{-7}$), and hemoglobin in RBCs ($K_a = 2.5 \times 10^{-7}$ for oxyhemoglobin; 6.3×10^{-9} for deoxyhemoglobin).

The effectiveness of weak acids as buffers depends on not only the dissociation constant but also $[A_{tot}]$, which is the sum of the dissociated (A^-) and undissociated (HA) forms: $[A_{tot}]$ mEq/L = [HA] + $[A^-]$. In this equation, $[A_{tot}]$ is an independent variable and [HA] and $[A^-]$ are dependent variables. In plasma, $[A_{tot}]$ represents the ionic equivalent of the plasma proteins and may be estimated via multiplication of the protein content by 0.24. Thus at a normal total protein of 70 g/L, $[A_{tot}]$ is 17 mEq/L. This value comprises $[A^-]$ of 15 mEq/L and [HA] of 2 mEq/L at pH = 7.4. Thus even though plasma proteins behave as weak acids, they are mostly dissociated (15/17) at normal arterial pH. The bicarbonate buffer system acts mainly through variations in total CO_2 content brought about by variations in P_{CO_2} and $[H^+]$ (Equation 21-7).

Bicarbonate Buffer System

The two components of the bicarbonate buffer system are hydration of CO_2 into carbonic acid (H_2CO_3) and the dissociation of carbonic acid into HCO_3^- and hydrogen ion, as follows:

$$H_2O + CO_2 \rightarrow H_2CO_3 \rightarrow H^+ + HCO_3^-$$

These two equations can be combined and solved for $[H^+]$ to yield an equation containing two constants and $[H_2O]$. All these constants may be incorporated into a single overall ionization constant (K'_a) to obtain the following:

$$[H^+] = \frac{K'_a[CO_2]}{[HCO_3^-]}$$

where $[CO_2]$ is the concentration of dissolved CO_2 and is related to the P_{CO_2} by the solubility constant for CO_2 (3.01×10^{-5} Eq/L/mm Hg). Substituting the solubility constant into the equation gives the following:

$$[H^+] = K'_a \times \frac{(3.01 \times 10^{-5}) \, P_{CO_2}}{[HCO_3^-] \, Eq/L}$$

For K'_a of 7.94×10^{-7} the single constant can be used, as follows:

$$K_c = (7.94 \times 10^{-7}) \times (3.01 \times 10^{-5})$$

Thus

$$[H^+] = (2.4 \times 10^{-11}) \times \frac{P_{CO_2}}{[HCO_3^-] \, Eq/L}$$

For P_{CO_2} expressed in mm Hg, $[HCO_3^-]$ in mEq/L and $[H^+]$ in nEq/L the following occurs:

$$[H^+] = 24 \times \frac{P_{CO_2}}{[HCO_3^-]}$$

This is Henderson's equation. P_{CO_2} is the independent variable of the bicarbonate buffer system, whereas $[H^+]$ and $[HCO_3^-]$ are both dependent variables. At a normal P_{aCO_2} of 40 mm Hg, if H^+ is 40 nEq/L, then $[HCO_3^-]$ is 24 mEq/L.

Because the SID concept rigorously defines the acid-base systems in terms of their dependent and independent components, it enables identification of the mechanisms that lead to changes in $[H^+]$ in plasma, cells, and interstitial fluid. Replacing base excess and anion gap with the variables [SID] and $[A^-]$ also clarifies some vague concepts, including the use of the Henderson-Hasselbalch equation to imply that $[H^+]$ is controlled by changes in $[HCO_3^-]$; the concept of protons being produced or eliminated; and concepts implying that $[HCO_3^-]$ may be produced, removed, retained (by the kidneys), or administered as a useful therapy.

Clinically, it is useful to obtain the total [SID] that satisfies the measured arterial $[H^+]$ and P_{CO_2} with graphs or solutions of the equations. The inorganic [SID] ($[Na^+]$ + $[K^+]$ − $[Cl^-]$) obtained from plasma electrolyte measurements then can be compared with the value of total [SID] for possible effects of other strong ions. A difference between the inorganic [SID] and total [SID] indicates the presence of unmeasured ions, such as lactate or ketoacids.

This exercise is similar to the calculation of the anion gap, except that $[A^-]$ is a variable rather than a constant.

Variations in the relative magnitude of the independent variables involved in control of acid-base status produce differing effects in different fluid compartments and tissues. In ICF, [SID] is large and dominated by a high $[K^+]$. Large protein and phosphate concentrations $[A_{tot}]$ also minimize the effects of reductions in [SID] resulting from falls in $[K^+]$ or accumulation of strong organic ions, such as lactate. In tissues, P_{CO_2} is high and increases by metabolism, but $[HCO_3^-]$ is low. Changes in P_{CO_2} influence $[H^+]$ in tissues much less than in plasma. Control of intracellular $[H^+]$ is achieved through buffering by A_{tot} and exchange of strong ions with extracellular fluid (ECF), thereby changing [SID], and through diffusion of CO_2 from the cell. In interstitial fluid and other ultrafiltrates of plasma, such as lymph or cerebrospinal fluid, $[H^+]$ is influenced only by changes in [SID] and P_{CO_2} because protein is virtually absent and the weak acid system does not have a role. In plasma, [SID] also tends to regulate the pH, but variations in P_{CO_2} may bring about large and rapid changes in arterial $[H^+]$.

Regulation of pH

For many years, partly because of the difficulty in the study of pH changes within tissues, acid-base physiology has dealt primarily with the status of the blood. The normal pH of arterial blood is 7.40, which is slightly higher than that of capillary and venous blood (about 7.36). The pH of most remaining ECF is virtually identical to that of capillaries and venous blood because H^+ can permeate across the endothelial barrier. The pH of ICF is lower and ranges from 6.8 to 7.2.

Changes in intracellular pH may not parallel the changes in extracellular pH. In some circumstances, changes in pH in the two compartments may be in opposite directions. The pH of neutrality varies inversely with temperature, increasing from 6.8 at 37° C to nearly 7.5 at 0° C. Extracellular pH is maintained at 0.6 to 0.8 pH units higher than the prevailing intracellular pH at any given temperature, thereby providing a sink for disposal of the acids produced by intracellular metabolism. Rahn and colleagues have proposed that in living systems, regulatory mechanisms attempt to keep intracellular pH at or very close to the neutrality of water, the pH at which $[H^+]$ = $[OH^-]$.[50] This hypothesis is based on the effects of temperature on tissue pH that parallel its effects on the fractional dissociation (pK_a) of the imidazole group of histidine in proteins. The fractional dissociation was termed *alpha*, and the control mechanism was called the *alphastat*.

The importance of this alphastat concept can be illustrated by the following example (see Figure 21-7). During exercise on a cold day, an individual's core temperature is 37° C, and intracellular and blood pH are 6.8 and 7.4, respectively. The intracellular P_{CO_2} is 40 mm Hg. In the exercising muscle, where the temperature is 41° C and P_{CO_2} is 48 mm Hg, intracellular and blood pH decrease to 6.7

and 7.35, respectively. However, in the skin, where the temperature is cooled to 25° C and intracellular P_{CO_2} is 22 mm Hg, intracellular and blood pH increase to 7.0 and 7.6, respectively. Despite these striking regional variations in pH and P_{CO_2}, the relative alkalinity, or the net charge of imidazole buffer, between cells and blood is maintained throughout the body.

Erythrocytes and Acid-Base Control

Erythrocytes buffer sudden changes in ions or P_{CO_2} and help maintain relatively constant conditions in plasma and ECF. The ECF composition of the erythrocyte lies between that of ICF and plasma. $[K^+]$ is not as high as in ICF, but $[Na^+]$ and $[Cl^-]$ are higher, although still well below plasma values. The erythrocyte [SID] is 60 mEq/L compared with 40 mEq/L in plasma and 130 mEq/L in ICF. The erythrocyte $[A_{tot}]$ (60 mEq/L) provided by hemoglobin also lies between plasma (20 mEq/L) and ICF (200 mEq/L). The R and T forms of hemoglobin also provide a variable K_a, which enables deoxyhemoglobin to buffer venous acidity more effectively. The carbonic anhydrase in the erythrocyte enables the hydration of CO_2 to proceed rapidly, and carbonate formation enhances CO_2 content without a comparable increase in $[H^+]$. Cell membrane transport systems also facilitate ion exchange between the plasma and erythrocyte while controlling erythrocyte volume.

When O_2 dissociates from hemoglobin, $[H^+]$ inside the erythrocyte decreases. As CO_2 enters the erythrocyte, this decrease in $[H^+]$ is offset by the ionization of carbonic acid. HCO_3^- moves from the cell, and Cl^- moves into the cell (chloride shift), which tends to increase plasma [SID] and leads to a rise in plasma $[HCO_3^-]$. At the same time, CO_2 forms carbamates very rapidly. This reaction is facilitated by deoxygenation of hemoglobin, which allows the αNH_2 groups of the β chain of deoxyhemoglobin to form carbamates. In addition to these reactions associated with the deoxygenation of hemoglobin and CO_2 content of venous blood, the erythrocyte can modulate rapid changes in plasma ion concentration.

Ventilation and Acid-Base Control

The Pa_{CO_2} is controlled mainly by changes in ventilation, as shown in the alveolar ventilation equation, which expresses the simple inverse relationship between Pa_{CO_2} and $\dot{V}A$. The equation is useful because neither metabolic rate nor ventilation needs to be measured to assess the adequacy of breathing in relation to metabolic demand. Pa_{CO_2} represents the balance between metabolic CO_2 production and ventilation. In tissues and venous blood, P_{CO_2} is regulated primarily by the balance between metabolism and blood flow. The extent to which arterial P_{CO_2} reflects the adequacy of ventilation also depends on carbonic anhydrase activity in allowing rapid equilibration of P_{CO_2} between pulmonary capillary blood and alveolar gas. Thus Pa_{CO_2} is increased by carbonic anhydrase inhibition.

The ventilatory responses to acid-base disorders of non-respiratory origin are extremely important in the regulation of $[H^+]$ because they change rapidly. In long-term responses to acid-base disturbances the response of the central medullary chemoreceptors is the most important factor in the ventilatory set point. The major effector is the $[H^+]$ in cerebrospinal fluid (CSF), and because CSF is protein free, P_{CO_2} and [SID] are the two important independent variables in central ventilation control.

Kidneys and Acid-Base Control

The kidneys influence acid-base status mainly by changing the [SID] of the plasma. In the glomerulus, Na^+ reabsorption from plasma ultrafiltrate in the tubules is an active process that lowers both $[Na^+]$ and osmolality in the tubules, leading to water reabsorption. This process in the distal tubule is controlled by antidiuretic hormone (ADH). Chloride reabsorption is mediated in part electrically and in part by an active process related to adenosine triphosphatase (ATPase)-driven membrane pumps on renal tubular cells. If Cl^- is reabsorbed less rapidly than Na^+, urine $[Cl^-]$ increases relative to $[Na^+]$, and urine [SID] falls and increases urine $[H^+]$. If Na^+ is less rapidly reabsorbed than Cl^-, the opposite is the case.

In the tubular lumen a decrease in [SID] and an increase in $[H^+]$ tends to increase P_{CO_2} because the tubule is partly closed to the circulation and the removal of CO_2 by the renal capillary blood flow may not keep pace with its production. The $[HCO_3^-]$ tends to fall with the increase in $[Cl^-]$, and when urine pH has fallen to less than 6, urine $[HCO_3^-]$ is very low. In this way, the excretion of Cl^- in excess of Na^+ and K^+ contributes to control of plasma [SID] and $[H^+]$. When $[H^+]$ has increased because of accumulation of organic anions such as lactate, the renal tubular cells can excrete the lactate, Cl^-, or both. Because the reabsorption of strong organic anions is less efficient, Cl^- is reabsorbed in preference to lactate, resulting in a very high urine [lactate] and low $[Cl^-]$. In this situation the kidney prevents a too-low urine pH by excreting more water and Na^+, if available, and excreting ammonia and phosphates, allowing reabsorption of Na^+ or excretion of Cl^- without an increase in urine $[H^+]$. Both effects tend to increase plasma [SID] and decrease plasma $[H^+]$. Because ammonia and phosphate excretion have limited capacities, adequate Na^+ and water delivery to the distal tubule in an organic acidosis is very important. The kidneys normally can adjust to water excretion between 0.5 and 25 L/day and sodium excretion between 0.05 and 25 g/day.

Evaluation of Acid-Base Disorders

The primary acid-base disorders may be considered in terms of abnormalities in the three acid-base variables capable of independent action: [SID], $[A_{tot}]$, and P_{CO_2} in arterial blood. Primary acid-base changes are modified by compensatory changes that must involve independent variables, such as changes in ventilation leading to changes in P_{CO_2} or movement of strong ions into cells or urine to modify [SID], to be effective.

Metabolic Acidosis

Processes that reduce [SID], such as increases in [Cl$^-$], tend to increase [H$^+$], leading to a primary metabolic acidosis (Box 21-4). A number of compensatory responses take place to minimize this effect. Reductions in [SID] may be offset by responses to increased [SID]; for example, in diabetic acidosis, dehydration may increase [Na$^+$], and more Cl$^-$ excretion in urine may help reduce plasma [Cl$^-$]. These two changes help compensate for the effects of the increase in plasma ketoacid concentration. In disease states such as uremic acidosis, these adaptive responses may not be available. Measurement of urinary electrolyte excretion may be helpful to assess the role of the kidneys in an acidosis. A tendency for [H$^+$] to increase also leads to an association of weak acids (plasma proteins, A$_{tot}$) and thus a reduction in [A$^-$], which may amount to 3 to 4 mEq/L (slightly more in cases of very severe acidosis). Increases in [H$^+$] also stimulate ventilation, leading to a decrease in PaCO$_2$. The effectiveness of this response depends on the ventilatory capacity, the efficiency of pulmonary gas exchange, and the ventilatory control mechanisms. If none of these physiologic mechanisms are impaired, the increase in [H$^+$] expected for a given reduction in [SID] may be used to identify the adequacy of the responses.

Normally the weak acid concentration [A$_{tot}$] is determined by the plasma protein concentration alone. The [A$_{tot}$] may increase if plasma proteins or other weak acids, such as phosphate, increase. Increases of more than 2 or 3 mEq/L in [A$_{tot}$] are uncommon, but because they act as weak acids, the effect an increase in [A$_{tot}$] is similar to a reduction in [SID]—a metabolic acidosis. The effects of increases in plasma proteins, such as in multiple myeloma, vary, depending on the isoelectric points of the class of globulin involved.

Metabolic Alkalosis

An increase in [SID], such as a decrease in [Cl$^-$], tends to reduce [H$^+$], producing a metabolic alkalosis. Common causes of primary metabolic alkalosis are shown in Box 21-5. The compensatory responses to an increase in [SID] may be considered in terms similar to those seen in low [SID] states. These are retention of Cl$^-$ by the kidneys in patients with normal renal function and occasional movement of Na$^+$ into the ICF. Although [H$^+$] may be defended by dissociation of weak acids with an increase in [A$^-$], this effect usually amounts to 1 mEq/L or less. Decreases in plasma [H$^+$] are usually accompanied by a reduction in ventilatory responsiveness, and PaCO$_2$ rises by about 1 mm Hg for each 10 mEq/L increase in [SID]. In some cases of metabolic alkalosis, severe loss of K$^+$ may accompany Cl$^-$ in the kidneys, leading to depletion of intracellular [K$^+$] and a fall in ICF [SID]—an intracellular acidosis complicating the extracellular alkalosis. This effect may lead to respiratory muscle weakness.

When plasma protein concentration is reduced, the [A$_{tot}$] is reduced, leading to a fall in [A$^-$]. The effects are similar to increases in [SID] of equimolar size—a metabolic alkalosis. Quantitatively, the effect may be assessed via multiplication of the total protein concentration in grams per liter by 0.24 [A$_{tot}$] and taking of 0.9 of this value

---

𝓑ox 21-4

Common Causes of Metabolic Acidosis

Increased Unmeasured Anions (Increased Anion Gap or Decreased SID)
  Ketoacidosis: diabetic, alcoholic, starvation
  Lactic acidosis: hypoxia, circulatory failure, drugs and toxins, enzyme defects
  Poisoning: salicylates, ethylene glycol, methanol
  Renal failure

Normal Unmeasured Anions (Normal Anion Gap or SID)
  Renal tubular acidosis, chronic pyelonephritis, obstructive uropathy
  Hypoaldosteronism
  Potassium-sparing diuretics (spironolactone)
  Diarrhea
  Pancreatic or biliary fistulas, ureterosigmoidostomy
  Carbonic anhydrase inhibitors: acetazolamide
  Excessive intake of ammonium chloride, cationic amino acids

---

𝓑ox 21-5

Common Causes of Metabolic Alkalosis

Associated with Chloride (Volume) Depletion (Chloride-Responsive)
  Vomiting, gastric drainage
  Diuretic therapy
  Posthypercapnic alkalosis

Associated with Hyperadrenocorticism (Chloride-Unresponsive)
  Cushing's syndrome
  Primary aldosteronism
  Bartter's syndrome

Excessive Alkali Intake
  Milk-alkali syndrome
  Ingestion of sodium bicarbonate

Severe Potassium Depletion

SID, Strong ion difference.

as [A$^-$] because A$_{tot}$ is about 90% dissociated in most situations. This value then may be added to [Cl$^-$] and [HCO$_3^-$] to identify the presence of any unmeasured anions. The major exception is an increase in immunoglobulin G (IgG) paraproteins in myeloma, which act as weak bases because of the basic amino acids lysine and arginine, which have isoelectric points close to pH = 9.0. They have a weak positive charge in the physiologic pH range, and [A$_{tot}$] and [A$^-$] appear falsely low in their presence.

Respiratory Acidosis

Respiratory acidosis is associated with an elevated PaCO$_2$ caused by alveolar hypoventilation or severe V̇A/Q̇ mismatch. Common causes of respiratory acidosis are shown in Box 21-3. The effect of an increase in PaCO$_2$ may be minimized by an increase in [SID]. Virtually the only compensatory mechanism that is effective and well tolerated is a reduction in plasma [Cl$^-$]. Acutely, this reduction occurs through a shift of Cl$^-$ into erythrocytes; over a longer time, excretion of Cl$^-$ in excess of Na$^+$ and K$^+$ in urine leads to a fall in plasma [Cl$^-$]. In general, [Cl$^-$] falls acutely by 1 mEq/L and in chronic states by 3 to 4 mEq/L for each 10-mm Hg increase in PaCO$_2$. These changes in [Cl$^-$] are accompanied by increases in [HCO$_3^-$] of similar magnitude. Increases in [SID] are effective in limiting increases in [H$^+$]. In the presence of superimposed metabolic acidosis, [SID] increases less than that expected for the rise in PaCO$_2$, or metabolic alkalosis, where [SID] increases more than expected. In recovery from ventilatory failure, resolution of the changes in [SID] also is time dependent. If the reduction in PaCO$_2$ toward normal occurs rapidly, the increase in [Cl$^-$] (posthypercapnic metabolic alkalosis) is delayed.

Respiratory Alkalosis

Respiratory alkalosis is associated with reductions in PaCO$_2$ caused by hyperventilation. Conditions that lead to this situation are shown in Box 21-6. Reductions in PaCO$_2$ tend to reduce [HCO$_3^-$] in plasma, but unless a decrease occurs in [SID], this reduction is quite limited and a marked fall in [H$^+$] results, especially in cases of acute hyperventilation. Reductions in [SID] minimize the fall in [H$^+$], and they are caused by two compensatory responses: (1) retention of Cl$^-$ through a fall in its renal excretion and (2) a small accumulation of lactate resulting from the stimulation of glycolysis in erythrocytes and liver. Retention of Cl$^-$ tends to characterize chronic states of hyperventilation, but increases in [La$^-$] (the concentration of lactate) may occur very rapidly. These compensatory changes are associated with increases in [H$^+$] toward normal and a fall in [HCO$_3^-$]. The usual reduction in total [SID] that results from an increase in both [Cl$^-$] and [La$^-$] accompanying an acute fall in PaCO$_2$ amounts to 1 to 2 mEq/L for each 10-mm Hg decrease in PaCO$_2$ and 3 to 4 mEq/L when hyperventilation is sustained for several days. The reductions in PaCO$_2$ and [H$^+$] in hyperventilation are accompanied by a surprisingly large increase in [CO$_3^{-2}$], predisposing to hypocalcemia and tetany.

Interpretation of Acid-Base Disorders

A major problem in the assessment of acid-base disorders results from the compensatory responses of the lungs and kidneys. As a rule of interpretation, the disorder is named based on the pH as the primary disorder (Table 21-7). For

Box 21-6

Common Causes of Respiratory Alkalosis

Associated with Normal Lungs
Anxiety
Fever
Drug overdose: salicylates, respiratory stimulants (such as strychnine)
CNS lesions: encephalitis, meningitis, tumor
Pregnancy
Sepsis
Liver cirrhosis
High altitudes

Associated with Ventilation/Perfusion Mismatch
Acute bronchial asthma
Pneumonia
Pulmonary vascular diseases: pulmonary embolism
Early diffuse lung parenchymal diseases (such as sarcoidosis or pulmonary fibrosis)
Pulmonary edema

CNS, *Central nervous system.*

Table 21-7

Classification of Acid-Base Disorders

Disorder	pH	Paco$_2$	HCO$_3^-$
Respiratory Acidosis			
Uncompensated	↓↓	↑↑	N
Partially compensated	↓	↑↑	↑
Fully compensated	N	↑↑	↑↑
Respiratory Alkalosis			
Uncompensated	↑↑	↓↓	N
Partially compensated	↑	↓↓	↓
Fully compensated	N	↓↓	↓↓
Metabolic Acidosis			
Uncompensated	↓↓	N	↓↓
Partially compensated	↓	↓	↓↓
Fully compensated	N	↓↓	↓↓
Metabolic Alkalosis			
Uncompensated	↑↑	N	↑↑
Partially compensated	↑	↑	↑↑
Fully compensated	N	↑↑	↑↑

↑, *Small increase;* ↓, *small decrease;* ↑↑, *large increase;* ↓↓, *large decrease;* N, *no change.*

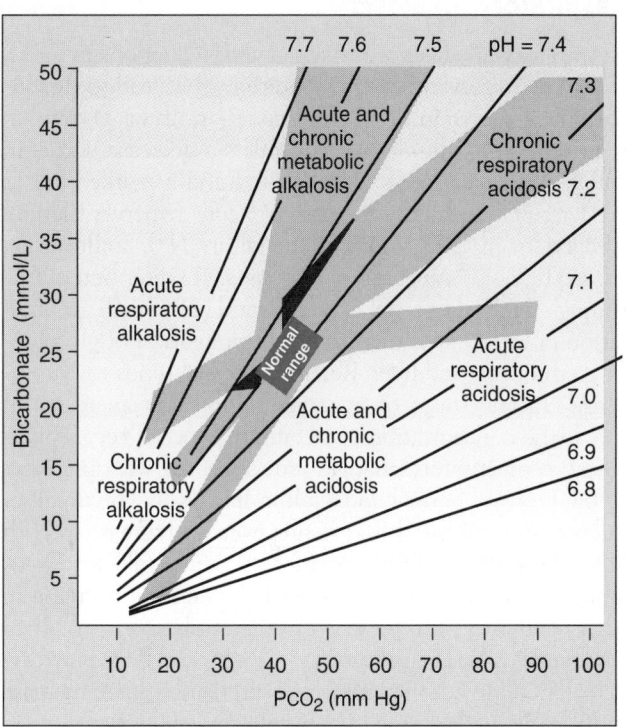

Expected Compensation for Acid-Base Disturbances*

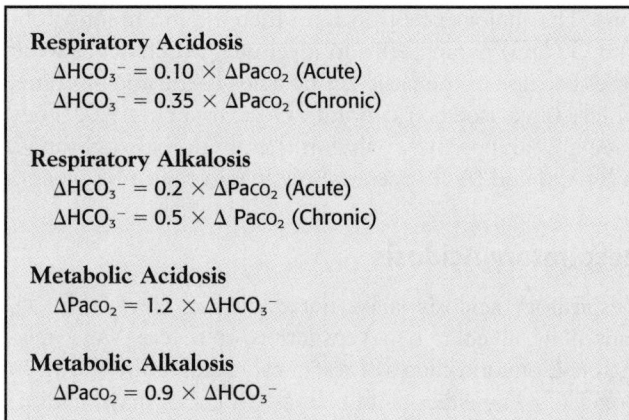

Respiratory Acidosis
$\Delta HCO_3^- = 0.10 \times \Delta Paco_2$ (Acute)
$\Delta HCO_3^- = 0.35 \times \Delta Paco_2$ (Chronic)

Respiratory Alkalosis
$\Delta HCO_3^- = 0.2 \times \Delta Paco_2$ (Acute)
$\Delta HCO_3^- = 0.5 \times \Delta Paco_2$ (Chronic)

Metabolic Acidosis
$\Delta Paco_2 = 1.2 \times \Delta HCO_3^-$

Metabolic Alkalosis
$\Delta Paco_2 = 0.9 \times \Delta HCO_3^-$

*If the acid-base status exceeds the expected level of compensation, a mixed acid-base disturbance is present.

Figure 21-21 Nomogram for uncomplicated respiratory or metabolic acid-base disorders in intact subjects. Each confidence band represents the mean 1 ± 2 SD for compensatory response of normal subjects or patients to a given primary disorder. *SD,* Standard deviation.

example, if a patient with chronic respiratory insufficiency has a pH of 7.25, a $Paco_2$ of 70 mm Hg, and a $[HCO_3^-]$ of 31 mEq/L, the acute event is most likely acute respiratory acidosis because $Paco_2$ is increased. However, the difficulty for the clinician is to determine whether the elevated bicarbonate is merely an appropriate renal compensation for hypercapnia or indicates the presence of a superimposed metabolic acid-base disorder.

The expected degree of compensation for an acid-base disorder can be calculated (Box 21-7). However, the most accurate method is the confidence band technique, as shown in Figure 21-21. In the previous example, inspection

of the confidence band marked "chronic respiratory acidosis" indicates that 95% of individuals with chronic elevation of Pco_2 to 70 mm Hg would have $[HCO_3^-]$ between 34 and 44 mEq/L because of renal compensation. Thus the $[HCO_3^-]$ of 31 mEq/L in the example cannot be interpreted as the sole result of an appropriate compensatory response to chronic hypercapnia. A second acid-base disorder, presumably metabolic acidosis, must be superimposed. On the other hand, if the hypercapnia in this patient is only recently present (1 to 2 days), the $[HCO_3^-]$ of 31 mEq/L would be too high for a purely compensatory response to acute respiratory acidosis. In this case the second acid-base disorder would be metabolic alkalosis. Similarly, if a patient with a metabolic acidosis resulting from poor diabetic control has a $Paco_2$ higher than expected, the presence of coexisting respiratory conditions (such as drugs or respiratory muscle weakness) that impair ventilatory capacity should be suspected. Thus acid-base data always should be interpreted in the context of clinical evaluation of the patient's condition, including factors of time, therapy, and the integrity of pulmonary and renal function.

References

1. Henderson LJ. Das Gleichgewicht Basen und Sauren im tierischen Organismus. Ergebn Physiol 1909;8:254.
2. Hasselbalch KA. Die Berechnung der Wasserstoffzahle des Blutes aus der freien und gebunden Kohlensaure desselben und die Sauerstoffbindung des Blutes als Funktion des Wasswestoffzahl. Biochem Z 1917;78:112.
3. Sanz MC. Ultramicromethods and standardization of equipment. Clin Chem 1957;3:406.
4. Astrup PA. Simple electrometric technique for the determination of carbon dioxide tension in blood and plasma, total content of carbon dioxide in plasma and bicarbonate content in 'separated' plasma at a fixed carbon dioxide tension. Scan J Clin Lab Invest 1956;8:33.
5. Siggaard-Andersen O, Engel OK, Jorgensen K, et al. A micromethod for determination of pH, carbon dioxide tension, base excess and standard bicarbonate in capillary blood. Scand J Clin Lab Invest 1960;12:172-176.
6. Severinghaus JW, Bradley AF. Electrodes for blood P_{O_2} and P_{CO_2} determinations. J Appl Physiol 1958;13:515-520.
7. Severinghaus JW, Weiskopf RB, Nishimura M, et al. Oxygen electrode errors due to polarographic reduction of halothane. J Appl Physiol 1971;31:640-642.
8. Allen E. Thromboangiitis obliterans: methods of diagnosis of chronic occlusive arterial lesions distal to the wrist with illustrative cases. Am J Med Sci 1929;178:237.
9. Wright I. Vascular diseases in clinical practice. Chicago: Year-Book; 1952.
10. National Committee of Clinical Laboratory Standards. Percutaneous collection of arterial blood for laboratory analysis. Approved Guideline H11-A, 5. Wayne, Pa: NCCLS; 1993.
11. Yoshimura H. Effects of anticoagulants on the pH of the blood. J Biochem (Tokyo) 1935;22:297.
12. Rahn H. Body temperature and acid-base regulation. Pneumologie 1974;151:87-94.
13. Severinghaus J. Respiration and hypothermia. Ann NY Acad Sci 1959;80:384.
14. Hansen J. Arterial blood gases. Clin Chest Med 1989;10:227-237.
15. Mahoney J, Hodgkin J, Van Kessel A. Arterial blood gas analysis. In: Burton G, Hodgkin J, Ward J, editors. Respiratory care: a guide to clinical practice. 4th ed. Philadelphia: Lippincott; 1997.
16. Perutz M. Molecular anatomy, physiology, and pathology of hemoglobin. In: Stamatayonnopoulos C, editor. Molecular basis of blood diseases. Philadelphia: WB Saunders; 1987.
17. Perutz M. Mechanisms of cooperativity and allosteric regulation in proteins. Quart Rev Biophys 1989;22:139-237.
18. Bunn H, Jandl J. Control of hemoglobin function within the red cell. N Eng J Med 1970;282:1414-1420.
19. Klocke R. Carbon dioxide transport. In: Farhi L, Tenney S, editors. Handbook of physiology. Section 3. Gas exchange. Bethesda, Md: American Physiological Society; 1987.
20. West J. Effect of slope and shape of dissociation curve on pulmonary gas exchange. Resp Physiol 1969;8:66-85.
21. Carter M. Carbonic anhydrase: isoenzymes, properties, distribution, and functional significance. Biol Rev 1972;47:465-513.
22. West J. Ventilation-perfusion inequality and overall gas exchange in computer models of the lung. Resp Physiol 1969;7:88-110.
23. Henry R. Multiple roles of carbonic anhydrase in cellular transport and metabolism. Ann Rev Physiol 1996;58:523-538.
24. Lindskog S. Structure and mechanism of carbonic anhydrase. Pharm Therap 1997;74:1-20.
25. Effros R, Chang R, Silnerman P. Acceleration of plasma bicarbonate conversion to carbon dioxide by pulmonary carbonic anhydrase. Science 1977;199:427-429.
26. Klocke R. Catalysis of CO_2 reaction by lung carbonic anhydrase. J Appl Physiol 1978;44:882-888.
27. O'Brasky J, Crandell E. Organ and species differences in tissue vascular carbonic anhydrase activity. J Appl Physiol 1980;49:211-217.
28. Knauf P. Anion transport in erythrocytes. In: Andreoli T, Hoffman J, Fanestil D, et al., editors. Physiology of membrane disorders. 2nd ed. New York: Plenum Press; 1986.
29. Tanner M. Molecular and cellular biology of the erythrocyte anion exchanger (AE1). Seminars in Hematol 1993;30:34-57.
30. Gros G, Rollema H, Forster R. The carbamate equilibrium of α- and ϵ-amino groups of human hemoglobin at 37° C. J Biol Chem 1981;256:5471-5480.
31. Klocke R. Mechanism and kinetics of the Haldane effect in human erythrocytes. J Appl Physiol 1973;35:673-681.
32. Bauer C. Reduction of the carbon dioxide affinity of human hemoglobin solutions by 2,3-diphosphoglycerate. Resp Physiol 1970;10:10-9.
33. Grant B. Influence of Bohr-Haldane effect on steady-state gas exchange. J Appl Physiol 1982;52:1330-1337.
34. Wagner P, Saltzman H, West J. Measurement of continuous distributions of ventilation-perfusion ratios: theory. J Appl Physiol 1974;36:588-599.
35. Wagner P, Laravuso R, Uhl R, et al. Continuous distributions of ventilation-perfusion ratios in normal subjects breathing air and 100% O_2. J Clin Invest 1974;54:53-68.

36. Dantzker D. Ventilation-perfusion inequality in lung disease. Chest 1987;91:749-754.

37. Wagner P, Dantzker D, Dueck R, et al. Ventilation-perfusion inequality in chronic obstructive lung disease. J Clin Invest 1977;59:203-216.

38. Cruz J, Hartley L, Vogel J. Effect of altitude relocations upon $AaDo_2$ at rest and during exercise. J Appl Physiol 1975;39:469-474.

39. Kuriyama T, Latham L, Horwitz L, et al. Role of collateral ventilation in ventilation-perfusion balance. J Appl Physiol 1984;56:1500-1506.

40. Roughton F, Forster R. Relative importance of diffusion and chemical reaction rates in determining rate of exchange of gases in human lung, with special reference to true diffusing capacity of pulmonary membrane and volume of blood in lung capillaries. J Appl Physiol 1957;11:290-302.

41. Sorbini C, Grassi V, Solinas E. Arterial oxygen tension in relation to age in healthy subjects. Respiration 1968;25:3.

42. Mellemgaard K. The alveolar-arterial oxygen difference: its size and components in normal man. Acta Physiol Scand 1966;67:10.

43. Gale G, Torre-Bueno J, Moon R, et al. Ventilation-perfusion inequality in normal humans during exercise at sea level and simulated altitude. J Appl Physiol 1985;58:978-988.

44. Dantzker D. Mechanisms of hypoxemia and hypercapnia. In: Bone R, editor: Critical care: a comprehensive approach. Park Ridge, Ill: American College of Chest Physicians; 1984.

45. Fowler W, Cornish E, Kety S. Analysis of alveolar ventilation by pulmonary N_2 clearance curves. J Clin Invest 1952;31:40-50.

46. Murray J. The normal lung. Philadelphia: WB Saunders; 1986.

47. Jones N. Determinants of breathing patterns in exercise. In: Whipp B, Wasserman K, editors. Exercise: pulmonary physiology and pathophysiology. New York: Marcel Dekker; 1991.

48. Douglas A, Jones N, Reed J. Calculation of whole blood CO_2 content. J Appl Physiol 1988;65:473-477.

49. Jones N. Acid-base physiology. In: Crystal R, West J, editors. The lung: scientific foundation. New York: Raven Press; 1991.

50. Rahn H, Reeves R, Howell B. Hydrogen ion regulation, temperature, and evolution. Am Rev Resp Dis 1975;112:165-172.

CHAPTER 22

Nutrition Assessment and Support

Randy S. Smith
James R. Mault

OBJECTIVES

1. Discuss the effects of nutritional status on the respiratory system.
2. Explain the principles of nutrition assessment.
3. Compare methods used to estimate nutrient needs and provide nutritional support for patients with acute or chronic lung disease.
4. Discuss the role of indirect calorimetry in nutrition assessment.
5. Describe nutrition therapies for acute and chronic lung disease.

$\mathcal{K}$EY TERMS

Anthropometry	Enteral Nutrition	Protein-Calorie Malnutrition (PCM)
Antioxidants	Indirect Calorimetry	Respiratory Quotient
Basal Metabolic Rate (BMR)	Nitrogen Balance	
Cell-Mediated Immunity	Parenteral Nutrition	

The human body requires an adequate supply of energy, protein, vitamins, and minerals to maintain an optimal state of health and normal physiology. Without these life-sustaining nutrients, organ system functions become compromised. The respiratory system is no exception. During periods of prolonged semistarvation and hypercatabolism, the diaphragm and other respiratory muscle groups are not spared, but rather may be broken down for use as a fuel source.[1-3] Caloric overfeeding, on the other hand, may also adversely affect lung function by increasing ventilatory demand and carbon dioxide production, which may result in hypercarbia and present problems for mechanically ventilated patients.[4] A careful assessment of the nutritional status of individuals with pulmonary disease is essential.

Effects of Nutrition on Respiratory Function

Muscle Compromise

When the body is faced with an energy deficit, it turns to its own reserves of glycogen, fat, and protein for the release of fuel. Initially protein is spared, because the body mobilizes and oxidizes fat to serve as the principal fuel source in starvation. However, if the deficit continues and undernutrition is prolonged, catabolism of muscle tissue occurs. In a stressed, critically ill patient, this muscle breakdown occurs within days as a result of the body's hypermetabolic response to injury. This circumstance has important implications for an individual with respiratory disease, because the diaphragm, intercostal muscles, and other accessory muscles make up part of the body's skeletal muscle pool and are preyed on in time of need.[5,6] Autopsy studies have shown that patients whose body weight was approximately 70% below their ideal weight for height had 43% to 60% less diaphragmatic muscle tissue than individuals at healthier weights.[5]

It also appears that, although **protein-calorie malnutrition (PCM)** affects all types of muscle fibers, it impairs fast-twitch fibers most profoundly, resulting in diminished contractile strength.[6-8] This effect is seen clinically as a decline in maximal inspiratory and expiratory pressures, vital capacity, and voluntary ventilation. Malnutrition also contributes to muscle weakness by depleting the body of phosphorus, which is essential for the production of adenosine triphosphate and 2,3-diphosphoglycerate, without which oxygen release to tissues is limited. This results in impairment of the expiratory muscles' contractility and endurance.[9,10] Magnesium deficiency also has been associated with muscle weakness and may hinder attempts at weaning from mechanical ventilation.[11] Malnutrition, however, is not the only precipitating factor. Hypophosphatemia and hypomagnesemia may be caused by gastrointestinal losses, the use of antacids and diuretics, and severe malabsorption conditions. With aggressive repletion of these minerals, diaphragmatic strength and contractility improve.

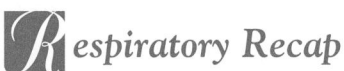espiratory Recap

Effects of Poor Nutrition on Respiratory Functions
Muscle compromise
Impaired immune function
Impaired surfactant production
Hypoalbuminemia
Overnutrition and obesity

Immune Function

The primary component of the immune system adversely affected by PCM is **cell-mediated immunity.**[1,12,13] However, secretory immunoglobulin A (IgA) antibody response, neutrophilic bactericidal capacity, and the complement system also are adversely affected.[14,15] Protein deficiency triggers a reduction in T4 helper cells and T8 cytotoxic cells and through these T cells impairs B-cell activity as well. With the reduction in IgA secretion, the lungs may be more susceptible to bacterial colonization and infection.[16] Indeed, in a study by Martin and colleagues,[12] protein-calorie malnutrition in rats was observed to adversely affect lung defenses by impairing macrophage recruitment to the lungs in response to the presence of infectious agents. This study also revealed the potential for malnutrition to disrupt the process by which the alveolar macrophage, an important barrier to invasion by inhaled organisms, is activated by the T lymphocyte, thus inhibiting antibacterial processes in the lung.

Nutritional compromise also is likely to result in deficiencies of the antioxidant vitamins A, C, and E and the mineral selenium, which play a role in the eradication of free radicals. Without the protective effects of these nutrients, oxidative damage to lung tissue is more likely. Other nutrients involved in enhancing immunity or protecting the body from free radical damage (or both) that may be depleted in malnutrition are zinc, iron, copper, folic acid, and vitamin B_6.

Surfactant Production

Severe starvation causes loss of pulmonary surfactant, which is essential to maintain alveolar stability and to reduce the work of breathing.[17] The size, number, and internal surface area of the alveoli are reduced. Lung lipid content also declines because of multiple factors associated with malnutrition, including alterations in elastin metabolism and a decrease in lipogenesis.[18] PCM has also been shown to reduce the number and size of the lamellar bodies of the granular alveolar pneumocytes, which are the storage sites for surfactant.[19]

Hypoalbuminemia

In a critically ill or malnourished patient, the serum albumin level is likely to be low. In critical illness this is a consequence of the body's metabolic response to injury, inflammatory damage, or sepsis because the synthesis of

TABLE 22-1

Objective Parameters of Malnutrition

Parameter	Mild Malnutrition	Moderate Malnutrition	Severe Malnutrition
Ideal body weight	80% to 90%	70% to 79%	<70%
Usual weight	80% to 95%	80% to 89%	<80%
Triceps skinfold thickness	40 to 50th percentile	30 to 39th	<30th
Serum albumin	2.8 to 3.4 g/dL	2.1 to 2.7 g/dL	<2.1 g/dL
Serum transferrin	150 to 200 mg/dL	100 to 149 mg/dL	<100 mg/dL
Serum prealbumin	12 to 17 mg/dL	7 to 11 mg/dL	<7 mg/dL

Modified from Dantzker DR, MacIntyre NR, Bakow ED, editors. Comprehensive respiratory care. Philadelphia: WB Saunders; 1995.

albumin is deferred to allow for the manufacture of other acute-phase proteins such as fibrinogen, haptoglobin, and ceruloplasmin.[20-22] Albumin is essential for the maintenance of plasma colloid oncotic pressure, which controls the movement of fluid from the interstitial space into the capillaries or intracellular space. When the serum albumin concentration is low, interstitial lung fluid increases, which may compromise lung function by increasing the risk of pulmonary edema.

Overnutrition and Obesity

Just as malnutrition and underweight can compromise respiratory effort, obesity also is likely to result in a decline in lung function. The mechanisms by which this may occur include a decrease in expiratory reserve volumes, a decline in maximal breathing capacities, an increase in both carbon dioxide production and retention, a decrease in maximal flow rates, and hypoxemia.[22-24] Weight loss in obese patients can improve lung function, presumably by reducing the work of breathing.

Nutrition Assessment

The components of a thorough nutrition evaluation are the patient history, a physical examination, anthropometric measurements, markers of visceral protein store status, and indicators of immune system function. Information from the patient's history should help determine the individual's baseline nutritional state and should reveal signs of nutrition compromise such as weight loss, anorexia, dysphagia, early satiety, nausea, or vomiting. A review of the patient's medications also is helpful to assess potential nutritional risk or the presence of nutrient deficiencies, because many medicines interfere with nutrient intake, metabolism, or absorption, or with all three.

Anthropometry is the study of human body measurements and components. It includes measurement of height, weight, body mass index, midarm muscle circumference, skinfold thicknesses, and skeletal breadths. Determination of an individual's weight as a percentage of usual weight and calculation of the percentage of weight loss over time are particularly important indices of nutritional risk and the extent of illness. Evaluation of weight as a percentage of ideal weight for height, with the Metropolitan Life Insurance Tables as a reference, also provides revealing data about the degree of nutritional risk. A weight loss of 10% or more of the usual body weight over a 6-month period or a body weight below 80% of ideal is considered a sign of significant nutritional risk and indicates a need for aggressive nutritional intervention.[25]

Biochemical assessment of nutritional status should accompany the physical and historical assessments. Along with other objective tests, laboratory measurements help reflect the status of a person's visceral and somatic body components and therefore the degree of nutritional risk (Table 22-1). The serum albumin, transferrin, and transthyretin

(prealbumin) levels, along with the retinol-binding protein level, are commonly used to assess the visceral protein stores (Table 22-2). The creatinine-height index may be used to reflect an individual's somatic protein stores, which would include skeletal muscle and adipose tissue. Studies of **nitrogen balance,** which involve a 24-hour urine collection and calculation of the difference between nitrogen intake and excretion, can help determine protein requirements and assess changes in visceral protein stores over time. However, interpretation of these values as indicators of nutritional status is difficult, because serum concentrations of proteins are affected by many factors, such as acute illness, infection, inflammation, stress, sepsis, hepatic disease, renal disease, malignancy, and hydration status.

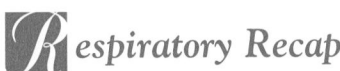

espiratory Recap

Components of Nutrition Assessment
Anthropometric measurements
Biochemical assessments

The ideal protein for use as a marker of nutritional status has a short half-life, a relatively small body pool, and a rapid rate of synthesis and remains unaffected by a disease or its severity. Albumin, transferrin, and transthyretin all have been used in attempts to fit this role.

Albumin, a protein synthesized by the liver, is required for the transport of molecules, maintenance of the vascular system, and prevention of edema.[26] Its body pool is large, and most of this protein (60%) is present in the extravascular space. The 40% found in the intravascular compartment functions primarily to maintain the plasma colloid oncotic pressure. Because of its abundance in the body and its long half-life (18 to 21 days), albumin does not respond quickly to acute changes in nutritional status. It more often reflects the severity of disease and the metabolic response to injury or infection and therefore can be used as an important prognostic indicator; low albumin levels have been associated with morbidity and mortality and with longer hospitalization.[27-29]

Transferrin is a β-globulin synthesized by the liver that functions as a transport protein for iron. Its biologic half-life is 8 to 10 days, and its body pool is small. It therefore may be a more sensitive indicator of protein status than

TABLE 22-2

Biochemical Measurements of Nutritional Status

Marker	Normal Range
Albumin	3.5 to 5 g/dL
Transferrin	200 to 400 mg/dL
Prealbumin	18 to 50 mg/dL
Retinol-binding protein	0.0372 ± 0.0073 g/L

the serum albumin level,[30] although its levels also may be affected by disease and should be interpreted with caution. Transferrin levels may be low with liver disease, after surgery or trauma, or with infection, even in patients with good nutritional status. Its serum levels may be elevated in individuals with iron deficiency anemia, acute hepatitis, dehydration, or acute blood loss.[31]

Transthyretin (thyroxine-binding prealbumin) is a carrier protein that aids in the transport of thyroxine and retinol-binding protein. It has a small body pool and a short half-life of 2 to 3 days. Transthyretin is not affected by iron deficiency, but decreased levels may be seen with zinc deficiency and with inflammation, hepatitis, or cirrhosis.[32] Increased levels are seen in patients with renal disease, presumably because of a decrease in protein breakdown by the kidneys.[33] Even so, changes and trends in the serum level of this protein can be monitored and used to assess acute changes in protein status and response to nutritional support.

Immune function measurements also can be used as objective markers of nutritional status. The measurements most commonly evaluate cell-mediated immunity, the immune system component most affected by malnutrition. A reduced total lymphocyte count, lack of delayed cutaneous hypersensitivity to antigens, and abnormal lymphocyte stimulation assay results all may reveal poor immune function. At least one study has shown that nutrition therapy for malnourished individuals with chronic obstructive pulmonary disease (COPD) resulted in improvements in these markers.[34]

Calculation of Energy Requirements

Equations Versus Measurements

The original work of Harris and Benedict in 1919 first described the amount of energy required to maintain the most basic bodily functions.[35] This amount of energy, expressed as kilocalories (kcal) per day, is known as the **basal metabolic rate (BMR).** The BMR has a fixed relationship with gender, weight in kilograms, height in centimeters, and age in years (Equation 22-1). The Ireton-Jones formula also is commonly used.[36] Energy needs may also be estimated with calories per kilogram of body weight (usually 25 to 35 kcal/kg) if other data are unavailable.

The use of equations to estimate energy expenditure and calculate needs has generated much discussion[37]; this approach most often has been criticized for overestimating needs, especially in patients with several stress or activity factors. The result may be administration of an excessive number of calories in an attempt to meet the estimations. The detrimental effects of gross overfeeding, particularly in patients with hypercarbic respiratory failure who require mechanical ventilation, have been studied extensively.[37-41] Providing excess calories may trigger an increase

in carbon dioxide production through lipogenesis,[40,42] which may increase the hypercarbia and deter attempts to minimize ventilatory support, prolonging the patient's dependence on the ventilator. Prolonged ventilation, in turn, may increase the risk of bacterial contamination and extend the patient's stay both in the intensive care unit and in the hospital.

In direct measurement of energy expenditure (direct calorimetry) an individual is placed in a sealed, thermally insulated chamber. The heat liberated from the individual is determined by measurement of the temperature change in water circulated through the walls of the chamber. Direct calorimetry is impractical in the clinical setting and is rarely performed even in research studies.

For clinical purposes, the most common technique to measure energy requirements is **indirect calorimetry,** which is based on the primary measurement of oxygen consumption ($\dot{V}O_2$). At the time of measurement, $\dot{V}O_2$ represents the actual rate of energy expenditure taking place for the measurement period.

$\mathcal{E}$QUATION 22-1

Equations Used to Estimate Energy Expenditure

Harris-Benedict Equation

BMR (men) = 66 + (13.7 × W) + (5.0 × H) − (6.8 × A)
BMR (women) = 655 + (9.6 × W) + (1.7 × H) − (4.7 × A)

where:

BMR = Basal metabolic rate
  W = Weight (kg)
  H = Height (cm)
  A = Age (years)

Ireton-Jones Formula

EEE (obese person) = [(606 × G) + (9 × W) − (12 × A)] + (400 × V) + 1444

where:

EEE = Estimated energy expenditure
  G = Gender (male = 1; female = 0)
  W = Actual body weight (kg)
  A = Age (years)
  V = Ventilator (present = 1; absent = 0)

EEE (ventilated person) = 1925 − (10 × A) + (5 × W) + (281 × G) + (292 × T) + (851 × B)

where:

EEE = Estimated energy expenditure
  A = Age (years)
  G = Gender (male = 1; female = 0)
  T = Trauma (present = 1; absent = 2)
  B = Burn (present = 1; absent = 0)
  W = Weight (kg)

Indirect Calorimetry Techniques

Indirect calorimetry (CPG 22-1) can be performed with one of several commercially available devices.[43] The complexity, capabilities, and cost of these devices range from simple and inexpensive with limited applications to extremely complex and expensive with broad applications (Table 22-3). These instruments measure $\dot{V}O_2$ by one of three methods. $\dot{V}O_2$ also can be determined with the Fick equation.

Closed-circuit rebreathing spirometry uses an airtight breathing circuit and a volume spirometer filled with oxygen. With inspiration, volume is drawn from the spirometer to the subject, and a portion of oxygen is consumed. The unused oxygen and the carbon dioxide produced are expired through a canister of sodium hydroxide crystals, which chemically extract all the carbon dioxide from the exhaled gas. The remaining gases return to the spirometer. Assuming that no air leak exists in the closed rebreathing circuit, the net volume loss from the system as recorded by the spirometer over time is the $\dot{V}O_2$. Carbon dioxide production ($\dot{V}CO_2$) can be measured in this system by measurement of the amount of carbon dioxide in exhaled gas before its removal by the sodium hydroxide crystals. Closed-circuit rebreathing spirometry can be used for mechanically ventilated patients by the adaption of a bag-in-a-box bellows chamber to the breathing circuit (Figure 22-1). With the patient's ventilator used for mechanical work, positive pressure is created in the chamber on the external surface of the bellows. As it collapses, the volume inside the bellows is directed to the patient via one-way valves. After the compressible volume of the breathing circuit has been compensated, this system delivers the same tidal volume, respiratory rate, and airway pressures as the baseline ventilator settings while maintaining a sealed breathing circuit to measure gas exchange.

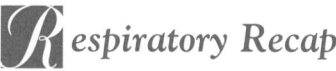 *espiratory Recap*

Indirect Calorimetry
Closed-circuit calorimetry
Open-circuit calorimetry
Combined open- and closed-circuit calorimetry

Open-circuit mixed exhaled gas analysis is another method used to measure $\dot{V}O_2$ and $\dot{V}CO_2$. The simplest example of this approach is the Douglas bag technique (Figure 22-2). In this configuration oxygen and carbon dioxide concentrations are measured in samples of inspired and expired gases. These concentrations can be precisely determined by mass spectrometry or more routinely by infrared carbon dioxide and paramagnetic or zirconium oxide oxygen analyzers. Accurate measurement of exhaled or inhaled minute volume is also required, usually by a precision volume pneumotachometer.

 CPG   22-1

Metabolic Measurement with Indirect Calorimetry during Mechanical Ventilation

Indications
In patients with known nutritional deficits or derangements
A number of nutritional risk and stress factors may considerably skew prediction by the Harris-Benedict equation, including neurologic trauma; paralysis; COPD; acute pancreatitis; cancer with residual tumor burden; multiple trauma; amputation; patients whose height and weight cannot be accurately determined; patients who fail to respond adequately to estimated nutritional needs; new patients receiving home TPN; patients unable to eat who require mechanical ventilation for longer than 5 days; transplant patients; morbidly obese patients; and severely hypermetabolic or hypometabolic patients.
To measure the O_2 cost of breathing in mechanically ventilated patients
To assess $\dot{V}O_2$ in mechanically ventilated patients to evaluate hemodynamic support

Contraindications
When a specific indication is present, no contraindications exist to the performance of metabolic measurement with indirect calorimetry unless short-term disconnection of ventilatory support to allow connection of measurement lines results in hypoxemia, bradycardia, or other adverse effects.

Hazards and Complications
Obtaining metabolic measurements with an indirect calorimeter is a safe, noninvasive procedure with few hazards or complications. However, under certain circumstances and with particular equipment, the following hazards or complications may be seen:
- Closed-circuit calorimeters may cause a reduction in alveolar ventilation because of increased compressible volume of the breathing circuit.
- Closed-circuit calorimeters may diminish the trigger sensitivity of the ventilator, resulting in increased work of breathing for the patient.
- Short-term disconnection of ventilatory support to allow connection of the indirect calorimetry apparatus may result in hypoxemia, bradycardia, or discomfort for the patient.
- Inappropriate calibration or system set up may produce erroneous values, resulting in incorrect patient management.

Modified from AARC clinical practice guideline. Respir Care 1994;39;1170-1175.
CPG, Clinical practice guideline; COPD, chronic obstructive pulmonary disease; TPN, total parenteral nutrition.

TABLE 22-3

Comparison of Gas Exchange Measurement Techniques

Technique	Complexity Level	Cost	Advantages	Limitations
Closed-circuit calorimetry	Medium	Moderate	Accuracy does not depend on FIO_2. Minimal calibration is needed.	Errors may be caused by circuit leaks. Work of breathing may be increased. Risk exists of CO_2 rebreathing.
Open-circuit calorimetry	High	High	Minimal work of breathing is required. Interface with ventilators is easily achieved. Technique is ideal for exercise measurements.	Accuracy is poor with FIO_2 >60%. Calibration drift is possible. Sampling error can occur.
Combined open- and closed-circuit calorimetry*	Low	Low	Accuracy does not depend on FIO_2. Minimal work of breathing is required. Device is portable and handheld.	Duration of measurement depends on size of scrubber cartridge. Accuracy of pneumotachometer is critical.
Reverse Fick equation	Medium	Low	Measurements are readily available with patients with pulmonary artery catheters.	Errors are possible in $\dot{Q}c$, Hb, and saturation values.

FIO_2, *Fractional inspired oxygen concentration;* FRC, *functional residual capacity;* CO_2, *carbon dioxide;* $\dot{Q}c$, *cardiac output.* Hb, *hemoglobin.*
Commercial device under development; advantages and disadvantages are theoretic.

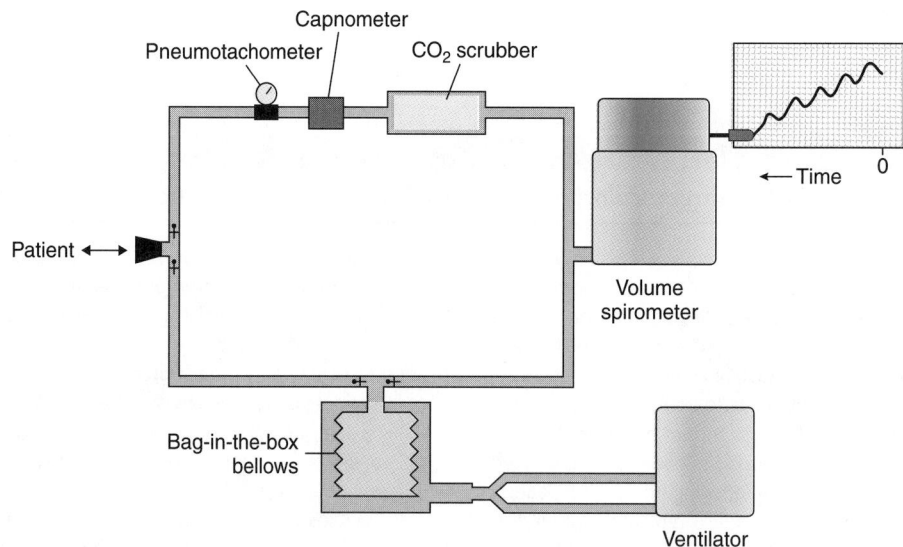

Figure 22-1 Closed-circuit rebreathing spirometry. (Modified from Dantzker DR, MacIntyre NR, Bakow ED, editors. Comprehensive respiratory care. Philadelphia: WB Saunders; 1995.)

$\dot{V}O_2$ is determined by subtraction of the volume of expired oxygen from the volume of inspired oxygen. Mixed exhaled gas analysis is a simple, accurate method of indirect calorimetry in relatively healthy individuals breathing room air. However, the accuracy of this technique requires precise knowledge of the inspired oxygen content (FIO_2). With mechanical ventilation, the FIO_2 delivered to the patient varies by 1% to 2% per breath. Although this variation has no clinical consequences, it can create significant error in the calculation of $\dot{V}O_2$. These problems are compounded by compression of gases being sampled by the analyzers. For these reasons, this method of indirect calorimetry generally is limited to patients who are spontaneously breathing in room air

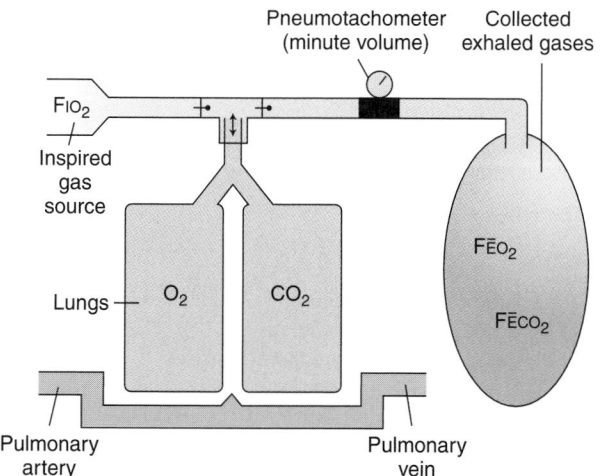

Figure 22-2   Open-circuit, mixed-exhaled gas analysis with the Douglas bag technique. (Modified from Dantzker DR, MacIntyre NR, Bakow ED, editors. Comprehensive respiratory care. Philadelphia: WB Saunders; 1995.)

and to those who are mechanically ventilated with an FIO_2 below 60%.

Combined open- and closed-circuit calorimetry[44] is a new technique that uses the closed-circuit measurement principle within an open-circuit architecture (Figure 22-3). With a bidirectional, high-precision pneumotachometer, inspired volume ($\dot{V}I$) is measured as the subject (or the mechanical ventilator) initiates a breath. Exhaled gases ($\dot{V}E$) flow via one-way valves through a carbon dioxide scrubber (where all exhaled carbon dioxide is removed) and exit through the pneumotachometer in the opposite direction ($\dot{V}E - \dot{V}CO_2$). $\dot{V}CO_2$ and the respiratory quotient can easily be determined by the addition of either a capnometer or a second pneumotachometer positioned immediately before the scrubber. This system can be easily adapted to a positive pressure ventilator circuit, and the $\dot{V}O_2$ can be measured continuously (for the life of the carbon dioxide scrubber) without any change in ventilator settings. Although this device is still under commercial development, by design it will be hand-held, inexpensive, and simple to operate and will allow measurements of gas exchange at any FIO_2.

As mentioned previously, the Fick equation also may be used to determine $\dot{V}O_2$ and the corresponding energy expenditure[42,45] (Equation 22-2). This technique requires the presence of a pulmonary artery catheter. The range of error for this calculation is significant when the individual errors of thermodilution, cardiac output, blood gas determinations, hemoglobin measurement, and estimation of the oxygen-carrying capacity of hemoglobin are added. For these reasons, the Fick method to calculate $\dot{V}O_2$ and energy expenditure should be regarded as only an approximation of the metabolic rate. This method does not allow for determination of $\dot{V}CO_2$ and the respiratory quotient.

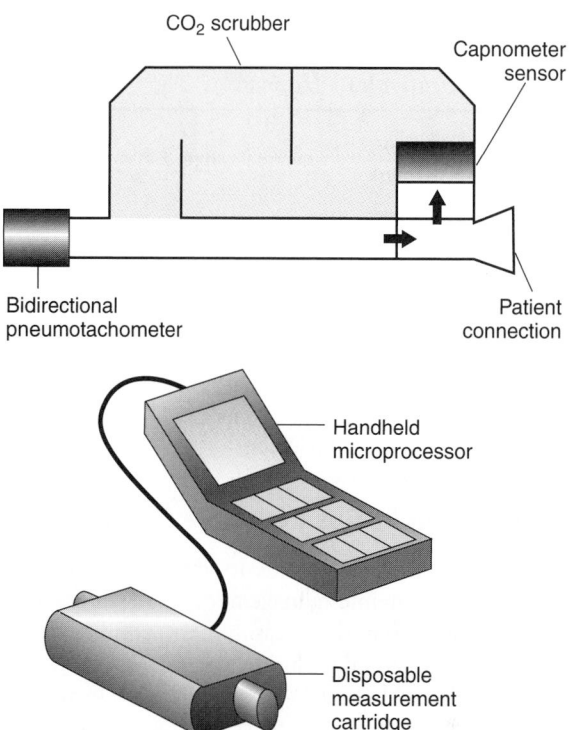

Figure 22-3   Combined open- and closed-circuit calorimetry. (Modified from Dantzker DR, MacIntyre NR, Bakow ED, editors. Comprehensive respiratory care. Philadelphia: WB Saunders; 1995.)

EQUATION 22-2

Calculation of Oxygen Consumption ($\dot{V}O_2$) with the Fick Equation

$$\dot{V}O_2 = \dot{Q}c \times C(a - \bar{v})O_2$$

where:

$\dot{V}O_2$ = Oxygen consumption
$\dot{Q}c$ = Cardiac output
$C(a - \bar{v})O_2$ = Difference between arterial and mixed venous oxygen content

To perform this calculation, an indwelling pulmonary artery catheter is required to determine the $\dot{Q}c$ (by thermodilution) and obtain a mixed venous blood sample (which must be obtained from the distal port of the catheter positioned in the pulmonary artery). An arterial blood sample also must be obtained. Blood gas analysis is performed on both samples, and the $C(a - \bar{v})O_2$ then is calculated, as follows:

$$C(a - \bar{v})O_2 = [(SaO_2 - S\bar{v}O_2) \times Hb \times 1.34] + [0.0031 \times (PaO_2 - P\bar{v}O_2)]$$

where:

$C(a - \bar{v})O_2$ = Difference between arterial and mixed venous oxygen content
SaO_2 = Oxygen saturation of arterial blood
$S\bar{v}O_2$ = Oxygen saturation of venous blood
Hb = Hemoglobin
PaO_2 = Partial pressure of arterial oxygen
$P\bar{v}O_2$ = Partial pressure of oxygen in mixed venous blood

EQUATION 22-3

Ventilatory Equivalent Ratios

$$\dot{V}eo_2 = \frac{\dot{V}_E \text{ (L/min)}}{\dot{V}o_2 \text{ (dL/min)}} \quad \text{(Normal range, 2.4 to 4)}$$

$$\dot{V}eco_2 = \frac{\dot{V}_E \text{ (L/min)}}{\dot{V}co_2 \text{ (dL/min)}} \quad \text{(Normal range, 3 to 4)}$$

where:

$\dot{V}_E$ = Minute ventilation
$\dot{V}o_2$ = Oxygen consumption
$\dot{V}eo_2$ = Ventilatory equivalent ratio for O_2
$\dot{V}eco_2$ = Ventilatory equivalent ratio for CO_2
$\dot{V}co_2$ = Carbon dioxide production

Interpretation of Gas Exchange Measurements

When gas exchange measurements are performed for nutritional or hemodynamic management, every effort must be made to ensure that the measurement conditions are at steady state.[46] Generally, during the measurement period the patient should be resting and recumbent. If the patient is mechanically ventilated, appropriate adjustments should be made to duplicate the patient's usual oxygen concentration, minute ventilation, and airway pressure. If the patient is breathing spontaneously, measurements should be taken only after the patient has adjusted to breathing through the mouthpiece or face mask, and the patient's respiratory effort is not influenced by the measurement device. After steady-state conditions have been confirmed, gas exchange measurements should be averaged over a period of at least 15 minutes. The patient's body temperature and other vital signs should be noted at the time of measurement as a reference for future studies.

After a measurement has been completed, the reliability of the resultant $\dot{V}o_2$ and $\dot{V}co_2$ values can be verified through the calculation of ventilatory equivalent ratios, $\dot{V}eo_2$ and $\dot{V}eco_2$ (Equation 22-3). Ventilatory equivalent values that fall below the normal range suggest that $\dot{V}o_2$ and $\dot{V}co_2$ are falsely high relative to minute ventilation. Values above the normal range suggest $\dot{V}o_2$ and $\dot{V}co_2$ are falsely low relative to minute ventilation. In either case, technical errors such as calibration mistakes, non-steady-state conditions, or tubing leaks may have occurred during the measurement period. After these factors have been corrected, the gas exchange measurement should be repeated.

After the results of a gas exchange measurement have been confirmed, the corresponding energy expenditure can be calculated. Energy metabolism is divided into several categories of metabolic activity, such as total energy expenditure (TEE) and resting energy expenditure (REE) (Equation 22-4). Hospitalized patients usually are resting and recumbent with minimal physical activity; therefore measurements of REE by indirect calorimetry accurately represent TEE for the purpose of guiding energy intake. If additional physical activity occurs, the energy intake should be adjusted accordingly.

EQUATION 22-4

Total Energy Expenditure and Resting Energy Expenditure

Total energy expenditure:

TEE = REE + AEE

where:

TEE = Total energy expenditure
REE = Resting energy expenditure
AEE = Energy expended by activity (exercise)

REE is further defined as follows:

REE = BMR + SDA

where BMR is the basal metabolic rate and SDA is the specific dynamic action (energy expenditure for metabolic processing of dietary intake).

With the use of the stoichiometry of aerobic pathways, a caloric equivalent has been derived for each class of foodstuffs. The caloric equivalent of a given energy substrate is the amount of heat (in kilocalories) liberated when the substrate is burned in 1 L of oxygen. Similarly, each class of foodstuffs has a unique respiratory quotient. The **respiratory quotient** is the ratio of carbon dioxide produced to oxygen consumed in the stoichiometric oxidation of a particular substrate (Table 22-4).

Through measurement of $\dot{V}o_2$, $\dot{V}co_2$, and urinary nitrogen excretion (in grams), the de Weir equation can be used to determine the REE (Equation 22-5).[44,47] If the measurement of urinary nitrogen excretion (Nu) and $\dot{V}co_2$ is unavailable, the REE can be accurately determined from $\dot{V}o_2$ alone with the use of an estimated respiratory quotient of 0.85 (to generate a value for $\dot{V}co_2$) and an estimated Nu of 10 g. On the basis of comparisons with continuous 24-hour gas exchange measurements, extrapolation of single 15- to 30-minute measurements of $\dot{V}o_2$ and $\dot{V}co_2$ to 24-hour values accurately describes daily energy requirements. Daily measurements are required because variability between days occurs.[48]

Protein Requirements

In both acute and chronic disease, to focus nutritional support efforts on the maintenance of protein stores is important. With prolonged inadequate nutrient intake, endogenous protein catabolism occurs, with most of the loss from muscle tissue. As mentioned previously, this includes the respiratory muscles, and weakness and fatigue are likely to result, causing increased difficulty breathing. Therefore providing patients with an adequate supply of nutrients for nitrogen building and endogenous protein sparing is important. It generally is suggested that 25 to 35 nonprotein calories per kilogram of body weight be provided to allow for metabolic utilization of 1 g of protein.[49] For most pa-

TABLE 22-4

Energy and Respiratory Values of Energy Substrates

Energy Substrate	Caloric Value (kcal/g)	Caloric Equivalent (kcal/L Oxygen)	Respiratory Quotient
Carbohydrate	4.1	5.05	1
Protein	4.1	4.46	0.82
Fat	9.3	4.74	0.71
Alcohol	7.1	4.86	0.6

EQUATION 22-5

de Weir Equation

REE (kcal) = $(3.581 \times \dot{V}_{O_2}) + (1.448 \times \dot{V}_{CO_2}) - (1.773 \times Nu)$

where:

$\dot{V}_{O_2}$ = Oxygen consumption (L/min)

$\dot{V}_{CO_2}$ = Carbon dioxide production (L/min)

Nu = Urinary nitrogen excretion

EQUATION 22-6

Calculation of Nitrogen Balance

$$\text{Nitrogen balance (g)} = \left[\frac{\text{24-Hour protein intake (g)}}{6.25} \right] - [\text{24-Hour urinary urea nitrogen (g)} + 4\text{ g}]$$

The 4 g added to the urinary urea nitrogen value is an estimate of insensible nitrogen loss (for example, from the feces, skin, and hair).

tients, in the absence of renal or liver disease, 1.2 to1.5 g of dietary protein per kilogram of body weight is recommended. Visceral protein stores are difficult to monitor, but attempts should be made to evaluate the adequacy of a feeding regimen, the response to nutrition therapy, and changes in protein status. Common tools include measurement of transferrin and transthyretin and 24-hour urine collections to calculate urinary urea nitrogen (UUN).

The UUN, or calculation of nitrogen balance, requires an accurate 24-hour urine collection and can be helpful in the assessment of a patient's response to nutrition therapy. The goal of nutritional support is to achieve positive nitrogen balance, which occurs when protein in the diet provides nitrogen in excess of its loss (Equation 22-6).[50] A negative nitrogen balance indicates protein catabolism, whereas a positive nitrogen balance reflects an anabolic state. The clinician should aim for a positive nitrogen balance of approximately 1 to 4 g a day. In certain diseases and conditions, however, this measurement may be misleading. In patients with renal disease, gastrointestinal fistulas, severe diarrhea, or other conditions that may involve excessive nitrogen loss, calculation of nitrogen balance is most likely to present the clinician with unreliable results and may not accurately reflect the patient's nutritional state.[51] It also should be kept in mind that in critically ill patients with infection, sepsis, or inflammatory disease and in those receiving steroid therapy, a positive nitrogen balance may not be achieved even with aggressive nutritional support. In these cases, only when the inflammatory process subsides and the patient's condition becomes less critical are improvements in protein stores reflected by serum protein levels and UNN studies.

Other Nutrient Considerations

Research on the possible benefits of antioxidants in disease and inflammatory processes has been increasing. Free radicals are constantly being produced as byproducts of normal metabolism and exposure to oxygen. These unstable molecules are highly reactive and can damage cellular components. **Antioxidants** such as β-carotene, α-tocopherol (vitamin E), and ascorbic acid (vitamin C) can help prevent lipid peroxidation triggered by free radicals and assist in the repair of tissue damaged by oxidative stress.[51] As such these vitamins have a potentially beneficial role in the treatment of acute lung injury and in the prevention of lung tissue damage over time. However, no specific recommendations have yet been made for antioxidant supplementation in respiratory disease.

Considerable attention has also been paid to the omega-3 fatty acids, which seem to play a role in protecting cells from damage associated with many inflammatory and autoimmune diseases. Their benefit appears to be related to their ability to reduce the number of arachidonic acid metabolites, which have inflammatory properties and are known to be involved in acute respiratory distress syndrome.[52,53] Moreover, they are precursors of prostaglandins, hormone-like compounds with antiinflammatory properties. Again, more research is needed before recommendations can be made for supplementation in patients with respiratory disease.

Nutritional Support Guidelines

The primary goal of nutrition therapy in patients with respiratory disease is to improve respiratory function through the prevention or minimization of the loss of muscle mass.[49] Other goals are to prevent infection, enhance the immune system, increase exercise tolerance, and improve the patient's quality of life.

Nutrition Delivery

The preferred and most convenient method of nutrient delivery is the oral route. However, it may be difficult for many individuals with severe respiratory disease to consume enough to maintain their weight and meet their increased nutrient needs. This may occur for several reasons, such as dyspnea on food preparation and consumption, early satiety, gastroesophageal reflux, bloating caused by air swallowing, nausea, and vomiting. Much of the gastrointestinal discomfort can be caused or exacerbated by medications commonly prescribed to treat respiratory symptoms and infection, including bronchodilators, anticholinergics, corticosteroids, antibiotics, and mucolytics. The reflux many patients experience may also be attributed to the effects of lung hyperinflation on the position of the stomach or an increase in abdominal pressure associated with coughing.

If oral intake is inadequate to meet daily energy needs despite the use of high-calorie, high-protein supplements and snacks, enteral delivery of nutrients by means of a feeding tube should be considered. This should also be the method of choice to feed patients requiring ventilatory support.

Enteral nutrition should always be considered when a patient has a functioning gastrointestinal (GI) tract. The benefits of enteral nutrient delivery are well documented.[54-57] Nutrients absorbed via the portal system with delivery to the liver may allow for better absorption and result in enhanced immune competence. The presence of nutrients in the gut prevents intestinal atrophy and maintains the absorptive capacity of the GI mucosa by directly nourishing the enterocytes, supporting epithelial cell repair and replication. Enteral nutrition also helps preserve normal gut flora and gastric pH, which may guard against bacterial overgrowth in the small intestine. Finally, nutrients, especially fats and proteins, stimulate feeding-dependent neuroendocrine activity, which results in the secretion of immunoglobulins. These substances, particularly secretory IgA, are important in the prevention of bacterial translocation and gut sepsis.[54] Although enteral nutrition is not entirely devoid of risk, if administered carefully and sensibly, it is safer than parenteral nutrition and considerably less expensive.

The route of delivery varies and may depend on the ease and availability of enteral access; the patient's risk of aspiration, tolerance to feedings, and clinical condition; and the length of time feeding is likely to be needed. Nasogastric or orogastric tubes often are used because they are easy to place at the bedside and usually are needed for medication administration. They are considered short-term feeding tubes (less than 3 to 4 weeks) and may be contraindicated in patients who have severe reflux or delayed gastric emptying or gastroparesis, or who are otherwise at high risk of aspiration. In these cases a feeding tube placed past the stomach into the small intestine should be considered. These tubes are also indicated for short-term tube feeding and allow for uninterrupted duodenal or jejunal feeding in patients with gastric dysmotility and large gastric residual volumes, which would otherwise prevent the administration of adequate nutrition support. In this case the feeding would be infused via the small bowel (enteric) tube, and a larger gastric tube could be used to decompress the stomach and allow for the drainage of gastric secretions. Presumably the more distal to the stomach the feeding is delivered, the less likely aspiration related to the feeding is to occur. Thus the optimal postpyloric tube placement is past the ligament of Treitz, or in the fourth portion of the duodenum.

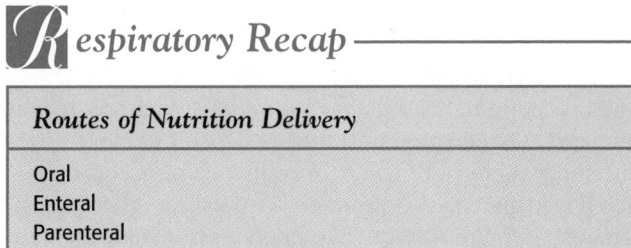

Respiratory Recap

Routes of Nutrition Delivery
Oral
Enteral
Parenteral

If a long-term feeding is anticipated, tubes can be placed through the skin into the stomach or small intestine by surgical, endoscopic, radiologic, or laparoscopic techniques. These tubes generally are more comfortable

TABLE 22-5

Composition of Select Enteral Formulas

Formula	Kcal/mL	Carbohydrate (g/mL)	Protein (g/mL)	Fat (g/mL)
Ensure Plus*	1.5	200	55	53
Boost High Protein†	1.06	140	61	23
Boost Plus†	1.5	190	61	57
Isocal†	1.06	138	34	44
Isocal HN†	1.06	123	44	46
Traumacal†	1.5	162	82	68
Deliver 2.0†	2.0	200	75	102
TwoCal HN*	2.0	217	84	91
Pulmocare*	1.5	106	63	93
Oxepa*	1.5	106	63	93
Respalor†	1.5	148	76	71

*Ross Products Division, Abbott Laboratories, Columbus, Ohio.
†Mead-Johnson Nutritionals, Evansville, Ind.

than the nasogastric, orogastric, or enteric tubes, and they can be removed or replaced as necessary.

Once a tube has been placed and is ready for use, the clinician must choose the feeding recipe or formula that best meets the individual's nutrition needs. Many enteral formulas are available (Table 22-5), and selection of the most cost-effective, beneficial product presents a great challenge to the clinical nutrition specialist. General purpose formulas are quite cost-effective, palatable, and well tolerated by most patients, except those individuals with malabsorption syndromes or other special conditions. These formulas generally provide 1 calorie (cal) per milliliter and are approximately 50% carbohydrate, 30% fat, and 15% to 20% protein.

Many specialized enteral nutrition formulas have been developed for patients with specific conditions, such as diabetes mellitus, hepatic disease, renal disease, and pulmonary disease. The composition of these formulas is different from that of more general formulas, and they tend to be higher in price. The formula designed for patients with pulmonary disease is based on the theory that through the provision of fewer calories from carbohydrate and more from fat, total carbon dioxide production will be decreased, reducing carbon dioxide retention. These formulas contain a higher percentage of calories from fat, or 40% to 55% of total calories. The carbohydrate sources, which include sucrose, maltodextrin, and hydrolyzed cornstarch, typically contribute less then 40% of total calories. The caloric density typically is 1.5 cal/mL, which reduces the amount of overall volume necessary to provide full nutritional support. This may be beneficial for patients at risk for the development of fluid overload and pulmonary edema. Studies that have shown positive outcomes with these specialty formulas have been criticized for their small sample sizes, and frequently reports of carbohydrate overfeeding have been based on studies with patients receiving excessive calorie loads (approximately 50 kcal/kg) via parenteral nutrition.[40,41,58,59] A recent study has concluded that when overall calories are not excessive, carbon dioxide production is more affected by total calories than by the percentage of carbohydrate calories.[39] The use of higher-priced specialized formulas for pulmonary patients therefore remains controversial, and more clinical trials are needed to support their efficacy.

Parenteral Nutritional Support

Intravenous delivery of substrate may be necessary when the GI tract is not functioning or if stimulation of the gastrointestinal or pancreatic systems would worsen the patient's condition. **Parenteral nutrition,** which bypasses the GI system, may be indicated for nutritional support in patients with severe pancreatitis, gastrointestinal fistulas, short bowel syndrome, prolonged ileus, and some cancers.[60] It should not be initiated if the expected duration of support is less than 7 days. Placement of a central or peripheral venous catheter is required for the infusion of nutrients

into the bloodstream; central venous access usually is preferred. Solutions with osmolarities above 600 to 900 mOsm/L may be infused, the volume of fluid is unrestricted, and support may continue for a longer period than with peripheral access. Complications involve in the placement of a central venous catheter include pneumothorax, arterial puncture, catheter malposition, catheter embolization, site infection, air embolus, thoracic duct injury, mediastinal injury, and cardiac injury.[61] The most common complication of percutaneously placed subclavian catheters is pneumothorax, with an incidence rate of 1% to 4%.[62] Pericardial tamponade, a lethal complication, has a mortality rate of 65% to 90%. Furthermore, the infusion of nutrients into the central circulation leaves the GI tract unstimulated, which can lead to gut atrophy, mucosal compromise, and a weakening of the gut barrier, which may increase the risk of bacterial contamination.

Nutritional Support in Chronic Respiratory Disease

The goals of nutrition therapy in acute respiratory disease are the same as for patients suffering from chronic disease. Maintaining nutritional status with an adequate energy, protein, vitamin, and mineral intake is essential. For individuals participating in pulmonary rehabilitation programs, poor nutrition may adversely affect their state of health and well-being in several ways. It decreases exercise tolerance, hinders the body's ability to regenerate healthy muscle tissue, increases susceptibility to infection, and ultimately may prevent successful progression through the program. These individuals need practical, simple guidelines to optimize their nutrient intake, such as those listed in Box 22-1.

Box 22-1

Nutritional Guidelines for Patients with Chronic Respiratory Disease

> Choose high-calorie, nutrient-dense foods.
> Plan for small, frequent meals or snacks rather than fewer large ones.
> Drink liquids between meals, not with them.
> Add fats to foods to increase calories and add dry milk powder to boost the protein content.
> Set alarm clocks as reminders to eat and keep your favorite foods visible.
> Avoid gas-forming foods (for example, cabbage, onions, and beans) that may cause bloating and indigestion.
> Use home-delivered meal services, frozen foods, and convenience foods to cut down on food preparation time.
> Supplement your food intake with medical nutritional products (for example, Ensure, Boost) if you are unable to consume an adequate diet.
> Review your medications and consult your physician about adjusting the dosage or type, if possible, of those that have an adverse effect on your food intake.

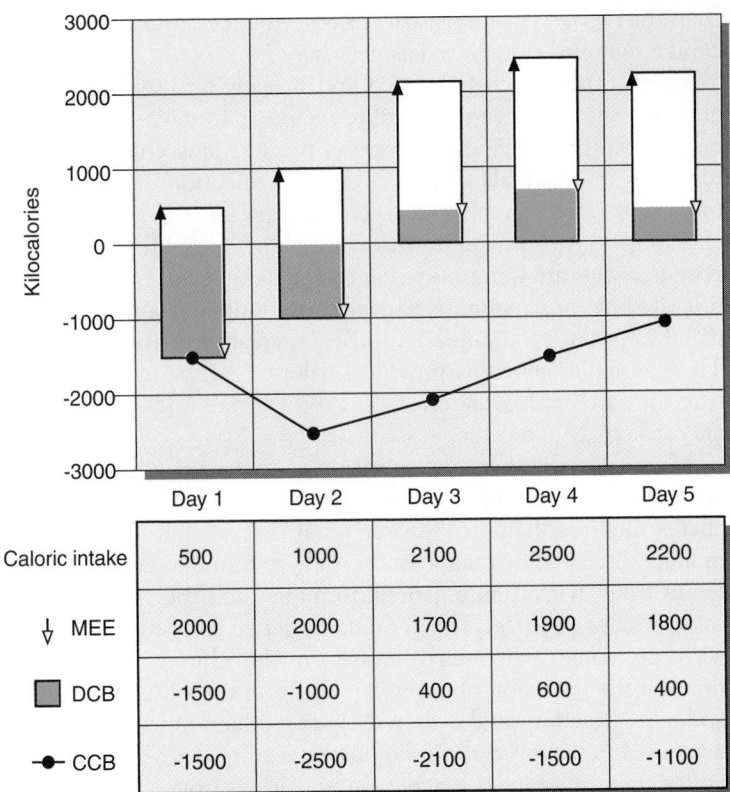

Figure 22-4 Daily tabulation of energy balance. Routine monitoring can be charted in graphic or tabular form as shown. After the measured energy expenditure (MEE) has been determined, the caloric intake is tabulated for the corresponding day. The daily caloric balance (DCB) is calculated by subtraction of the MEE from the caloric intake. The cumulative caloric balance (CCB) is the running sum of each successive DCB. CCB values are listed as total kilocalories since admission, but all other values are for kilocalories per 24 hours. (Modified from Dantzker DR, MacIntyre NR, Bakow ED, editors. Comprehensive respiratory care. Philadelphia: WB Saunders; 1995.)

	Day 1	Day 2	Day 3	Day 4	Day 5
↑ Caloric intake	500	1000	2100	2500	2200
↓ MEE	2000	2000	1700	1900	1800
▨ DCB	-1500	-1000	400	600	400
●— CCB	-1500	-2500	-2100	-1500	-1100

Nutritional Balance

As was emphasized at the beginning of this chapter, nutrition is a simple matter of supply and demand. After energy requirements have been determined through indirect calorimetry, the daily and cumulative caloric balances should be tabulated. The daily caloric balance is calculated by subtraction of the REE from the total energy (in kilocalories) administered per 24 hours. The cumulative caloric balance (CCB) results from the addition of the consecutive daily balances (Figure 22-4). The same format can (and should) be used to tabulate the daily and cumulative protein balances from measurements of total urinary nitrogen and protein intake. This approach to nutritional monitoring has shown significant value for the metabolic care of critically ill patients. Bartlett and colleagues[63] performed indirect calorimetry, tabulated the daily and cumulative caloric balances, and related these findings to outcome in critically ill patients with multiple organ failure. Of 57 patients studied in the surgical intensive care unit, 14 had a negative CCB of at least 10,000 kilocalories; 12 (86%) died. Twenty eight patients had a CCB of 0 to −10,000 kilocalories; of these, 11 (39%) died. In contrast, of 15 patients who were discharged with a positive CCB, only 4 (27%) died. The differences among these three groups were statistically significant ($p < 0.01$). Similar findings have more recently been demonstrated in a subgroup of critically ill patients with multiple organ fail-

ure who had acute renal failure.[64] Others also have shown benefit from the use of indirect calorimetry and protein balance measurements to guide the nutritional support of critically ill patients.[65]

KEY POINTS

- Respiratory function is affected by an individual's nutritional status, which also can affect muscle function, immunity, fluid balance, and surfactant production, in addition to other systems.
- Caloric overfeeding (more than 50 kcal/kg/day) should be avoided in patients with hypercarbic respiratory failure requiring mechanical ventilation, because it may result in increased hypercarbia and a prolonged ventilatory period.
- Indirect calorimetry is the most accurate method to determine energy expenditure in hospitalized patients.
- Enteral delivery of nutrients is preferred to parenteral nutrition, because it carries fewer risks of infection, may have a protective effect on the gastrointestinal mucosa, and is less costly.
- A complete nutrition assessment and subsequent support, if indicated, should be included in the plan of care for patients with acute or chronic lung disease.

References

1. DeMeo MT, Van De Graaff W, Gottlieb K, et al. Nutrition in acute pulmonary disease. Nutr Rev 1992;50:320-328.

2. Rochester DF. Malnutrition and the respiratory muscles. Clin Chest Med 1986;7:91-99.

3. Lewis MJ, Belman MJ. Nutrition and the respiratory muscles. Clin Chest Med 1988;9:337-348.

4. Herve P, Simmoneau G, Girard P, et al. Hypercapnic acidosis induced by nutrition in mechanically ventilated patients: glucose versus fat. Crit Care Med 1985;13:537-540.

5. Aurora NS, Rochester DF. Effect of body weight and muscularity on human diaphragm muscle mass, thickness, and area. J Appl Physiol 1982;52:64-70.

6. Kelsen SG, Ference M, Kappor S. The effect of prolonged undernutrition on structure and function of the diaphragm. J Appl Physiol 1985;58:1354-1359.

7. Lewis MI, Sieck GC, Fournier M, et al. Effect of nutritional deprivation on diaphragm contractility and muscle fiber size. J Appl Physiol 1986;60:596-603.

8. Lewis MI, Sieck GC, Fournier M, et al. The effect of undernutrition on diaphragmatic contractility and muscle fiber morphometry. Am Rev Respir Dis 1985;131(Suppl):A326.

9. Aubier M, Murciano D, Lecocguic Y, et al. Effect of hypophosphatemia on diaphragmatic contractility in patients with acute respiratory failure. N Engl J Med 1985;313:420-424.

10. Askanazi G, Mullen JL. Nutrition and acute respiratory failure. In: Fishman AP, editor: Pulmonary diseases and disorders. 2nd ed. Vol. 3. New York: McGraw-Hill; 1988.

11. Molloy DW, Dhingra S, Solven F, et al. Hypomagnesemia and respiratory muscle power. Am Rev Respir Dis 1984;129:497-498.

12. Martin TR, Altman LC, Alvares OF. The effects of severe protein-calorie malnutrition on antibacterial defense mechanisms in the rat lung. Am Rev Respir Dis 1983;128:1013-1019.

13. McMurray D, Loomis S, Casazza L, et al. Development of impaired cell-mediated immunity in mild and moderate malnutrition. Am J Clin Nutr 1981;34:68-77.

14. Chandra RK. Nutrition, immunity, and infection: present knowledge and future directions. Lancet 1983;1:688-691.

15. Edelman NH, Rucker RB, Peavy HH. NIH workshop summary. Nutrition and the respiratory system: chronic obstructive pulmonary disease. Am Rev Respir Dis 1986;134:347-352.

16. Martin TR. The relationship between malnutrition and lung infections. Clin Chest Med 1987;8:359-372.

17. Zamel N. Normal lung mechanics. In: Baum GL, Wolinsky E, editors. Textbook of pulmonary diseases. 4th ed. Boston: Little, Brown; 1989.

18. Sahebjami H. Nutrition and the pulmonary parenchyma. Clin Chest Med 1986;7:111-126.

19. Rothkopf NM, Stanislaus G, Haverstick L, et al. Nutritional support in respiratory failure. Nutr Clin Pract 1989;4:166-172.

20. Merritt RJ, Kalsh M, Roux LD, et al. Significance of hypoalbuminemia in pediatric oncology patients: malnutrition or infection? JPEN 1985;9:303-306.

21. Boosalis MG, Ott L, Levine AS, et al. Relationship of visceral proteins to nutritional status in chronic and acute stress. Crit Care Med 1989;17:741-747.

22. Doweiko JP, Nompleggi DJ. The role of albumin in human physiology and pathophysiology: albumin and disease states. JPEN 1991;15(Pt 3):476-483.

23. Said SI. Abnormalities of pulmonary gas exchange in obesity. Ann Intern Med 1960;53:1121-1129.

24. Barrer F, Reidenberg NM, Winters WL. Pulmonary function in the obese patient. Am J Med Sci 1967;254:785-796.

25. Buzby GT, Mullen JL. Nutritional assessment. In: Rombeau JL, Caldwell MD, editors. Clinical nutrition. Vol 1. Enteral and tube feeding. Philadelphia: WB Saunders; 1984.

26. Bedell GN, Wilson WR, Seebohm PM. Pulmonary function in obese persons. J Clin Invest 1958;37:1049-1060.

27. Rothschild MA, Oratz M, Schreiber SS. Albumin synthesis. N Engl J Med 1972;286:748-757.

28. Seltzer MH, Bastidas JA, Cooper DM, et al. Instant nutritional assessment. JPEN 1979;3:157-159.

29. Forse RA, Shizgal HM. Serum albumin and nutritional status. JPEN 1980;4:450-454.

30. Fletcher JP, Little JM, Gust PK. A comparison of serum transferrin and serum prealbumin as nutritional parameters. JPEN 1987;11:144-147.

31. Spiekerman AM. Proteins used in nutritional assessment. Clin Lab Med 1993;13:353-369.

32. Winkler MF, Gerrior SA, Pomp A, et al. Use of retinol-binding protein and prealbumin as indicators of the response to nutrition therapy. J Am Diet Assoc 1989;89:648-687.

33. Cano N, DiConstantanxo-Dufetel J, Calaf R, et al. Prealbumin-retinol–binding protein complex in hemodialysis patients. Am J Clin Nutr 1988;47:664-667.

34. Donahoe M. Nutrition support in advanced lung disease: the pulmonary cachexia syndrome. Clin Chest Med 1997;18:547-561.

35. Harris JA, Benedict FG. Standard basal metabolism constants for physiologists and clinicians: a biometric study of basal metabolism in man. Philadelphia: JB Lippincott; 1919.

36. Ireton-Jones CS, Turner WW Jr, Liepa GU, et al. Equations for estimating energy expenditures in burned patients with special reference to ventilatory status. J Burn Care Rehabil 1992; 13:330-333.

37. Ireton-Jones CS, Jones JD. Should predictive equations or indirect calorimetry be used to design nutrition support regimens? Predictive equations should be used. Nutr Clin Pract 1998; 13:141-143.

38. Askanazi J, Elwyn DH, Silverberg BS, et al. Respiratory distress secondary to a high carbohydrate load: a case report. Surgery 1980;87:596-598.

39. Covelli HD, Black JW, Olsen MS, et al. Respiratory failure precipitated by high carbohydrate loads. Ann Intern Med 1981;95:579-581.

40. Talpers SS, Romberger DJ, Bunce SB, et al. Nutritionally associated increased carbon dioxide production: excess total calories versus high proportion of carbohydrate calories. Chest 1992;102:551-555.

41. Askanzi J, Rosenbaum SH. Respiratory changes induced by the large glucose loads of total parenteral nutrition. JAMA 1990;234:1444-1447.

42. Grant JP. Nutrition care of patients with acute and chronic respiratory failure. Nutr Clin Pract 1994;9:11-17.

43. Branson RD. The measurement of energy expenditure: instrumentation, practical considerations, and clinical applications. Respir Care 1990;35:640-659.

44. Mault JR, inventor, assignee. Respiratory calorimeter with bidirectional flow monitor. US patent 5,179,958. 1993.

45. Cobean RA, Gentilello LM, Parker A, et al. Nutritional assessment using a pulmonary artery catheter. J Trauma 1992;33: 452-456.

46. McClave SA, Snider HL. Use of indirect calorimetry in clinical nutrition. Nutr Clin Pract 1992;7:207-221.

47. de Weir JB. New methods for calculating metabolic rate with special reference to protein metabolism. J Physiol 1949;109:1-9.

48. Vermeij CG, Feenstra BW, Van Lanscot JJ, Bruining HA. Day-to-day variability of energy expenditure in critically ill surgical patients. Crit Care Med 1989;17:623-626.

49. Christman JW, McCain RW. A sensible approach to the nutritional support of mechanically ventilated critically ill patients. Intensive Care Med 1993;19:129-136.

50. Bernard MA, Jacobs DO, Rombeau JL. Nutritional and metabolic support of hospitalized patients. Philadelphia: WB Saunders; 1986.

51. Sardesai VM. Role of antioxidants in health maintenance. Nutr Clin Pract 1995;10:19-25.

52. Wennberg AK, Nelson JL, DeMichele SJ, et al. Affecting clinical outcome in acute respiratory distress syndrome with enteral nutrition. Columbus, Ohio: Ross Products Division, Abbott Laboratories, 1997.

53. Seidner DL. Clinical uses for omega-3 polyunsaturated fatty acids and structured triglycerides. Support Line 1994;16:7-11.

54. Alverdy J. Effect of nutrition on gastrointestinal barrier function. Semin Respir Infect 1994;9:248-255.

55. Lord LM, Sax H. The role of the gut in critical illness. AACN Clin Issues Crit Care Nurs 1994;5:450-458.

56. Heyland DK, Cook DJ, Guyatt GH. Enteral nutrition in the critically ill patient: a critical review of the evidence. Intensive Care Med 1993;19:435-442.

57. Saito H, Trocki O, Alexander JW, et al. The effect of route of nutrient administration on the nutritional state, catabolic hormone secretion, and gut mucosal integrity after burn injury. JPEN 1987;11:1-7.

58. Jannace PW, Lerman RH, Dennis RC, et al. Total parenteral nutrition–induced cyclic hypercapnia. Crit Care Med 1988;16:727-728.

59. Amene PC, Sladen RN, Feely TW, et al. Hypercapnia during total parenteral nutrition with hypertonic dextrose. Crit Care Med 1987;15:171-172.

60. ASPEN Board of Directors. Guidelines for the use of parenteral and enteral nutrition in adult and pediatric patients. JPEN 1993;17:1SA-52SA.

61. Varow AJ, Civetta JM. Physiologic monitoring of the surgical patient. In: Schwartz S, editor. Principles of surgery. 6th ed. New York: McGraw-Hill; 1994.

62. Whitman ED. Complications associated with the use of central venous access devices. Curr Probl Surg 1996;33:311-378.

63. Bartlett RH, Dechert RE, Mault JR, et al. Measurement of metabolism in multiple organ failure. Surgery 1982;92:771-779.

64. Bartlett RH, Mault JR, Dechert RE, et al. Continuous arteriovenous hemofiltration: improved survival in surgical acute renal failure. Surgery 1986;100:400-408.

CHAPTER 23

Cardiac Assessment

Andrew Wang

CHAPTER **OUTLINE**

OBJECTIVES

1. Compare the similarity of symptoms and interaction between the respiratory and cardiovascular systems.
2. Describe the pathophysiology of cardiac dysfunction in an anatomic format.
3. Describe the changes in right heart function caused by respiratory disease and methods of assessment.
4. Describe tests of cardiac function, their use in clinical practice, and their advantages and disadvantages.

KEY TERMS

Afterload	Ejection Fraction (EF)	Stroke Volume
Angina	Electrocardiography (ECG)	Systolic Dysfunction
Cardiac Catheterization	Ischemia	Transesophageal Echocardiography
Cardiac Output	Myocardial Perfusion Imaging	(TEE)
Contractility	Preload	Valvular Heart Disease
Cor Pulmonale	Pulmonary Hypertension	Valvular Regurgitation
Diastolic Dysfunction	Radionuclide	Valvular Stenosis
Doppler	Radionuclide Angiocardiography	Ventriculography
Echocardiography	Stress Test	

Diseases of the respiratory and cardiovascular system interact in pathophysiology, symptomatology, treatment, and prognosis. Although primary diseases of either organ system may not involve the other, a significant interaction is more common. This interaction between the respiratory and cardiovascular systems often confounds the diagnosis of the primary problem and complicates its management.

nal dyspnea may suggest that the primary cause of dyspnea is ventricular dysfunction rather than a pulmonary disorder. The initial diagnostic step used to evaluate patients with symptoms of ventricular dysfunction should be determining whether **systolic dysfunction** (impaired contractility) or **diastolic dysfunction** (impaired filling) is the major pathophysiologic mechanism because therapeutic

Evaluation of Ventricular Function

Left Ventricular Systolic Dysfunction

The primary symptom of patients with left ventricular dysfunction is dyspnea, but additional symptoms of congestive heart failure such as orthopnea or paroxysmal noctur-

*R*espiratory Recap

Ventricular Dysfunction
Systolic function (impaired contractility)
Diastolic function (impaired filling)

411

interventions for these forms of ventricular dysfunction differ significantly. Although the history and physical examination are useful for differentiation of cardiac causes from respiratory causes of dyspnea, it may be more difficult to determine whether congestive heart failure is due to systolic or diastolic dysfunction without an imaging study of left ventricular function.

The left ventricle is a thick-walled, muscular, ellipsoid structure that ejects blood into the systemic circulation. The myocardial fibers of the left ventricle are arranged in a spiral fashion around a central cavity. During ventricular contraction, the myocardial fibers shorten and thicken, and the left ventricular cavity decreases both circumferentially and longitudinally. As the myocardial fibers shorten and the myocardial walls thicken during systole, the interventricular pressure rises and blood is ejected from the ventricle into the systemic circulation. Because of its greater muscle mass, the left ventricle is able to eject blood to the body despite the high **afterload,** or resistance, of the systemic circulation. The absolute volume of blood ejected during a single ventricular contraction is called the **stroke volume** of the ventricle, and the total blood volume ejected during a minute interval is the **cardiac output.**

The common measure of all imaging techniques for the evaluation of left ventricular systolic performance is the **ejection fraction (EF),** which is the percentage of blood pumped from the ventricle during a single cardiac contraction. The normal left ventricular ejection fraction is more than 50%. Ideally, left ventricular volume is determined at end-diastole (EDV) and end-systole (ESV), and the ejection fraction is calculated as a ratio:

$$EF = \frac{EDV - ESV}{EDV}$$

that is, the stroke volume of the left ventricle divided by the end-diastolic volume. Because of the complexity involved in the measurement of left ventricular volumes, left ventricular dimensions commonly are used in equations to calculate volume, with inherent assumptions about the geometry of the chamber.

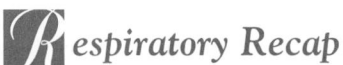 *espiratory Recap*

Ejection Fraction
The ejection fraction (EF) is the percentage of blood pumped by a single cardiac contraction. It often is used as a measure of contractility but is affected by afterload. The normal left ventricular ejection fraction is more than 50%.

Although the ejection fraction is often used as a measure of **contractility,** it must be understood that the ejection fraction is also affected by the afterload conditions (the systemic pressure against which ventricular contraction occurs), **preload** conditions (distending pressure in the left ventricle during diastole), heart rate, and certain medications. However, because the ejection fraction is an easily obtained, reproducible measure of left ventricular performance, its clinical application is universal. Furthermore, the severity of left ventricular dysfunction as measured by the ejection fraction is one of the important prognostic indicators of survival regardless of the cause of left ventricular dysfunction.[1-3]

If left ventricular systolic function is impaired, imaging studies also may help determine the cause of dysfunction. The ejection fraction provides a quantitative measure of *global* left ventricular function, but the left ventricle also can be divided into different segments (specifically, the anterior, inferior, lateral, and septal walls) for assessment of *regional* wall motion. Wall motion is qualitatively evaluated as normal, hypokinetic (decreased movement and thickening of the region during systole), akinetic (no movement or thickening), or dyskinetic (movement in the direction opposite to normal contraction). The overall pattern of wall motion abnormality suggests the cause of left ventricular systolic dysfunction. For instance, a disease such as viral myocarditis may affect all segments of the myocardium equally (a global process), whereas a myocardial infarction that occurred previously or **ischemia** in a specific coronary artery distribution results in a focal wall motion abnormality (a regional or localized process).

Specific Tests to Assess Left Ventricular Function

In general, **electrocardiography (ECG)** is an insensitive and nonspecific test used to evaluate ventricular function and cannot reliably differentiate systolic dysfunction from diastolic dysfunction. However, it is a simple and specific test to detect hypertrophy of either ventricular chamber. ECG evidence of left ventricular hypertrophy (LVH) is commonly found in patients with both systolic and diastolic dysfunction. ECG manifestations of LVH include an increase in voltage, a shift in the QRS axis, prolongation of depolarization, and repolarization abnormalities (characterized by changes in the ST segment and T waves in a direction opposite to the major QRS deflection). A number of QRS voltage criteria exist for the diagnosis of LVH (Figure 23-1). It is important to realize that the sensitivity of a single voltage criterion is approximately 50% or less, whereas specificity is much higher (85% to 95%).[4]

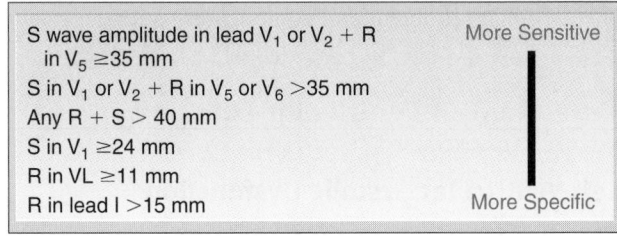

Figure 23-1   Commonly used electrocardiographic voltage criteria for the diagnosis of left ventricular hypertrophy.

Radionuclide angiocardiography is a very useful technique used to evaluate left ventricular function. It is a noninvasive method that involves intravenous injection of a radioisotope (most commonly technetium-99m because of its high spatial resolution and favorable radiation dosimetry) and the use of a γ-ray scintillation camera to detect the isotope's signal in the left ventricle. The isotope's signal can be detected by first-pass radionuclide angiocardiography or by equilibrium radionuclide angiography. The first-pass technique involves sampling of the radioactive signal for only seconds during the initial transit of the isotope through the left ventricle; the equilibrium technique involves repetitive sampling of the signal over several hundred heartbeats. Sampling of the signal occurs at several points in time in the cardiac cycle and is gated to the ECG (often called *multiple gated acquisition*, or MUGA, scanning). The equilibrium technique has a number of advantages over the first-pass technique; for example, multiple studies can be performed after a single radionuclide injection; regional wall motion can be assessed in numerous views; and the results are not invalidated by transient arrhythmia during sampling.

ℛespiratory Recap

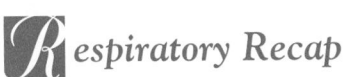

Tests to Assess Left Ventricular Function
Electrocardiography
Radionuclide angiocardiography
Echocardiography: M-mode, two-dimensional
Left ventriculography by cardiac catheterization

With radionuclide angiocardiography the left ventricular ejection fraction is calculated as follows:

$$\frac{\textbf{End-diastolic counts} - \textbf{End-systolic counts}}{\textbf{End-diastolic counts}}$$

because the radioactivity level at any point in the cardiac cycle in the chamber is proportional to volume (Figure 23-2). This method to determine the left ventricular ejection fraction correlates highly with findings obtained by contrast **ventriculography** (discussed later) over a wide range.[5,6] In addition to the ejection fraction, the equilibrium technique may be used to measure *regional* left ventricular function.[7] In this technique the left ventricular blood pool (as visualized by scintigraphy with angulated camera positions) is divided into several discrete regions that correlate with specific anatomic regions of the left ventricle.

Echocardiography uses ultrasonography to examine the heart structures and function. High-frequency ultrasound waves are transmitted through the chest, and the reflected sound wave energy is directly proportional to the difference between the density of the structure and its surroundings. By calibration of the velocity of sound waves

in the medium under examination, the time required for the ultrasound wave to be transmitted and returned to the transducer can be used to determine the distance of the structure from the transducer. Because of its portability and noninvasiveness (safety), echocardiography often is the primary test used in the assessment of ventricular function.

Echocardiography encompasses a number of ultrasound modalities, including M-mode and two-dimensional echocardiography. M-mode echocardiography is a basic one-dimensional technique in which the distance of the ultrasonic wave reflector (in this instance, a wall of the left ventricle) is recorded over time. The motion of the heart wall is seen as a line that moves toward and away from the transducer, but the information obtained is simply the depth of the structure as viewed along a single line (often described as an "ice pick" view). In two-dimensional echocardiography, the ultrasonic beam is moved in a sector or pie-shaped arc in a rapid and organized fashion controlled by a computer or microprocessor. In addition to information about the depth of the ventricular wall at various points in time, this technique provides better spatial orientation (a larger segment of the cardiac structure is visualized).

M-mode echocardiography allows the measurement of left ventricular thickness and thus is well suited to detect left ventricular hypertrophy. M-mode echocardiography can be used to measure the internal dimension of the left ventricle between the interventricular septum and the basal portion of the posterior wall (Figure 23-3). The difference between the end-diastolic and end-systolic dimensions, calculated as the fractional shortening, provides information about left ventricular systolic function. These dimensions can also be used to estimate

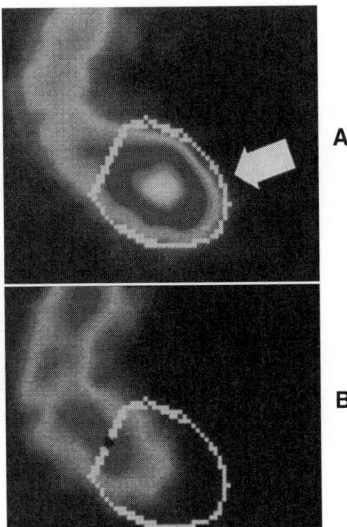

Figure 23-2 First-pass radionuclide (nuclear cardiology) study demonstrating normal left ventricular volume and function. The left ventricle is outlined *(arrow)* at corrected end diastole **(A)** and corrected end-systole **(B)**.

ventricular volume. However, because of the significant assumptions that must be made to estimate global left ventricular function and volume from a single dimension, M-mode echocardiography is less accurate than two-dimensional echocardiography to determine the ejection fraction, particularly with segmental wall motion abnormalities.[8,9]

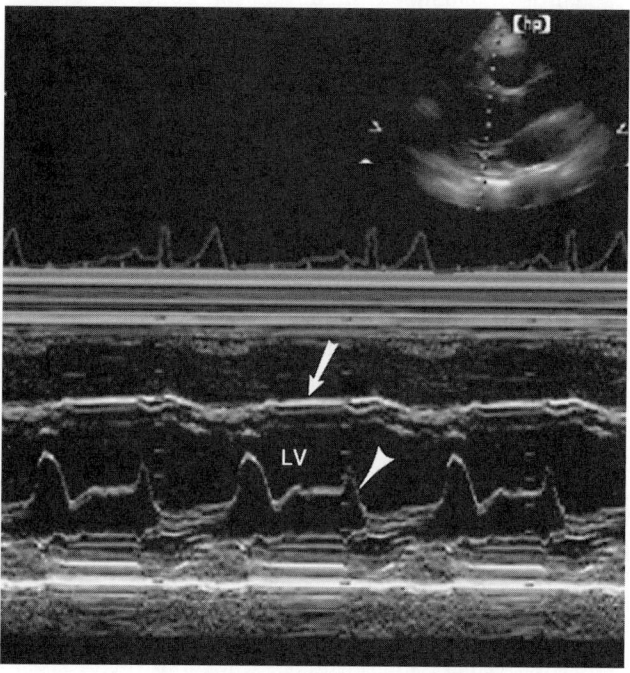

Figure 23-3 M-mode echocardiography of the left ventricle *(LV)* during three cardiac cycles. The two-dimensional echocardiographic image is depicted in the upper right corner. The white arrow points to the interventricular septum, and the arrowhead points to the anterior leaflet of the mitral valve, which opens during diastole.

Two-dimensional echocardiography allows visualization of the left ventricular internal chamber dimensions. By measurement of the area of the chamber in different views, ventricular volumes at end-diastole and end-systole can be calculated and the ejection fraction determined. Because two-dimensional echocardiography measurements allow visualization of ventricular wall motion in the planes of all three hemiaxes, fewer assumptions must be made regarding regional wall motion abnormalities compared with the M-mode technique. Thus the correlation between two-dimensional echocardiography and contrast ventriculography for both ventricular volumes and ejection fraction is better than for M-mode echocardiography.[10] In clinical practice, the ejection fraction often is estimated visually rather than calculated based on measurement of ventricular dimensions.[11,12] Although such estimates have been reported to correlate with other, more quantitative measures of ejection fraction when made by skilled observers,[12,13] this is a subjective interpretation and should be used carefully in clinical practice. In addition to the assessment of global performance of the left ventricle, two-dimensional echocardiography can evaluate regional wall motion (Figure 23-4). Because the two-dimensional echocardiographic examination of the heart uses different views of the heart, all regions of the left ventricle are visualized, and the uniformity and degree of wall motion may be assessed.

Left ventriculography performed during **cardiac catheterization** is the "gold standard" of cardiac imaging modalities, although the risks of the procedure are higher than in noninvasive methods. The left ventriculogram typically involves injection of a radiocontrast agent directly into the chamber through a catheter passed retrograde via the femoral artery and aorta into the left ventricle. The radiographic absorbency of the contrast agent

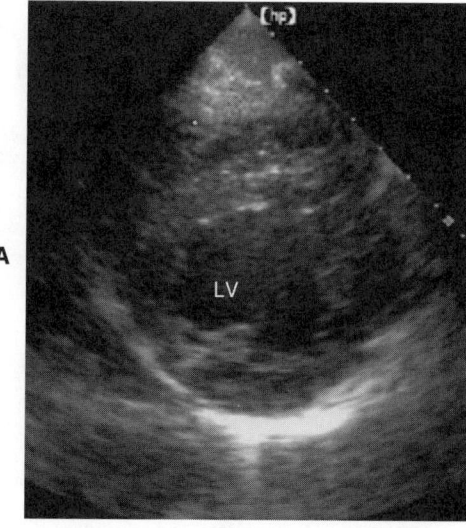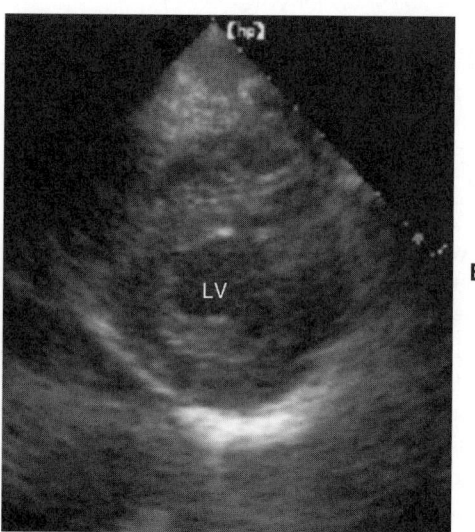

Figure 23-4 Two-dimensional echocardiography (short axis view) of the left ventricular cavity *(LV)* and surrounding myocardium during diastole **(A)** and systole **(B)**. Note that during systolic contraction, all regions of the left ventricular myocardium thicken and contract inwardly, reducing the size of the left ventricular cavity.

increases the radiographic density of the blood in the chamber so that the internal contours are visualized throughout cardiac contraction (Figure 23-5).

The determination of accurate left ventricular volumes depends on the quality of the image, the care with which the endocardial contour is traced, and the correction for magnification of the image. The end-diastolic and end-systolic endocardial contours are traced in two orthogonal views, and the left ventricular volumes are calculated by a number of methods (most commonly, the area-length method, which assumes the left ventricle to be ellipsoid) (see Figure 23-5). Similar to other methods used to assess left ventricular systolic function, regional wall motion abnormalities can be detected either qualitatively (by viewing of the segments of the left ventricle in orthogonal projections) or quantitatively (such as with the center line method, in which the contour of the left ventricle is divided into 100 different segments for which the motion, or shortening fraction, is compared to normal controls).

Cardiac catheterization techniques include other methods used to evaluate ventricular function. Cardiac output reflects forward blood flow from the heart into the peripheral vasculature and provides an overall assessment of cardiovascular function. Cardiac output, expressed in liters per minute, reflects the overall relationship of oxygen consumption and use throughout the cardiovascular system. Cardiac output can be calculated by a number of different techniques, including the Fick method, indicator dilution, and thermodilution. Although cardiac output depends on myocardial contractility, it also is affected by preload and afterload conditions of the left ventricle and therefore may not be a reliable indicator of systolic function. Systolic function can also be evaluated by hemodynamics derived from the left ventricular pressure-volume relationship (obtained from simultaneous pressure and angiographic volume measurements) or the rate of rise of left ventricular systolic pressure, but these measurements are used primarily for research studies.

Left Ventricular Diastolic Dysfunction

Symptoms of congestive heart failure (dyspnea on exertion, orthopnea, paroxysmal nocturnal dyspnea) can also occur with normal systolic function of the left ventricle. Diastolic dysfunction (impaired ventricular filling) increasingly is recognized as a cause of the symptoms of congestive heart failure[14,15] and may be present with or without systolic dysfunction. It is important to determine whether symptoms of heart failure are caused primarily by systolic or diastolic dysfunction, because the prognosis and management of the two disorders differ significantly.

Normally, blood flow into the left ventricle during diastole occurs in three phases: the first phase is a rapid, "passive" filling phase when left atrial pressure exceeds left ventricular diastolic pressure in early diastole (which accounts for the greatest volume of filling); the second phase is diastasis, or slow, passive filling; and the third phase is the late filling of atrial contraction. Diastolic function depends primarily on the pressure in the left ventricle during diastole and the properties of the left ventricular myocardium. Diastolic dysfunction refers to an abnormality

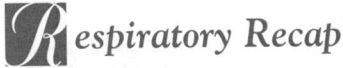

R̲espiratory Recap ————————

Tests to Evaluate Diastolic Function
Echocardiography Cardiac catheterization

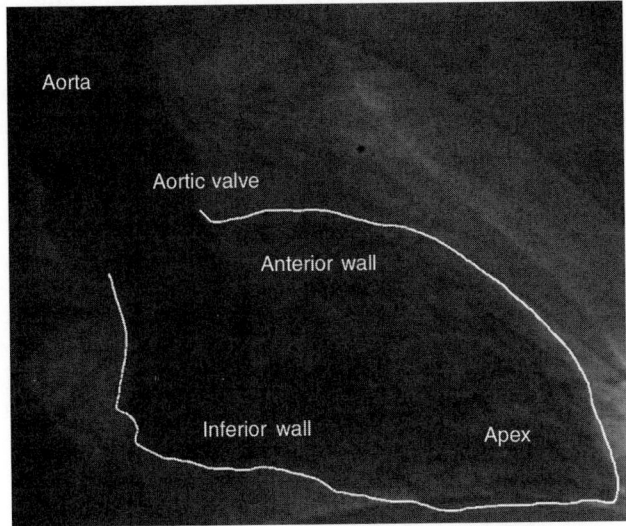
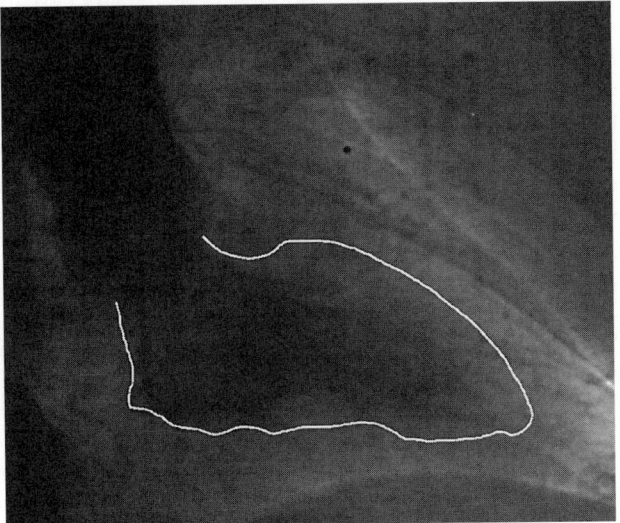

Figure 23-5 Left ventriculogram performed during cardiac catheterization. **A,** Left ventricular cavity at end-diastole. **B,** Left ventricle at end-systole, with normal contractility of all regions of the myocardium.

of filling of the left ventricle, usually caused by impaired relaxation or decreased compliance of the myocardium. In evaluations of diastolic function, it is important to understand that factors other than pathologic changes in the myocardium may affect filling of the left ventricle, including the patient's age, cardiac rhythm, heart rate, left ventricular EDV, and systolic function.

As mentioned previously, ECG is unable to differentiate systolic from diastolic dysfunction, but the changes of left ventricular hypertrophy may suggest the presence of diastolic dysfunction, because increased chamber thickness can increase chamber stiffness and reduce compliance. Radionuclide angiocardiography can determine a number of different indices of diastolic function, such as the peak filling rate and time to peak filling rate.[16] However, these measures have been evaluated primarily in research studies and are less useful in clinical practice.

Echocardiography is proving increasingly useful for the evaluation of diastolic dysfunction.[17,18] Two-dimensional echocardiography may reveal hypertrophy of the left ventricle, suggesting a cause for increased stiffness. Systolic function may be normal or hyperdynamic. Diastolic dysfunction often coexists with systolic dysfunction. **Doppler echocardiography**, which uses ultrasound waves to detect the velocity of blood flow in the heart, is more useful for the evaluation of left ventricular filling velocities.[19] Pulsed Doppler echocardiography of normal left ventricular inflow demonstrates two filling waves: early (E) filling wave and atrial contraction (A) wave. In patients with diastolic dysfunction, the ratio of E/A velocities may be altered as a result of abnormal left ventricular filling.

Again, cardiac catheterization with measurement of left ventricular hemodynamics is the gold standard used to evaluate diastolic function. Active relaxation of the left ventricle is evaluated as the rate of reduction of left ventricular pressure during early diastole. Ventricular compliance can be determined by simultaneous pressure and angiographic volume measurements. By alteration of preload conditions, the left ventricular pressure-volume loops are created and thus the end-diastolic pressure-volume relationship can be determined. However, these measurements not only require an invasive procedure, but they also can be technically challenging to obtain because simultaneous pressure and volume measurements are required.

Right Ventricular Function

Evaluation of right ventricular function is important to determine the effects and severity of pulmonary disease. For example, in patients with chronic obstructive lung disease, the pulmonary artery pressure may be elevated, resulting in hypertrophy and dilation of the right ventricle, a condition known as **cor pulmonale. Pulmonary hypertension** with chronic respiratory disease is a poor prognostic finding.[20,21] Right ventricular dysfunction, or right-sided heart failure, may be suspected in patients with lung disease by the findings of peripheral edema, elevated jugular venous pressure, hepatomegaly, and ascites.

The right ventricle is a thin-walled, crescent-shaped structure that ejects blood into the low resistance of the pulmonary vasculature. Because of its lower muscle mass, it is very compliant (able to accommodate an increase in volume without a significant increase in filling pressure).[22] However, it is very sensitive to an acute increase in afterload (pulmonary artery pressure), and right ventricular systolic dysfunction may develop. If pulmonary hypertension develops more slowly, the right ventricle may adapt by the process of hypertrophy so that the right ventricular ejection fraction remains normal at rest (but may decrease during exercise because of an increase in pulmonary artery pressure). A lack of increase in the cardiac output during exercise may result in the symptom of dyspnea. If the pulmonary artery pressure continues to increase over time, further elevation of the right ventricular systolic pressure and subsequently diastolic pressure occurs. The elevation in right ventricular diastolic (filling) pressure results in the signs of right-sided congestive heart failure, such as lower extremity edema, hepatomegaly, and ascites.

Analysis of right ventricular function is complicated by the complex, crescent-like shape of this chamber. Quantitative evaluation is difficult, and a gold standard for analysis has not been recognized. The ECG is less sensitive for the diagnosis of right ventricular hypertrophy (RVH) than for LVH because in the normal ECG, the larger muscle mass and electrical forces of the left ventricle mask right ventricular forces. In order for RVH to be evident on the electrocardiogram, the right ventricular forces must overcome the electrical forces of the left ventricle. These right ventricular forces are most apparent in the right precordial leads (V_1 and V_2). Although ECG criteria for RVH are insensitive, the commonly used ECG criteria for the diagnosis of RVH are very specific; they are: right axis deviation, 110 degrees or more; R/S ratio in lead V_1 more than 1; and R in V_1 7 mm or more.[23]

Characteristic electrocardiographic changes may occur with other pulmonary conditions, such as acute pulmonary embolism or obstructive lung disease. If an acute pulmonary embolus results in a significant increase in pulmonary arterial pressure, a number of electrocardiographic features suggestive of acute right ventricular strain may be present: (1) $S_1Q_3T_3$ (development of an S wave in lead I, and Q wave and T wave inversion in lead III)[24]; (2) rightward QRS axis shift[25]; (3) transient right bundle branch block[26]; and (4) T wave inversion in the right precordial leads (V_{1-2}). However, these changes are relatively insensitive and transient (as resolution or thrombolysis of the pulmonary embolus occurs).

Chronic obstructive lung disease also may cause characteristic electrocardiographic changes, which are thought to be due to hyperinflation of the lungs and a low position of the diaphragm. As a result, the heart becomes more vertical in the chest and rotates clockwise along its longitudinal axis. These spatial changes may be accompanied by hypertrophy or enlargement of the right atrium and ventricle. However, the classic ECG criteria of right ventricular hypertrophy were derived from patients with congenital heart disease[27] and are less accurate in patients with chronic obstructive lung disease,[28,29] probably because of the spatial changes mentioned previously. Other electrocardiographic abnormalities include right atrial abnormality, right axis deviation, low QRS voltage, T wave abnormalities in the right precordial leads (V_{1-2}), and leftward shift of the transitional zone.[29,30]

Respiratory Recap

Tests to Evaluate Right Ventricular Function	
Electrocardiogram	Echocardiography
Radionuclide angiography	Angiography

Radionuclide angiography is used to determine the ejection fraction of the right ventricle (normal value >45%). Different techniques have been used, and one method is similar to that used to measure left ventricular ejection fraction, in which the area of the right ventricle (as detected by scintigraphy) is drawn at end-diastole and end-systole.[31] Although first-pass and equilibrium techniques may be used, first-pass imaging allows for visualization of the right ventricle separate from left ventricular radioactivity.

Two-dimensional echocardiography provides valuable information about global right ventricular function even though a significant portion of the right ventricle is directly posterior to the sternum and thus may be difficult to image. Because of the complex shape of the chamber, a number of geometric assumptions and mathematic equations have been tested to measure the right ventricular volume and ejection fraction as compared with angiography. These comparative studies have demonstrated good correlation between methods.[32,33] In addition to quantitative assessment of right ventricular function and qualitative assessment of right ventricular size and wall thickness, Doppler echocardiography can be used to estimate the pulmonary artery systolic pressure (discussed below) and suggest if right ventricular dysfunction is caused by pressure overload or volume overload.

Finally, angiographic techniques used to measure left ventricular volume can be applied to the right ventricle. Despite the differences in geometric shape between the right and left ventricles, the calculation of right ventricular volume by the area-length method is accurate for right ventricular volume and comparable to that of measurements of the left ventricle.[34]

Evaluation of Valvular Function

Acquired or congenital heart disease may affect valve function. The normal valvular anatomy is shown in Figure 23-6. Hemodynamically, **valvular heart disease** can be differentiated into two types, stenotic lesions resulting from a decrease in the size of the valve orifice or impaired valve

opening, or regurgitant lesions caused by impaired valve closure. The two types may be present concurrently. Valvular heart lesions may remain stable for years or may increase in severity because of the underlying disease or degenerative changes. One caveat in the assessment and management of valvular heart disease is that the severity of the valvular lesion may not correlate with the symptoms or indicate the need for treatment, particularly if the valvular abnormality has progressed slowly and adaptive changes in cardiac function have occurred.

Respiratory Recap

Types of Valvular Heart Disease
Stenotic lesions
Regurgitant lesions

Normally, a valve opens when the pressure in the proximal chamber of the heart exceeds the pressure in the distal chamber. Although the pressure difference (gradient) is responsible for opening of the valve and blood flow across the valve, the normal valve gradient is minimal as blood flows between chambers of the heart. When diseases cause narrowing of the valve orifice, a higher pressure difference develops between the chambers of the heart that are separated by the stenotic valve. Stenotic valvular lesions result in pressure overload of the proximal or upstream heart chamber, eventually resulting in abnormal diastolic function and the symptoms and signs of heart failure.

The severity of **valvular stenosis** is determined by measurement of either the pressure gradient across the

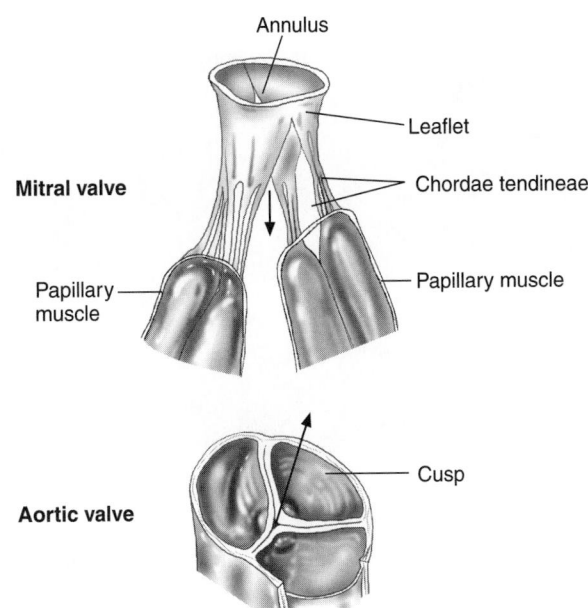

Figure 23-6 Normal cardiac valve anatomy. (Modified from Guyton AC, Hall JE. Textbook of medical physiology. 8th ed. Philadelphia: WB Saunders; 1991.)

valve or the valve area. The pressure gradient reflects not only the severity of stenosis but also depends on the rate of blood flow across the valve. If the amount of blood flow and the pressure gradient across the valve are known, the valve area can be calculated by hydraulic principles. In general, valve area measurements have been correlated with severity of disease for left-sided valvular lesions (mitral and aortic stenosis), but the clinical application of valve areas is less clear for the right-sided heart valves; therefore pressure gradients are used to express the severity of stenosis. Using mean gradients alone, "severe" stenosis may be defined as a measurement more than 50 mm Hg across the aortic or pulmonic valve, more than 10 mm Hg across the mitral valve, and more than 5 mm Hg across the tricuspid valve.

Valvular regurgitation is caused by abnormal or impaired valve closure. Normally, when pressure in the downstream chamber exceeds pressure in the upstream chamber, the leaflets of the interceding valve close and coapt to prevent regurgitation of blood flow into the proximal chamber. Acquired or congenital valvular disease may affect the valve leaflets, annulus, or subvalvular apparatus (in the case of the mitral and tricuspid valves), or all of these, resulting in abnormal valve closure. In such cases a proportion of the ventricular stroke volume flows backward rather than contributing to forward blood flow.

With aortic regurgitation, for instance, the total amount of blood ejected from the left ventricle during systole is elevated because the stroke volume is the sum of net forward flow to the systemic circulation during systole and retrograde flow of regurgitation during diastole (regurgitant volume). The amount of regurgitant volume (backward flow) determines the severity of regurgitation. The regurgitant fraction is another measure of severity and is calculated as the ratio of regurgitant volume to total forward flow. Chronic, severe regurgitation results in volume overload and dilation of the ventricle, and symptoms usually result from systolic dysfunction.

Specific Tests to Assess Valvular Function

Electrocardiography may offer clues to the presence of a valvular lesion. Pressure overload caused by a stenotic valve may result in changes of hypertrophy (for example, left ventricular hypertrophy with aortic stenosis or right ventricular hypertrophy with pulmonic stenosis), and volume overload may result in changes of chamber enlargement (for example, left atrial enlargement with chronic mitral regurgitation). However, these ECG changes are insensitive and nonspecific for the diagnosis of the particular valve lesion or its hemodynamic severity.

Radionuclide angiocardiography is less useful for the diagnosis of valvular lesions but can be used to assess the effect of valvular lesions on ventricular function. Decisions on when to repair or replace a valve, especially with regurgitant lesions, often are based on measures of ventricular volume and function,[35,36] because the preoperative left ventricular size and function are strong predictors of the ejection fraction after repair or replacement.

Echocardiography

Echocardiography is the most useful initial test to evaluate valvular function. Two-dimensional echocardiography allows visualization of valve leaflet anatomy and mobility. The appearance of thickened, calcified leaflets with poor mobility suggests valvular stenosis (Figure 23-7). In addition, with different angles of ultrasound transmission the

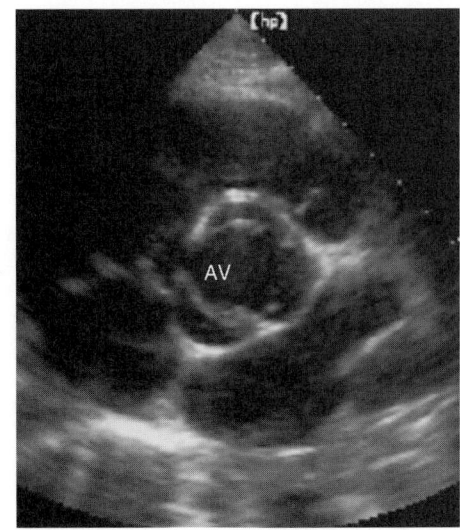
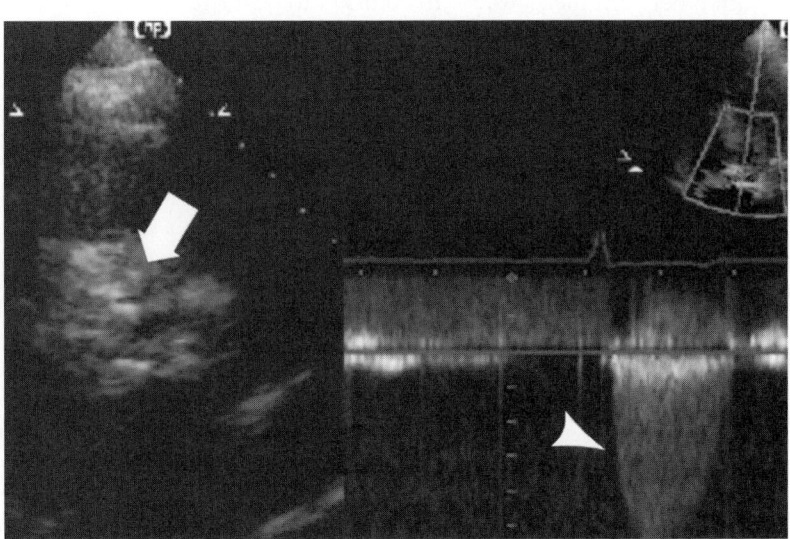

Figure 23-7 Two-dimensional echocardiography (short axis view). **A,** Normal aortic valve *(AV)* orifice. **B,** Calcified, stenotic aortic valve *(white arrow).* The continuous wave Doppler analysis across the aortic valve *(white arrowhead)* demonstrates a high-velocity jet (more than 4 m/second), which is consistent with severe aortic stenosis.

orifice of the valve can be visualized and measured by planimetry (tracing the valve orifice to determine its area). Finally, two-dimensional echocardiography is useful in evaluations of the sequelae of valve stenosis, such as left ventricular hypertrophy secondary to aortic stenosis or left atrial enlargement secondary to mitral stenosis.

ℛespiratory Recap

Tests to Assess Valvular Function	
Electrocardiography	Transesophageal
Radionuclide angiography	echocardiography
Echocardiography	Cardiac catheterization

Although no echocardiographic techniques can measure pressure gradients directly, Doppler echocardiography allows calculation of the pressure difference across a stenotic valve. Doppler ultrasound, as mentioned above, involves measurement of the velocity of intravascular blood flow. The Bernoulli equation expresses the relationship between blood flow velocity and pressure in a vessel (Equation 23-1). With a stenotic valve, Doppler echocardiography can be

ℰQUATION   23-1
Bernoulli Equation

In its modified form the difference in velocity between two points is accounted for as changes in pressure, as follows:

$$P_2 - P_1 = 4[(v_2)^2 - (v_1)^2]$$

where P_1 and v_1 are the pressure and velocity, respectively, at point 1 (proximal to the stenosis) and P_2 and v_2 are the pressure and velocity, respectively, at point 2 (at the stenosis). In most clinical situations this equation can be simplified further as follows:

$$\text{Pressure gradient} = 4(v_2)^2$$

ℰQUATION   23-2
Continuity Equation

The underlying principle of the continuity equation is that the amount of blood flow at two points is equal. Because flow in a cylinder is equal to the cross-sectional area of the cylinder and the velocity of flow at a single point, the continuity equation states the following:

$$A_1 \times v_1 = A_2 \times v_2$$

where A_1 and v_1 are the cross-sectional area and velocity of flow, respectively, at point 1 (proximal to the valve) and A_2 and v_2 are the cross-sectional area and velocity, respectively, at point 2 (at the valve orifice).

used to measure the peak or mean velocity of blood flow across the valve to calculate the peak or mean pressure gradient. This peak pressure gradient reflects the peak *instantaneous* pressure difference at any moment in time as blood flows forward through the valve (see Figure 23-7).

The area of the stenotic valve can be calculated with the continuity equation (Equation 23-2). This equation is not applicable when more than mild valvular regurgitation accompanies the stenotic lesion or when an intracardiac shunt is present, because the volume of blood flow at the two points is not constant in these situations.

Two-dimensional echocardiography is particularly useful to determine the cause of valvular regurgitation because it allows visualization of valve anatomy and function. For example, mitral regurgitation may be caused by a number of different processes, including dilation of the mitral annulus, prolapse of one or both leaflets, or subvalvular disease, such as rupture of chordae tendineae or a papillary muscle. Two-dimensional echocardiography is also useful in the assessment of secondary changes of valvular regurgitation, such as increased ventricular size and impaired systolic function, as an indication of when to intervene.

Color flow imaging, an extension of pulsed Doppler techniques, allows mapping of Doppler information simultaneously with two-dimensional echocardiography. In color flow imaging, the Doppler velocities (and therefore the direction of flow) are depicted along a color scale. The color flow image is then superimposed on the two-dimensional echo image. Color flow imaging of blood flow permits detection of valvular regurgitation, which is visualized as a color jet in a direction opposite to normal flow (Figure 23-8). Regurgitation of flow is best detected when the ultrasonic beam is parallel to the flow and the velocity

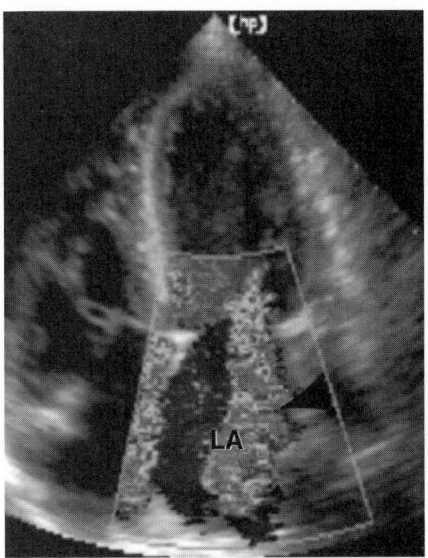

Figure 23-8   Doppler echocardiography demonstrating severe mitral regurgitation *(black arrowhead)*. The jet of mitral regurgitation is evident during systolic contraction of the left ventricle and fills a significant proportion of the left atrium *(LA)*.

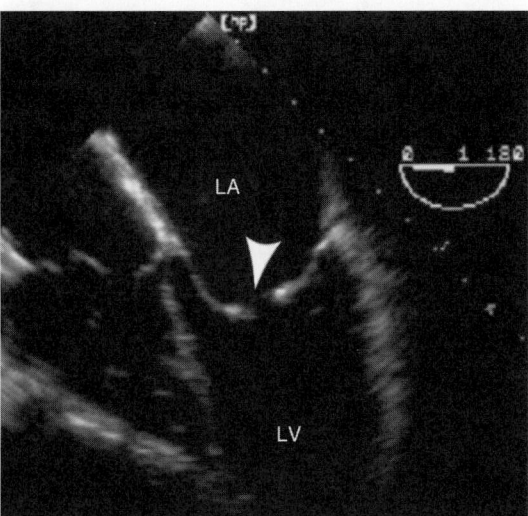

Figure 23-9 Transesophageal echocardiography demonstrating significant mitral stenosis. The left atrium *(LA)* and left ventricle *(LV)* are depicted, along with the stenotic mitral valve opening *(arrow)*.

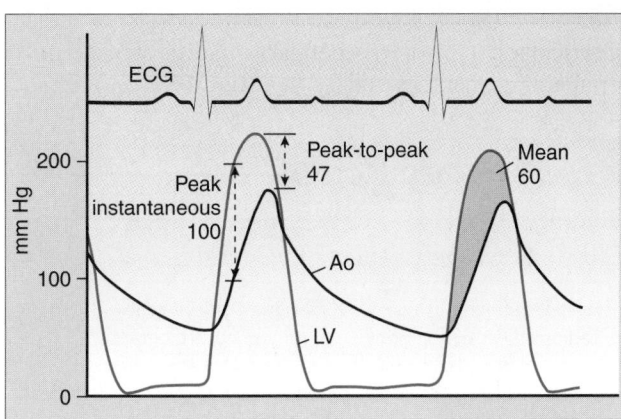

Figure 23-10 Terminology of pressure gradients measured in the evaluation of aortic stenosis. Note that the difference between the left ventricular *(LV)* and the aortic *(Ao)* pressures can be expressed in three ways: the maximum difference when pressures are measured at the same time (peak instantaneous = 100 mm Hg); the difference between the peak pressures (peak-to-peak = 47 mm Hg); and the average difference between pressures during systole (mean = 60 mm Hg).

displayed along the color scale is a function of the angle between the ultrasound waves and the direction of blood flow. The size or area of the regurgitant jet allows a semi-qualitative estimate of the severity of regurgitation but has significant limitations in the determination of quantifying regurgitation. These quantitative limitations include measurement variables (gain settings, frequency of ultrasound transmission) and physiologic variables (afterload, duration of the regurgitation, direction of the regurgitant jet). Newer color flow techniques have focused on measurement of the regurgitant orifice of the valve for more accurate quantification of the regurgitant fraction. However, simple color flow imaging remains the basic method because of the ease of obtaining this information.

Additional information can be gathered from the velocity of the jet of regurgitation as measured by Doppler echocardiography. For example, the pulmonary artery systolic pressure can be calculated from the velocity of tricuspid valve regurgitation.[37] The velocity of the tricuspid regurgitant jet reflects the driving pressure of the right ventricle as it ejects blood forward into the pulmonary artery during systole. The velocity of tricuspid regurgitation can be measured by Doppler echocardiography, and the pressure gradient between the right ventricle and right atrium can be calculated with the Bernoulli equation (pressure = 4 × peak velocity^2). The right ventricular systolic pressure is calculated by estimation of the right atrial mean pressure, which is added to the calculated pressure gradient. This provides the pulmonary artery systolic pressure because if pulmonary valve or right ventricular outflow obstruction is not a factor, the right ventricular systolic pressure is equal to the pulmonary artery systolic pressure. This measurement is particularly important in patients with pulmonary disease, in whom pulmonary hypertension may develop and progress, with implications for management and prognosis.

Transesophageal echocardiography (TEE), in which a smaller ultrasound transducer is passed posterior to the heart via the esophagus, allows closer investigation of valvular heart disease because of the proximity of the transesophageal probe to the heart and the absence of intervening anatomic barriers such as the thoracic ribs. TEE includes all aspects of transthoracic imaging, including two-dimensional, Doppler, and color Doppler techniques, and is useful in assessments of valve morphology and function. It is particularly advantageous in evaluations of both the mitral valve, because of this valve's posterior position (Figure 23-9), and prosthetic valves, which may be difficult to visualize by transthoracic echocardiography because of shadowing of the ultrasound beam.

Cardiac Catheterization

Cardiac catheterization is an invasive, accurate means to quantify valvular stenosis and regurgitation. The pressure gradient can be directly assessed with the use of fluid-filled or micromanometer catheters to measure the pressure in the distal and proximal heart chambers across the stenotic valve. The pressure gradient usually is expressed as the mean pressure difference between chambers (as measured by planimetry of the hemodynamic tracing), which closely correlates to the mean pressure difference obtained by Doppler echocardiography. With aortic or pulmonic valve stenosis, the pressure difference across the valve often is expressed as the *peak-to-peak* difference, which is the absolute difference in systolic pressure across the valve. It is important to note that this peak-to-peak gradient is not a true physiologic event because the peak pressures do not

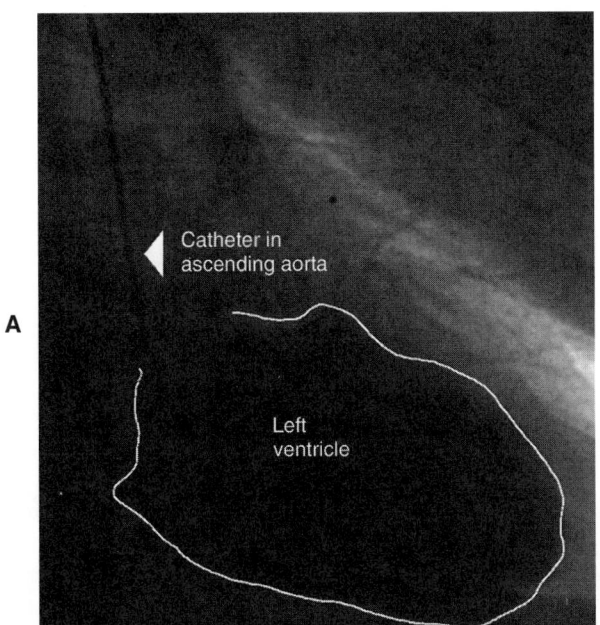
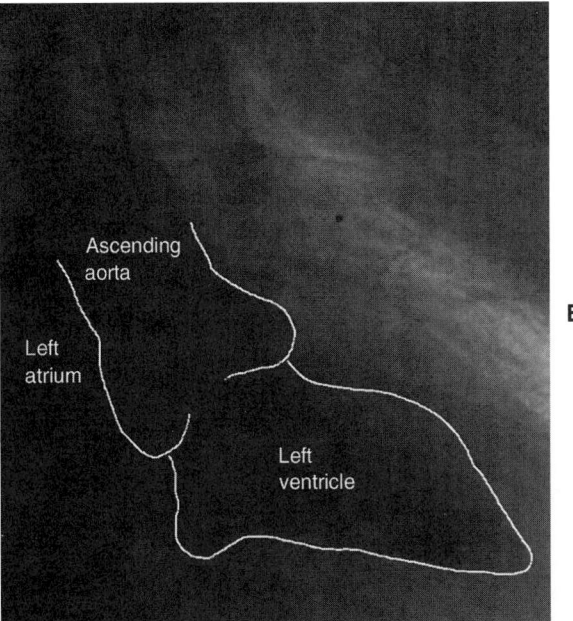

Figure 23-11   **A,** Left ventriculogram during diastole depicting normal left ventricular cavity size. **B,** Left ventriculogram during systolic contraction demonstrating normal left ventricular function with severe mitral regurgitation. Note the opacification of the left atrium during systole. The patient had a history of progressive dyspnea on exertion, and a loud heart murmur was detected on the physical examination.

occur simultaneously, unlike the peak instantaneous gradient described previously (Figure 23-10). This is an important point to consider when measurements of the aortic valve gradient are obtained by two different techniques, such as echocardiography and cardiac catheterization.

The pressure gradient across a stenotic valve is inversely related to the valve area. The best relationship between the mean pressure gradient and valve area is described by the Gorlin formula,[38] which is derived from hydraulic principles and applicable with aortic or mitral stenosis (Equation 23-3). Because the valve area is directly related to the measured cardiac output and inversely related to the *square root* of the mean pressure gradient, careful determination of the cardiac output is necessary for an accurate valve area. Furthermore, because the cardiac output as measured by the Fick or thermodilution methods reflects only the *forward* blood flow through the valve and not the additional regurgitant volume, the Gorlin formula underestimates the valve area if significant regurgitation of the valve is also present. With significant regurgitation and valvular stenosis, the angiographic cardiac output is required for accurate calculation of the valve area. The angiographic cardiac output is determined through measurement of the stroke volume of the ventricle (total volume of blood ejected from the left ventricle) during contrast ventriculography and multiplication by the heart rate.

The severity of regurgitation of a valve is determined by angiography during cardiac catheterization. A quantitative assessment can be performed by calculation of the ventricular end-diastolic and end-systolic volume. This difference in volume is the angiographic stroke volume, which, when multiplied by the heart rate, provides the to-

EQUATION 23-3

Gorlin Formula

The Gorlin formula has been simplified as follows:

$$\text{Valve area} = \frac{\text{Cardiac output}}{\sqrt{\text{Mean pressure gradient}}}$$

tal cardiac output of the ventricle. Subtraction of the *forward* cardiac output as determined by the thermodilution or Fick method yields the *regurgitant* volume of blood. The regurgitant fraction is the ratio of regurgitant volume divided by the total cardiac output.

A semiquantitative measure of regurgitation severity is more commonly used because calculation of the regurgitant fraction requires the challenge of calibrating ventricular volumes with angiography. For the semiquantitative method, radiocontrast is injected at a rate and volume sufficient to visualize the cardiac chamber (or great vessel) distal to the valve in question; the degree and rapidity of visualization of the proximal chamber determines the severity of regurgitation (Figure 23-11).[39] For instance, to detect the presence or evaluate the severity of mitral regurgitation, radiocontrast is injected into the left ventricle. The appearance of radiocontrast in the left atrium confirms the presence of mitral regurgitation, and the degree to which the left atrium is filled by contrast relative to the left ventricle allows grading of the condition's severity. Angiographic assessment of regurgitation typically is expressed on a scale of 0 to 4+, with 4+ representing severe regurgitation. One limitation of this method is the subjective nature of determining opacification by radiocontrast. Moreover, a number of variables other than the regurgitant volume of blood influence the evaluation of regurgitation by this method, including the pressure gradient driving the blood across the valve and the duration of the regurgitation.

Evaluation of the Coronary Circulation

The most common cause of abnormal coronary circulation is coronary artery disease caused by atherosclerosis. Significant coronary artery disease primarily affects the left ventricular chamber of the heart because of the relative mass of this chamber and the distribution of the coronary arteries. Therefore left ventricular diastolic dysfunction, systolic dysfunction, or mitral valve dysfunction may occur as a result of ischemia, and dyspnea is a common symptom of coronary artery disease.

Longitudinal, epidemiologic studies have revealed that patients with certain clinical characteristics, or *risk factors*, have a greater likelihood of developing coronary artery disease.[40,41] These risk factors include older age, tobacco use, hypertension, diabetes mellitus, hyperlipidemia, and a family history of premature coronary artery disease. The presence of risk factors and the clinical history of the patient's symptoms may suggest coronary artery disease, and a test for the purpose of diagnosis is then pursued.

With any test for the diagnosis of a disease, it is important first to consider Bayes' theorem. This concept states that when the prevalence of disease is known in patients similar to the patient in question (the pretest probability of disease) and the sensitivity and specificity of the test are known, the posttest probability that the disease is present can be calculated. A test is clinically useful if it changes the probability of disease to affect decision making. For example, if a 20-year-old patient with no risk factors for coronary artery disease undergoes an exercise stress test, the pretest probability of disease is so low that the test result will not significantly affect the posttest probability, even if the test has a high sensitivity and specificity. Conversely, a 70-year-old patient with multiple risk factors and a history consistent with **angina** has a relatively high pretest probability of coronary artery disease. Therefore the test result will not significantly alter the probability of a *diagnosis* of coronary artery disease, although it may offer *prognostic* information about the patient's likelihood of experiencing a cardiac event, such as a myocardial infarction.

Clinical tests used to evaluate the coronary circulation can be divided into two categories, anatomic or functional. Both types of tests provide diagnostic and prognostic information, and the rationale in the choice of one test over another is based on the information sought for treatment and the clinical scenario. Anatomic tests provide information on the presence, distribution, and severity of coronary artery disease. In some cases the anatomy of coronary artery disease provides important prognostic in-

formation. For instance, significant stenosis of the left main coronary artery or stenoses involving the proximal segments of all three coronary arteries are known to be associated with a decrease in long-term survival with medical therapy alone, indicating the need to consider revascularization either by percutaneous or surgical means.

With impaired coronary circulation, the supply of blood to the myocardial tissue may be unable to meet metabolic demands, and ischemia results. Major determinants of myocardial oxygen demand include the myocardial wall tension, contractility, and the heart rate. The physiologic basis for all functional tests is that impaired coronary blood flow, with resultant ischemia, results in a number of abnormalities of cardiac function. Furthermore, the response of the heart to ischemia is progressive (the ischemic cascade); therefore as ischemia persists, additional abnormalities of cardiac function develop.[42] The ischemic response is summarized in Figure 23-12. When blood flow via a coronary artery is diminished significantly, diastolic dysfunction of the left ventricle is the first demonstrable abnormality of cardiac function. Continued ischemia leads to systolic dysfunction, electrocardiographic changes, and finally, the symptom of angina. Prolonged lack of blood flow results in a myocardial infarction (myocardial cell death or necrosis).

Specific Tests to Assess Coronary Circulation

Electrocardiography is a simple, readily available technique that should be the first test performed in the diagnosis of coronary artery disease. However, up to one third of patients with coronary artery disease may have a normal ECG at rest; therefore this test is relatively insensitive for diagnostic purposes. Similar to the spectrum of clinical

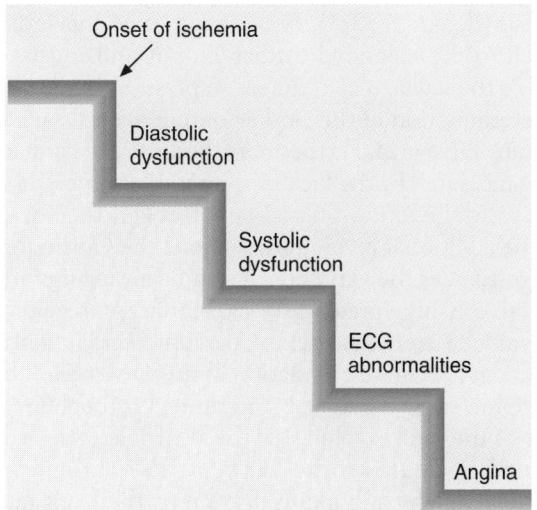

Figure 23-12 Ischemic cascade of cardiac dysfunction during coronary artery occlusion. *ECG,* Electrocardiographic. (Modified from Nesto RW, Kowalchuck GJ. The ischemic cascade: temporal sequence of hemodynamic, electrocardiographic and symptomatic expressions of ischemia. Am J Cardiol 1987;57:23C-27C.)

manifestations of coronary artery disease, a range of electrocardiographic changes may occur that may reflect ischemia, injury, or infarction, or all three.

Ischemia typically is manifested as changes in the T wave, which reflects abnormalities of repolarization of the myocardium. Displacement of the ST segment (depression or elevation) is an indicator of myocardial injury. The diagnostic feature of myocardial infarction, either acute or old, is the Q wave. The location of myocardial ischemia, injury, or infarction (that is, anterior, inferior, or lateral) often is suggested by the specific leads in which the abnormalities occur. The ability to localize the region of affected myocardium is limited for T wave changes and ST segment depression but greater for findings of ST segment elevation or Q waves. Furthermore, all the ECG changes mentioned may be apparent in conditions other than coronary artery disease, such as metabolic abnormalities, left ventricular hypertrophy, or chronic obstructive lung disease. For these reasons, such ECG abnormalities must be interpreted in the context of the individual patient's symptoms, history, and physical examination results.

Functional studies, specifically stress tests, of the coronary circulation use a stressor to induce an imbalance between the coronary blood supply and myocardial demand and a means to detect the ischemic response. The simplest and perhaps most informative stressor is exercise, because it provides additional evidence of the patient's functional status (exercise capacity). Typically, a target heart rate to be achieved during exercise is calculated based on the patient's age (85% to 90% of the predicted maximum heart rate), and attainment of the target heart rate is thought to represent an adequate stress. The rate-pressure product (peak heart rate multiplied by the peak systolic blood pressure during exercise) also provides information about the effectiveness of the exercise on increasing myocardial oxygen demand.

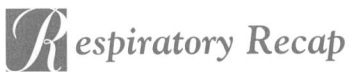

espiratory Recap

Tests to Assess Coronary Circulation
Electrocardiogram: ST segment changes
Exercise stress testing
Radionuclide angiocardiography
Echocardiography
Myocardial perfusion imaging
Coronary arteriography

Patients may be unable to exercise because of coexisting medical problems or may be unable to achieve an adequate heart rate response. In such cases a pharmacologic stressor, such as dobutamine, may be used to increase the myocardial oxygen demand. Dobutamine is a catecholamine with a β_1-adrenergic agonist effect, which increases the three main determinants of myocardial oxygen demand (heart rate, systolic blood pressure, and myocar-

dial contractility). Intravenous administration of dobutamine at increasing doses is used to increase the myocardial oxygen demand above the threshold of ischemia, similar to exercise. Both exercise and dobutamine may be used as a stressor in combination with different methods used to detect ischemia. Other pharmacologic agents include dipyridamole and adenosine, which result in vasodilation rather than a true ischemic response.

Markers of an ischemic response commonly used in clinical practice include ECG changes, systolic wall motion abnormalities, or myocardial perfusion changes. Electrocardiography is used in conjunction with exercise as a simple, readily available, and less expensive **stress test.** The most common ischemic response detected by electrocardiography is a change in the ST segment. The standard criterion for an abnormal result is horizontal or downsloping ST segment depression of 0.10 mV or more for 60 to 80 milliseconds or longer after the end of the QRS complex, either during or after exercise (Figure 23-13).[43] Other factors related to the presence and severity of coronary artery disease include the amount, time of appearance, duration, and number of leads with ST segment depressions.[43] In patients with ST segment depression at baseline, an additional 0.10 mV or more of ST depression should be present to improve the specificity of the test result. It is important to remember that ST segment depression does not localize the region of myocardial ischemia nor the coronary artery involved.

ST segment elevation is a less common finding during exercise stress testing, yet the site of ST segment elevation is relatively specific for the coronary artery involved in patients who have not had a previous Q wave myocardial infarction. ST segment elevation in ECG leads with evidence of previous Q wave infarction may reflect wall motion abnormality or a ventricular aneurysm. Exercise electrocardiography may not be diagnostic for ischemia in other clinical conditions that affect the interpretation of ST segment changes, such as left bundle branch block, ventricular paced rhythms, left ventricular hypertrophy, or treatment with digitalis. In these settings, another marker of ischemic response, such as wall motion or myocardial perfusion, should be used instead of electrocardiography alone.

In most studies the sensitivity (percentage of patients with the disease who have an abnormal test result) of exercise stress testing for the diagnosis of coronary artery disease is approximately 70%.[43] The specificity (percentage of patients without the disease who have a normal test result) of exercise stress testing is approximately 70% to 80%.[43] The sensitivity and specificity of exercise stress tests also depend on the number of vessels with significant disease. Therefore for the detection of multivessel coronary artery disease, the sensitivity is higher but the specificity is somewhat lower. The specificity of ECG abnormalities during exercise stress testing is lower in women, for reasons that are unclear. Other responses detected during exercise testing may increase the specificity of the test, including the presence of angina and hemodynamic

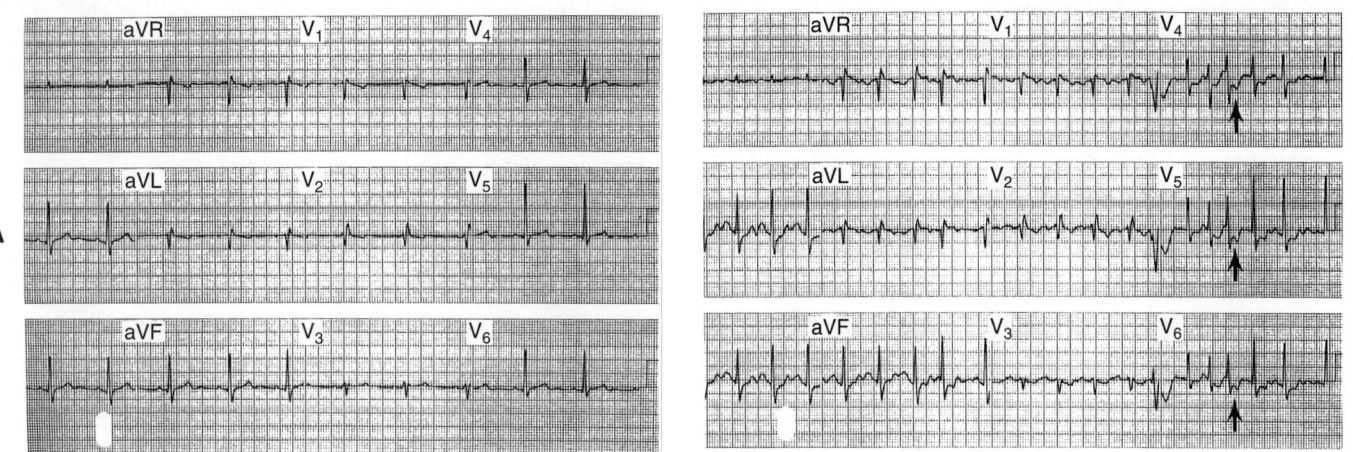

Figure 23-13   Electrocardiogram **(A)** at baseline and **(B)** during exercise treadmill test at peak heart rate, demonstrating ST segment depression in leads V_4 to V_6 *(arrows)* caused by myocardial ischemia.

changes (decrease in blood pressure). The presence of angina during exercise, the duration of exercise, and the degree of ST depression are prognostic indicators for patients with coronary artery disease.[44]

Other functional tests for the diagnosis of coronary artery disease use different markers of ischemia, such as left ventricular systolic dysfunction or perfusion abnormalities, in conjunction with ECG changes. These tests generally have the advantages of greater sensitivity with similar specificity and the ability to localize the region of ischemic myocardium. However, they are more complicated and expensive.

Radionuclide angiocardiography can be used in a manner similar to that for the determination of left ventricular function. The left ventricle is imaged both at rest and during peak exercise, and the normal response is an increase in the left ventricular ejection fraction of at least 5%. A decrease in the ejection fraction of more than 5% suggests the presence of significant coronary artery disease, and the ejection fraction during exercise provides important prognostic information. An increase in left ventricular volume during exercise may also be seen in patients with significant coronary disease. Furthermore, because regional wall motion of the left ventricle can be assessed, the region of ischemia is suggested by decreased contractility in that area.

Echocardiography, called *stress echo*, can also be used to detect wall motion abnormalities during exercise as a marker of ischemia. With a significant coronary artery lesion, the region of myocardium supplied by the artery may have normal contractile function at rest, seen as thickening and inward motion of the segment by echocardiography, but decreased function during exercise. Similarly, chronic ischemia may result in a wall motion abnormality or segmental hypocontractility at rest (known as *hibernating myocardium*) which, with exercise and more severe ischemia, becomes akinetic. The overall sensitivity and specificity, re-

spectively, for exercise echocardiography are 85% and 77%.[45] Echocardiography can be paired with either exercise or dobutamine as a stressor, because both can induce ischemia and subsequent wall motion abnormalities.

Myocardial perfusion imaging involves intravenous injection of a **radionuclide** agent, which accumulates in the myocardium in proportion to regional myocardial perfusion. Thallium-201 (a potassium analog) or technetium-99m is commonly used with similar results, although the latter compound has better imaging characteristics. The radioactive signal is detected by a γ-ray scintillation camera, and the image is acquired by planar or tomographic techniques. Tomographic imaging offers higher contrast resolution and avoids overlap of different segments of myocardium compared to the planar approach. The left ventricle can be divided into territories based on the coronary blood supply, and the relative perfusion of one territory is compared to other territories by perfusion imaging.

The comparison of perfusion images obtained at rest and exercise allows determination of whether perfusion is normal, decreased because of hypoperfusion during exercise (ischemia), or decreased because of a myocardial infarction during rest and exercise (Figure 23-14). A region of myocardium that is hypoperfused during exercise but appears normal at rest is called a *reversible perfusion defect*, and the change in perfusion over time is called *redistribution*. This abnormality is consistent with the presence of a significant lesion in the coronary artery that limits the increase in myocardial blood flow to that region normally seen during exercise. A region of myocardium that is hypoperfused both during exercise and at rest is called a *fixed perfusion defect* and is consistent with a myocardial infarction.

The sensitivity of perfusion imaging, or *scintigraphy*, is higher (approximately 85%), with comparable specificity, compared with electrocardiography alone.[45-47] The ability to predict accurately the number of diseased vessels and to identify specific ischemic regions is improved with tomo-

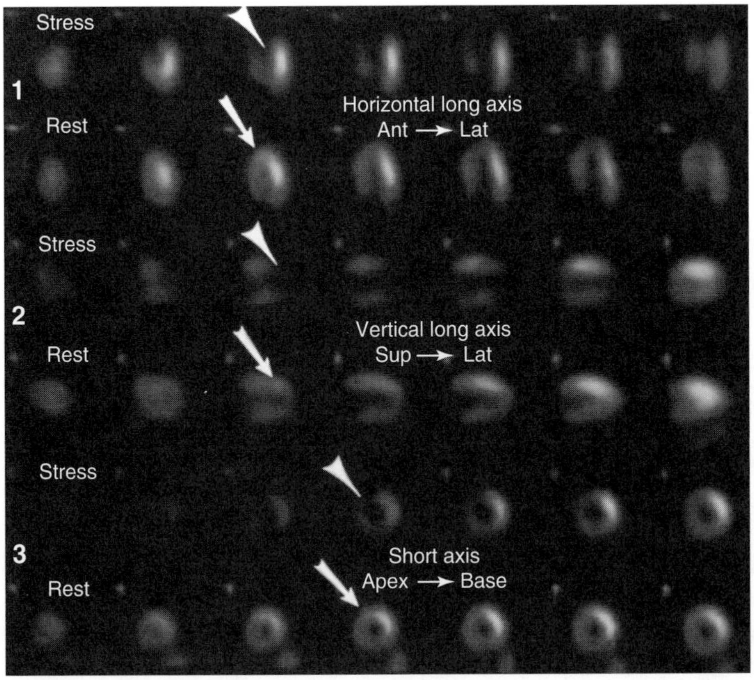

Figure 23-14 Nuclear cardiology perfusion imaging of the left ventricular myocardium during exercise and rest. The left ventricle is depicted in three different views[1-3] and during exercise and rest in each view. The perfusion images demonstrate hypoperfusion of the anterior, apical and septal regions during exercise (*white arrowheads*) which redistributes at rest (*white arrows*), consistent with myocardial ischemia in the distribution of the left anterior descending coronary artery.

graphic imaging. This ability to localize ischemia to a specific coronary artery distribution is very useful when revascularization is considered, such as percutaneous transluminal coronary angioplasty (PTCA) or coronary artery bypass grafting (CABG).

The information obtained from scintigraphy may have additional prognostic value. For instance, patients after myocardial infarction who have multiple, reversible perfusion defects, transient dilation of the left ventricle immediately after exercise, or increased pulmonary uptake of thallium-201 after exercise are at high risk of a cardiac event compared with patients who have only a single, fixed defect.[48] The most consistent predictor of a cardiac event seems to be the number of reversible perfusion defects induced either by exercise or by pharmacologic stress.[48-51]

Another useful aspect of scintigraphy is its clinical application in conjunction with vasodilator agents, such as adenosine or dipyridamole. With a significant coronary artery stenosis, the vascular bed distal to the stenosis is maximally dilated at rest to reduce vascular resistance and maintain adequate coronary blood flow to the myocardial area. When a vasodilator such as dipyridamole is administered, the vascular territory of a normal coronary artery dilates further, whereas the territory supplied by a diseased artery is nearly maximally dilated at rest. As a result, there is a relative decrease in perfusion to the region of the diseased artery compared with the normal artery, and this heterogeneous perfusion of the myocardium can be detected by scintigraphy. In actuality, this type of pharmacologic "stress" does not induce ischemia (as provoked by exercise or dobutamine), but rather is a test of coronary flow reserve. For this reason, vasodilator pharmacologic tests are not useful in tests with ischemic markers as

endpoints, such as wall motion abnormalities during exercise echocardiography.

In addition to their role in the diagnosis of coronary artery disease, functional tests provide significant prognostic information. These tests can determine the effect of coronary artery disease on the patient's functional capacity, electrocardiogram, left ventricular function, or myocardial perfusion; therefore they may be performed in patients known to have coronary artery disease. For instance, the evaluation of a patient who has experienced a recent myocardial infarction often includes a functional test (such as an exercise perfusion study) to assess for ischemia and define the patient's risk of a recurrent infarction. In such cases the functional test result is used to *risk stratify* the patient as having a high risk (presence of a partly reversible perfusion defect, or residual ischemia) or low risk (fixed perfusion defect, or infarction only) of a cardiac event in the near future. Functional tests also are commonly used for risk stratification of patients known to have coronary artery disease who are scheduled for noncardiac surgery to assess their risk of a perioperative myocardial infarction.

An abnormal functional test may suggest the presence of significant coronary artery disease and prompt further evaluation to confirm the condition and define the extent of disease. Coronary arteriography performed during cardiac catheterization is the gold standard anatomic assessment of the coronary circulation. In this procedure, radiocontrast is injected directly into the coronary arteries via a catheter passed retrograde through the aorta. As with left ventriculography, the radiographic density of blood is increased by the radiocontrast, allowing visualization of the internal contour of the epicardial coronary arteries (Figure 23-15). Angulation of the camera allows visual

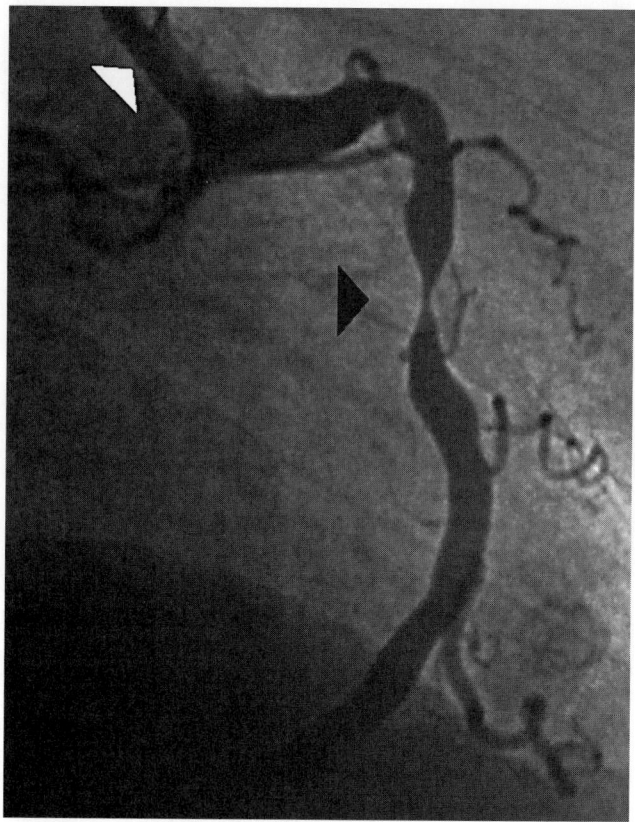

Figure 23-15 Right coronary angiogram of a patient with angina and an abnormal result on the exercise treadmill test. The white arrowhead points to the catheter in the ostium of the right coronary artery. The black arrowhead points to a 95% mid-right coronary artery stenosis.

separation of the branches and segments of the coronary arteries, and multiple views or projections are necessary to assess the presence and severity of a lesion.

In general, a 50% stenosis (a decrease in the coronary artery lumen diameter of more than 50%) is considered significant. However, despite demonstration of the anatomic presence of a coronary artery lesion by coronary arteriography, the functional significance of the lesion on coronary blood flow is less certain. A decrease in blood flow is not apparent during resting conditions until the artery is severely narrowed (90% of luminal diameter), but a less significant stenosis may limit blood flow during exercise. The effect of a stenosis on coronary blood flow depends not only on the severity of the stenosis but also on other factors, such as the extent of the lesion and its geometry, the presence of other lesions in series, the shape of the artery immediately proximal and distal to the narrowed segment, the blood flow velocity, and the presence of collateral circulation to the region of myocardium.

The degree of stenosis of a coronary artery can be quantitatively measured from the diameter of the lumen at the stenotic segment relative to a normal segment of coronary artery. More commonly, the degree of stenosis and its geometry are estimated visually in a qualitative manner. Because of the subjective nature of this assessment, interpretation may vary according to the observer and may be affected by factors such as the location of the stenotic lesion, the degree of stenosis, and the quality of the images.

KEY POINTS

- Assessment of cardiac function is an important element in the care of patients with symptoms of pulmonary disease or documented pulmonary conditions because of the overlap of symptoms between cardiac and pulmonary disease.
- Clinical tests such as electrocardiography, nuclear cardiology, echocardiography, and cardiac catheterization have an important role in the diagnosis and prognosis of cardiac conditions, and each test may be used to assess various elements of cardiac function.

- A single test can provide information about several elements of cardiac function, and the advantages and disadvantages of the specific test must be considered in the clinical context of the individual patient.
- The relative advantages and disadvantages of each test must be considered in the context of the individual patient and the clinical question to be answered.
- Tests of cardiac function may be used not only to help diagnose cardiac disease but also to evaluate the prognosis of patients with these conditions and guiding therapeutic interventions.

References

1. Anonymous. Risk stratification and survival after myocardial infarction. N Engl J Med 1983;309:331-336.
2. Gradman A, Deedwania P, Cody R, et al. Predictors of total mortality and sudden death in mild to moderate heart failure. J Am Coll Cardiol 1989;14:564.
3. Weiner DA, Ryan TJ, McCabe CH, et al. Prognostic importance of a clinical profile and exercise test in medically treated patients with coronary artery disease. J Am Coll Cardiol 1984;3:772-779.
4. Romhilt DW, Bove KE, Norris RJ, et al. A critical appraisal of the electrocardiographic criteria for the diagnosis of left ventricular hypertrophy. Circulation 1969;40:185-195.
5. Burow RD, Strauss HW, Singleton R, et al. Analysis of left ventricular function from multiple gated acquisition cardiac blood pool imaging. Circulation 1977;56:1024-1028.

6. Berman DS, Salel AF, DeNardo GL, et al. Clinical assessment of left ventricular regional contraction patterns and ejection fraction by high-resolution gated scintigraphy. J Nucl Med 1975;16:865-874.

7. Okada RD, Pohost GM, Nichols AB, et al. Left ventricular regional wall motion assessment by multigated and end-diastolic, end-systolic radionuclide left ventriculography. Am J Cardiol 1980;45:1211-1218.

8. Pombo JF, Troy BL, Russell RO Jr. Left ventricular volumes and ejection fraction by echocardiography. Circulation 1971;43:480.

9. Teichholz LE, Kreulen T, Herman MV, et al. Problems in echocardiographic volume determinations: echocardiographic-angiographic correlations in the presence or absence of asynergy. Am J Cardiol 1976;37:7.

10. Folland ED, Parisi AF, Moynihan PF, et al. Assessment of left ventricular ejection fraction and volumes by real-time, two-dimensional echocardiography: a comparison of cineangiographic and radionuclide techniques. Circulation 1979;60:760-766.

11. Amico AF, Lichtenberg GS, Reisner SA, et al. Superiority of visual versus computerized echocardiographic estimation of radionuclide left ventricular ejection fraction. Am Heart J 1989;118:1259-1265.

12. Martin RP. Real-time ultrasound quantification of ventricular function: has the eyeball been replaced or will the subjective become objective? J Am Coll Cardiol 1992;19:321-323.

13. Stamm RB, Carabello BA, Mayers DL, et al. Two-dimensional echocardiographic measurement of left ventricular ejection fraction: prospective analysis of what constitutes an adequate determination. Am Heart J 1982;104:136-144.

14. Dougherty AH, Naccarelli GV, Gray EL, et al. Congestive heart failure with normal systolic function. Am J Cardiol 1984;54:778-782.

15. Soufer R, Wohlgelernter D, Vita NA, et al. Intact left ventricular systolic function in clinical congestive heart failure. Am J Cardiol 1985;55:1032-1036.

16. Bonow RO, Bacharach SL, Green MV, et al. Impaired left ventricular diastolic filling in patients with coronary artery disease: assessment with radionuclide angiography. Circulation 1981;64:315.

17. Appleton CP, Hatle LK, Popp RL. Relation of transmitral flow velocity patterns to left ventricular diastolic function: new insights from a combined hemodynamic and Doppler echocardiographic study. J Am Coll Cardiol 1988;12:426-440.

18. Nishimura RA, Schwartz RS, Tajik AJ, et al. Noninvasive measurement of rate of left ventricular relaxation by Doppler echocardiography. Circulation 1989;79:357-370.

19. Cohen GI, Pietrolungo JF, Thomas JD, et al. A practical guide to assessment of ventricular diastolic function using Doppler echocardiography. J Am Coll Cardiol 1996;27:1753-1760.

20. Burrows B, Kettel LJ, Niden AH, et al. Patterns of cardiovascular dysfunction in chronic obstructive lung disease. N Engl J Med 1972;286:912.

21. Traver GA, Cline MG, Burrows B. Predictors of mortality in chronic obstructive pulmonary disease. Am Rev Respir Dis 1979;119:895.

22. Laks MM, Garner D, Swan HJC. Volumes and compliances measured simultaneously in the right and left ventricles of the dog. Circ Res 1967;20:565.

23. Chou TC. Electrocardiography in clinical practice. Philadelphia: WB Saunders; 1991.

24. McGinn S, White PD. Acute cor pulmonale resulting from pulmonary embolism: its clinical recognition. JAMA 1935;104:1473.

25. Kuo PT, VanderVeer JB. Electrocardiographic changes in pulmonary embolism with special reference to an early and transient shift of the electrical axis of the heart. Am Heart J 1950;40:825.

26. Durant TM, Ginsburg IW, Roesler H. Transient bundle branch block and other electrocardiographic changes in pulmonary embolism. Am Heart J 1939;17:423.

27. Goodwin JF, Abdin ZN. The cardiogram of congenital and acquired right ventricular hypertrophy. Br Heart J 1959;21:523.

28. Phillips RW. The electrocardiogram in cor pulmonale secondary to pulmonary emphysema: a study of 18 cases proven by autopsy. Am Heart J 1958;56:352.

29. Kilcoyne MM, Davis AL, Ferrer MI. A dynamic electrocardiographic concept useful in the diagnosis of cor pulmonale. Circulation 1970;42:903.

30. Wasserburger RH, Kelly JR, Rasmussen HK, et al. The electrocardiographic pentology of pulmonary emphysema. Circulation 1959;20:831.

31. Mancini GB, Peck WW, Slutsky RA. Analysis of phase-angle histograms from equilibrium radionuclide studies: correlation with semiquantitative grading of wall motion. Am J Cardiol 1985;55:535-540.

32. Ninomiya K, Duncan WJ, Cook DH, et al. Right ventricular ejection fraction and volumes after Mustard repair: correlation of two-dimensional echocardiograms and cineangiograms. Am J Cardiol 1981;48:317.

33. Kaul S, Tei C, Hopkins JM, et al. Assessment of right ventricular function using two-dimensional echocardiography. Am Heart J 1984;107:526.

34. Lange PE, Onnasch D, Farr FL, et al. Angiocardiographic right ventricular volume determination: accuracy, as determined from human casts and clinical application. Eur J Cardiol 1978,8:477-501.

35. Hochreiter C, Niles N, Devereux RB, et al. Mitral regurgitation: relationship of noninvasive descriptors of right and left ventricular performance to clinical and hemodynamic findings and to prognosis in medically and surgically treated patients. Circulation 1986;73:900-912.

36. Bonow RO, Lakatos E, Maron BJ, et al. Serial long-term assessment of the natural history of asymptomatic patients with chronic aortic regurgitation and normal left ventricular systolic function. Circulation 1991;84:1625-1635.

37. Yock PG, Popp RL. Noninvasive estimation of right ventricular systolic pressure by Doppler ultrasound in patients with tricuspid regurgitation. Circulation 1984;70:657-662.

38. Hakki AH, Iskandrian AS, Bemis CE, et al. A simplified valve formula for the calculation of stenotic cardiac valves. Circulation 1981;63:1050-1055.

39. Sellers RD, Levy MJ, Amplatz K, et al. Left retrograde cardioangiography in acquired cardiac disease. Am J Cardiol 1964;14:437-447.

40. Kannel WB, Gordon T. The Framingham Study: an epidemiologic investigation of cardiovascular disease. Vol. 12. Bethesda, Md: National Heart, Lung, and Blood Institute, National Institutes of Health; 1968.

41. The American Heart Association: Coronary risk handbook. New York: The Association; 1973.

42. Nesto RW, Kowalchuck GJ. The ischemic cascade: temporal sequence of hemodynamic, electrocardiographic, and symptomatic expressions of ischemia. Am J Cardiol 1987;57:23C-27C.

43. Gibbons RJ, Balady GJ, Beasley JW, et al. ACC/AHA guidelines for exercise testing: executive summary. A report of the American College of Cardiology/American Heart Association Task Force on Practice Guidelines (Committee on Exercise Testing). Circulation 1997;96:345-354.

44. Mark DB, Hlatky MA, Harrell FE, et al. Exercise treadmill score for predicting prognosis in coronary artery disease. Ann Intern Med 1987;106:793-800.

45. Maddahi J, Garcia EV, Berman DS, et al. Improved noninvasive assessment of coronary artery disease by quantitative analysis of regional stress myocardial distribution and washout of thallium-201. Circulation 1981;64:924.

46. Fleischmann KE, Hunink MG, Kuntz KM, et al. Exercise echocardiography or exercise SPECT imaging: a meta-analysis of diagnostic test performance. JAMA 1998;280:913-920.

47. Maddahi J, Abdulla A, Garcia EV, et al. Noninvasive identification of left main and triple vessel coronary artery disease: improved accuracy using quantitative analysis of regional myocardial stress distribution and washout of thallium-201. J Am Coll Cardiol 1986;7:53.

48. Gibson RS, Watson DD, Craddock GB, et al. Prediction of cardiac events after uncomplicated myocardial infarction: a prospective study comparing predischarge exercise thallium-201 scintigraphy and coronary angiography. Circulation 1983;68:321.

49. Brown KA, Boucher CA, Okada RD, et al. Prognostic value of exercise thallium-201 imaging in patients presenting for evaluation of chest pain. J Am Coll Cardiol 1983;1:994-1001.

50. Hendel RC, Layden JJ, Leppo JA. Prognostic value of dipyridamole-thallium scintigraphy for evaluation of ischemic heart disease. J Am Coll Cardiol 1986;7:464-471.

51. Kaul S, Finkelstein DM, Homma S, et al. Superiority of quantitative exercise thallium-201 variables in determining long-term prognosis in ambulatory patients with chest pain: a comparison with cardiac catheterization. J Am Coll Cardiol 1988;12:25-34.

CHAPTER 24

Imaging the Thorax

Michael A. Farrell
Paul W. Burrowes
Carl E. Ravin
Edward F. Patz, Jr.

CHAPTER OUTLINE

OBJECTIVES

1. Describe the normal chest radiograph.
2. Describe the indications, clinical utility, and radiographic findings on chest radiographs for thoracic abnormalities.
3. Compare imaging techniques to diagnose deep venous thrombosis.
4. List the indications for radiologic studies of the thorax, including computed tomography (CT), magnetic resonance imaging (MRI), and positron emission tomography (PET) imaging.

KEY TERMS

Air Bronchogram
Airspace Disease
Computed Tomography (CT)
Contrast Venography
Deep Sulcus Sign

Duplex Ultrasound
Extraalveolar Air
Magnetic Resonance Imaging (MRI)
Positron Emission Tomography (PET)
Pulmonary Angiography

Radiographic Opacity
Silhouette Sign
Ventilation/Perfusion (V̇/Q̇) Scan
Visceral Pleural Line

Conventional chest radiography is a powerful and essential tool for accurate evaluation of the thorax. Depending on the clinical scenario, chest films may reveal a number of unsuspected findings. The incidence of abnormalities on intensive-care-unit (ICU) chest radiographs is as high as 65%.[1] In a respiratory ICU, 45% of patients had a clinically unsuspected finding or device malposition on morning routine radiographs, and 38% of radiographs resulted in a change in management.[2] The information provided by this readily available, relatively inexpensive, low-risk procedure is almost unparalleled. When applied in appropriate situations and interpreted correctly, the chest radiograph often is diagnostically specific. In situations in which specificity is not possible, constructing a limited differential that will guide subsequent evaluation in an efficient manner is very often possible.

The Normal Chest Radiograph

A chest radiograph is produced by x-ray beams (energy) passing through the thorax and exposing a photographic plate or film. Conventionally the x-ray beam passes from posterior to anterior for the frontal view (PA projection) and from right to left for the lateral view. However, portable films in a bedrest patient often are taken with the x-ray beam entering from the anterior surface and exposing a photographic plate behind the patient's back (AP projection). Special positioning such as lateral decubitus and apical lordotic are used to better visualize the pleural space and the lung apices, respectively (Box 24-1).

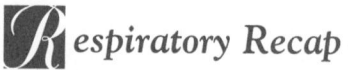*espiratory Recap*

Densities Seen on Chest Radiographs
Air: very radiolucent and appears black
Tissue: density of the mediastinum and vascular markings
Bone: density of ribs
Metal: very radiopaque (injected contrast materials are of this density)

Radiographic images for conventional studies occur because different structures within the thorax have different radiodensities (the ability to absorb x-ray energy). The amount of x-ray energy that penetrates an object depends on the density of the object. Air is the least radiodense and calcium (bone) is very radiodense. Thus air-filled structures appear black (heavily exposed photographic plate), whereas bones appear white (virtually unexposed photographic plate). Soft tissues in the thorax have varying radiodensities depending on the amounts of water, fat, and other components within them. Metal is very dense and therefore absorbs the most x-ray energy. For this reason, lead is commonly used to shield x-ray energy. Contrast occurs when two objects of different densities are side by side. Radiodense materials are sometimes injected into the body to improve contrast between anatomic structures (for example, arteriogram, bronchogram, or barium swallow).

In most thoracic diseases, the abnormalities produce radiodense processes within the lung or pleura, which often are termed *opacities*. On the other hand, emphysematous destruction of lung tissue reduces radiodensity in the lung regions of the chest radiograph. Abnormal vascular structures generally appear enlarged on the chest radiograph. However, proper anteroposterior alignment is important

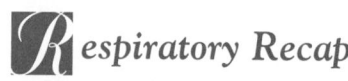*espiratory Recap*

Normal Chest Radiograph
Right hemidiaphragm higher than the left
Clear and sharp costophrenic angles
Left hilum higher than right
Air tracheogram midline under sternum
Aortic arch to left of spine
Heart toward left thorax
Gastric air bubble on left

Box 24-1

Chest Radiograph Positions

Posteroanterior (PA)
The PA position is the most commonly used position.
X-ray energy passes posterior to anterior through the chest of the patient, with the radiograph film anterior to the patient's chest.
The radiograph is taken with the patient upright, with maximal inspiration, and the scapulae are rotated away from the lung fields.

Anteroposterior (AP)
The AP position is commonly used for portable radiographs in the critical care unit.
X-ray energy passes anterior to posterior through the chest of the patient.
The heart size is magnified.
The quality of film is inferior to PA.

Lateral
X-ray energy passes laterally through the chest of the patient.
The later position allows visualization of the lung bases and lung parenchyma behind the heart.

Oblique
X-ray energy passes obliquely through the chest of the patient.
The oblique position is used to project abnormalities away from overlying structures.

Lordotic
The lordotic position provides a better view of the lung apex, lingula, and right middle lobe.

Expiratory
The expiratory position is used to demonstrate a small pneumothorax or unilateral airway obstruction.

Lateral Decubitus
The radiograph is taken with the patient in a side-lying position.
The lateral-decubitus position is used to identify the presence of free pleural fluid or confirm the presence of an air-fluid level in the lung.

in the assessment of vascular structures, which are rarely symmetric and can appear quite distorted if the x-ray beam is at an angle. In assessments of heart size, the clinician also must consider the distance of the heart from the photographic plate because the cardiac image will appear larger at a greater distance from the plate (the portable AP projection). To improve the quality of the chest radiograpy, the radiograph is taken at maximal inspiration.

Examination of the chest radiograph should include systematic inspection of the extrathoracic soft tissues, bony thorax, mediastinal contour, hilar region, pleural surfaces, vascular pattern, and lung fields. Figure 24-1 shows a normal chest radiograph with anatomic reference lines.

Airspace Diseases

The airspaces of the lung parenchyma are normally radiolucent structures. However, when they are filled with edema, pus, blood, or tumor cells, they become opacified **(airspace disease).** When gas is removed from the alveolar airspaces, as in atelectasis, a parenchymal opacity also may be created. The first step in radiographic interpretation of an airspace opacity is to confirm that it lies in the

lung parenchyma and not in the pleura, the extrapleural soft tissues, or the bones. The use of two radiologic signs, the **silhouette sign** and **air bronchogram,** may help localize a **radiographic opacity.** The mediastinum, heart, diaphragm, and vascular shadows in the lung are radiographically visible due to contrast with contiguous aerated lung. If the contiguous lung becomes opacified from any cause, the normal contrast between these structures is lost and the border between them is obliterated—the silhouette sign (Figure 24-2).[3] If vascular shadows within the lung are silhouetted, this localizes an opacity to the lung parenchyma. An air bronchogram occurs when the alveolar airspaces become filled with fluid, causing increased

ℛespiratory Recap

Presentation of Airspace Disease on Chest Radiograph
Parenchymal opacity is created.
Silhouette sign may occur.
Air bronchograms may occur.

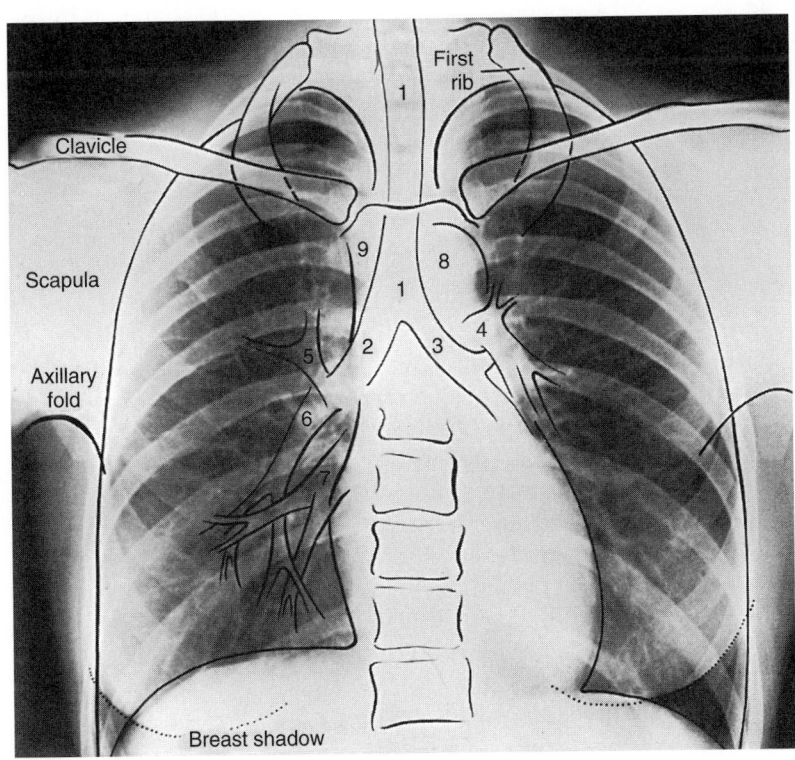

A

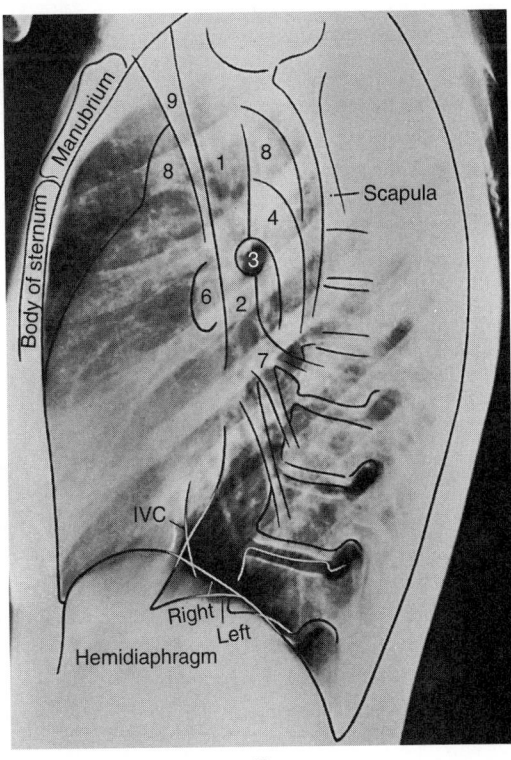

B

Figure 24-1 **A,** Posteroanterior projection of normal chest film showing the trachea *(1)*, right main bronchus *(2)*, left main bronchus *(3)*, left pulmonary artery *(4)*, right upper lobe pulmonary artery *(5)*, right interlobar artery *(6)*, right lower and middle lobe vein *(7)*, aortic knob *(8)*, and superior vena cava *(9)*. **B,** Lateral projection of normal chest film showing trachea *(1)*, right main bronchus *(2)*, left main bronchus *(3)*, left interlobar artery *(4; not visible this view [5])*, right main pulmonary artery *(6)*, confluence of pulmonary veins *(7)*, aortic arch *(8)*, and brachiocephalic vessels *(9)*. (From Fraser RS, Pare PD. Diagnosis of diseases of the chest. Philadelphia: WB Saunders; 1970.)

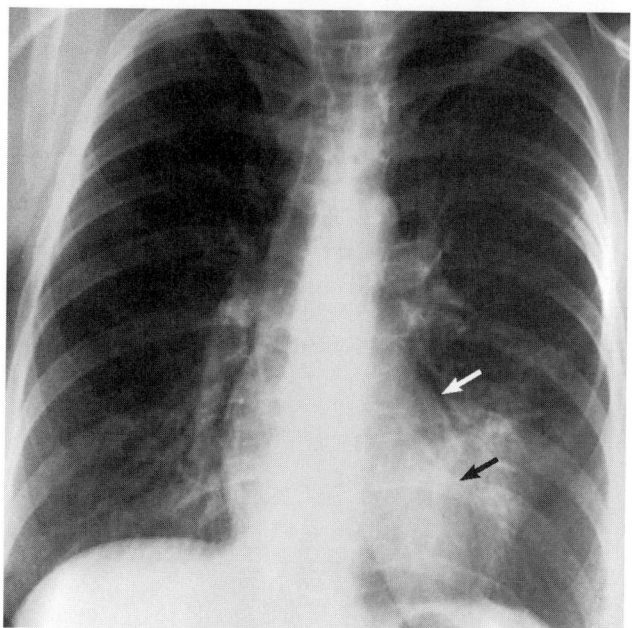

Figure 24-2 Posteroanterior chest radiograph demostrates a poorly defined opacity in the left lung that obliterates the normal sharp left heart border *(black arrow)* and localizes this consolidation to the lingular segment of the left upper lobe. Air bronchograms *(white arrow)* are visualized within the area of consolidation.

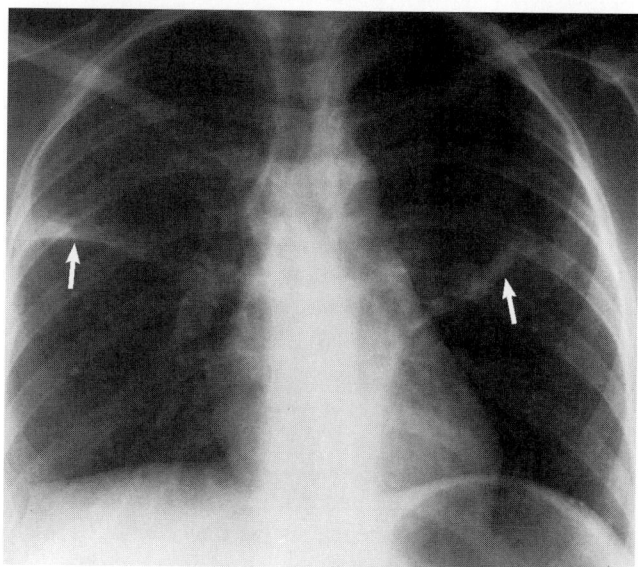

Figure 24-3 Posteroanterior chest radiograph shows bilateral linear opacities *(arrows)* representing subsegmental atelectasis.

contrast between the air-filled bronchi and adjacent fluid-filled lung parenchyma. This renders the bronchi lucent, projecting them as branching, tubular, air-filled structures. A radiographic abnormality that does not cause an air bronchogram or does not obscure vascular structures may be pleural or extrapleural in origin.

Once the opacity has been localized to the lung parenchyma, further differentiation between the various potential causes requires careful evaluation of the entire radiograph with attention given to the distribution of the disease, the evolution of the abnormality over time, and correlation with available clinical information. For example, in a postoperative patient, an abnormality localized only to the dependent portions of the lung may suggest a diagnosis of aspiration pneumonia. However, a peripheral, wedge-shaped opacity in the lower lobes would be more suggestive of a pulmonary infarct. When differentiating atelectasis from pneumonia, examination of serial radiographs often is invaluable because atelectasis may appear and disappear rapidly, whereas pneumonia generally takes days or weeks to resolve.

Atelectasis

Direct signs of atelectasis on the chest radiograph include displacement of fissures toward collapsed lung, increased radiopacity, and air bronchograms. Indirect signs of atelectasis on the chest radiograph include hemidiaphragm elevation, displacement of the mediastinum or hilum, and compensatory overinflation of the remainder of the ipsilateral lung.

Atelectasis most commonly occurs secondary to interruption of the normal communication between the alveoli and trachea. This frequently follows mucous plugging, but other causes, such as an obstructing tumor, always should be considered if atelectasis persists. If small airways obstruct, subsegmental opacities result, which often are described as discoid or platelike in appearance. They appear as thin, linear, horizontal or obliquely oriented opacities and frequently are seen in postsurgical patients at the lung bases (Figure 24-3). On the other hand, obstruction of large airways may result in lobar atelectasis, most commonly involving the left lower lobe (66%) or the right lower lobe (22%).[4] Involvement of the left lower lobe is particularly common after cardiac surgery because of paresis of the French nerve from stretching or cold cardioplegia.[5] Although a common cause of a focal parenchymal opacity, the displacement of an interlobar fissure is the only direct roentgenographic sign of atelectasis that truly confirms loss of lung volume.

Distinguishing atelectasis from pneumonia may be difficult and at times impossible, often requiring corroborative clinical information and follow-up radiographs. When atelectasis persists beyond the third or fourth postoperative day, pneumonia becomes more likely. In contrast to pneumonia, atelectasis may appear and clear very rapidly. Air bronchograms can be seen with pneumonia or atelectasis, although they are classically absent in atelectasis secondary to obstruction. Therefore absence of an air bronchogram in an area of persistent atelectasis may be helpful because therapeutic bronchoscopy may relieve the obstruction if it is caused by mucous plugging.

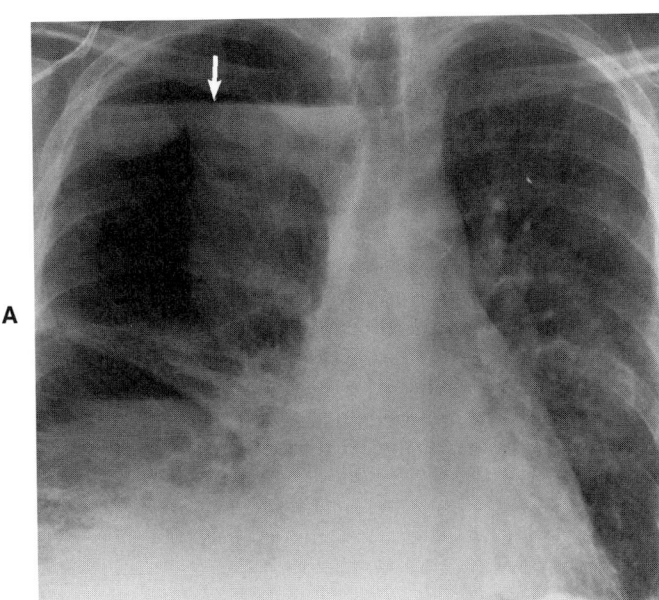 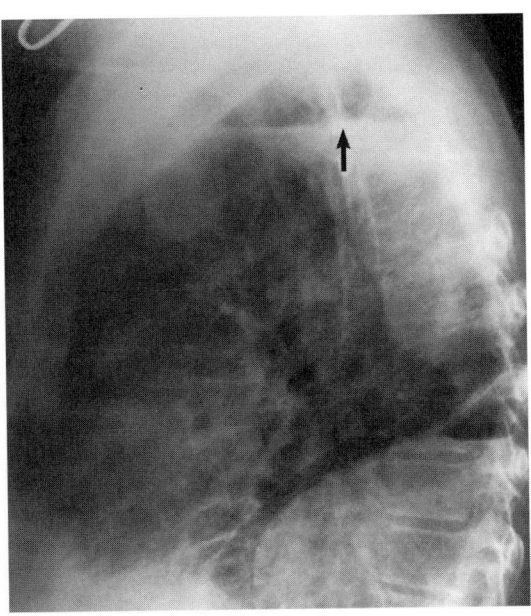

Figure 24-4 Posteroanterior **(A)** and lateral **(B)** chest radiographs show a complex right pleural collection with an air-fluid level *(arrows)* in the right apex. The fluid level is much longer in one dimension than the other, reflecting the configuration of the pleural space. The patient had the fluid, which was an empyema, drained.

Pneumonia

The distribution of aspiration pneumonia often helps arrive at the diagnosis. Supine patients have a predilection for the posterior segments of the upper lobes and the superior segments of the lower lobes—the dependent regions of the lung. Pneumonia can cause a wide variety of abnormalities on the chest radiograph, resulting in segmental or lobar homogenous opacities or scattered nonsegmental opacities. At times, an extensive and diffuse airspace process results. In pneumonia, as opposed to atelectasis, lung volume is generally preserved and findings persist for days to weeks. Air bronchograms may be present, and associated pleural effusions may occur.

Pneumonia is difficult to diagnose in the ICU because superimposed cardiopulmonary processes are frequently involved, such as chronic obstructive disease, heart failure, and acute respiratory distress syndrome (ARDS). In 29% of patients with ARDS, the diagnosis of pneumonia is missed.[6,7] A new focal parenchymal opacity in ICU patients may be secondary to atelectasis, pulmonary infarct, hemorrhage, or pneumonia. Correlation with additional clinical and laboratory information is important, along with evaluation on serial radiographs.

Aspiration pneumonia is a major cause of pneumonia in hospitalized patients, especially in the ICU. Factors predisposing to aspiration include reduced level of consciousness, esophageal disorders, presence of a tracheostomy tube, endotracheal intubation, and interference with function of the cardiac sphincter by a nasogastric tube.[8-10] Another factor to consider in aspiration is the common use of antacids and drugs to reduce gastric acid production and thus prevent stress ulcers in ICU patients. Antacids are known to increase the bacterial colonization of the stomach because they increase pH.[11,12] Occasionally, a necrotizing pneumonia, a lung abscess, or empyema may result after aspiration.[9]

On general chest radiographs, differentiating between a cavitated lung abscess and empyema with bronchopleural fistula may be difficult. Evaluation of an air-fluid level, if present, may help distinguish between the two. The length of the air-fluid level in a lung abscess is equal on frontal and lateral projections, whereas in empyema the pleural space air-fluid level usually is much longer in one projection than the other (Figure 24-4). At times, evaluation with **computed tomography (CT)** may be necessary to differentiate these two entities.[13,14]

Pulmonary Edema

Pulmonary edema, the most common diffuse process seen on chest radiographs, is classically divided into cardiogenic and noncardiogenic causes. Distinguishing the various causes of edema with a chest radiograph may be impossible because more than one mechanism is frequently involved.

Milne and colleagues have described several discriminating criteria for cardiogenic and noncardiogenic pulmonary edema.[15] In the capillary permeability (noncardiogenic) type, the edema often occurs peripherally and is not gravitationally distributed (Figure 24-5). Furthermore, the heart size often is normal, and peribronchial cuffing and septal lines usually are absent. In contrast, edema caused by increased hydrostatic pressure (cardiogenic) often is visible in connective tissue around the vessels and airways,

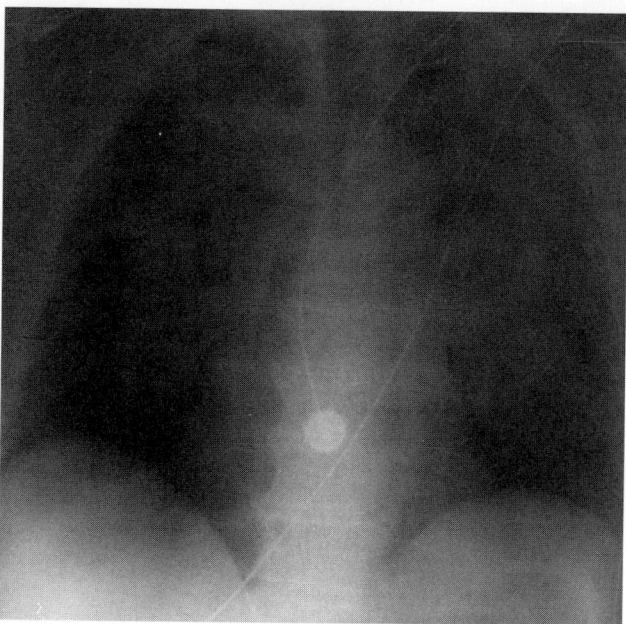

Figure 24-5   Anteroposterior chest radiograph shows bilateral heterogenous pulmonary opacities with normal cardiac size. The patient had inhaled cocaine and has findings consistent with noncardiogenic pulmonary edema.

presenting as peribronchial cuffing and blurring of vascular margins, and presenting as septal lines in the interlobar septa. The vascular distribution in an upright patient, unlike that seen in capillary permeability edema, is gravitationally affected, first involving the lower lobes. Other than in the acute setting, the heart size generally enlarges in hydrostatic edema. In renal failure or fluid overload, the heart size may be enlarged, with the distribution of pulmonary blood flow equalized between the upper and lower lobes but without the upper lobe redistribution seen in hydrostatic edema. Pleural fluid commonly appears in hydrostatic edema and fluid overload, but it is uncommon in capillary permeability edema. Despite these guidelines, in patients with severe pulmonary edema, only 87% of patients with hydrostatic edema and 60% of patients with increased permeability edema were correctly identified.[16]

Several factors complicate the diagnosis of pulmonary edema. Findings on low lung volume films may mimic pulmonary edema. Pulmonary vascular redistribution to the upper lobes, a useful sign of left ventricular failure in the upright position, becomes a normal finding in the recumbent position. In addition, if the patient has been supine, edema may not first occur in the lower lobes because of the loss of gravitational effect. In patients with emphysema or pulmonary emboli, edema often is asymmetric, occurring only where relatively normal perfusion exists.

ARDS is a specific clinical syndrome caused by diffuse lung injury from a variety of pulmonary and nonpulmonary conditions. Pleural effusions and septal lines may occur but are uncommon.[15] The pulmonary abnormality often persists for weeks or months, with 20% of survivors showing permanent radiographic abnormalities.[17] Because of the high ventilatory pressures often required in patients with ARDS, close monitoring is particularly important to detect complications of barotrauma, such as pulmonary interstitial emphysema, pneumomediastinum, and pneumothorax.[18-20]

Pulmonary Embolism

Many patients with pulmonary embolism (PE) have abnormal chest radiographs.[21] However, the findings are generally nonspecific and may be difficult to appreciate in a preexistent abnormal chest radiograph. The most common findings are platelike or discoid atelectasis, peripheral airspace consolidation, and pleural effusion. Other, less common abnormalities include enlargement of one or both pulmonary arteries secondary to large emboli, signs of right-sided heart failure, and hemidiaphragm elevation. Decreased vascularity in one lung causing a unilateral increase in radiographic lucency (Westermark's sign) suggests the presence of a large pulmonary embous.[22] A wedge-shaped peripheral infiltrate may be seen after a pulmonary embolus that occludes distal vessels in the pulmonary arterial tree (Hampton's hump). Emboli in the ambulatory patient are more frequent in the lower lobes because of increased blood flow in this region. However, this does not apply to patients in the ICU, in whom emboli more characteristically involve the posterior segments of both upper lobes and lower lobes because of supine positioning.

*R*espiratory Recap ———————

Imaging Techniques for Pulmonary Embolism
Ventilation/perfusion scan
Spiral CT
Pulmonary angiography

Traditionally, the initial investigation of PE has relied on **ventilation/perfusion ($\dot{V}/\dot{Q}$) scanning** to confirm or exclude the diagnosis. A normal $\dot{V}/\dot{Q}$ scan or the combination of a low-probability $\dot{V}/\dot{Q}$ scan and a low pretest probability reliably excludes a PE. The combination of a high-probability $\dot{V}/\dot{Q}$ and high clinical probability is associated with a 96% prevalence of PE.[23] Unfortunately, in the majority of patients, these criteria are not satisfied and results are inconclusive.

Many recent studies have demonstrated that contrast-enhanced spiral CT of the thorax is more sensitive and specific than radionuclide $\dot{V}/\dot{Q}$ scanning in the detection of PE.[24-26] It also is able to reveal nonembolic lesions presenting with symptoms similar to pulmonary embolus. Faster scanning times and the use of multiplanar reformatting have made it possible to depict noninvasively endoluminal clots in central, segmental, and subsegmental pul-

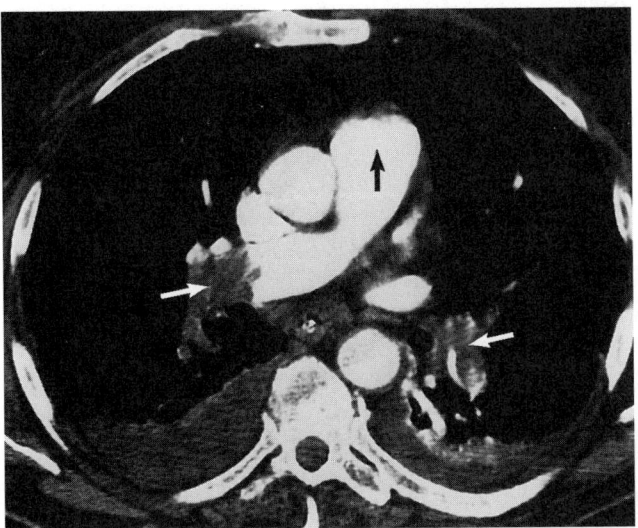

Figure 24-6 Axial spiral computed tomography (CT) image at the level of the right pulmonary artery demonstrates intravascular filling defects in the right main and left interlobar pulmonary arteries *(white arrows)* consistent with pulmonary embolism. Note the contrast in the main pulmonary artery *(black arrow).*

monary arteries. Signs of PE on CT include a central intravascular filling defect, eccentric tracking of contrast around a filling defect, or complete vascular occlusion (Figure 24-6).

The sensitivity and specificity of spiral CT in detection of PE to segmental level is approximately 90%.[24-26] The sensitivity is reduced in subsegmental vessels because of small size, adjacent consolidation, atelectasis, or pleural effusions and breathing artifact in dyspneic patients. However, isolated subsegmental emboli occur only in an estimated 10% of cases.[23] Even the diagnosis of subsegmental clot with **pulmonary angiography** is difficult, as demonstrated by the low agreement of 66% between two angiographers for subsegmental clot and 13% for three observers.[27,28] Spiral CT is particularly useful in assessment or exclusion of PE in patients with low or intermediate $\dot{V}/\dot{Q}$ scans.[24] CT scans are either positive or negative for PE in the majority of cases, whereas up to 73% of $\dot{V}/\dot{Q}$ scans are indeterminate for the diagnosis of PE. Because the majority of ICU patients have an abnormal chest radiograph, the likelihood of an indertiminate $\dot{V}/\dot{Q}$ scan is high. Therefore $\dot{V}/\dot{Q}$ scanning should be bypassed in these patients, who should be examined with CT.

The traditional gold standard for the diagnosis of PE is pulmonary angiography. In acute PE, intraluminal filling defects, peripheral occlusions, and wedge-shaped perfusion defects are visualized. Performing selective and superselective angiography improves the detection of small emboli.[29] Despite the low mortality (<1%) and low morbidity (2% to 5%) of pulmonary angiography, it is an invasive procedure. In one retrospective review of 214 patients with clinically suspected PE and indeterminate $\dot{V}/\dot{Q}$ study, only 26% of patients had a pulmonary angiogram.[30]

Pulmonary angiography should be considered in patients with an inconclusive CT or those with a negative CT and negative extremity Doppler ultrasound in whom subsegmental embolus is considered clinically important.[31] In selected patients, pulmonary angiography can be complemented by interventional procedures such as direct thombolysis or mechanical fragmentation of clot.

Radiographic resolution of PE varies and depends on the presence and size of lung necrosis. With complete infarction, the parenchymal opacity may resolve in weeks to months, with residual linear scarring or focal pleural thickening.[32] Without infarction, resolution usually occurs within several weeks, often without residual abnormality. With PE, resolution occurs from the periphery, unlike pneumonia. This has been likened to the melting of an ice cube. Occasionally, cavitation from either ischemic necrosis or infection occurs during the course of resolution.

Imaging the Lower Extremities for Deep Vein Thrombosis

As many as 50% of patients with leg symptoms are proven to have a diagnosis other than deep vein thrombosis (DVT), and the physical examination in patients with DVT is misleading in 50% of cases.[33] Therefore it is a difficult diagnosis to make clinically, and the physician must rely on imaging modalities. The common radiographic studies used in the diagnosis of DVT include **contrast venography, duplex ultrasound, magetic resonance imaging (MRI),** and iodine-125 fibrinogen uptake.

Respiratory Recap

Imaging Techniques for Deep Vein Thrombosis

Contrast venography
Duplex ultrasound
Magnetic resonance imaging
Iodine-125 fibrinogen uptake

Contrast Venography

Contrast venography is considered the gold standard for the diagnosis of DVT. It involves cannulation of a dorsal foot vein and injection of intravenous (IV) contrast to render the veins radiopaque. Therefore it is limited in patients with renal failure or allergies to iodinated contrast media. Contrast venography involves transport of the patient to the radiology department and therefore may be unsuitable in an intubated, unstable patient. It is very accurate in the diagnosis of calf, popliteal, and femoral vein thrombosis, but sensitivity is reduced in evaluation of the iliac and pelvic veins.

Duplex Ultrasound

Duplex ultrasound refers to the combination of real time B-mode and Doppler ultrasound. It is suitable for the ICU patient because the examination can be performed with a portable unit in the ICU. On real-time ultrasound, the normal vein is thin walled and compressible with an anechoic lumen. The *Doppler effect* refers to the fact that moving red blood cells reflect ultrasound impulses, and the pitch of the reflected signals depends on the velocity and direction of the blood flow. Using a spectrum analyzer, a Doppler waveform is produced, which is a graphic representation of venous blood flow.

The normal Doppler waveform is biphasic, increasing with expiration and decreasing with inspiration. Forward flow is increased by application of slight pressure to the distal veins, referred to as *augmentation*. Typically the veins are examined at 1- to 2-cm intervals from the inguinal ligament to the popliteal vein bifurcation. With the compression technique, the vein is compressed in a transverse plane with the transducer. In a vein containing thrombus, compressing and apposing the walls of the vein is not possible. If the vein is completely occluded, no Doppler signal occurs. Failure of augmentation implies obstruction of flow by thrombus above the site of examination. Color Doppler fills the lumen with color depending on the direction of flow in relation to the transducer and therefore can confirm the patency of a vein. It also aids in the localization of small vessels, particularly those in the calf, and is useful in the examination of the iliac vessels, which cannot be compressed easily.

Ultrasound has a sensitivity of more than 90% and a specificity of nearly 100% in the diagnosis of femoral and popliteal vein thrombosis.[34,35] It is less sensitive in the detection of iliac and calf vein thrombosis. However, the risk of embolization from isolated calf thrombus is very low and the major source of emboli is proximal DVT.[36-38] Up to 20% of calf vein thrombus propagates into the popliteal and femoral veins, which occurs before embolization.[38,39] Therefore in those patients in whom a high index of suspicion exists regarding DVT and whose initial ultrasound is normal, serial examination should be performed to look for propagation.[40]

Magnetic Resonance Imaging

MRI is extremely accurate in the diagnosis of DVT, particularly for those vessels above the knee, including the pelvic and iliac veins and vena cava. With gradient refocused image sequences, the veins are visualized as high-signal structures, eliminating the need for IV contrast material. In contrast to venography, MRI permits the evaluation of the upper extent of the thrombus and thus the potential risk of embolization. In comparison with contrast venography, MRI has a sensitivity of 95% and specificity of 100% in the detection of DVT in the thigh and an overall sensivity greater than 97% in the detection of thrombus above the knee. Some studies have suggested that it is more accurate than venography in evaluation of

the iliac veins.[41-43] Below the knee, the sensitivity is 87% with a specificity of 97%.[44]

MRI is limited by the difficulty in patient monitoring. It also requires the patient to be transported to the radiology department, and it is contraindicated in patients with a cardiac pacemaker. Its high cost cannot justify its use in the routine evaluation of femoral-popliteal venous thrombi. However, it should be considered in those patients in whom ultrasound is technically difficult because of leg swelling, obesity, and diagnostic uncertainty due to the presence of numerous collaterals and in patients in whom isolated pelvic thrombus is suspected.

Iodine-125 Fibrinogen Uptake

Fibrinogen is the precursor of fibrin. Radiolabeled fibrinogen is injected into a peripheral vein. In sites of active clot formation, it is transformed and deposited as radioactive fibrin. The extremities are scanned under a gamma camera at 24 and 72 hours for evidence of local accumulation. Sites of increased radioactivity correspond with areas of active fibrin clot formation. It is insensitive in the detection of iliofemoral venous thrombosis. This technique also has a

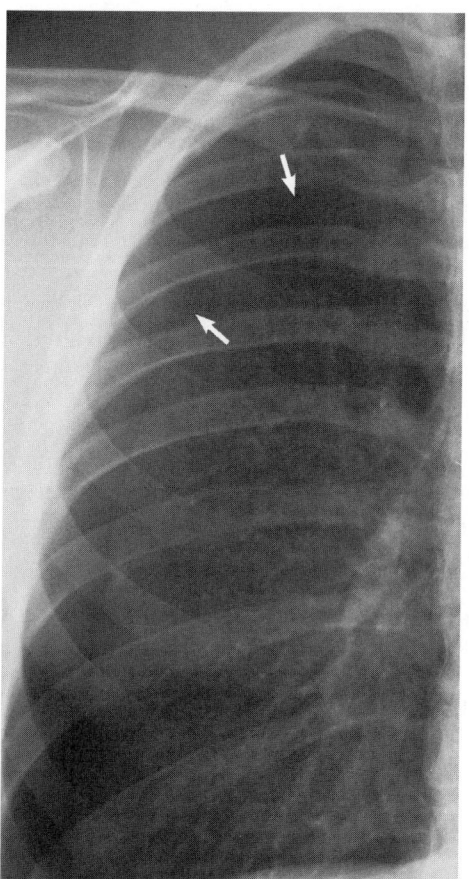

Figure 24-7   Posteroanterior chest radiograph shows the viseral pleural line *(arrows)* with lateral lucency consistent with a pneumothorax.

high false-positive rate caused by wounds and hematomas and a false-negative rate of 30%.[45-47] Since the introduction of ultrasound and MRI, it has had very limited clinical use.

Extraalveolar Air

Recognition of **extraalveolar air** is critical in thoracic imaging. Extraalveolar air includes pneumothorax, pneumomediastinum, and interstitial emphysema. Each is characterized by a distinctive radiographic appearance. Between 5% and 15% of patients receiving positive end–expiratory ventilation (PEEP) develop complications involving extraalveolar air.[48,49] Mechanical ventilation perpetuates an air leak and, if unrecognized and untreated, most patients develop a tension pneumothorax.[48]

Pneumothorax

The radiographic diagnosis of pneumothorax is established by identification of the **visceral pleural line** (Figure 24-7). This thin, white line represents the visceral pleura visualized between air in the pleural space laterally and air

in the aerated lung medially. Although other radiographic features are occasionally suggestive of pneumothorax, including the absence of vascular markings and increased lucency in the hemithorax, they often are misleading. Thus the specific diagnosis of pneumothorax generally requires identification of the visceral pleural line.

Visualization of the visceral pleura can be enhanced by exposure of the film in expiration. With expiration, the volume of the pneumothorax remains constant, whereas the volume of the hemithorax in which it is contained is reduced. Therefore the pneumothorax occupies proportionately more of the hemithorax, facilitating visualization. Perhaps of more importance is that the orientation of the visceral pleural line relative to the overlying ribs often is changed by exposure in expiration, again facilitating visualization. A skin fold may mimic the visceral pleural line, but whereas the visceral pleural line is a thin line with air on both sides, a skin fold is represented as an interface in which one edge is sharp but the medial edge gradually fades away (Figure 24-8).[50]

In patients radiographed in the upright position, free air in the pleural space generally collects over the apex of the lung. Most clinicians have been trained to look for air in this location when they suspect pneumothorax. In patients in the supine position, the highest portion of the thorax is generally the anterior costophrenic sulcus. Free air within the pleural space rises to this position, projecting over the upper abdomen and diaphragm. This results in a distinctive radiographic appearance that has been referred to as the **deep sulcus sign** of pneumothorax in the supine position (Figure 24-9).[51] If the pneumothorax is on

Figure 24-8   Posteroanterior chest radiograph shows an interface *(arrows)* rather than a true viseral line. Gradual fading exists from a sharp lateral margin medially. This represents a skin fold, although the appearance may mimic a pneumothorax.

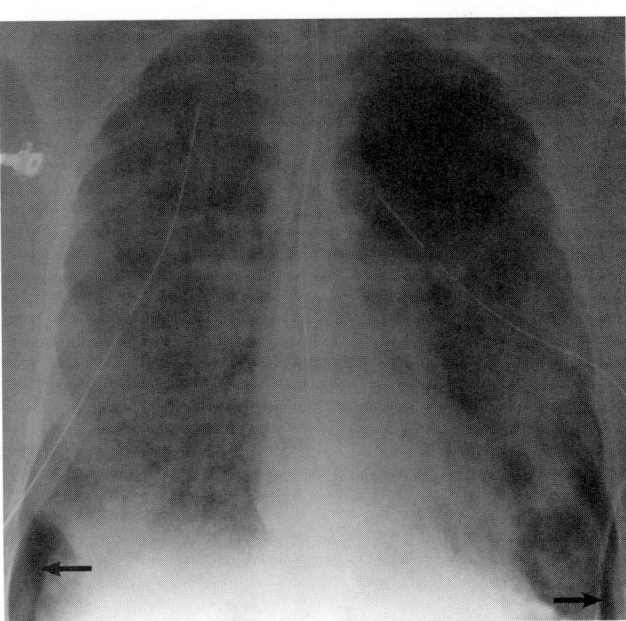

Figure 24-9   An anteroposterior supine radiograph shows air in the pleural space inferiorly in the anterior costophrenic sulcus, creating a deep sulcus bilatrally *(arrows)* consistent with bilateral pneumothoraces. Note the multiple cystic lucencies in the right lung, representing interstitial emphysema.

the left side, the apex of the heart and the pericardial fat pad often will be sharply outlined. In addition, the edge of the lung and the visceral pleural line also may be identified. However, in the supine projection, recognition of the deep sulcus and increased lucency over the upper abdomen is critical because direct visualization of the visceral pleura in this projection often is difficult.

In patients in the supine position, free fluid in the pleural space tends to layer posteriorly. Significant amounts of fluid create a generalized increased opacity over the affected hemithorax. When associated free air (hydropneumothorax) occurs in a supine projection, the ability to visualize the pneumothorax depends on the relative amounts of air and fluid.[52] If sufficient air is present within the pleural space to outline the pleura laterally, a sharp pleural line can be visualized. If the quantity of air is relatively small and the quantity of fluid relatively large, the lateral portion of the lung may not be visualized and no pleural line will be identified. The presence of an associated pneumothorax in this setting would be evident only on an upright or a decubitus film. Although it often is difficult to take radiographs of critically ill patients in the upright position, decubitus films can be obtained in these patients. Appropriate decubitus projection allows confirmation of the presence of either free air or free fluid in the pleural space if their presence is suspected from conventional views.

Interstitial Emphysema

The pathophysiology of extraalveolar air generally begins with the rupture of distal alveoli into the interstitial space

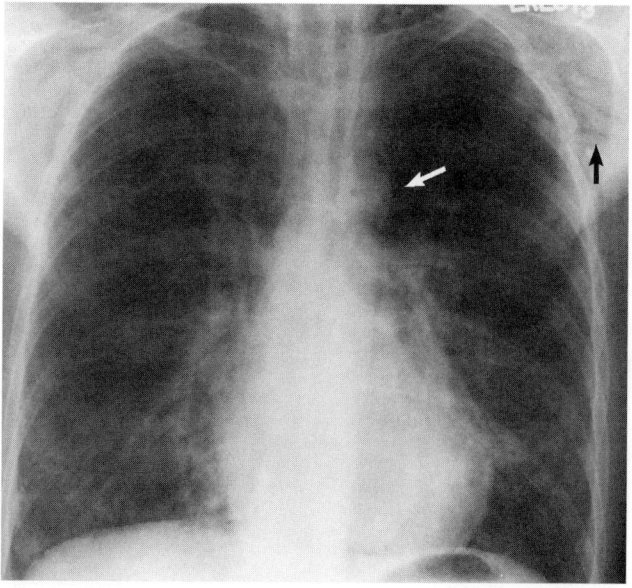

Figure 24-10 Posteroanterior chest radiograph shows lateral displacement of the mediastinal parietal pleura *(white arrow)* with a lucent region medially characteristic of pneumomediastinum. Note lucencies in the soft tissues, reflecting air dissecting through fascial and muscle planes *(black arrow)*.

and the subsequent dissection of air back toward the mediastinum or occasionally directly into the pleural space.

Radiographic recognition of this early stage of extraalveolar air, pulmonary interstitial emphysema, is possible.[53] In general, air dissects along bronchovascular bundles, producing a characteristic appearance of a pulmonary vessel surrounded by air. The radiographic recognition of this frequently portends impending pneumothorax, pneumomediastinum, or both. The radiographic appearance may suggest improvement because of increased lucency in the lungs, but the characteristic configuration of air surrounding an intrapulmonary vessel should indicate the correct diagnosis.

Pneumomediastinum

Air dissecting into the mediastinum creates a characteristic radiographic appearance. The air dissects through the mediastinal tissues, creating vertical linear streaks (Figure 24-10). Air can dissect superiorly into the neck, the muscles overlying the thorax, or both, and inferiorly into the abdomen, both intraperitoneally and extraperitoneally. Air dissecting through the mediastinum may outline the pulmonary artery in characteristic fashion on both frontal projections and lateral projections.

Evaluation of Support and Monitoring Equipment

Complications of tube or catheter placement are a significant cause of morbidity in hospitalized patients, and chest radiography should be routinely performed after the insertion of endotracheal tubes, chest drainage tubes, nasogastric tubes, and central venous catheters.

Endotracheal and Tracheostomy Tubes

Studies show as high as a 10% incidence of inappropriate positioning of endotracheal tubes. If the diameter of the cuff is more than 1.5 times the tracheal diameter, severe ulceration or tracheostenosis may result.

Endotracheal tubes have a radiopaque marker for radiographic assessment. Optimal positioning requires the top of the endotracheal tube to be approximately 4 to 6 cm above the carina with the neck in the neutral position. This limits accidental extubation with neck extension and inadvertent intubation of the right mainstem bronchus with neck flexion (Figure 24-11).[54] The tube diameter should be one half to two thirds that of the trachea lumen, and the inflated cuff should not cause bulging of the tracheal wall.

Esophageal intubation occasionally occurs. Clues on the chest radiograph include projection of the endotracheal tube beyond the carina and distention of the esophagus and stomach.

A tracheostomy tube should be midline, and the cuff should not cause the tracheal wall to bulge. Optimal positioning of the tip is one half to two thirds of the distance between the stoma and the carina. A malpositioned tube may produce ulceration, hemorrhage, and scarring. Prolonged hyperinflation of the cuff may lead to tracheomalacia, as with endotracheal cuff hyperinflation.

Chest Tubes

Chest radiographs should routinely be obtained after tube placement to detect malpositioning and potential complications such as pneumothorax and hemothorax. They often are inserted for the removal of intrapleural air or fluid. Chest tubes have a radiopaque line that is interrupted by a side hole proximal to the tip, which always should be seen medial to the inner margin of the ribs. Inadvertent insertion of the tube into the soft tissues may be suspected by silhouetting of the nonopaque wall of the tube by the adjacent soft tissue density. Normally, the nonopaque wall is rendered visible by surrounding lucent lung.[55] Optimal positioning of the tube depends on whether the air or fluid collection is free or loculated within the pleural space. CT can be very helpful in the direction of tube placement if pleural fluid is loculated. Intraparenchymal placement may be complicated by bronchopleural fistula, pulmonary laceration, and hematoma. Placement into a fissure is associated with a 29% rate of unsatisfactory drainage.[56]

Central Venous Catheters

Common malpositions of a central venous catheter include insertion into the internal mammary and azygous veins and insertion into the internal jugular vein in the case of subclavian line placement.

Central venous catheters usually are inserted through the subclavian or internal jugular vein. To monitor central venous pressure, the tip of the catheter must be intrathoracic and central to all venous valves (Figure 24-12). The location of the most proximal venous valve is approximately the medial margin of the first rib.[57] The optimal position for the distal tip of central lines is the junction of the brachiocephalic vein and superior vena cava or just proximal to the right atrium in the superior vena cava. Both the placement of catheter tips adjacent to the tricuspid valve and hypertonic instillation into the right atrium may produce arrhythmias.[8]

Swan-Ganz Catheter

Pulmonary artery catheters are used to monitor pulmonary artery wedge pressures. The optimal tip position is the right or left pulmonary artery, approximately 5 cm distal to the bifurcation of the main pulmonary artery. Placement of the tip into the right ventricle predisposes to arrhythmias and myocardial perforation. Placement too distal in the pulmonary artery may result in pulmonary infarction, hemorrhage, or rupture of the pulmonary artery.[58,59] The inflated cuff never should be seen on a radiographic study.

Intraaortic Balloon Pump

Intraaortic balloon pumps are increasingly used to maximize coronary artery perfusion and decrease cardiac after-

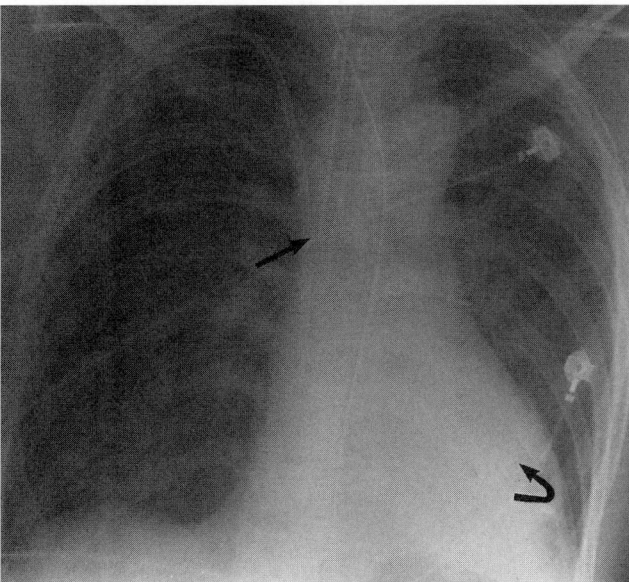

Figure 24-11   Anteroposterior radiograph shows the endotracheal tube postitioned in the right mainstem bronchus. The retrocardiac density and obscuration of the left hemidiaphragm *(curved arrows)* is caused by secondary left lower lobe collapse.

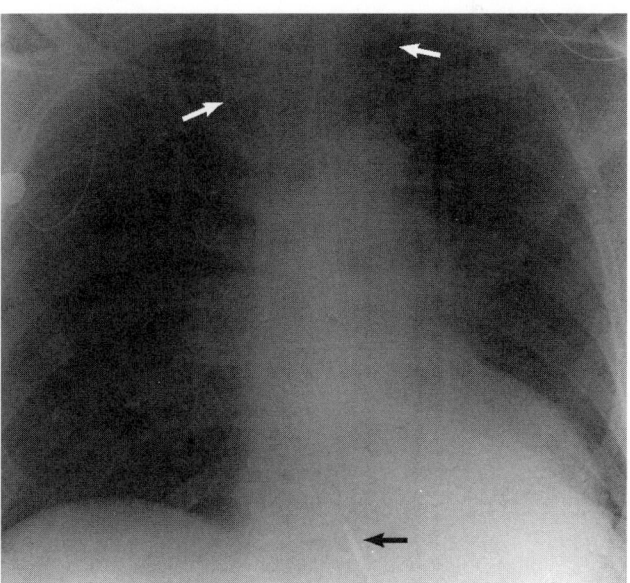

Figure 24-12   Posteroanterior chest radiograph shows a malpositioned central venous catheter. The right internal jugular catheter *(white arrows)* is inadvertently positioned in the left internal jugular vein instead of the superior vena cava. Note the malpositioned nasogastric tube in the distal esophagus *(black arrow)*.

load, usually in patients with cardiogenic shock or poor left ventricular function. The catheter tip is optimally placed just distal to the left subclavian artery.[58] The balloon inflates during diastole and deflates during systole. The major complication of the use of the intraaortic balloon pump is aortic dissection, although occlusion of abdominal vessels may occur if the balloon is placed too low. If the balloon is too high, occlusion of the great vessels may result.

Nasogastric Tube

The use of a nasogastric tube is associated with complications, the most common of which is malpositioning. The tip and the side hole of the tube should be below the level of the gastroesophageal junction to prevent gastroesophageal reflux. With known gastroesophageal reflux before tube placement, more distal placement of an enteric tube usually is necessary. Misplacement of the nasogastric tube into the airway may occur, with subsequent administration of fluids into the lung. Tracheal or bronchial perforation also may occur with resultant pneumomediastinum or pneumothorax.

Transvenous Pacemaker

Transvenous pacemakers are used either temporarily or permanently to treat arrhythmias. The pacing leads are generally placed in the right ventricle in unipolar systems and in the right atrium and right ventricle in bipolar systems. Electrode malpositioning frequently occurs. The electrode also may migrate over time, passing into the pulmonary artery or the coronary sinus. Perforation of the myocardium is an unusual complication and should be suspected when radiographs demonstrate the electrode tip projecting beyond the right ventricle apex. Breakage of a pacing wire is an infrequent but important complication.

Other Imaging Techniques of the Thorax

Although conventional chest radiography remains the fundamental imaging procedure for the chest, several other imaging modalities can provide significant additional information in appropriate clinical settings. These other technologies include CT, MRI, and more recently, positron emission tomography. Each modality has certain advantages and disadvantages, and therefore their indications depend on the clinical situation.

Patients with abnormalities related to the thorax always should be initially studied with plain chest radiography. Plain chest radiography is readily available, inexpensive, and often diagnostic. If this examination does not sufficiently identify the particular problem, several questions must be addressed before further studies are performed to take full advantage of current imaging techniques: What type of abnormality is expected? Can the suggested study provide the necessary information? What

will be done with the information? If all these questions can be appropriately answered, the additional study should be performed.

Computed Tomography

CT is the most common and readily available additional imaging modality for the thorax, with rapid scan times and exquisite anatomic information. New scanners with scan times of 0.4 seconds have made it possible to scan the thorax in a single breath hold, thereby eliminating breathing artifact. With advances including high-resolution imaging for the evaluation of interstitial lung disease (Figure 24-13) and helical technique, the applications for CT have increased and its diagnostic capabilities have been continuously refined.

Because CT provides exquisite anatomic detail of the thorax, it can be used for a number of different problems, including soft tissue or bony abnormalities, pleural abnormalities, lung parenchyma and interstitial disease, hilar or mediastinal pathology including the heart and great vessels, PE, and aortic dissection. These general categories include an entire spectrum of disease entities.

Depending on the clinical situation, studies should be tailored to answer specific questions. The field of view of an image can be changed to magnify or target regions of interest, different reconstruction algorithms can be employed for the evaluation of specific structures of different densities (Figure 24-14), and thin sections (1 to 2 mm) can be used to produce finer detail. In addition, IV contrast, which can be useful for delineating vascular structures, is required in certain situations such as aortic dissection (Figure 24-15) and the detection of PE. Approximately 100 to 150 mL of IV contrast usually is sufficient for most examinations. However, because most

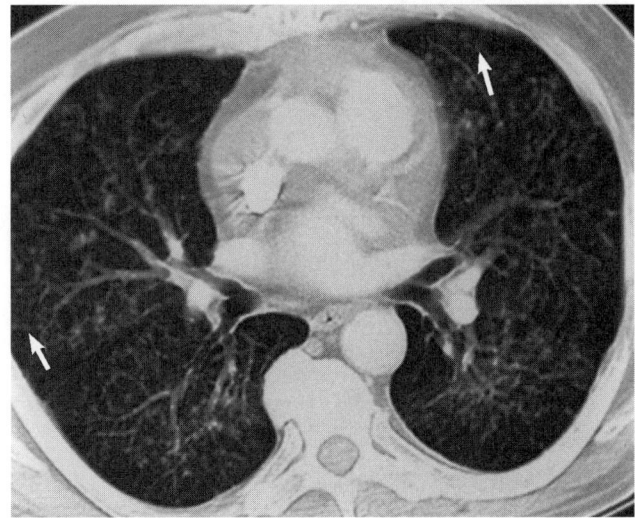

Figure 24-13   High-resolution computed tomography (CT) image of the lung parenchyma shows multiple small bilateral pulmonary nodules *(arrows)* in a heart transplant pateint with cytomegalus viral pneumonia.

CT studies of the thorax do not require IV contrast, the additional information does not justify the low but potential risk, cost, time, or patient discomfort.

However, CT uses ionizing radiation. Although no study to date has shown a significant risk with the present doses, exposure in some patient groups, including pregnant women and children, should be limited. CT is currently the most powerful additional imaging tool available to the radiologist. Current applications are numerous, although its clinical utility with the continuously improving technology has yet to be fully defined.

Magnetic Resonance Imaging

MRI also is a useful imaging tool in the thorax. With MRI, more clinical questions must be answered than with CT because MRI has a number of different technical parameters that must be determined to tailor each study.

MRI imaging takes advantage of a well-described phenomenon, nuclear magnetic resonance, in which nuclei with odd numbers of protons and a magnetic moment become aligned when placed in a strong magnetic field. These protons then can be excited to a more energetic state with the addition of a radio-frequency pulse. Once allowed to relax, excited protons emit a resonance signal that reflects the number of protons and their nuclear environment. Different relaxation signals are generated depending on the pulse sequence, the way in which the protons within the nuclei are excited.

In the body, the greatest source of odd-number protons, the hydrogen nuclei, are used to create a resonance signal. Although some signals have features suggestive of a particular disease process, signal characteristics often are nonspecific.

Once a resonance signal has been generated, the information can be mathematically transformed to produce an image. MRI provides accurate anatomic detail of the thorax. Its current indications include soft tissue and bone marrow pathology, complicated pleural and diaphragmatic diseases, hilar and mediastinal abnormalities (including congenital heart disease, cardiac abnormalities, and vascular pathology), PE, and aortic dissection.

The applications of MRI are numerous and although MRI often is complementary to CT, it has several advantages. The use of IV contrast for the intensive care patient usually is unnecessary. Patients with renal dysfunction often are better served by MRI because IV contrast, which can be nephrotoxic, usually is not required. On conventional (spin echo) MRI images, the vessels are seen as a signal void because the protons excited do not remain in the same plane being imaged (the blood is moving). This flow phenomenon thus creates the body's own internal vascular contrast. Additional pulse sequences (gradient-refocused images) that use different excitation patterns to produce bright signals within the vessels can be performed to demonstrate flowing blood (Figure 24-16). More recently, the introduction of contrast-enhanced three-dimensional gradient echo sequences with gadolinium contrast agents has allowed the accurate visualization of vessels, especially veins.[60] However, some structures lack sufficient free hydrogen nuclei for excitation, and thus a low signal is created. Cortical bone and lung parenchyma are the most notable areas in the chest. MRI has several other disadvantages, including limited patient monitoring capabilities and motion artifacts caused by cardiac and respiratory motion, which can obscure the images. MRI is contraindicated in patients with cardiac pacemakers. Despite these limitations, MRI offers information not available from other modalities. In addition, MRI, unlike CT, uses no ionizing radiation.

The full potential of MRI in pulmonary angiography continues to be actively pursued. On conventional,

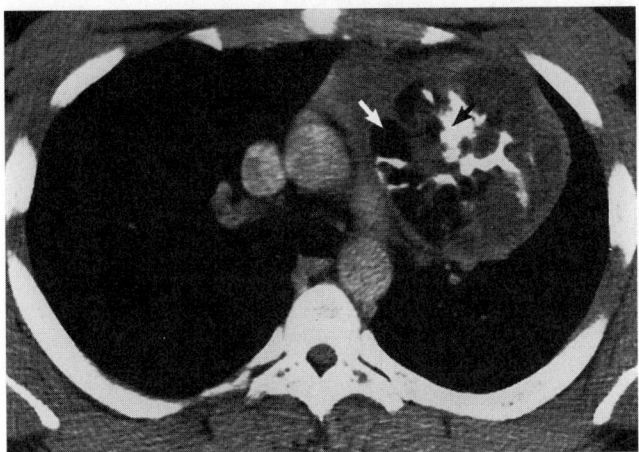

Figure 24-14   Axial computed tomography (CT) image demonstrates a heterogeneous anterior mediastinal mass. The mass contains low-attenuation material *(white arrow)* representing fat and high-attenuation material *(black arrow)* representing calcium. This appearace on CT is typical of a teratoma.

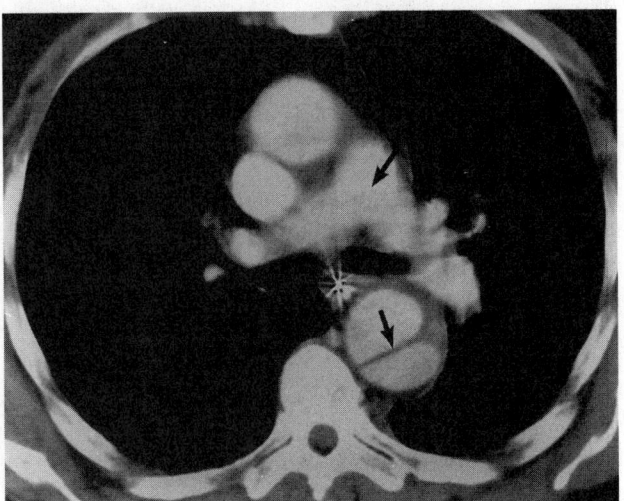

Figure 24-15   Spiral computed tomography (CT) of the mediastinum demonstrates an intraluminal flap within the descending aorta consistent with a type B aortic dissection. Note contrast in the main pulmonary artery *(large arrow)*.

nonenhanced spin-echo sequences, pulmonary emboli can be detected with different signal intensities, depending on the age of the clot. On gradient echo imaging and contrast-enhanced magnetic resonance (MR) angiography, emboli are visualized as filling defects within high-signal intensity vessels. The sensitivity and specificity of non-contrast MR angiography in the detection of pulmonary embolus ranges from 90% to 96% and 63% to 78%, respectively.[61,62] The sensitivity and specificity for contrast

enhanced MR angiography ranges from 70% to 87% and 97% to 100%, respectively.[63,64] Presently, MR angiography is a second line test if spiral CT is not available or is contraindicated and may obviate pulmonary angiography.

Another application of MRI in lung disease is the detection of pelvic and lower extremity venous thrombosis in patients at risk for PE. MRI has the added advantage of a high degree of accuracy in the assessment of the pelvic veins. MR venography also is an excellent imaging modality for evaluation of the veins of the thorax and upper extremities, where conventional venography and sonography are limited. It is 97% sensitive and 94% specific for the detection of central venous occlusion and has been shown to accurately predict successful central venous catheter placement in 100% of cases.[60,65]

Research continues to try to improve visualization of lung parenchyma. Imaging after inhalation of hyperpolarized gases such as xenon or helium have demonstrated promising initial results.[66]

Positron Emission Tomography

The newest imaging modality, **positron emission tomography (PET),** has become a recognized tool for the assessment of thoracic pathologic processes, in particular for tumor imaging. Previous PET investigations were performed almost exclusively on the brain, but now some of the same principles have been applied to thoracic abnormalities. Unlike CT and MRI, PET provides physiologic and metabolic information. This test, which focuses on the biochemical properties of cells, has the ability to analyze abnormalities quantitatively. Currently, the positron emitting agent most commonly used in the thorax is F18-fluorodeoxyglucose (FDG). Metabolically active cells take up and trap this D-glucose

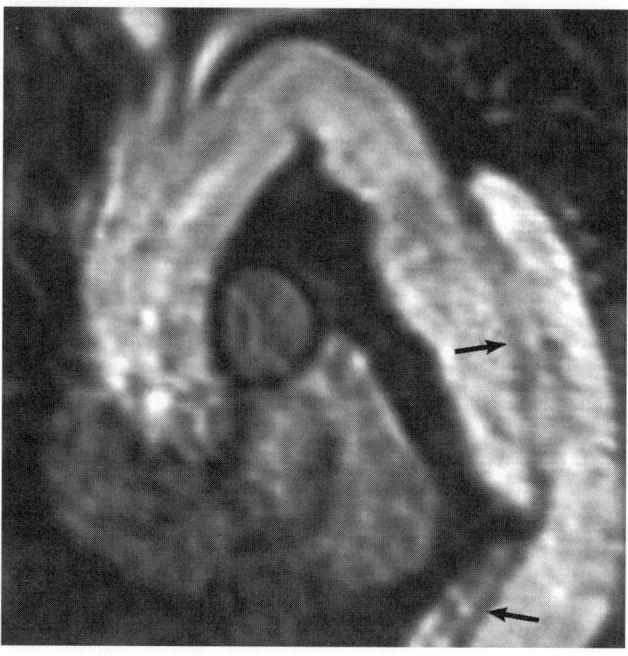

Figure 24-16 Oblique sagittal magnetic resonance imaging (MRI) image demonstatrates an intimal flap *(arrows)* separating the true and false lumen in this patient with aortic dissection.

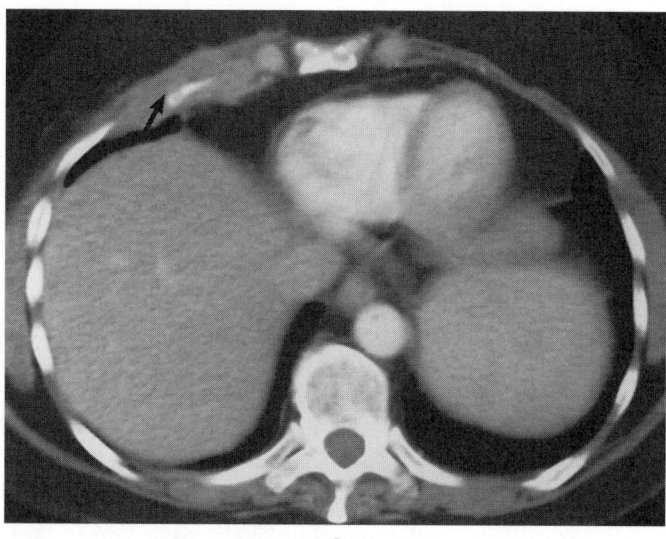 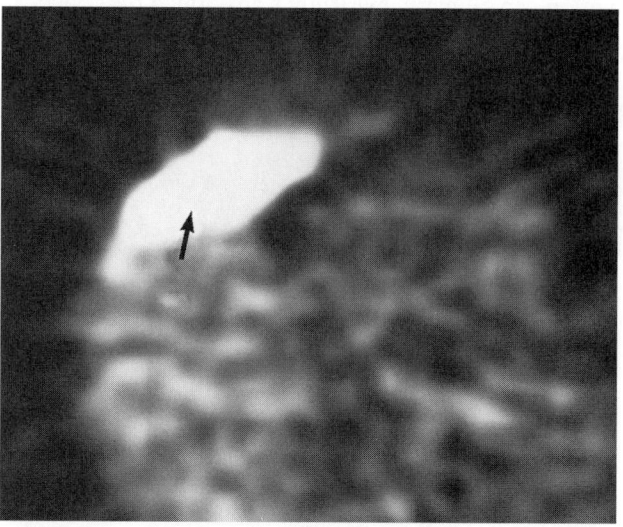

A	B

Figure 24-17 **A,** Axial computed tomography (CT) image at the lower thoracic level in a patient with right anterior chest wall pain. Nonspecific soft tissue thickening is noted, encasing the anterior ribs *(arrow)*. **B,** Axial F18-fluorodeoxyglucose–positron emission tomography (FDG-PET) image at the same level demonstrates intense activity *(arrow)* in the soft tissues, representing increased glucose metabolism. CT-guided biopsy revealed lymphoma.

analogue (Figure 24-17). The activity then can be measured and mapped to a specific region within the thorax. Data from multiple studies demonstrate that more metabolically active tumor cells show increased FDG uptake compared with normal tissues or a benign process.

Several indications for PET in the thorax exist: distinguishing benign and malignant focal pulmonary abnormalities including solitary pulmonary nodules, staging lung cancer, and differentiating fibrosis from tumor in patients treated for lung cancer. PET imaging has a sensitivity of approximately 95% for the detection of cancer in patients who have indeterminate lesions on CT. Evaluation of lesions less than 1 cm is limited by spatial resolution and may produce false-negative results.[67-69] The specificity of 85% with PET in these lesions is less than the sensitivity because some inflammatory processes such as granulomatous infection avidly accumulate FDG. PET has been shown to be more accurate than CT in determination of the presence or absence of intrathoracic metastatic nodal disease.[67,70] Intrathoracic and extrathoracic disease can be staged in a single examination with whole-body PET. This allows the detection of occult metastasis and alters treatment in up to 40% of cases.[71,72] As newer agents develop, this imaging technique should prove valuable in the management of cancer patients, although the role of PET in critically ill patients is limited at this time.

$\mathcal{K}$EY $\mathcal{P}$OINTS

- Chest radiography is an inexpensive imaging modality used to evaluate thoracic disease and monitor the position and complications of support apparatus.
- Airspace disease results in parenchymal opacification, the silhouette sign, and air bronchograms.
- Duplex sonography is the first line-imaging modality for the evaluation of lower limb DVT in the ICU patient. Patients in whom the technique is technically difficult or evaluation of the iliac vessels is required should be evaluated with conventional or MR venography.
- A common use of chest radiography in critically ill patients is the identification of tube and catheter position. These devices are radiopaque to facilitate their identification.
- Extraalveolar air includes pneumothorax, pneumomediastinum, and interstitial emphysema; each of these is characterized by a distinctive radiographic appearance.
- CT provides excellent anatomic detail and is useful in evaluation of the lung parenchyma, pleura, mediastinum and soft tissues. Spiral CT diminishes respiratory motion and slice misregistration and provides three-dimensional images of the thorax.
- Increasing evidence suggests that spiral CT is more accurate than ventilation/perfusion scanning in the diagnosis of PE.
- PET imaging uses physiologic rather than morphologic information to distinguish between benign and malignant diseases.

References*

1. Henschke CI, Pasternack GS, Schroeder S, et al. Bedside chest radiography; diagnostic efficacy. Radiology 1983;49:23-26.
2. Bekemeyer WB, Crapo RD, Calhoon S, et al. Efficacy of chest radiography in a respiratory intensive care unit. Chest 1985;88:691-696.
3. Felson G, Felson H. Localization of intrathoracic lesions by means of the posteroanterior roentgenogram: the silhouette sign. Radiology 1950;55:363.
4. Shevland JE, Hirleman MT, Hoang KA, et al. Lobar collapse in the surgical intensive care unit. Br J Radiology 1983;56:531-534.
5. Wilcox P, Baile EM, Hards J, et al. Phrenic nerve function and its relationship to atelectasis after coronary artery bypass surgery. Chest 1988;93:693-698.
6. Andrews CP, Coalson JJ, Smith JD, et al. Diagnosis of nosocomial bacterial pneumonia in acute diffuse lung disease. Chest 1981;80:254-258.
7. Roberts J, Barnes W, Pennoeh MHS, et al. Diagnostic accuracy of fever as a measure of postoperative pulmonary complications. Heart Lung 1982;17:139-144.
8. Swensen SJ, Peters SG, LeRoy AJ, et al. Radiology in the intensive care unit. Mayo Clin Proc 1991;66:396-410.
9. Finegold SM. Aspiration pneumonia. Rev Infect Dis 1991;13 (Suppl 9):S737-S742.
10. Torres A, Serra-Batlles J, Ros E, et al. Pulmonary aspiration of gastric contents in patients receiving mechanical ventilation: the effect of body position. Ann Intern Med 1992;116:540-543.
11. Sheld WM, Mandell GL. Nosocomial pneumonia: pathogenesis and recent advances in diagnosis and therapy. Rev Infect Dis 1991;13(Suppl 9):S743-S751.
12. Goodman LR, Putman CE. Critical care imaging. Philadelphia: WB Saunders; 1992.
13. Williford ME, Godwin JD. Computed tomography of lung abscess and empyema. Radiology Clin North Am 1983;21:575-583.
14. Snow N, Bergin KT, Horrigan TP. Thoracic CT scanning in critically ill patients: information obtained frequently alters management. Chest 1990;97:1467-1470.
15. Milne ENC, Pistolesi M, Miniati M, et al. The radiologic distinction of cardiogenic and noncardiogenic edema. Am J Roentgenol 1985;144:879-894.
16. Aberle DR, Wiener-Kronish JP, Webb WR, et al. Hydrostatic versus increased permeability pulmonary edema: diagnosis based on radiographic criteria in critically ill patients. Radiology 1988;168:73-79.
17. Aberle DR, Brown K. Radiologic considerations in the adult respiratory distress syndrome. Clin Chest Med 1990;11:737-754.
18. Suchyta MR, Clemmer TP, Elliott CG, et al. The adult respiratory distress syndrome: a report of survival and modifying factors. Chest 1992;101:1074-1079.
19. Shale D. The adult respiratory distress syndrome—20 years on. Thorax 1987;42:641-645.
20. Montgomery AB, Stager MA, Carrico CJ, et al. Causes of mortality in patients with the adult respiratory distress syndrome. Am Rev Respir Dis 1985;132:485-489.
21. Buckner CB, Walker CW, Purnell GL. Pulmonary embolism. J Thorac Imaging 1989;4:23-27.
22. Westermark N. On the roentgen diagnosis of lung embolism. Acta Radiology 1938;19:357.

*The entire issue of Respiratory Care, September 1999, is devoted to thoracic imaging in the ICU.

23. The PIOPED Investigators. Value of the ventilation/perfusion scan in acute pulmonary embolism: results of the Prospective Investigation of Pulmonary Embolism Diagnosis (PIOPED). JAMA 1990;263:2753-2759.

24. Goodman RL, Curtin JJ, Mewissen MW, et al. Detection of pulmonary embolism in patients with unresolved clinical and scintigraphic diagnosis: helical CT versus angiography. Radiology 1995;194:313-319.

25. Remy-Jardin MJ, Remy J, Deschildre F, et al. Diagnosis of acute pulmonary embolism with spiral CT: comparison with pulmonary angiography and scintigraphy. Radiology 1996;200:699-706.

26. Teigen CL, Maus TP, Sheedy PF, et al. Pulmonary embolism: diagnosis with contrast-enhanced electron beam CT and comparison with pulmonary angiography. Radiology 1995;194:313-319.

27. Stein P, Athanasoulis C, Alavi A, et al. Complications and validity of pulmonary angiography in acute pulmonary embolism. Circulation 1992;85:462-468.

28. Quinn M, Lundell C, Klotz T, et al. Reliability of selective pulmonary angiography in the diagnosis of pulmonary embolism. AJR 1987;149:469-471.

29. Stein P. Opinion response to acute pulmonary embolism: the role of computed tomographic imaging. J Thorac Imaging 1997;12:86-89.

30. Khorasani R, Gudas TF, Nikpoor N, et al. Treatment of patients with suspected pulmonary embolism and intermediate-probability lung scans: is diagnostic imaging underused? AJR 1997;169:1355-1357.

31. Goodman LR, Lipchik RJ. Diagnosis of acute pulmonary embolism: time for a new approach. Radiology 1996;199:25-27.

32. McGoldrick PJ, Rudd TG, Figley MM, et al. What becomes of pulmonary infarcts? Am J Roentgenol 1979;133:1039-1045.

33. Barnes RW, Wu KK, Hoak JC. Fallibility of the clinical diagnosis of venous thrombosis. JAMA 1975;234:605-607.

34. Cronan JJ, Dorfman GS, Scola FH, et al. Deep venous thrombosis: US assessment using vein compression. Radiology 1987;162:191-194.

35. Baxter GM, McKechnie S, Duffy P. Colour Doppler ultrasound in deep venous thrombosis: A comparison with venography. Clin Radiology 1990;42:32-36.

36. Kistner RL, Ball JJ, Nordyke RA, et al. Incidence of pulmonary embolism in the course of thrombophlebitis of the lower extremities. Am J Surg 1972;124:169-176.

37. Moser KM, LeMoine JR. Is embolic risk conditioned by location of deep venous thrombosis? Ann Intern Med 1981;94:439-444.

38. Philbrick JT, Becker DM. Calf deep vein thrombosis: a wolf in sheep's clothing? Arch Intern Med 1988;148:2131-2138.

39. Ginsberg JS. Management of venous thromboembolism. N Engl J Med 1996;335:1816-1828.

40. Hull RD, Raskob GE, Ginsberg JS, et al. A noninvasive strategy for the treatment of patients with suspected pulmonary embolism. Arch Intern Med 1994;154:289-297.

41. Carpenter JP, Holland GA, Baum RA, et al. Magnetic resonance venography for the detection of deep venous thrombosis: comparison with contrast venography and duplex Doppler ultrasonography. J Vasc Surg 1993;18:734-741.

42. Montgomery KD, Potter HG, Helfet DL. Magnetic resonance venography to evaluate the deep venous system of the pelvis in patients who have an acetabular fracture. J Bone Joint Surg Am 1995;77:1639-1649.

43. Evans AJ, Sostman HD, Witt YLA, et al. Detection of deep venous thrombosis: prospective comparison of MR imaging and sonography. J Magn Reson Imaging 1996:1:44-51.

44. Evans AJ, Sostman HD, Knelson MH, et al. Detection of deep venous thrombosis: prospective comparison of MR imaging with contrast venography. AJR 1993;161:131-139.

45. Comerota AJ, Katz ML, Grossi RJ, et al. The comparative value of noninvasive testing for diagnosis and surveillance of deep vein thrombosis. J Vasc Surg 1988;7:40-49.

46. Harris WH, Salzman EW, Athanasoulis C, et al. Comparison of 125I fibrinogen count scanning with phlebography for detection of venous thrombi after elective hip surgery. N Engl J Med 1975;292:665-667.

47. Moser KM, Brach BB, Dolan GF. Clinically suspected deep venous thrombosis of the lower extremities. JAMA 1977;237:2195-2198.

48. Pasternack G, O'Cain C. Thoracic complications of respiratory intensive care. In: Herman P, editor. Iatrogenic thoracic complications. New York: Springer-Verlag; 1983.

49. Westcott J, Cole S. Barotrauma. In: Herman P, editor. Iatrogenic thoracic complications. New York: Springer-Verlag; 1983.

50. Chiles C, Ravin CE. Radiographic recognition of pneumothorax in the intensive care unit. Crit Care Med 1986;14:677-680.

51. Gordon R. The deep sulcus sign. Radiology 1980;136:25-27.

52. Onikl G, Goodman PC, Webb WR, Brasch RC. Hydropneumothorax: detection on supine radiographs. Radiology 1984;152:31-34.

53. Unger JM, England DM, Bogust GA. Interstitial emphysema in adults: recognition and prognostic implications. J Thorac Imaging 1989;4:86-94.

54. Conrady PA, Goodman LR, Lainge F, et al. Alteration of endotracheal tube position: flexion and extension of the neck. Crit Care Med 1976;4:8-12.

55. Webb WR, Godwin JD. The obscured outer edge: a sign of improperly placed pleural drainage tubes. Am J Roentgenol 1980;131:1062-1064.

56. Mauser JR, Friedman PJ, Wing VW. Thoracostomy tube in an interlobar fissure: radiologic recognition of a potential problem. Am J Roentgenol 1982;139:1155-1161.

57. Ravin CE, Putman CE, McLoud TC. Hazards of the intensive care unit. Am J Roentgenol 1976;126:423-431.

58. Ovenfors CO. Iatrogenic trauma to the thorax. J Thorac Imaging 1987;2:18-31.

59. Landay MJ, Moot AR, Estrera AS. Apparatus seen on chest radiographs after cardiac surgery in adults. Radiology 1990;174:477-482.

60. Hartnell GG, Hughes LA, Finn JP, Longmaid HE. Magnetic resonance angiography of the central chest veins—a new gold standard? Chest 1995;107:1053-1057.

61. Grist TM, Sostman HD, MacFall JR, et al. Pulmonary angiography with MR imaging: preliminary clinical experience. Radiology 1993;189:523-530.

62. Erdman WA, Peshock RM, Redman HC, et al. Pulmonary embolism: comparison of MR images with radionuclide and angiographic studies. Radiology 1994;190:499-508.

63. Loubeyre P, Revel D, Douek P, et al. Dynamic contrast-enhanced MR angiography of pulmonary embolism: comparison with pulmonary angiography. AJR 1994;162:1035-1039.

64. Meaney J, Weg J, Chenevert T, et al. Diagnosis of pulmonary embolism with magnetic resonance angiography. N Engl J Med 1997;336:1422-1427.

65. Rose S, Gomes A, Yoon H. MR angiography for mapping potential central venous access sites in patients with advanced venous occlusive disease. AJR 1996;166:1181-1187.

66. Mugler JP, Dreihuys B, Brookerman JR, et al. MR imaging and spectroscopy using hyperpolarized 129Xe gas: preliminary human results. Magn Reson Med 1997;37:809-815.

67. Patz EF, Lowe VJ, Hoffman JM, et al. Focal pulmonary abnormalities: evaluation with F-18 fluorodeoxyglucose PET scanning. Radiology 1993;188:487-490.

68. Gupta NC, Frank AR, Dewan NA, et al. Solitary pulmonary nodules: detection of malignancy with PET with F18-2-fluoro-2-deoxy-D-glucose. Radiology 1992;184:441-444.

69. Scott WJ, Schwabe JL, Gupta NC, et al. Positron emission tomography of lung tumors and mediastinal lymph nodes using [F18] fluorodeoxyglucose. Ann Thorac Surg 1994;58:698-703.

70. Patz Jr EF, Lowe VJ, Goodman PC, et al. Thoracic nodal staging with positron emission tomography (PET) and F18-fluoro-2-deoxy-D-glucose in patients with bronchogenic carcinoma. Chest 1995;108:1617-1621.

71. Lewis P, Griffin S, Marsden P, et al. Whole-body ^{18}F-fluorodeoxyglucose positron emission tomography in preoperative evaluation of lung cancer. Lancet 1994;344:1265-1266.

72. Valk PE, Pounds TR, Hopkins DM, et al. Staging non-small cell lung cancer by whole-body positron emission tomographic imaging. Ann Thorac Surg 1995;60:1573-1582.

CHAPTER 25

Pulmonary Function Testing

Gul Gursel
Alexander B. Adams

CHAPTER **OUTLINE**

OBJECTIVES

1. Describe the general purposes of pulmonary function testing.
2. Define lung volumes and capacities.
3. Describe methods used to measure functional residual capacity (FRC).
4. State the American Thoracic Society (ATS) standards for the spirometry testing.
5. Identify the features of normal and abnormal spirometry tracings.
6. Recognize the common errors seen in spirometry testing.
7. Specify the spirometry values seen in tests of patients with normal lungs, obstructive disease, restrictive disease, air trapping, and hyperinflation.
8. Explain the importance of spirometry testing before and after bronchodilator use.
9. Explain the rationale of office spirometry.
10. Describe the importance of diffusion testing.
11. State the goals of the following specialized pulmonary function tests: bronchial challenge testing, airway resistance, respiratory muscle strength, ventilation distribution, and respiratory muscle coordination.

KEY TERMS

Air Trapping
Airway Resistance (R_{aw})
Body Plethysmography
FEV_1/FVC
Flow-Volume Loop
Forced Expiratory Volume (FEV)
Forced Vital Capacity (FVC)
Helium Dilution

Hyperinflation
Inductance Plethysmography (IP)
Lung Capacity
Lung Volumes
Maximum Expiratory Pressure (PE_{max})
Maximum Inspiratory Pressure (PI_{max})
Maximum Voluntary Ventilation (MVV)
Midflow Rate

Nitrogen Washout
Obstructive Lung Disease
Office Spirometry
Restrictive Lung Disease
Single-Breath Nitrogen Test
Sniff Test
Spirometry
Upper-Airway Lesions

Pulmonary function testing (PFT) routinely evaluates lung size, flow rates, and the diffusing capacity of the lungs. The tests can provide valuable information about the presence of ventilatory defects, degree of lung impairment, responsiveness to therapy, and possible effects on gas exchange. The tests themselves are not definitively diagnostic, but their results can be strongly suggestive of lung pathology. Testing requires clear instruction and encouragement; acceptable patient cooperation must be ensured before the test results are evaluated. The training of personnel conducting the tests should meet minimal criteria as recommended by the American Thoracic Society (ATS).[1] PFT has a long, rich history, and the tests regularly performed are relatively well standardized. This chapter describes the parameters commonly measured in the outpatient pulmonary function laboratory. The primary goal of testing in the outpatient setting is the detection of restrictive and/or obstructive lung defects. **Restrictive lung disease** is detected by measurement of reduced lung volumes. **Obstructive lung disease** is detected by measurement of reduced airflow rates from the lungs.

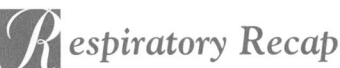

Respiratory Recap ──────────

Goals of Pulmonary Function Testing
To detect and assess the degree of restrictive lung disease
To detect and assess the degree of obstructive lung disease

Lung Volumes and Capacities

Lung size or **lung volumes** and the vital capacity were first measured systematically by Hutchinson in 1846.[2] When obstructive lung disease became more clearly defined in the 1960s, the emphasis of testing shifted to measurement of dynamic lung volumes or flows (timed measurements made during forced effort maneuvers). Nevertheless, for more than 100 years, PFT was primarily the measurement of static lung volumes. *Static* refers to volumes measured between the four resting or static positions: maximal inhalation, end inspiration, end expiration, and maximal exhalation. Despite the importance of the detection of obstructive disease related to cigarette smoking, the measurement of static lung volumes and lung capacities continues to contribute to the diagnosis of a restrictive process. Indications for the measurement of static lung volumes are shown in Box 25-1. The static lung volumes and lung capacities are compartments of the lungs that have expected sizes and relationships to each other.

A **lung capacity** is two or more lung volumes (Figure 25-1). Of the eight lung volumes and capacities, four provide the most useful information: vital capacity (VC), total lung capacity (TLC), functional residual capacity (FRC), and residual volume (RV). Static lung volumes are

Box 25-1

Indications for the Measurement of Lung Volumes and Capacities

1. To detect restrictive processes and differentiate between obstructive and restrictive disease patterns or mixed processes
2. To detect or quantify trapped gas (an increase in RV/TLC ratio)
3. To assess response to therapeutic intervention (such as drugs, radiation, transplantation, chemotherapy, or volume reduction surgery)
4. To quantify the presence and amount of unventilated lung (gas dilution versus plethysmographic methods)
5. To assess chronic diseases such as sarcoidosis, rheumatoid, or uremic lung diseases
6. To aid in the interpretation of other lung function tests

measured by volume spirometers or pneumotachometer-based spirometers (Figure 25-2). The patient is connected to the spirometer or pneumotachometer and instructed to perform maneuvers that measure the lung volumes and capacities. The four lung volumes include the following:

Respiratory Recap ──────────

Lung Volumes	
Tidal volume	Expiratory reserve volume
Inspiratory reserve volume	Residual volume

1. *Tidal volume* (VT) is the volume of gas inhaled or exhaled during normal breathing.
2. *Inspiratory reserve volume* (IRV) is the maximum volume of gas that can be inspired from the end of a normal inspiration.
3. *Expiratory reserve volume* (ERV) is the maximum volume of gas that can be expired from the end of a resting expiration.
4. *Residual volume* (RV) is the volume of gas remaining in the lungs after a maximal expiration. By definition, this volume cannot be exhaled.

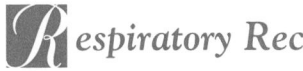

Respiratory Recap ──────────

Lung Capacities	
Vital capacity	Functional residual capacity
Inspiratory capacity	Total lung capacity

Figure 25-1   The volumes and capacities of the lungs. *IRV,* Inspiratory reserve volume; *ERV,* expiratory reserve volume; *RV,* residual volume; *VC,* vital capacity; *IC,* inspiratory capacity; *FRC,* function residual capacity; *TLC,* total lung capacity; *VT,* tidal volume.

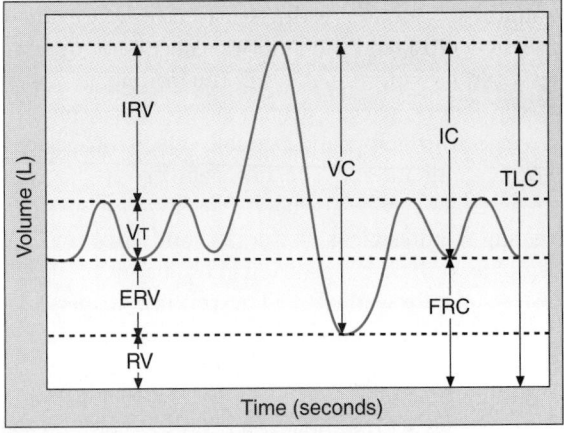

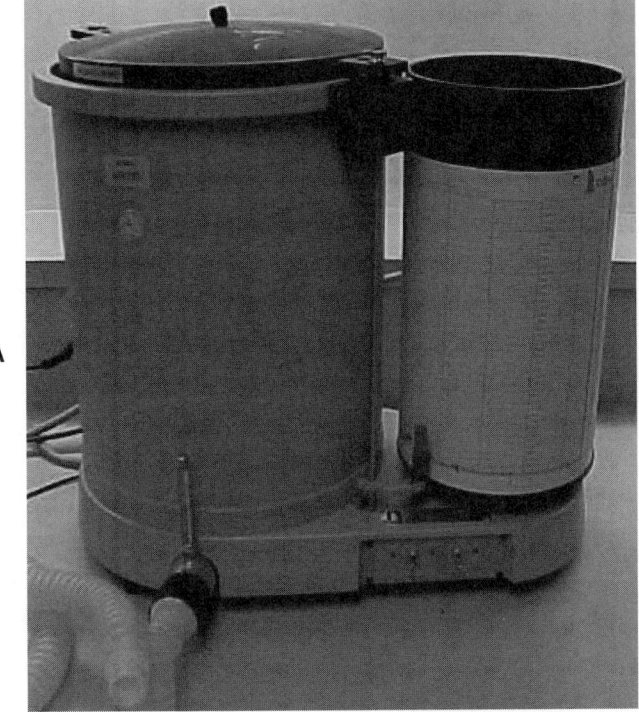

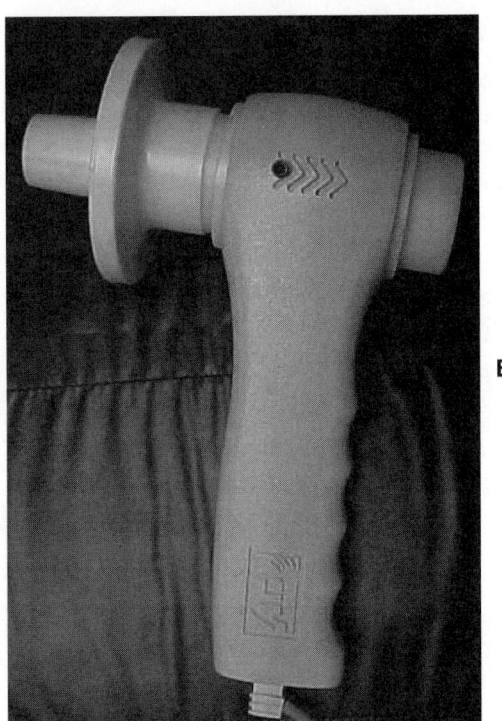

Figure 25-2   A, Spirometer. **B,** Pneumotachometer.

The four lung capacities include the following:

1. *Vital capacity* (VC) is the maximum volume of gas that can be exhaled from the lungs after a maximal inspiration (expiratory vital capacity) or inhaled from a point of maximal exhalation (inspiratory vital capacity). The VC includes the V_T, IRV, and ERV.
2. *Inspiratory capacity* (IC) is the maximum volume of gas that can be inspired from the normal end-expiratory position. The IC is the sum of V_T and IRV.
3. *Functional residual capacity* (FRC) is the volume of gas remaining in the lungs at the end of a resting expiration. The FRC is the sum of RV and ERV.
4. *Total lung capacity* (TLC) is the volume of gas in the lungs at the end of a maximal inspiration. The TLC is the sum of the 4 lung volumes (V_T, IRV, ERV, and RV).

Measurement of Lung Volumes

The subdivisions of the VC can be measured with a spirometer. The RV must be measured separately because the lungs cannot be emptied completely (zero lung volume). Thus FRC and TLC cannot be determined without knowledge of

*R*espiratory Recap

Methods to Measure FRC
Nitrogen washout
Helium dilution
Body plethysmography

CPG   25-1

Static Lung Volumes

Indications
Differentiate between obstructive and restrictive disease patterns.
Assess response to therapeutic interventions (such as drugs, transplantation, radiation, chemotherapy, or lobectomy).
Aid in the interpretation of other lung function tests.
Make preoperative assessments in patients with compromised lung function (known or suspected) when the surgical procedure is known to affect lung function.
Evaluate pulmonary disability.
Quantify the amount of nonventilated lung.

Contraindications
No absolute contraindications exist.
Relative contraindications for spirometry include hemoptysis of unknown origin, untreated pneumothorax, unstable cardiovascular status, or thoracic, abdominal, or cerebral aneurysms.

With respect to whole-body plethysmography, such factors as claustrophobia, upper body paralysis, obtrusive body casts, or other conditions that immobilize or prevent the patient from fitting into or gaining access to the body box are a concern. In addition, the procedure may necessitate stopping IV therapy or supplemental oxygen.

Hazards and Complications
Nosocomial infection may be contracted from improperly cleaned tubing, mouthpieces, and pneumotachygraphs.
Discomfort may be associated with the body box.
Ventilatory drive in susceptible subjects (such as CO_2 retainers) may be depressed as a consequence of breathing 100% oxygen during the nitrogen washout. Such patients should be carefully observed.
Hypercapnia and hypoxemia may occur during He-dilution FRC determinations as a consequence of failure to adequately remove CO_2 or add O_2.

Modified from AARC Clinical practice guideline: static lung volumes. Respir Care 1994;39:830-836.
CPG, Clinical practice guideline.

RV. Because zero lung volume cannot be measured with a spirometer, other methods must be used. Commonly, FRC is measured by a nonspirometric method. ERV is measured by a spirometer and subtracted from FRC to obtain a value for RV. The three most commonly used methods used to measure FRC are **nitrogen washout, helium dilution,** and **body plethysmography** (CPG 25-1).[3,4] A radiographic method has been developed but is not used routinely.

Nitrogen Washout

In this measurement method, the subject is switched from breathing room air ($\approx$21% O_2) to inhaling from a reservoir of 100% oxygen and exhaling through a nitrogen analyzer and spirometer. This is called an *open-circuit method* because rebreathing does not occur. The 100% oxygen dilutes the residual nitrogen during each breath (initially $\approx$79% N_2) until the nitrogen is washed out. All the nitrogen is measured as it is exhaled into the pool of exhaled gas. The FRC then can be calculated from the dilution formula (Equation 25-1). In practice, the procedure is terminated after 7 minutes. This method can underestimate the FRC with airway obstruction because noncommunicating lung regions are not allowed to wash out their nitrogen.

Inert Gas Dilution

Helium, argon, or neon can be used in this technique, although helium (He) usually is used. The patient is connected to the circuit and switched to breathing from a spirometer with a known volume containing helium of a

EQUATION   25-1

Measurement of FRC by Nitrogen Washout Technique

The FRC is calculated from the dilution formula, as follows:

$$C_1 \times V_1 = C_2 \times V_2$$

where:

V_1 = Functional residual capacity
C_1 = Nitrogen concentration in the lungs at the beginning of the procedure ($\approx$79%)
C_2 = Nitrogen concentration in the pooled exhaled volume
V_2 = Total exhaled volume from the washout

FRC then is calculated as follows:

$$FRC = \frac{C_2 \times V_2}{C_1}$$

Because all the nitrogen is not completely removed from the lung by 7 minutes (usually less than 1.5% remains), the final nitrogen percentage can be accounted for in the final calculation.

FRC, Functional residual capacity.

known concentration. This is called a *closed circuit method* because rebreathing occurs. The procedure is stopped when the He concentration falls to a new plateau or steady value. The rate of fall in He concentration (time to equilibrium) should be rapid; a slow rate can imply slow gas mixing or obstructive disease. The FRC measured by this method is then determined by the standard dilution calculation (Equation 25-2). Any leaks occurring during

TABLE 25-1

Standard Prediction Equations (Adults)

Parameter	Men	Women	Reference
VC	$0.0774 \times H - 0.0212 \times A - 7.75$	$0.0414 \times H - 0.0232 \times A - 2.198$	1
TLC	$0.0760 \times H - 6.69$	$0.0646 \times H - 5.44$	1
RV	Pred TLC − Pred FVC	Pred TLC − Pred FVC	
RV/TLC	Pred RV/Pred TLC	Pred RV/Pred TLC	
$FEV_1/FVC\%$	$-0.1314 \times H - 0.149 \times A + 110.23$	$-0.2145 \times H - 0.152 \times A + 124.48$	1
FEV_1	(Pred FEV_1/FVC) × pred FVC	(Pred FEV_1/FVC) × pred FVC	
FEF_{25-75}	$e^{(0.00811 \times H - 0.0096 \times A + 0.301)}$	$e^{(-0.012 \times A + 1.563)}$	1
FEF_{50}	$0.0684 \times H - 0.0366 \times A - 5.54$	$0.0321 \times H - 0.0240 \times A - 0.44$	2
PEF	$0.094 \times H - 0.035 \times A - 5.99$	$0.049 \times H - 0.025 \times A - 0.74$	2

H, Standing height in cm; A, age in years. If the patient is black or Asian, a correction is made by multiplication of the values by 0.85.
1, Miller A, Thornton JC, Warshaw R, et al. Mean and instantaneous expiratory flows, FVC and FEV₁: prediction equations from a probability sample of Michigan, a large industrial state. Bull Eur Physiopathol Respir 1986;22:589-597; 2, Miller A, Thornton JC, Warshaw R, et al. Single breath diffusing capacity in a representative sample of the population of Michigan, a large industrial state. Am Rev Respir Dis 1983;127:725-734.

EQUATION 25-2

Measurement of FRC by Helium Dilution Technique

The FRC measured by this method is determined by the standard dilution calculation, as follows:

$$C_1 \times V_1 = C_2 \times V_2$$

where:

C_1 = Initial helium concentration
V_1 = Spirometer volume
C_2 = Final helium concentration
$V_2 = V_1 + FRC$

Therefore

$$V_2 = \frac{C_1 \times V_1}{C_2}$$

Because

$$V_2 = V_1 + FRC$$

Therefore

$$FRC = \frac{C_1 \times V_1}{C_2} - V_1$$

FRC, Functional residual capacity.

the procedure will give a falsely high FRC. A correction (subtraction) for the mouthpiece volume is necessary.

Body Plethysmography

This technique (CPG 25-2) is based on Boyle's law, wherein the product of one pressure and volume (P_1V_1) of a gas will be equal to the product of another pressure and volume related to that gas (P_2V_2), or $P_1V_1 = P_2V_2$. In practice, the patient is placed inside a fixed-volume, air-sealed body box where the effects of excursion of the chest wall can be measured by small pressure changes in the box and airway. At the beginning of the test (end-expiration or FRC), the subject has an unknown volume of gas in the thorax (FRC). By occluding the airway and allowing the subject to decompress the chest by making an inspiratory effort, a new airway or lung pressure (P_1) and new body box pressures (P_2) are generated. The slope of change in airway and box pressures (P_1/P_2) is then used to calculate the missing volume (V_1 or FRC). The box volume (V_2) is known. The advantage of the body box technique is its speed. About 30 minutes or longer usually are required to measure FRC by helium dilution or nitrogen washout. FRC can be determined multiple times in 10 minutes by body plethysmography.

In patients with severe obstructive lung disease, the FRC actually may be overestimated by this technique, primarily because of inaccuracies in the measurement of lung or alveolar pressure at the mouth during airway occlusion. However, normal lungs show similar results with each FRC measurement method. The technique used to measure FRC is important because the gas dilution methods (He dilution and nitrogen washout) measure only communicating gas spaces. On the other hand, body plethysmography measures gas spaces, regardless of whether they are communicating (for example, bullae). Measuring He dilution or washout FRC in conjunction with body-plethysmography FRC can determine trapped gas because body-plethysmography FRC (total gas volume) minus the FRC measured by He dilution (communicating gas) equals the noncommunicating or trapped gas.

Interpretation

Measured static lung volumes and capacities are evaluated in comparison with predicted values. Prediction equations calculated from height, age, and gender exist for all pulmonary function parameters (Table 25-1).

CPG   25-2

Body Plethysmography

Indications

Measuring lung volumes to distinguish between restrictive and obstructive processes

Evaluating obstructive lung diseases such as bullous emphysema and cystic fibrosis, which may produce artifactually low results if measured by helium dilution or N_2 washout (an index of trapped gas [FRC plethysmograph/FRC He dilution] can be established)

Measuring lung volumes when multiple repeated trials are required or when the subject is unable to perform multibreath tests

Evaluating resistance to airflow

Determining the response to bronchodilators (R_{aw}, SG_{aw}, and V_{TG})

Determining bronchial hyperreactivity in response to methacholine, histamine, or isocapnic hyperventilation (V_{TG}, R_{aw}, and SG_{aw})

Following the course of disease and response to treatment

Contraindications

Mental confusion, muscular incoordination, body casts, or other conditions that prevent the subject from entering the plethysmograph cabinet or adequately performing the required maneuvers (such as panting against a closed shutter)

Claustrophobia that may be aggravated through entry into the plethysmograph cabinet

Presence of devices or other conditions, such as continuous IV infusions with pumps or other equipment that will not fit into the plethysmograph and should not be discontinued or that might interfere with pressure changes (for example, chest tube, transtracheal O_2 catheter, or ruptured eardrum)

Continuous oxygen therapy that should not be temporarily discontinued

Hazards and Complications

Excessive intrathoracic pressures caused by V_{TG} and R_{aw} measurements requiring the subject to pant against a closed shutter

Symptoms of claustrophobia caused by enclosure in the plethysmograph

Hypercapnia or hypoxia resulting from prolonged confinement in the plethysmograph chamber (an uncommon occurrence because of the limited length of the test and the fact that the plethysmograph must be vented periodically)

Transmission of infection through improperly cleaned equipment (for example, mouthpieces) or as a consequence of the inadvertent spread of droplet nuclei or body fluids (patient-to-patient or patient-to-technologist)

Modified from AARC Clinical practice guideline: body plethysmography. Respir Care 1994;39:1184-1190.
CPG, Clinical practice guideline.

Whereas measured values/predicted values would be expected to be 100%, normality usually is between 80% and 120% because of the variability of the measurements. Generally, reductions in lung volumes imply a restrictive lung disease process whereas elevations imply **air trapping** or **hyperinflation.**

The size of the TLC is determined by the ability of the respiratory muscles to enlarge the chest wall to its maximum volume configuration (in other words, to fill completely). A lower-than-expected TLC could result from an increase in stiffness of the lung or chest wall, respiratory muscle weakness, or a less than maximal effort by the patient. FRC is another important lung volume measurement. In healthy individuals, the size of the FRC is determined by the balance between the elastic recoil of the lungs, which acts in an expiratory direction and tends to reduce the lung volume, and that of the chest wall, which acts in an inspiratory direction, tending to expand the chest. The RV is normally about 25% of the TLC in healthy individuals and the FRC is normally 30% to 35% of TLC. Milder forms of airflow limitation have an elevated RV only, without a significant effect on TLC. Therefore the ratio may be greater than 25% without an elevation in TLC. An elevated RV, FRC, RV/TLC, or FRC/TLC then can be interpreted as air trapping. Because the variability in measurements of RV can be great, only

values of greater than 140% of predicted can be interpreted as abnormally high. An elevation in TLC is interpreted as hyperinflation. It is possible to have coexisting restrictive lung disease and air trapping, as seen in some cases of interstitial lung disease.

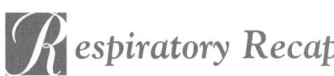

Respiratory Recap

Abnormal Lung Volumes and Capacities
Reduced lung volumes and capacities generally indicate restrictive disease.
Elevated residual volume or total lung capacity can indicate air trapping or hyperinflation

Table 25-2 provides examples of results from lung volume testing and their interpretations. The examples are from tests that were interpreted as normal and restrictive with presence of air-trapping and hyperinflation. Note that the values for each parameter must be evaluated in the context of the entire test. Interpretations are made considering the cooperation of the patient, actual values from the test, height and age, and smoking history.

TABLE 25-2

Examples of Predicted* and Actual Lung Volumes and Capacities

Patient A (Normal)			
Volume/ Capacity	Predicted Value	Actual Value	% Predicted
VC	3.25 L	2.62 L	81
TLC	5.09 L	4.57 L	90
RV	1.84 L	1.95 L	106
RV/TLC	35% L	45%	
FRC	2.98 L	2.84 L	95
ERV	0.89 L		
IC	1.37 L		

Patient B (Evidence of Air Trapping)			
Volume/ Capacity	Predicted Value	Actual Value	% Predicted
VC	2.88 L	1.20 L	42
TLC	4.50 L	3.62 L	80
RV	1.49 L	2.42 L	163
RV/TLC	33%	67%	
FRC	2.16 L	2.63 L	122
ERV	0.21 L		
IC	0.76 L		

Patient C (Evidence of Hyperinflation)			
Volume/ Capacity	Predicted Value	Actual Value	% Predicted
VC	3.51 L	1.44 L	41
TLC	5.49 L	6.95 L	127
RV	1.97 L	5.51 L	279
RV/TLC	36%	79%	
FRC	2.57 L	5.89 L	229
ERV	0.38 L		
IC	1.14 L		

*Predicted values for ERV and IC often are omitted and volumes do not necessarily add up to their respective capacities because the tests are performed independent of one another.

Spirometry

Spirometry is the most commonly performed pulmonary function test (CPG 25-3). The test is unique and repeatable if properly performed; the tracing is like an individual's fingerprint. The purpose of spirometry is to measure volume and flow, the volume of air an individual inhales or exhales as a function of time. Flow impairment defines an obstructive defect of lung function or the obstructive lung disease. Box 25-2 lists indications for spirometry. This test measures a forced expiratory vital capacity (FVC) maneuver in which the subject inhales maximally and then exhales as rapidly and completely as possible. The two methods used to display the FVC test are shown in Figure 25-3. In the volume-time curve, the spirometer records the vol-

BOX 25-2

Indications for Spirometry

To evaluate symptoms, signs, or abnormal laboratory tests
To measure the effects of other diseases on pulmonary function
To screen individuals at risk for pulmonary diseases (such as smokers and those with occupational exposures)
To assess preoperative risks
To assess prognosis (for example, lung transplant)
To assess health status before enrollment in strenuous physical activity programs

Monitoring
  To assess therapeutic interventions such as bronchodilator or steroid therapy
  To describe the course of diseases affecting lung function (such as obstructive airway, interstitial lung, or neuromuscular diseases)
  To monitor persons in occupations with exposure to injurious agents
  To monitor for adverse reactions to drugs with known pulmonary toxicity

Disability or Impairment Evaluations
  To assess patients as part of a rehabilitation program
  To assess risks as part of an insurance evaluation
  To assess individuals for legal reasons

Public Health
  To use for epidemiologic surveys

Derivation of Reference Equations

ume exhaled (y axis) plotted as a function of time (x axis). From this tracing, volumes at specific time intervals can be easily identified (**forced expiratory volume [FEV]**) at 0.5 seconds ($FEV_{0.5}$) and at 1, 2, and 3 seconds ($FEV_{1.0}$, $FEV_{2.0}$, $FEV_{3.0}$, respectively), and the ratio **FEV_1/FVC** can be calculated. The volume-time curve allows examination of the duration of the tracing and whether a plateau is achieved. In the flow-volume curve, the same maneuver plots flow (y axis) versus volume (x axis). From this tracing, flows of interest can be easily identified, such as the peak expiratory flow (PEF) and forced expiratory flow at 50% of FVC (FEF_{50}) or midflow. The flow-volume curve allows a closer examination of the early part of the effort. The validity of the FVC maneuver measurements depends largely on the cooperation and effort of the patient. For the results to be

Respiratory Recap

Spirometry
Is the most basic and commonly performed PFT
Requires a maximal effort to assess flow rates

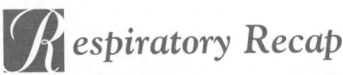

CPG   25-3

Spirometry

Indications

Detect the presence or absence of lung dysfunction suggested by history or physical signs and symptoms (such as age, smoking history, family history of lung disease, cough, dyspnea, or wheezing), the presence of other abnormal diagnostic tests (such as chest radiograph or arterial blood gas analysis), or both.

Quantify the severity of known lung disease.

Assess the change in lung function over time or after administration of or change in therapy.

Assess the potential effects or response to environmental or occupational exposure.

Assess the risk for surgical procedures known to affect lung function.

Assess impairment, disability, or both (for example, for rehabilitation, legal reasons, or military tests).

Contraindications

Hemoptysis of unknown origin (forced expiratory maneuver may aggravate the underlying condition)

Pneumothorax

Unstable cardiovascular status (forced expiratory maneuver may worsen angina or cause changes in blood pressure) or recent myocardial infarction or pulmonary embolus

Thoracic, abdominal, or cerebral aneurysms (danger of rupture caused by increased thoracic pressure)

Recent eye surgery (for example, cataract)

Acute disease process that might interfere with test performance (such as nausea or vomiting)

Recent surgery of thorax or abdomen

Hazards and Complications

Pneumothorax

Increased intracranial pressure

Syncope, dizziness, or lightheadedness

Chest pain

Paroxysmal coughing

Contraction of nosocomial infections

Oxygen desaturation caused by interruption of oxygen therapy

Bronchospasm

Modified from AARC Clinical practice guideline: spirometry. Respir Care 1996;41:629-636.
CPG, Clinical practice guideline.

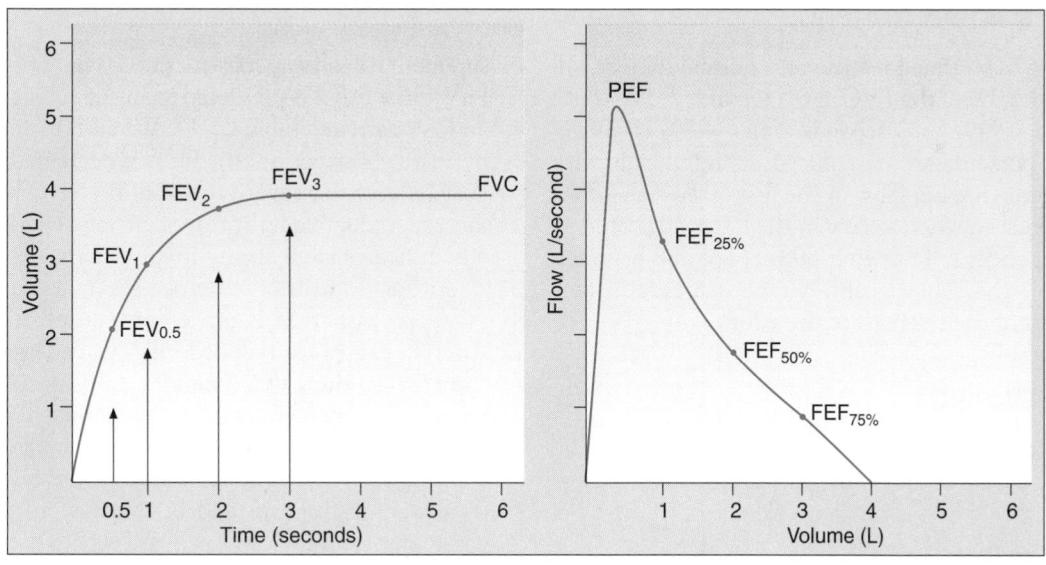

Figure 25-3   The volume-time curve is on the left, and the flow-volume curve is on the right. *FEV₁*, Forced expiratory volume in 1 second; *FEF₂₅%*, forced expiratory flow at 25% of forced vital capacity.

valid, the therapist must follow the ATS guidelines. The guidelines specify criteria for the forced maneuver and specifications for the spirometry equipment (Box 25-3).

Forced Vital Capacity

Vital capacity without a forced effort is called the *slow vital capacity (SVC)*, or relaxed vital capacity. In some subjects, SVC provides a more accurate determination of the VC than

the **forced vital capacity (FVC).** With severe airway obstruction, SVC values may be larger than FVC values by as much as 1 L. The difference between SVC and FVC reflects the trapping of air in the lungs when the effort is forced. Nevertheless, the FVC value in comparison with predicted values is most commonly examined in routine spirometry testing as an indicator of a restrictive disease process.

After the FVC maneuvers have been verified as acceptable, the details of the efforts can be further analyzed for

Box 25-3

ATS Recommendations for Spirometry Testing

Forced Expiratory Maneuver and Tracing

1. The patient is instructed to inhale completely, place the mouthpiece in the mouth, and exhale rapidly and completely. Vigorous coaching is helpful.
2. A minimum of three acceptable efforts is required, but not more than eight efforts should be made if the patient is becoming fatigued.
3. Acceptable efforts must have a rapid start, a good effort, no cough, no evidence of early termination, and no leak or physical obstruction such as glottic closure or tongue in the mouthpiece.
4. The best FVC, FEV_1, or PEF can be selected from different efforts. For FVC and FEV_1, the highest two values must repeat within 0.2 L.
5. The best FEF_{25-75} must be selected from the curve with the highest sum of FVC and FEV_1.
6. The patient can be sitting or standing. Nose clips are encouraged.
7. The back extrapolation method is used to determine the start of the test.
8. End-of-test criteria are a minimal exhalation time of 6 seconds and no change in exhaled volume for more than 1 second, or if the patient cannot exhale further.

Spirometry Equipment Performance

1. For a forced maneuver, the tracing must be able to display more than 15 seconds.
2. Volume accuracy must be $\pm$ 3% or $\pm$ 0.050 L, whichever is greater.
3. The equipment and circuitry must not have resistance greater than 1.5 cm H_2O/L/second.
4. Volumes and flows must be able to be corrected to BTPS.
5. A calibration with a 3-L syringe is required daily.
6. The spirometer must be able to measure volumes from 0.5 to 8 L and flows from 0 to 14 L/second.
7. Testing must be conducted within the temperature range of 17° to 40° C.
8. Hard copy tracings are required.
9. The recorder requirements include:
   a. For a volume-time display, the volume must be >10 mm/L and time must be >2 cm/second.
   b. For a flow-volume display, the volume must be >10 mm/L and flow must be >5 mm/L/second.
   c. The flow-volume ratio must be greater than 2:1.

From American Thoracic Society. Standardization of spirometry: 1994 update. Am J Respir Crit Care Med 1995;152:1107-1136.

interpretation. As a timed maneuver, a normal subject will exhale 50% to 60% of the FVC in 0.5 second, 75% to 85% in 1 second, ≈ 94% in 2 seconds, and ≈ 97% in 3 seconds. These percentages are reduced in individuals with obstructive lung disease. Flow in the first 50% of the FVC is effort dependent, whereas flow in the latter 50% of FVC is effort independent. Thus after 50% of VC has been exhaled (FEF_{50}), the subject cannot exceed a certain flow rate regardless of the strength of the effort.

FEV_1 and FEV_1/FVC

The FEV_1 is the volume of air exhaled in the first second of the FVC maneuver and is the most reproducible mea-

surement of airway obstruction. The normal value for FEV_1, like FVC, is predicted from the subject's height, age, and gender (see Table 25-1). When flow rates are slowed by airway obstruction, the FEV_1 is decreased by an amount that reflects the severity of the disease. The FEV_1 is the most reproducible indicator of airway obstruction and usually indicates large airway involvement.

Although restrictive processes may cause decreased FEV_1, a distinction is made between obstructive and restrictive causes for reduced FEV_1 values by referencing of the FEV_1 to the FVC. The FEV_1/FVC ratio usually is expressed as a percentage. In the normal adult, this ratio ranges from 75% to 85%, but it tends to decrease with increasing age. This ratio is a sensitive and reliable indicator of airway obstruction and is valuable in identifying the cause of a low FEV_1. A low FEV_1 with a normal ratio usually indicates a restrictive process, whereas a low FEV_1 and a decreased ratio signify an obstructive process.

Figure 25-4 displays normal, restrictive, and obstructive flow-volume curve patterns. The expiratory portion of the obstructive pattern, the **flow-volume loop,** demonstrates decreased flow rates for any given lung volume. Nonuniform emptying of the airway is reflected by a concave upward configuration of the curve. The flow-volume curve in the restrictive example appears relatively tall (preserved flow rates) but narrow (decreased lung volumes). Further definition of obstruction versus restriction components requires measurement of lung volumes.

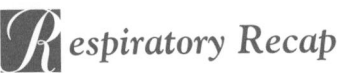espiratory Recap

FEV_1/FVC
The primary measures of flow in spirometry testing are FEV_1 and FEV_1/FVC.
FEV_1/FVC may indicate whether a reduced FEV_1 may be caused by restrictive disease.
Reduced FEV_1 and FEV_1/FVC indicate obstructive disease.
Reduced FEV_1 and normal or elevated FEV_1/FVC indicate restrictive disease.

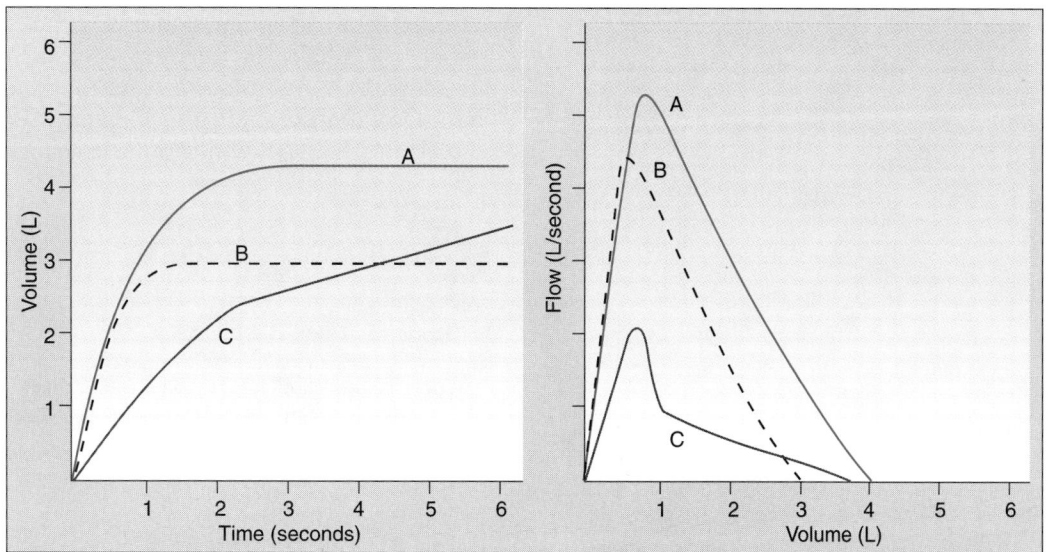

Figure 25-4 The volume-time curve is on the left, and the flow-volume curve is on the right, both showing a normal test (*A*), restrictive lung disease (*B*), and obstructive lung disease (*C*).

Midflow Rates

Other common measurements of maximum expiratory flow rates are FEF_{25-75}, FEF_{50}, FEF_{75}, and PEF. FEF_{25-75} is the average forced expiratory flow rate over the middle 50% of the FVC, whereas FEF_{50} is the flow rate precisely at mid-FVC (**midflow rate**) (see Figure 25-3). FEF_{50} and FEF_{25-75} are similar measurements, and both have been considered sensitive to early airway obstruction or small airway disease. Unfortunately, the variability of midflow measurements calls into question their usefulness. FEF_{75} is the flow after 75% of the FVC has been exhaled and may be a more precise indicator of small airway disease, but the values can be variable and the validity of the variable is questionable. PEF is the maximum flow rate attained during an FVC maneuver and usually is reported in liters per second. PEF can be easily measured with disposable, handheld devices. Although the PEF measurement is very dependent on patient effort, it can be a sensitive indicator of airway obstruction. For this reason the PEF is particularly valuable in home monitoring of patients with asthma. The serial monitoring of PEF can assess the adequacy of the medication regimen and detect exacerbation of the disease.

Tracing Quality

A careful examination of the quality of the spirometry tracing must precede any interpretation of the results. The standards for tracing quality and equipment specifications have been published by the ATS (see Box 25-3). This screening of tracing quality is best performed at the time of testing by the respiratory therapist.

Three acceptable efforts must be performed for the spirometry test to be valid. Four errors are commonly seen in the forced expiratory maneuver and require rejection of

the effort: delayed start, suboptimal effort, early cough, and early termination (Figure 25-5). These errors are relatively easy to distinguish. A delayed start is a pause or slow flow period before the peak flow is attained; the peak flow should occur promptly after the effort begins. This error will offset the timed parameters, $FEV_{0.5}$ and FEV_1. Therefore if a delayed start is identified, the effort must be rejected. A cough within the first second is easily identified as an abrupt change in flow rate during the maneuver. If the patient coughs slightly while bearing down (late cough), the tracing may be acceptable. A cough can alter any of the measured flow values, FEF_{50}, FEF_{75}, or PEF. Another error occurs when the patient disconnects early or stops pushing before the breath is entirely exhaled. This error, early termination, will underestimate VC and generate a falsely elevated FEV_1/FVC, thereby underestimating or not detecting an obstructive component. The patient must be instructed to keep pushing until the lungs are completely empty. A suboptimal effort can be detected by the lack of an elevated or sharp peak flow. A suboptimal effort also can underestimate all parameters. All these errors are correctable with coaching and patience, two keys to attaining good spirometry tracings. The patient must be clearly instructed to take the deepest breath and exhale as fast and long as possible. Most patients are ex-

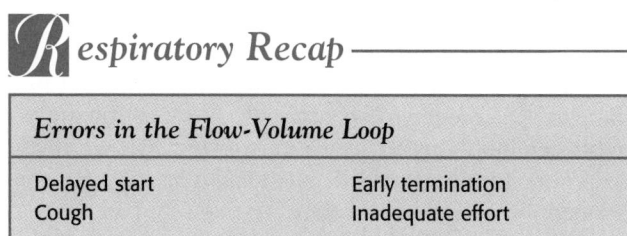

$\mathcal{R}$*espiratory Recap* ——————

Errors in the Flow-Volume Loop	
Delayed start	Early termination
Cough	Inadequate effort

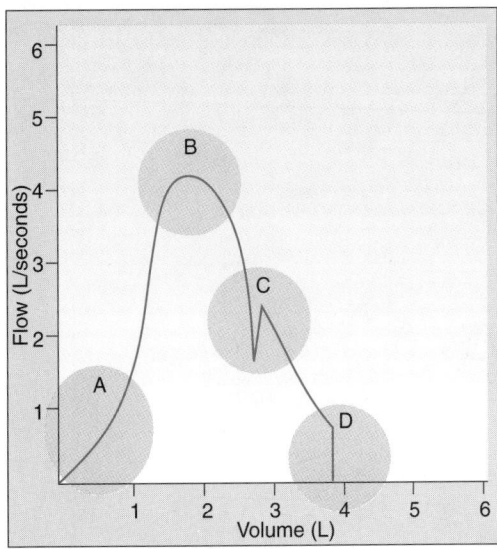

Figure 25-5 Common errors observed on flow-volume tracings: delayed start (*A*), suboptimal effort (*B*), cough (*C*), and early termination (*D*).

tremely cooperative and provide excellent tests with the proper instruction and coaching. However, some patients do have difficulties with the maneuvers. In these cases, re-instruction and a later attempt or a deferment of testing is always better than reporting of possibly questionable spirometry values. Although most modern spirometry systems have software algorithms to alert technicians to errors, the technicians must be aware of the ATS guidelines and the advantages or limitations of the system in use.

Maximum Voluntary Ventilation

The **maximum voluntary ventilation (MVV)** is the largest volume that can be moved in and out of the lungs by a maximal voluntary effort during a 12- to 15-second interval. This is a distinct, additional test that is now performed less frequently. A reduced MVV can evaluate pulmonary disability, but a low MVV can occur in obstructive, restrictive, neuromuscular, or heart disease. Spirometry and lung volume/capacity measurements further distinguish the type of pulmonary disability. In certain settings, MVV may have a role in the assessment of exercise capacity or breathing reserve.[5]

Bronchodilator Response

One important indication for spirometry is to determine whether airflow limitation is reversible. Will bronchodilator therapy be beneficial for the patients with airflow limitation? β-Adrenergic agents such as albuterol are the most commonly used medications to test bronchodilator response. Ideally, the patient should not take any prescribed bronchodilator before testing. Use of corticosteroids need not be discontinued. Spirometry should be

repeated 10 to 15 minutes after bronchodilator administration by inhaler or nebulizer. An increase in FEV_1 $\geq 12\%$ to 15% is considered significant and indicates reversibility. On occasion, the FVC increases after bronchodilator administration with little change in FEV_1.

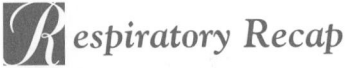

Respiratory Recap

Bronchodilator Response
A positive bronchodilator response is an increase in FEV_1 or FVC of greater than 15%. This response indicates airway reversibility.

Large Airway Obstruction

Obstructive lesions involving the major airway (carina to oropharynx) can be detected by changes in the flow-volume loop. If the lesion narrows the airway and decreases flow excessively during inspiration or expiration, it is categorized as a variable lesion. If the flow is decreased equally during inspiration and expiration, the lesion is fixed. A lesion above the thoracic outlet is extrathoracic, whereas a lesion between the thoracic outlet and the carina is intrathoracic.

Figure 25-6 shows three different patterns of large airway obstruction. With a variable extrathoracic obstruction such as vocal cord paralysis (Figure 25-6, *A*), the atmospheric pressure on inspiration exceeds intraluminal pressure, an inward collapse of the airway causes obstruction of flow, and the inspiratory portion of the curve is reduced. However, on expiration, intraluminal pressure is greater than atmospheric pressure and the airway remains patent. Thus the expiratory limb of the flow-volume curve is preserved.

In a variable intrathoracic obstruction such as tracheomalacia (see Figure 25-6, *B*), the intraluminal pressure on inspiration is greater than the pleural pressure and the airway remains patent. However, on expiration, the intraluminal pressure at the area of abnormality becomes less than the pleural pressure and the airway collapses, causing obstruction. The contour of the curve is normal during inspiration, but the expiratory limb of the curve is truncated, representing a reduction in airflow caused by obstruction. Therefore with an extrathoracic lesion, the expiratory flow is preserved whereas an intrathoracic le-

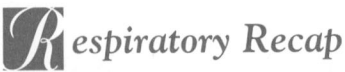

Respiratory Recap

Upper-Airway Lesions
Variable and fixed upper-airway lesions have distinct flow-volume loop patterns.

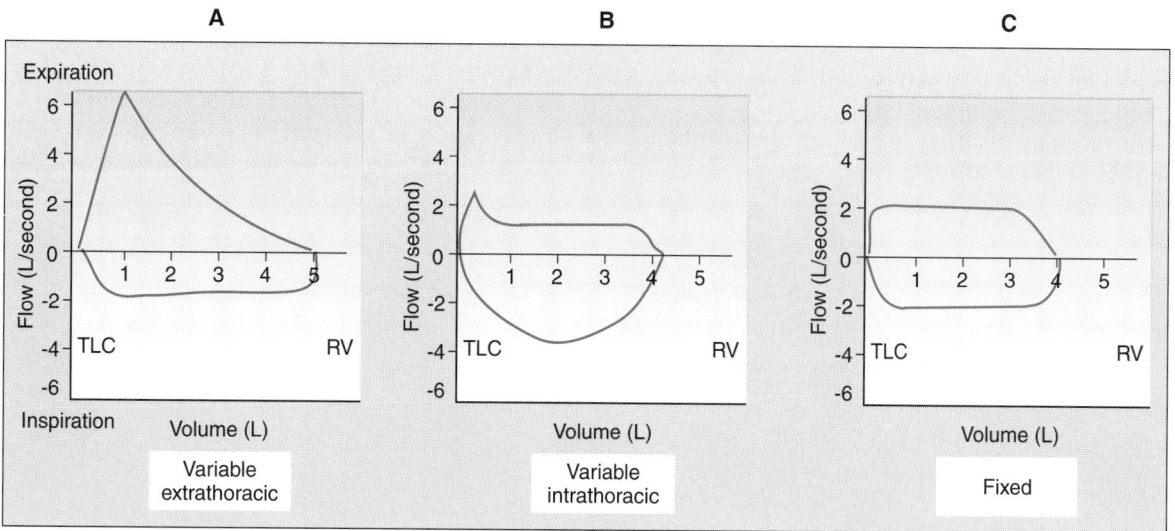

Figure 25-6 Upper-airway lesions on flow-volume curves. **A,** Variable extrathoracic obstruction. **B,** Variable intrathoracic obstruction. **C,** Fixed obstruction. *TLC,* Total lung capacity; *RV,* residual volume.

sion has a preserved inspiratory flow profile. A quantitative method used to identify the location of a variable lesion is to compare the forced expiratory midflow (FEF_{50}) with the forced inspiratory midflow (FIF_{50}). An extrathoracic lesion has a $FEF_{50}/FIF_{50} > 1$, and an intrathoracic lesion has a $FEF_{50}/FIF_{50} < 1$.

In a fixed intrathoracic or extrathoracic obstruction (such as tracheal stenosis, foreign body, or tumor), the intraluminal pressure remains constant during pleural and atmospheric pressure changes. Thus the flow-volume loop reflects a reduction in flow during both inspiration and expiration (see Figure 25-6, *C*).

Office Spirometry

Office spirometry testing was developed primarily to facilitate testing of all cigarette smokers more than 45 years old and those less than 45 years old with respiratory symptoms—nearly 60 million people.[6] However, the number of pulmonary function laboratories and their capacities to provide this testing are inadequate. The beneficial effects of smoking cessation on pulmonary function are now firmly established because smoking cessation is known to halt the rapid reduction in FEV_1 seen in smokers.[7,8] Furthermore, chronic obstructive pulmonary disease (COPD) can be detected at early stages in smokers with few symptoms.[7,8] The knowledge of spirometry testing results (and the opportunity to discourage smoking at that office visit) is expected to enhance smoking cessation rates. Therefore the National Lung Health Education Program (NLHEP) was formed to increase the awareness of lung health and develop office spirometry. Office spirometry will measure lung function to detect COPD and then provide a patient-doctor session for the purpose of encouraging smoking cessation.

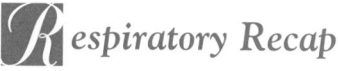

espiratory Recap

Office Spirometry

Introduced to facilitate testing of all smokers over 45 years old and those under 45 with respiratory symptoms.

A goal of office spirometry is to perform a less rigorously monitored spirometry test in primary care provider offices. The testing is relatively simple and affordable. Equipment to perform the testing could be modified by further automation to ease the requirements to validate a test. Therefore industry has been encouraged to manufacture spirometers that meet a different set of standards for office spirometry. Guidelines for office spirometry have been designed to shorten and simplify the testing sessions yet minimize the number of false-positive or false-negative tests. The current recommendations for office spirometry are:

1. The spirometers must report only the FEV_1, FEV_6, and FEV_1/FEV_6 ratios.
2. FEV_6 will replace FVC as an end of test criteria. Normal predicted values for FEV_6 are now available.[9] The FEV_6 shortens the testing session and avoids overexertion while attempting a FVC.
3. Airway obstruction will be detected when FEV_1/FEV_6 and FEV_1 are below the lower limit of normal as indicated (for example, by an asterisk) in the report.
4. The spirometer will display messages regarding the acceptability and reproducibility of the maneuvers.
5. The printout or hard-copy curves or tracings of testing is optional.

6. Alternatives to the use of 3-L calibration syringes can be developed.
7. FEV_1 and FEV_6 must be corrected to body temperature and pressure, saturated (BTPS).
8. Current recommendations to prevent cross-contamination should be followed.

Interpretation

Spirometry values are deceptively easy to obtain, yet the effort and cooperation by the patient must be excellent to interpret the results. The spirometry equipment must be meticulously maintained to be sure that equipment factors are not affecting the results. All technicians performing

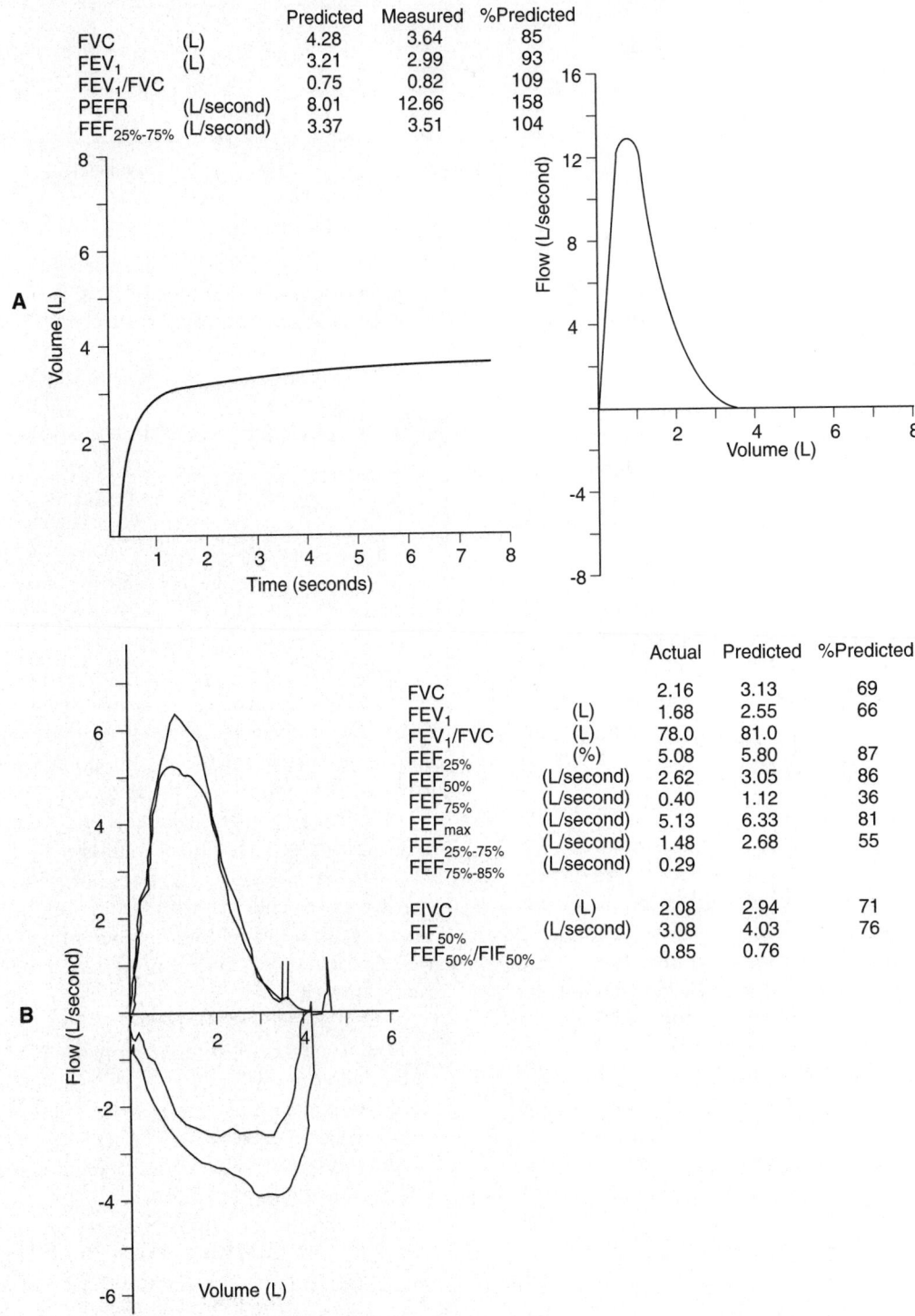

		Predicted	Measured	%Predicted
FVC	(L)	4.28	3.64	85
FEV_1	(L)	3.21	2.99	93
FEV_1/FVC		0.75	0.82	109
PEFR	(L/second)	8.01	12.66	158
$FEF_{25\%-75\%}$	(L/second)	3.37	3.51	104

		Actual	Predicted	%Predicted
FVC		2.16	3.13	69
FEV_1	(L)	1.68	2.55	66
FEV_1/FVC	(L)	78.0	81.0	
$FEF_{25\%}$	(%)	5.08	5.80	87
$FEF_{50\%}$	(L/second)	2.62	3.05	86
$FEF_{75\%}$	(L/second)	0.40	1.12	36
FEF_{max}	(L/second)	5.13	6.33	81
$FEF_{25\%-75\%}$	(L/second)	1.48	2.68	55
$FEF_{75\%-85\%}$	(L/second)	0.29		
FIVC	(L)	2.08	2.94	71
$FIF_{50\%}$	(L/second)	3.08	4.03	76
$FEF_{50\%}$/$FIF_{50\%}$		0.85	0.76	

Figure 25-7 Examples of spirometry tracings from patients. **A,** Normal. **B,** Restrictive lung disease.

the testing must strictly adhere to the policies and procedures used to obtain spirometry results, with particular attention to the quality of the tracings. The advantages of spirometry testing are the portability of the equipment and the relative ease to perform the tests.

The assessment and monitoring of restrictive and obstructive lung diseases requires spirometry information. The forced maneuvers provide the flow parameters FEV_1 and FEV_1/FVC. The FEV_1 and FEV_1/FVC are reproducible and valid measures used to assess the presence and degree of obstructive disease. A reduced FVC indicates a restrictive component. Lung volume/capacity studies are needed to provide additional information about a restrictive component of disease, such as a degree of air trapping or hyperinflation.

In addition to an initial assessment of obstructive or restrictive disease components, airway reversibility is an important part of spirometry testing. Also, **upper-airway lesions** can be identified by careful examination of the flow-volume curve. Examples of spirometry tracings interpreted as normal, obstructive disease, and restrictive disease are displayed in Figure 25-7.

Diffusing Capacity

The diffusing capacity of the lungs is the rate of gas diffusion across the alveolar-capillary membrane (CPG 25-4). A small concentration of CO is used in this test because its diffusing capacity (DLCO) is greater than that of oxygen. In North America, this test is commonly called the *diffusing capacity* (DLCO), whereas in Europe it is referred to as the *transfer factor* (TLCO).[10] The major factors influencing DLCO are the area and thickness of the alveolar-capillary membrane available for diffusion and pulmonary blood volume. Other factors that may alter DLCO but do not directly reflect the gas transfer properties of the lung are lung volume, anemia, inspired oxygen pressure, and carboxyhemoglobin level.

Respiratory Recap

> **Diffusion Testing**
>
> Diffusion testing measures the diffusing capacity of the lungs. The diffusing capacity indicates the quantity of gas that diffuses across the alveolar-capillary membrane.

Methods used to measure DLCO include the single breath with breath-holding technique, single-breath three-equation method, single breath with intrabreath analysis, rebreathing, and steady-state techniques.[4] The current choice for clinical use is the single breath with breath-holding DLCO, which is expressed as mL CO/min/mm Hg (normal is 25 mL CO/min/mm Hg). In this technique, the subject exhales to residual volume, then rapidly inhales a

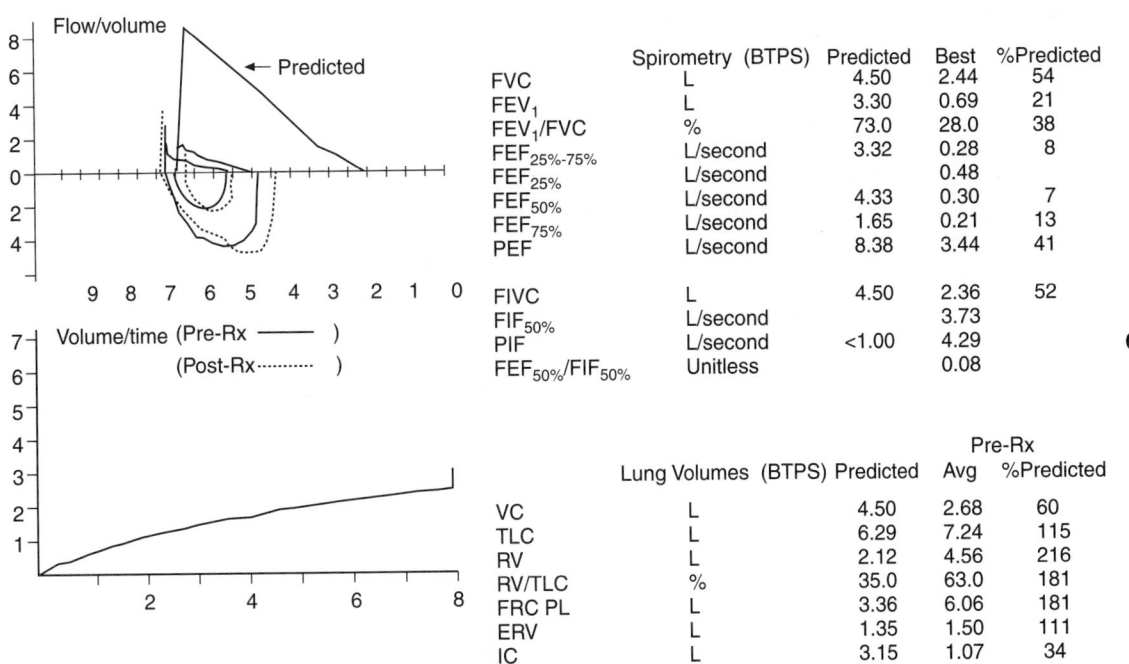

Spirometry (BTPS)		Predicted	Best	%Predicted
FVC	L	4.50	2.44	54
FEV$_1$	L	3.30	0.69	21
FEV$_1$/FVC	%	73.0	28.0	38
FEF$_{25\%-75\%}$	L/second	3.32	0.28	8
FEF$_{25\%}$	L/second		0.48	
FEF$_{50\%}$	L/second	4.33	0.30	7
FEF$_{75\%}$	L/second	1.65	0.21	13
PEF	L/second	8.38	3.44	41
FIVC	L	4.50	2.36	52
FIF$_{50\%}$	L/second		3.73	
PIF	L/second	<1.00	4.29	
FEF$_{50\%}$/FIF$_{50\%}$	Unitless		0.08	

			Pre-Rx	
Lung Volumes (BTPS)		Predicted	Avg	%Predicted
VC	L	4.50	2.68	60
TLC	L	6.29	7.24	115
RV	L	2.12	4.56	216
RV/TLC	%	35.0	63.0	181
FRC PL	L	3.36	6.06	181
ERV	L	1.35	1.50	111
IC	L	3.15	1.07	34

Figure 25-7—cont'd C, Obstructive lung disease. *FVC,* Forced vital capacity; *FEV₁,* forced expiratory volume in 1 second; *PEFR,* peak expiratory flow rate; *FEF₂₅%-₇₅%,* forced expiratory flow at 25% to 75% of FVC; *FIVC,* forced inspiratory vital capacity; *FIF,* forced inspiratory flow; *VC,* vital capacity; *TLC,* total lung capacity; *RV,* residual volume; *ERV,* expiratory reserve volume; *IC,* inspiratory capacity.

CPG 25-4

Single-Breath Carbon Monoxide Diffusing Capacity

Indications

Evaluation and follow-up of parenchymal lung diseases including idiopathic pulmonary fibrosis (IPF, also known as *usual interstitial pneumonitis* or *UIP*) and bronchiolitis obliterans organizing pneumonia (BOOP, or cryptogenic organizing pneumonia, COP), diseases associated with dusts such as asbestos, or drug reactions (for example, from amiodarone) or related to sarcoidosis; quantification of disability associated with interstitial lung disease

Evaluation and follow-up of emphysema and cystic fibrosis; differentiation among chronic bronchitis, emphysema, and asthma in patients with obstructive patterns; and quantification of impairment and disability

Evaluation of cardiovascular diseases (such as primary pulmonary hypertension, acute or recurrent thromboembolism, or pulmonary edema)

Evaluation of pulmonary involvement in systemic diseases (such as rheumatoid arthritis or systemic lupus erythematosus)

Evaluation of the effects of chemotherapy agents or other drugs (such as amiodarone or bleomycin) known to induce pulmonary dysfunction

Evaluation of pulmonary hemorrhage

Early indication of certain pulmonary infections (such as *Pneumocystis carinii* pneumonia)

Prediction of arterial desaturation during exercise in some patients with lung disease

Contraindications

Absolute contraindications: the presence of carbon monoxide toxicity or dangerous levels of oxyhemoglobin desaturation without supplemental oxygen

Relative contraindications: mental confusion or muscular incoordination preventing the subject from adequately performing the maneuver; inability to obtain or maintain an adequate lip seal on the instrument mouthpiece; a large meal or vigorous exercise immediately before the test; smoking within 24 hours of test administration (may have a direct effect on DLCO independent of the effect of COHb); decreased lung volumes that would not yield valid test results; devices that are improperly calibrated or maintained; the unavailability of a qualified operator

Hazards and Complications

Diffusion of the lungs for carbon dioxide-single breath (DLCOSB) requires breath-holding at total lung capacity (TLC); some patients may perform either a Valsalva (higher than normal intrathoracic pressure) or Müller (lower than normal intrathoracic pressure) maneuver. Either of these can result in alteration of venous return to the heart and pulmonary capillary blood volume.

Interruption of supplemental oxygen may result in oxyhemoglobin desaturation.

Transmission of infection is possible through improperly cleaned mouthpieces or as a consequence of the inadvertent spread of droplet nuclei or body fluids (patient-to-patient or patient-to-technologist).

Modified from AARC Clinical practice guideline: single-breath carbon monoxide diffusing capacity. Respir Care 1999;44:539-546.
CPG, Clinical practice guideline.

full breath of a test gas comprising about 0.3% CO and an inert gas such as 10% helium. The breath is held for 9 to 11 seconds and then exhaled rapidly into a collection bag or chamber. Measurements include the volume of inspired test gas, breath-hold time, and the inspired and expired alveolar gas concentrations for CO and the inert gas. A diffusion coefficient (DLCO/VA) can be calculated to provide normalization of DLCO for alveolar volume, but its value has been questioned.[11]

Usually, an increased DLCO is not a concern. However, some interesting causes of an increased DLCO include use of the supine position, exercise, asthma, obesity, polycythemia, intraalveolar hemorrhage, and left-to-right intracardiac shunts. Causes of decreased DLCO are listed in Box 25-4. Keep in mind that many technical and biologic variables can alter DLCO. Therefore measuring and interpreting the test requires very careful control of test quality.[12]

Specialized Pulmonary Function Tests

Several tests of specific aspects of lung function are performed in larger pulmonary function laboratories. These tests are not considered in the context of routine outpatient testing and can be useful to help further classify the cause, type, or degree of pulmonary disability.

Bronchial Challenge Testing

Bronchial challenge testing (BCT) determines the extent of airway hyperreactivity to a challenge (CPG 25-5). The most common indications for BCT are normal results of spirometry with either (1) a history suggesting asthma with occasional wheezing, chronic cough, night symptoms, or episodic chest tightness, (2) unexplained decrease in exercise tolerance, or (3) detection of the allergic and occupational agents which trigger symptoms.

CPG 25-5

Bronchial Provocation

Indications

Diagnose or confirm a diagnosis of airway hyperreactivity (asthma).

Follow changes in hyperresponsiveness.

Document the severity of hyperresponsiveness.

Determine who is at risk in the military or workplace.

Establish a control or baseline before a series of environmental or occupational exposures.

Contraindications

Relative contraindications are existence of ventilatory impairment at the time of the proposed challenge, FEV_1 <80% of previously recorded best value, $FEV_1/FVC\%$ <70%, FEV_1 <1.0 L in adults, significant response to the diluent (>10% fall in FEV_1 from baseline, upper- or lower-respiratory-tract infection within previous weeks, specific antigen exposure within previous week, exposure to high atmospheric pollution levels within previous week, pregnancy (the effect on the fetus is unknown).

Subject's inability to perform acceptable spirometry (based on ATS guidelines) at baseline, during postdiluent measurements (such as variability in FEV_1 > ±5%), or both.

Failure to withhold medications that may affect the bronchial reactivity test. Recommended periods for withholding medications are β_2-adrenergic aerosols, 12 hours; anticholinergic aerosols, 12 hours; disodium cromoglycate, 8 hours; oral β_2-adrenergic agonists, 12 hours; theophyllines, 48 hours; H_1-receptor antagonists, 48 hours; antihistamines, 72 to 96 hours. Corticosteroids (inhaled or oral) have been shown to decrease hyperresponsiveness. Duration of effect is unknown but may be prolonged. β-blockers may increase response, but duration of effect is unknown. Managing physician should be consulted before test is performed.

Other factors that may confound results include ingestion of cola drinks, chocolate, and other agents containing caffeine or theobromines; smoking; or occupational exposure to antigens.

Hazards and Complications

Bronchoconstriction, hyperinflation, or severe coughing

Hazards associated with spirometry, such as dizziness, light-headedness, or chest pain

Systemic hypotension and flushing from histamine

Possible exposure of technicians to provocative substances

Modified from AARC Clinical practice guideline: bronchial provocation. Respir Care 1992;37:902-906.
CPG, Clinical practice guideline.

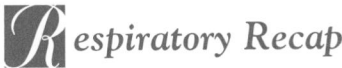

Respiratory Recap

Methacholine Challenge Test

The methacholine challenge test is indicated when results from spirometry are normal yet the history suggests airway reactivity.

BCT requires careful and detailed standardization.[13] Methacholine and histamine are bronchoconstricting agents that act directly and predominantly on smooth muscle in the airway. Other stimuli of airway reactivity depend on the involvement of cellular or neurogenic mechanisms, indirectly leading to smooth muscle contraction and possibly inflammatory changes in the airway wall (for example, nonisotonic aerosols, cold or dry air, or exercise). Inflammatory mechanisms predominate after challenge with sensitizing agents, particularly during late asthmatic reactions (such as allergens or occupational sensitizers). Therefore methacholine or histamine is used most frequently in BCT. It is not surprising that the results of the different challenge tests are only weakly correlated because each test probably provides different and comple-

Box 25-4

Causes of Decreased DlCO

Obstructive lung diseases

Cystic fibrosis

Interstitial lung diseases

Fibrogenic dusts (asbestosis)

Drug reactions (amiodarone, bleomycin)

Pulmonary involvement in systemic diseases

Progressive systemic sclerosis

Rheumatoid arthritis

Wegener's granulomatosis

Cardiovascular diseases

Chronic renal failure

Primary pulmonary hypertension

Acute and recurrent pulmonary thromboembolism

Fat embolization

Chronic hemodialysis

Acute and chronic ethanol ingestion

Cigarette smoking

Emphysema

Parenchymal lung diseases

Sarcoidosis

Biologic dusts (allergic alveolitis)

Idiopathic

Systemic lupus erythematosus

Mixed connective tissue disease

Dermatomyositis-polymyositis

Inflammatory bowel disease

Acute myocardial infarction

Mitral stenosis

Pulmonary edema

Diseases associated with anemia

Marijuana smoking

Cocaine freebasing

Bronchiolitis obliterans with organizing pneumonia

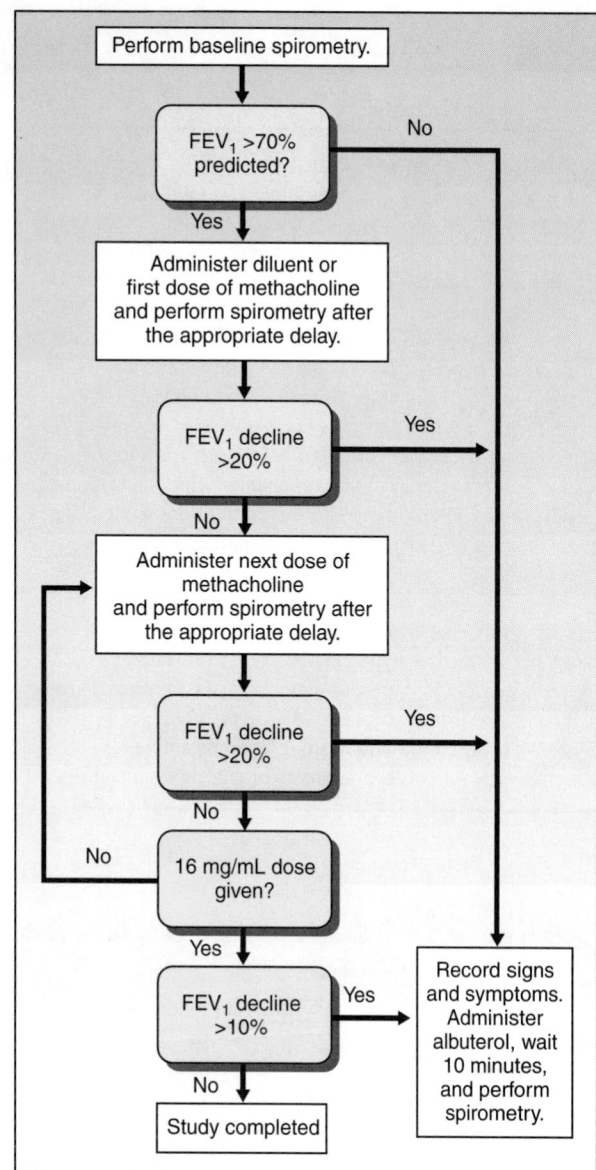

Figure 25-8 Algorithm for performance of methacholine challenge testing. *FEV₁*, Forced expiratory volume in 1 second. (Modified from Crapo RO, Casaburi R, Coates AL, et al. Guidelines for methacholine and exercise challenge testing—1999. Am J Respir Crit Care Med 2000;161:309-329.) *TLC,* Total lung capacity; *RV,* residual volume.

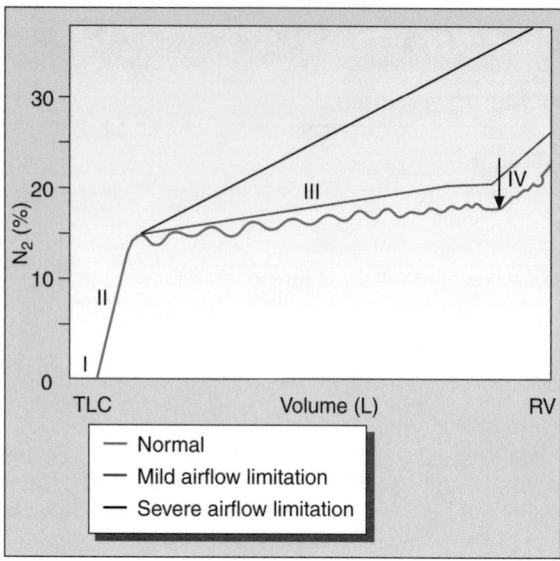

Figure 25-9 Single-breath nitrogen (N₂) test for distribution of ventilation with normal lung function, mild obstructive lung disease, and significant maldistribution of ventilation. *TLC,* Total lung capacity; *RV,* residual volume.

after exercise challenge should not exceed a 10% fall from the baseline value.

Airway Resistance

Airway resistance (R_{aw}) measurements can complement other tests evaluating airway responsiveness to bronchial provocation or bronchodilation. R_{aw} is the pressure difference developed per unit flow as gas flows in or out of the lungs and is normally 2.4 cm H_2O/L/second at 0.5 L/second. The most common method used to assess R_{aw} is the interrupter method in a body plethysmograph.[18] R_{aw} and FRC usually are measured in the same testing session when flow and pressure changes are being measured during panting and the flow is then interrupted by an airway occlusion. Conductance (G_{aw}) is the reciprocal of R_{aw} and is the flow generated per unit of pressure drop across the airway.

Ventilation Distribution

The simplest test of ventilation distribution is the **single-breath nitrogen test.** This test involves a maximal inspiration of 100% oxygen followed by a slow exhalation to RV. The slow, complete exhalation is directed by a one-way valve through a nitrogen meter and into a spirometer. The nitrogen meter continuously records the nitrogen concentration of the expired gas and simultaneously plots the expired nitrogen concentration against expired volume on an x-y plotter.[23] The normal curve has four important portions (Figure 25-9). Phase I is dead space gas, phase II is mixed gas (dead space and alveolar), phase III is alveolar gas, and phase IV is closing volume.

mentary information on the multiple pathways leading to airway reactivity.[14]

The most frequently performed BCT uses methacholine by a standardized protocol (Figure 25-8). The lung function measurement of reactivity is a 20% reduction in FEV₁, signifying a reaction. Standardized bronchoprovocation tests also may be performed by challenging with exercise, cold air, hypertonic or hypotonic aerosols, or allergens.[15-17] The majority of the standardized bronchoprovocation tests have reference values that differ from each other; for example, a reduction in FEV₁

For many years, phase III has been recognized as an index of nonuniform ventilation. The slope of phase III is normally 1% to 2.5% nitrogen per liter expired. This value increases in older adults. The onset of phase IV is considered an indication of the onset of airway closure in the dependent regions and often is called the *closing volume*. With the onset of obstructive lung disease, closing volume and the slope of phase III are increased. If the distribution of ventilation becomes nonuniform, the slope of phase III becomes steeper. In advanced obstructive disease, phase IV becomes lost in the very steep slope of phase III. In obstructive lung disease, the distribution of ventilation worsens because regional differences in airway resistance and airspace compliance affect the rate at which airspace empties and fills. In fact, this maldistribution may be an earlier manifestation of obstructive lung disease than spirometric changes.

Respiratory Muscle Strength

The most useful and practical test of respiratory muscle strength is the **maximum inspiratory (PI_{max}) and expiratory (PE_{max}) pressures.** PI_{max} is measured from RV and is the greatest subatmospheric pressure that can be developed during inspiration against an occluded airway. PE_{max} is the highest pressure that can be developed during a forceful expiratory effort against an occluded airway. PE_{max} is measured from TLC. The serial evaluation over time of PI_{max} and PE_{max} can provide insight as to the progression or regression of muscle weakness. Normal values for PI_{max} and PE_{max} are -84 cm H_2O and $+188$ cm H_2O in a 65-year-old male.[19]

The maximum transdiaphragmatic pressure (PDI_{max}) test provides the measurement of the strength of the diaphragm and is the best index of diaphragmatic intramuscular tension, the pressure developed across the diaphragm, and is the method of choice for the diagnosis of severe diaphragmatic weakness and bilateral diaphragmatic paralysis. It requires the simultaneous measurement of esophageal (Pes) and gastric pressures (Pga) by use of balloon catheters placed in the midesophagus and in the stomach, respectively. Pdi is calculated as the difference between Pga and Pes, measured at isotime during a maximal voluntary effort. A $Pdi_{max} >100$ cm H_2O is not associated with muscle weakness and thus cannot be the cause of ventilatory failure.[20] Another method used to measure the pressure generating capacity of diaphragm is the **sniff test.**[21] Values more negative than -80 cm H_2O represent a good force and respiratory muscle weakness is unlikely to be present. The major advantages of this test are that it is practical and easy.

Phrenic nerve stimulation consists of a supramaximal bilateral stimulation of the phrenic nerves (electrically or magnetically) at the neck with surface electrodes that results in a single brisk diaphragmatic contraction (twitch) pressure.[22] Measurement of the time interval from nerve stimulation until the beginning of the compound muscle action potential (CMAP) provides the phrenic nerve velocity of conduction. Absence of CMAP indicates phrenic nerve transaction or neuromuscular junction failure.

Respiratory Muscle Coordination

Muscle coordination can be assessed with respiratory **inductance plethysmography (IP).**[24,25] With the use of this system, rib cage and abdominal bands or magnetometers are used to obtain noninvasive, simultaneous recordings of the volume displacement of each of the two compartments. IP can monitor occurrence of apnea, hyperpnea, and irregular, rapid, shallow patterns of breathing. Nonsynchronous and paradoxical thoracoabdominal movements can be identified through a variety of experimental and clinical conditions. When well calibrated, IP can measure tidal volume and minute ventilation within 5% to 10% of the values obtained through measurements at the mouth by spirometry.

𝒦EY 𝒫OINTS

- Decreases in lung volumes and capacities generally indicate restrictive lung disease.
- Increases in residual volume and RV/TLC indicate air trapping, whereas an increase in TLC indicates hyperinflation.
- Although spirometry testing is relatively simple to perform, the obtaining of a valid test requires attentive, vigorous coaching and careful scrutiny of the tracings.
- Spirometry evaluates the forced expiratory maneuvers, which allows evaluation of flow rates from the lungs.
- Reductions in flow rates (FEV_1 and FEV_1/FVC) indicate obstructive disease.
- A reduction in FVC or FEV_1 with a normal FEV_1/FVC indicates restrictive lung disease.
- An examination of the flow-volume curve can detect the presence of an upper-airway lesion.
- Office spirometry, an abbreviated version of outpatient spirometry testing, has been recommended to facilitate the testing of all smokers over 45 years of age.
- Diffusing capacity testing evaluates disturbances in the gas exchange diffusion area (the alveolar capillary membrane).
- Specialized pulmonary function tests are used to evaluate airway reactivity, airway resistance, respiratory muscle strength and coordination, and distribution of ventilation.

References

1. Gardner RM, Clausen JL, Epler G, et al. Pulmonary function laboratory personnel qualifications. Am Rev Respir Dis 1986; 134:623-624.

2. Hutchinson J. On the capacity of the lungs, and on the respiratory functions, with a view of establishing a precise and easy way of detecting disease by the spirometer. Med Chir Trans 1846;29:137.

3. Hyatt RE, Scanlon PD, Nakamura M. Interpretation of pulmonary function tests: a practical guide. Philadelphia: Lippincott-Raven; 1997.

4. Ruppel GE. Manual of pulmonary function testing, 6th ed. St Louis: Mosby; 1994.

5. Weisman IM, Zeballos RJ. An integrated approach to the interpretation of cardiopulmonary exercise testing. Clin Chest Med 1994;15:421-425.

6. Ferguson GT, Enright PL, Buist AS, Higgins MW. Office spirometry for lung health assessment in adults: a consensus statement from the National Lung Health Education Program. Respir Care 2000;45:513-530.

7. Enright PL, Johnson LR, Connett JE, et al. Spirometry in the lung health study: methods and quality control. Am Rev Respir Dis 1991;143:1215-1223.

8. Anthonisen NR, Connett JE, Kiley JP, et al. Effects of smoking intervention and the use of an inhaled anticholinergic bronchodilator on the rate of decline in FEV_1: the lung health study. JAMA 1997;277:246-253.

9. Hankinson JL, Odencranz JR, Fedan FB. Spirometric reference values from a sample of the general U.S. population. Am J Respir Crit Care Med 1999;159:179-187.

10. Cotes JE, Chinn DJ, Quanjer PH, et al. Standardization of the measurement of transfer factor (diffusing capacity): official statement of the European Respiratory Society. Eur Respir J 1993;6(Suppl 16):41-52.

11. Crapo RO. Carbon monoxide diffusing capacity (transfer factor). Sem Respir Crit Care Med 1998;19:335-345.

12. American Thoracic Society. Single-breath carbon monoxide diffusing capacity (transfer factor) recommendations for a standard technique—1995 update. Am J Respir Crit Care Med 1995;152:2185-2198.

13. Sterk PJ. Bronchoprovocation testing. Sem Respir Crit Care Med 1998;19:317-323.

14. Crapo RO, Casaburi R, Coates AL, et al. Guidelines for methacholine and exercise challenge testing—1999. Am J Respir Crit Care Med 2000;161:309-329.

15. Smith CM, Anderson SD. Inhalation provocation tests using nonisotonic aerosols. J Allergy Clin Immunol 1989;84:781-900.

16. Cockroft DW, Murdock KY, Kirby J, et al. Prediction of airway responsiveness to allergen from skin sensitivity to allergen and airway responsiveness to histamine. Am Rev Respir Dis 1987;135:264-267.

17. Inman MD, Watson R, Cockroft DW, et al. Reproducibility of allergen-induced early and late asthmatic responses. J Allergy Clin Immunol 1995; 95:1191-1195.

18. Bates JHT, Milic-Emili J. The flow interruption technique for measuring respiratory resistance. J Crit Care 1991;6:227-238.

19. Sandqvist L, Kjellmer I. Normal values for the single-breath nitrogen elimination test in different age groups. Scand J Clin Lab Invest 1960;12:131-135.

20. Enright PL, Kronmal RA, Manolio TA, et al. Respiratory muscle strength in the elderly: correlates and reference values. Cardiovascular health study research group. Am J Respir Crit Care Med 1994;149(2 Pt 1):430-438.

21. Bellemare F, Grassino A. Effect of pressure and timing of contraction on human diaphragmatic fatigue. J Appl Physiol 1982;53:1190-1195.

22. Miller JM, Moxham J, Green M. The maximal sniff in the assessment of diaphragmatic function in man. Clin Sci 1985; 69:91-96.

23. Similowski T, Fleury B, Launois S, et al. Cervical magnetic stimulation: a new painless method for bilateral phrenic nerve stimulation in conscious humans. J Appl Physiol 1989;67:1311-1318.

24. Tobin MJ. Monitoring respiratory mechanics in spontaneously breathing patients. In: Tobin MJ, editor. Principles and practice of intensive care monitoring. New York: McGraw Hill; 1998.

25. Tobin MJ, Perez W, Guenther SM, et al. Does rib cage abdominal paradox signify respiratory muscle fatigue? J Appl Physiol 1987;63:851-860.

CHAPTER 26

Hemodynamic and Gas Exchange Monitoring

James E. Ramage, Jr.

CHAPTER OUTLINE

OBJECTIVES

1. Discuss the clinical importance of monitoring heart rate and rhythm.
2. Compare noninvasive and invasive techniques used to monitor arterial blood pressure.
3. Discuss the roles of arterial blood pressure, central venous pressure, and pulmonary artery pressure in hemodynamic monitoring.
4. Describe the structure of the pulmonary artery catheter.
5. Compare techniques used to measure respiratory rate and pattern.
6. Explain how blood gas monitors measure blood gases and pH.
7. Discuss the operating principles, clinical usefulness, and limitations of transcutaneous monitoring, pulse oximetry, and capnography.
8. Describe methods used to monitor tissue perfusion.
9. Describe the operating principles of sensors and transducers used for monitoring.
10. Describe methods of signal transmission in monitors.
11. Describe techniques used for signal processing in monitors.

KEY TERMS

Analog-to-Digital Converter	Fick Equation	Oxygen Extraction Ratio (O_2ER)
Arterial Blood Pressure	Fractional Saturation	Photoplethysmography
Beer-Lambert Law	Functional Saturation	Piezoelectric Plethysmography
Bioimpedance	Gastric Tonometry	Pulmonary Artery Catheter (PAC)
Capnogram	Holter Monitor	Pulmonary Artery Wedge Pressure
Capnography	Impedance Pneumography	(PAWP)
Capnometry	Invasive	Pulse Oximetry
Central Venous Pressure (CVP)	Mass Spectrometer	Raman Spectroscopy
End-Tidal P_{CO_2} ($P_{ET}CO_2$)	Oxygen Consumption	Respiratory Inductance
Fiberoptic Plethysmography	Oxygen Delivery	Plethysmography (RIP)

$\mathcal{K}$EY TERMS—cont'd

Spectrophotometry	Thermistors	Transcutaneous Monitoring
Strain Gauge	Thermocouples	Transducer
Telemetry	Thermodilution	Wheatstone Bridge

Monitoring can be defined as a continuous or nearly continuous evaluation of a patient's physiologic functions to guide management decisions, including when therapeutic interventions are warranted and assessment of those interventions. Monitoring can be **invasive** or noninvasive, and it is an important aspect of the care of patients with cardiopulmonary disease.

Hemodynamic Monitoring

A list of hemodynamic variables and their normal ranges are presented in Table 26-1.

Cardiac Rate and Rhythm

As one of the four vital signs, the heart rate provides a readily accessible bedside measure of the patient's cardiovascular status. With electrocardiographic (ECG) techniques, cardiac rhythms can be displayed, transmitted to a central monitoring area, printed, and stored for later review.

$\mathcal{T}$ABLE 26-1

Normal Ranges for Certain Hemodynamic Measurements

Variable	Units	Normal Range
Systolic blood pressure (SBP)	mm Hg	100 to 140
Diastolic blood pressure (DBP)	mm Hg	60 to 90
Mean arterial pressure (MAP)	mm Hg	70 to 105
Pulmonary artery systolic pressure (PASP)	mm Hg	15 to 30
Pulmonary artery diastolic pressure (PADP)	mm Hg	4 to 12
Mean pulmonary artery pressure (MPAP)	mm Hg	9 to 16
Right ventricular systolic pressure (RVSP)	mm Hg	15 to 30
Right ventricular end-diastolic pressure (RVEDP)	mm Hg	0 to 8
Central venous pressure (CVP)	mm Hg	0 to 8
Pulmonary artery wedge pressure (PAWP)	mm Hg	2 to 12
Cardiac output (CO)	L/min	Varies with size of patient

From Nelson LD. The new pulmonary artery catheters: right ventricular ejection fraction and continuous cardiac output. Crit Care Clin 1996;12:795.

The heart rate is controlled by electrical impulses that arise regularly at the sinus node in the right atrium. The normal resting heart rate is 50 to 90 beats/min. It accelerates during exercise and slows during sleep as a result of the direct influence of the autonomic nervous system on the sinus node. During exercise or with pain or anxiety, for example, the sympathetic nerves act on the sinus node to increase the heart rate. Parasympathetic, or *vagal*, effects slow the rate. Cardiac *arrhythmias* (excessively fast or slow rates and irregular rhythms) frequently occur during the course of critical illness, especially during cardiopulmonary failure, myocardial infarction, and toxic overdose.

The heart rate can be estimated at the bedside by counting of the peripheral pulses, and the radial pulse is most commonly used for this purpose. It is counted for 15 to 30 seconds and multiplied to equal beats per minute. However, obtaining an accurate pulse in critically ill patients can be difficult. In hypotensive patients, the only palpable pulses may be over the carotid or femoral arteries. In patients with cardiac arrhythmias, peripheral pulses may vary in intensity because of poor transmission of the irregular beats. In these cases the apical heartbeat should be auscultated to obtain an accurate measurement.

With ECG electrodes, cardiac electrical activity can be detected at the skin surface and processed to display the heart rate and waveforms. The electrodes are applied to the chest and extremities in standardized arrays (Figure 26-1). In the past, electrodes were made of brass plates coated with a conducting paste held against the skin by straps or suction cups. Modern electrodes have a silver–silver chloride metal contact button or wafer secured to the skin surface with an adhesive foam or plastic backing. The electrode array is connected directly to the bedside monitor or ECG machine or is plugged into a radio transmitter that sends the signals to a central telemetry console.

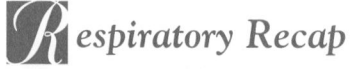

$\mathcal{R}$*espiratory Recap*

Cardiac Monitoring
Bedside ICU monitors measure the heart rate and detect arrhythmias. Telemetry is used for cardiac monitoring outside the ICU. Holter monitors are used for ambulatory patients.

Cardiac monitoring is performed in a variety of settings. For almost every patient in the intensive care unit (ICU),

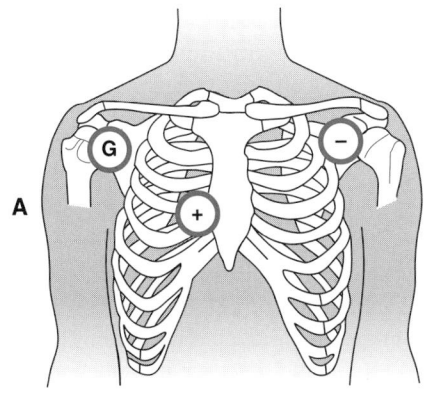

Figure 26-1 **A,** Electrode placement for three-lead array. **B,** Cardiac rate and rhythm recorded from a single ECG lead. **C,** Respiratory impedance plethysmography tracing obtained from the same electrode array.

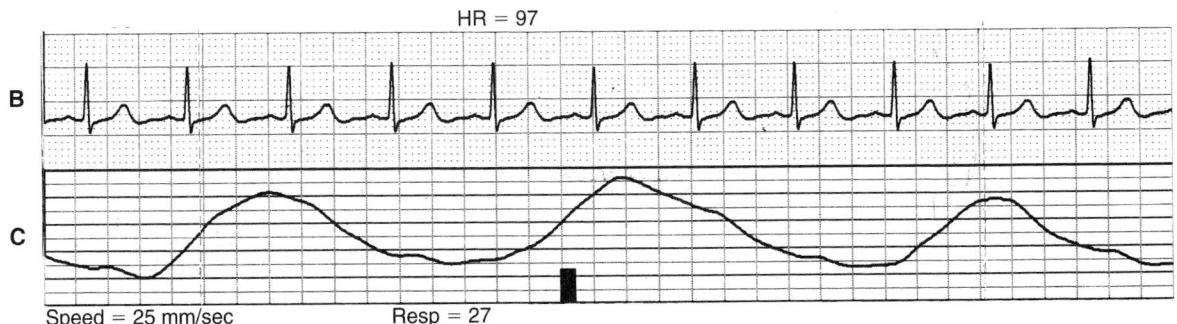

the heart rate and rhythm are displayed on a bedside monitor. These systems accurately measure the heart rate; identify dangerous arrhythmias, such as ventricular tachycardia and fibrillation; and recognize episodes of myocardial ischemia. They are equipped with audio and visual alarms that can trigger the printing of a rhythm strip or freeze the monitor screen for immediate review. Cardiac monitoring has improved the prognosis for patients admitted to the coronary care unit with acute myocardial infarction.[1] The impact in noncardiac units has been studied less extensively. In these other settings, cardiac monitors may provide an early warning system for patients with labile respiratory or neurologic disorders, allowing earlier intervention and perhaps reducing the severity of complications.

On hospital telemetry units, patients wear small electronic boxes to transmit the ECG to central monitoring stations; this has allowed early transfer of otherwise stable patients from the ICU to the comfort and convenience of private rooms. The patient's electrodes are connected by wires to a small radio transmitter at the bedside that encodes the ECG signals into radio frequency waves and transmits them to strategically placed antennas, then on to the receiving unit, where they are decoded for display and analysis. A specific VHF (54 to 216 MHz) or UHF (407 to 806 MHz) radio frequency is assigned to each monitored patient; these frequencies avoid channels or frequencies used by local television stations and other devices that also operate in the VHF and UHF spectra. Cellular phones do not operate in these frequency ranges and do not pose a problem for telemetry units.

A **Holter monitor** is a portable device that continuously records the heart rate and rhythm for ambulatory patients over several days. Even longer recording periods are possible if the patient activates the recording only during symptomatic events. Other ambulatory monitoring systems allow the patient to transmit the cardiac rhythm directly to the clinician over telephone lines with a modem.

Arterial Pressure

The **arterial blood pressure** is another of the four vital signs. Monitoring techniques for this vital sign include intermittent manual determinations with *sphygmomanometry*, automated, noninvasive devices, and indwelling arterial cannulas that provide continuous pressure measurements and waveform graphics.

Intravascular pressure is determined by blood flow and vascular tone or resistance, or pressure = flow × resistance. The arterial waveform consists of peak, or *systolic*, blood pressure corresponding to cardiac contraction, an anacrotic and dicrotic notch, and a nadir, or *diastolic*, blood pressure. The *anacrotic notch* is a reflected pressure wave that rebounds from the peripheral vessels. The *dicrotic notch* represents closure of the aortic valve. In the peripheral vessels a normal increase in elasticity and resistance results in a peaked and narrower waveform. Systolic pressure in the radial artery, therefore, is about 6 mm Hg higher than a simultaneous measurement in the brachial artery. This difference diminishes in patients with inelastic arteries, such as the elderly or those with vascular disease.[2,3]

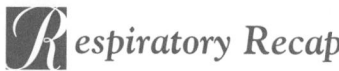

Respiratory Recap

Arterial Blood Pressure

Automated noninvasive systems are based on oscillometry or photoplethysmography; invasive systems use transducers attached to an intraarterial catheter.

Noninvasive methods used to measure blood pressure generally use a blood pressure cuff, which is gradually inflated around an extremity to a pressure above the systolic pressure and then slowly deflated while the artery is auscultated for *Korotkoff* sounds. The first and last of the five Korotkoff sounds represent systolic and diastolic blood pressure, respectively. Automated noninvasive blood pressure monitors program inflation and deflation of the cuff at selected intervals. Most of these systems are based on *oscillometry* and use a sensitive transducer to measure not only total cuff pressure but also the minute oscillations in the cuff caused by the pulsating vessel. The systolic and diastolic pressures are recognized by changes in oscillation intensity (Figure 26-2). These devices are available with

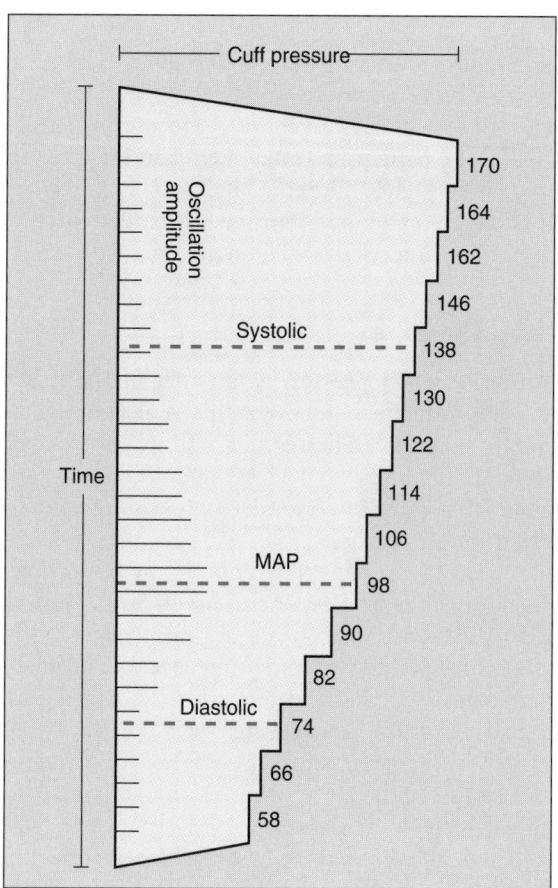

Figure 26-2 Noninvasive blood pressure measurements are derived from analysis of oscillation amplitude during a programmed cuff inflation-deflation cycle. (Modified from materials courtesy Critikon LLC, Tampa, Fla.)

programmable blood pressure intervals, memory, display, and print features. Portable units are available for use on hospital wards and plug-in modules for multifunctional critical care monitors. Manual and automated cuff measurements correlate well with simultaneous intraarterial values. However, in adults the first Korotkoff sound do not appear until 4 to 15 mm Hg below the intravascular systolic pressure, and the fifth sound disappear 3 to 6 mm Hg above the intravascular diastolic pressure.[2]

Photoplethysmography is another noninvasive method that uses a small finger cuff and a technique similar to pulse oximetry. A light source and detector are built into the cuff to measure the absorption of a specific wavelength of light passed across the arterial bed of the finger. The cuff inflates to eliminate the pulsatile component of absorption. At this point, cuff pressure equals intraarterial pressure, and the result displayed.

Noninvasive systems have certain limitations and complications. Poor-fitting cuffs may lead to measurement errors. Larger cuffs must be used with obese patients, because undersized cuffs can result in an overestimation of arterial pressure. In hypotensive, edematous, or vasoconstricted patients, automated systems may not be able to detect weakly transmitted blood pressure sounds. Programmable noninvasive systems have also been associated with ulnar palsies and extremity ischemia when used with frequent inflation-deflation cycles.

Intraarterial monitoring is indicated for critically ill patients with extremes of blood pressure requiring aggressive resuscitation efforts or titration of potent vasoactive agents. Small catheters, usually 18- or 20-gauge, are inserted into the radial, femoral, axillary, or brachial artery (in descending order of preference) based on ease of access and relative frequency of complications. The cannula is connected to a bedside pressure transducer, usually with a stopcock to allow intermittent arterial blood sampling.[4]

Some systematic differences exist between invasive and noninvasive pressure measurements. Normally, the intraarterial systolic pressure is 10% to 20% higher and the diastolic pressure lower in distal extremities because of changes in the elasticity and caliber of the arteries. This effect, known as *distal pulse amplification*, causes a widened pulse pressure without affecting mean arterial pressure. For patients who are rewarming after cardiopulmonary bypass or receiving vasopressors for septic shock, measurements obtained from the radial artery have been shown to underestimate central (femoral artery) pressures. Failure to recognize this phenomenon may lead to the inappropriate use of vasoactive agents.[5]

Intraarterial monitoring is associated with several well-recognized complications, including injury to the artery or adjacent nerves, bleeding, and ischemia and infection of the extremity. The radial artery generally is favored for placement of the indwelling cannulas because of its accessibility and the presence of vascular collateral circulation to the hand. The ulnar and brachial arteries are avoided, if possible, because of their tenuous and variable collateral blood flow.[4]

Central Venous Pressure

The **central venous pressure (CVP),** which is measured in the superior vena cava, is used to estimate intravascular volume status. Single-lumen or multilumen catheters are positioned in the superior vena cava via the subclavian or internal or external jugular vein to permit CVP monitoring and venous blood sampling. The femoral vein is also a commonly used access site, especially during emergencies. Although they cannot be reliably stabilized in the thoracic cavity, femoral catheters positioned in the common iliac vein or inferior vena cava have been shown to provide a reasonable estimate of CVP, at least in the absence of increased abdominal pressure or vena caval injury.[6]

In adults, central venous catheters usually measure 7 Fr (about 2.3 mm) in diameter and 16 to 20 cm in length. They are constructed of biocompatible plastics, most commonly polyethylene, Teflon, and polyurethane. All intravascular catheters are designed with certain important properties, including flexibility, a smooth surface, thromboresistance, lack of kink memory, and chemical stability.[7]

The CVP waveform has two major positive waves, *a* and *v*, which correspond to right atrial and ventricular contractions. To minimize respiratory effects, the CVP is always measured at end-exhalation at the midpoint of the *a* wave, which can be identified during the PR interval of a simultaneously recorded ECG strip. A normal CVP reading is 0 to 8 mm Hg, with a mean of 3 to 4 mm Hg.[8]

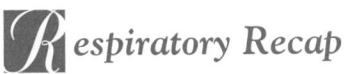
Respiratory Recap

Central Venous Pressure

CVP is measured in the superior vena cava.
The CVP reading is used to estimate intravascular volume status.
Central venous catheters can be used to obtain blood samples for laboratory analysis.

The CVP is particularly useful in volume-depleted states. Low values guide fluid and blood volume replacement in bleeding or hypovolemic patients. However, a normal or elevated CVP correlates poorly with intravascular volume status, especially for patients with heart and lung disease, and cannot be used reliably to guide therapy.

Central venous catheters are also used to monitor venous blood chemistries intermittently or continuously. Samples may be drawn periodically from the ports for laboratory analysis. Automated systems allow blood to be withdrawn through a dedicated port at clinician-selected intervals for bedside blood gas analysis, with the remainder of the sample flushed back to the patient to minimize losses. Venous pH and base deficit monitoring is helpful in the management of patients with metabolic acidosis, especially diabetic ketoacidosis.

Central venous catheterization is associated with several well-recognized complications. Mechanical complications related to insertion of the catheter include pneumothorax, bleeding, and injury to nerves, vessels, or the thoracic duct. Fewer complications are seen when the operator is skilled and ultrasound is used to identify the venous anatomy.[9] Malpositioned catheters can cause cardiac arrhythmias, valvular injury, chamber perforation, and cardiac tamponade. Increased risks of air embolism and thromboembolism are also factors. Infection can develop at the insertion site, sometimes resulting in bacteremia, especially with prolonged use. Antimicrobial-coated catheters have been developed to reduce the incidence of infectious complications.

Pulmonary Artery Catheters

The Swan-Ganz, or **pulmonary artery catheter (PAC),** is inserted through a central venous access sheath into the pulmonary artery (PA). It provides pressure measurements, cardiac output determinations, and mixed venous blood analysis. Special pulmonary artery catheters have been developed to allow cardiac pacing and mixed venous oximetry, as well as continuous measurement of cardiac output and the right ventricular ejection fraction. The PAC can be used to manage a wide variety of clinical problems,[8,10-13] but in randomized control trials, few of these have been established as indications that improve the outcome.[14]

The pulmonary artery catheter is inserted through one of the central veins with the percutaneous Seldinger technique and an introducer sheath. It usually is placed in the internal jugular or subclavian vein, although the femoral or cephalic vein also may be used. The internal jugular vein is convenient for intraoperative monitoring, because the catheter remains readily accessible to the anesthesiologist. In the ICU, where a pulmonary artery catheter may remain in place for longer periods, subclavian sites are easier to stabilize and keep sterile. The cephalic or femoral vein frequently is used in catheterization laboratories because it is easily accessible, the procedure is short term, fluoroscopy is available, and complications at these sites are uncommon.

The catheter has a balloon at the tip that is inflated with air, which allows blood flow to direct the catheter through the right ventricle into the pulmonary artery. The right internal jugular vein or the left subclavian vein may be the easiest site to use in difficult access conditions, such as pulmonary hypertension. These approaches take advantage of the predesigned curve of the catheter. Fluoroscopy may be necessary when the cephalic or femoral site is used because of the tortuous vascular pathway to the pulmonary artery. The standard adult thermodilution PAC is usually 7 to 7.5 Fr and approximately 110 cm long, with a balloon capacity of 1.5 mL. Smaller catheters are available for pediatric patients. From the internal jugular or subclavian vein in adults, the catheter generally is properly positioned at 45 to 60 cm.[10]

Pulmonary artery catheters have three or four ports for pressure measurements, thermodilution injections, and medication infusion. A proximal port 30 cm from the tip resides in the right atrium–superior vena cava, and a distal port is positioned at the tip in the pulmonary artery. The catheter tip balloon can be inflated intermittently to allow wedging in the distal pulmonary artery. The **pulmonary artery wedge pressure (PAWP)** provides an estimate of left atrial and left ventricular end-diastolic or filling pressure (LVEDP). Each anatomic position produces a characteristic waveform (Figure 26-3).

Respiratory Recap

Pulmonary Artery Catheters

PACs are used to measure the pulmonary artery pressure and the pulmonary artery wedge pressure.
Thermodilution catheters measure cardiac output.
Oximetry catheters measure the mixed venous oxygen saturation.
Blood samples from pulmonary artery catheters are used to measure mixed venous blood gases..

The right atrial (RA) pressure is similar to the CVP in the adjacent superior vena cava, because these structures are contiguous without interrupting valves. Normal RA pressure is 0 to 6 mm Hg. The right ventricular (RV) and pulmonary artery systolic pressure (RVSP and PASP) and diastolic pressure (RVDP and PADP) represent the peak and trough of these waveforms, respectively. Normal RV pressures are 17 to 30 mm Hg systolic and 0 to 6 mm Hg diastolic. Normal PA pressures are 15 to 30 mm Hg systolic, 4 to 12 mm Hg diastolic, and mean of 9 to 16 mm Hg. The RVSP usually equals the PASP, because the pulmonary valve is open during right ventricular contraction. During diastole the valve closes, and the PADP remains higher than the RVDP as the right ventricle relaxes and fills from the right atrium.[8,10,13]

The pulmonary artery wedge pressure is similar to the CVP and RA waveform. It has a positive *a* and *v* wave. The PAWP *a* wave occurs during the R wave of a simultaneously recorded ECG. The normal PAWP is 2 to 12 mm Hg. The midpoint of the *a* wave at end-exhalation is used to estimate the PAWP value. The PADP often approximates the PAWP, unless pulmonary vascular resistance is elevated (precapillary pulmonary hypertension). Recognizing this relationship can reduce the number of balloon inflations and catheter manipulations.

Bedside ICU monitors have internal computation software to smooth the waveforms and discard artifactual swings caused by patient coughing or movements. The average pressure values are then calculated and displayed. Special care must be taken to obtain accurate values for subsequent hemodynamic calculations. The pressure waveforms should be printed and inspected directly to confirm the computer-generated data. Measurements are taken at the end-exhalation point in the respiratory cycle

(*function residual capacity*, or FRC) to minimize the effect of airway pressure on the waveforms.

Catheters are equipped with thermistors, located 3.5 to 4 cm from the tip, which allow measurement of cardiac output by **thermodilution.** When a saline bolus (V) of known temperature ($T°_0$) is injected proximally and its temperature is measured as it passes the distal portion of the catheter ($T°_B$), cardiac output can be calculated from the following mathematic relationship: [10]

$$\text{Cardiac output} = \frac{[V(T°_B - T°_0) \times K]}{\int T°_B(t)}$$

where K is a constant based on the design of the catheter, and t is time. The thermistor tip must be in the pulmonary artery for an accurate measurement. Five mL of iced saline (or 10 mL of room temperature saline) is injected at end-exhalation to reduce the effect of intrathoracic pressure on cardiac output. The procedure is repeated three to five times to obtain an average value.

To obtain accurate and reproducible pressure measurements, the bedside clinician must zero the catheter. The pressure transducer is leveled at the midaxillary line, or *phlebostatic position*, in the fourth intercostal space, preferably with the patient in the supine position. A stopcock adjacent to the transducer is opened to air, and the monitor is adjusted to display zero. The skin may be marked at this point to ensure reproducibility. Disposable pressure transducers need only a single point calibration (zero), because they are manufactured with a specified linear response through the physiologic range. Reusable pressure transducers require intermittent two-point calibration, because their response characteristics may change over time. Two-point (external) calibration is performed by application of a known pressure at the upper end of the expected measurement range. External calibration requires more time and skill but should be used periodically to confirm the linearity and compatibility of any type of transducer, disposable or reusable, with the bedside monitor unit. Once calibration is complete, the transducer must remain at the zero reference level relative to the patient to measure pressure accurately. For example, if the transducer is moved 20 cm below the zero reference site, the measured pressure will be falsely increased by 20 cm H_2O.

The catheter must also be properly positioned in the pulmonary artery. After insertion, placement should be confirmed by a chest radiograph. If the distance between the proximal injector port and the thermistor is altered (for example, by catheter looping in the right ventricle), the cardiac output calculations will be incorrect. The catheter also tends to migrate outward into the pulmonary artery as it warms to body temperature. Distal positioning increases the risk of PA rupture during balloon inflation. As a precaution, the operator should always observe the PA pressure waveform as the balloon is slowly inflated. If the PAWP waveform is observed before two thirds of the balloon volume has been inflated (for example, 1 mL in

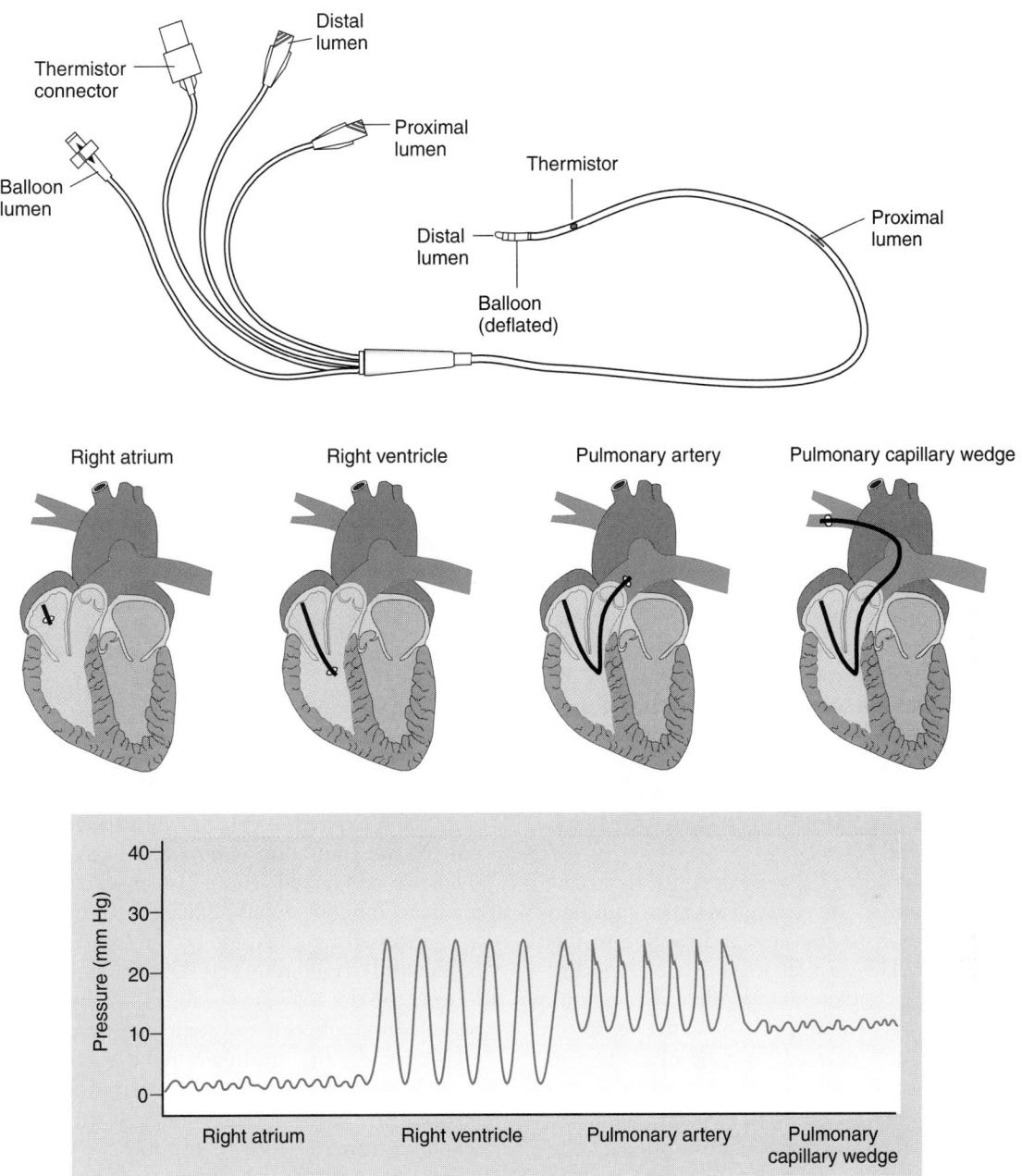

Figure 26-3   Conventional pulmonary artery catheter and characteristic pressure waveforms.

the 1.5-mL capacity balloon), the inflation should be aborted and the catheter's position reassessed. Position-monitoring catheters have been developed to more precisely determine the tip's position. In these catheters an infusion port has been placed 10 cm from the distal end. If this port produces an RV waveform, the tip is positioned no more than 10 cm beyond the pulmonary valve.[10]

If the PAWP is to provide an accurate estimate of left atrial and left ventricular end-diastolic pressure, there must be an uninterrupted column of blood between the catheter tip and the left atrium after balloon inflation. This condition depends on the relative values of pulmonary artery, venous, and alveolar pressures. Three zones

have been described based on vascular and alveolar pressure and the effect of gravity and the patient's position (Table 26-2). In zone III, the pulmonary artery and venous pressures both exceed the alveolar pressure, ensuring an uninterrupted column of blood from the pulmonary wedge position to the left atrium. The distal tip of the catheter must reside in zone III for accurate PAWP estimates of left atrial pressure and LVEDP. If the catheter is in zones I or II, the alveolar pressure exceeds the pulmonary venous pressure and the PAWP will actually reflect the alveolar pressure. Fortunately, with the patient in the supine position, zone III characteristics are found in all but the most anterior lung regions.[12]

TABLE 26-2

Verifying the Position of the Pulmonary Artery Catheter

Parameter	Zone III	Zone I or II
Respiratory variation of PAWP	$<\frac{1}{2}\Delta P_{ALV}$	$>\frac{1}{2}\Delta P_{ALV}$
PAWP contour	Cardiac ripple	Unnaturally smooth
Catheter tip location	Level of left atrium or below	Above level of left atrium
PEEP trial	$\Delta PAWP <\frac{1}{2}\Delta PEEP$	$\Delta PAWP >\frac{1}{2}\Delta PEEP$
PADP	PADP > PAWP	PADP < PAWP

From Marini JJ. Crit Care Clin 1986;3:551.
PAWP, Pulmonary artery wedge pressure; P_{ALV}, alveolar pressure PEEP, positive end-expiratory pressure; PADP, pulmonary artery diastolic pressure.

BOX 26-1

Indications for Pulmonary Artery Catheterization

Differentiation of shock syndromes
  Evaluation of intravascular volume, cardiac output, and oxygen transport
  Pulmonary embolism
  Pericardial tamponade
Determination of type of pulmonary edema (cardiogenic or permeability type)
Evaluation of complicated myocardial infarction
  Valvular dysfunction (for example, acute mitral regurgitation)
  Right ventricular dysfunction
  Ventricular septal defect
Evaluation of chronic congestive heart failure
  Constrictive pericarditis
  Cardiomyopathy
  Valvular lesions
Evaluation of chronic pulmonary hypertension
Trending of response to titrated hemodynamic therapy (for example, inotropes or vasodilators)
Volume challenge or diuresis

The pulmonary artery catheter has many possible uses, including differentiating shock states, determining intravascular volume status and cardiac performance, and monitoring interventions such as volume challenges, diuresis, and the infusion of vasoactive agents (Box 26-1). The analysis of complex hemodynamic disorders is beyond the scope of this discussion. However, certain cardiopulmonary disorders are associated with characteristic hemodynamic profiles (Table 26-3).[15,16]

Catheters introduced in 1980 were designed to provide continuous mixed venous oximetry. Two fiberoptic bundles at the tip are used to transmit and receive specific wavelengths of light. The wavelengths are chosen according to the reflectance characteristics of deoxyhemoglobin and oxyhemoglobin. As the red cells pass the sensor on the catheter tip, light is beamed into the blood and reflected back to the sensor. The mixed venous oxyhemoglobin saturation ($S\bar{v}O_2$) is calculated from the amount of light reflected at each wavelength. The oxyhemoglobin saturation of mixed venous blood decreases with anemia, arterial hypoxemia, and low cardiac output, because peripheral oxygen extraction increases to compensate for decreased oxygen availability. These catheters may be particularly useful in cardiac surgery and trauma patients in unstable condition, in whom the hemoglobin level and cardiac output can change abruptly.

Catheter systems have also been developed to provide continuous cardiac output ($\dot{Q}c$) measurements. Two strategies have been used, the Fick principle and thermodilution technology. With the Fick principle, three separate technologies were brought together at the bedside to provide on-line $\dot{Q}c$ determinations. Rearranging the **Fick equation** to calculate cardiac output gives the following equation:

$$\text{Cardiac output} = \frac{\text{Oxygen consumption}}{\text{Arterial} - \text{Mixed venous oxygen content}}$$

Oxygen consumption is measured through analysis of inspired and expired oxygen in the ventilator circuit. Arterial oxygen saturation is obtained from continuous pulse oximetry, and mixed venous oxygen saturation from a PAC equipped for continuous mixed venous oximetry. The data are processed by a bedside computer to calculate cardiac output and oxygen transport. Unfortunately, this system relies on the accuracy and stability of three separate technologies and suffers if any component fails to perform.

Thermodilution catheters have been reengineered to provide near continuous $\dot{Q}c$ determinations. Instead of reliance on a proximal injectate, a heating filament or coil several centimeters long is built into the catheter proximal to the thermistor (see Figure 26-3). The surrounding blood is heated with pulses of thermal energy, and the temperature changes are sensed downstream at the thermistor. This process is repeated every 10 to 30 seconds, and an updated cardiac output is displayed. Because of the time required to complete the measurements, the displayed cardiac output represents an average value from the previous 3 to 4 minutes and is essentially near real-time and not continuous.[10,11]

Advances in the design of thermodilution catheters also enabled the measurement of right ventricular function. The injector port was modified to disperse the injectate more uniformly into the cardiac chambers, and a rapidly responding thermistor was incorporated to sense beat by beat temperature changes. With beat to beat temperature, cardiac index, and heart rate values, the right ventricular ejection fraction and right ventricular end-diastolic volume index (RVEDVI) are calculated by a ded-

TABLE 26-3

Characteristic Hemodynamic Profiles of Certain Cardiopulmonary Disorders

Condition	CVP/RA	PAP	PAWP	CO	SVR	PVR
Hypovolemic shock	↓	↓	↓	↓	↑	Normal
Cardiogenic shock	↑	↑	↑	↓	↑	Normal
Septic shock	Normal or ↓	Normal or ↑	Normal or ↓	↑	↓	Normal or ↓
Pulmonary embolism	↑	↑	Normal	↓	↑	↑

CVP/RA, Central venous and right atrial pressures; PAP, pulmonary artery pressure; PAWP, pulmonary artery wedge pressure; CO, cardiac output; SVR, systemic vascular resistance; PVR, pulmonary vascular resistance.

icated microprocessor. The RVEDVI has been used to predict responses to volume challenge in certain critically ill patients.[11]

Although these new catheters accurately measure cardiac and oxygen transport variables under most circumstances, no clinical outcome studies yet exist to support their use. They are significantly more expensive than conventional PACs, although they may reduce certain personnel and laboratory costs.

The potential overuse or abuse of the PAC has been a focus of concern. A consensus panel was convened in 1997 to review the literature supporting *routine* use of the catheter in certain clinical settings.[14] Few quality studies have described a favorable impact on patient outcomes. These studies have been difficult to conduct for many reasons, particularly the complexity and variability of critical care patients and the reluctance of attending physicians to randomize these types of patients. A recent retrospective analysis that suggests a higher mortality rate in a group of patients managed with PACs indicates the need for further quality research in this area. However, use of the catheter is indispensable for differentiation of complex shock states in individual patients in whom the CVP may not correlate with intravascular volume status and for whom clinical assessment of cardiac performance may be inaccurate. It also is useful in the management of acute respiratory distress syndrome (ARDS) and multiple organ dysfunction syndrome, in which conflicting organ support goals require complex tradeoffs (for example, volume challenge versus diuresis). The PAC also has the potential to improve cost-effectiveness in certain clinical settings by facilitating communication among staff members, ensuring accurate physiologic assessment and rapid response to critical hemodynamic changes, and allowing prompt restoration of homeostasis to prevent organ injury and improve outcomes.

Use of the PAC may result in the mechanical and infectious complications observed with any central venous access. In addition, the PAC further increases the risk of cardiac valvular injury, arrhythmias and heart block, pulmonary artery rupture, catheter knotting, and endocarditis.[8,10]

Thoracic Bioimpedance

It has been recognized that the impedance to a very small alternating current (AC) passed across the chest varies with the blood flow through the thoracic cavity. By placing an array of electrodes around the thorax to transmit and receive this type of current, cardiac output can be estimated. $\dot{Q}c$ measurements derived in this way have correlated well with thermodilution studies. This method is essentially free of complications and relatively inexpensive. It is not completely understood, however, and the effect of various diseases and interventions is unknown, perhaps rendering it unreliable.

Soluble Gas Technique

Soluble gases can be used to measure the pulmonary capillary blood flow, which is an approximation of cardiac output in the absence of significant intrapulmonary or cardiac shunting. When gases of moderate solubility such as acetylene (C_2H_2) or carbon dioxide (CO_2) are inhaled, they are taken up by the capillary blood as it passes by the alveoli. A dilute concentration of a soluble gas (for example, 0.3% C_2H_2) is delivered to the lungs, and analysis of its concentration in exhaled gas during a slow exhalation or rebreathing allows calculation of the pulmonary capillary blood flow.

These methods have been used with cardiopulmonary exercise studies and mechanical ventilation to provide noninvasive measurement of cardiac output. Cardiopulmonary exercise equipment is available commercially with C_2H_2 and CO_2 cardiac output technology. Unfortunately, soluble gas methods have not proved useful in the ICU, because critically ill patients generally have marked ventilation-perfusion abnormalities, which adversely affect this technique.

Respiratory Monitoring

Respiratory Rate and Pattern

The respiratory rate is also one of the four vital signs. It is a core component of ICU monitoring, because respiratory rate slowing (*bradypnea* or *apnea*) or acceleration (*tachyp-*

nea) may warn of clinical deterioration or impending respiratory arrest. In sleep laboratories sophisticated respiratory rate and pattern monitoring are required during polysomnography. Respiratory (apnea) monitors are also used for infant studies in the home.

The respiratory rate is easily measured at the bedside by counting chest excursions for 30 to 60 seconds and multiplying to obtain breaths per minute. However, several hospital-based studies have shown this method to be remarkably inaccurate. The reason for this is not completely clear, although perhaps staff members underestimate the importance of this vital sign! Fortunately, a number of other methods are available to monitor this important parameter accurately.[1]

During sleep studies, temperature and pressure probes can be used to measure the rate and pattern of airflow. Disordered breathing, hypopneas, and apneas are characterized in this way. **Thermistors** and **thermocouples** detect bidirectional airflow at the nose and mouth by sensing the temperature difference between inspired room air and exhaled air that has been warmed to body temperature (Figure 26-4). The ability of these devices to detect airflow diminishes if the room air temperature approaches body temperature. Likewise, if the sensor touches skin and rises to body temperature, airflow cannot be detected. Other limitations of thermally based sensors are (1) they cannot be calibrated in terms of airflow and provide only qualitative information; (2) moisture condensing on the probe compromises temperature sensing capabilities; and (3) loss of signal may occur if the sensor becomes dislodged from the airstream.[17]

$\mathcal{R}$ *espiratory Recap*

Techniques to Measure the Respiratory Rate

Counting by inspection at the bedside
Nasal temperature and pressure sensing devices
Impedance pneumography
Respiratory inductance plethysmography
Fiberoptic plethysmography
Piezoelectric plethysmography

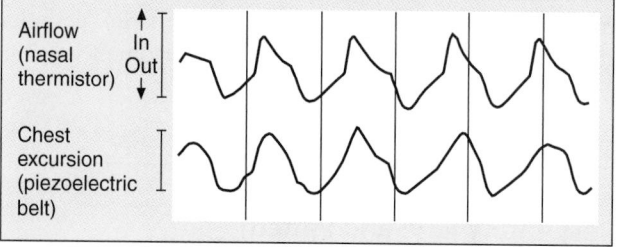

Figure 26-4 Airflow and chest and abdominal excursion waveforms are used to monitor respiratory rate and pattern during sleep studies. (Modified from materials courtesy Pro-Tech Services, Woodinville, Wash.)

Nasal air pressure transducers also provide a qualitative measurement of airflow and allow detection of certain types of airway obstruction during sleep studies. An airflow cannula is positioned under the nose to pick up respiratory pressure changes. The pressure signal is transmitted the length of the catheter to a transducer element inside a battery-powered unit, where it is amplified, filtered, and sent to the DC or AC input of a polygraph. These devices can pick up the high-frequency pressure pulses that occur with snoring, which can be seen riding on top of the relatively slow sinusoidal breathing waveform, eliminating the need for a separate snore sensor. The typical working range for a nasal pressure transducer is ± 25 cm H_2O, which allows it to be used inside a nasal mask during continuous positive airway pressure (CPAP) ventilation. Events characterized by flow limitation may be more easily recognized with a nasal pressure cannula. Otherwise, nasal pressure transducers share the same limitations as thermally based designs.[17]

With **impedance pneumography,** the respiratory rate and excursion can be measured by use of two electrodes placed on the chest wall. A high-frequency (20 to 100 Hz) and low-ampere AC current (less than 100 μa) is passed between the electrodes on the chest surface (this is, of course, a current too small to be felt by the patient). The strength of the current when it reaches the receiving electrode varies according to the *impedance*, or effective resistance of the tissue between the electrodes. During chest expansion, as the distance between the electrodes increases, impedance increases, causing the current to decrease. The change in current is electronically processed to calculate the respiratory rate (see Figure 26-1). During normal tidal breathing, the signal can also be calibrated to measure tidal volume. However, volume measurements deteriorate with patient movement or a change in position. Moreover, an obstructive apnea cannot be detected with this method, because the chest wall continues to move despite cessation of airflow. These systems usually are configured as a plug-in module for bedside monitoring of the respiratory rate in the ICU. They use the same electrodes that generally are applied to the patient for cardiac rhythm monitoring. Infant home apnea monitors are based on this relatively inexpensive technology.[1,18]

The most accurate method for indirect measurement of tidal volume is **respiratory inductance plethysmography (RIP).** Inductance sensors use a circuit of coiled wire woven into an elastic band and excited by an AC current. *Inductance* results from alternating electrical currents that create magnetic fields around themselves and the changes in those magnetic fields that alter other electrical currents they encounter. During tidal breathing, the bands stretch and relax. As the belt is displaced during chest expansion, changes in the magnetic fields around the wire coils result in changes in the excitation current. Variations in the excitation current caused by the expansion and contraction of the belt are electronically processed to provide a display of the ventilatory pattern, rate, and change in volume.

When rib cage and abdominal bands are used simultaneously, respiratory motion is described more completely, resulting in tidal volume measurements that correlate well with spirometry ($\pm 10\%$). RIP is stable and comfortable despite patient movement, which makes it suitable for use in sleep laboratories. This noninvasive technique has also been used in the ICU to monitor noninvasive ventilation and to conduct studies of the effect of positive end-expiratory pressure (PEEP) on the functional residual capacity. Because it is more expensive than impedance pneumography, its use in the ICU usually is reserved for cases in which noninvasive measurements of tidal volume or changes in FRC are desired.[1,19,20]

A modification of inductance plethysmography, **fiberoptic plethysmography,** uses optical fibers woven into elastic belts. Light is passed through the fibers into a photodetector. When rib cage or abdominal displacements stretch the elastic belt, large changes in light transmission through the fibers result. The change in light transmission is electronically processed to provide data similar to RIP discussed above. This technique has the advantage of being free of electrical interference and electrically safe for patients. It also is more sensitive than conventional RIP to small changes in lung volume. Clinical experience with this device currently is limited.[21]

To simplify the plethysmography apparatus, the wire coils have been removed from the elastic belts and replaced by a piezoelectric buckle (**piezoelectric plethysmography).** This reduces the cost and allows for belts that can be adjusted to different-size patients. The buckle encloses a sensor, which generates a voltage in response to stretch passed through the ends of the belts. The sensor is not calibrated, however, and provides only a qualitative record of chest or abdominal movement, hence the term *effort belts.* These devices are also commonly used in sleep laboratories (see Figure 26-4). Effort belts based on piezoelectric sensors do not require a battery. As with all belt-type transducers, the quality and interpretability of the respiratory signal are affected if the belt loosens or slips out of the original position.

Rib cage and abdominal belts with mercury strain gauges have been phased out because of the hazard of mercury exposure. Most modern mechanical ventilators have integrated airflow transducers designed to monitor and display the respiratory rate. End-tidal CO_2 monitors also display respiratory rate data.

Point of Care Testing

Samples for blood gas analysis traditionally are drawn from the patient, prepared and packaged for delivery to the blood gas laboratory, transported to the laboratory, and analyzed, and the results are reported back to the patient care unit. This system can result in preanalytic and postanalytic error and considerable delay in test results. Interest has been increasing in point of care (POC) testing, in which blood gases are measured at or near the site of patient care.

POC testing has proved to be accurate and useful despite concerns about regulatory, managerial, and quality issues. POC testing devices are portable, and some are hand-held. They typically require only a few drops of blood for testing. The blood is introduced into a single-use disposable cartridge, which is put into the portable analyzer (Figure 26-5). The cartridge chosen determines the tests that will be run (for example, blood gases, electrolytes, hematocrit, glucose, blood urea nitrogen, creatinine, or ionized calcium). A calibrant solution automatically calibrates the sensor, after which the blood sample is drawn over the biosensors. The POC analyzer calculates, displays, and stores the results. The POC testing device can communicate with the central laboratory or hospital information system for reporting and archiving of results.

The role of POC testing is evolving and will continue to expand. However, the issues of cost and regulation must be addressed before it comes into more widespread use. Quality control and quality assurance also must be appropriately addressed, but these goals typically are achieved by following the manufacturer's recommendations for use of the device. Cost is more difficult to address. The cost of the basic unit and the cost of the single-use cartridges must be balanced against a quicker test turnaround time (possibly resulting in faster treatment and better patient outcomes), the lower overhead (compared to the central laboratory), and the smaller blood volume required for testing (resulting in lower transfusion requirements).

Optical Blood Gas Monitors

Optically based systems that use an intraarterial sensor (Neotrend and Paratrend 7) have been developed to provide continuous measurement of arterial blood gases.[22] The sensor is placed through an arterial cannula and rests

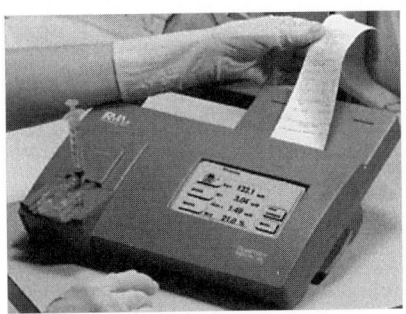

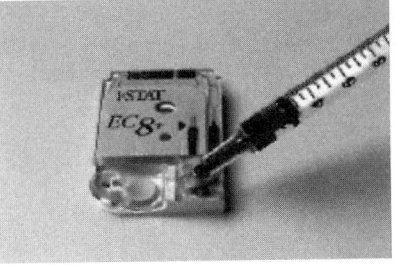

Figure 26-5   A, Point of care blood gas analyzers. Note that these are small and can be handheld. **B,** A few drops of blood are placed on a cartridge for analysis.

inside the artery (Figure 26-6). It is constructed from microporous polyethylene and has four miniature filaments (the outside diameter is less than 0.5 mm). One filament is a thermocouple to measure temperature. The other three are pH, oxygen pressure (PO_2), and carbon dioxide pressure (PCO_2) sensors. The pH sensor (range of 6.8 to 7.8, ±0.03 units) contains a red dye sensitive to pH in its distal section. The dye is yellow-orange at low pH and turns dark red as the pH increases. The device transmits green light down the length of the fiberoptic filament through the dye to a mirror at its end, where it is reflected back to a detector. The amount of green light returned is proportional to the hydrogen ion concentration [H^+]. The PCO_2 sensor (range of 10 to 80 mm Hg, ±3 mm Hg) works on a similar principle. The red dye is dissolved in a bicarbonate buffer inside a gas-permeable membrane. As CO_2 molecules diffuse through the membrane, they react with the buffer to create hydrogen ions, causing a similar color change in the dye. The PO_2 sensor (range of 20 to 500 mm Hg, ±5% [under 120 mm Hg] or ±10% [120 to 500 mm Hg]) is not an optical sensor but a miniature version of the Clark electrode with two ultrathin silver wires in a potassium chloride electrolyte solution encased in a polyethylene tube. The 0% to 90% response time (t_{90}) of the entire system is 15 seconds or less at 37° C. It has been found to be accurate and reliable in human studies. Several other optical systems have been developed for continuous intraarterial blood gas monitoring but are not commercially available or have been withdrawn from the market.[23]

Transcutaneous Blood Gas Monitoring

Transcutaneous O_2 and CO_2 monitoring ($PTCO_2$ and $PTCCO_2$) uses measurements at the skin surface to provide estimates of PaO_2 and $PaCO_2$ (CPG 26-1). This type of monitoring has been widely used with neonates, infants, small children, and patients with arterial insufficiency. The devices warm the skin to induce hyperemia, then electrochemically measure oxygen and carbon dioxide partial pressures at the skin surface, providing a noninvasive means of continuously monitoring arterial oxygenation and ventilation. They have been particularly useful in neonates and infants, in whom arterial sampling is technically difficult. Also, because intact circulation is a prerequisite for successful hyperbaric oxygen therapy, candidates with peripheral vascular disease often are screened with transcutaneous O_2 monitors.

Transcutaneous electrodes use the same principle as blood gas electrodes to measure PO_2 and PCO_2 at the skin surface. The transcutaneous oxygen electrode uses the polarographic technique. The anode is surrounded by heat-

---

CPG 26-1

Transcutaneous Blood Gas Monitoring for Neonatal and Pediatric Patients

Indications
To monitor the adequacy of arterial oxygenation or ventilation, or both
To quantitate the response to diagnostic and therapeutic interventions as evidenced by values for the transcutaneous partial pressure of oxygen ($PTCO_2$) or the transcutaneous partial pressure of carbon dioxide ($PTCCO_2$), or both

Contraindications
Transcutaneous monitoring may be relatively contraindicated in patients with poor skin integrity or those who are allergic to adhesive.

Hazards and Complications
$PTCO_2$ and $PTCCO_2$ monitoring are considered safe procedures. However, because of device limitations, false-negative and false-positive results may lead to inappropriate treatment. Also, tissue injury, such as erythema, blisters, burns, and skin tears, may occur at the measuring site.

Limitations
$PTCO_2$ is an indirect measurement of the partial pressure of arterial oxygen (PaO_2) and, like PaO_2, does not reflect oxygen delivery or oxygen content. Complete assessment of oxygen delivery requires knowledge of the hemoglobin, saturation, and cardiac output values. $PTCCO_2$ is an indirect measurement of the partial pressure of arterial carbon dioxide ($PaCO_2$), but knowledge of delivery and content is not necessary to use $PTCCO_2$ as an indicator of the adequacy of ventilation.

Technical
The procedure may be labor intensive, although newer designs have made it quicker and simpler.
A prolonged stabilization period is required after electrode placement.
Manufacturers state that electrodes must be heated to produce valid results; however, clinical studies suggest that valid results may be obtained with $PTCCO_2$ electrodes operated at lower than recommended temperatures or with no heat. The theoretic basis for mandatory heating of the $PTCO_2$ electrode has been established.
Improper calibration is possible and may be difficult to detect.

Clinical
Hyperoxemia (PaO_2 over 100 mm Hg)
Hypoperfused state (shock, acidosis)
Improper electrode placement or application
Use of vasoactive drugs
Nature of the patient's skin and subcutaneous tissue (skinfold thickness, edema)

Modified from AARC Clinical practice guideline: transcutaneous blood gas monitoring for neonatal and pediatric patients. Respir Care 1994;39:1176-1179. CPG, *Clinical practice guideline.*

ing coils, and the platinum cathode is centered inside the anode ring. The heating coil induces local hyperemia to arterialize the skin surface. A flat membrane separates the electrode from the skin. Oxygen diffuses from the blood vessels to the skin surface and through the membrane into the electrode. Transcutaneous carbon dioxide electrodes use a similarly flat glass membrane permeable to CO_2. A pH electrode is positioned behind the membrane in a bicarbonate buffer. Carbon dioxide diffuses from the skin through the membrane and reacts with the buffer to produce a change in [H^+]. Similar to the P_{CO_2} blood gas electrode, the P_{TCCO_2} electrode detects changes in [H^+] but is calibrated to display P_{CO_2}. The response times (t_{90}) for the P_{TCCO_2} and P_{TCO_2} electrodes are 45 seconds and 12 seconds, respectively.

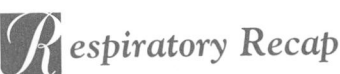 *espiratory Recap*

Transcutaneous Blood Gas Monitors
Warmed electrodes are placed on the skin to measure the P_{TCO_2} and P_{TCCO_2}, which are used to estimate the Pa_{O_2} and Pa_{CO_2}. The electrodes operate on the same principles as blood gas electrodes.

Because a prolonged stabilization time is required after the electrode is placed on the patient, **transcutaneous monitoring** should be continuous and displayed in a trend mode. Spot checks are not appropriate. A discrepancy between arterial and transcutaneous measurements may result with hyperoxia, hypoperfusion, vasoactive drugs, and increased skinfold thickness or edema. This discrepancy has led to the description of a P_{TCO_2}/Pa_{O_2} *index* to characterize hypoperfusion or shock states. A low P_{TCO_2}/Pa_{O_2} index correlates with a low cardiac index and reduced oxygen delivery.

Transcutaneous monitoring is relatively contraindicated in patients with poor skin integrity or allergy to adhesive. Tissue injury can occur at the measuring site (for example, erythema, blisters, burns, and skin tears). In an effort to avoid burns, several centers have documented that the electrodes can be operated at room temperature or at least at lower than recommended temperatures with satisfactory results.[23]

Pulse Oximetry

Pulse oximetry noninvasively measures the oxyhemoglobin saturation of arterial blood. It is used in nearly every medical setting, from the operating room to home care (CPG 26-2). The ability to rapidly detect changes in the arterial oxygen saturation noninvasively undoubtedly ranks as one of the most important technologic advances in modern respiratory care.

The first oximeter to continuously monitor oxygen levels was developed in 1935. It was improved over time, but

oximetry did not gain widespread acceptance until the invention of the *pulse oximeter*,[24,25] which works on the principle that the pulsatile component of the absorption signal was related to arterial blood. The static components of absorption related to tissue and venous blood could be mathematically eliminated, and the calibration process simplified.

Oximetry is based on **spectrophotometry,** or the process by which substances are identified by their absorption (also called *extinction*) of specific wavelengths in the electromagnetic spectrum. The various hemoglobin molecules absorb wavelengths between 500 and 1000 nm in the infrared and visible light regions. The **Beer-Lambert law** defines the relationship between the concentration of a substance and the amount of light (I) transmitted through it, as follows:

$$I_{out} = I_{in} \times e^{-A}$$

and

$$A = L \times C \times \epsilon$$

where L is the optical path length, C is the concentration of the substance, e is the base of the natural logarithm (2.7183), and ϵ is the absorption of the particular wave-

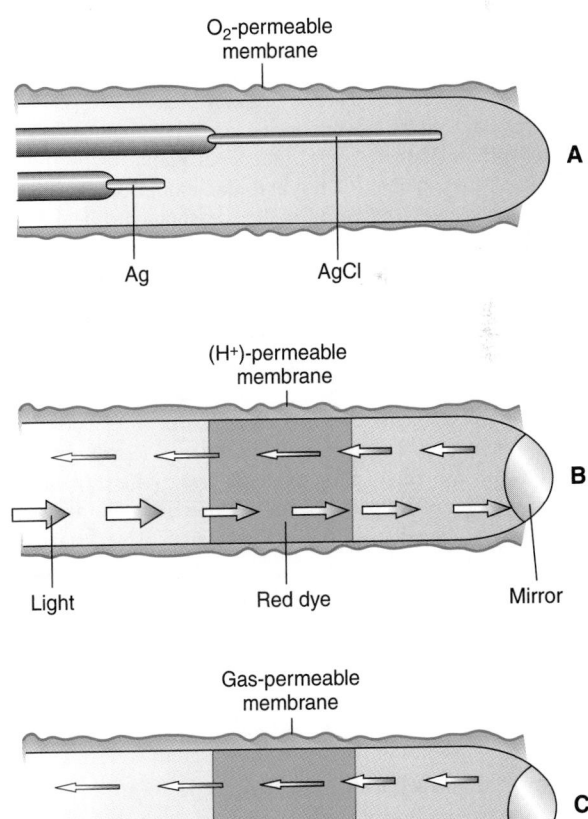

Figure 26-6   Intraarterial sensors. **A,** Oxygen pressure (P_{O_2}). **B,** pH level. **C,** Partial pressure of carbon dioxide (P_{CO_2}). (Modified from materials courtesy Diametrics Medical, St. Paul, Minn.)

CPG 26-2

Pulse Oximetry

Indications

To monitor the adequacy of arterial oxyhemoglobin saturation

To quantitate the response of arterial oxyhemoglobin saturation to therapeutic intervention or to a diagnostic procedure, such as bronchoscopy

To comply with regulations or recommendations

Contraindications

A need for continuous measurement of pH, partial pressure of arterial carbon dioxide ($Paco_2$), total hemoglobin, or abnormal hemoglobins may be a relative contraindication to pulse oximetry.

Hazards and Complications

Pulse oximetry (Spo_2) is considered a safe procedure. However, because of device limitations, false-negative results for hypoxemia or false-positive results for normoxemia or hyperoxemia may lead to inappropriate treatment. Also, tissue injury may occur at the measuring site as a result of probe misuse; such injuries may include pressure sores from prolonged application or electrical shock and burns caused by the substitution of incompatible probes between instruments.

Limitations

Factors, agents, or situations that may affect readings, limit precision, or limit the performance or application of a pulse oximeter include motion artifact, abnormal hemoglobins (primarily carboxyhemoglobin [COHb] and methemoglobin [metHb]), intravascular dyes, exposure of the measuring probe to ambient light during measurement, low perfusion states, skin pigmentation, nail polish or nail coverings (with a finger probe), inability to detect saturations below 83% with the same degree of accuracy and precision seen at higher saturations, and inability to quantitate the degree of hyperoxemia present; hyperbilirubinemia has been shown *not* to affect the accuracy of Spo_2 readings.

To validate pulse oximeter readings, the correlation between Spo_2 and arterial oxyhemoglobin saturation (Sao_2) obtained by direct measurement should be assessed; these measurements initially should be performed simultaneously and then periodically reevaluated in relation to the patient's clinical state.

To help ensure consistency of care based on Spo_2 readings, the proper probe must be selected and placed appropriately. For continuous, prolonged monitoring, the high- and low-limit alarms are set appropriately; the specific manufacturer's recommendations are followed; the device is applied and adjusted correctly to monitor response time and electrocardiographic coupling; the strength of the plethysmograph waveform or the pulse amplitude is assessed; and the device is checked to ensure that it is detecting an adequate pulse.

Spo_2 results should be documented in the patient's medical record and should detail the conditions under which the readings were obtained: date, time of measurement, and pulse oximeter reading; the patient's position, activity level, and location during monitoring (the physician's order determines the patient's activity level); the inspired oxygen concentration or supplemental oxygen flow, specifying the type of oxygen delivery device; the type of probe and the placement site; the model of the device (if more than one type is available for use); the simultaneously obtained arterial pH, partial pressure of arterial oxygen (Pao_2), and $Paco_2$ values and directly measured saturations of COHb, metHb, and oxyhemoglobin (O_2Hb) (if direct measurement was not simultaneously performed, an additional, one-time statement must be made explaining that the Spo_2 reading has not been validated by comparison to directly measured values); the stability of readings (length of observation time and range of fluctuation; for continuous or prolonged studies, review of the recording may be necessary); the patient's clinical appearance, a subjective assessment of perfusion at the measuring site (for example, signs of cyanosis or lowered skin temperature); and the correlation between the patient's heart rate as determined by pulse oximeter and that obtained by palpation and use of an oscilloscope.

When there is a disparity between the Spo_2 and Sao_2 readings and the patient's clinical presentation, possible causes should be explored before results are reported. Monitoring at alternative sites or appropriate substitution of instruments or probes may resolve the discrepancies. If not, the pulse oximetry results should not be reported; rather, a statement describing the corrective action should be included in the patient's medical record, and direct measurement of arterial blood gas values should be requested. The absolute limits that constitute unacceptable disparity vary with the patient's condition and the specific device. Clinical judgment must be exercised.

Modified from AARC Clinical practice guideline: pulse oximetry. Respir Care 1991;36:1406-1409.
CPG, Clinical practice guideline.

length used. A separate wavelength is required for each substance to be identified. Commercial pulse oximeters use two wavelengths, red (660 nm) and infrared (940 nm), at which oxyhemoglobin (oxyHb) and deoxyhemoglobin (deoxyHb) have different absorption characteristics (Figure 26-7). Red and infrared light-emitting diodes (LEDs) in the oximeter probe serve as light sources. Because oxyHb and deoxyHb differ in light absorption at each wavelength, the amount of red and infrared light transmitted is related to oxygen saturation. A photodiode positioned on the opposite side of the probe serves as the photodetector. To identify the oxygen saturation of arterial blood only, the device relies on the pulsatile nature of arterial flow. During systole, a new volume of blood enters the arteriolar bed, and light absorption increases. During diastole, absorption decreases to a minimal level (Figure 26-8). Measuring pulsatile absorption eliminates the effects of nonpulsatile components such as tissue, bone, and

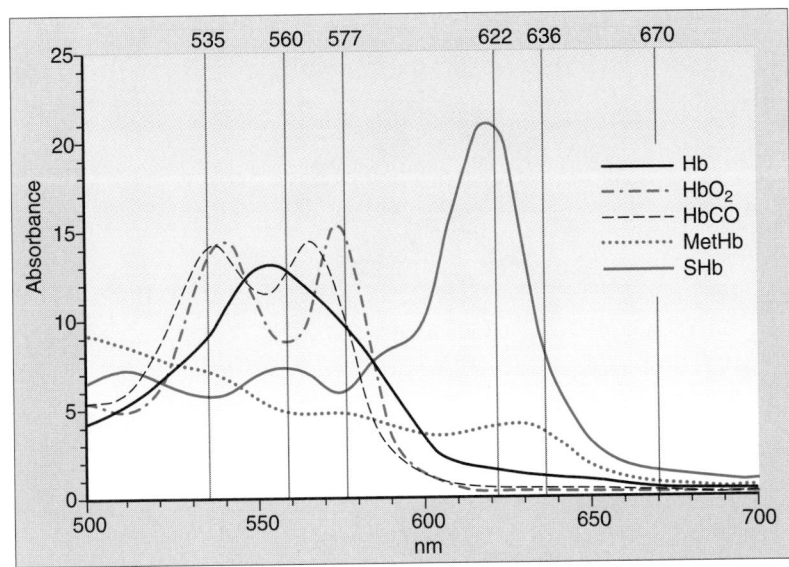

Figure 26-7 Absorption spectra for different types of hemoglobin molecules. (Modified from Radiometer Medical A/S. Blood gas, oximetry, and electrolyte systems reference manual. Copenhagen: The Company; 1996.)

venous blood. Oxygen saturation (SpO_2) is related to the ratio of minimum and maximum absorption at each wavelength, as follows:

$$SpO_2 = f\ \frac{\ln(min/max)_{red}}{\ln(min/max)_{infrared}}$$

The function f is determined by the physical properties of the LEDs. A calibration curve is plotted for the pulse-added absorption at the two wavelengths and stored in a software algorithm. Devices vary by manufacturer in the type of LED, photodiode, and microprocessor used. Because the SpO_2 calculation is based on a constantly updated signal ratio, the system is self-zeroing. Also, because all computations are performed by internal software and there are no critical parts to drift, no calibration is required.[25,26]

Most pulse oximeters use *transmittance spectrophotometry*, sending light through the arterial bed to a photodetector on the opposite side (Figure 26-9). Reflectance pulse oximeter sensors have been developed with the light source and detector on the same side of the arterial bed, which increases the number of practical sampling sites.

In general, pulse oximeter measurements have a 95% confidence interval (±4%) at oxygen saturations (SpO_2) above 75%. They are less accurate below an SpO_2 of 70%. The calibration curves are developed from studies on healthy volunteers and vary by manufacturer, depending on the range of concentrations achieved by the volunteers and the accuracy of the gold standard, usually a cooximeter. One reason for poor accuracy at lower saturations is the 660-nm LED. A slight shift in emitted wavelength or *center frequency* from the LED can result in significant error. Center frequency represents the dominant frequency in the emitted light. Even though it is specified as one wavelength (660 nm), the LED emits a range of frequencies around this central frequency. During use of the instrument, the LED may shift slightly off center frequency. The extinction coefficient (*absorption curve*) for

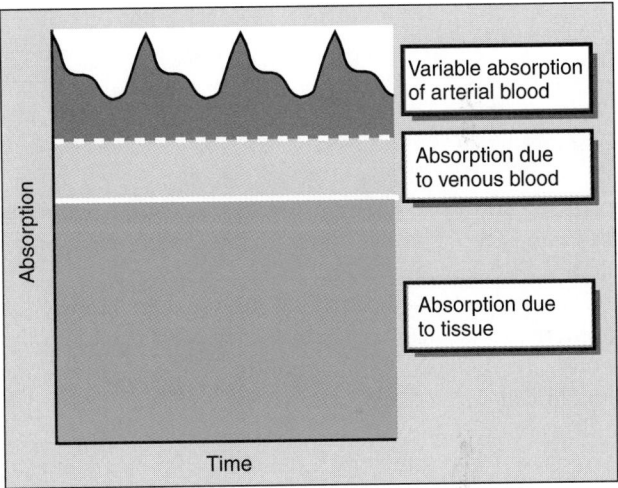

Figure 26-8 Dynamic and static light absorption during pulse oximetry. (Modified from materials courtesy Novametrix Medical Systems, Wallingford, Conn.)

reduced hemoglobin is relatively steep at this wavelength, therefore a slight shift results in a substantial change in absorption. The error is magnified by the increased levels of deoxyHb in the lower SpO_2 ranges. Strategies to improve performance at lower saturations include improved LED

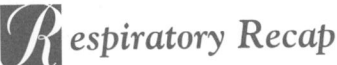espiratory Recap

Pulse Oximetry
Pulse oximetry measures oxygen saturation with a variation of the Beer-Lambert law.
Accuracy is ±4% and can be affected by abnormal hemoglobins, dyes (external and internal), motion, and low perfusion.

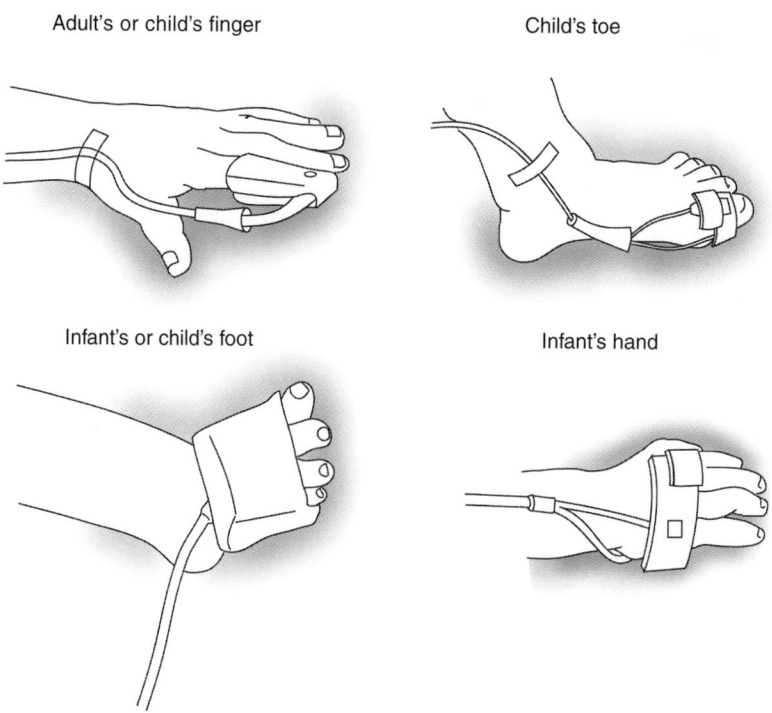

Adult's or child's finger

Child's toe

Infant's or child's foot

Infant's hand

Figure 26-9   Oximetry sensors.

quality control and a design that tracks center frequency shifts and feeds the data back to the microprocessor for mathematic compensation.[25-29]

Pulse oximetry is indicated whenever there is a need to monitor the adequacy of oxyHb saturation or to follow responses to therapeutic intervention. It is recognized that the clinical signs of hypoxemia (skin color and respiratory and heart rate) are inaccurate. The American Society of Anesthesiologists, the Joint Commission on Accreditation of Healthcare Organizations (JCAHO), and the Society of Critical Care Medicine have published standards and guidelines to monitor oxygenation in the operating room and in patients receiving oxygen therapy or undergoing procedures that may interfere with airway protection.[25,30]

Pulse oximetry is used universally for intraoperative and postoperative monitoring and has been demonstrated to reduce the frequency and duration of low saturation states. The value of SpO_2 monitoring has also been demonstrated during high-risk transports, such as operating room to recovery room and ICU to operating room or radiology department.[25] In the ICU, SpO_2 monitoring can be used to rapidly respond to desaturation events and to titrate inspired oxygen concentrations during mechanical ventilation. It is also used to monitor procedures that may adversely affect oxygenation, such as intubation, suctioning, dialysis, bronchoscopy, central venous access, and pulmonary artery catheterization. Pulse oximetry has been associated with a reduction in arterial blood gas measurements, providing cost savings without compromising outcomes.[29-31]

In neonatal and pediatric care, pulse oximeters appear to have replaced transcutaneous oxygen monitors for protection against hypoxemia. Pulse oximetry has the advantage

of self-calibration and overall ease of use. However, pulse oximetry is inaccurate in the flat portion of the oxyhemoglobin dissociation curve (95% to 100% saturation range) and may not protect against complications of hyperoxia (retrolental fibroplasia). In neonates, it is important to set the high saturation alarm in the 92% to 95% range.[32]

The availability of portable, battery-powered units has resulted in the common practice of spot-checking hospitalized patients during clinical care or oxygen therapy. Although this practice may enhance oxygen therapy, allowing weaning or discontinuation of unnecessary oxygen prescriptions, it has some potential problems. It provides no direct information about the $PaCO_2$ and may not accurately reflect the PaO_2 because of changes in the shape and position of the oxyhemoglobin dissociation curve. The spot-check also may not represent the patient's baseline if a recent change has occurred in the fractional inspired oxygen concentration (FiO_2) or activity.

In the ambulatory setting, oximetry is routinely used during bronchoscopy, clinical exercise, and sleep studies. During cardiac catheterization, it is helpful during long procedures, especially in patients with poor cardiopulmonary function.

Pulse oximetry may be used to prescribe long-term home oxygen therapy under Medicare guidelines (SpO_2 of 85% or lower). This use has been questioned in a study comparing arterial blood gas determinations and pulse oximetry. Only 80% of patients with a resting PaO_2 of 55 or lower had a concomitant SpO_2 of 85% or lower. The remaining 20% of this cohort would have been inappropriately denied home oxygen therapy if the decision had been based on oximetry alone. Pulse oximetry, therefore, should not be the primary method used to determine home oxygen needs; rather, it is an alternative when arterial blood gas determinations are unavailable.[25]

Pulse oximetry has become so widely used in prehospital care and emergency departments that it has been called the fifth vital sign. However, certain problems are unique to these settings, including motion artifact and an increased incidence of carboxyhemoglobinemia (carbon monoxide poisoning).[31,33]

Pulse oximetry is limited by several factors. The technique only measures the percentage of oxyHb relative to the sum of oxyHb and deoxyHb. The term **functional saturation** (SpO_2) is used to represent the amount of hemoglobin bound to oxygen expressed as a percentage of the amount of hemoglobin available for oxygen binding, as follows:

$$Spo_2 = \frac{oxyHb}{(oxyHb + deoxyHb)} \times 100\%$$

SpO_2 provides an accurate measure of oxygen saturation if dysfunctional hemoglobins, notably carboxyhemoglobin (COHb) and methemoglobin (metHb), are present only in negligible concentrations. In contrast, **fractional saturation** represents oxyHb expressed as a percentage of the total amount of hemoglobin, as follows:

$$\text{Fractional } Sao_2 = \frac{oxyHb}{(oxyHb + deoxyHb + COHb + metHb + Other\ Hb)} \times 100\%$$

SpO_2 overestimates the fractional oxyHb saturation when there are increased amounts of abnormal hemoglobin. Because the light absorption characteristics of COHb are similar to those of oxyHb, for example, the oximeter overestimates oxyHb saturation by an amount roughly equal to the COHb level. The effects of other Hb types are more complicated. Fortunately, fetal hemoglobin (HbF), which constitutes 69% of the hemoglobin in a newborn infant, and adult hemoglobin behave similarly. Clinical studies have confirmed a good agreement between SpO_2 and simultaneous cooximetry in newborns.[31,32]

Skin pigmentation, nail polish, or nail coverings may affect SpO_2 measurements. Black, blue, or green nail polish causes an underestimation of SpO_2, and these materials should be removed before a probe is placed. Darker skin pigmentation has been shown to affect the accuracy of SpO_2 in at least one study. Because of possible PaO_2 underestimation in darkly pigmented patients, it has been recommended that oxygen therapy be titrated to a target SpO_2 of 94% or higher in these patients. Intravascular dyes (methylene blue and indocyanine green) also cause an underestimation of SpO_2. Hyperbilirubinemia has not been shown to affect accuracy. The absorption peak for bilirubin (460 nm) is below that used in pulse oximetry. Xenon and fluorescent lighting have been shown to affect certain probes; this can be prevented by shielding.[28,29,31]

The accuracy of pulse oximetry diminishes with motion artifact and low perfusion states. Moving the patient or probe can distort the transmitted light signal before it reaches the photodiode. If the pulsatile absorption is small relative to nonpulsatile absorption, accuracy and precision may also deteriorate. Many monitors display the pulse as a waveform or moving bar, often enlarging it for display purposes; however, it may not directly correspond to the quality of the pulse signal. The ECG and pulse oximetry heart rates should also agree, but this does not guarantee a quality SpO_2 measurement. Engineers have developed *digital oximetry* to improve upon these limitations. With an **analog-to-digital converter,** the pulsatile waveform can be digitally encoded to provide enhanced resolution. This digital technique improves the processing of small signals and allows data validation. Each detected pulse can be compared to recent pulse waveforms to ensure integrity and consistency. Validation routines discard distorted or artifactual signals, increasing the reliability of results and reducing the number of nuisance alarms.[27,28]

Pulse oximetry is a safe procedure. Tissue injury may result from inappropriate probe application or electrical shock and burns from substitution of incompatible probes between instruments. Inappropriate substitution of pulse oximetry for other monitoring techniques or the unavailability of trained personnel are relative contraindications to its use. A need for pH, $PaCO_2$, and dyshemoglobin measurements always requires blood gas analysis and cooximetry.[30]

Capnography

Capnometry and capnography are noninvasive techniques that measure the carbon dioxide levels in expired gas (CPG 26-3). In the mid-1970s, mass spectroscopy was adapted to provide expired CO_2 measurements to assist in the management of mechanically ventilated patients. Less costly infrared systems were developed for clinical use by the 1980s, and affordable systems became widely available for use in the operating room and ICU.[34,35]

Capnometry refers to the numeric display of PCO_2 measurements taken from the airway. When the PCO_2 is plotted against time and displayed graphically as a waveform, it is called **capnography.**

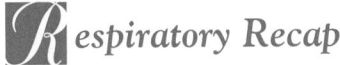

espiratory Recap

Capnography
Capnography uses either mainstream or sidestream sampling. The CO_2 level is measured by infrared absorption, mass spectrometry, or colorimetric techniques. End-tidal PCO_2 often is an imprecise reflection of $PaCO_2$. Capnography is useful in the detection of esophageal intubation.

Two airway sampling systems are used in capnometry, *mainstream* sensors and *sidestream* sensors. The *mainstream* capnometer is placed in the airway, usually inserted into a ventilator circuit. Infrared light is passed across the airstream to a photodetector. Improvement in analyzer

CPG 26-3

Capnometry and Capnography during Mechanical Ventilation

Indications

To evaluate exhaled CO_2, especially end-tidal CO_2, which is the maximum partial pressure of CO_2 exhaled during a tidal breath (just before the beginning of inspiration) and is designated $PetCO_2$

To monitor the severity of pulmonary disease and evaluate the response to therapy, especially therapy intended to improve the ratio of dead space to tidal volume (V_D/V_T) and the matching of ventilation to perfusion ($\dot{V}/\dot{Q}$), and possibly to increase coronary blood flow

To ensure that tracheal rather than esophageal intubation has taken place (low or absent cardiac output may negate its use for this indication)

To continuously monitor the integrity of the ventilatory circuit, including the artificial airway

To evaluate the efficiency of mechanical ventilatory support through determination of the difference between the arterial partial pressure of carbon dioxide ($PaCO_2$) and the $PetCO_2$, reflecting CO_2 elimination.

To monitor the adequacy of pulmonary and coronary blood flow

To monitor inspired CO_2 when CO_2 gas is administered therapeutically

To graphically evaluate the ventilator-patient interface; evaluation of the capnogram may be useful in the detection of rebreathing of CO_2, obstructive pulmonary disease, waning neuromuscular blockade (curare cleft), cardiogenic oscillations, esophageal intubation, cardiac arrest, or contamination of the monitor or sampling line with secretions or mucus

Contraindications

There are no absolute contraindications to capnography in mechanically ventilated adults provided the data obtained are evaluated in light of the patient's clinical condition.

Hazards and Complications

Capnography with a clinically approved device is a safe, noninvasive test associated with few hazards. With mainstream analyzers, use of too large a sampling window may introduce an excessive amount of dead space into the ventilator circuit. Care must be taken to minimize the amount of additional weight placed on the artificial airway by the sampling window or, in the case of a sidestream analyzer, by the sampling line.

Limitations

The composition of the respiratory gas mixture may affect the capnogram, depending on the measurement technology used.

The infrared spectrum of CO_2 has some similarities to the spectra of oxygen and nitrous oxide.

High concentrations of either or both of those gases may affect the capnogram, therefore, a correction factor should be incorporated into the calibration of any capnograph used in such cases.

The reporting algorithm of some devices (primarily mass spectrometers) assumes that the only gases present in the sample are those that the device is capable of measuring. When a gas that the mass spectrometer cannot detect (such as helium) is present, the reported values of CO_2 are incorrectly elevated in proportion to the concentration of helium present.

The breathing frequency may affect the capnograph. High breathing frequencies may exceed the response capabilities of the capnograph. In addition, a breathing frequency above 10 breaths/min has been shown to affect devices differently.

The presence of Freon (used as a propellant in metered dose inhalers) in the respiratory gas has been shown to artificially increase the CO_2 reading of mass spectrometers (that is, to show an apparent increase in the CO_2 concentration). A similar effect has not yet been demonstrated with Raman or infrared spectrometers.

Contamination of the monitor or sampling system by secretions or condensate, use of a sample tube that is too long, a sampling rate that is too high, or obstruction of the sampling chamber can lead to unreliable results.

Modified from AARC Clinical practice guideline: capnometry and capnography during mechanical ventilation. Respir Care 1995;40:1321-1324. CPG, Clinical practice guideline.

technology and miniaturization have resulted in the development of low dead space, lightweight, and durable mainstream sensors. Because they are positioned in the airway, they may be adversely affected by the accumulation of moisture, secretions, and debris. Mainstream designs are best suited to patients with artificial airways and are available as stand-alone units or plug-in components for multifunctional ICU monitors.

The *sidestream* capnometer uses small-bore tubing to aspirate gas from or adjacent to the airway. The tubing conducts the respiratory gases to a remote measuring chamber for analysis. Moisture and secretions must be removed from the tubing with traps, filters, purging, or reverse flow maneuvers before the sample enters the analysis cell. Some tubing is designed to be water vapor permeable, allowing moisture to escape by diffusion and evaporation. There is always an analysis delay when sidestream monitors are used because of the time required to move the sample from the airway to the sensor. The delay depends on the length of the tubing, its diameter, and the rate at which the gas is aspirated. Sidestream capnometers are easier to use in spontaneously breathing patients. The sample port is simply positioned in the airstream so as not to be contaminated by ambient air.[34-37]

Most CO_2 analyzers are based on infrared absorption. They are relatively inexpensive and are found in most cap-

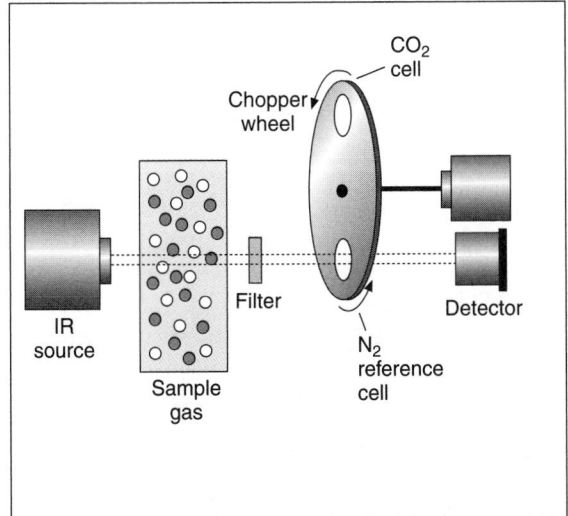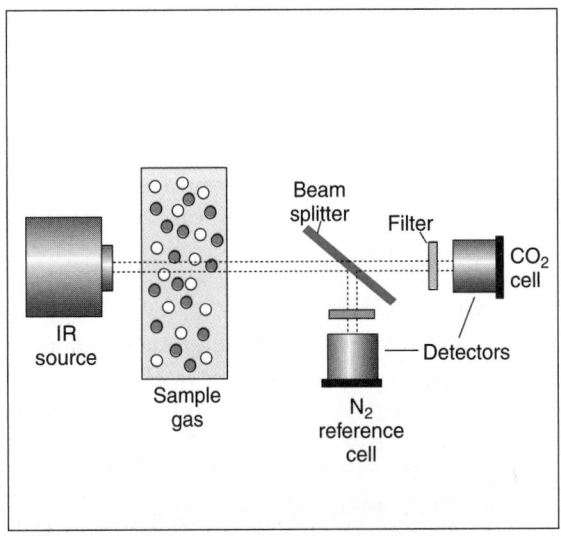

Figure 26-10   Carbon dioxide (CO_2) sensors using the single beam design have a rotating chopper wheel to pass cells containing carbon dioxide and nitrogen gas through the light path. The newer solid-state, split-beam design eliminates moving parts. (Modified from materials courtesy Novametrix Medical Systems, Wallingford, Conn.)

nometers, indirect calorimeters, and pulmonary exercise systems. In a conventional analyzer, infrared light (IR) is passed through a sample cell containing gas from the patient. The IR light is also passed through a reference sample containing gas of known concentration and absorption. The transmitted IR light excites a photodetector, which generates an electrical signal. An electrical circuit repeatedly compares signals from the sample, reference cell, and dark current (the current before and after the light signals). This strategy continually corrects for drift and improves precision. *Single beam* systems use one beam of light and a rotating chopper wheel to pass the sample and reference cells through the light source (Figure 26-10). *Double* or *split beam* systems divide the light with mirrors into separate sample cell and reference cell beams.[35]

The CO_2 infrared absorption peak (4.26 μm) lies between two peaks for water and very close to a peak for nitrous oxide (Figure 26-11). The latter poses an interference problem during the administration of nitrous oxide (N_2O) as an anesthesia gas. Correction factors and filters can be used to address this problem. Conventional infrared analyzers must be calibrated regularly. Room air (zero) and 5% CO_2 are used to perform a two-point calibration. Accuracy should be ±12% or ±4 mm Hg, whichever is larger. The response time (t_{90}) is approximately 100 ms.[35-38] Solid-state engineering has resulted in the development of a simplified CO_2 analyzer, now commercially available (Novametrix), which eliminates moving parts and allows self-zeroing and calibration features. This analyzer has an accuracy of ±4 mm Hg at a P_{CO_2} of 0 to 40 mm Hg; ±5% at a P_{CO_2} of 41 to 70 mm Hg; and a t_{90} of less than 60 ms.[27]

Until recently, the infrared radiation technique used for capnography was the nondispersive blackbody technology

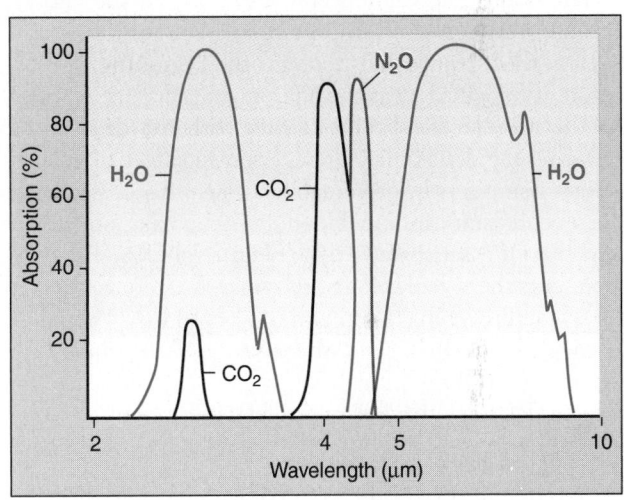

Figure 26-11   Carbon dioxide absorption spectra. (Modified from Decker M, Strohl K. Pulse oximetry. Biophysical measurement series: respiration. Redmond, Wash: SpaceLabs Medical; 1994.)

described previously. Molecular correlation spectroscopy has recently become available. This technique operates at room temperature and uses a radiation source that emits only CO_2-specific radiation. The CO_2 specificity and sensitivity of the emitter-detector combination allows for use of a small sample cell (15 μL) and a small flow rate.[39]

The **mass spectrometer** is also used to measure respiratory and anesthetic gases. Multichannel units are available to monitor several patients simultaneously. A mass spectrometer aspirates sample gas into a vacuum chamber, where it is ionized by an electron beam. The charged molecules are accelerated through a magnetic field and disperse according to their mass and charge. This dispersion allows them to be separated before they reach a panel of detectors. Because even molecules of similar mass (N_2O and CO_2) ionize to different species (N_2O^+ and CO_2^+), this technique allows accurate measurement of several gases. Mass spectrometers have the advantage of being able to measure all respiratory gases breath by breath and are the most accurate analyzers in clinical use. However, they generally are too expensive and cumbersome for use outside the operating room or research settings. Their response time also may increase to over 80 seconds if they are shared among several operating suites or if the sampling tubing reaches excessive lengths.[37]

Another method that can be used to measure CO_2 in capnographs is **Raman spectroscopy.** When ultraviolet or visible light strikes gas molecules, energy is absorbed and reemitted at the same wavelength and direction. A small fraction of the absorbed energy is remitted at new wavelengths in a phenomenon known as *Raman scattering.* Raman scattering results in reemission at a longer wavelength to produce a red-shifted spectrum. The wavelength shift and amount of scattering can be used to measure the constituents of a gas mixture.

The traditional **capnogram** plots P_{CO_2} on the vertical axis and time on the horizontal axis. During inhalation, P_{CO_2} at the airway equals zero. At the beginning of exhalation, it remains low as the anatomic dead space empties. As the alveolar gas begins to mix with the dead space, CO_2 rises rapidly. A plateau, representing alveolar gas, develops, rising gently, presumably because of CO_2 added to the alveoli from capillary blood during exhalation (Figure 26-12, A). Peak exhaled P_{CO_2} or end-tidal CO_2 ($P_{ET}CO_2$) represents the alveolar P_{CO_2}. Alveolar P_{CO_2} equals arterial P_{CO_2} when the ventilation/perfusion ratio ($\dot{V}/\dot{Q}$) equals 1. As $\dot{V}/\dot{Q}$ approaches zero, the alveolar P_{CO_2} equals the mixed venous P_{CO_2}. In high $\dot{V}/\dot{Q}$ regions or dead space, the alveolar P_{CO_2} approaches inspired P_{CO_2} (zero).

A normal volume-based capnogram is shown in Figure 26-13. It is displayed with the P_{CO_2} on the vertical axis and the volume on the horizontal axis. At the beginning of exhalation, the P_{CO_2} remains zero as gas from the anatomic dead space leaves the airway (phase I). The capnogram then rises sharply as alveolar gas mixes with dead space gas (phase II). The capnogram then forms a plateau during most of exhalation (phase III). Phase III represents gas flow from the alveoli and therefore is called the *alveolar plateau.* The P_{CO_2} at end-exhalation is the **end-tidal P_{CO_2}** ($P_{ET}CO_2$). As shown in Figure 26-13, airway dead space volume (that is, anatomic dead space), alveolar dead space volume, and the volume of exhaled CO_2 ($\dot{V}_{CO_2}$) can be determined from the volume-based capnogram. The determination of alveolar dead space requires knowledge of the Pa_{CO_2} in addition to the exhaled capnogram. The angle between phase II and phase III is referred to as the alpha angle and is normally 100 to 110 degrees. As the slope of phase III increases, the alpha angle also increases. The slope of phase III is determined by the $\dot{V}/\dot{Q}$ of the lungs. Patients with airway obstruction, such as in chronic obstructive pulmonary disease (COPD) and asthma, show an increase in the alpha angle. Other factors that may affect the alpha angle include the response time on the capnometer, the sweep speed of the device, and the patient's respiratory cycle time. The alpha angle may also change with changes in cardiac output.

In a patient with stable ventilation and perfusion ratios, end-tidal CO_2 is determined by the production of CO_2, its subsequent delivery to the lungs by cardiac output, alveolar ventilation, and proper sampling and equipment performance. An increase in the $P_{ET}CO_2$ may be seen in sepsis, bicarbonate administration, an increased metabolic rate, muscular paralysis, obstructive lung disease, rebreathing, or leaks in the ventilator circuit. A decrease in the $P_{ET}CO_2$ may be seen in pulmonary hypoperfusion, cardiac

A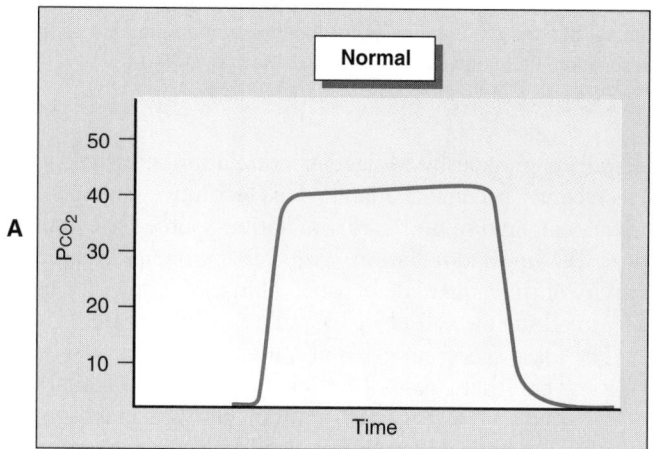

B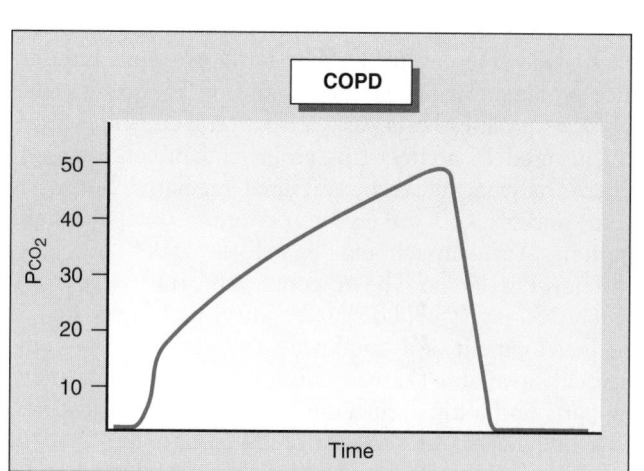

Figure 26-12 **A,** Normal capnogram rises sharply (as dead space is eliminated) during exhalation to a relatively flat plateau before returning to zero with the next inhalation. Normally, inspired gas does not contain any carbon dioxide (CO_2). **B,** With chronic obstructive pulmonary disease (COPD), the obstructed regions of the lung empty CO_2 later in exhalation, resulting in a rising plateau phase.

arrest, hyperventilation, endotracheal cuff leaks, ventilator disconnects, and esophageal intubations.

The capnographic waveform can be inspected for specific abnormalities or patterns. In patients with airways obstruction, the slope of the alveolar plateau increases because of inhomogeneous alveolar emptying (see Figure 26-12, B). Regions of the lung with delayed emptying caused by increased resistance (long time constants) continue to add CO_2 to expired gas during the latter part of exhalation. Rebreathing previously exhaled gas is characterized by an increase in both inspired and expired CO_2. This can be caused by a malfunctioning exhalation valve, excessive mechanical dead space, or depletion of CO_2 absorbent in anesthesia circuits. The curare cleft has been described in patients recovering from neuromuscular paralysis. The capnogram may also be used when hemodynamic measurements are performed to identify end-exhalation in the respiratory cycle.[35-38]

End-tidal CO_2 measurements are used clinically for four main reasons: (1) to ensure that the tracheal tube or mask ventilates the lungs; (2) to estimate the $PaCO_2$; (3) to detect changes in pulmonary blood flow or dead space ventilation; and (4) to detect the addition of excess CO_2 to the systemic circulation.[37]

Because the lungs excrete large amounts of CO_2, whereas levels in the esophagus are essentially zero, the presence of CO_2 in exhaled gas usually indicates an adequate patient-airway interface. An elevated $PETCO_2$ does not always assure proper endotracheal tube placement, however, because the tube could be in the main stem bronchus or in the pharynx and still serve as conduit for exhaled CO_2. Esophageal intubation generally results in a very low $PETCO_2$. Falsely elevated readings may occur, however, if preintubation bag-valve-mask ventilation has forcefully insufflated the stomach with respiratory gases or the patient has ingested bicarbonates. The elevated value

should diminish with subsequent breaths. Even with proper endotracheal tube placement, the $PETCO_2$ may remain deceptively low with cardiogenic shock.[37,38,40]

In the operating room, end-tidal CO_2 monitoring represents the standard of care for monitoring of the integrity of the ventilatory circuit and evaluation of the ventilator-patient interface.[33] In the emergency department and critical care unit, capnometers and disposable CO_2 indicators increasingly are used to verify tracheal intubation. Small, inexpensive, colorimetric carbon dioxide indicators contain a pH-sensitive dye that undergoes a color change in the presence of CO_2 (Figure 26-14). These single-use devices are especially helpful in prehospital settings, in which tracheal intubation and verification can be especially difficult.

Even though the $PETCO_2$ approximates the $PaCO_2$ in normal individuals, capnometry cannot routinely be used as a substitute to measure arterial PCO_2. Most critically ill patients have ventilation-perfusion abnormalities, particularly an increased ratio of dead space to tidal volume (V_D/V_T), resulting in a significant $PaCO_2 - PETCO_2$ difference ($P[a - ET]CO_2$). Even patients whose $P(a - ET)CO_2$ is calibrated by simultaneous arterial blood gas and capnometry measurements do not remain stable enough over time to render the measurement a reliable estimate of $PaCO_2$. One important exception, however, may be closed head injuries. Many of these patients have isolated head injuries and undergo a period of hyperventilation therapy. Often they are young, with relatively normal lungs and a narrow $P(a - ET)CO_2$. Titrating mechanical hyperventilation by $PETCO_2$ can reduce the number of arterial blood gas determinations required to manage these patients.

Because the end-tidal CO_2 is partly determined by the amount of blood flow returning to the lungs from the systemic circulation, it has been used to verify the effectiveness of cardiopulmonary resuscitation (CPR). Adequate

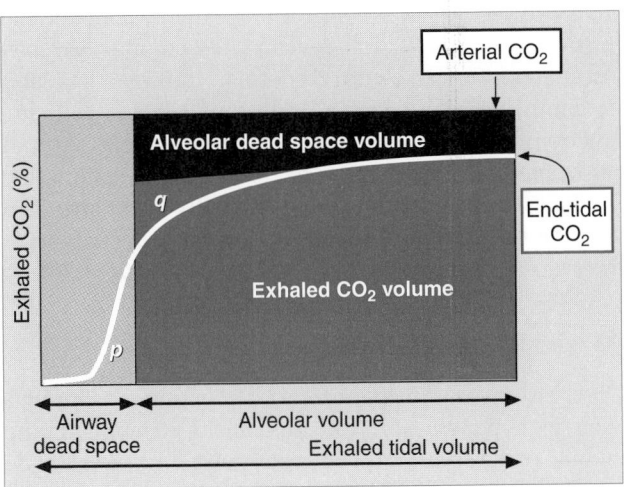

Figure 26-13 Volume-based capnogram. Note that the area under the capnogram is carbon dioxide production. Also note that the volume-based capnogram allows determination of anatomic dead space, alveolar volume, and alveolar dead space.

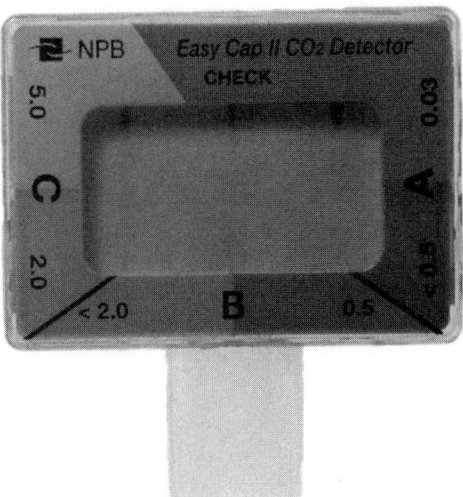

Figure 26-14 Colorimetric carbon dioxide sensor designed to confirm endotracheal intubation. The device fits between the endotracheal tube and the manual bag-valve device. (From Hess DR. Managing the artificial airway. Respir Care 1999;44(7):759-772.)

CPR is associated with increasing PETCO₂ levels. It has been suggested that if end-tidal CO₂ does not rise above 10 mm Hg after 20 minutes of pulseless resuscitation, the prognosis is so poor that CPR should be terminated. If used carefully in the prehospital setting, this strategy might reduce the number of futile resuscitations or transports. Because pulmonary embolism is also associated with decreased cardiac output, as well as an increased V_D/V_T, PETCO₂ measurements have been studied in this setting. More research is needed before these measurements could reduce the need for or improve upon noninvasive nuclear medicine studies.[35,36,41]

End-tidal CO₂ monitoring can reliably detect large increases in systemic production. This is most helpful in the operating room, where sudden increases in CO₂ production may indicate malignant hyperthermia. Early recognition allows prompt therapy and a reduction in complications.[37]

Capnometry has also been proposed as a means to determine optimum PEEP during mechanical ventilation and as an adjunct to weaning. In patients with ARDS, for example, excessive levels of PEEP theoretically increase V_D/V_T and $P(a - ET)CO_2$. Unfortunately, this approach has not proved reliable enough for routine use in ICU patients. As a noninvasive monitor of the weaning process, capnometric measurements of the respiratory rate and elevated PETCO₂ have also been unreliable, with some studies reporting good correlations with PaCO₂ and others finding the technique insensitive to hypercarbia and weaning failure. A multifunctional monitor combining accurate flow and volume measurements with capnography and pulse oximetry (volumetric capnography) has been developed for ventilator management and weaning.[27] The role of capnography, however, remains to be defined in the critical care unit.

Currently capnometry is indicated to verify intubation of the trachea and esophagus. It may allow early recognition of malignant hyperthermia in the operating room and early termination of CPR in the field. The capnogram may be used to identify the end-exhalation point in the respiratory cycle for hemodynamic measurements, assess patient recovery from neuromuscular agents, and monitor airway obstruction.[34-41]

Technology has recently become available that uses partial rebreathing in conjunction with volumetric capnography to noninvasively measure cardiac output. A differential form of the Fick equation is used to calculate cardiac output. In brief, partial rebreathing decreases CO₂ elimination, and the concentration of CO₂ in the pulmonary artery increases. By measurement of the CO₂ production and end-tidal PCO₂ with and without rebreathing, cardiac output is calculated as:

$$\dot{Q}c = \frac{\Delta \dot{V}CO_2}{S \Delta P_{ET}CO_2}$$

where $\dot{Q}c$ is cardiac output, $\Delta \dot{V}CO_2$ is the difference in $\dot{V}CO_2$ with and without rebreathing, S is the slope of the CO₂ dissociation curve, and $\Delta P_{ET}CO_2$ is the difference in end-tidal PCO₂ with and without rebreathing.

Multiple Inert Gas Elimination Technique

The multiple inert gas elimination technique (MIGET) is a research technique developed to study ventilation-perfusion relationships. Eight inert gases of different solubilities, such as sulfur hexafluoride, pentane, and acetone, are dissolved in a solution for intravenous infusion. This solution is infused at a constant rate into a subject's vein, then exhaled gases and arterial and mixed venous blood are periodically sampled. Expired gases and tonometered blood are analyzed by mass spectrometry. Elimination of the gases through the exhaled air depends on ventilation-perfusion ratios and the solubility of each gas. The data are fitted to a 50-compartment mathematic lung model. The distribution of high and low $\dot{V}/\dot{Q}$ regions, dead space ventilation, and shunt can be calculated. With this technique, remarkable insight has been provided into the pathophysiology of many lung diseases. Studies have included normal subjects and patients with ARDS, pulmonary embolism, fibrosis, and COPD.

Monitoring Tissue Perfusion

A continuous supply of oxygen must reach the tissues for cells to function normally. Every cell has pathways that allow the uptake of oxygen and storage of energy as adenosine triphosphate (ATP). Fuel molecules such as glucose are oxidized or burned in the process. The most efficient pathway involves a series of oxidative-reduction reactions in the mitochondria called *oxidative phosphorylation*, or the Krebs cycle. When sufficient oxygen is present, 38 moles of ATP per mole of glucose are generated by the cycle. The last reaction in this series is the reduction of oxygen to form H₂O, catalyzed by cytochrome a,a₃ (cyt a,a₃). If an oxygen supply is lacking, ATP is produced by another pathway called *anaerobic glycolysis*. In this pathway only 2 moles of ATP per mole of glucose are produced, along with lactate and H₂O. This is an insufficient amount of energy to sustain most cells for more than a short period. In this setting, an *O₂ debt* develops, which must be repaid before function can return to normal. If oxygen availability diminishes past a critical value and persists, cells stop functioning properly and organ failure develops. A number of methods, in addition to the physical examination, can be used to obtain measured and derived parameters to describe the state and adequacy of oxygen availability to the tissues (Box 26-2).

Physical Examination

Observation and palpation of the extremities provide clues to hypoperfusion and ischemia. Pertinent findings include pallor, cyanosis, decreased pulse intensity, and decreased temperature. Tachycardia (heart rate over 100 beats/min) follows loss of 15% to 30% (750 to 1500 mL) of the blood volume. An increased rate and depth of respiration (Kussmaul pattern) develops during acidosis as minute volume increases to eliminate CO_2. Changes in mental status, such as stupor or confusion, result from decreased cerebral blood flow. Hourly urine output is a reflection of intravascular fluid and blood volume. The physical examination is central to the management of critically ill patients; however, it is recognized that by itself, it provides an incomplete picture of organ perfusion and tissue oxygenation.[15,16]

Oxygen Transport and Utilization

In the critical care unit and clinical exercise laboratory, a measure of energy utilization often is required to estimate metabolic status or work output. Oxygen consumption ($\dot{V}O_2$) is the rate of oxygen uptake by the body. Under resting conditions it is approximately 220 to 250 mL/min in adults. It rises during periods of metabolic stress, such as exercise, fever, sepsis, or injury. Most often the total $\dot{V}O_2$ is measured, although each organ system has an individual or regional $\dot{V}O_2$ that contributes in part to the global measurement.

Respiratory Recap

Measures of Tissue Perfusion	
Oxygen transport and use	Gastric tonometry
Lactate and base deficit	Near-infrared spectroscopy

In clinical practice, oxygen consumption is calculated via either respiratory gas analysis (indirect calorimetry) or the Fick equation. Respiratory gas analysis usually is performed with a commercial metabolic cart or exercise system by use of an algorithm based on the following equation:

$$\dot{V}O_2 = (\dot{V}_I \times FIO_2) - (\dot{V}_E \times FEO_2)$$

where $\dot{V}_I$ is inspired minute ventilation, $\dot{V}_E$ is expired minute ventilation, FIO_2 is the fractional concentration of oxygen in inspired air, and FEO_2 is the fractional concentration of oxygen in expired gas. The cart uses a flowmeter or pneumotachometer to measure minute volume, and gas analyzers to measure oxygen and carbon dioxide in respired gases. In the ICU, the study usually is conducted over a 15- to 30-minute period during steady-state conditions. During exercise studies, $\dot{V}O_2$ can be measured breath by breath with rapid-response gas analyzers.

The Fick equation relates $\dot{V}O_2$ to cardiac output and arterial and mixed venous oxygen content, where $\dot{V}O_2$ is the product of the cardiac output and the arteriovenous oxygen content difference, as follows:

$$\dot{V}O_2 = \dot{Q}c \times (CaO_2 - C\bar{v}O_2)$$
$$CaO_2 = (SaO_2 \times Hb \times 1.34) + (0.0031 \times PaO_2)$$
$$C\bar{v}O_2 = (S\bar{v}O_2 \times Hb \times 1.34) + (0.003 \times P\bar{v}O_2)$$

where $\dot{V}O_2$ is oxygen consumption, $\dot{Q}c$ is cardiac output, CaO_2 is arterial oxygen content, $C\bar{v}O_2$ is oxygen content of

Box 26-2

Methods to Determine Tissue Oxygenation

Noninvasive Methods
Mental status
Skin temperature
Heart rate
Urine output
Pulse oximetry
Transcutaneous oxygen pressure
Near-infrared spectroscopy

Invasive Methods
Arterial blood sampling (PaO_2, SaO_2, base deficit)
Mixed venous blood sampling ($P\bar{v}O_2$, $S\bar{v}O_2$, lactate level)
Oxygen availability
Oxygen extraction ratio
Gastric tonometry

PaO_2, *Partial pressure of arterial oxygen*; SaO_2, *arterial oxygen saturation*; $P\bar{v}O_2$, *partial pressure of oxygen in mixed venous blood*; $S\bar{v}O_2$, *oxygen saturation of mixed venous blood.*

mixed venous blood, SaO_2 is arterial oxygen saturation, Hb is hemoglobin, and $S\bar{v}O_2$ is mixed venous oxyhemoglobin saturation.

Cardiac output usually us measured with a thermodilution PAC. Arterial and mixed venous blood samples are required for blood gas and hemoglobin measurement. The contribution of dissolved oxygen is small and ignored except under hyperbaric conditions. The amount of oxygen bound to hemoglobin is represented by 1.34 mL of O_2 per 1 g Hb (1.34, 1.36, or 1.39 can be used). It is multiplied by 10 to allow $\dot{V}O_2$ to be expressed in milliliters per minute. In the ICU, respiratory gas analysis is preferred when available because it collects and averages data over a steady-state interval, measures regional pulmonary $\dot{V}O_2$, and is independent of *linked variables* (see below). The Fick estimate represents only those few minutes when the cardiac output and blood samples are obtained and does not include pulmonary $\dot{V}O_2$. Nevertheless, it still correlates well with respiratory gas analysis under steady-state resting conditions.[42,43]

Before the development of dye-indicator dilution techniques, the $\dot{V}O_2$ measurements obtained by respiratory gas analysis were combined with arterial and mixed venous blood sampling values at the time of right and left cardiac catheterization to calculate cardiac output. Today, the metabolic carts using respiratory gas analysis are used primarily to conduct pulmonary exercise studies and to measure the resting energy expenditure (indirect calorimetry) for nutritional support calculations.

Oxygen delivery (DO_2) is the rate of oxygen transport to the peripheral tissues. It is also referred to as O_2 *availability* or O_2 *transport*. It is determined by the cardiac output (CO) and arterial oxygen content (CaO_2). The arterial oxygen content depends on the Hb concentration and the amount of oxygen bound to each gram of hemoglobin, as follows:

$$Do_2 \text{ (mL/min)} = \dot{Q}c \text{ (L/min)} \times Cao_2 \times 10$$

In normal individuals, cardiac output can increase two to four times to meet increased demand during exercise or to compensate for decreases in oxygen or hemoglobin. Oxygen delivery often is expressed as an *index* (Do_2I), dividing by body surface area (BSA) to account for individuals of different sizes. For a normal cardiac index of 3 L/min/m², a hemoglobin value of 12 g/dL, and an Sao_2 of 96%, the Do_2I equals 500 mL/min/m² (Table 26-4).[43]

Mixed venous blood sampled from the pulmonary artery represents blood combined from all the capillary beds in the body. It is mixed in the right heart but has not been reoxygenated in the lungs. The mixed venous oxyhemoglobin saturation ($S\bar{v}o_2$) can be used to track changes in arterial oxygenation (Sao_2), cardiac output ($\dot{Q}c$), and hemoglobin (Hb). The Fick equation can be rearranged in terms of $S\bar{v}o_2$, as follows:

$$S\bar{v}o_2 = Sao_2 - \left(\frac{\dot{V}o_2}{\dot{Q}c \times Hb \times 1.34} \right)$$

Values of 70% to 75% are considered normal. A $S\bar{v}o_2$ of 65% has been used as a resuscitation target in critically ill patients. To measure $S\bar{v}o_2$, a heparinized blood sample must be drawn from the distal port of a conventional PAC for blood gas analysis. Oximetric PACs are designed with fiberoptic sensors at the distal tip to measure the $S\bar{v}o_2$ continuously, eliminating the need for repeated blood sampling. A mixed venous blood sample is required periodically, however, for calibration purposes.

The **oxygen extraction ratio (O_2ER)** is a derived parameter relating the amount of oxygen removed by the peripheral tissues to the amount contained in the arterial blood, or global oxygen consumption divided by oxygen availability, as follows:[43]

$$O_2ER = \frac{\dot{V}o_2}{Do_2} = \frac{Cao_2 - C\bar{v}o_2}{Cao_2}$$

where $\dot{V}o_2$ is oxygen consumption, Do_2 is oxygen delivery, Cao_2 is the arterial oxygen content, and $C\bar{v}o_2$ is the oxygen content in mixed venous blood. Normally, when oxygen needs are stable, the body adapts to decreases in arterial content by extracting more oxygen. In disease, the ability of certain regions of the body to extract oxygen may be deranged. The cells may fail to take up oxygen from the capillaries, or oxygen may fail to reach certain tissues because of microvascular shunts or obstruction, such as is observed in sepsis and trauma.[44]

TABLE 26-4

Derived Hemodynamic and Oxygen Transport Variables

Term	Derivation	Normal Range
Mean arterial pressure (MAP)	$MAP = DBP + \frac{1}{3}(SBP - DBP)$	70 to 105 mm Hg
Mean pulmonary artery pressure (MPAP)	$MPAP = PADP + \frac{1}{3}(PASP - PADP)$	9 to 16 mm Hg
Cardiac index (CI)	$CI = \dfrac{\dot{Q}c}{BSA^*}$	2.8 to 4.2 L/min/m²
Stroke volume (SV)	$SV = \dfrac{\dot{Q}c}{HR}$	Varies with body size
Stroke index (SI)	$SVI = \dfrac{CI}{HR}$	30 to 65 mL/beat/m²
Systemic vascular resistance index (SVRI)	$SVRI = \dfrac{(MAP - CVP)}{CI} \times 80$	1600 to 2400 dyne × s × cm⁵/m²
Pulmonary vascular resistance index (PVRI)	$PVRI = \dfrac{(MPAP - PAWP)}{CI} \times 80$	250 to 430 dyne × s × cm⁵/m²
Arterial oxygen content (Cao_2)	$Cao_2 = (Sao_2 \times Hb \times 1.34) + (0.0031 \times Pao_2)$	16 to 22 mL/dL
Oxygen delivery (Do_2)	$Do_2 = \dot{Q}c \times Cao_2 \times 10$	500 to 650 mL/min/m²
Oxygen consumption ($\dot{V}o_2$)	$\dot{V}o_2 = \dot{Q}c \times (Cao_2 - C\bar{v}o_2) \times 10$	110 to 150 mL/min/m²
Oxygen extraction ratio (O_2ER)	$\dfrac{\dot{V}o_2}{Do_2}$	0.22 to 0.3

Modified from Nelson LD. Crit Care Clin 1996;12:795-818.
Body surface area (BSA) = Weight (kg) × Height (cm) × 0.007184.
DBP, *Diastolic blood pressure;* SBP, *systolic blood pressure;* PADP, *pulmonary artery diastolic pressure;* PASP, *pulmonary artery systolic pressure;* $\dot{Q}c$, *cardiac output;* HR, *heart rate;* CVP, *central venous pressure;* PAWP, *pulmonary artery wedge pressure;* Sao_2, *arterial oxygen saturation;* Hb, *hemoglobin;* Pao_2, *partial pressure of arterial oxygen;* C\bar{v}o_2, *mixed venous oxygen content.*

Regional cerebral tissue perfusion can be studied by an adaptation of the Fick equation. Standard arterial oxygen delivery measurements (DO_2) and *jugular bulb* venous blood gas analysis are used to calculate cerebral O_2ER. Cerebral mixed venous blood is obtained by insertion of a special catheter in the jugular bulb at the base of the internal jugular vein. Similar to systemic O_2ER, an increase in central nervous system (CNS) extraction implies inadequate cerebral oxygen delivery.

During exercise, tissue energy needs increase. Glucose and other fuels are burned, and oxygen consumption rises. Oxygen delivery and extraction increase proportionately. An increase in DO_2 results primarily from increases in cardiac output as stroke volume and heart rate increase. The increase in O_2ER results from capillary recruitment (the capillaries open up, or *dilate*, to perfuse muscle tissue) and from the increased cellular uptake of oxygen molecules. At higher levels of exercise, an *anaerobic threshold* is reached when cardiac output and extraction are maximized. Further effort results in anaerobic glycolysis, acidosis, and the production of lactate. The normal maximum extraction or *critical O_2ER* is 50% to 80%.

In normal resting individuals, if oxygen delivery decreases, oxygen consumption remains stable because oxygen extraction increases to make up the difference. If oxygen delivery falls below the level of maximum extraction, tissue oxygen consumption must fall, which culminates in anaerobic glycolysis and lactic acidosis. This point is called *critical DO_2* (DO_2-crit), the point where lactate levels start to rise. The critical DO_2 ranges from 5 to 10 mL/kg/min.

The relationship between $\dot{V}O_2$ and DO_2 in critical illness is complicated and controversial. In animal models of sepsis and critically ill patients, increases in DO_2-crit and decreases in O_2ER-crit, have been observed. In these conditions an otherwise normal DO_2 may be below DO_2-crit and insufficient for body needs. Efforts to increase the DO_2 under these circumstances should result in an increase in $\dot{V}O_2$. This has been called *pathologic dependence of O_2 consumption on O_2 delivery*. It may result from the body's failure to redistribute capillary blood flow to tissues or organs with the greatest need.

These observations have been vigorously challenged, partly because of the difficulty in accurate measurement of energy demands ($\dot{V}O_2$) in critical illness. Metabolic carts provide the best independent $\dot{V}O_2$ estimate but are cumbersome and still relatively imprecise ($\pm 10\%$). When the Fick relationship is used to calculate $\dot{V}O_2$ and DO_2, the same variables (cardiac output, hemoglobin, and arterial saturation) are shared in both the $\dot{V}O_2$ and DO_2 equations. This *mathematic coupling* or *linking* of variables magnifies the random and systematic error in any one of the variables and can create the false appearance of $\dot{V}O_2 - DO_2$ dependency. This has cast doubt on the use of pathologic dependence theories to guide patient care.[43,44]

End Points in Resuscitation

The observations that $\dot{V}O_2$ may be pathologically dependent on DO_2 and that decreases in $\dot{V}O_2$ correlate with ICU mortality led to strategies to increase DO_2 to supranormal levels in an attempt to improve outcomes. A low $\dot{V}O_2$ implied an unpaid oxygen debt, which left unaddressed could lead to multiple organ failure and death. Through study of the clinical differences between survivors and nonsurvivors, protocols were developed to guide management. The preselected goals were a cardiac index over 4.5 L/min/m², a DO_2 over 600 mL/min/m², and a $\dot{V}O_2$ over 170 mL/min/m². These values generally were achieved by red cell transfusion, volume challenges, and administration of inotropic agents. Numerous studies have addressed this strategy, and current data do not support the use of supranormal oxygen transport variables as end points for resuscitation.[44]

Lactate is the end point molecule in anaerobic glycolysis. It is produced from pyruvate by the enzyme lactate dehydrogenase (LDH). Ordinarily, sufficient oxygen is present in normal individuals, and pyruvate is converted to acetyl-CoA, entering the Krebs cycle and mitochondria to produce 38 moles of ATP. In the absence of sufficient oxygen, pyruvate is converted to lactate, H_2O, and 2 moles of ATP per mole of glucose. The accumulation of lactate has been used as a marker for oxygen debt and a guide for resuscitation. Moreover, the time required to normalize serum lactate in critically ill patients has been correlated with organ failure and survival. Lactate may persist in the circulation, however, because of impaired clearance rather than ongoing oxygen debt. This may occur in liver or kidney failure, because the liver normally accounts for about 50% and the kidney for about 30% of lactate metabolism.

Serum lactate usually is drawn from the mixed venous blood, iced, and transported to the laboratory. The turnaround time is 1 to 2 hours. New multichannel analyzers available for stat-lab or ICU use can measure lactate with a turnaround of about 90 seconds. Based on current evidence, serial lactate determinations are used in many centers as an end point for shock resuscitation.[44]

The base deficit is the amount of base, such as bicarbonate, required to titrate a liter of whole blood to a pH of 7.4 when the sample is fully saturated with oxygen at 37° C and the PCO_2 is 40 mm Hg. This value is automatically calculated from the arterial blood gas by most arterial blood gas analyzers. It correlates fairly well with serum lactate in shock and provides an estimate of tissue acidosis. Severely abnormal base deficits at the time of ICU admission have been associated with mortality. A worsening base deficit also correlates with uncontrolled hemorrhage in trauma patients. The base deficit has the advantage of being easily measured and available to any ICU with an arterial blood gas analyzer. For these reasons, it has been adopted by many centers as an end point for resuscitation.[44]

Gastric Tonometry

The measurements and strategies discussed above provide global estimates of tissue perfusion with arterial and mixed venous blood sampling. Important regional perfusion deficits may be masked by the averaging effect of blood mixing in the circulation. Under conditions of stress, the gut is one of the first regional capillary beds to suffer as blood is redirected to the brain, heart, and kidneys. It also has a unique microvascular anatomy that makes it particularly sensitive to hypoxia. **Gastric tonometry** is a technique that measures CO_2 in the gastric lumen with a catheter placed in the stomach. The intraluminal P_{CO_2} is used to calculate the gastric or intestinal pH (pH_i) with the Henderson-Hasselbalch equation, as follows:

$$pH_i = 6.1 + \log \frac{HCO_3^-}{\alpha \times \text{Tonometer } P_{CO_2}}$$

where α is 0.03, the solubility of CO_2 in plasma, and HCO_3^- is the mucosal concentration of bicarbonate. The arterial HCO_3^- is used to estimate the mucosal HCO_3^-. In the tonometer's original design, a balloon holding 2 to 3 mL of saline was attached to a nasogastric tube and placed in the stomach. Saline was introduced, and over an equilibration period of 30 to 90 minutes, the mucosal CO_2 diffused into the saline. The saline was withdrawn and run through an arterial blood gas analyzer to measure P_{CO_2}. A simultaneous arterial blood sample was required to calculate the plasma HCO_3^-. A new automated system uses air instead of saline, pumping it in and out of the balloon, as an infrared analyzer measures P_{CO_2}. An updated value is available every 10 to 15 minutes. Other designs use recirculating air, balloonless tonometers, and fiberoptic CO_2 sensors. Complications usually are minor and are related to the placement of a small-bore gastric tube (for example, sinusitis, aspiration, and esophageal injury or perforation).

Gastric tonometry has been studied in a variety of conditions, such as aortic aneurysm repair and major trauma, in which patients are at risk of intestinal ischemia. A low gastric pH_i has been associated with postoperative complications, failure to wean from mechanical ventilation, increased ICU costs, and mortality. This technique is being investigated in critically ill patients in an attempt to develop improved resuscitation and management strategies.[45]

Near-Infrared Spectroscopy

Near-infrared spectroscopy (NIRS) is a noninvasive optical technique that measures the absorption of near-infrared light by tissues to study regional O_2 availability and consumption. It can measure blood flow, relative amounts of oxyhemoglobin and deoxyhemoglobin, and the redox state of cytochrome a,a_3 (cyt a,a_3) at the end of the mitochondrial electron transport chain. In the presence of adequate amounts of O_2, cyt a,a_3 donates its electron (and is oxidized) to an oxygen molecule (which is reduced) to form ATP and water. Under anaerobic conditions, when there is insufficient O_2 to receive electrons, cyt a,a_3 remains in a re-

duced state. Measuring the redox state (whether cyt a,a_3 is reduced or oxidized) determines the adequacy of O_2 delivery to the tissue being monitored.

Near-infrared light (700 to 1000 nm) is beamed through or reflected from an accessible target organ, such as the brain, or extremity and collected by an optical analyzer. Complex and deep tissues such as skin, bone, and muscle can be studied, because the only light-absorbing molecules, or *chromophores*, that vary with changes in oxygenation are hemoglobin, myoglobin, and cyt a,a_3. This promising technique remains a research tool until certain technical challenges can be overcome. It provides unique clinical information about tissue perfusion and cellular function not available with other methods.[46]

Monitoring Principles and Technology

Respiratory therapists are confronted with a diverse array of monitoring technologies. To make informed decisions about equipment purchases, use, and maintenance, they must understand the engineering principles behind these systems. Cardiopulmonary monitoring technology relies on sensing devices to measure biophysical parameters and signal transmission to central processing units and may involve sophisticated display and storage functions, as well as dynamic interfaces with other computer networks.

Sensors and Transducers

A sensor is a device designed to detect and respond to changes in its physical or chemical environment. A good sensor responds in a predictable way to the quantity being studied. Sensors usually are designed so that these biophysical effects change a parameter in an electrical circuit. In respiratory care these are biophysical variables, such as blood pressure or oxygen concentration. Based on their electrical behavior, sensors are divided into two types. *Active sensors* generate their own current in response to a change in the parameter being measured; these include thermocouples, piezoelectric elements, and pH probes. *Passive sensors* require an external source of energy, such as a battery; these include bioelectrodes, hot-wire anemometers (flowmeters), thermistors, and strain gauges. Sensors usually are supported by *conditioning equipment*, such as electronic circuitry, power supplies, and temperature con-

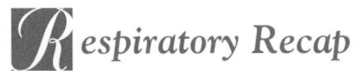

$\mathcal{R}$*espiratory Recap*

Sensors and Transducers	
Bioelectrodes	Diodes
Thermistors	Strain gauges
Thermocouples	Pressure transducers
Piezoelectrics	Wheatstone bridge

trollers. A **transducer** is a type of passive or active sensor that converts one form of energy directly into another. In most medical uses this involves conversion of mechanical energy into electrical energy (for example, pressure or ultrasound transducers).[47]

Bioelectrodes are a class of sensors that detect ionic (charged molecule) movements. They change these ionic currents into electronic (electron) conduction that can be processed in electrical circuits. Human tissue is made up of cells that contain ionic solutions. All the electrical activity in the human body is actually ionic, involving sodium (Na^+), potassium (K^+), calcium (Ca^{+2}), magnesium (Mg^{+2}), chloride (Cl^-), and other charged molecules. For example, ionic movements in the heart result in charge gradients or potentials that can be detected at the skin surface. These potentials are electronically processed to generate the electrocardiogram.

A bioelectrode allows the transfer of ions from the body surface through a chemical reaction to a detector. Electrodes are constructed from metal compounds with properties that allow them to participate in these reactions. Not all materials are suitable, because metals can be toxic to biologic tissue, and body fluids can be corrosive to the electrode. The noble metals (gold and platinum), some tungsten alloys, and silver–silver chloride (Ag–AgCl) usually are used. The Ag–AgCl electrode is most often used for ECG recording. It is placed in contact with the skin through a conducting electrolyte gel or paste to improve contact and reduce irritation. The AgCl is plated on the Ag wire and is in contact with the skin, allowing a two-way exchange of Ag^+ and Cl^- ions between the skin and metal. A charge gradient builds in the Ag wire portion of the electrode, creating a potential difference, also known as an electrode potential or *half-cell potential*. Usually two or more electrodes are applied to the body, and the potential or voltage difference between two is measured and amplified. The surface ECG signal is about 1 to 2 mV, and the electroencephalogram (EEG) scalp potentials are about 50 μV.[47]

A thermistor, as its name suggests, is a thermally dependent resistor. If the electrical resistance decreases with increasing temperature, the device has a negative temperature coefficient (NTC), and conversely a rise in resistance with increasing temperature defines a thermistor with a positive temperature coefficient (PTC). NTC types are more common. Both types are nonlinear when used over large temperature ranges. Over a limited range, as in clinical uses, the thermistor can assumed to be fairly linear. Some materials used in the manufacture of thermistors include oxides of cobalt, nickel, copper, iron, titanium, strontium, and manganese. Most of the thermistors used for airflow detection are in the form of small beads with a glass or epoxy protective coating.[19]

Because a thermistor is a passive device, its changing resistance is detected by the application of a small voltage, which in turn causes a small current to flow. The circuitry providing power to the thermistor usually is designed to produce a relatively constant current so that the thermistor

output becomes a varying voltage. The actual current may come from the polygraph or monitor that has been designed to work with a particular thermistor or from a small in-line module housing a battery and circuitry. A low current is used to reduce the effects of self-heating, which reduce the sensitivity of the thermistor. Although it is desirable to maximize the exposed surface area so that the sensor remains in the path of flowing air, the mass of the sensor is minimized for faster response to airflow changes.[19,47]

A thermocouple is an active sensor used to measure temperature. When two dissimilar materials, usually metals or semiconductors, are joined, a small voltage develops across their junction. This voltage is sensitive to temperature. In practice, one of the junctions is kept at a reference temperature, and the other is exposed to the temperature to be measured. It usually is impractical to choose the same two metals for the interconnecting cable conductors, therefore two new junctions are formed when the connecting cable (for example, copper wire) is attached, creating three important thermal junctions (Figure 26-15). The output becomes a function of the temperature and contacting materials at all three junctions. To measure the thermoelectric voltage changes produced by a sensing junction in the airstream, it is important that the temperature at the other two junctions remain relatively constant, usually insulated in the body of the sensor, and that the connecting material at these junctions be chosen to produce only small thermal voltages. About two dozen different combinations of conductors are used in thermocouples, including chromel, constantan, iron, and copper.

The differences between thermistors and thermocouples, other than their theory of operation, are minimal. Thermocouples are simpler to operate because they produce their own voltage and therefore can be plugged directly into most polygraphs or EEG machines. No batteries are required. Their output also is very linear with temperatures over the human physiologic range. Thermistors do allow greater control of the sensor output level, or *gain*, because increasing the level of the current source results in a higher output voltage at a given temperature.[19,47,48]

Piezoelectric materials are widely encountered in bioengineering designs. They are used to record heart sounds, measure pressure and displacements, and create ultrasound for therapeutic and diagnostic purposes. These crystalline piezoelectric materials generate an AC voltage at the frequency of an applied mechanical force, or conversely, an applied AC electrical potential produces a physical deformation at the applied frequency (see Figure 26-15). The piezoelectric phenomenon occurs in asymmetric crystal lattices. When the lattices are mechanically distorted, a charge reorientation takes place, causing a relative displacement of negative and positive charges. Surface charges of opposite polarity develop on opposing sides of the crystal, producing a potential difference that can be measured with a voltmeter.

Many different piezoelectric materials can be found in biomedical devices. Some of the more common are quartz,

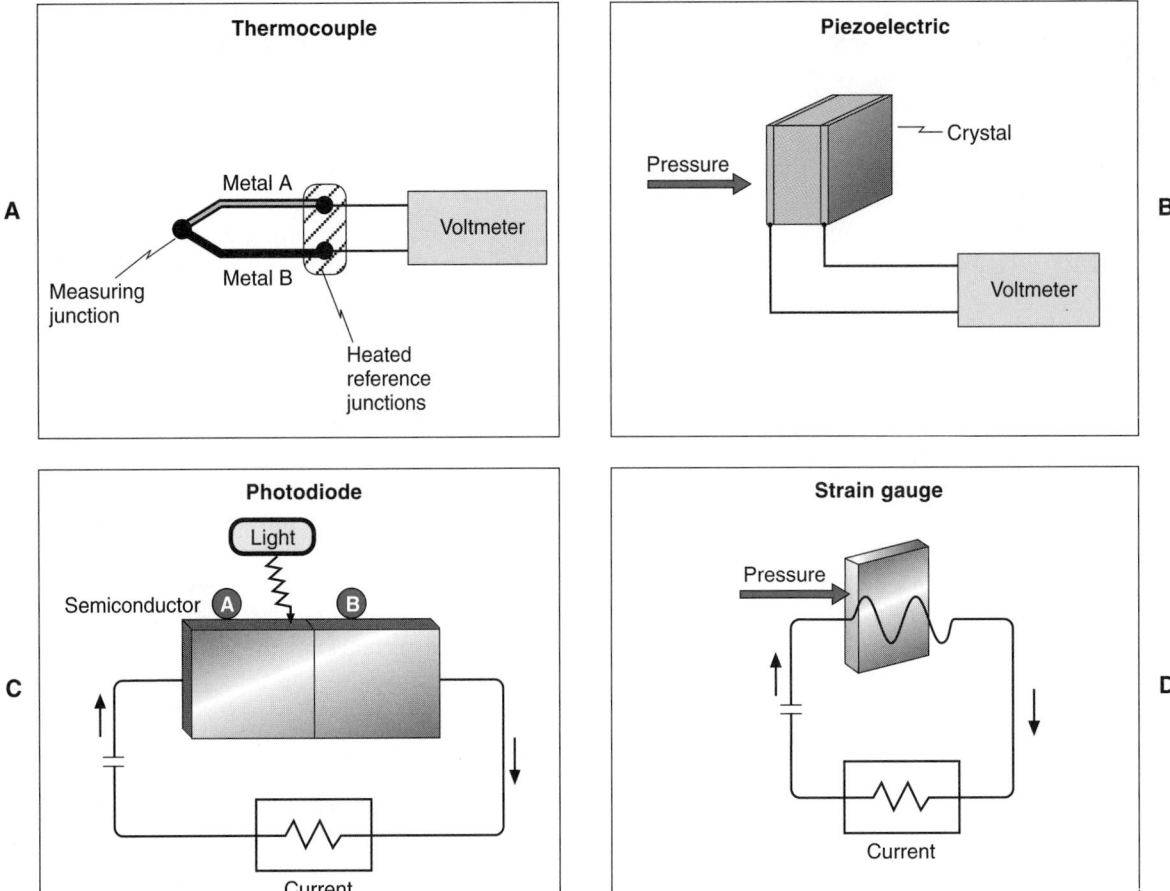

Figure 26-15 Biophysical sensors interact with the environment to produce a change in an electrical circuit. Active sensors such as thermocouples **(A)**, piezoelectric crystals **(B)**, and photodiodes **(C)** generate small electrical potentials, or currents, when stimulated. **D,** Strain gauges are passive sensors that change the resistance of a circuit supplied by an external current source.

Rochelle salts, and tourmaline. Synthetic polymeric materials such as polyvinyl fluoride and polyvinylidene fluoride also have piezoelectric properties. Depending on the use intended, synthetic films may have advantages over the natural and ceramic materials, which are brittle, stiff, and difficult to produce in large amounts. Although synthetics provide less transducing power, they can be cut or stamped into almost any shape and are light, flexible, and resistant to stress fatigue and abrasion. They also operate over a broader range of frequencies and respond to a wider degree of mechanical stress.[19,48]

Diodes are electronic devices that function like one-way valves. They are constructed from dissimilar semiconductors joined at a junction. The valve allows current to flow in only one direction. A *light-emitting diode* (LED) is designed to emit light at certain wavelengths in response to an input current. Conversely, a *photodiode* is a diode with a junction designed to be stimulated by photons of specific wavelengths (see Figure 26-15). The junction causes an excitation, or *bias current,* to rise or fall depending on the light intensity. The properties of these ubiquitous circuit elements are determined by the semiconductors used and a process called *doping.* Doping involves the

addition of impurities such as phosphorus or boron to the silicon or gallium semiconductor substrate. In a photodiode, the junction can be doped to respond to specific or broad wavebands of light. For example, in pulse oximeter probes three diodes are used, a single photodiode capable of detecting a very wide range of optical wavelengths and two LEDs, one emitting a narrow band of light at 660 nm and the other at 940 nm. The photodiode recognizes light from one of the two LEDs at a time by a process known as *time-division multiplexing.* The photodiode does not know which LED is shining on it, causing it to generate an electrical response, but the microprocessing unit does, because it knows which LED is turned on at any given moment. The microprocessor turns the two LEDs on and off at very high rates, about 1000 times a second. This gives the red LED the appearance of always being on because the infrared LED is always, of course, invisible to the eye. The flaw inherent in time division multiplexing is that the monitor assumes that the signal from the photodiode is exclusively generated by the LED it turned on at that time. If light from another source, particularly another pulsed source, including fluorescent light, is being detected by the photodiode at the same time, the monitor cannot distinguish between the light it is generating and the light from the external source. It is essential, therefore, that oximetry sensors be optically shielded with opaque material.[48,49]

The unique Capnostat solid-state CO_2 analyzer also is a broad waveband photodetector made from lead selenide that changes its resistance to current flow in response to infrared light. It is not a diode, however, because there are no discrete junctions. Optical filters and mirrors are placed downstream from the sample cell to split the beam, passing one wavelength band from inside the CO_2 spectrum and one outside the spectrum (reference) to adjacent detectors (see Figure 26-10). The photodetector response to a known concentration of CO_2 is stored in the monitor memory, which allows the system to electronically self-calibrate.[49]

The **strain gauge** is a sensor that changes its electrical resistance in response to an applied force. The force may tend to shorten or lengthen the element. Metals or semiconductors usually are used and bonded to a deformable diaphragm (see Figure 26-15). Most physiologic pressure transducers are based on this design.

The pressure transducer is a device that converts mechanical into electrical energy. Pressure monitoring devices such as intraarterial cannulas and pulmonary artery catheters are fluid filled and connected to the transducer by semirigid, noncompliant tubing. Pressure is physically defined as force applied on an area. Mechanical forces at the catheter-blood interface are transmitted back through the continuous column of fluid to the transducer, a fluid-filled dome and diaphragm containing a strain gauge. As the diaphragm is deflected by the movement of the fluid column, the electrical resistance of the strain gauge changes. The strain gauge is connected to a Wheatstone bridge or similar electronic circuit to process the signal and display the results.

Intravascular pressure monitoring systems require tubing and connectors designed for their specific use. The shape of the pressure waveform is determined by the *dynamic response*, or the way the entire system reacts to a mechanical impulse. The dynamic response, in turn, is determined by the *harmonic* or *natural resonant frequency* and *damping* characteristics of the entire system (cannula to transducer). Fluid-filled systems have a natural resonant frequency governed mainly by the length and composition of the pressure tubing. If the repetitive changes in pressure are similar to this natural frequency, the system vibrates, or *resonates*, causing the signal to be overamplified. This falsely elevates the pressure readings. Pressure transducers, therefore, are designed for use with a specified narrow gauge, relatively stiff tubing that is usually less than 87.5 to 112.5 cm long. In general, the resonant frequency should be at least five times the physiologic frequency to avoid resonance and ensure good fidelity. This would correspond to a resonant frequency of 10 to 20 Hz (cycles or vibrations/second) if pressure signals were measured at adult heart rates of 60 to 120 beats/min.

Damping is the loss of the physiologic signal as the result of loss of mechanical energy in the system. This usually is caused by air bubbles contaminating the fluid-filled

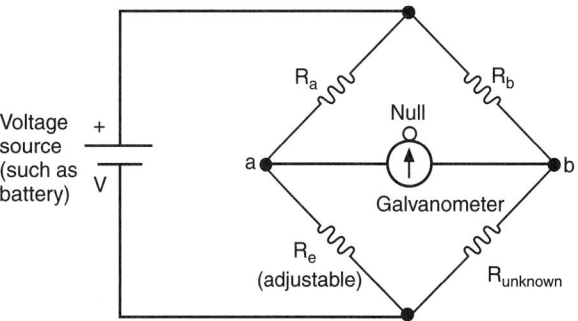

Figure 26-16 Wheatstone bridge circuit is used to measure electrical resistance changes in strain gauges built into pressure transducers. Solid-state bridge circuits have replaced the classic galvanometer and resistor array.

column. When the bubbles are compressed, energy is lost and the transmitted force is diminished. Damping may also result from kinking, loose connections, blood clots in the tubing, and measurements attempted above the natural frequency. Excessive damping causes a flattening of the waveform.[13]

The most straightforward way to use a passive sensor is to apply a voltage with a battery and measure the resulting change in current as the electrical resistance of the sensor changes in response to its environment. The current changes usually are very small, however, and difficult to measure accurately. Consequently, a *bridge circuit* is used to improve the quality of the measurement, based on the **Wheatstone bridge** concept (Figure 26-16). The bridge has four separate arms, or *resistors*, connected in a circuit. When a voltage is applied across the bridge, a potential develops across the other two corners of the circuit depending on the individual resistances. The *null condition* exists when the resistances *balance* and the output voltage is zero. In its original design, one of the arms was used to measure an unknown resistance. The other arms included known and adjustable resistors (R_a, R_b, and R_c). A voltage was placed across the bridge that included the unknown resistor, such as the strain gauge in a pressure transducer. When the resistors were adjusted to balance the bridge, the unknown resistance could be calculated. This strategy worked for static measurements but was too slow for dynamic or rapidly changing biologic systems. In biomedical uses, transducers usually are connected to other electronic components to form a modification of the Wheatstone bridge circuit. The wires connecting the sensor or transducer to the monitor unit complete a circuit that contains one or more arms of the bridge. In most monitor designs, the bridge is *balanced* and the *null condition* prevails when no stimulus is applied; the transducer is then at *zero baseline*. The parameter being measured generates a change in the resistance of the circuit at the sensor and unbalances the bridge. The unbalanced bridge, in turn, produces an output voltage proportional to the value of the applied stimulus.[48,49]

All sensing elements must be *calibrated,* or compared to a standard. The response of the sensor and electronics to a standard input is recorded, and a calibration plot or curve is generated. Some sensors are calibrated at the manufacturer (for example, ECG electrodes and oximetry probes) and then self-calibrate with monitor software and solid-state electronics. Standard external inputs are required to calibrate mechanical systems (pressure transducers and respiratory inductance bands) and chemical systems such as blood gas analyzers. One-, two-, or multiple-point calibrations may be required. A *one-point* calibration involves the inputting of a single standard, usually zero, atmospheric pressure, or a single known concentration of the gas or liquid analyte. The response of the system is presumed to follow a known curve, usually linear, after calibration at this one point. Disposable pressure transducers, for example, have a standard sensitivity of 5 μV/V/mm Hg, allowing a one-point (zero) calibration. The transducer response is then linear through its designated range. *Two-point* or *multiple-point* calibrations use several known inputs along the desired measurement range to define the calibration curve. Multiple calibration points are necessary for systems in which the response of the sensor may change with use or environmental conditions. Reusable pressure transducers require two-point calibrations, because the flexibility of the diaphragm (strain gauge) changes over time. Multiple-point calibrations are also usually required for analyzers based on chemical reactions such as blood gas and electrolyte systems.

Signal Transmission

Many portable and bedside units are *hardwired* with electrical wires to connect the sensor to the processing unit. These wires are used to detect a voltage arising between two points, such as ECG leads, or to conduct a small current sent by the monitor. All wires and connections are insulated to avoid interference from stray electrical signals and to prevent contact with other conductors, causing shorting or grounding. Moreover, the entire patient circuit must be insulated or separated from the bedside electrical circuitry in some way to avoid accidental electrical shock. This is accomplished by special inductance circuits inside the monitor or by optical connectors at the module-monitor interface.

Two types of currents are encountered in analyzers and monitoring systems. *Direct current* (DC) involves a one-way flow of electrons away from the cathode (positive terminal) to the anode (negative terminal). Direct current energy can be supplied by chemical batteries, solar cells, thermocouples, or DC generators. The ionic or electrolyte-based reactions in the human body generate very small voltages and DC currents. DC circuits are described by Ohm's Law: $V = I \times R$, where V is the voltage (volts), or driving force; I is the current (amperes), or flow of electrons; and R is resistance (Ohms). *Alternating currents* (AC) involve the to and fro movement of electrons in wires in response to an alternating voltage. Most electrical energy is generated and transmitted via AC current. The analysis of AC currents is more complex. In an AC current, the overall resistance is called impedance. **Bioimpedance,** for example, is the opposition encountered by an AC current sent between two electrodes placed on the body.[48]

Data transmission to a remote location is called **telemetry,** or measurement at a distance. Electrical signals can be transmitted through the air as radio waves or over telephone-type lines. When radio waves are used to broadcast data, such as the cardiac rhythm, the transmitter changes, or *modulates*, a high-frequency carrier wave to superimpose the data. The receiving unit *demodulates*, or reverses, the process to decode the carrier wave and retrieve the data. In cardiac telemetry the carrier wave is in the VHF or UHF (very high or ultrahigh frequency) spectrum used by television channels. Two familiar systems are used to encode data on radio carrier waves: amplitude modulation (AM), and frequency modulation (FM), similar to AM and FM radio stations. In the AM system, the *amplitude* of the carrier wave is varied according to changes in the data. In the FM system, the *frequency* is varied. The modulated signal is actually a complicated wave containing several *sidebands*. The carrier wave frequency plus its sidebands represents its *bandwidth*. FM bandwidths are 200 kHz wide (about 20 times wider than AM bandwidths), resulting in less noise or stray radio wave interference from nearby frequencies and therefore greater *fidelity*. Each telemetry patient is assigned to a specified bandwidth or channel.

Early home cardiac telemetry used telephone lines to transmit audio signals through telephone-like devices. A carrier audio tone was modulated to encode the ECG information. For a single ECG lead, the voltage deflections changed the frequency or pitch of the tone (FM). The sequence of musical tones was actually audible to the ear and sent directly through the earpiece of a telephone handset. The telephone on the receiving end listened to the tone and decoded it, changing it back to voltage deflections to trace the ECG on a paper strip. This was one of the first modulator-demodulator units, or *modems*, used in clinical medicine.

When several different signals must be telemetered, time division multiplexing is used. A timer in the transmitter circuit allows sampling of each separate input for a specified time interval in rotation (for example, ECG lead I, II, III, AVL, and so on) and then repeats the process over and over (Figure 26-17). The timer is synchronized with the receiver so that it can decode the carrier signal into the separate components.[48]

Signal Processing

Analog data are the output of a device that is *analogous* to the system being measured. For example, the current from a sensor causes a galvanometer needle to move across a calibrated scale. During transmission, however, electrical analog signals are susceptible to deterioration by stray electrical noise and attenuation in long cables. To maintain signal integrity over long distances and extreme conditions, almost all analog signals in medical monitoring systems are now electronically converted to digital format by an analog-to-

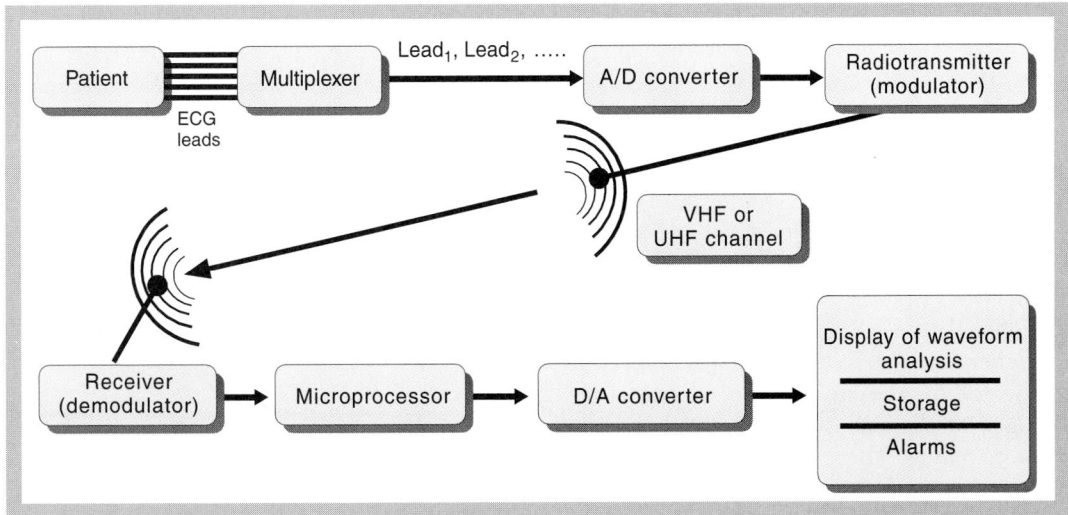

Figure 26-17   Telemetry system.

digital (A to D) converter. A digital signal is discrete, using binary digits (a string of 0's and 1's), or *bits*, to code the analog signal. An analog-to-digital converter samples the analog signal at very short intervals and assigns a digit to the analog value at each time point. After transmission the digital information can be converted back to analog for display, for example, on a video monitor (see Figure 26-17). Digital data can be inspected for errors and artifact and discarded, if necessary, by the monitoring system. Additional information can be coded into digital transmissions, such as ECG lead identification. Early computers were based on analog designs but were soon replaced by faster, more accurate digital computers. All modern computers, including personal computers (PCs), are digital.[48]

Respiratory Recap

Components of Signal Processors	
Analog-to-digital converters	Storage media
Microprocessors	Alarms
Displays and monitors	Power sources

Modern monitoring units or systems are small, dedicated computers with microprocessors or central processing units (CPUs). They have most of the components familiar to PC technology, including memory and software designed to receive signals from the sensor and analog-to-digital converter; they also rapidly perform complex calculations, then display, store, or transmit the data. In most microprocessor-controlled monitoring systems, the integrity of the electrical circuitry, including the sensor, modular plug-in interfaces, and power supplies, is checked each time the system is turned on by internal software routines.

Microprocessor-based monitoring systems all require some type of input device, such as push buttons or a keyboard, to allow custom programming by the user. New generation monitoring systems may interface with bedside notebook computers, which have a mouse or keyboards or allow the monitor screen itself to be used as a touchpad.

One of the first electromechanical analog display devices was the galvanometer, which uses a needle rotating in front of a calibrated scale or face. The base of the needle is attached to a magnet that is suspended on an axle inside a wire coil connected to the sensor. As the sensor causes current changes in the coil, the magnetic field around the axle changes, and the needle rotates or points to a value on the scale. These devices are still used in oxygen analyzers. The *cathode-ray oscilloscope* represents another prototype display design. A cathode-ray tube generates a small controlled spot where a beam of electrons strike a fluorescent screen. The vertical position of the beam, up or down, is proportional to input voltages from the sensor or transducer. When a sweep generator moves the spot horizontally across the screen, waveforms are generated. Hemodynamic waveforms were first displayed with this device. If the sweep generator is replaced by rolling graph paper and the voltages are used to deflect a heated pen, *strip-recordings* result.

Newer microprocessor or computer-based systems have a number of display capabilities. With LEDs or liquid crystal displays (LCDs), the numeric results and waveforms are displayed for ease of visual inspection. Larger systems use *monitors*, in this context meaning a video display device similar to TV screens, based on the cathode-ray tube. They function in a manner similar to PC systems, using video *drivers* (software) and *controllers* (hardware) to provide multiple channels of data and waveforms. The software allows programming of alarms, color, size, custom displays, and freeze options.

Online printer modules can provide paper copies of graphic data or formatted reports. Original strip chart recorders rolled graph paper from a spool at a specified speed, usually 25 mm/second under a pen deflected up and down by the electrical potentials inputted from the sensors. The pen could write on the paper with pencil or ink or could be heated to burn the tracing into the graph paper. A polygraph is a multichannel strip recorder. These early devices required cumbersome zeroing and calibration with each use. Modern printers are microprocessor-controlled, internally calibrated systems that use an array of pens to reproduce or print the tracing, along with graph lines and additional data, such as the date and the patient's name, on chemically treated blank paper. The pens are electrically heated to generate a focused chemical reaction on the paper. Measurements can be stored on various media for later analysis. The array of available storage media has evolved from the first spools or cassettes of magnetic tape to diskettes, hard drives, and writeable compact discs of enormous capacity.

By definition a monitor is a physiologic analyzer or sensor plus an alarm appropriate to the clinical setting. Audio and visual alarms may be used. Advanced units store information as to the cause of the alarm for later review. Many systems have default alarm ranges that may need to be adjusted if used in different patient populations. An alarm's integrity and ranges should be verified frequently. There is a danger that systems that alarm too frequently will be tuned out by caregivers. The proliferation of monitoring devices has created a noise problem for critical care areas, causing interference with clinical care and disrupting patient sleep cycles. Studies are underway on the critical care work environment to find ways to manage the intrusion of alarms. Fortunately, despite the increasing numbers of alarms, clinical staff have been found to adapt quickly, developing an ear for the characteristic ring of the most important monitors.

Microprocessors require electrical power. All larger systems use 120-V AC wall output as their primary power source or as backup for portable units. Rechargeable 9- to 15-V lead-acid batteries are used to power portable systems, such as pulse oximeters. Monitor performance can deteriorate with battery fatigue. A fully charged battery has a specified lifetime. Recharging times may be substantial, such as 4 hours for 1 hour of operating time. These parameters are provided in the technical manuals and differ from product to product. In addition, small coin-type lithium batteries of about 3 V are required to power the internal computer memory and clocks in microprocessor-controlled units. These have a longer lifetime but may fail unexpectedly and confuse the user, because the other larger and more visible power sources will still be charged.[26-28]

The critical care clinician now can assemble a system of monitoring devices at the bedside using modular components. One patient may need pulmonary artery pressure monitoring, another, capnography. The modules are plugged in and immediately configured for calibration and use by the central microprocessor. With the concept of *open architecture*, products from different manufacturers can be interfaced with personal computers and operating platforms. This allows monitoring systems to download measured parameters into documentation or clinical software to generate paperless medical records. Data from several patients can be loaded into data bases to create custom reports, and these data bases can be used to perform outcome and performance analysis in units and among institutions.

ℋEY 𝒫OINTS

- The heart rate can be measured by counting of the peripheral pulse or use of bedside cardiac monitors, telemetry units, or Holter monitors.
- Arterial blood pressure can be measured noninvasively or invasively.
- The central venous pressure is a useful guide to fluid and blood volume replacement.
- The pulmonary artery catheter is used to measure the pulmonary artery pressure, wedge pressure, cardiac output, mixed venous oxygen saturation, and right ventricular ejection fraction.
- The respiratory rate and pattern can be monitored through observation of chest wall motion, monitoring of nasal airflow, and measurement of chest wall motion.
- Intraarterial blood gas monitors measure blood gases and pH continuously.
- Point of care (POC) analyzers allow blood gases to be measured at the bedside with a few drops of blood.
- Transcutaneous P_{O_2} and P_{CO_2} are measured with a heated electrode placed on the skin.
- Pulse oximetry measures oxygen saturation by passing two wavelengths of light through a pulsating vascular bed.
- The accuracy of pulse oximetry is ±4%; a number of factors can affect the accuracy and performance of pulse oximetry.
- Capnometry measures the concentration of carbon dioxide exhaled from the lungs.
- Although capnography can be useful for such purposes as detection of esophageal intubation, end-tidal P_{CO_2} may not be an accurate reflection of Pa_{CO_2}.
- Tissue perfusion can be assessed by monitoring of oxygen transport and utilization, the lactate level, and the base deficit and by gastric tonometry and infrared spectroscopy.
- Sensors detect and respond to changes in the physical and chemical environment.
- Transducers convert one form of energy into another.
- A monitor senses a physiologic signal and transmits it to a processing unit, which displays it in a usable format.

References

1. Curley FJ, Smyrnios NA. Routine monitoring of critically ill patients. J Intensive Care Med 1990;5:153-174.

2. Perloff D, Grim C, Flack J, et al. Human blood pressure determination by sphygmomanometry. Circulation 1993;88:2460-2467.

3. Reeves RA. Does this patient have hypertension? How to measure blood pressure. JAMA 1995;273:1211-1218.

4. Clark VL, Kruse JA. Arterial catheterization. Crit Care Clin 1992;8:687-697.

5. Dorman T, Breslow MJ, Lipsett PA, et al. Radial artery pressure monitoring underestimates central arterial pressure during vasopressor therapy in critically ill surgical patients. Crit Care Med 1998;26:1646-1649.

6. Agee KR, Balk RA. Central venous catheterization in the critically ill patient. Crit Care Clin 1992;8:677-686.

7. Arrow multi-lumen central venous catheter care: nursing care guidelines. Reading, Pa: Arrow International; 1996.

8. Voyce SJ, Rippe JM. Pulmonary artery catheters: an update. J Intensive Care Med 1990;5:175-192.

9. Randolph AG, Cook DJ, Gonzales CA, et al. Ultrasound guidance for placement of central venous catheters: a meta-analysis of the literature. Crit Care Med 1996;24:2053-2058.

10. Ermakov S, Hoyt JW. Pulmonary artery catheterization. Crit Care Clin 1992;8:773-806.

11. Nelson LD. The new pulmonary arterial catheters: right ventricular ejection fraction and continuous cardiac output. Crit Care Clin 1996;12:795-818.

12. Marini JJ. Hemodynamic monitoring with the pulmonary artery catheter. Crit Care Clin 1986;3:551-572.

13. Amin DK, Shah PK, Swan HJC. The technique of inserting a Swan-Ganz catheter. J Crit Illness 1993;8:1147-1156.

14. Pulmonary Artery Catheter Consensus Conference. Consensus statement. Crit Care Med 1997;25:910-925.

15. American Heart Association. Advanced cardiac life support. Dallas: The Association; 1997.

16. American College of Surgeons. Advanced trauma life support. Chicago: The College; 1998.

17. Margulis L. Personal communication. December 1999.

18. Yount J. Impedance pneumography. Biophysical measurement series: respiration. Redmond, Wash: SpaceLabs Medical; 1994.

19. Myrabo K. Airway monitoring of adult, pediatric, and neonatal patients. Biophysical measurement series: respiration. Redmond, Wash: SpaceLabs Medical; 1994.

20. Cohen KP, Ladd WM, Beams DM, et al. Comparison of impedance and inductance ventilation sensors on adults during breathing, motion, and simulated airway obstruction. IEEE Trans Biomed Eng 1997;44:555-565.

21. Davis C, Mazzolini A, Murphy D. A new fiberoptic sensor for respiratory monitoring. Australas Phys Eng Sci Med 1997;20:214-219.

22. Diametrics Medical Co. Paratrend 7 operating instructions. St Paul: The Company; 1998.

23. AARC Clinical Practice Guideline. Transcutaneous blood gas monitoring for neonatal and pediatric patients. Respir Care 1994;39:1176-1179.

24. Decker M, Strohl K. Pulse oximetry. Biophysical measurement series: respiration. Redmond, Wash: SpaceLabs Medical; 1994.

25. Welch JP, DeCesare R, Hess D. Pulse oximetry: instrumentation and clinical applications. Respir Care 1990;35:584-601.

26. Nonin Medical, Inc. Onyx instruction manual. Plymouth, Minn: The Company; 1995.

27. Novametrix Medical Systems. CO₂SMO user's manual. Wallingford, Conn: The Company; 1998.

28. Nellcor Puritan Bennett. N-3000 pulse oximeter service manual. Pleasanton, Calif: The Company; 1998.

29. Rodriguez RM, Light RW. Pulse oximetry in the ICU. J Crit Illness 1998;13:247-252.

30. AARC Clinical Practice Guideline. Pulse oximetry. Respir Care 1991;36:1406-1409.

31. Wahr JA, Tremper KK. Noninvasive oxygen monitoring techniques. Crit Care Clin 1995;11:199-217.

32. Grieve SH, McIntosh N, Laing IA. Comparison of two different pulse oximeters in monitoring preterm infants. Crit Care Med 1997;25:2051-2054.

33. Hampson NB. Pulse oximetry in severe carbon monoxide poisoning. Chest 1998;114:1036-1041.

34. Morley TF. Capnography in the intensive care unit. J Intensive Care Med 1990;5:209-223.

35. Hess D. Capnometry and capnography: technical aspects, physiologic aspects, and clinical applications. Respir Care 1990;35:557-576.

36. Rodriguez RM, Light RW. Capnography in the ICU. J Crit Illness 1998;13:372-378.

37. Stock C. Noninvasive carbon dioxide monitoring. Crit Care Clin 1988;4:511.

38. Cohen N. Capnography and gas monitoring. Biophysical measurement series: respiration. Redmond, Wash: SpaceLabs Medical; 1994.

39. Colman Y, Krauss B. Microstream capnography: a new approach to an old problem. J Clin Monit 1999;15:403-409.

40. AARC Clinical Practice Guideline. Capnography/capnometry during mechanical ventilation. Respir Care 1995;40:1321-1324.

41. Levine RL, Wayne MA, Miller CC. End-tidal carbon dioxide and outcome of out of hospital cardiac arrest. N Engl J Med 1997;337:301-306.

42. Baigorri F, Russell JA. Oxygen delivery in critical illness. Crit Care Clin 1996;12:971-994.

43. Vincent JL. Determination of oxygen delivery and consumption versus cardiac index and oxygen extraction ratio. Crit Care Clin 1996;12:995-1006.

44. Porter JM, Ivatury RR. In search of optimal end points of resuscitation in trauma patients: a review. J Trauma 1998;44:908-914.

45. Taylor DE, Gutierrez G. Tonometry: a review of clinical studies. Crit Care Clin 1996;12:1007-1018.

46. Simonson SG, Piantadosi CA. Near-infrared spectroscopy: clinical applications. Crit Care Clin 1996;12:1019-1029.

47. Carr JJ, Brown JM. Introduction to biomedical equipment technology. 2nd ed. Englewood Cliffs, NJ: Prentice Hall; 1993.

48. Smith RJ, Dorf RC. Circuits, devices, and systems. 5th ed. New York: John Wiley & Sons; 1992.

49. Terry R. Personal communication. January 1999.

CHAPTER 27

Exercise Assessment

Frank C. Sciurba
Sanjay A. Patel

CHAPTER **OUTLINE**

OBJECTIVES

1. Describe the advantages of exercise testing has over traditional pulmonary function testing.
2. Describe the normal physiologic responses of the respiratory, cardiac, skeletal muscle and peripheral and pulmonary vascular systems to exercise.
3. List the primary physiologic measurements obtained during exercise testing.
4. Discuss the indications for exercise testing.
5. Describe the physiologic indices of cardiac, pulmonary, and metabolic function obtained during exercise testing.
6. Interpret exercise testing results.
7. List the characteristics of ventilatory limitation to exercise.
8. List the most important indicators of cardiovascular limitation to exercise.
9. List indicators that suggest abnormal gas exchange during exercise.
10. Discuss the significance of the lactate threshold in exercise test interpretation and its effect on ventilatory parameters.

KEY TERMS

Carbon Dioxide Production ($\dot{V}CO_2$)	Oxygen Delivery	Timed Walk Test
Exercise Testing	Oxygen Extraction	Ventilatory Equivalent
Lactate	Oxygen Pulse	Work Rate
Oxygen Consumption ($\dot{V}O_2$)	Respiratory Exchange Ratio (RER)	

Exercise testing measures physiologic reserve and functional capacity that cannot be determined from resting measurements. Standard parameters commonly considered for cardiopulmonary function, such as forced expiratory volume in 1 second (FEV_1) and cardiac ejection fraction, often correlate poorly with symptoms or exercise capacity. Changes in these resting parameters after an intervention often do not reflect functional improvements. Exercise testing not only delineates the reserve of each contributing subcomponent of respiration but also permits assessment of functional status through determination of maximal power output and oxygen consumption.

The physiology of exercise assessment is known to respiratory therapists and physicians familiar with the principles of intensive care medicine. In fact, the intensive care unit in many ways represents a resting exercise laboratory in that patients have exhausted their cardiovascular, ventilatory, mechanical, and gas exchange reserves. The physiologic observations (respiratory pattern, heart rate, lactic acidosis, arterial and mixed venous blood gas) in patients with respiratory failure or cardiogenic shock are similar to those seen in subjects at maximal exertion. The indication for most exercise testing is for cardiac ischemic disease. The emphasis in this chapter, however, is on the principles of maximal exercise testing with expiratory gas analysis to directly or indirectly assess the cardiovascular, ventilatory, mechanical, and gas exchange response to the metabolic stress of exertion.

Normal Exercise Physiology

Respiration and Exertion

The **oxygen consumption ($\dot{V}O_2$)** at rest is approximately 3.5 mL/kg/min. With slow walking, $\dot{V}O_2$ is 8 to 10 mL/kg/min (the minimal requirements to perform simple daily activity). At maximal exertion, $\dot{V}O_2$ increases to 30 mL/kg/min in a sedentary 70 year old and more than 80 mL/kg/min in a young, elite athlete.[1,2] At rest the skeletal muscles account for less than 40% of $\dot{V}O_2$. However, this percentage rises to greater than 80% at higher levels of exertion. Such variations in metabolic demand require the integrated response of multiple organ systems, a concept that is demonstrated by the equations describing $\dot{V}O_2$ (Equation 27-1). The maximum $\dot{V}O_2$ ($\dot{V}O_{2max}$) depends on genetics, level of conditioning, and presence of disease. At rest, humans are capable of maintaining homeostasis under all but the most severe internal disease conditions or in the most extremes of physical environments. However, abnormal cardiopulmonary reserve is commonly exposed during exertion, when the increased metabolic demands delineate the limits to the systems' response.

Oxygen Delivery

The rise in heart rate is the most important factor contributing to the increases in cardiac output ($\dot{Q}c$) during exertion. Stroke volume increases only during the initial

EQUATION 27-1

Oxygen Consumption

Oxygen consumption is commonly represented by the Fick equation, as follows:

$$\dot{V}O_2 = \dot{Q}c \times (CaO_2 - C\bar{v}O_2)$$

where:

$\dot{V}O_2$ = Oxygen consumption
$\dot{Q}c$ = Cardiac output
CaO_2 = Oxygen content of arterial blood
$C\bar{v}O_2$ = Oxygen content in mixed venous blood

Another way to represent this value permits better isolation of the components that contribute to oxygen delivery and oxygen extraction, as follows:

$$\dot{V}O_2 = \text{Oxygen delivery} \times \text{Tissue extraction rate}$$

Therefore the maximum capacity of an individual for oxygen consumption is determined by the maximal values for the parameters represented in the following equation:

$$\dot{V}O_{2max} = fc_{max} \times \text{Maximum stroke volume} \times C\bar{v}O_2 \times$$
$$\text{Maximum muscle extraction rate}$$

where:

$\dot{V}O_{2max}$ = Maximum oxygen consumption
fc_{max} = Maximum heart rate
$C\bar{v}O_2$ = Oxygen content in mixed venous blood

phase of exercise, after which the entire increase in $\dot{Q}c$ is related to increases in heart rate. An increase in stroke volume is an important component of the increase in $\dot{Q}c$ and $\dot{V}O_2$ induced by aerobic training. The heart rate is higher for any given power output with exercise that uses smaller muscle mass. Therefore heart rate during arm exercise is greater than during bicycle exercise, which is greater than during treadmill exercise for any given power output.

The hemoglobin concentration is directly associated with the oxygen-carrying capacity and in turn **oxygen delivery.** The low pH and increased temperature of exercising muscle results in shifts of the oxyhemoglobin dissociation curve to the right. This shift (the Bohr effect) facilitates the unloading of oxygen into the contracting muscle. The circulation responds to exercise with an increase in blood flow to active skeletal muscle, maintaining blood flow to the brain and decreasing blood flow to the kidneys and gastrointestinal tract. Vasoconstriction of the spleen increases circulating blood volume. Peripheral vascular resistance decreases, but blood pressure rises because of disproportionate increases in $\dot{Q}c$.

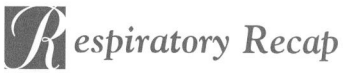

Respiratory Recap

Determinants of Oxygen Consumption
Oxygen delivery: cardiac output and oxygen-carrying capacity
Oxygen extraction by skeletal muscles

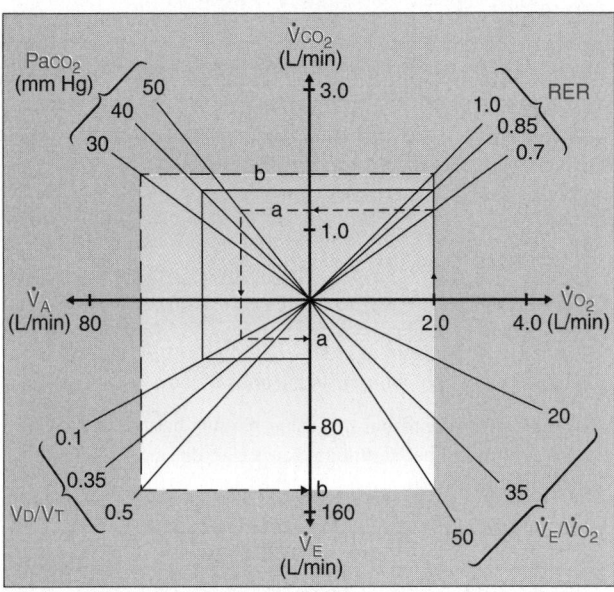

Figure 27-1 Impact of respiratory exchange ratio (RER), partial pressure of carbon dioxide ($Paco_2$; influenced by central drive), and dead space to tidal volume ratio (V_D/V_T) on minute ventilation ($\dot{V}_E$) requirement for a given level of metabolic work ($\dot{V}o_2$; oxygen consumption). Note that $\dot{V}_E$ requirements for a given level of metabolism may increase substantially (*dashed arrow*) compared with normal values (*solid arrow*), with abnormal variation in the basic physiologic variables. Note the combination of determining variables leading to a reduced $\dot{V}_E$ (*arrow a*) or a markedly high $\dot{V}_E$ (*arrow b*). $\dot{V}_A$, Alveolar ventilation; $\dot{V}_E/\dot{V}o_2$, ratio of minute ventilation to oxygen consumption; $\dot{V}co_2$, carbon dioxide production. (Modified from Whipp BJ, Pardy RL. In: Fishman AP, editor. Handbook of physiology: the respiratory system. Vol III. Mechanics of breathing. Part 2. Bethesda, Md: American Physiological Society; 1986. pp. 605 629.)

Oxygen Extraction

The skeletal muscle must efficiently use the oxygen supplied through the circulation to support cellular production of adenosine triphosphate (ATP) for muscle contraction. **Oxygen extraction** from the blood is improved with endurance training through increases in muscle mitochondrial density, capillary density, and metabolic enzymes. Short-term intense exercise can occur without the use of oxygen through a release of high-energy phosphate from creatinine phosphate in the exercising muscle and through anaerobic glycolysis resulting in lactate production.

Increases in blood **lactate** also occur during incremental exercise tests at approximately 60% of $\dot{V}o_{2max}$. This lactate rise is important in the evaluation of the respiratory system because the carbon dioxide generated through bicarbonate buffering of lactic acid and the subsequent acidemia act as independent stimulants to increase minute ventilation disproportionate to cellular metabolism during exercise. Although this phenomenon is commonly referred to as the *anaerobic threshold*, increasing evidence suggests that it is unrelated to anaerobic metabolism. Probable mechanisms for the rise in lactate include in-

EQUATION 27-2

Minute Ventilation Requirements

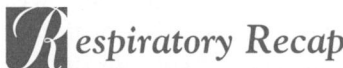

$$\dot{V}_E = \frac{0.86 \times \dot{V}co_2}{Paco_2 \times (1 - V_D/V_T)}$$

where:

$\dot{V}_E$ = Minute ventilation
$\dot{V}co_2$ = Carbon dioxide production
$Paco_2$ = Partial pressure of arterial carbon dioxide
V_D/V_T = Ratio of dead space to tidal volume

creases in glycogenolysis and glycolysis because of abrupt rises in serum catecholamines and glucagon; recruitment of fast-twitch glycolytic muscle fibers; and shifts in blood flow from the liver, which removes lactate from the circulatory system through gluconeogenesis. Hence, the term *lactate threshold (LT)* rather than *anaerobic threshold* is used in this text to describe the lactic acidosis associated with incremental exercise testing.

Respiratory Recap

Physiologic Responses to Exercise
Respiratory system: increased minute ventilation
Cardiovascular system: increased cardiac output and blood pressure
Peripheral circulation: decreased systemic vascular resistance
Blood: facilitation of oxygen delivery
Skeletal muscle: increased glycolysis

Ventilation and Gas Exchange

Increases in minute ventilation ($\dot{V}_E$) during exertion are necessary to maintain arterial blood gas and acid-base homeostasis. The $\dot{V}_E$ required depends on the central set point for $Paco_2$ that is influenced by vagal and humoral input, carbon dioxide production ($\dot{V}co_2$), and dead space, a concept illustrated in Figure 27-1 and Equation 27-2.

Measured Indices

Traditional cardiopulmonary exercise testing (CPX) involved staged steady-state maneuvers and analysis of expired gas collected in large compliant balloons. Advances in rapid-response gas analyzers and microprocessor technology now enable analysis of CO_2, O_2, and flow of the expired gas of the exercising subject to determine the value of the various metabolic parameters over shorter periods of time, allowing even breath-by-breath determinations.[3] Analysis of the exercise response is determined from the relationships among variables calculated from these sig-

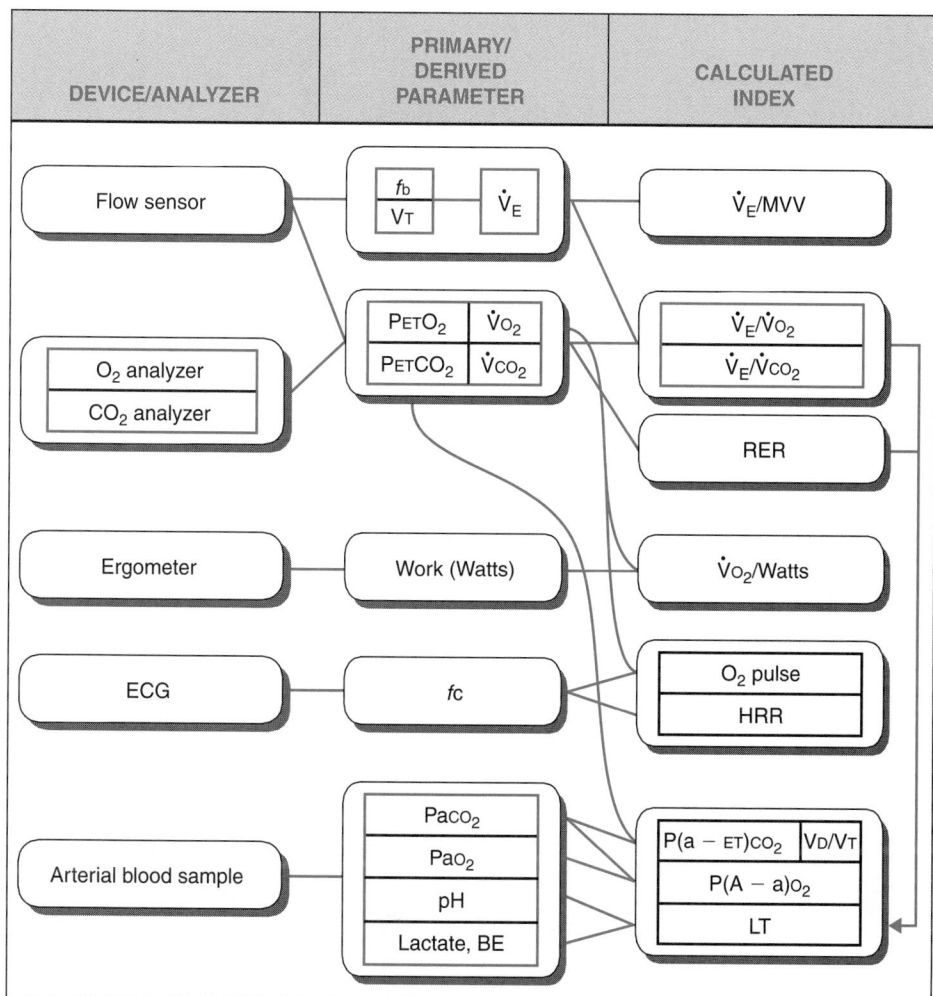

Figure 27-2 Schematic illustration demonstrating the relationship among direct signal measurements and derived parameters and calculated indices used in exercise assessment. *ECG,* Electrocardiogram; *fb,* breathing frequency (respiratory rate); *fc,* heart rate; *VT,* tidal volume; $\dot{V}_E$, minute ventilation; $P_{ET}O_2$, partial pressure of end-tidal oxygen; $P_{ET}CO_2$, partial pressure of end tidal carbon dioxide; $\dot{V}_{O_2}$, oxygen consumption; $\dot{V}_{CO_2}$, carbon dioxide production; Pa_{CO_2}, partial pressure of arterial carbon dioxide; Pa_{O_2}, partial pressure of arterial oxygen; *BE,* base excess; $\dot{V}_E/MVV$, ratio of minute ventilation to maximum voluntary ventilation; $\dot{V}_E/\dot{V}_{O_2}$, ratio of minute ventilation to oxygen consumption; $\dot{V}_E/\dot{V}_{CO_2}$, ratio of minute ventilation to carbon dioxide production; *RER,* respiratory exchange ratio; $\dot{V}_{O_2}/Watts$, ratio of oxygen consumption to work rate; *HRR,* heart rate reserve; $P(a-_{ET})_{CO_2}$, difference between arterial and end-tidal P_{CO_2}; V_D/V_T, ratio of dead space to tidal volume; $P(A-a)_{O_2}$, difference between alveolar and arterial P_{O_2}; *LT,* lactate threshold. (Modified from Whipp BJ, Pardy RL. In: Fishman AP, editor. Handbook of physiology: the respiratory system. Vol III. Mechanics of breathing. Part 2. Bethesda, Md: American Physiological Society; 1986. pp. 605-629.)

nals, along with the electrocardiogram (ECG) signal, and blood gas and blood pressure measurements.

Figure 27-2 shows the relationship among physiologic signals and derived and calculated indices used to describe or interpret the response to exercise. Some of the terms represent overlapping or redundant concepts and are the offshoots of varying paradigms from different groups of researchers. Although many variations in exercise modalities and protocols are performed in different laboratories, this chapter focuses on the interpretation of protocols involving bicycle ergometry, with incrementation in workload every minute until the subject reaches exhaustion. This technique has gained the greatest acceptance. Such protocols generally include 1 to 2 minutes of unloaded pedaling and an incrementation of work rate either in a continuous ramp or in increments that result in symptom limitation between 8 and 12 minutes.

Oxygen Consumption

$\dot{V}_{O_2}$ is the most important parameter obtained during exertion. Many other variables derived during exercise testing are plotted as a function of $\dot{V}_{O_2}$ to measure the appropriateness of their responses throughout exertion (Figure

27-3). At maximal exertion, this function is called $\dot{V}_{O_{2max}}$ and represents an individual's cardiopulmonary fitness and level of conditioning. In healthy individuals and those with cardiac abnormalities, the $\dot{V}_{O_{2max}}$ represents the level of work at which symptoms become overwhelming due to the limits of oxygen delivery and oxidative capacity.

If the individual stops exercise at levels below the maximal capacity for oxygen transport and use, the designation $\dot{V}_{O_{2peak}}$ is used. Such a situation occurs with dyspnea from lung disease or with pain from orthopedic or peripheral vascular disease. $\dot{V}_{O_{2max}}$ is reported as a percentage of predicted normal values (Table 27-1) or is adjusted for weight as milliliters per kilograms per minute. Normal $\dot{V}_{O_{2max}}$ percentage is greater than 84%. Differences in exercise protocol may result in differences in $\dot{V}_{O_{2max}}$. Treadmill exercise results in values approximately 10% higher than those achieved with cycle ergometry. Protocol durations that are too short or too long may decrease maximal achieved values.

Carbon Dioxide Production

During low-level exertion, **carbon dioxide production** ($\dot{V}_{CO_2}$) reflects the amount of CO_2 produced in the mito-

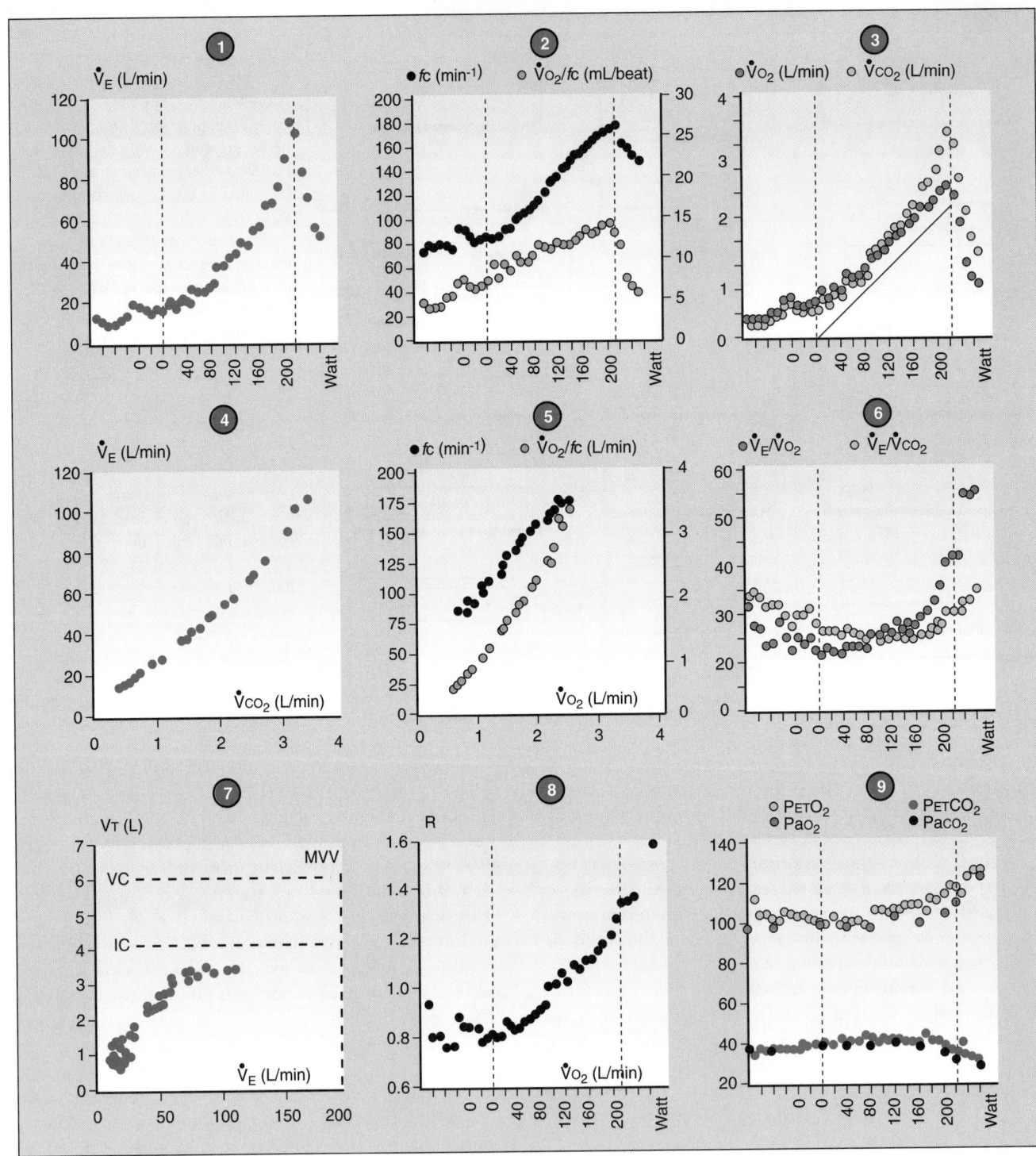

Figure 27-3 Graphic relationship of various parameters of exercise response. $\dot{V}_E$, Minute ventilation; fc, heart rate; $\dot{V}_{O_2}$, oxygen consumption; $\dot{V}_{CO_2}$, carbon dioxide production; $\dot{V}_E/\dot{V}_{O_2}$, ratio of minute ventilation to oxygen consumption; $\dot{V}_E/\dot{V}_{CO_2}$, ratio of minute ventilation to carbon dioxide production; $P_{ET}O_2$, partial pressure of end-tidal oxygen; $P_{ET}CO_2$, partial pressure of end tidal carbon dioxide; Pa_{O_2}, partial pressure of arterial oxygen; Pa_{CO_2}, partial pressure of arterial arbon dioxide; V_T, tidal volume. (Modified from Wasserman K. Diagnosing cardiovascular and lung pathophysiology from exercise gas exchange. Chest 1997;112:1091-1101.)

TABLE 27-1

Predictive Equations for Maximum Oxygen Consumption

Author	Equation
Hansen	Men: mL/min = $(50.75 - 0.372A) \times W$
	Women: mL/min = $(22.78 - 0.17A) \times (W + 43)$
Jones	Men: L/min = $0.046H - 0.021A - 4.31$
	Women: L/min = $0.046H - 0.021A - 4.93$
Blackie	Men: L/min = $0.0142H - 0.0494A + 0.00257W + 3.015$
	Women: L/min = $0.0142H - 0.0115A + 0.00974W + 0.651$
Fairbarn	Men: L/min = $0.023H - 0.031A + 0.0117W - 0.322$
	Women: L/min = $0.0158H - 0.027A + 0.00899W + 0.207$

A, *Age;* W, *weight;* H, *height.*

chondria as a metabolic byproduct and increases with increases in $\dot{V}O_2$. As exercise becomes more intense, however, a disproportionate amount of CO_2 is generated to buffer lactic acid with bicarbonate. This reaction is catalyzed by carbonic anhydrase, as follows:

$$Na^+HCO_3^- + H^+La^- = Na^+La^- + H_2O + CO_2$$

With moderate exertion, $\dot{V}_E$ is most closely linked to $\dot{V}CO_2$, which is expected to maintain a normal $PaCO_2$. However, the precise mechanisms linking these parameters are not clearly known. When the bicarbonate buffering capacity is exceeded at higher levels of exertion, the acidemic stimulus to the medullary receptor and carotid bodies results in stimulation of $\dot{V}_E$ at levels disproportionate to the level of $\dot{V}CO_2$. This relative hyperventilation results in decreased $PaCO_2$ at higher levels of exertion. CO_2 output from the lungs does not always reflect $\dot{V}CO_2$ at the muscle because a significant capacity exists to store CO_2 in the blood and tissues. Ultimately, CO_2 output depends on appropriate matching of alveolar ventilation to $\dot{V}CO_2$.

Respiratory Exchange Ratio

The **respiratory exchange ratio (RER)** is the ratio of $\dot{V}CO_2$ to $\dot{V}O_2$ ($\dot{V}CO_2/\dot{V}O_2$). During steady-state exercise at moderate to low levels of exertion, the RER reflects the respiratory quotient (RQ), which is the ratio of $\dot{V}CO_2$ to $\dot{V}O_2$ in the mitochondria. The actual value depends on the relative contributions of fat versus carbohydrate as the mitochondrial fuel. The RQ of fat is 0.7 and that of carbohydrate is 1.0. Exercise at the limits of $\dot{V}O_2$ is achieved predominantly with carbohydrate metabolism; thus RQ is approximately 1.0. However, endurance athletes are capable of shifting the RQ downward by increasing fat metabolism. The RQ can never be greater than 1.0 during exertion.

The RER, on the other hand, can differ significantly from the RQ for the following reasons. During periods of relative hypoventilation or hyperventilation, when the PCO_2 is rising or falling, the RER respectively underestimates and overestimates the RQ. Furthermore, at higher levels of exertion, an RER greater than 1.0 reflects the increased CO_2 generated from bicarbonate buffering of lactic acid, which is independent of the metabolism at the muscle. On this basis the RER has been used as one determinant of the LT (see Figure 27-3, panel 8).

Minute Ventilation

The $\dot{V}_E$ for a given level of metabolism depends on central respiratory drive (PCO_2 set point) and dead space. The plot of $\dot{V}_E$ as a function of $\dot{V}O_2$ can be compared with normal response ranges to provide a rough determination of the appropriateness of the respiratory response (Figure 27-4). Maximum values of $\dot{V}_E$ achieved during exertion are normally less than 70% of a healthy individual's ventilatory capacity; thus ventilatory capacity is almost never the cause of exercise limitation in a healthy individual. The exception to this idea can be observed in elite athletes capable of conditioning the metabolic capacity to such a level that it challenges the limits of the ventilatory system.[4] In contrast to the cardiac and skeletal muscles, little or no capacity exists to increase the ventilatory capacity through aerobic training.

$\dot{V}_E$ is commonly compared with the maximum voluntary ventilation (MVV) to assess the ventilatory reserve (VR). VR is commonly expressed in absolute terms (MVV − $\dot{V}_E$) or as $\dot{V}_E$ as a percentage of MVV ($\dot{V}_E$/MVV%). The normal range is wide but has been reported as 38 ± 22 L/min for absolute VR and 72 ± 15 for $\dot{V}_E$/MVV% (Figure 27-5). Criticism of this method includes the measurement of the MVV under conditions at rest (maximum coached air flow in and out for 12 seconds extrapolated to 1 minute), which differs with respect to the flow-versus-volume characteristics of ventilation during true exercise.[1] In addition, the MVV may decrease during exercise in cases of exercise-induced bronchospasm, congestive heart failure, or respiratory muscle weakness and reflect a falsely high determination of ventilatory reserve. Nonetheless, in the absence of a valid and simple alternative technique, comparison of $\dot{V}_E$ with MVV continues to be an essential exercise in the assessment of the VR.

Respiratory Pattern: Tidal Volume and Respiratory Rate

The initial rise in $\dot{V}_E$ is largely affected by a rise in tidal volume (V_T). In healthy young individuals with significant ventilatory mechanical reserve, the V_T begins to plateau midway through a maximal exercise maneuver at approximately 55% of the vital capacity and may even decrease at maximal exercise (Figure 27-6). Hence, the increasing $\dot{V}_E$ that accompanies increasing levels of severe exertion is affected by increasing inspiratory and expiratory flow rates, thus shortening the respiratory cycle time and increasing the respiratory rate. This pattern minimizes

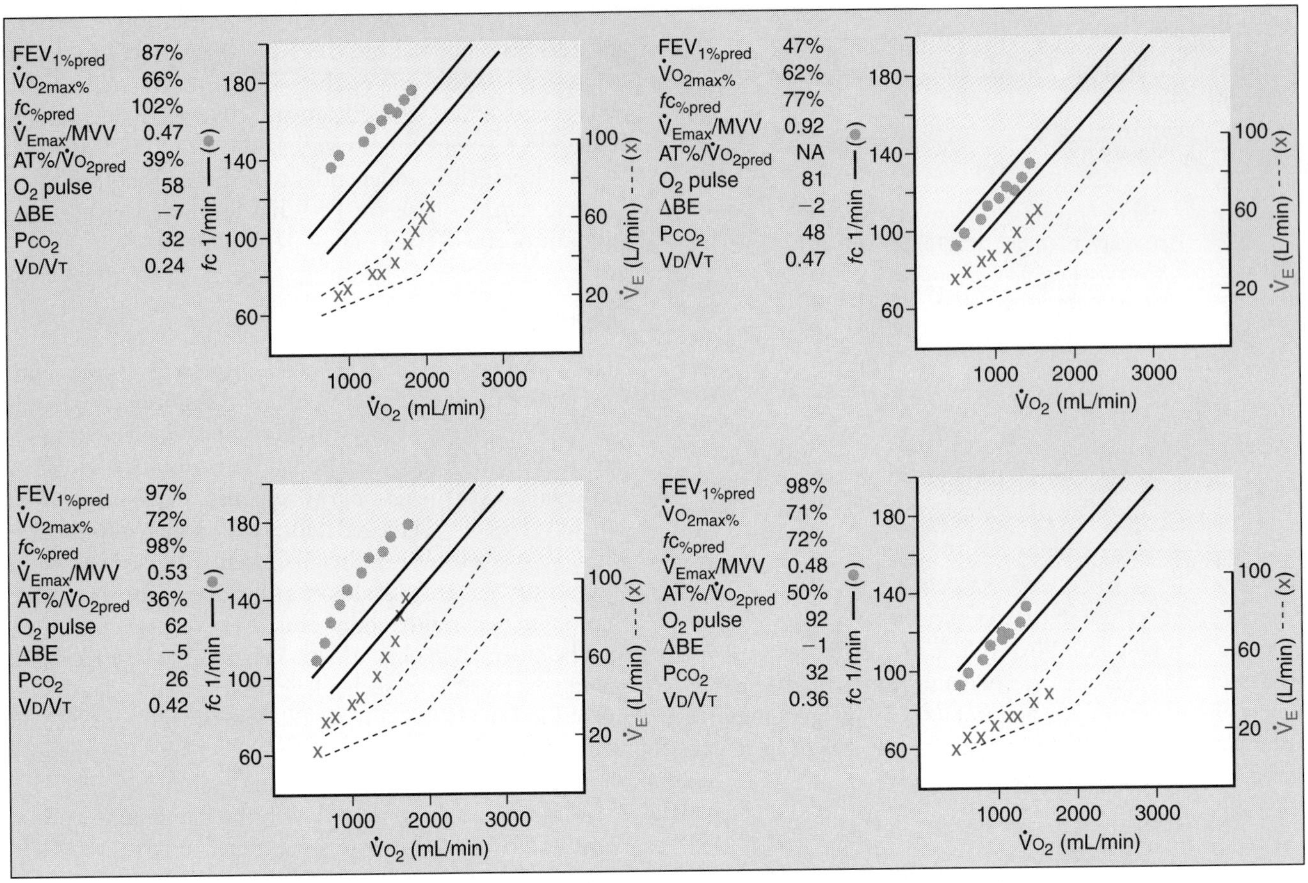

A

FEV$_{1\%pred}$	87%
$\dot{V}O_{2max\%}$	66%
$fc_{\%pred}$	102%
$\dot{V}_{Emax}$/MVV	0.47
AT%/$\dot{V}O_{2pred}$	39%
O$_2$ pulse	58
ΔBE	−7
PCO_2	32
V$_D$/V$_T$	0.24

B

FEV$_{1\%pred}$	47%
$\dot{V}O_{2max\%}$	62%
$fc_{\%pred}$	77%
$\dot{V}_{Emax}$/MVV	0.92
AT%/$\dot{V}O_{2pred}$	NA
O$_2$ pulse	81
ΔBE	−2
PCO_2	48
V$_D$/V$_T$	0.47

C

FEV$_{1\%pred}$	97%
$\dot{V}O_{2max\%}$	72%
$fc_{\%pred}$	98%
$\dot{V}_{Emax}$/MVV	0.53
AT%/$\dot{V}O_{2pred}$	36%
O$_2$ pulse	62
ΔBE	−5
PCO_2	26
V$_D$/V$_T$	0.42

D

FEV$_{1\%pred}$	98%
$\dot{V}O_{2max\%}$	71%
$fc_{\%pred}$	72%
$\dot{V}_{Emax}$/MVV	0.48
AT%/$\dot{V}O_{2pred}$	50%
O$_2$ pulse	92
ΔBE	−1
PCO_2	32
V$_D$/V$_T$	0.36

Figure 27-4 Graphic showing heart rate (*fc*) and minute ventilation ($\dot{V}_E$) as a function of maximum oxygen consumption ($\dot{V}O_{2max}$) during incremental bicycle ergometry. The solid and dashed lines represent the normal ranges for heart rate and minute ventilation, respectively. Key pulmonary function and exercise parameters are listed in each table. **A,** The typical response in an individual with an abnormal cardiovascular response and cardiovascular limitation to exertion. **B,** The typical response in an individual with an abnormal ventilatory and gas exchange response to exertion with a pure ventilatory limitation to exertion. **C,** The typical response in an individual with combined cardiovascular and ventilatory abnormalities during exertion but with predominant cardiovascular limitation and normal resting spirometry (FEV$_1$%), as with pulmonary vascular disease. **D,** The typical response in an individual who has not achieved a maximal physiologic response in either cardiovascular or ventilatory parameters but who otherwise exhibits a normal cardiovascular and gas exchange response to exertion, as occurs in a submaximal exercise response. *FEV$_{1\%pred}$,* Percent of predicted forced expiratory volume in 1 second; fc$_{\%pred}$, percent of predicted heart rate; $\dot{V}_E$/*MVV,* ratio of minute ventilation to maximum voluntary ventilation; *AT%/$\dot{V}O_{2pred}$,*ratio of the anaerobic threshold to predicted oxygen consumption; Δ*BE,* change in base excess; PCO_2, partial pressure of carbon dioxide; V$_D$/V$_T$, ratio of dead space to tidal volume.

Figure 27-5 Minute ventilation as a function of work rate in healthy individuals and those with chronic obstructive pulmonary disease (COPD). The dark area represents alveolar ventilation; the light area represents dead space ventilation. Note that the dead space volume is greater in cases of COPD compared with healthy cases. Healthy individuals have a significant reserve in ventilation at maximal exercise. Individuals with COPD approach the mechanical limits of ventilation not only because the limit (represented by MVV) is lower but also because of a greater proportion of dead space ventilation at any given level of work.

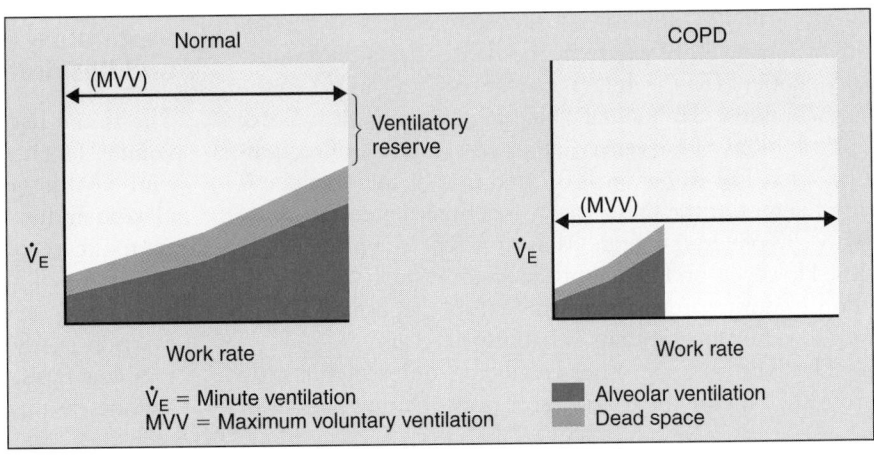

$\dot{V}_E$ = Minute ventilation
MVV = Maximum voluntary ventilation

Alveolar ventilation
Dead space

the elastic work of breathing. In healthy individuals, maximum breathing frequency averages 40/min, but it may exceed 50/min in conditioned individuals with higher ventilatory demands or in persons with restrictive lung disease. Erratic or nonphysiologic breathing patterns may indicate an anxiety disorder or intentional malingering.

Exercise Inspiratory Capacity and End-Expiratory Lung Volume

The end-expiratory lung volume (EELV) in healthy individuals decreases toward residual volume with exertion. However, individuals with chronic obstructive pulmonary disease (COPD) increase their EELV, resulting in further impingement on inspiratory capacity (IC; Figure 27-7). This measure is a sensitive indicator of early disease,[5] and dyspnea has been found to correlate closely with measurements of exercise EELV.[6] The maneuver is based on the assumption that total lung capacity (TLC), measured at rest,

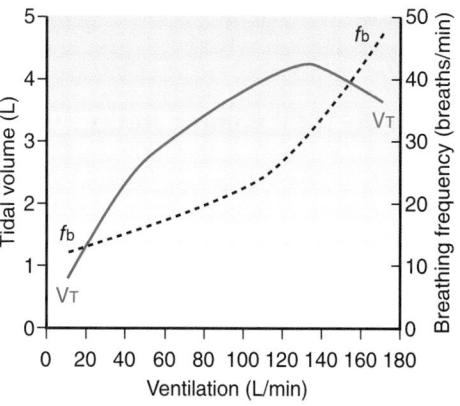

Figure 27-6 Response of tidal volume (Vᴛ) and respiratory rate (fb) to increasing levels of minute ventilation. Note that initial increases in ventilation are largely related to increases in tidal volume, whereas increases in minute ventilation near maximal exertion are largely due to increases in respiratory rate.

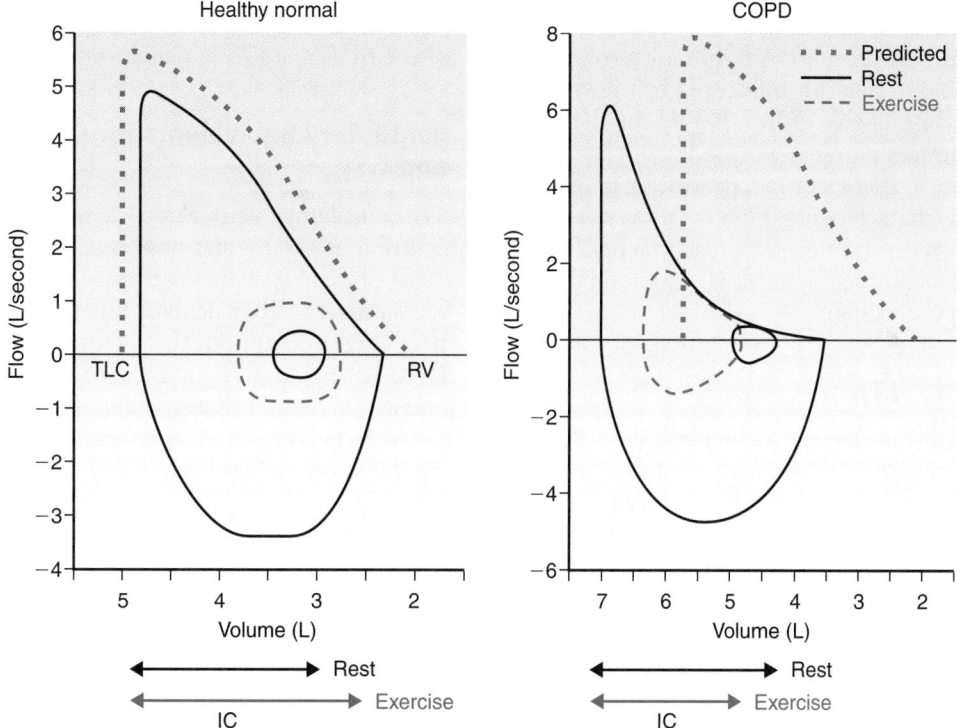

Figure 27-7 Flow-volume loops during rest and exercise relative to maximal flow volume loops in healthy subjects and individuals with chronic obstructive pulmonary disease (COPD). In healthy subjects, tidal volume increases from rest to exertion by both increasing end inspiratory lung volume and lowering end-expiratory lung volume. Because of the latter response the inspiratory capacity (IC) normally increases during exertion. In contrast, individuals with COPD can maintain adequate flow rates to increase minute ventilation by both increasing end-inspiratory and end-expiratory lung volumes, with a resulting decrease in inspiratory capacity as the exercise loop begins to impinge on total lung capacity (TLC). *RV,* Residual volume. (Modified from O'Donnell DE. Assessment of bronchodilator efficacy in symptomatic COPD: is spirometry useful? Chest 2000;117:428-478.)

does not change during exertion. Multiple IC maneuvers can be performed throughout exertion, and EELV then is calculated as the difference between TLC and IC.

Dead Space to Tidal Volume Ratio

The ratio of dead space to tidal volume (VD/VT), an important parameter of gas exchange, represents the proportion of each breath that is not in contact with alveoli receiving adequate perfusion and thus has not equilibrated with capillary $PaCO_2$. This ratio represents both the anatomic dead space (upper airway and bronchi) and physiologic dead space (high $\dot{V}/\dot{Q}$). Although absolute dead space rises normally during exertion, the VD/VT should be less than 0.35 at rest and less than 0.25 at maximal exertion.

As shown in Equation 27-3, an arterial blood sample is necessary to calculate dead space. Consider a theoretic lung with absolutely no perfusion (that is, 100% dead space), in which the expired CO_2 is zero. In this case the VD/VT is 1. The other extreme is a theoretic perfectly matched ventilation, in which case the VD/VT is zero. One weakness with the use of the VD/VT ratio to represent parenchymal disease is that it is influenced by the ventilatory pattern. Because of the 150 to 200 mL of anatomic dead space, respiratory patterns with shallow VTs have a greater proportion of dead space independent of parenchymal gas exchange characteristics. Finally, in the computation of the dead space and the VD/VT, subtraction of the dead space of the measuring device used to perform the gas analysis is an important step.

PetCO₂ and P(a − ET)CO₂

In healthy individuals the end-tidal PCO_2 (PetCO$_2$) is used as an estimate of the $PaCO_2$. Both the $PaCO_2$ and the PetCO$_2$ remain unchanged at moderate levels of exertion. However, they both drop during the hyperventilation associated with the LT. Even with healthy lungs, small differences exist between the $PaCO_2$ and the PetCO$_2$. The normal P(a − ET)CO$_2$ difference is 2 to 3 mm Hg at rest and becomes negative at maximal exertion (−4 mm Hg). In diseases of the lung associated with significant increases in physiologic dead space, the PetCO$_2$

may differ considerably from the $PaCO_2$. In these situations, values greater than 10 mm Hg during maximal exertion can be recorded.

PaO₂ and P(A − a)O₂

PaO_2 does not change significantly during exercise in healthy individuals. However P(A − a)O$_2$ does increase significantly with exertion. Because of significant variability in the RER during exercise, the unabridged computation of the alveolar air equation should be used (Equation 27-4). Both the resting and exercise P(A − a)O$_2$ values increase with aging. One series of middle-aged to elderly men demonstrated resting values of 13 ± 7 mm Hg, which increased to 19 ± 9 mm Hg at maximal exertion.[7]

PetO₂

End-tidal PO_2 (PetO$_2$) is commonly plotted as a function of increasing workload. Values rise during hyperventilation associated with lactic acidosis, and thus PetO$_2$ can be one of the factors used in the noninvasive determination of the LT (Figure 27-3, panel 9).

Ventilatory Equivalents for Carbon Dioxide and Oxygen

The **ventilatory equivalent** is commonly reported during exertion at the LT and has been used as an indirect estimate of dead space in the absence of arterial blood gas measurements to calculate VD/VT. Unfortunately, the necessary assumption that ventilatory drive and thus $PaCO_2$ is in a normal range is commonly incorrect.[8] Increases in the ventilatory equivalent for carbon dioxide ($\dot{V}_E/\dot{V}CO_2$) and ventilatory equivalent for oxygen ($\dot{V}_E/\dot{V}O_2$) can be associated with psychogenic hyperventilation, malingering, metabolic acidosis or other causes of increased ventilatory drive. Normal values for $\dot{V}_E/\dot{V}CO_2$ and $V_E/\dot{V}O_2$

ℰQUATION 27-3
Physiologic Dead Space

$$VD/VT = \frac{PaCO_2 - P\bar{E}CO_2}{PaCO_2}$$

where:

VD/VT = Ratio of dead space to tidal volume
$PaCO_2$ = Partial pressure of arterial carbon dioxide
$P\bar{E}CO_2$ = Partial pressure of mixed exhaled carbon dioxide

---

ℰQUATION 27-4
Unabridged Alveolar Gas Equation

$$P(A-a)O_2 = (FIO_2 \times [PB - PH_2O]) - \left(PaCO_2 \times \left[FIO_2 + \frac{1 - FIO_2}{RER}\right]\right) - PaO_2$$

where:

P(A − a)O$_2$ = Difference between the partial pressure of alveolar and arterial oxygen
PB = Barometric pressure
FIO_2 = Fraction of inspired oxygen
PH_2O = Partial pressure of water vapor
$PaCO_2$ = Partial pressure of arterial carbon dioxide
RER = Respiratory exchange ratio
PaO_2 = Partial pressure of arterial oxygen

at LT are less than 34 and 31, respectively. Plots of $\dot{V}_E/\dot{V}CO_2$ and $\dot{V}_E/\dot{V}O_2$ as a function of $\dot{V}O_2$ are commonly used in the detection of the LT (see Figure 27-3, panel 6). Both values initially fall and then plateau up to moderate levels of exertion. In cases of early lactic acidosis, during which time bicarbonate buffering results in increasing CO_2 production but not in acidemia (the iso-capneic buffering period), the $\dot{V}_E/\dot{V}O_2$ rises while the $\dot{V}_E/\dot{V}CO_2$ remains constant. With increasing academia the $\dot{V}_E/\dot{V}CO_2$ increases.

Lactate, Base Excess, and Lactate Threshold

The LT is more commonly referred to as the *anaerobic threshold,* although substantial scientific evidence discussed previously supports causes other than anaerobiosis for the rise in lactate concentration during exertion. Nonetheless, the onset of lactic acidosis does have clinical utility independent from its physiologic source. Conditions associated with decreases in oxygen delivery, such as deconditioning or cardiovascular pathologic processes, are unquestionably associated with early onset of lactic acidosis and the lowering of the LT. Furthermore, the consequences of lactic acidosis on the stimulation of ventilation independent of skeletal muscle $\dot{V}CO_2$ are well known.

The gold standard used to determine the LT is through serial measurements of arterial lactate, a process requiring arterial line placement and multiple gas analyses. The plot of log [lactate] versus log $\dot{V}O_2$ is used to determine the threshold $\dot{V}O_2$ at which lactate begins to rise. Because changes in lactate are associated with equimolar changes in base excess (BE; the change in bicarbonate adjusted for changes due to respiratory compensation of $PaCO_2$), the ΔBE can be used as a more readily accessible surrogate to lactate. Arterial blood gas samples are commonly drawn at rest and maximal exertion to minimize the invasiveness and expense of repeated collection. As a general rule if BE falls to less than −1, the individual likely has surpassed the LT; if values fall to less than −3, these indicate maximal cardiovascular effort.

Many of the previously discussed variables have been used in the noninvasive detection of the LT. The V-slope method ($\dot{V}CO_2$ versus $\dot{V}O_2$; see Figure 27-3, panel 5) has recently gained the greatest acceptance in LT determination. The $\dot{V}_E/\dot{V}O_2$ and $\dot{V}_E/\dot{V}CO_2$ as a function of $\dot{V}O_2$, as discussed previously and shown in Figure 27-3, panel 6, also are useful. In respiratory conditions such as COPD, increased tissue stores of CO_2 associated with hypoventilation may make the noninvasive determination of LT impossible.[9] Normal LT occurs at 50% to 60% of $\dot{V}O_{2max}$, but the confidence limits extend as low as 40% in groups of individuals without known disease. LT can be protocol dependent and varies with rate of incrementation and type of exercise, with cycle ergometry resulting in values approximately 10% lower than those seen with treadmill exercise.

Heart Rate

Although the heart rate (fc) response to exertion varies considerably in healthy individuals, heart rate normally approaches the predicted maximum: fc predicted = 220 − age. Heart rate reserve (fc predicted − fc) should be less than 15, and fc% of predicted should be greater than 90%. Values outside these ranges should raise the suspicion of noncardiovascular limitations to exertion, such as those associated with ventilatory mechanical limitation or submaximal effort. On the other hand, identification of significant metabolic acidosis in the presence of a large heart rate reserve may indicate chronotropic insufficiency (as with β-blocker, calcium-channel blocker, or conduction system abnormalities or heart transplantation); however, it also may reflect large-extremity ischemia if associated with symptoms of claudication.

Heart Rate–Oxygen Consumption Relationship and Oxygen Pulse

fc may be plotted as a function of $\dot{V}O_2$ to assess the appropriateness of its response. Elevations in the fc-versus-$\dot{V}O_2$ slope are associated with abnormal stroke volume because heart rate must increase to maintain $\dot{Q}c$ for a given $\dot{V}O_2$. Hemoglobin, SaO_2, and peripheral muscle function independently affect the body's ability to increase $\dot{V}O_2$ and may result in increases in the fc-versus-$\dot{V}O_2$ slope independent of stroke volume. The O_2 pulse ($\dot{V}O_2/fc$) is another way to represent this concept. Although maximal O_2 pulse has been considered the noninvasive surrogate to stroke volume, influences of pathologic processes exist in the blood and muscle as well (Equation 27-5). Normal values for O_2 pulse are determined by the ratio of $\dot{V}O_2$-predicted to fc-predicted. Normal values are greater than 80%.

Cardiac Output

Direct measurements of cardiac output ($\dot{Q}c$) require a level of sophistication beyond that of most exercise laboratories.[10] The gold standard for $\dot{Q}c$ assessment is the direct Fick method, which requires invasive placement of a pulmonary artery catheter. A mixed venous gas is sampled from the pulmonary artery catheter, arterial blood is sampled, and

EQUATION 27-5

Oxygen Pulse

$$O_2 \text{ pulse} = \frac{\dot{V}O_{2max}}{fc_{max}} = \text{Stroke volume}_{max} \times Cao_2 \times$$
$$\text{Muscle extraction rate}_{max}$$

where:

$\dot{V}O_{2max}$ = Maximum oxygen consumption
Cao_2 = Oxygen content of arterial blood
fc_{max} = Maximum heart rate

EQUATION 27-6

Fick Equation

$$\dot{Q}c = \frac{\dot{V}_{O_2}}{Ca_{O_2} - C\bar{v}_{O_2}}$$

where:

$\dot{Q}c$ = Cardiac output
$\dot{V}_{O_2}$ = Oxygen consumption
Ca_{O_2} = Oxygen content of arterial blood
$C\bar{v}_{O_2}$ = Oxygen content of mixed venous blood

$\dot{V}_{O_2}$ measurements are made from expired gas. $\dot{Q}c$ then is calculated from the Fick equation (Equation 27-6). This technique is reliable during submaximal steady-state exercise, but its use is limited because of its invasive nature and inaccuracy in non-steady–state exercise.

Acetylene and other inert gas rebreathing methods used to assess $\dot{Q}c$ follow the assumption that after rebreathing, the rate of disappearance of the inert soluble gas is directly proportional to the flow of blood past the lungs. The technique is accurate and simple to perform at maximal exercise in healthy individuals but is inaccurate in persons with gas-exchange abnormalities caused by lung disease. Recently Doppler echocardiography has shown promise as a noninvasive accurate technique to measure beat-by-beat changes in $\dot{Q}c$. The downside of this technique is its expense and the requirement of trained personnel, although recent advances may improve access to this technology.

Work Rate

Many of the previously discussed parameters can be plotted as a function of the externally applied **work rate.** In the case of a bicycle ergometer the changes in workload are precisely known (Watts). A commonly used unit of work during treadmill exercise is a met. One met is a simple unit that approximates the resting $\dot{V}_{O_2}$ (3.5 mL/kg). In reality, changes in treadmill speed and grade produce different external loads in individuals of different body sizes and efficiencies.

Oxygen Consumption–Work Rate Relationship

The relationship between oxygen consumption and work rate ($\Delta\dot{V}_{O_2}/\Delta$Watts) reflects the change in the internal metabolic demand of exercise for a given change in external load and thus remains relatively constant under most circumstances (approximately 10mL/min/Watt). This value cannot be determined for treadmill exercise, in which the external load depends on the individual's walking efficiency, nor is it valid during the few couple of minutes of cycle ergometry during unloaded pedaling, when $\dot{V}_{O_2}$ and actual workload depend on an individual's limb mass, coordination, and motor efficiency. Values less than 8.8 mL/min/Watt may be associated with significant impairments in oxygen delivery or use, such as severe cardiac disease or myopathy. Sudden drops in this value dur-

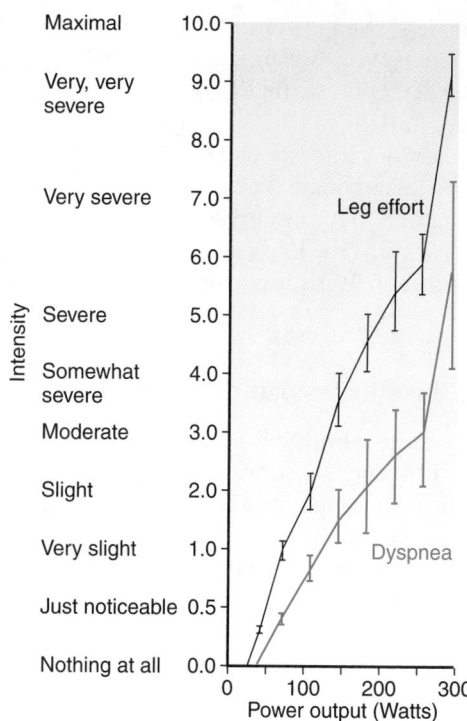

Figure 27-8 Subjective measurement of leg effort and sense of dyspnea measured by the Borg scale in healthy individuals during incremental bicycle ergometry exercise. (Modified from Kearon MC, Summers E, Jones NL, et al. Effort and dyspnea during work of varying intensity and duration. Eur Respir J 1991;4:917-925.)

ing an exercise study may indicate cardiac ischemia. If this value is consistently less than 10 in all patients tested in a given laboratory, the calibration of the ergometer should be questioned.

Ratings of Perceived Exertion

Subjects stop exercising because they achieve intolerable symptoms; thus the sense of effort is an important factor limiting exercise.[11] The Borg ratings for dyspnea and leg effort (Figure 27-8) offer a validated technique to assess symptoms during exertion.[12]

Timed Walk Tests

Timed walk tests focus primarily on functional performance.[13] They are generally easy to perform, and patients usually prefer them to other forms of exercise testing because the exercise is familiar to them and the tests allow patients to set their own pace (including rests) and adaptive maneuvers (for example, pursed-lip breathing). A timed walk test generally involves a request for the patient walk over a measured course for a set duration of time (for example, 6 or 12 minutes). Patients are encouraged to go as far as they can, and supplemental oxygen is provided as necessary. The protocol used for the National Emphysema Treatment Trial is depicted in Box 27-1, and predicted normal values are given in Box 27-2.[14]

Box 27-1

*Six-Minute Walk Test Procedures**

Walk Course
Course should be unobstructed, flat, and indoors.
If testing site is moved, configuration should remain constant.

Patient Preparation
Prewalk bronchodilator should be administered at least 15 minutes in advance.
Oxygen supplementation should be provided as necessary.
The test should take place 2 hours after the last meal.
The patient should sit at rest at least 10 minutes before the test.
The patient should wear comfortable clothes and shoes.

Procedure
Instruct the patient to cover as much ground as possible.
Allow the patient to slow down or rest as needed (included in the 6 minutes).
Ask the patient not to talk or carry oxygen.
Provide the patient with encouragement and the time remaining at each 1-minute mark.
At the end of 6 minutes, ask the patient to stop. Then perform the following:
  Record the distance traveled.
  Record dyspnea (Borg scale).
  Record the patient's heart rate, blood pressure, and Sp_{O_2} (optional).

Sp_{O_2}, *Oxygen saturation measured by pulse oximetry.*
From the National Emphysema Treatment Trial (ongoing).

Walk test distance has a fair correlation with maximal exercise tolerance[15] but a very strong correlation with an individual's ability to perform activities of daily living and quality of life. Indeed, this latter correlation makes the timed walk test attractive in the evaluation of novel therapies, such as lung volume reduction surgery. In a study of individuals who had experienced heart failure, a 20 to 40 m change correlated with clinically important improvements in quality of life.[16] Walk tests do not determine maximal exercise capabilities, nor do they routinely record ventilatory or cardiovascular responses. However, blood pressure, f_c, FEV_1, and pulse oximetry (or arterial blood gas) can be determined at the end of the walk test to further define the exercise response.

Indications for Clinical Cardiopulmonary Exercise Testing

Unexplained or Disproportionate Dyspnea

When routine history, physical, and basic pulmonary function and blood tests fail to determine the cause of dyspnea, CPX can help document impairment and distinguish abnormal cardiopulmonary physiologic responses from inor-

Box 27-2

Prediction Equations for Healthy Subjects for 6-Minute Walk (in Meters)

Men: $(7.57 \times H^*) - (502 \times A) - (1.76 \times W^*) - 309^\dagger$
Women: $(2.11 \times H^*) - (2.29 \times W^*) - (5.78 \times A) + 667^\dagger$

From Enright PL, Sherrill DL. Reference equations for the 6 minute walk in healthy adults. Am J Resp Crit Care Med 1998;158:1384-1387.
H, Height; A, age; W, weight.
**Height is in centimeters; weight is in kilograms.*
†For the lower limit of normal, subtract 153 for men and 139 for women.

ganic causes associated with anxiety or even malingering.[17,18] A normal study can serve to reassure the individual and avoid expensive and invasive testing. An abnormal study may direct the work-up toward more invasive testing, such as right or left heart catheterization, pulmonary angiography, lung biopsy, or muscle biopsy or indicate specific therapy, such as exercise training, bronchodilator use, or angiotensin-converting enzyme (ACE)-inhibitor use. Because of the wide variation of normal values, serial tests in the case of persistent or progressive symptoms may be necessary to document progression of an abnormal physiologic response. CPX can help determine the relative contributions of cardiovascular and ventilatory abnormalities to exercise impairment in individuals with known disease. Such determinations can direct therapy toward the appropriate organ system.

Assessment of Intervention

CPX has shown promise for research and clinical use in the assessment of physiologic and functional change associated with an intervention. Exercise testing not only offers greater insight into specific physiologic changes than resting testing, but it also allows assessment of the integrated response of varying effects of the intervention on the system. For example, in the assessment of exercise response to lung volume reduction surgery, a given individual may demonstrate increased V_T and lower respiratory rates, lower V_D/V_T, and increased IC associated with less dynamic hyperinflation. However, an earlier-onset LT and decreased O_2 pulse due to simultaneous excision of the pulmonary vascular bed may balance the beneficial pulmonary mechanical effects and result in no change in $\dot{V}_{O_{2max}}$ or maximum Watts. Another example can be observed in the treatment of an individual with sarcoidosis with oral corticosteroids, in which case decreased exercise $P(A - a)_{O_2}$ and reduction in V_D/V_T after therapy are balanced by decreased muscle oxygen extraction and weight gain due to the myopathic and lipid-accumulating side effects of steroids. Exercise testing has been used to document the effects of bronchodilators in individuals with COPD,[19,20] immunosuppressive therapy in those with idiopathic pulmonary fibrosis (IPF),[21] lung transplantation in those with COPD, lung volume reduction surgery,[22] and prostacyclin therapy in individuals with primary pulmonary hypertension (PPH).[23]

Prognosis

Measurements of $\dot{V}O_{2max}$ are predictive of *survival* in individuals with cystic fibrosis (CF) and congestive heart failure (CHF). According to one study, CF subjects with $\dot{V}O_{2peak}$ values less than 59% of predicted were more than three times as likely to die as those with values greater than 82% of predicted, whereas measures of resting pulmonary function did not independently correlate with survival.[24] Individuals with cardiomyopathy awaiting heart transplantation who have $\dot{V}O_{2peak}$ values greater than 14 mL/min/kg demonstrate a 94% 1-year survival rate, compared with 70% survival in those individuals with values less than 14 mL/min/kg.[25] Based on these data, individuals with values for $\dot{V}O_{2peak}$ less than 14 mL/min/kg are prioritized higher in considerations for heart transplantation.

$\dot{V}O_{2peak}$ measurements have been used *to assess preoperative risk* before thoracotomy in individuals with cardiopulmonary disease. The rationale for its use includes its dependence on the pulmonary vasculature and pulmonary mechanics. CPX mimics the hypermetabolism and tachycardia of the perioperative state and represents an objective evolution of stair-climbing techniques traditionally used by surgeons. CPX should be reserved to include patients with relatively preserved functional status, those with resectable lung lesions, and those who do not have acceptable FEV$_1$ and diffusing capacity values by use of traditional criteria, or conversely, those patients who meet FEV$_1$ criteria but appear to have disproportionate disabilities.

One study reported a 29% mortality rate and 43% morbidity rate in individuals undergoing lobectomy or pneumonectomy with $\dot{V}O_{2peak}$ values less than 10 mL/min/kg. Both individuals in this group who underwent pneumonectomy died. Individuals with $\dot{V}O_{2peak}$ values greater than 10 mL/min/kg demonstrated no mortalities, and no individuals with $\dot{V}O_{2max}$ values greater than 20 mL/min/kg sustained any morbidity or death. Other investigators have demonstrated low morbidity rates with CPX testing in individuals otherwise considered high risks for thoracotomy by use of traditional criteria.[26,27] Table 27-2

presents risk stratification based on the $\dot{V}O_{2peak}$ value and extent of the operation.

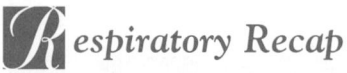

espiratory Recap

Indications for Exercise Testing

Unexplained or disproportionate dyspnea
Assessment of the impact of an intervention
Determination of prognosis
Disability assessment
Determination of a pulmonary rehabilitation prescription

Other investigators have examined CPX measurements used to assess risk in elderly individuals undergoing non-thoracic (abdominal) surgery. In this study a low LT (<11 mL/min/kg) was associated with an 18% mortality rate, in contrast to less than a 1% mortality rate in individuals with values greater than 11 mL/min/kg.[28]

Disability Assessment

Although clear guidelines to determine disability are lacking, resting pulmonary function measurements clearly do not adequately predict functional status. In a group of subjects studied who met American Thoracic Guidelines for respiratory disability, 48% had slight or no disability measured by use of CPX testing.[29] One standard commonly used to determine disability is to compare $\dot{V}O_2$ measurements in the laboratory to published energy requirements for different jobs.[30] The average energy requirement on the job should not exceed 50% of an individual's maximal work capacity.

Pulmonary Rehabilitation

CPX testing before pulmonary rehabilitation is recommended to define safety and determine exercise prescription.[31] CPX permits supervised observation of cases of potential ischemia, arrhythmia, hypotension, and hemoglobin oxygen desaturation. Although optimum exercise intensity

TABLE 27-2

Risk Stratification Based on Type of Procedure and Maximum $\dot{V}O_2$

| Procedure | $\dot{V}O_2max$ (mL/kg/min) | | | |
	<10	10 to 15	15 to 20	>20
Pneumonectomy	High risk*	High risk	Moderate risk	Low risk
Lobectomy	High risk	Moderate risk	Low risk	Low risk
VATS/wedge	Moderate risk	Low risk	Low risk	Low risk

$\dot{V}O_{2max}$, *Maximum oxygen consumption;* VATS/wedge, *video-assisted thoracic surgery/wedge resection.*
High risk = avoid surgery; moderate risk = consider alternatives; low risk = proceed with surgery.

is not well defined in respiratory patients, individuals who do not reach the LT are known to be able to train at a higher percentage of maximal exercise tolerance than those who reach the LT threshold.[32] Although some advocate that beneficial effects of pulmonary rehabilitation can be gained with lower-intensity work, evidence suggests that higher-work-intensity training results in greater reductions in lactic acidosis and ventilation requirements.[33]

Exercise-Induced Asthma

Assessment for exercise-induced asthma (EIA) can be performed as an add-on to CPX or as a separate diagnostic maneuver. If performed as an add-on to routine CPX testing, spirometry measurements are made before and then every 5 minutes for 20 minutes after a maximal exercise maneuver.[34] A drop in FEV_1 of greater than 15% is considered diagnostic. If the testing is performed as a stand-alone procedure, the work rate is incremented until the subject achieves an exercise heart rate of 80% of the maximum predicted value and continues at this pace for 6 to 10 minutes. Spirometry is again performed.

Testing for EIA in the laboratory is only moderately sensitive because conditions may not mimic the cold and dry air conditions or the pattern of ventilation present under field conditions. If EIA is still suspected after a negative exercise challenge, methacholine inhalation challenge testing is a highly sensitive (albeit less specific) tool to assist in diagnosis.

Interpretative Strategies in Cardiopulmonary Exercise Testing

Although CPX has earned a position as a tool that complements other information available to the physician, much of standard practice is not firmly based on evidence but rather on sound physiologic principles. Many interpretative strategies have been proposed.[35-37] Tests should ideally be interpreted in the context of other clinical data; for example, a borderline low LT and **oxygen pulse** may represent deconditioning in a sedentary elderly individual, but such findings in an endurance athlete may represent a significant cardiovascular pathologic process.

Maximal Exercise Capacity

The first question that should be answered is whether an individual has a normal exercise capacity. A $\dot{V}O_{2max}$ of greater than 84% of predicted indicates a normal physiologic capacity to perform metabolic work. In obese or otherwise inefficient individuals, significant discrepancies may exist between their physiologic capacity to perform work ($\dot{V}O_{2max}$) and the actual work performed on their environment or power output, which may be abnormally decreased (Figure 27-9). Furthermore, in obese individuals $\dot{V}O_{2max}$ adjusted for weight (mL/min/kg) may be decreased

into the mild (<25 mL/min/kg) or even severe (<15 mL/min/kg) disability range in the setting of normal $\dot{V}O_{2max}$% predicted, which is calculated based on height or lean body mass.

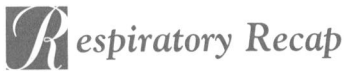

Respiratory Recap

> **Interpretative Strategies for CPX**
>
> Is the subject's maximal exercise capacity abnormal?
> What is the major limiting factor to maximal exertion: cardiac, ventilatory, gas exchange, or combined?
> Are abnormalities present in the cardiovascular and ventilatory gas exchange response?

Limiting Factor to Maximal Exertion

Cardiovascular limitation to exercise occurs when the cardiac and peripheral vascular components of the Fick equation are maximized; thus further increases in $\dot{V}O_2$ cannot occur, resulting in unbearable symptoms that lead to exercise termination ($\dot{V}O_{2max}$). Indicators of cardiovascular limitation include a heart rate reserve (HRR) of less than 15 beats/min or a heart rate greater than 90% of predicted. In addition, a drop in BE or a lactate increase of more than 3 in the case of chronotropic insufficiency can indicate cardiovascular limitation. Healthy individuals exhibit a cardiovascular limitation to exercise; abnormalities need not be present in the cardiovascular system.

Ventilatory limitation occurs when an individual approaches the mechanical limits of the respiratory system,

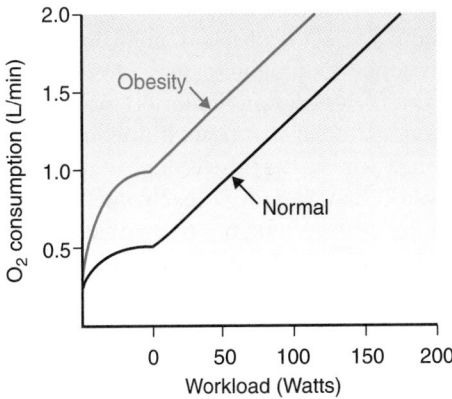

Figure 27-9 Maximal oxygen consumption as a function of workload in normal-weight compared with obese individuals during incremental bicycle ergometry. Note that maximal oxygen consumption and slope of oxygen consumption as a function of workload are similar between normal-weight and otherwise physiologically healthy obese individuals. The inefficiencies of pedaling and mass of the lower extremities influence the higher oxygen consumption during unloaded pedaling in obese individuals.

Box 27-3

Abnormalities in Exercise Testing

Cardiovascular Response

Parameters indicating an abnormal cardiovascular response include low LT, elevated heart rate-versus-work rate relationship, decreased oxygen pulse, and decreasing $\Delta \dot{V}O_2/\Delta Watts$ with increasing workload. In general, abnormalities in cardiovascular response are associated with a decrease in maximal exercise tolerance. The differential diagnosis for isolated abnormalities in the cardiovascular response include any condition that affects the delivery or use of oxygen, including severe deconditioning, left or right heart systolic or diastolic dysfunction, anemia, hemoglobinopathy, carboxyhemoglobin myopathy, or peripheral shunt.

Ventilation

Parameters indicating an abnormal ventilation response include $\dot{V}_{Emax}/MVV$ of greater than 75%, VR of less than 11 L/min, and a rising $Paco_2$.

Gas Exchange

Parameters indicating an abnormal gas exchange response include increased V_D/V_T, abnormally widened $P(A - a)o_2$, a decrease in Pao_2 or Spo_2, elevated $\dot{V}_E/\dot{V}o_2$ at LT, and increased $P(a - ET)co_2$. Because most healthy individuals have a large ventilatory reserve at maximal exertion, significant abnormalities in ventilatory mechanics and gas exchange may be present without an associated ventilatory limitation. The finding of abnormalities in gas exchange supports the presence of and quantifies the magnitude of overt or occult parenchymal lung disease or airways disease.

Combined Abnormalities

Abnormalities in both the cardiovascular and ventilatory parameters may be characteristic of disease processes, such as primary pulmonary vascular disease. In other cases the response pattern helps subcategorize disease. For example, although COPD is primarily associated with significant deficits in gas exchange, abnormalities in the cardiovascular parameters may indicate the presence of secondary pulmonary hypertension, myopathy, or left ventricular comorbidity. Whereas subjects with idiopathic pulmonary fibrosis have qualitatively similar findings, that disease process is characterized by more profound arterial desaturation and rapid respiratory rates, which often exceed 60/min at maximal exertion. More subtle abnormalities in gas exchange can be observed in subjects with cardiomyopathy, in whom abnormalities in cardiovascular response are prominent. Disproportionate symptoms in individuals can be more clearly understood through observation, for example, of the synergistic effects of early lactic acidosis on an individual with ventilatory mechanical and gas exchange abnormalities.

$\Delta \dot{V}o_2/\Delta Watts$, *Oxygen consumption/work rate relationship;* $Paco_2$, *partial pressure of arterial carbon dioxide;* $\dot{V}_{Emax}$, *maximum minute ventilation;* MVV, *maximal voluntary ventilation;* V_D/V_T, *ratio of dead space to tidal volume;* $P(A - a)o_2$, *difference between alveolar and arterial Po2;* Spo_2, *oxygen saturation measured by pulse oximetry;* $\dot{V}_E/\dot{V}o_2$, *ventilatory equivalent for oxygen;* LT, *lactic threshold;* $P(a - ET)co_2$, *difference between arterial and end-tidal Pco2;* COPD, *chronic obstructive pulmonary disease.*

resulting in intolerable dyspnea that leads to exercise termination; thus $\dot{V}o_2$ cannot increase further despite significant reserves in the cardiovascular system ($\dot{V}o_{2peak}$). Indicators of ventilatory limitation include $\dot{V}_{Emax}/MVV$ of greater than 0.75 or VR of less than 11 L/min. Although tidal flow-volume loop analysis may provide a more specific indicator of ventilatory limitation, no specific criteria have been validated at this time. Individuals demonstrating ventilatory limitation nearly all have abnormalities in ventilatory mechanics and gas exchange. Exceptions include the elite athlete, who has trained the cardiovascular system to challenge the limits of the capacity for the ventilatory system, and the individual with increased ventilatory drive, as may occur in cases of severe acute or chronic metabolic acidosis.

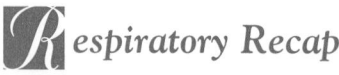

Indicators of Cardiovascular Limitation

Heart rate reserve: <15 beats/min
Heart rate: >90% of predicted

espiratory Recap

Indicators of Ventilatory Limitation

V_{Emax}/MVV: >75%
Ventilatory reserve: <11 L/min

Gas exchange limitations, particularly hypoxemia leading to intolerable dyspnea, are commonly considered a separate category of exercise limitation. Actually the impairment in oxygen delivery associated with hypoxemia and the elevation in $\dot{V}_E$ associated with dead space abnormalities may contribute to premature cardiovascular and ventilatory limitations.

A combined limitation occurs when both cardiovascular and ventilatory parameters approach physiologic limits. In such cases, symptoms from both processes likely contribute to exercise termination.

A submaximal response occurs when neither cardiovascular nor ventilatory system parameters approach their physiologic limits; in such cases the study is considered to be submaximal. This finding may be a valid measure of exercise capacity if symptoms arise from peripheral muscle weakness or musculoskeletal pain, but the values are less meaningful if exercise is terminated due to a lack of effort, dry mouth, or sore buttocks.

Abnormalities in the Cardiovascular and Ventilatory/Gas Exchange Response

Abnormalities in the various cardiovascular and ventilatory/gas exchange parameters can occur independent of whether these disturbances ultimately limit maximal exertion. Patterns of response in a given clinical setting can provide physiologic understanding and assist in the refining of a differential diagnosis (Box 27-3). On the other hand, strict interpretation algorithms are difficult to apply to CPX because the importance of any given parameter depends on its relationship to other parameters and the specific clinical scenario. Although conclusive studies are currently unavailable, a normal exercise physiologic response is likely to significantly decrease the likelihood of a serious pathologic process. Abnormal responses, on the other hand, rarely provide a specific diagnosis without corroboration with clinical data.

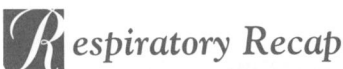
espiratory Recap

Abnormal Response to Exercise
Abnormal Cardiovascular Response
Low LT
Elevated heart rate/workload relationship
Decreased oxygen pulse
Decreased $\Delta\dot{V}O_2/\Delta$Watts with increased workload
Abnormal Ventilatory/Gas Exchange Response
Increased V_D/V_T, which does not decrease appropriately with exercise
Widened $P(A - a)O_2$
Decrease in PaO_2 or SpO_2
Elevated $\dot{V}_E/\dot{V}O_2$ at LT
Increased $P(a - ET)CO_2$

Safety Issues

After a maximal exercise maneuver, the patient must continue to pedal with unloaded or low resistance on the bicycle to maintain venous return. This action is especially important for patients with primary or secondary pulmonary hypertension who have a poorly compliant right ventricle and are particularly prone to postexercise hypotension and syncope. In these situations a very serious physiologic cascade can occur, with inadequate preload leading to inadequate $\dot{Q}c$, yielding underperfusion of the cardiac conducting system and bradycardia. The ensuing decrease in $\dot{Q}c$ may lead to a drop in mixed venous oxygen saturation and hypoxia-induced increases in pulmonary vascular resist-

Box 27-4

Criteria for Exercise Test Termination

Chest pain suspicious of angina
Evolving mental confusion or lack of coordination
Evolving lightheadedness
ECG evidence of ischemia or serious arrhythmia or conduction system abnormality (evolving complex ventricular ectopy, sustained SVT, new LBBB, second- or third-degree heart block)
Blood pressure: systolic >250 mm Hg; diastolic >120 mm Hg
Fall in systolic blood pressure >20 mm Hg
Chronotropic insufficiency in absence of β-blockers
SpO_2 <80%
Inability to sustain cadence above 40 rpm
Subject's request to stop despite encouragement because of symptoms of dyspnea, leg or global fatigue, or otherwise

ECG, Electrocardiogram; SVT, supraventricular tachycardia; LBBB, left bundle branch block; SpO₂, oxygen saturation measured by pulse oximetry.

ance, thus furthering $\dot{Q}c$ deterioration, which may continue in a spiral that leads to death. A rule in this author's laboratory is that an individual is either pedaling or are rapidly assisted off the bicycle into a reclining chair, with a capability for leg elevation if necessary. The patient who says, "Just give me 1 second to sit here, and I will be all right," is potentially on the verge of a serious complication. Criteria for exercise termination are listed in Box 27-4.[3]

Key Points

- Cardiopulmonary exercise testing permits delineation of the physiologic subsystems responsible for exercise limitation.
- The normal physiologic response to exercise includes alterations in cardiac output, ventilation, peripheral circulation, hemoglobin oxygen affinity, and cellular metabolism.
- Important indications for exercise testing include diagnosis of unexplained dyspnea, determination of prognosis and risk, and responses that follow interventions, such as pulmonary rehabilitation.
- No standard interpretative strategies exist for cardiopulmonary exercise tests. A global strategy involves definition of the physiologic systems responsible for exercise limitation and subsequent determination of the abnormal responses within these systems.

References

1. Johnson BD, Badr MS, Dempsey JA. Impact of the aging pulmonary system on the response to exercise. Clin Chest Med 1994;15:229-246.

2. Johnson B, Saupe K, Dempsey J. Mechanical constraints on exercise hyperpnea in endurance athletes. J Appl Physiol 1992;73:874-886.

3. Zeballos R, Weisman I. Behind the scenes of cardiopulmonary exercise testing. Clin Chest Med 1994;15:193-213.

4. Dempsey JA. Is the lung built for exercise? Med Sci Sports Exerc 1986;18:143.

5. Babb T, Viggiano R, Hurley B, et al. Effect of mild-to-moderate airflow limitation on exercise capacity. J Appl Physiol 1991; 70:223-230.

6. O'Donnell DE, Webb KA. Exertional breathlessness in patients with chronic airflow limitation: the role of lung hyperinflation. Am Rev Respir Dis 1993;148:1351-1357.

7. Hansen J, Sue D, Wasserman K. Predicted values for clinical exercise testing. Am Rev Respir Dis 1984;129(Suppl):S49-S55.

8. Resnikoff J, Covin R, Harper P, et al. Cardiopulmonary exercise testing (CPET) in the evaluation of dyspnea: the need for routine invasive testing. Am J Respir Crit Care Med 1994;151 (Suppl 4):A548.

9. Belman MJ, Botnick WC, Shin JW. Inhaled bronchodilators reduce dynamic hyperinflation during exercise in patients with chronic obstructive pulmonary disease. Am J Respir Crit Care Med 1996;153:967-975.

10. Warburton DER, Haykowsky MJF, Quinney HA, et al. Reliability and validity of measures of cardiac output during incremental to maximal aerobic exercise. Part I. Conventional techniques. Sports Med 1999;1:23-41.

11. Mahler D, Horowitz M. Clinical evaluation of exertional dyspnea. Clin Chest Med 1994;15:259-269.

12. Jones N, Killian, KJ. Mechanisms of disease: exercise limitation in health and disease. N Engl J Med 2000;343:632-641.

13. Guyatt GW, Sullivan MJ, Thompson PJ, et al. The 6 minute walk: a new measure of exercise capacity in patients with chronic heart failure. Canadian Medical Association Journal 1985;132:919-923.

14. Enright PL, Sherrill DL. Reference equations for the 6 minute walk in healthy adults. Am J Resp Crit Care Med 1998;158: 1384-1387.

15. Mottram CD. Exercise testing. Respir Care Clin N Am 1997; 3:247-272.

16. O'Keefe ST, Lye M, Donnellan C, et al. Reproducibility and responsiveness of quality of life assessment and six minute walk test in elderly heart failure patients. Heart 1998;80:377-382.

17. Martinez F, Stanopoulos I, Acero R, et al. Graded, comprehensive, cardiopulmonary exercise testing in the evaluation of dyspnea unexplained by routine evaluation. Chest 1994;105: 168-174.

18. Sue DY, Oren A, Hansen JE, et al. Diffusing capacity for carbon monoxide as a predictor of gas exchange during exercise. N Engl J Med 1987;316:1301-1306.

19. Belman MJ, Epstein LJ, Doornbos D, et al. Noninvasive determinations of the anaerobic threshold: reliability and validity in patients with COPD. Chest 1992;102:1028-1034.

20. O'Donnell DE. Assessment of bronchodilator efficacy in symptomatic COPD: is spirometry useful? Chest 2000;117:428-478.

21. Watters L, Schwarz M, Cherniack R, et al. Idiopathic pulmonary fibrosis.: pretreatment bronchoalveolar lavage cellular constituents and their relationships with lung histopathology and clinical response to therapy. Am Rev Respir Dis 1987;135: 696-704.

22. Sciurba FC. Early and long-term functional outcomes following lung volume reduction surgery. Clin Chest Med 1997;18:259-276.

23. Higenbottam TW, Spiegelhalter DJ, Scott JP, et al. Survival in primary pulmonary hypertension (PPH): a comparison of vasodilator treatment and heart-lung transplantation, with the Mayo Clinic retrospective analysis of survival. Am Rev Respir Dis 1989;139:A265.

24. Nixon P, Orenstein D, Kelsey S, et al. The prognostic value of exercise testing in patients with cystic fibrosis. N Engl J Med 1992;327:1785-1788.

25. Mancini D, Eisen H, Kussmaul W, et al. Value of peak exercise oxygen consumption for optimal timing of cardiac transplantation in ambulatory patients with heart failure. Circulation 1991;83:778-786.

26. Morice RC, Peters EJ, Ryan MB, et al. Exercise testing in the evaluation of patients at high risk for complications from lung resection. Chest 1992;101:356-361.

27. Bolliger C, Jordan P, Soler M, et al. Exercise capacity as a predictor of postoperative complication in lung resection candidates. Am J Respir Crit Care Med 1995;151:1472-1480.

28. Older P, Smith R, Courtney P, et al. Preoperative evaluation of cardiac failure and ischemia in elderly patients by cardiopulmonary exercise testing. Chest 1993;104:663-664.

29. Cotes J, Zejda J, King B. Lung function impairment as a guide to exercise limitation in work-related lung disorders. Am Rev Respir Dis 1988;137:1089-1093.

30. Passmore R, Durnin JV. Human energy expenditure. Physiol Rev 1955;35:801-840.

31. Roca J, Whipp BJ, Agusti AGN, et al. Clinical exercise testing with reference to lung diseases: indications, standardization and interpretation strategies. European Respir J 1997;10:2662-2689.

32. Punzal PA, Ries AL, Kaplan RM, et al. Maximum intensity exercise training in patients with chronic obstructive pulmonary disease. Chest 1991;100:618-623.

33. Casaburi R, Patessio A, Ioli F, et al. Reductions in exercise lactic acidosis and ventilation as a result of exercise training in patients with obstructive lung disease. Am Rev Respir Dis 1991;143:9-18.

34. Cypcar D, Lemanske RF. Asthma and exercise. Clin Chest Med 1994;15:351-368.

35. Weisman I, Zeballos R. An integrated approach to the interpretation of cardiopulmonary exercise testing. Clin Chest Med 1994;15:421-445.

36. Wasserman K. Diagnosing cardiovascular and lung pathophysiology from exercise gas exchange. Chest 1997;112:1091-1101.

37. Wasserman K, Hansen J, Sue D, et al. Principles of exercise testing and interpretation. Philadelphia: Lea & Febiger; 1994.

CHAPTER 28

Fiberoptic Bronchoscopy

Sharona Sachs

CHAPTER **OUTLINE**

OBJECTIVES

1. Compare rigid and flexible fiberoptic bronchoscopy.
2. Discuss the roles of patient selection, patient preparation, and sedation in the performance of flexible fiberoptic bronchoscopy.
3. Describe the bronchoscopic techniques of airway exam, bronchoalveolar lavage, bronchoscopic washing, bronchial brushing with nonprotected brush, bronchial brushing with protected brush, endobronchial biopsy, transbronchial needle aspiration, and transbronchial biopsy.
4. Discuss patient selection, patient preparation, and sedation for rigid bronchoscopy.
5. Describe the technique of rigid bronchoscopy.
6. Describe the technique of laser bronchoscopy.
7. Describe the following diagnostic indications for bronchoscopy: suspected carcinoma, pneumonia, lobar atelectasis, suspected foreign body aspiration, interstitial lung disease, hemoptysis, cough, and trauma.
8. Describe the following therapeutic indications for bronchoscopy: intubation, brachytherapy, and stent placement.
9. List complications of bronchoscopy.

KEY TERMS

Brachytherapy
Bronchoalveolar Lavage (BAL)
Bronchoscopic Washing
Endobronchial Biopsy
Flexible Fiberoptic Bronchoscopy (FOB)

Laser Bronchoscopy
Nonprotected Bronchial Brush
Protected Specimen Brush (PSB)
Rigid Bronchoscopy
Tracheobronchial Stents

Transbronchial Biopsy (TBBx)
Transbronchial Needle Aspiration
  (TBNA)

The practice of bronchoscopy dates to the late 1890s, when Gustav Killian first visualized the larynx and trachea under local anesthesia with the use of a hollow metal tube and a light source. In 1905, Chevalier Jackson elaborated on this design to develop the rigid bronchoscope, a modification of which is still in use today. Professor Jackson popularized the use of the rigid bronchoscope, training primarily thoracic surgeons and otorhinolaryngologists in its use.[1] The advent of flexible fiberoptic bronchoscopy significantly simplified the technique, which is the most commonly used in clinical practice. Fiberoptic bronchoscopy is commonly performed by pulmonary physicians, thoracic surgeons, and intensivists with the assistance of a respiratory therapist (CPG 28-1). This chapter covers the clinical and technical aspects of bronchoscopy.

The Bronchoscope

The basic design of the rigid scope (Figure 28-1) limited the applications of bronchoscopy for several decades. The instrument is comprised of a hollow, stainless-steel tube with a light source incorporated along its shaft (currently fiberoptic), an angled distal end to facilitate insertion through the larynx, a variety of proximal ports

---

CPG 28-1

Fiberoptic Bronchoscopy Assisting

Indications

The presence of lesions of unknown etiology on the chest radiograph film or the need to evaluate recurrent or persistent atelectasis or pulmonary infiltrates

The need to assess patency or mechanical properties of the upper airway

The need to investigate hemoptysis, persistent unexplained cough, localized wheeze, or stridor

Suspicious or positive sputum cytology results

The need to obtain lower respiratory tract secretions, cell washings, and biopsies for cytologic, histologic, and microbiologic evaluation

The need to determine the location and extent of injury from toxic inhalation or aspiration

The need to evaluate problems associated with endotracheal or tracheostomy tubes (tracheal damage, airway obstruction, or tube placement)

The need for aid in performing difficult intubations

The suspicion that secretions or mucus plugs are responsible for lobar or segmental atelectasis

The need to remove abnormal endobronchial tissue or foreign material by forceps, basket, or laser

The need to retrieve a foreign body (although under most circumstances, rigid bronchoscopy is preferred)

Contraindications

Absolute contraindications include absence of consent from the patient or patient's representative unless a medical emergency exists and the patient is not competent to give permission; absence of an experienced bronchoscopist to perform or closely and directly supervise the procedure; lack of adequate facilities and personnel to care for such emergencies as cardiopulmonary arrest, pneumothorax, or bleeding; inability to adequately oxygenate the patient during the procedure.

The danger of a serious complication from bronchoscopy is especially high in patients with the disorders listed, and these conditions usually are considered absolute contraindi-

cations unless the risk-benefit assessment warrants the procedure: coagulopathy or bleeding diathesis that cannot be corrected, severe obstructive airway disease, severe refractory hypoxemia, and unstable hemodynamic status including dysrhythmias.

Relative contraindications (or conditions involving increased risk) include lack of patient cooperation; recent myocardial infarction or unstable angina; partial tracheal obstruction; moderate-to-severe hypoxemia or any degree of hypercarbia; uremia and pulmonary hypertension (possible serious hemorrhage after biopsy); lung abscess (danger of flooding the airway with purulent material); obstruction of the superior vena cava (possibility of bleeding and laryngeal edema); debility, advanced age, and malnutrition; respiratory failure requiring mechanical ventilation; disorders requiring laser therapy, biopsy of lesions obstructing large airways, or multiple transbronchial lung biopsies; and known or suspected pregnancy because of radiation exposure.

The safety of bronchoscopic procedures in asthmatic patients is a concern, but the presence of asthma does not preclude the use of these procedures.

Hazards and Complications

Adverse effects of medication used before and during the bronchoscopic procedure

Hypoxemia

Hypercarbia

Wheezing

Hypotension

Laryngospasm, bradycardia, or other vagally mediated phenomena

Mechanical complications such as epistaxis, pneumothorax, or hemoptysis

Increased airway resistance

Death

Infection hazard for health care workers or other patients

Cross-contamination of specimens or bronchoscopes

From AARC Clinical practice guideline: fiberoptic bronchoscopy assisting. Respir Care 1993;38:1173-1178.
CPG, Clinical practice guideline.

for oxygen insufflation, and distal ports for ventilation because the instrument is intended to occupy most of the airway diameter. Lengths vary up to 40 cm and external diameters up to 8 mm. Optical telescopes allow visualization of the lobar and segmental bronchi, but the size and rigidity of the instrument limit airway examination. Because of these constraints, the primary indications for bronchoscopy initially were foreign body aspiration and retrieval, and in the 1940s through the 1960s, identification of endobronchial tuberculosis or proximal endobronchial malignancies and evaluation of massive hemoptysis.

In the late 1960s, flexible bronchoscopes using fiberoptic technology were introduced. The **flexible fiberoptic bronchoscopy (FOB)** consists of a control unit (head) and soft, flexible shaft (Figure 28-2). The shaft contains a hollow internal operating channel used to suction secretions and collect specimens and a working channel for installation of solutions (saline, lidocaine) and passage of instruments. The control unit is attached to a light source and also can be fitted with a camera for dynamic or still photography. It contains instrumentation for focusing, a lever to flex the tip, and the opening that leads to the internal operating channel. The primary advantage of the flexible scope lies in its shaft, which has an external diameter of 3.5 to 6 mm (smaller sizes are available for infants and children) and a tip that can rotate through 310 degrees, controlled by guide wires that run through the shaft. In addition, the introduction of fiberoptic technology, with afferent and efferent glass fibers running the length of the shaft, has dramatically improved the resolution of images obtained. In the most recent technologic advance, fiberoptics have been replaced by videoscopes with high-resolution microchips for imaging. The endoscope itself has been progressively refined, with ultrathin scopes that allow visualization of the more distal airways in selected patients and scopes with specialized working channels for therapeutics such as laser.

Flexible Fiberoptic Bronchoscopy

There are several key elements to a successful bronchoscopic procedure. Although the technical proficiency of the operator is clearly of major importance, a number of other factors come into play. These include patient selection and preparation, adequacy and appropriateness of anesthesia, and an understanding of the indications and expected yields for the various bronchoscopic maneuvers, both diagnostic and therapeutic. Major indications for fiberoptic bronchoscopy are outlined in Box 28-1.

BOX 28-1

Indications for Fiberoptic Bronchoscopy

Diagnostic
  Suspected malignancy
    Unexplained radiographic volume loss
    Lung/mediastinal mass
    Nonresolving infiltrate
    Nonresolving atelectasis
    Unexplained hoarseness, vocal cord paralysis, or cough
    Mediastinal staging
    Abnormal sputum cytology
    Unexplained hemoptysis
  Infection
    Nonresolving pneumonia
    Exclusion of opportunistic infection
    Evaluation of ventilator-associated pneumonia
  Foreign body aspiration
  Interstitial lung disease
  Hemoptysis
  Trauma

Therapeutic
  Intubation
  Brachytherapy
  Stent placement

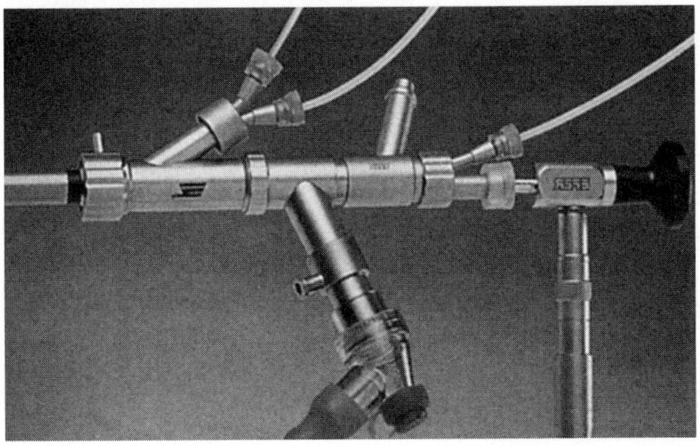

Figure 28-1 Rigid bronchoscope demonstrating numerous attachments and portals at the proximal end. (From Prakash UBS. Bronchoscopy. In: Albert RK, Spiro SG, Jett JR. Comprehensive respiratory medicine. Philadelphia: WB Saunders; 1999.)

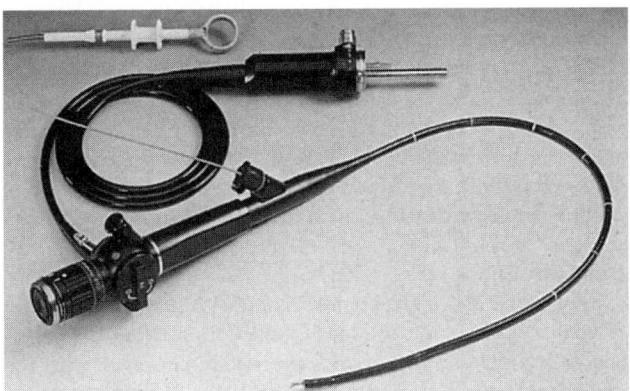

Figure 28-2 Flexible bronchoscope with biopsy forceps introduced through its working channel. (From Prakash UBS. Bronchoscopy. In: Albert RK, Spiro SG, Jett JR. Comprehensive respiratory medicine. Philadelphia: WB Saunders; 1999.)

Patient Selection

The ideal patient for awake fiberoptic bronchoscopy is able to understand and cooperate with the procedure and is free of major comorbid diseases—in particular, ischemic or arrhythmic heart disease, bleeding diathesis (coagulopathy, thrombocytopenia, or uremia), or respiratory insufficiency. Although bronchoscopy can be performed in patients who fall short of this ideal, the risk of the procedure increases and the options for invasive diagnostic manipulations decrease in proportion to the impairment of the patient's mental or physical status. The history and physical examination obtained should be directed toward ascertaining the presence and severity of such comorbidity, documenting previous anesthesia and associated complications, and defining ways in which the timing or the nature of the procedure can be modified to minimize risk.

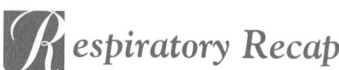*espiratory Recap*

Factors Necessary for Successful FOB
Patient selection
Patient preparation
Sedation

A number of conditions can be prospectively identified and treated to minimize risk. For example, although bronchoscopy has been safely carried out in asthmatic patients, it is associated with a significant drop in FEV_1 and PaO_2.[2] If being performed electively, the procedure therefore should be deferred until bronchospasm is effectively controlled. In the same way, older adults in particular have been noted to develop electrocardiographic evidence of ischemia during bronchoscopy, especially when the procedure is prolonged.[3] Patients with a history of active cardiac ischemia or recent myocardial infarction should have the procedure delayed until their cardiac status is stabilized if bronchoscopy is planned for elective diagnosis. In addition, such patients should be carefully monitored during the procedure and should have the duration of the procedure minimized. Increased intracranial pressure (ICP) has been anecdotally cited as a relative contraindication to bronchoscopy because the increase in intrathoracic pressure induced by bronchoscopy-associated cough may abruptly raise ICP and precipitate transtentorial herniation. When this issue was retrospectively studied, no increase in neurologic complications was found in patients undergoing bronchoscopy in the presence of space-occupying central nervous system lesions, although pretreatment with steroids to decrease cerebral edema was recommended.[4] The contraindications and relative contraindications to bronchoscopy and biopsy are outlined in Box 28-2. Although bronchoscopy has few absolute contraindications, the risk/benefit ratio changes for each patient and should be individually assessed, with

Box 28-2

Contraindications to Fiberoptic Bronchoscopy and Transbronchial Biopsy

Absolute
Inability to maintain adequate oxygenation
Operator inexperience
Inadequate facilities
Lack of informed consent

Relative/Increased Risk
Active ischemic heart disease
Active cardiac arrhythmia
Refractory hypoxemia
Resting hypercarbia
Bleeding diathesis
Debilitated or uncooperative patient
Active bronchospasm

every effort made to optimize the conditions under which the procedure is performed.

In addition to history and physical examination, a number of screening laboratory studies directed toward detection of the comorbid conditions previously outlined have been advocated. These studies include a platelet count to exclude thrombocytopenia, a creatinine and blood urea nitrogen level to exclude uremia, and coagulation studies to rule out a coagulopathy. In the current era of cost containment, the utility of these studies in asymptomatic patients has been reevaluated. In a retrospective review of 305 bronchoscopies with biopsy, Kozak and Brath found that routine coagulation studies were not useful in the prediction of bleeding complications.[5] If history does not reveal a bleeding diathesis, and history and physical exam do not suggest liver disease, renal insufficiency, or cardiopulmonary compromise, no standard requirement for preprocedure laboratory screening exists. Conversely, in a frail-appearing patient with an uncertain cardiopulmonary baseline, screening evaluation might include an electrocardiogram and arterial blood gas in addition to the blood work outlined previously.[6,7]

Patient Preparation

Once the appropriate patient is selected, the procedure begins when informed consent is obtained. Each aspect of the procedure, from the initial application of topical anesthesia to introduction of the bronchoscope through the nose or mouth, vocal cords, and distal airways, should be explained. The sensations that the patient should anticipate—including the sensation of upper-airway closure that is sometimes experienced as topical anesthesia takes effect, pressure at the nares as the bronchoscope is introduced, and most importantly, the strong desire to cough as the bronchoscope is manipulated through the airway—should be reviewed. The patient should be reassured about the steps that will be taken to maximize comfort, including continued topical anesthesia to alleviate cough throughout the procedure and IV sedation to alleviate anxiety as needed. Because of the risk of aspiration, the patient should be fasting except for medication past midnight for a planned morning procedure or fasting except for a light liquid breakfast for a planned afternoon procedure.

The risks of the procedure, tailored specifically to the maneuvers planned for the individual patient, must be reviewed. Risks include those associated with anesthesia and those associated with the procedure itself. Without transbronchial biopsy (TBBx), the risk of serious procedure-related complications is approximately 0.1%. When TBBx is performed, the risk of serious complications increases to 1% to 5%. Pneumothorax is one such serious adverse effect; it occurs with a reported incidence between 0.4% and 5.5%. Hemorrhage—defined as greater than 50 mL of blood loss—occurs in up to 4% of normal patients, up to 25% of immunosuppressed patients, and up to 45% of uremic patients when TBBx is obtained.[8-14] By contrast, in a study by Weiss and colleagues, bronchoscopy and bronchoalveolar lavage without biopsy were performed with relative safety in thrombocytopenic patients.[15]

Cardiopulmonary events are more rare, with cardiovascular complications including vasovagal reactions (2.4%), arrhythmias (0.9%), and ischemic changes (0.2%). Pulmonary complications include clinically significant bronchospasm or airway obstruction (0.4%). Death is a very rare complication, occurring in about 0.1% of patients.[14] More common complications include transient hypoxemia, with PaO_2 drops of 20 mm Hg on average[16]; transient fever, which typically peaks within 4 to 8 hours of the procedure and subsides within 24 hours (20%)[17]; and trivial hemoptysis. Modest hypoxemia often is obviated by supplemental oxygen, which is generally delivered during each procedure.[18] If the patient has marked hypoxemia before the procedure, refractory hypoxemia becomes a more significant problem. Most pulmonologists advocate elective intubation before bronchoscopy if the patient requires more than 50% oxygen to maintain a PaO_2 of 65 mm Hg. Similarly, any degree of hypercarbia (PcO_2 >45 mm Hg) suggests a significant risk of progressive ventilatory failure with the procedure and warrants consideration of elective intubation before endoscopy.

Sedation

After the patient has been counseled and informed consent has been obtained, premedication and topical anesthesia are initiated. Premedication typically includes narcotics such as meperidine or codeine—with or without potentiating and antiemetic agents such as hydroxyzine, phenergan, or droperidol—and antisialagogues such as atropine, glycopyrrolate, and scopolamine. The antisialagogues minimize secretions to optimize visualization and offer vagolytic properties to offset the vagal response often observed with tracheal manipulation. Narcotics depress the laryngeal cough reflex and alter the respiratory pattern to facilitate deeper, slower breathing, which assists in the introduction of the bronchoscope into the tracheobronchial tree. The disadvantages of narcotics lie in unwanted side effects of cardiorespiratory depression, especially in older patients, and the lack of amnestic and anxiolytic properties. The disadvantage of the antisialagogues lies in their propensity to precipitate arrhythmias and, in the case of scopolamine, a tendency to induce delirium. The intramuscular (IM) route is typically used to create a more gradual and sustained effect and to reduce the arrhythmogenic potential of antisialagogues. IM premedication usually is administered between 30 and 90 minutes before the planned procedure, with typical doses, onset and duration of action, and therapeutic and side effects outlined in Table 28-1.[16,19]

Unless a patient is considered unusually susceptible or fragile, continuous monitoring for arrhythmias, hemodynamic stability, and oxygen saturation does not need to be instituted before premedication. Such monitoring, however, is a standard accompaniment to the procedure itself and is particularly important if further IV sedation is to be used during the bronchoscopy. Standard monitoring includes continuous pulse oximetry, continuous electrocardiographic monitoring, and periodic blood pressure measurement (frequency determined by both the patient's condition and amount of sedation planned). IV access is typically established before the procedure.[6]

Topical anesthesia is initiated just before the procedure and can be accomplished by a variety of means. Nebulized 4% lidocaine can be delivered through a face mask to anesthetize the entire airway. This approach requires a lead time of approximately 20 minutes. Another approach that is effective and may be less time consuming is to have the patient sniff and gargle with viscous lidocaine to anesthetize the nasopharynx and anterior pharynx, and then deliver 4% lidocaine solution by atomizer to the posterior oropharynx and nasopharynx.[20-22] Whichever approach is used, careful attention must be paid to the total dose of lidocaine delivered to the upper and lower airways during the procedure because the serum concentration after topical administration may be up to 50% of that achieved by IV bolus.[8] The maximal recommended dose is 4 mg/kg of lean body weight, or about 300 mg. This dose should be adjusted downward in patients with significant hepatic or cardiac disease.

Entry into the nasopharynx can be facilitated by the application of topical vasoconstrictors such as 4% cocaine or 0.5% phenylephrine, both of which decrease local bleeding and mucosal edema. These can be applied with a cotton-tipped applicator, which at the same time assesses the patency of the nasopharynx and adequacy of topical anesthesia. After this initial topical treatment, the procedure can be performed with 1% or 2% lidocaine adminis-

TABLE 28-1

Commonly Used Drugs in Awake Fiberoptic Bronchoscopy

	Drug Dose	Time of Onset	Duration of Action	Therapeutic Effect	Potential Adverse Effect
Narcotic					
Morphine	2 to 10 mg	5 to 10 min IV 30 to 60 min IM	1 to 6 hr	Analgesia, sedation, antitussive	Respiratory depression, hypotension, bronchospasm, nausea, urinary retention, chest wall rigidity, decreased seizure threshold
Fentanyl	50 to 100 μg	1 to 2 min IV 10 to 15 min IM	30 to 60 min	Analgesia, sedation, antitussive	Same as morphine; less bronchospasm
Codeine	30 to 60 mg	30 to 120 min IM; IV not recommended	4 to 8 hr	Analgesia, sedation, antitussive	Same as morphine
Meperidine	50 to 100 mg	3 to 5 min IV	1 to 4 hr	Analgesia, sedation, antitussive	Same as morphine; more potential decrease in seizure threshold
Benzodiazepine					
Midazolam	0.5 to 2 mg initial*; 1 to 5 mg total	1 to 5 min IV 15 min IM	2 to 6 hr	Amnesia, sedation	Respiratory depression, hypotension, bronchospasm, paradoxical excitation
Lorazepam	1 to 4 mg	20 to 30 min IM 5 to 20 min IV	6 to 8 hr	Amnesia, sedation	Same as midazolam
Potentiating Agents					
Hydroxyzine	25 to 100 mg	15 to 30 min IM; should not be administered IV	4 to 6 hr	Sedation, anxiolysis	Drowsiness, anticholinergic effects, not well tolerated in older adults
Droperidol	2.5 to 10 mg	5 to 30 min IM, IV	2 to 4 hr; up to 12 hr	Sedation, anxiolysis, antiemetic	Extrapyramidal, hypotension, respiratory depression
Antisialogogues					
Atropine	0.4 to 0.6 mg	30 to 60 min IM	4 to 6 hr	Inhibition of secretions	Impaired GI motility, tachycardia, orthostatic hypotension, contraindicated in glaucoma
Glycopyrrolate	4.4 μg/kg	20 to 40 min IM	1 hr	Inhibition of secretions	Same as atropine
Scopolamine	0.3 to 0.65 mg	10 min IV, 30 to 60 min IM	20 to 60 min; may last several days	Inhibition of secretions, amnesia	Same as atropine, blurred vision

Modified from Reed AP. Preparation of the patient for awake flexible fiberoptic bronchoscopy. Chest 1992;101:244-253 and Lacy CF, Armstrong LL, Ingram NB, et al. Drug information handbook. 6th ed. Cleveland: Lexi-Comp Inc; 1998.

IV, Intravenous; IM, intramuscular; GI, gastrointestinal.

*Initial dose should be given slowly over a minimum of 2 minutes IV; subsequent doses should be given in small increments and at intervals of at least 2 to 3 minutes. Concomitant administration with narcotics requires a minimum of 30% dose reduction.

All drugs and doses are suggested doses based on normal renal and hepatic function. Alterations in renal or hepatic function, extremes of age, debility, or drugs that are coadministered may dramatically affect doses required. Careful individualization of drug regimen and dose is required.

tered in 2-mL aliquots through the bronchoscope as it is advanced. Typically, the vocal cords are pretreated, as are the carina, right and left mainstem bronchi, and major bronchial orifices as they are approached.

Many bronchoscopists advocate further IV sedation during the procedure for all or some patients. Commonly used agents are benzodiazepines for their amnestic and anxiolytic properties and narcotics to decrease the cough reflex and promote hyperpnea. Short-acting agents are optimal, with midazolam favored as a benzodiazepine and either morphine or fentanyl favored as a narcotic.[23,24] Propofol also has been used by some operators[25]; it does not yet have a standard indication in conscious sedation. As outlined in Table 28-1, cardiorespiratory depression is the major side effect of agents typically used in conscious sedation. The use of such agents requires careful patient selection, close monitoring during the procedure, and protracted postprocedure recovery. When these drugs are used, their specific reversal agents, naloxone for narcotics and flumazenil for benzodiazepines, should be readily available.

Flexible Fiberoptic Bronchoscopy Techniques

Airway Exam

The standard approach for the introduction of the flexible bronchoscope is transnasal. Alternatively, in a patient with unfavorable nasal anatomy, the bronchoscope can be introduced through the mouth (with a bite block in place), through a tracheostomy (a number 6 or larger with inner cannula removed is required), or through an endotracheal tube (the tube must be at least 1.5 mm larger than the bronchoscope; generally, a number 8 or larger endotracheal tube is required). The nasal and, to a slightly lesser extent, oral approaches allow visualization of the anatomy of the posterior nasopharynx and larynx—the eustachian tubes, base of the tongue, epiglottis, aryepiglot-

tic folds, and vocal cords. All approaches allow examination of the trachea, carina, mainstem bronchi, and sequentially, the distal airways to the level of fourth-order bronchi. The bronchoscope is lubricated with lidocaine gel and introduced under direct vision into the preanesthetized nare, or alternatively, through a mouthpiece into the posterior hypopharynx. While visualization of the upper-airway lumen is maintained, the tip of the bronchoscope is flexed downward to direct it toward the glottis.

*R*espiratory Recap

Fiberoptic Bronchoscopy Techniques	
Airway exam	Protected bronchoscopic
Bronchoalveolar lavage	brushing
Bronchoscopic washing	Endobronchial biopsy
Nonprotected broncho-	Transbronchial needle
scopic brushing	aspiration
	Transbronchial biopsy

After evaluation of the upper airway, the vocal cords are examined for abnormalities of structure or function. The patient is instructed to phonate (typically saying the letter *e*) to test for normal vocal cord mobility. Paralysis of the left true vocal cord is the most common abnormality seen. It is manifested as inability to abduct the left cord (Figure 28-3) and, in the setting of malignancy, is a critical finding because it provides valuable staging information. Left vocal cord paralysis in the setting of bronchogenic carcinoma strongly suggests involvement of the recurrent laryngeal nerve as it traverses the mediastinum, a finding that denotes extensive mediastinal lymph node involvement and therefore unresectable malignancy.

A systematic approach and knowledge of normal anatomy are vital in the evaluation of upper and lower tract structures (Figure 28-4).[26] The quality of the mucosa

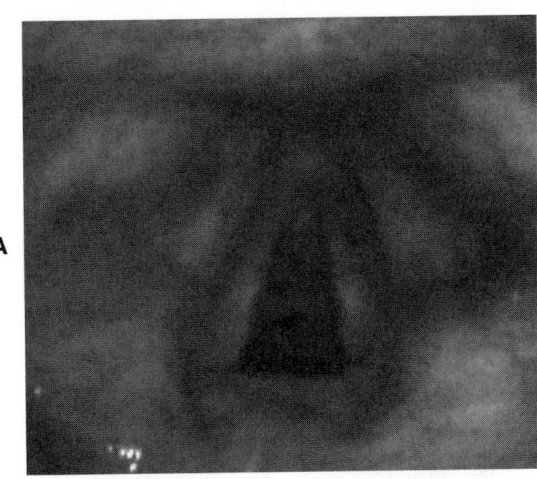
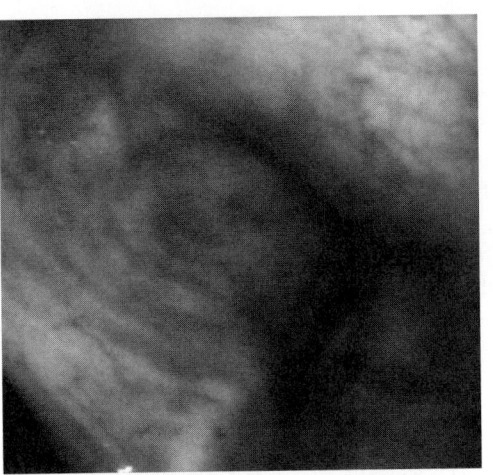

Figure 28-3 **A,** Normal vocal cord position and appearance. **B,** True left vocal cord paralysis.

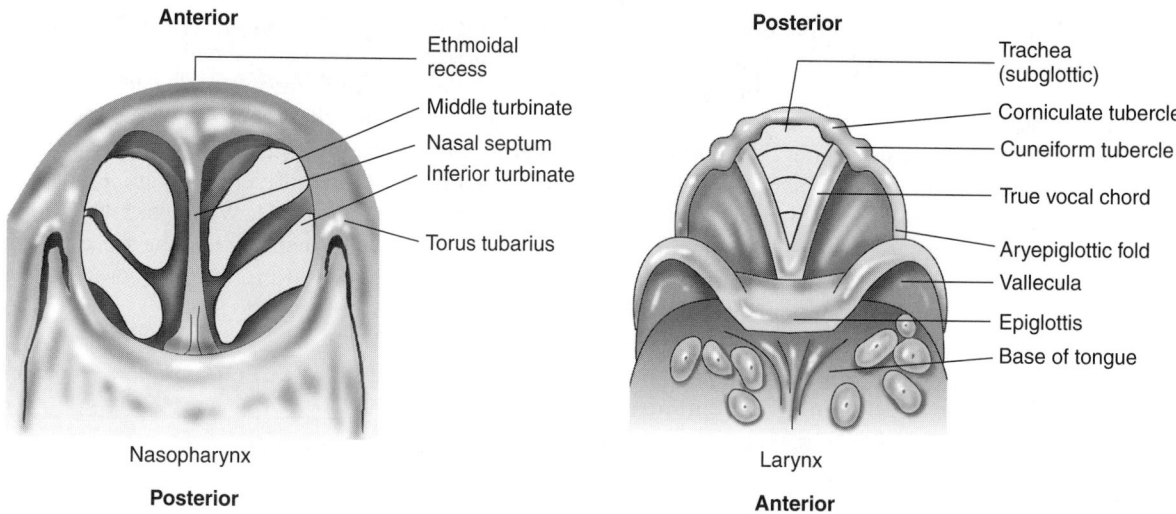

Figure 28-4 Normal nasopharyngeal and laryngeal structures as they appear to the bronchoscopist (facing patient). (Modified from Murray JF, Nadel JA, editors. Textbook of respiratory medicine. 2nd ed. vol 1. Philadelphia: WB Saunders; 1994.)

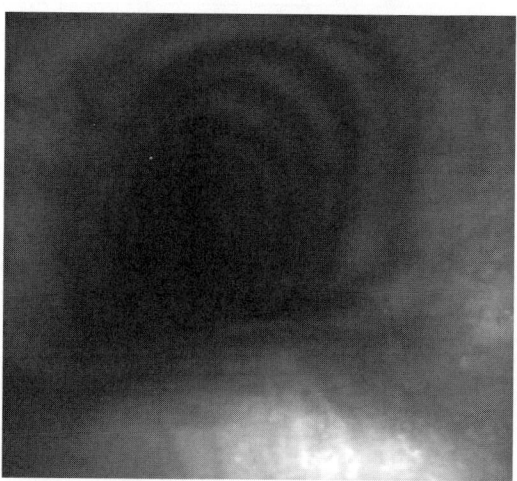

Figure 28-5 Normal tracheal anatomy with the anterior cartilaginous wall and the posterior membranous wall.

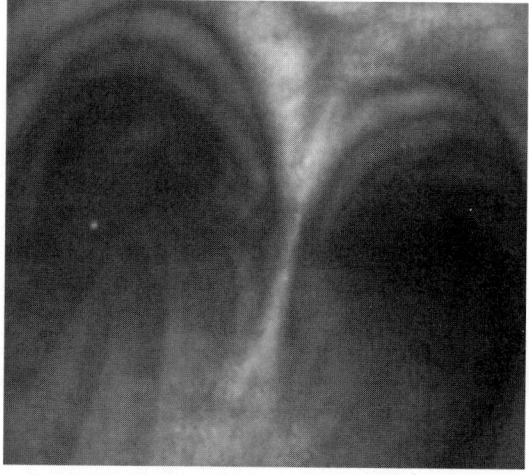

Figure 28-6 Normal-appearing main carina with smooth, regular overlying mucosa and a sharply defined bifurcation.

and presence of mucosal lesions can provide important diagnostic clues—is the hypopharynx inflamed, as may be seen with severe gastroesophageal reflux disease, or irregularly invaginated with so-called cobblestoning, as can be seen with sarcoid or lymphoma?

Examination of the trachea includes evaluation of mucosal pallor, inflammation, or ulceration; tracheal contour (trachea deformed or displaced?); and mobility, as well as exclusion of endotracheal neoplasms or foreign bodies. The normal trachea has well-defined cartilaginous rings anteriorly and a highly organized series of connective tissue and smooth muscle fibers that define the posterior (membranous) tracheal wall (Figure 28-5). With advancing age, the tracheal cartilage becomes more prominent because the overlying mucosal epithelium atrophies. Masses that occupy the anterior mediastinum may displace

the anterior or lateral trachea, and esophageal neoplasms may displace or ulcerate into the posterior trachea.

The carina is the next structure to be examined. The carina is the first major bifurcation of the conducting airways, the site at which the trachea divides into the right and left mainstem bronchi. The normal carina is a sharply angled structure with a smooth, regular mucosal covering (Figure 28-6). When the lymph nodes that occupy the subcarinal space in the mediastinum become enlarged because of involvement with inflammatory or neoplastic disease, the normal architecture of the carina becomes disrupted. Instead of its normal sharp, smooth border, the carina can become splayed or deformed (Figure 28-7). When tumor involves the submucosal layer of the tracheobronchial tree, the mucosal covering of the carina can become irregular and appear inflamed (Figure 28-8).

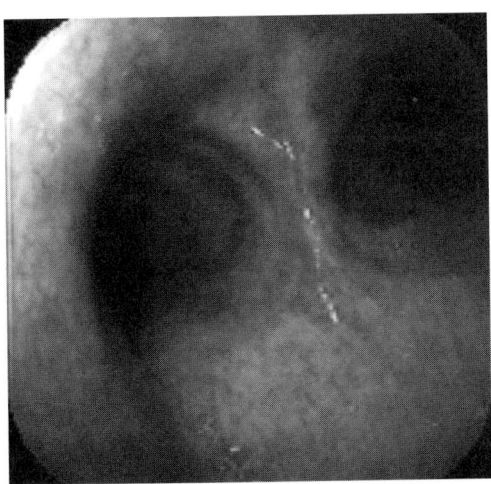

Figure 28-7   The normal carinal architecture is disrupted by the presence of a deforming subcarinal tumor; the carinal bifurcation is splayed rather than sharply defined.

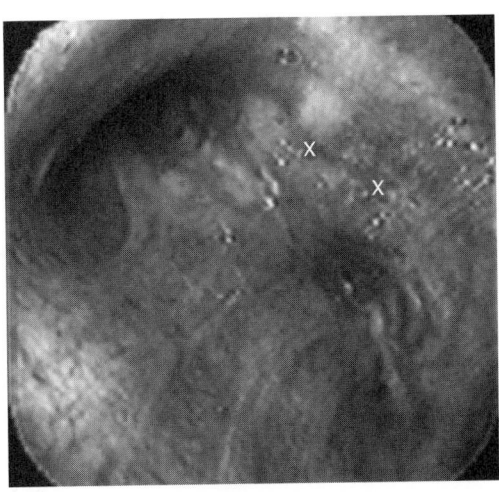

Figure 28-8   The normally smooth mucosal covering of the carina is disrupted by a submucosally infiltrating tumor.

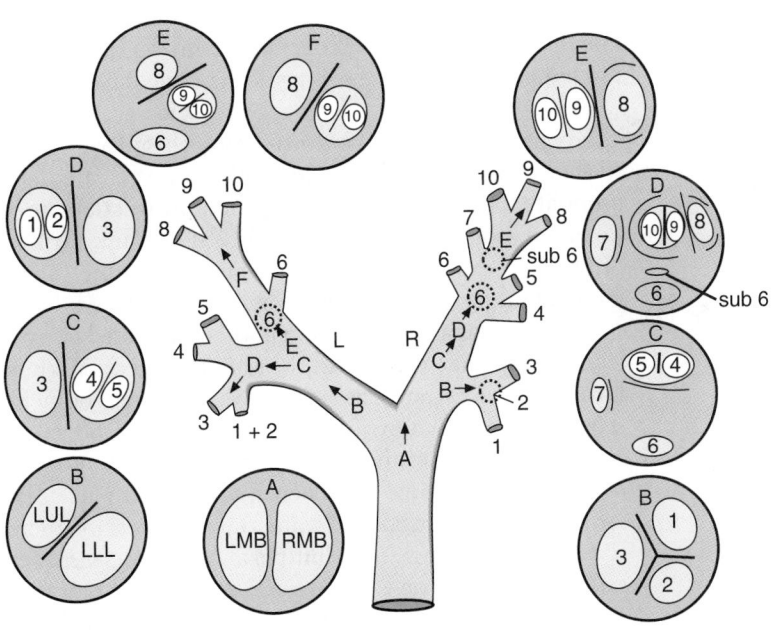

Figure 28-9   Normal endobronchial anatomy with accepted nomenclature depicted to the subsegmental level as viewed by the bronchoscopist at each point identified by letter or arrow. (Modified from Zavala DC. Flexible fiberoptic bronchoscopy: a training handbook. Iowa City: University of Iowa Department of Publications; 1978.)

After examination of the carina, the right and left bronchial trees are sequentially evaluated. Traditionally, if an examination is being performed for a focal abnormality, the airway examination begins on the opposite side to assure a complete and systematic evaluation. Regardless of where the exam is initiated, the most important elements are a systematic approach and a sound knowledge of normal endobronchial anatomy and nomenclature (Figure 28-9).[27] Orientation is defined and maintained by reference to the carina. Each bronchial division is examined to the subsegmental level, with notation made of anatomic variation, mucosal abnormality (Figure 28-10), presence of endobronchial tumors (Figure 28-11), or extrinsic compression of bronchial orifices (Figure 28-12). After each bronchial division is examined, biopsy, brush, or lavage samples are taken at directed sites, if indicated, and the bronchoscope is removed.

Complications related to airway exam alone are not separately reported in the literature, so their incidence is difficult to assess. Extrapolating from the reported complications of bronchoscopy without biopsy, complications include a 2.4% incidence of vasovagal reactions, a 0.9% incidence of cardiac arrhythmias, a 0.2% incidence of electrocardiographic abnormalities (not all patients were monitored, so incidence may be underestimated), a 0.4% incidence of bronchospasm and airway obstruction, a 0.2% incidence of nausea and vomiting, and a less than 0.1% incidence of aphonia and psychotic reactions. Transient fever, which typically occurs within 8 hours of the procedure and resolves within 24 hours, is a common event, occurring in up to 20% of patients who undergo bronchoscopy without biopsy.[9,14] In two large studies of major complications, half of the life-threatening compli-

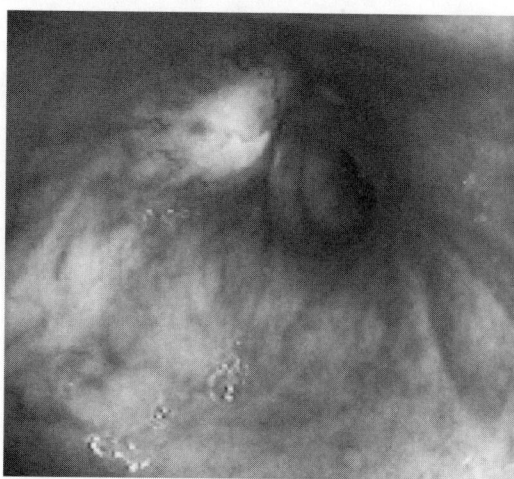

Figure 28-10 Normal smooth mucosa replaced by submucosally infiltrating tumor.

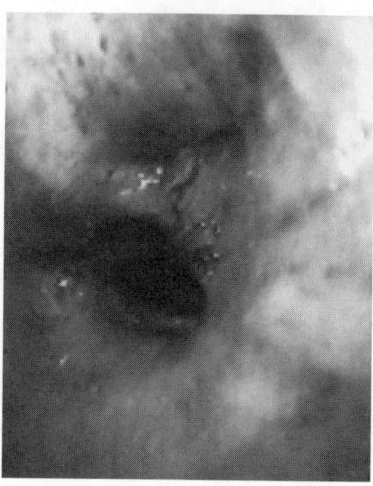

Figure 28-12 Bronchus extrinsically compressed by tumor.

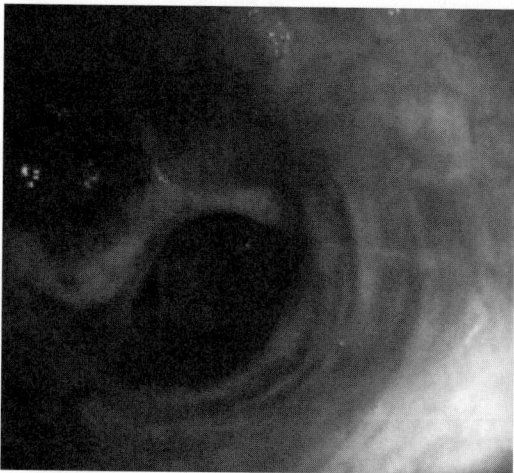

Figure 28-11 Bronchus occluded by exophytic obstructing tumor.

cations reported were associated with premedication or topical anesthesia.[8,10,11]

Bronchoalveolar Lavage

Bronchoalveolar lavage (BAL) is the method traditionally used to sample the cellular and microbiologic components of the alveolar space. It has been used as a research tool to establish the biochemical and cellular characteristics associated with a number of disease states such as sarcoid, idiopathic pulmonary fibrosis, and asthma. However, its primary use in everyday clinical practice is for cytologic and microbiologic sampling, and under specialized conditions, for pulmonary toilet in diseases such as pulmonary alveolar proteinosis.

When a specific radiographic abnormality is present, the bronchoscope is directed to that segmental orifice for lavage. In the presence of diffuse radiographic disease, either the right middle lobe or the lingula is selected for lavage because of ease of intubation and occlusion so that

recovery of lavage fluid is maximized. A complete airway examination precedes any diagnostic maneuver. If other manipulations such as TBBx are planned, BAL is performed first to minimize soiling of the sample by blood.

After the segment to be lavaged is selected, the bronchoscope is advanced to a third- or fourth-order bronchus so that it is completely wedged and a seal is created. Appropriate topical anesthesia and patient instruction are vital at this point to minimize cough and maximize volume of lavage fluid recovered. Room-temperature sterile buffered saline is the standard solution introduced. Before initiation of lavage, the suction port is connected to a collection trap that is reserved for sample collection alone. Lavage aliquots and techniques vary among bronchoscopists. Usually, a syringe containing 20 to 60 mL of saline is attached to the working channel of the bronchoscope after the scope has been wedged into place. The saline is rapidly introduced while the patient is instructed to refrain from coughing. Multiple aliquots can be sequentially introduced (up to 200 to 300 mL) before aspiration, or alternatively, lavage fluid can be suctioned back after each 20- to 60-mL instillation. Some bronchoscopists advocate immediate withdrawal of lavage fluid, while others encourage patients to take 1 or 2 deep breaths to promote enhanced mixing of the fluid within the subsegment. When suction is applied, care must be taken not to use overly vigorous or prolonged suction, which induces wall trauma and collapses the distal airway, interfering with lavage recovery. In normal lungs, the volume of lavage fluid recovered should be 50% to 60% of that instilled. In patients with severe disease, especially chronic obstructive pulmonary disease, recovered volumes are reduced to 10% to 40%.[28]

After lavage is complete, the bronchoscope is withdrawn and the orifice examined for untoward effects such as bleeding, which are rare with BAL alone. More than one segment can be sampled with BAL, although the total volume of saline instilled during one procedure should not exceed 300 mL and the samples should be processed separately. If the sample is to be transported to the laboratory within 1 hour, it can be maintained at room temperature. However, if a substantial delay in processing is anticipated, then the sample should be maintained on ice or refrigerated to prevent bacterial overgrowth and enhance cellular viability.

Routinely performed BAL carries the potential disadvantage of contamination of the sample with upper-airway secretions that limit the utility of routine bacterial cultures unless they are specially processed. Meduri and colleagues have introduced a specially designed catheter for so-called protected BAL. This catheter has a distal plug and distally inflatable balloon. The plugged catheter is passed into the segmental bronchus to be lavaged. The plug, which protects the tip from contamination as it passes through the working channel and proximal airways, is then dislodged. The distal balloon is inflated and the segment isolated by the inflation rather than wedging of the bronchoscope. Lavage is performed through the catheter. Samples collected by this method may be more suitable for routine bacterial culture because they are more likely to be representative of lower tract flora.[29]

Complications specifically related to BAL are unusual. Hypoxemia is the most common complication. In mechanically ventilated patients undergoing BAL as part of the evaluation of severe lung injury, the incidence of desaturation below 90% has been reported as less than 5%.[30] In nonintubated patients, the development of hypoxemia often can be predicted from preprocedure oxygen saturation. As mentioned, when hypoxemia is modest, the patient usually can be supported with supplemental O_2. When hypoxemia is severe (PaO_2 <65 on 50% oxygen), elective intubation for bronchoscopy may be necessary.[30]

Rarely, bleeding can complicate BAL. The incidence of this complication in thrombocytopenic patients has been shown to be minimal.[15] When significant bleeding occurs, it tends to be in the setting of significant immunocompromise.[12,13] Pneumothorax is an extremely rare complication of BAL that has been reported exclusively in intubated patients and presumably relates to increased airway pressures from the combination of positive pressure ventilation and BAL.[30]

Bronchoscopic Washing

Bronchoscopic washing is designed to sample the airway rather than the alveolar space. It has a more limited application than BAL. It can be useful in cytologic sampling when a patient has an exophytic lesion that obstructs a lobar or segmental orifice. Under these conditions, washing typically will be used in conjunction with other diagnostic methods such as bronchoscopic brushing or endobronchial biopsy. Some bronchoscopists advocate washing a lesion before any other manipulation. This approach minimizes contamination of the sample with blood, which can interfere with cytologic interpretation, and assesses bleeding risk by evaluating how easily the lesion bleeds with suction alone before invasive biopsy. Others advocate washing after invasive biopsy techniques, believing that recovery of viable malignant cells is maximized after the brush or forceps disrupts the surface of the tumor. An alternative use for bronchoscopic wash is for patients in whom volume of fluid recovered from BAL is inadequate. When wash is collected in this setting, it must be understood that it is useful only for isolation of strictly pathogenic organisms such as mycobacteria or endemic mycoses because secretions obtained by this method are invariably contaminated by upper-airway flora.[30]

As in BAL, the suction apparatus is fit with a collection trap reserved for the wash sample alone. The bronchoscope is placed in close proximity to the lesion (or placed nonocclusively in the segment of interest in the case of microbiologic sampling), and sterile buffered saline is introduced in 5- to 10-mL aliquots. These are suctioned after each instillation. About three or four instillations are typically performed, with the lesion observed for bleeding after each aliquot is suctioned. Care must be taken to apply suction when the bronchoscope is adjacent to but not directly abutting the lesion, to minimize trauma to the lesion and consequent bleeding.

Bronchoscopic Brushing—Nonprotected Brush

A standard **nonprotected bronchial brush** is used for cytologic sampling of proximal airways and central tumors under direct vision or peripheral lesions under fluoroscopic guidance. A catheter with a brush at its distal end (Figure 28-13) is introduced through the working channel of the bronchoscope. The brush can be open or enclosed within an open-ended sheath, through which it is advanced and retracted at the bronchoscopist's request. The open-ended sheath does not protect the sample from upper-airway contamination but does prevent material collected from becoming dislodged as the brush is withdrawn through the bronchoscope. When proximal airways or central tumors are to be sampled, the brush is advanced through the tip of the bronchoscope, placed adjacent to the site of interest, and vigorously advanced back and forth in short strokes under direct vision to entrap dislodged cells and tissue. The brush (withdrawn into its sheath if this type of brush is used) is then removed and may be processed in two ways. The contents of the bristles can be smeared directly onto glass slides that are fixed by immediate immersion into 95% alcohol or application of fixative spray. Alternatively, the entire brush can be placed in sterile saline solution and vigorously agitated to dislodge its contents. The first, "dry" method is suited to cytologic analysis or microbiologic staining for acid fast bacilli, fungi, or viral inclusions. The second, "wet" method allows culture of the specimen for pathogens. As is the case with BAL, a specially designed protected brush is required to collect meaningful, routine bacterial culture data.

A brush also may be used to sample peripheral tumors. Used in conjunction with biopsy techniques, a brush offers sampling of a wider area than focal biopsy. The lesion of interest is located with the use of fluoroscopy and the bron-

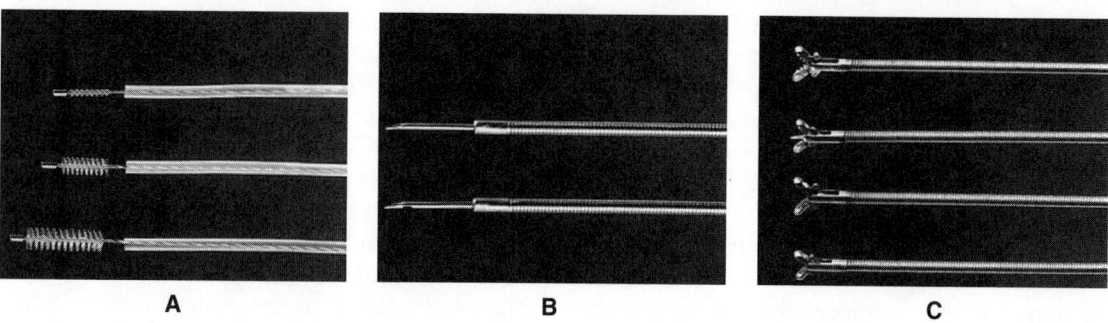

Figure 28-13 Instruments used for bronchoscopy. **A,** Brushes; **B,** needles; **C,** biopsy forceps. (From Prakash UBS. Bronchoscopy. In: Albert RK, Spiro SG, Jett JR. Comprehensive respiratory medicine. Philadelphia: WB Saunders; 1999.)

choscope advanced to the appropriate segmental orifice. The brush is then advanced under fluoroscopic guidance until it is abutting the lesion. Fluoroscopic observation is continued as the brush is advanced back and forth within the lesion. Fluoroscopy is then discontinued, the brush removed, and the sample processed as outlined previously.

Bronchoscopic Brushing—Protected Brush

When bronchoscopic brushing is being performed to identify specific pathogens in a suspected bacterial pneumonia, special care must be taken to assure that the bacteria recovered reflect lower tract pathogens rather than upper tract contaminants. Although special handling of the sample is recommended, a specially designed brush also is required. The **protected specimen brush (PSB)** is enclosed within two telescoping catheters, the outer of which is occluded at its tip by a biodegradable plug. The catheter tip is thus protected from contamination as it is advanced through the working channel and proximal airways. When the segment of interest is reached, the plug is dislodged, the inner catheter advanced, and the brush directed into the distal airway through the inner catheter. The brush itself is also specially designed with a denser population of bristles and a more flexible head to maximize retrieval of secretions. After the specimen is collected, the brush is withdrawn into the inner catheter, which is then withdrawn into the outer catheter, and the entire apparatus is removed through the bronchoscope. The outer catheter is wiped clean with 70% alcohol and cut distal to the inner catheter by use of a sterile technique. The inner catheter is then advanced, wiped clean in an identical fashion, and cut distal to the brush. Finally, the brush is advanced, sterilely cut, and placed into sterile saline for immediate specialized handling.

Because application of the brush involves rather vigorous manipulation of bronchial mucosa, brushing carries a slightly higher risk of induced bleeding compared with lavage or wash, especially if friable tumors are being sampled. In rare instances, when peripheral tumors are sampled, pneumothorax also may complicate the procedure. However, brushing is the least invasive biopsy method and offers a useful adjunct to needle or forceps biopsy, as well as a surrogate for these in patients at high risk of bleeding complications.

Endobronchial Biopsy

Endobronchial biopsy is the method used to sample endoscopically visible exophytic central tumors or mucosal ulceration, irregularity, or infiltration. It is of more questionable benefit in the addressing of extrinsically compressing lesions that impinge on but do not occupy the bronchial lumen. A variety of forceps sizes and designs are available, including a cupped tip forceps with a cutting edge, an alligator forceps with a toothed jaw, and a needle forceps with a sharp prong positioned between the jaws to assist in fixing the forceps to laterally or eccentrically placed lesions. In general, the choice of forceps is based on individual preference; no consistent difference in diagnostic yield is reported.[31] The smaller forceps often are preferred to approach upper lobe and superior segment lesions because they are more flexible than larger instruments and easier to manipulate through a bronchoscope maintained in extreme flexion.[32]

The biopsy forceps (see Figure 28-13) is advanced through the working channel of the bronchoscope in the closed position and opened under direct vision once the tip of the bronchoscope has been cleared. The open forceps is then placed in direct contact with the lesion and the jaws closed by the bronchoscopy assistant on request by manipulation of a lever at the proximal end of forceps outside the working channel. The forceps is gently shaken in the closed position by the bronchoscopist to dislodge the largest possible sample, and the closed forceps and sample are removed together through the working channel. The sample is then dislodged from the opened forceps, often with the assistance of a probe, and placed in the appropriate medium (formalin for histologic processing, sterile saline for microbiologic culture). When exophytic or submucosally infiltrating tumors are sampled, multiple biopsies should be attempted from the same exact site because the initial biopsy bite of the outer layer may sample either the necrotic edge of tumor or normal overlying mucosa, respectively. In general, multiple biopsies (three to six) should be attempted to maximize yield.[33]

The major complication of endobronchial biopsy is bleeding, although significant hemorrhage occurs less often with this procedure than with TBBx.[12] Some bronchoscopists advocate pretreatment of biopsy sites with 2 mL of epinephrine, diluted 1:10,000, especially if the site is a highly vascular-appearing or friable tumor. The value of this intervention has not been prospectively proven. Another, more common practice is to treat with topical epinephrine once bleeding has occurred. This practice is limited to patients without significant underlying cardiovascular or cerebrovascular disease, tachycardia, or hypertension because the topically administered epinephrine is systemically absorbed. In general, when used, the dose is limited to 6 mL of 1:10,000 solution.[12] Other measures to control bleeding include wedging of the bronchoscope over the bleeding site, limiting of suction so as not to dislodge freshly formed clot, and if bleeding continues, intubation of the patient for airway control and placement of the patient with the bleeding side dependent to protect the nonbleeding lung from aspirated blood. Often the magnitude of bleeding is difficult to assess because the bronchoscope tip becomes soiled by blood and vision is obscured. Unless the bronchoscope is being used for tamponade, it can be removed to the level of the carina and the tip can be flexed against the anterior wall of the trachea and rubbed up and down for cleaning.

Transbronchial Needle Aspiration

Transbronchial needle aspiration (TBNA) is one of the evolving innovations in bronchoscopic diagnosis. Its indications are growing and include staging of mediastinal lymph nodes in suspected bronchogenic lung cancer, diagnosis of submucosally infiltrating or extrinsically compressing tumors, approach of endobronchial tumors with necrotic or friable outer layers, and increasingly, diagnosis of peripheral nodules.[34-40] The first generation of flexible needles was adapted by Ko Pen Wang from the rigid needles used for gastrointestinal endoscopic sclerotherapy. They are used to obtain cytologic specimens. The needles vary in size from 19 to 22 gauge, in length from 1 to 1.3 cm, and in design from fixed to retractable, plastic to metal, and with and without stylet.[41]

Regardless of the specific needle design, the procedure for cytologic aspiration is basically the same. The apparatus (see Figure 28-13) consists of a long, flexible plastic catheter attached to a needle that is retracted within the tubing and protected by a metal spring. The sheathed needle is passed through the working channel of the bronchoscope after the site of interest is visualized. The catheter is advanced through the scope so that the tip is clearly seen and directed toward the target site. The needle must never be exposed outside the plastic catheter while within the bronchoscope, or the scope could be severely damaged. Once the catheter tip is well outside the scope, the needle is exposed and the catheter advanced so that the needle is well embedded in the site (typically through the wall of the bronchus or trachea for nodal sampling, or through an endobronchial/submucosal tumor). Once the needle is planted (Figure 28-14), the bronchoscopy assistant applies suction at the proximal end of the catheter. Suction is typically achieved through attachment of a 60-mL syringe filled with 2 mL of saline to the proximal end and withdrawal of the plunger on request. Aspiration of blood at this point indicates inadvertent cannulation of a blood vessel and should result in removal of the needle, retraction of the needle into the plastic catheter under direct endoscopic vision, and observation of the site. Such vessel puncture rarely results in significant bleeding with the small-gauge needles used.[42] Although sometimes unavoidable, this complication can be minimized by a detailed three-dimensional understanding of mediastinal structures in relation to the tracheobronchial tree. Because blood obscures further cytologic diagnosis, the catheter should be withdrawn from the bronchoscope and flushed or replaced before subsequent aspiration attempts.

If no blood is aspirated, then suction should be maintained for 1 to 2 minutes as the needle is gently advanced back and forth to maximize recovery of cells. If no resistance is felt when the syringe plunger is withdrawn, the needle is not adequately fixed in tissue and should be repositioned under direct vision. This difficulty is common when the needle is deflected by cartilaginous structures as it is passed through the tracheal or bronchial wall or when the position of the lesion requires a perpendicular approach. Entry of the needle into the lesion is sometimes facilitated by having the patient cough to enhance apposition of the needle to tissue. After the sample is obtained, the needle is removed from the aspiration site and retracted under direct vision outside the bronchoscope channel. The needle/catheter system is withdrawn from the bronchoscope and flushed with saline for recovery of the sample.

Cytologic sampling by bronchoscopic needle aspiration has inherent limitations. In the case of mediastinal node sampling, false-positive results can be obtained if malignant cells from the tracheobronchial tree contaminate the tip of the bronchoscope. This confounding effect is especially likely if the primary malignancy is in close proximity to the site at which the node is to be sampled or if other bronchoscopic maneuvers, including full endobronchial exam, are conducted before TBNA. In the latter case, performance of TBNA occurs as soon as the bronchoscope is introduced into the tracheobronchial tree, before any other endoscopic manipulation can minimize false-positive results. In that case, false-positive results may still occur from contaminated secretions that have migrated into the proximal airways with coughing. More prevalent than false-positive results are false-negative results caused by the small sample size and blind nature of the technique when mediastinal nodes or extrinsically compressive lesions are sampled. Cytologic results are difficult to inter-

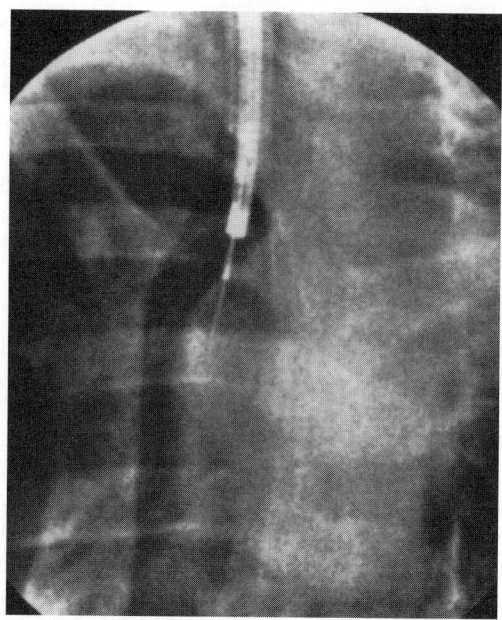

Figure 28-14   Bronchoscopic needle aspiration of a right paratracheal lymph node. (From Prakash UBS. Bronchoscopy. In: Albert RK, Spiro SG, Jett JR. Comprehensive respiratory medicine. Philadelphia: WB Saunders; 1999.)

pret with confidence without definitive reference to the site from which they were obtained. They also require specialized laboratory pathology expertise for appropriate interpretation. For all these reasons, the development of a needle apparatus capable of obtaining histologic samples has been of extensive interest.

Wang, mentioned previously as adapting the first generation of flexible needles, has popularized such a TBNA biopsy needle. This needle consists of a 1.5-cm, 18- or 19-gauge needle that is flat tipped and has a cutting edge tapering inward within which a smaller 20- or 21-gauge, 0.5-cm needle with a beveled tip is housed. The smaller gauge needle is attached to a guidewire and can be advanced or withdrawn by manipulation of the guidewire at the proximal end of the catheter system. When both needles are deployed, cytologic and core histologic biopsy samples are obtained.

The flat-tipped larger needle is passed through the working channel of the bronchoscope with the smaller needle retracted. When the tip of the larger needle is visible past the tip of the bronchoscope, the smaller needle is advanced and locked into place. The needle is then advanced into the target site by quick thrusting of the catheter or advancement of the bronchoscope and catheter together. Aspiration is performed to exclude inadvertent entry into a vessel. When the entire length of the needle is embedded in the bronchial wall, the smaller needle is retracted into the larger needle and sustained suction applied by a locking syringe. The larger needle is partially withdrawn and repositioned at different angles within the node while suc-

tion is applied. The needle is then withdrawn, the site observed, and the needle/catheter system withdrawn from the bronchoscope. The catheter is flushed with saline for recovery of both the cytologic sample and the tissue fragment from the larger cutting needle, which is then transferred to formalin.

In the hands of experienced operators, the incidence of significant bleeding with needle aspiration is negligible. When peripheral masses are sampled, rare incidences of pneumothorax have been reported, although these have occurred primarily in the setting of combined TBNA and TBBx. The overall incidence of both bleeding and pneumothorax observed with TBNA is significantly less than that seen with either TBBx or transthoracic needle aspiration, the traditional approaches to peripheral parenchymal lesions.[40,42,43]

Transbronchial Biopsy

Transbronchial biopsy (TBBx) is the primary bronchoscopic technique used to evaluate the alveolar compartment. It is used to sample peripheral parenchymal masses, diagnose a select number of specific interstitial lung diseases, and obtaining tissue specimens for culture or documentation of tissue invasion/microorganism pathogenicity. To optimize yield and safety, the procedure requires biplane fluoroscopy in addition to standard bronchoscopic equipment. Any forceps used for endobronchial biopsy can be used for TBBx. Before the introduction of the bronchoscope, the patient's chest is fluoroscopically assessed to localize the lesion if a specific mass is being biopsied or to select a zone for visualization in the case of diffuse lung disease. The bronchoscopy is then performed and the orifice of the segment of interest is visualized.

The closed forceps is passed under direct vision into the orifice of the selected segment. Once the instrument passes through the orifice, fluoroscopy is initiated and the forceps is advanced under fluoroscopic guidance into the area to be biopsied. If a focal mass is the target, either the patient or the C-arm of the fluoroscope is rotated to confirm that the forceps and the lesion are within the same three-dimensional plane. The biopsy forceps is then opened, advanced slightly (ideally, this will produce fluoroscopically visible deformation of the lesion), and closed.

Throughout the advance of the forceps, the patient is monitored for pleuritic pain or profound cough (suggesting that the pleura is being irritated), and the pleural margins visible in the 2-dimensional view are avoided. If the patient develops pain, resistance to advance is felt by the bronchoscopist, or the closed forceps has migrated to the extreme periphery, the forceps is withdrawn 1 to 2 cm before biopsy. When diffuse lung disease is being sampled, the most peripheral site at which the patient is asymptomatic, no resistance is felt, and the forceps does not directly abut the pleura is selected.

After the biopsy bite is taken, the forceps is jiggled in the closed position to free the sample, and then the forceps and the tissue sample are removed through the working channel. The bronchoscope is kept in place at the segmental orifice to monitor for bleeding. If no significant bleeding is observed, the process is repeated. A total of four to six biopsy specimens has been cited as producing optimal diagnostic yield.[31,44]

Some bronchoscopists advocate timing the biopsy with the respiratory cycle so that the forceps is closed at end-expiration, facilitating collapse of a larger portion of lung tissue into the forceps. However, when biopsy specimens collected at different times in the respiratory cycle have been compared, no difference in yield was found.[31,45] Some bronchoscopists perform TBBx for diffuse disease without fluoroscopic guidance, believing that the bronchoscopist's sensitivity to the sensation of resistance and patient's report of symptoms are sufficient to avoid violating the pleura. Most studies cite a significantly lower incidence of pneumothorax when fluoroscopy is used, suggesting that this should be the standard approach whenever feasible.[31]

TBBx significantly increases the frequency and severity of procedure-related complications. Depending on the way morbidities are grouped (major versus minor, or unspecified), TBBx results in a 10- to 22-fold increase in complications, although the overall rate remains low.[9,31] The mortality rate for bronchoscopy involving TBBx is reported at around 0.2%, the incidence of pneumothorax is reported at between 4% and 5.5%, and the incidence of mild to severe hemorrhage is cited at about 9%, with major hemorrhage occurring in 1.3%.[7,46]

The primary complications are bleeding—although life-threatening hemorrhage is rare in patients without hemostatic disorders—and pneumothorax. Patients at increased risk of bleeding include persons with known coagulopathies, pulmonary hypertension (mean pulmonary artery pressure above 15 mm Hg), or thrombocytopenia; those requiring mechanical ventilation; and anecdotally, patients with acquired immunodeficiency syndrome (AIDS).[31] Patients at increased risk of pneumothorax include those on mechanical ventilators, those with emphysema, and anecdotally, those undergoing biopsies for pneumocystis.[47,48]

When significant bleeding is observed from the orifice of the segment biopsied, the bronchoscope should be positioned in the opening of the segment and *kept in place* without suctioning for several minutes to tamponade the bleeding site and isolate it from the rest of the lung to prevent endobronchial soiling. In the rare instance that this maneuver proves ineffective, the airway should be secured with an endotracheal tube, the patient placed bleeding side dependent, and ideally, back-up with **rigid bronchoscopy** and surgical intervention readily available.

After every bronchoscopy with TBBx, either fluoroscopy, chest radiograph, or both should be performed immediately postprocedure to exclude procedure-related pneumothorax. If a pneumothorax develops, the patient can be clinically observed in hospital on oxygen or tube thoracostomy can be performed immediately to evacuate the extraalveolar air, depending on the patient's clinical stability and the size of the pneumothorax.

Rigid Bronchoscopy

Patient Selection

The principles outlined for the selection of patients for flexible fiberoptic bronchoscopy also apply to the selection of patients for rigid bronchoscopy. In addition, bronchoscopic indication plays an important role. Rigid bronchoscopy may be superior to flexible bronchoscopy in the assessment of patients with massive hemoptysis, the removal of aspirated foreign bodies (especially in children), and the performance of **laser bronchoscopy** or dilatation of tracheobronchial strictures. It also may be advantageous in cases in which bronchoscopy is required for retrieval of large volumes of tenacious secretions, necrotic debris, or large biopsy specimens.[49] Because rigid bronchoscopy often involves general anesthesia, cardiovascular stability should be optimized. In addition, although rigid bronchoscopy affords the opportunity to ventilate the patient, it also may induce significant laryngospasm and bronchospasm so that preoperative optimization of the patient with obstructive lung disease is desirable. Because of the need for significant neck extension for placement of the rigid scope, patients with limitations to neck extension or jaw opening are poor candidates for rigid bronchoscopy.

> ### Age-Specific Angle
>
> Rigid bronchoscopy is superior to flexible bronchoscopy for removal of foreign bodies in children.

Especially when manipulations such as laser resection are planned, preoperative chest radiograph, blood work including arterial blood gases and coagulation studies, and electrocardiograms are generally performed. When laser tumor resection is planned, it is important to have recent chest radiographs demonstrating previous airway patency because restoration of airway patency is unlikely if the involved lung has been atelectatic for more than 1 month.[50] Preoperative flexible bronchoscopy to determine that the luminal occlusion is endobronchial rather than extrinsic and to delineate its location and length is required. Extrinsic compression of the tracheobronchial tree is not amenable to laser treatment. Best results are obtained with tracheal or mainstem lesions, and least-favorable results are obtained with upper lobe or segmental lesions, extensive submucosal disease, total obstruction, or long, tapering occlusions. If tumor resection is planned, a ventilation/perfusion scan may be useful to assess perfusion to the involved lung because malignant occlusion of the pulmonary artery obviates the benefit of relieving high-grade tumor-related atelectasis.[50]

Patient Preparation

Rigid bronchoscopy requires the patient to be positioned with the cervical spine extended and exerts a significant amount of pressure on the soft tissues of the oropharynx and larynx. Because of the degree of discomfort imposed, the procedure is usually performed under general anesthesia. Alternatively, it can be performed with deep IV anesthesia with the patient maintaining spontaneous ventilation. As with flexible bronchoscopy, the entire procedure should be explained to the patient and informed consent obtained. In particular, patients should be forewarned about postprocedural soreness of the mouth and throat, which is more severe than that associated with FOB. The complications of the procedure itself (see "Complications") and general anesthesia, if used, should be reviewed.

Sedation

Before the introduction of the bronchoscope, the patient is premedicated with a short-acting benzodiazepine, narcotic, or both and often with an anticholinergic agent such as atropine. The hypopharynx and larynx are locally anesthetized. Choice of agents for deep anesthesia vary depending on the preferences of the bronchoscopist, age of the patient, and indication for bronchoscopy. Not uncommonly, neuromuscular blockade is used in conjunction with general anesthesia. Continuous ventilation can be provided through the side port of the rigid scope.[49]

Technique

After anesthesia has been initiated, dental guards and eye shields are placed and the patient's head is extended in the "sniff" position. The bronchoscopist places one hand over the teeth and gums to protect these structures and help guide the introduction of the scope. With the other hand, the lubricated tip of the scope, held almost vertically, should be introduced into the right side of the mouth, with the tongue pushed aside. The bronchoscope should be advanced through the pharynx with progressively more horizontal positioning until the epiglottis is visualized. The epiglottis should be lifted with the distal beveled tip so that the vocal cords are visualized. The bronchoscope should be rotated 90 degrees to the right as the vocal cords are approached. With the center of the field of vision focused on the left vocal cord, the scope should be gently advanced through the cords and rotated an additional 90 degrees. The bronchoscope also may be introduced with a standard straight laryngoscope. This is especially advanta-

geous in the pediatric population to facilitate selection of the appropriately sized scope. After the bronchoscope is in place, the mouth is packed with wet gauze to fix the position of the scope and minimize ventilatory leaks. To examine the right bronchial tree, the head is turned to the left and the bronchoscope may need to be shifted to the left side of the mouth. Lateral-viewing optical telescopes are placed through the scope and the head is raised or lowered to facilitate examination. Examination of the left tracheobronchial tree is more difficult and requires movement of the scope to the right side of the mouth and often, progressive, gentle repositioning of the head to the right. Depending on the indication, a variety of forceps, suction catheters, bougies, stents, lasers, and cryotherapy probes then can be advanced through the open scope.[49]

Laser Bronchoscopy

The technique of laser resection deserves detailed mention in the context of rigid bronchoscopy. Although laser technology is available with FOB, therapeutic laser remains one of the most common indications for rigid bronchoscopy in the adult population. The wider diameter of the working channel, which allows for simultaneous visualization, laser use, and suctioning; the rigidity of the scope, which can stent open the airway in the setting of high-grade occlusions; and the beveled tip, which can both assist in resection and provide tactile feedback, all render rigid endoscopy advantageous in laser resection. Laser technology is best applied to symptomatic, centrally located, unresectable, endobronchial malignancies; appropriately located benign tumors without extrabronchial involvement (such as papillomas); luminal obstructions such as webs or tracheal granulomas; and noninflammatory tracheal stenoses.[51] Of the laser technologies available, Nd-YAG has the widest application in tracheobronchial therapeutics. It is delivered through flexible quartz fibers that allow the laser beam to be brought into close proximity to the lesion, enhancing accuracy. Unlike CO_2 laser, which works by vaporization, Nd-YAG works by photocoagulation. Absorption is color dependent, with paler tissues absorbing more energy. Considerable scatter to surrounding tissue occurs depending on the duration and amount of energy supplied. The laser fiber should be greater than 1 cm past the tip of the scope and 4 to 10 mm from the lesion. The optical telescope (which provides better depth perception than that obtained with FOB), laser fiber, and suction catheter are passed through the scope in proximity to each other. Noncontinuous pulses of 20 to 40 watts in 0.5-second to 1-second periods are delivered. Initially, low-power pulses are delivered to photocoagulate the lesion. The beveled tip of the rigid bronchoscope then can be used to core out the tumor, along with biopsy forceps. Larger bore suction catheters can be introduced to remove tumor fragments, blood, and debris. The laser then can be used to photocoagulate the residual tumor bed. Conservative margins should be left because additional "die-back" effect occurs after initial treatment. When laser resection is performed, conventional ventilation may be superior to jet ventilation because jet tends to disturb the tissue bed and may force tissue fragments distally.[50,51]

When laser is used, the FIO_2 must be <0.40 to avoid the catastrophic complication of endobronchial fire. If the procedure is performed with a flexible bronchoscope or an endotracheal tube, adequate distance must be maintained between the laser tip and these flammable structures. Noncontinuous rather than continuous laser pulses are preferred to avoid the so-called "popcorn" effect, in which protracted application allows for the build-up of a pocket of steam in underlying tissue, which then may explode, causing extensive uncontrolled tissue damage. Close attention must be paid to the proximity of the mediastinal vessels (innominate artery anterior to the lower third of the trachea, aortic arch superior and posterior to the left mainstem bronchus, and left pulmonary artery circumferentially at the origin of the left upper lobe), and the ways in which anatomic relationships may be distorted by tumor.[50,51]

Complications

A variety of anatomic and physiologic complications have been reported in association with rigid bronchoscopy, with incidence and scope of complications varying depending on the endoscopic manipulations performed. Damage to the teeth and upper airway may occur, as may trauma to the lower tract mucosa, resulting in hemorrhage; airway occlusion; or perforation, with consequent subcutaneous emphysema or tension pneumothorax. Arrhythmias, bradycardia, and diastolic hypertension have been reported. In general, the modification of anesthetic techniques and the use of continuous pulse oximetry to detect desaturation have markedly reduced cardiac complications.[50] Systemic air embolization is a rare intraoperative complication. Perhaps the most dreaded complication is endobronchial fire, which has been reported as a complication of laser therapy when FOB and endotracheal tubes are used. The technical measures outlined—low inspired oxygen concentration, low power, noncontinuous pulses, adequate distance between laser and flammable structures—are all designed to minimize this risk. Should fire occur, all flammable structures should be rapidly removed, the airway reinspected and debrided if necessary, and antibiotics, steroids, and bronchodilators administered.[51]

Intraprocedural and postprocedural laryngospasm and bronchospasm have been reported, either in association with positioning of the rigid scope itself, in the context of procedure-related bleeding, or with laser procedure-generated smoke. Postprocedural upper-airway obstruction from laryngeal edema or laryngospasm has been reported, as has postoperative hypoxia from bleeding, retention of debris or secretions, and anesthesia-related respiratory depression. Noncardiogenic edema and localized hyperinflation are rare postoperative occurrences.[24,50,51]

Bronchoscopic Indications: Diagnostic

Suspected Carcinoma

Bronchoscopy has a variety of roles in the evaluation of suspected carcinoma. Starting with an airway exam, bronchoscopy can determine the presence of endobronchial tumor, which may be suggested by radiographic volume loss, postobstructive pneumonitis, or postobstructive hyperinflation; a localized wheeze; hemoptysis; or new cough. The procedure also can provide important staging information. Coincident oropharyngeal and nasopharyngeal lesions can be excluded. Vocal cord paralysis, indicative of recurrent laryngeal nerve entrapment by bulky mediastinal disease, can be assessed. Carinal deformation can be documented and subcarinal nodes subsequently sampled for staging. Additionally, precise staging with regard to endobronchial extent of tumor can be achieved, and in the case of peripheral nodules, albeit rarely, radiographically unsuspected endobronchial disease can be discovered.

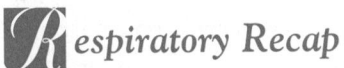

Respiratory Recap

Diagnostic Indications for Bronchoscopy	
Suspected carcinoma	Interstitial lung disease
Pneumonia	Hemoptysis
Lobar atelectasis	Cough
Suspected foreign body aspiration	Trauma

Endobronchial biopsy and brush have an excellent yield for endoscopically visible tumors. When exophytic tumor is present, the yield is up to 96%, with negative results based mainly on uninterpretable necrotic material. When all types of lesions are taken into account, yield is 86% to 96%.[52] Extrinsically compressing lesions are difficult to access with endobronchial biopsy, and these, as well as friable tumors and bulky endobronchial masses that may have a necrotic edge, benefit from needle aspiration, which obtains deeper samples with less tissue trauma. Endobronchial biopsy also has been evaluated for staging of the main carina because this may determine resectability in some patients. When endobronchial biopsy of the carina was routinely performed in one series, the overall yield was 13.8%. The yield ranged from 4.7% in patients with visually normal structures to 40% in patients with morphologic or mucosal distortion.[53]

TBNA has enhanced the yield of bronchoscopy in the diagnosis of primary lung cancer and contributed a great deal to preoperative staging. Needle aspiration has increased the diagnostic yield by up to 14% when added to wash, brush, and forceps biopsy.[43] When TBNA has been added to TBBx, brush, and wash in the diagnosis of peripheral masses, it has raised the yield from 48% to 69% and has been associated with less bleeding than TBBx.[39,40] In submucosal or peribronchial tumors, the combination of forceps biopsy and TBNA resulted in a significantly higher yield than forceps alone (89% versus 55%); the addition of wash and brush further improved diagnostic yield (to 97%).[38] TBNA of mediastinal nodes has been the sole means of diagnosis in up to 42% of patients with small-cell lung cancer.[37,54]

TBNA of the carina has proved to be a significant advance in nonoperative staging of the mediastinal extent of disease. Traditionally, most patients with evidence of malignant involvement of the subcarinal lymph nodes and all patients with involvement of mediastinal lymph nodes contralateral to the primary tumor are considered surgically unresectable for cure. Noninvasive methods used to assess lymph node involvement, such as chest computed axial tomography (CT), have an overall sensitivity of about 94%, a specificity of 79%, and an accuracy of 85%.[35] More definitive tissue diagnosis has previously relied on operative techniques such as mediastinoscopy or thoracotomy. The advent of TBNA has made nonoperative mediastinal sampling possible.

In a significant number of patients, carinal TBNA has proven to be the only bronchoscopic evidence of unresectability.[37] Positive carinal or paratracheal TBNA correlate most strongly with endoscopic evidence of extrinsic compression or distortion or radiographic evidence of lymphadenopathy.[34,35,37] Correlation also is noted with right-side location of the primary tumor and central location of disease.[54] Patients with no radiographic evidence of mediastinal disease by chest CT rarely have positive TBNA. However, up to 36% of patients with normal endoscopic exams have positive cytology on aspiration.[34] Because a significant percentage of false-negative findings from TBNA result from inadequate sampling, the presence of an on-site cytopathologist to assess the adequacy of the specimen significantly enhances the diagnostic yield of TBNA. An expert interpretation of a rapid stain of the cytologic contents of the aspirate spares unnecessarily repeated sampling and redirects biopsy site when appropriate.[55]

TBBx is the more traditional approach to the diagnosis of peripheral lesions. The yield of TBBx is determined by the size of the lesion, its distance from the hilum, and to a lesser extent, the number of bronchi that can be seen leading into it on CT of the chest when available. The overall yield is about 48%, with lower yields (about 27%) for lesions less than 2 cm in diameter or less than 2 cm from the carina and higher yields (71%) for tumors larger than 2 cm or within 2 to 6 cm of the hilum on chest radiograph.[56]

Pneumonia in the Immunocompetent Host

The utility of bronchoscopy in the diagnosis of pneumonia is intimately related to the immune status of the host, the index of suspicion for associated endobronchial disease

based on radiographic findings, and the specific techniques used to obtain and process the bronchoscopic sample.

The indications for bronchoscopy for diagnosis of an acute community-acquired pneumonia (CAP) in an immunocompetent host remain limited. Approximately 60% of such pneumonias do not have a specific microbiologic etiology identified when standard sputum and blood culture techniques are used. When bronchoscopy is added as a diagnostic modality, particularly when performed before antibiotic therapy, the specific etiologic agent is identified more frequently. However, this specific identification rarely results in a change in therapy compared with the empiric antibiotic choice that would be made based on knowledge of the pathogens typically implicated in CAP.[30] Bronchoscopy has a more defined role in cases in which the clinical or radiographic findings suggest endobronchial obstruction, atypical (mycobacterial or nonbacterial) infection, or a noninfectious etiology.

Feinsilver and colleagues have studied the characteristics associated with high diagnostic yield in patients undergoing bronchoscopy for delayed resolution of a presumed CAP. They confirmed the previously described observation that in the absence of radiographic or clinical findings suggestive of endobronchial obstruction, endobronchial malignancy is rarely encountered. In their series, multilobar pneumonia, age less than 55 years, and nonsmoking status correlated positively with specific bronchoscopic diagnosis, most commonly of unusual pathogens such as tuberculosis, actinomycosis, cytomegalovirus, or *Pneumocystis carinii (PCP)*. Of the 40% of patients ultimately found to have a specific alternative diagnosis, bronchoscopy was diagnostic in 86%, with malignancy being found in about 11%. Pneumocystis was found in about 8% of patients, none of whom were previously thought to be infected with human immunodeficiency virus (HIV). Patients who had comorbid diseases known to be associated with delayed recovery, such as chronic obstructive lung disease, diabetes, or alcoholism, rarely received an alternative diagnosis on the basis of bronchoscopy. These findings led to the recommendation that patients with nonresolving pneumonias be examined for underlying immune defects, including age, comorbidity, or HIV positivity, even in the absence of risk factors. If significant comorbidities are found, the authors recommend that bronchoscopy be deferred.[57]

Pneumonia in the Immunocompromised Host

Because of the wide variety of opportunistic infections that affect patients with serious immunosuppression, an empiric choice of therapy is frequently not possible. In addition, depending on the etiology of immunosuppression (HIV, malignancy, drug induced, collagen vascular disease), a variety of noninfectious diagnoses may merit consideration, such as recrudescent malignancy, hemorrhage, or noninfectious pneumonitis. Bronchoscopy has been closely evaluated to determine its role in providing specific diagnostic information. The highest yield for bronchoscopy occurs in patients with suspected infectious disease. In their evaluation of patients with focal or diffuse radiographic abnormalities, Matthay and colleagues reported a specific diagnostic yield of 84%.[58] In patients with diffuse pulmonary infiltrates undergoing bronchoscopy with BAL, brushing, and TBBx, Williams and colleagues reported an overall sensitivity of about 77% for all diagnoses, which rose to 90% if only infectious diagnoses were considered. When no evidence of infection at bronchoscopy existed, the predictive value of a negative procedure (for infection) was 94.4%. Interestingly, in Williams' study, TBBx added little to brush and BAL, an important consideration given the frequent incidence of thrombocytopenia and bleeding complications in such patients.[59]

The role of bronchoscopy in the evaluation of patients with HIV has evolved over time. Bronchoscopy with either BAL alone or TBBx and BAL has had high yield for a variety of infectious diagnoses (PCP, up to 94%; cytomegalovirus, 67%; mycobacterium avium intracellulare, 62%) and very low yield for noninfectious diagnoses (for example, Kaposi's sarcoma or nonspecific pneumonitis). More than one pathogen often is isolated, and correct identification of all pathogens has been made in about 65% of patients.[60] In patients with moderate disease severity in whom the clinical suspicion for PCP is high, decision analyses have suggested that a trial of empiric therapy with delayed bronchoscopy for nonresponders is superior to early bronchoscopy in terms of morbidity and cost, with no effect on clinical outcome.[61] In patients in whom the pre-bronchoscopy diagnosis is unclear (those in whom prophylactic therapy for PCP has been given or the clinical presentation is atypical) or those with severe clinical compromise in whom specific diagnosis for directed therapy is urgently required, early bronchoscopy remains a critical part of the diagnostic evaluation. In patients in whom the principal diagnostic considerations are noninfectious, early consideration should be given to open lung biopsy.

Ventilator-Associated Pneumonia

The development of nosocomial pneumonia in mechanically ventilated patients is a common and serious complication. Ventilator-associated pneumonia (VAP) develops in up to 25% of patients, carrying a high mortality.[62,63] Accurate diagnosis of this process presents an ongoing challenge for several reasons. A high incidence of heavy bacterial colonization of the endotracheal tube and tracheobronchial tree occurs following prolonged (>6 days) intubation. Culture of deep suction samples from intubated patients has a notoriously poor correlation with pathogens recovered from the lung parenchyma.[62] The presence of the tube may stimulate secretions or contribute to a tracheobronchitis without lower tract infection. Therefore purulence or volume of secretions is nonspecific and culture of tracheal samples is unreliable in the prediction of the presence or specific identity of lower respiratory tract pathogens. In addition, a number of

conditions that mimic pneumonia can afflict critically ill patients, such as pulmonary edema, hemorrhage, or adult respiratory distress syndrome. Thus the typical findings of progressive radiographic disease, fever, and leukocytosis do not necessarily reflect pneumonia, and the presence and bacterial content of purulent secretions does not reliably distinguish between tracheobronchitis and lower-tract infection.[30]

A variety of bronchoscopic techniques have been extensively evaluated with regard to their abilities to reliably detect the presence of pneumonia and identify the causative pathogen. The PSB and BAL have gained the widest acceptance, although their roles are still controversial. The PSB is designed to minimize contamination of the sample from the upper respiratory tract. In a number of studies, this technique has been combined with quantitation of bacterial cultures to define a bacterial count cut-off that reliably correlates with VAP. In a study by Chastre and colleagues, PSB reliably identified the presence and etiologic organism in VAP when the bacterial culture count was >10³ colony-forming units (compared with a standard of autopsy or blood culture confirmation) and reliably excluded VAP when the bacterial count recovered was below this cut-off.[64] Other investigators have confirmed a high percentage of true-positive results using this cut-off but with variable false-positive and false-negative results.[62] Duration of previous antibiotic therapy has consistently lowered the diagnostic utility of the procedure.[62,65] Other limitations include the need for specialized expertise in the performance of quantitative counts (not universally available) and the delay in processing (results unavailable for 24 to 48 hours).

Because of these limitations, modified BAL techniques have been examined for diagnostic utility. BAL offers the advantage of a wider sampling area but a standard disadvantage of contamination from the upper respiratory tract. Two variations in technique have been proffered to minimize contamination—specialized processing, which looks at recovery of intracellular bacterial organisms, and modified instrument design, with a "protected BAL catheter."

Chastre and colleagues suggest that BAL fluid be cyto-centrifuged and then microscopically examined for the presence of intracellular organisms. Theoretically, these organisms would reflect lower-tract pathogens rather than incidentally sampled, upper-tract colonizers. In their study, the presence of intracellular organisms in more than 25% of cells correlated with the presence of pneumonia and the pathogen ultimately identified by PSB; conversely, presence of organisms in less than 15% of cells correlated with a noninfectious diagnosis. The cell count and differential did not have discriminative value, nor did BAL culture, which was disproportionately representative of upper-tract rather than lower-tract flora.[64,65] This method has had variable reproducibility and also been shown to be negatively affected by previous antibiotic use.[65] It offers the advantage of rapid availability but also requires specialized expertise in processing.

A special balloon-tipped BAL catheter has been designed to minimize contamination of the catheter and lavage fluid by transit through the upper airway or endotracheal tube. In one study of both intubated and nonintubated patients with a gold standard of agreement with blood or pleural fluid cultures or PSB samples, quantitative bacterial cultures collected with this technique had a sensitivity of 97% and a specificity of 92%.[29] The role of this technique and the quantitative cut-off for microbiologic samples when it is used is currently under further investigation.

Lobar Atelectasis

When bronchoscopic yield has been evaluated purely on the basis of prebronchoscopy radiographic findings, lobar atelectasis is the radiographic finding associated with the highest incidence of a positive bronchoscopic diagnosis. Nearly 90% of patients in one such study had a specific diagnosis established on the basis of the procedure.[66] In an otherwise healthy person with normal ability to clear secretions, lobar atelectasis is strongly suggestive of an endobronchial mass lesion or extrinsic compression of the tracheobronchial tree by mediastinal mass lesions. Alternatively, in the appropriate clinical setting, it may indicate an aspirated foreign body. Therefore an airway exam, with appropriate biopsy techniques based on the lesion visualized, would be expected to be high yield.

A role for bronchoscopy also has been suggested in patients with impaired mucociliary clearance who develop lobar atelectasis on the basis of retained secretions. Bronchoscopy for pulmonary toilet often is requested to facilitate resolution of high-grade atelectasis presumed secondary to mucous plugging. In clinically stable patients with modest FiO_2 requirements, bronchoscopy has not been shown to be superior to nebulized aerosol and chest physiotherapy protocols to expedite radiographic resolution or improve gas exchange.[67] For selected patients, including those in whom conservative measures have failed, those with distorted airway architecture, and those with grossly impaired gas exchange caused by atelectasis such that rapid mechanical intervention is urgently indicated to forestall respiratory failure, bronchoscopy may have a role.

Suspected Foreign Body Aspiration

Bronchoscopy remains an important part of the diagnosis and therapy of aspirated foreign bodies. The absence of appropriate history or visualization of a radiopaque object does not exclude this diagnosis. Radiographic findings of persistent atelectasis or localized hyperinflation (especially evident on inspiratory and expiratory chest radiographs) suggest the diagnosis. When the diagnosis is suspected on clinical or radiographic grounds, either flexible or rigid bronchoscopy can be performed. The flexible bronchoscope can be used for diagnosis and therapeutics, with application of a basket extraction device through the working channel of the scope. FOB offers the advantage of not requiring general anesthesia and allowing visualization of more distal airways. Rigid bronchoscopy is preferred by some because of the wider range of extraction devices that can be applied, the ability to ventilate the patient during the procedure if necessary, and the ability to provide rapid suctioning in the event that attempted extraction incites substantial bleeding.[32,49] The rigid bronchoscope remains the instrument of choice for extraction in the pediatric population.[32,68]

Interstitial Lung Disease

The yield of TBBx in patients with diffuse interstitial lung disease depends on the diagnosis under consideration. TBBx has a high yield in the diagnosis of sarcoidosis (60% to 90%), even in the absence of radiographically demonstrable parenchymal disease; lymphangitic or bronchoalveolar cell carcinoma; and pulmonary alveolar proteinosis. TBBx can be specific but relatively insensitive for such diagnoses as eosinophilic granuloma and lymphangioleiomyomatosis. Most importantly, in the diagnosis of the spectrum of nonspecific inflammatory conditions, TBBx has been shown to be nondiagnostic or misdiagnostic when compared with open-lung biopsy samples in the majority of cases.[69] TBBx is a reasonable and high yield procedure when diagnoses such as sarcoid, infection, or malignancy are clinically likely. When diagnoses such as idiopathic pulmonary fibrosis or vasculitis are the primary considerations, open or video-assisted thoracoscopic lung biopsy may be the diagnostic procedure of choice.

Hemoptysis

The role of bronchoscopy in the evaluation of the patient with hemoptysis remains somewhat controversial and depends in part on the amount of bleeding, its time course, and associated clinical and radiographic data. Bronchoscopy has a potential role in localizing bleeding in the event that surgical intervention or vascular embolization is required and rendering a specific diagnosis. The factors associated with a high specific diagnostic yield for endobronchial malignancy include focal radiographic abnormalities, male sex, age greater than 40, and greater than 40 pack/year history of tobacco use.[70] For patients with a single episode of submassive bleeding without radiographic abnormalities or significant smoking history, the diagnostic yield is less certain, and the decision regarding whether to perform bronchoscopy remains individualized.

The timing of bronchoscopy in patients with nontrivial hemoptysis also is a subject of controversy. Multiple studies have shown that early bronchoscopy (performed within 48 hours of bleeding) is significantly more effective in the localization of a bleeding site; however, this localization has not materially impacted on either ultimate diagnosis or therapy.[71] Because localization may be crucial in the supportive management of a patient who develops recurrent or massive hemoptysis, many advocate early bronchoscopy to facilitate localization if urgent intervention is required.

Finally, the optimal instrument for bronchoscopy in the evaluation of hemoptysis is open to debate. Advocates of rigid bronchoscopy cite the markedly superior suctioning capability of the rigid scope and its ability to ventilate the patient during the procedure. Its disadvantage is that general anesthesia and an operating room are required, which impose a delay in procedure and limit availability. Flexible FOB is more rapidly and readily available but markedly limited in its ability to suction blood, maintain adequate visualization in the face of obscuring blood, and prevent asphyxiation. When FOB is used in the setting of massive hemoptysis, endotracheal intubation should be performed first to secure the airway, facilitate selective intubation to protect the nonbleeding lung, and allow for repeated reintroduction of the bronchoscope should vision become obscured by blood. The procedures often are complementary, with FOB carried out for initial localization and possible diagnosis while rigid endoscopy is being arranged. Likewise, the flexible FOB can be passed through the rigid scope for more distal airway examination.[71]

Cough

Bronchoscopy has an established diagnostic role when persistent cough is present with localizing findings such as hemoptysis, abnormal chest radiograph, or localized wheeze.[72] However, when persistent cough is the sole finding, bronchoscopy has not proven to be a high-yield early diagnostic procedure. In the absence of localized abnormalities, most chronic cough is attributable to chronic bronchitis, postnasal drip, asthma, or gastroesophageal reflux disease.[73,74] Therefore diagnostic and empiric therapeutic efforts should be first directed toward these diagnoses before bronchoscopy is considered. In one study of patients undergoing bronchoscopy for evaluation of chronic cough refractory to diagnostic and therapeutic efforts directed at the common diagnoses outlined above, 28% had a bronchoscopic diagnosis established. None of these diagnoses were malignant, and few resulted in successful therapy. Diagnoses ranged from broncholithiasis to upper-airway or tracheal malformations or stenoses. Female sex and age greater than 50 years were predictive of positive bronchoscopic findings. The authors concluded that bronchoscopy might have a role in carefully selected patients, although the diagnoses established in such cases often were more difficult to treat.[73]

Trauma

Either penetrating or blunt trauma to the chest can be associated with tracheal and bronchial injuries in 2% to 3% of cases.[75] Blunt trauma following high-speed motor vehi-cle accidents is especially associated with such injuries. These occur as a result of compression of the thorax, causing a so-called straddle injury with shearing of the mainstem bronchus from the carina; compression of the chest wall causing a sudden increase in intratracheal pressure and a tracheal blowout fracture; or rapid deceleration causing shearing of the trachea at the cricoid cartilage or the carina. Bronchoscopy is required for the exclusion of such injuries and should be performed in the setting of chest trauma accompanied by mediastinal or deep cervical emphysema, especially between mandible and clavicle; massive air leak through a chest tube, especially with incomplete reexpansion of the underlying lung; otherwise unexplained persistent atelectasis indicating lobar bronchial fracture; and any of these findings or the appropriate mechanism of injury accompanied by unexplained hemoptysis.[76]

Bronchoscopic Indications: Therapeutic

Intubation

Fiberoptic intubation is indicated in situations in which direct laryngoscopy does not allow successful visualization of the glottic opening or is contraindicated. Patients in whom direct laryngoscopy is contraindicated include those with small oral aperture (congenital, related to burns or scarring) or oropharyngeal tumor or trauma, those with temporomandibular joint disease, those with laryngeal or neck trauma, or those with abnormal cervical spine anatomy such that neck extension or flexion is either limited or contraindicated (rheumatoid arthritis with atlantoaxial instability, ankylosing spondylitis, or cervical spinal stenosis or fracture. Contraindications to fiberoptic intubation include life-threatening airway compromise that does not permit the delay inherent in equipment assembly, copious oropharyngeal secretions or bleeding that obscures vision, or significant upper-airway edema or infection. A lubricated endotracheal tube of an internal diameter at least 2 mm greater than the bronchoscope is passed over the bronchoscope. The bronchoscope is then introduced through the mouth and oropharynx until the glottic opening is visualized. The bronchoscope is advanced through the vocal cords and into the proximal tra-

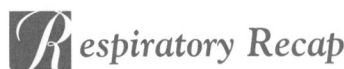

espiratory Recap

Therapeutic Indications for Bronchoscopy
Intubation Brachytherapy Stent placement

chea. The endotracheal tube is then gently advanced over the bronchoscope and positioned under direct vision.

Brachytherapy

Brachytherapy entails the endobronchial placement of encapsulated radionuclide in close proximity to an endobronchial malignancy. Currently, several techniques are available, the majority of which use FOB. Polyethylene catheters marked for length are threaded through the working channel of the bronchoscope and bronchoscopically placed in proximity to the tumor. The bronchoscope is then withdrawn and reinserted for bronchoscopic confirmation of catheter position. Radiopaque guidewires then can be threaded through the catheter for radiographic confirmation. The catheter is then afterloaded with radionuclide. A variety of radionuclides and dosing schedules are available. After treatment, the catheter is manually removed. Often, multiple bronchoscopies are required for scheduled serial treatments.

Brachytherapy is used primarily for palliation, although there are occasional applications with curative intent. The indication for palliative treatment is symptomatic biopsy-proven potentially radioresponsive malignancy causing airway compromise that has received maximal-dose external beam radiation. More rarely, brachytherapy is used as an adjunct to curative radiotherapy, to intensify dose, or to surgical resection, if the surgical margin reveals residual malignancy. Contraindications to brachytherapy include known fistulization to extrabronchial sites, lack of biopsy confirmation of malignancy, and if treatment is undertaken for palliation, lack of symptoms (such as postobstructive pneumonitis, intractable cough, dyspnea, or hemoptysis). If the airway is completely occluded or the patient is too ill to undergo bronchoscopy, the procedure is not feasible. Major complications are life-threatening hemoptysis, usually related to tumor proximity to the great vessels, and fistulization to the mediastinum. Less-frequent complications include pneumothorax, radiation bronchitis, radiation-related stenosis, and bronchospasm.[77] Subjective or objective palliation is reported in 50% to 90% of patients, with major complication rates reported to be about 10%.[77]

Stent Placement

Bronchoscopic placement of **tracheobronchial stents** may be indicated as a temporizing or palliative measure in a variety of patients. Such patients include those with either malignant extrinsic or endobronchial obstruction in whom other interventions such as laser or radiation have been unsuccessful or contraindicated, those with benign tracheobronchial stenosis from inflammatory disease, those with postintubation or posttransplant anastomotic strictures, those with tracheomalacia, or those with tracheoesophageal fistulization. Bronchoscopy is initially indicated to assess the lesion's location, extent, and severity; to mea-

sure the exact length and luminal diameter of the obstructed segment; and to assess the distance from vocal cords and carina, especially if complex stent placement or surgical intervention is being considered. Based on the anatomy and underlying disease, a decision then can be made regarding surgical versus endoscopic management.

If the obstruction is deemed appropriate for endoscopic stenting, a decision then must be made regarding the stent design (silicone or metal, specific shape) and mode of insertion (rigid or flexible bronchoscopy). Silicone stents are generally placed by rigid bronchoscopy, especially if long tracheal segments requiring tracheostomy and T- or inverted Y-shaped stents are required. Disadvantages of silicone stents include a greater propensity for migration, mucoid impaction of the stented segment because of the reduced mucociliary clearance within the solid-walled stent, and frequently the requirement for rigid bronchoscopy.

A variety of self-expanding metal stents originally designed for vascular or gastrointestinal endoscopic use have been adapted for rigid or flexible bronchoscopic use. These consist of braided tubular mesh or continuously looped zigzagged stainless steel wire of a variety of lengths and diameters, which are compressed into narrow cylinders within cartridges of various designs and placed either through a hollow catheter or over a guide wire, generally under fluoroscopic guidance. Metal stents tend to be partially or fully self-expanding, obviating the need for present dilatation. The disadvantage of metal stents is that they are extremely difficult to remove endoscopically and run a greater risk of bronchial or vascular injury because the struts may be sharp. If mesh stents are used, tumor may grow through the meshwork and reocclude the stented segment. In addition, granulation tissue may form and become occlusive.[78]

Future Directions

One of the primary limitations to conventional bronchoscopy in the diagnosis of malignant disease remains localization of lesions that cannot be directly visualized by the bronchoscopist—that is, peribronchial tumors or lymph nodes and peripheral lesions. Hurter and Hanrath pioneered the development of ultrasound–guided bronchoscopy in the early 1990s.[79] This technique applies the technology of endovascular ultrasound to the tracheobronchial tree. A catheter with an ultrasound transducer surrounded by a fluid-filled chamber to enhance signal transmission is threaded through the working channel of the scope after the scope has been positioned in the location of interest. The lesion is localized, the catheter removed, and the position marked. The appropriate biopsy instrument is then inserted. This system has been used to evaluate central peribronchial lesions, in which ultrasonographic transmission is limited by the difficulty of achieving a wide area of apposition (resulting in a pie-shaped, partial image), as well as peripheral lesions, in which the smaller bronchial diameter allows for 360 degrees of visualization. Ultrasound is purported to distinguish between normal bronchial wall (three distinct echo layers) and that invaded by tumor (in which this architecture is violated); assist in identification and characterization of lymph nodes (normal, less than 1 cm and with a characteristic echo-rich center; abnormal, larger and with distorted internal architecture and well-defined margins); distinguish between extrabronchial mass lesions and surrounding normal lung by their different echo characteristics; and localize vascular structures so that they can be avoided during biopsy. In a preliminary study by Steiner and colleagues, ultrasound proved helpful in the avoidance of vascular structures and the selection of biopsy site, especially in the case of peripheral lesions.[80] The dominant limitations to bronchoscopic ultrasound at this point remain cost, enhanced adaptation of ultrasound technology to this application, and increase in length of procedure.

Enhanced localization for diagnosis and treatment also has been attempted in the form of photodynamic therapy. This technique uses photosensitizing agents (primarily porphyrin-based agents) and fluorescent detection devices that exploit the different photosensitizing uptake and flu-orescence characteristics of normal and malignant tissue. Patients are pretreated with the photosensitizer and then undergo bronchoscopy with a specialized light source designed to deliver photons in the appropriate absorption spectrum.

This technique has been used in the diagnosis of subtle lesions beyond the resolution of standard endoscopic visualization. Directed endobronchial biopsy confirmation is then undertaken. Because photosensitizers form toxic oxygen-free radicals when exposed to light of the appropriate wavelength, this technique also has been used in therapy of carcinoma in situ or obstructing lesions in patients who are not resectional candidates. Preliminary studies suggest that photodynamic therapy may be a viable alternative for selected patients with nonbulky carcinoma in situ. Patients with obstructing advanced tumors fare less well, with only partial responses and complications including hemorrhage (especially when tumor extends beyond the bronchus), secretion retention requiring follow-up toilet bronchoscopy, pneumonia, and abscess.[81] More extensive study of the appropriate patient population and refinements of both photosensitizing agents and detection devices is under way.

𝒦EY 𝒫OINTS

- Factors necessary for a successful FOB include proper patient selection, patient preparation, and appropriate anesthesia.
- Common FOB techniques include airway examination, bronchoalveolar lavage, bronchoscopic washing, non-protected bronchoscopic brushing, endobronchial biopsy, transbronchial needle aspiration, and TBBx.
- Rigid bronchoscopy may be superior to flexible bronchoscopy in the assessment of patients with massive hemoptysis, the removal of foreign bodies, the per-formance of laser bronchoscopy, and the performance of dilation of tracheobronchial strictures.
- Diagnostic indications for bronchoscopy include suspected carcinoma, pneumonia, lobar atelectasis, suspected foreign body aspiration, interstitial lung disease, hemoptysis, and cough.
- Therapeutic indications for bronchoscopy include endotracheal intubation, brachytherapy, and stent placement.

References

1. Jackson C. Bronchoscopy: past, present and future. N Engl J Med 1928;199:759-763.
2. Djukanovic R, Wilson JW, Lai CKW, et al. The safety aspects of fiberoptic bronchoscopy, bronchoalveolar lavage, and endobronchial biopsy in asthma. Am Rev Respir Dis 1991;143:772-777.
3. Matot I, Kramer MR, Glantz L, et al. Myocardial ischemia in sedated patients undergoing fiberoptic bronchoscopy. Chest 1997;112:454-458.
4. Bajwa MK, Henein S, Kamholz SL. Fiberoptic bronchoscopy in the presence of space-occupying intracranial lesions. Chest 1993;104:101-103.
5. Kozak EA, Brath LK. Do "screening" coagulation tests predict bleeding in patients undergoing fiberoptic bronchoscopy with biopsy? Chest 1994;106:703-705.
6. Prakash UB, Offord KP, Stubbs SE. Bronchoscopy in North America: the ACCP survey. Chest 1991;100:1668-1675.
7. Prakash UB, Stubbs SE. The bronchoscopy survey: some reflections. Chest 1991;100:1660-1667.
8. Fulkerson WJ. Medical intelligence: fiberoptic bronchoscopy. N Engl J Med 1984;311:511-515.
9. Pereira W Jr., Kovnat DM, Snider GL. A prospective cooperative study of complications following flexible fiberoptic bronchoscopy. Chest 1978;73:813-816.
10. Credle WF Jr., Smiddy JF, Elliott RC. Complications of fiberoptic bronchoscopy. Am Rev Respir Dis 1974;109:67-72.
11. Suratt PM, Smiddy JF, Gruber B. Deaths and complications associated with fiberoptic bronchoscopy. Chest 1976;69:747-751.
12. Cordasco EM Jr., Mehta AC, Ahmad M. Bronchoscopically induced bleeding: a summary of nine years' Cleveland Clinic experience and review of the literature. Chest 1991;100:1141-1147.

13. Zavala DC. Pulmonary hemorrhage in fiberoptic transbronchial biopsy. Chest 1976;70:584-588.

14. Van Gundy K, Boylen CT. Fiberoptic bronchoscopy: indications, complications, contraindications. Postgraduate Med 1988; 83:289-294.

15. Weiss SM, Hert RC, Gianola FJ, et al. Complications of fiberoptic bronchoscopy in thrombocytopenic patients. Chest 1993;104:1025-1028.

16. Reed AP. Preparation of the patient for awake flexible fiberoptic bronchoscopy. Chest 1992:101:244-253.

17. Witte MC, Opal SM, Gilbert JG, et al. Incidence of fever and bacteremia following transbronchial needle aspiration. Chest 1986;89:85-87.

18. Milman N, Faurschou P, Grode G. Pulse oximetry during fibreoptic bronchoscopy in local anaesthesia: frequency of hypoxemia and effect of oxygen supplementation. Respiration 1994; 61:242-347.

19. Lacy CF, Armstrong LL, Ingrim NB, et al. Drug information handbook, 6th ed. Cleveland: Lexi-Comp Inc; 1998.

20. Keane D, McNicholas WT. Comparison of nebulized and sprayed topical anaesthesia for fibreoptic bronchoscopy. Eur Respir J 1992;5:1123-1125.

21. Foster WM, Hurewitz AN. Aerosolized lidocaine reduces dose of topical anesthetic for bronchoscopy. Am Rev Respir Dis 1992;146:520-522.

22. Graham DR, Hay JG, Clague J, et al. Comparison of three different methods used to achieve local anesthesia for fiberoptic bronchoscopy. Chest 1992;102:704-707.

23. Williams TJ, Nicoulet I, Coleman E, et al. Safety and patient acceptability of intravenous midazolam for fiberoptic bronchoscopy. Respir Med 1994;88:305-307.

24. Plummer S, Hartley M, Vaughn RS. Anaesthesia for telescopic procedures in the thorax. Br J Anaesth 1998;80:223-234.

25. Clarkson K, Power CK, O'Connell F, et al. A comparative evaluation of propofol and midazolam as sedative agents in fiberoptic bronchoscopy. Chest 1993;104:1029-1031.

26. Golden JA, Wang KP, Keith FM. Bronchoscopy, lung biopsy and other diagnostic procedures. In: Murray JF, Nadel JA, editors. Textbook of respiratory medicine. 2nd ed. vol 1. Philadelphia: WB Saunders; 1994.

27. Zavala DC. Flexible fiberoptic bronchoscopy: a training handbook. Iowa City: University of Iowa Department of Publications; 1978.

28. Reynolds HY. State of art: Bronchoalveolar lavage. Am Rev Respir Dis 1987;135:250-263.

29. Meduri GU, Beals DH, Maijub AG, et al. A new bronchoscopic technique to retrieve uncontaminated distal airway secretions. Am Rev Respir Dis 1991;143:855-864.

30. Baselski VS, Wunderink RG. Bronchoscopic diagnosis of pneumonia. Clin Microbiol Rev 1994;7:533-558.

31. Shure D. Transbronchial biopsy and needle aspiration. Chest 1989;95:1130-1138.

32. Zavala DC. Flexible fiberoptic bronchoscopy. In: Simmons DH, editor. Current pulmonology. Boston: Houghton Mifflin; 1980.

33. Shure D, Asterita RW. Bronchogenic carcinoma presenting as an endobronchial mass—optimal number of biopsy specimens for diagnosis. Chest 1983;83:865-867.

34. Wang KP, Brower R, Haponik EF, et al. Flexible transbronchial needle aspiration for staging of bronchogenic carcinoma. Chest 1983;84:571-576.

35. Schenk DA, Bower JH, Bryan CL, et al. Transbronchial needle aspiration staging of bronchogenic carcinoma. Am Rev Respir Dis 1986;134:146-148.

36. Shure D, Fedullo PF. The role of transcarinal needle aspiration in the staging of bronchogenic carcinoma. Chest 1984;86:693-699.

37. Utz JP, Patel AM, Edell ES. The role of transcarinal needle aspiration in the staging of bronchogenic carcinoma. Chest 1993;104:1012-1016.

38. Shure D, Fedullo PF. Transbronchial needle aspiration in the diagnosis of submucosal and peribronchial bronchogenic carcinoma. Chest 1985;88:49-51.

39. Wang KP, Haponik EF, Britt EJ, et al. Transbronchial needle aspiration of peripheral pulmonary nodules. Chest 1984;86:819-823.

40. Shure D, Fedullo PF. Concise clinical study: transbronchial needle aspiration of peripheral masses. Am Rev Respir Dis 1983;128:1090-1092.

41. Mehta AC, Ahmad M, Nunez C, et al. Newer procedures using the fiberoptic bronchoscope in the diagnosis of lung cancer. Cleve Clin J Med 1987;54:195-203.

42. Wang KP. Flexible transbronchial needle aspiration biopsy for histologic specimens. Chest 1985;88:860-863.

43. Salathe M, Soler M, Bolliger CT, et al. Transbronchial needle aspiration in routine fiberoptic bronchoscopy. Respiration 1992;59:5-8.

44. Milman N, Faurschou P, Munch EP, et al. Transbronchial biopsy through the fibre optic bronchoscope: results and complications in 452 examinations. Respir Med 1994;88:749-753.

45. Shure D, Abraham JL, Konopka R. How should transbronchial biopsies be performed and processed? Am Rev Respir Dis 1982;126:342-343.

46. Herf SM, Suratt PM, Arora NS. Deaths and complications associated with transbronchial biopsy. Am Rev Respir Dis 1977;115:708-711.

47. Milligan SA, Luce JM, Golden J, et al. Transbronchial biopsy without fluoroscopy in patients with diffuse roentgenographic infiltrates and the acquired immunodeficiency syndrome. Am Rev Respir Dis 1988;137:486-488.

48. Papin TA, Grum CM, Weg JG. Transbronchial biopsy during mechanical ventilation. Chest 1986;89:168-170.

49. Helmers RA, Sanderson DR. Rigid bronchoscopy: the forgotten art. In: Mathur PN, Beamis JF Jr, editors. Clinics in chest medicine: Interventional pulmonology. vol 16. no 3. Philadelphia: WB Saunders; 1995.

50. Ramser ER, Beamis JF Jr. Laser bronchoscopy. In: Mathur PN, Beamis JF Jr, editors. Clinics in chest medicine: interventional pulmonology. vol 16. no 3. Philadelphia: WB Saunders; 1995.

51. Dumon, JF, Meric B, Guillen JC, et al. Endoscopic Nd-YAG laser resection in bronchology. In: Martini N, Vogt-Moykopf I, editors. Thoracic surgery: frontiers and uncommon neoplasms. vol 5. St Louis: Mosby; 1989.

52. Loddenkemper R, Schoenfeld N. Role of endoscopy in the preoperative assessment of bronchial carcinoma. Monaldi Arch Chest Dis 1994;49:138-143.

53. Shure D, Fedullo PF, Plummer M. Carinal forceps biopsy via the fiberoptic bronchoscope in the routine staging of lung cancer. West J Med 1985;142:511-513.

54. Harrow E, Halber M, Hardy S, et al. Bronchoscopic and roentgenographic correlates of a positive transbronchial needle

aspiration in the staging of lung cancer. Chest 1991;100: 1592-1596.

55. Davenport RD. Rapid on-site evaluation of transbronchial aspirates. Chest 1990;98:59-61.

56. Stringfield JT, Markowitz DJ, Bentz RR, et al. The effect of tumor size and location on diagnosis by fiberoptic bronchoscopy. Chest 1977;72:474-476.

57. Feinsilver SH, Fein AM, Niederman MS, et al. Utility of fiberoptic bronchoscopy in nonresolving pneumonia. Chest 1990;98:1322-1326.

58. Matthay RA, Farmer WC, Odero D. Diagnostic fibreoptic bronchoscopy in the immunocompromised host with pulmonary infiltrates. Thorax 1977;32:539-545.

59. Williams D, Yungbluth M, Adams G, et al. The role of fiberoptic bronchoscopy in the evaluation of immunocompromised hosts with diffuse pulmonary infiltrates. Am Rev Respir Dis 1985;131:880-885.

60. Stover DE, White DA, Romano PA, et al. Concise clinical study: diagnosis of pulmonary disease in acquired immune deficiency syndrome (AIDS). Am Rev Respir Dis 1984;130:659-662.

61. Tu JV, Biem J, Detsky AS. Bronchoscopy versus empirical therapy in HIV-infected patients with presumptive *Pneumocystis carinii* pneumonia: a decision analysis. Am Rev Respir Dis 1993;148:370-377.

62. Allen RM, Dunn WF, Limper AH. Subspecialty clinics: Pulmonary and critical care medicine: diagnosing ventilator-associated pneumonia: the role of bronchoscopy. Mayo Clin Proc 1994;69:962-968.

63. Meduri GU. Ventilator-associated pneumonia in patients with respiratory failure: a diagnostic approach. Chest 1990;97:1208-1219.

64. Chastre J, Fagon JY, Soler P, et al. Diagnosis of nosocomial bacterial pneumonia in intubated patients undergoing ventilation: comparison of the usefulness of bronchoalveolar lavage and the protected specimen brush. Am J Med 1988;85:499-506.

65. Meduri GU, Chastre J. The standardization of bronchoscopic techniques for ventilator-associated pneumonia. Chest 1992;102S:557S-564S.

66. Su WJ, Lee PY, Perng RP. Chest radiographic guidelines in the selection of patients for fiberoptic bronchoscopy. Chest 1993;103:1198-1201.

67. Marini JJ, Pierson DJ, Hudson LD, et al. Acute lobar atelectasis: a prospective comparison of fiberoptic bronchoscopy and respiratory therapy. Am Rev Respir Dis 1979;119:971-978.

68. Castro M, Midthun DE, Edell ES, et al. Flexible bronchoscopic removal of foreign bodies from pediatric airways. J Bronchol 1994;1:92-98.

69. Wall CP, Gaensler EA, Carrington CB, et al. Comparison of transbronchial and open biopsies in chronic infiltrative lung diseases. Am Rev Respir Dis 1981;123:280-285.

70. O'Neil KM, Lazarus AA. Hemoptysis: indications for bronchoscopy. Arch Intern Med 1991;151:171-174.

71. Patel SR, Stoller JK. The role of bronchoscopy in hemoptysis. In: Wang KP, Mehta AC, editors. Flexible bronchoscopy. Cambridge, Mass: Blackwell Science; 1995.

72. Utz JP, Prakash UBS. Indications for and contraindications to bronchoscopy. In: Prakash UBS, editor. Bronchoscopy. New York: Raven Press; 1994.

73. Sen RP, Walsh TE. Fiberoptic bronchoscopy for refractory cough. Chest 1991;99:33-35.

74. Irwin RS, Corrao WM, Pratter MR. Chronic persistent cough in the adult: the spectrum and frequency of causes and successful outcome of specific therapy. Am Rev Respir Dis 1981;123:413-417.

75. Iwasaki M, Kaga K, Ogawa, et al. Bronchoscopy findings and early treatment of patients with blunt tracheobronchial trauma. J Cardiovasc Surg 1994;35:269-271.

76. Calhoon JH, Grover FL, Trinkle JK. Chest trauma: approach and management. In: Buchalter SE, McElvein RB, editors. Clinics in chest medicine: thoracic surgical considerations for the pulmonologist. vol 13. no 1. Philadelphia: WB Saunders; 1992.

77. Villanueva AG, Lo TCM, Beamis JF Jr. Endobronchial brachytherapy. In: Mathur PN, Beamis JF Jr, editors. Clinics in chest medicine: interventional pulmonology. vol 16. no 3. Philadelphia: WB Saunders; 1995.

78. Colt HG, Dumon JF. Airway stents: present and future. In: Mathur PN, Beamis JF Jr, editors. Clinics in chest medicine: interventional pulmonology. vol 16. no 3. Philadelphia: WB Saunders; 1995.

79. Hurter TH, Hanrath P. Endobronchial sonography: feasibility and preliminary results. Thorax 1992;47:565-657.

80. Steiner RM, Liu JB, Goldberg BB, et al. The value of ultrasound-guided fiberoptic bronchoscopy. In: Mathur PN, Beamis JF Jr, editors. Clinics in chest medicine: interventional pulmonology. vol 16. no 3. Philadelphia: WB Saunders; 1995.

81. Edell ES, Cortese DA. Photodynamic therapy: its use in the management of bronchogenic carcinoma. In: Mathur PN, Beamis JF Jr, editors. Clinics in chest medicine: interventional pulmonology. vol 16. no 3. Philadelphia: WB Saunders; 1995.

CHAPTER 29

Sleep Assessment

Joseph B. Khoury
Rodney A. Radtke

CHAPTER OUTLINE

Stages of Sleep
  Non-REM Sleep
  REM Sleep
Normal Physiology during Sleep
  Progressive Reduction in Ventilation
  Changes in Respiratory Muscle Activity and Tone

Changes in Upper Airway Muscle Tone
  Potential Pathophysiologic Effects
Monitoring Techniques
  Sleep Technologists
  Polysomnogram
Sleep Scoring

OBJECTIVES

1. Discuss the stages of wakefulness and sleep, including non-REM and REM sleep.
2. Discuss the normal physiologic changes that occur during sleep, including the progressive reduction in ventilation, changes in ventilatory muscle activity, and changes in upper airway and ventilatory muscle tone.
3. Describe the various monitoring techniques used in the field of sleep medicine.
4. List the key components of a full and partial polysomnogram.
5. Describe the role of sleep technologists, including respiratory therapists, in overnight polysomnography.
6. Describe the diagnostic features of obstructive apnea, central apnea, and mixed apnea and explain the terms commonly used with these conditions.
7. Explain the common terms used during scoring of a sleep study, including *apnea/hypopnea index, respiratory distress index, arousal index, upper airway resistance syndrome, obesity hypoventilation syndrome, obstructive sleep apnea syndrome, central sleep apnea syndrome,* and *periodic limb movement syndrome.*

KEY TERMS

Apnea	Mixed Apnea	Respiratory Disturbance Index
Apnea/Hypopnea Index (AHI)	Multiple Sleep Latency Testing (MSLT)	Sleep Cycle
Arousal Index	Non-REM Sleep	Sleep-Disordered Breathing
Central Apnea	Obstructive Apnea	Sleep Efficiency
Continuous Positive Airway Pressure	Periodic Leg Movements of Sleep	Sleep Latency
(CPAP)	Polysomnography (PSG)	Sleep Staging
Hypopnea	REM Sleep	

The field of sleep medicine is relatively new, given the only recent understanding and awareness of sleep disorders. Sleep medicine encompasses a number of different medical and psychiatric disorders, ranging from insomnia to sleep **apnea** syndromes, discussed in detail in subsequent sections of the chapter. In fact, the revised International Classification of Sleep Disorders, published by the American Sleep Disorders Association, now recognizes more than 80 separate diagnoses.[1]

Assessment of any patient with complaints that may arise from a sleep disorder begins with a thorough history and physical examination. Often a sleep questionnaire, including a sleep log of the previous 1 or 2 weeks, also is useful. If a sleep disorder is suspected, diagnostic tests are needed to identify the specific disorder and the severity of the problem. These tests include overnight diagnostic **polysomnography (PSG),** overnight nasal **continuous positive airway pressure (CPAP)** titration studies, overnight oximetry studies, and **multiple sleep latency testing (MSLT).**

Stages of Sleep

During sleep different levels of electroencephalographic (EEG) states correlate with different physiologic states, including wakefulness, rapid eye movement sleep **(REM sleep),** and **non-REM sleep.** Each of these physiologic states is subdivided into stages that reflect different levels of consciousness.

Wakefulness encompasses two EEG states, awake and drowsy. The awakened state is characterized by low-voltage, fast-frequency waves,[2] as shown in Figure 29-1. When a person becomes drowsy, the EEG pattern shifts to show α-rhythm. α-Waves (8 to 12 Hz) are seen when the eyes close and disappear when the eyes open. From the drowsy stage, the person moves into non-REM sleep.

 espiratory Recap

Stages of Wakefulness
Awake
Drowsy

Non-REM Sleep

Non-REM sleep is divided into four stages based on EEG patterns (see Figure 29-1). Stages 1 and 2 are considered light sleep, and stages 3 and 4 are called *deep sleep* or *slow-wave sleep*. Stage 1 sleep is characterized by 3- to 7-Hz θ-waves, and stage 2 is marked by sleep spindles and K complexes. Stages 3 and 4 are defined by slow waves (0.5 to 2 Hz) with a large amplitude (over 75 μV). Stage 3 is defined as having at least 50% slow waves and stage 4 as having at least 90% slow waves.[3]

REM Sleep

REM sleep is defined by the presence of rapid eye movements on electrooculography (EOG). These eye movements have a sharp slope and a frequency over 1 Hz, in contrast to the slow eye movements of non-REM sleep. REM sleep also is characterized by an EEG pattern similar to that of wakefulness and a marked reduction in muscle tone.

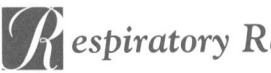 *espiratory Recap*

Stages of Sleep
Non-REM sleep (stages 1 through 4)

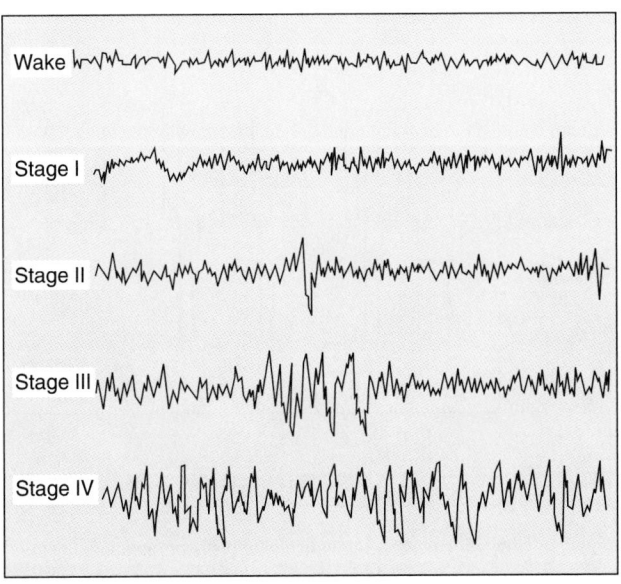

Figure 29-1 Electroencephalographic patterns during various stages of sleep.

Sleep is characterized not only by the above stages but also by a repetitive, ordered pattern of these stages throughout the night or sleep episode; this is referred to as the **sleep cycle.** The body makes the transition from an awakened state to stage 1 of non-REM sleep. The EEG pattern then fluctuates between stages 1 and 2 before progressing to slow-wave sleep. Finally, a period of REM sleep occurs, from which the EEG returns to stage 1 sleep, and the cycle begins again. Each cycle lasts approximately 90 to 110 minutes, with a total of four to six cycles per night. Sleep cycles that occur early in the night have a higher proportion of slow-wave sleep, whereas those occurring later have a higher proportion of REM sleep. A *sleep histogram* (Figure 29-2) is an easy way to visualize an entire night's sleep and the sleep cycles.[4]

Normal Physiology during Sleep

Major changes occur during sleep in many organ systems. The most important of these are the neurologic and respiratory systems. Respiratory physiology is affected by sleep stages in a number of ways, including changes in the direct neurologic control of ventilation, in ventilatory muscle tone, and in certain neurochemical reflexes that maintain homeostasis of the respiratory system. To better understand these changes, it is important to understand normal waking respiratory physiology.

Progressive Reduction in Ventilation

In wakefulness the control of ventilation is shared by cortical input, brain stem centers, peripheral chemoreceptors, and intrapulmonary baroreceptors. The brain stem centers

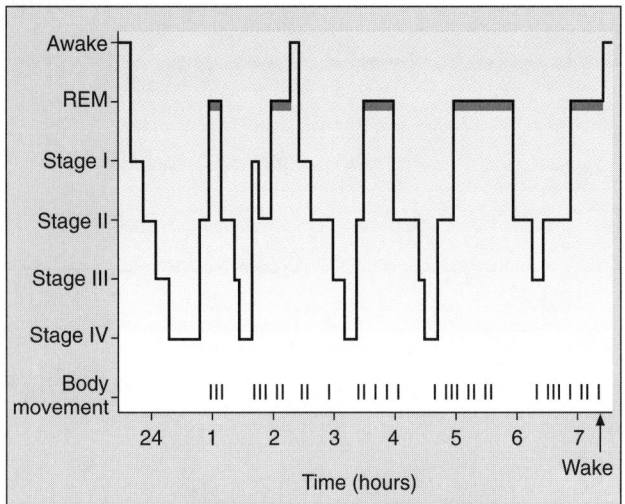

Figure 29-2   Typical sleep histogram.

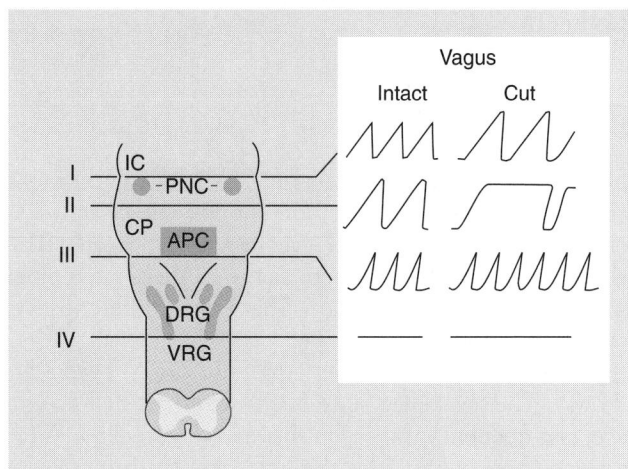

Figure 29-3   Breathing patterns resulting from transection of the spinal cord at various levels. *IC,* Inferior colliculus; *PNC,* pneumotaxic center; *CP,* cerebellar peduncle; *APC,* apneustic center; *DRG,* dorsal respiratory group; *VRG,* ventral respiratory group.

important in the maintenance of ventilation include the pneumotaxic center and the apneustic center. Animal models show that transection of the brain stem above the apneustic center does not affect normal breathing, whereas transection below this area causes a pattern of slow inspiration. Transection farther down the brain stem, below the pneumotaxic center, causes regular gasping breathing. Transection at the pontomedullary junction causes respiratory arrest[5] (Figure 29-3). The clinical implication of these neuroanatomic regions is apparent in patients with traumatic spinal cord injury or brain stem stroke.

The function of ventilation is to maintain the partial pressure of carbon dioxide (PCO_2) and the partial pressure of oxygen (PO_2) within certain physiologic boundaries. The main mechanisms for minute by minute control of ventilation, therefore, are the responses to hypoxia and hypercapnia. Hypoxemia has been shown to stimulate ventilation through the carotid body chemoreceptors.[6,7] This response, which is nonlinear, becomes especially prominent when the arterial oxygen pressure (PaO_2) falls below 60 mm Hg. However, the ventilatory response to a rising arterial carbon dioxide pressure ($PaCO_2$) is linear (Figure 29-4).[8] This latter response is mediated through carotid body and central nervous system (CNS) chemoreceptors in the medulla.[6,9]

Ventilation is reduced in both non-REM and REM sleep because of a decrease in the tidal volume, which lowers the minute ventilation. In non-REM sleep the minute ventilation is reduced by 0.5 to 1.5 L/min,[10-12] whereas in REM sleep the reduction typically is about 1.5 L/min.[11-13] The factors responsible for these ventilatory changes are not well understood, but four major events occur. First, the body's metabolic rate slows during sleep, causing a reduction in the amount of CO_2 produced. Because excretion of CO_2 is accomplished primarily through exhalation, a concomitant reduction in ventilation occurs. Second, the brain stem input responsible for maintaining ventilation is diminished. Third, the response of

the PO_2 and PCO_2 chemoreceptors is reduced. In fact, the hypercapnic ventilatory response in sleep is reduced by 20% to 50% in sleep.[14-16] An increase in PCO_2 therefore is required to stimulate ventilation (Figure 29-5).[16] Fourth, airway resistance increases significantly as a result of phasic changes in the tone of upper airway muscles during sleep that cause a reduction in tidal volume and minute ventilation. These changes in muscle tone in turn depend on the sleep stage.

Changes in Respiratory Muscle Activity and Tone

The changes in the tone of the respiratory muscles during sleep are particularly important. During wakefulness the muscles involved in ventilation and maintenance of upper airway patency show both background activity (*tonic activity*) and contraction with inspiration (*phasic activity*). In non-REM sleep the tonic activity of the intercostal muscles is constant compared with wakefulness, but the phasic activity is increased. In contrast, the diaphragm shows no significant change during non-REM sleep, consequently the tidal volume is more dependent on the rib cage musculature during non-REM sleep than during wakefulness.[17]

The tone of these ventilatory muscles is significantly different in REM sleep from that seen in non-REM sleep. In REM sleep the intercostal muscles lose almost all phasic and tonic activity, and the diaphragm loses its background tonic activity. The phasic activity of the diaphragm, however, is preserved. The tidal volume in REM sleep, therefore, is almost entirely produced by the activity of the diaphragm. The loss of all tonic activity in the ventilatory apparatus is reflected in a decrease in the functional residual capacity[18,19] and can lead to hypoxemia during REM sleep.

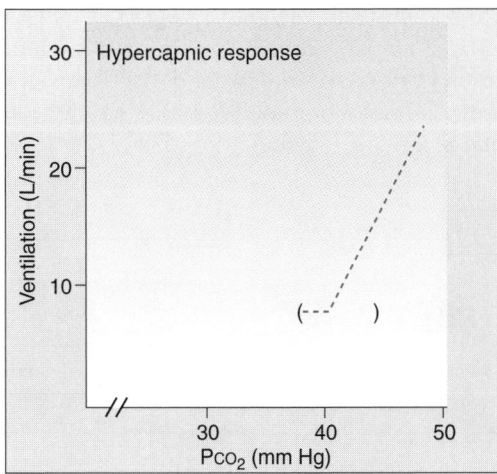
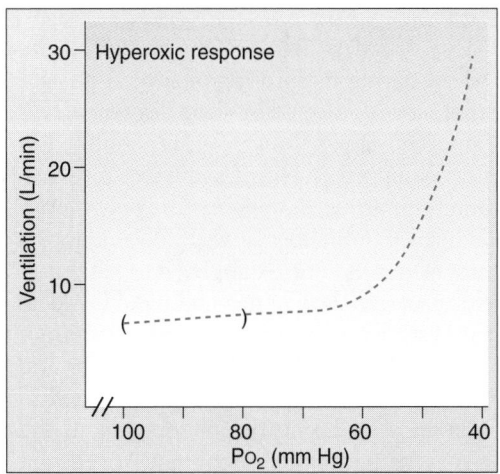

Figure 29-4   Normal ventilatory response to changing levels of Pa_{O_2} and Pa_{CO_2} during the awake state.

Changes in Upper Airway Muscle Tone

The upper airway muscles that maintain oropharyngeal and palatopharyngeal airway patency are the genioglossus muscle, the infrahyoid muscle group (sternohyoid, omohyoid, and sternothyroid), and the palatal muscle group (levator veli palatini, palatoglossus, and tensor veli palatini).[20] These muscles also show significant changes in tone during sleep. The tonic and phasic activity of the genioglossus muscle is reduced in non-REM sleep and even further reduced in REM sleep.[21,22] Similarly, the activity of the palatal muscle group is diminished in non-REM sleep and much further reduced during REM sleep.[23] The infrahyoid muscle group also shows decreased activity, but some research notes increased inspiratory bursts in relation to hypercapnia.[24] The overall effect of these changes is a progressive reduction in upper airway tone and in the airway space. This most certainly plays a role in the development of airway obstruction during sleep, especially because many obese patients already have airway narrowing caused by increased fat deposition in the airway structures.

Potential Pathophysiologic Effects

During sleep the combined effects of the reduced drive to breathe and increased airway resistance cause a slight increase in the Pa_{CO_2} in normal individuals. In patients with underlying lung disease (both obstructive disease, such as chronic obstructive pulmonary disease [COPD], and restrictive disease, such as pulmonary fibrosis), these factors can cause significant hypercapnia and hypoxemia, exacerbating underlying condition. Even in patients without underlying lung disease, complete obstruction of the upper airway can occur, leading to significant periods of apnea. This obstructive apnea can occur throughout the night, in severe cases more than 100 times an hour. Long-standing obstructive sleep apnea may cause significant heart disease and stroke.

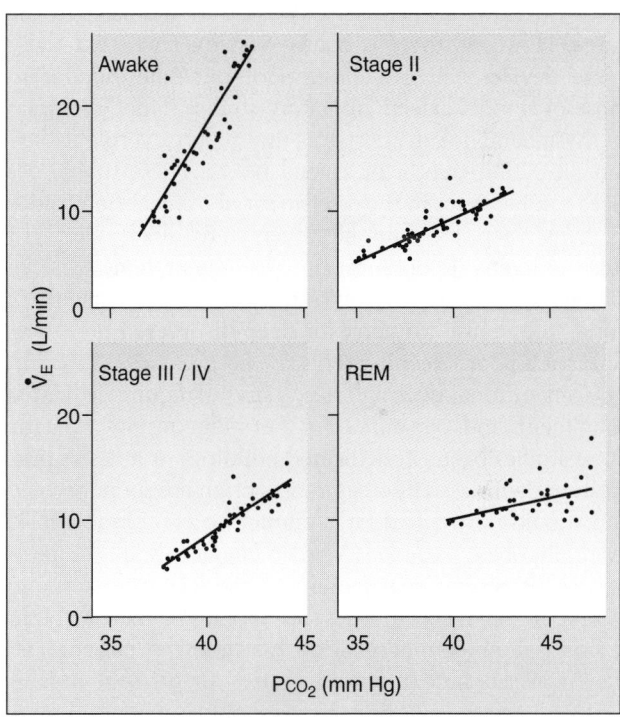

Figure 29-5   Normal ventilatory response to changing levels of Pco_2 during sleep.

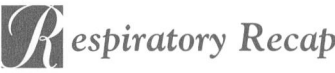 *espiratory Recap*

Physiologic Changes during Sleep	
Reduction in ventilatory muscle tone	Reduced muscle tone in upper airways
Alterations in neurochemical reflexes	Reduction of the airway space
Reduced drive to breathe	Increased airway resistance
	Reduced ventilation

Monitoring Techniques

Assessment of sleep disorders involves observation of the patient during sleep during monitoring of several physiologic variables that may be affected by sleep disorders. This test, known as an *overnight polysomnogram,* is performed in specialized centers equipped to monitor numerous neurologic, cardiac, and respiratory parameters. The polysomnogram can be modified in a number of ways, depending on the patient's circumstances. For example, if a patient is known to have obstructive sleep apnea and nasal CPAP is thought to be the best treatment, an overnight polysomnogram with titration of the CPAP may be performed to find the optimum CPAP settings; this is commonly referred to as a *CPAP titration study.* A diagnostic polysomnogram and CPAP titration may be performed in the same overnight study; this often is called a *split study.* Recent technologic advances in monitoring and recording devices have made overnight home PSG a realistic possibility. Similarly, some machines now can perform CPAP titration studies in the home. However, there is controversy over whether these home devices can provide patient outcomes similar to those of standard sleep laboratory studies. Finally, oxygen plethysmographs can now store and report overnight oxygen saturation trends for several hours. These simple devices can be useful in the assessment of oxygenation trends in many sleep disorders. However, stand-alone overnight pulse oximetry is no substitute for comprehensive sleep studies. Moreover, the low sensitivity and specificity of stand-alone pulse oximetry for **sleep-disordered breathing** makes it a poor screening tool.

Conventional overnight sleep studies require dedicated equipment and personnel for optimum results. Usually these studies occur in dedicated buildings or areas of hospitals and clinics. The sleep rooms often are soundproofed and should have a bed large enough to comfortably hold morbidly obese patients. A video camera should be positioned to observe the patient while asleep, and sound monitors and recording devices should be in the rooms both to allow communication between the patient and staff members and to record snoring or other sounds or speech during sleep. These rooms should also have climate control, light control, and a soft decor to promote sleep.

Sleep Technologists

Sleep technologists are trained professionals who are integral to the process of overnight PSG. In many hospitals respiratory therapists function as sleep technologists (CPG 29-1). Patients typically arrive 60 to 90 minutes before their usual bedtime, and the sleep technologist reviews the procedural aspects of the study while attaching the monitoring equipment to the patient. Sleep technologists also review the patient's history and medications before the study. They are in constant communication with the patient through both video surveillance and audio intercoms. Technologists also are responsible for placing any of

a variety of equipment chosen for the test, which can include EEG and electrocardiographic (ECG) electrodes and monitoring equipment for oxygen plethysmography, respiratory effort, airflow, and electromyography (EMG). The technologist should be able to immediately correct any technologic malfunction that occurs during the study.

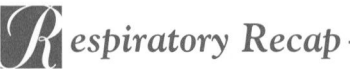
Respiratory Recap

Sleep Technologists
Respiratory therapists often function as sleep technologists. Sleep technologists are integral to the process of overnight PSG.

Polysomnogram

The minimum monitoring requirements to score sleep studies adequately are a two-channel EEG, a one-channel EOG, and a one-channel EMG. The more comprehensive study, however, uses many other techniques to provide the reviewer with additional information. These techniques include an expanded EEG montage, respiratory effort or airflow monitors (or both), oxygen saturation monitoring, an ECG channel, and one or two channels for recording of leg movement.

The EEG often is expanded to include at least four channels; this allows for more accurate assessment of sleep stages, which is crucial to accurate diagnosis of sleep disorders. Expanding the EEG montage makes identification of sleep stages, sleep spindles, vertex waves, REM sleep, and α-rhythm easier and allows for more accurate **sleep staging.** The international 10-20 system of EEG electrode placement is shown in Figure 29-6.[25]

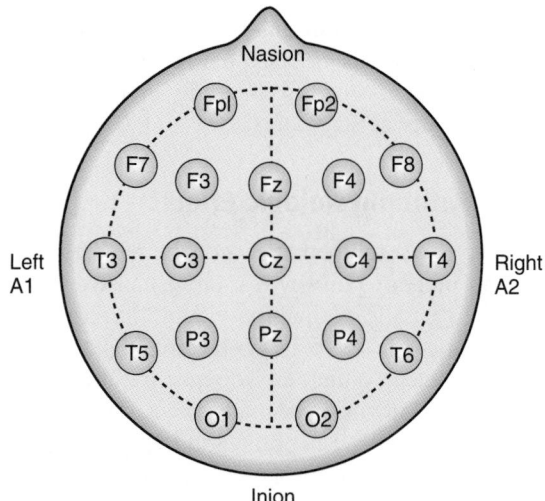

Figure 29-6 Electrencephalographic electrode placement. (Modified from Chokroverty S, editor. Sleep disorders medicine: basic science, technical considerations, and technical aspects. 2nd ed. Boston: Butterworth-Heinemann; 1999.)

The EOG typically is a two-channel montage that allows identification of eye movement. Because there is a difference in electrical potential in the eye in an anteroposterior direction, eye movements can be recorded and used to define different sleep stages.[26] The two-channel EOG allows recognition of phasic rapid eye movements, or REM. These eye movements are the hallmark of REM sleep, which has significant physiologic implications in the respiratory system.

The EMG usually is a one-channel measurement that records tonic and phasic muscle activity in either the submental (chin) muscle or the anterior tibialis muscle of the lower leg. The polysomnogram frequently records a signal in both these muscles. The submental muscle channel is important in the recognition of REM sleep, which results in marked dampening of the signal. The anterior tibialis signal is used to diagnose a sleep disorder known as periodic limb movements of sleep.

The methods used to monitor ventilation and respiratory effort are crucial in PSG, because most sleep studies are ordered when obstructive sleep apnea is suspected. The devices used to monitor ventilation are the most technically difficult aspects of a sleep study. To distinguish obstructive apnea from mixed or central apneic events,

both airflow and respiratory effort must be recorded. Briefly, an **obstructive apnea** is defined as a reduction in airflow to less than 90% of baseline despite persistent respiratory effort. A **central apnea** is a reduction in airflow in concert with no ventilatory effort, and a **mixed apnea** has features of both a central event and an obstructive event.

Airflow most often is measured with thermistors or thermocouplers. A thermistor uses small glass beads or wires with an electrical resistance that changes with temperature changes. Thermocouplers consist of two different types of metals in electrical contact with each other. The signal between the two metals varies as a function of temperature. Both these methods depend on the fact that an exhaled breath is at body temperature (37° C). The breath warms the thermocoupler or thermistor and changes the electrical signal from the device.[27,28] Thermocouplers and thermistors are attached to the patient's face below each nostril and the mouth, because the passage of air during the night varies between the nose and the mouth. The nasal measurements typically are combined and displayed as one reading on the polysomnogram.

CO_2 detectors also can be used to monitor airflow during the night. A small cannula is inserted just inside the nostril

---

CPG 29-1

Polysomnography

Indications

For patients with chronic obstructive pulmonary disease (COPD) whose awake partial pressure of arterial oxygen (Pao_2) is over 55 mm Hg but whose illness is complicated by pulmonary hypertension, right heart failure, polycythemia, or excessive daytime sleepiness

For restrictive ventilatory impairment that occurs secondary to chest wall and neuromuscular disturbances when the illness is complicated by chronic hypoventilation, polycythemia, pulmonary hypertension, disturbed sleep, morning headaches, or daytime somnolence and fatigue

For disturbances in respiratory control in patients whose awake partial pressure of arterial carbon dioxide ($Paco_2$) is over 45 mm Hg or whose illness is complicated by pulmonary hypertension, polycythemia, disturbed sleep, morning headaches, or daytime somnolence and fatigue

For nocturnal cyclic bradyrhythmias or tachyarrhythmias, nocturnal abnormalities of atrioventricular conduction, or ventricular ectopy that appear to increase in frequency during sleep

For excessive daytime sleepiness or insomnia

For snoring associated with observed apneas or excessive daytime sleepiness or both

For other symptoms of sleep-disordered breathing as described in the International Classification of Sleep Disorders

For symptoms of sleep disorders described in the International Classification of Sleep Disorders.

Contraindications

No absolute contraindications to PSG exist when indications are clearly established. However, risk-benefit ratios should be assessed if medically unstable patients are to are transferred from the clinical setting to a sleep laboratory for overnight PSG.

Hazards and Complications

Skin irritation may occur as a result of the adhesive used to attach electrodes to the patient. At the conclusion of the study, adhesive remover is used to dissolve the adhesive on the patient's skin. Adhesive removers (for example, acetone) should be used only in well-ventilated areas. The integrity of the polysomnographic equipment's electrical isolation must be certified by engineering or biomedical personnel qualified to make such assessment. The adhesive used to attach EEG electrodes should not be used to attach electrodes near the patient's eyes and should always be used in well-ventilated areas. Because collodion and acetone are highly inflammable, they should be used with caution, especially in patients requiring supplemental oxygen. Collodion should be used with caution in patients with reactive airways disease and in small infants. Patients with parasomnias or seizures may be at risk of injury related to movements during sleep. Institution-specific policies and guidelines describing personnel responsibilities and appropriate responses should be developed.

Modified from AARC Clinical practice guideline: polysomnography. Respir Care 1995;40:1336-1343.
CPG, Clinical practice guideline; EEG, electroencephalographic; EOG, electrooculogram; EMG, electromyelogram; ECG, electrocardiogram; PSG, polysomnography.

to sample CO_2 throughout the study. A mask may be used to sample the CO_2 content from both nostrils and the mouth. The cannula or mask is connected to an infrared device or mass spectrometer for measurement of the CO_2 level. This method is more accurate than the use of temperature-sensing devices, but the significant increase in cost and technical expertise has limited its use in most sleep centers.[29]

Laryngeal sound monitors record the sound produced from the throat during ventilation. A small stethoscope is taped over the larynx, and the sound recorded is converted to a signal representing airflow.[30] This method is now used when automatically titrating CPAP devices to detect airflow.

The most technically demanding method used to monitor airflow is pneumotachography. This is also the most accurate method, and the only one that truly quantifies ventilation throughout sleep. A tight-fitting face mask is placed on the patient, and a flow-to-pressure transducer is fitted to the mask.[31] The transducer causes significant resistance to airflow and therefore can cause the patient discomfort. Although this method is quite accurate, it can also disrupt sleep and affect the polysomnogram adversely.

Monitoring of the ventilatory effort requires a method of measurement separate from that used for airflow. The importance of these monitors cannot be understated. They define the category of sleep apnea, if present, and therefore greatly affect the type or course of treatment selected. Ventilation most often is monitored with *strain gauges*, which are distensible tubes filled with packed graphite or mercury. The electrical resistance of these compounds is directly related to the length of the tube and inversely related to the cross-sectional area of the tube. The strain gauge is placed over the point of largest chest circumference on inspiration to most accurately monitor effort. The resistance is greatest with inspiration, because it increases the length of the tube while decreasing its diameter.[32] This change in resistance is recorded on the polysomnogram. A second strain gauge should also be placed around the abdomen, because this provides additional information about inspiratory effort and can reflect paradoxical breathing patterns sometimes seen during periods of obstructive sleep apnea. Although these strain gauges are inexpensive and are accurate qualitative measures of ventilatory effort, they require careful positioning and are sensitive to artifact created by patient movement.

A more invasive monitoring device is the esophageal pressure monitor. This monitor is a small catheter with a balloon tip or pressure transducer on the tip that is passed through the nose or mouth into the middle or distal esophagus. The pressure changes measured by this catheter reflect pleural pressure, which is the most accurate measure of ventilatory effort.[33] The obvious problem with this method is its invasiveness and discomfort to the patient.

Impedance pneumography is a technique that involves placement of two electrodes to the chest and the application of a high-frequency signal to the chest wall through the electrodes.[34] The measured impedance between the two electrodes varies as a function of chest wall position. This method is reliable and less sensitive to patient movement than strain gauges.[35] As with strain gauges, two channels should be used to measure both chest and abdominal wall excursion.

Inductive plethysmography is a relatively new method of ventilatory effort monitoring. A wire is sewn into a mesh or elastic band that is placed around the patient's chest (or abdomen). A current is applied to the wire, and the inductance of the wire loop is monitored. As the loop of wire increases with expansion of the chest or abdominal wall, the inductance of the wire changes and is displayed on the polysomnogram.[36] The distinct advantage of this method is that it provides a quantitative measure of ventilatory effort.

Arterial oxygenation is also an important parameter measured during an overnight polysomnogram. It is useful in judgment of the severity of apneic periods, in diagnosis of **hypopnea** (a reduction in airflow to 50% to 90% of baseline), and in monitoring of patients with cardiopulmonary disease. Pulse oximetry is the most commonly used technique to assess a patient's oxygenation status during sleep. Transcutaneous oxygen tension may also be used and frequently is used in infants.[37] However, no studies have shown a significant advantage over pulse oximetry.

Respiratory Recap

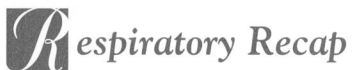

Components of a Polysomnogram	
Electroencephalogram (EEG)	Ventilatory effort
Electrooculogram (EOG)	measurement
Electromyelogram (EMG)	Pulse oximetry
Airflow measurements	Electrocardiogram (ECG)

The ECG is another parameter typically monitored during an overnight sleep study. Arrhythmias in association with sleep-disordered breathing have been described. Common types include bradycardia-tachycardias during an apneic event, premature ventricular contractions (PVCs), and sinus pauses.[38,39] The ECG itself consists of two leads placed over the precordium; however, this limited montage does not allow for assessment of ischemic changes. Any suspicion of a serious cardiac pathologic condition therefore should be evaluated outside the setting of the polysomnogram.

Sleep Scoring

An overnight polysomnogram is more than simple monitoring of all the previously discussed parameters. It must be interpreted as a cohesive test, with attention given to the way each parameter changes in relation to the others. Only by reviewing the test in this fashion can the polysomnographer devise a clinically relevant diagnosis or treatment plan.

A sleep study is scored in several categories. The first is an analysis of the sleep stages. **Sleep efficiency** is defined as the amount of time the patient was asleep per EEG criteria divided by the total recording time. **Sleep latency** is defined as the time from lights-out to when the patient falls asleep. The percentage of time the patient spent in the various stages of sleep also is recorded. By extracting this information from the EEG recording, the polysomnographer can recognize a pattern that may be characteristic for certain disorders.

The next element that is assessed is the number of awakenings or arousals a patient had throughout the night. An *awakening* is defined as a return in the patient's EEG to an awakened state for at least one epoch of recording, or 30 seconds. An *arousal* is not a return to the awakened state but a change in the EEG sleep stage to a different level of consciousness that is not as deep. For example, a patient in slow-wave sleep (stages 3 and 4) who abruptly moves into stage 1 sleep has undergone an arousal. Awakenings and arousals are important because they often accompany or are caused by other pathologic conditions, such as sleep-disordered breathing, restless leg syndrome, psychiatric disorders, and other medical conditions such as gastroesophageal reflux or sinusitis. The number of awakenings or arousals also may reflect the severity of the associated condition. The **arousal index** is the total number of arousals divided by time; this number is expressed in arousals per hour.

Another important parameter recorded in sleep scoring is leg movement. The EMG of the anterior tibialis muscle should be silent while the patient is asleep, except during awakenings or arousals. Pathologic repetitive myoclonic contractions can cause frequent arousals or awakenings and daytime symptoms such as excessive sleepiness. When these myoclonic jerks do cause these EEG findings, the diagnosis of **periodic leg movements of sleep** should be considered.

Respiratory Recap

Terms Related to Cessation of Airflow	
Apnea	Mixed apnea
Central apnea	Obstructive hypopnea
Obstructive apnea	Apnea/hypopnea index

The overwhelming reason to order sleep studies is to diagnose sleep-disordered breathing problems, which include obstructive sleep apnea syndrome and central sleep apnea syndrome (Figure 29-7). The diagnostic criteria for these disorders involve the ventilatory pattern and its relationship to oxygen saturation and awakenings and arousals. The definition of an obstructive apnea is a cessation or reduction in airflow to less than 90% of baseline for at least 10 seconds with persistent respiratory effort. These events often are associated with other physiologic alterations captured by the polysomnogram, which may include significant oxygen desaturation, cardiac arrhythmias, and awakenings or arousals. Airflow obstruction may also occur that does not cause apnea but causes a less marked reduction in airflow; this is called an *obstructive hypopnea*, which is a reduction in airflow to 50% to 90% of baseline despite persistent respiratory effort. A few apneic episodes may occur during sleep in normal individuals, especially during REM

sleep. Because normal young adults have about six to eight REM periods a night, up to 10 apneas during sleep would not be cause for concern. These events must be associated with oxygen desaturation or an EEG arousal to be considered pathologic and be scored in the polysomnogram. A central apnea is a cessation of airflow to less than 90% of baseline as a result of absence of respiratory effort. These events often are seen in patients with neurologic disease or advanced cardiopulmonary disease. A mixed apnea is an apneic event that has features of both a central apnea and an obstructive apnea. These events are most likely obstructive events in their physiologic etiology.

To define the degree of sleep-related breathing disturbance, several parameters have been created that are derived from the polysomnogram. The first value is simply the absolute number of apneas or hypopneas scored throughout the study. This can be useful information but does not give a sense of the degree of severity of disease with relation to the amount of sleep. The **apnea/hypopnea index (AHI),** which is also called the **respiratory disturbance index,** is a better indicator of pathologic sleep-related breathing. This index is a calculated value; it is derived from the total number of apneas plus hypopneas divided by the total amount of sleep throughout the study. It is expressed in terms of events per hour and normally is fewer than five. The severity of sleep apnea syndrome is divided into mild, moderate, and severe based on the apnea/hypopnea index. Although no studies have validated these categories, most polysomnographers use indices of five to 20 events per hour, 20 to 40 events per hour, and more than 40 events per hour, respectively.[3]

Similarly, the degree of arousal and awakening is most commonly expressed in terms of the *arousal index*. This value is derived from the data gathered during the polysomnogram and is simply the number of arousals divided by the total sleep time. This is expressed in arousals per hour and normally should be fewer than 15.[3] Like the apnea/hypopnea index, the arousal index is considered moderately elevated with more than 20 arousals per hour and markedly elevated with more than 40 per hour.

Although these indices are useful in the assessment of the degree of sleep disturbance, they must be used in the context of the entire study. The patient's position during a sleep study can significantly alter these indices, as can the sleep stage. Most important, the positioning of a patient during the polysomnogram can lead to a falsely low apnea/hypopnea index even with severe disease. As discussed previously, the collapse of the upper airway can be caused by many factors, which can lead to airway obstruction and apnea. For some patients, upper airway collapse occurs when lying supine but not when on the side. If a patient is allowed to sleep only on the side during a study, the severity of disease can be markedly underrepresented. For this reason, sleep technicians usually are instructed to make the subject sleep supine for some portion of the study. The apnea/hypopnea index frequently is subdivided into supine and on the side values; this allows the interpreter to comment as to the positional nature of the illness.

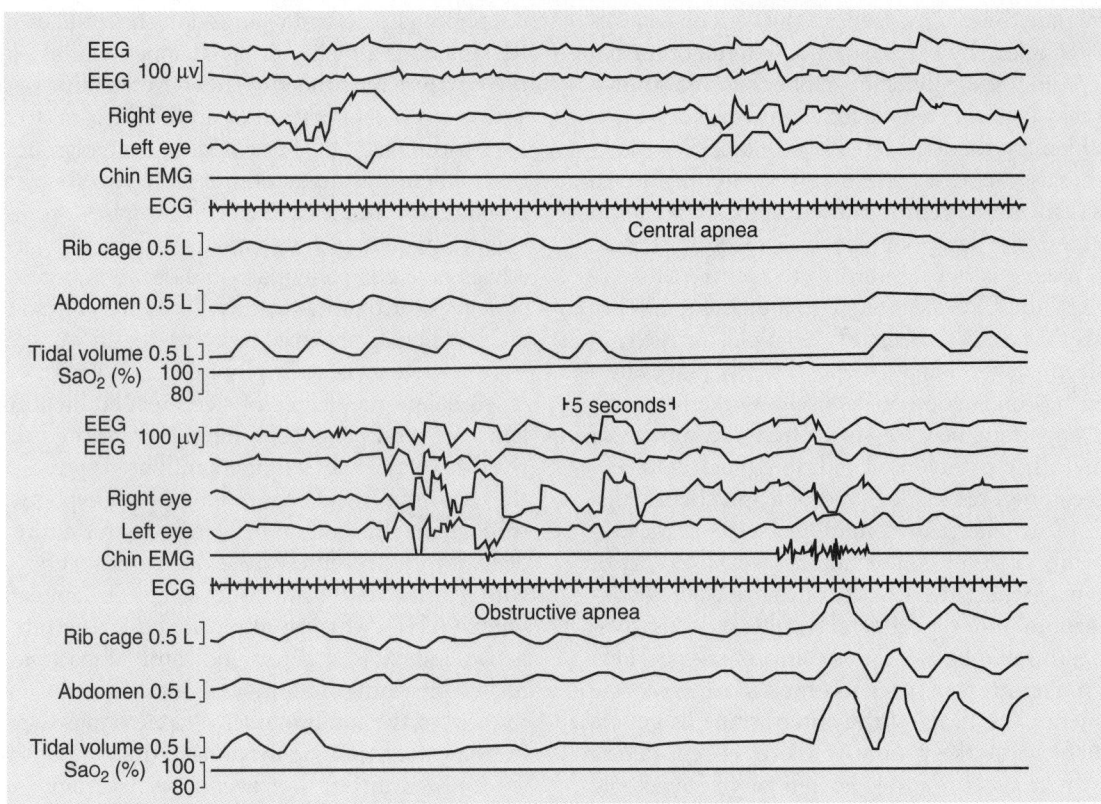

Figure 29-7   Polysomnographic study showing the distinction between central apnea *(top)* and obstructive apnea *(bottom)*. *EEG,* Electroencephalogram; *EMG,* electromyogram; *ECG,* electrocardiogram. (Modified from Phillioson EA, Bowes G. Sleep disorders. New York: McGraw-Hill; 1982.)

The sleep stage can also affect the apnea/hypopnea index. Specifically, REM sleep causes the most significant decrease in upper airway muscular tone, and upper airway collapse may be more pronounced during REM sleep for this reason. Some patients who do not have any obstructive sleep apnea during non-REM sleep may have significant events during REM sleep. Others may simply have increasing events during REM sleep. For this reason, the apnea/hypopnea index also is subdivided into the AHI in non-REM sleep and the AHI in REM sleep.

Like the apnea/hypopnea index, the arousal index is affected by several factors. The most important of these is position. Many patients exhibit snoring, frequent arousals, and possibly oxygen desaturation without frank apnea. This constellation of findings has recently been called *upper airway resistance syndrome.* This syndrome can lead to pathologic hypersomnolence similar to sleep apnea, most likely because of the degree of sleep disruption. Pathophysiologically the syndrome is due to collapse of the upper airway that does not cause complete occlusion and apnea. Many patients have a positional nature to their arousals, such that they worsen when supine because of the increased upper airway collapse. Therefore the arousal index often is subdivided into that when the patient is supine and that when the patient is on the side.

KEY POINTS

- There are many types of sleep disorders, but by far the most common is sleep-disordered breathing.
- The relationship between the respiratory system and the brain is not completely understood.
- Control of ventilation during sleep differs in many important ways from control during wakefulness.
- Although newer technology makes home sleep studies and overnight pulse oximetry possible, the laboratory-based polysomnogram remains the gold standard for diagnosis of sleep-disordered breathing.
- Sleep technologists are trained professionals who are integral to the process of overnight PSG. In many hospitals respiratory therapists function as sleep technologists.

References

1. American Sleep Disorders Association. The international classification of sleep disorders. Rochester, Minn: The Association; 1997.
2. Hauri P. The sleep disorders. Kalamazoo, Mich: Scope; 1983.
3. Radtke R. Sleep disorders: laboratory evaluation. In: Daly DD, Pedley TA, editors. Current practice of clinical electroencephalography. 2nd ed. New York: Raven Press; 1990.

4. Kales A, Kales J. Recent findings in the diagnosis and treatment of disturbed sleep. N Engl J Med 1974;209:487-499.

5. Berger AJ, Mitchell RA, Severinghausen JW. Regulation of respiration. N Engl J Med 1974;297;92-97,138-143, 194-201.

6. Whipp BJ, Wasserman K. Carotid bodies and ventilatory control dynamics in man. Fed Proc 1980;39:2668-2673.

7. Hornbein TF. The relationship between stimulus to chemoreceptors and their response. In: Torrance TW, editor. Arterial chemoreceptors. Oxford, England: Blackwell; 1968.

8. White DP. Central sleep apnea. Med Clin North Am 1985; 69:1205-1219.

9. Loeschcke HH. Central chemosensitivity and the reaction therapy. J Physiol (London) 1982;3321-3324.

10. Bulow K. Respiration and wakefulness in man. Acta Physiol Scand Suppl 1963;59:1.

11. Douglas NJ, White DP, Pickett CK, et al. Respiration during sleep in normal man. Thorax 1982;37:840-844.

12. Hudgel DW, Martin RJ, Johnson B, et al. Mechanics of the respiratory system and breathing during sleep in normal humans. J Appl Physiol 1984;56:133-137.

13. Tabachnik E, Muller NL, Bryant AC, et al. Changes in ventilation and chest wall mechanics during sleep in normal adolescents. J Appl Physiol 1981;51:557-564.

14. Robin ED, Whaley RD, Crump CH, et al. Alveolar gas tension, pulmonary ventilation, and blood pH during physiologic sleep in normal subjects. J Clin Invest 1958;37:981.

15. Goethe B, Altose MD, Gotham MD, et al. Effect of quiet sleep on resting and CO_2-stimulated breathing in humans. J Appl Physiol 1981;50:724-730.

16. Douglas NJ, White DP, Weil JV, et al. Hypercapnic ventilatory response in sleeping adults. Am Rev Respir Dis 1982;126: 758-762.

17. Phillipson EA, Bowes G. Control of breathing during sleep. In: Fishman AF, Cherniack NS, Widdicombe JG, editors. Handbook of physiology. Vol 2. The respiratory system. Bethesda, Md: American Physiologic Society; 1986.

18. Hudgel DW, Devadatta P. Decrease in functional residual capacity during sleep in normal humans. J Appl Physiol 1984; 57:1319-1322.

19. Tusiewicz K, Moldofsky H, Bryan AC, et al. Mechanics of the rib cage and diaphragm during sleep. J Appl Physiol 1977; 43:600-602.

20. Pansky B. Review of gross anatomy. New York: Macmillan; 1984.

21. Sauerland EK, Harper RM. The human tongue during sleep: electromyographic activity of the genioglossus muscle. Exp Neurol 1976;51:160-170.

22. Bartlett D Jr, Leiter JC, Knuth SL. Control and actions of the genioglossus muscle. In: Issa FG, Surrat PM, Remmers JE, editors. Sleep and respiration. New York: John Wiley & Sons; 1990.

23. Tangel DJ, Mezzanotte WS, Sandberg EJ, et al. Influence of sleep on tensor palatini EMG and upper airway resistance in normal men. J Appl Physiol 1991;70:2574-2581.

24. Van Lunteren E. Role of mammalian hyoid muscles in the maintenance of pharyngeal patency. In: Issa FG, Surrat PM, Remmers JE, editors. Sleep and respiration. New York: John Wiley & Sons; 1990.

25. Jasper HH. The 10-20 electrode system of the International Federation. Electroencephalogr Clin Neurophysiol 1958;10:371.

26. Keenan SA. Polysomnographic technique: an overview. In: Chokroverty S, editor. Sleep disorders medicine. Boston: Butterworth-Heinemann; 1999.

27. Broughton RJ. Polysomnography: principles and applications in sleep and arousal disorders. In: Niedemeyer E, Lopes de Silva F, editors. Electroencephalography. Baltimore: Urban & Schwarzenberg; 1988.

28. Block AJ, Cohn MA, Conway WA, et al. Indications and standards for cardiopulmonary sleep studies. Sleep 1985;8:371-391.

29. Howard GF. Laboratory assessment of sleep and related functions. In: Riley TL, editor. Clinical aspects of sleep and sleep disturbance. Boston: Butterworth-Heinemann; 1985.

30. Krumpe PE, Cummisky JM. Use of laryngeal sound recordings to monitor apnea. Am Rev Resp Dis 1980;122:797-801.

31. Sullivan WJ, Petters GM, Enright PL. Pneumotachographs: theory and clinical applications. Respir Care 1984;29:736-749.

32. Sackner MA. Diagnostic techniques in pulmonary disease. New York: Marcel Dekker; 1980.

33. Hurewitz AN, Sidhu U, Bergofsky EH, et al. How alterations in pleural pressure influence esophageal pressure. J Appl Physiol 1984;56:1162-1169.

34. Ashutosh K, Gilbert R, Auchincloss JH, et al. Impedance pneumography and magnetometer methods for monitoring tidal volume. J Appl Physiol 1974;37:964-966.

35. Pacela AF. Impedance pneumography: a survey of instrumentation techniques. Med Biol Eng 1966;4:1-15.

36. Cohn M. Respiratory monitoring during sleep: respiratory inductive plethysmography. In: Guilleminault C, editor. Sleeping and waking disorders: indications and techniques. Menlo Park, Calif: Addison-Wesley; 1982.

37. Schoemaker WC, Vidyasagar D. Physiological and clinical significance of $PtcO_2$ and $PtcCO_2$ measurements. Crit Care Med 1981;9:689-690.

38. Miller WP. Cardiac arrhythmias and conduction disturbance in the sleep apnea syndrome: prevalance and significance. Am J Med 1982;73:317-321.

39. Guilleminault C, Connolly SJ, Winkle RA. Cardiac arrhythmias and conduction disturbance during sleep in 400 patients with sleep apnea syndrome. Am J Cardiol 1983;52:490-494.

CHAPTER 30

Infant Apnea Monitoring

Bruce E. Estrem

CHAPTER OUTLINE

Infant Apnea
Diagnosing Apnea with Multichannel Recordings
Managing the Infant with Apnea
Guidelines for Home Apnea Monitoring
Problems in Home Apnea Monitoring

Discontinuation of Home Apnea Monitoring
Technical Aspects of Apnea Monitors
Other Types of Monitors
Role of the Respiratory Therapist in Apnea Monitoring

OBJECTIVES

1. List causes of infant apnea.
2. Discuss the management of the infant with apnea.
3. Discuss guidelines for home apnea monitoring.
4. Discuss problems associated with home apnea monitoring.
5. Describe the technical aspects of apnea monitors.
6. Discuss the role of the respiratory therapist in apnea monitoring.

KEY TERMS

Apnea
Apparent Life-Threatening Event (ALTE)
Apnea of Infancy
Apnea of Prematurity (AOP)
Central Apnea
Documented Event Monitoring (DEM)

Durable Medical Equipment (DME)
Infant Apnea Program
Mixed Apnea
Münchausen Syndrome by Proxy
National Association of Apnea Professionals (NAAP)

Obstructive Apnea
Pathologic Apnea
Periodic Breathing
Pneumogram
Polysomnogram
Sudden Infant Death Syndrome (SIDS)

Home breathing monitoring of newborns has been a widely accepted form of care for more than 20 years and has become increasingly popular. Approximately 45,000 babies are monitored annually.[1] Such home-based monitoring has been called *sudden infant death (SIDS) monitoring, apnea monitoring, cardiopulmonary monitoring, documented monitoring,* and *infant home monitoring.*

Infant Apnea

Sudden infant death syndrome (SIDS) was recognized in the 1800s but did not receive close attention until 1972, when a medical paper reported that two of five infants with documented prolonged sleep apnea had died of SIDS.[2] As a result, in the 1970s a great deal of attention was paid to the relationship between **apnea,** or the cessation of respiratory airflow, and SIDS. Over the next three decades, the use of monitors in the home to detect apnea expanded.[3] Although many hypotheses have been formu-

lated to explain why SIDS remains the foremost medical cause of death during the first year of life after the neonatal period, some facts have become known (Box 30-1). SIDS is a definitive medical entity that can be diagnosed only by a medical investigation at autopsy. It occurs in one to two infants per 1000 live births[4] and shows no predilection for race, nationality, or geography.

The evidence suggests that home monitoring of *low-risk* (asymptomatic) SIDS patients does not reduce, prevent, or affect the incidence of death, and therefore it is not rec-

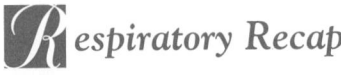

Respiratory Recap

Diagnoses Appropriate for Home Apnea Monitoring	
Pathologic apnea	Apparent life-threatening
Periodic breathing	event
Apnea of prematurity	Apnea of infancy

Box 30-1

Important Facts about Sudden Infant Death Syndrome

SIDS Is Not

Hereditary	Preventable, in most cases
Contagious	Predictable
Caused by smoking	

Box 30-2

Definitions Associated with Apnea

Apnea is cessation of respiratory airflow. The respiratory pause may be central or diaphragmatic (that is, no respiratory effort is made), obstructive (usually caused by upper airway obstruction), or mixed. Short episodes of central apnea (15 seconds or less) are considered normal at all ages.

Pathologic Apnea
An abnormal respiratory pause that lasts 20 seconds or longer or is associated with cyanosis; abrupt, marked pallor or hypotonia; or bradycardia

Periodic Breathing
A breathing pattern that includes three or more respiratory pauses longer than 3 seconds with less than 20 seconds of respiration between pauses; can be a normal event

Apnea of Prematurity (AOP)
Periodic breathing with pathologic apnea in a premature infant; usually ends by 37 weeks' gestation but occasionally persists for several weeks past term

Apparent Life-Threatening Event (ALTE)
An episode that is frightening to the observer and is characterized by some combination of apnea (central or obstructive), color change, marked change in muscle tone (limpness), choking, or gagging; previously used terms that have been abandoned include *aborted crib death* and *near-miss SIDS*

Apnea of Infancy
An unexplained episode of cessation of breathing lasting 20 seconds or longer, or a shorter respiratory pause associated with bradycardia, cyanosis, pallor, and/or marked hypotonia; generally refers to infants older than 37 weeks' gestational age at the onset of pathologic apnea and should be reserved for infants for whom no specific cause of an ALTE can be identified

Box 30-3

Causes of Apnea

Decreased oxygen delivery: hypoxemia, anemia, shock, cardiac shunting
Cardiac arrhythmia
Central nervous system disease: asphyxia and cerebral edema, hemorrhage, seizures, congenital defects
Drugs: maternal narcotics, fetal narcotics, poisoning, intentional administration of medicine (sedatives, antihistamines, analgesics), alcohol
Metabolic diseases: hypoglycemia, hypocalcemia, hyponatremia, dehydration, hyperammonemia
Thermal instability
Idiopathic apnea of prematurity
Intentional injury: child abuse, Münchausen syndrome by proxy
Gastroesophageal reflux
Central hypoventilation syndrome

whose birth weight is less than 1500 g. The prevalence is higher at lower gestational ages and may be the result of an immature respiratory control system, manifested by frequent periodic breathing, decreased ventilatory response to carbon dioxide (CO_2), and depression of respiration caused by hypoxemia.[7] Approximately half of all apneic episodes in premature infants involve some degree of upper airway obstruction, which indicates that respiratory muscle output and coordination are also disturbed.

Other types of apneic episodes may occur secondary to environmental surroundings or to other disease processes, which could include infection, central nervous system disorders, decreased metabolic oxygen delivery (heart or circulatory disorders), drugs, metabolic diseases, thermal instability, and gastroesophageal reflux (GER) (Box 30-3). Some research has linked GER to apnea through bronchospasm and laryngospasm secondary to acid irritation of the esophagus.[8,9]

Resolution of apnea of prematurity or apnea of infancy is determined by maturation of the respiratory control center, which appears to be most delayed in infants delivered at the youngest gestational age. Data suggest that maturation of respiratory control occurs in tandem with other measures of physiologic maturity, including coordination of suck and swallow and regulation of temperature.[10] Resolution of other types of apnea depends on treatment of the underlying disease process that includes apnea as a symptom.

Diagnosing Apnea with Multichannel Recordings

The diagnosis of apnea or other sleep disorders can be verified with one of many types of recording devices. These recordings may last from 8 to 24 hours or longer, depending on the device's storage capacity. The type and amount

ommended.[5] Diagnoses appropriate for the use of home apnea monitors are pathologic apnea, periodic breathing, **apnea of prematurity (AOP)**, **apparent life-threatening event (ALTE)**, and **apnea of infancy.** The National Institutes of Health established definitions for these categories during a consensus conference in October 1986,[6] and these definitions remain the international standards (Box 30-2).

Apnea of prematurity (AOP) occurs in approximately 50% of preterm infants born before 32 weeks gestation

of information recorded is based on the number of recording channels available. Historically, event recorders document two channels, which include the patient's cardiac (ECG) signal and chest wall motion (breathing). Other channels may be added to include pulse oximetry, nasal-oral airflow, esophageal pH or pressure, capnography, chest and abdominal strain gauge, snoring microphone, electroencephalography (EEG), eye movement, leg and intercostal muscle movements, torso position, video surveillance, and sound recording.[11]

Documented event monitoring (DEM) is a digital recording of chest wall impedance (channel 1), heart rate (channel 2), and oxygen saturation (channel 3). The duration of recording is limited only by the device's memory capacity. Indications for DEM include the following:

- To evaluate monitor alarms or to verify the presence or absence of events of central apnea, bradycardia, and oxygen desaturation
- To define the relationship between events (for example, central apnea associated with bradycardia and/or desaturation)
- To document compliance with home monitor use
- To evaluate isolated events of oxygen desaturation
- To evaluate the effectiveness of methylxanthine treatment

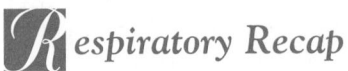

Respiratory Recap

Values Measured in Documented Event Monitoring
Channel 1: Chest wall impedance
Channel 2: Heart rate
Channel 3: Oxygen saturation

A **pneumogram** (Figure 30-1) is a 12- to 24-hour recording of the heart rate (channel 1), respiratory impedance (channel 2), oxygen saturation (channel 3), nasal-oral airflow (channel 4), and esophageal pH (channel 5). Indications for a pneumogram include the following:

- To record the heart rate, respiratory rate, oxygen desaturation, and airflow thermistry for detection of central apnea, obstructive apnea, bradycardia, oxygen desaturation
- To evaluate baseline oxygen saturation
- To determine whether oxygen desaturation is associated with periodic breathing
- To quantitate periodic breathing

Respiratory Recap

Values Measured in a Pneumogram
Channel 1: Heart rate
Channel 2: Respiratory impedance
Channel 3: Oxygen saturation
Channel 4: Nasal-oral airflow
Channel 5: Esophageal pH

A multichannel respiratory recording (sleep study) is an 8- to 24-hour comprehensive recording that includes all pneumogram variables plus capnography, chest and abdominal strain gauges, esophageal pH or pressure, and a snoring microphone. Indications include the following:

- To distinguish central apnea from obstructive apnea
- To screen for obstructive sleep apnea (OSA) or upper airway resistance syndrome (UARS)
- To define the relationship between apnea, bradycardia, desaturation, and GER (pH probe)
- To evaluate saturation of oxygen-dependent infants and children
- To evaluate changes in treatment with respiratory disease (for example, adjustment or discontinuation of oxygen or tracheostomy decannulation)
- To evaluate the function of phrenic pacemakers
- To evaluate the respiratory status or positioning requirement for patients at high risk of airway obstruction (for example, those with craniofacial anomalies or GER)
- To further evaluate patients with abnormal DEM or pneumogram results

A **polysomnogram** is an 8- to 24-hour comprehensive recording done in the special diagnostics laboratory. In addition to all the multichannel respiratory variables, EEG, electrooculography (EOG), and electromyography (EMG) electrodes are used to determine sleep states and leg and intercostal muscle movements. Polysomnograms typically are performed on children and adults but not on infants. Indications include the following:

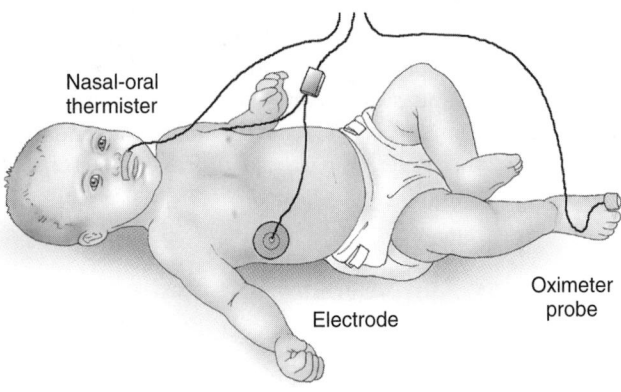

Figure 30-1 Positioning of equipment on the patient for pneumogram monitoring. (Modified from Pediatric Home Service. Apnea monitoring. Roseville, Minn: Pediatric Home Service; 1994.)

- To provide definitive diagnosis of OSA or narcolepsy
- To evaluate sleep state disturbances
- To determine the effectiveness of OSA treatment or to refine treatment (such as addition of continuous positive airway pressure [CPAP] or mask ventilation)
- To evaluate the relationship of sleep disturbances to seizures or GER
- To document the presence or absence of OSA in patients with enlarged tonsils or adenoids
- To document the absence of OSA after ear, nose, and throat or craniofacial surgery
- To evaluate other abnormalities

Clinicians assess a patient based on a review of the information provided by the recording device. However, programs differ in the way the data are analyzed, scored, and interpreted. Even with the corroboration of an observer during the study, physiologic data can be difficult to interpret because of movement artifact, scoring guidelines that may vary from institution to institution, and the amount of data collected (that is, the number of channels used). Even with the assistance of algorithms and computerized scoring systems, analysis first requires the consensus of the criteria used by the computer.[12]

Apnea is defined as the cessation of airflow. When airflow has stopped for 20 seconds or longer and is accompanied by bradycardia, with a heart rate reduction of 20% below baseline, or oxygen saturation below 80%, it may be considered **pathologic apnea.** When data gathered during a study are analyzed, the terms used to define apnea are *central apnea, obstructive apnea, mixed apnea,* and *periodic breathing* (Figure 30-2).[13] **Central apnea** is loss of diaphragmatic and other respiratory muscle function, resulting in cessation of respiratory effort. Short periods of apnea, 15 seconds or less, can be normal at any age.[14] **Obstructive apnea** is cessation of airflow despite continuous chest or abdominal wall movement. **Mixed apnea** is the combination of central and obstructive apnea. **Periodic breathing** is a pattern of regular respiration of up to

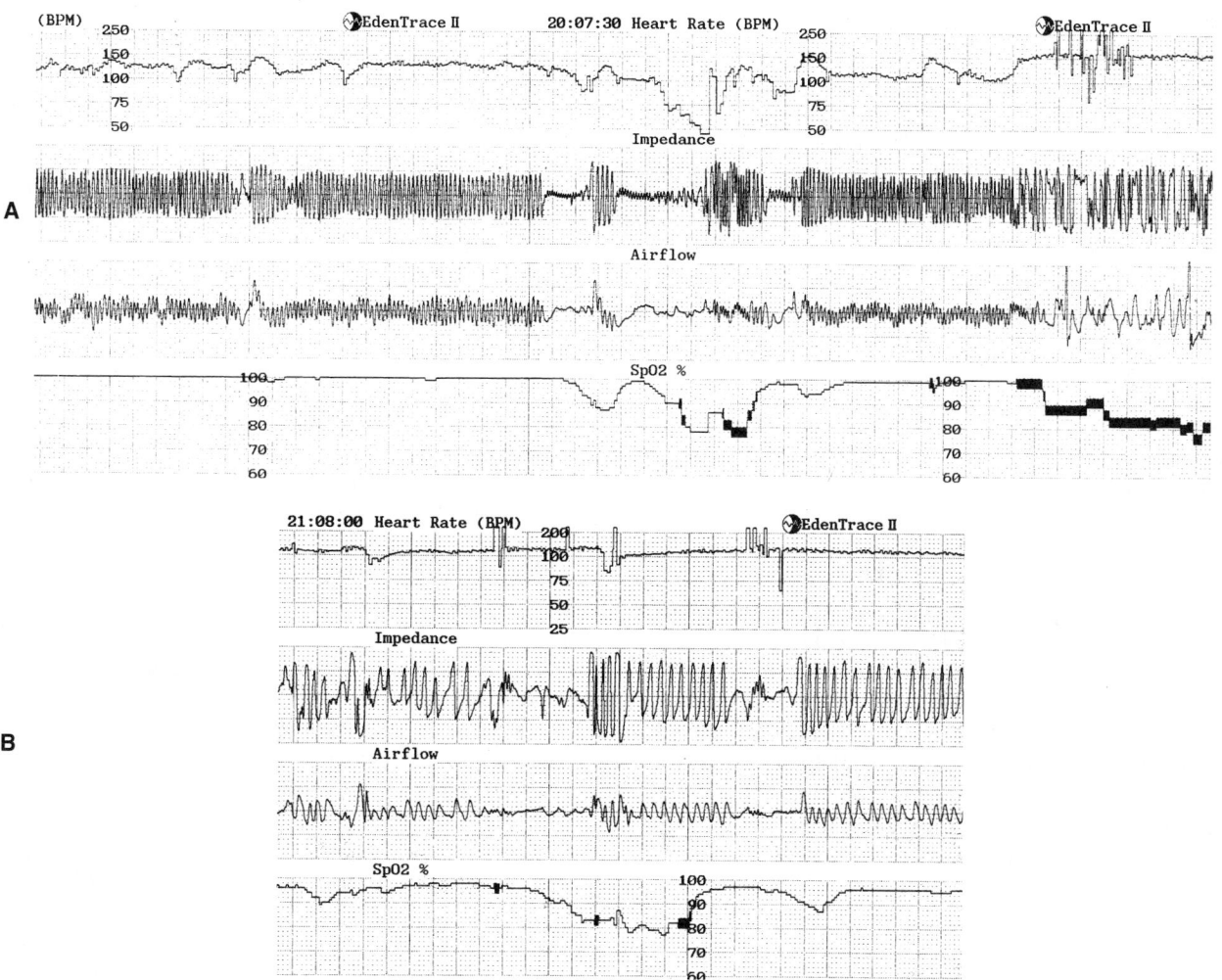

Figure 30-2 Four-channel pneumogram recording showing an 11-second episode of central apnea **(A)** followed by a 20-second period of mixed apnea and two obstructive events **(B)**.

Continued

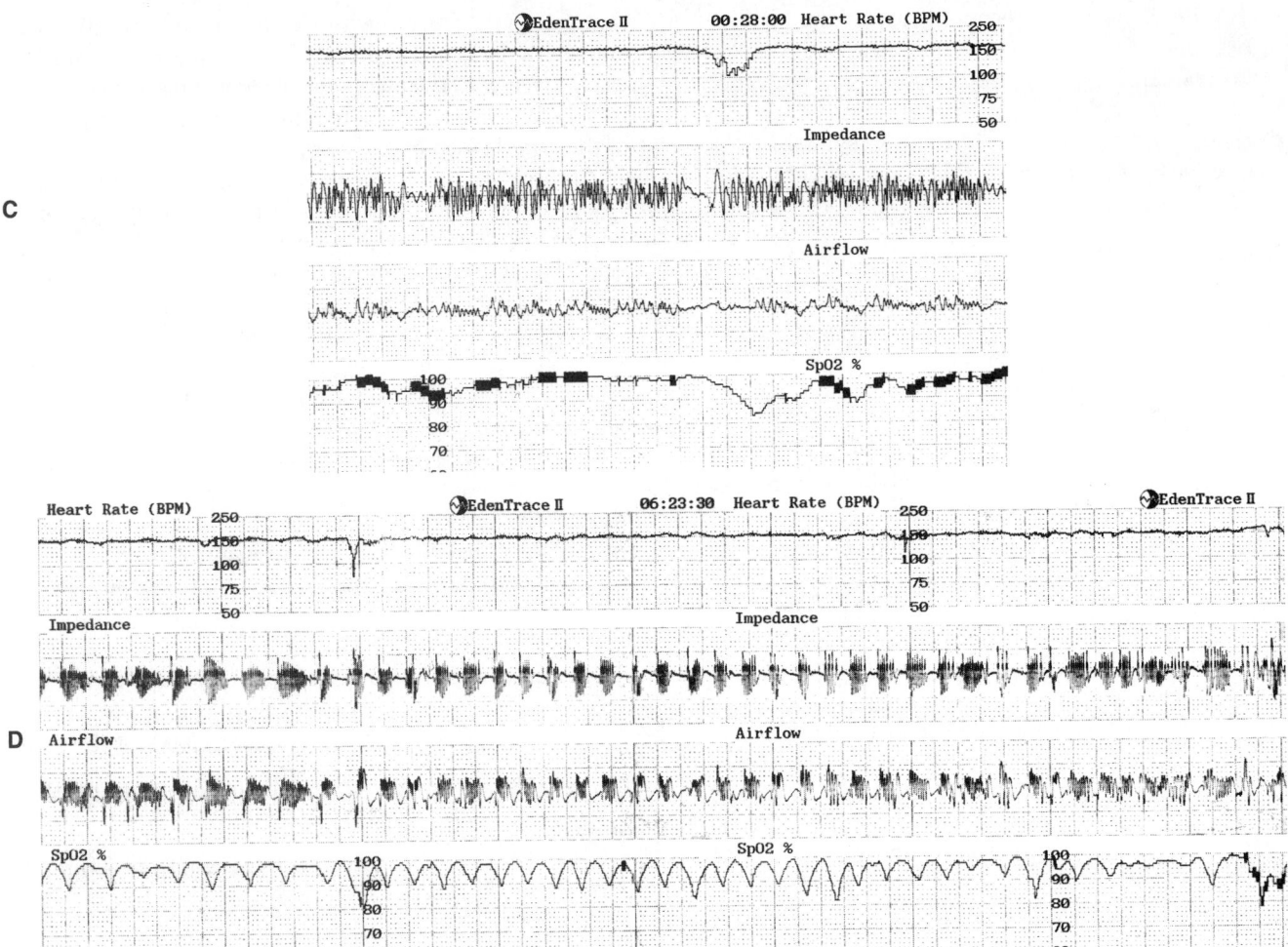

Figure 30-2—cont'd   Mixed apnea **(C)** and periodic breathing **(D)**. (Courtesy Pediatric Home Service, Roseville, Minn.)

20 seconds followed by apneic periods of no more than 10 seconds occurring three times or more in succession. This may be a normal event for some patients.

Managing the Infant with Apnea

After diagnosis through an appropriate study, an individual care plan for the patient is formulated. Several considerations must be taken into account, including the patient's medical history, age, social environment, and geographic location after discharge. Guidelines have been developed to establish a care plan for home-monitored patients.[13,15-17] For example, a home monitor should not be prescribed without appropriate evaluation or follow-up. The purpose of monitoring is to detect untoward physiologic events. Monitoring does not prevent SIDS, and apnea without associated significant bradycardia or desaturation is inconsequential.[18]

The most common diagnoses for home monitoring[5,18] are AOP, ALTE, sibling of an infant who died of SIDS, and GER. Other less common diagnoses are bronchiolitis, respiratory syncytial virus (RSV) infection, pertussis, seizures,

airway anomalies, airway foreign body, sepsis (viral or bacterial), and metabolic disorders. Specific guidelines have been established to evaluate the most commonly monitored patients; these guidelines involve determination of the type of test or tests to be performed and the specific scoring criteria for each test; elimination of unnecessary admissions or evaluations through use of outpatient clinics and overnight home testing and recording; reductions in the length of stay for patients who need to be admitted to the sleep laboratory for testing or who have not previously been discharged; and reductions in parental stress through detailed explanations of what is to be done and in what time frame. A flowchart has been formulated to visually represent the course of care and available options (Figure 30-3). Similar guidelines have been established for AOP patients.

Infants whose postconceptual age is under 34 weeks are evaluated with a 12-hour, three-channel pneumogram. If the infant tests positive for AOP, methylxanthines may be used. Theophylline is used only in the hospital because of its short half-life and the required increased frequency of administration. If methylxanthines have been recommended, the parents receive in-depth instruction on its use and dosage before discharge. Caffeine is given at a

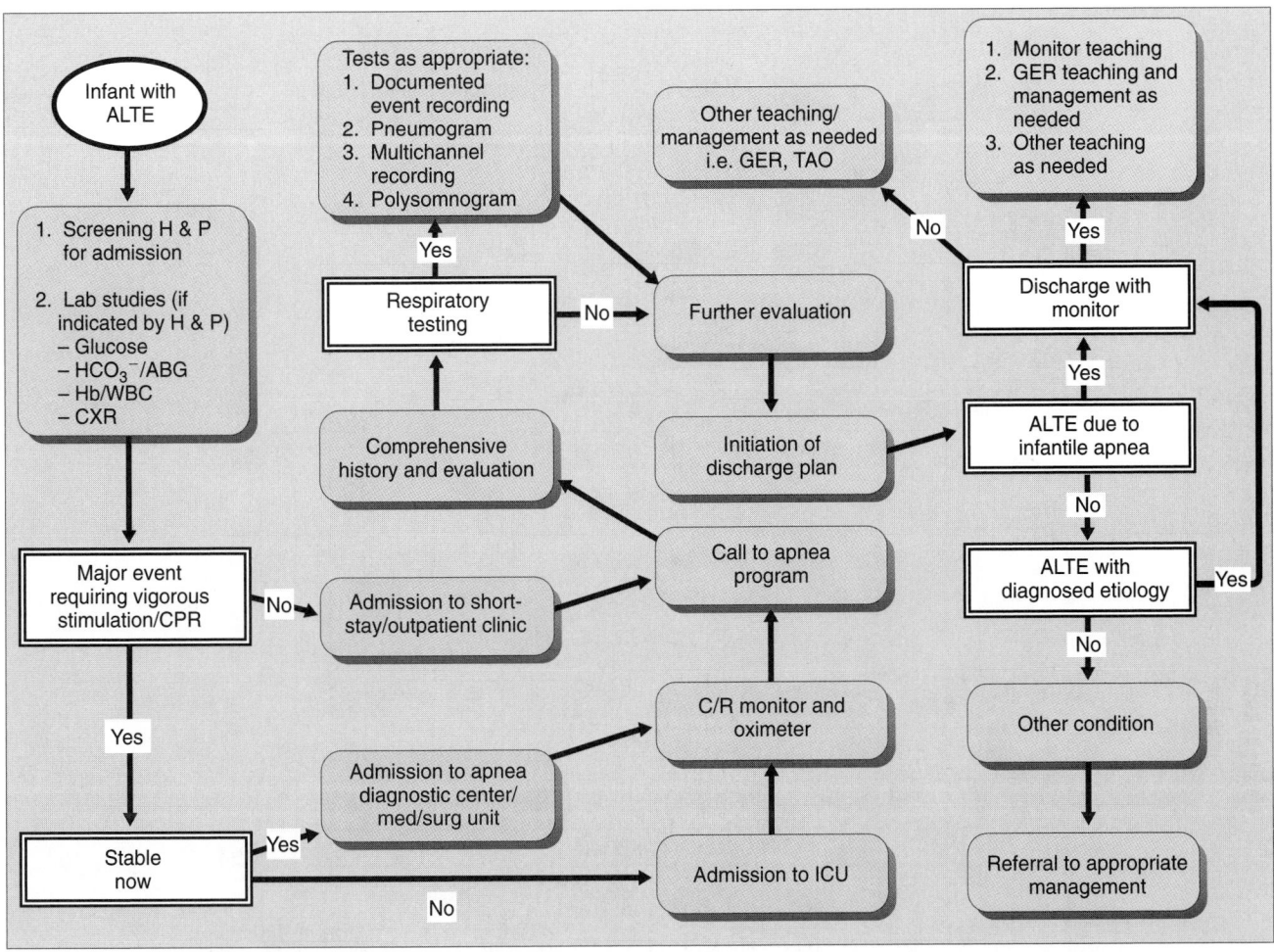

Figure 30-3 Flowchart for management of an apparent life-threatening event. *H & P,* History and physical exam; *WBC,* white blood cell; *CXR,* chest x-ray; *CPR,* cardiopulmonary resuscitation; *ALTE,* apparent life-threatening event; *GER,* gastroesophageal reflux; *ABG,* arterial blood gas. (Modified from Children's Hospitals and Clinics. A parent guide to home monitoring: infant apnea program. St. Paul, Minn: Children's Hospitals and Clinics; 1994.)

loading dose of 30 mg/kg and a maintenance dosage of 6 mg/kg/day to maintain a serum caffeine level of 8 to 20 μg/mL. Levels below 3.5 μg/mL are subtherapeutic and do not positively affect the patient's breathing patterns, heart rate, or saturation. This practice is in line with recommendations made by Miller and Martin.[19] Experience has shown that when caffeine administration is discontinued, the serum caffeine level falls into the subtherapeutic range in only 7 days, therefore reevaluation of the serum caffeine level after discontinuation typically is not needed. In addition, the maintenance of a therapeutic serum caffeine level in patients older than 44 weeks postconceptual age is difficult because of maturing metabolic rates. All infants requiring methylxanthine therapy in the home also require home monitoring.

Siblings of infants who died of SIDS but who have no medical symptoms are considered low risk for SIDS and are not recommended for monitoring.[16] Counseling should be offered to the parents, with information available from the American Sudden Infant Death Institute. Home monitoring is recommended for SIDS siblings only when parents exhibit extreme anxiety. SIDS is an uncommon diagnosis in two or more siblings; if this situation arises, other possibilities should be considered, including infanticide, **Münchausen syndrome by proxy,** or other diagnoses not usually considered in siblings.[20] Documented monitoring becomes even more important in this situation to provide the ordering physician with as much information as possible about alarms or events in the home and compliance with home monitor use.

Because documented monitors have the greatest potential to provide accurate and objective data about alarm conditions, rather than reliance on the observations of the primary care provider, all home monitors should be capable of capturing and storing significant events for later analysis, as well as compliance data (Figure 30-4).[21] Documenting monitors with phone modem downloading capabilities allow for timely evaluation of reported events. The

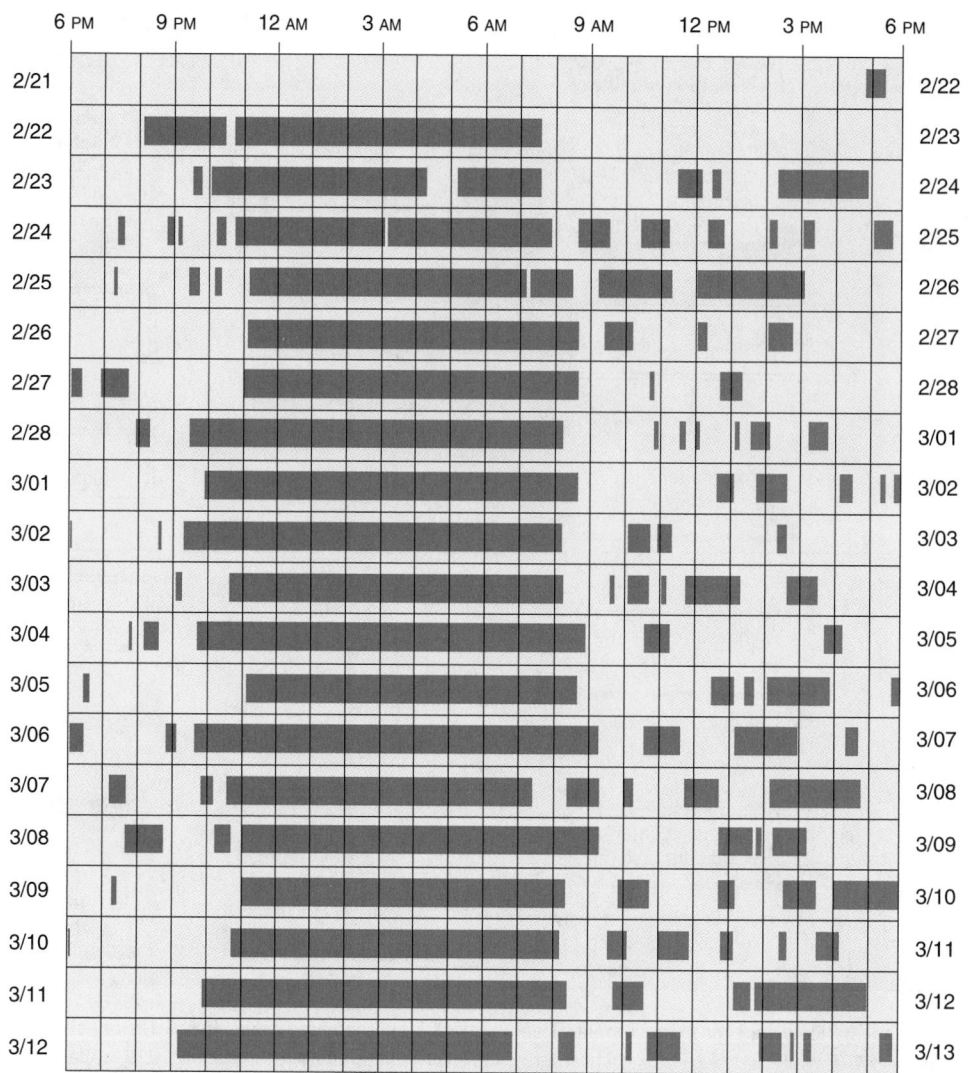

Figure 30-4   Typical compliance report for use of a home apnea monitor. (Modified from Children's Hospitals and Clinics. A parent guide to home monitoring: infant apnea program. St. Paul, Minn: Children's Hospitals and Clinics; 1994; and Pediatric Home Service. Apnea monitoring. Roseville, Minn: Pediatric Home Service; 1994.)

most significant events recorded at home occur within the first month of monitoring.[15] Access to the clinical information, and more than likely capture of one or more of those events electronically, has an immediate effect on the care and management of the patient.

Documented monitors have also reduced the overall time a patient requires a monitor. Hunt[17] reports that the use of documented monitors permits discontinuation of the home monitor a median of 6.6 weeks sooner and reduces the number of unnecessary diagnostic studies compared with patients using undocumented monitors. This analysis indicates that the total cost per patient of using documented monitors is actually less than that of nondocumented monitors. Some insurance providers do not recognize the potential long-term cost savings of documented monitor use, and the equipment provider and apnea program instructors need to educate insurance case managers in the benefits of documented monitors.

Enrollment of the patient in a managed apnea program has shown promise in reduction of the overall time that home monitors are used (Table 30-1).[21,22] Managed apnea programs have the benefit of close evaluation of the patient's progress, growth, and development and also compliance with use and offer consultation services for the patient's primary physician, who may have limited experience with monitored patients. In managed programs, the information from the documented monitor commonly is downloaded on a routine basis.

Guidelines for Home Apnea Monitoring

Proper instruction for home monitor use should emphasize two points: (1) use and application of the monitor and related equipment and (2) the proper response to an alarm, including training in cardiopulmonary resuscita-

TABLE 30-1

Duration of Monitoring with and without an Apnea Management Program

Diagnosis	Patients Enrolled in Management Program (Days)	Patients Not Enrolled in Management Program (Days)
Apnea of prematurity	67	100
Apparent life-threatening event	69	91
Gastroesophageal reflux	70	82
Sibling of child who died of sudden infant death syndrome	163	187

tion (CPR). Other areas covered include how and when to administer methylxanthines; how and when the recording device is downloaded; when the monitor is to be used and when it is acceptable not to connect the child; where to place the monitor to reduce the potential for electrical interference; and how to complete the alarm record log sheet (Figure 30-5).

Full, accurate information consistent with the family's learning style should be provided, including the treatment of apnea, the advantages and limitations of monitoring, and the specifics of the infant's condition. Before discharge the patient's family should be able to explain or demonstrate the following[23]:

- Why the monitor is recommended
- The prognosis of the underlying condition and the goals to be achieved before the monitor is discontinued
- How to use the monitor
- How to attach the monitor correctly to the infant
- Where to place the monitor and how to care for the unit at home
- What each alarm and signal emitted by the monitor means
- When to use the monitor and when it is acceptable not to use it
- When to call for help and who should be called for particular problems (for example, clinical questions, emergencies, supplies or equipment malfunction)

Respiratory Recap

Points to Cover in Family Education for Home Apnea Monitoring

Technical aspects of home monitoring	Appropriate monitor use
	Alarm response
Rationale for home monitoring	Record keeping
	Infant cardiopulmonary
Apnea and its relationship to SIDS	resuscitation
	Aid of the obstructed infant

- How to properly assess the infant's pulse and respiration
- How to respond to monitor alarms
- CPR appropriate to the patient's age
- How to monitor the patient when not at home (for example, during car travel, stroller walks, or other means of travel)

The **National Association of Apnea Professionals (NAAP)** suggests that organizations that provide care for infants with apnea and related disorders should not release monitors for use at home until they are reasonably satisfied that at least one of the infant's caregivers is capable of performing the steps listed above. Inability of the caregivers to learn about monitoring and care of the infant with a high-risk condition is sufficient grounds to delay discharge or temporary placement in foster care.[23]

Specific operating instructions, including how to set the alarm parameters, program the memory device, and maintain the equipment, should be obtained from the manufacturer of the selected device. The manufacturer's recommendations for parent education usually accompany the monitor, although slight variations may be made to accommodate the patient's specific needs. In most circumstances the child is linked to the monitor either with reusable carbon electrodes secured by a belt wrapped around the child's torso or by adhesive electrodes that secure without a belt (Figure 30-6). It is important to secure the lead wires that attach the electrode to the patient cable, ensuring that the wire and electrode connected to the right and left side of the torso are in the sockets of the patient cable labeled "right axillary" and "left axillary." Failure to attach the equipment correctly may result in false cardiac alarms.

Respiratory Recap

Placement of Apnea Monitor Electrodes

1. Secure lead wires to cable correctly.
2. Place electrodes on opposite sides of torso.
3. Adjust electrode position to area of greatest respiratory movement.

CHILDREN'S HOSPITALS AND CLINICS—St. Paul, Minn.

Date •																				
< Time AM/PM •																				
Number of beeps •																				
BABY																				
Awake																				
Asleep																				
Feeding																				
Position:																				
On back																				
On stomach																				
On side																				
Sitting																				
Normal color																				
Pale																				
Dusky																				
Blue																				
Red/purple																				
Normal breathing																				
Shallow breathing																				
No breathing																				
Couldn't tell																				
LIGHTS																				
Apnea																				
Heart rate slow																				
Heart rate fast																				
RESPONSE																				
A None—baby fine																				
B None—baby observed to self-correct																				
C Touch																				
D Gentle stimulation																				
E Vigorous stimulation																				
CPR																				
Obstructed airway																				
INITIALS																				

Figure 30-5 Monitoring record.

Placement of the electrodes on the patient is very important. The electrodes should be positioned slightly below the midnipple line, aligned with the midaxillary area. The electrodes must be on opposite sides of the torso, or false apnea alarms may result. One suggestion is to look at the patient's breathing pattern and observe the patient's chest movements during normal resting respiration, and then position the electrodes over the area that is moving. If the child is predominantly an abdominal breather, the electrodes may need to be moved down. If the child

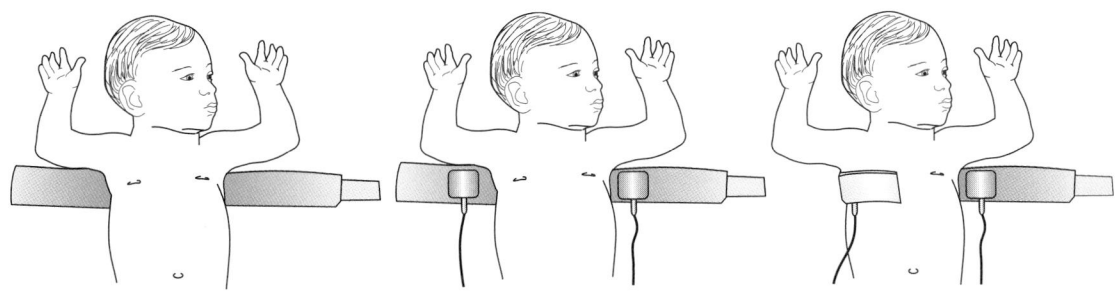

Figure 30-6   Preparing the baby for monitoring. (Modified from Children's Hospitals and Clinics. A parent guide to home monitoring: infant apnea program. St. Paul, Minn: Children's Hospitals and Clinics; 1994; and Pediatric Home Service. Apnea monitoring. Roseville, Minn: Pediatric Home Service; 1994.)

breathes with upper torso movement, placement higher on the chest wall may be warranted. A ground wire, usually connected with an adhesive electrode to the leg, is optional and reserved for patients experiencing significant electrical interference or for use during diagnostic studies.

The times the monitor is to be in use should be discussed in detail and should follow the patient's specific care plan. Parents and other care providers should be instructed to keep the child connected to the monitor at all times unless the child is in direct observation by the care provider. Time on the monitor should include all sleep times (naps, night, or any unexpected sleep), car rides, stroller walks, or other times when the care provider could be distracted by events, including siblings, phone calls, or household activities. Parents should understand that the purpose of the monitor is to constantly evaluate the child for unexpected physiologic events. The monitor watches the child when they are unable to do so.

Home apnea monitors consist of audible and visual human and mechanical alarms to alert the care provider of an event. During response training, the instructor must emphasize that all alarms, mechanical or human, must be acted on with the intention to correct a potentially life-threatening event. Human alarms include apnea, bradycardia, tachycardia, and, on some monitors, slow breath rate. Equipment alarms include low or insufficient battery power, parameter or on/off tampering, and loose wire or patient disconnect; a loose wire or patient disconnect is by far the most common alarm. Troubleshooting guidelines should be demonstrated in detail during instruction on the use of the equipment.

Respiratory Recap

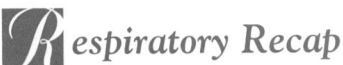

Types of Monitor Alarms
Human alarms
Equipment alarms

Alarm response training must be completed before the patient is discharged from the hospital or leaves the outpatient clinic (Figure 30-7). The care provider must be able to attend to the child within 10 seconds of the onset of the alarm.[14]

The patient should be observed for color in good lighting. If the infant's color is normal, chest movement and air passage through the nose should be observed. The infant's activity level should also be assessed, including movement, sleeping, eating, stretching, wakefulness, or alertness. If a patient assessment reveals the child to be normal, then troubleshooting of the monitor and electrode connections may be warranted. If the patient assessment reveals the child to be in distress, pale, blue, or in some other way of abnormal appearance, the child should be gently stimulated. If the response is not positive, more vigorous stimulation should be performed, including rubbing the patient's back, tapping the bottom of the feet, and loud, vocal stimulation. Age-appropriate CPR should begin if the patient does not respond to aggressive stimulation.[14]

Respiratory Recap

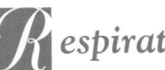

Responses to an Apnea Alarm
1. Rehearse response plan before hospital discharge.
2. Observe infant.
3. Assess infant's activity.
4. Stimulate infant if indicated.
5. Begin CPR if indicated.

A 24-hour-a-day contact number must be available to the caregiver in the event that questions and problems arise. The caregiver should understand whom and when to call for emergency or nonemergency assistance. This information can save frustration and ensure the most appropriate health care for the infant as needed.[6,14] It also is recommended that a member of the apnea program do a phone call follow-up 24 to 48 hours after discharge.[14] A regular and routine follow-up program should be established that may involve phone calls, downloading of documented monitors, and clinic visits or home visits by either the equipment provider or an apnea program team member. During these visits the team member should discuss clinical, technical, and social issues related to moni-

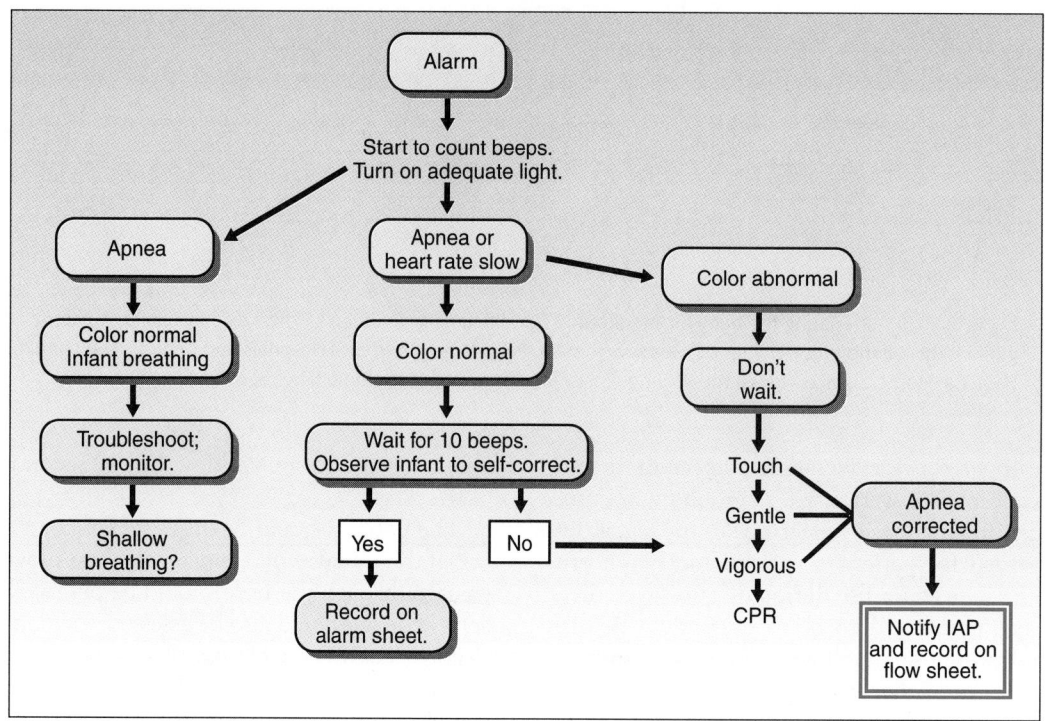

Figure 30-7 Alarm response flowchart. (Modified from Children's Hospitals and Clinics. A parent guide to home monitoring: infant apnea program. St. Paul, Minn: Children's Hospitals and Clinics; 1994.)

Box 30-4

Common Problems in Home Monitoring

Inability to initially distinguish real from false alarms
Increased incidence of false alarms as the infant matures
Monitor malfunction
Increased number of alarms during intercurrent illness
Difficulty finding day care for monitored infants
Skin irritation caused by electrodes
Psychologic reliance of family on monitor

toring. The stress on the family, one of the most important problems associated with home monitoring, usually is greatest during the first few weeks of monitoring. Frequent contact during this period may reduce some of this stress.

Problems in Home Apnea Monitoring

The technical aspects of home monitoring have improved greatly in the past two decades. Monitors have become smaller, have developed larger memory capabilities for documented monitoring, and have a longer battery life. Although this makes it easier for families to incorporate monitors into daily living, stress remains one of the most difficult problems with monitoring. Common problems associated with home monitoring are listed in Box 30-4.[17] All these factors can increase the level of stress incurred by the family.

According to Spinner and colleagues,[13] the family stress level peaks in the first 2 weeks, with the first night at home being the most difficult. Parents find they cannot do simple things such as shower or vacuum and be aware of the monitor. Use of devices that enhance the monitor, such as audible nursery intercoms, may help. During the initial instruction, caregivers should be taught that if routine activities interfere with their ability to hear and respond to the alarm, schedules should be arranged to correct those situations. A capable caregiver must be available at all times, including during showers, vacuuming, laundry, dishes, or other loud household activities. Compiling an informal list of parents enrolled in the apnea program who are willing to offer support and advice to new enrollees may be a helpful tool in coping with family stress.

Discontinuation of Home Apnea Monitoring

Before monitoring is discontinued, two questions must be addressed: (1) Is the patient clinically ready to be discontinued? and (2) Is the family psychologically ready to terminate monitoring? Most parents are ready to discontinue monitoring on the physician's recommendation if, since the time of original education, the protocols to end use of the monitor have been clearly defined and explained. In some cases the parents make the request to discontinue monitoring (sometimes prematurely) because of their comfort level with the patient's condition. Other parents,

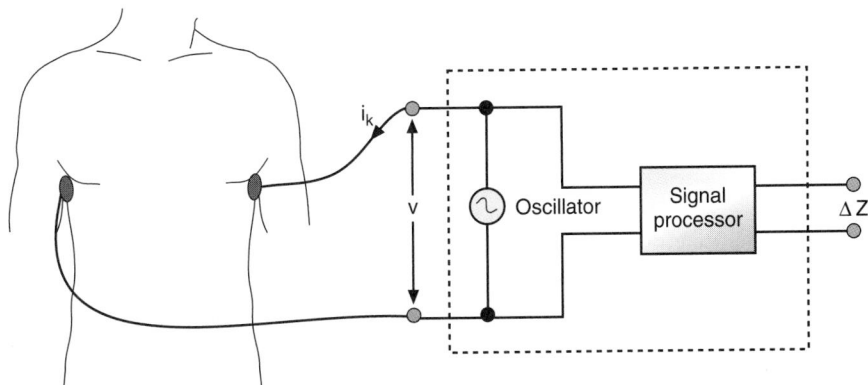

Figure 30-8   Placement of a single pair of electrodes to apply a constant current and to pick up the change in voltage associated with respiratory activity. (Modified from Baker L. Principles of the impedance technique. Eng Med Biol 1989;8:11-15.)

despite proper education and preparation for discontinuation, are unwilling to end monitoring. In such cases a gradual reduction in monitor usage may be helpful.

The criteria used to consider discontinuation should be based on the patient's clinical condition. For most patients the following criteria are used:

- Methylxanthine administration has been discontinued.
- No significant clinical alarms have sounded for the past 4 to 6 weeks.
- Normal values have been seen on follow-up of the cardiorespiratory recording (downloaded from a documented monitor).
- The patient is not ill at the time of discontinuation.
- Both parents agree on the discontinuation date in conjunction with the recommendations of the physician or the **infant apnea program** or both.

Patients given caffeine typically have the medication discontinued 2 weeks after discharge from the hospital or clinic. If the patient does not experience a significant clinical alarm during the 2 weeks after cessation of methylxanthines, a recording pulse oximeter is added at night to record saturation values by the documented monitor for 7 days. The monitor's data are then downloaded and the data analyzed. If no clinical events have occurred during that period, discontinuation of the monitor is recommended.

It becomes very important for the apnea program staff to contact the family throughout the weaning process to support the caregiver and answer any questions. If at any point the patient experiences a significant clinical event during the apnea weaning process, monitoring is continued for 1 more month. Discontinuation is revisited at the end of that month.[21]

Technical Aspects of Apnea Monitors

Transthoracic electrical impedance apnea monitors are the most commonly used monitors. They generally are most efficient at identifying and sounding an alarm for central apnea. However, situations occur in which breathing is detected during apparent apnea (false negative) and other cases in which apnea is detected even though the infant is breathing (false positive). The former case often is related to cardiogenic artifact, a significant problem with impedance monitors, or to motion artifact caused by active or passive infant movement.[6]

The electrical impedance of biologic tissues and the changes in impedance that accompany physiologic activity are complex subjects. Materials such as blood and muscle are poor conductors, relative to materials classified as conductors (for example, copper), at the frequencies most often used to measure physiologic activity.[24] By determining the electrical resistance of the different materials, monitors have been developed to measure changes of voltage as measured through the material. The question arises as to what is actually the physical source (or sources) of the impedance signal. The most general, but correct, answer is anything that changes the current density distribution between the voltage-sensing electrodes.

For impedance changes accompanying respiratory activity, several possibilities come to the forefront: the increased resistance of the lung tissue as it fills with air; the change in the circumference of the thorax as it expands and relaxes, the change in the conduction pathway associated with the downward movement of the diaphragm; and the large, highly conductive liver mass. Albisser and Carmichael[25] state that the geometric factors of chest circumference and interelectrode distance made significantly larger contributions to changes in thoracic impedance than did changes in lung resistance.

In more simplistic terms, electrodes placed on the chest wall opposite each other measure the distance between the two points by measuring the electrical resistance of the material through which the signal passes. As the chest wall expands and contracts, the distance between the electrodes changes, thus a change in voltage is detected. A microprocessor in the monitor processes the change in voltage to detect a breath (Figure 30-8). Programming the microprocessor to detect electrical signals from the heart results in the cardiac signal seen on the monitor. When electrodes are positioned improperly, the change in voltage may not be detected, or the cardiac signal may be misinterpreted as too fast or too slow. For these reasons, proper placement of the electrodes cannot be overemphasized.

Documented monitors have a data storage capacity similar to that of computers. Data are constantly received from the monitor and stored digitally. Storage is activated by user programmed markers. In essence, the memory device is always looking at data. When an event triggers the automatic saving of information, the device digitally records a predetermined time before the event and the event itself and concludes with a predetermined time after resolution of the event. Because the information is digital, the data can be downloaded by computer directly to the unit or by phone modem from the patient's home.

Other Types of Monitors

Oxygen saturation monitors, capnography, esophageal pH monitors, airflow thermistry, acoustic monitors (for snoring or intertracheal breath sounds), motion and body position monitors, and cardiac monitors all are used clinically to gather physiologic data. The most recognized limitation to cardiorespiratory monitoring is the inability to identify obstructive apnea that occurs secondary to the chest wall motion that continues during this type of event. Monitors that sense airflow thermistry, oxygen saturation, and breath sounds can detect both central and obstructive apnea, but their use is limited by cost and their relative difficulty for the care provider.

Pulse oximeters are widely used for patients with tracheostomies or those being mechanically ventilated. When a patient becomes obstructed or disconnected from the ventilator, the oxygen saturation and pulse deteriorate rapidly, resulting in an audible and visual alarm. Proper functioning of this type of monitor relies on many physical and physiologic factors. Because pulse oximeters calculate oxygen saturation based on hemoglobin levels and blood perfusion to the probe site, patients with poor distal perfusion may not be good candidates for this type of monitor.[19] Ambient light and excessive motion also can result in inaccurate information.

Capnography has advantages in terms of evaluating the degree of hypoventilation or hyperventilation, but currently home use is limited. Unless the patient has a tracheostomy, the end-tidal CO_2 value must be obtained by a sidestream sampler, which requires a nasal cannula for the patient. Because most infants are nasal breathers, use of a nasal sensing device may actually create an obstruction. The literature also suggests that the accuracy of capnography is highly dependent on the length of the tubing, particularly if coupled with low sampling flow rates.[26] The cost of home capnography also is a limiting factor.

Esophageal pH monitoring has great benefit in the detection of the effects of GER. The use of outpatient pH monitoring is gaining popularity for all age groups, especially for patients diagnosed with gastric insufficiency. GER may be a contributing factor to apnea, but it is not the only cause. Esophageal pH information has successfully been incorporated into multichannel diagnostic studies but should not be considered the only form of diagnostic tool or monitoring device for patients suspected of having apnea.

Airflow thermistry is an invaluable tool for diagnostic testing to differentiate between obstructive and central apnea. Air passing over the sensors causes a change in temperature, resulting in breath detection. Currently the technologic development of this type of monitor has not advanced to the point of serving as a sole method of monitoring. Possible obstruction of the nasal passages in nasal-breathing infants should always be a safety consideration with this device.

Acoustic monitoring uses sound signals as indicators of respiration. This technology is incorporated into some adult polysomnographic equipment to monitor for snoring. The movement of air through the air passages during normal respiration generates an acoustic signal that can be detected from the surface of the body at suitable sites with the aid of a microphone applied to the skin. Such acoustic signals have the potential to indicate respiration and cardiac sounds, but further work is required to develop a monitor appropriate for home use.[13,27]

Motion and position monitors are used in multichannel polysomnograms. Work is being done to further develop monitors that rely on body and breathing motion during sleep to detect periods of apnea. Use of these types of monitors is focused on adults and adolescents with sleep disorders and obstructed sleep apnea.

Cardiac monitors used as a diagnostic tool outside the clinical environment allow the medical team to record and evaluate a patient during normal living activities. Sometimes referred to as Holter monitors, these devices can record electrical activity produced by the heart and store and transmit the data to a designated location at predetermined intervals. These devices do not monitor a patient's respiratory status and typically are used for detailed evaluation of patients diagnosed with varying degrees of cardiac disease.

Role of the Respiratory Therapist in Apnea Monitoring

Respiratory therapists have many opportunities to use their professional skills in the area of cardiorespiratory (apnea) monitoring. These roles range from acute care clinicians to work in private sector equipment manufacturing (Table 30-2).

The acute care respiratory therapist may be involved with assessment and initial observation of a significant clinical event, which may include assisting with the birth of a premature or other high-risk neonate or responding to parents in the emergency room reporting an ALTE. In many small community hospitals, the respiratory therapist assumes many tasks after initial observations have been reported.

TABLE 30-2

Responsibilities of Respiratory Therapists in Home Apnea Monitoring

Setting	Responsibilities
Acute care	Initial observation
	Discharge planning
	Medical research
Home care	Instruction and initial set up
	Follow-up after discharge
	Home visits
	Equipment maintenance
Manufacturer	Research and development
	Technical support
	Sales and marketing
Insurance case management	Prior authorization
	Claims management

Most candidates for home monitoring require some type of diagnostic study, which may range from a simple three-channel event recording to a complete polysomnogram with video and sound evaluation. The selected evaluation tool is implemented by the respiratory therapist, including setting up, supervising, and performing the study and interpreting the information gathered. It is not unusual for the respiratory therapist to scan and score the information from the study, highlight clinically significant events, and present the findings to the managing physician for final diagnosis. Most managing pulmonologists or neonatologists rescan the information, paying particularly close attention to the areas highlighted by the respiratory therapist.

When a diagnosis has been established, the monitoring discharge team begins the planning process. This team, often referred to as the *apnea monitor program*, may consist of the following members:

- *The primary care physician* is available for consultation and ultimately responsible for the child's care. This physician directly or indirectly (through a close working relationship with the other team members) dictates and signs all orders pertaining to use of the monitor.
- *Staff nurses or a respiratory therapist (or both)* provide education, support, and follow-up care. Most successful programs have a nurse or respiratory therapist available 24 hours a day to answer questions, provide supportive advice, or troubleshoot unexpected problems.
- *A social worker* provides counseling and support network information and investigates insurance coverage or public assistance programs.
- *The home equipment company respiratory therapist* provides equipment used in the home, equipment training, and in-home follow-up care.[13]

The initial discussion with the family about home monitoring can be done by any of the team members except the home care respiratory therapist. As mentioned before, family stress is one of the primary problems with home moni-

toring. The initial contact sets the tone for the following months with the family and goes a long way toward reducing the amount of stress family members experience. It is important to remember that most families have limited experience with medical care. The realization that their child requires home monitoring, although it is technologically very simple to perform, often causes considerable anxiety.

Before discharge, the acute care respiratory therapist may also be involved in the education and training of the patient's primary care providers. This education includes how to use the monitor, the appropriate alarm response, and information about patient follow-up after discharge.

Because medical equipment and pharmaceutical manufacturers must have a substantial amount of clinical data before submitting a product for approval to the U.S. Food and Drug Administration (FDA), many acute care facilities have research laboratories that require the skills of respiratory therapists. Research may include the effectiveness of new medications or dosages, new monitoring techniques, comparison of computer-scoring software to the clinicians' scoring techniques, and other tasks. Many research projects involve retrospective studies of previous activities and data collection, which require detailed clinical knowledge of monitor use.

Home care respiratory therapists perform many duties in relation to monitoring. Clinically, the home care respiratory therapist instructs and educates the care provider in much the same manner as the acute care staff. Many hospitals do not have home monitor programs that assist in the management and discharge planning of the monitored patient. Some studies reflect that many physicians order monitors for home use for the sole purpose of limiting their own liability exposure.[28] When a monitor program is not available, the home care respiratory therapist performs many of the same duties as the respiratory therapist involved with hospital-based apnea programs.

Initial instruction may involve review of what the monitor program has previously instructed or performance of all of the instruction normally provided by a hospital-based program. Postdischarge follow-up ranges from phone discussion to home visits. It often is the home care respiratory therapist who downloads information from documented monitors. The home care respiratory therapist also has the responsibility of performing overnight diagnostic studies in the patient's home or of providing equipment and staff training for smaller acute care facilities so that diagnostic studies may be performed without transferring the patient to another hospital.

Because most of the equipment used by the patient outside the hospital is on lease or loan from a home care or **durable medical equipment (DME)** provider, the respiratory therapist is involved with the maintenance and repair of that equipment. One of the primary responsibilities of the DME provider is to replace broken or malfunctioning equipment used by the home care patient. The ability to successfully resolve problems of malfunctioning equipment by telephone conversation, thus preventing an unexpected visit to the home, is a skill gained through experience. Providing quality care in a cost-effective manner is of utmost importance.

Manufacturers of the equipment used by health care providers employ an ever-increasing number of respiratory therapists. Clinicians are involved with research and development of new and existing products, technical support for those products, and education of clinicians in the use of the equipment. Respiratory therapists also play an important role in sales and marketing. Areas of projected growth, in relation to monitoring, are scoring software, telemonitoring, alternative site diagnostic studies, and development of other monitors, such as CO_2, oxygen saturation, and acoustic monitors that are as cost-effective and easy to use as cardiorespiratory monitors.

Insurance case management has become a major component of the provision of quality care in a cost-effective manner. Respiratory therapists are involved with both private insurance providers and state-funded organizations to continually manage how insurance dollars are distributed. Although the need for a home monitor usually is supported by an abnormal diagnostic study or a witnessed event, many cases are reviewed by respiratory therapists employed by insurance providers to ensure that use of a monitor is warranted for specific patients. A successful program requires an understanding of the clinical use of home monitors and of the protocols for discontinuation of use.

KEY POINTS

- A home monitor should not be prescribed without appropriate evaluation, caregiver education, and follow-up.
- The purpose of monitoring is to detect untoward physiologic events.
- Monitoring does not prevent SIDS.
- Apnea without associated significant bradycardia or desaturation is inconsequential.
- Most apnea monitors use the electrical impedance technique

References

1. Speer M. Use and abuse of apnea monitors. Tex Med 1996; 92:54-55.
2. Steinschneider A. Prolonged apnea and sudden infant death syndrome: clinical and laboratory observations. Pediatrics 1972;50: 646-654.
3. Sheridan MS, editor. The NAAP handbook of infant apnea and home monitoring. Waianae, Hawaii: National Association for Apnea Professionals; 1992.
4. Brouillette R, Weese-Mayer D, Hunt C. Breathing control disorders in infants and children. Hosp Pract 1990;8:82-103.
5. Carrol J, Marcus C, Laughlin G. Disordered control of breathing in infants and children. Pediatr Rev 1993;14:51-65.
6. National Institute of Health Consensus Development Conference on Infantile Apnea and Home Monitoring. NIH Pub No

7. 87-2905. Bethesda, Md: US Department of Health and Human Services; 1987.
7. Bancalari E. Control of breathing and apnea in the premature infant. Fourteenth Conference on Apnea of Infancy. Annenberg Center for Health Sciences, Rancho Mirage, Calif., January 1996.
8. Walsh JK, Farrell MK, Keenan WJ, et al. Gastroesophageal reflux in infants: relation to apnea. J Pediatr 1981;99:197-201.
9. Orenstein S, Orenstein D. Gastroesophageal reflux and respiratory disease in children. J Pediatr 1988;112:847-857.
10. Eichenwald E, Aina A, Stark A. Apnea frequently persists beyond term gestation in infants delivered at 24 to 28 weeks. Pediatrics 1997;100:357-358.
11. Therapeutics and Technology Subcommittee of the American Academy of Neurology. Assessment: techniques associated with the diagnosis and management of sleep disorders. Neurology 1992;42:269-275.
12. Corwin M, Lister G, Silvestri JM, et al. Agreement among raters in assessment of physiologic waveforms recorded by a cardiorespiratory monitor for home use. Pediatr Res 1998;44:682-690.
13. Spinner S, Gibson E, Wrobel H, et al. Recent advances in home infant apnea monitoring. Neonatal Network 1995;14:39-43.
14. Whitaker S. The art and science of home infant apnea monitoring in the 1990s. J Obstet Gynecol Neonatal Nurs 1995; 24:84-89.
15. Cote A, Hun C, Brouillette RT, et al. Frequency and timing of recurrent events in infants using home cardiorespiratory monitors. J Pediatr 1998;132:758-759.
16. Spitzer A, Fox W. Infant apnea. Pediatr Clin North Am 1986;33:561-581.
17. Hunt C. Sudden infant death syndrome and subsequent siblings. Pediatrics 1995;95:430-432.
18. Children's Hospitals and Clinics. A parent guide to home monitoring: infant apnea program. St Paul, Minn: Children's Hospitals and Clinics; 1994.
19. Miller M, Martin R. Apnea in infancy: progress in diagnosis and implications for management. Neonatal Respiratory Diseases. Vol. 8. No. 1. Boston: Tufts University School of Medicine; 1998.
20. Foreman D, Farsides C. Ethical use of covert videoing techniques in detecting Münchausen syndrome by proxy. Br Med J 1993;307:611-613.
21. Gibson E, Spinner S, Cullen JA, et al. Documented home apnea monitoring: effect on compliance, duration of monitoring, and validation of alarm reporting. Clin Pediatr 1996;35:506-513.
22. Pediatric Home Service. Apnea monitoring. Roseville, Minn: Pediatric Home Service; 1994.
23. National Association of Apnea Professionals: Guidelines for the provision of services to families using infant apnea monitors (neonatal). Intensive Care May/June 1996;10-15.
24. Baker L. Principles of the impedance technique. Med Biol Eng 1989;8:11-15.
25. Albisser AM, Carmichael AB. Factors in impedance pneumography. Med Biol Eng 1974;12:599-605.
26. Kirpalani H, Kechagias S, Lerman J. Technical and clinical aspects of capnography in neonates. J Med Eng Technol 1991;15:154-161.
27. Ajmani A, Mazumdar J, Jarvis D. Spectral analysis of an acoustic respiratory signal with a view to developing an apnoea monitor. Australas Phys Eng Sci Med 1996;19:46-52.
28. Hickson G, Cooper W, Campbell P, et al. Effects of pediatrician characteristics on management decisions in simulated cases involving apparent life-threatening events. Arch Pediatr Adolescent Med 1998;152:383-387.

PART IV

Respiratory Therapeutics

CHAPTER 31

Medical Gases—Manufacture, Storage, and Delivery

Allan B. Saposnick

OBJECTIVES

1. Describe the physical properties, chemical symbols, and uses of air, oxygen, carbon dioxide, helium, nitric oxide, nitrous oxide, and nitrogen.
2. Describe the processes for production of various medical gases.
3. Compare and contrast gaseous and liquid storage methods.
4. Describe the production, safety features, types, and uses of medical gas cylinders.
5. Discuss the established safety systems for the various equipment connections to ensure delivery of a specific gas, such as oxygen.
6. Calculate the duration of flow from a gas cylinder.
7. Describe the design, use, and troubleshooting of various bulk gas supply systems.
8. Explain appropriate actions to take if a failure occurs in a bulk oxygen delivery system.

KEY TERMS

Air Liquefaction	Dewar	Medical Gas Cylinders
American Standard Safety System (ASSS)	Diameter-Index Safety System (DISS)	Nitric Oxide (NO)
Carbogen	Food and Drug Administration (FDA)	Nitrogen (N$_2$)
Carbon Dioxide (CO$_2$)	Fractional Distillation of Liquefied Air	Nitrous Oxide (N$_2$O)
Compressed Gas Association (CGA)	Heliox	Pin-Index Safety System (PISS)
Cryogenic Liquid	Helium (He)	United States Pharmacopoeia/National
Department of Transportation (DOT)	Hydrostatic Testing	Formulary (USP/NF)

Many therapeutic and diagnostic procedures routinely used in respiratory therapy involve the use of one or more medical gases. The respiratory therapist must have a thorough understanding of the properties of medical gases, their safe handling, and their use. In addition, the therapist must know when and how to troubleshoot equipment malfunction to ensure medical gas delivery as needed by patients.

Properties and Manufacture of Medical Gases

Flammability

All medical gases can be classified as either nonflammable or inflammable. A nonflammable gas does not burn. Examples include nitrogen, oxygen, helium, air, nitrous oxide, and carbon dioxide. However, some nonflammable gases such as oxygen, air, and nitrous oxide, support combustion. An inflammable gas is one that burns and is potentially explosive. The terms *inflammable* and *flammable* are used interchangeably. Propane and natural gas, although not used for medical purposes, are examples of flammable gases. For safety, flammable gases are rarely used medically. Table 31-1 lists the properties of medical gases.

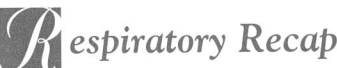espiratory Recap

Gas Flammability
Nonflammable gases do not burn, but some support combustion.
The terms *flammable* and *inflammable* are used interchangeably.
Inflammable gases burn and are rarely used for medical purposes.
Oxygen is a nonflammable gas; it does not burn and will not explode.
Oxygen supports combustion, making burning brighter, hotter, and faster.

Air

Air, at normal atmospheric conditions, is an odorless, colorless, transparent, tasteless mixture of gases and water vapor that is nonflammable and supports combustion. Air is composed of about 78% nitrogen and 21% oxygen by volume. The remaining 1% consists of extremely small amounts of chemically inert trace and rare gases, such as argon, neon, helium, krypton, and xenon. Table 31-2 shows the precise composition of air.

Dry air at standard temperature and pressure (STPD; 21.1° C, 760 mm Hg) has a density of 1.2 kg/m³. Air is used as the standard to measure the specific gravity of other gases and is assigned the value of 1. Air can be manufactured by a precise mixing of nitrogen and oxygen. More commonly, however, atmospheric air is filtered, compressed, and stored in cylinders or directly delivered through a central piping system, a procedure detailed later in this chapter. The **Compressed Gas Association (CGA)** specifies grades of gaseous air, A through J, with J being the medical grade. Medical-grade compressed air contains 19.5% to 23.5% oxygen, no water vapor, and minimum amounts of hydrocarbons and other impurities.

Oxygen

Scheele and Priestly announced the discovery of oxygen in 1774 within 3 months of each other, with Scheele's being first. Carl Scheele, a Swedish apothecary, called the gas "fire air," whereas England's Joseph Priestly called it "dephlogisticated air." A year later, France's Antoine Lavoisier gave the gas the name *oxygen*, meaning "acid generator."

Properties The element oxygen exists in molecular form (O_2) in the atmosphere and in combination with other elements in a great number of compounds. At standard temperature and pressure (STP), oxygen is a colorless, transparent, odorless, tasteless gas, only slightly heavier than air, with a specific gravity of 1.051 and a density of 1.326 kg/m³ at STPD. About 50% of the earth's crust by weight is oxygen, and the gas makes up 20.9% by volume of the atmosphere and 23.2% by weight. Oxygen is not very soluble in water. At STP, 3.3 mL of oxygen dissolves in 100 mL of water, which, however, is enough to sustain all aquatic life.

Gaseous oxygen can be liquefied when its temperature is lowered to −297.3° F (−182.9° C), its boiling point. Liquid oxygen has a pale-blue color and is 1.1 times heavier than water. Oxygen remains in the liquid state as long as its temperature remains below the boiling point. However, if pressure is applied, oxygen maintains its liquid state up to its critical temperature, −181.4° F (−118.6° C). The pressure necessary to maintain oxygen as a liquid at its critical temperature is 731.4 pounds per square inch, absolute (psia), referred to as the *critical pressure*.

Molecular oxygen, O_2, is formed when two oxygen atoms combine by sharing two electrons in their outer orbital shell. This unique molecular bonding characteristic gives oxygen a paramagnetic property—that of being attracted to a magnet—that can be used to determine oxygen concentration in a gas mixture.

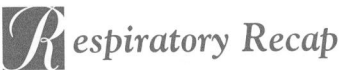espiratory Recap

Properties of Oxygen
Oxygen is a colorless, transparent, odorless, tasteless, nonflammable gas, only slightly heavier than air at STP.
Only 3.3 mL of oxygen dissolves in 100 mL of water at STP.
Gaseous oxygen can be liquefied when its temperature is lowered to −297.3° F (−182.9° C).
Liquid oxygen has a pale-blue color and is 1.1 times heavier than water.
Oxygen stays in the liquid oxygen state as long as its temperature remains below the boiling point.
O_2 forms when two oxygen atoms combine by sharing two electrons in their outer orbital shell.
FIO_2 in air is 0.2095 and remains constant with changes in altitude.
PO_2 varies depending on the PB.

The concentration or fraction (FIO_2) of oxygen in the air is 0.2095 and remains constant even to altitudes of 60 miles. The partial pressure of oxygen (PO_2), however, varies greatly depending on the barometric pressure (PB). At sea level, where the PB averages 760 mm Hg, the PO_2 is 159 mm Hg. The PO_2 can be calculated for any PB with the following calculation:

$$PO_2 = PB \times FIO_2$$

TABLE 31-1
Physical Properties of Commonly Used Medical Gases

Property	Air	Oxygen	Carbon Dioxide	Helium	Nitric Oxide	Nitrous Oxide	Nitrogen
Symbol	Air	O_2	CO_2	He	NO	N_2O	N_2
Color	Colorless	Colorless	Colorless	Colorless	Colorless	Colorless	Colorless
Odor	Odorless	Odorless	Odorless/pungent	Odorless	Faint metallic	Odorless/sweet	Odorless
Taste	Tasteless	Tasteless	Tasteless/slightly acidic	Tasteless	Tasteless	Tasteless/sweet	Tasteless
Life support	Supports life	Supports life	Does not support life	Does not support life	Does not support life	Does not support life	Does not support life
Flammability	Nonflammable; supports combustion	Nonflammable; supports combustion	Nonflammable	Nonflammable	Nonflammable	Nonflammable; supports combustion	Nonflammable
Molecular weight	28.975	31.999	44.01	4.003	30.006	44.013	28.013
Percent by volume of air	—	20.946	0.0335	0.000524	—	—	78.084
Percent by weight of air	—	23.2	0.045	—	—	—	75.5
Partial pressure (ATPD)	—	158 mm Hg	0.25 mm Hg	—	—	—	1.75 mm Hg
Viscosity*	182.7×10^{-6}	201.8×10^{-6}	148×10^{-6}	194.1×10^{-6}	—	—	—
Density*	1.2 kg/m³	1.326 kg/m³	1.833 kg/m³	0.1656 kg/m³	1.245 kg/m³	1.947 kg/m³	1.153 kg/m³
Specific gravity	1	1.1049	1.524	0.138	1.04	1.529	0.967
Boiling point	−194.3° C	−182.9° C	−29° C	−268.9° C	−151.8° C	−88.56° C	−195.9° C
Critical temperature	−140.7° C	−118.6° C	31.1° C	−267.9° C	−92.9° C	36.5° C	−146.9° C
Critical pressure	547 psia	731.4 psia	1076.6 psia	33 psia	949.4 psia	1054 psia	493 psia
Triple point	—	218.8° C at 0.220 psia	−56.6° C at 60.4 psia	—	—	−90.83° C at 12.74 psia	−210° C at 1.81 psia
Solubility in water†	0.0292	0.0489	0.9	0.0094	0.0734	1.3	0.023
State in cylinder	Gas	Liquid or gas	Liquid and gas	Gas	Gas	Liquid and gas	Liquid or gas

Modified from Langenderfer R, Branson R. Compressed gases: manufacture, storage, and piping systems. In: Branson R, Hess D, Chatburn R. Respiratory care equipment. 2nd ed. Philadelphia: Lippincott Williams & Wilkins; 1999.

ATPD, Atmospheric temperature and pressure, dry.
All values at 21.1° C and 1 atmosphere
†*At 0° C.*

TABLE 31-2

Composition of Room Air

Component	% by Volume	% by Weight
Nitrogen	78.084	75.5
Oxygen	20.946	23.2
Argon	0.934	1.33
Carbon dioxide	0.0335	0.045
Hydrogen	0.00005	—
Neon	0.001818	—
Helium	0.000524	—
Methan	0.0002	—
Krypton	0.000114	—
Nitrous oxide	0.00005	—
Xenon	0.0000087	

From Compressed Gas Association. Handbook of compressed gases. 4th ed. Boston: Kluwer Academic; 1999.

Equation 31-1 illustrates several examples of PO_2 calculations.

Support of Combustion

Oxygen is a nonflammable gas; that is, it does not burn. However, oxygen vigorously accelerates and supports combustion. The higher the concentration of oxygen, the hotter, faster, and brighter the burn. Burning (combustion) commonly occurs in air at 21% oxygen. If a burning match is exposed to an atmosphere containing 42% oxygen, however, it will burn twice as hot, bright, and fast as it did in room air. The oxygen does not actually burn but supports the combustion of the burning items. In concentrations greater than 21%, oxygen not only supports combustion but it also accelerates the burning process. In the presence of high concentrations of oxygen, certain combustible items, especially petroleum-based products (for example, oil, grease) can easily and violently ignite with great force from a spark, friction, pressure, or impact.

Manufacture

Photosynthesis Oxygen is produced naturally by all green land and aquatic plants through photosynthesis, a process in which chlorophyll-containing plants, in the presence of sunlight, convert carbon dioxide and water into glucose and release oxygen, as a byproduct, into the atmosphere. Equation 31-2 demonstrates the photosynthesis formula.

Electrolysis of Water An electric current passed through water causes the water to separate into its component parts—hydrogen and oxygen—with hydrogen bubbling off at the cathode in a 2:1 ratio to the oxygen at the anode. This process, electrolysis of water, is impractical for the commercial production of oxygen.

Fractional Distillation of Liquefied Air The two major components of air—oxygen and nitrogen—are produced in bulk commercial quantities by a process first described in 1907 by Karl von Linde. The process, **fractional distillation of liquefied air,** relies on the Joule-Kelvin principle, which

EQUATION 31-1

Effects of Altitude on Barometric Pressure and Partial Pressure of Oxygen

Altitude (Feet)	P_B (mm Hg)	P_{O_2} (mm Hg)
Sea level	760	159
5000	630	132
10,000	523	109
20,000	349	73
30,000	226	47

At 1 atmosphere (760 mm Hg), the P_{O_2} is 159 mm Hg. The partial pressure for any P_B can be calculated with the following formula:

$$P_{O_2} = P_B \times F_{IO_2}$$

Changes in P_{O_2} are most often encountered during ascent to a higher altitude. At an altitude of 30,000 feet (P_B = 226 mm Hg), P_{O_2} decreases by 70%, as follows:

$$P_{O_2} = 226 \text{ mm Hg} \times 0.21$$
$$P_{O_2} = 47.5 \text{ mm Hg}$$

These changes in P_{O_2} account for the need to pressurize aircraft during high-altitude flights and explain why the normal PaO_2 is variable according to geography.

Modified from Langenderfer R, Branson R. Compressed gases: manufacture, storage, and piping systems. In: Branson R, Hess D, Chatburn R. Respiratory care equipment. 2nd ed. Philadelphia: Lippincott Williams & Wilkins; 1999.
P_B, Barometric pressure; P_{O_2}, partial pressure of oxygen; F_{IO_2}, fraction of oxygen in the air; PaO_2, partial pressure of oxygen in arterial blood.

EQUATION 31-2

Photosynthesis Formula

$$6\ CO_2 + 6\ H_2O + \text{Sunlight} + \text{Chlorophyll} \rightarrow C_6H_{12}O_6 + 12\ O_2$$

states that when gases under pressure are released into a vacuum, the gas molecules tend to lose their kinetic energy. In the vacuum the reduction in kinetic energy causes a decrease in temperature and a reduction in the cohesive forces between the molecules, leading to liquefaction.

An **air liquefaction** plant is a large, complex industrial site that somewhat resembles a small oil refinery. The actual fractional distillation process consists of multiple stages and steps, as shown in Figure 31-1. The process begins with atmospheric air being drawn through filters and scrubbers to remove airborne contaminants, then compressed and cooled in several stages to 2000 pounds per square inch, gauge (psig) and −50° F. Along the way, water vapor in the air freezes and is removed. The air then is cooled further to −265° F at a pressure of 200 psig, then allowed to expand to 90 psig in a separator, where partial liquefaction takes place. The liquefied air from the separator is pumped to the top of the fractional distillation column. As it flows down the column, the nitrogen boils off and can be captured and stored in the gaseous or liquid state. Oxygen collects at the bottom of the column in liquid form. This liquid oxygen still contains a number of trace gas contaminants, primarily argon and krypton. It is further distilled to recover the argon. Distillation continues with careful control of temperature and pressure until the remaining liquid exceeds 99.0% oxygen, the standard of purity required by the **United States Pharmacopoeia/National Formulary (USP/NF)** for medical-grade oxygen.

Respiratory Recap

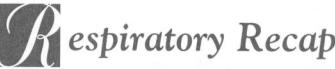

Ways to Produce Oxygen	
Photosynthesis	Fractional distillation of air
Electrolysis of water	Molecular filtration

Another method used to produce oxygen is molecular filtration. This process is used widely in respiratory home care with oxygen concentrator devices.

Carbon Dioxide

Carbon dioxide (CO_2) is a naturally occurring compound found in the atmosphere in a concentration of approximately 0.03%. At STP, CO_2 is a colorless, transparent, odorless to pungent aroma, tasteless or slightly acid-tasting gas with a specific gravity of 1.522, making it $1\frac{1}{2}$ times heavier than air. CO_2 is nonflammable and does not support combustion or animal life. It can be obtained from the burning of fossil fuels (coal, oil, natural gas, coke), from natural springs, through heating of limestone, and as a byproduct of the fermentation process. CO_2 is processed and refined to a purity of 99% or higher for medical use.

CO_2 can simultaneously exist as a solid, liquid, and gas at $-56.6°$ C ($-70°$ F) and 60.4 psig, referred to as the *triple point*. Solid CO_2 (dry ice), at room temperature and normal atmospheric pressure, turns from its solid state directly to a gas without first becoming a liquid. This phenomenon is known as *sublimation*. Because its critical temperature is 31° C (87.8° F), pressurized cylinders of CO_2 contain both liquid and gas.

CO_2 is rarely used therapeutically. It has been used to treat hiccups (singultus), atelectasis, and cerebrovascular conditions. Because it does not support life, CO_2 must be mixed with O_2 if it is to be administered via inhalation, with the usual mixtures being 90% O_2 to 10% CO_2 or 95% O_2 to 5% CO_2. CO_2/O_2 mixtures are frequently referred to as **carbogen.** Today, CO_2 mixtures are used primarily in the calibration of capnographs, blood gas analyzers, and other laboratory and diagnostic equipment.

Helium

Helium (He) is a rare gas naturally occurring in the atmosphere in extremely small amounts (0.000524% by

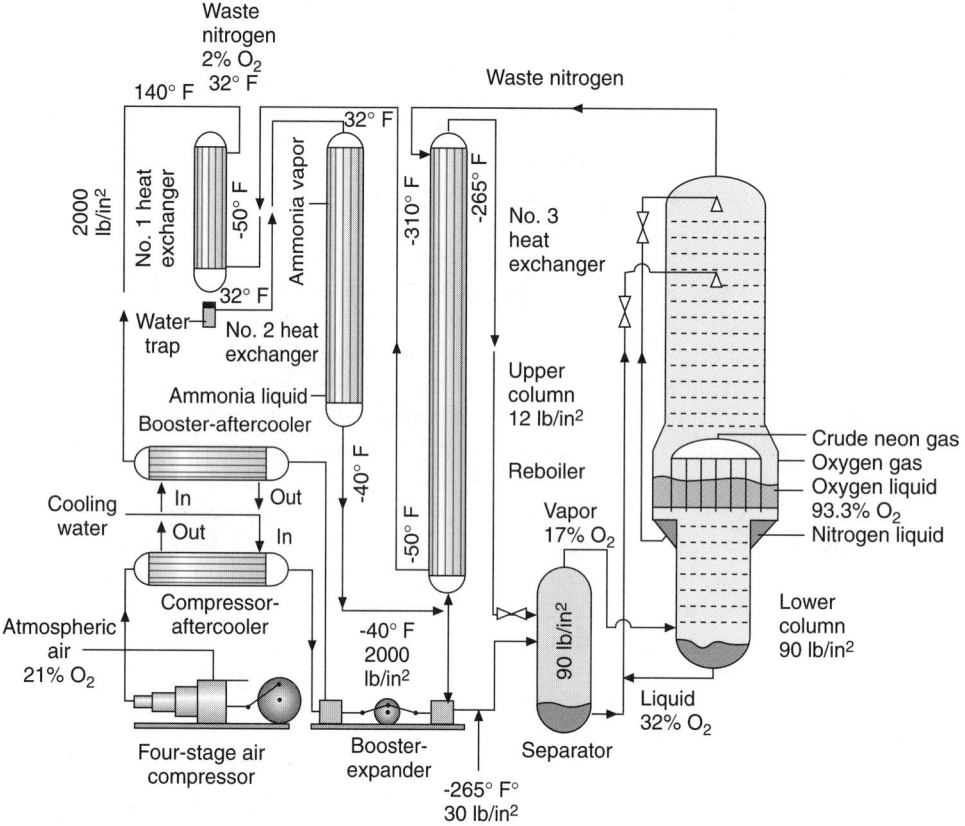

Figure 31-1 Diagrammatic representation of the process of fractional distillation of liquefied air.

volume). It is colorless, transparent, odorless, tasteless, nonflammable; does not support combustion or life; and is chemically and physiologically inert. Helium is the second-lightest element (hydrogen being lighter), with an extremely low density (0.165 kg/m^3) and specific gravity (0.138), slightly more than one-eighth that of air. The commercial source of helium is natural gas, where it can be found in concentrations up to 2%.

The low-density property of helium makes it useful in the treatment of airway obstruction; it helps decrease the work of breathing, resulting in a less turbulent flow and increased flow through narrowed airways. Because helium is an inert, non–life-supporting gas, it must be mixed with at least 20% O_2. He/O_2 mixtures are often referred to as **heliox.** Helium in low concentrations also is used in the pulmonary function laboratory in tests to determine lung volumes and diffusing capacity.

Nitric Oxide

Nitric oxide (NO) is a colorless, tasteless gas with a slight metallic odor. This nonflammable, and non–life-supporting gas that supports combustion and is toxic is found in the atmosphere in extremely small amounts (10 to 100 parts per billion) as an air pollutant byproduct of combustion. Nitric oxide is extremely unstable and in air rapidly becomes nitrogen dioxide (NO_2), a highly toxic substance. Nitric oxide is produced in the reaction of sulfur dioxide with nitric acid and through the oxidation of ammonia at temperatures above 500° C in the presence of platinum as a catalyst. Nitric oxide is purified to 99.0%, diluted with medical-grade nitrogen to concentrations from 100 to several thousand parts per million (ppm) and delivered in specially cleaned, high-pressure aluminum cylinders.

Nitric oxide is naturally synthesized in human tissue and plays an important role in vascular smooth muscle relaxation, inhibition of platelet aggregation, neurotransmission, and immune regulation. The inhalation administration of nitric oxide in very low concentrations (5 to 80 parts per million [ppm]) causes selective pulmonary vascular dilation, which has lead to the use of nitric oxide to treat persistent pulmonary hypertension of the newborn (PPHN) and other diseases characterized by hypoxemia and pulmonary hypertension.

Nitrous Oxide

Nitrous oxide (N$_2$O) is a colorless, odorless and tasteless gas, although it is sometimes described as having a slightly sweet taste and aroma. It is a dense compound (1.947 kg/m^3) with a specific gravity of 1.529, just more than 50% heavier than air and heavier than CO_2. N_2O is nonflammable and supports combustion to a greater degree than air but less than O_2. N_2O does not support life and if inhaled in high concentrations without sufficient oxygen, causes asphyxia. Because the critical temperature of N_2O is 36.5° C (97.7° F), cylinders contain both liquid and gas. N_2O is manufactured by the thermal decomposition of ammonium nitrate.

In 1799 Sir Humphry Davy inhaled N_2O and wrote that it had "absolutely intoxicated me." A year later, after further experimentation, he suggested that N_2O "seems capable of destroying physical pain, it may probably be used with advantage in surgical operations." N_2O affects the central nervous system. After a few breaths are taken, it may induce symptoms resembling alcoholic intoxication, including dizziness and giddiness. That reaction of some individuals resulted in N_2O being referred to colloquially as "laughing gas." In the early 1900s, N_2O mixed with oxygen began to be used as an anesthetic, a medical application that continues today.

Nitrogen

Nitrogen (N$_2$) is the major component of the atmosphere, 78% by volume. It is a colorless, transparent, odorless, tasteless gas that is slightly less dense than air. N_2 is nonflammable and does not support combustion or life. It is produced in large quantity, along with O_2, during fractional distillation of liquefied air and used to provide the zero-point reference in some oxygen analyzers and as a diagnostic gas in pulmonary function testing. In addition, because N_2 does not support combustion, it is also used to power pneumatic instruments in the operating room.

Storage and Distribution of Medical Gases

Medical gases can be stored and transported in the gaseous state or as liquefied gas **(cryogenic liquid)** in various-sized cylinders and in bulk containers. High-pressure **medical gas cylinders** are available from small, lightweight units containing a few cubic feet of gas to large cylinders of several hundred cubic feet. Containers of liquefied gas, such as oxygen, can be portable, containing a few liters or gallons to several hundred gallons in a container mounted in a delivery vehicle or several thousand gallons in a tanker truck or railway car. Bulk liquid oxygen storage vessels, such as those found at most hospitals, contain from 500 to 10,000 gallons. Oxygen and other medical gases from bulk storage containers are distributed through a piping system throughout the hospital, where needed.

Numerous federal, state, and local statutes, as well as industry standards and guidelines regulate the storage, transport, distribution, and use of medical gases. The government agencies and private organizations and their areas of responsibilities and expertise are described in Box 31-1.

Medical Gas Cylinders

Manufacture Federal regulation of the construction of cylinders used to transport compressed gas began in 1948 under the jurisdiction of the U.S. Interstate Commerce Commission (ICC). In 1968 that responsibility was given to the U.S. **Department of Transportation**

$\mathcal{B}$ox 31-1

Regulatory and Standards Organizations in the Manufacture, Storage, and Distribution of Medical Gases

ANSI—American National Standards Institute: a private, not-for-profit organization that coordinates U.S. private-sector voluntary standards development

ASME—American Society of Mechanical Engineers: organization that issues design, mechanical, and structural standards for items such as components of central piping systems

ASTM—American Society for Testing and Materials: a not-for-profit organization that aids in the development and publication of voluntary consensus standards for medical devices and many consumer products

CGA—Compressed Gas Association: industry technical trade organization that has developed numerous safety standards involving cylinders, fittings, and connections

CSA—Canadian Standards Association: an independent Canadian organization that recommends standards for the safety, quality, and performance of equipment

DOT—(U.S.) Department of Transportation: federal body that regulates cylinder manufacture and testing and the transport of hazardous materials, including compressed gases and cryogenic liquids

EPA—(U.S.) Environmental Protection Agency: government agency that establishes standards and administers regulations concerning potential and actual environmental hazards

FDA—(U.S.) Food and Drug Administration: an agency of the Department of Health and Human Services (HHS) that enforces regulations and standards concerning the purity of medical gases and their manufacture, packaging, and labeling

HHS—(U.S.) Department of Health and Human Services: the principal government agency dealing with health and social services, with the following subsets: FDA, Centers for Disease Control and Prevention (CDC), National Institutes of Health (NIH), and Health Care Financing Administration (HCFA), which administers Medicare and Medicaid

ICC—(U.S.) Interstate Commerce Commission: a government bureau that before 1967 set and administered the regulations currently the domain of the DOT

ISO—International Standards Organization: a worldwide agency coordinating and establishing technologic standards in manufacturing and safety

NFPA—(U.S.) National Fire Protection Association: a private independent agency that recommends standards related to fire and safety, which are routinely adopted as regulations by state and local government building and safety codes

NIOSH—(U.S.) National Institute for Occupational Safety and Health: a part of the CDC responsible for conducting research and making recommendations for the prevention of work-related disease and injury

OSHA—(U.S.) Occupational Safety and Health Administration: an agency of the Department of Labor that establishes and enforces standards of safety in the workplace

TC—Transport Canada: Canadian government agency that administers regulations concerning manufacture and testing of compressed gas cylinders and their distribution

USP/NF—United States Pharmacopoeia/National Formulary: a not-for-profit private organization founded to develop officially recognized quality standards for drugs, including medical gases

Z-79—A committee of ANSI that establishes standards for oxygen and respiratory and anesthesia equipment and devices

(DOT). In Canada since 1980, Transport Canada (TC) has set cylinder standards. DOT regulations specify that high-pressure medical gas cylinders be of seamless construction from high-quality steel, chromium-molybdenum alloy, or aluminum. Steel cylinders are produced by one of two methods. One involves the pressing of a mass of soft steel into a tubular form, and with heat, shaping and sealing of the bottom and formation of the shoulder and neck at the outlet end. Hot steel also can be spun to form a seamless cylinder. Aluminum cylinders are produced by extrusion with an alloy often containing a blend of magnesium and silicon. Aluminum cylinders are as much as 40% lighter than steel. Another type of construction available for cylinders is up to 70% lighter than steel, the composite cylinder. Composite cylinders are manufactured when a thin-walled aluminum cylinder is overwrapped with multiple layers of carbon, fiberglass, or Kevlar fibers in an epoxy resin wrap. Steel and aluminum cylinders have flat bottoms, whereas composite cylinder bottoms are rounded. Composite cylinders are only available in small sizes, up to 22 cubic feet of gas (623 liters), whereas steel and aluminum are available in a wide range of sizes as described in Figure 31-2 and Table 31-3.

Cylinder Marking   Figure 31-3 shows the typical DOT required markings found permanently struck into the shoulder of all cylinders. In Canada the mark "TC" would replace the "DOT." The DOT specifications to which the cylinder was manufactured are indicated as DOT 3A, seamless carbon-steel; DOT 3AA, seamless heat-treated, tempered alloy-steel; or DOT 3AL, seamless cylinders made from specified aluminum alloys. The service pressure in psig immediately follows the DOT specification marking and is 2015 for most medical gas cylinders. Cylinders may be filled to 10% more than the service pressure, most being filled to 2200 psig. Also found struck into the cylinder are the name or mark of the manufacturer, the serial number of the cylinder, and the original hydrostatic test date followed by the date(s) of subsequent tests.

Cylinder Testing   The DOT and TC require that cylinders be tested at regular intervals to ensure that they remain safe for filling to their specified pressures. For steel medical cylinders (3A, 3AA) the test must be repeated at least once every 10 years and for aluminum (3AL) every 5 years. The cylinder exterior is inspected for signs of damage from rust, corrosion, dents, or deep scarring. After the valve is removed, the interior is inspected for signs of rust,

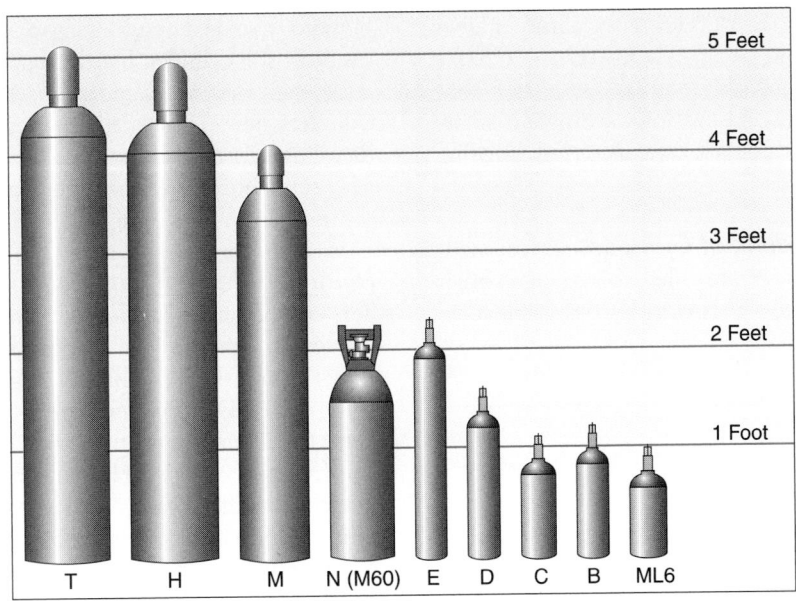

Figure 31-2   Size and letter designation of medical gas cylinders.

$\mathcal{T}$ABLE 31-3

Physical Characteristics of Common-Sized Aluminum and Steel Cylinders

	B or M6	ML6	C or M9	D	E	N or M60	M or MM	D	E	M	H	T
	Aluminum							**Steel**				
Service pressure (psig)	2216	2015	2015	2015	2015	2216	2216	2015	2015	2015	2265	2400
Height without valve (inches)	11.6	7.7	10.9	16.5	25.6	23	35.75	16.75	25.75	43	51	55
Diameter (inches)	3.2	4.4	4.4	4.4	4.4	7.25	8	4.2	4.2	7	9	9.25
Weight without valve empty (pounds)	2.2	2.9	3.7	5.3	7.9	21.7	38.6	7.9	11.3	58	117	139
Capacity at Listed Pressure at STPA												
Oxygen (cubic feet)	6	6	9	15	24	61.4	122	15	24	110	250	300
Oxygen (L)	170	170	255	425	680	1738	3455	425	680	3113	7075	8490

STPA, *Standard temperature and pressure, atmospheric.*

corrosion, and scaling and then hydrostatically tested to a pressure at least five-thirds its normal working pressure. For most cylinders that would be a test pressure of 3358 psi (2015 × ⅝).

The **hydrostatic testing** (Figure 31-4) process measures the expansion characteristic of the cylinder when it is exposed to internal pressures two-thirds greater than normal. This process is done through total suspension of the cylinder in a tank of water and pumping of water into the cylinder. The increased pressure causes the cylinder to expand. The amount of this expansion is measured by the water displaced. The amount of elastic expansion is di-

rectly related to the cylinder-wall thickness. As the wall thickness diminishes over time due to normal wear, the cylinder expands more during hydrostatic testing, eventually failing the test and being removed from service before becoming unsafe.

Cylinder Color-Coding and Labeling   A standard color-coding system for medical gas cylinders was suggested by the CGA and adopted by the U.S. Department of Commerce on recommendation of the Bureau of Standards. A slightly different international color-coding scheme exists as shown in Table 31-4. In addition to the color code, each medical gas cylinder must feature a label meeting the U.S. **Food and Drug Administration (FDA)** specifications indicating the gas contained, ensuring that it meets USP specifications, and noting warnings and dangers and that a prescription is necessary for dispensing (Figure 31-5).

Safe Storage and Handling of Cylinders
Most medical gas cylinders of all sizes are filled to the same high pressure—2200 psi. This pressure involves a formidable force

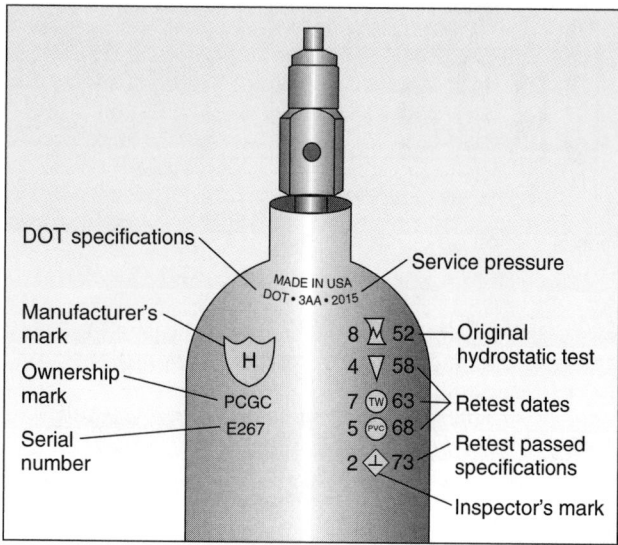

Figure 31-3 Typical cylinder markings required by the U.S. Department of Transportation.

of more than a ton pushing against every square inch of the inside of the cylinder. For this reason and because cylinders are shaped awkwardly and steel cylinders are quite heavy, all cylinders must be treated with care in handling. Careless handling can result in serious—even fatal—accidents. Box 31-2 summarizes the recommendations of the CGA for safe practices in the handling and storing of cylinders.

Filling of Medical Gas Cylinders
Medical gas cylinders can be refilled and reused, many being in continuous use for 30 or more years. Because oxygen is dispensed by prescription, the FDA has set strict controls over its packaging. The FDA regulates the filling of medical gas cylinders by issuing current good manufacturing practices (GMP) enforced by biannual on-site inspection. All refillers of medical gases—whether commercial operations filling hundreds of cylinders a day or small home medical equipment dealers filling just several dozen a week—must register with the FDA and comply with the GMP, regulations that ensure the following:

- Only safe, clean (inside and out), properly labeled cylinders are refilled.
- The gas meets USP/NF standards of purity and is traceable to its origin.
- Each batch of refilled cylinders is identified by lot number and is traceable if necessary for a recall.
- Only properly trained individuals using certified equipment are involved in the refilling process.

The process consists of four elements: (1) cylinder prefill check, (2) cylinder filling, (3) postfill procedures, and (4) documentation, all of which are described in Box 31-3.

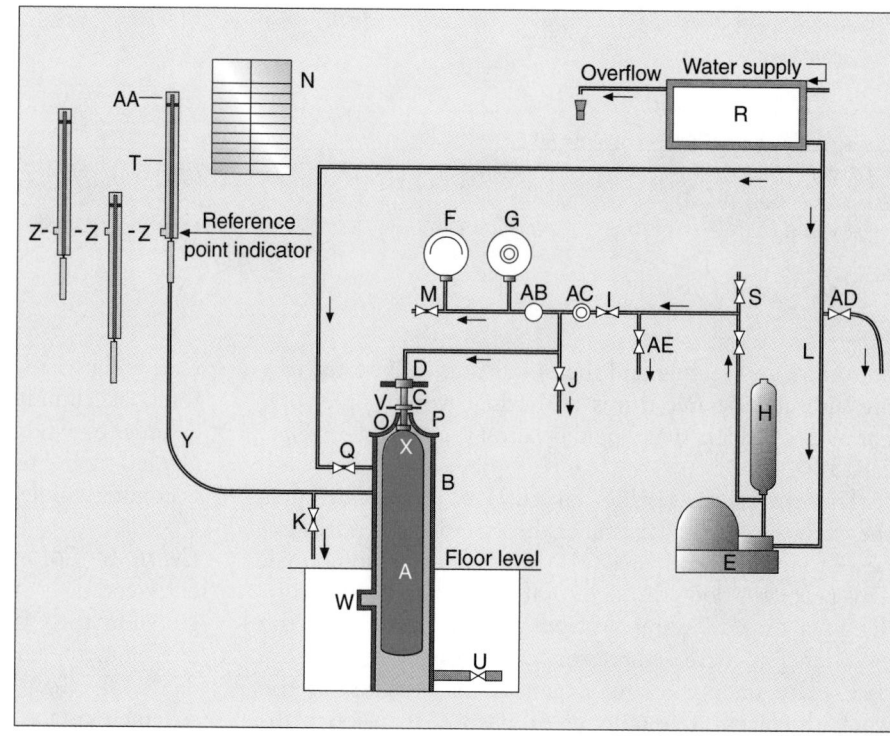

Figure 31-4 Hydrostatic testing system for compressed gas cylinders. *A,* Cylinder being tested; *B,* water jacket; *C, D, O, P, V,* cylinder connection and water jacket cover assembly; *E,* hydraulic pressure source; *F,* pressure indicating gauge; *G,* pressure recording gauge; *H,* pressure surge chamber; *I, J, K, L, M, Q, U, AD, AE,* valves; *N,* test data sheet; *R,* water reservoir; *S,* safety relief valve; *T,* burette calibrated in cubic centimeters; *W,* safety blowout port. (Modified from Keith BR. Health care facilities handbook. 4th ed. Quincy, Mass: National Fire Protection Agency; 1993.)

Filling cylinders with gaseous oxygen, usually referred to as *transfilling,* can be done with a supply source of oxygen gas or liquid oxygen. Transfilling gas to gas is appropriate for filling of small-size cylinders (E, C, D, etc.) from a supply of large-size cylinders (H, K, T, etc.) and the number of cylinders to be filled at one time is 40 or less. Figure 31-6 shows a typical gas-to-gas transfilling manifold system. The cylinders to be refilled first are individually inspected to ensure that they have no visible damage; are within the test date; and contain the proper color-coding, valve, and label. After attachment to the manifold, the empty cylinders are evacuated by a vacuum pump to −25 inches Hg to ensure the removal of all residual gas, impurities, and moisture. Then the first cylinder from the supply-side bank is opened, and its gas flows equally into all the empty cylinders until equilibrium is reached. That supply cylinder is turned off and the next cylinder in the supply bank opened. This process, known as *cascade filling,* proceeds until the filling cylinders reach 2000 to 2200 psig at 70° F. Gas flow into the cylinders is restricted to a maximum rate of 200 psi per minute to prevent overheating due to recompression in the filling cylinders.

When large numbers of cylinders of any size are to be filled regularly, liquid oxygen is used as the source. As with gas-to-gas transfilling, the cylinders first are inspected and evacuated, after which liquid oxygen that has been converted to gas by passing through a vaporizing unit is pumped into the cylinders at the controlled rate of 200 psi per minute until the cylinders are full.

Transfilling a single small cylinder from a larger full cylinder is a procedure that is potentially dangerous and should not be performed. The transfilling adapters do not generally contain a flow limiter to prevent rapid filling, which allows for a rapid buildup of heat caused by recom-

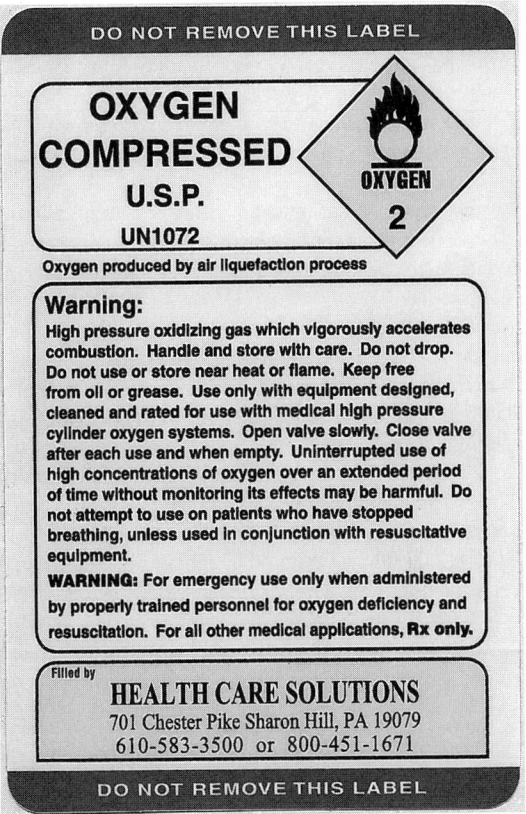

Figure 31-5 Typical medical gas cylinder label containing all wording required by the U.S. Food and Drug Administration.

TABLE 31-4

Color Codes and Purity of Medical Gases

Gas	Chemical Symbol	Purity*	Color Code U.S.	International
Oxygen	O_2	99.0	Green	White
Air	—	99.0	Yellow	Black and white
Nitrogen	N_2	99.0	Black	Black
Nitrogen/oxygen†	N_2/O_2	99.0	Black and green	Pink
Carbon dioxide	CO_2	99.0	Gray	Gray
Carbon dioxide/oxygen†	CO_2/O_2	99.0	Gray and green	Gray and white
Helium	He	99.0	Brown	Brown
Helium/oxygen†	He/O_2	99.0	Brown and green	Brown and white
Nitrous oxide	N_2O	97.0	Blue	Blue
Nitric oxide/nitrogen†	NO/N_2	99.0	Teal and black	Teal and black
Cyclopropane‡	C_3H_6	99.0	Orange	Orange
Ethylene‡	C_2H_4	99.0	Red	Red

*United States Pharmacopoeia/National Formulary standards.
†Labels should always be checked for the percentage of each gas.
‡Flammable anesthetic gas (rarely used).

Box 31-2

Safe Cylinder Storage and Handling

Storage

Cylinder storage must be in compliance with NFPA standards and all local, state, and federal regulations.

Cylinders must be stored in a cool, dry, fire-resistant enclosure that has good ventilation to prevent accumulation of gas if leaks occur.

Cylinder storage areas must be protected from the elements to prevent exposure to rain, snow, ice, and temperatures above 125° F.

Cylinder storage areas must be locked and secured from access and tampering by all unauthorized persons and should not be located near flammable or combustible substances.

Segregated locations within the cylinder storage area must be clearly labeled for full and empty cylinders to prevent their co-mingling.

Flammable gases must not be stored with gases that support combustion.

Large cylinders must be stored upright, with their protective caps screwed on tightly, and secured by a chain or other restraint mechanism to prevent their falling over.

Small cylinders may be stored upright or horizontally. In either position, they must be secured in racks, holders, or carts.

Cylinder storage areas must be clearly posted with signs inside and out indicating no smoking; no open flames; no combustible materials; no oil or grease, etc.

Transport and Handling

Cylinders must be transported on an appropriate cart secured with a restraining chain or strap. They must never be dragged, rolled, or slid.

Large cylinders must be transported with their protective caps screwed on tightly.

A cylinder should never be lifted by its protective cap.

Cylinders should be transported and handled only by properly trained personnel.

Cylinders must never be handled with oily or greasy hands, gloves, or clothing.

Petroleum-based products and lubricants must never be used on cylinder valves, regulators, fittings, or connections. Oxygen and petroleum-based products coming into contact under pressure may cause an explosive oxidation reaction.

Cylinders and cylinder valves should always be treated with care and respect.

NFPA, *National Fire Protection Association.*

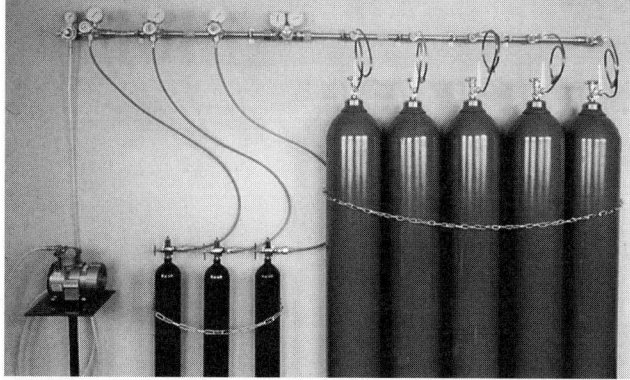

Figure 31-6 Example of a transfilling manifold. Shown on the right are the large full supply cylinders connected by "pigtails" to the manifold header. In the center are the smaller cylinders to be refilled. At the left is the vacuum pump used to evacuate the small cylinders before refilling takes place.

pression and a potentially hazardous condition if any oxidizable particles are present.

Cylinder Valves Each gas cylinder has a valve threaded tightly into its neck to control the turning on and off of gas flow from the cylinder. Small cylinders, sizes A through E, use a four-sided rectangular post valve, whereas larger cylinders feature a faucetlike valve with a threaded outlet. Most high-pressure medical gas cylinders use a direct-acting valve, as shown in Figure 31-7, in which turning of the handle moves the stem up or down, thereby raising or lowering the seat and allowing gas to flow from the cylinder or to stop the gas flow.

Because the pressure in a closed cylinder is directly related to the temperature (Gay-Lussac's law), all cylinder valves have pressure-relief safety devices that allow for the controlled release of excessive pressure from the cylinder if it is exposed to high temperatures, thus preventing an explosive rupturing. Most smaller cylinders that use a post valve have either a frangible copper disc that fractures if the cylinder pressure exceeds approximately 3022 psi (1½ times the normal filling pressure) or a fusible lead alloy plug that melts if the temperature reaches 208° F to 220° F, or a combination of frangible disc and fusible plug. The pressure safety relief on a large cylinder valve may be a spring-loaded device in which the spring pressure holds the safety valve outlet closed. However, if the gas pressure in the cylinder exceeds the spring tension, the outlet will open, allowing gas to escape and causing the pressure to lower to a safe level; the safety valve then will close. Figure 31-8 illustrates examples of cylinder valve pressure-relief safety devices.

Safety-Indexed Connection Systems

The American Standards Association, working in conjunction with the CGA, has established several safety systems to ensure that a device intended to dispense a specific gas, such

Box 31-3

Refilling Cylinders

Cylinder Prefill Checks

Before any cylinder to be refilled is placed on the transfilling manifold, the following must be completed:

Each cylinder valve is opened and any residual gas slowly vented into the atmosphere.

As oxygen cylinders vent, the gas should be carefully sniffed for any odors. If an odor is present, the cylinder is removed from service.

Each cylinder is checked for the last hydrostatic test date. Any found to exceed DOT retest criteria must be removed from service and retested before being refilled.

A visual inspection of the exterior of each cylinder and valve is conducted to detect signs of physical damage, such as dents and deep scratches or gouges. Any suspicious cylinders are removed from service and retested.

Aluminum cylinders are checked for a yellowing discoloration of the exterior surface, a sign that the cylinder has been exposed to excessive temperatures and must be retested and repainted.

A ring test is conducted on all steel cylinders by a gentle striking of the center of the cylinder with a lightweight hammer. The resulting sound should be bell-like, sharp, and clear. A dull or flat sound suggests a weakening of the steel wall, often due to interior rust. Such cylinders should be removed from service and retested.

Each cylinder must have a current label meeting FDA and DOT regulations. The label must be intact and completely readable.

The cylinder should be cosmetically acceptable and clean.

Cylinder Filling

The cylinders to be refilled are attached to the manifold.

The cylinders are evacuated with a vacuum pump to draw at least -25 inches Hg, after which the vacuum pump is turned off.

Gas from the supply source then is allowed into the cylinders at a controlled flow, permitting a filling rate of no more than 200 psig per minute.

One cylinder of the group being filled is monitored for temperature with a thermometer mounted on its surface. Temperatures should not exceed 100° F.

Gas is allowed to flow or is pumped into the cylinders until the permitted full pressure is attained. Because the temperature affects the volume of gas in the cylinder at the time of filling, the full pressure is corrected for temperature so that an accurate volume is present at STP.

Postfill Procedures

The valves of the filled cylinders are closed and the cylinders removed from the manifold.

The valve of each cylinder is sprayed with a leak test solution approved for use with oxygen and observed for bubbling (indicating a leak) at such points as the valve outlet, safety relief device, and valve stem. All leak test solution then is wiped from the valve.

In the case of oxygen, one cylinder is selected from the filled group, and its gas is tested with an FDA-approved and calibrated analyzer. The gas must meet the minimum purity standard of the USP/NF—99% in the case of oxygen. If purity is below the minimum standard, that cylinder may not be released, and every cylinder in that group must be assayed before release.

A lot number label is attached to each cylinder and is used to track each cylinder in the batch if a recall is necessary.

The cylinders are placed in the full cylinder storage area.

Documentation

Each of the previously listed steps are checked off as completed on the cylinder transfilling log. The log must be signed by the individual who filled the cylinders and co-signed by the supervisor. Documentation of the filling process is required to meet the GMP of the FDA.

A record must be kept of the daily calibration, according to manufacturer specifications, of the FDA-approved oxygen analyzer.

The manifold and its valves and gauges must be inspected and cleaned according to an established schedule and then documented.

Pressure gauges, thermometers, and analyzers must be recalibrated in accordance with manufacturer requirements and then documented.

DOT, *Department of Transportation;* FDA, *Food and Drug Administration;* USP/NF, *United States Pharmacopoeia/National Formulary;* GMP, *good manufacturing practices.*

as oxygen, can only be connected to a source of that gas. An oxygen regulator can only be attached to an oxygen cylinder. It will not attach to a cylinder of nitrous oxide or helium or anything other than oxygen. Three indexed safety systems are available for medical gases: the American Standard Compressed Gas Cylinder Outlet and Inlet Connections, usually referred to as the American Standard Safety System (ASSS); the Pin-Index Safety System (PISS); and the Diameter-Index Safety System (DISS).

American Standard Safety System

The threaded outlets of the faucetlike valves found on large sized cylinders (larger than E) conform to the **American Standard Safety System (ASSS).** This system uses a combination of the following factors specific for each gas or gas combination:

- Diameter of the outlet in thousandths of an inch
- Number of threads per inch
- Whether it has right-handed or left-handed threads
- Whether the threads are external or internal
- The shape of the mating nipple on the corresponding regulator

A large high-pressure oxygen cylinder has an outlet that meets the following specification: 0.903-14-RH-Ext. Its

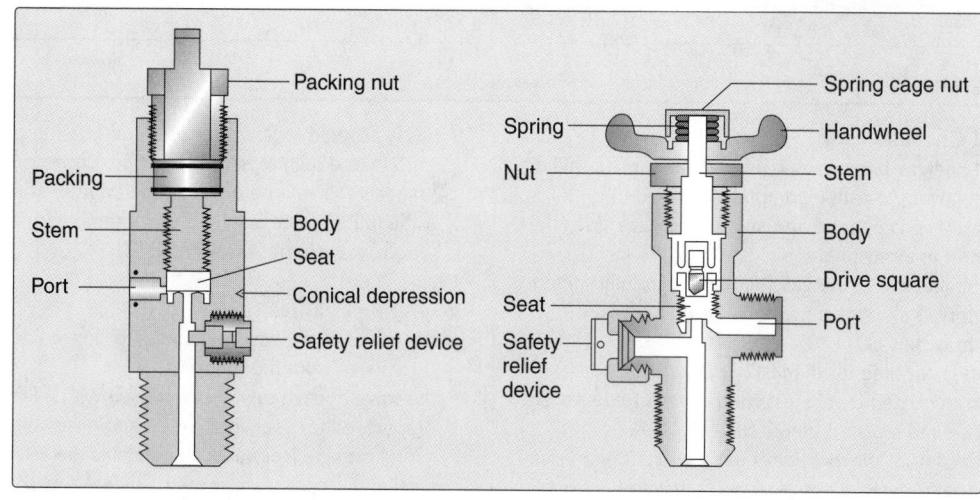

Figure 31-7 Direct-acting cylinder valve.

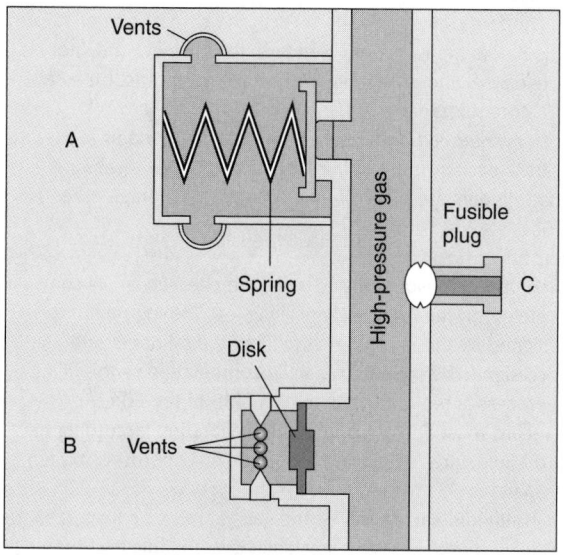

Figure 31-8 Cylinder valve-pressure relief safety devices. *A,* Spring loaded device. When gas pressure exceeds the spring tension, the spring is compressed to the left, allowing gas to escape through the vents. When gas pressure is reduced to normal, the spring tension re-closes the valve. *B,* Frangible disk. When gas pressure exceeds safe limits, the disc ruptures, allowing all the contents of the cylinder to escape into the atmosphere through the vents. *C,* Fusible plug. If the temperature inside or outside the cylinder exceed safe limits, the plug melts, allowing all the gas in the cylinder to safely escape. (Modified from Branson RD, Hess DR, Chatburn RL. Respiratory care equipment. 2nd ed. Philadelphia: Lippincott Williams & Wilkins; 1999.)

outlet diameter is 0.903 inch, with 14 threads to the inch, the connections will screw on with a turn to the right, and the threads are external. This configuration also is referred to by the CGA's designation CGA 540. Figure 31-9 illustrates selected ASSS valve outlets and connections.

Pin-Index Safety System High-pressure medical gas cylinders, size E and smaller, use another indexing system known as the **Pin-Index Safety System (PISS).** This system uses a specific combination of two holes in the post valve just below the gas outlet for each gas or gas mixture. Any regulator or device intended to connect to the valve has pins that correspond to the holes, allowing for a proper connection. The pin index for oxygen is 2-5, which is also referred to as a CGA 870. Figure 31-10 illustrates various gas pin indexes, and Figure 31-11 shows the connecting of a pin-indexed regulator to the post valve.

Diameter-Index Safety System The PISS and ASSS systems are designed for use on high-pressure cylinders. The **diameter-index safety system (DISS)** was designed by the CGA for low-pressure (under 200 psig) connections and fittings. It consists of a system of specific diameter-threaded "male" outlets that mate with a corresponding "female" nut and nipple. Different diameters, thread pitch, and nipple configurations are assigned to various gases and gas mixtures. The common oxygen DISS connection (CGA 1240) has a

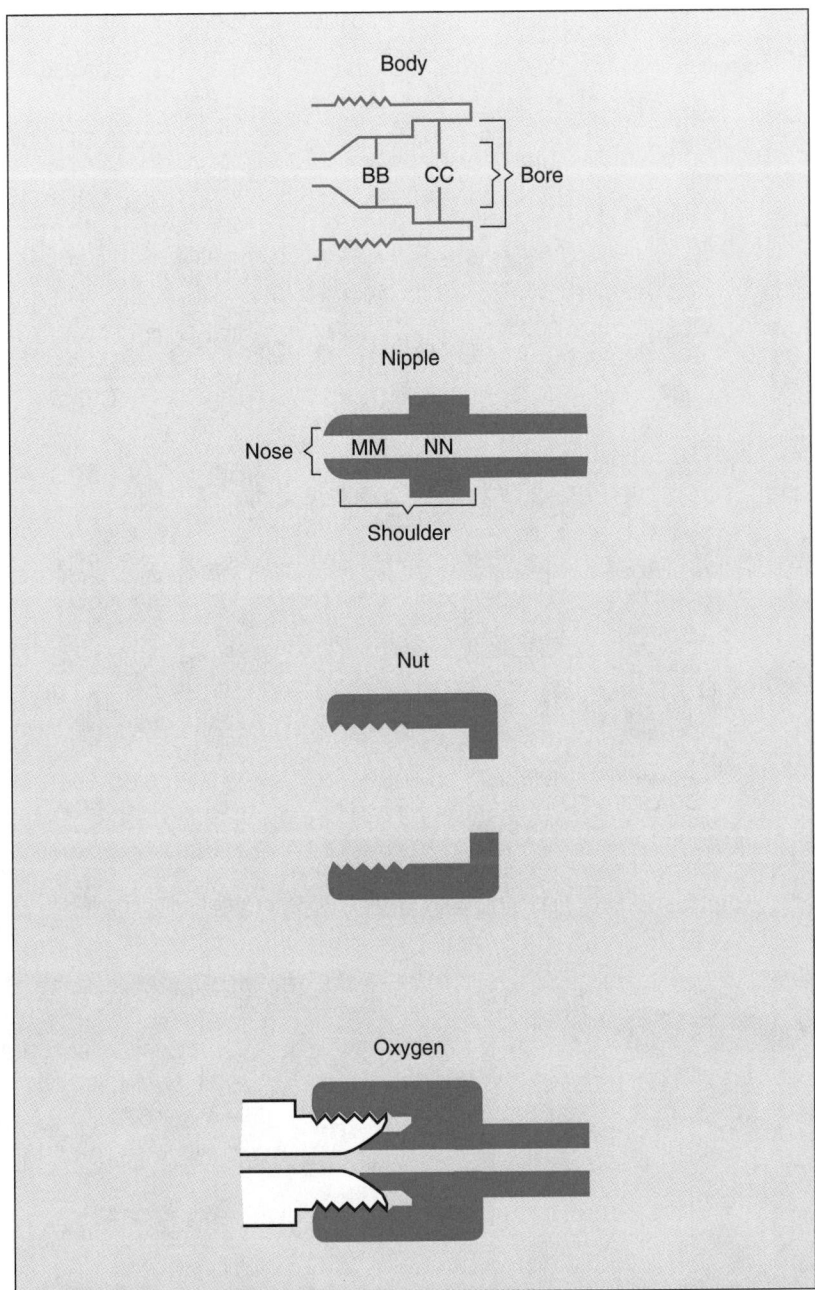

Figure 31-9   Valve outlet connections for large cylinders showing use of nut, thread, and nipple to set specifications for different gases. (Modified from Dorsch JA, Dorsch SE. Understanding anesthesia equipment. 3rd ed. Baltimore: Williams & Wilkins; 1994.)

diameter of $^9/_{16}$ of an inch and 18 threads to the inch, often indicated as $^9/_{16}$ − 18. It is found for example at the outlet of an oxygen flow meter, the inlet to a bubble humidifier, and the threaded connection at the end of an oxygen hose. Figure 31-12 illustrates the use of all three indexed safety systems.

Calculating Duration of Flow from a Gas Cylinder

Being able to calculate how long the contents of any size cylinder will last at a specified flow is important (for ex-

ample, how many cylinders are needed during transport of a patient). This simple calculation requires knowledge of how many liters of gas are in the cylinder and the prescribed liters per minute flow rate. Dividing the contents of the cylinder (in liters) by the rate of flow (in liters per minute) provides the time (in minutes) available. Table 31-5 lists the duration of flow of various-sized cylinders at flows from $^1/_2$ to 6 L/min.

Table 31-3 lists specifications for the most commonly used sizes of medical gas cylinders, including the contents

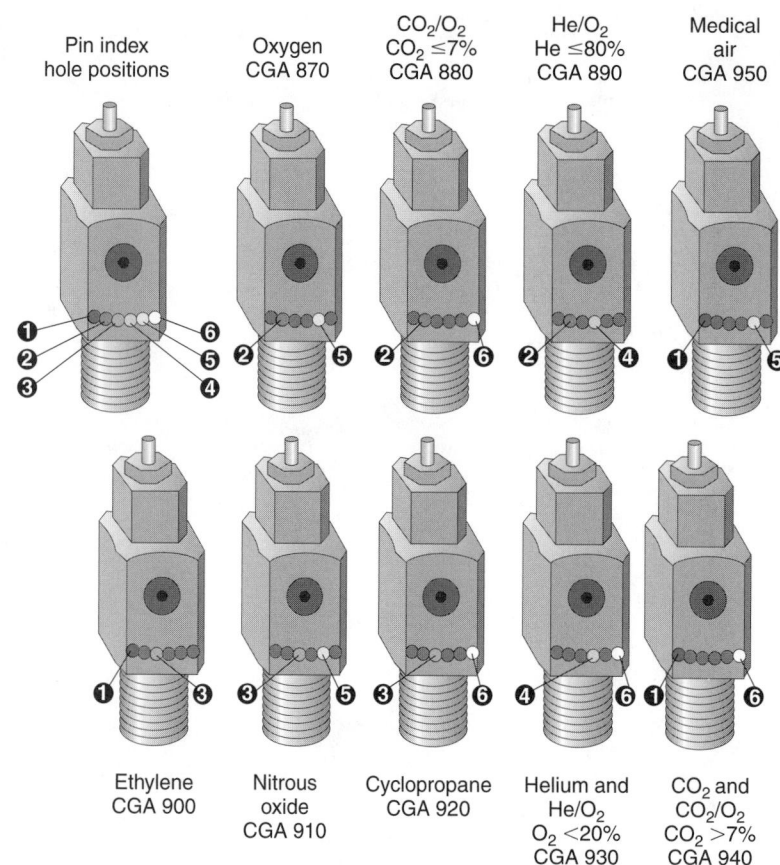

Figure 31-10   The Pin-Index Safety System (PISS) for small-cylinder valves.

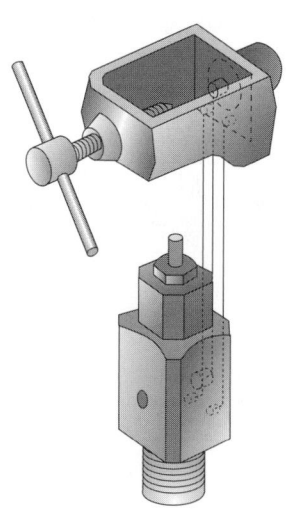

Figure 31-11   Yoke connector showing the alignment of the pins on the yoke with the holes on the post valve of small cylinders (size E and smaller). (Modified from Barnes TA, editor. Core textbook of respiratory care practice. 2nd ed. St Louis: Mosby; 1994.)

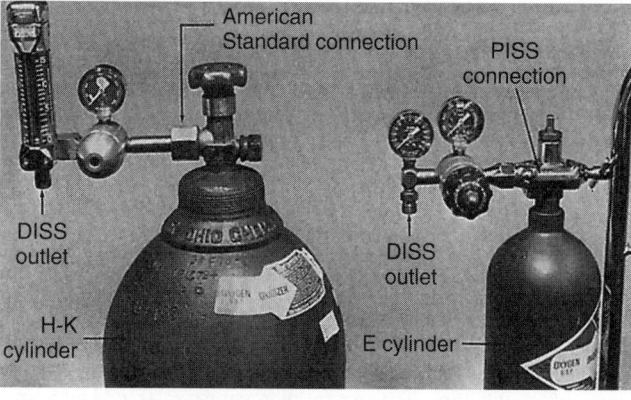

Figure 31-12   Examples of the three indexed safety systems: the American Standard Safety System (ASSS) for high-pressure connections to large-size cylinders; the Pin-Index Safety System (PISS) that uses a yoke with specifically spaced pins to mate with matching holes on the post valve of small cylinders (size E and smaller); and the Diameter-Index Safety System (DISS) used at low-pressure (less than 200 psig) connections and fittings. (From Scanlan CL, Wilkins RL, Stoller JK. Egan's fundamentals of respiratory care. 7th ed. St Louis: Mosby; 1999.)

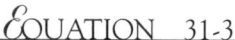EQUATION   31-3

Conversion Factor for E Cylinder

$$\frac{22\ \text{Cubic feet of gas} \times 28.3\ \text{L/ft}^3}{2200\ \text{psig}} = 0.28\ \text{L/psig}$$

of a full cylinder in cubic feet and liters of gas at 70° F and 2200 psig. However, if the cylinder is not full, a further calculation must be made to determine its contents in cubic feet or liters. The volume of gas in any cylinder is directly related to the pressure in the cylinder. If, for example, a full E cylinder contains 622 L (22 cubic feet) at

TABLE 31-5
Duration of Use of Oxygen from Selected Cylinder Sizes

Size Cylinder	Liters Full	½	1	1½	2	2½	3	4	5	6
B or ML6	170	5.6	2.8	1.9	1.4	1.1	0.9	0.7	0.5	0.4
C	255	8.5	4.25	2.8	2.1	1.7	1.4	1	0.8	0.7
D	425	14	7	4.7	3.5	2.8	2.3	1.7	1.4	1.1
E	680	22.7	11.3	7.5	5.6	4.5	3.7	2.8	2.2	1.9
N (M60)	1738	58 (2.4 days)	29	19.3	14.5	11.5	9.6	7.25	5.8	4.8
M	3455	115 (4.8 days)	57.5 (2.4 days)	38.4 (1.6 days)	28.8	23	19	14.3	11.5	9.5
H	7075	235.8 (9.8 days)	118 (4.9 days)	78.6 (3.25 days)	59 (2.5 days)	47 (1.9 days)	39 (1.6 days)	29.5	23.5	19.6
T	8490	283 (11.8 days)	141.5 (5.9 days)	94.3 (3.9 days)	70.75 (2.9 days)	56.6 (2.4 days)	47.1 (1.9 days)	35.3 (1.5 days)	28.3	23.5

NOTE: *Although these times are accurate, they represent use of a cylinder until it is empty. In actual practice a cylinder would be changed before it emptied.*

2200 psig, at a pressure of 1100 psig it will have one-half that volume (311 liters) and at 550 psig, 155.5 L. Because one cubic foot holds 28.3 L, the number of liters in any number of cubic feet can be determined by multiplication by 28.3.

Respiratory Recap

Determining Duration of Flow

Such calculations are necessary to determine how long an oxygen supply will last when a patient is transported.

For compressed gas cylinders, duration of flow is calculated by use of the actual pressure in the cylinder, the conversion factor for the size of the cylinder, and the oxygen flow rate.

For cylinders containing liquefied gas the weight of the cylinder is used to infer the amount remaining because the gauge shows a constant pressure.

To make the calculation easier, conversion factors are commonly used. The conversion factor can be determined for any cylinder via multiplication of the cubic feet of gas in the full cylinder by 28.3 and division of that product by 2200 psig (the pressure in a full cylinder). For example, the calculation of the conversion factor for an E cylinder is illustrated in Equation 31-3.

The conversion factors for a number of cylinder sizes are presented in Table 31-6. The duration of flow can be accurately calculated by multiplication of the actual pressure in the cylinder (psig) by the conversion factor for that size cylinder and division of that product by the prescribed flow rate (liters per minute). Equation 31-4 provides such an example.

EQUATION 31-4
Calculation of Duration of Flow

When an E cylinder of oxygen is used with 1600 psig at a flow rate of 4 L/min, the duration of flow is calculated as follows:

$$\frac{1600 \text{ psig} \times 0.28 \text{ L/psig}}{4 \text{ L/min}} = 112 \text{ minutes}$$

TABLE 31-6
Cylinder Conversion Factors

Cylinder Size	Conversion Factor		
	O₂,Air, O₂/N₂	O₂/CO₂	He/O₂
D	0.16	0.20	0.14
E	0.28	0.35	0.23
G	2.41	2.94	1.93
H or K	3.14	3.84	2.50

O_2, *Oxygen;* N_2, *nitrogen;* CO_2, *carbon dioxide;* He, *helium.*

The previously described relationships are valid for cylinders containing only compressed gas. In the case of cylinders containing liquefied gases, such as nitrous oxide and carbon dioxide, the contents are directly related to the net weight—the weight of the contents minus the weight of the cylinder. For example, knowing that the weight of the liquid in the full cylinder is 30 pounds, it follows that when the weight decreases by 15 pounds, one-half the contents would have been used. A pressure gauge on a cylinder with liquefied gas shows a constant pressure, the vapor

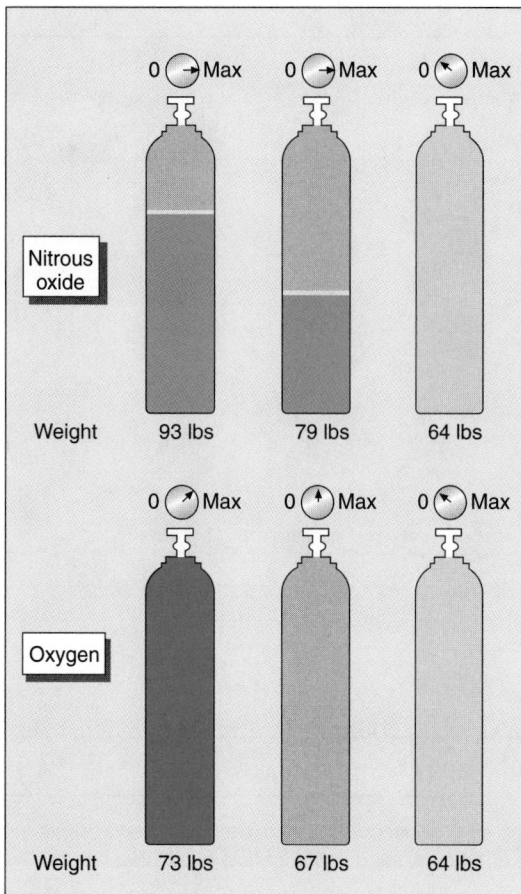

Figure 31-13 The relationship among cylinder weight, pressure, and contents. A gas stored partially in liquid form, such as nitrous oxide, shows a constant pressure, its vapor pressure (as long as the temperature remains constant), until all the liquid has vaporized to gas. At that point the gas volume in the cylinder becomes directly related to the cylinder pressure. A nonliquefied gas shows a steady decline in pressure as the gas is used. Both, however, show a steady decline in weight as gas is used. (Modified from Dorsch JA, Dorsch SE. Understanding anesthesia equipment. 4th ed. Baltimore: Williams & Wilkins; 1994.)

pressure of that gas, and bears no relationship to the contents. However, when all the liquid in the cylinder has vaporized to gas, the direct relationship between pressure and gas content comes into play, a concept that is illustrated in Figure 31-13.

Central Medical Gas Distribution and Vacuum Systems

Most hospitals and many other health care facilities, such as skilled nursing homes, rehabilitation centers, and outpatient surgical or diagnostic clinics commonly feature piped medical gas distribution systems for oxygen, air, and vacuum. Depending on usage, systems for nitrous oxide and occasionally for nitrogen and other gases are centrally distributed from a bulk source. Central oxygen, air, and

vacuum piping systems have made these commodities as common as water faucets and available at every bedside and other locations throughout most health care facilities. As with water and electricity distribution systems, little thought is given to the design, function, maintenance, or complexity of the system until something goes wrong and alternative systems must be used.

Bulk Supply Systems

Oxygen piping systems are supplied from a central source of liquid oxygen or a combination of liquid and gas, or only from cylinders of gaseous oxygen. The volume of gas used and the costs of supply dictate the choice of the supply source. Three central bulk supply systems are used: alternating supply systems (1) with or (2) without a reserve emergency supply and (3) continuous supply systems.

Alternating Supply Systems   Alternating supply systems are used in smaller facilities to supply oxygen or specialty gases, such as nitrous oxide and nitrogen. Figure 31-14, A, shows the arrangement of an alternating supply system without a reserve supply. It consists of two banks of cylinders, each of which contains at least two cylinders, or as many as 20, usually size H or the larger T. Each cylinder is connected by a flexible "pigtail" pipe, containing a one-way check valve that allows flow from the cylinder only to a high-pressure header and a pressure regulator. The combination of the header with its pigtails, valves, and regulator is often referred to as a *manifold*.

Gas flows from one bank of cylinders, the supply bank, through its manifold valve and regulator, where the pressure is reduced to 100 to 200 psig, and then to the main line pressure regulator, where it is further reduced to 50 to 55 psig and proceeds through the main shut-off valve and into the piping system. Flow continues until the pressure in the supply bank approaches 100 to 200 psig, which activates the changeover switch, automatically opening the valve from the second bank of cylinders, which now becomes the supply bank, and closing the valve from the first bank. The switch-over process also activates an alarm usually located in a manned location, such as security, maintenance, or the central telephone operator area, to alert the responsible party that one bank is empty and needs to be refilled or replaced.

An alternating supply system with an emergency reserve supply is shown in Figure 31-14, B. This system is similar to that in the previous description but adds a third gas supply as an emergency reserve in case either the primary and/or secondary supply fail. The system depicted in Figure 31-14, B, shows liquid vessels being used as the primary and secondary sources of the oxygen supply. Banks of cylinders of gaseous oxygen also can be used. Oxygen vendors can supply liquid oxygen in various-sized containers, often referred to as *vessels* or **dewars** (named for Scottish chemist and physicist Sir James Dewar, its inventor), which have a capacity of several hundred liters of liquid oxygen. Because 1 L of liquid oxygen yields 861 L of

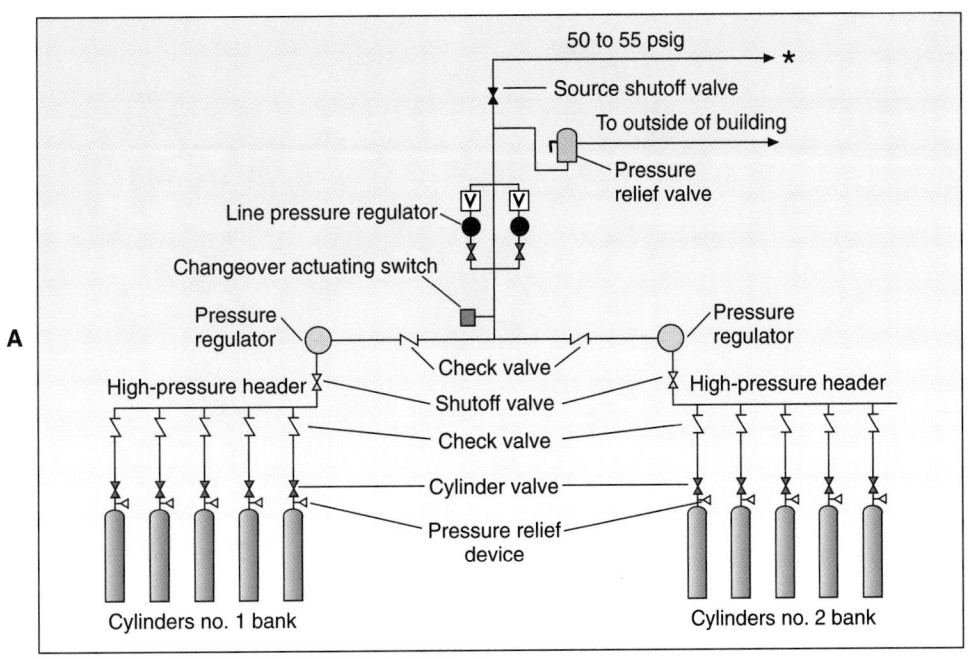

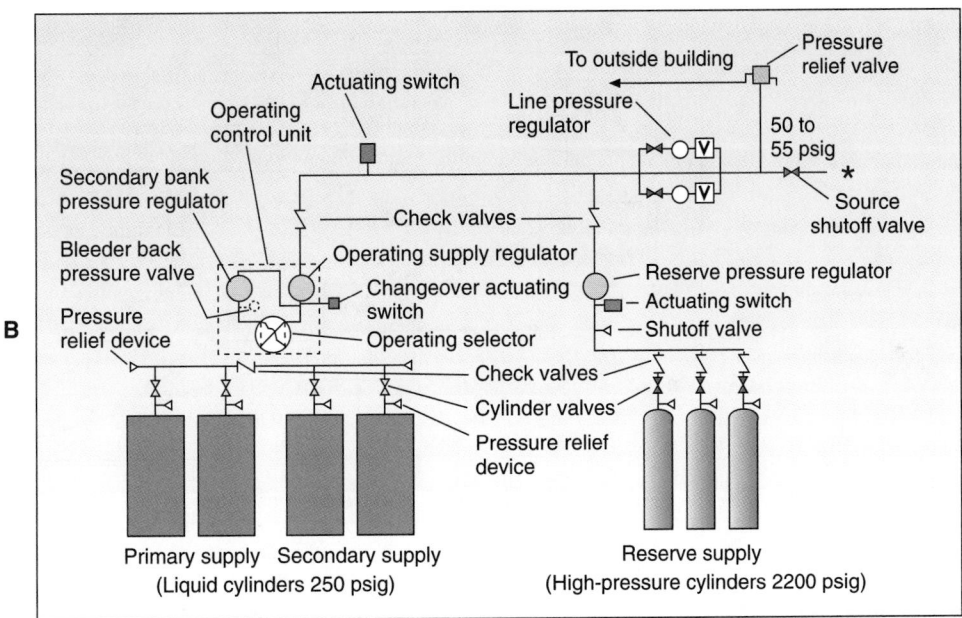

Figure 31-14 **A,** Schematic illustration of a typical alternating cylinder supply system without an emergency reserve supply. **B,** Schematic illustration of a typical alternating cylinder supply system with an emergency reserve supply. (Modified from NFPA 99C. Standard on Gas and Vacuum Systems. 1999 ed. Quincy, Mass: National Fire Protection Association; 1999.)

gaseous oxygen, a dewar containing 200 liquid L of oxygen delivers more than 172,000 L of oxygen gas, equivalent to the contents of 25 H cylinders. Refilling or exchanging one liquid dewar of oxygen is much more cost effective than handling and exchanging 25 H cylinders.

Continuous Supply Systems

Acute care facilities use an enormous amount of oxygen daily. As an example, 50 patients using oxygen at 2 L/min require a total of 144,000 L of oxygen gas in 24 hours, the equivalent of 21 H cylin-

ders a day and 625 a month. A large active facility may require many times more. To satisfy this demand a bulk liquid oxygen storage system is used. Containers for the bulk supply of liquid oxygen, referred to as *stand tanks*, are available in sizes ranging from as small as 500 gallons to 6000 gallons or more. Because 1 gallon of liquid oxygen is equal to 3.785 L of liquid oxygen and 1 L of liquid converts to 861 L of gaseous oxygen, a 500 gallon tank can deliver 1.6 million L of gas and a 6000-gallon vessel, 19.5 million L of gaseous oxygen.

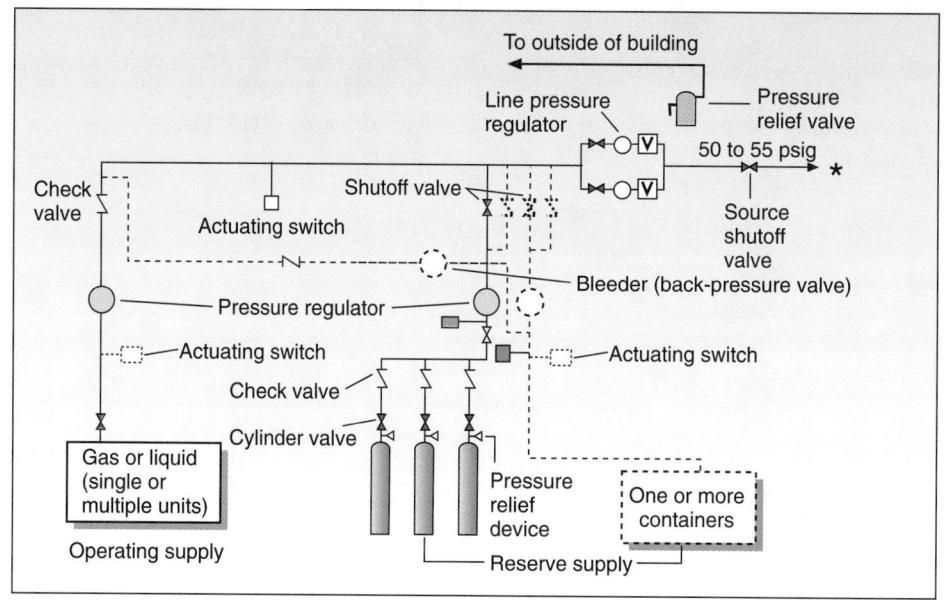

Figure 31-15 Schematic illustration of a typical bulk liquid oxygen supply system. (Modified from NFPA 99C. Standard on Gas and Vacuum Systems. 1999 ed. Quincy, Mass: National Fire Protection Association; 1999.)

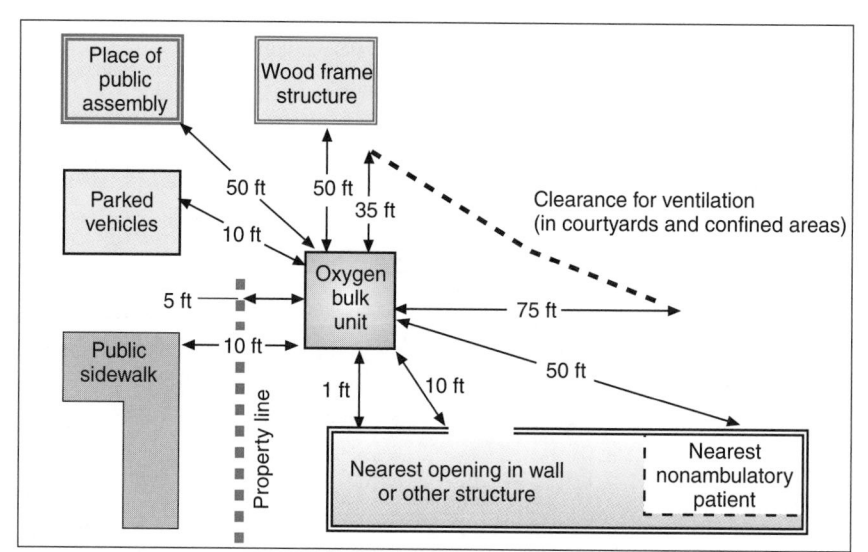

A

Figure 31-16 National Fire Protection Association standards for placement of a bulk liquid oxygen supply system. **A,** Distances to structures and public exposures. **B,** Distances to sources of ignition. (Modified from NFPA 99C. Standard on Gas and Vacuum Systems. 1999 ed. Quincy, Mass: National Fire Protection Association; 1999.)

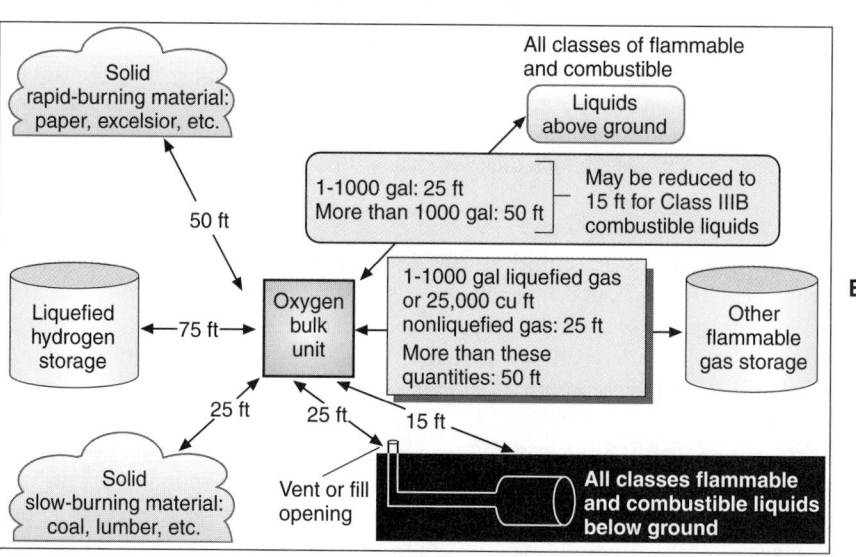

B

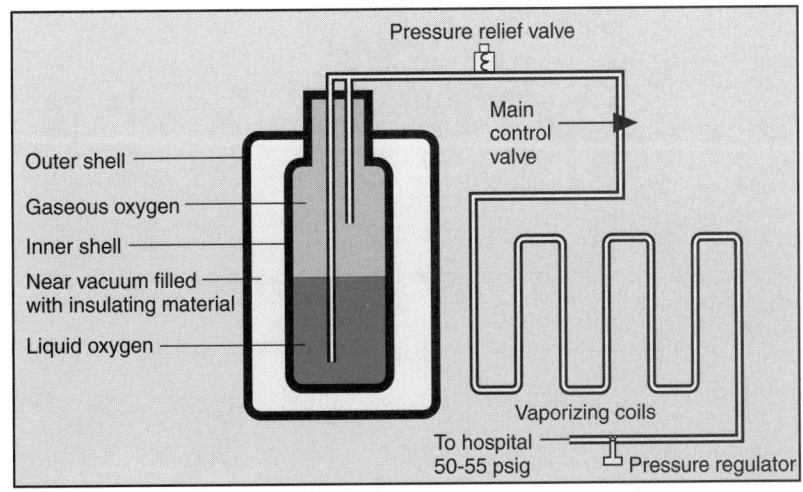

Figure 31-17 Diagram of a stationary bulk liquid oxygen storage system. (Modified from Branson RD, Hess DR, Chatburn RL. Respiratory care equipment, 2nd ed. Philadelphia: Lippincott Williams & Wilkins; 1999.)

Because the boiling point of liquid oxygen is −297.3° F, liquid oxygen must be stored in a container resembling a thermos bottle to keep heat transfer to a minimum and maintain the liquid state. All liquid storage containers, from small portable units for individual patient use to the largest stand tanks, are similarly designed and constructed, as shown in Figure 31-17. The liquid oxygen is held in an inner stainless-steel vessel surrounded by an outer exterior shell. Between the inner vessel and the outer shell is an insulation-filled space on which a vacuum is drawn. The inner reservoir contains oxygen both as a liquid and as a gas. As oxygen is needed in the facility, liquid oxygen flows from the reservoir and is quickly converted to gas through exposure to ambient temperature as it passes through the vaporizing coils. So much heat is necessary for this vaporization process that the vaporizer plates are kept extremely cold and are frequently coated with ice as a result of moisture in the air condensing and freezing on them. The pressure of the gas is regulated to enter the facility at 50 to 55 psig. If the liquid in the vessel warms up too much and some boils off as gas, thereby increasing the gas pressure, the pressure-relief valve will open, allowing a controlled release of pressure. This release of gas causes the remaining gas in the vessel to expand, and according to Gay-Lussac's Law, lowers the temperature in the vessel and helps maintain the liquid

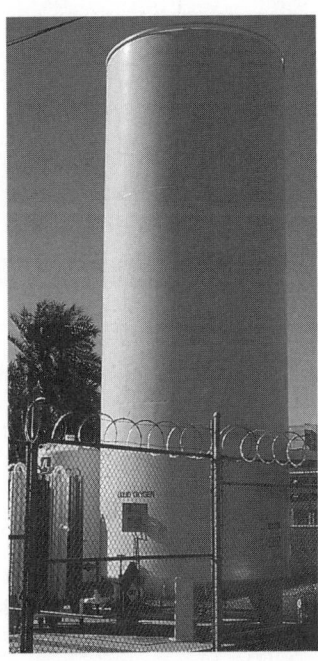

Figure 31-18 A 5000-gallon bulk liquid oxygen stand tank.

between its boiling point and critical pressure so that most of the contents remains in the liquid state.

The National Fire Protection Association (NFPA) issues standards concerning the placement, construction, and maintenance of bulk vessels and piping systems that are widely adopted by local and state regulatory authorities. Figure 31-15 is a schematic illustration of a typical bulk liquid oxygen system; Figure 31-16 illustrates the NFPA standards for placement of a bulk liquid oxygen stand tank; Figure 31-17 is a diagram of a stationary bulk oxygen storage tank; and Figure 31-18 shows an actual unit.

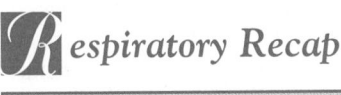

espiratory Recap

Bulk Gas Systems
Alternating supply systems
without an emergency reserve supply
with an emergency reserve supply
Continuous supply systems

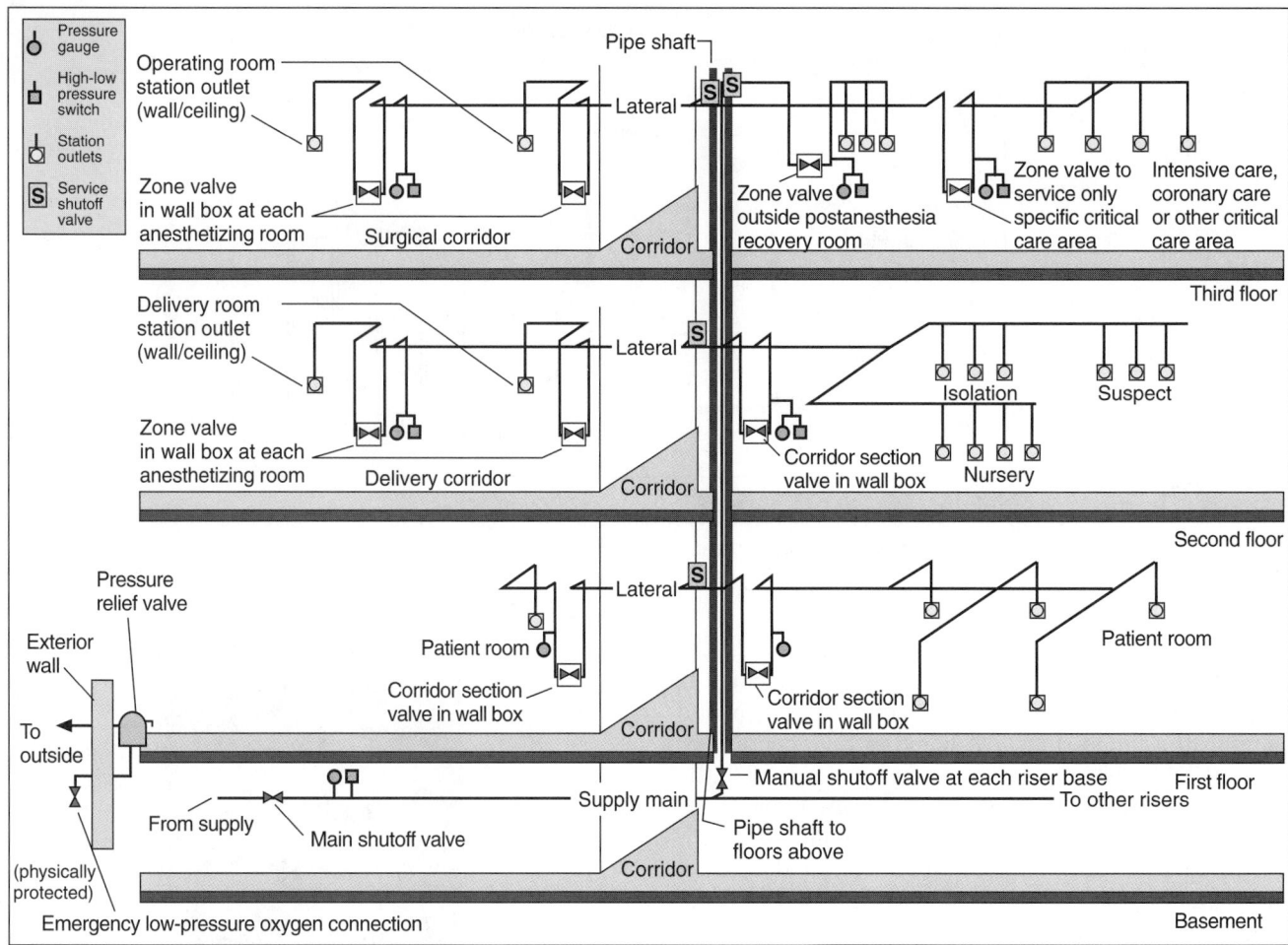

Figure 31-19 General schematic illustration of a central medical gas piping system showing locations of shut-off valves, pressure gauges, and alarm pressure switches. (Modified from NFPA 99C. Standard on Gas and Vacuum Systems. 1999 ed. Quincy, Mass: National Fire Protection Association; 1999.)

Gas Piping Systems

Gases stored in bulk supplies are distributed throughout the facility via a system of pipes, valves, and outlets, as shown in Figure 31-19. The entire system must meet the standards of the NFPA for construction, installation, testing, and maintenance. The pipe must be type K or L seamless copper tubing specially cleaned to remove all traces of oxidizable material. Engineering studies determine the size (diameter) pipe required to maintain 50 psig and maximum flows throughout the system. In most cases the pipe decreases in diameter size the further it is from the main. Each pipe must be clearly labeled at regular intervals to indicate the gas contained. All joints and fittings are sweat-soldered with silver solder.

The piping system, or an addition to an existing system, is blown clean with oil-free dry air or nitrogen before any outlets are attached to dislodge and eliminate debris, such as solder, flux, and metallic fillings. When construction is completed, the entire system is pressurized to a minimum of 150 psig with oil-free dry air or nitrogen. Every fitting, connection, valve, and outlet is individually inspected for leaks. The system then must hold that pressure for at least

24 hours. The blowing-clean and leak-testing procedure is conducted on each of the piping systems—oxygen, air, nitrous oxide, and any others. Before any piping system can be put into use, the test gas must be purged and the gas supply for that system attached. Then every outlet must be tested to ensure that it functions properly, that flow and pressure meet specifications, and that the correct gas is present by analysis.

Valves A primary supply shut-off valve must exist, where the main distribution pipe leaves the bulk supply and, in the case where the bulk supply is located outside the building, a main shut-off valve should exist, where the main supply pipe enters the facility. From the main line, pipes extend laterally and usually further branch into zones serving groups of patient rooms or other service areas. Risers proceed vertically from the main line to service upper floors.

A shut-off valve must be located at the beginning of each lateral branch and at the base of each riser. Additionally, zone valves are placed in strategic locations so as to isolate specific areas in case of fire, maintenance, or

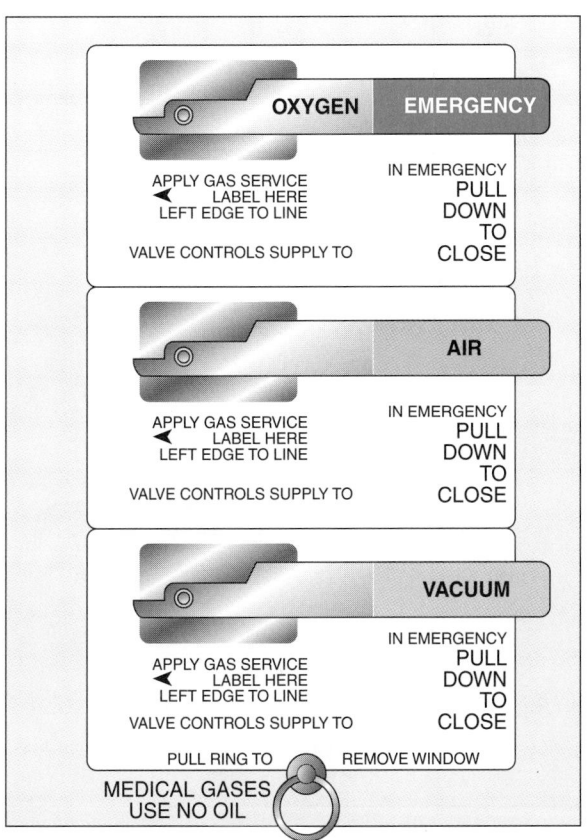

Figure 31-20 Zone shut-off valves for oxygen, air, and vacuum in a common box recessed in the wall. (Modified from Cairo JM, Pilbeam SP. Mosby's respiratory care equipment. 6th ed. St Louis: Mosby; 1999.)

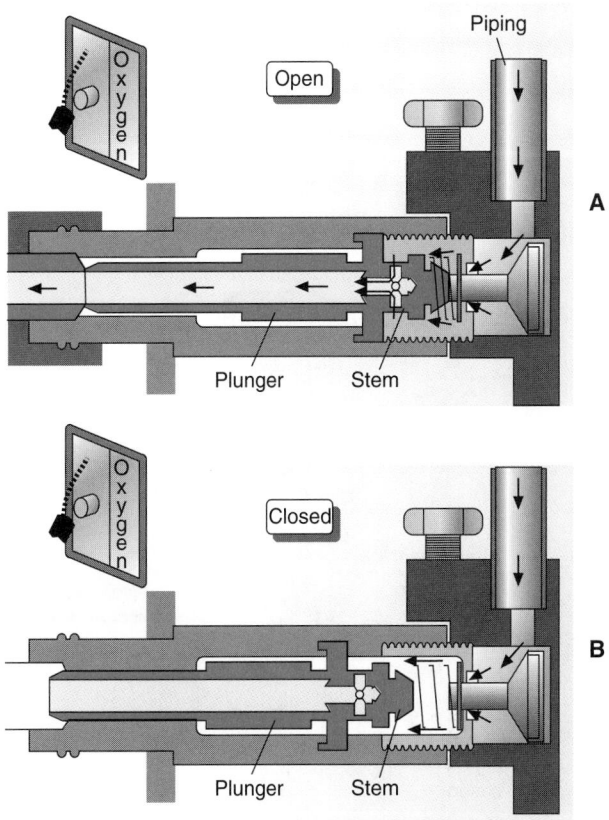

Figure 31-21 An in-wall Diameter-Index Safety System (DISS) type of station outlet showing the outlet **(A)** in use with a connector screwed on, engaging the plunger and pushing it forward to activate flow from the piping system. Unscrewing the DISS connector from the threaded outlet **(B)** causes the internal spring to push the stem and plunger assembly outward and the flow to cease. (Modified from Cairo JM, Pilbeam SP. Mosby's respiratory care equipment. 6th ed. St Louis: Mosby; 1999.)

construction. Zone valves are frequently grouped so that several gases may be controlled from the same box, as shown in Figure 31-20. In addition to groups of patient rooms, zone valves would be located to control gas flow to nurseries, each intensive care unit, the emergency department, recovery rooms, and other necessary areas. Each anesthetizing location (operating rooms, special procedures room, for example) must have its own dedicated shut-off valve. All shut-off valves must be easily accessible, clearly marked to indicate the area being controlled, and protected from tampering.

Gauges and Alarms Each gas distribution system must have an automated continuous-monitoring and alarm system to alert personnel to changes in the system such as the following:

- The normal operating pressure has increased or decreased.
- The liquid oxygen supply has reached a low level.
- Switch-over has occurred from the primary to the secondary bank.
- Moisture in the piped air system has exceeded an acceptable level.

A master set of alarms should be located in two locations within the facility to ensure rapid response to any sit-

uation. The master alarms must be located in areas that are manned 24 hours a day. The alarms must have both an audible and a visual signal that cannot be manually canceled but turns itself off when the situation is corrected. Certain critical areas of the hospital, such as the operating rooms, recovery room, intensive care units, nurseries, and emergency department, should have line-pressure gauges and audible/visual alarms for high and low system pressure. Area alarms are frequently located next to or as part of the zone valves.

Station Outlets The station outlet is the working end of the gas distribution piping system. It is where the gas can be accessed and used by delivery devices, such as flow meters and ventilators. Outlets, like cylinders, must be color-coded and labeled for the gas they deliver and have indexed fittings that allow connection to compatible delivery devices only. Two safety systems are in common use: the DISS and the quick-connect system.

A DISS-type station outlet is shown in Figure 31-21. As the female nut and nipple is manually tightened onto

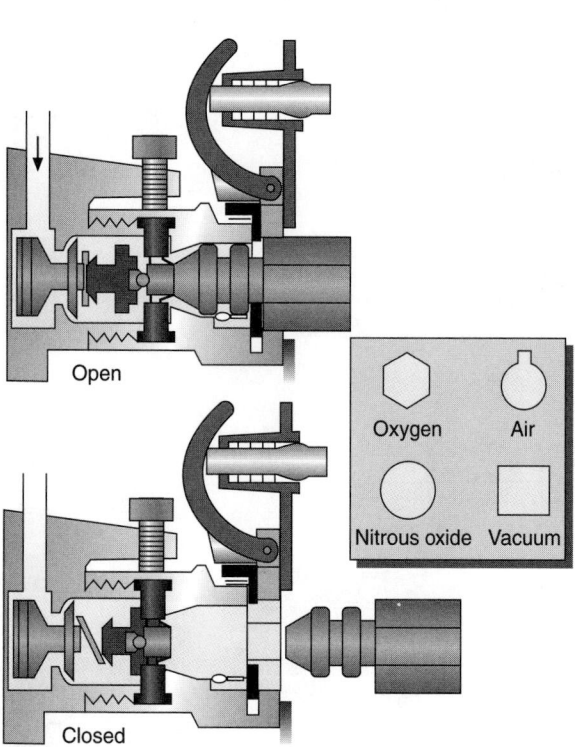

Figure 31-22 Example of a typical quick–connect-type station outlet showing, in the outlet-open position, the adapter inserted and locked in the outlet, pushing the stem inward and activating flow from the piping system. In the outlet-closed position, the adapter has been released from the outlet by pressing of the release button, located just above the outlet opening, which releases the adapter and causes the internal spring to push the adapter from the outlet and move the stem into the closed position, stopping flow. Also illustrated are examples of differing shapes for various gas services. Availability of different shapes prevents connection of a gas adapter into an outlet of another gas. (Modified from Cairo JM, Pilbeam SP. Mosby's respiratory care equipment. 6th ed. St Louis: Mosby; 1999.)

the outlet, it makes contact with the plunger, which moves it forward until it seats on the stem, allowing gas to flow from the piping system. An example of a quick-connect outlet is shown in Figure 31-22. The internal mechanism of the two outlet systems is similar. Instead of the tightening of a screw fitting to engage the plunger, a "male" adapter is inserted into the outlet to push the plunger against the seat and allow air flow. Once inserted, the adapter is locked in place and a release mechanism, such as the pressing of a button or twisting of a collar, must be activated to remove the adapter from the outlet. Manufacturers of quick-connect outlet stations have designed adapters that are usable only in their brand of outlet. A representative sample of quick-connect adapters is shown in Figure 31-23. All manufacturers design their adapters so that only an adapter made for oxygen can fit into an oxygen outlet. That adapter would be physically incompatible with an air, nitrous oxide or vacuum outlet.

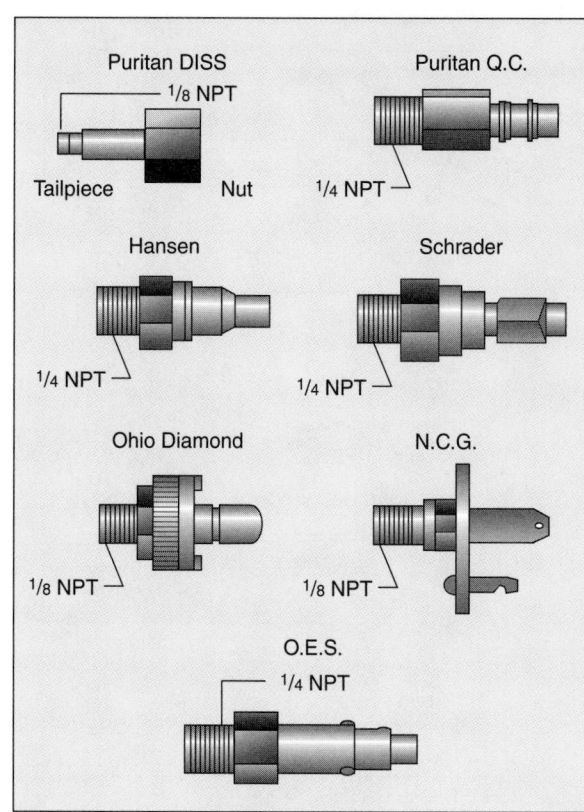

Figure 31-23 Examples of various quick-connect adapters from different manufacturers and suppliers. (Modified from Cairo JM, Pilbeam SP. Mosby's respiratory care equipment. 6th ed. St Louis: Mosby; 1999.)

Central Compressed Medical Air Distribution System

Compressed medical-grade air is commonly used as the source gas to aerosolize medications, activate large-volume nebulizers, and mix with oxygen in ventilators and blenders to provide a specific FIO_2. The central air distribution system is similar to the oxygen system in the layout of the piping, valves, alarms, and station outlets. The source of the compressed air may be banks of cylinders, but this scenario would be practical only in the case of a very small facility or a facility with a very minimal need for compressed air.

In most cases the bulk source of the air comes from dual central compressors, as shown in Figure 31-24. The compressors can operate together or alternate, but in either case each must be able to supply the full demands of the facility for compressed air when the other needs maintenance. For medical use the compressors must deliver oil-free air. The compressors used for central systems are usually of the piston or centrifugal/rotary type. Piston compressors use carbon or Teflon rings to create the seal against the cylinder wall and eliminate the need for an oil lubricant. High-pressure rotary compressors use a liquid sealant, usually water, between the impeller blades and the housing, again eliminating the need for oil lubrication.

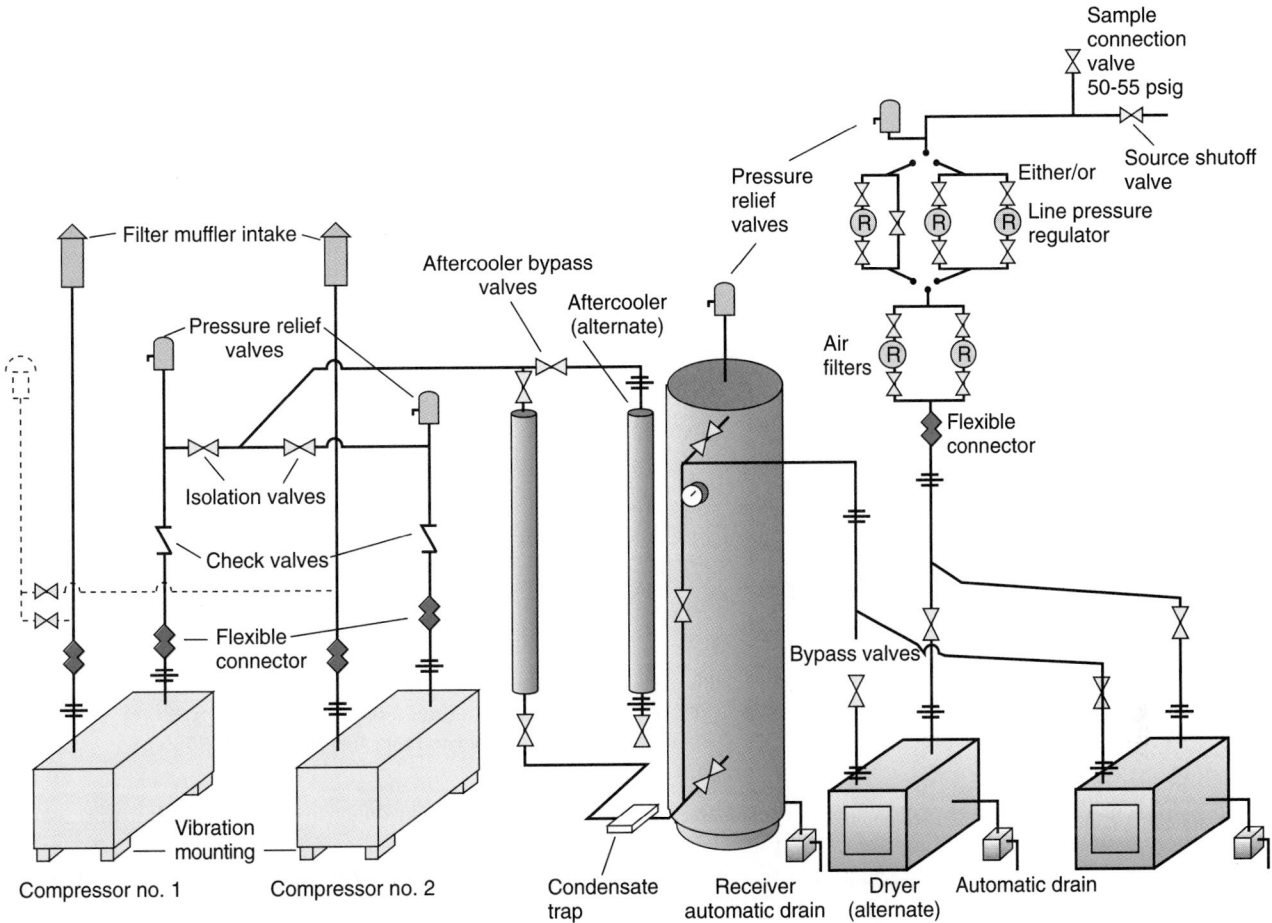

Figure 31-24 Schematic illustration of a typical central medical compressed air supply system with two compressors and dryers, either of which can be used simultaneously or alternately. (Modified from Cairo JM, Pilbeam SP. Mosby's respiratory care equipment. 6th ed. St Louis: Mosby; 1999.)

The source of air being drawn into the compressor, by NFPA standards, must come from an intake located outside the building above the roof and in a location where the air is free from particulates, odors, engine exhausts, and vacuum system discharges. The air is filtered, compressed, and passed through an aftercooler, where cooling causes water vapor to condense and be removed. The air then is stored in a large tank, called a *reservoir* or *receiver*. Air is stored in the receiver tank at a pressure higher than the 50 to 55 psig required in the facilities piping system, allowing the air to flow in a steady stream from the line pressure regulator. In addition, the compressor turns off when a sufficient supply of air is stored in the reservoir, thus minimizing wear, and additional water vapor condenses in the tank and is eliminated.

After leaving the reservoir the air passes through a dryer to remove any remaining water vapor. Removal of water vapor, water droplets, and humidity from the compressed air supply is important to prevent microbial growth (bacteria, fungi, molds) within the piping system. Water in the air supply causes serious damage to ventilators, blenders, and other devices. Alarm systems to monitor dew point (humidity) and carbon monoxide in the main air supply are required as of the 1999 NFPA standards. The compressed air

delivered to the station outlets, although it is dry, oil-free and clean, is not sterile, and appropriate filters should be used between the air supply and delivery devices.

Central Piped Vacuum System

Common in health care facilities is the finding of a vacuum outlet alongside most oxygen station outlets. Vacuum is routinely used in oral/nasal/tracheal suctioning and to apply suction to nasogastric and gastrostomy tubes and chest tubes. As with other central piping systems, medical vacuum systems must conform to NFPA standards, which are similar to those set up for medical gases and compressed air concerning valves, gauges, and alarms. The piping used may be seamless-type K, L, or M copper tubing or stainless-steel tubing or galvanized steel pipe. Because the same type and size of copper tubing can be used for all central piping systems and the pipes are frequently positioned side-by-side in pipe shafts, each pipe *must* be clearly labeled with the contained gas at required intervals.

The central source of the vacuum, as with air systems, involves two or more pumps designed to operate alternately or simultaneously, each being capable of supply-

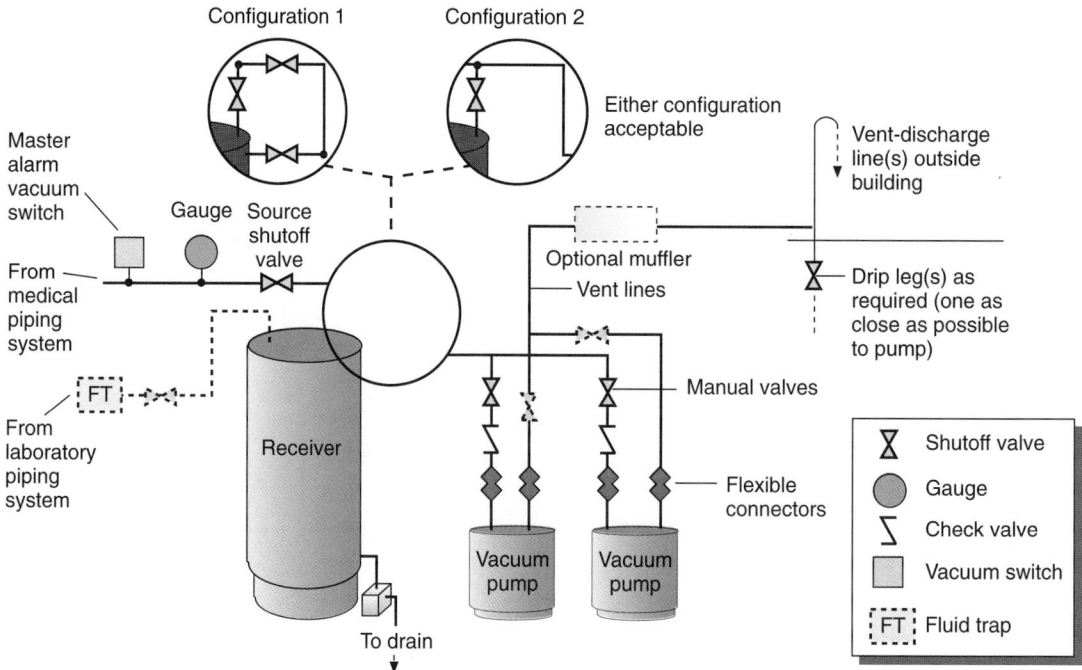

Figure 31-25 Schematic illustration of a typical central vacuum system source. (Modified from NFPA 99C. Standard on Gas and Vacuum Systems. 1999 ed. Quincy, Mass: National Fire Protection Association; 1999.)

ing the full peak demand if the other fails or requires maintenance. Figure 31-25 is a diagram of a typical central vacuum source. A receiver tank located between the piping system and the vacuum source collects fluids and debris to prevent damage to the vacuum pumps. The exhaust from the vacuum pumps must be discharged outside the facility and located so as to minimize environmental contamination. The exhaust must not be near any door or window, and care must be taken not to locate it near any intakes for ventilation or compressed air systems.

The vacuum in a central system is maintained at a subambient pressure between 380 and 760 mm Hg (15 to 30 in Hg; 203 to 407 in H_2O). This supply line pressure must be reduced to a safe clinical level (20-200 mm Hg) at the station outlet through attachment of a pressure-reducing valve and a vacuum regulator to the outlet ahead of any patient suction device.

KEY POINTS

- Examples of nonflammable gases, which do not burn, include nitrogen, oxygen, helium, air, nitrous oxide, and carbon dioxide.
- Some nonflammable gases support combustion, such as oxygen, air, and nitrous oxide.
- The terms *inflammable* and *flammable* can be used interchangeably.
- A flammable gas is rarely used for medical purposes because it burns and can be explosive.
- At standard temperature and pressure, oxygen is a colorless, transparent, odorless, tasteless gas, only slightly heavier than air, that makes up approximately 50% of the earth's crust by weight and 20.9% by volume of the atmosphere.
- Oxygen is produced by photosynthesis, electrolysis of water, and fractional distillation of liquefied air.

- Carbon dioxide is a naturally occurring compound found in the atmosphere in a concentration of about 0.03% and is rarely used today for medical purposes.
- Helium/oxygen mixtures are often referred to as *heliox*.
- Nitric oxide is naturally synthesized in human tissue, playing an important role in vascular smooth muscle relaxation, inhibition of platelet aggregation, neurotransmission, and immune regulation.
- Nitrous oxide is a colorless, odorless, tasteless gas, referred to as "laughing gas," that can be used with oxygen as an anesthetic.
- Nitrogen is a colorless, transparent, odorless, tasteless gas that is slightly less dense than air and the major component of the atmosphere, 78% by volume.

$\mathcal{K}$EY $\mathcal{P}$OINTS—cont'd

- Medical gases can be stored and transported in the gaseous state or as liquefied gas in various-sized cylinders and in bulk containers.
- Cylinder markings, color-coding, labeling, standardized testing, valves, and connection indexing systems help ensure the safe use and handling of medical gas cylinders.

- During patient transport, the duration of flow for a medical gas cylinder must be calculated to determine how many cylinders are needed.
- Most hospitals and many other health care facilities have piped medical gas distribution systems for oxygen, air, and vacuum.

Recommended Reading

Branson RD, Hess DR, Chatburn RL. Respiratory care equipment. 2nd ed. Philadelphia: Lippincott Williams & Wilkins; 1999.

Cairo JM, Pilbeam SP. Mosby's respiratory care equipment. 6th ed. St Louis: Mosby; 1999.

Dorsch JA, Dorsch SE. Understanding anesthesia equipment. 4th ed. Baltimore: Williams & Wilkins; 1994.

NFPA 99C. Standard on Gas and Vacuum Systems. 1999 ed. Quincy, Mass: National Fire Protection Association; 1999.

Compressed Gas Association: Handbook of compressed gases. 4th ed. Boston: Kluwer Academic; 1999.

CHAPTER 32

Oxygen Therapy: Administration and Management

Allan B. Saposnick
Dean R. Hess

CHAPTER OUTLINE

OBJECTIVES

1. Describe the operation of pressure-reducing regulators.
2. Compare flow control devices.
3. Discuss the effect of downstream resistance on the accuracy of flow control devices.
4. Describe the operation of an oxygen concentrator.
5. Discuss the use of home oxygen systems.
6. Compare low-flow and high-flow oxygen delivery systems.
7. Calculate the FIO_2 delivered by a nasal oxygen cannula.
8. Describe the operation of oxygen-conserving devices.
9. Discuss the limitations of hoods, tents, and incubators.
10. Describe the principles of oxygen analysis.

KEY TERMS

Air-Entrainment Mask	Nonrebreathing Mask	Oxygen Tent
Air-Oxygen Blender	Oxygen Cannula	Partial-Rebreathing Mask
Bourdon Gauge Flowmeter	Oxygen Catheter	Regulator
Demand-Oxygen Conserver	Oxygen Analyzer	Sieve Bed
Flowmeter	Oxygen Concentrator	Thorpe Tube Flowmeter
Flow Restrictor	Oxygen Hood	Transtracheal Catheter
Incubator	Oxygen Mask	

The therapeutic use of oxygen has a history of little more than 100 years, and the acceptance and use of oxygen to treat hypoxic conditions dates to the 1940s and 1950s. In the second half of the twentieth century, oxygen-administering devices became smaller, lighter, safer, more accurate and reliable, easier to use, and more comfortable for the patient. Oxygen administration is a common procedure performed by respiratory therapists (CPG 32-1 and CPG 32-2).

This chapter presents technical issues related to the administration of oxygen.

Pressure-Regulating Devices

Gas-powered respiratory therapy equipment in the United States is designed and calibrated to operate with an inlet gas pressure of 50 pounds per square inch, gauge (psig). Central piping systems have pressure-reducing valves within the system that regulate and maintain the pressure at a constant 50 psig. Ventilators, blenders, and **flowmeters** can be connected directly to the station outlets without further need for pressure control. When cylinders of gas are used, the pressure in a full cylinder may be 2200 psig and must be reduced to the standard and safe working pressure of 50 psig through attachment of a high–pressure-reducing valve, called a **regulator,** to the cylinder outlet. High-pressure regulators can be direct-acting or indirect-

acting; can be configured in single or multiple stages; and can be preset or adjustable.

Figure 32-1 illustrates the basic components and operating functions of a direct-acting, single-stage, preset high–pressure-reducing regulator. The regulator is connected to the cylinder by a pin-indexed or American Standard fitting. The high-pressure source of gas enters at the inlet, usually passing through a fine-sintered brass filter to remove any debris. A pressure gauge is positioned at the inlet to indicate the pressure in the cylinder, which is directly related to the volume of gas in the cylinder. The

 CPG 32-1

Oxygen Therapy in the Acute Care Hospital

Indications

Documented hypoxemia: in adults, children, and infants older than 28 days, Pao_2 <60 mm Hg or Sao_2 <90% in subjects breathing room air or with Pao_2 and/or Sao_2 below desirable range for specific clinical situation; in neonates, Pao_2 <50 mm Hg and/or Sao_2 <88%

An acute care situation in which hypoxemia is suspected (substantiation of hypoxemia being required within an appropriate period of time after initiation of therapy)

Severe trauma

Acute myocardial infarction

Short-term therapy (for example, postanesthesia recovery)

Contraindications

No specific contraindications to oxygen therapy exist when indications are judged to be present.

Hazards and Complications

With PaO_2 ≥60 mm Hg, ventilatory depression may occur in spontaneously breathing individuals with elevated $Paco_2$.

With Fio_2 ≥0.5, absorption atelectasis, oxygen toxicity, and/or depression of ciliary and/or leukocytic function may occur.

In premature infants with Pao_2 >80 mm Hg oxygen therapy should not be performed because of the possibility of retinopathy of prematurity.

Increased Pao_2 can contribute to closure or constriction of the ductus arteriosus, a possible concern in infants with ductus-dependent heart lesions.

Supplemental oxygen should be administered with caution to individuals suffering from paraquat poisoning and those receiving bleomycin.

During laser bronchoscopy, minimal levels of supplemental oxygen should be used to prevent intratracheal ignition.

Fire hazard is increased in the presence of increased oxygen concentrations.

Bacterial contamination associated with certain nebulization and humidification systems is a possible hazard.

From AARC Clinical practice guideline: oxygen therapy in the acute care hospital. Respir Care 1991;36:1410-1413.
CPG, *Clinical practice guideline.*

 CPG 32-2

Oxygen Therapy in the Home or Extended Care Facility

Indications

Documented hypoxemia: In adults, children, and infants older than 28 days, indications include Pao_2 ≤55 mm Hg or Sao_2 ≤88% in subjects breathing room air, or Pao_2 of 56 to 59 mm Hg or Sao_2 or Spo_2 ≤89% in association with specific clinical conditions (for example cor pulmonale, congestive heart failure, or erythrocythemia with hematocrit >56%).

Some patients may not qualify for oxygen therapy at rest but do qualify during ambulation, sleep, or exercise. Oxygen therapy is indicated during these specific activities when Sao_2 falls to ≤88%.

Contraindications

No absolute contraindications to oxygen therapy exist when indications are present.

Hazards and Complications

In spontaneously breathing hypoxemic patients with chronic obstructive pulmonary disease, oxygen administration may lead to an increase in $Paco_2$.

Undesirable results or events may result from noncompliance with physicians' orders or inadequate instruction in home oxygen therapy.

Complications may result from use of nasal cannulas or transtracheal catheters.

Fire hazard is increased in the presence of increased oxygen concentrations.

Bacterial contamination associated with certain nebulizers and humidification systems is a possible hazard.

Possible physical hazards can be posed by unsecured cylinders, ungrounded equipment, or mishandling of liquid oxygen (resulting in burns). Power or equipment failure can lead to an inadequate oxygen supply.

From AARC Clinical practice guideline: oxygen therapy in the home or extended care facility. Respir Care 1992;37:918-922.
CPG, *Clinical practice guideline.*

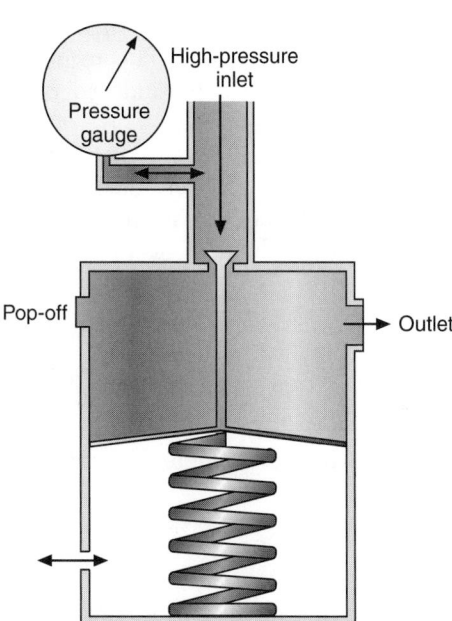

Figure 32-1   Diagram of a direct-acting, single-stage, preset, high–pressure-reducing regulator illustrating the basic operating components and functions. (Modified from Scanlan CL, Wilkins RL, Stoller JK. Egan's fundamentals of respiratory care. 7th ed. St Louis: Mosby; 1999.)

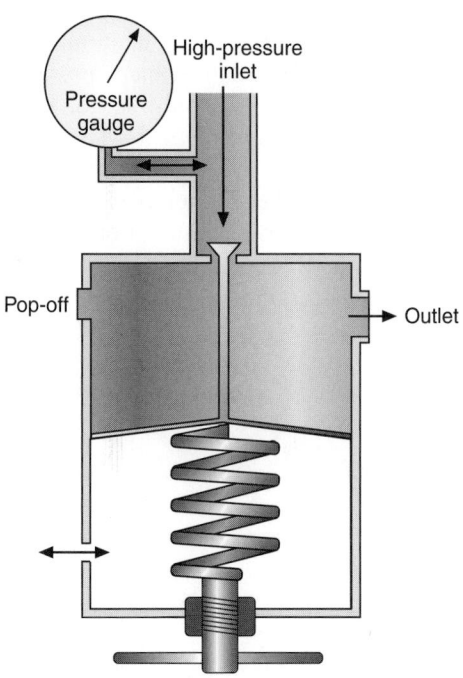

Figure 32-2   Diagram of an adjustable, direct-acting, single-stage, high-pressure reducing regulator. (Modified from Scanlan CL, Wilkins RL, Stoller JK. Egan's fundamentals of respiratory care. 7th ed. St Louis: Mosby; 1999.)

body of the regulator is divided into two chambers by a flexible diaphragm—a high-pressure chamber and a chamber open to ambient pressure. A spring is attached to the ambient-pressure side of the diaphragm. A valve stem is attached to the high-pressure side of the diaphragm, and its end is positioned in the high-pressure inlet. In the regulator the very high pressure from the cylinder is exerted on a very small area of the valve stem, which is balanced by the much larger area of the diaphragm.

The tension of the spring exerts a preset pressure on the diaphragm and moves the valve stem to hold the high-pressure inlet open. When the gas outlet is open, the high-pressure inlet remains open and a balance is maintained between the flow through the outlet and the pressure at the high-pressure inlet. This balance between the force of the spring upward on the diaphragm and the gas pressure above the diaphragm maintains a near-constant outlet pressure, usually preset at 50 psig. When the outlet is closed, pressure increases in the chamber above the diaphragm until it exceeds that of the spring, causing the diaphragm to move downward, pulling the valve stem down and closing the high-pressure inlet.

Adding an adjustment screw to the base of the spring allows the force on the ambient side of the diaphragm to be increased, which in turn increases the outlet pressure. Figure 32-2 shows an adjustable, single-stage, direct-acting, high–pressure-reducing regulator. The external pressure adjustment control is operated by hand. Some adjustable regulators (Figure 32-3) require the removal of a

protective nut to gain access to the adjusting screw, which usually requires an Allen wrench to turn. A pressure relief (pop-off) valve is part of the high-pressure chamber. If a malfunction occurs, allowing excessive pressure to develop, this safety valve will open and vent the pressure, preventing a rupture of the diaphragm or regulator body. Modern regulator design has added a second spring, allowing regulators to become more compact because the size of the diaphragm can be diminished.

For most respiratory therapy applications the single-stage regulator is adequate. For applications in which more precise control of pressure and flow are necessary a multistage regulator is used by connection of two or more single-stage regulators in series (Figure 32-4). The first stage reduces the high pressure from the cylinder to a preset intermediate pressure of 500 to 700 psig. The next stage, or stages, further reduces the pressure until the 50 psig outlet pressure is reached. Each stage of a multi-

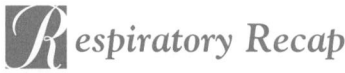

*R*espiratory Recap ⸺⸺⸺⸺⸺⸺

Regulators
Can be direct-acting or indirect-acting
Reduce pressure in single or multiple stages
Reduce pressure to a preset level or require manual adjustment
Are available in single stage or multistage

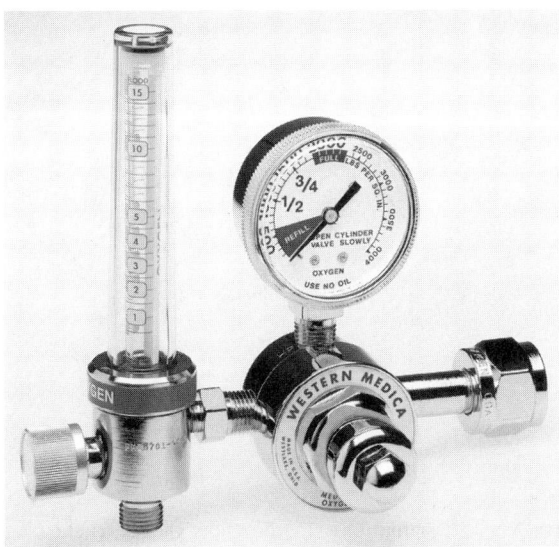

Figure 32-3   Example of an adjustable regulator that requires the removal of the protective nut to gain access to the adjustment Allen screw. (Courtesy Western Medica, Westlake, Ohio.)

stage regulator must have a safety pressure relief valve. The gradual reduction of pressure in two or more stages allows for better pressure control than can be attained in a single stage and a smoother flow. These qualities may be important when precise instrumentation is being used, such as in research applications. Multiple-stage regulators are larger, heavier, and more expensive than the more common single-stage units.

Flow Control Devices

Once the gas pressure has been reduced to the safe working pressure of 50 psig, a device to control the rate of flow usually is needed. Flow control may be handled automatically or internally when the 50 psig gas supply is connected directly to devices such as blenders or ventilators. However, when oxygen or gas mixtures are administered directly to the patient via mask or cannula, for example, a method to meter the flow is necessary. Flow control devices can be categorized as follows:

- Flow restrictor: A preset inlet pressure with a fixed outlet orifice
- Bourdon gauge flowmeter: An adjustable inlet pressure with a fixed outlet orifice
- Thorpe tube flowmeter: A preset inlet pressure with adjustable outlet orifice

Flow Restrictors

A **flow restrictor** (Figure 32-5) is a specific-size orifice that allows a specific flow of gas to pass, provided the inlet pressure is a constant 50 psig. The outlet flow is calculated by the following equation:

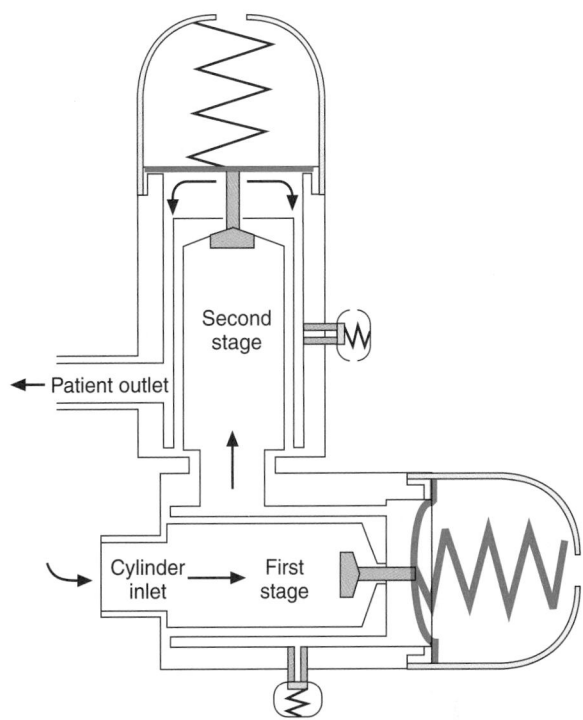

Figure 32-4   Diagram of a multistage, preset regulator. (Modified from Cairo JM, Pilbeam SP. Mosby's respiratory care equipment. 6th ed. St Louis: Mosby; 1999.)

$$\dot{V} = \frac{P_1 - P_2}{R}$$

where $\dot{V}$ is the flow per unit of time (liters per minute), P_1 is the inlet pressure (50 psig), P_2 is the outlet pressure (atmospheric), and R is the resistance to gas flow through the orifice. Any change to the $P_1 - P_2$ relationship alters the accuracy of the output flow, which occurs if the inlet pressure varies from the 50 psig or if increased resistance is present downstream from the orifice outlet, creating a back-pressure.

Flow restrictors are uncomplicated, require no maintenance (because they have no moving parts), can be used in any position, and do not allow accidental changing of the flow. However, when a flow change is necessary, the single-flow flow restrictor must be removed and replaced by another with an orifice delivering the appropriate flow. This concern is addressed through the use of an adjustable flow restrictor that allows the selection of one of a number of orifices, depending on the flow required. Adjustable, multi-orifice flowmeters in combination with an indirect, single-stage, preset regulator are commonly used on small cylinders in home care or patient transport because of their compact and lightweight configuration (Figure 32-6).

Bourdon Gauge Flowmeters

The **Bourdon gauge flowmeter**, like the flow restrictor, has a fixed outlet orifice. However, the inlet pressure is made variable through combination of the fixed outlet orifice with an adjustable pressure regulator. Increases in the

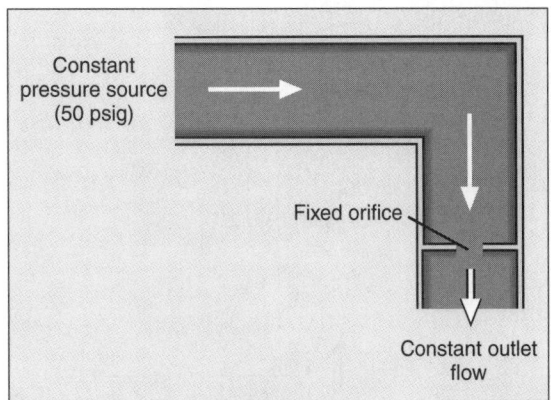

Figure 32-5 Diagram of a fixed-orifice flow restrictor. (Modified from Scanlan CL, Wilkins RL, Stoller JK. Egan's fundamentals of respiratory care. 7th ed. St Louis: Mosby; 1999.)

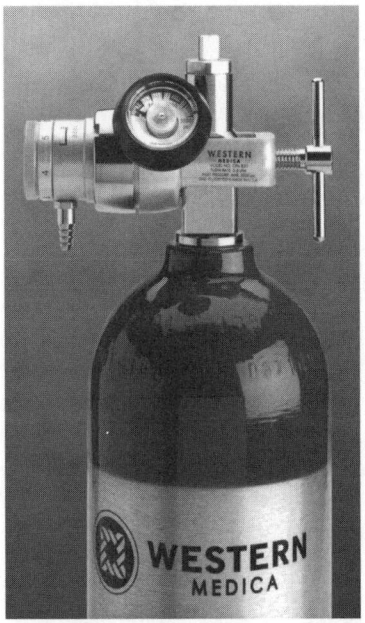

Figure 32-6 A compact, indirect, single-stage, preset regulator with an adjustable, multiorifice flowmeter. (Courtesy Western Medica, Westlake, Ohio.)

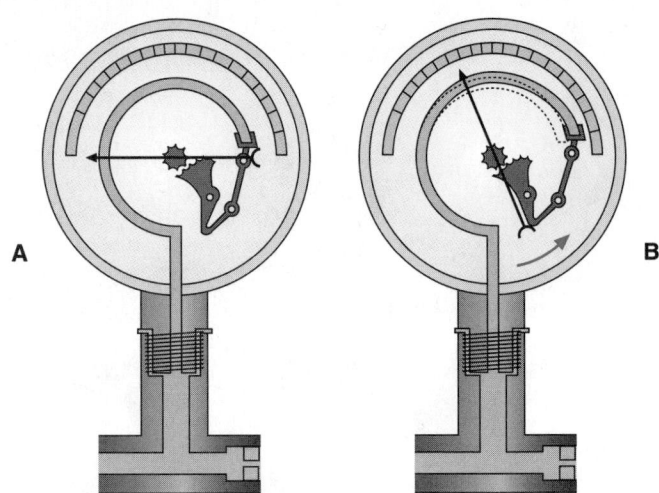

Figure 32-7 Diagram of a Bourdon flow gauge (**A**) showing the hollow pressure tube and gearing mechanism in an unpressurized state and (**B**) pressurized showing how the increase in pressure causes straightening of the tube and movement of the indicator needle. (Modified from Ward JJ. Equipment for mixed gas and oxygen therapy. In: Barnes TA, editor. Core textbook of respiratory care practice. 2nd ed. St Louis: Mosby; 1994.)

gear system and an indicator needle pointing to the calculated output flow for that pressure. Bourdon gauge flowmeters are commonly used in combination with adjustable high–pressure-reducing valves (Figure 32-8). The gauge closest to the cylinder is calibrated to indicate the pressure contents of the cylinder. The Bourdon gauge, which indicates the flow, is located after the adjustable pressure source and before the fixed outlet orifice.

Similar to the flow restrictors, Bourdon gauge flowmeters have a fixed outlet orifice size, making outlet flow accuracy dependent on the maintenance of the relationship of the inlet pressure to the outlet pressure ($P_1 - P_2$). As long as the outlet flow is unrestricted, both flow control devices deliver accurate flow rates. However, when resistance is added downstream of the fixed outlet orifice, such as the addition of a long length of tubing and respiratory equipment, the outlet pressure (P_2) rises and the actual outlet flow is decreased. The Bourdon gauge (Figure 32-9) measures inlet pressure, which remains constant, and although the actual outlet flow is diminished due to the in-

inlet pressure create a proportional increase in the outlet flow. The change in pressure is displayed on the Bourdon gauge face, which has been calibrated in liters per minute corresponding to the predictable flows at the variable inlet pressures. The Bourdon gauge (Figure 32-7) is positioned between the pressure source and the fixed orifice. The gas pressure is transmitted to the gauge through a hollow tube. As the pressure increases, the closed distal end of the curved hollow tube is straightened. It is linked to a

*R*espiratory Recap

Flow Restrictors and Bourdon Gauges

These devices provide accurate flow as long as the outlet is unrestricted.
Downstream resistance reduces outlet flow, causing the devices to overestimate the delivered flow.

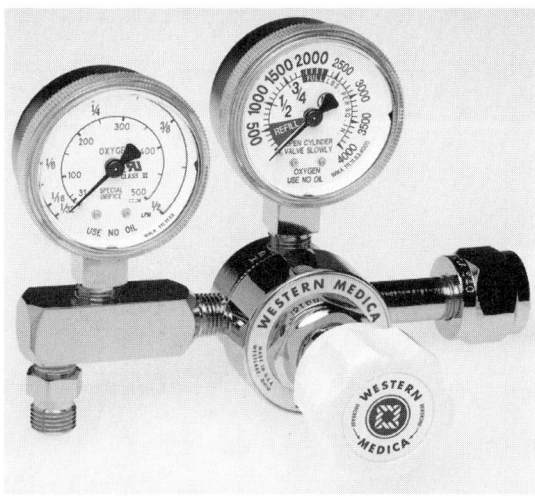

Figure 32-8   A single-stage, adjustable regulator with two Bourdon gauges. The gauge to the right, closest to the connection to the gas source, is calibrated in pounds per square inch (psi), indicating the contents of the cylinder. The Bourdon gauge, closest to the outlet, is calibrated in liters per minute. Flow is set by a turn of the knob to increase or decrease the regulator pressure and thus the outlet flow through the fixed orifice. (Courtesy Western Medica, Westlake, Ohio.)

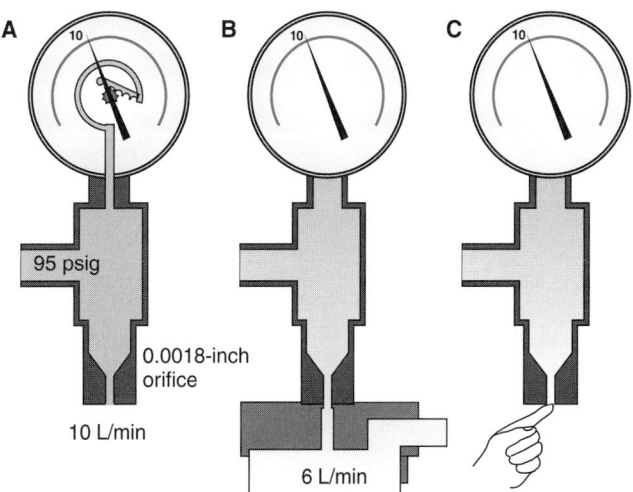

Figure 32-9   Diagrams of a Bourdon gauge illustrating (**A**) that with a constant inlet pressure and a known fixed outlet orifice size a predictable outlet flow is achieved and is indicated on the gauge face. Adding resistance downstream of the fixed outlet orifice (**B**) causes flow to be diminished, yet the gauge reading remains unchanged because it measures the pressure before the resistance. If the outlet orifice is completely obstructed (**C**), allowing no flow, the gauge continues to read a flow even though none is present because it continues to read preobstruction pressure. (Modified from materials courtesy Nellcor Puritan Bennett, Pleasanton, Calif.)

creased resistance downstream, the gauge reading remains unchanged, indicating a higher-than-actual outlet flow. In fact, if the outlet were completely obstructed, the gauge would continue to show flow when in fact none would be present.

Thorpe Tube Flowmeters

Unlike flow resistors and Bourdon gauges, pressure-compensated **Thorpe tube flowmeters** display the actual outlet flow in the face of downstream resistance. As long as the inlet pressure remains constant, the pressure-compensated Thorpe tube flowmeter displays correct readings of outlet flow. For this reason, these devices are the most common type used for flow control and flow measurement in hospitals for direct, quick-connect application to piped outlet stations.

A Thorpe tube flowmeter consists of a clear, tapered glass tube with a diameter that is larger at the top than at the bottom. The tube has graduated markings calibrated to indicate flow (usually liters per minute or milliliters per minute). A float in the glass tube and a needle valve control flow (Figure 32-10). When the needle valve is opened, gas flows from the pressure source. Gas entering the bottom of the Thorpe tube creates a pressure differential significant enough to lift the float. As the float rises in the tapered tube, the diameter of the tube increases (equivalent to an increase in the outlet orifice size) and more gas is able to flow around the float. Eventually the float stabilizes when the upward forces of the pressure differential across the float equal the downward force of gravity.

The location of the needle valve in the Thorpe tube flowmeter is important. It can be located distal to the Thorpe tube or proximal to the Thorpe tube. Placing the needle valve distal to the Thorpe tube creates a pressure-compensated flowmeter. With increasing back-pressure applied to the outlet of the flowmeter, the float drops, reflecting the decrease in outlet flow. A non-pressure–compensated Thorpe tube flowmeter, on the other hand, has the needle valve located proximal to the Thorpe tube. When a flow-restricting device is attached, increasing downstream resistance, pressure is increased within the Thorpe tube, forcing the float downward and providing a reading lower then the actual flow.

The pressure-compensated Thorpe tube flowmeter is preferred for clinical applications. It provides an accurate display of flow, provided it is in a vertical position and the inlet pressure is constant. Determining whether a Thorpe tube flowmeter is pressure compensated can be done when the needle valve is closed and the flowmeter

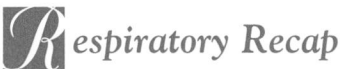
*R**espiratory Recap***

Back–Pressure-Compensated Flowmeters
Only back–pressure-compensated Thorpe tubes provide an accurate display of flow with downstream resistance.

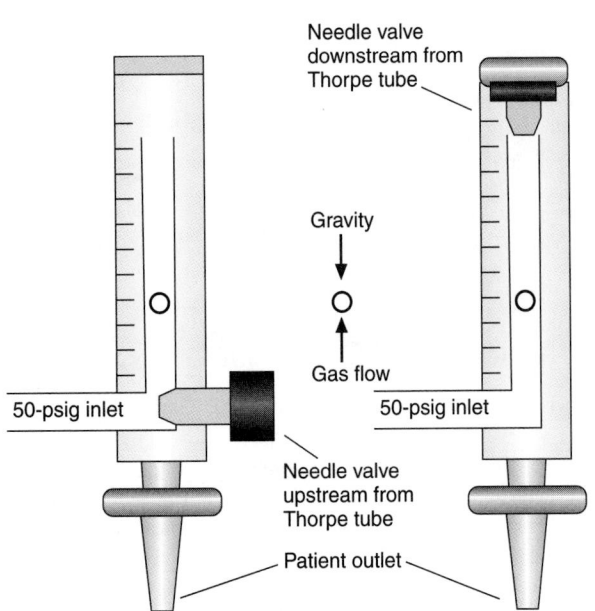

Figure 32-10 Diagram of a flowmeter (*left*) in which the needle valve is placed before the Thorpe tube (non-pressure–compensated) and flowmeter (*right*) with the needle valve placed after the Thorpe tube (back–pressure-compensated). (Modified from Cairo JM, Pilbeam SP. Mosby's respiratory care equipment. 6th ed. St Louis: Mosby; 1999.)

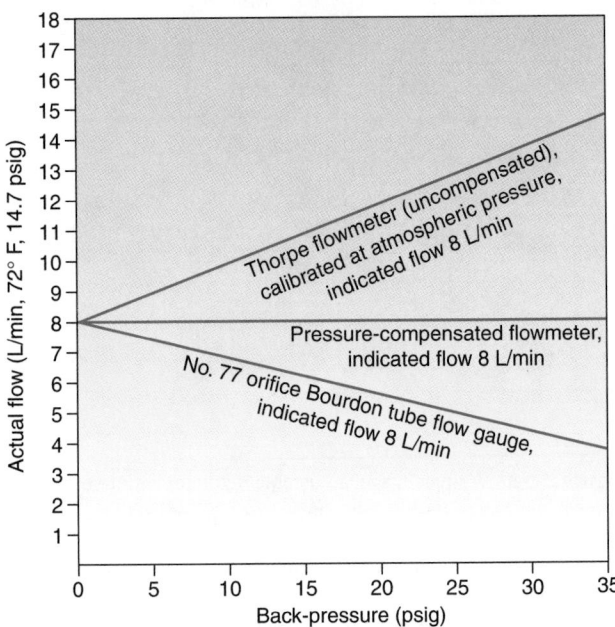

Figure 32-11 Comparison of the accuracy of a pressure-compensated and noncompensated Thorpe tube flowmeter and a Bourdon gauge when faced with increasing levels of downstream back-pressure. The pressure-compensated Thorpe tube's indicated flow is the actual flow regardless of back-pressure. With a noncompensated Thorpe tube, actual flow is higher than the indicated flow at increasing downstream pressure. With the Bourdon gauge, indicated flow is progressively higher than actual flow as back-pressure increases. (Modified from McPherson SP, Spearman CB: Respiratory therapy equipment. 5th ed. St Louis: Mosby; 1995.)

subsequently pressurized as the cylinder valve is opened or it is connected to a station outlet. If the Thorpe tube flowmeter is pressure compensated, the float jumps to the top of the tube and then falls back as gas rushes in and fills the tube to the needle valve. Figure 32-11 compares the accuracy of compensated and uncompensated Thorpe tube flowmeters and the Bourdon gauge flowmeter at various levels of downstream resistance (for example, back-pressure).

Most Thorpe tube flowmeters commonly used in respiratory therapy use a ball as the float, although the float may assume various shapes and configurations. Sighting the float at eye level is important. A ball float is read through the center of the ball, whereas most other floats are read at the top surface.

Oxygen Sources

Oxygen can be distributed by cylinder or through a bulk-supplied piping system. Oxygen also can be separated from the air by oxygen concentrators and used by individual patients in their homes or in subacute or long-term care facilities. Liquid oxygen can be supplied in containers that are easily delivered to the home care patient or health care facility.

Oxygen Concentrators

Oxygen concentrators (Figure 32-12) were introduced in the early 1970s as a means to produce low flows (0.5 to 5.0 L/min) of high-purity oxygen (90% to 95%) from room air. The first concentrators were as large as an office desk, weighed hundreds of pounds, were noisy, and generated a lot of heat. Today most concentrators are about 2 cubic feet, 50 pounds, quiet, and very reliable. Because they operate reliably for extended periods of time, require minimum care and maintenance, and use a standard 110-volt current, oxygen concentrators are the most widely used sources of oxygen in the home and extended care facilities. Oxygen concentrators produce oxygen from room air by either molecular adsorption of nitrogen or filtration of air through a membrane.

The most commonly used technique is the molecular sieve, also referred to as the *pressure swing adsorption (PSA) method* (Figure 32-13). Room air is drawn through one or more filters by an oil-less air compressor, where it is compressed to a pressure of 15 to 25 psig and passed through an air-cooled heat exchanger before entering the sieve columns, often called **sieve beds.** Each sieve bed (at

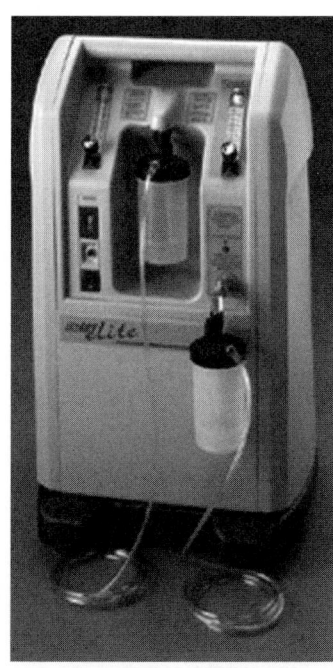

Figure 32-12 An oxygen concentrator. Concentrators are available that can provide up to 3, 5, 6, and 10 L/min of oxygen all at concentrations of between 90% and 97%. The concentrator shown has an optional second flow outlet, allowing two patients to receive oxygen therapy from the same machine as long as the combined total outlet flow is 6 L/min or less. (Courtesy AirSep Corporation, Buffalo, N.Y.)

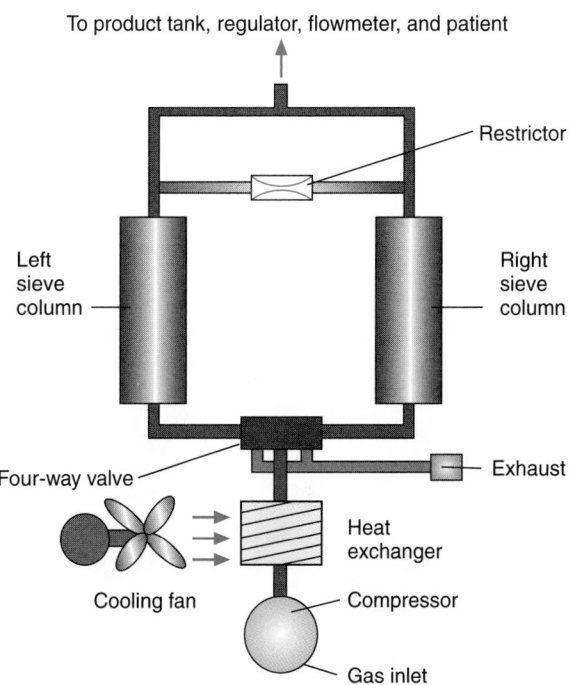

Figure 32-13 A schematic representation of the major components of a standard dual sieve bed concentrator using the pressure swing adsorption method of oxygen production.

least two must be present) is filled with a porous crystalline aluminosilicate material called *zeolite,* a naturally occurring substance that is artificially synthesized for use in concentrators to contain microscopically sized pores that allow oxygen to pass, thus the name *molecular sieve.* Zeolite actually holds nitrogen in the air pumped through it by adsorption to its large surface area. If the zeolite is properly packed in the sieve column and the air passing through it is properly pressurized, the oxygen exiting can achieve concentrations of 92% to 97% at 6 L/min or less.

Zeolite surfaces are quickly covered with nitrogen, as well as moisture and other gases and contaminants, and the sieve bed must be purged every 12 to 20 seconds through alternate pressurization of one sieve bed while the other is purged. A microprocessor controls the sequence of cycling of a series of valves, triggered by either pressure or time, allowing air to flow through one sieve bed. A small portion of the oxygen exiting that bed is directed to the product tank for patient use while the rest is shunted to the opposite sieve bed and back-flushes the nitrogen through the exhaust. This cycle through which the pressure swings from one sieve bed to the other is repeated 3 to 5 times per minute. Oxygen is stored in the product tank so that the flow to the patient is unaffected by the sieve bed pressure swings. The outlet pressure is set by a

regulator between the product tank and the flowmeter and is generally between 5 and 10 psig, requiring a flowmeter calibrated for this low inlet pressure.

R̄espiratory Recap

Oxygen Concentrators
Produce 90% to 97% oxygen
Use a zeolite molecular sieve
Cause nitrogen adsorption from air

An internal design modification of the oxygen concentrator was introduced in the mid-1990s with the goal to eliminate or reduce the number of pneumatic fittings, valves, solenoids, and electronics. The concentrator still uses PSA technology but instead of two large sieve beds, twelve shorter beds of smaller diameter are used. In place of the valves sequencing flow from one sieve bed to the other, a disk with flow channels rotates on top of the package of sieve beds (Figure 32-14), directing the compressed room air through four columns and pressurizing four others, while purging the other four. When the device is fitted with the smaller set of sieve beds, up to 95% oxygen is available at 5 L/min, whereas the larger package delivers at least 90% at 10 L/min.

An oxygen analyzer is a frequent optional component of many newer concentrators. They use new oxygen analysis technology that is reliable for years of use and does not require calibration. If the oxygen concentration decreases to between 90% and 85%, a visual and/or audible signal is triggered, alerting the user to a below-normal concentration. If outlet concentration drops below 85%, a visual and audible alarm is activated, alerting the patient to switch to

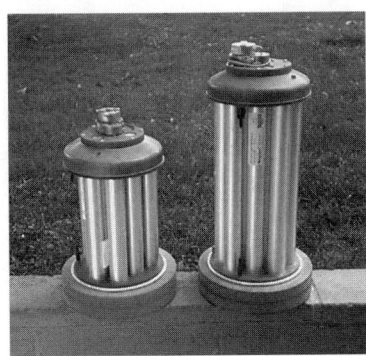

Figure 32-14 Carousel of twelve small-diameter sieve beds with a rotating cap directing airflow through various combinations of sieves. The smaller set can produce up to 5 L/min of oxygen, whereas the larger unit produces up to 10 L/min. (Courtesy SeQual Technologies, San Diego, Calif.)

a backup cylinder until the home medical equipment supplier can correct the problem. All oxygen concentrators have an audible electricity supply interruption alarm, loud enough to alert the patient or caregiver even during the night that the concentrator has stopped and the alternative emergency backup supply must be put into use.

A recent innovation in concentrators is the ability of several concentrators to fill cylinders with oxygen gas while simultaneously providing oxygen flow to the patient (Figure 32-15). The concentrator produces 92% to 96% oxygen and can supply 1 to 4 L/min to the patient and 0.5 to 2 L/min to the booster pump to fill the cylinder. To fill one cylinder to 2000 psi takes 6 to 10 hours, depending on the cylinder's capacity. Another innovative device (Figure 32-16) takes the 5 L/min output from any concentrator, delivers up to 4 L/min to the patient, refrigerates a portion of the remainder, and stores it as a liquid. It can produce up to 1.2 L of liquid oxygen every 24 hours, enough to fill a standard portable liquid oxygen unit.

The oxygen concentrators described to this point use PSA through a molecular sieve to produce a flow of oxygen. Almost all concentrators in general use are of this type. However, another process separates oxygen from air for use by individual patients. This concentrator (Figure 32-17), frequently called a *membrane oxygenator* or *oxygen enricher*, uses a vacuum pump to draw filtered room air

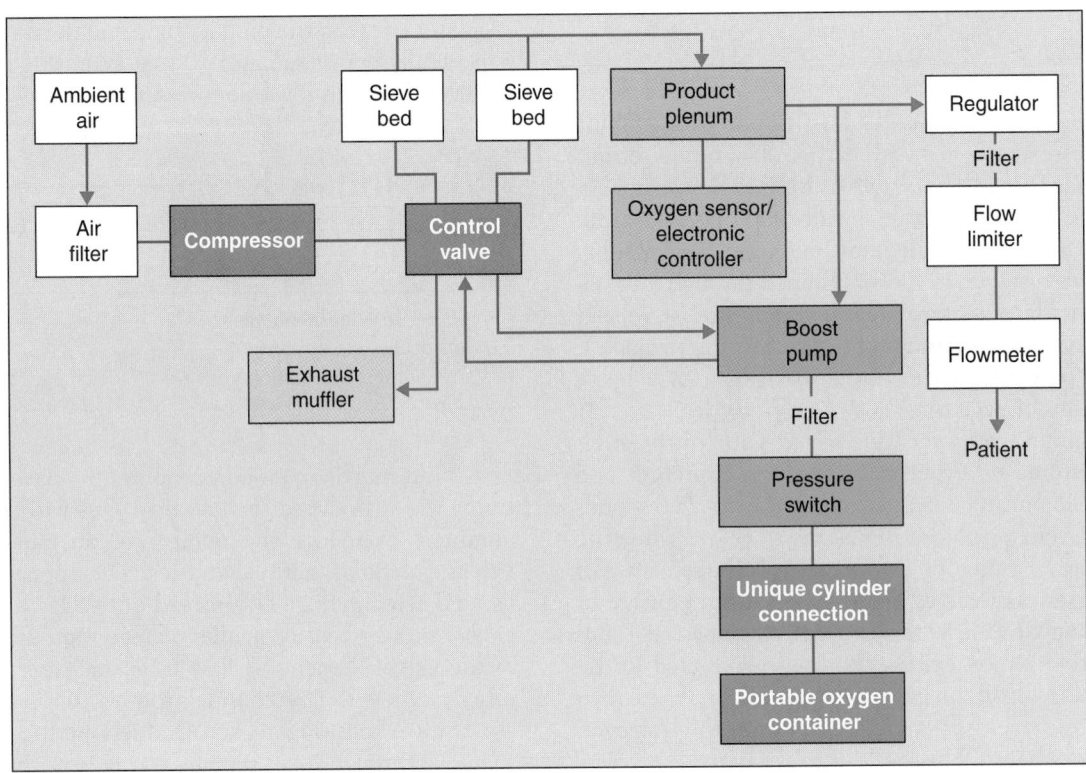

Figure 32-15 Schematic illustration of an oxygen concentrator that has the capability of filling E-size and smaller cylinders with gaseous oxygen while simultaneously supplying up to 3 L/min of 92% to 96% oxygen to the patient. (Modified from materials courtesy Chad Therapeutics, Chatsworth, Calif.)

through a set of very thin plastic membranes. Water vapor and oxygen readily diffuse through this membrane at a greater rate then nitrogen, creating a flow of up to 10 L/min of 40% oxygen. This type of oxygen concentrator has not found wide acceptance because it is considerably more expensive then the sieve-bed type and can produce only a maximum outlet concentration of 40% oxygen. However, the oxygen produced is well humidified.

Liquid Oxygen Systems

Liquid oxygen systems have been available for use in the home since the early 1970s. Liquid oxygen may be the home oxygen delivery modality of choice, rather then cylinders or a concentrator, when the patient requires high flow rates (>5 to 6 L/min) or is extremely mobile. The home liquid oxygen system consists of two parts—the stationary base reservoir and the smaller portable unit (Figure 32-18). Liquid reservoirs are available in a number of sizes, with capacities from 12 to 60 L, with the 40 L unit being the most common. Portable units have capacities of 0.5 to 1.2 L of liquid oxygen.

The design and construction of the home care stationary liquid reservoir is similar to that of large bulk tanks used by hospitals. The thermos-bottle type of construction consists of an inner vessel containing the liquid oxygen and the space between the inner vessel and the outer shell that is an insulation-filled vacuum. The reservoir serves as the primary source of oxygen while the patient is at home. A standard oxygen Diameter-Index Safety System (DISS) outlet is used because outlet pressure is usually 20 to 22 psig (although some older units may be 50 psig), connected to

either a variable orifice flow restrictor or a pressure-compensated Thorpe tube flowmeter. Most reservoirs provide a flow of 0.25 to 15 L/min.

When the flowmeter is opened, oxygen gas in the reservoir above the liquid, at a pressure of 22 psig, flows through the economizer valve to the patient. As long as oxygen gas in the reservoir has a pressure greater than atmospheric pressure, the economizer valve remains open. When gas pressure is too low to meet the flow demand, the economizer valve closes, causing liquid oxygen to flow up the withdrawal tube and through the vaporizing and

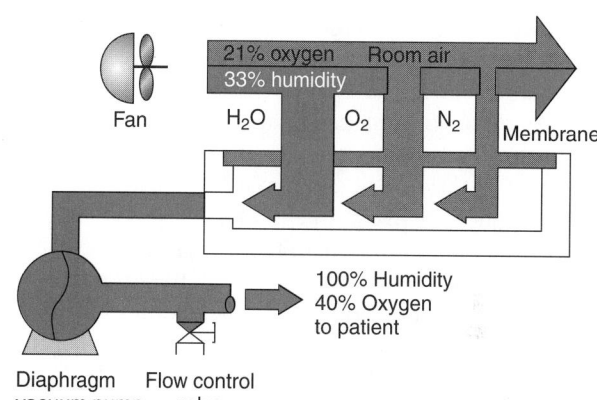

Figure 32-17 Schematic illustration of the operating concept of the membrane oxygen enrichment type of concentrator. A vacuum on one side of a thin plastic membrane allows oxygen in the room air to diffuse through it at a more rapid rate than nitrogen, creating oxygen enriched gas output. (Modified from materials courtesy Oxygen Enrichment Co., Schenectady, N.Y.)

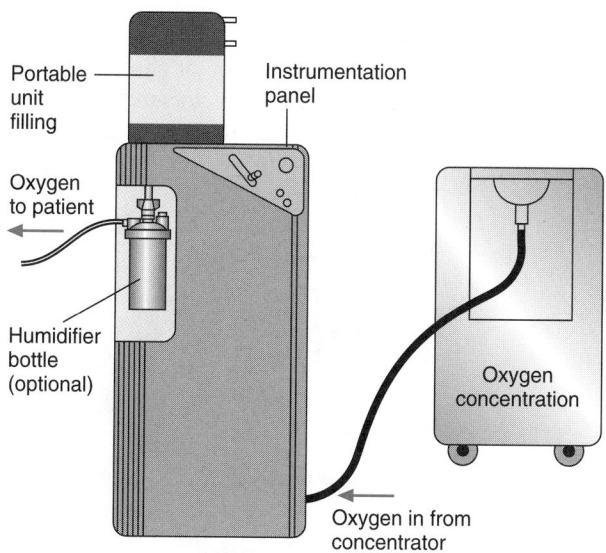

Figure 32-16 Diagrammatic representation of a system that takes the output from any 5 L/min oxygen concentrator and converts the gaseous oxygen to liquid oxygen and fills a portable liquid oxygen unit while still providing up to 3 L/min to the patient. (Modified from materials courtesy In-X Corporation, Denver, Colo.)

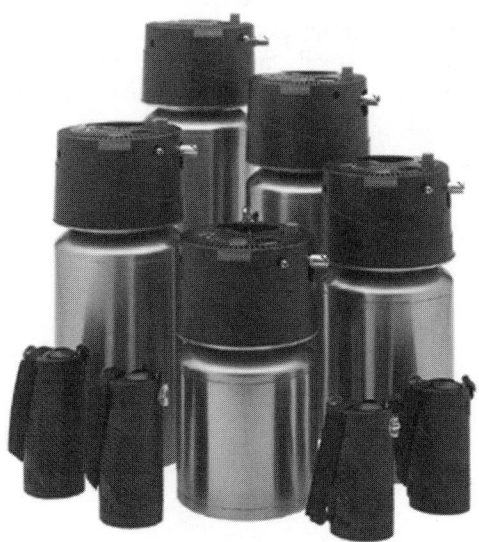

Figure 32-18 Stationary liquid oxygen reservoirs are available in many sizes to meet different patient needs. Also shown are several sizes of portable liquid oxygen units that are refilled from the reservoirs. (Courtesy Caire Inc., Burnsville, Minn.)

warming coils, changing to the gaseous state before delivery through the flowmeter.

An advantage of liquid oxygen is that the active ambulatory patient can fill a portable liquid unit from the stationary reservoir whenever necessary. The portable unit is a smaller version of the reservoir, weighing from 5 to 15 pounds when full, depending on capacity and construction. To fill the portable unit the user couples it to the reservoir with quick-connect fittings and opens the vent valve on the portable unit, allowing liquid to flow into it. Filling time is less than 2 minutes. The portable unit then is ready to be carried by a shoulder strap or in a small wheeled cart to supply oxygen up to 12 hours, depending on flow rate, respiratory rate, and whether a conserving device is used.

Unlike the oxygen concentrator, liquid reservoirs must be regularly refilled. The supplier can deliver a full reservoir to the patient regularly based on usage, exchanging the full unit for the nearly empty one. Reservoirs also can be easily refilled at the patient's home from a liquid vessel mounted in the supplier's delivery truck. The delivery technician takes the reservoir to the truck after first placing the patient on oxygen from the portable unit. A fill hose is connected from the truck's liquid tank to the quick-connect fitting on the reservoir and the vent valve opened to allow liquid to flow into the reservoir, filling it in 10 to 15 minutes.

Oxygen-Administering Devices

Classification of Oxygen Delivery Systems

Oxygen therapy systems generally are categorized as either low-flow or high-flow devices that provide variable-performance or fixed-performance outcomes concerning the fractional concentration of inspired oxygen (FIO_2). Low-flow devices, such as the nasal oxygen cannula, deliver oxygen at flow rates usually no greater than 6 to 8 L/min, which is insufficient to meet the normal inspiratory flow

demand of 30 L/min. The additional required flow is inhaled from the room air. The FIO_2 performance of low-flow devices varies from breath to breath and minute to minute, depending on the tidal volume and respiratory rate. Thus low-flow devices provide variable-performance. High-flow devices, however, satisfy the patient's full inspiratory flow demand and thus maintain a fixed FIO_2 unaffected by changes in respiratory rate or pattern. Air-entrainment devices (masks and large volume nebulizers) are examples of high-flow, fixed-performance oxygen delivery systems.

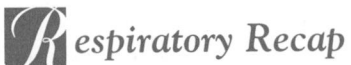

Respiratory Recap ——————————

Oxygen Delivery Systems
Low flow, variable performance
High flow, fixed performance

Low-Flow Devices

Nasal Oxygen Catheter   Nasal **oxygen catheters** (Figure 32-19) were widely used as the standard low-flow oxygen delivery system of choice until the late 1960s. Although still available, nasal oxygen catheters are rarely used today, having been replaced by the nasal oxygen cannula. The nasal oxygen catheter is a soft, pliable plastic tube about 12 inches long with a series of small holes at the distal end and a fitting at the other end to connect it to the oxygen supply tubing. Nasal oxygen catheters for adults are 12 or 14 F (3.96 mm and 4.72 mm outside diameter [OD]), whereas those for pediatric use are 8 and 10 Fr (Fr = French size). The catheter is inserted in either nostril and advanced along the floor of the nasal cavity into the nasopharynx until the tip is located just behind the uvula. The catheter is held in place to the nose or

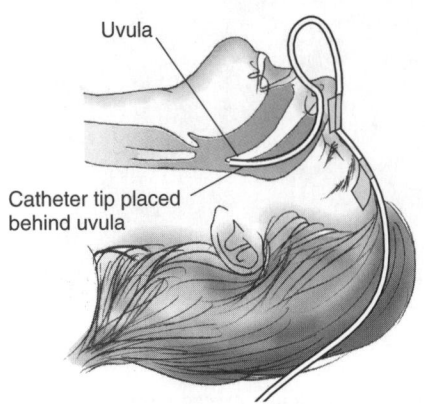

Figure 32-19 A nasal catheter for oxygen administration. (Modified from Scanlan CL, Wilkins RL, Stoller JK. Egan's fundamentals of respiratory care. 7th ed. St Louis: Mosby; 1999.)

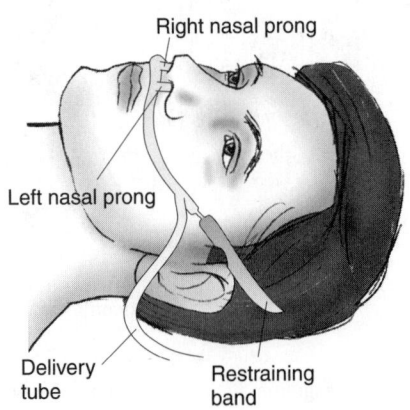

Figure 32-20 A nasal cannula for oxygen administration. (Modified from Scanlan CL, Wilkins RL, Stoller JK. Egan's fundamentals of respiratory care. 7th ed. St Louis: Mosby; 1999.)

cheek with tape. At flow rates of 1 to 5 L/min the delivered FIO_2 ranges from 0.22 to 0.35.

Nasal Oxygen Cannula

The nasal **oxygen cannula** is the most widely used device to administer low-flow oxygen to infants, children, and adults in the hospital and the home. The oxygen cannula consists of a delivery tube that ends in two short prongs, each about one-half inch long and made of soft, pliable plastic. Cannula prongs are available curved or straight, tapered to a flair or nontapered. Most patients best tolerate the curved, nontapered configuration because it directs the flow toward the nasopharynx rather than at the roof of the nasal cavity. The cannula is easily applied, well tolerated by most patients when used with flow rates of 6 L/min or less, and held in place with an elastic band around the head (Figure 32-20) or more commonly with the delivery tubing looped over the ears and held in place and an adjustable slide placed under the chin. When oxygen is delivered by nasal cannula to an adult, the expected delivery may be an FIO_2 of 0.24 at 1 L/min and up to about 0.40 at 5 to 6 L/min. Calculating the theoretic FIO_2 delivered by the nasal oxygen cannula is possible at any oxygen flow rate, assuming a constant tidal volume, inspiratory-expiratory ratio, inspiratory time, and respira-

tory rate, as illustrated in Equation 32-1. The FIO_2 from a nasal cannula can be variable even though the oxygen flow remains constant. For that reason regular assessment of the patient's response to the oxygen therapy is important.

Nasal cannulas are available in sizes appropriate for infants, toddlers, and children. Because of their small tidal volumes, the oxygen flow rate to infants and young children must be precisely controlled by use of a pressure-compensated Thorpe tube flowmeter with a scale of 0 to 2 L/min in increments of $\frac{1}{4}$ or $\frac{1}{16}$ L/min. A flow of 0.25 L/min by nasal cannula to an infant can achieve an FIO_2 of 0.35, and more than 0.60 at 1 L/min is possible. The maximum flow to a nasal cannula for an infant is 2 L/min.

Age-Specific Angle

A flowmeter with a scale of 0 to 2 L/min in increments of $\frac{1}{4}$ to $\frac{1}{16}$ L/min is used with an oxygen cannula for infants.

Simple Mask

The simple **oxygen mask** is used when a higher FIO_2 is needed than can be attained with a nasal cannula or when a cannula is not appropriate (because of nasal obstruction), such as in emergency situations and during and after minor surgical procedures. The simple oxygen mask is a disposable plastic product available in infant, child, and adult sizes with a length of small-diameter oxygen supply tubing connected to the base of the mask (Figure 32-21). These masks are available in two designs, both fitting over the bridge of the nose, and often are held in place with a malleable aluminum strip (also helping to minimize leakage toward the eyes). They cover the nose and mouth down to the lower lip, or to under the chin, and are held in place by an elastic band around the head.

ℰQUATION 32-1

Estimation of FIO_2 from Nasal Cannula

Cannula flow	6 L/min
100% oxygen provided	100 mL/second
Tidal volume	500 mL
Mechanical reservoir	None
Anatomic reservoir	50 mL
Respiratory rate	20/min
Inspiratory time	1 second
I:E ratio	1:2

Volume of Oxygen Inspired

Approximately 50 mL is inspired from the anatomic reservoir (volume of nasopharyngeal cavity).

Approximately 100 mL is inspired from oxygen flow.

Because 150 mL of 100% oxygen is inspired, the remainder of tidal volume is room air (350 mL), with 21% of the 350 mL (70 mL) being the amount of O_2 in room air inspired.

The volume of oxygen inspired = 50 mL + 100 mL + 70 mL = 220 mL.

$$FIO_2 = \frac{220 \text{ mL } (O_2)}{500 \text{ mL (tidal volume)}} = 0.44$$

If tidal volume is decreased to 250 mL, the FIO_2 increases to 0.64.

If tidal volume is increased to 1000 mL, the FIO_2 decreases to 0.32.

Similar mathematic approaches can be used to calculate the effects of changes in oxygen flow or inspiratory time.

I:E ratio, Inspiration to expiration ratio.

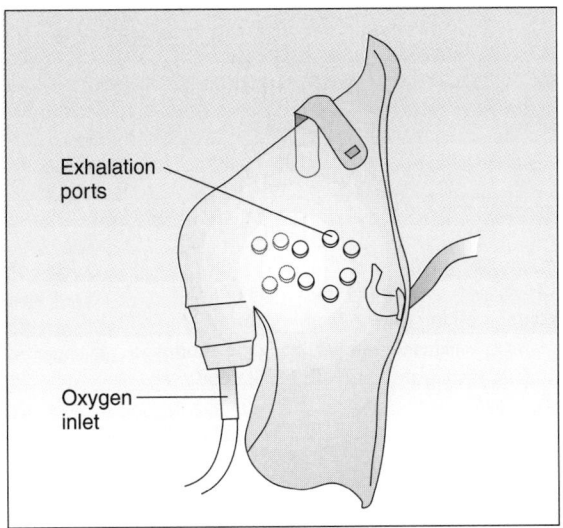

Figure 32-21   Simple oxygen face mask. (Modified from Scanlan CL, Wilkins RL, Stoller JK. Egan's fundamentals of respiratory care. 7th ed. St Louis: Mosby; 1999.)

The simple mask increases the inspired oxygen concentration by acting as an oxygen reservoir, adding a volume in an adult mask of 100 to 200 mL, which is inhaled at the beginning of inspiration. The patient also inhales room air through a series of small holes in the mask. Because the mask accumulates carbon dioxide during exhalation, the oxygen flow rate must be sufficient to wash out the mask and prevent the rebreathing of carbon dioxide. A general recommendation is that a minimum flow of 5 L/min should be used. The simple mask is a low-flow, variable-performance oxygen delivery system capable of providing an FIO_2 of from 0.3 to 0.6 at flows of 5 to 10 L/min, depending on the size of the mask and the patient's respiratory pattern. All oronasal masks present the same problems involving claustrophobic feelings for some patients, speech muffling, and difficulty with eating and drinking.

Partial-Rebreathing Mask

The **partial-rebreathing mask** (Figure 32-22, A) is a simple mask with the addition of a 300- to 600-mL reservoir bag. The oxygen supply tube is positioned between the mask and the reservoir bag. The oxygen flow is set at a rate sufficient to keep the bag at least partially inflated throughout inspiration. This flow rate varies depending on the patient's respiratory pattern but is usually between 8 and 15 L/min.

During inspiration the patient inhales oxygen from the reservoir bag, partially deflating it, and draws in an additional volume of air through the mask ports. The first part of exhalation, usually about a third of the tidal volume, fills the bag, and the remaining two-thirds exits the mask through the mask ports. The first third of exhalation that goes into the reservoir bag is high in oxygen and low in carbon dioxide. This portion is the volume that is rebreathed, along with additional oxygen and some room air, on the next inspiration. FIO_2 in the range of 0.4 to 0.7 is delivered with oxygen flows of 8 to 15 L/min, depending on the respiratory pattern.

Nonrebreathing Mask

The **nonrebreathing mask** (Figure 32-22, B) takes the partial-rebreathing mask and adds a one-way valve between the bag and the mask and another one-way valve over one or both mask ports. All the patient's exhaled volume is directed from the mask through the mask ports. The valve positioned between the mask and bag prevents exhaled gases from entering the bag. During exhalation the bag fills completely with 100% oxygen. At the beginning of inspiration the mask port valves are sucked closed, preventing the drawing in of room air, the bag valve opens, and the patient inhales the 300 to 500 mL of oxygen from this reservoir, along with additional oxygen volume from the supply source. The oxygen flow must be set at a rate high enough to prevent the bag from emptying more than halfway.

If this system were perfect, delivery of 100% oxygen would theoretically be possible. However, these inexpensive disposable masks cannot provide an airtight fit on the face, and their valves are simple rubber or vinyl disks that don't provide a perfect seal. However, at flows of 10 to 15 L/min, an FIO_2 of 0.6 to 0.8 is achievable. The nonrebreathing mask has a valve on only one of the exhalation ports. Most manufacturers supply the mask this way to allow the patient to inhale room air if the oxygen supply flow becomes inadequate.

Oxygen-Conserving Devices

The majority of oxygen is wasted when it is delivered in a continuous flow by nasal cannula. All of the oxygen flow during the expiratory phase of the respiratory cycle and during any pause between breaths is wasted. Only during the initial period of inspiration is the supplemental flow of oxygen needed. This first part of inspiration gets down to the alveoli and participates in gas exchange; the rest of the inspired air and supplemental oxygen fills the anatomic dead space and is exhaled without contributing to respira-

Figure 32-22 **A,** Partial-rebreathing mask. **B,** Nonrebreathing mask. (Modified from Scanlan CL, Wilkins RL, Stoller JK. Egan's fundamentals of respiratory care. 7th ed. St Louis: Mosby; 1999.)

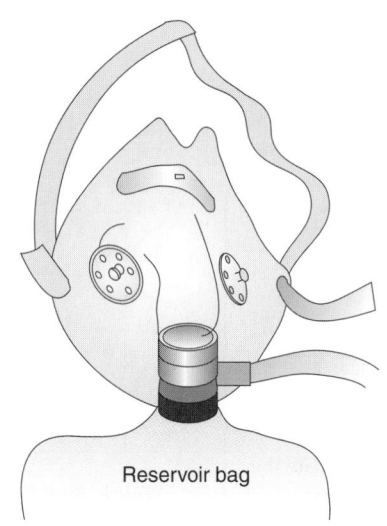

Reservoir bag

A

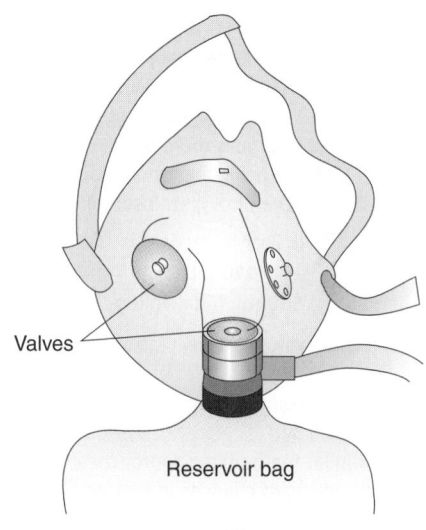

Valves

Reservoir bag

B

tion. Oxygen-conserving devices save oxygen by either allowing a decrease in the continuous rate of flow of oxygen through the use of a reservoir, providing oxygen flow only during inspiration, or providing only an appropriate-volume bolus of oxygen at the beginning of inspiration.

The patient's physiologic need for oxygen changes with varying levels of activity. Oxygen administered at 2 L/min to a patient who is awake and at rest in a chair may easily maintain an oxyhemoglobin saturation of greater than 90%. However, mild exertion may necessitate an increase in the flow to 3 L/min to maintain the greater-than-90% saturation, and 4 L/min may be necessary at even greater exertion levels. Often, providing higher-liter flow is necessary during sleep to prevent desaturation. Patients who require oxygen while at rest to maintain an acceptable saturation level must be tested while performing their normal daily activities to determine whether higher doses of oxygen are necessary to maintain saturation on exertion, a concept that is especially true when any type of oxygen-conserving device is used.

Reservoir Cannula

Two styles of reservoir cannulas exist (Figure 32-23)—the moustache type and the pendant. Both are worn like the standard nasal cannula. When the patient exhales, a small, expandable membranelike reservoir bag fills with oxygen from the supply source. The moustache-style reservoir holds about 20 mL of oxygen, whereas the pendant can hold up to 40 mL and an additional 20 mL in its tubing leading to the nasal prongs. At the beginning of inspiration in both types of reservoir cannulas, a high-concentration bolus of oxygen of from 20 mL to 40 mL is drawn in from the reservoir, undiluted with room air. Theoretically, no additional oxygen flow is necessary during inspiration. However, flow does continue, and both types of reservoir cannulas function as do standard cannulas during the remaining portion of inspiration. During exhalation the oxygen flow washes out the pendant tubing dead space and refills the reservoir bag of both types of reservoir cannulas.

Because the small-volume, high-concentration bolus of oxygen is delivered at the very beginning of inspiration, an FIO_2 comparable to that delivered by a standard cannula can be maintained, but at a flow rate that can be reduced by as much as 75%. Continuous assessment of oxyhemoglobin saturation by pulse oximetry is necessary to determine the actual oxygen flow required at rest and various levels of exertion to maintain a satisfactory oxygen saturation measured by pulse oximetry (SpO_2). For most patients a 50% savings in the amount of oxygen used is generally realized; or a patient's portable system lasts twice as long; or a smaller and lighter portable system lasts as long as a larger system at the higher flow rate.

Reservoir cannulas have been available since the 1980s, but their acceptance by patients has never been high due to their appearance. The moustache cannula has a very obtrusive appearance because of the placement of the reservoir under the nose. Moving the reservoir to a pendant at chest level has solved part of that objection, but the tubing from the pendant and the nasal prongs are larger in diameter and heavier than that of a standard cannula, often leading to patient complaints and noncompliance.

Transtracheal Catheter

The **transtracheal catheter** has been commercially available since the early 1980s. It is a small-diameter, usually 9 Fr (2.97 mm OD) Teflon catheter, surgically inserted into the trachea between the second and third tracheal rings. The catheter is connected to a small flange and held in place by an adjustable chain (Figure 32-24). Oxygen supply tubing connects directly to the catheter and delivers oxygen into the midtrachea. Because oxygen is continuously delivered directly into the

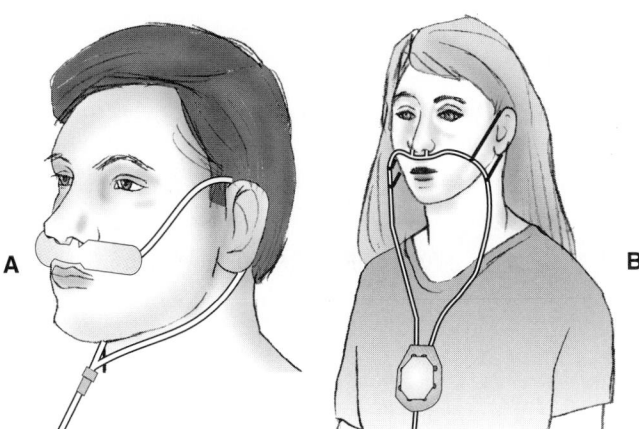

Figure 32-23 A, The moustache-style reservoir cannula. **B,** The pendant-type reservoir cannula. (Modified from Scanlan CL, Wilkins RL, Stoller JK. *Egan's fundamentals of respiratory care.* 7th ed. St Louis: Mosby; 1999.)

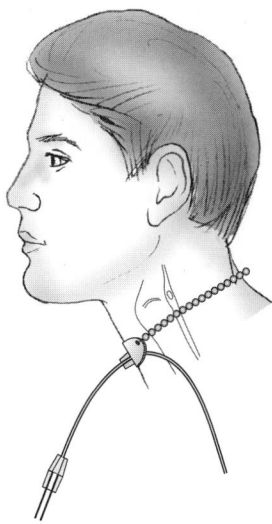

Figure 32-24 Transtracheal oxygen catheter in place. (Modified from Scanlan CL, Wilkins RL, Stoller JK. *Egan's fundamentals of respiratory care.* 7th ed. St Louis: Mosby; 1999.)

trachea, during exhalation and the pause between breaths the anatomic reservoir fills with oxygen that is inhaled at the beginning of the next breath with less dilution from room air. This filling permits a reduction in the oxygen flow rate by about 50% without an effect on the FIO_2.

In addition to the positive oxygen-conserving effect of the transtracheal catheter, patients also may find the catheter inconspicuous and able to be easily covered with a scarf, blouse, or shirt collar. On the other hand, the transtracheal catheter features a number of disadvantages that have hindered its widespread acceptance. Insertion of the catheter involves a minor surgical procedure usually conducted in an outpatient surgical unit of a hospital via a sterile procedure. Complications of the initial catheter placement can include infection, bleeding, and subcutaneous emphysema. The catheter must be replaced at least every 90 days, usually in the physician's office, before it becomes cracked, kinked, or mucus encrusted. Transtracheal catheters are not covered by some major medical insurance plans. In addition, the catheter must be cleaned regularly to prevent mucus buildup and possible obstruction through the instillation of saline and insertion of a cleaning wire into the lumen of the catheter.

Demand-Oxygen Conservers

As the name implies, **demand-oxygen conservers** supply a flow of oxygen only when it is needed, on demand at the initiation of inspiration. The conserver is placed between the oxygen supply and the delivery device, which can be a nasal catheter, nasal cannula, or transtracheal catheter. Demand-oxygen conservers have gained widespread acceptance in recent years, especially in home care. They offer a number of advantages over continuous-flow systems. Their use extends the oxygen supply by a factor of at least two and to as much as five to seven times, depending on the type of con-

server used, patient activity, respiratory rate, and inspiration to expiration (I:E) ratio. They can be used on stationary liquid oxygen reservoirs, on liquid portables, and on any size oxygen cylinder, which decreases the frequency of deliveries from once a week to every 2 or 3 weeks, an advantage for both the patient and the supplier. Patients need to store fewer cylinders in their homes; the contents of each cylinder last much longer than with other devices, allowing greater freedom and mobility without the need to transport extra backup cylinders. Patients unable to handle the weight of one size cylinder can use a smaller, lighter cylinder, and with the conserving device the smaller volume of oxygen lasts as long as the larger cylinder without the conserver. These advantages may lead to more compliant use of oxygen, especially outside the home. Patients also report less nasal drying because the oxygen flow is intermittent rather than continuous.

Several types of demand-oxygen conservers exist, including continuous inspiration, pulsed bolus, and hybrid combinations of pulse and continuous. Figure 32-25 illustrates a patient breathing flow pattern and compares it with the delivery flow patterns of continuous-oxygen and that of the pulsed-bolus, continuous-inspiration, and hybrid oxygen-conserving devices.

Continuous Inspiration Conserver

The continuous inspiration conserver supplies oxygen flow throughout the inspiratory phase of respiration and can realize a 2:1 to 3:1 savings in oxygen use compared with continuous flow. These conservers operate pneumatically, without batteries or electronics. When the patient begins an inspiration, creating a negative pressure in the supply tubing, this action causes a demand valve to open and supply a continuous flow of oxygen at the patient's prescribed flow setting until inspiration ends. A switch allows the patient to turn off the demand conserver function and change to continuous flow. This type of pneumatic demand valve system requires the use of a double-lumen nasal cannula—one channel through

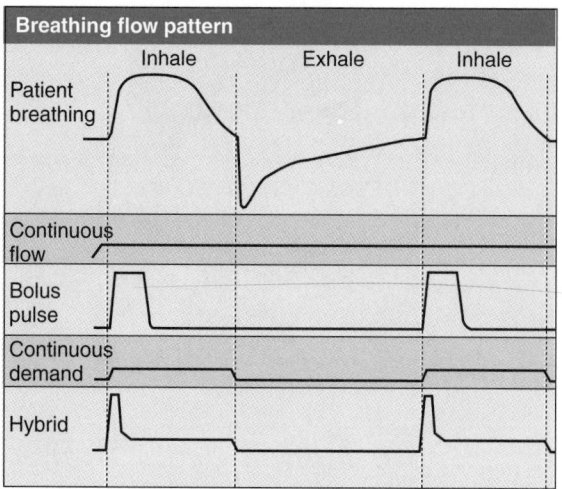

Figure 32-25 Graphic depiction of the oxygen delivery patterns from mechanical conserving devices compared with continuous oxygen flow and the ways they interact with the normal respiratory cycle. (Modified from McCoy R. Economics drives oxygen conserving device popularity. Adv Manag Respir Care 2001;10:59-60.)

*T*ABLE 32-1

Set FIO_2, Minimum Flow Requirements, Outputs, and Entrainment Ratios for Air-Entrainment Masks

FIO_2 Setting	Minimum Oxygen Flow (L/min)	Entrainment Ratio (Oxygen:Air)	Total Flow (L/min)
0.24	4	1:25	104
0.28	4	1:10	44
0.31	6	1:7	48
0.35	8	1:5	48
0.40	8	1:3	32
0.50	12	1:1.7	32
0.60	12	1:1	24
0.70	12	1:0.6	19

From Branson RD. The nuts and bolts of increasing arterial oxygenation: devices and techniques. Respir Care 1993;38:672-686.

which the demand valve is activated and the second channel to carry the oxygen flow to the nasal prongs.

Pulsed Conserver

The pulsed conserver delivers a pulsed bolus or dose of oxygen at the beginning of inspiration and then remains off until activated again by inspiratory demand at the initiation of the next breath. The inspiratory effort opens a valve that releases the bolus of oxygen of a volume equivalent to the patient's prescribed liter flow. At a 2-L/min setting the bolus is generally between 30 mL and 36 mL. Pulsed conservers are somewhat more sophisticated then the wholly pneumatic continuous-inspiration type and use electronic controls requiring a power source, usually a rechargeable or replaceable battery. A standard nasal cannula is used with this type of conserver. The ability to optionally switch the conserver to continuous flow is a built-in feature. If the conserver's electronics fail, the unit's valve automatically opens to provide a continuous flow of oxygen, usually at 2 L/min. Oxygen savings of 3:1 to 4:1 are attainable with this conserver system compared with continuous oxygen flow.

ℛespiratory Recap

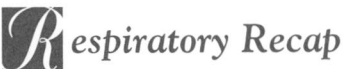

Oxygen-Conserving Devices
Bolus of oxygen from a reservoir at the beginning of inspiration Oxygen flow only during inspiration Measured-bolus dose of oxygen at the beginning of inspiration Bolus of oxygen at the beginning of inspiration and continuing flow throughout inspiration

A variation on the pulsed conserver involves a fixed-volume bolus of oxygen delivered on selected breaths depending on the prescribed liter flow. A patient prescribed a continuous flow of 1 L/min would, with this type of conserver, receive a pulsed dose of oxygen on every fourth breath. Thus a 2 L/min order gets a bolus every other breath; 3 L/min, three of every four breaths; and 4 L/min, each breath. At the 1-L/min setting, oxygen savings of sixfold to sevenfold, compared with continuous-flow oxygen, can be achieved.

ℰQUATION 32-2

Air-to-Oxygen Ratios and Determination of Air and Oxygen Flows

---

Air:oxygen ratio $= \dfrac{1.0 - \text{FIO}_2}{\text{FIO}_2 - 0.21}$

Suppose an FIO_2 of 0.4 is desired, and the calculation is as follows:

Air:oxygen ratio $= \dfrac{1.0 - 0.4}{0.4 - 0.21} = \dfrac{0.6}{0.2} = 3{:}1$

If a total flow of 60 L/min is required, an air flow of 45 L/min and an oxygen flow of 15 L/min will produce an FIO_2 of 0.4.

Hybrid Pulse/Continuous Conserver

The hybrid pulse/continuous conserver delivers a fixed-volume bolus of oxygen, 12 to 15 mL, at the beginning of each breath and follows with a continuous flow throughout the remaining inspiratory cycle. An oxygen savings of twofold to threefold can be achieved, depending on the I:E ratio, over full continuous flow delivery.

High-Flow Devices

Air-Entrainment Masks

An **air-entrainment mask** consists of the mask, a jet nozzle, and entrainment ports. Oxygen is delivered through the jet nozzle, which increases its velocity. This gas at high velocity entrains ambient air into the mask because of the viscous shearing forces between the gas traveling through the nozzle and the stagnant ambient air. The FIO_2 depends on the nozzle size and the size of the entrainment ports. Commercially available systems use interchangeable jets, adjustable entrainment ports, or a combination of these (Figure 32-26). Obstruction of the entrainment port or the downstream flow decreases entrainment and increases FIO_2. To deliver a fixed FIO_2, the flow to the mask must exceed the patient's peak inspiratory flow, which may be difficult to achieve with a high FIO_2 setting (Table 32-1).

Mixture of Air and Oxygen

Two flowmeters, one air and one oxygen, can be used to deliver precise oxygen concentrations. Gas should be humidified before it is delivered to the patient via a variety of patient interfaces (Figures 32-27) at flows exceeding the patient's peak inspiratory flow. Calculating FIO_2 from known flow rates of air and oxygen is illustrated in Equation 32-2. **Air-oxygen blenders** (Figure 32-28) use 50-psig sources of air and oxygen to deliver precise FIO_2 values. Blenders are compact and convenient but expensive compared with the use of

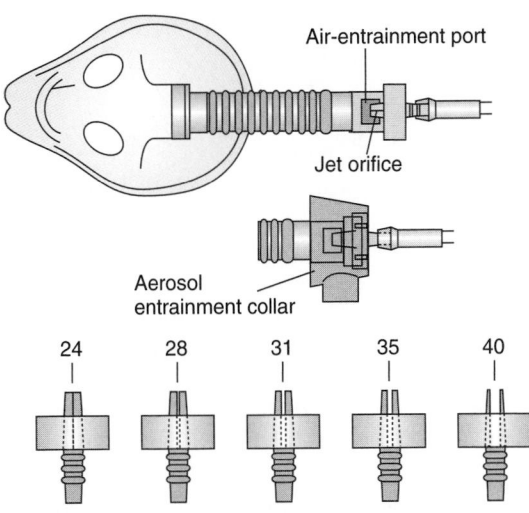

Figure 32-26 Diagram of an air-entrainment mask that uses variable jet orifice sizes to change FIO_2. (Modified from Kacmarek RM. Methods of oxygen delivery in the hospital. Prob Respir Care 1990;3:563-574.)

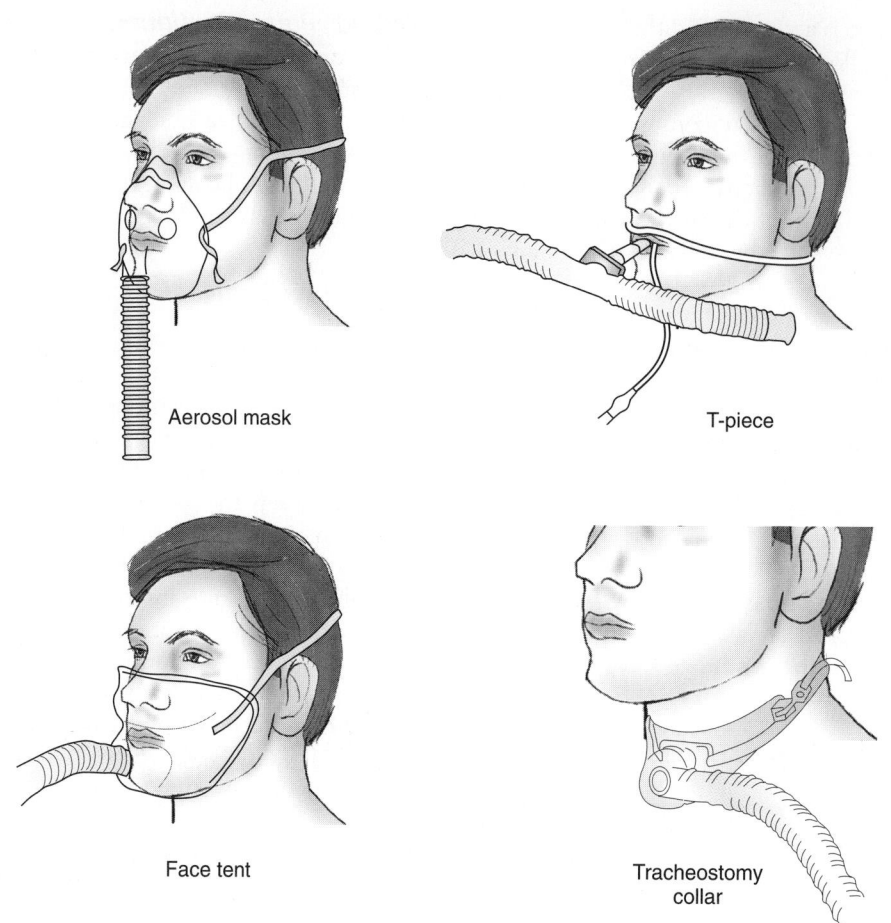

Aerosol mask

T-piece

Face tent

Tracheostomy collar

Figure 32-27 Patient interfaces for a high-flow oxygen delivery system. (Modified from Fink JR, Hunt GE. Clinical practice of respiratory care. Philadelphia: Lippincott Williams & Wilkins; 1999.)

two flowmeters. The principal component of a blender is the proportioning module, where air and oxygen are metered to produce the desired FIO_2. Clockwise movement of the control knob decreases FIO_2 by increasing the area for gas from the air source to flow to the outlet, whereas counterclockwise movement increases FIO_2 by allowing greater oxygen flow and less air flow.

Oxygen Enclosures

Placing the patient into an oxygen-enriched environment is one of the early methods of oxygen administration. Adult oxygen tents, infant incubators, and pediatric croup tents were all introduced between the mid-1920s and the 1940s. The adult tent was widely used for both oxygen administration and high-humidity therapy through the 1960s. Today enclosures are used primarily in infant and pediatric applications and include hoods, incubators, and croup tents.

Hoods The **oxygen hood** (Figure 32-29) is a round or rectangular, bottomless, clear rigid plastic device with a half-moon shaped cutout that allows it to be placed over the infant's neck and enclose the entire head. Hoods are

available in a variety of sizes and shapes to accommodate a full range of neonates and infants. By enclosing only the infant's head, the body is accessible for medical and nursing care procedures. Oxygen is delivered to the hood through either a blender with a heated humidifier or a heated air-entrainment nebulizer. Providing a minimum flow of 6 to 8 L/min is necessary to prevent the accumulation of carbon dioxide. Flows as high as 15 L/min may be necessary to maintain an adequate FIO_2.

Frequent or continuous monitoring of the oxygen concentration within the hood is necessary. Most hood designs include a deflector to prevent the incoming gas flow from being directed at the infant's head, which may cause excessive heat loss and cold stress, leading to increased oxygen consumption. For these same reasons, the gas supply should be heated to 30° C or higher, depending on the infant's size and gestational age. The method used to provide gas flow and humidification should not produce high noise levels (>65 decibels); such levels may be harmful to the neonate.

Incubators The **incubator** is designed to totally enclose the infant within an environment where the temperature, oxygen concentration, and humidity can be con-

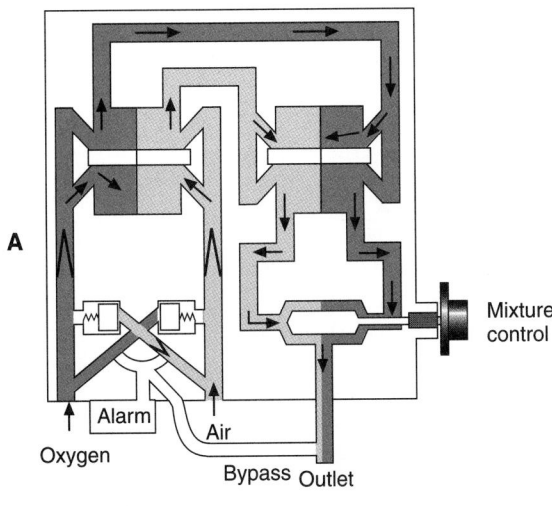

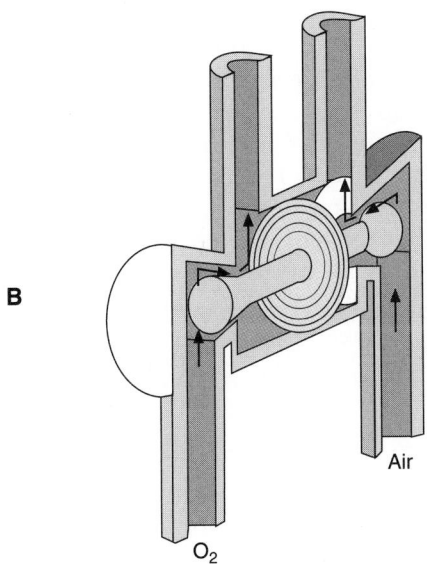

Figure 32-28 A, Schematic illustration of an air-oxygen blender. **B,** Proportioning valve in an air-oxygen blender. (Modified from Ward JJ. Equipment for mixed gas and oxygen therapy. In: Barnes TA, editor. Core textbook of respiratory care practice. 2nd ed. St Louis, Mosby; 1994.)

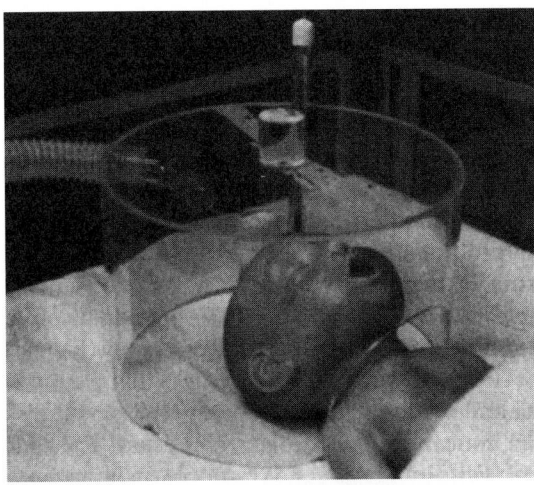

Figure 32-29 A typical infant oxygen hood. (From Scanlan CL, Wilkins RL, Stoller JK. Egan's fundamentals of respiratory care. 7th ed. St Louis: Mosby; 1999.)

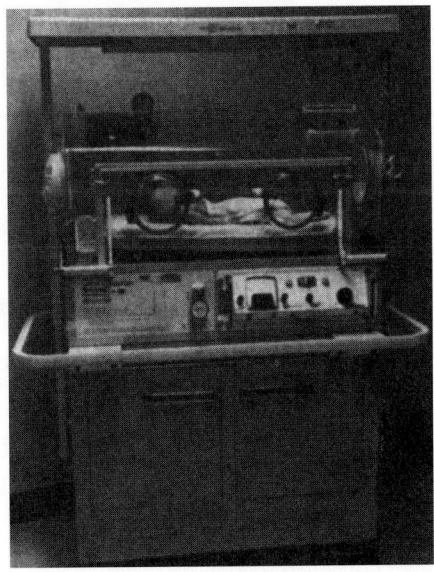

Figure 32-30 An infant incubator. (From Scanlan CL, Wilkins RL, Stoller JK. Egan's fundamentals of respiratory care. 7th ed. St Louis: Mosby; 1999.)

trolled (Figure 32-30). The patient is placed entirely within the incubator under a clear, rigid plastic enclosure. Access to the infant is gained by tilting of the entire cover, which causes a loss of the controlled environment. Whenever possible, a more appropriate method is to use one or more of the several portholes. When the incubator is closed, the temperature within can be maintained within narrow limits by thermostatic servo-controls.

Oxygen can be supplied to the incubator through its air-entrainment inlet designed to limit the incoming oxygen concentration to 40%. If a higher FIO₂ is needed, the air-entrainment ports can be blocked, causing a red warning flag to alert personnel that 100% oxygen is being delivered into the incubator. Humidified oxygen from a blender or air-entrainment system could be the primary source of gas flow to the incubator. In either case, the large internal volume of the incubator and the necessity to open it for patient access

makes maintenance of a consistent oxygen environment difficult and requires that the oxygen concentration be monitored frequently or continuously. To maintain a more stable FIO₂ in infants requiring supplemental oxygen, the

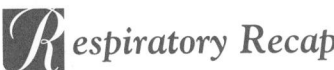

espiratory Recap

Oxygen Enclosures
Hoods
Incubators
Tents

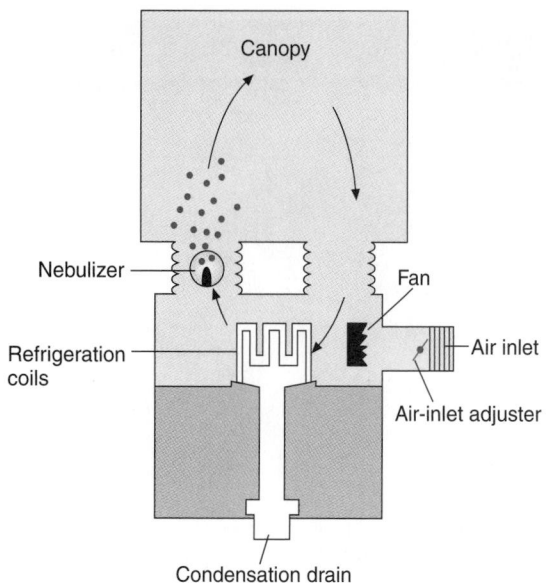

Figure 32-31   Schematic illustration of an oxygen tent. (Modified from Scanlan CL, Wilkins RL, Stoller JK. Egan's fundamentals of respiratory care. 7th ed. St Louis: Mosby; 1999.)

oxygen hood is commonly used within the incubator. Since the introduction of efficient servo-controlled radiant heating infant warmers, which can be used in conjunction with the oxygen hood, the use of incubators has waned.

Tents   With the introduction of inexpensive, efficient, disposable nasal cannulas and masks, the use of the inefficient and expensive electric refrigerated adult **oxygen tent** diminished and stopped being used by the late 1960s. The large internal volume of the canopy necessary to enclose an adult in a hospital bed and the frequent need to open the canopy for patient access made the achievement and maintenance of an oxygen concentration less than 50% difficult, even with flows of 12 to 15 L/min.

The croup tent, however, encloses the young pediatric patient under a lightweight clear plastic canopy supported over a frame (Figure 32-31). A large-volume aerosol generator powered by high-flow oxygen or air (8 to 12 L/min),

Age-Specific Angle

Hoods, incubators, and tents are used to administer oxygen to infants and children.

creates an ice-cooled circulation through the canopy. Cystic fibrosis patients who use this treatment are generally older, requiring a larger canopy and more efficient means of cooling and circulation.

Oxygen Analyzers

Oxygen analyzers are used to measure the concentration of oxygen administered to patients. Polarographic analyzers use a Clark electrode to measure oxygen. Although it actually measures PO_2, the polarographic analyzer usually displays the percent oxygen. These devices are accurate at any altitude, provided the instrument is calibrated at that altitude. Calibration is usually accomplished by exposure of the electrode to room air (21% oxygen) or 100% oxygen. An external power source is required, usually provided by a battery, which makes these analyzers portable. The inability to calibrate the analyzer usually means that the electrolyte in the electrode needs to be changed.

The galvanic cell analyzers, like the polarographic analyzers, use an electrochemical principle. Although the electrode responds to changes in PO_2, the analyzer usually displays the percent oxygen. The analyzer is calibrated with either room air (21% oxygen) or 100% oxygen. Unlike polarographic analyzers, galvanic cell analyzers do not require an external power source.

Paramagnetic analyzers use the Pauling principle, which is based on oxygen being a paramagnetic gas. A Wheatstone bridge oxygen analyzer uses the principle of thermoconductivity. Oxygen, being of higher molecular weight, cools the wire more than nitrogen. The Wheatstone bridge principle of oxygen analysis depends on the ability of oxygen to cool a heated wire.

In the zirconium analyzer, an electric potential is developed across heated zirconium oxide that is proportional to the PO_2. The cell must be heated to 700° C to 800° C, which requires substantial time for thermal stabilization, as well as considerable thermal insulation.

$\mathcal{R}$*espiratory Recap*

Oxygen Analyzers	
Polarographic	Thermoconductivity
Galvanic	Zirconium
Paramagnetic	

$\mathcal{K}$EY $\mathcal{P}$OINTS

- Pressure-reducing regulators are either single stage or multistage and feature fixed or adjustable pressure outlets.
- Flow control devices are flow restrictors, Bourdon gauges, or Thorpe tubes.
- Back-pressure–compensated Thorpe tubes are accurate regardless of downstream resistance.
- Oxygen concentrators are commonly used to provide home oxygen therapy.
- Portable liquid oxygen systems can be used to provide ambulatory oxygen therapy.
- Nasal catheters, nasal cannulas, simple masks, partial-rebreathing masks, and nonrebreathing masks are low-flow oxygen delivery devices.

- The F_{IO_2} from a low-flow oxygen delivery device is determined by the oxygen flow, reservoir volume, and inspiratory flow of the patient.
- Oxygen-conserving devices decrease the amount of oxygen waste and thus decrease the cost of therapy or extend the duration of a portable oxygen delivery system.
- High-flow oxygen delivery systems meet the entire inspiratory needs of the patient.
- Hoods, incubators, and tents are oxygen enclosure devices.
- Oxygen analyzers use polarography, galvanic cells, the Pauling principle, or thermoconductivity to measure oxygen concentration.

Recommended Reading

Branson RD, Hess DR, Chatburn RL. Respiratory care equipment. 2nd ed. Philadelphia: Lippincott Williams & Wilkins; 1999.

Cairo JM, Pilbeam SP. Mosby's respiratory care equipment. 6th ed. St Louis: Mosby; 1999.

Branson RD. The nuts and bolts of increasing arterial oxygenation: devices and techniques. Respir Care 1993;38:672-686.

Barnes TA. Equipment for mixed gas and oxygen therapy. Respir Care Clin N Am 2000;6:545-595.

CHAPTER 33

Hyperbaric Oxygen

David A. Desautels

CHAPTER OUTLINE

OBJECTIVES

1. Discuss the history of hyperbaric oxygen therapy.
2. Describe the physics of hyperbaric oxygen.
3. Compare diving diseases encountered during compression, while at pressure, and during decompression.
4. Discuss the use of decompression tables during hyperbaric therapy.
5. List indications and contraindications of hyperbaric oxygen therapy.
6. Describe the primary effects and secondary benefits of hyperbaric oxygen therapy.
7. Discuss the use of hyperbaric oxygen for the following conditions: carbon monoxide poisoning, clostridial myonecrosis (gas gangrene), crush injury, compartment syndrome, acute traumatic ischemias, enhancement of healing in selected problem wounds, necrotizing soft tissue infections, refractory osteomyelitis, radiation tissue damage (osteoradionecrosis), compromised skin grafts and flaps, thermal burns, and cranial abscess.
8. Discuss important aspects of the hyperbaric oxygen treatment.
9. Discuss issues related to drug therapy in the hyperbaric oxygen chamber.
10. Compare the use of multiplace and monoplace hyperbaric oxygen chambers.
11. Discuss issues related to maintenance and safety of hyperbaric oxygen chambers.

KEY TERMS

Arterial Gas Embolism	Carbon Monoxide Poisoning	Decompression
Barotrauma	Compression	Decompression Sickness (DCS)

KEY TERMS—cont'd

Decompression Tables	Inert Gas Necrosis	Oxygen Toxicity
Gas Gangrene	Monoplace Chamber	Unit Pulmonary Toxicity Dose
Hyperbaric Oxygen	Multiplace Chamber	(UPTD)
Hyperoxygenation	Osteoradionecrosis	

Hyperbaric oxygen, as defined by the Hyperbaric Oxygen Therapy Committee of the Undersea and Hyperbaric Medical Society, is treatment in which a patient breathes 100% oxygen (O_2) intermittently while the pressure of the treatment chamber is increased to a point higher than sea level pressure (that is, <1 atmosphere absolute).[1] Hyperbaric chambers are available from several manufacturers. This chapter describes the physiologic and technical aspects of hyperbaric oxygen.

History

The use of pressurized air dates to 1662 when Henshaw built a pressurized chamber he called a "domicilium."[2] He used this device to treat acute diseases with increased pressure and chronic diseases with decreased pressure. The use of O_2 in combination with increased pressure was impossible because this period was 112 years before Joseph Priestly discovered "dephlogisticated air" (O_2) and before Thomas Beddoes described the first medicinal use of O_2.[3] In France in the 1830s, air chambers capable of treating up to 50 patients at one time flourished across Europe and attracted people from as far away as the United States.

John Smearton (circa 1791) used a diving bell to fashion a caisson in the repair of the Henham Bridge in England. He later used the first real caisson to construct the Ramsgate Bridge.[2] *Caisson*, a French word, is a munitions carrier, compartment, or sunk-panel in a pressurized compartment that keeps water out as workers construct bridge footings or tunnels. Difficulties arose in the use of caissons when these workers returned to the surface and experienced decompression sickness, often referred to as "the bends." The colloquial bends came from the stilted manner in which these workers walked while on the surface. Only while they were under pressure did they feel comfortable. During the building of the Brooklyn Bridge (1860-1870), workers were subjected to pressures of 79 feet of sea water (fsw). During this operation, 110 cases of decompression sickness (bends) were reported.[4]

In the United States a chamber was patented but never built by Daniel Kelly in 1876[5]; a chamber then was built by Orval J. Corning in New York in 1891. In 1921, Cunningham first built a chamber 10 feet in diameter and 88 feet long. Not satisfied with the product, in 1928 he built a five-story chamber, which was 64 feet in diameter. He used the chamber to treat hypertension, diabetes, syphilis, and cancer. Because he and the American Medical Association (AMA) did not agree on these uses for hyperbaric oxygen, he was eventually put out of business and the chamber was sold for scrap.

The major new beginnings of hyperbaric medicine began in Amsterdam with the use of large chambers to perform open-heart procedures under pressure. The first of these chambers, built in 1959, extended the time a heart could be left open from 3 to 27 minutes. A short time later, in 1960, I. Boerema wrote his paper "Life Without Blood," in which he demonstrated that life could be sustained in a hyperbaric environment without hemoglobin. Soon thereafter the heart/lung bypass machine was developed, and performance of surgery under pressure no longer was necessary.

In 1963 the U.S. Air Force, led by Dr. Jefferson Davis, began using hyperbaric oxygen at Brooks Air Force Base in San Antonio, Texas. Until this time, military use of hyperbaric chambers was limited to the treatment of diving accidents by the U.S. Navy. On occasion, civilian clinicians asked for and received assistance from the U.S. Navy in treating non-diving–related problems. However, Davis and his Air Force team began using clinical hyperbaric oxygen therapy in the United States.

Six physicians from the United States Navy's Underwater Swimmers School formed the Undersea Medical Society in 1967. They oversaw the use of hyperbaric oxygen therapy through a special committee formed in 1976 called the *Hyperbaric Oxygen Therapy Committee*, which still today regularly reviews the scientific literature regarding the appropriate use of hyperbaric oxygen, publishing its results every 3 years. Not until 1986 did the Undersea Medical Society incorporate the term *hyperbaric* into its name to become the *Undersea and Hyperbaric Medical Society (UHMS)*.

Physics

Respiratory care involves the administration of O_2 at increased partial pressures to patients who might be hypoxic breathing room air. Hyperbaric oxygen therapy involves O_2 concentrations much greater than those attainable at sea level. To understand hyperbaric oxygen therapy, several types of pressure must be understood.

Atmospheric pressure is the weight of the air column from sea level to the outer limits of the atmosphere. This weight can be expressed as 14.7 pounds per square inch (psi; the weight of the atmospheric column on a square inch at sea level), 760 mm Hg, or 1033.4 cm of water (cm H_2O). Atmospheric pressure is a standard in hyperbaric measures.

Gauge pressure is the pressure indicated on a pressure gauge. At atmospheric pressure, with no load on the pressure gauge, it reads zero and is expressed in pounds per square inch, gauge (psig). Once a load is applied to the pressure gauge, it is added to the atmospheric pressure to equal absolute pressure. For example, if 2250 psi is read on a gauge attached to an air cylinder, the absolute pressure is 2264.7 psi.

Hydrostatic pressure is the weight of water expressed in psi, mm Hg, cm H_2O, or any of the other measures of pressure. Hydrostatic pressure also can be related to atmospheric pressure. One cubic foot of sea water weighs 64 pounds. If the terms are changed to psi by division by the conversion factor to change cubic feet to square inches (144), 0.445 psi is obtained. This conversion means that for each foot of depth a person descends in this sea water, a pressure of 0.445 psi is added. At a depth of 33 fsw the equivalent of 1 atmosphere is attained. For each 33 fsw a person descends into the ocean, an additional atmosphere of pressure can be added (Table 33-1).

The gas laws have important implications during hyperbaric oxygen therapy (Equation 33-1). If a mixture of gases is contained in a fixed volume and temperature, the total pressure of the mixture is equal to the sum of the pressures,[6] a concept known as *Dalton's law* that profoundly affects the patients and clinicians in hyperbaric chambers. Individuals are exposed to increasing partial pressures as the chamber is compressed and decreasing par-

tial pressures as the chamber is decompressed. Increases and decreases in O_2, nitrogen (N_2), and carbon dioxide (CO_2) pressures can cause problems. Although the majority of these problems are physiologic, some are physical, such as the increased fire risk.

Boyle's law states that the volume of a gas varies inversely with pressure at any given temperature.[6] Boyle's law affects everything entering and leaving a hyperbaric chamber. As chamber pressure increases, volume decreases and vice versa, affecting equipment and physiology during compression and decompression of the chamber. Charles' law states that the volume of a gas at constant pressure varies directly with the absolute temperature,[6] which affects the operation of the hyperbaric chamber during compression and decompression. Gay-Lussac's law states that the pressure of a gas varies directly with the absolute temperature when the volume is kept constant.[6] It affects the operation of the hyperbaric chamber during compression and decompression. The combined gas law uses Boyle's, Charles' and Gay-Lussac's laws to calculate the changes in pressure, temperature, and volume.

Pascal's law states that the pressure applied to an enclosed liquid is transmitted uniformly and undiminished to all parts of the liquid.[7] This law affects everything compressed in a hyperbaric chamber and explains why the sinuses and ears hurt as compression occurs. The pressure is transmitted uniformly throughout the body to the middle ears and sinuses, creating pain when it reduces the size of the air space to maintain an even pressure through the system. Henry's law states that the solubility of a gas in a liquid is directly proportional to the partial pressure of the gas overlying the liquid.[6] In the hyperbaric environment this law affects the rate at which gases move into or from solution, which can produce diving diseases, such as decompression sickness.

$\mathcal{R}$espiratory Recap

Physical Principles Important to Hyperbaric Therapy	
Dalton's law	Combined gas law
Boyle's law	Pascal's law
Charles' law	Henry's law
Gay-Lussac's law	

$\mathcal{T}$ABLE 33-1

Comparison of Various Measures of Pressure Used During Hyperbaric Therapy

Atm Abs	fsw	psig	psi, Absolute	mm Hg	cm H_2O
1	0	0	14.7	760	1033.6
2	33	14.7	29.4	1420	2067.2
3	66	29.4	44.1	2280	3100.8
4	99	44.1	58.8	3040	4134.4
5	132	58.8	73.5	3800	5168.0
6	165	73.5	88.2	4560	6201.6

Atm abs, Atmospheres absolute; fsw, feet of sea water; psig, pounds per square inch, gauge; psi, absolute, pounds per square inch, absolute; mm Hg, millimeters of mercury; cm H₂O, centimeters of water.

Diving Diseases

Diving diseases occur on **compression** (barotrauma), at pressure (inert gas narcosis and O_2 toxicity), and on **decompression** (arterial gas embolism and decompression sickness).

Diseases Encountered during Compression

Barotrauma is an all-inclusive term used in hyperbaric medicine to describe injuries of body air spaces due to a pressure differential. As Boyle's law states, as the environmental pressure increases, the body air space decreases in volume. During compression this pressure may cause lung, middle ear, sinus, or dental barotrauma. A pressure differential occurs when the individual exposed to the increasing pressure fails to equalize body cavity pressure with ambient pressure. As stated in Pascal's law, pressure is transmitted to the body air space as the surrounding pressure is increased. In the lungs, pressure is equalized at each breath if no breath-holding is present, as in the case of free diving or free ascending from increased pressure.

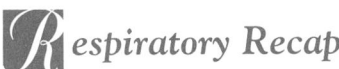espiratory Recap

Classification of Diving Diseases
Encountered during *compression*
Encountered at *pressure*
Encountered during *decompression*

In the ear the eustachian tube must be opened to allow pressurized gas into the middle ear. Otherwise, pressure against the eardrum is greater than that of the middle ear, and the eardrum is pushed inward, causing the individual great pain. Clearing the ears may be done in several ways, with the most common being the Valsalva maneuver, which involves a forcible exhalation against a closed glottis. This action increases pressure in the eustachian tubes, allowing equalization of the pressure on the inside of the tympanic membrane with the outside surrounding environment. Once the pressure is equalized, the individual no longer feels any discomfort. Most people have experienced this situation in an airplane or in swimming to the bottom of a pool. Individuals not properly trained wait until experiencing pain before they begin clearing their ears, which results in injury to the ear, one of the most common adverse affects of hyperbaric oxygen therapy.

If the pressure is not equalized in a timely manner, a problem called "trapped door" can result. Once the trapped-door effect has occurred, the individual must be decompressed through a slight reduction in the pressure until normal equalization can be attained. If a decongestant is used to assist the individual and the decongestant has a rebound effect, the patient must be held at pressure because decompression would result in a reverse barotrauma, causing an outward rupture of the eardrum. If the individual is unconscious, equalization of pressure with the inner ear is accomplished through surgical puncture of the eardrum before hyperbaric therapy is initiated. The sinuses are affected in the same way. The Valsalva maneuver used to clear the ears also equalizes the pressure in the sinuses. Reverse barotrauma and trapped door also are similar. A faulty dental filling can cause gas to accumulate behind the filling during compression, causing dental barotrauma. During decompression, as pressure behind the filling is exceeded, the filling is explosively removed from its placement.

Barotrauma is not limited to body air spaces. Any device, instrument, apparatus, or medication with an air space that is placed into a hyperbaric chamber is affected by Boyle's law. Implosions or explosions can result from the glass, membrane, plug, or wall of the equipment being overcome by the pressure differential. If a glass vial is sealed at sea level, atmospheric pressure and then taken to increased pressures, eventually the increasing pressure on the outside of the vial is sufficient to overcome the tensile strength of the glass, causing the vial to implode. The reverse is true if a device is taken inside the hyperbaric chamber, opened, and then sealed at that pressure. As the pressure inside the chamber is reduced to return to ambient atmospheric pressure, the pressure differential becomes great enough to cause the device to explode. For these reasons, the facility's safety director must approve all items entering a hyperbaric chamber.

Diseases Encountered at Pressure

Inert gas narcosis, which is analogous to the feeling of intoxication, seldom occurs with routine hyperbaric oxygen therapy. A pressure greater then 60 fsw must occur to cause this problem, which may occur in multiplace chambers (which treat more than one individual at a time) treating divers for arterial gas embolism at depths of 165 fsw. Attendants working in chambers equipped to treat divers to this depth need practice dives to ensure that they can experience inert gas narcosis and gain competence caring for divers at this depth. Some individuals are not capable of providing quality care at this depth. Inert gas necrosis is self-limiting, and no effects remain after decompression.

Two forms of **oxygen toxicity**—pulmonary and cerebral—can occur in the hyperbaric chamber. Pulmonary O_2 toxicity, described by Lorrain Smith in 1899, affects the lungs and results from the breathing of O_2 at concentrations greater than 40% at sea level. Cerebral O_2 toxicity, first described by Paul Bert in 1878, is unique to hyperbaric oxygen therapy and is caused by the breathing of 100% O_2 at pres-

$\mathcal{E}$QUATION   33-1

Gas Laws Important in Hyperbaric Oxygen Therapy

Dalton's Law

$$k = P_1 + P_2 + P_3 + \ldots P_n$$

where *P* is pressure, and *k* is a constant.

Boyle's Law

$$k = PV$$

where:

k = Constant
P = Pressure
V = Volume

Charles' Law

$$k = \frac{V}{T}$$

where:

k = Constant
V = Volume
T = Absolute temperature

Gay-Lussac's Law

$$k = \frac{P}{T}$$

where:

k = Constant
P = Pressure
T = Temperature

Combined Gas Law

$$k = \frac{PV}{T} \text{ or } \frac{P_1V_1}{T_1} = \frac{P_2V_2}{T_2}$$

where:

k = Constant
P = Pressure
V = Volume
T = Temperature

sures greater than two atmospheres absolute (atm abs). The greater the pressure, the shorter the time required for symptoms, including nausea, facial fasciculations, and grand mal seizures. The seizures are self-limiting in the hyperbaric environment and should not necessitate the cessation of therapy. However, in the diving environment, seizures usually result in death by drowning.

Monitoring the O_2 dose an individual requires for treatment is important to determine how much is in excess. The **unit pulmonary toxicity dose (UPTD)** serve to not only determine when a patient may be in trouble from O_2 toxicity but also helps in the calculation of the dose of O_2 when treatment tables are intermixed during treatment of a large number of patients in a multiplace chamber. On each treatment table listed in this chapter, the number of UPTDs is listed. A rough calculation of UPTD is 1 minute of 100% O_2 at 1 atm abs.

Diseases Encountered on Decompression

Robert Boyle first recognized **decompression sickness (DCS)** when he saw bubbles in the eye of a pit viper in 1667. DCS is considered a primary use for hyperbaric oxygen therapy. It was once the only indication for hyperbaric therapy but now accounts for a small percentage of the patients receiving this therapy. Because of Henry's law, breathing of increased partial pressures of N_2 causes more of this gas to dissolve in the tissues. If the ambient pressure decreases too rapidly, the gas comes from physical solution and forms a gas, much like a warm and shaken soda. Bubbles formed by these gases create symptoms dependent on where they form.

Separated into categories, decompression sickness can be type I, which is pain only (usually in or around the joints), or type II, which is neurologic. Type II symptoms can include tingling, numbness, paresthesia, paralysis, and death. The differentiation is important because each type requires a different treatment protocol. The hyperbaric staff members should have a working knowledge of the nationwide Divers Alert Network (DAN), which is available to assist with the treatment of DCS. Hyperbaric oxygen therapy is the primary treatment for DCS. Recompression may shrink the bubble size, allowing it to enter the circulation and be expelled by respiration. The most effective therapy is provided by increased O_2, which helps heal damaged tissue. Although many treatment tables have been developed, the primary one is for treatment of decompression sickness (Figure 33-1).

Arterial gas embolism occurs from pulmonary overpressurization. If the pressure in the lungs exceeds the integrity of the lung parenchyma, the lung tears and the air escapes in to one of several places. If it vents into the pleura, it results in a pneumothorax. If it vents into the mediastinum, pneumomediastinum or subcutaneous emphysema occurs. In the worst-case scenario, it can tear into pulmonary vessels, resulting in air being carried to the heart. If it enters the right side of the heart and proceeds to the lungs, effective filtration occurs and large quantities of air can be absorbed. If air enters the left side of the heart, it is sent out the aorta and, in the upright individual, to the carotid artery in the brain. In the brain the bubble moves through the vessel until the body can no longer tolerate its size, plugging the vessel and preventing blood flow beyond that point. Depending on the location in the brain, this plugging can cause severe consequences, including death.

Arterial gas embolism has not occurred in the hyperbaric environment. However, it often occurs in self-contained underwater breathing apparatus (SCUBA) divers who panic while diving. A diver breathing compressed gas at increased pressure must breathe normally or exhale as the pressure is reduced around that diver during ascent. For example, if a diver should panic at a depth of 33 fsw, twice the volume of gas is contained in the lungs as at the surface. If this volume is not vented during ascent, the volume of the lungs will be twice as great at the surface. The SCUBA diver is a dramatic example of Boyle's law. The lungs can

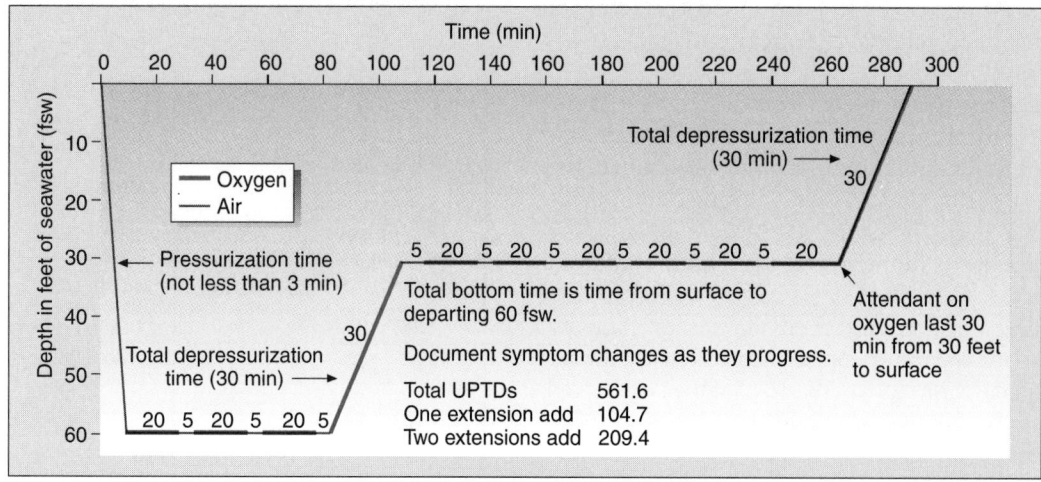

Figure 33-1   Treatment table for decompression sickness. *UPTDs,* Units pulmonary toxicity dose.

tear from an over-pressure as low as 90 mm Hg, which is the equivalent of breathing from a SCUBA tank at 4 fsw and ascending without exhaling. Treatment for arterial gas embolism requires a hyperbaric chamber capable of compression to 6 atm abs and the ability to administer nitrox, a mixture of 50% O_2 and 50% N_2, which is the highest dose of O_2 used in any treatment (Figure 33-2).

Decompression Tables

Decompression tables should not be confused with Treatment Tables. Decompression tables are a schedule of depths at which any person exposed to increased pressure must stop for a prescribed period of time to prevent decompression sickness.

Gases move in and from the various body tissues at different rates. O_2 moves into and from the tissues quickly, whereas N_2 moves very slowly. Each tissue absorbs and releases gases at its own rate, which is generally determined by its vascularity. Very vascular tissue moves the gases quickly. These decompression stops allow the gas the same amount of time to emerge from the tissue as it did for the gas to enter into solution. In addition to vascularity, the pressure and length of exposure determine the amount of gas absorbed. The higher the pressure and the longer the time, the more gas is absorbed. The slower the absorption, the longer the time necessary to release gas from the tissue. Even after the diver returns to atmospheric pressure, the tissues are over-saturated with gases. The primary culprit is N_2, which requires fivefold as much time to absorb into fatty tissue as it does for lean or vascular tissue. If the diver avoids the decompression stops and ascends directly to the surface, N_2 becomes oversaturated in the body's tissue and gas emerges from physical solution and forms a gas.

At extreme pressures, even limited exposures can take an inordinate amount of time to desaturate. For example, for a relatively short dive to a deep depth in a commercial

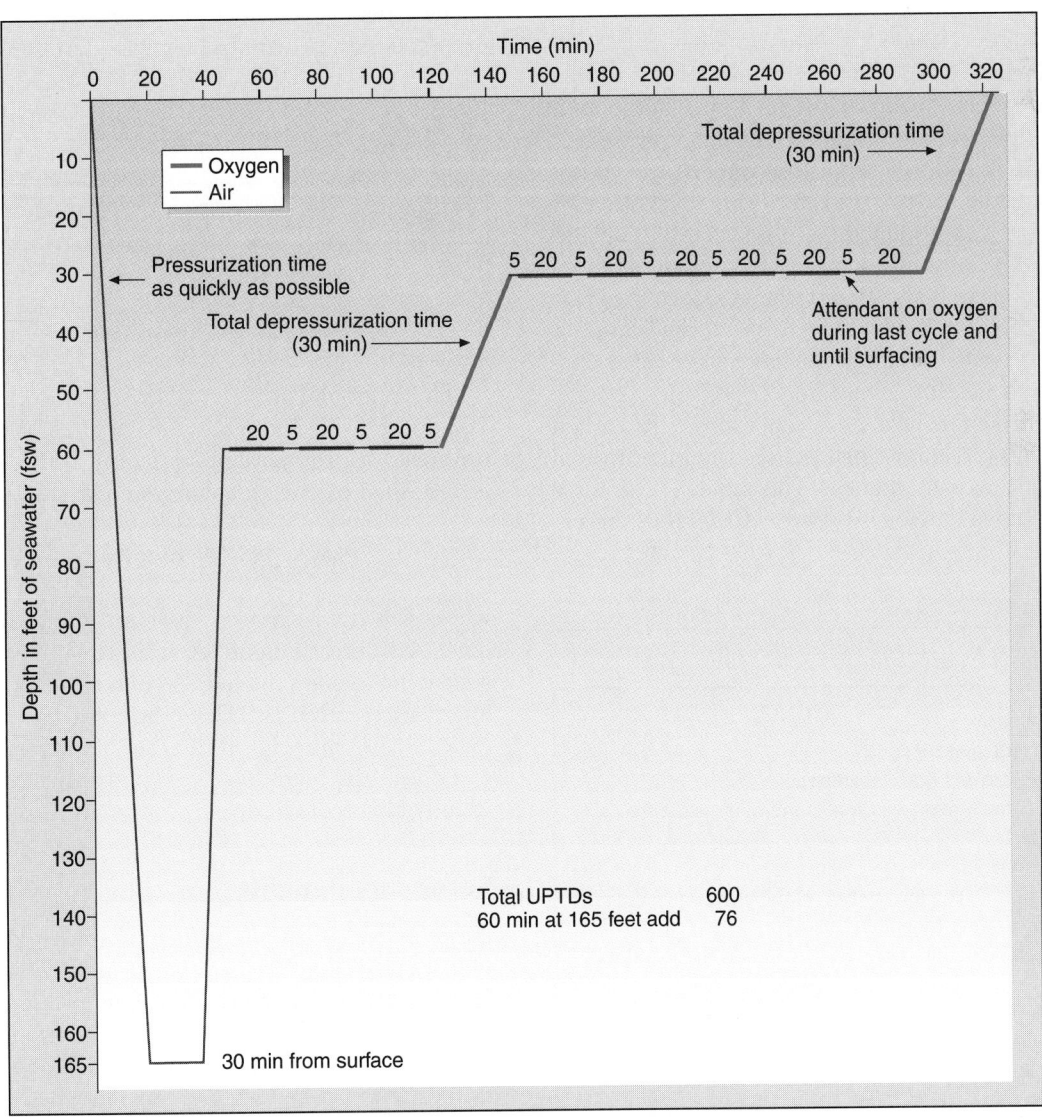

Figure 33-2 Treatment table for air embolism. *UPTDs,* Units pulmonary toxicity dose.

oil field the diver takes weeks to desaturate. Hyperbaric technologists entering the chamber with patients are exposed to increased pressure each day. Because residual N_2 remains in a vascular tissue for long periods of time, absorption escalates in attendants who work daily in hyperbaric chambers. Eventually the tissue N_2 becomes excessive, and decompression sickness occurs; sickness can be prevented, however, with regular breaks in the routine of daily dives or a reduction in the total exposure.

Indications and Contraindications for Hyperbaric Oxygen Therapy

The UMHS, through the Hyperbaric Oxygen Therapy Committee, specifies the indications for hyperbaric therapy.[8] Through solid scientific investigation of these indications, the committee has established a foundation for the appropriate use of hyperbaric oxygen therapy, which is acceptable to most third-party payers. Currently accepted indications are listed in Box 33-1.

Patients with the extremely debilitating diseases listed in Box 33-1 often have other problems that complicate the use of hyperbaric oxygen therapy. Untreated pneumothorax is the only absolute contraindication to the use of hyperbaric oxygen therapy. In addition, the use of hyperbaric oxygen is not indicated while the patient is receiving chemotherapy drugs, especially doxorubicin (Adriamycin), cisplatin (Platinol), and bleomycin sulphate, which produce peroxides in levels toxic to body systems when exposed to hyperbaric oxygen conditions. However, this contraindication is considered relative to how much the therapy is needed. Protocols prohibit a pregnant female from hyperbaric exposure, but if the pregnant female has been exposed to carbon monoxide (CO) poisoning, then the fetus must be treated with hyperbaric oxygen therapy. The same is true for a chronic obstructive pulmonary disease (COPD). If the pa-

Box 33-1

Indications for Hyperbaric Oxygen Therapy

Air or gas embolism
Carbon monoxide poisoning
Clostridial myonecrosis (gas gangrene)
Crush injury, compartment syndrome, and other acute traumatic ischemias
Decompression sickness
Enhancement of healing for selected problem wounds
Exceptional blood loss (anemia)
Necrotizing soft tissue infections (subcutaneous tissue, muscle, fascia)
Osteomyelitis (refractory)
Radiation tissue damage (osteoradionecrosis)
Skin grafts and flaps (compromised)
Thermal burns
Adjunctive hyperbaric oxygen in intracranial abscess

tient requires hyperbaric oxygen therapy to treat osteoradionecrosis, therapy should proceed with special precautions during ascent. Relative contraindications for hyperbaric therapy are listed in Box 33-2.

Rationale and Mechanisms of Action of Hyperbaric Oxygen Therapy

Primary Effects

Hyperbaric oxygen therapy is considered the primary therapy for only two diseases—DCS and arterial gas embolism. The mechanism of action is twofold—bubble reduction and **hyperoxygenation.** Bubble reduction is directly related to pressure (Boyle's law). In both air embolism and DCS, pressure-volume changes are of primary importance in the establishment of the treatment protocol. The greater the pressure, the smaller the volume and diameter of the bubble in the circulation and tissues. Hyperbaric oxygen therapy decreases the bubble size in the circulation and tissues, thereby improving circulation.

Respiratory Recap

Hyperbaric Oxygen: Primary Therapy
Decompression sickness
Arterial gas embolism

The normal PaO_2 at sea level (1 atm abs) is 90 to 100 mm Hg. At 3 atm abs, a PaO_2 of 1800 mm Hg is not unusual with the patient breathing 100% O_2. This idea is described by the alveolar gas equation, as follows[9]:

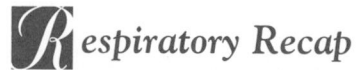

$$PAO_2 = [P_B - P_{H_2O}] \times FiO_2 - \frac{PaCO_2}{R}$$

where R is the respiratory quotient. From the PaO_2 at sea level, with breathing of 100% O_2 (673 mm Hg), for each additional atm abs the full 760 mm Hg is O_2. For example, a patient breathing 100% O_2 at 3 atm abs should have a PaO_2 of 2193 mm Hg. In the case of DCS and arterial gas embolism, the high-dose O_2 is probably more therapeutic than bubble reduction.

Secondary Benefits

Exposure to a high-pressure environment alters the individual's physiology in many ways. In the case of secondary benefits, all are related to O_2 at high pressure.

O_2 under pressure causes vasoconstriction in normal arteries that are not already ischemic. Blood vessel reduction of 25% can be seen at 3 atm abs when the individual is breathing 100% O_2. This effect can minimize edema formation while maintaining oxygenation.

Polymorphonuclear leukocytes and macrophages are one of the body's major lines of defense against bacterial infections and require O_2 for their antibiotic activity. In many cases O_2 tensions above the 30 to 40 mm Hg levels activate the patient's leukocyte response in both aerobic and anaerobic infections. When the partial pressure of O_2 surrounding bacteria increases beyond 1.3 atm abs, bacterial growth can be inhibited (known as the *bacteriostatic effect*).

Delivery of high-pressure 100% O_2 inhibits the growth of anaerobes and some aerobes, which produce toxins (toxin inhibition and inactivation). Toxins can destroy cell membranes, producing tissue necrosis. The progressing cell and tissue destruction establishes anaerobic conditions in an ever-enlarging area of tissue. Bacterial multiplication causes increased levels of toxins and the death of the host unless the condition is properly treated.

ℛespiratory Recap

Hyperbaric Oxygen: Secondary Benefits	
Vasoconstriction	Neovascularization
Bacteriostasis	Hyperoxygenation
Toxic inhibition and inactivation	

Tissue O_2 tensions of 30 to 40 mm Hg are necessary for fibroblastic synthesis of collagen and the subsequent development of a collagen matrix for capillary budding into avascular areas. Increasing abnormally low tissue tensions to a higher level stimulates fibroblastic activity. Hyperbaric oxygen therapy helps provide tissue viability by providing support through collagen deposition and capillary budding (neovascularization and angiogenesis).

Hemoglobin carries the majority of the O_2 in the red blood cell (RBC). However, a limited amount of hemoglobin is carried in the plasma. Hyperbaric oxygen therapy adds 2.3 mL/dL per atmosphere to the plasma. At 3 atm abs, the hemoglobin could be removed from a patient and normal saline substituted for the blood. Breathing 100% O_2 at 3 atm abs would make available 6.9 mL/dL O_2 dissolved in plasma, which is adequate oxygenation for metabolic needs.

Clinical Use of Hyperbaric Oxygen

Carbon Monoxide Poisoning

Carbon monoxide poisoning is the most common type in the United States. Thousands of cases are reported annually, and more are not correctly diagnosed. Use of 100% O_2 by mask is the emergency treatment, and hyperbaric oxygen therapy should be the primary treatment. Time is

crucial to a successful outcome. As in most emergent diagnoses treated in the hyperbaric chamber, the first 6 hours are the golden period for treatment.

CO binds to hemoglobin with an affinity 240 times greater than O_2. The half-life of CO in tissue is 5 hours and 20 minutes if air is breathed. This time is reduced to 80 minutes if 100% O_2 is breathed and to 23 minutes if 100% O_2 is breathed at 3 atm abs. Hyperbaric oxygen can sustain life while CO is off-loading from the hemoglobin. Hyperbaric oxygen also causes a decrease in cerebral edema and helps heal ischemic tissue during this recovery. Laboratory measurements of carboxyhemoglobin levels have not proven useful because of the dosing exposure and delay to treatment. The clinical picture is the most accurate, and psychometric tests are useful in some instances. The important point of laboratory tests is to prevent delay. If a test such as magnetic resonance imaging (MRI) requires hours to complete, the therapy should be begun instead. Treatment for CO poisoning requires a special treatment table, which incorporates the hemoglobin half-life (Figure 33-3).

Clostridial Myonecrosis (Gas Gangrene)

Fortunately, **gas gangrene** is infrequently encountered in the civilian population. The distinct smell and dramatic turn of events once hyperbaric oxygen therapy is used makes this disease one of the most rewarding to treat. It is caused by the anaerobic bacterium *Clostridium perfringens* that is common in soil and the intestine. Progression of the disease is rapid, moving at the rate of up to 6 inches per hour. The α-toxin this bacterium produces liquefies muscle in its path. Once hyperbaric oxygen therapy is initiated, the disease is stopped, leaving a distinct bronzing appearance to the skin. Often radical amputation is required to stop the progression of the disease. However, if hyperbaric oxygen therapy is used first, a more accurate diagnosis and level of amputation are determined. One hyperbaric treatment does not kill this spore-forming bacterium, and the proper protocol calls for seven

ℬox 33-2

Contraindications for Hyperbaric Oxygen Therapy

Upper respiratory infection
Chronic obstructive pulmonary disease
Seizure disorder
Thoracic surgery
Spontaneous pneumothorax
Emphysema with carbon dioxide retention
Viral infection
Congenital spherocytosis
History of optic neuritis
History of spontaneous pneumothorax
Uncontrolled high fever
Chronic sinusitis
Pregnancy

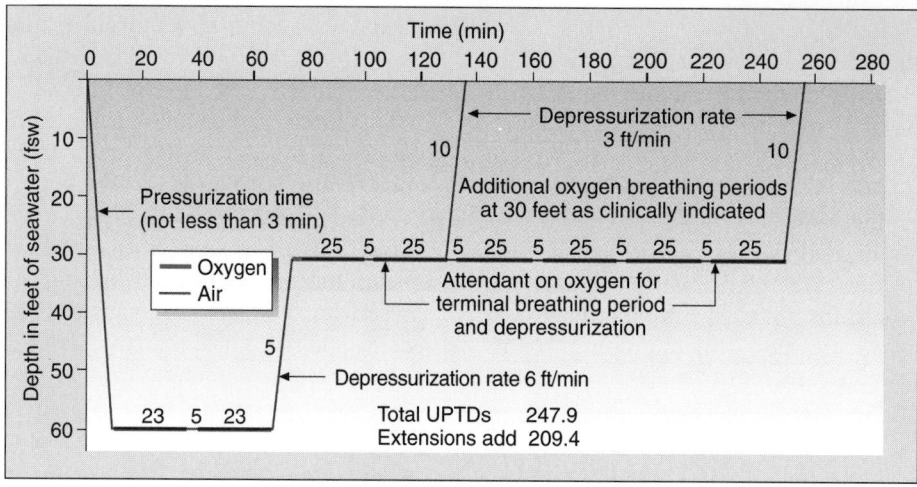

Figure 33-3   Carbon monoxide treatment table. *UPTDs,* Units pulmonary toxicity dose.

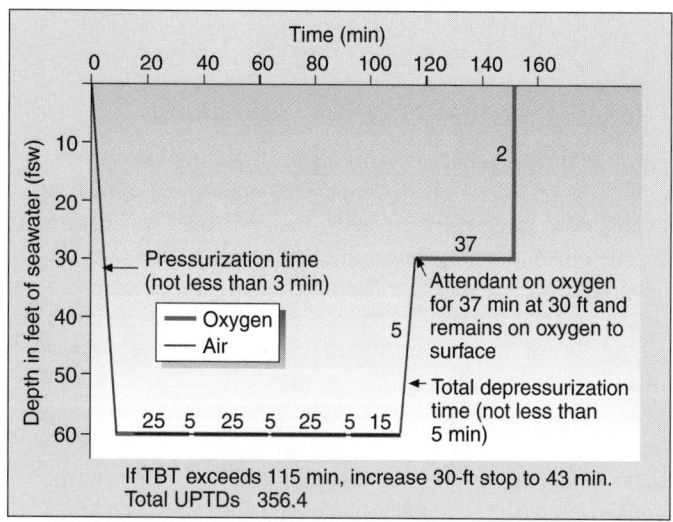

Figure 33-4   Gas gangrene treatment table. *TBT,* Total bottom time; *UPTDs,* units pulmonary toxicity dose.

treatments within 3 days. Individuals with gas gangrene are extremely toxic. Therefore the hyperbaric technologist must be alert for symptoms of O_2 toxicity during treatment (Figure 33-4). Therapy is a three-pronged approach of hyperbaric oxygen therapy, antibiotics, and surgery.[10]

Crush Injury, Compartment Syndrome, and Other Acute Traumatic Ischemias

Traumatic amputations, crush injuries, and similar conditions that cause severe hypoxic damage and tissue insult can result in a secondary injury called a *reperfusion injury.* Although physiology would normally indicate that hyperbaric oxygen therapy is the exact opposite of the recommended treatment, hyperbaric oxygen therapy in fact is exactly what the injury requires. Amputated arms, legs, digits, and other appendages that have been traumatically

removed have been successfully replaced through the use of hyperbaric oxygen therapy. Indications include degloving injuries, in which the skin spins on the fascia, closed muscle lacerations, and ear evulsions.

Enhancement of Healing in Selected Problem Wounds

Fibroblasts do not proliferate if the pressure gradient to O_2 does not reach 30 mm Hg or greater. Given a wound with significant impedance to the diffusion of O_2 through the tissue, if the patient is breathing air at sea level, the gradient can fall from 90 mm Hg to less than 30 mm Hg at the wound site. Because wounds require O_2 levels greater than 30 mm Hg to heal, the wound worsens. However, if the O_2 gradient is 2193 instead of 90, significant levels of O_2 can penetrate the tissue and help the wound heal.

The first phase of wound healing, the vascular-hemostatic phase, lasts from the time of injury to 4 days. The second phase, the inflammatory phase, also lasts about 4 days. This phase can create a barrier to O_2 transport by reducing the blood flow as much as 20%. The third phase, the proliferate phase, lasting from 1 to 3 weeks, is the time during which collagen is produced. Collagen production depends on appropriate O_2 tissue levels to create the matrix of the scar. In addition, capillary budding and increased tissue perfusion occur during this phase. The fourth and final phase of wound healing is the remodeling phase, which occurs within 3 weeks to months. During this phase the tensile strength of the new scar develops. Impedance to any and all phases can occur from diabetes, radiation, and immune deficiencies.

In an uncompromised host the healing cascade progresses without incident; only in the compromised host is hyperbaric oxygen required. Whether O_2 can be delivered at all then must be determined. The degree of circulation can be determined by arteriograms, transcutaneous O_2, or Doppler monitors. Measuring with and without O_2 can

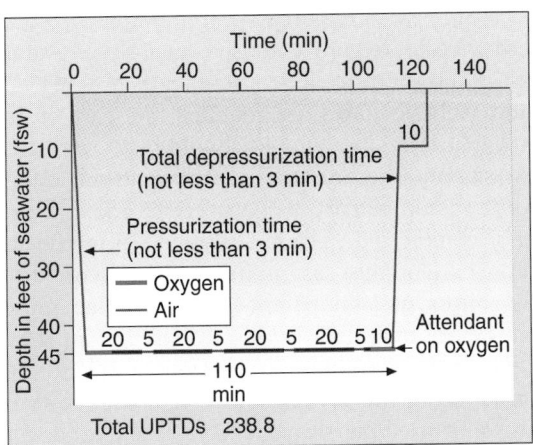

Figure 33-5 Wound healing treatment table. *UPTDs,* Units pulmonary toxicity dose.

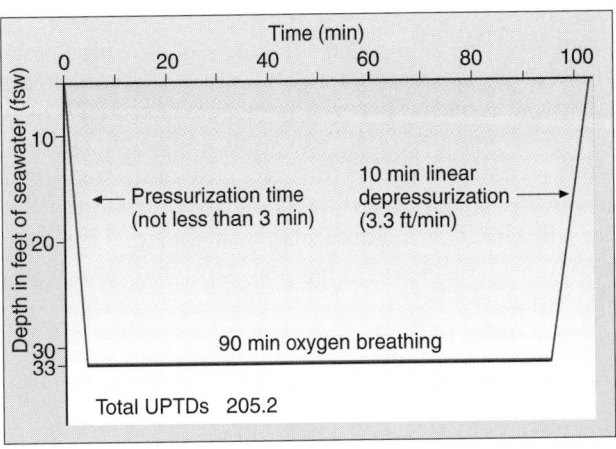

Figure 33-6 Wound healing treatment table for 33 fsw (monoplace). *UPTDs,* Units pulmonary toxicity dose.

help determine how well the O_2 can be delivered. Hyperbaric oxygen therapy does not help individuals without the proper circulation to deliver the O_2 in the first place.

Treatment tables for problem and compromised wounds are known as "Texas tables" after those developed by Dr. Jefferson Davis while in the U.S. Air Force in San Antonio, Texas (Figure 33-5). Many variants to this table are used. Some use 20-minute O_2 breathing periods with 5-minute air breaks, whereas others use 30-minute O_2 periods with 10-minute air breaks; still others use 45-minute O_2 breathing periods with 15-minute air breaks. The objective is to attain the equivalent of 90 minutes of O_2 at 3 atm abs. The reason 2.4 atm abs is used in multiplace chambers is because the mask used does not always deliver 100% O_2. To compensate, Davis decided to take the worst-case scenario and go to a greater depth. Monoplace chambers, which are compressed with 100% O_2 and therefore do not require masks, use a different table (Figure 33-6).

Necrotizing Soft Tissue Infections

Necrotizing soft tissue infections are similar to gas gangrene in that they can be gas forming and devastating. This type of infection can take the form of necrotizing fasciitis, a nonclostridial myonecrosis, crepitant anaerobic cellulites, or Fournier's disease. In nonmedical publications, soft tissue necrotizing infections are often referred to as "flesh-eating bacteria" and can lead to death if not aggressively treated. The treatment table of choice is that of the problem wound table, but treatments are administered twice daily (see Figure 33-5 or Figure 33-6).

Refractory Osteomyelitis

Hyperbaric oxygen therapy is only used for chronic refractory osteomyelitis. Osteomyelitis is defined as *chronic* if it

has existed for 6 months or longer and *refractory* once it has been treated unsuccessfully with two courses of intravenous (IV) antibiotics. Then hyperbaric oxygen therapy is adjunctive to an additional course of antibiotics and ongoing aggressive debridement. The treatment table of choice is the same as that for the problem or compromised wound (see Figure 33-5 or Figure 33-6).

Radiation Tissue Damage (Osteoradionecrosis)

The most researched and best success rate of hyperbaric oxygen therapy beyond that of diving diseases is that of **osteoradionecrosis.** In fact, it has been successful enough that hyperbaric oxygen therapy is used prophylactically by most oral surgeons anticipating surgery for patients who have received more than 6500 rads of radiation during their course of treatment. Left untreated, osteoradionecrosis is a debilitating, painful, and costly disease that deforms the individual significantly.

Radiation leaves the irradiated tissue hypoxic, hypoperfused, and hypocellular. Hyperbaric oxygen therapy induces angiogenesis and fibroplasias after approximately eight treatments. O_2 measurements of the irradiated tissue compared with the healthy tissue demonstrate a curve similar to the oxyhemoglobin dissociation curve because the damaged tissue becomes oxygenated. Nothing occurs for the first 8 days, after which time the O_2 increases exponentially until about day 23, when the O_2 level reaches an asymptote. Although the O_2 level never reaches beyond 80% to 90% of normal, it does maintain that level up to 4 years—the limit of the study. The treatment table used is the problem and compromised wound healing (Texas) table (see Figure 33-5 or Figure 33-6). This treatment is administered 30 times unless the patient continues to smoke, which further compromises healing and requires a much longer period to heal. Prophylactic therapy should include the full course of this therapy regimen before surgery is attempted.

Compromised Skin Grafts and Flaps

Hyperbaric oxygen therapy is helpful for skin flaps for which treatment has been unsuccessful. A 28% greater take of split-thickness grafts exists with hyperbaric oxygen therapy, with 64% of patients having a 90% to 100% healing rate, as opposed to 16% in control subjects. Unfortunately, reimbursement is not received until traditional therapy has failed, even if the clinician is certain that the flap will fail. The treatment table of choice is the same as that of problem and compromised wounds (see Figure 33-5 or Figure 33-6).

Thermal Burns

Treatment of thermal burns is one of the newer uses for hyperbaric oxygen therapy. As previously discussed, hyperbaric oxygen therapy reduces edema and fights infection. In addition, because it promotes wound healing, it reduces fluid loss and scarring. Although hyperbaric oxygen therapy for thermal burns has had tremendous difficulty in gaining support in routine care, studies have shown a significant cost savings over standard treatment.[11] The treatment table of choice is the same as that of problem and compromised wounds (see Figure 33-5 or Figure 33-6).

Cranial Abscess

The treatment of cranial abscess is the newest treatment to be added to the UHMS list of diseases to be treated with hyperbaric oxygen therapy. However, this therapy has been used often and for some time worldwide. The significant morbidity and mortality of cranial abscess and the high risk-to-benefit ratio of hyperbaric oxygen therapy is good reason for its use. The treatment table of choice is the same as that of problem and compromised wounds (see Figure 33-5 or Figure 33-6).

Patient Care

Patient care begins with a thorough evaluation. Because of the checkered past of hyperbaric oxygen therapy, all persons involved with hyperbaric medicine must be diligent in treating only those diseases approved by the Hyperbaric Oxygen Therapy Committee of the UHMS. Inappropriate use lessens the credibility not only of the unit but also of the entire field.

Depending on the wishes of the medical director, patients might come directly into the unit for consultation or be required to visit via physician referral. Either method has its advantages and disadvantages. With the former the patient volume might be higher, but adherence to legitimate criteria may be more difficult. The latter requires the hyperbaric physician to be the first line of defense for the colds, sniffles, and headaches of all the hyperbaric patients.

Initial assessment must review active medical problems, medications, and allergies. A systems review with detailed emphasis on the ears, sinuses, cardiopulmonary systems, and social history is required for routine patients. Diving accident victims require extensive neurologic exams. In the case of a wound-healing patient, extensive wound history and diabetic status are required. As part of quality wound care, serial photographs should begin with the initial assessment. A recent chest x-ray film to rule out pneumothorax should be part of the safety protocol before the patient is compressed. As a final step in written documentation the patient must sign an informed consent. If the patient is a minor, an adult parent or legal guardian must give consent before treatment begins. All things are the same for pediatric patients—dose, indications, and barotrauma.

Instruction of the patient must begin with initial contact and be carried out through the assessment, documentation, and orientation phases and then beyond discharge. Throughout contact with the patient, the hyperbaric personnel should not compare the chamber to diving. Many patients develop a fear of the chamber, suspecting that they will be lowered under the water to receive treatment. Such fears should be allayed from the outset and continued throughout the treatment regime. Pamphlets, videos, booklets, and hands-on orientation help make the patient familiar with hyperbaric therapy. In addition, the patient's family should be included as much as possible. Pamphlets written to educate the patient and family should include information about the chamber, foot care, diabetes management, and diet (high protein diets being helpful for wound-healing patients). All pamphlets should be printed in a variety of languages as well.

Hyperbaric Oxygen Treatment

The hyperbaric oxygen treatment itself should begin with as much physical and psychologic support as possible. In the beginning, such support is a function of the hyperbaric technologist. After an initial period the patient's social interaction is as much a part of healing as the wound dressings and hyperbaric oxygen treatments themselves. The attendant must continue to teach and explain each step of the operation as it proceeds.

Before entering the hyperbaric chamber, patients must remove all clothing, cosmetics, hair spray, and jewelry and don cotton scrubs and foot covers for fire safety. Thus the control is in the hands of the attendant, not the patient. Directly before the treatment begins, the attendant should remind the patient to use the bathroom (because the procedure can last 2 hours). As the patient enters the chamber, the attendant should check the pockets for harmful materials. For example, many smokers are unaware that they may be carrying lethal devices, such as lighters or matches. If the door to the chamber is low, the attendant should remind the patient to "watch your head." Stretcher patients must be transferred to the hyperbaric gurney; during this transfer the attendant should use safe back dynamics for protection during patient lifting, the action accounting for the largest number of injuries in the hyperbaric facility. Once in the chamber, the patient should settle in while the attendant explains what will happen as the chamber is compressed—noise, increased temperature, and pressure on the ears. The attendant should again explain how to clear the ears. Failure to maintain equal pressure can result in a "trapped door" effect, as previously described. If this effect happens, the operator must decompress the chamber slightly before further compression can continue.

Rapport should be established with the patient, with an introduction by the attendant before each treatment session to determine why the patient is being treated, the treatment number, the patient's general feeling of well-being, patient history, clinical findings, and laboratory results. Vital signs should be obtained for all patients entering the chamber and about midway through the treatment. If the patient is critically ill, monitoring should mirror that given in the intensive care unit (ICU).

Drugs

Any drug brought into a hyperbaric chamber with excessive air in its sealed container can cause problems. Ampules, vials, blood tubes, and glass bottles have the potential to implode or explode and should not be taken into the chamber if possible. Even if the container does not explode, a laboratory technician could later open a blood collection tube that was filled under pressure.

Medication in plastic vials and Viaflex bags are preferred. If a glass vial or bottle is required, it must be vented to prevent disaster. All IV administration sets reduce the air space on compression (making the counting of drops impossible); then on decompression the air space expands. If the hyperbaric attendant compensates for the air space on compression, the air can expand into the IV tubing, creating potential air in the IV line.

Other mechanical problems are not as evident. Oral and IV administration is safe under pressure inside the hyperbaric chamber. However, subcutaneous and intramuscular (IM) injections should not be administered under pressure. Because high-dose O_2 causes vasoconstriction, the medication can become loculated, leading to erratic drug absorption. This effect often leads to added doses of medication while the patient is under pressure, only to have excessive amounts of medication absorbed once decompression has occurred.

Chemotherapy drugs are contraindicated while a patient is undergoing hyperbaric oxygen therapy. These drugs include cisplatin (Platinol), doxorubicin (Adriamycin), acetazolamide (Diamox), disulfiram (Antabuse), and reserpine (Serpasil). Drugs that depress respiration, or any drugs that increase $PaCO_2$, can potentially increase seizure activity and induce cerebral O_2 toxicity. Some drugs that increase the seizure risk are amphetamines, antidepression medications, and norepinephrine or epinephrine. Diazepam (Valium) is the drug of choice to control seizures. It acts faster than phenytoin (Dilantin), which can be used

prophylactically for patients who are febrile, toxic from gas gangrene, or taking steroids. Phenobarbital possesses more seizure-suppressant activity relative to its respiratory-depressant activity, which makes it most effective in the prevention of O_2 convulsions. Vitamin E is also recommended to prevent seizures, but no supporting data exists. Insulin requirements might be decreased under pressure. However, whether glucometers function accurately in hyperbaric chambers is questionable because the test procedure involves an O_2 process.

In the haste to help patients clear their ears during compression, oxymetazoline (Afrin) nasal spray is sometimes used. Afrin used in excess can lead to dependence, with ongoing congestion when the drug is not used; thus its use should be limited as much as possible. If a patient is dependent, the individual should be encouraged to use it in one nostril only for 3 days. Once that nostril is cleared, the medication should be stopped. Medications that have been found to function appropriately under pressure include antihypertensive drugs, neuromuscular relaxers, and lidocaine.

Hyperbaric Systems

According to the National Fire Protection Association (NFPA), three types of hyperbaric chambers exist—Class A, human, multiple occupancy; Class B, human, single occupancy; and Class C, animal, no human occupancy. Chambers for humans have been loosely interpreted as multiplace chamber (many persons, more than one lock) and monoplace chambers (single occupant, single lock). However, in recent years chambers have been constructed to accommodate many persons within a single-lock chamber. For purposes of this chapter, a **multiplace chamber** is defined as a chamber for more than one person that has more than one lock (not including a medical lock), and a **monoplace chamber** is designed for one person with one lock. Most multiplace chambers are compressed with air, whereas most monoplace chambers are compressed with 100% O_2.

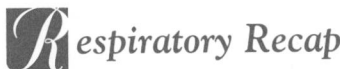 *espiratory Recap*

Types of Hyperbaric Chambers
Class A: human, multiple occupancy
Class B: human, single occupancy
Class C: animal, no human occupancy

The systems that support these chambers are different by both design and code. Multiplace chambers require separate utility support, such as compressors, O_2 supply, fire deluge systems, control consoles, seating, patient delivery system, patient monitoring system, and supplemental air breathing systems. Monoplace chambers require so little support equipment that they can be portable, with O_2

being the only required utility. Thus monoplace chambers can be mass produced, whereas multiplace chambers are individually designed and built.

Operation of the Multiplace Chamber

The multiplace chamber (Figures 33-7 and 33-8) is a complex system composed of the chamber, chamber support equipment, patient support equipment, and monitoring equipment. The multiplace chamber is the chamber of choice in the care of critically ill patients. The operation of the chamber should be without incident and without complications, and for this reason, start-up and shut-down checklists must be followed. The chamber always must be ready for emergencies and evaluated for such readiness before each compression. Operators and attendants should have their own separate checklists to complete before each treatment.

Treatment Procedures

Once all checklists have been completed, the operator announces to the inside attendant that compression is about to begin. The attendant announces this to the patients inside the chamber and reminds them to equalize the pressure in their ears. Patient notification should be performed whenever anything is about to take place outside the chamber that can be heard inside. Loud noises inside a hyperbaric chamber can be frightening to patients, even though such noises may be routine to the operator and attendant. The patients should be notified before the operator ventilates the chamber. Although most chambers have continuous ventilation through the chamber, additional venting is needed for O_2 accumulation, increased CO_2 levels, and odor reduction. Operators outside the chamber should take their queue from the inside attendant who requests ventilation and not question the reason.

When treatment pressure is reached, the attendant places masks or hoods on the patient to breathe supple-

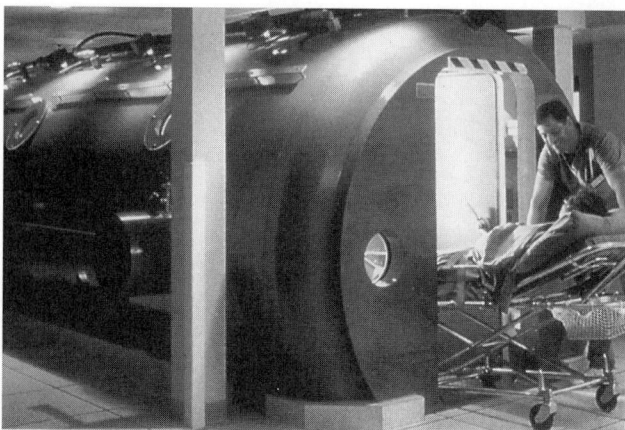

Figure 33-7 Multiplace hyperbaric chamber. (Courtesy Perry Baromedical Services, Riviera Beach, Fla.)

mental O_2. If the chamber accommodates several patients, the order in which the patients are placed on O_2 is important and the same order is used throughout the treatment. The first patient on O_2 should be the first patient off O_2 in this procedure. Once breathing O_2, the patient should be encouraged to avoid talking because the facial movement distorts the mask and reduces the O_2 concentration. Silent games, such as chess, checkers, or cards, can be played during these periods. Patient interaction is important to total well-being and should be encouraged.

Once the treatment is completed, decompression-to-surface pressure results in a decrease in the temperature (Gay-Lussac's law). The attendant should be ready with blankets to warm the patients. The blankets should *not* be warmed in the microwave and sent into the chamber via the medical lock. Heat energy contained in the blanket may erupt by spontaneous combustion once the item is inside the chamber at increased O_2 pressure. The attendant should remember to check IV chambers, catheter pilot tubes, and endotracheal tube cuffs for pressure during decompression if they have been filled with air instead of liquid during compression.

Patients breathe 100% O_2 during the treatment and therefore do not accumulate much additional N_2 in their tissues. The attendant breathes air during the treatment and should be decompressed, just as divers decompress after a sport dive. Because of this and other physiologic changes taking place, the attendant and patients should be cautioned not to cross their legs, adjust to an awkward position, cough or sneeze, or hold the breath. Once at surface pressure, the patients should be instructed to rise slowly because pressure changes in the middle ear can cause transient vertigo.

While under pressure the patient is not completely isolated from atmospheric pressure. In multiplace chambers both personnel locks and medical locks are present and can be used to send medications, food, personnel, and other necessities from the surface to the inside of the chamber, or vice versa. In addition, the personnel entry lock may be used as a comfort station for patients to use a commode.

Treatment tables are very precise regarding O_2 breathing periods. Therefore beyond the operation of valves and other controls, one of the most important functions of the operator is that of timekeeper and documenter. The operator tells the attendant precisely when the patient is to breathe O_2, when to breathe air, when decompression is taking place, and when medications are due. An operator's job can be even more complex if additional patients have different O_2 breathing schedules or if the patient is critically ill or other ancillary functions are required. The operator not only notifies but also records each change in status and medication.

Emergency Procedures

Loss of Primary Air If the dedicated compressor fails and the support compressors are inadequate to maintain pressure in the reservoir that serves as a capacitor, the compression of the chamber or its ventilation is compromised. The patient is not in any imminent danger, but the treatment cannot be completed.

Loss of Backup Air Supply
Backup air supplies are usually air cylinders near the chamber. Changing the cylinders corrects this situation.

Contamination of Primary Air
The attendant inside the chamber is the only one at risk for the contamination of primary air because the patients are breathing O_2. However, such contamination has occurred in the O_2 system as well when one supplier delivered liquid N_2 to the liquid O_2 storage tank. The full-face masks used in case of fire are always on and charged, with a separate air supply.

Loss of Primary Oxygen Source
The primary O_2 source is always backed up with a redundant supply. Therefore loss of the primary O_2 source is inconsequential.

Loss of Backup Oxygen Supply
The first order of priority is to remove the patient from the O_2 breathing device. As in the case of the backup air system, backup O_2 supplies are usually cylinders near the chamber. Changing the cylinders corrects this situation.

Rapid Increase in Chamber Pressure
Few situations can cause the rapid increase of the chamber pressure. If the input or compression valve becomes frozen open, the chamber will continue to compress. The short-term solution is to open the decompression valve.

Rapid Decrease in Chamber Pressure
Few examples of rapid decompression exist with chambers designed since the early days of hyperbaric medicine. One example is a broken window or view port. The first response is to remain clear of the source of decompression. Once the chamber has decompressed to atmospheric pressure, a plug may be placed in the view port and treatment of those affected instituted.

Fire Inside chamber
A fire inside a hyperbaric chamber is devastating. Prevention is of utmost importance through diligent fire prevention by staff members, patients, and hospital personnel. Multiplace chambers have water deluge systems throughout the chambers and locks. Activation buttons are at strategic spots inside the chamber and at the operator's console. Activation of the water deluge button should be linked to the hospital fire system and local fire station, which can notify the location of the fire. If an individual suspects a fire, that person should not hesitate to activate the sprinkler system. Fires can spread quickly under increased O_2 pressure.

The protocol for the attendant inside the chamber is somewhat different. The first response is to place a full-face air mask (which is always ready for use during operations) over the face and then over the faces of the patients. The reason for the mask is to prevent asphyxiation, which has taken more lives than fires in hyperbaric chambers. The attendant's second priority is to turn off the O_2 supply and pick up the on-board, hand-line fire hose. The order of priority of the operator outside the chamber is to first activate the water deluge button and then turn off the O_2 supply. Although the order of this sequence of events seems reversed, it is determined by the proximity of the buttons and valves and the ease with which a button can be pressed as opposed to the time taken to turn a valve. Routine hospital fire protocols then take effect, such as evacuation of the area and closing of doors.

Fire in Facility Outside Chamber
When smoke or fire is outside the chamber but nearby and patients are under pressure, the first priority of the hyperbaric staff members is to protect the patients inside the chamber. Emergency decompression is instituted, and patients are evacuated by the best route.

The operator must remain on site instead of leaving immediately, a task that can become difficult if the smoke is dense. Therefore the NFPA states that an air-breathing apparatus be available to the operator—a long hose with a full-face air mask. Logic would suggest that a self-contained breathing apparatus (SCBA) be available. However, if SCBA is used, the Occupational Safety and Health Administration (OSHA) requires that all personnel must be

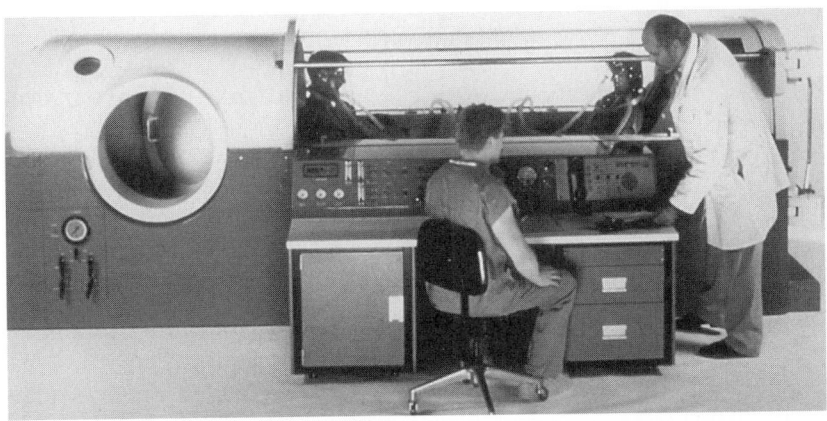

Figure 33-8   Two-person hyperbaric chamber. (Courtesy Perry Baromedical Services, Riviera Beach, Fla.)

involved in a respiratory program that requires expensive regular physical exams of all personnel, including pulmonary function tests, stress tests, and mask fit tests (obviating beards and glasses on personnel).

Oxygen Toxicity Seizure

Cerebral O_2 toxicity manifests as a seizure. If a seizure occurs under pressure inside the chamber, the attendant should remove the O_2 breathing device from the patient and protect the patient from harm. The seizure many seem threatening, and the tendency is to abort the treatment. However, the protocol defined by the U.S. Navy states that the patient continue treatment 15 minutes after becoming stable.

Cardiopulmonary Arrest

Cardiopulmonary arrest is handled exactly the same under pressure as it is on the surface. The only difference is that the cardiac arrest team is not allowed to enter the chamber until surface pressure has again been attained. The chamber may not be immediately returned to the surface pressure, depending on the threat to the well-being of the others in the chamber with the arresting patient, a practice that can be frustrating to all at the surface but remains the safest procedure. A physician who has been qualified to be compressed in the chamber can be locked in to assist as needed. The point is not to panic and jeopardize the health of the other patients.

Barotrauma on Pressurization or Depressurization

Barotrauma can occur on compression as well as decompression. The most common barotrauma in hyperbaric exposure is to the eardrum, which can be prevented through slow compression while the patient is watched. Compression should cease with any sign of ear problems.

Suspected Pneumothorax

The only true contraindication to compression in a hyperbaric chamber is a pneumothorax. If a pneumothorax is suspected, the first response is to hold pressure and administer O_2. Pressure should not be increased or decreased. The hyperbaric physician then should be locked in to evaluate the situation. Portable chest x-rays are unavailable, so diagnosis is done with clinical signs. Once a diagnosis is made, the physician inserts a chest tube before chamber pressure can change. Once the tube is in place, treatment may continue as before.

Loss of Communication

Loss of communication means that the intercom has failed. In most cases a backup phone is available, but if not, hand signals and note-writing can suffice.

Loss of Power

Hyperbaric chambers should be on the critical branch for electricity if the main source fails. Backup electricity maintains operations without difficulty. However, hyperbaric chambers do not require electricity for most of their critical operations, allowing most functions to continue without incident.

Omitted Decompression

Omitted decompression is a serious hazard for personnel working in hyperbaric chambers. Most operations are routine and feature built-in decompression with the protocol. Personnel can experience decompression with a new procedure, changes in routines, or mistakes that omit decompression. If decompression tables must be calculated, several individuals should calculate them independently and verify them against one another. If such calculations are not possible, the U.S. Navy has special tables to follow for omitted decompression.

Accidental Activation of Fire Suppression System

Perhaps the most frequent accident occurring in the hyperbaric chamber is accidental activation of the fire deluge system. In such instances, those in the chamber will be soaked. The wetness is only a problem for wound-care patients because the wounds can be contaminated by the water which has remained stagnant in the system since the last time it was used.

Operation of the Monoplace Chamber

The monoplace chamber (Figure 33-9) is purchased from chamber manufacturers (Box 33-3). Support equipment is built into the chamber body, and the chamber is easily transportable. Monoplace chambers can be installed in reconditioned patient care rooms with little difficulty. A large-diameter tube to deliver slightly higher pressure than normal and an equally large tube to carry the exhausted O_2 to the outside of the building are the only necessary structures. Cost of the monoplace chamber itself is roughly one-tenth the cost of a multiplace chamber. Add the support equipment and the building codes to install a multiplace chamber, and a monoplace chamber is one-twentieth the time, at one-twentieth the cost, with one-twentieth the training. One of the major drawbacks to monoplace chambers is the inability to perform hands-on care of the patient. However, this obstacle has not deterred any mono-

---

$\mathcal{B}$OX 33-3

Manufacturers of Hyperbaric Chambers

Perry Baromedical Services, 275 West 10th Street, Box 10297, Riviera Beach, FL 33404; (407) 840-0395

Reimers Engineering, 6314-K Gravel Avenue, Alexandria, VA 22310; (703) 922-0606

Environmental Tectonics Corporation, County Line Industrial Park, Southampton, PA 18966-3877; (215) 355-9100

Gulf Coast Hyperbarics, P.O. Box 9737, Panama City, FL 32407; (904) 784-7159

Hyperbaric Oxygen Therapy Systems, 980 F Street, Chula Vista, CA 92010; (619) 691-1121

Sechrist Industries, 4225 East La Palma Avenue, Anaheim, CA 92807; (714) 579-8400

place facilities from successful placement of complex patients inside the monoplace chamber.

Treatment Procedures

Checklists must be used with the monoplace chamber. However, only the physician and operator need be present for its operation. The operator notifies the patient via the communication system when compression is about to begin and again reminds the patient how to equalize the pressure in the ears. The patient is able to see the operator at all times, which provides comfort enough to the patient that some prefer the monoplace chamber.

Monoplace chambers are most often compressed with O_2, which negates the need for a respiratory apparatus to be placed on the patient's face, thus reducing the confinement anxiety in monoplace chambers. Some monoplace chamber manufacturers compress the chamber with air or leave the operator the option of air or O_2. If the option for compression with air is selected, then a respiratory device must be placed on the patient before that individual enters the chamber. When a chamber is compressed with 100% O_2, treatments are shorter and not at such high pressure as with the multiplace chamber.

Emergency Procedures

Loss of Primary Oxygen Source
In monoplace chambers compressed with 100% O_2, the loss of primary O_2 results in the decompression of the chamber and the inability to continue the treatment. If a secondary source is available, a quick change to the secondary supply provides the pressure to continue treatment.

Fire Inside Chamber
A fire inside a monoplace chamber is deadly. Operators can only save themselves and others by evacuating the area as quickly as possible. As Gay-Lussac's law indicates, as the temperature caused by the fire increases, so does the pressure. Once pressure attains blow-off pressure, high pressure is exhausted or parts from the chamber are projected in all directions with deadly force.

Fortunately fires in monoplace chambers have been few in the United States, a credit to the hyperbaric technologists and manufacturers. Training has reinforced prevention. Valuable lessons have been learned through tragic accidents in other countries, one of which is to restrict patients from taking anything inside with them. Four major accidents have occurred when children brought sparking toys into the chamber, four in which patients brought hand warmers into the chamber, and one in which the operator allowed the patient's friends to compromise safety. In this accident an operator allowed an unconscious diver to be placed into the monoplace chamber in his street clothes. On regaining consciousness the patient reached into his pocket and lit a cigarette.

Fire in Facility Outside Chamber
In the monoplace chamber the patient does not accumulate N_2 in the tissue. Therefore the patient can be brought to the surface quickly and evacuated without much difficulty because the device on which the patient lies inside the chamber also serves as the gurney for transportation.

Oxygen Toxicity Seizure
A cerebral O_2 toxicity seizure inside a monoplace chamber can be frightening for the operator. The important thing to remember is that if the patient is seizing and the glottis is suspected of being locked, the patient should *not* be decompressed. Attempts to quickly decompress the patient could result in a fatal case of arterial gas embolism. The operator must wait patiently until the seizure has ended and then bring the patient to the surface.

Cardiopulmonary Arrest
The worst thing about a cardiopulmonary arrest in the monoplace chamber is that the operator is unable to reach the patient. However, the patient's tissues are loaded with O_2 and therefore can tolerate cardiopulmonary arrest for much longer periods

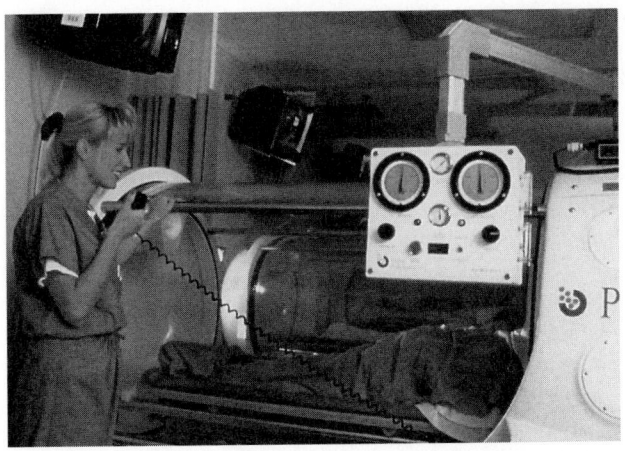
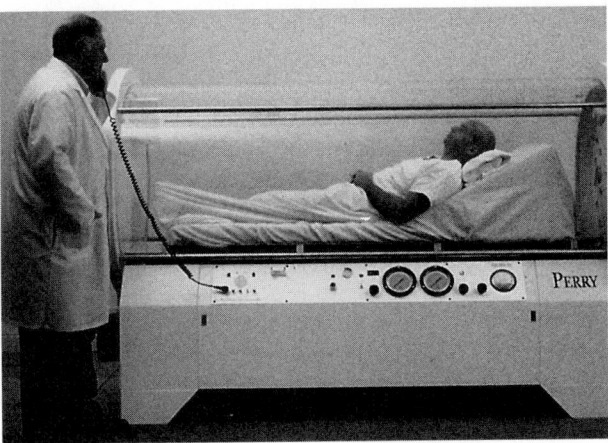

Figure 33-9 Two examples of a monoplace hyperbaric chamber. (Courtesy Perry Baromedical Services, Riviera Beach, Fla.)

without assistance. The caution in such a case is that once the patient reaches the surface, all clothing and sheets must be removed from the patient and that patient taken a safe distance from the chamber before defibrillation is attempted. Otherwise, the clothing saturated with O_2 could catch fire if defibrillation causes a spark.

Suspected Pneumothorax

If a pneumothorax is suspected, the physician and operator have a significant dilemma. If the patient is decompressed, the pneumothorax will grow larger. Yet the patient cannot remain under pressure without treatment. The only alternative is to bring the patient to the surface as quickly as possible and be ready to treat the pneumothorax as soon as the patient reaches surface.

Loss of Communication

Monoplace chambers are usually made of acrylic. Therefore the operator and patient can see each other and communicate with hand signals or writing paper.

Loss of Power

Loss of power in a monoplace results only in loss of communication.

Equipment in the Hyperbaric Chamber

When any equipment is taken into the hyperbaric chamber, two concerns must be considered. Is it a fire risk, and are any air spaces contained in the device? Only essential equipment should be taken into the chamber. Periodic checks should be made that the equipment in the chamber functions properly and that additional equipment has not found its way inside. Respiratory equipment is required to deliver the O_2 critical to the therapy. Either air or 100% O_2 is delivered to the patient. Therefore gas-mixing devices are usually not necessary. The only exception is when a critically ill patient desaturates with O_2 concentrations below 40%. A Built-In Breathing System (BIBS) delivers the gas (O_2, air, or nitrox) at a pressure of 50 psi greater than ambient. If the patient is at a pressure of 165 fsw, the pressure in the chamber is 88.1 pounds per square inch, absolute (psia). Therefore to deliver gas (air or nitrox) at that depth the pressure to the system must be 138.1 psia.

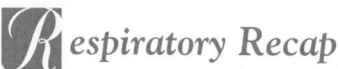 *espiratory Recap*

Equipment Concerns
Fire risk
Air spaces contained in the devices

Methods used to deliver gas mixtures to the patient inside the hyperbaric chamber include demand mask, hood, T-tube, or tracheostomy collar. Each gas delivery device

must include an overboard dump system, which is a reverse demand system that scavenges the exhaled gas and exhausts it outside the chamber and outside the building. In this way the chamber, which is compressed with air, is not contaminated with the high exhaled O_2 to prevent fire risk. A special precaution must be taken when this apparatus is connected to the patient, especially when a tracheostomy tube is connected. If the system is not protected with an over-pressure valve, the lungs could be exposed to the differential pressure of the depth of the chamber. Although it did not involve the lungs, in a famous accident a diver was sitting on the commode when the outside worker opened the valve to clean the toilet while it was under pressure. The toilet and diver experienced the pressure differential from inside to outside the chamber. The vacuum eviscerated the diver, and a surgeon had to remove the majority of his intestines inside the chamber.

The ventilator used in the hyperbaric chamber may be either volume or pressure controlled.[12] Small transport ventilators seem ideal for the hyperbaric chamber, but Boyle's law alters the delivered tidal volume and respiratory rate, making the ventilator too erratic to operate in the chamber. Some hyperbaric operators have placed the pneumatic components of sophisticated ventilators on the inside of the chamber, leaving the electronics on the outside and a pass-through penetrator conducting the pneumatics inside the chamber. The problem with this configuration is that the therapist on the inside is unable to regulate the ventilator because the controls are on the outside. With the monoplace chamber, time-cycled, pressure-limited ventilators are designed to function specifically with the hyperbaric chamber (Figure 33-10). These ventilators have limited capabilities and are difficult to use to ventilate critically ill patients. Before a patient with an artificial airway is placed into the chamber, air is removed from the cuff and an equal volume of saline placed into the cuff.

Cardiac monitors operate the same as the more sophisticated ventilators, with functions inside and controls outside. This configuration is frustrating for the clinician inside the chamber, who is unable to see the electrocardiographic (ECG) pattern during care of the patient. At one time the ideal setup involved the ECG pickup leads on the patient fed to the outside of the chamber for the physician to read; the signal then was sent back into the chamber to a low-voltage system, and the clinician was able to read patterns on the liquid plasma screen. However, after the fire in Japan in 1996, the manufacturer retracted the monitor and denied its use in hyperbaric chambers.

Battery-operated devices, such as IV pumps and portable cardiac monitors, are safe and work fine if they are not charged while inside the chamber. Thus battery-operated devices that charge when plugged in cannot be used to plug into electricity inside the chamber (something that should not be available anyway). Batteries cannot be changed while under pressure inside the chamber; therefore devices that operate for only 2 hours are not acceptable because most treatments take longer than 2 hours. Lithium batter-

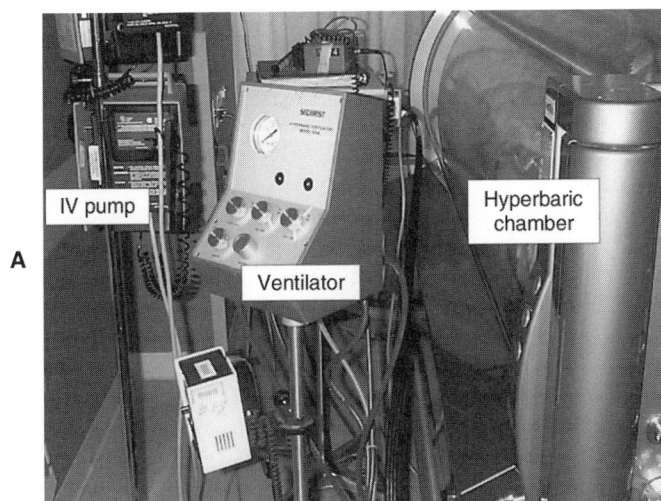 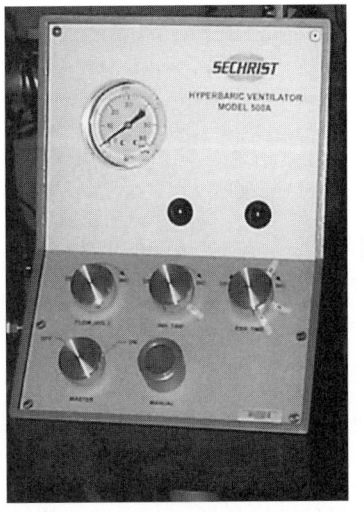

Figure 33-10 A, Time-cycled, pressure-limited ventilator used with the monoplace hyperbaric chamber. **B,** Close-up view of the ventilator.

ies are not allowed inside high-O_2 environments because of the potential for "runaway" charging from cell to cell and the toxic gas produced when O_2 combines with lithium.

The manufacturer should be consulted before cardiac pacemakers, internal defibrillators, and other implanted devices are used under pressure. For example, the Medtronic pacemaker has been tested under pressure and approved for use to 100 fsw. If this device or another is taken to untested pressures, the resultant pressure increase may cause the device to cease functioning or even malfunction.

Maintenance of Hyperbaric Chambers

Maintaining the hyperbaric facility is the responsibility of the entire team. If maintenance is required, only qualified personnel are allowed to repair the equipment. Once repairs are made, the safety director should evaluate the repair and direct a test compression when necessary before operations resume.

Preventive Maintenance

Preventive maintenance is specific to the type, model, and chamber. When a program is established, a preventive maintenance schedule is developed. Specific procedures are performed before each treatment, daily, weekly, monthly, quarterly, semiannually, and annually. Every maintenance operation and preventive maintenance procedure must be documented and retained indefinitely (Box 33-4).

Chamber Safety

Many organizations monitor the safety of hyperbaric chambers either directly or indirectly. Some of these organizations set rules, whereas other enforce them. All

chamber personnel should be informed about who these organizations are and how they influence the industry. As an overview of each organization's relations to individual chambers, chambers are only bound to the rules that apply at the time of manufacture. Therefore if a chamber is designed and manufactured under the rules for 1996, no agency can establish rules in 1997 that can put the chamber out of business. To understand who makes the rules, the following terms must be defined[13]:

- *Law* is a rule that must be obeyed, or some form of punishment will follow. Enforcement is by government agency.
- *Code* contains *only* mandatory provisions and uses the word *shall* to indicate requirements and in a form generally suitable for adoption into law.
- *Standard* contains mandatory provisions and uses the word *shall* to indicate requirements. Nonmandatory provisions, which use the word *should*, are placed in the appendix.
- *Recommended practice* is similar in content and structure to a code or standard but uses only nonmandatory provisions with the word *should* in the body of the text to indicate recommendations.
- *Guidelines* are advisory or informative in nature and contain only nonmandatory provisions.
- *Associations, societies,* and *organizations* have no power to police or enforce.
- *Federal, state, county,* and *local governments* enforce the law.
- *Medicare, Medicaid,* and *third-party payers* have the ability to deny payment.
- *Insurance companies* affect rates by various criteria.

To develop codes, standards, and guidelines, an organization usually enrolls in the American National Standards Institute (ANSI). Rules established by ANSI regarding consensus voting, publication of intent to establish rules, and

Box 33-4

Routine Preventive Maintenance of the Hyperbaric Facility

After Each Procedure
Perform operator checklist.
Perform attendant checklist.

Daily
Perform operator checklist.
Perform attendant checklist.

Weekly
Order oxygen and air cylinders.
Check liquid oxygen level and record in log.
Inspect viewports for chips, cracks, and crazing.
Drain bilges.
Inspect oxygen masks and hoses for holes, cuts, and dry rot;
   check straps.
Inspect resuscitation bag.
Clean inner and outer lock of chamber.
Inspect communication wires for wear; check functions of
   channels; clean earmuffs and headband.
Inspect firefighting masks in entry and main locks; dust and
   clean as needed.
Clean support equipment area.

Monthly
Check SCBA equipment; check air pressure; dust and clean
   units.
Break down oxygen mask regulators and clean.
Inspect oxygen and air mask hoses.
Check fire suppression hand lines for operation.
Check fire suppression system on bypass.
Inspect door seals in monoplace, main, entry, and medical
   locks.
Lubricate door seals in monoplace, main, entry, and medical
   locks.
Dust top of chamber and equipment.
Clean bilges.
Check filter regulator element.
Calibrate oxygen analyzer.
Ensure ventilator functions properly.
Ensure all monitors function properly.
Check all penetrators.
Turn on and test all IV pumps.
Drain fire suppression system deluge tank.

Quarterly
Check valves for function; turn on and off to verify operation of
the following:
   Main lock air supply valve
   Main lock overboard dump valve
   Main lock sprinkler valve
   Main lock fire suppression system valve
   Main lock fire sprinkler test valve
   Main lock over-pressure valve
   Main lock exhaust valve
   Main lock hand line valve
   Entry lock exhaust air valve
   Entry lock fire sprinkler test valve
   Entry lock fire sprinkler bypass valve
   Entry lock oxygen supply valve
   Entry lock air supply valve
   Entry lock hand line valve
Inspect and clean chamber lighting; change bulbs as
   necessary.
Schedule air samples.
Activate fire suppression system.
Drain and refill fire suppression system deluge tank.

Semiannually
Pressure-test entry and main locks; ensure pressure holds for
   2 hours.
Calibrate depth gauges on monoplace and multiplace
   chambers.
Take blood pressure cuffs and suction to biomedical engineer-
   ing for calibration and preventive maintenance.
Check atmosphere control; clean strainer and replace if necessary.
Check water level in fire suppression system deluge tank.
Check fire suppression system in the entry and main locks for
   operation at 45, 60, and 165 fsw.
Check hand lines in entry and main locks for operation at 45,
   60, and 165 fsw.

Annually
Visually inspect inside of deluge, hand line, and control air
   tanks.
Paint deluge tank as needed.
Calibrate gauges.

SCBA, *Self-contained breathing apparatus;* IV, *intravenous.*

many other criteria allow organizations to create codes, standards, or guidelines. Many organizations, such as the American Society of Mechanical Engineers (ASME), NFPA, and
Compressed Gas Association (CGA) set codes, standards, or
guidelines for hyperbaric medicine. However, none of these
organizations can enforce the rules. Only governmental
agencies, such as the Food and Drug Administration (FDA)
and OSHA can enforce the rules they set down.

UHMS is not a member of ANSI. Therefore it can neither write nor enforce codes, standards, or guidelines. However, through education, research, and a strong commit-

ment to ethics, UHMS has established its credibility to provide guidelines. In 1962, an ad hoc committee on hyperbaric oxygenation was appointed under the Committee on
Shock of the Division of Medical Sciences of the National
Academy of Science-National Research Council to evaluate the usefulness of hyperbaric oxygen.[14] This committee
published documents substantiating the use of hyperbaric
oxygen in 1963 and again in 1966.[15] On November 4, 1976,
the UMS (the organization's name before UMHS was
adopted in 1986) formed a Committee on Hyperbaric Oxygen, which published the first *Hyperbaric Oxygen Report* on

May 12, 1977.[16] This report has been revised every 3 years since. Through its objective presentation of data, Medicare, Medicaid, and other third-party payers have used this document as a guideline for reimbursement.

Publications from the UHMS establish further guidelines for such things as the design and fabrication of a multiplace chamber,[17] use of monoplace chambers,[18] fitness to dive,[19] and use of decompression tables.[20] Many criteria are established during intense workshops held at the international scientific meeting annually. Therefore although the UHMS is not a coding or standards-establishing society, it nevertheless has been effective in establishing guidelines through objective criteria developed with a long history of credibility. In addition to fire and pressure safety, chamber safety considerations include the following:

- *Structural integrity:* Structural integrity comes from the engineering design and manufacture. The agency that oversees the design and manufacture of hyperbaric chambers, is ASME through a section designated as Pressure Vessels for Human Occupancy (PVHO). A member of ANSI, the ASME/PVHO has representatives from manufacturing, insurance agencies, special interests, and end users. Through an elaborate process, consensus must be attained before standards are written.
- *Gas purity:* Gas purity is defined by the CGA and the U.S. Pharmacopoeia. The FDA recognizes the U.S. Pharmacopoeia, which defines the amount of hydrocarbons, water, CO, CO_2, and other gases that can be present in compressed air to qualify for specific classification. Compressed air in a hyperbaric chamber, which is to be used to pressures greater than 125 fsw, must meet or exceed the specifications for grade E air. A wise move is to have the compressed air entering the hyperbaric chamber tested at least quarterly by a third party.
- *Oxygen delivery and control:* O_2 delivery and control specifications are designated by the NFPA. The maximum O_2 concentration allowed in a multiplace chamber is 23.5%.
- *Ventilation control:* Ventilation control also is established by the NFPA. Determined by the number of occupants, a minimum ventilation rate of 3 actual cubic feet per minute of air per chamber occupant not using an overboard-dump breathing device must be maintained during operation.
- *Electrical components:* The electrical components, such as maximum allowable voltage, wattage, or amperes (amps), is set by the NFPA. In Class A (multiplace) chambers, circuits not in fixed conduits shall not exceed 28 volts and 0.5 amps. In Class B (monoplace) chambers, circuits are restricted to ECG leads, and communications and must not exceed 28 volts and 0.5 watts.
- *Materials:* Materials allowed within the hyperbaric chamber are set by the NFPA.
- *Fire prevention:* Fire prevention standards are set by the NFPA, which has been instrumental in preventing fire deaths in hyperbaric chambers in North America since their standards were established.

- *Crew performance and procedures:* Crew performance and procedures are established primarily by individual hospitals. However, many national organizations have begun writing standards for their countries. In the United States the UHMS has provided guidelines in their multiplace and monoplace documents.
- *Crew qualification:* Crew qualifications are being addressed by the National Board of Diving and Hyperbaric Medical Technology (NBDHMT); however, certification for the majority of technologists in the field will take some time.

Establishing a Hyperbaric Department

The UHMS and the ASME/PVHO have recommendations regarding the design of a hyperbaric chamber.[21,22] Once the chamber has been designed and built, a strategic plan should be developed regarding operation of the program. An official organizational structure involving the administration and physician hierarchy should be in place for the governance of the department. However, an advisory group consisting of all the departmental leaders with whom the hyperbaric department will work is invaluable. Advice from the physical therapy, social services, diabetes management, wound care, critical care, nutrition, nursing, pharmacy, respiratory care, orthotics, information services, and administration departments also is invaluable. A group meeting of as many of these persons as possible to assist in development of the situation analysis is helpful. When the department is new, this group can help assist in determining the strengths, weaknesses, opportunities, and threats to the program. Also advisable is to keep this group as an ongoing committee and a functional part of the team, especially until flow charts can be developed to determine the movement of patients through the process. Meeting with as many physician groups as possible to create a referral base is paramount to survival. Parts of the strategic plan include a business plan, a marketing plan, a reimbursement plan, a budget plan, a staffing plan, an information services plan, an equipment plan, an education plan, a policy and procedure plan, an orientation plan, and an emergency plan. Along with the strategic plan, a mission, vision, and value statement should be reached.

Staffing

Although staffing is unique to each facility, a few basic rules should be followed. A monoplace chamber must be staffed with at least a hyperbaric physician and an operator. Some method must exist to relieve these persons periodically because an operator *cannot* leave the side of the monoplace chamber or be distracted from its operation. In the operation of a multiplace chamber, a hyperbaric physician, a supervisor, an operator, and an attendant should be inside the chamber with the patient. In cases in which a critically ill patient is in the chamber, a nurse and a respiratory therapist should be with the patient if that individual is on a ventilator. Additional personnel, such as a secretary, clinical coordinator, educator, and wound specialist, can be added depending on the needs of the department.

Forms and Records

Forms and records should be determined by the hospital and the Joint Commission for the Accreditation of Healthcare Organizations (JCAHO). A special form resembling a certificate for the completion of treatment may help improve patient relations. In addition, patient education literature printed in several languages can be helpful.

𝒦EY 𝒫OINTS

- The history of hyperbaric oxygen dates to the 17th century.
- The gas laws, Pascal's law, and Henry's law are important in the understanding of hyperbaric oxygen therapy.
- Diving diseases can occur during compression, at pressure, and during decompression.
- Decompression tables are used to determine the amount of time an individual can be exposed to increased pressure.
- The primary effects of hyperbaric oxygen therapy are related to bubble reduction and hyperoxygenation.
- Secondary effects of hyperbaric oxygen therapy are related to vasoconstriction, bacteriostasis, toxic inhibition and inactivation, neovascularization, and hyperoxygenation.
- Hyperbaric oxygen is used to treat CO poisoning, clostridial myonecrosis (gas gangrene), crush injury, compartment syndrome, and acute traumatic ischemias and to enhance healing in selected problem wounds, necrotizing soft tissue infections, refractory osteomyelitis, radiation tissue damage (osteoradionecrosis), compromised skin grafts and flaps, thermal burns, and cranial abscesses.
- Hyperbaric oxygen therapy can be administered with a multiplace chamber or a monoplace chamber.

References

1. Undersea and Hyperbaric Medical Society. Hyperbaric oxygen therapy: a committee report. Kensington, Md: The Society; 1999.
2. Jacobson JH. The historical perspective of hyperbaric therapy. Ann NY Acad Sci 1965;117:651-670.
3. Beddoes T, Watt J. Considerations of the medicinal use of factitious airs, and on the manner of obtaining them in large quantities. 1st ed. Part II. Bristol, England: Bulgin and Rossier; 1794.
4. McCallum RI, editor. Decompression of compressed air workers in civil engineering. Newcastle upon Tyne: Oriel Press; 1967.
5. Haux G. Wie aus der HB die HBO wurde. Germany; 1997.
6. Epstein LI, Kuzava BA. Basic physics in anesthesiology. Chicago: Year-Book; 1976.
7. Greenwood ME. An illustrated approach to medical physics. 2nd ed. Philadelphia: FA Davis; 1966.
8. Undersea and Hyperbaric Medical Society. Hyperbaric oxygen therapy: a committee report. Kensington, Md: The Society; 1999.
9. Shapiro BA, Harrison RA, Walton JR. Clinical application of blood gases. 2nd ed. Chicago: Year-Book; 1977.
10. Demello FJ, Haglin JJ, Hitchcock CR. Comparative study of experimental *Clostridium perfingens* infection in dogs treated with antibiotics, surgery, and hyperbaric oxygen. Surgery 1973;73:936-941.
11. Ray CS, Green B, Cianci P. Hyperbaric oxygen therapy in burn patients: cost-effective adjuvant therapy. Abstract presented at the Undersea and Hyperbaric Medical Society Annual Meeting. San Diego, Calif; 1991.
12. Blanch PB, Desautels DA. Deviations in function of mechanical ventilators during hyperbaric compression. Respir Care 1991;36:803-814.
13. Davison W. Codes and standards in hyperbaric medicine. Presented at Undersea and Hyperbaric Medical Society Annual Meeting. West Palm Beach, Fla; 1994.
14. National Academy of Sciences-National Research Council, Committee on Hyperbaric Oxygenation. Fundamentals of hyperbaric medicine. Pub no 1298. Washington, DC: The Academy; 1966.
15. Undersea and Hyperbaric Medical Society. Hyperbaric oxygen therapy: a committee report. Kensington, Md: The Society; 1996.
16. Undersea and Hyperbaric Medical Society. Hyperbaric oxygen therapy: a committee report. Kensington, Md: The Society; 1986.
17. Undersea and Hyperbaric Medical Society. Guidelines for clinical multiplace hyperbaric facilities. Kensington, Md: The Society; 1994.
18. Weaver LK, Strauss MB. Monoplace hyperbaric chamber safety guidelines. Kensington, Md: Undersea and Hyperbaric Medical Society; 1997.
19. Weaver LK, Vorosmarti J. Fitness to dive. Kensington, Md: Undersea and Hyperbaric Medical Society; 1990.
20. Vann RD. The physiological basis of decompression. Kensington, Md: Undersea and Hyperbaric Medical Society; 1989.
21. Undersea and Hyperbaric Medical Society, Chairman Desautels DA. Guidelines for clinical multiplace hyperbaric facilities: report of the hyperbaric chamber safety committee of the undersea and hyperbaric medical society. Kensington, Md: The Society; 1994.
22. American Society of Mechanical Engineers. Safety standard for pressure vessels for human occupancy: an American national standard. ASME PVHO-1-1997. New York, NY; The Society; 1997.

Recommended Reading

The Undersea Hyperbaric Medical Society (UHMS): www.uhms.org.
American College of Hyperbaric Medicine (ACHM): www.hyperbaricmedicine.org
Baromedical Nurses Association (BNA): www.hyperbaricnurses.org
National Board of Diving and Hyperbaric Medical Technology (NBDHMT): (504) 366-8871.

CHAPTER 34

Humidity and Aerosol Therapy

James B. Fink
Dean R. Hess

CHAPTER OUTLINE

OBJECTIVES

1. Describe the normal gas warming and humidification functions of the upper airway.
2. List the goals of aerosol therapy.
3. Compare the advantages and disadvantages of active and passive humidifiers.
4. Compare heated and unheated humidifiers.
5. Compare condensers, hygroscopic condensers, and hydrophobic condensers.
6. List the indications for bland aerosol therapy.
7. Define *mass median aerodynamic diameter* and *geometric standard deviation*.
8. Describe the effects of inertial impaction, gravitational sedimentation, and diffusion on aerosol deposition in the lungs.
9. Compare jet nebulizers, ultrasonic nebulizers, pressurized metered dose inhalers, and dry powder inhalers for aerosol drug administration.
10. Distinguish between spacers and valved holding chambers.
11. Discuss issues involved in the selection of a device for aerosol delivery.
12. Discuss issues pertinent to aerosol drug delivery during mechanical ventilation.

KEY TERMS

Active Humidifier	Inertial Impaction	Passover Humidifier
Aerosol	Isothermic Saturation Boundary (ISB)	Pressurized Metered Dose Inhaler (pMDI)
Artificial Nose	Jet Nebulizer	
Bland Aerosol Therapy	Large-Volume Nebulizer	Respirable Range
Bubble Humidifier	Mass Median Aerodynamic Diameter (MMAD)	Spacer
Dry Powder Inhaler (DPI)		Ultrasonic Nebulizer (USN)
Geometric Standard Deviation (GSD)	Nebulizer	Valved Holding Chamber
Gravitational Sedimentation	Neutral Thermal Environment	
Humidity Therapy	Passive Humidifier	

Administration of humidity and aerosol therapy are common tasks for the respiratory therapist. Humidification of inspired gas is particularly important in the care of mechanically ventilated patients, and many respiratory drugs are administered as aerosols. The selection of appropriate devices for humidity and aerosol production may have an important impact on the outcome of the patient's condition.

Humidity

The interface between air and the lungs is mediated through the fluid lining of secretions in the airway. Water in inspired gas is essential to a healthy respiratory tract. Administration of dry, cold gas bypassing the upper airway can change the balance of the fluid lining the airways and may result in either short-term or irreversible structural damage of the airway.[1-5] Exposure of the airway to cold, dry air from the ambient environment increases mucus production and thickening of secretions, reduces the motility of the cilia, and increases airway irritability. Administration of dry gases via an endotracheal tube can damage the tracheal epithelium.[3] **Humidity therapy** is the addition of water to gas delivered to the airway.

The nose is an efficient active humidifier, which adds heat and humidity to the inspired gas. The respiratory mucosa lining the sinuses, trachea, and bronchi assist in heating and humidifying inspired gas.[2] The respiratory mucosa is covered by secretions produced by mucus glands, goblet cells, and transudation of fluid through cell walls (Figure 34-1). Heat is transferred from capillary beds close to the surface of the mucosa. The nasal mucosa is particularly well suited for this function, having the highest concentration of mucus glands in the airway and a rich vascular bed close to the surface that provides heat and water. The turbinates and conchae provide a convoluted path for gas to travel, creating turbulent flow and a large surface area for contact with respiratory gases. This large surface area gives up heat and moisture to inspired gas and efficiently recovers heat and water on exhalation.

Normal Heat and Moisture Exchange

By the time inspired gas reaches the lung parenchyma, it is fully saturated at body temperature (44 mg/L at 37° C; Figure 34-2). The point at which this occurs is known as the **isothermic saturation boundary (ISB)**, which is approximately 5 cm below the carina at the level of the third-generation airways.[1] Above the ISB, temperature and humidity fall during inspiration and rise during exhalation. Below the ISB, temperature and relative humidity do not fluctuate. A drop in environmental temperature and humidity, mouth breathing, an increase in tidal volume, or endotracheal intubation (which bypasses the upper airway) moves the ISB deeper into the lungs, although it never reaches the level of the respiratory bronchioles or alveoli.

At the end of inspiration, the temperature of the nasal mucosa is 31° C or lower because of heat loss caused by turbulent convection and loss of the latent heat of vaporization. As inspired gas warms, water vapor is transferred by evaporation from the mucosal lining through the latent heat of vaporization. Warming and humidification continue until the inspired gas is fully saturated at body temperature. Although the latent heat of vaporization remains as water vapor and does not contribute to warming of gases, the loss of latent heat of vaporization does cause the mucosa to cool. During exhalation, heat is transferred from exhaled gas to the cooler tracheal and nasal mucosa by convection. As these gases cool, their capacity to hold water vapor diminishes, and condensation occurs. Water accumulates on the tracheal surfaces, where it is reabsorbed by the mucus. Heat is transferred back to the mucosa, resulting in warming and rehydration. Latent heat and water

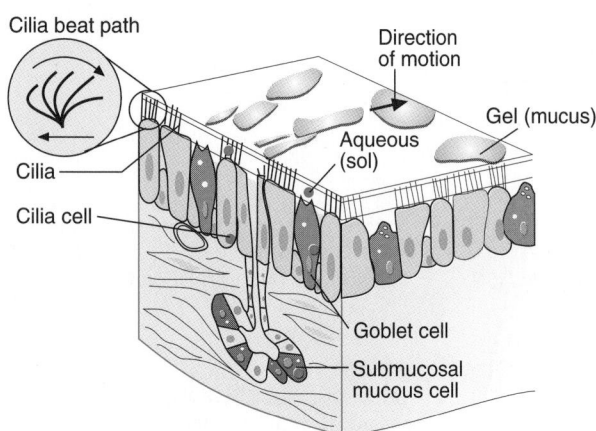

Figure 34-1 Cellular, aqueous, and mucus components of the airway mucosa. (Modified from Williams R, Rankin N, Smith T, et al. Relationship between the humidity and temperature of inspired gas and the function of the airway mucosa. Crit Care Med 1996;24:1920-1929.)

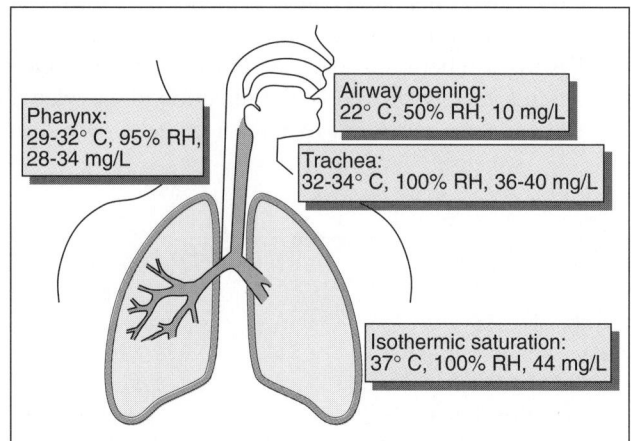

Figure 34-2 Normal temperature and humidity of gas at various points along the respiratory tract. RH, Relative humidity.

are held until the next inspiration. With mouth breathing, the flow is more laminar, requiring heat transfer by radiation. Because air is a poor conductor of heat, the mouth is less efficient than the nose at heating inspired air.

ℛespiratory Recap

Normal Heat and Moisture Exchange
The upper airway is an effective heat and moisture exchanger. The isothermic saturation boundary (ISB) is the point at which inspired gas reaches body temperature and humidity. Breathing dry gas moves the ISB deeper into the respiratory tract.

Primiano and colleagues[6] measured temperature and water vapor continuously at the oropharynx during oral and nasal breathing of room air at 22° C with a relative humidity (RH) of 15% to 39%. At the pharynx, the temperature difference between inspired and expired gas was 4° C during nose breathing and 7° C during mouth breathing. The inspired gas temperature increased 5° C during mouth breathing and 9° C during nose breathing. During inspiration with nose breathing, the RH was 95% at the oropharynx; this measurement was 75% during mouth breathing. On exhalation, the RH was nearly 95% at the pharynx and 90% at the airway opening. This suggests that the normal airway can condition inspired gas to add humidity with either nose or mouth breathing. However, more heat and moisture are lost with exhalation in mouth breathing than with exhalation in nose breathing. Even with mouth breathing, the ISB is not typically lower than the third generation of the bronchi.

Heat and moisture normally are lost from the mucosa above the ISB, from a surface area of approximately 300 cm² that is covered by 240 μL of airway lining fluid 8 μm deep. With normal tidal volume for an adult male, 22 μL of water and 61 J of heat are required to condition each breath from normal ambient conditions to 100% RH at body temperature. The water and heat losses per breath are 15 μL and 42 J, respectively. Over a 24-hour period, these losses total 250 mL of water and 726 kJ.[5]

When dry, cold gases are inhaled, the ISB is shifted deeper into the respiratory tract, and ciliary function and mucus production are compromised. Bypassing the upper airway eliminates the normal efficient mechanisms used to retain heat and humidity in the lungs.[7] Recruitment of airways that are less efficient for humidification changes their mucosal characteristics. The lower gas temperature farther down the airways reduces ciliary activity within 10 minutes. Once compromised, ciliary function can take several weeks to recover. Respiratory secretions become thicker, contributing to mucus plugging and inability to maintain normal bronchopulmonary hygiene. When absolute humidity drops below 24 mg/L in the inhaled gas, the beat frequency of the cilia is reduced.

Goals of Humidity Therapy

The primary goal of humidity therapy is to maintain normal physiologic conditions by providing adequate heat and humidity to inspired gas to approximate normal inspiratory conditions. Administration of heat and humidity is also advocated, with less supporting data, for the treatment of hypothermia, reactive airway response to cold air, and thickened secretions.

Medical gases are processed to remove all water vapor. When this gas is delivered to the nose and mouth, ideally it should be heated and humidified to normal ambient room air conditions (22° C at 50% RH or an absolute humidity of 10 mg/L). For gas delivered to the trachea through an endotracheal or tracheotomy tube, heat and humidity should be 32° to 35° C at 100% RH (absolute humidity of 36 to 40 mg/L).[7]

For premature and newborn infants, a **neutral thermal environment** should be maintained, with adequate warmth and humidity to minimize insensible heat and water loss. Low-birth-weight infants provided adequate heat and humidity showed a reduced morbidity rate compared with infants breathing colder and dryer inspired gas.[8] The body loses considerable heat through normal ventilation. For hypothermic patients, rewarming and reduction of further heat loss can be facilitated by heating the inspired gases[9]; however, this technique is less useful than other warming treatments (for example, wrapping the patient in blankets and warming intravenous solutions). Many asthmatic individuals develop increased airway resistance when they breathe cold air.[10] Airway hyperreactivity to cold inspired gas is associated with a shift of the ISB to more distal airways, with associated stimulation of mast cells in that area. This response can be diminished by warming of the inspired gases and provision of gas humidified with at least 20 mg/L of water at 23° C.

ℛespiratory Recap

Goals of Humidity Therapy
To provide adequate heat and humidity to the inspired gas To treat hypothermia To prevent airway response to cold air To aid removal of thick secretions

Heated humidity has been used in the treatment of patients with thick, tenacious secretions. However, no studies have reported a benefit from the use of external humidifiers to try to improve the character and mobilization of thick secretions. The most effective method to improve the character of pulmonary secretions is systemic hydration. Most patients with an artificial airway require humidification of inspired gas to prevent the formation of thick, tenacious secretions. However, there is no evidence to support the use of humidity therapy (that is, cool mist or heated aerosol) for patients with an intact upper airway. Cool (colder than room temperature) humidified gases and aerosols commonly are used in the treatment of upper airway inflammation caused by croup, epiglottitis, and swelling resulting from extubation.[11] The cold gas promotes localized peripheral vasoconstriction, thereby reducing swelling and relieving the discomfort associated with upper airway inflammation.

Excessive humidity is defined as a level greater than 100% RH at body temperature. The water volume of a vapor stream is 20 to 50 μL of water per liter of air and is unlikely to cause overhumidification. To exceed that water volume, gas temperatures would have to be grossly in excess of body temperature. Humidification of inspired gas reduces insensible water loss from the airway but is unlikely to add significant water to the body. Inspired gas warmer than 45° C may cause thermal injury to the airway.[5]

Devices Used for Humidification

A humidifier adds molecular water to gas (CPG 34-1).[12-16] An **active humidifier** adds water or heat or both to the inspired gas. A **nebulizer** produces an **aerosol,** or suspension of particles in gas. A **passive humidifier** uses exhaled heat and moisture to humidify inspired gas; heat and moisture exchangers (HMEs) are passive humidifiers. The American National Standards Institute (ANSI) recommends that heated humidifiers have a water output level of at least 30 mg/L (100% RH at 30° C).[17] This is considered the minimum level of humidity to avoid mucosal damage and inspissation of secretions for patients who have a bypassed upper airway (that is, an endotracheal or a tracheostomy tube). The Emergency Care Research Institute (ECRI) recommends that active humidifiers have an output of 37 mg of water per liter of inspired gas (85% RH at body temperature or 100% RH at 34° C).[18] Active heated water humidifiers are the devices of choice for intubation, tracheostomy, and long-term mechanical ventilation. The ANSI recommends a water output of 10 mg/L for unheated humidifiers[17]; this provides approximately 50% RH at 22° C ambient conditions, which enhances the dissipation of static electricity to prevent fires. This humidity level is thought to be the lowest acceptable level to minimize mucosal damage to the upper airway in a variety of environments.

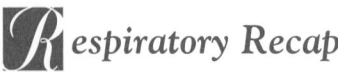

espiratory Recap

Types of Humidifiers
Active humidifiers add water or heat (or both) to inspired gas. *Passive* humidifiers use exhaled heat and moisture to humidify inspired gas.

Active Humidifiers

In a **bubble humidifier,** dry gas is directed toward the bottom of a water-filled reservoir, where the stream of gas is broken up (diffused) into bubbles, which gain humidity as they rise through the water (Figure 34-3, C). This commonly is accomplished with a tube that directs gas beneath the surface of the water; with a tube that has small holes along its length; or with a tube that is attached to a diffuser made of plastic foam, sintered metal, or mesh that breaks the stream of gas into small bubbles. Bubble humidifiers typically are not heated and are used with simple oxygen delivery devices. The higher the gas flow through a bubble humidifier, the lower the vapor content and temperature of the gas leaving the device. Commercially available bubble humidifiers are capable of humidifying dry medical gas to an absolute humidity of 10 to 20 mg/L at flows of 2 to 10 L/min. Bubble humidifiers are most efficient at flows of 5 L/min or less.[19] When flows greater than 10 L/min are required, other humidifying options should be considered. At flows under 10 L/min, bubble humidifiers are safe for extended single patient use without risk of infection.[20] Heating the reservoir improves the efficiency of these humidifiers; however, the small-bore tubing used to connect the humidifier to the administration appliance is easily obstructed by condensate as the humidified gas cools en route to the patient. Low flow, unheated bubble humidifiers typically have a gravity or spring-loaded pressure relief valve to protect against obstructed or kinked tubing and an alarm that sounds when a pressure of 2 psi or higher develops in the humidifier.

The addition of humidity to low flow medical gas is not supported by any objective criteria, and eliminating the use of humidifiers for low flow oxygen reduces the cost of routine oxygen administration.[21] Humidification of the inspired gas should be considered for patients who complain of discomfort associated with nasal dryness or irritation. However, such humidification may best be accomplished by devices that are more efficient than simple bubble humidifiers. Topical application of water-based lubricants to the nostrils may be a reasonable first response to complaints of dryness.

Heated bubble humidifiers (Figure 34-3, D) are used with intubated patients. These humidifiers can accommodate flow rates of 10 to 120 L/min and use tubing with a 22-mm inside diameter (ID). Use of corrugated, 22-mm ID tubing between the humidifier and the patient minimizes the tendency of condensate to pool at the lowest part of the tubing, occluding the path of the gas to the patient. At high flows bubble humidifiers produce aerosols that may transmit bacteria from the humidifier's reservoir to the patient.

A **passover humidifier** directs gas over the surface of a body of water (Figure 34-3, A and B). The passover wick humidifier (Figure 34-3, E) incorporates a wick of absorbent paper or cloth that draws water from the reservoir and becomes saturated; the wick comes in contact with the gas stream. A passover/barrier humidifier uses a hydrophobic barrier that allows water molecules but not

CPG 34-1

Humidification During Mechanical Ventilation

Indication

Humidification of inspired gas during mechanical ventilation is mandatory when an endotracheal or tracheostomy tube is present.

Contraindications

There are no contraindications to the provision of physiologic conditioning of inspired gas during mechanical ventilation. A heat and moisture exchanger (HME) is contraindicated under some circumstances.

   Use of an HME is contraindicated for patients with thick, copious, or bloody secretions.

   Use of an HME is contraindicated for patients with an expired tidal volume less than 70% of the delivered tidal volume (for example, those with large bronchopleurocutaneous fistulas or incompetent or absent endotracheal tube cuffs).

   Use of an HME is contraindicated for patients with a body temperature below 32° C.

   Use of an HME may be contraindicated for patients with high spontaneous minute volumes (over 10 L/min).

   An HME must be removed from the patient circuit during aerosol treatments when the nebulizer is placed in the circuit.

Hazards and Complications

Hazards and complications associated with the use of humidification devices include the potential for electrical shock (heated humidifier); hypothermia (HME or heated humidifier); hyperthermia (heated humidifier); thermal injury to the airway from heated humidifiers; burns to the patient and tubing meltdown if heated wire circuits are covered or circuits and humidifiers are incompatible; underhydration and impaction of mucous secretions (HME or heated humidifier); hypoventilation or alveolar gas trapping (or both) caused by mucus plugging of airways (HME or heated humidifier); possible increased resistive work of breathing caused by mucus plugging of airways (HME or heated humidifier); possible increased resistive work of breathing through the humidifier (HME or heated humidifier); possible hypoventilation caused by increased dead space (HME); inadvertent overfilling, resulting in unintentional tracheal lavage (heated reservoir humidifier); potential for burns to caregivers from hot metal (heated humidifier); inadvertent tracheal lavage from pooled condensate in patient circuit (heated humidifier); elevated airway pressures caused by pooled condensation (heated humidifier); patient-ventilator dyssynchrony and improper ventilator performance as a result of pooled condensation in the circuit (heated humidifier); ineffective low-pressure alarm during disconnection as a result of resistance through an HME.

When disconnected from the patient, some ventilators generate a high flow through the patient circuit that may aerosolize contaminated condensate, putting both the patient and clinician at risk for nosocomial infection (heated humidifiers).

Monitoring

The humidification device should be inspected visually during the patient-ventilator system check, and condensate should be removed from the patient circuit as necessary. HMEs should be inspected and replaced if secretions have contaminated the insert or filter. The following variables should be recorded during equipment inspection:

   Humidifier setting (temperature setting or numeric dial setting or both). During routine use on an intubated patient, a heated humidifier should be set to deliver an inspired gas temperature of 33° ±2° C and should provide a minimum of 30 mg/L of water vapor.

   Inspired gas temperature. If a heated humidifier is used, this value should be monitored as near the patient's airway opening as possible. Specific temperatures may vary with the patient's condition, but the inspiratory gas temperature should not exceed 37° C at the airway threshold.

   Alarm settings (if applicable). The high temperature alarm should be set no higher than 37° C, and the low temperature alarm should be set no lower than 30° C.

   Water level and function of automatic feed system (if applicable).

   Quantity and consistency of secretions. Characteristics should be noted and recorded. When an HME is being used, if secretions become copious or appear increasingly tenacious, a heated humidifier should replace the HME.

When a heated-wire patient circuit is used with an infant to prevent condensation, the temperature probe should be located outside the incubator or away from the direct heat of the radiant warmer.

Modified from AARC Clinical practice guideline: humidification during mechanical ventilation. Respir Care 1992;37:887-890.
CPG, Clinical practice guideline.

droplets to cross from the water reservoir into the gas stream.

A **jet nebulizer** (Figure 34-4) uses a jet of compressed gas that passes through a restricted orifice, creating a low-pressure area near the tip of a narrow tube. Fluid is drawn from a reservoir and sheared or shattered into droplets by the airstream. Jet nebulizers incorporate baffles to minimize aerosol exiting particle size and use the aerosol in the device to maximize surface contact with the gas. Jet nebulizers deliver 26 to 35 mg of water per liter when unheated and 33 to 55 mg of water per liter when heated.[11] Because jet nebulizers pose a risk of infection from bacteria that

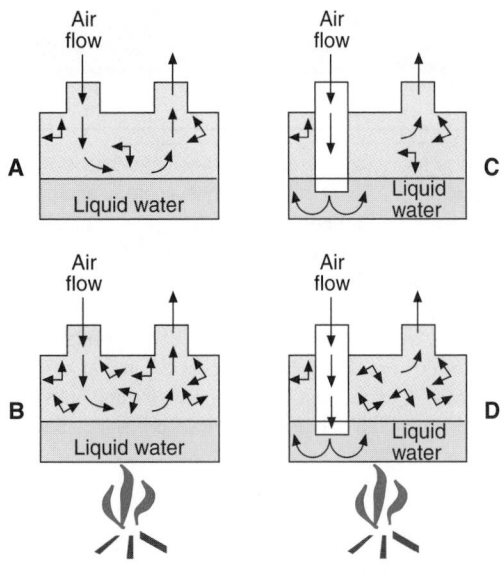

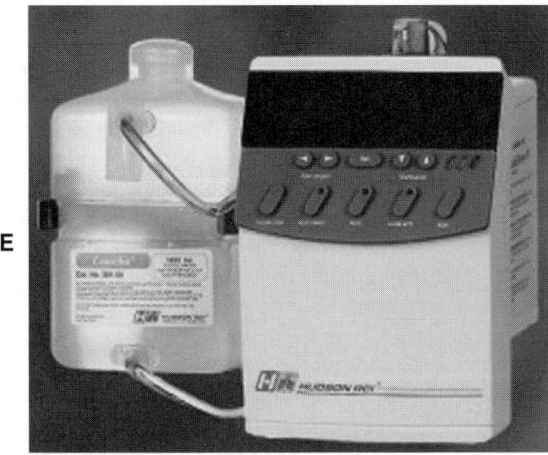

Figure 34-3 **A,** Passover humidifier. **B,** Heated passover humidifier. **C,** Bubble humidifier. **D,** Heated bubble humidifier. **E,** Commercially available heated wick humidifier. (**A-D,** Modified from Peterson BD. Heated humidifiers. Respir Care Clin North Am 1998;4:243-260; **E,** Courtesy Hudson RCI, Temecula, Calif.)

might colonize the reservoir, they should always be filled with sterile fluids and changed daily, and residual fluids should be discarded before refilling.

In active humidification systems, water must be added as the inspired gases are humidified. Systems used to replace the water in the humidifier should ensure continuity of therapy and minimize disruption of gas flow to the patient. Continuous feed systems are desirable because the water is replenished without operator intervention or interruption of gas flow to the patient. These systems often rely on gravity, usually consisting of a mounted reservoir external to the humidifier mechanism and most commonly with flotation controls and level-compensated reservoirs.

Intermittent feed systems have major disadvantages compared with continuous feed systems. Changing the water level in a fixed volume container changes the compressible volume in both the humidifier and the ventilator,

resulting in fluctuations in the delivered tidal volume. This problem is of greatest concern for mechanically ventilated newborns and pediatric patients. Open intermittent feed systems are more susceptible to contamination of the reservoir. With humidifiers that do not have alarms for low water levels, the humidifier chamber must be checked regularly or it can become empty, reducing the humidity and temperature of gas delivered to the patient.

Humidifier heaters most commonly use controllers to regulate electrical power to the heater element. The most basic units do not monitor the temperature of the heater, providing power to the heating element based on the setting of the temperature control knob rather than the patient's airway temperature. Active humidifiers use one of six types of heating elements: a heating plate located under the reservoir; a curved, often flexible element wrapped around the humidifier chamber; a yolk or collar between the water reservoir and the active mechanism of the nebulizer; a plate or rod immersed in the water reservoir; a set of wires or elements that heat an absorbent wick or tubes containing water; or a compartment of Sodasorb, which chemically reacts with exhaled carbon dioxide.

Servo-controlled humidifiers monitor the temperature of gas delivered to the patient, adjusting the power to the heating elements according to the temperature monitored by a thermistor probe placed downstream from the humidifier, near the patient's airway connection. When the temperature at the patient's airway is lower than desired, the controller supplies more power to the heater. As this distal temperature nears or exceeds the set temperature, power to the heating system is reduced. Thermistor probes are best placed in the inspiratory limb of the ventilator circuit, far enough from the patient that the temperature of the exhaled gas is not detected. Heated humidifiers should have alarms and an alarm-activated heater shutdown function. The sensor probe in the inspiratory limb must be located outside the heated environment to allow the heated wire controller to maintain the desired temperature and water content of inspired gases (Figure 34-5). Selection of an active humidifier should be based on performance, cost, safety, and ease of use.

Age-Specific Angle

The temperature probe of a humidifier should not be placed inside an incubator, because the surrounding air temperature affects humidifier function.

As heated and humidified gas cools, its ability to hold water vapor declines, and condensation (rain out) occurs. The amount of condensate is affected by the ambient temperature, gas flow, and the patient's airway temperature and by the length, diameter, and thermal mass of the tubing between the humidifier and the patient. In a traditional ventilator circuit, the humidifier is heated to 50° C or higher, and saturated gas contains more than 80 mg of water per liter. As the gas cools to 35° C en route to the

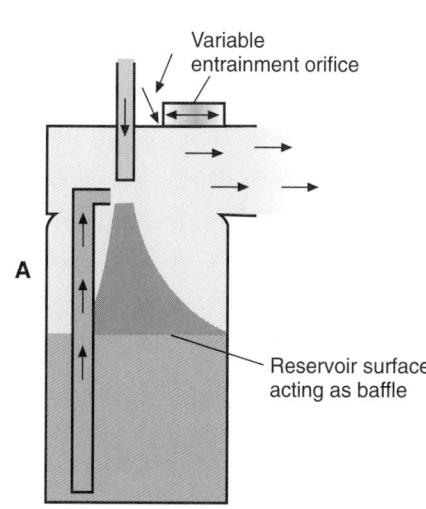

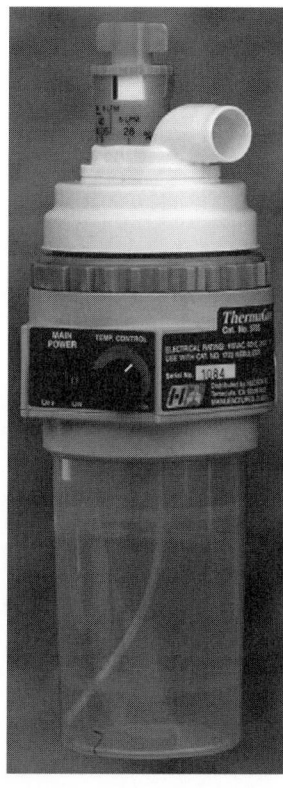

Variable
entrainment orifice

A

Reservoir surface
acting as baffle

Figure 34-4 **A,** Schematic drawing of large-volume jet nebulizer. **B,** Commercially available heated nebulizer. (**A,** Modified from Cohen N, Fink J. Humidity and aerosols. In: Eubanks DH, Bone RC, editors. Principles and applications of cardiorespiratory care equipment. St. Louis: Mosby; 1994; **B,** Courtesy Hudson RCI, Temecula, Calif.)

patient, it can hold only 40 mg of water per liter; therefore any amount over that condenses in the tubing. The circuit must be drained frequently to prevent pooling condensate from obstructing the gas flow or inadvertently pouring into the patient's airway.

Often the ventilator circuit, and subsequently condensate, becomes contaminated with bacteria from the patient within the first hour that the patient is attached to the ventilator.[11] The tubing should be positioned such that drainage is away from the patient's airway to avoid accidental lavage of the airway. Condensate presents a risk to the staff and should always be treated and disposed of as contaminated waste. Water traps placed in dependent positions in both the inspiratory and expiratory limbs drain condensate from the ventilator circuit, reducing the obstruction to gas flow. Water traps should minimize changes in circuit compliance and allow emptying without disrupting ventilation of the patient.

Techniques used to reduce the formation of condensate include an increase in the thermal mass of the circuit, use of a coaxial circuit with the inspiratory limb surrounded by the expiratory limb, or addition of heated wires to the circuit.[12] Increasing the passive thermal mass of the circuit with thick tubing or wrapping the tubing with insulating material insulates the gas inside the tubing from ambient air. Surrounding the inspiratory limb of the circuit with the expiratory limb in a coaxial manner uses the patient's exhaled gas as a heated air bath surrounding the inspiratory limb; however, this principle is of limited use for ventilator circuits because of concerns about a possible increase in imposed airway resistance.

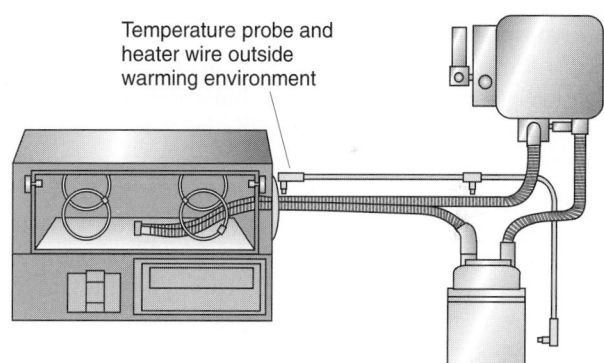

Temperature probe and
heater wire outside
warming environment

Figure 34-5 Temperature probe is positioned outside the incubator when a heated humidification system is used. (Modified from Peterson BD. Heated humidifiers. Respir Care Clin North Am 1998;4:243-260.)

Placing heated wires in the inspiratory and expiratory tubing of the ventilator circuit heats the gas in the circuit, reducing the temperature differential between humidifier and patient. The humidifier operates at a lower temperature with heated wire circuits than it does with conventional circuits. The humidifier's RH control regulates the temperature differential between the humidifier and the circuit temperature. When the humidifier is cooler than the gas in the inspiratory limb, the absolute humidity remains the same although the relative humidity is decreased, and the circuit has no condensate (Figure 34-6). When no condensate is visible in the cir-

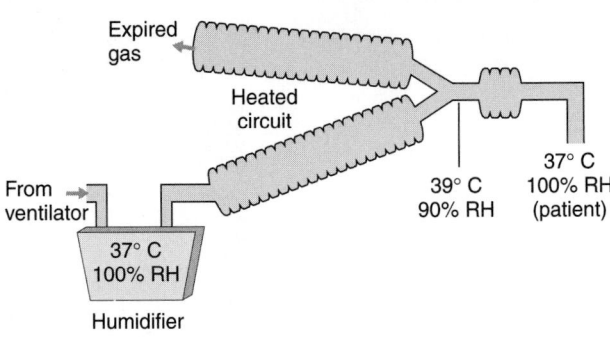

Figure 34-6 Appropriate settings for heated wire circuit to ensure that gas delivered to the patient is 100% body humidity. *RH,* Relative humidity.

Figure 34-7 Settings too low for heated wire circuit; gas delivered to the patient will be too dry. *RH,* Relative humidity.

cuit, it is impossible to know if the gas is being humidified without direct humidity measurements. To ensure humidification of the inspired gas, the temperature differential should be adjusted to the point that condensation forms near the patient's airway; this is the most reliable indicator that gas is fully saturated. If no condensate is visible, the relative humidity could be anything from zero to 99%, and the clinician has no way of knowing what it is without using a hygrometer. If the humidity control is set incorrectly, dry gas can be delivered to the patient's airway, resulting in mucus obstruction of the airway (Figure 34-7).[13,14]

ℜespiratory Recap

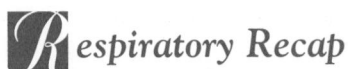

> **Assessment of Adequate Humidity Delivery**
>
> The delivered relative humidity is 100% if condensate is seen in the delivery tubing near the patient's airway.

Passive Humidifiers

A heat and moisture exchanger (HME), or **artificial nose,** is a passive humidifier. The HME captures exhaled heat and moisture and transfers part of that heat and humidity to the next inspired breath (Figure 34-8). The ideal HME should add minimal dead space, weight, and resistance to the airway, should incorporate standard connections, and

should operate at 70% efficiency or higher. In this case efficiency is defined as the ratio of the humidity of exhaled gas to the humidity returned to the patient by the HME.[15]

Artificial noses include condensers, hygroscopic condensers, and hygrophobic condensers. Condenser humidifiers are constructed of metallic gauze, corrugated metal, or parallel metal tubes that provide high thermal conductivity. The condenser cools to room temperature during inspiration. During exhalation, saturated gas cools as it contacts the condenser, water condenses and collects on the elements of the condenser, and the temperature of the condenser core rises. On the next inspiration cool, dry air is warmed by the condenser through evaporation of water from the surface. Condenser humidifiers usually are only about 50% efficient.

Hygroscopic condenser humidifiers contain materials of *low thermal conductivity* (meaning that heat from conduction and the latent heat of condensation are not dissipated), such as paper, wool, or foam, that are impregnated with a hygroscopic chemical such as calcium chloride or lithium chloride. During exhalation, warm saturated gas precipitates water on the cool condenser element while water molecules bind to the salt without transition from vapor to liquid state. During inspiration the lower water vapor pressure in the inspired gas liberates water molecules from the hygroscopic compound without a fall in temperature from vaporization. The efficiency of these devices can be as high as 70%.

Hydrophobic condenser humidifiers use a water-repellent element with a large surface area and low thermal conductivity. During exhalation the condenser temperature rises to

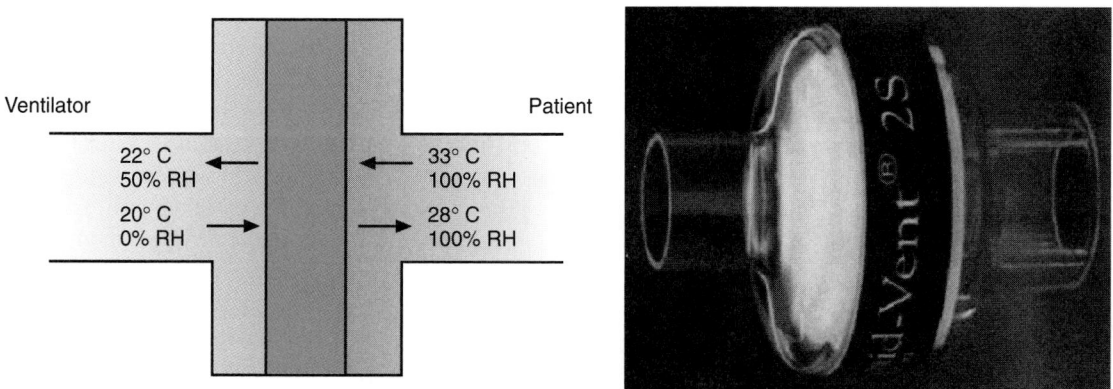

Figure 34-8 Heat and moisture exchanger. *RH,* Relative humidity (Photo courtesy Hudson RCI, Temecula, Calif.)

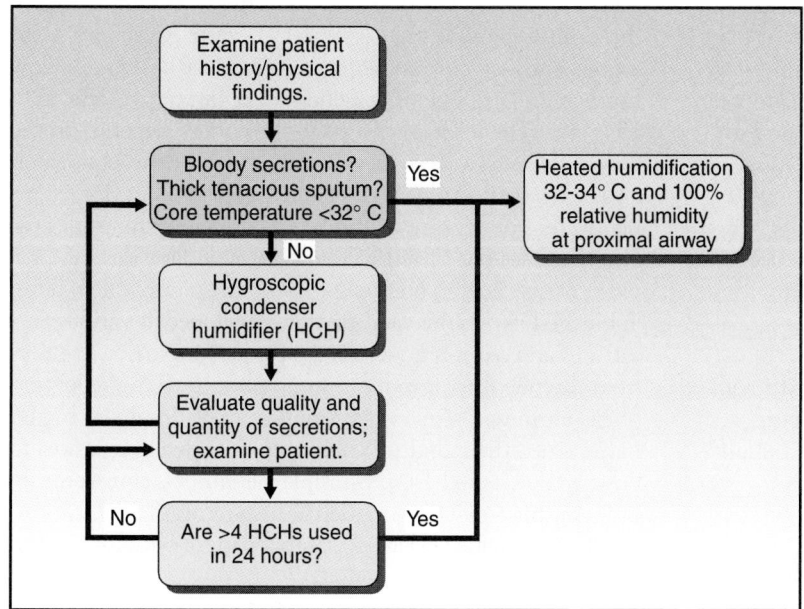

Figure 34-9   Clinical algorithm for use of heat and moisture exchanger. (Modified from Branson RD, Campbell RS. Humidification in the intensive care unit. Respir Care Clin North Am 1998;4: 305-320.)

about 25° C. On inspiration cool gas and evaporation cools the condenser to about 10° C. This large temperature shift results in more water condensation in the humidifier on exhalation, and this water is used to humidify the next inspiration. These devices are about 70% efficient. Hydrophobic humidifiers can also serve as efficient microbiologic filters.

The efficiency of HMEs declines as the tidal volume, inspiratory flow, or fractional inspired oxygen concentration (FIO_2) increases. Resistance through the HME increases as the water load of the device increases. When the HME is dry, resistance across the device is minimal, but after several hours of use, resistance may increase as water is absorbed onto a hygroscopic HME.[16] The increased work of breathing imposed by HMEs may not be well tolerated by patients with already high work of breathing or underlying lung disease.[22-24] Use of HMEs also increases me-

chanical dead space. Although HMEs increase the minute ventilation requirement and work of breathing, these drawbacks can be overcome by use of a low level of pressure support ventilation.

The HME forms a barrier between the patient and the ventilator circuit.[25] However, the value of the HME as a filter, in terms of patient outcomes and the safety of the health care provider, has not been established. HMEs are an inexpensive alternative to humidifiers.[26,27] They may be the device of choice for adult patients who do not have complex humidification needs. A clinical algorithm can be used to guide the use of HMEs (Figure 34-9). Although manufacturers recommend these devices be changed daily, current evidence suggests that they can be safely used for at least 48 hours.[28] The choice of an appropriate HME should be based on efficiency, dead space, weight, and cost.

ℛespiratory Recap

Contraindications for HME use include the presence of thick, copious, or bloody secretions; a large leak around an endotracheal tube, such as might occur with a large bronchopleural fistula or leaking endotracheal tube cuff; a body temperature below 32° C; and a minute ventilation greater than 10 L/min. Hazards associated with use of HMEs include underhydration, impaction of pulmonary secretions, increased resistive work of breathing, mucus plugging of the airways, increased dead space, and hypothermia. During aerosol administration HMEs must be removed from the patient circuit unless the aerosol generator is placed between the HME and the patient.

Bland Aerosol Therapy

Bland aerosol therapy provides humidification with solutions such as saline for therapeutic and diagnostic purposes. Large-volume pneumatic nebulizers and ultrasonic nebulizers are commonly used for these purposes. Large-volume pneumatic nebulizers, which have reservoir volumes greater than 100 mL, are commonly used to aerosolize solutions such as normal saline (0.9% NaCl), half normal saline (0.45% NaCl) and distilled water for prolonged periods. They are primarily indicated to provide humidification of medical gases for patients with bypassed upper airways, as treatment of upper airway inflammation with cold mist for local vasoconstriction, and to induce sputum production, most often for diagnostic purposes. There is little evidence to support the use of bland aerosols to hydrate a dehydrated patient. Fluid administration by the oral or intravenous route is better for hydration of secretions and presents less risk. For delivery of humidified inspired gases, a **large-volume nebulizer** offers little advantage over alternative methods such as heated wick humidifiers.

The total gas flow delivered through large-volume nebulizers depends on the design of the delivery system. Some of these units provide the desired FIO_2 with oxygen as a gas source and air entrainment (Figure 34-10). Oxygen flow through the jet nebulizer generally is limited to less than 15 L/min. The total flow of gas to the patient depends on the flow of driving gas and the size of the aperture through which air is entrained. Any back-pressure in this system (for example, water condensate in the tubing) reduces the total flow and increases the FIO_2. By definition, high flow devices provide enough flow to meet the patient's inspiratory flow rates. Table 34-1 shows the total gas flow developed at various FIO_2 settings and oxygen flows. As the set FIO_2 increases, the flow from the nebulizer is reduced in proportion to the reduction of gas entrained. An inspiratory flow of 30 L/min or higher may exceed the nebulizer's ability to provide enough flow to ensure the desired FIO_2. Multiple nebulizers, connected in tandem, may meet the patient's inspiratory flow. Unfortunately, to provide an FIO_2 of 0.9 to a patient with an inspira-

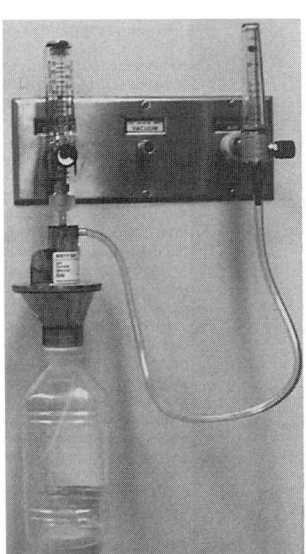 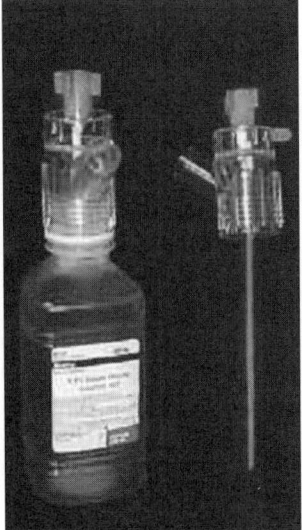

Figure 34-10 Two examples of closed dilution nebulizers. The primary gas is delivered to the jet and limited to about 40 L/min. The secondary gas flow may reach 80 L/min. The combination of oxygen flow and airflow determines the oxygen concentration and flow to the patient. (Courtesy LDH and B&B Medical Technologies, Orangevale, Calif.)

𝒯ABLE 34-1

Total Gas Flow at Various FIO_2 Settings and Oxygen Flows*

FIO_2	Airflow	/	Oxygen Flow	Total Flow 10 L/min	Total Flow 15 L/min
0.24	25	/	1	260	390
0.30	8	/	1	90	135
0.35	4.6	/	1	46	69
0.40	3.2	/	1	32	48
0.60	1	/	1	20	30
0.70	0.6	/	1	16	24
0.80	0.34	/	1	13.4	20
0.90	0.14	/	1	11	16
1	0	/	1	10	15

FIO_2, Fractional inspired oxygen concentration.
*Values given for a large-volume jet nebulizer.
Air:Oxygen = $(1 - FIO_2)$: $(FIO_2 - 0.21)$
Backslash (/) in third column from left represents a ratio.

tory flow of 60 L/min, four nebulizers would be required, which is both unwieldy and expensive. A more rational alternative is the use of high flow, closed dilution nebulizers.

Device Selection for Humidity Therapy

Selection of an appropriate humidification device should include consideration of the following questions:

- What source, temperature, and humidity of gas is the patient breathing?
- What is the point of entry of gas into the airway?
- What is the rate of inspiratory flow or minute volume?
- Does the patient have an intact or a bypassed upper airway?
- Is the endotracheal or tracheotomy tube cuffed or uncuffed?
- Does the patient have normal or diseased lungs?
- Is there evidence of increased, thick secretions or a humidity deficit?
- Are special needs imposed by dead space or the patient's size, age, ability to tolerate administration, or sensitivity to changes in the work of breathing?

Table 34-2 compares the relative attributes of common humidification systems.

Aerosol Drug Administration

Aerosol drug therapy has a number of advantages: a smaller dose can be targeted to the site of action; the onset of action occurs more quickly; and the therapeutic effect is achieved with fewer systemic side effects.[29] When aerosolized drugs are delivered directly to the airways, systemic absorption is limited, systemic side effects are minimized, and a high therapeutic index is achieved compared with systemic administration. In contrast, a variety of medications, including peptides and other macromolecules, can be targeted to the lung parenchyma for systemic administration across the alveolar-capillary membrane into the pulmonary vascular bed. Aerosol devices can deliver a wide variety of medications, from bronchodilators to insulin, and many types of devices are used, including nebulizers, pressurized metered dose inhalers (pMDIs), and dry powder inhalers (DPIs).[30] For medical use, aerosol generators produce respirable particles with a **mass median aerodynamic diameter (MMAD)** of 1 to 5 μm.[31]

Basic Concepts of Aerosol Therapy

An aerosol is composed of particles suspended in air. The time that particles can remain suspended depends on their low terminal settling velocity (v_t), or the velocity at which the aerosol particles fall in air because of gravity, a value related to the size and density of the particle. The geometric size of the particles is commonly expressed as the MMAD. The deposition of inhaled aerosols onto airway surfaces varies with the size of the particles. For example, the v_t of a 5-μm water droplet is 0.074 cm/second, almost 22 times greater than a 1-μm water droplet but one fourth that of a 10-μm water droplet. Half the mass of particles in an aerosol is less than the MMAD and the other half is greater. Relatively few particles larger than the median particle diameter comprise the mass above the MMAD, with a much greater

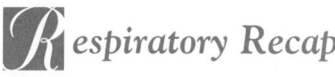
espirata **Recap**

Characterization of Aerosols
Mass median aerodynamic diameter (MMAD)
Geometric standard deviation (GSD)

TABLE 34-2

Comparison of Common Humidification Systems

Parameter	Bubble Humidifiers*	Passover Humidifiers†	Unheated Nebulizers	Heated Nebulizers	Heat and Moisture Exchangers
Output (mg/L)	15-20	30-50	15-30	20-40	19-32
Temperature (°C)	10-20	30-40	10-20	22-28	22-30
Flow limitation	Yes	No	Yes	Yes	Yes
Retains body heat	No	Yes	No	Yes	Yes
Infection risk	Yes	No	Yes	Yes	No
Potential for overheating	No	Yes	No	Yes	No
Potential for overhydration	No	No	Yes	Yes	No
Potential for underhydration	Yes	No	Yes	No	Yes
Increases work of breathing	Yes	No	Yes	Yes	Yes
Possible electrical hazard	No	Yes	No	Yes	No

*Unheated.
†Heated.

number of particles less than the median required to reach comparable mass. **Geometric standard deviation (GSD)** is a measure of the magnitude of variation of particle size distribution. A monodisperse aerosol, in which all particles are basically the same size, has a GSD under 1.2, whereas a heterodisperse aerosol, with a wider range of particle sizes, has a GSD more than 1.2. Most therapeutic aerosols are heterodisperse.

Inertia is the tendency of an object with mass, once it is in motion, to travel in a straight line. The greater the mass and velocity of a particle, the greater the inertia that keeps the particle in motion. **Inertial impaction** is the primary mechanism of deposition of aerosol particles 5 μm or larger and an important mechanism for particles as small as 2 μm. As aerosol is inhaled and the stream of gas is diverted in the airway, particles tend to continue along their initial trajectory, impacting and depositing on the airway. The higher the inspiratory flow, the greater the velocity and inertia of the particles, increasing the tendency of smaller particles to impact and deposit in airways. Turbulent flow, complex passageways, bifurcation of the airways, and inspiratory flows greater than 30 L/min increase the impaction of particles larger than 2 μm in the larger airways.

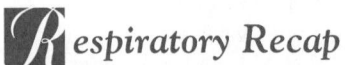espiratory Recap

Primary Factors Affecting Aerosol Deposition
Inertia
Gravity
Diffusion

Gravitational sedimentation occurs when aerosol particles settle out of suspension because of gravity. The greater the mass of the particle, the faster it settles. Very small particles (those less than 0.5 μm in diameter) do not settle at all. Holding the breath for 4 to 10 seconds after inhalation of an aerosol lengthens the residence time for particles in the lungs, increasing the time for deposition through gravitational sedimentation, especially in the last 6 generations of the airway. Breath holding increases deposition of aerosol by as much as 10% with up to a fourfold increase in peripheral distribution. This marginal increase in deposition may explain why breath holding has not been demonstrated to significantly improve the clinical response to aerosolized medications conducted to targeted airways.

Diffusion, or brownian movement, is the primary mechanism of deposition of particles less than 3 μm in the airway. As gas reaches the distal regions of the lungs, gas flow stops. Aerosol particles bouncing against air molecules and each other deposit on contact with the airway surfaces. Preferential deposition for particles 0.5 to 3 μm is divided between the central and peripheral airways. *Coalescence,* the attraction of particles to each other, occurs when particles come within a distance 25 times or less their diameter.

Aerosol droplets in the **respirable range** (1 to 5 μm MMAD) are more likely to deposit in the lower respiratory tract than are larger or smaller particles. For particles larger than 0.5 μm, the depth of penetration into the lungs is inversely proportional to the particle size. Particles between 0.1 and 1 μm are so small a significant proportion of those that enter the lungs may be exhaled. Particles larger than 5 μm impact in the upper airway before reaching the lower respiratory tract.

Aerosol Deposition, Targeting, and Translocation

Once an aerosol deposits on the airway, it must translocate across the mucus barrier and retain bioactivity to be effective as a therapeutic agent. The optimum site of action depends on the agent administered. Bronchodilators and steroids must reach the epithelium to be effective. Aerosolized antibiotics and mucolytics are most effective when dispersed in infected airway secretions at sites of maximum airway obstruction. Gene transfer therapy must not only access the epithelium through the mucous barrier but also must then gain access to the submucous glands or basal (progenitor) cells of the epithelium.

Particle charge, solubility, and size and the biophysical properties of secretions all affect the ability of an aerosol to penetrate the mucous barrier. Turbulent flow and airway obstruction affect the airway deposition pattern. Other factors that limit efficacy, especially of macromolecules, include binding to constituents of mucus, including mucin and deoxyribonucleic acid (DNA), and the breakdown of bioactive molecules by proteases and other enzymes. Molecular weight and particle diffusion through mucus are inversely related. The antibiotic diffusion barrier represented by mucin may be significant in vitro, particularly for nebulized antibiotics. Translocation of macromolecules can be further compromised by the hypersecretion that accompanies inflammation and chronic pulmonary disease. These secretions can act as a barrier to the penetration of any aerosol.

Factors that promote translocation of medicated aerosols to the airway include an effective surfactant layer and increased particle retention time. Mucus discontinuity in the airway may assist deposition and translocation. The translocation of particles through the mucous layer depends partly on the presence of bronchial surfactant. Pulmonary surfactant promotes the displacement of some particles from air to the aqueous phase. The extent of particle immersion depends on the surface tension of the surface active film. For particles smaller than 100 μm, the surface tension force is several orders of magnitude greater than forces related to gravity.

Factors Affecting Drug Dose Distribution

Dosing of aerosolized medication is imprecise. It is unclear how much drug is delivered to targeted areas of the lung with progressive disease states and during acute exacerbations. These factors reduce aerosol deposition in the respiratory tract to as little as 1% of the medication dose placed in a nebulizer, regardless of whether the patient is breathing spontaneously or is mechanically ventilated. There is no established correlation between tidal volume and aerosol effectiveness. Theoretically, larger breaths capture more aerosol, but this relationship has not been shown clinically. This may be the result of partitioning of the tidal volume, which is regulated both by the delivered volume and by the airway dimensions. High inspiratory flow increases aerosol impaction in larger airways, whereas low inspiratory flow may result in a reduced amount of medication being available for inhalation from a dry powder inhaler.

Humidity also influences the delivery of aerosol medications. This has been well demonstrated with ventilator circuits, in which humidity can result in a 40% or greater reduction in aerosol delivered to the lungs. Droplets of solution evaporate or grow, depending on the water content and temperature of the gas, and powder can clump or aggregate in high humidity.

Drug formulations dictate, in part, which aerosol options are available for delivery of a specific medication. Most solutions can be nebulized if the medication is *soluble* (corticosteroids are an exception), but the physical characteristics of the solution (or suspension) can affect particle size and nebulizer output. Furthermore, some macromolecules may not enter suspension well and can be shattered into nonbioactive forms by the force of air required to generate an aerosol.

Because of development costs, many aerosol medications initially are developed as nebulizer solutions and later reformulated for pMDIs or DPIs. Theoretically, if a particle can be milled to a respirable size while retaining bioactivity, it can be delivered by a pMDI or DPI. However, development costs are greater for these devices than for nebulizer solutions. Currently DPI formulations in the United States are limited to a few preparations, but it is expected that a greater variety of DPI medications and devices will become available. A greater variety of formulations are available for pMDIs then for any other type of aerosol generator system, with more being developed for the new hydrofluororalkene-based pMDIs.

Aerosol Generators

Jet Nebulizers

Pneumatic jet nebulizers use the Bernoulli principle to drive a high-pressure gas through a restricted orifice across the top of a capillary tube, with the bottom of the tube immersed in the solution (Figure 34-11).[32] An aerosol is formed when the jet stream shears fluid from the capillary tube and drives the particles against a solid or liquid surface that acts as a baffle. Impaction against a baffle removes larger particles from suspension and allows them to return to the reservoir, whereas smaller particles remain suspended in the gas and travel from the nebulizer. Nebu-

lizers produce smaller particle sizes by use of baffles such as one-way valves, often at the cost of a lower total drug output per minute than the same nebulizer without baffling, thereby requiring more time to deliver a standard dose of medication. Baffles that do not allow medication to return to the reservoir may also reduce the total drug available to the patient. A number of factors affect the delivery of aerosols by nebulizer (Box 34-1). The technique for the use of a medication nebulizer is shown in Box 34-2.

An effective small-volume pneumatic nebulizer should deliver more than 50% of its total dose as aerosol in the respirable range (1 to 5 μm MMAD) in 10 minutes or less of nebulization time. Nebulizer performance varies with fill volume, flow, gas density, and nebulizer model.[33] The amount of drug nebulized increases as the fill volume increases. The residual volume of solution (dead volume) that remains in commercial small-volume nebulizers varies from 0.5 to 1.5 mL, depending on the specific device. Therefore increasing the fill volume allows a greater proportion of the medication to be nebulized. For example, with a 1-mL residual volume, a fill of 2 mL provides only 50% of the nebulizer charge available for nebulization. However, a fill of 4 mL makes 3 mL, or 75%, of the medication available for nebulization. Droplet size and

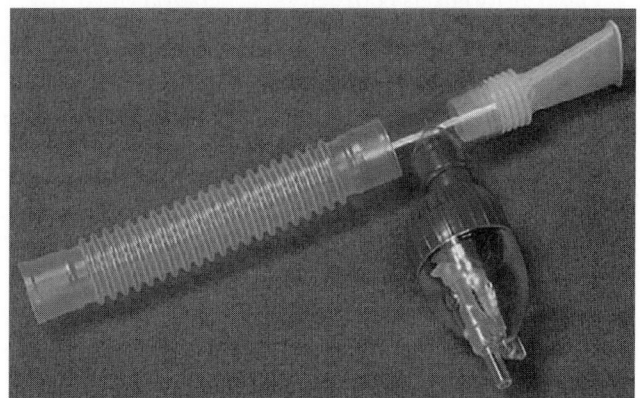

A

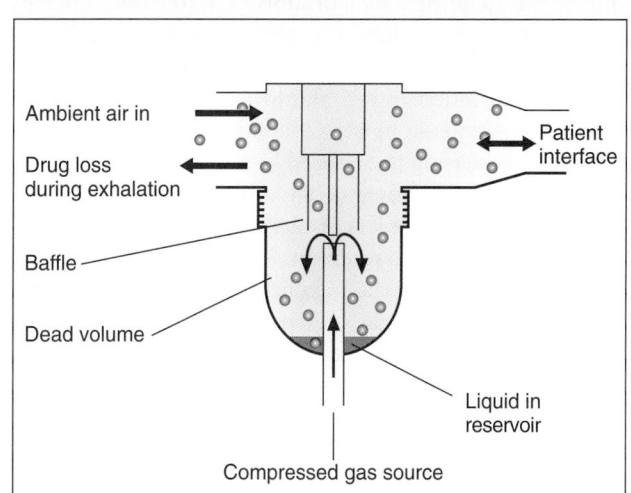

B

Figure 34-11   **A,** Small-volume jet nebulizer for drug delivery. **B,** Schematic drawing of a small-volume jet nebulizer.

Box 34-1

Factors That Affect Aerosol Delivery by Nebulizer

Technical Factors
Manufacturer
Flow
Fill volume
Solution characteristics
Characteristics of driving gas
Designs to enhance output
Continuous versus intermittent delivery

Patient Factors
Breathing pattern
Nose versus mouth breathing
Characteristics of gas
Airway obstruction
Positive pressure delivery
Artificial airway and mechanical ventilation

Box 34-2

Technique for Use of a Small-Volume Nebulizer

1. Assemble the apparatus.
2. Mix the medication according to the prescription and add it to the nebulizer.
3. Ensure that the fill volume is 4 to 6 mL.
4. If the nebulizer is to be operated continuously, add 6 inches of aerosol tubing (50 mL) or other reservoir.
5. Attach the gas source, ensuring that the gas flow meets the nebulizer's specifications.
6. Help the patient into an upright position. (The patient may be sitting or reclining against some pillows.)
7. If a mouthpiece or mask is used, encourage the patient to breathe through the mouth.
8. If the patient has an artificial airway or a bypassed upper airway (that is, an endotracheal tube or a tracheostomy), make sure the nebulizer is not putting undue pressure on the airway.
9. Encourage the patient to take normal, comfortable breaths, with occasional deep breaths; use low inspiratory flow rates.
10. Periodically tap the nebulizer to return impacted particles to the reservoir.
11. Assess the patient for comfort, adverse effects, and response throughout the treatment.
12. When the nebulizer begins to sputter and stops nebulizing, remove it from the patient. Clean and disinfect it, replace it, or rinse it with sterile water and allow it to air dry; store it properly between treatments.

Modified from Fink JB. Aerosol device selection: evidence to practice. Respir Care 2000;45:874-885.

nebulization time vary inversely with flow. Within the design limits of the nebulizer, the higher the flow to the nebulizer, the smaller the particle size generated and the shorter the time required to nebulize the full dose.[33]

Gas density effects both aerosol generation and delivery of aerosol to the lungs. This is most evident with low-density helium-oxygen mixtures.[34] A carrier gas of lower density produces less turbulent flow, reducing aerosol impaction losses during inspiration and improving delivery of aerosol to the lungs. However, when helium-oxygen is used to drive a jet nebulizer, aerosol output is reduced, requiring a twofold increase in flow to produce a comparable respirable aerosol output per minute. Consequently, helium-oxygen mixtures may increase the percentage of aerosol available to the lungs but impairs the production of the aerosol by the nebulizer. Humidity and temperature affect the particle size and concentration of drug remaining in the nebulizer. Evaporation of water and adiabatic expansion of gas reduce the temperature of the aerosol more than 5° C below the ambient temperature. Aerosol particles entrained into a warm and water-saturated gas stream may increase in size. These larger particles tend to coalesce, increasing the MMAD.

Clinicians and patients commonly tap a nebulizer periodically to shake droplets of medication from the walls of the nebulizer into the reservoir. However, in one study albuterol delivery from the nebulizer stopped with the onset of inconsistent nebulization (sputtering).[35] Aerosolization past the point of initial jet nebulizer sputter is ineffective and should indicate an end the treatment. Because the nebulizer selected affects aerosol delivery, a nebulizer should be chosen that reliably delivers specific medications.[32] When a compressor is used to power the nebulizer, the performance of the compressor is also important.

Nebulizers commonly are operated continuously; that is, throughout the patient's respiratory cycle. This wastes the aerosol produced during the expiratory phase. A typi-

cal inspiration to expiration ratio of 1:3 results in 75% of the aerosol emitted from the nebulizer being lost to the atmosphere. This is a major factor in the poor efficiency associated with pneumatic nebulizers. If 50% of the nominal dose is emitted, 50% in the respirable range, and 25% of that is inhaled by the patient, then 12.5% of the nominal dose is inhaled by the patient and 20% of that is exhaled. This correlates with the 10% deposition observed with in vivo measurements.

A reservoir on the expiratory limb of the nebulizer conserves drug by collecting some of the nebulizer output that otherwise would be wasted to the atmosphere.[32] A reservoir can be created through placement of 15 cm of aerosol tubing on the expiratory side of the nebulizer. As an alternative, commercial devices such as simple bag reservoirs (Figure 34-12) provide a greater volume reservoir in which the smaller aerosol particles remain in suspension for inhalation and larger particles rain out.

Vented nebulizer systems (Figure 34-13) allow the patient to inhale additional air through the nebulizer, increasing drug delivery on inspiration. The inlet vent closes on exhalation, and aerosol exits via a one-way valve in the mouthpiece. This design reduces aerosol waste and increases the inhaled dose by as much as 50% without increasing the treatment time.

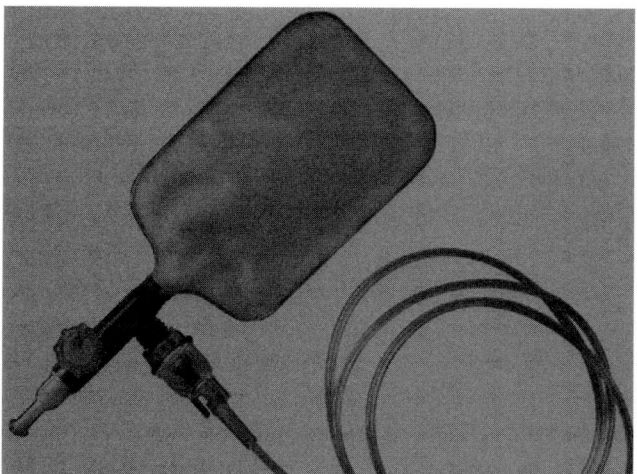

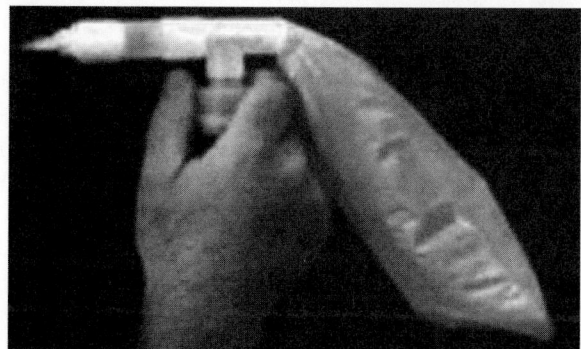

Figure 34-12 Nebulizers with reservoir bag to capture aerosol during expiratory phase. (*Top* courtesy WestMed Inc., Tucson, Ariz., and Piper AeroTee, Hudson RCI, Temecula, Calif.).

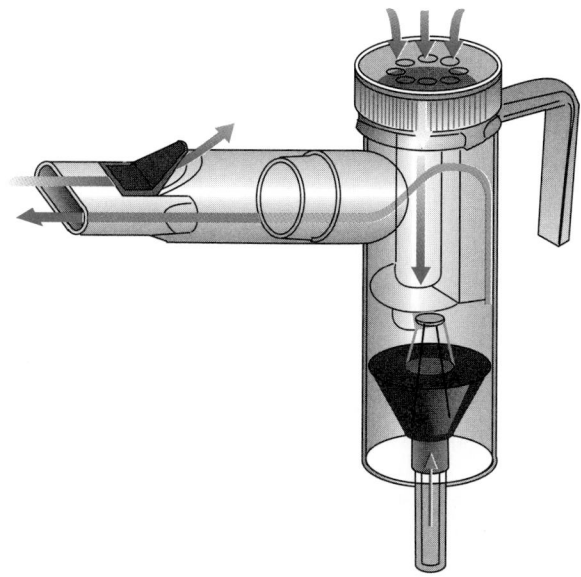

Figure 34-13 Vented breath-enhanced nebulizer. (Modified from photo courtesy Pari, Midlothian, Va.)

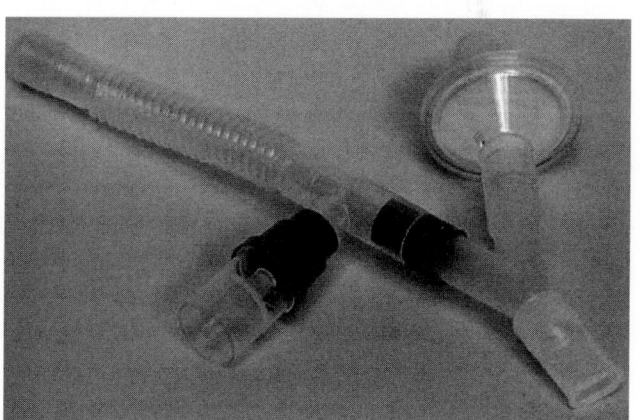

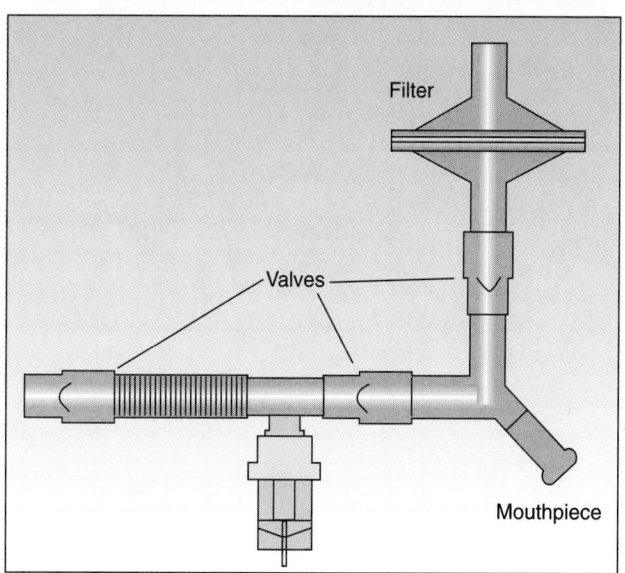

Filter

Valves

Mouthpiece

Figure 34-14 **A,** Respigard nebulizer for pentamidine administration. **B,** Schematic drawing of Respigard nebulizer. (**A,** Courtesy Marquest, Totowa, N.J.)

Breath-actuated nebulization synchronizes aerosol generation with inspiration, increasing the amount of drug available for inspiration by up to fourfold. The inhaled aerosol per breath is similar, but the amount of drug inhaled and treatment time increase by a factor of four. Inspiratory phase nebulization can be accomplished with a thumb control port that allows the patient to manually direct gas to the nebulizer only on inspiration. This improves the efficiency of the nebulizer if the patient has good hand-breath coordination. More effective systems do not require hand-breath coordination and operate by the synchronizing of aerosol production to the patient's inspiratory phase. The Medic Aid Halolite system uses a microprocessor and pneumotachometer to regulate nebulization during the first half of inspiration, monitoring the inspiratory time of the first three breaths and creating a template for nebulization during inspiration of subsequent breaths. The Monaghan AeroEclipse is a pneumatic breath-actuated nebulizer that responds to the patient's inspiratory flow, producing aerosol during inspiration and ending nebulization when the inspiratory flow drops below a threshold.

Some nebulizers are valved and have expiratory filters (Figure 34-14); these are designed specifically for the delivery of pentamidine. The filter minimizes ambient contamination with the aerosol and the patient's exhaled gases. These nebulizers also produce very small particles to enhance parenchymal deposition.

Plastic nebulizers may show degradation of performance after many uses. A study of disposable nebulizers reported that repeated use did not alter performance as long as proper cleaning was performed.[36] Nebulizers should be cleaned and disinfected or rinsed with sterile water between uses and air dried. Contamination of nebulizer solutions is related to storage of multiple-dose solutions at room temperature and reuse of syringes to measure the solution. Refrigerating solutions and disposing of syringes every 24 hours eliminates bacterial contamination.

For patients who cannot use a mouthpiece, the nebulizer can be fitted to an appropriate mask. No difference in clinical response has been found between mouthpiece and close-fitting mask treatment; therefore patient compliance and preference should guide selection of the device.[37] However, mouth breathing enhances medication delivery to the airways in adults. Crying is a long exhalation preceded by a very short and rapid inhalation; this completely prevents lower airway deposition of an aerosol. Thus aerosols should never be administered to a crying child. It is more efficient to deliver medication by close-fitting mask when the child is asleep. Blow-by, in which the practitioner directs the aerosol from the nebulizer toward the patient's nose and mouth, is not supported by empiric evidence; aerosol deposition studies suggest that virtually no drug enters the airway.

The small particle aerosol generator (SPAG) is a jet-type aerosol generator used to administer ribavirin (Figure 34-15). It uses a secondary drying chamber that reduces the MMAD to 1.2 μm with a GSD of 1.4. The SPAG reduces the 50 psi of line pressure medical gas to 26 psi, connected to two flowmeters that control flow to the nebulizer and the drying chamber. The aerosol generated in the medication reservoir enters the long cylindric drying chamber, where additional flow of dry gas reduces the size of the aerosol particles through evaporation. The flow to the nebulizer is adjusted to a maximum of 7 L/min, with a total flow from both flowmeters of 15 L/min. The administration of ribavirin has highlighted concerns about second-hand exposure of health care workers to aerosol, resulting in recommendations that open air administration be avoided.[38] To help protect staff members, ribavirin administration should be limited to a negative-pressure, single-patient room with six air exchanges per hour. Procedures used to reduce the release of ribavirin into the environment include containment of the aerosol with a canopy over the delivery device (Figure 34-16),[39] use of a scavenging system, and filtering of the expiratory limb of the circuit of a mechanically ventilated patient. Practices that reduce caregiver exposure include the turning off of

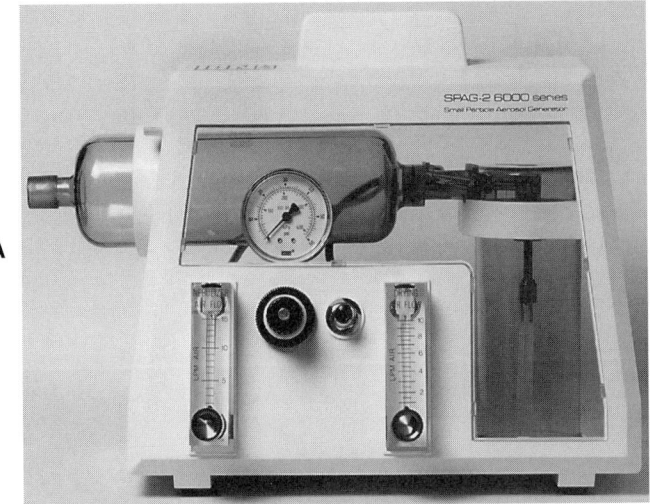

A

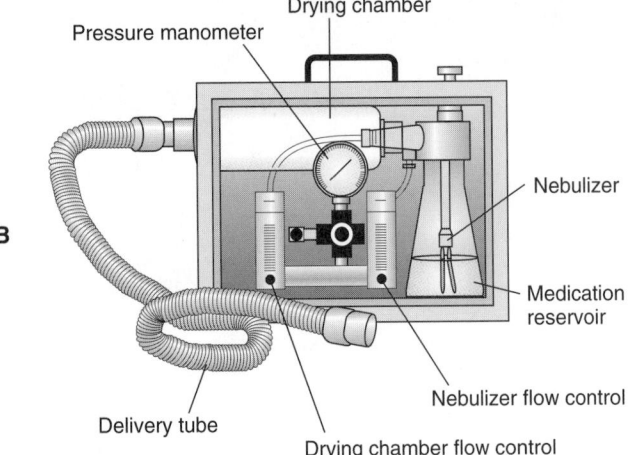

B

Figure 34-15 A, Small particle aerosol generator (SPAG) for ribavirin administration. **B,** Schematic drawing of a SPAG. (**A,** Courtesy ICN Pharmaceuticals, Costa Mesa, Calif.; **B,** Modified from Scanlan CL, Wilkins RL, Stoller JK. Egan's fundamentals of respiratory care. 7th ed. St Louis: Mosby; 1999.)

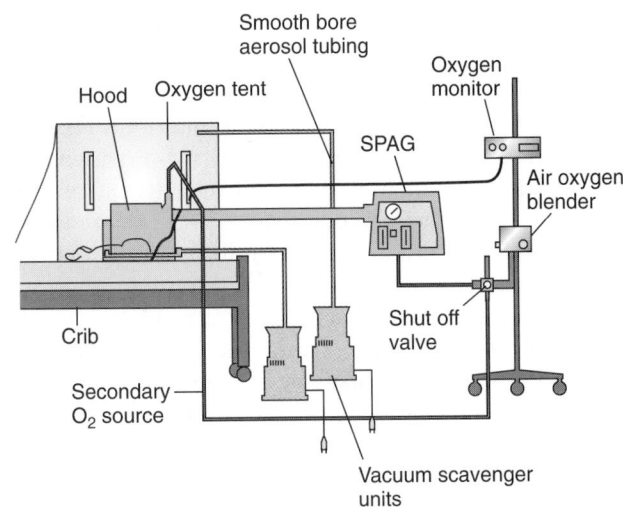

Figure 34-16 Scavenging system for ribavirin administration. (Modified from Kacmarek RM, Kratohvil J. Evaluation of a double-enclosure double-vacuum unit scavenging system for ribavirin administration. Respir Care 1992;37:37-45.)

the nebulizer 5 minutes before opening the tent or 1 minute before disconnecting the ventilator and the use of personal protective equipment, including goggles, a respirator, gown, and gloves. Administrative policies should prevent pregnant or lactating women and staff members who have had reactions to the drug from coming into contact with ribavirin. Caution must be used when ribavirin is administered during mechanical ventilation because of the drug's tendency to occlude filters, valves, and endotracheal tubes. Tandem filters placed in series in the expiratory limb of the ventilator reduce expiratory valve occlusion but require frequent changing. Aerosol from the SPAG is entrained into the ventilator circuit distal to the output of the humidifier through a one-way valve.[40] A high-pressure alarm in the circuit alerts the clinician to an excessive baseline pressure should expiratory occlusion occur.

If the symptoms of a patient with acute exacerbation of asthma are not relieved with standard bronchodilator dosing, other dosing strategies can be used. The frequency of administration commonly is increased to an hourly basis, then every 15 to 20 minutes if symptoms are not relieved. As an alternative, continuous nebulization can be provided at a controlled rate of medication delivery.[32] Doses of albuterol between 7.5 and 15 mg/hour have proved effective in treating acute exacerbations of asthma. One strategy is to use an intravenous infusion pump to deliver a premixed bronchodilator solution into a jet nebulizer (Figure 34-17). Another strategy is to use a large-volume nebulizer that delivers a consistent output of medication at a specific flow. Albuterol solution and saline are mixed in the reservoir, and the nebulizer is operated at a flow recommended by the manufacturer to deliver the desired dose. The aerosol can be delivered with a mask or in-line with a ventilator circuit. For patients with moderately severe asthma, continuous or intermittent therapy has a similar effect with either low- or high-dose β-agonists.

Ultrasonic Nebulizers

The **ultrasonic nebulizer (USN)** uses a piezoelectric crystal that vibrates at a high frequency to convert electricity to sound waves, creating standing waves in the liquid immediately above the transducer and disrupting the liquid's surface, forming a geyser of droplets (Figure 34-18). Because electronics are not readily sterilized, disposable medication cups with a flexible diaphragm are commonly used, with the sound waves communicated through a layer of water acting as a couplant. USNs are capable of greater aerosol output (0.4 to 5 mL/min) with greater aerosol density than conventional jet nebulizers. Particle size is determined by frequency, and output by the amplitude of the signal. Within limits, the particle size is inversely proportional to the frequency and is not user adjustable. Two USNs from the same manufacturer can operate at different frequencies (1.24 to 2.25 MHz), producing a range of MMADs (2.5 to 6 μm).

Large-volume USNs, which are used primarily for bland aerosol therapy or sputum induction, incorporate air blowers

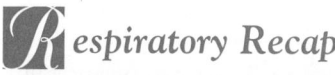

R̶espiratory Recap

Aerosol Medication Delivery Devices
Jet nebulizer
Ultrasonic nebulizer (USN)
Pressurized metered dose inhaler (pMDI)
Metered dose inhaler with spacer or holding chamber
Dry powder inhaler (DPI)

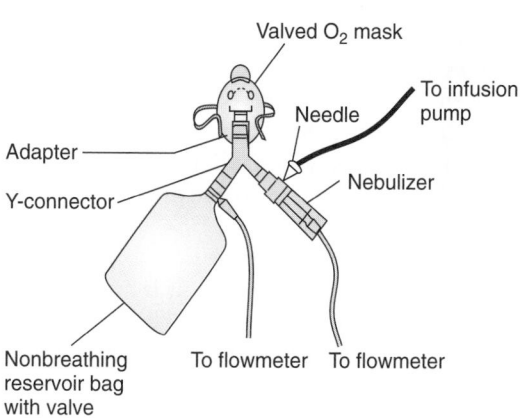

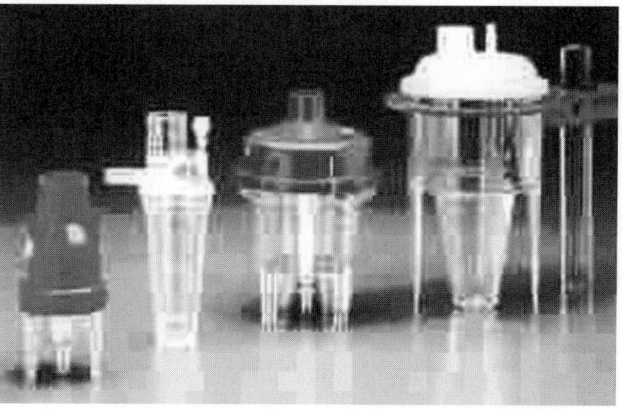

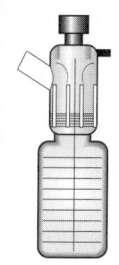

A   **B**   **C**

Figure 34-17   Delivery systems for a continuous aerosolized bronchodilator include continuous infusion of medications into a standard small-volume nebulizer **(A)** and commercially available large-volume nebulizers such as the HEART nebulizer **(B)** and the closed dilution HOPE nebulizer **(C)**. **(A,** Modified from Moler FW, Johnson CE, Van Laanen C, et al. Continuous versus intermittent nebulized terbutaline: plasma levels and effects. Am J Respir Crit Care Med 1995;151:602-606; **B,** Courtesy WestMed, Inc., Tucson, Ariz. **C,** Modified from materials courtesy Band B Medical Technologies, Inc., Orangevale, Calif.)

In figure A labels: Valved O₂ mask, Needle, To infusion pump, Adapter, Nebulizer, Y-connector, Nonbreathing reservoir bag with valve, To flowmeter, To flowmeter

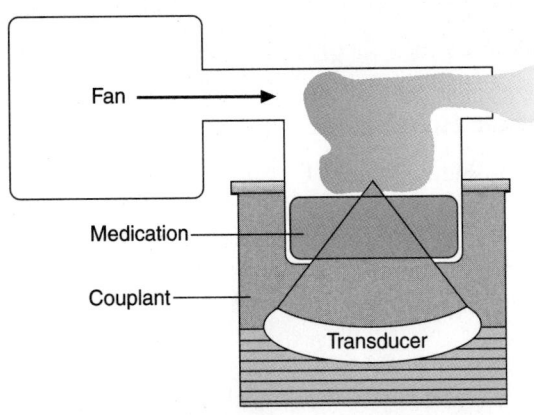

Figure 34-18 Schematic drawing of an ultrasonic nebulizer. (Modified from Cohen N, Fink J. Humidity and aerosols. In: Eubanks DH, Bone RC. Principles and applications of cardiorespiratory care equipment. St Louis: Mosby; 1994.)

to carry the mist to the patient. An inverse relationship exists between the aerosol density emitted by the USN and the flow of gas through the nebulizer. Because of the energy required, the temperature of the solution in a USN increases by as much as 15° C over 15 minutes. As the temperature rises, the drug concentration also rises, increasing the likelihood of undesirable side effects such as denaturing proteins.

Small-volume ultrasonic nebulizers are available for aerosol drug delivery.[41] These systems may or may not use a water-filled couplant compartment, with the medication placed in a cup or directly onto the transducer connected to a battery-powered power source. The patient's inspiratory flow draws aerosol from the nebulizer into the lungs. As the USN operates, the aerosol remains in the medication cup or chamber until a flow of gas pushes or pulls the aerosol from the nebulizer. If a USN creates aerosol continuously, the patient draws aerosol from the nebulizer during inspiration and clears aerosol from the chamber during exhalation, with aerosol collecting in the chamber between end expiration and through inspiration. If exhalation is diverted away from the medication chamber, there is minimal waste to atmosphere and more drug available for inhalation.

Small-volume USNs may have less dead volume than small-volume nebulizers. The contained portable power source provides convenience and mobility. However, the advantages of ultrasonic nebulizers may be offset by their high cost relative to standard jet nebulizers. USNs have been promoted for administration of a wide variety of formulations ranging from bronchodilators to antiinflammatory agents and antibiotics, but they generally have proved less effective than other delivery devices, especially with suspensions.[42]

Overhydration has been associated with prolonged bland aerosol treatment by use of an USN in children and patients with renal insufficiency. The high-density aerosol from USNs may precipitate bronchospasm. An acoustic power output above 50 watts/cm[2] has been associated with disruption of the structure of some molecules. USNs re-

cently have drawn attention for the administration of aerosols during mechanical ventilation because they do not require the addition of a driving gas flow to the circuit.[43] Disadvantages of the USN in the ventilator circuit include weight, position dependency, a tendency to heat medications, and the need for water couplants.

Not all USNs that use piezoelectric crystals have the same characteristics as the classic ultrasonic nebulizers. A new type of nebulizer, the Aerodose (Aerogen, Inc., Sunnyvale, Calif.) is a hand-held, battery-operated, breath-actuated nebulizer that produces precision aerosols. It uses a piezoelectric element to rapidly move a domed aperture plate, creating a pumping action. The Aerodose does not heat medication and can effectively deliver large and small molecules and suspensions.

Pressurized Metered Dose Inhalers

The **pressurized metered dose inhaler (pMDI)** is the most commonly prescribed method of aerosol delivery.[44] Pressurized MDIs are used to administer bronchodilators, anticholinergics, antiinflammatory agents, and steroids. In the United States more formulations are available by pMDI than by other aerosol delivery systems. When properly used, pMDIs are at least as effective for drug delivery as other nebulizers.[30] For this reason, pMDIs often are the preferred method used to deliver bronchodilators to both spontaneously breathing and mechanically ventilated patients.[30]

A pMDI consists of a pressurized canister containing a drug in the form of a micronized powder or solution that is suspended with a mixture of propellants, surfactant, preservatives, flavoring agents, and dispersing agents. The concentrations of the dispersing agents are equal to or greater than that of the medication, and dispersing agents may be associated with coughing and wheezing. The active drug accounts for about 1% of the contents of the pMDI. As much as 80% by weight of the spray from the pMDI is composed of a propellant, commonly a chlorofluorocarbon (CFC), such as Freon. Adverse reactions to CFCs are extremely rare. Because of international agreements to ban CFCs, new pMDIs are in development that use environmentally friendly propellants. The best developed of the new propellants are the hydrofluororalkenes (HFAs), such as HFA133a.[44]

In a pMDI the mixture is released from the canister through a metering valve and stem that fit into an actuator boot, and the device is designed and tested by the manufacturer to work with a specific medication formulation (Figure 34-19). Small changes in the actuator's design can change the characteristics and output of the aerosol.[44] The metering valve volume varies from 30 to 100 μL and contains 20 μg to 5 mg of drug. The volume emitted by the pMDI is 15 to 20 mL after volatilization of the propellant.[45] Lung deposition ranges from 10% to 25% of the nominal dose in adults, with intersubject variability largely technique dependent. When proper technique and an effective accessory device are used, the pMDI delivers substantially more of the dose of medication to the lungs than a jet nebulizer.

Metered dose inhaler

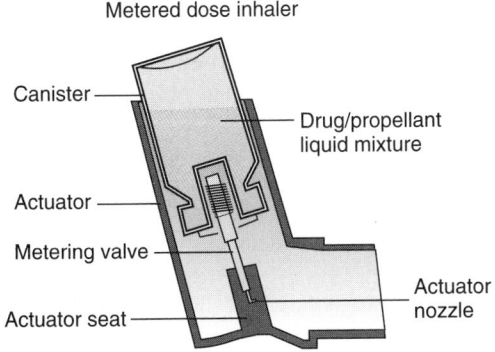

A

Metered valve function

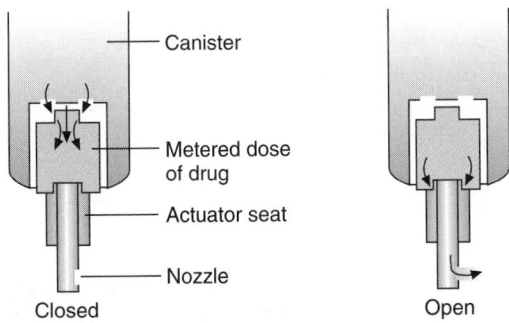

Closed   Open

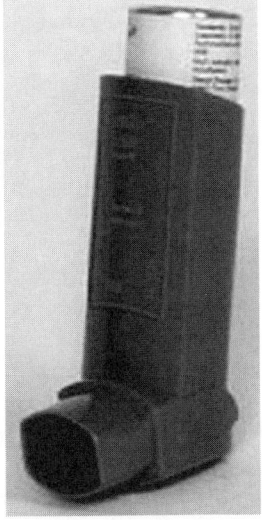

B

Figure 34-19 **A,** Schematic drawings of a metered dose inhaler. **B,** Actual metered dose inhaler. (Drawings modified from Rau JL Jr. Respiratory care pharmacology. 5th ed. St. Louis: Mosby; 1998.)

The nominal dose of medication with the pMDI is much smaller than that with a nebulizer. The amount of albuterol from a pMDI exiting the actuator nozzle is 100 μg with each actuation or 90 μg from the opening of the actuator boot; this is how pMDI aerosol actuations are characterized in the United States. Thus a dose of two to four actuations (200 to 400 μg nominal dose) usually is used. In ambulatory patients, 10% deposition may deliver a dose of 20 to 40 μg for an effective bronchodilation response.

Effective use of the pMDI is technique dependent. As many as two thirds of patients who use pMDIs and health professionals who teach pMDI use do not perform the procedure properly.[46] The steps to administer a bronchodilator with a pMDI are listed in Box 34-3.[47] Good patient instruction can take 10 to 30 minutes and should include demonstration, practice, and confirmation of the patient's performance (demonstration placebo units are available for this purpose). Repeated instruction improves performance.[48] Infants, young children, the elderly, and patients in acute distress may not be able to use a pMDI effectively. A cold Freon effect can occur when the aerosol plume reaches the back of the mouth and the patient stops inhaling. The pMDI can be used as often as every 30 seconds without affecting its performance. A new pMDI or one that has not been used recently should be actuated several times before use to prime the metering chamber properly.

The pMDI should always be stored with the cap on, both to prevent foreign objects from entering the boot and to reduce humidity and microbial contamination. Pressurized MDIs should always be discarded when empty to avoid administration of propellant without medication. Although it has been suggested that pMDIs can be tested for drug remaining by floating of the canister in water, this technique is no longer recommended by manufacturers; it is difficult to interpret; and it poses the risk of changing the device's performance. It is easier and more accurate for the patient to note when the medication was started, the number of doses to be taken each day, and the number of doses in the canister and from this information to calculate a discard date. For example, if a canister has 200 actuations (this information is always indicated on the canister label) and four puffs are taken each day, the canister

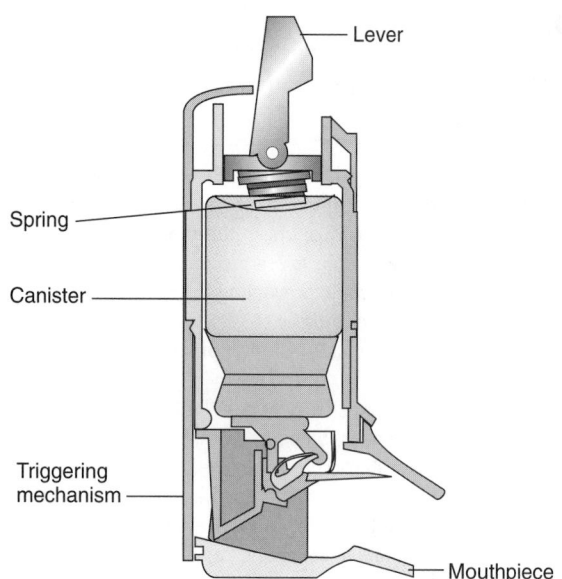

Figure 34-20 Schematic drawing of breath-actuated metered dose inhaler. (Modified from materials courtesy 3M Corp., St. Paul, Minn.)

Box 34-4

Technique for Use of a Pressurized Metered Dose Inhaler with a Spacer or Valved Holding Chamber

1. Warm the pressurized metered dose inhaler (pMDI) canister to hand or body temperature.
2. Assemble the apparatus and make sure no objects are present in the device that could be aspirated or could obstruct outflow.
3. Shake the canister vigorously and hold it vertically.
4. Place the holding chamber in the mouth (or place the mask completely over the nose and mouth); breathe through the mouth.
5. Breathe normally and actuate at the beginning of inspiration. Small children and infants should continue to breathe through the device for five or six breaths. Larger breaths with breath holding may be encouraged in patients who can cooperate. Observe that the valve opens with inhalation.
6. Allow 30 seconds between actuations.

Modified from Fink JB. Aerosol device selection: evidence to practice. Respir Care 2000;45:874-885.

should be discarded 50 days or 7 weeks after the start date. This discard date should be written on the canister label on the day the canister is started.

The Autohaler (3M Corp., St. Paul, Minn.) is a flow-triggered pMDI designed to reduce the need for hand-breath coordination by firing in response to the patient's inspiratory effort (Figure 34-20). To use the Autohaler, the patient cocks a lever on top of the unit that spring loads the canister against a vane mechanism. When the patient's inspiratory flow exceeds 30 L/min, the vane moves, allowing the canister to be pressed into the actuator, firing the pMDI. In the United States this device is available only with the β-agonist pirbuterol. The flow required to actuate the device may be too great for some small children to generate, especially during acute exacerbations of disease.

Spacers and Valved Holding Chambers

Spacers and valved holding chambers are accessory devices that reduce oropharyngeal deposition of drug, ameliorate the bad taste of some medications, eliminate the cold Freon effect and, in the case of valved holding chambers, reduce the need for hand-breath coordination.[42] These devices reduce the pharyngeal dose of aerosol from the pMDI tenfold to fifteenfold. This reduces the total body dose from swallowed medications, which is an important consideration with steroid administration.

A **spacer** is a simple open-ended tube or bag that with sufficiently large device volume provides space for the pMDI plume to expand by allowing the CFC propellant to evaporate. To perform this function, a spacer must have an internal volume of more than 100 mL and provide a distance of 10 to 13 cm between the pMDI nozzle and the first wall or baffle. Smaller, inefficient spacers can reduce the res-

piratory dose by 60% and offer no protection against poor coordination of actuation and breathing pattern. Spacers with internal volumes greater than 100 mL generally provide some protection against early firing of the pMDI, although exhalation immediately after the actuation clears most of the aerosol from the device, wasting the dose.

A **valved holding chamber** (usually 140 to 750 mL in volume) allows the plume from the pMDI to expand and incorporates a one-way valve that permits the aerosol to be drawn from the chamber during inhalation only, diverting the exhaled gas to the atmosphere and not disturbing remaining aerosol suspended in the chamber (Figure 34-21). Patients with small tidal volumes may empty the aerosol from the chamber with five to six breaths except when there is an exceptionally large dead space. A valved holding chamber can also incorporate a mask for use with an infant, a child, or a patient unable to use a mouthpiece because of size, age, coordination, or mental status. With infants these masks must have minimal dead space and must be comfortable on the child's face, and the chamber must have a valve that opens or closes with the low inspiratory flow generated by the patient. The optimal technique for use of a valved holding chamber is shown in Box 34-4. The high oropharyngeal drug deposition with steroid pMDIs can increase the risk of oral yeast infections (thrush). Rinsing the mouth after steroid use can reduce this problem, but most pMDI steroid aerosol impaction occurs deeper in the pharynx, which is not easily rinsed. For this reason, steroid MDIs should always be used in combination with a valved holding chamber.

The belief that a jet nebulizer is better than a pMDI if the patient is not able to inhale with optimum technique is not supported by data. A patient who cannot perform an

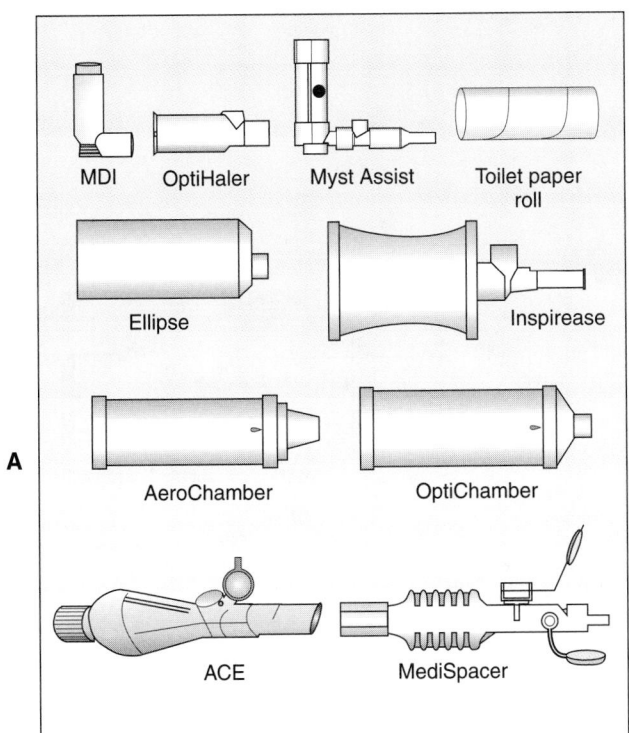

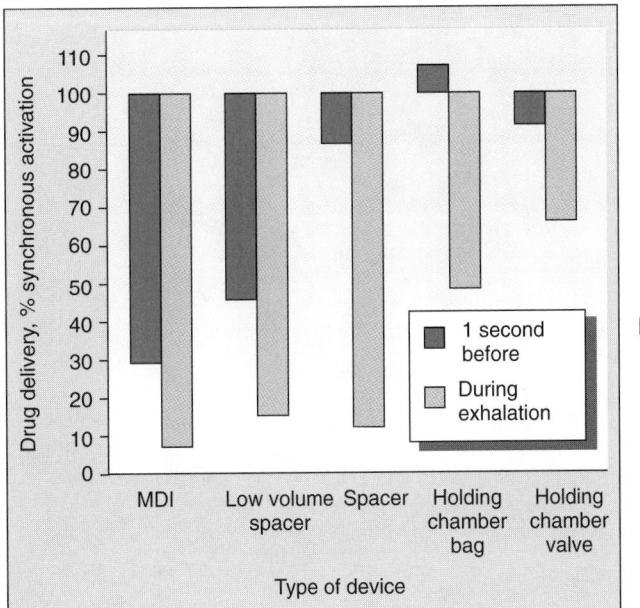

Figure 34-21   **A,** Devices used to deliver aerosol by pressurized metered dose inhaler (pMDI). **B,** In vitro comparison of albuterol delivery to the airway during tidal breathing with a pMDI alone and with low-volume spacers (OptiHaler, Myst Assist), large-volume spacers (toilet paper roll, Ellipse), a holding chamber bag (Inspirease), and valved holding chambers (AeroChamber, Optichamber, ACE, and MediSpacer). Actuation of the pMDI synchronized with the beginning of the breath (100%) was compared with actuation 1 second before the beginning of the breath and actuation during exhalation. The low volume spacers offered no advantage over the pMDI alone, whereas both spacers and holding chambers offered protection against actuating 1 second before the breath. Only the valved holding chambers delivered 70% or more of the dose when the pMDI was actuated during exhalation. (**A** and **B,** Modified from Wilkes W, Fink JB, Dhand R. J Aerosol Med 2001 [in press].)

optimal maneuver with a pMDI probably will be unable to perform an optimum maneuver with a jet nebulizer. Although optimum technique is always preferred, it often is difficult to attain with an infant, a small child, or a severely dyspneic patient. In such cases an alternative may be to increase the pMDI or nebulizer dosage.

Particles containing drug deposit in spacers and holding chambers cause a whitish buildup on the inner chamber walls. This residual drug poses no risk to the patient but may be rinsed off periodically. After a chamber or spacer is washed with tap water, it is less effective for the next 40 puffs, until the static charge in the chamber (which attracts small particles) is once again reduced. Use of regular dish soap reduces or eliminates this static charge. To reduce static charge on the device, which reduces drug delivery to the patient, the valved holding chamber or spacer should never be towel dried after cleaning. It is also important to instruct patients to actuate only one dose, not several doses, into the holding chamber and to inhale the drug from the chamber immediately after the pMDI is actuated.

Accessory devices either use the manufacturer-designed boot that comes with the pMDI or incorporate a universal canister adapter to fire the pMDI canister. Different formulations of pMDI drugs operate at different pressures and have different size orifices in the boot designed by the manufacturer for use exclusively with that pMDI. The output characteristics of a pMDI change if an adapter with a different size orifice is used. For this reason, spacers or holding chambers with universal canister adapters should be avoided and only those with a universal boot adapter should be used.

Dry Powder Inhalers

Dry powder inhalers (DPIs) create aerosols by drawing air through a dose of powdered medication (Figure 34-22). The powder contains micronized drug particles (less than 5 μm MMAD) with larger lactose or glucose particles (over 30 μm in diameter) or micronized drug particles bound into loose aggregates.[49] Micronized particles adhere strongly to each other and to most surfaces. Adding the larger particles of the carrier diminishes cohesive forces in the micronized drug powder so that separation into individual respirable particles (*deaggregation*) occurs more

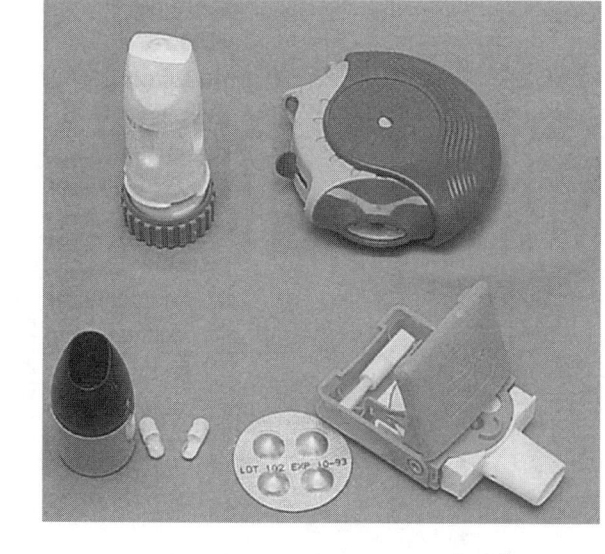

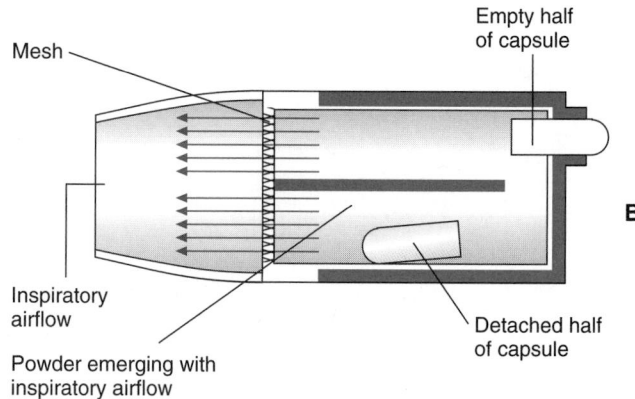

Mesh

Empty half
of capsule

Inspiratory
airflow

Powder emerging with
inspiratory airflow

Detached half
of capsule

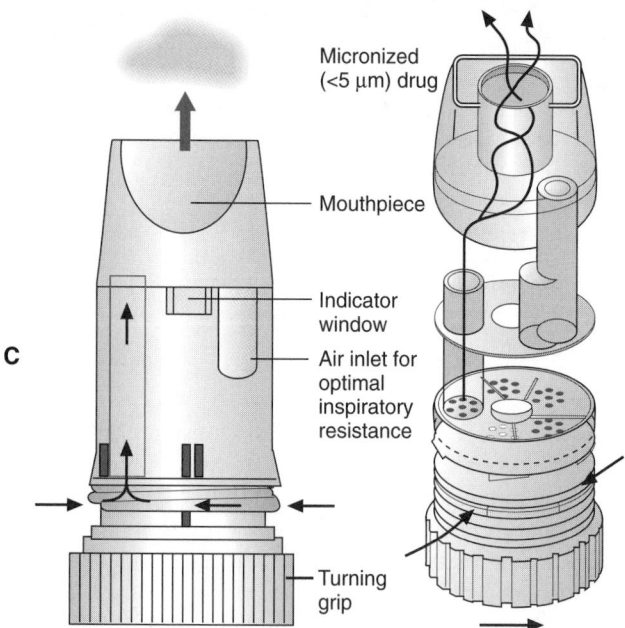

Micronized
(<5 µm) drug

Mouthpiece

Indicator
window

Air inlet for
optimal
inspiratory
resistance

Turning
grip

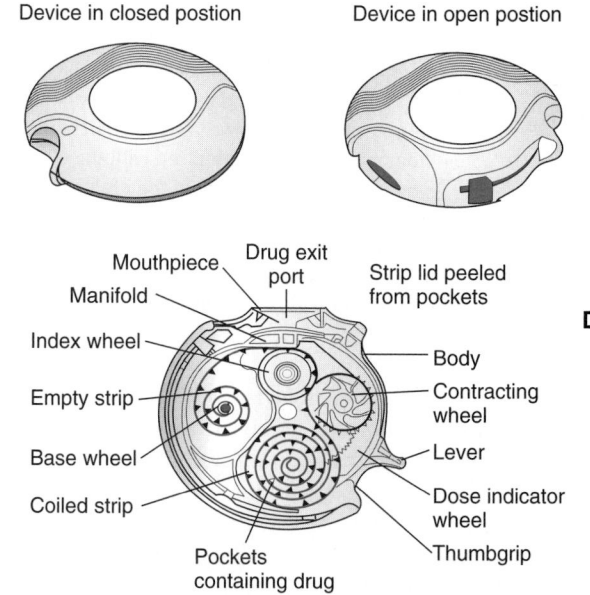

Device in closed postion

Device in open postion

Mouthpiece

Drug exit
port

Manifold

Strip lid peeled
from pockets

Index wheel

Body

Empty strip

Contracting
wheel

Base wheel

Lever

Coiled strip

Dose indicator
wheel

Thumbgrip

Pockets
containing drug

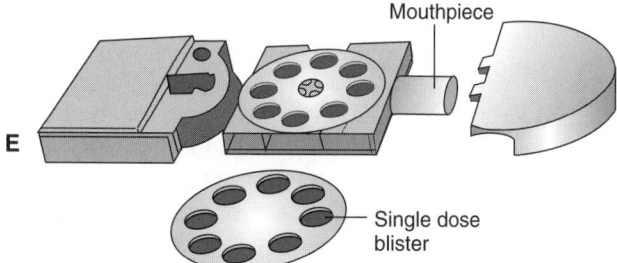

Mouthpiece

Single dose
blister

Figure 34-22 **A,** Dry powder inhalers. **B,** Rotahaler. **C,** Turbuhaler.
D, Diskus. **E,** Diskhaler. (**A,** Modified from Spiro S, MacCochran G.
Delivery of medication to the lungs. In: Albert R, Spiro S, Jett J, edi-
tors. Comprehensive respiratory medicine. St Louis: Mosby; 1999;
B-E, Modified from Dhand R, Fink JB. Dry powder inhalers. Respir
Care 1999;44:940-951.)

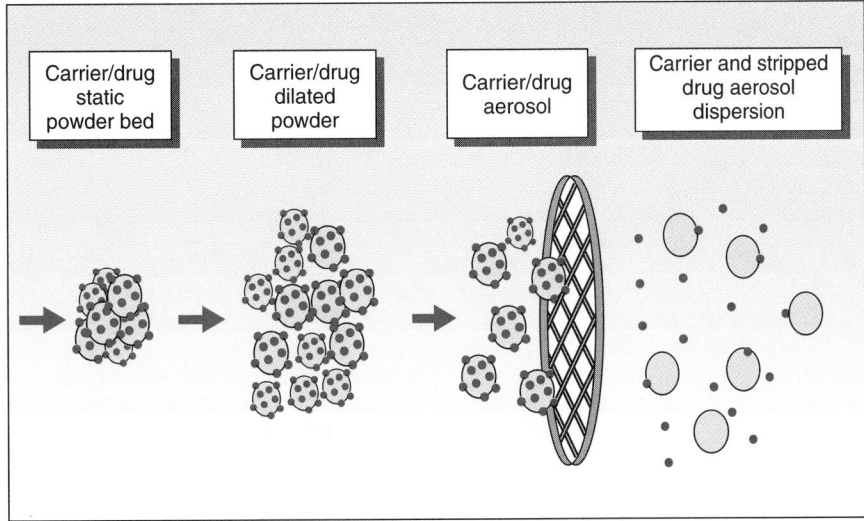

Figure 34-23   Aerosolization of dry powder. (Modified from Dhand R, Fink JB. Dry powder inhalers. Respir Care 1999;44:940-951.)

readily. Thus the carrier particles aid the flow of the drug powder from the device. Carriers also act as fillers by adding bulk to the powder when the unit dose of a drug is very small. The drug particles usually are loosely bound to the carrier and are stripped from the carrier by the energy provided by the patient's inhalation (Figure 34-23). The release of respirable particles of the drug requires inspiration at relatively high flow (30 to 120 L/min).[50,51] A high inspiratory flow results in pharyngeal impaction of the larger carrier particles that make up the bulk of the aerosol. The oropharyngeal impaction of carrier particles gives the patient the sensation of having inhaled a dose.

The internal geometry of the DPI device influences the resistance offered to inspiration and the inspiratory flow required to deaggregate and aerosolize the medication. Devices with higher resistance require a higher inspiratory flow to produce a dose. Inhalation through high-resistance DPIs may improve drug delivery to the lower respiratory tract compared with pMDIs[52] provided the patient can reliably generate the required flow rate. High-resistance devices have not been shown to improve either deposition or bronchodilation compared with low-resistance DPIs. DPIs with several components require correct assembly of the apparatus and/or priming of the device to ensure aerosolization of the dry powder. Some DPIs require periodic brushing to remove any residual powder that has accumulated in the device.

DPIs produce aerosols in which most of the drug particles are in the respirable range, with the distribution of particle sizes differing significantly among various DPIs. High ambient humidity causes the dry powder to clump, creating larger particles that are not as effectively aerosolized.[53] Air with a high moisture content is less efficient at deaggregating particles of dry powder than dry air, such that high ambient humidity increases the size of drug particles in the aerosol and may reduce drug delivery to the lungs. High ambient humidity also can result from exhalation into a DPI;

from bringing of a DPI into a warm indoor environment from the cold outdoors or a cold car, causing condensation to form inside the device; or from just being used in a warm, humid environment. Newer DPIs contain individual doses that are better protected from humidity. Humidity also can accumulate if the DPI is stored with the cap off.

Because the energy from the patient's inspiratory flow disperses the drug powder, the magnitude and duration of the patient's inspiratory effort influences aerosol generation from a DPI.[54] Failure to perform inhalation at a sufficiently fast inspiratory flow reduces the dose of the drug emitted by the DPI and increases the distribution of particle sizes within the aerosol. Research on active DPI delivery devices is underway. These devices use either a small motor and impeller or compressed gas propulsion to disperse the powder. With active DPIs, aerosol production and airway deposition are less influenced by the patient's inspiratory flow than with DPIs that rely solely on patient effort for aerosol production.

Breath coordination is also important during use of a DPI. Exhalation into a DPI blows out the powder from the device and reduces drug delivery. Moreover, the humidity in the exhaled air reduces subsequent aerosol generation. For these reasons, patients must be instructed not to exhale into a DPI. Because DPIs are breath actuated, they reduce the problem of coordinating inspiration with actuation. Using a DPI differs in important respects from the technique used to inhale drugs from a pMDI (Box 34-5). Although DPIs are easier to use than pMDIs, as many as 25% of patients may use DPIs improperly.[55] DPIs are critically dependent on inspiratory airflow to generate the aerosol; therefore they should be used with caution, if at all, in a very young or ill child, the weak, the elderly, and those with altered mental status. Patients may need repeated instruction before they can master the use of a DPI, and periodic assessment is necessary to ensure that patients continue to use optimum technique.

Box 34-5

Technique for Use of Dry Powder Inhalers

Rotahaler
1. Insert the capsule into the device.
2. Twist the device to break the capsule.
3. Keep the device level while inhaling the dose.
4. Hold the breath for 4 to 10 seconds.
5. Remove the device from the mouth and exhale.
6. Store the device in a cool, dry place.

Diskhaler
1. Remove the mouthpiece cover.
2. Pull out the tray.
3. Place the disk on the wheel (numbers up).
4. Rotate the disk by sliding the tray in and out.
5. Lift the back of the lid until it is fully upright so that the needle pierces both sides of the blister.
6. Keep the device level while inhaling the dose.
7. Hold the breath for 4 to 10 seconds.
8. Remove the device from the mouth and exhale.
9. Once a week, brush off any powder remaining in the device.
10. Store the device in a cool, dry place.

Diskus
1. Open the device.
2. Slide the lever.
3. Keep the device level while inhaling the dose.
4. Hold the breath for 4 to 10 seconds.
5. Remove the device from the mouth and exhale.
6. Store the device in a cool, dry place.

Turbuhaler
1. Twist and remove the cover.
2. Hold the inhaler upright (mouthpiece up).
3. Turn the grip right, then left until it clicks.
4. Inhale the dose (the inhaler may be held upright or horizontal).
5. Hold the breath for 4 to 10 seconds.
6. Remove the device from the mouth and exhale.
7. Replace the cover and twist to close.
8. Store the device in a cool, dry place.

Modified from Dhand R, Fink J. Dry powder inhalers. Respir Care 1999;44:940-951.

Selection of an Aerosol Delivery Device

Each type of aerosol delivery device has advantages and disadvantages (Table 34-3; CPGs 34-2 and 34-3). The choice of device often is determined by patient preference or clinician bias. In some cases the choice of device is dictated by the drug to be delivered (for example, antibiotics are available only for nebulizer delivery). Whenever possible, patients should use only one type of aerosol delivery device. The technique for the use of each device is different, and repeated instruction is necessary to ensure that the patient uses the device appropriately. Using different devices can be confusing for patients and may reduce their compliance with therapy.

For most patients the pMDI (often with a valved holding chamber) is a convenient, cost-effective aerosol delivery device. The jet nebulizer is a convenient but not mandatory device when high doses are needed and when the patient has difficulty mastering the use of a pMDI. A DPI can be considered as an alternative to a pMDI for patients who can generate inspiratory flow rates greater than 30 to 60 L/min and who are unable to use a pMDI effectively.

To improve compliance, aerosol therapy should be administered with some easily remembered activity of daily living. For twice daily administration, medications can be kept with the toothbrush and inhaled just before teeth brushing. This also reduces aerosol corticosteroid deposition in the oropharynx. It is always best to avoid regular use of medication at school, because the inconvenience can significantly reduce compliance and may be an embarrassment to some children. However, rescue medication must be available at school or day care or the caretaker's home. It helps to prepare written guidelines for use of the medication, and the guidelines must be distributed to all places where the child stays, such as home, school, or the residences of both parents in cases of divorce or separation.

Lack of response to inhaled asthma medication can be related to a number of factors, including incorrect inhalation technique, inhalation from an empty canister, failure to take preventive medications as prescribed, a change in the patient's environment, or perhaps misdiagnosis. For example, children who have aspirated a foreign body or who have gastroesophageal reflux disease or psychogenic wheeze have a poor response to asthma therapy, and infants with tracheomalacia or bronchopulmonary dysplasia may even worsen after inhaling a bronchodilator aerosol because of increased dynamic airway collapse.

Age-Specific Angle

Dry powder inhalers (DPIs) are not recommended for patients with acute bronchospasm or children under 6 years of age.

TABLE 34-3

Advantages and Disadvantages of Various Aerosol Delivery Devices

Device	Advantages	Disadvantages
Jet nebulizer	Patient coordination is not required. High doses can be given. No chlorofluorocarbon (CFC) is released.	System is expensive. Device is not portable; a pressurized gas source is required. More time is required for aerosol administration. Contamination is possible. Preparation of the device is required before treatment. Not all medications can be used with this device. Device is less efficient (more wasteful) than others.
Ultrasonic nebulizer (USN)	Patient coordination is not required. High doses can be given. No CFC is released. Device has a small dead volume. Device is quiet. Delivery is faster than with a jet nebulizer. Less drug is lost during exhalation.	Device is expensive. Contamination is possible. System is prone to malfunction. Not all medications can be used with this device. Preparation of the device is required before treatment.
Metered dose inhaler (MDI)	System is convenient. Device is less expensive than a nebulizer. Device is portable. No drug preparation is required. Device is difficult to contaminate. Treatment time is shorter than with a nebulizer.	Patient coordination is essential. Patient actuation is required. Large pharyngeal deposition occurs. High doses are difficult to deliver. Not all medications can be used with this device. Many of these devices use CFC propellants.
Metered dose inhaler with holding chamber	Less patient coordination is required. Less pharyngeal deposition occurs.	Device is more complex for some patients. System is more expensive than an MDI alone. Device is less portable than an MDI.
Dry powder inhaler	Less patient coordination is required. Propellant is not required. Device is breath activated.	System requires moderate to high inspiratory flow. Some units are single dose. High pharyngeal deposition is possible. Not all medications can be used with this device. High doses are difficult to deliver.

From AARC consensus statement: aerosols and delivery devices. Respir Care 2000;45:589-596.

Because most therapeutic aerosols are administered in the home, patient education and adherence to written medication and action plans are crucial. Standard nebulizers and pMDIs have no intrinsic mechanism for tracking use or compliance. With the pMDI this includes no mechanism to track how many doses remain in the canister. If accurately completed, medication diaries can help track medication use and the use of rescue medications in conjunction with monitoring of prescription refill records. Numerous devices are entering the market that can directly track use and monitor compliance. These include electronic devices integrated with the nebulizer that track the number of breaths taken, the size of the breaths, and the duration and frequency of treatment, as well as simple counting devices attached to the pMDI actuator boot.

More sophisticated devices allow monitoring both of pMDI use and expiratory maneuvers for later transmission to the caregiver. Some of the new DPI devices contain a built-in counter that advances each time a dose is loaded (Figure 34-24). These devices also give a visual signal when only a few doses are left.

Aerosol Delivery during Mechanical Ventilation

Aerosolized drugs are often administered to mechanically ventilated patients (CPG 34-4).[56-59] The ventilator circuit typically is a closed system that is pressurized during operation, requiring the nebulizer or pMDI to be attached with

CPG 34-2

Selection of an Aerosol Delivery Device for Neonatal and Pediatric Patients

Indication

An aerosol delivery system is indicated when a medication approved for inhalation is prescribed.

Contraindications

Contraindications associated with specific medications may exist, and pharmaceutical information should be consulted for relative contraindications.

A metered dose inhaler (MDI) or dry powder inhaler (DPI) should not be used for patients known to be allergic to medication preservatives or for patients unable to perform the respiratory maneuver required to disperse and deliver the drug.

Hazards and Complications

Aerosol delivery

Malfunction of the device or improper technique may result in underdosing; overuse may result in overdosing.

Specific pharmacologic agents may cause adverse side effects.

Inadequate patient training can lead to misuse of aerosol delivery devices prescribed for use in the home.

Small-volume nebulizer (SVN)

Continuous nebulizer flow increases tidal volume and associated pressure during volume-targeted ventilation.

Continuous flow creates a bias flow in the ventilator circuit and may interfere with patient triggered modes of ventilation.

Continuous flow of aerosol may damage the expiratory flow transducers found in some ventilators.

Continuous flow of gas from a flowmeter or compressor to an in-line nebulizer used with a continuous flow ventilator may result in an excess of flow and may cause an increase in airway pressure and/or expiratory retard or positive end-expiratory pressure (PEEP).

Continuous flow of gas from a flowmeter or compressor to an in-line nebulizer used with a ventilator may result in a variable fractional inspired oxygen concentration (F_{IO_2}).

Aerosol particles may deposit and crystallize on expiratory mechanisms and may create inadvertent expiratory resistance or PEEP.

Medication reservoirs may become contaminated and can be a source of infection.

Diluents that are not isotonic may increase airway reactivity.

Metered dose inhaler (MDI)

The volume of gas discharged with actuation of the canister or inhaler may add a clinically important volume to tidal volume, particularly in neonates.

Additional dead space volume can occur when a spacer device is placed at the end of an artificial airway.

The volume of gas discharged from the MDI may affect the F_{IO_2}.

Inappropriate patient use may result in underdosing or overdosing.

Reactions to propellants and other additives may occur, including coughing and wheezing.

Chlorofluorocarbons may contribute to ozone depletion.

Oropharyngeal impaction from a corticosteroid supplied in MDI form may cause local side effects.

Dry powder inhaler (DPI)

The dry powder may cause airway irritation.

A reaction to lactose or glucose carriers may occur.

Large-volume nebulizer

Side effects may occur at any time during continuous nebulization; frequent assessment is required.

Medication reservoirs may become contaminated and can be a source of infection.

Modified from AARC Clinical practice guideline: selection of an aerosol delivery device for neonatal and pediatric patients. Respir Care 1995;40:1325-1335. CPG, Clinical practice guideline.

CPG 34-3

Aerosol Delivery Devices

Indication

Aerosol delivery devices are required when medications must be administered as an aerosol to the lower airways; such medications include the following drug classifications: β-adrenergic agents, anticholinergic agents (antimuscarinics), antiinflammatory agents (for example, corticosteroids), mediator-modifying compounds (for example, cromolyn sodium), and mucokinetics.

Contraindications

There are no contraindications to the administration of aerosols by inhalation.

Contraindications related to a specific medication may exist; the package insert should be consulted for these product-specific contraindications.

Hazards and Complications

Malfunction of the device or improper technique may result in underdosing or overdosing.

Complications of a specific pharmacologic agent may occur.

Cardiotoxic effects of Freon have been reported as an idiosyncratic response that may be a problem with excessive use of a metered dose inhaler (MDI).

Freon may affect the environment by its effect on the ozone layer.

Repeated exposure to aerosols has been reported to produce asthmatic symptoms in some caregivers.

Modified from AARC Clinical practice guideline: aerosol delivery devices. Respir Care 1992;37:891-897. CPG, Clinical practice guideline.

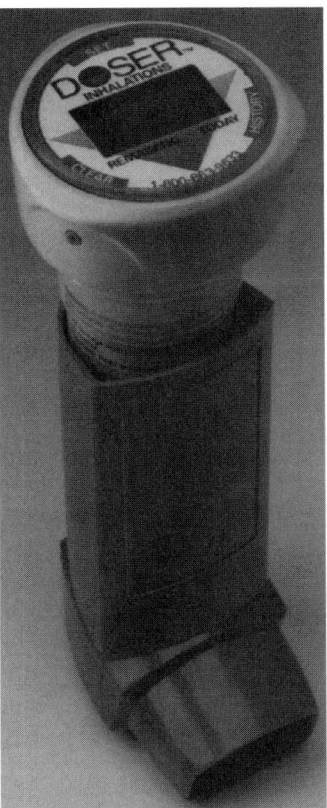

Figure 34-24 Doser device attached to a metered dose inhaler to determine the number of actuations of the inhaler.

$\mathcal{B}$OX 34-6

Technique for Aerosol Delivery by Nebulizer during Mechanical Ventilation

1. Fill the nebulizer with the drug solution to the optimum fill volume.
2. Place the nebulizer in the inspiratory line at least 30 cm from the patient's Y-piece.
3. Ensure that the airflow through the nebulizer is 6 to 8 L/min. The nebulizer may be operated continuously or only during inspiration (the latter method has proved more efficient for aerosol delivery). Some ventilators provide inspiratory gas flow to the nebulizer. Continuous gas flow from an external source also can be used to power the nebulizer.
4. Ensure that the tidal volume is adequate (500 mL or higher in adults). Use a duty cycle over 0.3 if possible.
5. If necessary, adjust the minute volume, sensitivity trigger, and alarms to compensate for additional airflow through the nebulizer.
6. Turn off the flow-by or continuous flow on the ventilator and remove the heat and moisture exchanger.
7. Check the nebulizer for adequate aerosol generation throughout its use.
8. Disconnect the nebulizer when all the medication has been nebulized or when no more aerosol is being produced. Store the nebulizer under aseptic conditions.
9. Reconnect the ventilator circuit and reinstate the original ventilator and alarm settings.

Modified from Fink JB, Tobin MJ, Dhand J. Respir Care 1999;44:53-69.

$\mathcal{B}$OX 34-7

Technique for Use of a Pressurized Metered Dose Inhaler during Mechanical Ventilation

1. Minimize the inspiratory flow rate during administration.
2. Aim for an inspiratory time (excluding the inspiratory pause) of over 0.3 of total breath duration.
3. Make sure the ventilator breath is synchronized with the patient's inspiration.
4. Shake the pressurized metered dose inhaler (pMDI) canister vigorously.
5. Place the canister in the actuator of a cylindric spacer situated in the inspiratory limb of the ventilator circuit. With pMDIs it is preferable to use a spacer that remains in the ventilator circuit so that the circuit need not be disconnected for each bronchodilator treatment. Although bypassing the humidifier can increase aerosol delivery, it prolongs the treatment and requires disconnection of the ventilator circuit.
6. Actuate the pMDI to synchronize with the precise onset of inspiration by the ventilator.
7. Allow passive exhalation.
8. Repeat actuations at 20- to 30-second intervals until the total dose has been delivered.

Modified from Fink JB, Tobin MJ, Dhand J. Respir Care 1999;44:53-69.

connectors that maintain the integrity of the circuit during operation. With mechanical ventilation the inspiratory flow pattern and respiratory rate are different from those of spontaneous respiration, and this may influence aerosol delivery to the lower respiratory tract. The techniques used to deliver aerosolized bronchodilators during mechanical ventilation by nebulizer and pMDI are presented in Boxes 34-6 and 34-7. A number of factors affect aerosol delivery during mechanical ventilation (Figure 34-25).

Abrupt angles in the ventilator circuit, such as the 90-degree connector often are used to connect the ventilator circuit Y-piece to the endotracheal tube. This results in points of impaction and turbulence not found in the normal airway. Although the endotracheal tube is narrower than the trachea, its smooth interior surface may create a more laminar flow path than the structures of the glottis and larynx and may be less of a barrier to aerosol delivery than the ventilator circuit. Deposition of aerosol in the endotracheal tube and ventilator circuit is thought to significantly reduce the fraction of aerosol delivered to the lower respiratory tract. Until recently, the consensus was that the efficiency of aerosol delivery to the lower respiratory tract in mechanically ventilated patients was much lower that that in ambulatory patients.[59] However, it has been reported that twice as much aerosol from the pMDI deposits in the ventilator circuit as in the endotracheal tube under both dry and humidified conditions, raising some doubt that the en-

CPG 34-4

Selection of a Device for Administration of a Bronchodilator and Evaluation of the Response to Therapy in Mechanically Ventilated Patients

Indication

Aerosol administration of a bronchodilator and evaluation of the response are indicated whenever bronchoconstriction or increased airway resistance is documented or suspected in mechanically ventilated patients.

Contraindications

Some assessment maneuvers may be contraindicated for patients in extremis (for example, a prolonged inspiratory pause for patients with high auto-PEEP).

Certain medications may be contraindicated in some patients; the package insert should be consulted for these product-specific contraindications.

Hazards and Complications

Specific assessment procedures may have inherent hazards or complications (for example, inspiratory pause or expiratory pause).

Inappropriate selection of a device or inappropriate use of a device and/or technique variables may result in underdosing.

Device malfunction may result in reduced drug delivery and may compromise the integrity of the ventilator circuit.

Complications may arise from specific pharmacologic agents. Higher doses of β-agonists delivered by an MDI or nebulizer may cause adverse effects secondary to systemic absorption of the drug or propellants. The potential for hypokalemia and atrial and ventricular dysrhythmias may exist with high doses in critically ill patients.

Aerosol medications, propellants, or cold, dry gas that bypasses the natural upper respiratory tract may cause bronchospasm or irritation of the airway. Although the efficiency of aerosol delivery from an MDI can be increased by actuating of the canister into a narrow-gauge catheter with the catheter positioned at the end of the endotracheal tube, a study in rabbits has shown that this technique produces necrotizing inflammation and mucosal ulceration, probably caused by the topical effect of the oleic acid used for its surfactant property and the chlorofluorocarbons (CFCs); therefore such administration is not recommended. Further study of the practice is needed.

The aerosol device or adapter used and the technique of operation may affect ventilator performance characteristics or alter the sensitivity of the alarm systems.

Addition of gas to the ventilator circuit from a nebulizer may increase volumes, flows, and peak airway pressures, thereby altering the intended pattern of ventilation. Ventilator setting adjustments made to accommodate the additional gas flow during nebulization must be reset at the end of the treatment.

Addition of gas from a nebulizer into the ventilator circuit may result in the patient's becoming unable to trigger the ventilator during nebulization, leading to hypoventilation.

At least one early anecdotal report described cardiac toxicity caused by CFCs used as propellants in MDIs. Adverse cardiac effects are unlikely to occur with the doses recommended in clinical practice because of the short half-life of CFCs in the blood (less than 40 seconds), particularly when at least a short interval is maintained between doses.

Modified from AARC Clinical practice guideline: selection of a device for administration of a bronchodilator and evaluation of the response to therapy in mechanically ventilated patients. Respir Care 1999;44:105-113.
CPG, Clinical practice guideline.

dotracheal tube is the primary barrier to aerosol.[60] Aerosol impaction in the endotracheal tube can reduce the efficiency of aerosol delivery in children,[56] but the efficiency of aerosol delivery beyond the endotracheal tube does not vary between tube sizes that measure internal diameters of 7 to 9 mm.

Ventilator circuits are designed to heat and humidify the inspired gas. Humidity can increase particle size and reduce deposition during mechanical ventilation. Humidification of inhaled gas reduces aerosol deposition by approximately 40%, probably because of an increase in particle loss in the ventilator circuit.[61] Some experts have proposed bypassing of the humidifier during aerosol administration. However, some nebulizers require as long as 35 minutes to complete aerosolization,[62] and inhalation of dry gas for this length of time can damage the airway. In addition, disconnection of the ventilator circuit, which is required to bypass the humidifier, interrupts ventilation, and may increase the risk of ventilator-associated pneumonia.

Placement of a jet nebulizer 30 cm from the endotracheal tube is more efficient than placement between the inspiratory limb and the patient Y-piece because the inspiratory ventilator tubing acts as a spacer for the aerosol to accumulate between breaths.[63-65] Addition of a spacer between the nebulizer and the endotracheal tube modestly increases aerosol delivery.[66] Operating the nebulizer only during inspiration is more efficient for aerosol delivery than continuous aerosol generation.[64,65]

Because the pMDI cannot be used with the actuator designed by the manufacturer, a third-party actuator is required (Figure 34-26). The size, shape, and design of these actuators affect the amount of respirable drug available to the patient and may vary with different pMDI formulations.[67] A pMDI with a spacer in the inspiratory limb of the ventilator circuit produces a fourfold to sixfold greater delivery of aerosol than pMDI actuation into a connector attached directly to the endotracheal tube or into an in-line device that lacks a chamber. When an elbow adapter

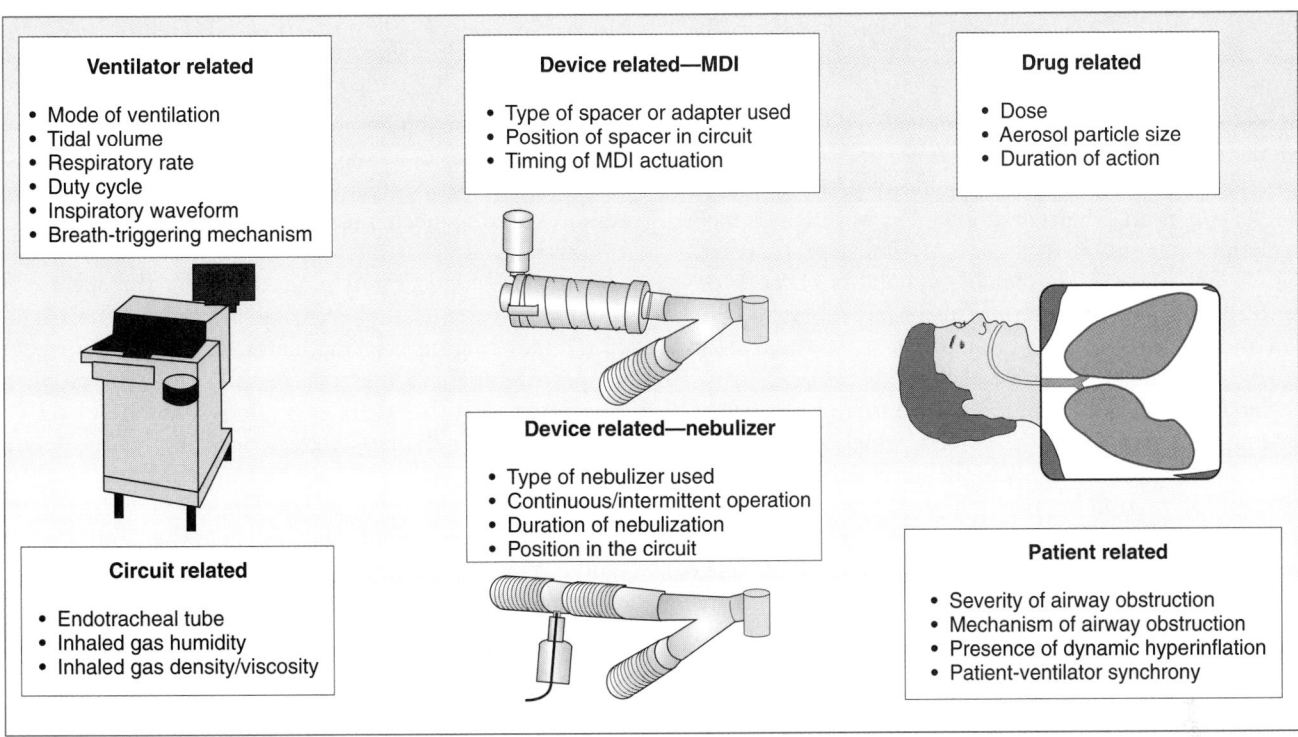

Figure 34-25   Factors that affect delivery of aerosols during mechanical ventilation. (Modified from Dhand R, Tobin MJ. Bronchodilator delivery with metered-dose inhalers in mechanically ventilated patients. Eur Respir J 1996;9:585-595.)

connected to the endotracheal tube is used, actuation of the pMDI out of synchrony with inspiratory airflow delivers very little aerosol to the lower respiratory tract.[68] This may explain the lack of therapeutic effect with this type of adapter in some studies after administration of very high doses of aerosol from a pMDI.[69]

Aerosol can be delivered during patient-triggered ventilation provided the patient is breathing in synchrony with the ventilator. Albuterol deposition has been reported to be more than 20% higher during simulated spontaneous breaths than with controlled breaths of equivalent tidal volume. For efficient aerosol delivery to the lower respiratory tract, the tidal volume of the ventilator-delivered breath must be larger than the volume of the ventilator tubing and endotracheal tube. Tidal volumes of 500 mL or greater in adults are associated with adequate aerosol delivery, but the higher pressures required to deliver larger tidal volumes can be detrimental to the lungs. During mechanical ventilation, delivery of a large tidal volume,[70] use of an end-inspiratory pause,[71] and use of a slow inspiratory flow[72] have little effect on aerosol delivery and deposition. Aerosol delivery by nebulizer is directly correlated with higher inspiratory time, because longer inspiratory times allow a higher proportion of the aerosol generated by the nebulizer to be inhaled with each breath. Because nebulizers generate aerosol over several minutes, longer inspiratory times have a cumulative effect in improving aerosol delivery. However, pMDIs produce aerosol only over a portion of a single inspiration, and the mechanism by which longer inspiratory times increase aerosol

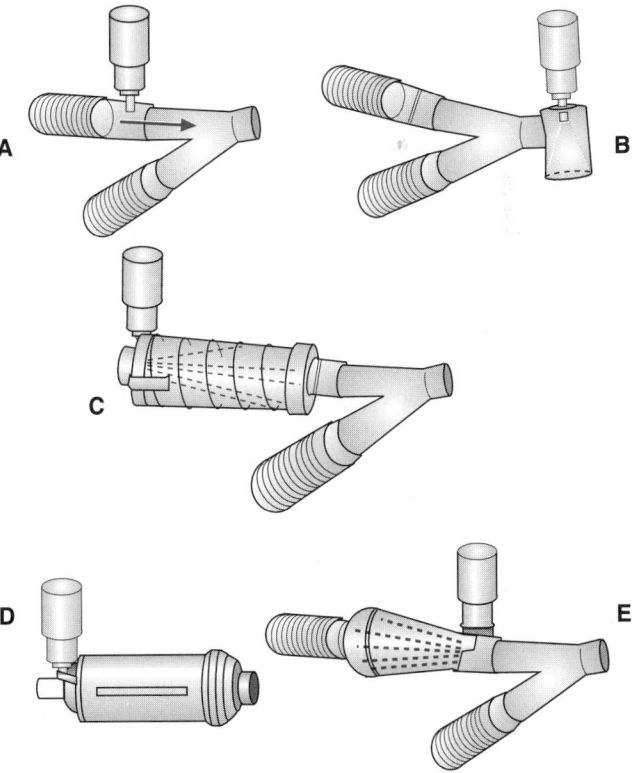

Figure 34-26   Devices to adapt a metered dose inhaler to a ventilator circuit. **A,** In-line device. **B,** Elbow device. **C,** Collapsible chamber device. **D,** Chamber device. **E,** Chamber device in which aerosol is directed retrograde into the ventilator circuit. (Modified from Dhand R, Tobin MJ. Bronchodilator delivery with metered-dose inhalers in mechanically ventilated patients. Eur Respir J 1996;9:585-595.)

delivery is unclear. Aerosol particles that deposit in the ventilator tubing may be swept off the walls and entrained by longer periods of inspiratory flow. Approximately 5% of the nominal dose of albuterol administered by a pMDI is exhaled in mechanically ventilated patients,[60] whereas less than 1% is exhaled by ambulatory patients using a pMDI. The mean exhaled fraction (7%) with nebulizers in mechanically ventilated patients is similar to that with pMDIs, but there is considerable variability between patients. Helium-oxygen mixtures also affect aerosol deposition and in vitro modeling has reported a 50% increase in deposition of albuterol from a pMDI.[73]

Nebulizers placed in-line in the ventilator circuit can become contaminated with bacteria, which are then carried as microaerosols directly to the lower respiratory tract. Such contamination has been reported even after a single use of a nebulizer.[74] The federal Centers for Disease Control and Prevention (CDC) recommend that nebulizers be sterile at the start of nebulization, and that they be removed from the ventilator circuit after each use, disassembled, cleaned with sterile water, rinsed, and air dried. Care should be taken to store the nebulizer aseptically between uses. When the collapsible chamber spacer remains in the ventilator circuit between treatments, condensate collects inside it.[75] Care must be taken to prevent the condensate in the spacer from being washed into the patient's respiratory tract when the spacer is pulled open during use. When a noncollapsible spacer chamber is used to actuate a pMDI, it should be removed from the ventilator circuit between treatments. No studies have demonstrated contamination problems with administration of aerosol from a pMDI during mechanical ventilation.

Leaving a pMDI noncollapsible chamber device in-line is not practical because of the increased compressible volume it adds to the circuit. Depending on the FiO_2 and the propellant gas volume, an in-line pMDI actuation theoretically may result in a hypoxic gas mixture to an infant receiving a tidal volume less than 100 mL. It is possible to deliver a pMDI aerosol medication to an intubated neonate, especially those medications available only in pMDI preparations. If a chamber adapter is used, the infant must be removed from the circuit, the chamber placed in-line, and the infant reattached to the circuit before the pMDI medication is administered. The large dead space volume created through placement of a spacer or chamber at the end of the endotracheal tube must also be considered during administration of pMDI medications to an infant.

Studies that have examined the dose response to bronchodilators in mechanically ventilated patients found effects with administration of 2.5 mg of albuterol via a standard nebulizer even under less than optimum conditions or with four actuations (400 μg) with a pMDI.[76-79] Although the efficiency is greater with a pMDI and spacer, the dose delivered with the nebulizer is greater because of the higher nominal dose placed into the nebulizer.[78] In the routine clinical setting, higher doses of bronchodilators may be needed for patients with severe airway obstruction or if the technique of administration is not optimal. When

the technique of administration is carefully executed, most mechanically ventilated patients in stable condition who have chronic obstructive pulmonary disease (COPD) achieve near-maximum bronchodilation after administration of four puffs of albuterol with a pMDI or 2.5 mg with a nebulizer. Dosing requirements for infants and small children during mechanical ventilation have not yet been established.

Nebulizers and pMDIs produce similar therapeutic effects in mechanically ventilated patients. The use of pMDIs for routine bronchodilator therapy in ventilator-supported patients is preferred because of several problems associated with the use of nebulizers. The rate of aerosol production by nebulizers varies considerably, not only in nebulizers from different manufacturers but also in different batches of the same brand. The gas flow driving the nebulizer produces additional airflow in the ventilator circuit, requiring adjustment of tidal volume and inspiratory flow when the nebulizer is in use. When patients are unable to trigger the ventilator during assisted modes of mechanical ventilation (because of the additional nebulizer gas flow), hypoventilation can result.[80] Aerosol delivery by pMDI is easy to administer, involves less personnel time, provides a reliable dose of the drug, and is free of the risk of bacterial contamination. When pMDIs are used with a collapsible cylindric spacer, the ventilator circuit need not be disconnected with each treatment; thus reducing the risk of ventilator-associated pneumonia.

𝒦ᴇʏ 𝒫ᴏɪɴᴛs

- The upper airway is an efficient humidifier.
- The primary goal of humidity therapy is to maintain normal physiologic conditions by providing heat and humidity in the inspired gas.
- Humidifiers can provide active or passive humidification.
- Active humidifiers may be heated or unheated.
- Heated circuits can be used to maintain heat and humidity in gas delivery.
- The humidity delivery device should be assessed for condensate near the patient.
- HMEs are effective humidification devices for many mechanically ventilated patients.
- Bland aerosol therapy is used to deliver saline or water for therapeutic and diagnostic purposes.
- The MMAD of aerosols for medical purposes should be 1 to 5 μm.
- Devices used to deliver therapeutic aerosols include jet nebulizers, ultrasonic nebulizers, metered dose inhalers, metered dose inhalers with a spacer or holding chamber, and dry powder inhalers.
- The metered dose inhaler is an effective aerosol medication delivery device even in small children and mechanically ventilated patients.

References

1. Shelley MP, Lloyd GM, Park GR. A review of the mechanisms and the methods of humidification of inspired gas. Intensive Care Med 1988;14:1-9.
2. Irlbeck D. Normal mechanisms of heat and moisture exchange in the respiratory tract. Respir Care Clin North Am 1998;4:189-198.
3. Branson RD. The effects of inadequate humidity. Respir Care Clin North Am 1998;4:199-214.
4. Rankin N. What is optimum humidity? Respir Care Clin North Am 1998;4:321-328.
5. Williams RD. Effects of excessive humidity. Respir Care Clin North Am 1998;4:215-228.
6. Primiano FP Jr, Montague FW Jr, Saidel GM. Measurement system for water vapor and temperature dynamics. J Appl Physiol 1984;56:1679-1685.
7. Chatburn RL, Primiano FP. A rational basis for humidity therapy. Respir Care 1987;32:249-253.
8. Tarnow-Mordi WO, Reid R, Griffiths P, et al. Low inspired gas humidity and respiratory complications in very low birth weight infants. J Pediatr 1988;114:438.
9. Anderson S, Herbring BG, Widman B. Accidental profound hypothermia. Br J Anaesth 1970;42:653.
10. Greenspan JS, Wolfson MR, Shaffer TH. Airway responsiveness to low inspired gas temperature in preterm neonates. J Pediatr 1991;118:443-445.
11. Hill TV, Sorbello JG. Humidity outputs of large reservoir nebulizers. Respir Care 1987;32:225-260.
12. Peterson BD. Heated humidifiers. Respir Care Clin North Am 1998;4:243-260.
13. Miyao H, Hirokawa T, Miyasaka K, et al. Relative humidity, not absolute humidity, is of great importance when using a humidifier with a heating wire. Crit Care Med 1992;20:674-679.
14. Miyao H, Miyasaka K, Hirokawa T, et al. Consideration of the international standard for airway humidification using simulated secretions in an artificial airway. Respir Care 1996;41:43-49.
15. Wilkes AR. Heat and moisture exchangers: structure and function. Respir Care Clin North Am 1998;4:261-279.
16. Ploysongsang Y, Branson D, Rashkin MC, et al. Effect of flow rate and duration of use on the pressure drop across six artificial noses. Respir Care 1989;343:902-907.
17. American National Standards Institute. American national standards for nebulizers and humidifiers. Washington, DC: The Institute; 1979. p. Z79.9.
18. Emergency Care Research Institute. Heated humidifiers. Health Devices 1987;16:223-250.
19. Darin J, Broadwell J, MacDonnell R. An evaluation of water vapor output from four brands of unheated prefilled humidifiers. Respir Care 1981;27:41.
20. Seigel D, Romo B. Extended use of prefilled humidifier reservoirs and the likelihood of contamination. Respir Care 1990;35:806-810.
21. American College of Chest Physicians. National Heart, Lung, and Blood Institute National Conference on Oxygen Therapy. Respir Care 1984;29:922.
22. Iotti GA, Olivei MC, Palo A, et al. Unfavorable mechanical effects of heat and moisture exchangers in ventilated patients. Intensive Care Med 1997;23:399-405.
23. LeBourdelles G, Mier L, Fiquet B, et al. Comparison of the effects of heat and moisture exchangers and heated humidifiers on ventilation and gas exchange during weaning trials from mechanical ventilation. Chest 1996;110:1294-1298.
24. Pelosi P, Solca M, Ravagnan I, et al. Effects of heat and moisture exchangers on minute ventilation, ventilatory drive, and work of breathing during pressure-support ventilation in acute ventilatory failure. Crit Care Med 1996;24:1184-1188.
25. Hedley RM, Alt-Graham J. A comparison of the filtration properties of heat and moisture exchangers. Anaesthesia 1992;47:414-420.
26. Branson RD, Davis K. Evaluation of 21 passive humidifiers according to the ISO 9360 standard: moisture output, dead space, and flow resistance. Respir Care 1996;41:736-743.
27. Branson RD, Davis K Jr, Brown R, et al. Comparison of three humidification techniques during mechanical ventilation: patient selection, cost, and infection considerations. Respir Care 1996;41:809-816.
28. Hess D. Prolonged use of heat and moisture exchangers: why do we keep changing things? Crit Care Med 2000;28:1667-1668.
29. Newhouse MT, Dolovich MB. Control of asthma by aerosols. N Engl J Med 1986;315:870-874.
30. AARC Consensus statement: aerosols and delivery devices. Respir Care 2000;45:589-596.
31. Dolovich M. Physical principles underlying aerosol therapy. J Aerosol Med 1989;2:171-178.
32. Hess DR. Nebulizers: principles and performance. Respir Care 2000;45:609-622.
33. Hess D, Fisher D, Williams P, et al. Medication nebulizer performance: effects of diluent volume, nebulizer flow, and nebulizer brand, Chest 1996;110:498-505.
34. Hess DR, Acosta FL, Ritz RH, et al. The effect of heliox on nebulizer function using a beta-agonist bronchodilator. Chest 1999;115:184-189.
35. Malone RA, Hollie MC, Glynn-Barnhart A, et al. Optimal duration of nebulized albuterol therapy. Chest 1993;104:1114-1118.
36. Standaert TA, Morlin GL, Williams-Warren J, et al. Effects of repetitive use and cleaning techniques of disposable jet nebulizers on aerosol generation. Chest 1998;114:577-586.
37. Lowenthal D, Kattan M. Face masks versus mouthpieces for aerosol treatment of asthmatic children. Pediatr Pulmonol 1992;14:192-196.
38. Harrison R. Reproductive risk assessment with occupational exposure to ribavirin aerosol. Pediatr Infect Dis J 1990;9(Suppl):S102-S105.
39. Kacmarek RM, Kratohvil J. Evaluation of a double-enclosure double-vacuum unit scavenging system for ribavirin administration. Respir Care 1992;37:37-45.
40. Adderly RJ. Safety of ribavirin with mechanical ventilation. Pediatr Infect Dis J 1990;9(Suppl):S112-S114.
41. Phillips GD, Millard FJL. The therapeutic use of ultrasonic nebulizers in acute asthma. Respir Med 1994;88:387-389.
42. Nakanishi AK, Lamb BM, Foster C, et al. Ultrasonic nebulization of albuterol is no more effective than jet nebulization for the treatment of acute asthma in children. Chest 1997;97:1505-1508.
43. Thomas SH, O'Doherty MJ, Page CJ, et al. Delivery of ultrasonic nebulized aerosols to a lung model during mechanical ventilation. Am Rev Respir Dis 1993;148:872-877.
44. Fink JB. Metered dose inhalers, dry powder inhalers, and transitions. Respir Care 2000;45:623-625.
45. Hess D, Daugherty A, Simmons M. The volume of gas emitted from five metered dose inhalers at three levels of fullness. Respir Care 1992;37:444-447.
46. Guidry GG, Brown WD, Stogner SW, et al. Incorrect use of metered dose inhalers by medical personnel. Chest 1992;1010:31-33.
47. Kacmarek RM, Hess D. The interface between patient and aerosol generator. Respir Care 1991;36:952-972.

48. Johnson DH, Robart P. Inhaler technique of outpatients in the home. Respir Care 2000;45:1182-1187.

49. Dhand R, Fink JB. Dry powder inhalers. Respir Care 1999; 44:940-951.

50. Engel T, Heinig JH, Madsen F, et al. Peak inspiratory flow rate and inspiratory vital capacity of patients with asthma measured with and without a new dry powder inhaler device (Turbuhaler). Eur Respir J 1990;3:1037-1041.

51. Pederson S, Hansen OR, Fuglsang G. Influence of inspiratory flow rate upon the effect of a Turbuhaler. Arch Dis Child 1990;65:308-310.

52. Svartengren K, Lindestad PA, Svartengren M, et al. Added external resistance reduces oropharyngeal deposition and increases lung deposition of aerosol particles in asthmatics. Am J Respir Crit Care Med 1995;152:32-37.

53. Rajkumari NJ, Byron PR, Dalby RN. Testing of dry powder aerosol formulations in different environmental conditions. Int J Pharmacol 1995;113:123-130.

54. Timsina MP, Martin GP, Van der Kolk H, et al. The effect of inhalation flow on the performance of a dry powder inhalation system. Int J Pharmacol 1992;81:199-203.

55. Kesten S, Elias M, Cartier A, et al. Patient handling of a multidose dry powder inhalation device for albuterol. Chest 1994;105:1077-1081.

56. Fink JB, Dhand R. Bronchodilator therapy in mechanically ventilated patients. Respir Care 1999;44:53-69.

57. Dhand R, Tobin MJ. Bronchodilator delivery with metered dose inhalers in mechanically ventilated patients. Eur Respir J 1996;9:585-595.

58. Dhand R, Juran A, Tobin MJ. Bronchodilator delivery by metered dose inhaler in ventilator-supported patients. Am J Respir Crit Care Med 1995;151:1827-1833.

59. Dhand R. Special problems in aerosol delivery: artificial airways. Respir Care 2000;45:636-645.

60. Fink JB, Dhand R, Grychowski J, et al. Reconciling in vitro and in vivo measurements of aerosol delivery from a metered dose inhaler during mechanical ventilation and defining efficiency-enhancing factors. Am J Respir Crit Care Med 1999;159:63-68.

61. Fink JB, Dhand R, Duarte AG, et al. Deposition of aerosol from a metered dose inhaler during mechanical ventilation: an in vitro model. Am J Respir Crit Care Med 1996;154:382-387.

62. McPeck M, O'Riordan TG, Smaldone GC. Choice of mechanical ventilator: influence on nebulizer performance. Respir Care 1993;38:887-895.

63. Hughes JM, Saez J. Effects of nebulizer mode and position in a mechanical ventilator circuit on dose efficiency. Respir Care 1987;32:1131-1135.

64. O'Riordan TG, Greco MJ, Perry RJ, et al. Nebulizer function during mechanical ventilation. Am Rev Respir Dis 1992; 145:1117-1122.

65. O'Riordan TG, Palmer LB, Smaldone GC. Aerosol deposition in mechanically ventilated patients: optimizing nebulizer delivery. Am J Respir Crit Care Med 1994;149:214-219.

66. Harvey CJ, O'Doherty MJ, Page CJ, et al. Effect of a spacer on pulmonary aerosol deposition from a jet nebulizer during mechanical ventilation. Thorax 1995;50:50-53.

67. Fuller HD, Dolovich MB, Turpie FH, et al. Efficiency of bronchodilator aerosol delivery to the lungs from the metered dose inhaler in mechanically ventilated patients: a study comparing four different actuator devices. Chest 1994;105:214-218.

68. Diot P, Morra L, Smaldone GC. Albuterol delivery in a model of mechanical ventilation: comparison of metered dose inhaler and nebulizer efficiency. Am J Respir Crit Care Med 1995;152: 1391-1394.

69. Manthous CA, Hall JB, Schmidt GA, et al. Metered dose inhaler versus nebulized albuterol in mechanically ventilated patients. Am Rev Respir Dis 1993;148:1567-1570.

70. Mouloudi E, Katsanoulas K, Anastasaki M, et al. Bronchodilator delivery by metered dose inhaler in mechanically ventilated COPD patients: influence of tidal volume. Intensive Care Med 1999;25:1215-1221.

71. Mouloudi E, Katsanoulas K, Anastasaki M, et al. Bronchodilator delivery by metered dose inhaler in mechanically ventilated COPD patients: influence of end-inspiratory pause. Eur Respir J 1998;12:165-169.

72. Mouloudi E, Prinianakis G, Kondili E, et al. Effect of inspiratory flow rate on β_2-agonist–induced bronchodilation in mechanically ventilated COPD patients. Intensive Care Med 2001; 27:42-46.

73. Good M, Fink JB, Dhand R, et al. Improvement in aerosol delivery with helium-oxygen mixtures during mechanical ventilation. Am J Respir Crit Care Med 2001;163:109-114.

74. Craven DE, Lichtenberg DA, Goularte TA, et al. Contaminated medication nebulizers in mechanical ventilator circuits: a source of bacterial aerosols. Am J Med 1984;77:834-838.

75. Waugh JB, Waugh JB. Water accumulation in metered dose inhaler spacers under normal mechanical ventilation conditions. Heart Lung 2000;29:424-428.

76. Thomas SHL, O'Doherty MJ, Fidler HM, et al. Pulmonary deposition of a nebulized aerosol during mechanical ventilation. Thorax 1993;48:154-159.

77. Dhand R, Duarte AG, Jubran A, et al. Dose response to bronchodilator delivered by metered dose inhaler in ventilator-supported patients. Am J Respir Crit Care Med 1996;154: 388-393.

78. Marik P, Hogan J, Krikorian J. A comparison of bronchodilator therapy delivered by nebulization and metered dose inhaler in mechanically ventilated patients. Chest 1999;115: 1653-1657.

79. Duarte AG, Momii K, Bidani A. Bronchodilator therapy with metered dose inhaler and spacer versus nebulizer in mechanically ventilated patients: comparison of magnitude and duration of response. Respir Care 2000;45:817-823.

80. Beaty CD, Ritz RH, Benson MS. Continuous in-line nebulizers complicate pressure support ventilation. Chest 1989; 96:1360-1363.

CHAPTER 35

Secretion Clearance Techniques

James B. Fink
Dean R. Hess

CHAPTER OUTLINE

OBJECTIVES

1. Describe the mechanism of normal mucus transport in the lungs.
2. Describe the use of bland aerosol for sputum induction.
3. Demonstrate the techniques of nasotracheal suctioning, mechanical insufflation-exsufflation, postural drainage, manually assisted coughing, active cycle of breathing, autogenic drainage, incentive spirometry, intermittent positive pressure breathing, positive expiratory pressure, Flutter valve, Percussionaire, ThAIRapy Vest, and the Hayek oscillator.
4. List indications, contraindications, hazards, and precautions for nasotracheal suctioning, mechanical insufflation-exsufflation, postural drainage, manually assisted coughing, active cycle of breathing, autogenic drainage, incentive spirometry, intermittent positive pressure breathing, positive expiratory pressure, Flutter valve, Percussionaire, ThAIRapy Vest, and the Hayek oscillator.
5. Compare the advantages and disadvantages of various secretion clearance techniques.

KEY TERMS

Active Cycle of Breathing (ACB)	Forced Expiratory Technique (FET)	High-Frequency Oscillation of the Chest Wall (HFOCW)
Autogenic Drainage (AD)	High-Frequency Oscillation of the Airway (HFOA)	Huff Coughing
Bland Aerosol		Incentive Spirometry (IS)
Chest Physiotherapy (CPT)		

Difficulty in clearing airway secretions is a symptom of many conditions that compromise lung function. In normal lungs, mucociliary activity, breathing, and coughing are the primary mechanisms used to remove secretions. With disease, changes in volume and character of secretions, dyskinesia of the cilia, and instability of the airway reduce the ability to clear secretions from the airway. Difficulty with secretion clearance commonly occurs at the end of life.[1]

Efforts to clear secretions range from mechanical aspiration to postural drainage (PD) and breathing maneuvers. A variety of breathing maneuvers and mechanical devices have been used to assist patients in mobilizing secretions from the lower respiratory tract. For more than 50 years, PD, percussion, and vibration commonly have been advocated for secretion management. Breathing maneuvers such as active cycle of breathing (ACB), forced expiratory technique (FET), huff coughing, and autogenic drainage (AD) have been used alone or with devices providing positive airway pressure (PAP), high-frequency oscillation of the airway (HFOA), and high-frequency oscillation of the chest wall (HFOCW). This chapter explores how these maneuvers and devices function, their theoretic benefit, and their clinical benefit in the treatment of patients.

Normal Mechanisms of Mucociliary Transport

Secretions from the submucosal glands and surface secretory cells cover the ciliated epithelium of the airway (Figure 35-1). The relatively thin and watery sol layer, through which the cilia normally beat, arises from serous cell secretions. The thicker, superficial gel layer is formed from the more viscous secretions contributed by mucous cells and surface goblet cells, possibly enriched by components from the sol layer as water evaporates. This gel layer traps and holds dust, pollens, contaminants, and microorganisms. In the central airways, the majority of the secretory capacity is attributed to submucosal glands rather than surface secretory cells.

The cilia beat in a coordinated wavelike motion through the sol layer, with the tips of the cilia extending to the gel layer, propelling it toward the pharynx during the forward power stroke. This action is followed by a return recovery stroke in which the cilia return to their starting position, closer to the cell surface and at a slower speed.[2] The normal respiratory tract produces about 100 mL of mucus per day, some of which is absorbed as the secretions converge on the trachea, the remainder being expelled from the respiratory tract and swallowed.

Mucociliary transport is dependent on the rheologic properties of mucus.[3,4] The interaction of mucus and airflow can alter these properties. Mucous gel properties are primarily dependent on the concentration and molecular characteristics of the mucous glycoproteins (mucins). In lung diseases, deoxyribonucleic acid (DNA) and actin fibers resulting from infection and inflammation can contribute additional cross-linking to the mucous gel. The purulent sputum from adult patients with cystic fibrosis (CF) has higher elasticity and viscosity than nonpurulent sputum.[5] Sputum from adult CF patients has higher viscoelasticity compared with tracheal mucus from normal human subjects.

Effect of Cough on Mucus Rheology

Cough and other high-airflow maneuvers reduce the cross-linking of mucus when airflow linear velocities are high enough (3 L/second in the trachea) to cause wave formation in the mucus layer.[6] Reduced mucus viscosity during the cough maneuver may improve sputum clearance. Mucus acts as a low-viscosity fluid during the short time of the rapidly changing, turbulent airflow associated with effective cough but resumes its high-viscosity character after cessation of the cough and does not flow backward under the influence of gravity. Airflows associated with tidal breathing have no effect on mucus viscoelasticity.

Cephalad Airflow Bias

Cephalad airflow bias is responsible for the movement of mucus in airways during normal ventilation.[7,8] Airway diameters normally increase on inspiration and narrow on expiration. The narrowing of airways on exhalation increases the velocity and shearing forces in the airway, creating a cephalad airflow bias with tidal breathing. This bias is amplified during coughing, when increased transmural pressure causes the airways to fold and constrict, increasing airflow velocity even further.[9]

Cough

In healthy individuals the mucociliary escalator is the primary mechanism of mucus clearance from the lung. In acute airway diseases leading to ciliary dysfunction and/or mucus hypersecretion, cough is the primary mechanism for mucus clearance from the central airways, and cepha-

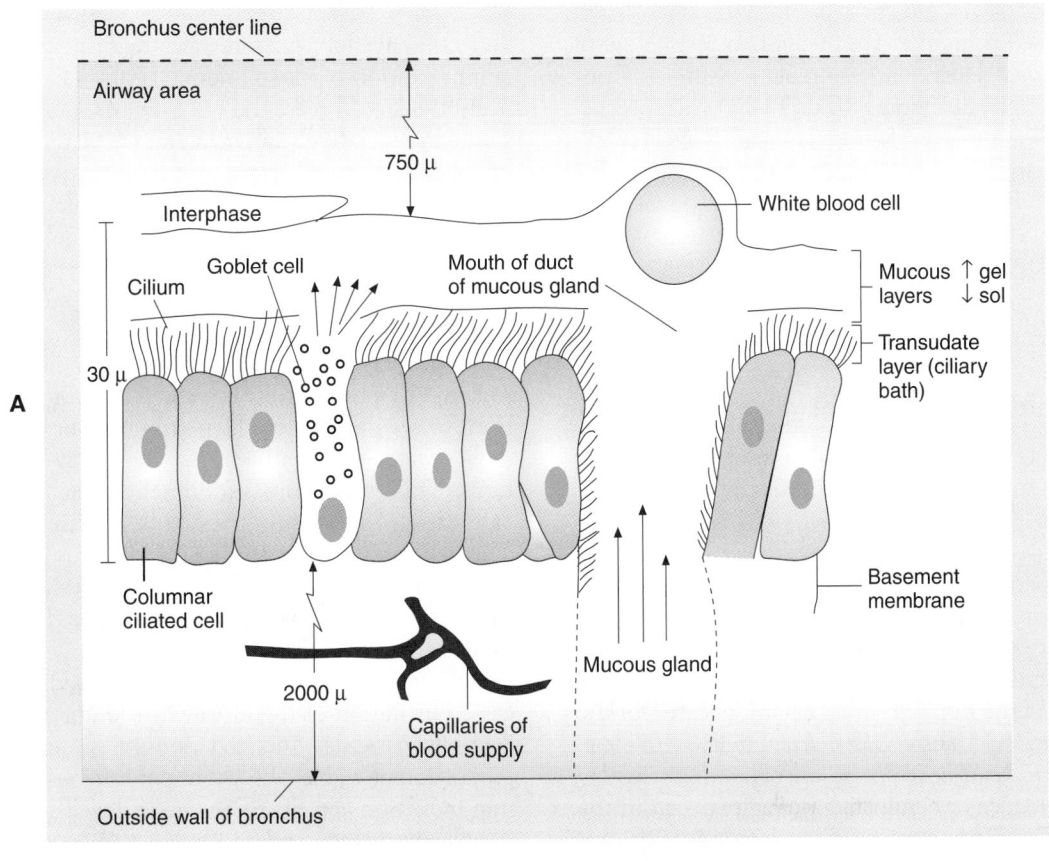

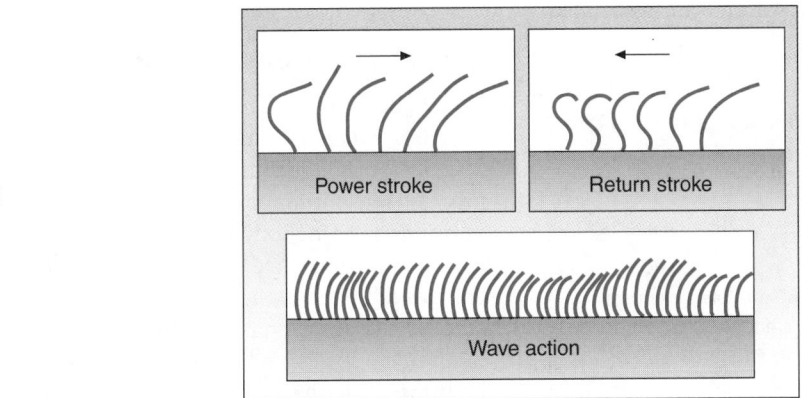

Figure 35-1   A, Drawing of the surface of a typical ciliated epithelium. **B,** Drawing of cilia at each phase of beat cycle.

lad airflow contributes increasingly to peripheral airway clearance. In chronic airway diseases involving mucus hypersecretion, these latter mechanisms become the major mechanisms responsible for keeping the airways patent.

Cough is one of the most common respiratory symptoms for which patients seek medical attention.[10] During a normal cough the expiratory airflow rises to a maximum along with narrowing of the intrathoracic airways. The narrowing of the airways is a product of high airflows and pressure differentials across the lung. Airflow velocity varies inversely with the cross-sectional area of the airways, creating high linear velocities, increased turbulence, high shearing forces within the airway, and high kinetic energy.

These forces shear secretions and debris from the airway walls, propelling them toward the central and upper airway, where they are expectorated or swallowed. In chronic obstructive pulmonary disease (COPD), narrowing airways may close prematurely, trapping gas, reducing expiratory flow rates, and limiting the effectiveness of the cough.

Gravity

Clinicians have used gravity to mobilize secretions since the 1930s. Postural drainage (PD) has been shown to be of clinical benefit for some patients under very specific circumstances. However, gravity is not a primary mechanism for normal mucociliary transport because the viscosity of the normal mucous blanket is sufficient to resist flow of mucus into gravity-dependent terminal bronchioles. Conventional **chest physiotherapy (CPT)**—PD with percussion and/or vibration—results in significantly greater expectoration than no treatment in patients with CF.[11] Conventional CPT has become the standard to which all other bronchial hygiene techniques are compared.

Treatment of Thick Secretions

Role of Humidity and Aerosol

Humidification of inspired gas **(bland aerosol)** has been advocated for treatment of thick, tenacious secretions, whether the patients have intact upper airways (CPG 35-1). This practice is highly suspect based on available evidence. No studies have reported a benefit of external humidifiers in improving the character and mobilization of thick secretions. The most effective method used to improve the character of pulmonary secretions is systemic hydration. Nonetheless, humidification of the inspired air has been advocated for the patient with tenacious secretions that are difficult to clear. For patients with an artificial airway, use of humidity therapy is indicated to reduce or eliminate a humidity deficit in the airway. Heated humidifiers are more efficient for such a purpose than are ambient or cool aerosol and are associated with less risk of bronchospasm.

CPG 35-1

Bland Aerosol Administration

Indications
   The presence of upper airway edema (cool bland aerosol): laryngotracheobronchitis, subglottic edema, postextubation edema, postoperative management of the upper airway
   The presence of a bypassed upper airway
   The need for sputum specimens

Contraindications
   Bronchoconstriction
   History of airway hyperresponsiveness

Hazards and Complications
   Bronchospasm
   Infection
   Overhydration
   Patient discomfort
   Caregiver exposure to droplet nuclei of *Mycobacterium tuberculosis* or other airborne contagion produced as a consequence of coughing, particularly during sputum induction

*Modified from AARC Clinical practice guideline: bland aerosol administration. Respir Care 1993;38:1196-1200.
CPG, Clinical practice guideline.*

Aerosol for Sputum Induction

Aerosols have long been used to treat thick secretions with administration of mucokinetic agents. The most effective agent used to decrease the viscosity of sputum is water. Unfortunately relatively large volumes of water are required to dilute secretions. Water is not an effective agent in that aerosols of water decrease in size as they warm in the airway, delivering little if any water to the gel layer. Aerosols of bland solutions, such as distilled water and hypertonic saline, are used to stimulate cough and secretion production. Such therapy has been used for diagnostic sputum induction.[12] Hypertonic saline (for example, 3% to 10% sodium chloride [NaCl]) is widely used for **sputum induction** for several reasons. Hypertonic saline on the mucosa moves water via osmosis from the airway into the secretions. This action causes a bronchorrhea, diluting the secretions and increasing their bulk to ease expectoration. The delivery of hypertonic saline by ultrasonic nebulizer is used to induce sputum for the diagnoses of *Pneumocystis carinii*, tuberculosis, and *Legionella* species. Because sputum induction is often repeated over 3 days, dosages of hypertonic saline should be limited to 10 mL/day to avoid excessive irritation of the airway or sodium overload in susceptible patients. Induced sputum contains a higher proportion of viable cells than spontaneous sputum.[12] Sputum induction appears to be safe and well tolerated for patients with asthma and COPD.[13]

Aerosol Deposition and Airway Secretions

To be effective as a therapeutic agent, an aerosol medication must efficiently deposit in the airway and then translocate across the mucous barrier, retaining bioactivity in this process. The optimal site of action depends on the agent administered. Bronchodilators and steroids need to reach the epithelium to be effective. Aerosolized antibiotics and mucolytics are effective when dispersed in infected airway secretions at sites of maximal airway obstruction. Mucus is a nonhomogeneous, adhesive, viscoelastic gel consisting of high-molecular-weight, cross-linked glycoproteins mixed with serum, cellular proteins, lipids, and water. An inverse relationship exists between molecular-weight particle diffusion through mucus.[14] The antibiotic diffusion barrier represented by mucin may be significant in vitro, particularly for nebulized antibiotics.[15] Translocation of macromolecules can be further compromised by the hypersecretion that accompanies inflammation and chronic pulmonary disease. These secretions can be a barrier to the penetration of any aerosol.

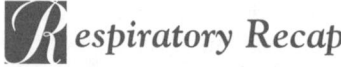

Treatment of Thick Secretions
Humidity
Mucoactive medications

Mucoactive Medications

Sputum is expectorated mucus mixed with inflammatory cells, cellular debris, polymers of DNA and F-actin, and bacteria. Recombinant human deoxyribonuclease (dornase alfa) was the first approved mucoactive agent for the treatment of CF.[16] Efficacy of dornase alfa has not been demonstrated for therapy of acute exacerbations of CF lung disease or for the treatment of other chronic airway diseases. Acetylcysteine (N-acetyl-L-cysteine sodium; Mucomyst) has long been administered by aerosol based on its demonstrated ability to break down disulfide bonds that provide stability to the mucoprotein network in mucus. This medication has never been approved for inhalation use, and little data supports its efficacy when it is nebulized. Mucomyst is an irritant to the airway that is capable of inducing bronchospasm, and patients tend to be nauseated by its smell and taste.

Aspiration of Secretions

When secretions in the airway cannot be effectively expelled with a cough, mechanical aspiration may be required. Mechanical aspiration, or suctioning, of secretions is an invasive procedure involving a catheter placed in the airway, attached to a negative pressure (vacuum) controlled through a regulator.

Suctioning

Patients with artificial airways almost always require assistance with secretion removal by suctioning. Some indications for suctioning include direct evidence of secretions in the airway, coarse or diminished breath sounds, unexplained increases in ventilator pressure during volume ventilation or decreases in tidal volume during pressure ventilation, and unexplained deterioration in blood gases. Suctioning can cause hypoxemia, which is prevented or minimized by preoxygenation for several minutes before suction.[17] The suction catheter should remain in the airway for less than 15 seconds. Patients may experience less hypoxemia if hyperinflation is performed between suctioning attempts, but this action may be harmful for patients prone to air-trapping, alveolar overdistention, elevated intracranial pressure (ICP), or poor cardiac output.

When secretions are exceptionally thick and tenacious, sterile saline can be instilled to loosen secretions and promote a cough. The available evidence, however, suggests that routine saline instillation does not increase recovery of secretions from the lungs and may worsen oxygenation.[18] A prudent approach is to use saline instillation only when evidence of sputum retention is present after suctioning attempts without saline. In-line catheters, which allow suctioning without opening of the ventilator circuit, are becoming increasingly popular because they allow maintenance of ventilation and oxygenation during suctioning. Changing these catheters on an as-needed basis, rather than daily, significantly reduces costs and causes no increase in the rate of nosocomial pneumonia.[19]

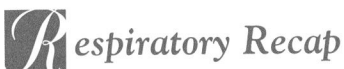 *espiratory Recap*

> **Aspiration of Secretions**
>
> Suctioning through an artificial airway
> Nasotracheal suctioning
> Bronchoscopy

Nasotracheal Suctioning

Some patients without artificial airways may need suctioning of bronchial secretions. To remove secretions from the upper airway, oropharyngeal suction may be performed with a Yankauer tip or suction catheter. To remove secretions from the lower respiratory tract, nasotracheal suction is performed (CPG 35-2). The **nasotracheal suction** procedure is outlined in Figure 35-2. Patients

 CPG 35-2

Nasotracheal Suctioning

> **Indications**
> Inability to clear secretions
> Audible evidence of secretions in the large/central airways that persist in spite of patient's best cough effort
>
> **Contraindications**
> Occluded nasal passages
> Nasal bleeding
> Epiglottitis or croup
> Acute injury of head or facial or neck injury
> Coagulopathy or bleeding disorder
> Laryngospasm
> Irritable airway
> Upper respiratory tract infection
>
> **Hazards and Complications**
> Mechanical trauma to upper airway
> Hypoxia/hypoxemia
> Cardiac dysrhythmias/arrest
> Bradycardia
> Increase in blood pressure
> Hypotension
> Respiratory arrest
> Uncontrolled coughing
> Gagging/vomiting
> Laryngospasm
> Bronchospasm
> Pain
> Nosocomial infection
> Atelectasis
> Misdirection of catheter
> Increased intracranial pressure

Modified from AARC Clinical practice guideline: nasotracheal suctioning. Respir Care 1992;37:898-901.
CPG, Clinical practice guideline.

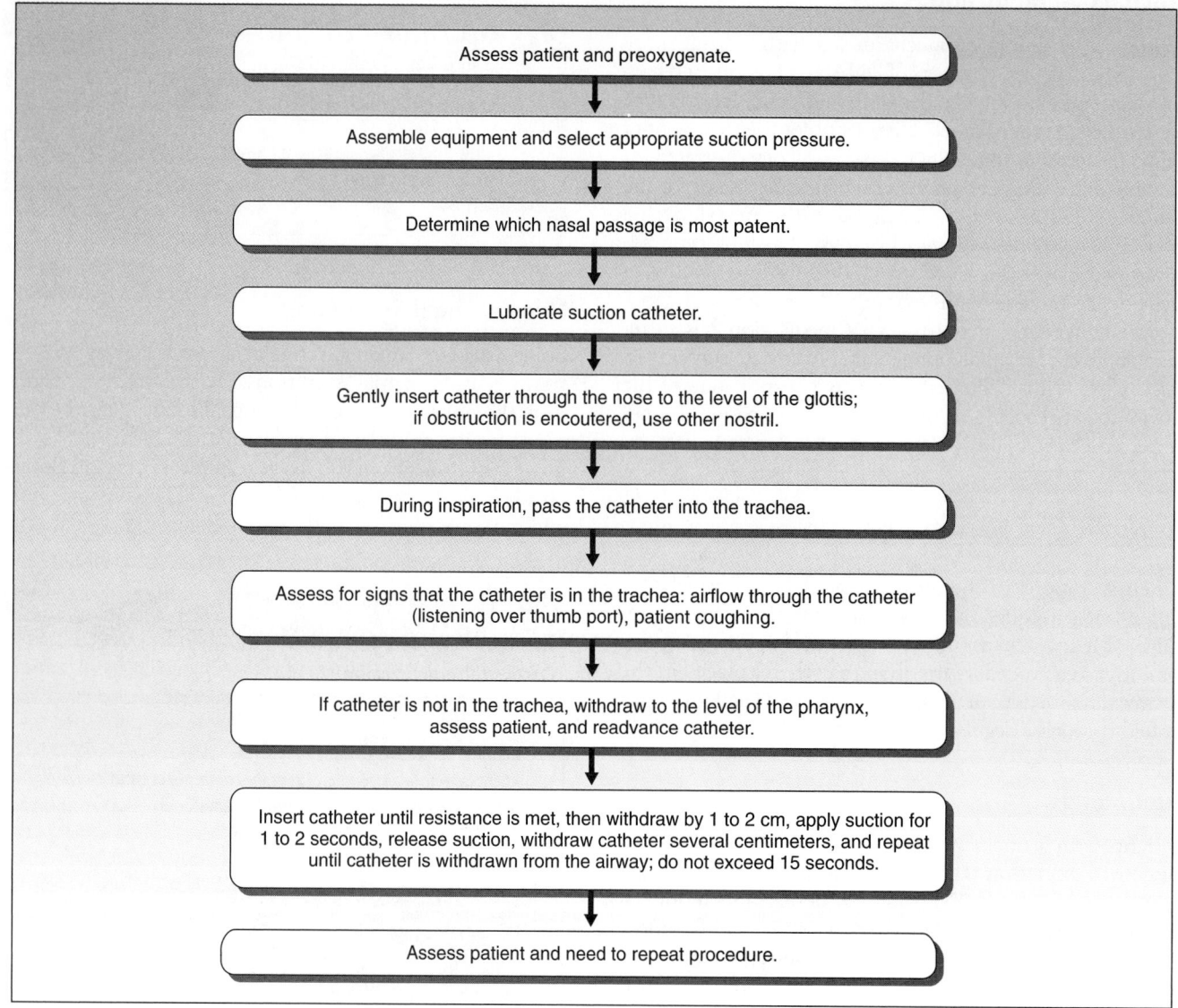

Figure 35-2   Procedure for nasotracheal suctioning.

who require frequent nasotracheal suction may benefit from placement of a nasal airway to reduce the trauma of repeated catheter insertion. Many patients respond to nasopharyngeal insertion of the catheter with a cough, which effectively removes secretions. Topical anesthetics and decongestants are rarely needed for nasotracheal suctioning. However, when patient discomfort, bleeding, or nasal edema prevent effective suctioning, these options should be considered.

Bronchoscopy

Therapeutic bronchoscopy is used for removal of foreign bodies from the airway, treatment of focal atelectasis, and airway occlusion secondary to secretions. A frequent therapeutic use of the bronchoscope is removal of retained secretions. In hospitalized patients with new atelectasis or col-

lapse of a lung segment, bronchoscopy has a role after CPT and suctioning have failed.[20,21] An exception is the patient who is hypoxic in spite of oxygen supplementation, in whom it is determined that relief of the obstruction might relieve the hypoxemia.[22] Although there is limited evidence to support routine use of bronchoscopy for secretion removal clearance, there is less dispute over the role it has in securing secretions from the airway for diagnostic testing.

Bronchoalveolar Lavage

The mini-bronchoalveolar lavage (mini-BAL) is performed with a catheter with a radiopaque coudé-type tip that allows the operator to direct the catheter to specific areas of the lungs. Evidence suggests that BAL performed by respiratory therapists has results comparable to bronchoscopy and is less costly.[23]

Mechanical Insufflation-Exsufflation

The mechanical insufflation-exsufflator is a device (Figure 35-3) that inflates the lungs with positive pressure followed by a negative pressure to simulate a cough.[24] Treatment consists of five cycles of **mechanical insufflation-exsufflation (MIE)** followed by 20 to 30 seconds of normal breathing, with repetitions until secretions are cleared. For each cycle the inspiratory pressure is 25 to 35 cm H_2O for 1 to 2 seconds, followed by an expiratory pressure of 30 to 40 cm H_2O for 1 to 2 seconds. Combining manual abdominal thrusts with expiration can help to increase expiratory flow expulsion of secretions. This procedure has been shown to be effective in patients with neuromuscular disease.[24] The MIE can be used with an oronasal mask or attached to an artificial airway.

Postural Drainage

Postural drainage (PD) consists of patient positioning so that secretions drain from specific segments and lobes of the lung toward gravity-dependent central airways, where they can be more readily removed with cough or mechanical aspiration (CPG 35-3). This action is accomplished by positioning of the patient so that the affected lung segments are superior to the carina, with each position maintained for 5 to 10 minutes (Figure 35-4). Typically, 11 to 12 positions are identified to drain all areas of the lungs, requiring at least 1 hour for a complete session.

In the treatment of acutely ill patients with unilateral lung disease, placement of the good lung down promotes matching of ventilation with areas of perfusion.[25] For critically ill patients, the use of beds that automatically rotate the patient from side to side are commonly used, but the cost-effectiveness of these beds is unclear.[26] Because turning may have deleterious effects, each change in position should be evaluated for patient tolerance. When a lung with atelectasis or consolidation is in the dependent position, the resultant shunt can produce significant hypoxemia. Prone positioning of these patients can result in significant improvement in arterial oxygenation.[27]

PD is used in the treatment of acute and stable CF, bronchiectasis, and other conditions characterized by excessive sputum production that the patient has difficulty clearing or expectorating.[28-32] PD has no benefit in conditions presenting with scant secretions (for example, viral pneumonia, postoperative coronary artery bypass). The indications for PD are largely limited to patients diagnosed with CF or bronchiectasis, and those who produce more than 30 mL of secretions/day and have difficulty clearing them. Drainage positions for less than 5 to 10 minutes fail to show improvement. Sputum production of less than 25 mL/day is insufficient to justify the application of PD therapy. Some patients have productive coughs with spu-

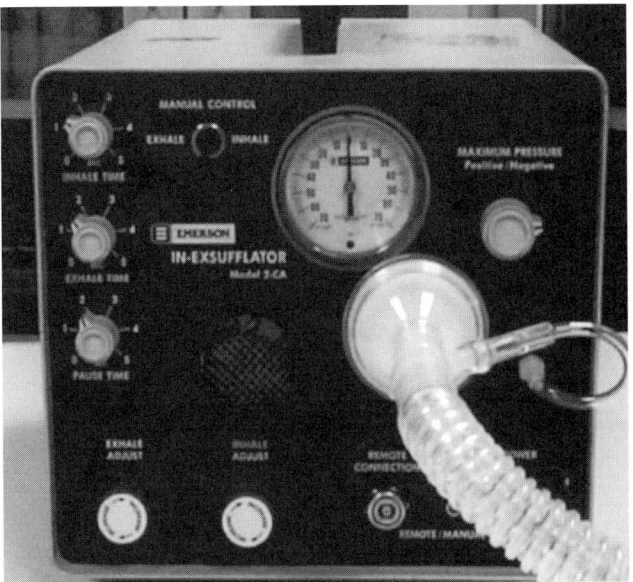

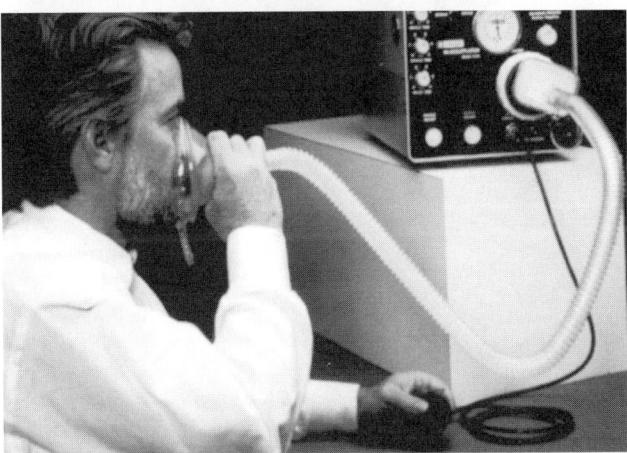

Figure 35-3 Mechanical In-Exsufflator. (Courtesy JH Emerson Co., Cambridge, Mass.)

tum production from 15 to 30 mL/day (occasionally as high as 70 or 100 mL/day) without use of PD. If PD does not increase sputum production in a patient who produces more than 30 mL/day of sputum without PD, the continued use of PD is not indicated. On the other hand, improved ease of clearing secretions during and immediately after PD supports continuation of therapy.

Conventional CPT is overused in many hospitals, and efforts to reduce its unnecessary use have been successfully implemented without adversely affecting patient outcomes.[33] Patient satisfaction with conventional CPT is less than with other bronchial hygiene techniques.[34]

External Manipulation of the Thorax

Percussion therapy is a technique involving rapid clapping, cupping, or striking of the external thorax directly over the lung segment being drained, with either cupped

Text continued on p. 674

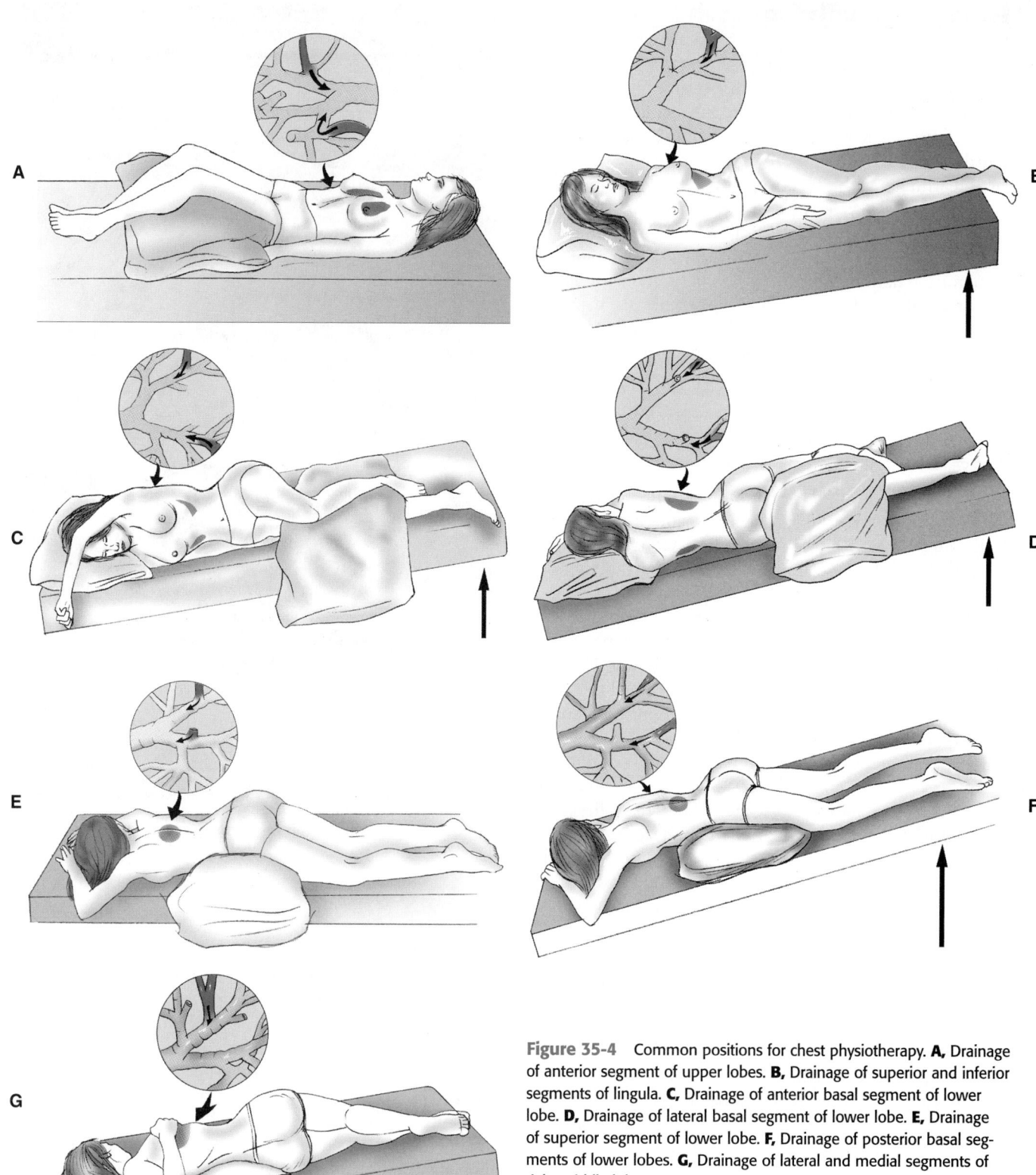

Figure 35-4   Common positions for chest physiotherapy. **A,** Drainage of anterior segment of upper lobes. **B,** Drainage of superior and inferior segments of lingula. **C,** Drainage of anterior basal segment of lower lobe. **D,** Drainage of lateral basal segment of lower lobe. **E,** Drainage of superior segment of lower lobe. **F,** Drainage of posterior basal segments of lower lobes. **G,** Drainage of lateral and medial segments of right middle lobe.

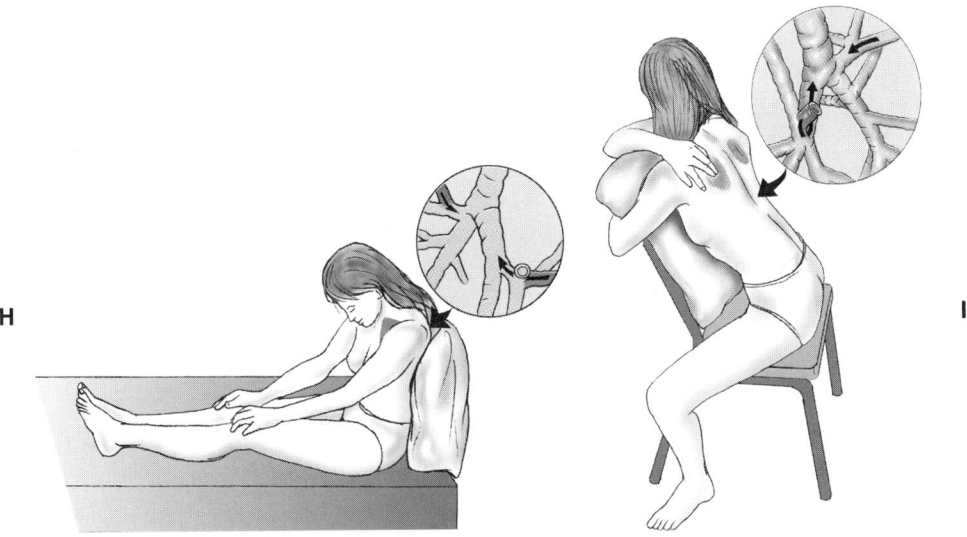

Figure 35-4—cont'd   H, Drainage of apical segment of upper lobe. **I,** Drainage of posterior segment of upper lobe. (Modified from Scanlan CL, Wilkins RL, Stoller JK. Egan's fundamentals of respiratory care. 7th ed. St Louis: Mosby; 1999.)

 CPG   35-3

Postural Drainage Therapy

Indications

Turning: Inability or reluctance of patient to change body position (for example, mechanical ventilation, neuromuscular disease, drug-induced paralysis), poor oxygenation associated with position (for example, unilateral lung disease), potential for or presence of atelectasis, presence of artificial airway

Postural drainage (PD): Evidence or suggestion of difficulty with secretion clearance, difficulty clearing secretions with expectorated sputum production greater than 25 to 30 mL/day (adult), evidence or suggestion of retained secretions in the presence of an artificial airway, presence of atelectasis caused by or suspected of being caused by mucous plugging, diagnosis of diseases such as cystic fibrosis, bronchiectasis, or cavitating lung disease; presence of foreign body in airway

External manipulation of the thorax: Sputum volume or consistency suggesting a need for additional manipulation (for example, percussion and/or vibration) to assist movement of secretions by gravity in a patient receiving PD

Contraindications

The decision to use PD therapy requires assessment of potential benefits versus potential risks. Therapy should be provided for no longer than necessary to obtain the desired therapeutic results.

All positions are contraindicated for intracranial pressure (ICP) greater than 20 mm Hg; head and neck injury until stabilized (absolute); active hemorrhage with hemodynamic instability (absolute); recent spinal surgery (for example, laminectomy) or acute spinal injury; acute spinal injury or active hemoptysis; empyema; bronchopleural fistula; pulmonary edema associated with congestive heart failure; large pleural effusions, pulmonary embolism; aged, confused, or anxious patients who do not tolerate position changes; rib fracture, with or without flail chest; and surgical wound or healing tissue.

The Trendelenburg position is contraindicated for ICP greater than 20 mm Hg; patients in whom increased ICP is to be prevented (for example, neurosurgery, aneurysms, eye surgery); uncontrolled hypertension; distended abdomen; esophageal surgery; recent gross hemoptysis related to recent lung carcinoma treated surgically or with radiation therapy; and uncontrolled airway at risk for aspiration (tube feeding or recent meal). Reverse Trendelenburg is contraindicated in the presence of hypotension or vasoactive medication.

External manipulation of the thorax is contraindicated with subcutaneous emphysema, recent epidural spinal infusion or spinal anesthesia; recent skin grafts, or flaps, on the thorax; burns, open wounds, and skin infections of the thorax; recently placed transvenous pacemaker or subcutaneous pacemaker (particularly if mechanical devices are to be used); suspected pulmonary tuberculosis; lung contusion; bronchospasm; osteomyelitis of the ribs; osteoporosis; coagulopathy; complaint of chest-wall pain.

Hazards and Complications

Hypoxemia
Increased ICP
Acute hypotension
Pulmonary hemorrhage
Pain or injury to chest wall
Vomiting and aspiration
Bronchospasm
Dysrhythmias

Modified from AARC Clinical practice guideline: postural drainage therapy. Respir Care 1991;36:1418-1426.
CPG, Clinical practice guideline.

hands or a mechanical device (Figure 35-5, A).[35,36] Percussion has been advocated to assist secretion mobilization by shaking loose secretions, similar to the shaking of ketchup from a bottle. Vibrating the chest wall over the draining area with a fine tremorous action also has been used to assist mobilization of secretion during PD. **Vibration therapy** is manually performed by pressing in the direction that the ribs and soft tissue of the chest normally move during exhalation (Figure 35-5, B). Some evidence suggests that vibration for up to an hour can increase movement of secretions,[37] but conclusive evidence has yet to prove the efficacy of this procedure. Percussion and vibration appear to be relatively ineffective and do not add to the effectiveness of the combination of coughing, breathing exercises, and PD.[38-42] No evidence exists that percussion alone, without positioning of the patient, is of any value.

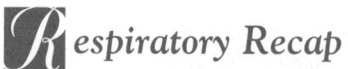

Respiratory Recap

Conventional Chest Physiotherapy
Postural drainage External manipulation of the thorax: percussion and vibration

Although the clinical efficacy of percussion and vibration is ill defined and questionable, the complications or hazards are better understood. Patients should be evaluated for a variety of conditions that may be exacerbated by performance of percussion or vibration to the thorax: irregularities of the skin (such as burns, open wounds, skin infections, and recent skin grafts), subcutaneous emphysema, recently placed transvenous pacemaker or subcutaneous pacemaker, or recent epidural spinal infusion of anesthetic of the spinal type. Percussion and vibration are difficult for patients to apply without assistance. Whether vibration or percussion are effective for mobilization of secretions, the application of these procedures, especially with mechanical vibrators and percussors, might feel good to the patient. This possibility might prove to be the most convincing reason to consider application of the techniques during PD therapy sessions.

Contraindications for Postural Drainage and Percussion

Placing the patient in a head down or Trendelenburg position effects both hemodynamics and interaction of physical forces between the thorax and the abdomen. With the head down, there is increased blood flow to the head. Therefore the Trendelenburg position should be avoided in patients with ICP more than 20 mm Hg (for example, those who have neurosurgery, aneurysms, eye surgery), uncontrolled hypertension, or gross hemoptysis (related to recent lung carcinoma treated surgically or with radiation therapy).[43] Shifting of abdominal and thoracic contents with gravity in the Trendelenburg position may be deleterious in patients at risk for aspiration, distended abdomen, or recent esophageal surgery. Reverse Trendelenburg may be hazardous for patients with hypotension or those receiving vasoactive medication.

Percussion, far from being benign, offers substantial additional risk and shows little benefit. Because percussion is intended to loosen secretions, it is contraindicated for patients with suspected pulmonary tuberculosis and resectable tumors of the thorax or neck. The concern is that percussion might shake loose or "break up" cysts and tumors, thereby spreading bacteria or cancerous cells to other parts of the body. (Small lipomas and sebaceous cysts are not contraindications for percussion.) Percussion has been associated with precipitating and increasing bronchospasm, resulting in increased wheezing, airway closure, and dyspnea. Potential damage to the thorax from percussion makes osteoporosis and osteomyelitis of the ribs, as well as complaints of chest pain, relative contraindications to this therapy. Lung contusion and coagulopathies may be aggravated by percussion, resulting in increased bruising or bleeding within the chest wall or lung.

Hazards and Complications of Postural Drainage Therapy

During PD therapy, care should be taken to identify hypoxemia, bronchospasm, acute hypotension, increased intracranial pressure, pulmonary hemorrhage (blood in the sputum), pain/injury to the tissue, and vomiting with risk of aspiration. To minimize risk of vomiting and aspiration,

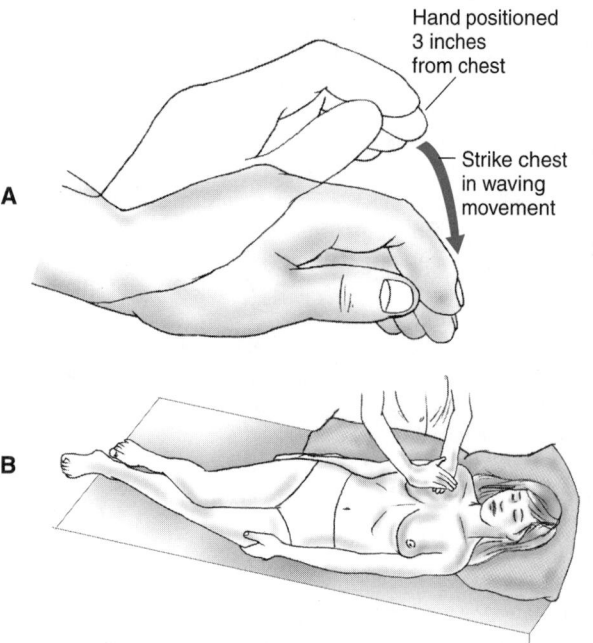

Hand positioned
3 inches
from chest

Strike chest
in waving
movement

A

B

Figure 35-5   **A,** Movement of cupped hand at wrist to percuss chest. **B,** Chest vibration. (Modified from Scanlan CL, Wilkins RL, Stoller JK: Egan's fundamentals of respiratory care. 7th ed. St Louis: Mosby; 1999.)

therapy should be performed before meals or more than 1 hour after meals. For patients receiving tube feedings, feedings should cease 1 hour before and during therapy. For patients with a history of bronchospasm, bronchodilators are commonly administered before PD therapy. PD therapy is time intensive, requiring the patient and caregiver to set aside 30 to 60 minutes three to four times each day and to have special equipment such as a tilt table. This time commitment is a major obstacle to prescription adherence by the patient.

Conventional CPT has been suggested as the most stimulating and disturbing procedure in mechanically ventilated patients and thus should not be administered to patients with poor cardiopulmonary reserve.[44] In mechanically ventilated patients, CPT may be accompanied with manual hyperinflation. This practice is discouraged, however, because it may result in dangerously high airway pressures and tidal volumes in patients with acute lung injury.[45] Given the potential for hazard, the time required for therapy, and the paucity of evidence to support its use,[46] it is necessary to use prudence in any decision involving whether to use CPT. In patients with CF, tolerance for CPT may be improved when combined with noninvasive pressure support ventilation.[47]

Clockwise Rotation for a Complete Postural Drainage

A technique used to perform a complete PD session with minimal movement of the patient is the clockwise rotation of the patient, with each rotation draining a different segment of the lung. Each position should be maintained for 5 to 10 minutes as tolerated, with the patient being encouraged to deep breathe and cough during and between positions. This technique starts with the patient flat on his or her back and proceeds through eight partial turns in a clockwise direction (Figure 35-6). The general procedure for CPT is shown in Figure 35-7.

Deep Breathing and Coughing

The normal mechanism for lung expansion and bronchial hygiene is spontaneous deep breathing (including yawn and sigh maneuvers) and an effective cough. Instructing and encouraging the patient to take sustained deep breaths (Figure 35-8) is among the safest, most effective, and least expensive strategies to keep the lungs expanded and secretions moving.[48] The negative intrathoracic pressure generated during spontaneous deep breathing tends to better inflate the less compliant, gravity-dependent areas of the lung than do mechanical methods relying on lung inflation by application of positive airway pressure. A deep breath is a key component for a normal effective cough.

An effective cough is a vital component of bronchial hygiene therapy. The normal cough involves the taking of a deep breath, closure of the glottis, and compression of

abdominal and thoracic muscles (generating pressures in excess of 80 mm Hg), followed by an explosive release of gas as the glottis opens (Figure 35-9). In addition to mobilizing and expelling secretions, the high pressures generated during a cough may be an important factor in reexpanding lung tissue. Comparable pressures generated by positive pressure applied to the airway have been associated with barotrauma, which does not appear to be a problem with controlled cough maneuvers (CPG 35-4). The normal cough maneuver can be extremely painful for the patient (especially after upper abdominal surgery), and it has been reported to dislodge central venous catheters.[49] Paroxysms of uncontrolled coughing have been associated with neurologic symptoms[50] and gastroesophageal reflux.[51]

In the patient with unstable airways, high pressures and flow combine in the dynamic compression of the airways, trapping gas and secretions, rendering the cough ineffective. A variety of breathing techniques enhance cephalad airflow bias. In patients with CF and chronic bronchitis, directed cough and ACB have been shown to be as effective in mobilizing secretions and increasing lung volumes as PD with percussion and vibration.[52-61]

For patients unable to generate an effective cough, sharp forced exhalations without glottis closure (**huff coughing**) appear to be the maneuver of choice.[59-61] Huff coughing is a **forced expiratory technique (FET)** that is performed through sharp exhalation from high to mid lung volumes through an open glottis. The individual takes in a slow, deep breath, followed by a 1- to 3-second breath hold, and then performs short, quick forced exhalation with the glottis open. The subject may be instructed to say the word *huff* during exhalation. Small children are sometimes instructed to flap their arms (with hands near their shoulders, rotating their elbows from a position horizontal to the shoulder down to their lateral chest wall) as they perform the huff cough. This technique has been referred to as the *chicken (flapping wings) breath* to focus on the expiratory maneuver, associating positive reinforcement and play with the huff technique.

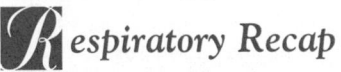

*R*espiratory Recap

Coughing	
Huff coughing	Active cycle of breathing
Forced expiratory technique	Autogenic drainage
Manually assisted coughing	

Manually Assisted Coughing

Manually assisted coughing involves thrusts with hands and arms positioned on the patient's abdomen, coordinated with expiration (Figure 35-10). Compression of the lateral aspect of the chest also can be effective. Often this technique is augmented with manual hyperinflation for patients with limited vital capacity (VC; <1.5 L). This

Text continued on p. 678

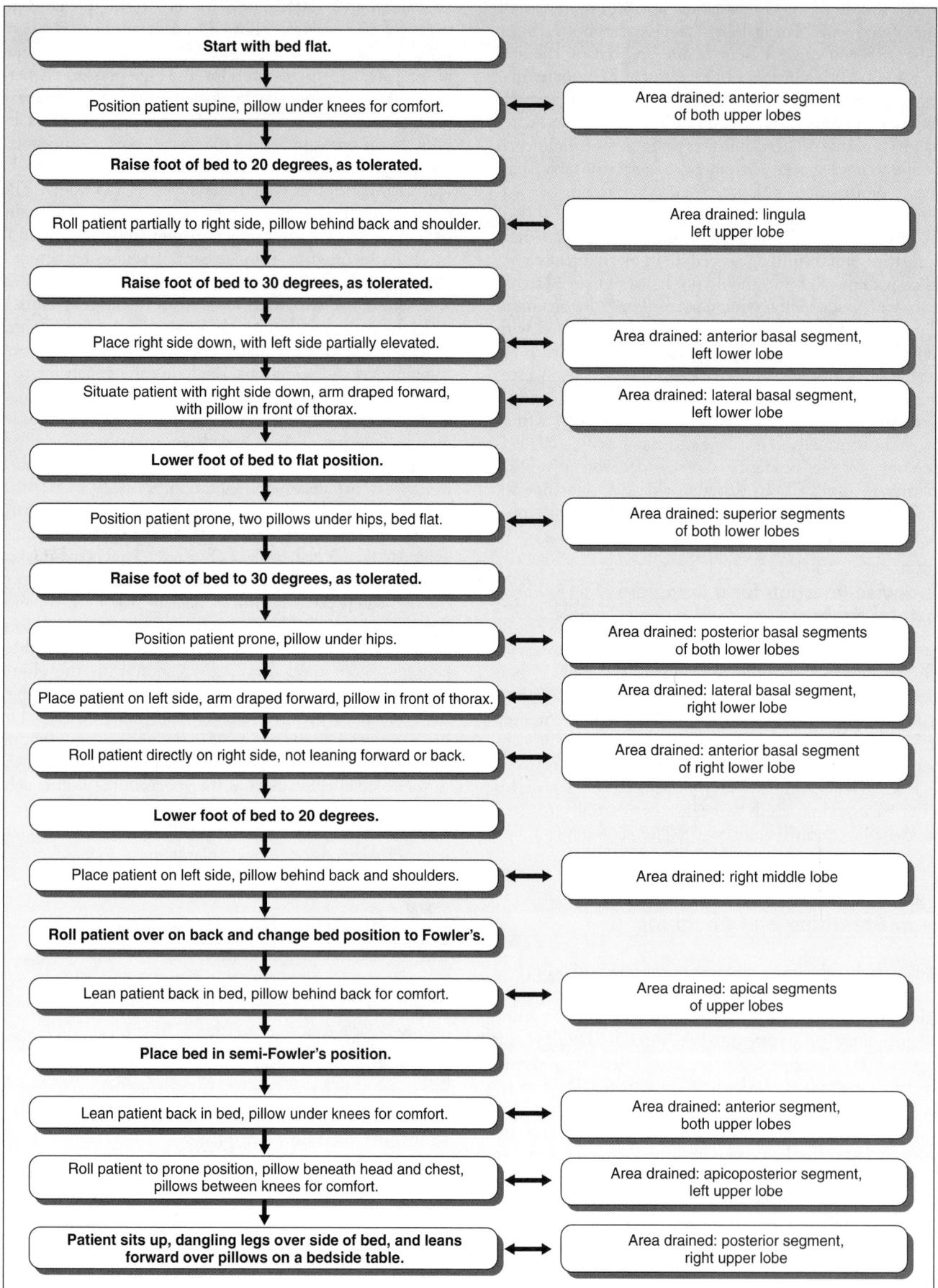

Figure 35-6 Clockwise rotation for complete postural drainage.

Assess patient and need for chest physiotherapy.

↓

Gather appropriate equipment: bed or table that can assume range of positions, pillows to support patient, light towel to cover chest percussion area, tissues or basin for secretions, mechanical percussor or vibrator (optional).

↓

Explain therapy to patient and instruct patient in proper cough techniques.

↓

Assist patient to each position and maintain for 5 to 10 minutes.

↓

Assess patient response in each position; modify position if necessary.

↓

Perform chest percussion and vibration over the affected area if necessary.

↓

Encourage patient to take slow deep breaths and cough between positions; note character of cough and secretions.

↓

Document procedure and response to therapy in the medical record; communicate adverse effects to physician.

Figure 35-7 Procedure for chest physiotherapy.

Instruct patient to take three to five slow deep breaths, inhaling through the nose, exhaling through pursed lips, and using diaphragmatic breathing.

↓

Ask patient to take a deep breath and hold for 1 to 3 seconds.

↓

Exhale from mid lung volumes to low lung volumes to clear secretions from periphery.

↓

Take in a normal breath and contract the abdominal and chest wall muscles with the mouth (and glottis) open while whispering the word *huff*.

↓

Repeat several times.

↓

As secretions enter the larger airways, exhale from high to mid lung volumes to clear secretions from more proximal airways.

↓

Repeat maneuver two to three times.

↓

Take several relaxed diaphragmatic breaths before the next cough.

↓

Document procedure and patient response in the medical record.

Figure 35-8 Directed cough technique.

CPG   35-4

Directed Cough

Indications

The need to aid in the removal of retained secretions from central airways (with the suggestion that forced expiratory technique [FET] at lower lung volumes may be effective in preferentially mobilizing secretions in peripheral airways whereas larger volumes facilitate movement in the central airways lacking validation)

The presence of atelectasis

As prophylaxis against postoperative pulmonary complications

As a routine part of bronchial hygiene in patients with cystic fibrosis, bronchiectasis, chronic bronchitis, necrotizing pulmonary infection, or spinal cord injury

As an integral part of other bronchial hygiene therapies such as postural drainage (PD) therapy, positive expiratory pressure (PEP) therapy, and incentive spirometry (IS)

The need to obtain sputum specimens for diagnostic analysis

Contraindications

Directed cough is rarely contraindicated. The contraindications listed must be weighed against potential benefit in deciding to eliminate cough from the care of the patient. The following listed contraindications are relative:

Inability to control possible transmission of infection from patients suspected or known to have pathogens transmittable by droplet nuclei (for example, *Mycobacterium tuberculosis*)

Presence of an elevated intracranial pressure or known intracranial aneurysm

Presence of reduced coronary artery perfusion, such as in acute myocardial infarction

Acute unstable head, neck, or spine injury

Possibly manually assisted directed cough with pressure to the epigastrium in presence of increased potential for regurgitation/aspiration (for example, unconscious patient with unprotected airway), acute abdominal pathologic process (abdominal aortic aneurysm, hiatal hernia, or pregnancy), a bleeding diathesis, untreated pneumothorax

Possibly manually assisted directed cough with pressure to the thoracic cage in presence of osteoporosis, or flail chest

Hazards and Complications

Reduced coronary artery perfusion

Reduced cerebral perfusion

Incontinence

Fatigue

Headache

Paresthesia

Bronchospasm

Muscular discomfort

Barotraumas

Cough paroxysms

Chest pain

Rib or costochondral junction fracture

Incisional pain or evisceration

Anorexia or vomiting and retching

Visual disturbances including retinal hemorrhage, central line displacement, and gastroesophageal reflux

Modified from AARC Clinical practice guideline: directed cough. Respir Care 1993;38:495-499.
CPG, Clinical practice guideline.

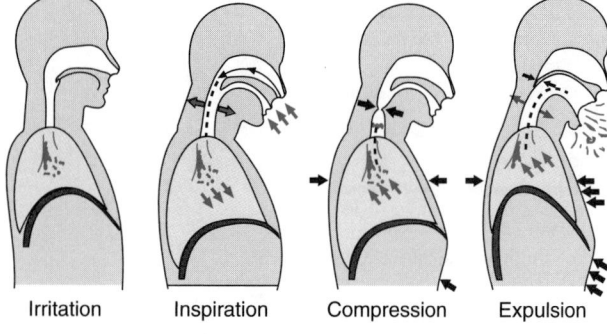

Irritation   Inspiration   Compression   Expulsion

Figure 35-9   The cough reflex.

technique requires a cooperative patient, good coordination between patient and clinician, and a clinician with sufficient physical strength to reliably perform the maneuver. Efficacy is limited for patients with significant scoliosis and osteoporosis of the rib cage. This technique is used most commonly in patients with neuromuscular disease or quadriplegia and is sometimes called *quad coughing*.

Active Cycle of Breathing

The **active cycle of breathing (ACB)** techniques are a combination of breathing control, thoracic expansion control, and forced expiration technique (Figure 35-11). Breathing control is described as gentle breathing with the lower chest. With the upper chest and shoulders relaxed, the subject breathes at normal tidal volume and rate. The patient should feel a swelling around the waist on inspiration, which subsides while breathing out. Breathing control is the default maneuver between the more active techniques.

Thoracic expansion exercises are simply large breaths with active inspiration (involving both diaphragm and rib cage musculature) and relaxed expiration. Increasing lung volume increases flow through small airways and collateral ventilation channels, increasing the volume of gas available to help mobilize secretions on expiration. This is limited to three or four deep breaths to avoid fatigue and hyperventilation.

The FET consists of one or two forced expirations or huffs, combined with a period of controlled breathing.[62-64]

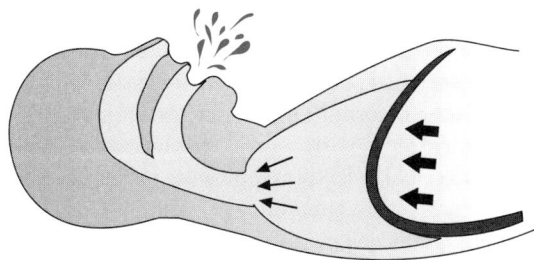

Figure 35-10   To produce manually assisted (quad) coughing, external abdominal pressure is applied under the diaphragm during exhalation following maximal inspiration, resulting in an increased expiratory flow and secretion clearance.

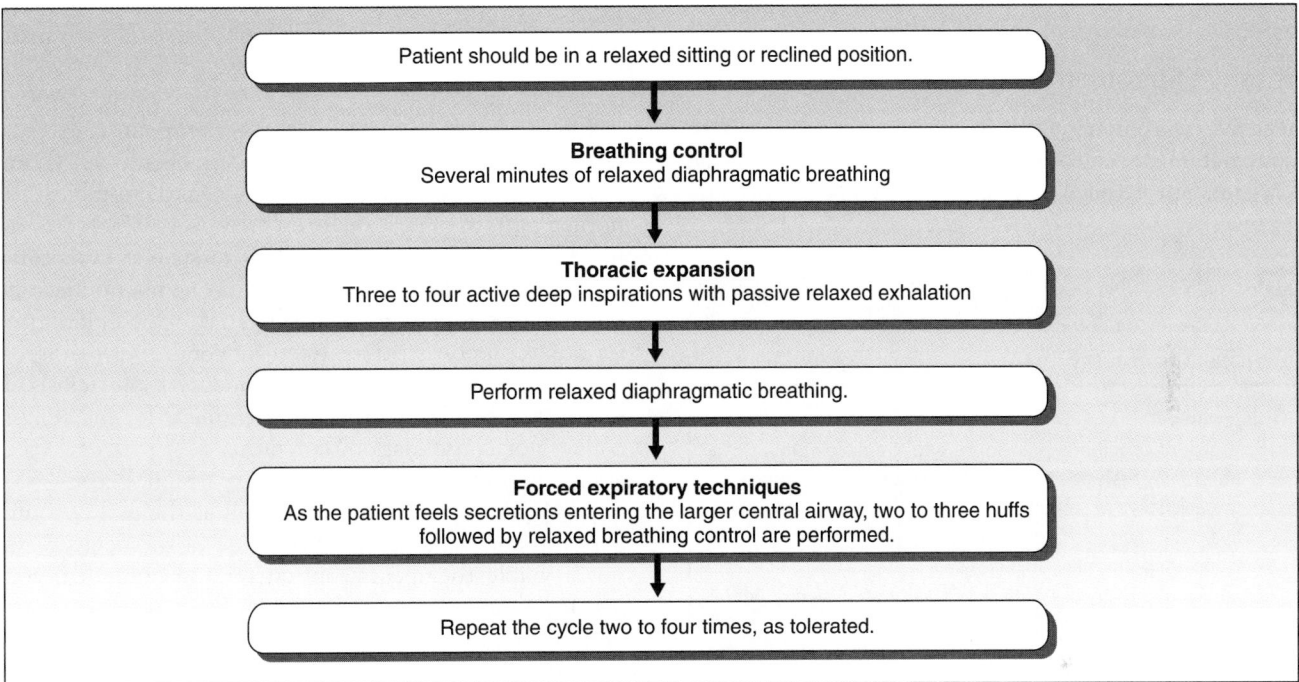

Patient should be in a relaxed sitting or reclined position.

Breathing control
Several minutes of relaxed diaphragmatic breathing

Thoracic expansion
Three to four active deep inspirations with passive relaxed exhalation

Perform relaxed diaphragmatic breathing.

Forced expiratory techniques
As the patient feels secretions entering the larger central airway, two to three huffs followed by relaxed breathing control are performed.

Repeat the cycle two to four times, as tolerated.

Figure 35-11   Active cycle of breathing technique.

A normal breath is taken in, and then the air is squeezed out by contraction of the chest wall and abdominal muscles. The mouth and glottis are kept open. The huff should not be a violent or explosive exhalation. Some people find that physical compression of the chest wall helps during the huff cough.

The ACB can be taught to parents for use with children from the age of about 2 years, with children performing the technique independently from about age 8 or 9. Patients should be encouraged to exercise; often they will find that shorter ACB sessions are required as a consequence of exercising.

Autogenic Drainage

Autogenic drainage (AD) aims to achieve the highest possible airflow in the different generations of bronchi to move secretions without forced expirations (Figure 35-12).[65,66] AD may be as effective as PD in mobilizing secretions for patients with CF. This technique depends on staged breathing at different lung volumes, starting with small tidal breaths from expiratory reserve volume (ERV), repeated until secretions are

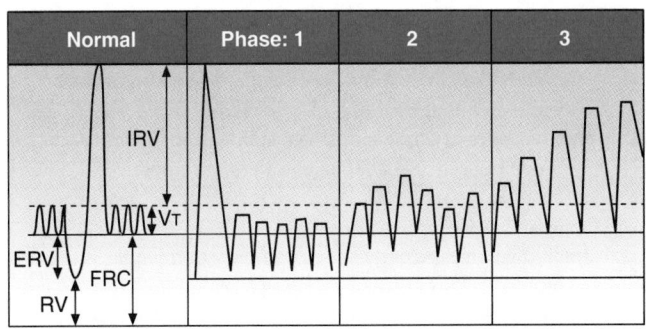

Figure 35-12   Spirogram of lung volumes during phases of autogenic drainage. *ERV,* Expiratory reserve volume; *RV,* residual volume; *FRC,* functional residual capacity; *IRV,* inspiratory reserve volume; *VT,* tidal volume. (Modified from Hardy KA. A review of techniques, indications, and recommendations. Respir Care 1994;39:440-452.)

felt gathering in the central airways. At that point the cough is suppressed, and a larger tidal volume is taken for a series of 10 to 20 breaths, followed by a series of larger (approaching VC) breaths, followed by several huff coughs. Although this technique has been shown to be effective, it requires a great deal of patient cooperation and is only recommended for patients older than 8 years of age and in those who have a good sense of their own breathing. Several studies have reported similar secretion clearance with AD and PD.[67,68]

Exercise

Exercise causes increased sputum production compared with rest.[69,70] Exercise appears to augment bronchial hygiene and should be encouraged, as tolerated; however, it should not substitute for other bronchial hygiene regimens.

Incentive Spirometry

Incentive spirometry (IS) is a technique designed to mimic natural sighing or yawning maneuvers, also referred to as *sustained maximal inspiration* (CPG 35-5).[71] Because

CPG 35-5

Incentive Spirometry

Indications
 Presence of conditions predisposing to the development of pulmonary atelectasis such as upper abdominal surgery, thoracic surgery, surgery in patients with chronic obstructive pulmonary disease (COPD)
 Presence of pulmonary atelectasis
 Presence of a restrictive lung defect associated with quadriplegia and/or dysfunctional diaphragm

Contraindications
 Patient cannot be instructed or supervised to ensure appropriate use of the device.
 Patient cooperation is absent, or patient is unable to understand or demonstrate proper use of the device.
 Incentive spirometry (IS) is contraindicated in patients unable to deep breathe effectively (for example, with vital capacity less than about 10 mL/kg or inspiratory capacity less than about one third of predicted).
 The presence of an open tracheal stoma is not a contraindication but requires adaptation of the spirometer.

Hazards and Complications
 Ineffective unless closely supervised or performed as ordered
 Inappropriate as sole treatment for major lung collapse or consolidation
 Hyperventilation
 Barotraumas
 Discomfort secondary to inadequate pain control
 Hypoxia secondary to interruption of prescribed oxygen therapy
 Exacerbation of bronchospasm
 Fatigue

Modified from AARC Clinical practice guideline: incentive spirometry. Respir Care 1991;36:1402-1405.
CPG, Clinical practice guideline.

postoperative patients often adopt a pattern of rapid, shallow breathing, they should be encouraged to take 5 to 10 deep breaths every hour. Incisional pain and splinting may make those breaths painful after upper abdominal surgery, so IS provides patients with sensory feedback to quantify the depth of the breath. IS should provide patients with an objective comparison to the volumes (of flows) they were generating preoperatively, with the goal of attaining or returning to that preoperative volume, in spite of the pain experienced. In addition, the IS device instruction should include recording how long breaths are to be held, how many times the breaths were attempted, and how many times the patient succeeded in meeting his or her volume goals (Figure 35-13).

Objectives of IS are to increase transpulmonary pressure and inspiratory volumes to near-preoperative VC, improve inspiratory muscle performance, and reestablish the normal pattern of periodic deep breathing. When the sustained maximal inspiration (SMI) maneuver is repeated on a regular basis, airway patency may be maintained and lung atelectasis prevented and reversed.[72-73] IS is indicated for use as prophylactic treatment of conditions predisposing to the postoperative development of atelectasis. It should not be used as the sole treatment for major lung collapse or consolidation, but rather as a part of a more comprehensive program of lung reexpansion. Because SMI requires patient cooperation, as well as the ability to understand and demonstrate proper use of the device, IS is not a viable therapeutic option for the obtunded, confused, or uncooperative patient. IS is not the therapeutic option of choice for the patient who cannot spontaneously generate a VC greater than 10 mL/kg or inspiratory capacity (IC) more than one third of predicted. For these patients, options such as intermittent positive pressure breathing (IPPB) or positive airway pressure (PAP) should be considered.

Respiratory Recap

Deep Breathing Assistance
Mechanical insufflation-exsufflation
Incentive spirometry
Intermittent positive pressure breathing

As with many therapeutic modalities in respiratory care, IS is ineffective unless performed frequently and properly, making compliance a critical issue. If the patient experiences pain during deep inspiratory efforts, pain management or alternative options such as PAP should be considered. Although most IS devices are used with a mouthpiece, they may be adapted for use with an open tracheal stoma or artificial airway.

Evidence suggests that deep breathing alone, without mechanical aides, may be as beneficial as IS in preventing or reversing pulmonary complications, and controversy exists concerning overuse of IS. If the patient can take deep breaths without IS, he or she should be encouraged to do so at regular intervals. Deep breathing, coughing, and IS work best as shared tasks among all clinicians in the surgical units, with each clinician providing frequent reminders to the patient.

The need for IS should focus on factors including surgical procedures involving the upper abdomen or thorax, conditions predisposing to development of atelectasis (for example, immobility, poor pain control, and abdominal binders), and the presence of neuromuscular disease involving the respiratory muscles. Outcome assessment should include improvement of atelectasis (for example, decreased respiratory rate, improved breath sounds, normal chest x-ray films and improved PaO_2), increased VC to preoperative values (in absence of lung resection), and improved inspiratory muscle performance.

A volume displacement IS device is a cylindrical bellows that is displaced upward as the patient breathes in, with a scale on the side of the container to indicate volume goals (Figure 35-14). These units are bulky, requiring a lot of space at the patient bedside and on the hospital supply shelves. The volumetric incentive spirometer combines a quasi volume displacement indicator (takes less space) and flow indicator (to encourage slow inspirations). The other type of IS device is a simple flow-oriented device. Although the underlying premise of IS is to take slow deep breaths, many hospitals have adopted IS flow-oriented devices for space and cost reasons.[74]

These devices usually direct the patient's inspiratory flow through a tube to lift one or more light balls (or disks). The higher the patient's inspiratory flow, the higher the ball is raised or the greater the number of balls that are raised. The longer the flow is maintained, the larger the volume, so the patient is encouraged to take slow deep breaths. Unfortunately, high flows can be generated (with low volumes) to raise the flow indicator to target levels without the patient meeting therapeutic volume or breath-holding objectives. Although flow-oriented IS devices impose an additional work of breathing,[75] it is unclear whether this additional workload is deleterious or a beneficial part of the therapy.

Successful use of IS devices depends on patient education and compliance. Although there are no clinically important differences among IS devices,[76] a reduced frequency

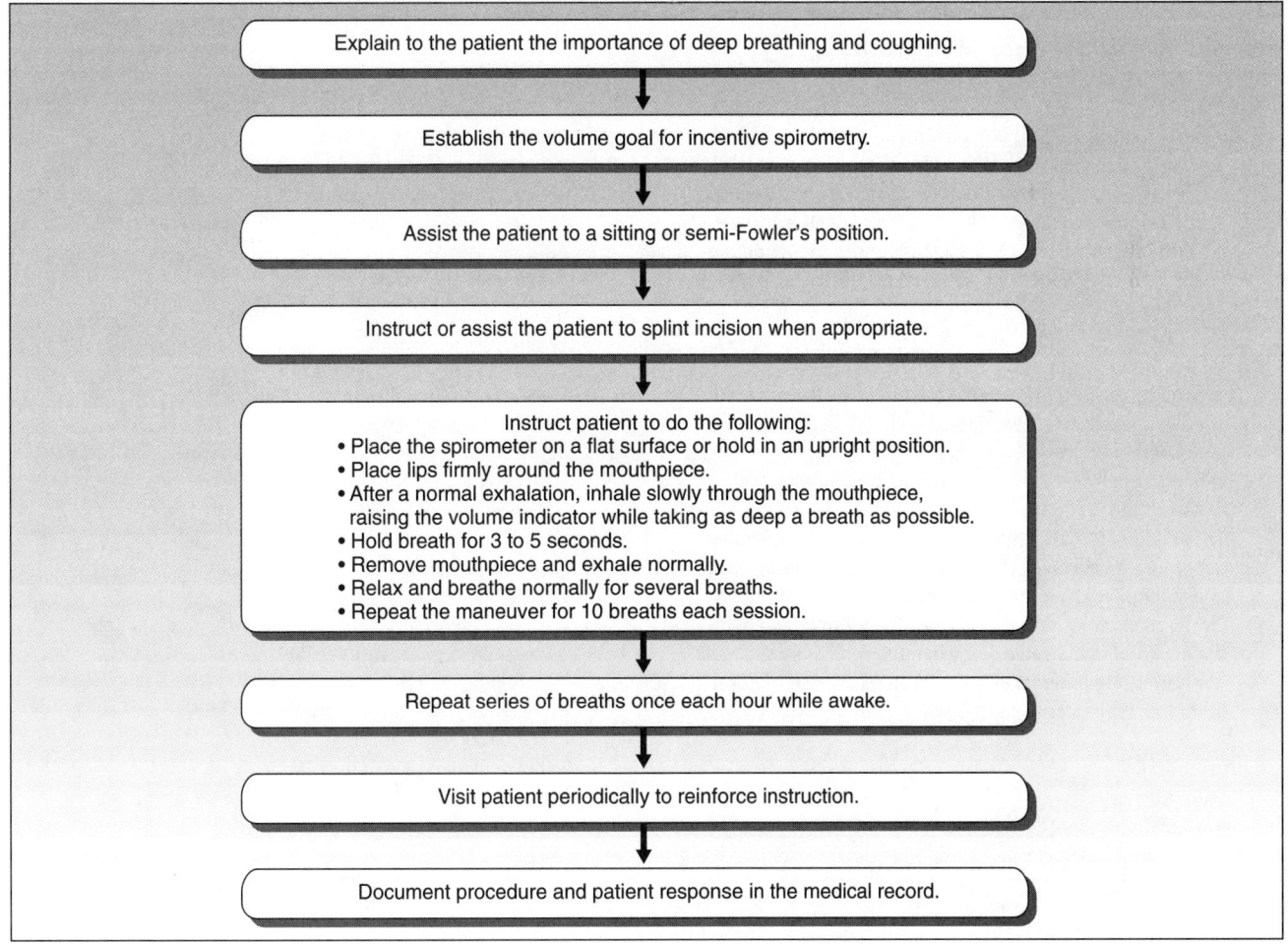

Figure 35-13   Incentive spirometry procedure.

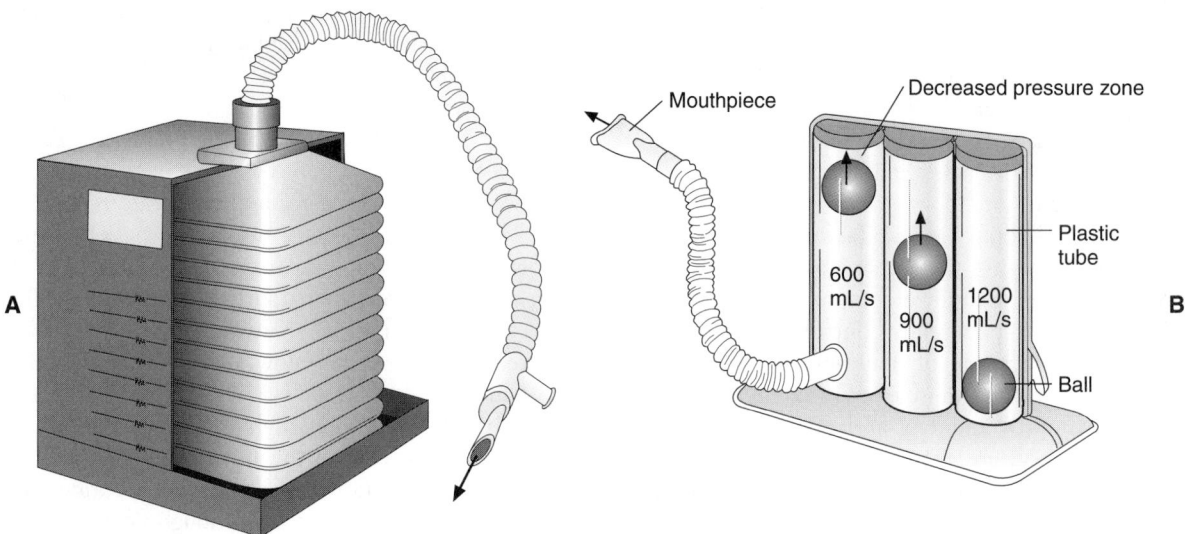

Figure 35-14 **A,** Volume-oriented incentive spirometer. **B,** Flow-oriented incentive spirometer. (Modified from Eubanks DH, Bone RC. Comprehensive respiratory care. St Louis: Mosby; 1985.)

 CPG 35-6

Intermittent Positive Pressure Breathing

Indications

The need to improve lung expansion; the presence of clinically important pulmonary atelectasis when other forms of therapy have been unsuccessful (incentive spirometry [IS], chest physiotherapy [CPT], deep breathing exercises, positive airway pressure) or the patient cannot cooperate; inability to clear secretions adequately because of pathologic process that severely limits the ability to ventilate or cough effectively; and failure to respond to other modes of treatment

The need for short-term ventilatory support for patients who are hypoventilated as an alternative to tracheal intubation and continuous ventilatory support

The need to deliver aerosol medication. Intermittent positive pressure breathing (IPPB) may be used to deliver aerosol medications to patients with fatigue as a result of ventilatory muscle weakness (for example, failure to wean from mechanical ventilation, neuromuscular disease, kyphoscoliosis) or chronic conditions in which intermittent ventilatory support is indicated (for example, ventilatory support for home care patients and the more recent use of nasal IPPV for respiratory insufficiency)

Contraindications

Pneumothorax
Intracranial pressure (ICP) >15 mm Hg
Hemodynamic instability

Recent surgery to face or mouth or skull
Tracheoesophageal fistula
Recent esophageal surgery
Active hemoptysis
Nausea
Air swallowing
Active untreated tuberculosis
Radiographic evidence of bleb
Singultations (hiccups)

Hazards and Complications

Increased airway resistance
Barotrauma
Nosocomial infection
Hypocarbia
Hemoptysis
Hyperoxia when oxygen is the gas source
Gastric distention
Impaction of secretions associated with inadequately humidified gas mixture
Psychologic dependence
Impedance of venous return
Exacerbation of hypoxemia
Hypoventilation
Increased mismatch of ventilation and perfusion
Air trapping

Modified from AARC Clinical practice guideline: intermittent positive pressure breathing. Respir Care 1993;38:1189-1195.
CPG, Clinical practice guideline.

of use decreases their efficacy.[77] IS is comparable in therapeutic effect to deep breathing exercises, coughing, early mobilization, and IPPB in the postoperative patient.[78-81] IS is also comparable to CPT after abdominal surgery,[82] whereas mounting evidence suggests that IS may not have a viable role in treatment of patients who have had thoracic surgery and have healthy lungs.[83]

Intermittent Positive Pressure Breathing

Intermittent positive pressure breathing (IPPB) is short-term or episodic mechanical ventilation for the primary purpose of assisting ventilation and providing short-duration hyperinflation therapy (CPG 35-6). IPPB is usually administered with pneumatically driven, pressure-triggered, and pressure-cycled ventilators (Figure 35-15). IPPB was first described in 1947. In the 1950s, it gained popularity as a method to treat and prevent postoperative atelectasis. In the 1960s, IPPB became a popular therapy for patients with pulmonary disease. In the 1970s, IPPB came under scrutiny both scientifically and by health care payers. Although IPPB has been used as a method for administration of aerosolized medication, it has no advantage over nebulizers or metered dose inhalers (MDIs). In fact, it

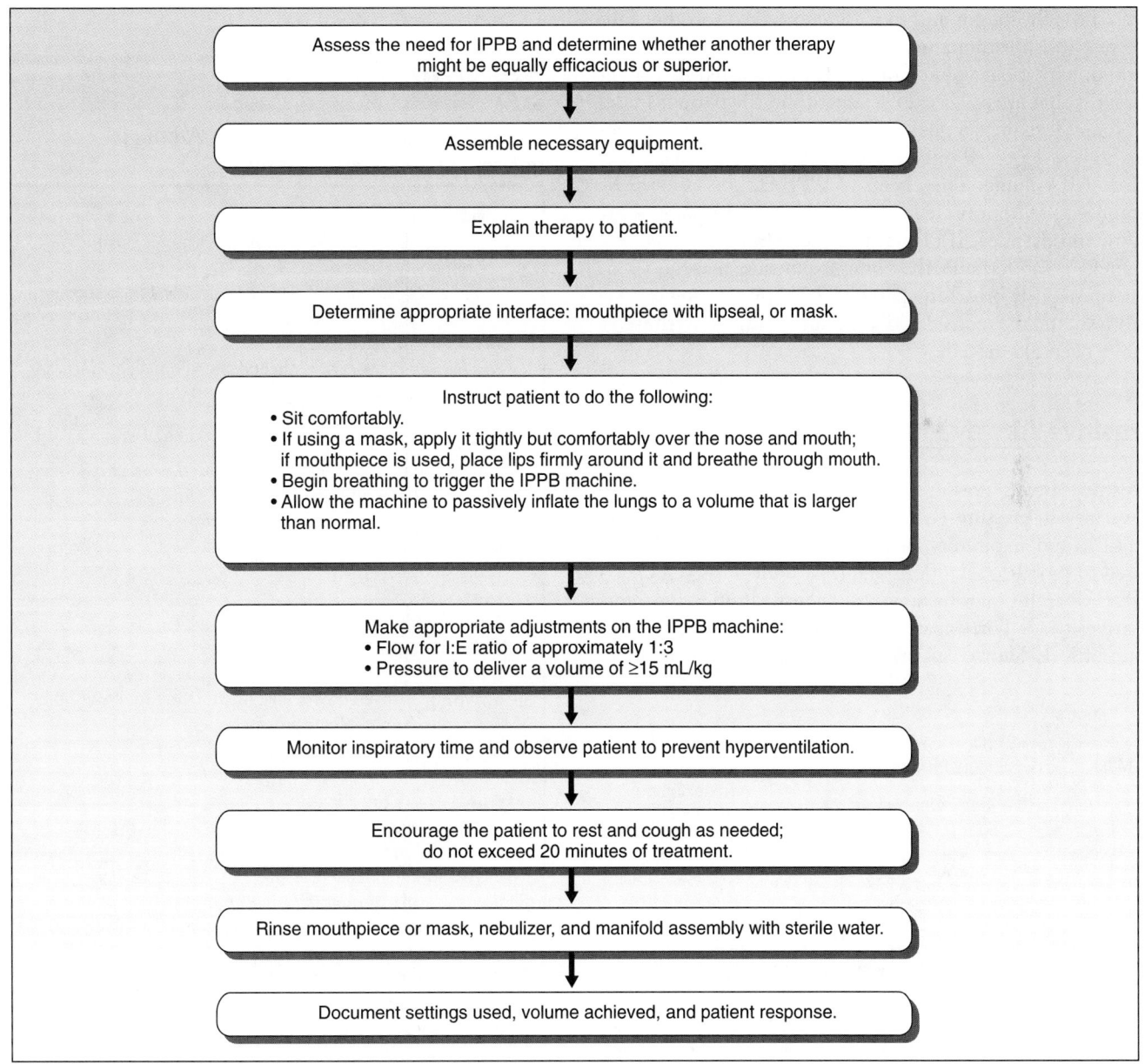

Figure 35-15 Procedure for intermittent positive pressure breathing (IPPB) therapy.

has been demonstrated that aerosols administered with IPPB deposit 32% less of the drug in the lungs than a hand-held nebulizer.[84] All of the mechanical effects of IPPB are short-lived, lasting an hour or less after the treatment. Efficacy of IPPB for ventilation and aerosol delivery is technique dependent (for example, coordination, breathing pattern, selection of appropriate inspiratory flow, peak pressure, inspiratory hold). Efficacy is dependent on the design of the device (for example, flow, volume, pressure capability) and on the aerosol output and particle size.

Assessment of the need for IPPB should include evidence of atelectasis, reduced pulmonary function precluding an effective cough, neuromuscular disorders, or kyphoscoliosis with decreased lung volumes. IPPB may be applicable in situations of fatigue or muscle weakness with impending respiratory failure, in the presence of acute severe bronchospasm, and in COPD exacerbation that fails to respond to other therapy. IPPB should be volume oriented, with tidal volume during IPPB adjusted to deliver breaths that are at least 25% larger than the patient's tidal volume. It may be argued that IPPB should target volumes as high as 15 to 20 mL/kg, approximating a normal effective sigh volume. The effects of IPPB can be assessed by improved secretion clearance, breath sounds, chest x-ray film, and dyspnea. IPPB has not been shown to have any benefit greater than other lung expansion techniques in spontaneously breathing patients.[85] Its use for lung expansion should be considered only after other alternatives have been exhausted.

Positive Airway Pressure

Positive airway pressure (PAP) includes continuous positive airway pressure (CPAP), positive expiratory pressure (PEP), and expiratory positive airway pressure (EPAP), used to mobilize secretions and treat atelectasis (CPG 35-7). PAP techniques have proven to provide effective alternatives to CPT in expanding the lungs and mobilizing secretions. Evidence suggests that PAP therapy is more effective than IS and IPPB in the management of postoperative atelectasis[86,87] and as an adjunct to enhance the benefits of aerosol bronchodilator delivery.[88,89] Cough and other airway clearance techniques are essential components of PAP therapy.

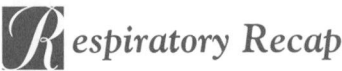

Respiratory Recap

Positive Airway Pressure Techniques
Continuous positive airway pressure
Expiratory positive airway pressure
Positive expiratory pressure

CPG 35-7

Use of Positive Airway Pressure Adjuncts to Bronchial Hygiene Therapy

Indications
To reduce air trapping in asthma and chronic obstructive pulmonary disease
To aid in mobilization of retained secretions (in cystic fibrosis and chronic bronchitis)
To prevent or reverse atelectasis
To optimize delivery of bronchodilators in patients receiving bronchial hygiene therapy

Contraindications
Patients unable to tolerate the increased work of breathing
Intracranial pressure greater than 20 mm Hg
Hemodynamic instability
Recent surgery to face or mouth or skull
Acute sinusitis
Epistaxis
Esophageal surgery
Active hemoptysis
Nausea
Known or suspected tympanic membrane rupture or other middle ear pathologic process
Untreated pneumothorax

Hazards and Complications
Increased work of breathing that may lead to hypoventilation and hypercarbia
Increased intracranial pressure
Cardiovascular compromise
Air swallowing with increased likelihood of vomiting and aspiration
Claustrophobia
Skin breakdown and discomfort from mask
Pulmonary barotrauma

Modified from AARC Clinical practice guideline: use of positive airway pressure adjuncts to bronchial hygiene therapy. Respir Care 1993;38:516-521. CPG, Clinical practice guideline.

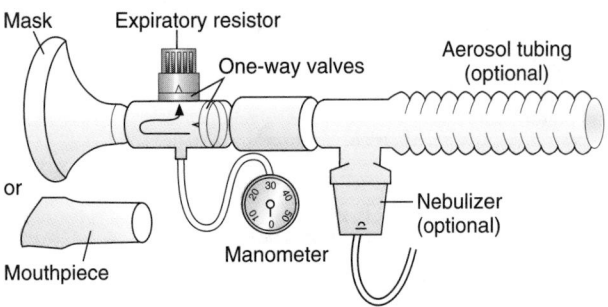

Figure 35-16 Equipment for positive expiratory pressure therapy. (Modified from Malmeister MJ, Fink JB, Hoffman GL. Positive expiratory pressure mask therapy: theoretical and practical considerations and a review of the literature. Respir Care 1991;36:1218-1229.)

CPAP is the application of a positive airway pressure to the spontaneously breathing patient throughout the respiratory cycle at pressures of 5 to 20 cm H_2O. EPAP applies positive pressure to the airway, much like CPAP, but only during the expiratory phase. Unlike CPAP, patients generate subatmospheric pressures during inspiration. **Positive expiratory pressure (PEP)** consists of positive pressure generated as a patient exhales through a fixed orifice resistor generating pressures ranging from 10 to 20 cm H_2O (Figure 35-16).[90] The fixed orifice resistor (which differentiates PEP from EPAP) only generates pressure when exhaled flow is high enough to generate back pressure. EPAP, using a threshold resistor, does not produce the same mechanical or physiologic effects as PEP with a fixed orifice. Threshold resistors exert a predictable, quantifiable, and constant force at the expiratory limb of a circuit. A true threshold resistor maintains constant pressure in the circuit, independent of changing flows. Relatively few CPAP devices are true threshold resistors in that they offer some flow resistance once the valve is open. Because the patient must breathe to subatmospheric pressures on inspiration, EPAP and PEP may require more breathing effort than CPAP.

Rationale for Continuous Positive Airway Pressure

Pursed-lip breathing is a procedure that many patients with COPD have taught themselves to relieve air trapping caused by collapse of unstable airways during expiration. The resistance at the mouth during a pursed-lip exhalation transmits back pressure to splint the airways open, preventing compression and premature closure (much like the fixed orifice resistor). Pursed-lip breathing represents a functional predecessor to modern strategies used to apply PEP to the airway.

The prophylactic and therapeutic use of intermittent mask CPAP has been shown to be as effective as IS after thoracic or upper abdominal surgery, and it is an effortless and less painless type of postoperative respiratory care.[91-93] By preventing the collapse of expiratory airways, CPAP may facilitate a homogenous distribution of ventilation throughout the lungs, via collateral interbronchiolar channels.[94,95]

Positive Expiratory Pressure Administration Techniques

PEP therapy is performed with the patient seated comfortably and with elbows resting on a table (Figure 35-17). Equipment consists of a soft transparent mask or mouthpiece, T-assembly with a one-way valve, a variety of fixed orifice resistors (or adjustable expiratory resistor), and a manometer. The mask is applied tightly but comfortably over the mouth and nose. The subject is instructed to relax while performing diaphragmatic breathing, inspiring a volume of air larger than normal tidal volume but not to

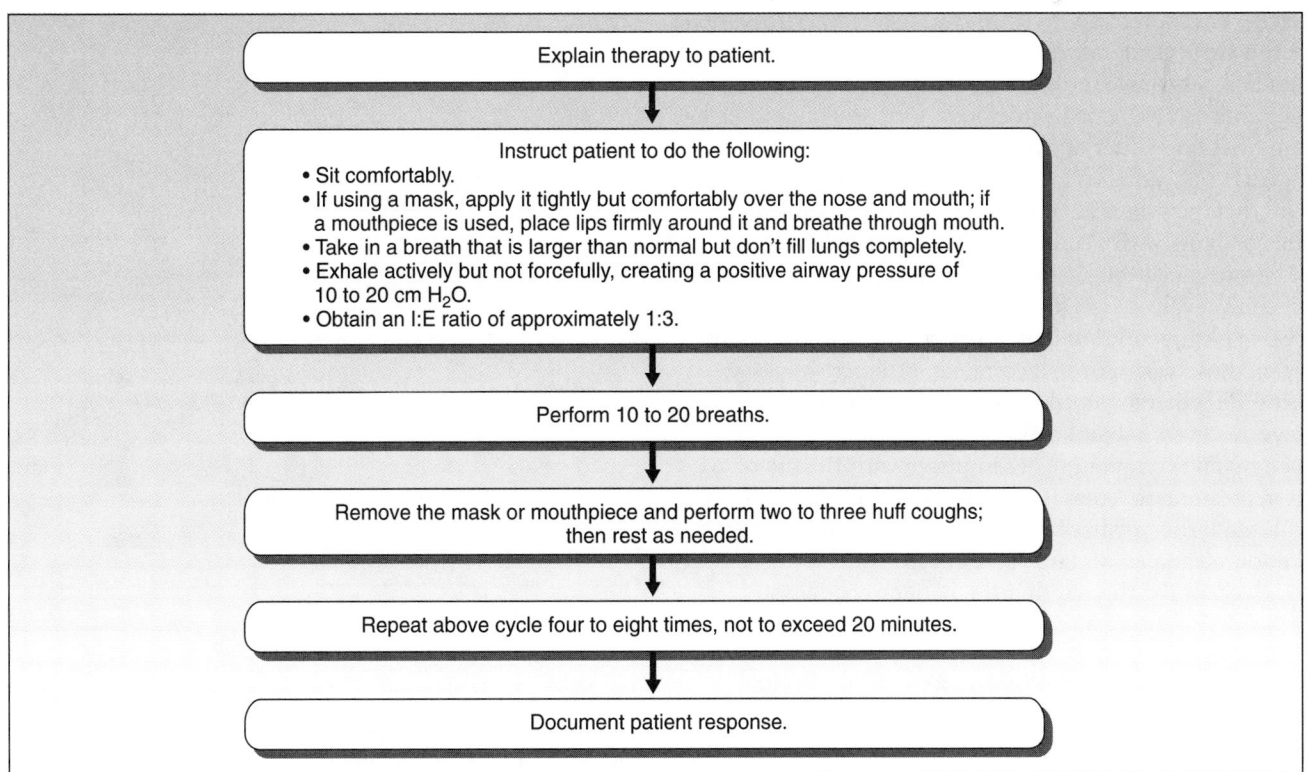

Figure 35-17   Technique for positive expiratory pressure therapy.

the level of total lung capacity, through the one-way valve. Exhalation to functional residual capacity (FRC) is active but not forced, through the resistor chosen to achieve a PAP of 10 to 20 cm H_2O during exhalation. A series of 10 to 20 breaths are performed with the mask or mouthpiece in place. The mask (or mouthpiece) is then removed, and the patient performs several coughs to raise secretions. This sequence of 10 to 20 breaths, followed by huff coughing, is repeated four to six times per PEP therapy session. Because of its secretion-clearing effects in patients with CF, PEP may be superior to standard CPT in this patient population. Each session requires 10 to 20 minutes and may be performed one to four times per day as needed. For lung expansion, patients should be encouraged to take 10 to 20 breaths every hour while awake.

Selection of a resistor with an appropriate orifice size is critical to proper technique. The therapeutic goal is to achieve a PEP of 10 to 20 cm H_2O, with an inspiration to expiration (I:E) ratio of 1:3 to 1:4. When a fixed orifice is used, most adults achieve this pressure range with an orifice of 2.5 to 4.0 mm in diameter. A manometer is placed in line to measure the expiratory pressure while the appropriate-sized orifice is selected. Once the proper resistor orifice has been determined, the manometer may be removed from the system. Selection of a resistor with too large an orifice produces a short exhalation, with failure to achieve the proper expiratory pressure. Too small an orifice prolongs the expiratory phase, elevates the pressure above 20 cm H_2O, and increases the work of breathing. Performing a PEP session for more than 20 minutes may lead to fatigue. During periods of exacerbation, individuals are encouraged to increase the frequency with which PEP is performed, rather than extending the length of individual sessions. Aerosol therapy may be performed simultaneously with or just before a PEP session, either by hand-held nebulizer or MDI.

Although no absolute contraindications to the use of PEP therapies have been reported, common sense dictates that patients with acute sinusitis, ear infection, epistaxis, or recent facial, oral, or skull injury or surgery should be carefully evaluated before a decision is made to initiate PEP mask therapy. Patients experiencing active hemoptysis or those with unresolved pneumothorax should avoid using PEP therapy until these acute pulmonary problems have resolved. Complications such as barotrauma or hemodynamic compromise are intuitive with the use of positive pressure; no complications have been reported when PEP mask therapy has been used for lung expansion or secretion clearance, in large part because of the techniques involved in the therapy and the patient population.

High-Frequency Techniques

High-frequency oscillation of the airway (HFOA) in the conducting airways is used in a variety of techniques designed to enhance clearance of secretions. HFOA can be generated by devices providing the oscillations at the air-

way opening or on the chest wall. The oscillations can be mechanically generated and administered to the patient or self-generated by expiration through an oscillatory device. HFOAs can influence mucus clearance through a variety of mechanisms, including alteration of mucus rheology, enhanced mucus-airflow interaction, and reflex mechanisms.

HFOA reduces the viscosity of sputum in vitro.[96] Shearing at the air-mucus interface could be a significant factor in the enhanced tracheal mucus clearance during HFOA.[97] Although the mechanism for the reduction in viscoelasticity is unknown, likely possibilities involve the cooperative unfolding of the physical entanglements between the primary network of mucous glycoproteins and other structural macromolecules, the rupture of cross-linking bonds such as disulfide bridges, or the fragmentation of larger molecules such as DNA or F-actin, which are present as byproducts of infection and can increase mucus viscoelasticity because of their interactions with glycoproteins.

High-frequency oscillation of the chest wall (HFOCW) has been shown to increase tracheal mucus clearance rates and to correlate with improved ventilation. HFOCW may improve secretion clearance by a combination of three possible mechanisms. First, it may reduce the viscoelastic and cohesive properties of mucus,[98,99] thus making it more easily

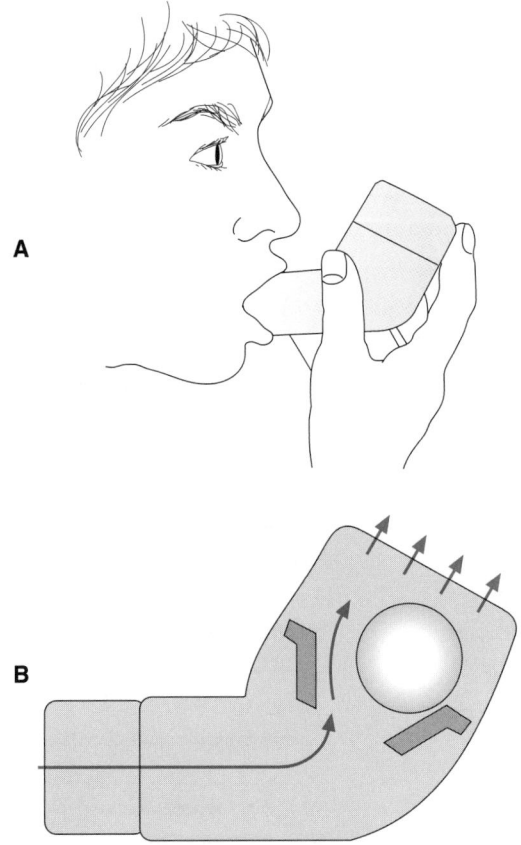

Figure 35-18 A, Position of Flutter valve in patient's mouth. **B,** During exhalation, the position of the steel ball is the result of an equilibrium between the pressure of the exhaled gas, the force of gravity on the ball, and the angle of the cone where the contact with the ball occurs. As the steel ball rolls and bounces up and down, it creates oscillations in the airway.

clearable by the air-liquid interactions associated with cephalad airflow velocity bias. Second, HFOA may reinforce the interaction with the cilia or the natural harmonics of the chest wall. Third, HFOCW may stimulate the release of fresh secretions by a vagal reflex mechanism, the fresh secretions being more easily mobilized by airflow interactions.

Flutter Valve

The Flutter mucus clearance device combines the techniques of PEP with HFOA at the airway opening. A pipe-shaped device with a steel ball in the bowl is loosely covered by a perforated cap (Figure 35-18). The weight of the ball serves as a PEP device (approximately 10 cm H_2O), whereas the internal shape of the bowl allows the ball to flutter, generating oscillations of about 15 Hz (2 to 32 Hz), varying with the position of the device. The proposed mechanism of effect includes shearing of mucus from the airway wall by oscillatory action; stabilization of airways, preventing premature airway closure; facilitation of cepha-

lad flow of mucus; and changes in mucus rheology. The procedure for Flutter therapy is shown in Figure 35-19.

Although the Flutter has been available for several years, little has been published on its efficacy. In one study,[100] the amount of sputum expectorated by patients with CF was more than three times the amount expectorated with either voluntary cough or PD. Another study reported that Flutter valve therapy was an acceptable alternative to conventional CPT in hospitalized patients with CF.[101] However, conflicting results have been reported in other studies.[102-106]

Percussionaire

Intermittent percussive ventilation (IPV) of the lungs is a therapeutic form of CPT with the use of a pneumatic device called a *Percussionator*. IPV was designed to treat atelectasis, enhance the mobilization and clearance of retained secretions, and deliver nebulized medications to the distal airways.[107] With IPV the patient breathes through a mouthpiece that delivers high-flow minibursts at rates of more than 200 cycles per minute (Figure 35-20). During these percussive bursts of gas into the airway a continuous airway pressure is maintained while the pulsatile percussive intra-airway pressure rises progressively. Each percussive cycle is programmed by holding of a thumb button for 5 to 10 seconds for the percussive inspiratory cycle, followed by release of the button for exhalation. Treatments of approximately 20 minutes are recommended by the manufacturer. Impaction pressures of 25 to 40 psig (pounds per square inch, gauge) are delivered with a frequency from less than

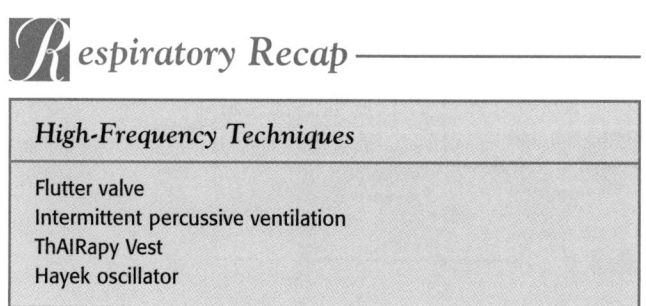

℟ *espiratory Recap* ———————

High-Frequency Techniques
Flutter valve
Intermittent percussive ventilation
ThAIRapy Vest
Hayek oscillator

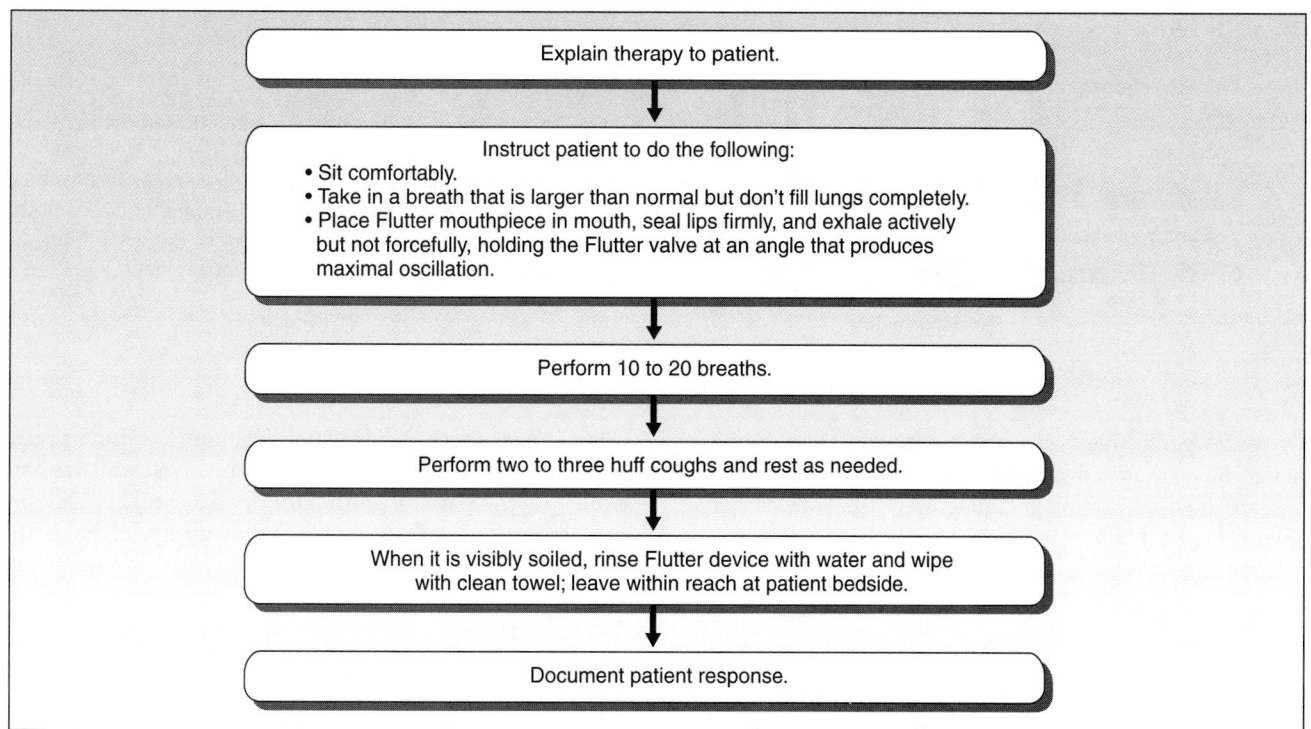

Explain therapy to patient.

Instruct patient to do the following:
• Sit comfortably.
• Take in a breath that is larger than normal but don't fill lungs completely.
• Place Flutter mouthpiece in mouth, seal lips firmly, and exhale actively but not forcefully, holding the Flutter valve at an angle that produces maximal oscillation.

Perform 10 to 20 breaths.

Perform two to three huff coughs and rest as needed.

When it is visibly soiled, rinse Flutter device with water and wipe with clean towel; leave within reach at patient bedside.

Document patient response.

Figure 35-19   Technique for Flutter valve therapy.

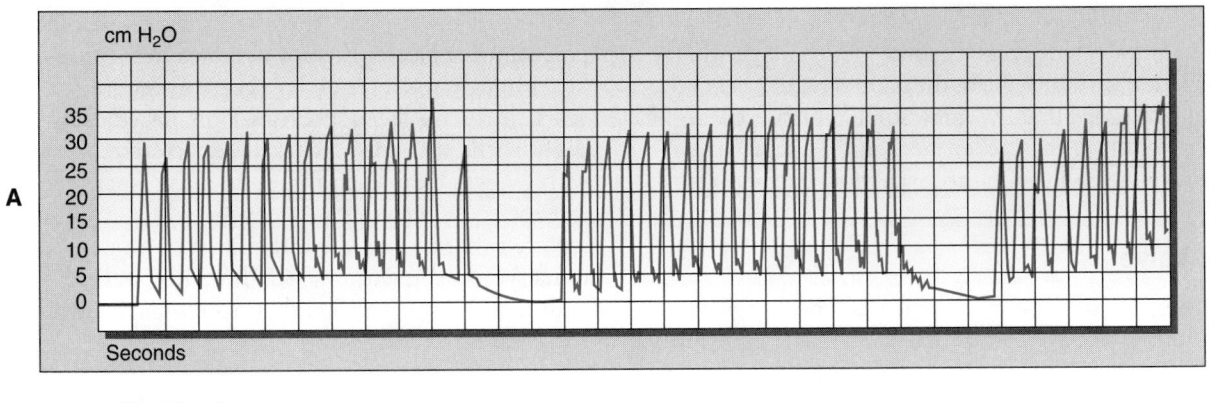

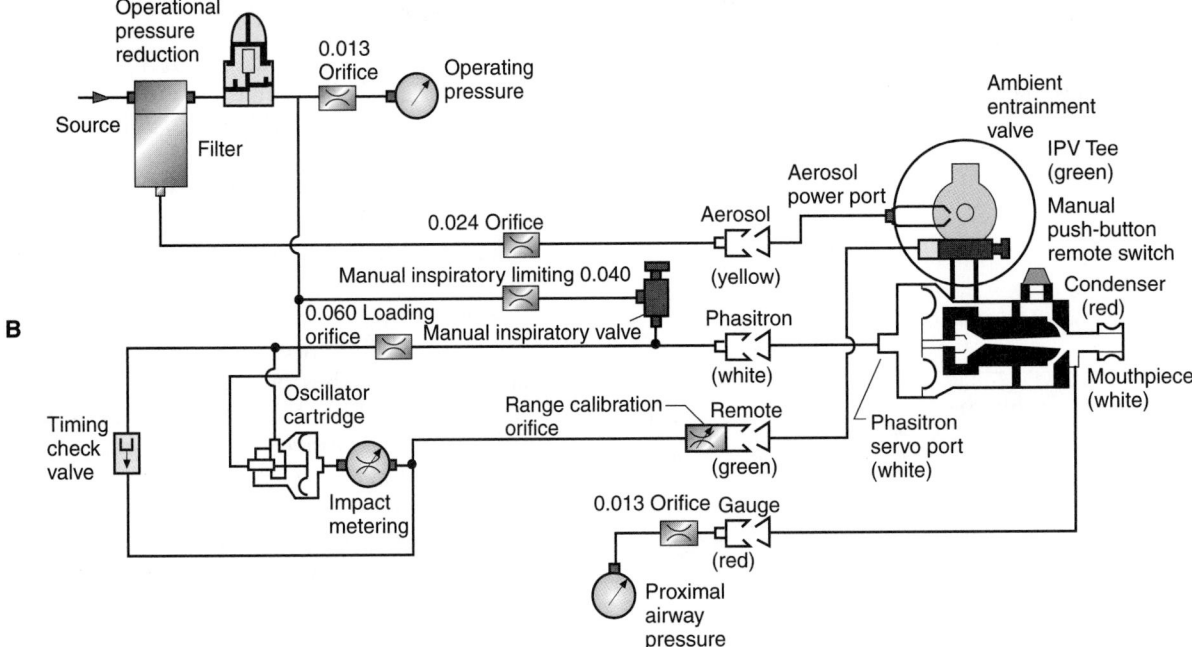

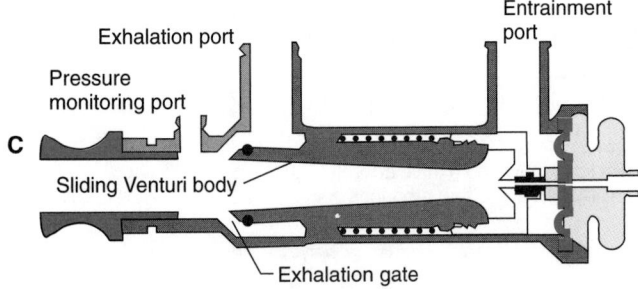

Figure 35-20 **A,** Airway pressure pattern seen during intermittent percussive ventilation (IPV) therapy. **B,** Internal schematic of the IPV ventilator. **C,** The phasitron, which is the heart of the IPV ventilator, is a sliding Venturi that directs both inspiratory and expiratory gas at the airway. (Modified from materials courtesy Percussionaire, Sandpoint, Idaho.)

100 to 225 percussive cycles per minute at 40 psig. Several studies have reported comparable results with IPV and standard CPT.[108-110] The manufacturer lists sore ribs, fatigue, stress, and irritation as potential side effects.

ThAIRapy Vest

The ThAIRapy Vest (Advanced Respiratory, St. Paul, Minn.) consists of a large-volume, variable-frequency air pulse delivery system attached to a nonstretchable inflatable vest worn by the patient that extends over the entire

torso down to the iliac crest (Figure 35-21). Pressure pulses that fill the vest and vibrate the chest wall are controlled by the patient (with a foot pedal) and applied during expiration or the entire respiratory cycle. Pulse frequency is adjustable from 5 to 25 Hz, with pressure in the vest varying from 28 mm Hg at 5 Hz to 39 mm Hg at 25 Hz. In theory, these vibrations to the chest wall cause transient increases in airflow in the lungs, to improve gas-liquid interactions and the movement of mucus. The frequency of oscillations (cycles per second) and flow bias (inspiratory versus expiratory) are important in determin-

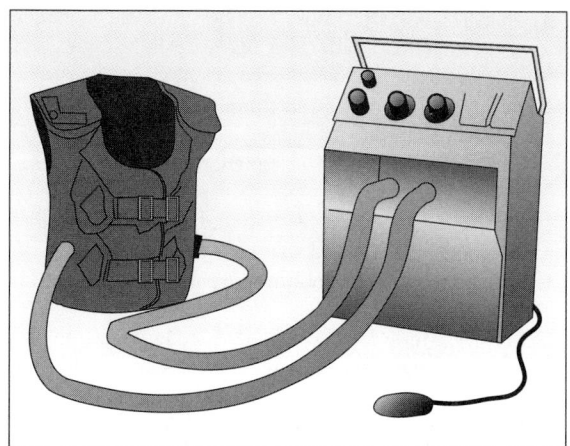

Figure 35-21 The ThAIRapy Vest airway clearance system is a portable device consisting of an inflatable vest connected by hose to an air-pulse generator. The generator rapidly inflates and deflates The Vest, compressing and releasing the chest wall. This process moves mucus towards the larger airways where it can be cleared. (Modified from materials courtesy Advanced Respiratory, St. Paul, Minn.)

ing effectiveness.[111, 112] ThAIRapy has been reported to be effective for secretion clearance in patients with CF.[113-115] Conjecture that this device has a role in lung expansion for patients other than those with CF in the acute care settings has not been empirically established.

Hayek Oscillator

The Hayek oscillator is an electrically powered, microprocessor-controlled, noninvasive oscillator ventilator that uses an external flexible chest enclosure (cuirass) to apply negative and positive pressure to the chest wall to deliver noninvasive oscillation to the lungs (Figure 35-22). The negative pressure generated in the cuirass causes the chest wall to expand for inspiration, whereas positive pressure compresses the chest to produce a forced expiration. Both inspiratory and expiratory phases may be active and not reliant on passive recoil of the chest. Expiratory pressure can be positive, atmospheric, or negative, allowing ventilation to occur above, at, or below the patient's normal FRC. Success has been reported with this device as a method of ventilatory support.[116] Four adjustable parameters with the Hayek include frequency range (to 999 oscillations per minute),

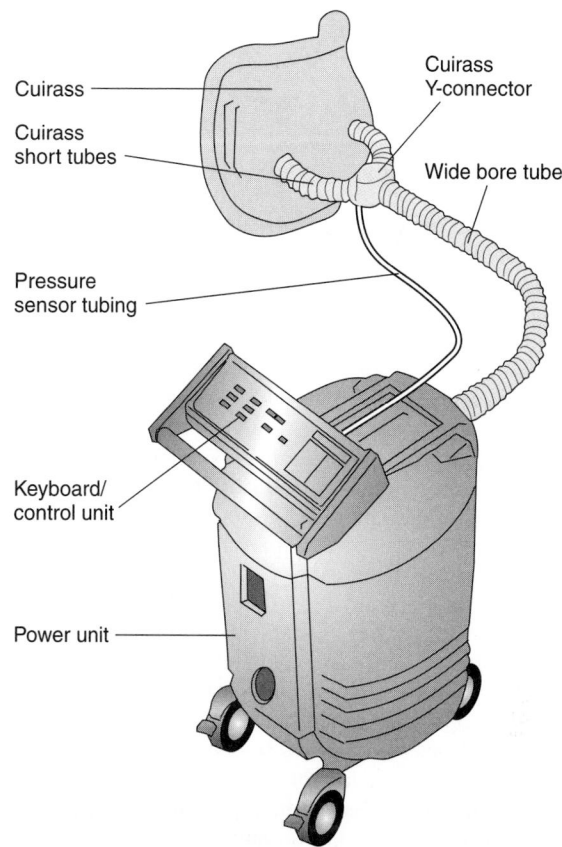

Figure 35-22 Schematic drawing of the Hayek oscillator. (Modified from materials courtesy Breasy Medical Equipment, Stamford, Conn.)

I:E ratio (6:1 to 1:6), inspiratory pressure, and expiratory pressure (-70 to $+70$ cm H_2O).

Clinicians' anecdotal observations of spontaneous expulsion of secretions during high-frequency ventilation has led to the development of several discrete secretion management program recommendations in which the chest is oscillated through two sets of cycles: several minutes at a high frequency of up to 999/minute (usually 600 to 720/minute) at an I:E ratio of 1:1 followed by 60/90 cycles per minute at an I:E ratio of 5:1. The setting can be changed according to the patient's need. Reports of efficacy of this or similar protocols for secretion management with the Hayek have yet to be published. It has been reported that high-frequency oscillation applied via the airway or via the chest wall and CPT have comparable augmenting effects on expectorated sputum.[117]

$\mathcal{K}$EY $\mathcal{P}$OINTS

- Mucociliary transport is responsible for normal clearance of secretions from the lower respiratory tract.
- Cough is responsible for secretion clearance in cases of acute and chronic respiratory disease.
- Humidification of the inspired gas has little effect on secretion clearance.
- Bland aerosols are most commonly used for induced sputum.
- Airway suctioning, nasotracheal suction, and bronchoscopy are used to mechanically clear secretions from the lower respiratory tract.
- Conventional chest physiotherapy consists of postural drainage, percussion, and vibration.
- Active cycle of breathing techniques consist of breathing control, thoracic expansion control, and forced expiratory technique.
- Autogenic drainage aims to achieve the highest possible airflow in different generations of bronchi to move secretions.
- Incentive spirometry is used to facilitate deep breathing in postoperative patients.
- Intermittent positive pressure breathing is used for short-term hyperinflation therapy.
- Positive expiratory pressure therapy consists of positive pressure generated as a patient exhales through a fixed orifice generator, producing pressures of 10 to 20 cm H_2O.
- High-frequency techniques for secretion clearance include the Flutter valve, intermittent percussive ventilation, and external chest wall compression.

References

1. Sorenson HM. Managing secretions in dying patients. Respir Care 2000;45:1355-1362.
2. Sleigh MA. Ciliary function in transport of mucus. Eur J Respir Dis 1983;128(Suppl 64):287-289.
3. King M. Viscoelastic properties of airway mucus. Fed Proc 1980;39:3080-3085.
4. King M. Rheological requirements for optimal clearance of secretions: ciliary transport versus cough. Eur J Respir Dis 1980;110(Suppl):39-45.
5. King M. Is cystic fibrosis mucus abnormal? Pediatr Res 1981;15:120-122.
6. King M, Kelly S, Cosio M. Alteration of airway reactivity by mucus. Respir Physiol 1985;62:47-59.
7. Gross D, Zidulka A, O'Brien C, et al. Peripheral mucociliary clearance with high frequency chest wall compression. J Appl Physiol 1985;58:1157-1163.
8. Warwick WJ. Mechanisms of mucus transport. Eur J Resp Dis 1983;127(Suppl 64):162-167.
9. Camner P. Studies on the removal of inhaled particles from the lungs by voluntary coughing. Chest 1981;80(Suppl 6):824-827.
10. Irwin RS, Madison JM. The diagnosis and treatment of cough. N Engl J Med 2000;343:1715-1721.
11. Thomas J, Cook DJ, Brooks D. Chest physical therapy management of patients with cystic fibrosis. Am J Respir Crit Care Med 1995;151:846-850.
12. Pizzichni MM, Popov TA, Efthimiadis A, et al. Spontaneous and induced sputum to measure indices of airway inflammation in asthma. Am J Respir Crit Care Med 1996;154:866-869.
13. Bhowmik A, Seemungal TA, Sapsford RJ, et al. Comparison of spontaneous and induced sputum for investigation of airway inflammation in chronic obstructive pulmonary disease. Thorax 1998;53:953-956.
14. Desai MA, Mutlu M, Vadgama P. A study of macromolecular diffusion through native porcine mucus. Experientia 1992;48:22-26.
15. Bolister N, Basker M, Hodges NA, et al. The diffusion of beta-lactam antibiotics through mixed gels of cystic fibrosis–derived mucin and *Pseudomonas aeruginosa* alginate. J Antimicrob Chemother 1991;27:285-293.
16. Wilmott RW, Amin RS, Colin AA, et al. Aerosolized recombinant human DNase in hospitalized cystic fibrosis patients with acute pulmonary exacerbations. Am J Respir Crit Care Med 1996;153:1914-1917.
17. Hess D. Managing the artificial airway. Respir Care 1999;44:759-772.
18. Raymond SJ. Normal saline instillation before suctioning: helpful or harmful? A review of the literature. Am J Crit Care 1995;4:267-271.
19. Kollef MH, Prentice D, Shapiro SD. Mechanical ventilation with or without daily changes of in-line suction catheters. Am J Respir Crit Care Med 1997;156:466-472.
20. Jaworski A, Goldberg SK, Walkenstein MD, et al. Utility of immediate postlobectomy fiber-optic bronchoscopy in preventing atelectasis. Chest 1988;94:38-43.
21. Marini JJ, Pierson DJ, Hudson LD. Acute lobar atelectasis: a prospective comparison of fiber-optic bronchoscopy and respiratory therapy. Am Rev Respir Dis 1979;19:971-978.
22. American Thoracic Society Medical Section of the American Lung Association Guidelines for fiber-optic bronchoscopy. Am Rev Respir Dis 1987;136:1066.
23. Kollef MH, Bock KR, Richards RD, et al. The safety and diagnostic accuracy of minibronchoalveolar lavage in patients with suspected ventilator-associated pneumonia. Ann Intern Med 1995;122:743-748.
24. Bach JR. Update and perspective on noninvasive respiratory muscle aids. Part 2. The expiratory aids. Chest 1994;105:1538-1544.
25. Zack MB, Pontoppidan H, Kazemi H. The effect of lateral positions on gas exchange in pulmonary disease: a prospective evaluation. Am Rev Respir Dis 1974;110:49-55.
26. Hess D, Agarwal NN, Myers CL. Positioning, lung function, and kinetic bed therapy. Respir Care 1992;37:181-197.
27. Curley MA. Prone positioning of patients with acute respiratory distress syndrome: a systematic review. Am J Crit Care 1999;8:397-405.
28. Oberwaldner B. Physiotherapy for airway clearance in paediatrics. Eur Respir J 2000;15:196-204.
29. van der Schans C, Prasad A, Main E. Chest physiotherapy compared to no chest physiotherapy for cystic fibrosis. The Cochrane Database of Systematic Reviews. Vol 4; 2000.
30. Jones AP, Rowe BH. Bronchopulmonary hygiene physical therapy for chronic obstructive pulmonary disease. The Cochrane Database of Systematic Reviews. Vol 4; 2000.

31. van der Schans C, Prasad A, Main E. Conventional chest physiotherapy compared to any form of chest physiotherapy for cystic fibrosis. The Cochrane Database of Systematic Reviews. Vol 4; 2000.

32. Flenady VJ, Gray PH. Chest physiotherapy for preventing morbidity in babies being extubated from mechanical ventilation. The Cochrane Database of Systematic Reviews. Vol 4; 2000.

33. Alexander E, Weingarten S, Mohsenifar Z. Clinical strategies to reduce utilization of chest physiotherapy without compromising patient care. Chest 1996;110:430-432.

34. Oermann CM, Swank PR, Sockrider MM. Validation of an instrument measuring patient satisfaction with chest physiotherapy techniques in cystic fibrosis. Chest 2000;118:92-97.

35. Murphy MB, Concannon D, Fitzgerald MX. Chest percussion: help or hindrance to postural drainage? Irish Med J 1983; 76:189-190.

36. Sutton PP, Lopez-Vidriero MT, Pavia D, et al. Assessment of percussion, vibratory shaking and breathing exercises in chest physiotherapy. Eur J Respir Dis 1985;66:147-152.

37. Pavia D, Thomson ML, Phillipakos D. A preliminary study of the effect of a vibrating pad on bronchial clearance. Am Rev Respir Dis 1976;113:92-96.

38. Maxwell M, Redmond A. Comparative trial of manual and mechanical percussion technique with gravity-assisted bronchial drainage in patients with cystic fibrosis. Arch of Dis Child 1979;54:542-544.

39. Holody B, Goldberg HS. The effect of mechanical vibration physiotherapy in arterial oxygenation in acutely ill patients with atelectasis or pneumonia. Am Rev Respir Dis 1981;124: 372-375.

40. Wollmer P, Ursing K, Midgren B, et al. Inefficiency of chest percussion in the physical therapy of chronic bronchitis. Eur J Respir Dis 1985;66:233-239.

41. van der Schans CP, Peris DA, Postma DS. Effect of manual percussion on tracheobronchial clearance in patients with chronic airflow obstruction and excessive tracheobronchial secretion. Thorax 1986;41:448-452.

42. Radford R, Barutt J, Billingsley JG, et al. A rational basis for percussion-augmented mucociliary clearance. Respir Care 1982;27:556-563.

43. Tyler ML. Complications of positioning and chest physiotherapy. Respir Care 1982;27:458-466.

44. Krause MF, Hoehn T. Chest physiotherapy in mechanically ventilated children: a review. Crit Care Med 2000;28: 1648-1651.

45. Clarke RCN, Kelly BE, Convery PN, et al. Ventilatory characteristics in mechanically ventilated patients during manual hyperventilation for chest physiotherapy. Anaesthesia 1999; 54:936-940.

46. Wallis C, Prasad A. Who needs chest physiotherapy? Moving from anecdote to evidence. Arch Dis Child 1999;80:393-397.

47. Fauroux B, Boule M, Lofaso F, et al. Chest physiotherapy in cystic fibrosis: improved tolerance with nasal pressure support ventilation. Pediatrics 1999;103:658-659.

48. Partridge C, Pryor J, Webber B. Characteristics of the forced expiratory technique. Physiotherapy 1989;75:193-194.

49. Jacobs WR, Zaroukian MH. Coughing and central venous catheter dislodgement. JPEN 1991;15:491-493.

50. Stern RC, Horwitz SJ, Doerslock CF. Neurologic symptoms during coughing paroxysms in cystic fibrosis. J Pediatr 1988; 112:909-912.

51. Ing AJ, Ngu MC, Breslin AB. Chronic persistent cough and gastroesophageal reflux. Thorax 1991;46:479-483.

52. Pryor JA, Webber BA. An evaluation of the forced expiration technique as an adjunct to postural drainage. Physiotherapy 1979;65:304-307.

53. Pryor JA, Webber BA, Hodson ME et al. Evaluation of the forced expiration technique as an adjunct to postural drainage in the treatment of cystic fibrosis. Br Med J 1979;2:417-418.

54. Bateman JRM, Newman SP, Daunt KM, et al. Is cough as effective as chest physiotherapy in the removal of excessive secretions? Thorax 1981;36:683-687.

55. DeBoeck C, Zinman R. Cough versus chest physiotherapy: a comparison of the acute effects on pulmonary function in patients with cystic fibrosis. Am Rev Respir Dis 1984;129: 182-185.

56. Webber BA, Hofmeyer JL, Morgan MDL, et al. Effects of postural drainage, incorporating the forced expiration technique, on pulmonary function in cystic fibrosis. Br J Dis Chest 1986; 80:353-359.

57. Bain J, Bishop J, Olinsky A. Evaluation of directed coughing in cystic fibrosis. Br J Dis Chest 1988;82:138-148.

58. Hie T, Pas BG, Roth RD, et al. Huff coughing and airway patency. Respir Care 1979;24:710-713.

59. Sutton PP, et al. Assessment of the forced expiration technique, postural drainage, and directed coughing in chest physiotherapy. Eur J Respir Dis 1983;64:62-68.

60. Hardy KA. A review of airway clearance: new techniques, indications, and recommendations. Respir Care 1994;39:440-452.

61. Pryor JA, Webber BA, Hodson ME, et al. Evaluation of the forced expiration technique as an adjunct to postural drainage in the treatment of cystic fibrosis. Br Med J 1979;2:417-418.

62. Hasani A, Pavia D, Agnew JE, et al. Regional lung clearance during cough and forced expiration technique (FET): effects of flow and viscoelasticity. Thorax 1994;49:557-561.

63. Hasani A, Pavia D, Agnew JE, et al. Regional mucus transport following unproductive cough and forced expiration technique in patients with airways obstruction. Chest 1994;105:1420-1425.

64. Chevaillier J. Autogenic drainage (AD). In: Lawson D, editor. Cystic fibrosis: horizons. Chichester, England: John Wiley; 1984. p. 235.

65. Schom MH. Autogenic drainage: a modern approach to physiotherapy in cystic fibrosis. J R Soc Med 1989:82(Suppl 16):32-37.

66. Miller S, Hall DO, Clayton CB, et al. Chest physiotherapy in cystic fibrosis. A comparative study of autogenic drainage and the active cycle of breathing techniques with postural drainage. Thorax 1995;50:165-169.

67. Giles DR, Wagener JS, Accurso FJ, et al. Short-term effects of postural drainage with clapping vs autogenic drainage on oxygen saturation and sputum recovery in patients with cystic fibrosis. Chest 1995;108:92-94.

68. Sahl DL, Bilton D, Dodd M, et al. Effect of exercise and physiotherapy in aiding sputum expectoration in adults with cystic fibrosis. Thorax 1989;44:1006-1008.

69. Zach MS, Purrer B, Oberwaldner B. Effect of swimming on forced expiration and sputum clearance in cystic fibrosis. Lancet 1981;ii:1201-1203.

70. Bilton D, Dodd M, Webb AK. Evaluation of exercise as an adjunct to physiotherapy in the treatment of cystic fibrosis in the treatment of cystic fibrosis. Thorax 1989;44:859.

71. Bartlett RH, Krop P, Hanson EL, et al. Physiology of yawning and its application to postoperative care. Surg Forum 1970; 21:223-224.

72. Craven JL, Evans GA, Davenport PJ, et al. The evaluation of incentive spirometry in the management of postoperative pulmonary complications. Br J Surg 1974;61:793-797.

73. Scuderi J, Olsen GN. Respiratory therapy in the management of postoperative complications. Respir Care 1989;34:281-291.

74. Dohi S, Gold MI. Comparison of two methods of postoperative respiratory care. Chest 1978;73:592-595.

75. Mang H, Obermayer A. Imposed work of breathing during sustained maximal inspiration: comparison of six incentive spirometers. Respir Care 1989;34:1122-1128.

76. Lederer DH, Vandewater JM, Indech RB. Which breathing device should the postoperative patient use? Chest 1980;77:610-613.

77. Rau JL, Thomas L, Haynes RL. The effect of method of administering incentive spirometry on postoperative pulmonary complications in coronary bypass patients. Respir Care 1988;33:771-778.

78. Celli BR, Rodriguez KS, Snider GL. A controlled trial of intermittent positive pressure breathing, incentive spirometry, and deep breathing exercises in preventing pulmonary complication after abdominal surgery. Am Rev Respir Dis 1984;130:12-15.

79. Jenkins SC, Soutar SA, Loukota JM, et al. Physiotherapy after coronary artery surgery: are breathing exercises necessary? Thorax 1989;44:634-639.

80. Stiller K, Montarello J, Wallace M, et al. Efficacy of breathing and coughing exercises in the prevention of pulmonary complications after coronary artery surgery. Chest 1994;105:741-747.

81. Dull JL, Dull WL. Are maximal inspiratory breathing exercises better or incentive spirometry better than early mobilization after cardiopulmonary bypass? Phys Ther 1983;63:655-659.

82. Hall JC, Tarala R, Harris J, et al. Incentive spirometry versus routine chest physiotherapy for prevention of pulmonary complications after abdominal surgery. Lancet 1991;337:953-956.

83. Gooselink R, Schever K, Cops P, et al. Incentive spirometry does not enhance recovery after thoracic surgery. Crit Care Med 2000;28:679-683.

84. Dolovich MB, Killian D, Wolff RK, et al. Pulmonary aerosol deposition in chronic bronchitis: intermittent positive pressure breathing versus quiet breathing. Am Rev Respir Dis 1977;115:397-402.

85. The IPPB Trial Group. Intermittent positive pressure breathing therapy of chronic obstructive pulmonary disease: a clinical trial. Ann Intern Med 1983;99:612-620.

86. Paul WL, Downs JB. Postoperative atelectasis: intermittent positive pressure breathing, incentive spirometry, and facemask positive end-expiratory pressure. Arch Surg 1981;116:861-863.

87. Ricksten SE, Bengtsson A, Soderberg C, et al. Effects of periodic positive airway pressure by mask on postoperative pulmonary function. Chest 1986; 89:774-781.

88. Andersen JB, Klausen NO. A new mode of administration of nebulized bronchodilator in severe bronchospasm. Eur J Respir Dis 1982;63(Suppl):97-100.

89. Frischknecht-Christensen E, Norregaard O, Dahl R. Treatment of bronchial asthma with terbutaline inhaled by cone-spacer combined with positive expiratory pressure mask. Chest 1991;100:317-321.

90. Mahlmeister MJ, Fink JB, Hoffman GL, et al. Positive-expiratory-pressure mask therapy: theoretical and practical considerations and a review of the literature. Respir Care 1991;36:1218-1230.

91. Katz JA. PEEP and CPAP in perioperative respiratory care. Respir Care 1984;29(Suppl 6):614-623.

92. Branson RD, Hurst JM, DeHaven CB. Mask CPAP: state of the art. Respir Care 1985;30:846-857.

93. Branson RD. PEEP without endotracheal intubation. Respir Care 1988;33:598-610.

94. Andersen JB, Qvist H, Kann T. Recruiting collapsed lung through collateral channels with positive end-expiratory pressure. Scan J Respir Dis 1979;60:260-266.

95. Andersen JB, Jespersen W. Demonstration of intersegmental respiratory bronchiole in normal lungs. Eur J Respir Dis 1980;61:337-341.

96. King M, Zidulka A, Phillips DM, et al. Tracheal mucus clearance in high-frequency oscillation: effect of peak flow rate bias. Eur Respir J 1990;3:6-13.

97. Dasgupta B, Tomkiewicz RP, Boyd WA, et al. Effects of combined treatment with rh DNase and airflow oscillations on spinability of cystic fibrosis sputum in-vitro. Pediatr Pulmonol 1995;20:78-82.

98. Tomkiewicz RP, Biviji AA, King M. Effects of oscillating air on the rheological properties and clearability for mucus gel simulant. Biorheology 1994;124:689-693.

99. van Henstum M, Festen J, Buerskens C, et al. No effect of oral high frequency oscillation combined with forced expiration maneuvers on tracheobronchial clearance in chronic bronchitis. Eur Respir J 1990;3:14-18.

100. Konstan MW, Stern RC, Doershuk CF. Efficacy of the Flutter device for airway mucus clearance in patients with cystic fibrosis. J Pediatr 1994;124:689-693.

101. Gondor M, Nixon PA, Mutich R, et al. Comparison of Flutter device and chest physical therapy in the treatment of cystic fibrosis pulmonary exacerbation. Pediatr Pulmonol 1999;28:255-260.

102. Mahesh VK, McDougal JA, Haluszka L. Efficacy of the Flutter device for airway mucus clearance in patients with cystic fibrosis. J Pediatr 1996;128:16.

103. Pryor JA, Webber BA, Hodson, ME, et al. The Flutter VRP1 as an adjunct to chest physiotherapy in cystic fibrosis. Respir Med 1994;88:677-681.

104. Homnick DN, Anderson K, Marks JH. Comparison of the Flutter device to standard chest physiotherapy in hospitalized patients with cystic fibrosis: a pilot study. Chest 1998;114:993-997.

105. App EM, Kieselman R, Reinhardt D, et al. Sputum rheology changes in cystic fibrosis lung disease following two different types of physiotherapy: Flutter vs autogenic drainage. Chest 1998;114:171-177.

106. Girard JP, Terki N. The Flutter VRP1: a new personal pocket therapeutic device used as an adjunct to drug therapy in the management of bronchial hygiene. J Investig Allergol Clin Immunol 1994;4:23-27.

107. McInturff SL, Shaw LI. Intrapulmonary percussive ventilation. Respir Care 1985;30:884-885.

108. Natale JE, Pfeifle J, Homnick DN. Comparison of intrapulmonary percussive ventilation and chest physiotherapy. Chest 1994;105:1789-1793.

109. Homnick DN, White F, de Castro C. Comparison of effects of an intrapulmonary percussive ventilator to standard aerosol and chest physiotherapy in treatment of cystic fibrosis. Pediatr Pulmonol 1995;20:50-55.

110. Newhouse PA, White F, Marks JH, et al. Clin Pediatr 1998;37:427-432.

111. King M, Phillips DM, et al. Tracheal mucus clearance with high-frequency chest wall compression. Am Rev Resir Dis 1983;128:511-515.

112. King M, Zidulka A, Phillips DM, et al. Tracheal mucus clearance in high-frequency oscillation: effect of peak flow rate bias. Eur Respir J 1990;3:6-13.

113. Hansen L, Warwick W. High frequency chest compression system to aid in clearance of mucus from the lung. Biomed Instru Tech 1990;24:289-294.

114. Kluft J, Beker L, Castagnino M, et al. A comparison of bronchial drainage treatments in cystic fibrosis. Pediatric Pulmonol 1996;22:271-274.

115. Arens R, Gozal D, Omlin KJ, et al. Comparison of high frequency chest compression and conventional chest physiotherapy in hospitalized patients with cystic fibrosis. Am J Respir Crit Care Med 1994;150:1154-1157.

116. Spitzer SA, Fink G, Mittelman M. External high-frequency ventilation in severe chronic obstructive pulmonary disease. Chest 1993;104:1698-1701.

117. Scherer TA, Barandun J, Martinez E, et al. Effect of high-frequency oral airway and chest wall oscillation and conventional chest physical therapy on expectoration in patients with stable cystic fibrosis. Chest 1998;113:1019-1027.

CHAPTER 36

Airway Management

Robert A. May
Pamela L. Bortner

CHAPTER **OUTLINE**

OBJECTIVES

1. Compare oropharyngeal and nasopharyngeal airways.
2. Demonstrate the techniques for inserting oropharyngeal and nasopharyngeal airways.
3. Describe the construction of an endotracheal tube.
4. Describe the technique for orotracheal and nasotracheal intubation.
5. Demonstrate the technique used to secure an endotracheal tube.
6. Demonstrate the technique used to measure cuff pressure.
7. Compare conventional and percutaneous dilational tracheostomy.
8. Compare various designs of tracheostomy tubes.
9. Compare conventional and closed suction catheters.
10. Describe techniques used to prevent complications from suctioning.
11. Discuss the important points of extubation and decannulation.

KEY TERMS

Airway Cuff
Bite Block
Decannulation
Endotracheal Intubation
Endotracheal Tube

Extubation
Laryngeal Mask Airway
Nasopharyngeal Airway
Nasotracheal Intubation
Oropharyngeal Airway

Orotracheal Intubation
Speaking Valve
Suction Catheter
Tracheostomy Tube

Airway management is an important aspect of respiratory care (CPG 36-1). It involves the insertion of oropharyngeal airways, nasopharyngeal airways, endotracheal tubes, and tracheostomy tubes, as well as all aspects of the care of patients with artificial airways.

Oropharyngeal Airways

The **oropharyngeal airway** is designed to be inserted into the mouth between the lips and teeth. It extends from the lips to the pharynx, following the natural curvature of the

CPG 36-1

Management of Airway Emergencies

Indications

Conditions requiring management of the airway, in general, are impending or actual airway compromise, respiratory failure, and the need to protect the airway. Specific conditions include but are not limited to airway emergency before endotracheal intubation, obstruction of the artificial airway, apnea, acute traumatic coma, penetrating neck trauma, cardiopulmonary arrest and unstable dysrhythmias, severe bronchospasm, severe allergic reactions with cardiopulmonary compromise, pulmonary edema, sedative or narcotic drug effect, foreign body airway obstruction, choanal atresia in neonates, aspiration, risk of aspiration, severe laryngospasm, and self-extubation.

Conditions requiring emergency tracheal intubation include but are not limited to persistent apnea, traumatic upper airway obstruction (partial or complete), accidental extubation of a patient unable to maintain adequate spontaneous ventilation, obstructive angioedema (edema involving the deeper layers of the skin, subcutaneous tissue, and mucosa), massive uncontrolled upper airway bleeding, coma with potential for increased intracranial pressure, infection-related upper airway obstruction (partial or complete, such as epiglottitis in children or adults, acute uvular edema, tonsillopharyngitis or retropharyngeal abscess, or suppurative parotitis), laryngeal and upper airway edema, neonatal- or pediatric-specific conditions (perinatal asphyxia, severe adenotonsillar hypertrophy, severe laryngomalacia, bacterial tracheitis, neonatal epignathus, obstruction from abnormal laryngeal closure caused by arytenoid masses, mediastinal tumors, congenital diaphragmatic hernia, thick and/or particulate meconium in amniotic fluid), and absence of airway protective reflexes, such as cardiopulmonary arrest or massive hemoptysis.

When airway control is not possible by other methods, surgical placement of an airway (needle or surgical cricothyrotomy) may be required.

Conditions in which endotracheal intubation may not be possible and in which alternative techniques may be used include but are not limited to restriction of endotracheal intubation by policy or statute; situations in which endotracheal intubation is not immediately possible; and failed intubation in the presence of risk factors associated with difficult tracheal intubations, such as a short or bull neck, protruding maxillary incisors, receding mandible, reduced mobility of the atlantooccipital joint, temporomandibular ankylosis, congenital oropharyngeal wall stenosis, anterior osteophytes of the cervical vertebrae associated with diffuse idiopathic skeletal hyperostosis, large substernal and/or cancerous goiters, Treacher Collins syndrome, Brailsford-Morquio syndrome, or endolaryngeal tumors.

Contraindications

Aggressive airway management (intubation or establishment of a surgical airway) may be contraindicated if the patient's desire not to be resuscitated has been clearly expressed and documented in the patient's medical record or other valid legal document.

Hazards and Complications

Failure to establish a patent airway

Failure to intubate the trachea

Failure to recognize intubation of the esophagus

Upper airway trauma, laryngeal and esophageal damage

Aspiration

Cervical spine trauma

Unrecognized bronchial intubation

Eye injury

Vocal cord paralysis

Problems with endotracheal tubes (cuff perforation, cuff herniation, pilot tube–valve incompetence, tube kinking during biting, inadvertent extubation, tube occlusion)

Bronchospasm

Laryngospasm

Dental accidents

Dysrhythmias

Hypotension and bradycardia caused by vagal stimulation

Hypertension and tachycardia

Inappropriate tube size

Bleeding

Mouth ulceration

Specific problems arising from nasal intubation (nasal damage, including epistaxis; tube kinking in the pharynx; sinusitis; and otitis media)

Tongue ulceration

Tracheal damage (tracheoesophageal fistula, tracheal innominate fistula, tracheal stenosis, and tracheomalacia)

Pneumonia

Laryngeal damage with consequent laryngeal stenosis, laryngeal ulcer, granuloma, polyps, or synechiae

Specific problems arising from surgical cricothyrotomy or tracheostomy (stomal stenosis, innominate erosion)

Specific problems arising from needle cricothyrotomy (bleeding at the insertion site with hematoma formation, subcutaneous and mediastinal emphysema, esophageal perforation)

Modified from AARC Clinical practice guideline: management of airway emergencies. Respir Care 1995;40:749-760. CPG, Clinical Practice Guideline.

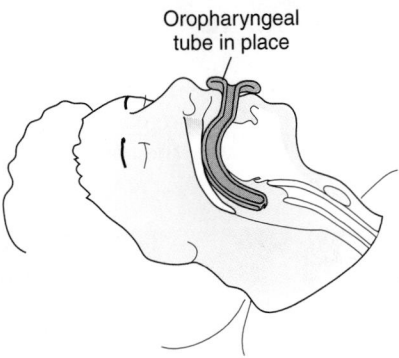

Figure 36-1 Oropharyngeal airway in place.

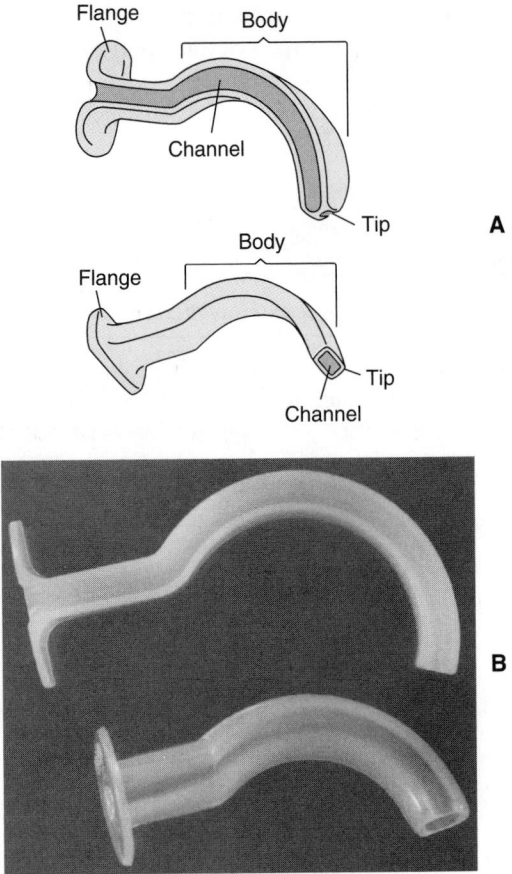

Figure 36-2 Berman **(A)** and Guedel **(B)** oropharyngeal airways.

tongue, without entering the larynx or esophagus (Figure 36-1). Oropharyngeal airways are made of metal, plastic, or rubberlike materials and are relatively rigid. The device generally consists of a flange, a bite portion (body), and an air channel. The *flange* at the mouth opening prevents the airway from falling back into the mouth and becoming an obstruction. It also provides a means to stabilize the airway in place against the lips or teeth. The *bite portion*, which fits between the teeth or gums, is straight and firm enough to prevent the patient from closing the air channel by biting down. The *air channel,* or curved portion, extends upward and backward along the curve of the tongue, pulling it and the epiglottis away from the posterior pharyngeal wall to provide a patent air passage.

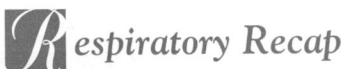

*R*espiratory Recap

Oropharyngeal Airways
Prevent upper airway obstruction
May be used as a bite block
May make bag-valve-mask ventilation more effective
Should not be used in semicomatose or alert patients

Oropharyngeal airways are designed to prevent the patient's tongue from falling backward into the hypopharynx and partly or completely obstructing the upper airway. Use of an oropharyngeal airway may be indicated during spontaneous, manual, or mouth-to-tube ventilation. Oropharyngeal airways allow ready access to the mouth and pharynx for suctioning, and they may be inserted instead of a bite block to prevent a patient from biting an oral **endotracheal tube.** These airways also may help in providing bag-valve-mask ventilation, for example, in a patient who is edentulous or who has facial trauma that causes the cheeks to collapse, making an airtight mask seal impossible. It is important to note that because of its position in the pharynx, an oropharyngeal airway may gag a semicomatose or an alert patient, which could induce vomiting and increase the risk of aspiration.

Types of Oropharyngeal Airways

The Berman airway (Figure 36-2) has a flange at the oral end, a rigid support beam through the center, and open sides; there is no hollow center for air passage.[1] The open sides allow suctioning and serve as air channels. The center may have openings for suctioning should the airway become lodged sideways in the mouth. The advantages of the Berman airway are ease of cleaning and the fact that the dual side air channels are less likely to be obstructed by mucus or foreign bodies. Because the Berman airway is uniformly rigid over its full length, it has an advantage over the Guedel airway in resistance to occlusion by the patient's bite.[2]

The Guedel airway (see Figure 36-2) has a large flange at the oral end and a supportive bite, and the curved portion that follows the curve of the tongue is made of a semirigid material. The Guedel airway differs from the Berman airway in that it is reinforced only in the bite region. This may pose a problem if the patient should bite down on the Guedel airway before it is completely inserted, causing an unreinforced portion to occlude the airway and preventing complete insertion. The Guedel airway also differs from the Berman airway in that it has an enclosed tubular channel to facilitate air exchange and suctioning.

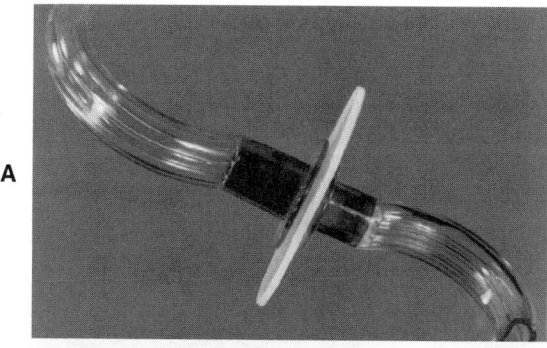

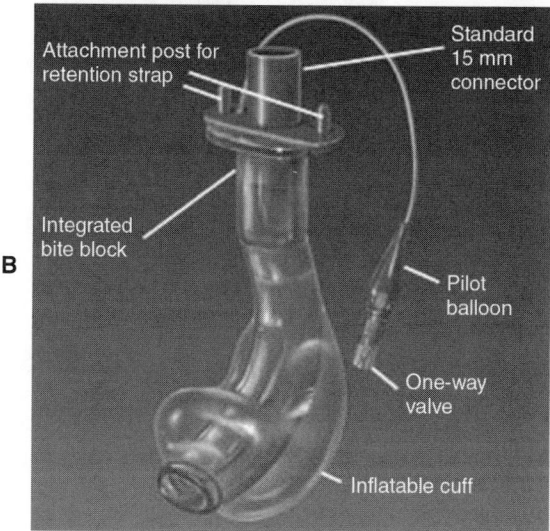

Figure 36-3   **A,** S-tube airway. **B,** Cuffed oropharyngeal airway (COPA). (**A,** From Bortner PL, May RA. Artificial airways and tubes. In: Eubanks DH, Bone RC, editors. Principles and applications of cardiorespiratory care equipment. St Louis: Mosby; 1994; **B,** Courtesy Mallinckrodt, Inc., St Louis, Mo.)

The S-tube oropharyngeal airway (Figure 36-3) is similar to the Guedel airway except that it allows the user to connect two units to form one double-ended tube for mouth-to-airway ventilation. The central flange is reversible to facilitate use of either the short or the long end as the airway while the other end is used as a mouthpiece for the rescuer. However, the adequacy of the S-type airway for this type of ventilation is questionable. The cuffed oropharyngeal airway (COPA) inserts as does a standard oropharyngeal airway but has a cuff to position the tongue and epiglottis properly (see Figure 36-3).[3] The COPA, which has a standard 15-mm connector to attach a breathing circuit, is primarily used during administration of anesthesia.

Insertion of Oropharyngeal Airways

To insert an oropharyngeal airway, the intubator stands at the patient's head, hyperextends the head and neck, and uses the cross-finger technique to open the mouth (Figure 36-4). One method of insertion is to turn the airway 180 degrees from its resting position as it is passed

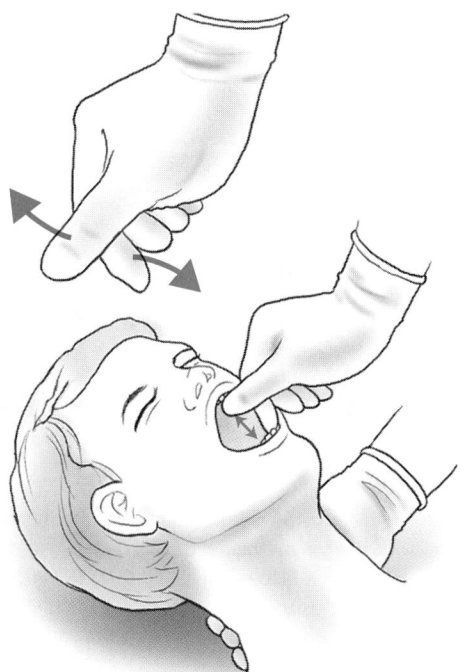

Figure 36-4   Cross-finger technique to open the mouth.

over the tongue to avoid pushing the tongue back into the pharynx. When the tip of the airway reaches the uvula, the airway is rotated 180 degrees so that the tip is positioned behind the tongue and facing the larynx. In the second method, a tongue blade is used to hold the tongue in position. The airway can be inserted from the lateral aspect of the mouth and rotated 90 degrees to the position in which it will rest (Figure 36-5). Once it is in place, the airway should be assessed for proper size and position through determination of whether it allows unobstructed breathing.

Complications of Oropharyngeal Airways

Vomiting and aspiration are risks when an oral airway is used. If the patient bites the endotracheal tube, sedation or use of neuromuscular blocking agents may be indicated, or a bite block may be inserted. If the oropharyngeal airway selected is too large, its tip may press the epiglottis against the posterior pharyngeal wall or the larynx, obstructing both the device and the patient's physiologic airway. If the airway is inserted improperly or is too small, the tongue may be pushed against the posterior pharynx, causing obstruction. Obstruction also can be caused by foreign objects or other material, such as vomitus or secretions. Laryngospasm and coughing can be induced in an awake patient or by insertion of an oropharyngeal airway that is too long and consequently comes into contact with the epiglottis or vocal cords.

Another problem with oral airways is dental damage. Teeth can be broken or torn forcibly from the mouth as the patient bites down on the oral airway. Oral airways should

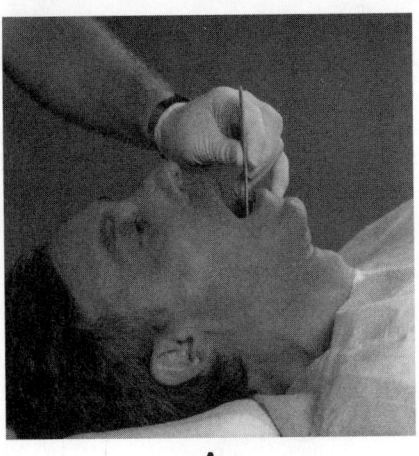
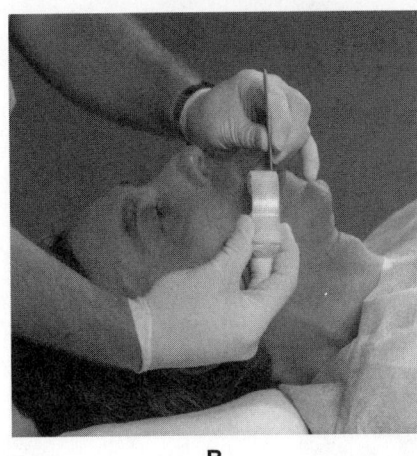
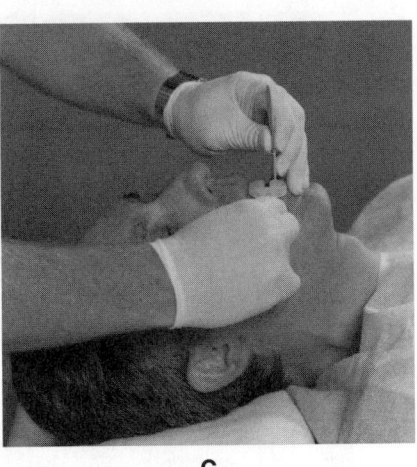

A   **B**   **C**

Figure 36-5   Insertion of an oropharyngeal airway. **A,** The tongue is displaced downward and anterior with the tongue blade. **B,** The oropharyngeal airway is inserted from the lateral aspect of the mouth along the tongue blade until the tip reaches the base of the tongue. **C,** The airway is rotated 90 degrees to its final resting position in the posterior of the pharynx. (From Bortner PL, May RA. Artificial airways and tubes. In: Eubanks DH, Bone RC, editors. Principles and applications of cardiorespiratory care equipment. St Louis: Mosby; 1994.)

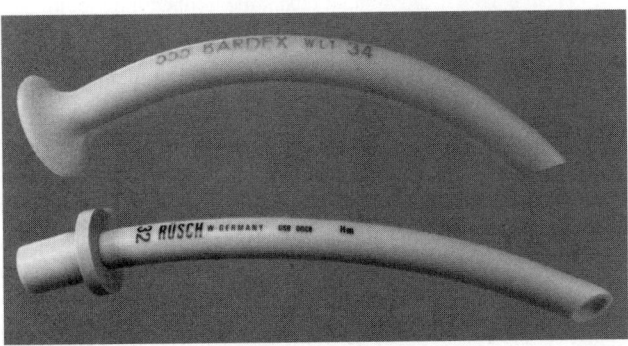

Figure 36-6   Nasopharyngeal airways. (From Bortner PL, May RA. Artificial airways and tubes. In: Eubanks DH, Bone RC, editors. Principles and applications of cardiorespiratory care equipment. St Louis: Mosby; 1994.)

ened endotracheal tube. All types have some degree of flange at the nasal end to facilitate insertion and prevent accidental aspiration of the tube. The proper length of airway can be determined by measurement of the distance from the tip of the nose to the meatus of the ear or from the tip of the nose to the tragus of the ear plus 2 cm.

*R*espiratory Recap ——————

Nasopharyngeal Airways
May be used to bypass an upper airway obstruction Aid passage of a bronchoscope Reduce trauma caused by repeated nasotracheal suctioning

be used judiciously if the patient has disease or decay of the teeth or caps, crowns, or other dental appliances. In such cases use of a nasopharyngeal airway or bite block may be indicated.[4] When the oral airway is in place, the lip may be damaged if it is pinched between the teeth and the airway, or continuous chewing motions by a comatose patient may damage the tongue. Pressure necrosis of the tongue can occur if the airway is left in place for a prolonged period.

Nasopharyngeal Airways

The **nasopharyngeal airway** (Figure 36-6) is an alternative to the oropharyngeal airway. Nasopharyngeal airways are inserted into the nose and directed along the floor of the nose parallel to the hard palate. They are curved to follow the anatomy of the nasopharynx so that the tip rests behind the tongue, just above the epiglottis. These airways are made of plastic or rubber and resemble a short-

The nasopharyngeal airway is an alternative to the oropharyngeal airway to provide a patent airway. In some situations the mouth cannot be opened, or an oral airway does not relieve the obstruction. In these cases a nasopharyngeal airway is better tolerated and more comfortable in a semiawake patient than an oral airway. A nasopharyngeal airway also eliminates the risk of trauma of the tongue and teeth seen with oral airways. Nasopharyngeal airways are used as aids to perform fiberoptic bronchoscopy; they provide easy access to the trachea for nasotracheal suction; and they protect the nasopharyngeal mucosa from the traumatic effects of repeated suctioning.[5] Nasopharyngeal airways have also proved useful in the management of airway problems seen with Pierre Robin syndrome.[6]

Types of Nasopharyngeal Airways

The Bardex nasopharyngeal airway has a large flange at the nasal end and a bevel at the pharyngeal end, whereas

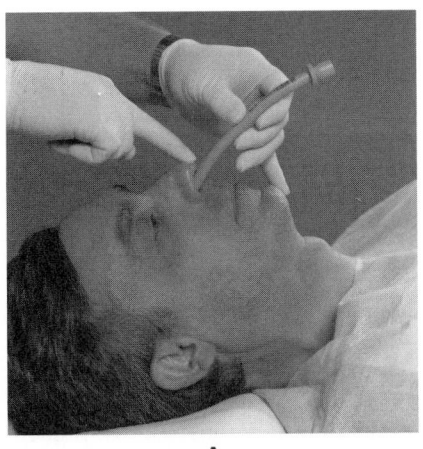
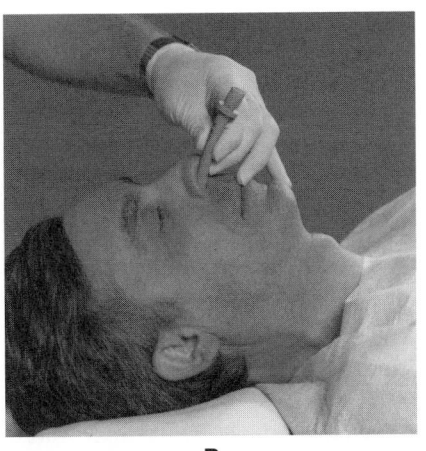
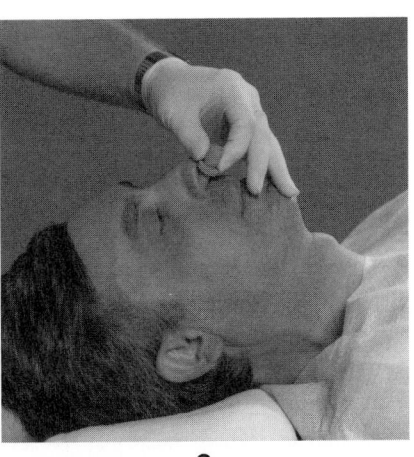

A   **B**   **C**

Figure 36-7   Insertion of a nasopharyngeal airway. **A,** The nasopharyngeal airway is initially directed through the naris in a slightly upward direction. **B,** After passing through the naris, the airway should be advanced along the plane parallel to the floor of the nasal cavity. **C,** The airway should come to rest with the flange at the external naris. (From Bortner PL, May RA. Artificial airways and tubes. In: Eubanks DH, Bone RC, editors. Principles and applications of cardiorespiratory care equipment. St Louis: Mosby; 1994.)

the Rusch nasopharyngeal airway has a firm flange at the nasal end and a short bevel at the pharyngeal end. The Linder airway is made of soft plastic and has a bubble-tip introducer with a smooth, rounded tip for easier insertion. With the Linder airway the complete assembly is placed through the nostril, and once it is in position, the air in the distal balloon and the introducer are removed.[7]

Insertion of Nasopharyngeal Airways

The nasopharyngeal airway first should be lubricated with a water-soluble gel. It is then introduced into the naris, and the end is pointed parallel to the hard palate. It is advanced gently to prevent trauma and bleeding (Figure 36-7). If resistance is met, the airway is redirected. If excessive resistance is met, the attempt is made through the other nostril, or a smaller airway is chosen. If the nasopharyngeal airway is too long, laryngospasm may occur. If it is too short, complete airway patency will not be achieved. All oral and nasal airways should be clearly marked with the inside diameter (ID) and the outside diameter (OD) to aid selection of the proper tube.

Complications of Nasopharyngeal Airways

Laryngospasm and coughing can be induced by insertion of a nasopharyngeal airway that is too long and comes into contact with the epiglottis or vocal cords. Nosebleeds can occur from insertion of a nasopharyngeal airway, particularly if it is too large. These airways should be used with caution in patients undergoing anticoagulation therapy. Improper insertion of nasopharyngeal airways may damage the turbinate, and insertion of a nasopharyngeal airway into a patient who is draining blood or cerebrospinal fluid may cause infection. Prolonged use of this airway may result in sinus infections. In patients with severe facial or

head trauma, insertion of a nasopharyngeal airway may result, in rare cases, in cranial vault intubation, the risk being greatest in patients with basilar skull fractures.

History of Intubation

The use of tracheotomy to relieve upper airway obstruction dates to Asclepiad's first surgical tracheostomy in approximately 100 BC. Even several hundred years earlier, crude attempts to open airways had been made with swords or other instruments.[8,9] In the mid-1600s Robert Hooke performed an experiment in which he kept animals alive by blowing air into their lungs with a bellows by use of a tracheotomy.[10] In the early 1700s Friedrich Trendelenburg fitted an inflatable cuff to a **tracheostomy tube,** creating the prototype for current airway devices.[8,9] In the 1880s MacEwen,[11] O'Dwyer,[12] and Fell[13] all described the use of **endotracheal intubation** for delivery of positive pressure ventilation. The fundamental design of current endotracheal tubes was established in 1941 by Murphy.[14] In 1971 Grillo and colleagues[15] studied low-pressure, high-compliance cuffs and showed that these devices caused less frequent and less severe tracheal injury than the standard high-pressure tubes. This work was the foundation for endotracheal tubes in common use today.

Selection and Training of Personnel

Understanding the concepts of airway management and becoming proficient in the techniques used to establish and maintain a patent airway are paramount in the practice of respiratory care. The airway can easily be taken for granted, and at times a simple maneuver to reestablish a patent airway may be life-saving. It is universally accepted that ensuring an *airway* is the first concern in life support protocols.

A logical sequence can be followed in the evaluation and establishment of an airway. The respiratory therapist must be able to determine the adequacy of an airway and, when appropriate, implement corrective action to establish patency of an airway. Not only may a simple maneuver be life-saving, but it also is an attempt to implement an incorrect maneuver may be life-threatening. It is imperative that airway patency be reevaluated properly after any interventional technique to determine if the corrective action has indeed improved the situation. All these techniques are performed under time pressure, because compromise of oxygen uptake has serious consequences.

Because of the significant impact airway management can have on the patient's outcome, guidelines should be established that address which personnel should perform endotracheal intubation and under what circumstances, and how the training of these individuals should be accomplished. The literature offers very little guidance in the medicolegal aspects of who should manage the airway, and regional practices vary from locale to locale. The standard of care usually prevails but is very poorly defined. In the surgical areas, anesthesiologists and certified registered nurse anesthetists manage the airway. In the nonhospital setting, most regions are comfortable with paramedics performing endotracheal intubation. Because most hospitals have code teams, and respiratory therapists are part of the team, it makes sense that respiratory therapists should manage the airway in the absence of more highly trained personnel.

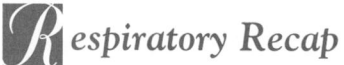espiratory Recap

---

Health Care Workers Who Perform Endotracheal Intubation

Anesthesia personnel (anesthesiologists and nurse anesthetists)
Critical care and emergency physicians
Paramedics
Respiratory therapists

The National Board for Respiratory Care (NBRC) includes endotracheal intubation in its examination outline for registered respiratory therapists. Most respiratory therapy training programs instruct their students in the technique of endotracheal intubation.[16] Although many studies have tried to determine failure rates by category of personnel, no universal conclusions have resulted. Anesthesia personnel have the highest skill level, but in the hospital setting, the practitioner with the highest level of experience and training outside the operating room probably is the respiratory therapist. The anesthesiologist and the operating room provide a logical means to implement a program that uses the skills of respiratory therapists in

acute airway management.[17,18] Initial training is given by the anesthesiologist, followed by 10 to 15 supervised intubations in the operating room. Trained respiratory therapists should perform 10 intubations a year to be requalified or should undergo a repeat training course in the operating room. Because the requirement for intubation outside the operating room is low and varies, training may need to be limited to supervisors or designated members of the code team to achieve continued competence.

Indications for Endotracheal Intubation

The indications for endotracheal intubation are numerous, many requiring emergency intubation and others allowing a more structured, relaxed approach. Specific conditions that require emergency tracheal intubation are listed in Box 36-1. Generally accepted indications include establishment and maintenance of a patent airway, protection of the airway from aspiration, application of positive pressure to the airway, facilitation of clearance of secretions, and delivery of high oxygen concentrations.[19,20]

Establishment of a patent airway is the most basic intervention in all of health care and probably the most important. Without an adequate airway, meaningful survival is impossible. Establishment of an airway has retained its position as the first step in cardiopulmonary resuscitation for decades because all other treatment is futile unless a patent airway exists. However, because of the development of new techniques and equipment, endotracheal intubation may not necessarily be the first step to establish the airway; use of the **laryngeal mask airway** or the Combitube may precede or replace it. Nevertheless, endotracheal intubation remains the gold standard used to establish an airway.

Aspiration of foreign objects into the airway can result in significant morbidity and mortality. Although not 100% effective, placement of an endotracheal tube in the trachea minimizes the risk of aspiration. Aspiration also can occur during insertion or removal of the endotracheal tube, and strong evidence suggests that aspiration of pharyngeal secretions occurs with the high-volume, low-pressure endotracheal tube cuffs, resulting in ventilator-associated pneumonia.[1,21] Unquestionably, in a patient with compromised upper airway reflexes and function, the risk of aspiration is lower with an endotracheal tube in place.

Ever since the development of positive pressure ventilation, the endotracheal tube has been the mainstay for delivery of this type of ventilation. However, the use of noninvasive positive pressure ventilation (NPPV) and mask continuous positive airway pressure (CPAP) has increased, and these can be accomplished without the use of an endotracheal tube in some patients.[22-25] The need for endotracheal intubation to deliver positive pressure ventilation will always exist, although practitioners certainly can be more selective and avoid intubation in some cases. Even when used by skilled clinicians, NPPV will fail in 25% of cases and intubation will be required.[26]

Box 36-1

Indications for Emergency Intubation

Persistent apnea
Traumatic upper airway obstruction
Accidental extubation of a patient unable to maintain adequate spontaneous ventilation
Obstructive angioedema
Massive uncontrolled upper airway bleeding
Coma with potential for increased intracranial pressure
Infection-related upper airway obstruction (for example, epiglottitis, acute uvular edema, tonsillopharyngitis or retropharyngeal abscess, supportive parotitis)
Laryngeal and upper airway edema
Absence of airway protective reflexes
Cardiopulmonary arrest
Massive hemoptysis
Neonatal or pediatric disorders (for example, perinatal asphyxia, severe tonsillar hypertrophy, severe laryngomalacia, bacterial tracheitis, neonatal epignathus, obstruction from abnormal laryngeal closure caused by arytenoid masses, mediastinal tumors, congenital diaphragmatic hernia, thick and/or particulate meconium in the amniotic fluid)

From Hess DR. Indications for translaryngeal intubation. Respir Care 1999;44:604-609.

Facilitation of the evacuation of pulmonary secretions by suctioning through an endotracheal tube is a common indication for endotracheal intubation. The requirements of positive pressure ventilation and pulmonary toilet often coexist, and as the need for each declines, the need for the endotracheal tube also declines. Secretion clearance can be accomplished with deep breathing, coughing, and chest physiotherapy. Positive expiratory pressure techniques also enhance mobilization of pulmonary secretions. Determination of the appropriate time for extubation depends on the patient's ability to perform these airway maintenance procedures.

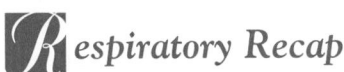

Respiratory Recap

Indications for Endotracheal Intubation
To bypass an upper airway obstruction
To protect the airway from aspiration
To apply positive pressure ventilation
To aid clearance of secretions
To deliver high oxygen concentrations

When high oxygen concentrations are required, placement of an endotracheal tube may be necessary. Most oxygen delivery devices fall well short of a 100% oxygen concentration because of air entrainment caused by poorly fitting devices or inadequate flow delivery.[27] Tight-fitting masks work well for high oxygen delivery if the inspiratory flows are high enough, but patients find these devices uncomfortable and often remove them, dropping the inspired oxygen concentration (FIO_2) to dangerous levels. Often when high oxygen concentrations are needed, administration is required for several hours, therefore positive pressure may be used to reduce the levels of inspired oxygen. NPPV and mask CPAP can be used in some situations and may avert the need for endotracheal intubation.

Difficult Airways: Assessment and Strategy

Intubation will remain the mainstay to secure a patent airway and increasingly will be performed by nonanesthesia health care workers as outlined in emergency protocols. Of significant concern is the difficult airway. Health care workers who do not intubate regularly may not have the experience to recognize, evaluate, or manage a patient with a difficult airway. The American Society of Anesthesiologists (ASA) Task Force on Management of the Difficult Airway has described a difficult airway as one that a conventionally trained anesthesiologist cannot manage without systemic oxygen desaturation despite increased inspired oxygen tension and without signs of hypercapnia, including hypertension, tachycardia, and other secondary evidence of ventilatory inadequacy.[28] Conventionally trained individuals have average skills for their specialty, which implies that the person is not a regional expert but has performed hundreds of tracheal intubations for operative anesthesia care. In emergency situations an individual with much less experience than a conventionally trained anesthesiologist may have to perform endotracheal intubation and may encounter a difficult airway. For this reason, training in the recognition and management of a difficult airway must occur concomitantly with training in basic intubation.

The incidence of difficult direct laryngoscopy and intubation is reported to be 1.5% to 15%, and impossible intubation during anesthesia has been reported in fewer than 1% of patients studied.[29-31] Figure 36-8 and Table 36-1 present a difficulty class scale based on visualization of airway structures during direct laryngoscopy. Table 36-2 presents a difficulty class scale based on structures visualized during an oropharyngeal examination. Any laryngoscopy is complicated by tissue trauma, failed attempts, esophageal intubation, cardiovascular and respiratory instability, and aspiration of gastric or esophageal contents. Prediction of the ability to perform direct laryngoscopy and intubation is also associated with structural and anatomic factors (Table 36-3). It must be noted that although many of these factors seem obvious, some are subtle and often are not appreciated in an emergency situation. The ASA task force has recommended preintubation assessment as a guide to plan intubation; use of awake techniques if direct laryngoscopy is likely to be difficult; selection of alternative airways and techniques in a methodical fashion when direct laryn-

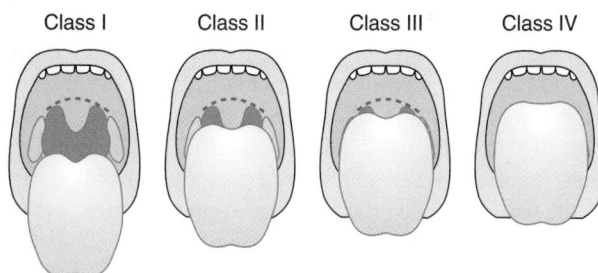

Class I   Class II   Class III   Class IV

Figure 36-8 Pictorial representation of the Samsoon and Young modification of the Mallampati classification based on the ability to see oropharyngeal structures. Decreased ability to see oropharyngeal structures is associated with increased difficulty in intubation. (Modified from Samsoon GLT, Young JRB. Anesthesiology 1987;42:487-490.)

*T*ABLE 36-1

Visualization Class Based on Structures Visible on Direct Laryngoscopy

Class	Visible Structures
I	Supraglottic structures
	Laryngeal inlet
	Vocal cords
II	Epiglottis
	Laryngeal inlet
	Posterior aryepiglottic folds
III	Epiglottis only
IV	Epiglottis not visible

From Watson CB. Prediction of difficult intubation: methods for successful intubation. Respir Care 1999;44:777-796.

*T*ABLE 36-2

Oropharyngeal Class Based on Structures Visible during the Oropharyngeal Examination

Class	Visible Structures
I	Tongue
	Hard palate
	Soft palate
	Uvula
	Posterior pharynx
II	Tongue
	Hard palate
	Soft palate
	Part of the uvula and the posterior pharynx
III	Tongue
	Hard palate
	Soft palate
	Posterior pharynx not visible
IV	Anterior tongue
	Hard palate

From Watson CB. Prediction of difficult intubation: methods for successful intubation. Respir Care 1999;44:777-796.

goscopy is unexpectedly difficult; and use of an airway management algorithm (Figure 36-9) to improve the outcome.

Endotracheal Intubation

Endotracheal intubation is the establishment of an artificial airway by placement of a tube through the mouth or nose, through the glottis, and into the trachea.[32] This procedure can be performed electively under preplanned conditions or on an emergency basis if respiratory failure occurs. The type of endotracheal tube and the placement technique are determined by the factors dictating its use. Instrumentation of the airway stimulates intense reflexive responses in all individuals except severely obtunded patients. For this reason, preplanning is imperative whenever possible, including a combination of topical application of local anesthetics, establishment of an intravenous line, intravenous sedation, general anesthesia, electrocardiographic monitoring, oximetry, suction capability, and availability of various types of equipment to meet unforeseen circumstances. In a true emergency, establishing an airway precludes many of the above procedures. However,

if ventilation can be performed with a bag-valve-mask system while some of this equipment is gathered, the chances of successful intubation increase.

Anatomy of the Upper Airway

An understanding of the basic anatomy and physiology of the airway is paramount to airway management, regardless of the technique used. The airway consists of five regions: the nose and nasopharynx, oral cavity and oropharynx, hypopharynx, larynx, and tracheobronchial tree (Figure 36-10).

The nose and nasopharynx region consists of the nasal cavity, turbinates, nasal septum, and adenoids. Warming, humidification, and filtering of inspired air are the primary functions of the nasopharyngeal structures, which are well suited to these tasks because of the region's large mucosal surface area and rich blood supply. If the nose is bypassed with an endotracheal tube, these important functions are lost and must be substituted artificially. The vascular supply to the area is received from the ethmoid artery and the maxillary artery. Sensory innervation is supplied by the trigeminal nerve through the pterygopalatine branches of the maxillary division. Openings to the paranasal sinuses also are present in the nasal cavity, and drainage of these sinuses may be interrupted if they are occluded by an endotracheal tube or nasogastric tube. Endotracheal intubation also interferes with the sense of olfaction.

The oral cavity and oropharynx consist of the teeth, tongue, buccal mucosa, faucial pillars, hard palate, soft palate, uvula, tonsils, and posterior pharyngeal wall. Func-

TABLE 36-3

Complicating Anatomic Factors in Intubation

Factor	Common Condition	Primary Problem
Disproportionate soft tissues	Lingual hypertrophy	Oversized tongue
	Down syndrome	Mass effect
	Lingual tonsillar hypertrophy	Redundant soft tissue
	Marked obesity	Swelling
	Supraglottic inflammation	Torsion
	Previous neck dissection	Deviation
	Expanding neck hematoma	Obstructive edema
Distorted anatomy	Peritonsillar abscess	Lateral compression and risk of rupture
	Pharyngeal mass and brachial cleft cyst	Deviated larynx or trachea
	Thyroid tumor or goiter	Bony incongruity and disproportionate anatomy
	Developmental craniofacial anomalies	
	Spinal subluxation or osteophytes	Extrinsic mass effect
	Maxillofacial trauma	Displacement or bleeding or both
Inadequate jaw mobility	Temporomandibular joint (TMJ) dysfunction	Fixed or limited motion
	Short mandibular ramus	Inadequate hinge length
	Trauma	Trismus or locked jaw or both
	Malignant hyperthermia	Masseter tetanus and generalized rigidity
	Myotonic crisis	Rigidity, trismus, tetanus
	Neuroleptic-malignant syndrome	
	Drug intoxication	
	Infections	
Inadequate neck mobility	Degenerative cervical arthritis	Fused or irregular intervertebral joints
	Morbid obesity	Tissue limits movement
	Facial or neck burn scarring	Fusion and contractures
	Dwarfism	Short, thick neck
	Hydrocephalus	Limited neck extension
	Cranial dysplasia	Inadequate space
	Cervical meningomyelocele	External fixation
	Cervical trauma	Fractures
	Fractures	Hematoma
	Thoracic kyphosis	Limited cervical extension

From Watson CB. Prediction of difficult intubation: methods for successful intubation. Respir Care 1999;44:777-796.

tionally these structures are important for mastication, taste, phonation, and humidification and warming of inspired gas. As swallowing occurs, the soft palate closes the entrance to the nasopharynx. The area has a rich mucosal blood supply, and innervation is complex, involving mandibular branches of the trigeminal nerve, the facial nerve, and the glossopharyngeal nerve. The mandible houses the tongue, and the temporomandibular joint (TMJ) determines the ability to mobilize these structures. Reduced mobility of the TMJ may make direct laryngoscopy difficult or impossible. Teeth may also form obstructions to direct laryngoscopy, depending on their position and shape. Dental appliances should be removed during intubation attempts to prevent damage.

Below the oropharynx and above the larynx is the hypopharynx. This area contains the epiglottis and the opening to the esophagus. It is an extension of the oropharynx and the position where a laryngeal mask airway (LMA) seats. The larynx is a complex structure composed of nine cartilages, seven muscles, and the vocal ligaments (Figure 36-11). The space between the vocal cords is the glottis; in adults this is the narrowest part of the upper airway, whereas in children the narrowest point is the cricoid ring. The vocal cords protect the lower airway from aspiration of

Age-Specific Angle

In adults the glottis is the narrowest point of the upper airway, whereas in children the cricoid ring is the narrowest point.

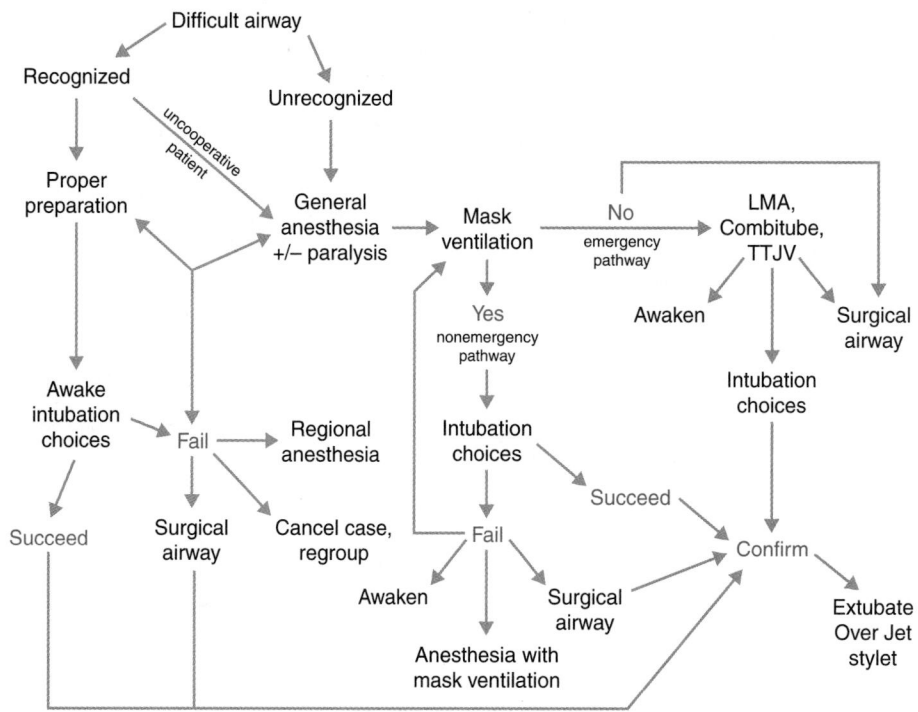

Figure 36-9 Algorithm for a difficult airway, devised by the American Society of Anesthesiologists. (Modified from Benumof JL. Laryngeal mask airway and the ASA difficult airway algorithm. Anesthesiology 1996;84:686-699.)

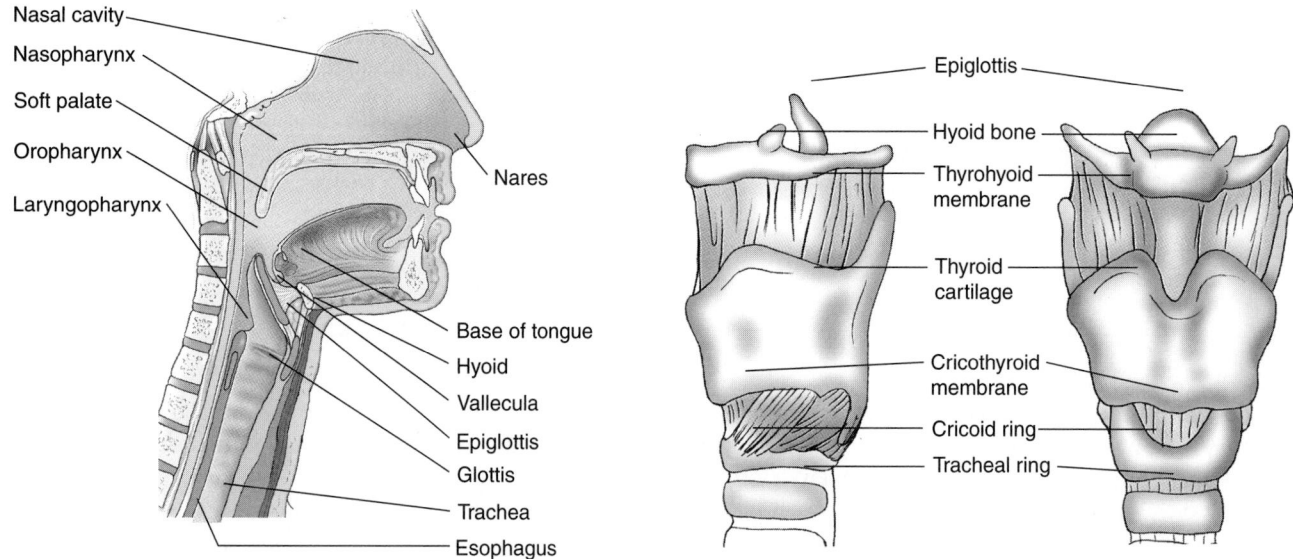

Figure 36-10 Anatomy of the upper airway.

Figure 36-11 Anatomy of the larynx.

foreign objects and produce phonation. The cartilaginous structures and complex muscle groups of the larynx are responsible for the intricate vocal abilities of human beings. With nerve or muscle damage, the vocal cords may not open, causing airway obstruction, or may be unable to close, which leaves the lower airway unprotected.

The trachea is inferior to the larynx, starting just below the cricoid ring. C-shaped cartilaginous rings connected

by fibromuscular tissue extend approximately 10 to 12 cm to where the trachea bifurcates into the left and right mainstem bronchi at the carina. The carina usually is located at the level of the fourth thoracic vertebra. Posteriorly the tracheal cartilages are open, and the wall is formed by a longitudinal fibromuscular band that allows expansion into the trachea as food traverses the esophagus en route to the stomach.

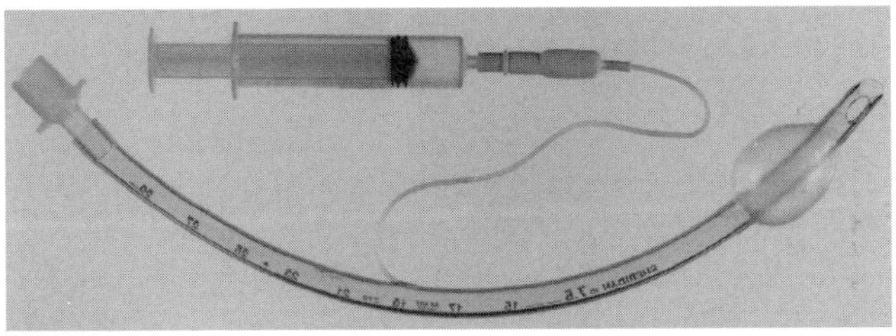

Figure 36-12 Endotracheal tube. (From Bortner PL, May RA. Artificial airways and tubes. In: Eubanks DH, Bone RC, editors. Principles and applications of cardiorespiratory care equipment. St Louis: Mosby; 1994.)

Endotracheal Tubes

The construction of endotracheal tubes is dictated by the standards of the American Society for Testing and Materials (ASTM; Figure 36-12).[33,34] The tubes usually are made of polyvinyl chloride (PVC). PVC is rigid, to facilitate insertion of the tube, but becomes softer at body temperature. The material used in endotracheal tubes is implant tested (that is, it does not react with tissue), and it is smooth, to facilitate passage of a **suction catheter.** The distal end of the tube is beveled and rounded to minimize trauma on insertion. Many endotracheal tubes also have a Murphy eye near the distal tip, which allows the passage of gas if the end of the tube becomes occluded by secretions or the wall of the patient's airway. Near its distal end the tube has a cuff, which can be inflated by a pilot tube that extends past the proximal end of the tube and terminates with a pilot balloon and spring-loaded valve. A radiopaque line is molded into the tube to allow visualization of the tube on radiography. The tube's ID and OD measurements (in millimeters) are marked on it, as are the distance from the distal tip (in centimeters), the manufacturer's name, whether the tube is for oral or nasal use (an oral tube has a 45-degree angle at the tip, a nasal or oral-nasal tube has a 60-degree angle), and an indication that the tube material has been implant tested (IT). The proximal end of the tube is fitted with a standard 15-mm OD connection for respiratory and anesthesia equipment. By convention, the size of the endotracheal tube is given by its ID measurement.

Respiratory Recap

Components of a Typical Endotracheal Tube	
Cuff	Radiopaque line
Pilot balloon	Proximal 15-mm connector

Many variations in the design of the endotracheal tube can be seen. The anode tube has a steel reinforcing wire that is wound spirally within the wall of the tube. This allows the tube to be made of a softer material, yet prevents kinking when the tube must be bent at an angle to clear the surgical field. The Endotrol allows the practitioner to control the direction of the distal tip of the endotracheal tube during intubation by pulling a loop near the tube's proximal end. A flexible, spiral stainless steel tube called the Laser-Flex can be used for laser surgery. Tubes for selective endobronchial intubation (Figure 36-13) are used during thoracic surgery (such as pneumonectomy), independent lung ventilation, or bronchospirometry. The Evac tube allows continuous aspiration of subglottic secretions (Figure 36-14), which has been shown to reduce the risk of ventilator-associated pneumonia.[35-37]

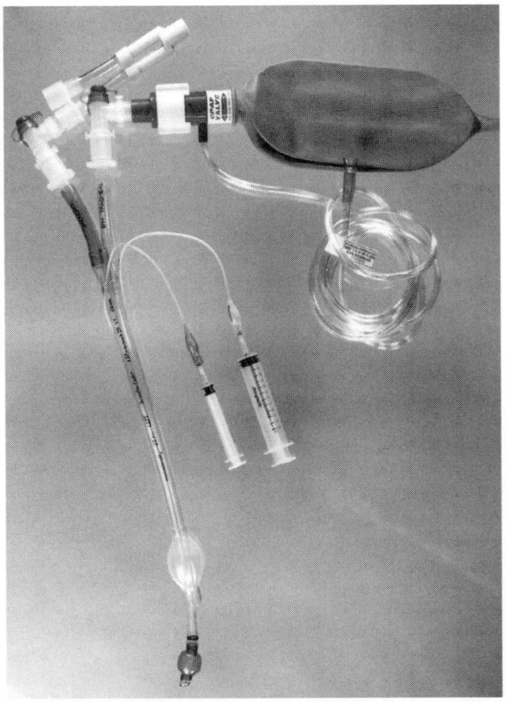

Figure 36-13 Double-lumen endotracheal tube used for endobronchial intubation. (From Bortner PL, May RA. Artificial airways and tubes. In: Eubanks DH, Bone RC, editors. Principles and applications of cardiorespiratory care equipment. St Louis: Mosby; 1994.)

Technique for Orotracheal Intubation

Once it has been determined that endotracheal intubation is required, proper preparation must follow. Each institution should have an emergency airway kit designed by the health care workers most likely to use it. It is important to have all supplies assembled and in working order before manipulation of the airway. A difficult airway may be encountered unexpectedly, or a marginal airway may deteriorate rapidly, leaving little time to obtain an item from elsewhere.

The intubation process is approached calmly. Frantic and rushed attempts often result in failure and worsening of the situation. Some method of oxygenation must be provided while the following preparatory steps are taken:

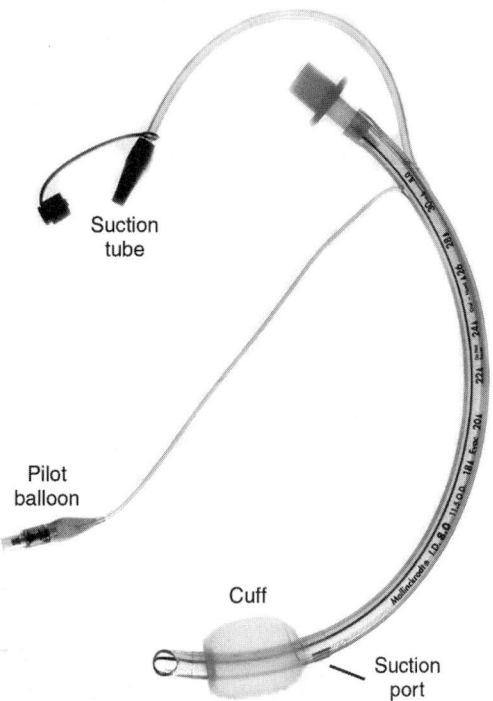

Figure 36-14   Endotracheal tube designed to allow continuous aspiration of subglottic secretions. (From Hess DR. Managing the artificial airway. Respir Care 1999;44:759-772.)

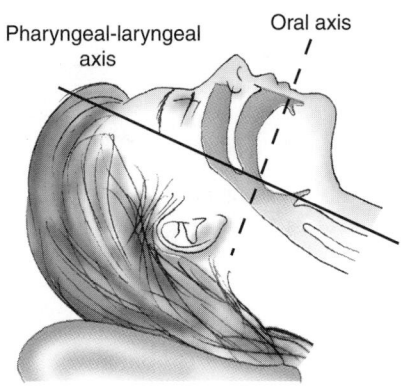

Figure 36-15   Sniffing position for endotracheal intubation.

1. Obtaining a brief history is important, and the few seconds this requires may prevent surprises during the process.
2. Positioning is a key aspect of preparation. The patient should be positioned as optimally as possible within the limits of the environment. Some positioning tips include moving the bed away from the wall and raising its height, bringing the patient as close to the head of the bed as possible to limit the amount of reaching, adjusting the patient into an even supine position, and placing a folded blanket or towels under the head to achieve the sniffing position (Figure 36-15), which aligns the oral, pharyngeal, and laryngeal axes for optimum visualization of the larynx. In essence, this is flexion of the lower cervical spine and extension of the upper cervical spine. However, this position is contraindicated in a patient with a confirmed or suspected neck injury. In such cases an assistant should maintain the head and neck in a neutral position as intubation is attempted.
3. Suction must be ready, preferably with a tonsil-tip suction apparatus, and a functioning intravenous line must be in place before any attempts at intubation are made.
4. Sedation or neuromuscular blocking agents may be necessary in a responsive patient to facilitate the intubation process. However, abolishing spontaneous ventilation shortens the available intubation time, eliminates airway reflexes, and further compromises airway patency.

When all preparations are complete, the procedure can be started. **Orotracheal intubation** is most commonly performed with a laryngoscope. The laryngoscope is composed of a handle and a blade. The handle may be made of metal or plastic, may be disposable or nondisposable, and may have a detachable or permanently affixed blade (Figure 36-16). Batteries in the body of the handle provide power to a lighting device in the blade or the handle. When the lighting mechanism is in the handle, a fiberoptic bundle in the blade transmits light to the distal end of the blade. The fiberoptic laryngoscope has several advantages over the traditional type. Because the light bulbs are in the handle in fiberoptic laryngoscopes, they do not contact the patient and cannot be dislodged in the airway. Also, fewer bulbs are needed because a laryngoscopy set with a handle and several blades requires only one light bulb, whereas the older system requires a bulb in each blade. The proper function of the handle and its light bulb and batteries must be determined before use.

Laryngoscope blades vary in construction and are available in several shapes and sizes. The three standard blades are the curved (MacIntosh) blade, the straight (Wisconsin) blade, and the straight with a slightly curved tip (Miller) blade. Many specialty blades also are available, all designed for the occasional unusual circumstance that requires a minor variation of these standard blades. The operator's preference, training, and experience determine which blade is used. Most clinicians choose the blade they have used most often, but an experienced intubator is comfortable with all three types, so that when one does not work, an alternative is available. Nearly all blades come in sizes 0 through 4, a range that accommodates neonates up through large adults.

The laryngoscope is introduced into the mouth from the right side, displacing the tongue to the left. This maneuver is used with either a curved or straight blade to prevent the tongue from reducing visualization of the glottis. As the posterior pharyngeal wall comes into view, the intubator looks for the epiglottis (Figure 36-17). When the

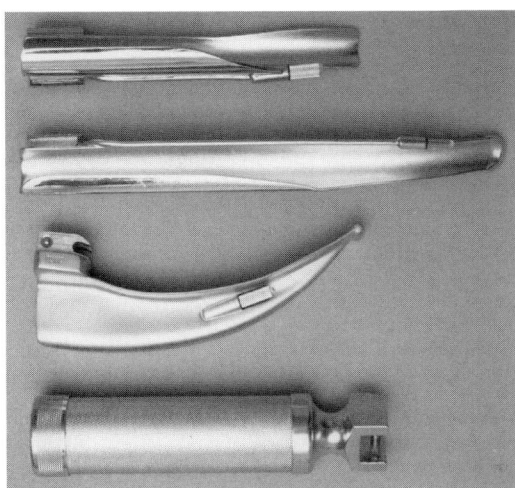

Figure 36-16   Laryngoscope handle *(bottom)* and blades. *Top,* Wisconsin blade. *Middle,* Miller blade. *Second from bottom,* MacIntosh blade. (From Bortner PL, May RA. Artificial airways and tubes. In: Eubanks DH, Bone RC, editors. Principles and applications of cardiorespiratory care equipment. St Louis: Mosby; 1994.)

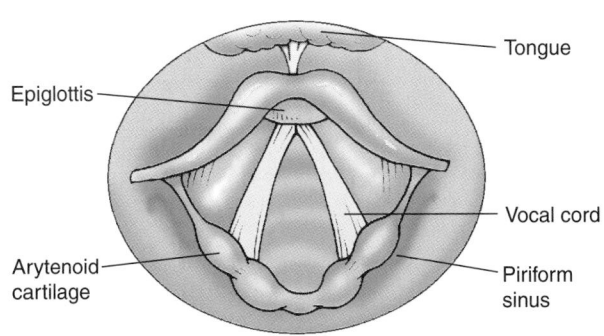

Figure 36-17   View of the glottis with the laryngoscope in the vallecula.

epiglottis can be seen, and a curved blade is used, the laryngoscope is gently readjusted to place the tip of the blade into the vallecula (the junction of the base of the tongue and the epiglottis) (Figure 36-18). If a straight blade is used, the laryngoscope is readjusted to lift the tip of the epiglottis (Figure 36-19). The proper motor action of readjustment of the laryngoscope is to direct a force on a vector caudally and anteriorly without a prying action. Using the laryngoscope in a prying action increases the likelihood of dental damage during the procedure. The above maneuvers usually bring the glottis into view, with the opening into the lower airway between the vocal cords (see Figure 36-17). With spontaneous ventilation, the appropriately sized endotracheal tube is introduced gently between the vocal cords during inspiration. If difficulty is encountered with passing the tube into the trachea, a stylet can be used to change the tube's curvature.

In adults, a 7- to 7.5-mm ID endotracheal tube is used for women and an 8- to 8.5-mm ID tube for men. The tube is advanced 2 to 4 cm below the level of the vocal cords into the trachea, and bilateral breath sounds are then verified. Correct placement is then checked by other means, such as measurement of expired carbon dioxide, negative auscultation of air movement over the epigastrium, and chest radiograph. As a general rule, the tube should be secured at the 21-cm mark (at the teeth) in women and at the 23-cm mark in men.[38] The tube is secured to the upper lip and maxilla, and another check is made for bilateral breath sounds. An appropriate oxygen delivery and ventilation system is then connected.

As described previously with difficult airways, direct visualization of the laryngeal structures sometimes is inadequate or even impossible. Repeated attempts at intubation can cause trauma, can make subsequent attempts even

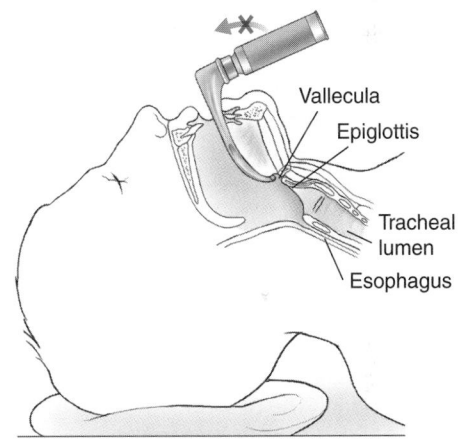

Figure 36-18   Position of the laryngoscope with a curved blade.

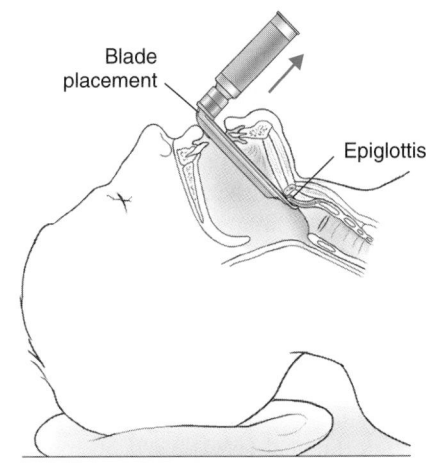

Figure 36-19   Position of the laryngoscope with a straight blade.

more difficult, and also can interfere with ventilation. A disciplined approach must be used, including the abandonment of attempts that could make a bad situation worse. The difficult airway algorithm (see Figure 36-9) presents a problem-based approach to proceeding in this situation.

ℛespiratory Recap

Equipment Required for Endotracheal Intubation	
Correct size endotracheal tube	Stylet
Lubricant	Carbon dioxide detector
Suction	Bag-valve-mask
Syringe	Oxygen
Laryngoscope	Sedative agents
	Tape to secure tube

Technique for Nasotracheal Intubation

Nasotracheal intubation generally is used for specific indications and has some special characteristics compared with orotracheal intubation.[39] Nasotracheal intubation is useful when access to the mouth is unavailable, as in oral surgery or oral trauma, or when the mouth cannot be opened adequately, as in trauma, TMJ dysfunction, or mandibular fixation. Some experts feel that a nasotracheal tube is more easily tolerated. Because the lips are not distorted, communication with the patient and oral care are easier. In addition, uncooperative patients often bite on an orotracheal tube, causing occlusion of the tube and difficulty with mechanical ventilation. However, the development of sinusitis often is associated with nasotracheal intubation. Although the nasotracheal tube may be easier to secure, it is more difficult to suction secretions through this tube. A nasotracheal tube is more stable because of the immobility of the nose and maxilla, in contrast to mandibular movement, which can affect an orotracheal tube. Because movement of the endotracheal tube in the trachea is one of the determining factors in airway trauma from intubation, nasotracheal intubation may be less likely to cause tracheal injury.

For nasotracheal intubation, as with orotracheal intubation, equipment for oxygen delivery, manual ventilation, and suction is required. A Magill forceps and a fiberoptic laryngoscope also are useful. When access to the mouth is difficult, spontaneous breathing should not be suppressed, but light sedation is beneficial. A topical anesthetic spray or jelly and a vasoconstricting spray are applied to the nares and nasopharynx to minimize sensation, trauma, and bleeding. The nasal passage can be gently dilated with lubricated, soft nasopharyngeal airways to facilitate introduction of the firmer and larger endotracheal tube. The endotracheal tube should be inserted with an initial upward motion until it just passes into the naris and then continued on a course parallel to the palate with firm, gentle pressure. As the tip of the tube reaches the

posterior wall of the nasopharynx, resistance is met. Slightly increasing the gentle pressure usually causes the tip to deflect downward. If it does not, rotating the tube slightly usually works. It is important not to use excessive force, or a false passage may be created in the pharyngeal wall, causing trauma and bleeding. As an alternative, the other naris can be tried. As the tube is directed toward the glottis, the intubator should listen for air passing in and out of the tube. As long as air is heard, the tube should be superior to the larynx. The tube is inserted into the glottis during inspiration, and as it passes the cords, a cough usually is produced. If the tube does not blindly pass into the glottis, it can be directed fiberoptically or directly with a Magill forceps and laryngoscope if the mouth can be opened (Figure 36-20). When the tube has been inserted to the appropriate depth, verification of breath sounds, carbon dioxide measurement, and verification of placement by chest radiograph should be performed.

Nasotracheal intubation may be contraindicated in some cases. Alternate techniques should be seriously considered for cases involving a suspected basilar skull fracture, nasal fracture, nasal polyps, epistaxis, coagulopathy, or planned thrombolysis.[40] Nasotracheal intubation with a basilar skull fracture is very controversial, although several studies have not shown an increase in the complication rate with this condition.[40] Epistaxis is the most common complication of nasotracheal intubation and usually can be easily managed in patients with normal coagulation processes. Because the tube causes mucosal trauma and edema, the opening to the maxillary sinuses may become occluded, with subsequent development of sinusitis. Purulent drainage may or may not be evident, but sinus radiographs or computed tomography (CT) scans of the sinuses can aid in the diagnosis.[41]

Laryngeal Mask Airway

The laryngeal mask airway (LMA; Figure 36-21) has evolved over a relatively short time into wide use both for routine management of the airway during general anes-

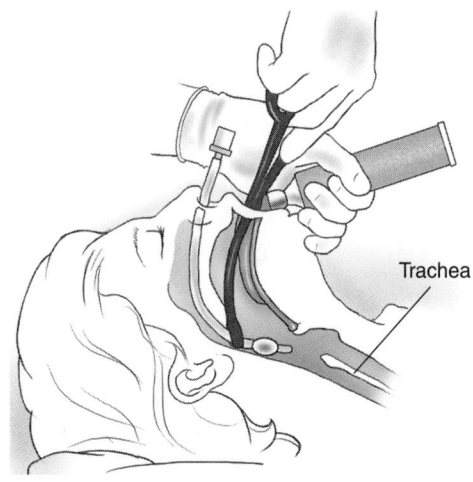

Figure 36-20 Use of a laryngoscope and Magill forceps to manipulate a nasally placed endotracheal tube through the glottis.

thesia and as an emergency airway adjunct for difficult airways. Dr. Archie Brain of the LMA Anaesthetic Centre at England's Royal Berkshire Hospital began developing the LMA in 1981, modifying more than 100 prototypes to achieve the current LMA.[42] This device provides access to the upper airway with minimal potential for involving the upper gastrointestinal tract. The LMA allows more direct ventilation than bag-mask ventilation by isolating the laryngeal structures from the esophageal structures in most cases. Ventilation provided by an LMA generally is superior to bag-mask ventilation. The LMA does not provide the same level of airway protection and security as an endotracheal tube. On the other hand, it does not require instrumentation of the laryngeal or tracheal structures and is relatively easy to place. With as little as a few hours of training, successful placement can occur in 95% of attempts. One study reviewed the use of the LMA in 11,910 patients and reported successful placement in 99.8% of cases. A total of 44 (0.37%) critical incidents occurred, the most common being regurgitation (0.03%), vomiting (0.017%), aspiration (0.009%), laryngospasm (0.07%), and bronchospasm (0.025%).[43]

The LMA is available in a range of sizes, from neonate to large adult. A #5 LMA is used for large adults, and sizes #3 and #4 are most often appropriate for small to average-sized adult. Basically, the LMA is a large-bore tube with a small inflatable mask at its distal end made of medical-grade silicone, latex-free rubber. A locking valve inflation port and tube allow inflation of the mask after it has been inserted and placed. The proximal end has the standard 15-mm adapter for connection to a ventilating or gas delivery device. Early generation LMAs were reusable and expensive, but disposable models are now in production. The shape and design of this device, which has been refined over the past two decades and many prototypes, allows it to form a seal around the glottic opening while excluding the esophageal opening from the airway. This facilitates optimum ventilation with little risk of gastric insufflation or regurgitation. The risk of aspiration is not eliminated, but there is little evidence that this complication occurs with significant incidence.

The LMA has made a significant contribution to the management of the difficult airway. When attempts at intubation fail, an LMA is inserted and rescues an otherwise bad situation. Introduction of a fiberoptic bronchoscope down the lumen of an appropriately placed LMA nearly always reveals the glottic opening in plain view. Threading a small endotracheal tube over the bronchoscope through the LMA lumen accomplishes intubation in this otherwise difficult circumstance. The widespread use of this technique and its inclusion in the difficult airway algorithm prompted the development of a special intubating LMA that has found its way onto most difficult airway carts. Its rigid, preformed, and larger lumen makes passage of an endotracheal tube through it much easier. It also has special endotracheal tubes and pushers that allow removal of the LMA after successful endotracheal intubation. In contrast, removal of the standard LMA after placement of an endotracheal tube is cumbersome and risky.

Complications of Endotracheal Intubation

A number of complications have been associated with endotracheal intubation (Box 36-2).[44,45] These have been temporally classified as complications that occur during the intubation procedure, those that occur while the endotracheal tube is in place, those that occur during and immediately after extubation, and those that occur late after extubation. The risk of complications associated with endotracheal intubation is reduced by meticulous attention to care of the airway in intubated patients.

Securing the Endotracheal Tube

Securing the endotracheal tube is an extremely important aspect of airway management. The rate of unplanned extubation (accidental extubation or self-extubation) has been reported as 2% to 13%.[46-58] Although reintubation is not necessary in every case of unplanned extubation, it is more likely than with planned extubation. Unplanned extubation may result in serious complications, and deaths have been reported. Factors that contribute to unplanned extubation include chronic respiratory failure, orotracheal intubation, lack of intravenous sedation, and securing of the endotracheal tube with only thin adhesive tape.

The traditional method used to secure an endotracheal tube is to apply benzoin to the skin and secure the tube with adhesive tape (Figure 36-22).[59] Tape 2.5 cm wide is cut long enough to go around the circumference of the patient's head one and one half to two times. A second piece of tape is cut long enough to fit over the midportion of the first piece, thus preventing the tape from sticking to the patient's neck. The tape is then placed around the patient's neck. The skin surface is dried, and tincture of benzoin is placed on both of the patient's cheeks where the tape will come into contact with the skin. The tape is pulled snug against the patient's neck and applied on the patient's cheeks to the edge of the endotracheal tube. The remaining tape is split longitudinally so that at least 5 cm of tape is available to be wrapped around the endotracheal tube at the lips. Later removal of the tape can be facilitated if the end of the

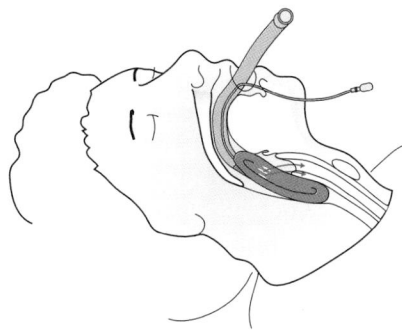

Figure 36-21   Laryngeal mask airway placed in the upper airway.

Box 36-2

Complications of Intubation

During the Intubation Procedure
Cardiac arrest
Nasal and oral trauma
Pharyngeal and hypopharyngeal trauma
Laryngeal and tracheal trauma
Main bronchus intubation
Pulmonary aspiration
Esophageal intubation

While the Endotracheal Tube is in Place
Nasal and oral ulceration (oral cellulitis)
Sinus effusions and sinusitis
Otitis
Laryngeal injury
Tracheal injury
Pulmonary complication
Self-extubation
Mechanical problems with the tube or cuff
Patient discomfort

During and Immediately after Extubation
Sore throat
Stridor
Hoarseness
Odynophagia
True vocal cord immobility
Pulmonary aspiration
Cough

Late Complications after Extubation
Laryngeal injury
Stenosis
Granuloma formation
Tracheal injury
Stenosis

From Stauffer JL, Silvester RC. Complications of endotracheal intubation, tracheostomy, and artificial airways. Respir Care 1982;27:417-434.

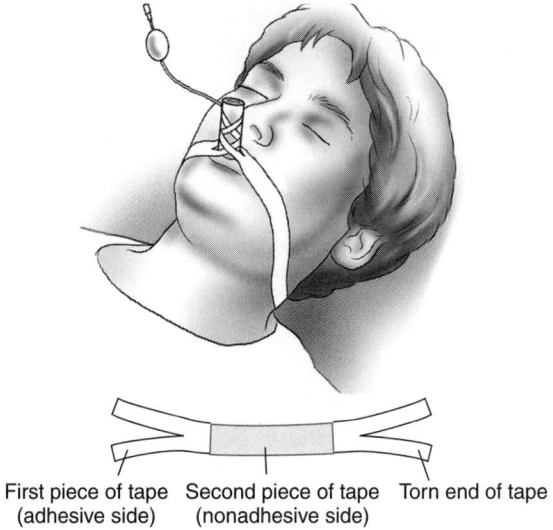

First piece of tape   Second piece of tape   Torn end of tape
(adhesive side)   (nonadhesive side)

Figure 36-22   Use of adhesive tape to secure the endotracheal tube.

Respiratory Recap

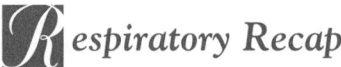

Means to Secure Endotracheal Tubes

Adhesive tape
Twill tape
Commercially available devices

Adhesive tape can pose some problems. Mouth care is difficult when too much tape is used. When an oral airway is added for stabilization and to prevent the patient from biting the tube, airway care becomes even more difficult. The patient's oral cavity and lips and the skin around the mouth must be carefully observed for signs of complications. The skin around the mouth of debilitated or immunosuppressed patients may become excoriated by tape on the face. In addition, the tape has been shown to promote bacterial growth. Although there are methods of securing tape for patients with beards and moustaches, it has been shown that these methods create problems with tube stabilization.[60]

Twill tape is another common means to secure the endotracheal tube.[59] With this method, a 1-m length of twill tape is folded in half and looped around the endotracheal tube. The ends are brought through this loop and tightened around the tube. One end of the twill tape is passed around the patient's head below one ear and the other end is passed above the other ear. The two ends are tied in a bow on the cheek. This technique sometimes is repeated with a second piece of twill tape so that two ties are used to secure the endotracheal tube.

Tube movement is considered a major cause of airway trauma. Movement of the tube against the tracheal mucosa causes a raking motion along the soft tissues of the airway. The contact is greatest at pressure points of the lips, posterior pharynx, and posterior of the glottis and at the site of

tape is folded back on itself to form a tab. Some clinicians wrap both ends of the split tape around the tube, whereas others wrap one piece around the tube and pass the other piece over the lip and fasten it to the contralateral cheek. The tape is applied snugly but not so tight as to cause breakdown of the facial skin. The advantage of this method is that tape passes completely around the neck, which is preferable to techniques in which one or two pieces of tape are used to tape the tube to the patient's cheeks. A similar method can be used for nasally placed tubes. The endotracheal tube, gastric tube, and oral airway (if present) should be taped separately. In this way, one device can be repositioned or removed without affecting the other. The tube should not be taped to the mandible, because this increases the likelihood of tube movement if the jaw is moved.

the cuff.[60-62] In adults the tip of the endotracheal tube should be positioned 3 to 7 cm above the carina when the neck is in a neutral position.[60] Flexion of the neck causes the distal tip to move toward the carina, and extension of the neck causes the tube to move toward the glottis (Figure 36-23). If the tube advances too far distally, it may enter a mainstem bronchus (usually the right).[63] If the tube moves proximally with the cuff inflated, laryngeal damage may occur. Displacement into the esophagus or pharynx may result in gastric insufflation and inadequate lung ventilation.

Several studies have evaluated various methods and devices used to secure endotracheal tubes. One study[64] compared conventional adhesive tape with a commercial tube holder and reported that patients with the tube holder had less endotracheal tube displacement. Another study compared four securing methods: adhesive tape, twill tape, adhesive tape with a bite block, and twill tape with a bite block. Results showed that the adhesive tape and twill tape methods were better used to perform oral hygiene than the methods that included the bite block.[61] The two bite block methods also were associated with a higher incidence of extubation or near-extubation. Of the four methods, twill tape was most preferred by patients because it caused less skin irritation and was more comfortable than adhesive tape. Nurses preferred adhesive tape because it was easy to use. In a similar study,[62] a comparison of three types of commercial endotracheal tube holders and a standard method with waterproof tape were evaluated. Findings showed that the SecureEasy device (Respironics, Pittsburgh, Pa.) was associated with the fewest unplanned extubations. Both the SecureEasy and Dale devices (Dale Medical, Plainville, Mass.) had low rates of facial and lip breakdown. The major disadvantage of the SecureEasy was its hindrance of mouth care. No one retention device has been universally accepted. The ideal method would allow minimal tube migration, would be comfortable for the patient, would allow oral hygiene, and would preserve skin integrity; it also would be easy to apply and would require minimal maintenance time from nurses or respiratory therapists.[65,66]

The endotracheal tube should be repositioned in the mouth periodically to allow provision of mouth care and to prevent pressure sores of the lips, gums, and mouth.[59] Two people should be present when the endotracheal tube is unsecured for this care. One person is responsible for maintaining the tube's position, and the other person is responsible for providing mouth care and resecuring the tube. In some units it is also common practice to trim the excess endotracheal tube length. This may reduce the risk of tube malposition or kinking. However, it is important to ensure that the tube is properly positioned before it is trimmed. A swivel connector should be used between the endotracheal tube and the breathing circuit, and the breathing circuit should be supported so that it does not promote tube movement.

Bite Blocks

A **bite block** is placed between the teeth to prevent the patient from biting an orotracheal airway or from biting

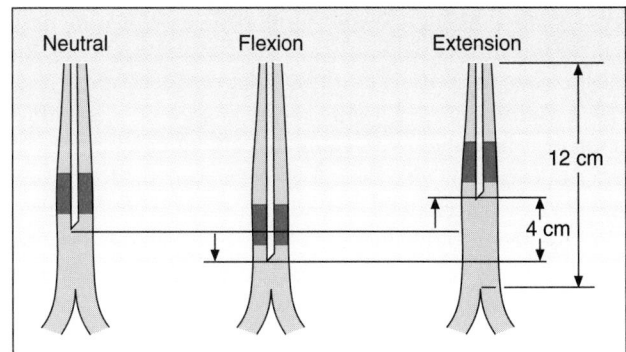

Figure 36-23   Movement of the distal portion of the endotracheal tube in the trachea with flexion and extension of the neck. (Modified from Conrardy PA, Goodman LR, Lainge F, et al. Alteration of endotracheal tube position: flexion and extension of the neck. Crit Care Med 1976;4:8-12.)

the tongue or lips, causing bleeding and trauma to the mouth. The material should be tough but not rigid and may have channels for air passage. A variety of materials and adaptations of other airways have been used as bite blocks. Oropharyngeal airways are sometimes used but may damage the teeth. Also, the complications of oropharyngeal airways when endotracheal tubes are in place for prolonged periods are problematic. Oral airways have been modified for this purpose by removal of the pharyngeal portion.[66] An airway gag was developed for patients receiving electroconvulsive therapy. The device, a wedge-shaped piece of surgical rubber, consists of a body with air channels, a flange, and a tongue depressor and retractor that hold the tongue in place but do not extend into the pharynx deep enough to induce a gag reflex.[67]

Bite blocks are used to prevent a patient from occluding an oral endotracheal tube by biting it and in unconscious patients to prevent biting of the lips or tongue. A genuine bite block designed for dental surgery and placed between the molars rather than the front teeth is the most easily tolerated device and offers greater protection to the dentition. As a safety feature, a long string is fixed to the block on one end and to the patient's gown or face on the other. In the event the bite block becomes displaced into the patient's oropharynx or larynx, it can easily be removed by pulling the string.

Tracheostomy

Advantages and Disadvantages of Tracheostomy

The primary reason used to perform a tracheostomy is to maintain a secure airway in patients who require long-term ventilation. Although tracheostomy is the preferred method, there is much controversy over when it should be performed.[68] A tracheostomy should be performed only after the clinical benefits and risks for the individual patient have been considered, not because a certain number of days of intubation have elapsed.

Compared with endotracheal intubation, a tracheostomy has the advantages of lowering airway resistance, causing less tube movement in the trachea, affording greater patient comfort, and allowing the patient to swallow secretions and nourishment. The patient can communicate by moving the lips and can even talk with the aid of special tracheostomy tubes and devices. If accidental decannulation occurs, the tube can be reinserted into the mature stoma more easily than reintubation with an endotracheal tube can be accomplished after accidental extubation. Because the tracheostomy tube is shorter than an endotracheal tube, more of the airway below the cuff may be suctioned with greater efficiency. Tracheostomy also avoids the oral, nasal, pharyngeal, and laryngeal complications of translaryngeal intubation.

A tracheostomy also has disadvantages. It is a surgical procedure and has greater morbidity and mortality risks than endotracheal intubation. Additional risks include incisional hemorrhage, subcutaneous emphysema, pneumothorax, and pneumomediastinum. Tracheal stenosis is common, and a permanent scar is unavoidable. As with endotracheal intubation, the tracheostomy tube bypasses normal defense mechanisms and impedes an effective cough because the glottis is bypassed. Many of the complications experienced during conventional tracheostomy may be avoided if the surgery is performed by a skilled surgeon as an elective procedure under optimum conditions when the patient's airway has already been stabilized, rather than at the bedside as an emergency effort.[36]

Percutaneous Dilational Tracheostomy

Percutaneous dilational tracheostomy (PDT) is a comparatively new procedure that is less traumatic than the conventional surgical method.[69] It can be performed safely and expeditiously at the bedside without the risk and cost of transportation to the operating room.[70-74] The patient is positioned with the neck extended, and the skin in the area of puncture and incision is infiltrated with a local anesthetic with epinephrine. A small incision is made midway between the cricoid cartilage and the sternal notch, and a 14-gauge cannula is inserted into the trachea between the first and second tracheal rings. A guide wire is introduced into the trachea under direct bronchoscopic observation, and the stoma is dilated with increasing sizes of specially designed plastic dilators by use of the Seldinger catheter-over-wire technique. Once the dilation is complete, an appropriately sized tracheostomy tube is inserted over a small dilator and placed in position in the trachea.

The advantages of PDT are that it can be performed at the bedside in the intensive care unit, eliminating the risks involved in moving a high-risk patient to the operating room, and it greatly reduces the potential for hemorrhage. A point that should be considered in PDT selection is that the dilation creates an opening that fits tightly around the tracheostomy tube for several days, rather than the large, secured opening created during a conventional tracheotomy. A mature tract does not form for 2 weeks, and

attempted reinsertion of the tracheotomy tube before maturation can lead to bleeding, tracheal injury, and death. If accidental decannulation occurs, the patient should be reintubated orally to control the airway. Once the airway is secure, the tract can be explored, the guide wire and dilators replaced, and the tracheotomy tube reinserted. Longer term problems with PDT, such as tracheal stenosis, have not yet been seen. PDT, when done properly, has proved to be a safe, cost-effective procedure. Compared with open tracheostomy procedures, PDT has a lower incidence of pneumothorax, bleeding complications, and stenosis.[70-74]

Tracheostomy Tubes

Metal Tracheostomy Tubes

Metal tracheostomy tubes of various types were used throughout the nineteenth century to relieve upper airway obstruction. In the early 1930s Chevalier Jackson developed a systematic approach to the management of airway obstruction that became universally accepted. This approach made tracheostomy with double-lumen silver tubes the standard for treatment of airway obstruction.[75]

Silver has long been used in the manufacture of tracheostomy tubes because the metal walls can be kept very thin, which is an advantage when the inner cannula is used. Silver was selected for construction of the tracheostomy tube because it is nonreactive when in contact with human tissue. The disadvantages of silver for tracheostomy tubes are that it is expensive and rigid. The curved shape does not conform well to the trachea, which can lead to compression damage along the tracheal wall and even erosion of major vessel walls.

The Jackson tracheostomy tube is constructed completely of silver. It has a rigid outer cannula with an attached fixed neck plate and a rigid inner cannula. These metal tracheostomy tubes are cuffless, but a rubber, reusable, high-pressure cuff can be added to prevent leaks during mechanical ventilation. The size of the metal tubes is identified by the Jackson system,[76] which uses the outer tube diameter. Disadvantages of metal tracheostomy tubes are their narrow ID, the rigid structure of the neck plate, and the lack of a 15-mm adapter for connection to most ventilatory devices. Problems associated with the reusable high-pressure cuffs are nonuniform expansion along the tracheal wall, lack of cuff strength, and the danger of the cuff slipping over the end of tracheostomy tube, causing airway occlusion. Metal tracheostomy tubes are available in pediatric and adult sizes. However, because of the improvements in material design, clinical use of metal tracheostomy tubes is almost nonexistent.

Current Construction

Tracheostomy tubes may be made of metal, rubber, silicone, Teflon, polyethylene, and PVC materials.[33] Like endotracheal tubes, tracheostomy tubes must satisfy ASTM requirements. Because the tubes are in direct contact with body tissue, the ideal material is nontoxic and determined by implant testing. Modern plastic tracheostomy tubes (Figure 36-24) are available in sizes 2.5 to 11.5 mm according to their ID. On most tracheostomy tubes the manufacturer should mark the ID and the OD as a guide for the user. Besides materials, standard requirements cover surface characteristics, dimensions, tolerances, cuff characteristics, and labeling of tubes and packages.

The shape of the tracheostomy tube should conform as closely as possible to the anatomy of the airway. Two main types of tracheostomy tubes are available—those that are curved and those that are angled to fit the trachea at one end and the area between the skin and the trachea at the other end (Figure 36-25). Curved tracheostomy tubes usually have an inner cannula that can be removed for cleaning while the outer cannula remains in place. The outer cannula may have a window, or fenestration, to allow for speech when the inner cannula is removed. Because the trachea is mostly straight, the curved tracheostomy tube often does not conform to the shape of the trachea, which

may allow compression of the membranous part of the trachea, and the tip may traumatize the anterior portion. These tubes may also damage the area of the stoma.

Angled tracheostomy tubes enter the trachea in a way that may cause less pressure damage at the stoma. Because the tube portion that extends into the trachea is straight and conforms more closely to the anatomy of the airway, the angled tracheostomy tube is well centered in the trachea and causes less pressure necrosis along the tracheal wall. One disadvantage of angled tubes is that they generally are difficult to fit with an inner cannula. An extra-long tracheostomy tube is used for a patient with a large neck.

Uncuffed Tracheostomy Tubes

Standard uncuffed tracheostomy tubes have the same basic design as those described previously. On the flange attachment of some uncuffed adult tracheostomy tubes, *UNCUFFED* designates it is as uncuffed, and *FEN* indicates that the tube is fenestrated. If the tracheostomy tube chosen uses a removable inner cannula, the package of the inner cannula should have the size and make of the tube into which it is intended to fit. Uncuffed tracheostomy tubes are used primarily in pediatric patients, in whom the cricoid ring is narrower than the glottis. Because the tissues anterior to the trachea in infants are thinner and the laryngeal and tra-

ℛespiratory Recap ———————

Tracheostomy Tube Shapes
Curved
Angled
Extra-long

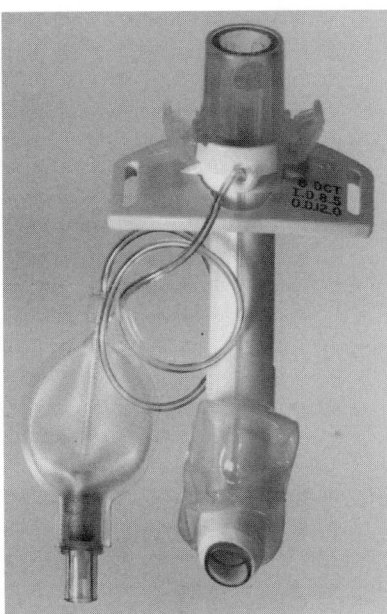

Figure 36-24   Standard cuffed tracheostomy tube. (From Bortner PL, May RA. Artificial airways and tubes. In: Eubanks DH, Bone RC, editors. Principles and applications of cardiorespiratory care equipment. St Louis: Mosby; 1994.)

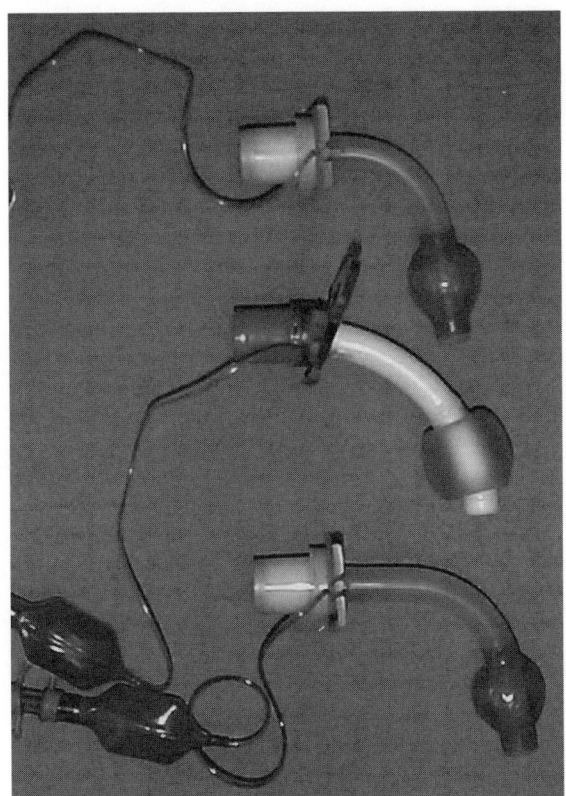

Figure 36-25   Examples of angled *(top),* curved *(center),* and extra-long *(bottom)* tracheostomy tubes.

cheal cartilages are softer, use of cuffed tracheostomy tubes in infants and children up to 6 years of age makes them susceptible to tracheal deformation. In children, especially infants, the shape of the neck plate of the tracheostomy tube is important. The usual straight neck plate does not fit well because of anatomic differences between infants and adults. The newer, flexible, soft, swivel neck flange on most current tracheostomy tubes solves this problem.

Age-Specific Angle

Uncuffed tracheostomy tubes are used primarily for pediatric patients.

Uncuffed tracheostomy tubes are intended to allow a small leak during ventilation. Unfortunately, some clinicians tend to use a tube that fits rather snugly to reduce this leak. The large stomal opening required to accommodate the tube increases the chances of stomal stenosis. Silastic tubes with a single lumen that do not require an inner cannula are available for pediatric patients.

In adults uncuffed tracheostomy tubes are used primarily after laryngectomy and in patients with neuromuscular disease who need frequent suctioning but not mechanical ventilation. Uncuffed tubes have also been used as a method of weaning from the tracheostomy tube. Progressively smaller diameters of uncuffed tubes are used to allow suctioning and maintenance of the stoma while allowing the patient to adapt to the normal airway. The absence of a cuff on a tracheostomy tube does not help prevent aspiration, and this type of tube should not be used in unconscious patients or those in whom airway defenses have been lost.

Cuffed Tracheostomy Tubes

Like the uncuffed standard tracheostomy tubes, the typical cuffed tracheostomy tube is composed of outer and inner cannulas. The outer cannula forms the primary structure of the tube and also has the cuff assembly attached to its distal end. On most tracheostomy tubes, a removable inner cannula with a standard 15-mm adapter attaches securely into place at the proximal end of the outer cannula to provide a point of attachment for humidification and ventilation systems. During normal use it is kept in place inside the outer cannula but can be removed for cleaning. Also at the proximal end are the inflation tube and pilot balloon with spring-loaded valve assembly for cuff inflation and deflation. An obturator with a rounded tip is placed into the outer cannula before insertion of the tracheostomy tube. The rounded obturator tip extends beyond the distal end of the tube far enough to round the otherwise blunted end; this minimizes trauma to the mucosa of the tracheal wall during insertion of the tube. The tubes have a radiopaque marker on the distal tip to provide confirmation of the tube's position on radiographs.

Tracheostomy tubes are constructed primarily of PVC or other synthetic materials and are tissue compatible as determined by acceptable implant test methods. The Shiley tracheostomy tube is an example of a modern tracheostomy tube system. It is disposable and offers the practitioner a variety of tube models ranging from a standard system similar to the silver tracheostomy tube to one with single and double fenestrations and pressure-limiting automatic relief valves that limit the internal cuff pressure to approximately 25 mm Hg. As mentioned above, some tracheostomy tubes have a radiopaque marker on the distal tip of the outer cannula to provide confirmation of tube positioning on radiographs.

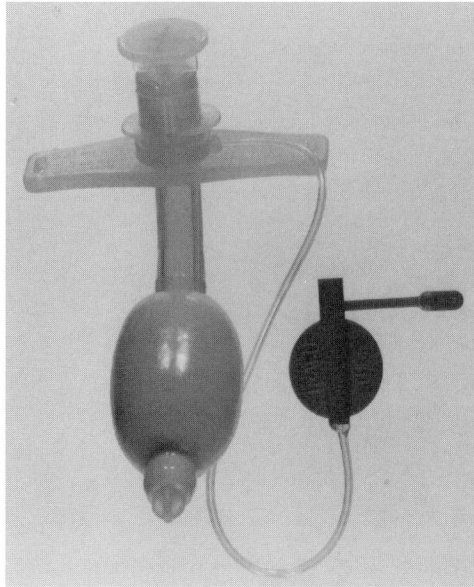 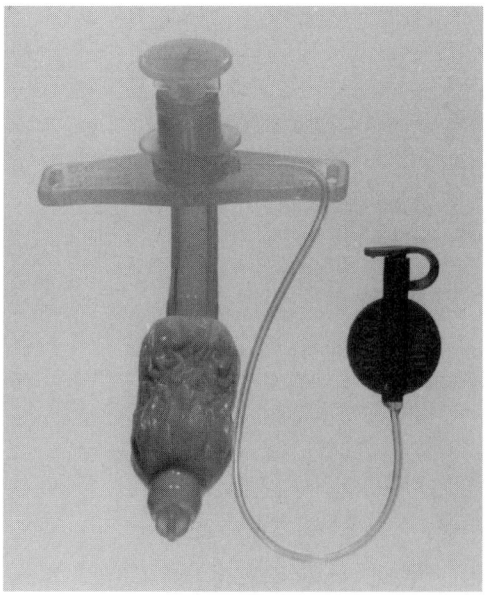

Figure 36-26   Foam cuff tracheostomy tube with the cuff inflated *(left)* and deflated *(right)*. (From Bortner PL, May RA. Artificial airways and tubes. In: Eubanks DH, Bone RC, editors. Principles and applications of cardiorespiratory care equipment. St Louis: Mosby; 1994.)

The use of cuffs has been associated with many types of complications. Efforts to limit these problems have resulted in numerous recent developments in the size and shape of tube cuffs. Design characteristics believed to be important are the cuff volume and the diameter of the cuff when fully expanded at atmospheric pressure.[77] Another controversy in the selection of the proper tracheostomy tube involves the choice of a single-lumen tube or a tube with an inner cannula. The Shiley tracheostomy tube has an inner cannula that can be removed for cleaning, whereas the Portex Soft Seal and the Bivona tracheostomy tube (Bivona Medical Technologies, Gary, Ind.) are single lumen tubes. Careful consideration must be given to each clinical situation in the selection of a tracheostomy tube. Some important factors are the cuff pressure necessary to achieve minimal leak, the transmission of pressure to the tracheal walls, the ability to monitor intracuff pressure, and the simplicity of the tube's design for optimal clinical use.

Foam Cuff Tracheostomy Tubes

The Bivona foam cuff, designed by Kamen and Wilkinson, consists of a large diameter, high residual volume cuff composed of polyurethane foam covered by a silicone sheath.[78] This cuff was designed to address the problem of high lateral tracheal wall pressures that lead to complications such as tracheal necrosis and stenosis. Before insertion, air in the cuff is evacuated by a syringe attached to the pilot port, which makes the foam contract (Figure 36-26). This allows insertion of the tracheostomy tube. Once the tube is in place, the syringe is removed to allow the cuff to re-expand until it is stopped by the tracheal wall. The pilot tube remains open to the atmosphere so that the intracuff pressure is at ambient levels. The open pilot port also permits compression and expansion of the cuff during the ventilatory cycle, which allows intermittent perfusion of the tracheal tissue in contact with the tube without loss of volume during ventilation. The degree of foam expansion is a determining factor in the amount of pressure exerted on the tracheal wall. As the foam expands further, lateral tracheal wall pressure increases. However, when the device is used properly, this pressure rarely exceeds 20 mm Hg.

When a foam cuff tracheostomy tube is selected, the proper size is important to maintain a seal and still benefit from the pressure-limiting advantages of the foam-filled cuff. If the tube is too small, the foam will inflate to its unrestricted size and the cuff may leak, causing loss of ventilation and loss of protection against aspiration. If the tube is too large, the foam is unable to expand properly to provide the desired cushion, with resultant increased pressure against the tracheal wall. If air is injected into the cuff to increase the lateral wall pressure and provide a seal, the purpose and pressure-limiting benefits of the foam cuff are defeated, and the cuff may leak, which can result in a loss of ventilator volume during inspiration. The manufacturer recommends periodic cuff deflation in order to assess the integrity of the cuff and prevent the silicone sheath from adhering to the tracheal mucosa.

Fenestrated Tracheostomy Tubes

A fenestrated tracheostomy tube can be useful in the assessment of a patient's readiness to be decannulated, and it allows the patient to talk when the tube is occluded and the cuff deflated. The fenestrated tracheostomy tube is similar in construction to a regular tracheostomy tube, with the addition of an opening in the posterior portion of the tube above the cuff (Figure 36-27). Fenestrated tubes are composed of a tracheostomy tube with a fenestration, a removable inner cannula, and a plastic plug. When the inner cannula is removed, the cuff deflated, and normal air passage occluded with the plug, the patient can inhale and exhale through the fenestration and around the tube. This allows for assessment of the patient's ability to breathe through the normal oral/nasal route (preparing the patient for decannulation) and permits air to pass by the vocal cords, creating phonation.

Health care workers must be properly trained in the use of fenestrated tracheostomy tubes. If the patient has been receiving humidified, oxygen-enriched air via the tube, an alternate source must be provided, such as a nasal cannula. Also, before the proximal end is blocked, the cuff must be completely deflated by evacuating all of the air. The tracheal cap is then put in place to allow the patient to breathe through the fenestrations and around the tube. If the cuff is left inflated during the capping procedure, airway resistance will be excessive, and the patient will experience respiratory distress. The patient must be observed carefully for aspiration of secretions or oral fluids while the

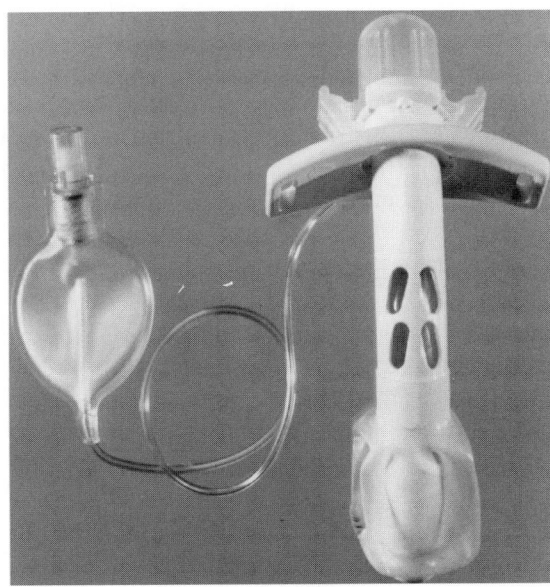

Figure 36-27   Fenestrated tracheostomy tube. (From Bortner PL, May RA. Artificial airways and tubes. In: Eubanks DH, Bone RC, editors. Principles and applications of cardiorespiratory care equipment. St Louis: Mosby; 1994.)

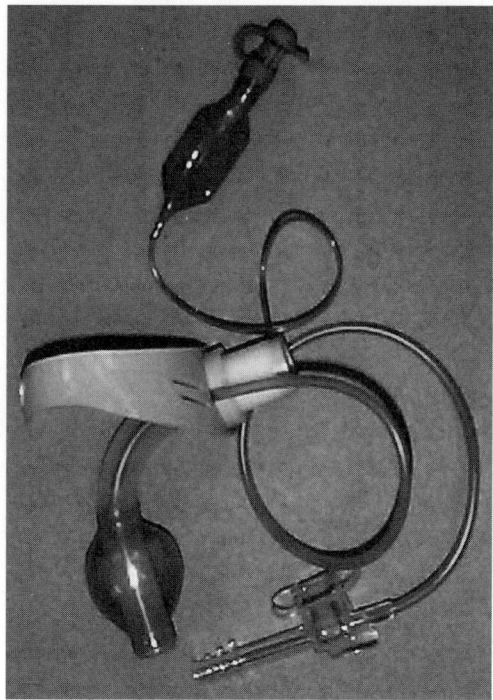

Figure 36-28   Portex speaking tracheostomy tubes.

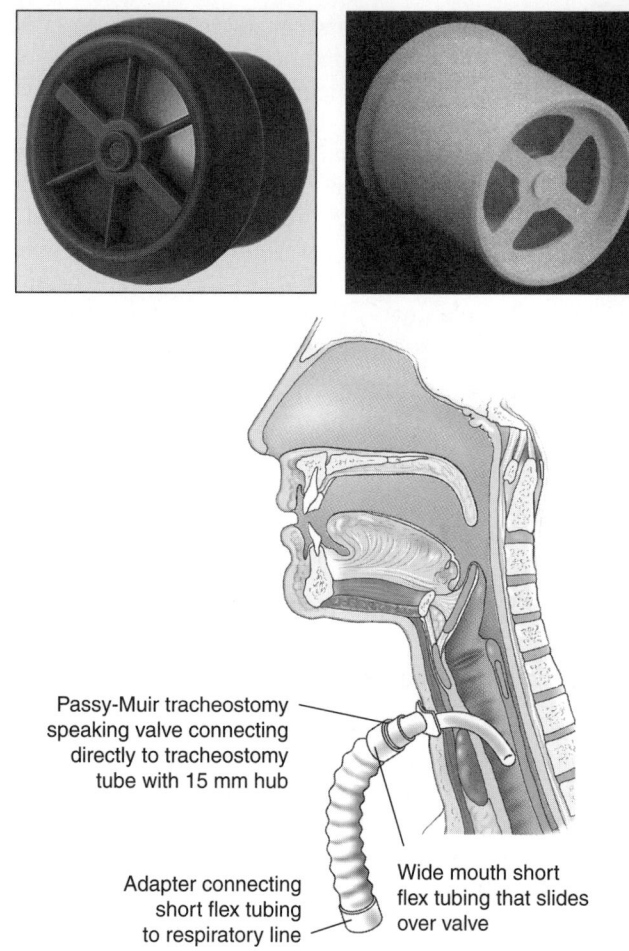

Passy-Muir tracheostomy
speaking valve connecting
directly to tracheostomy
tube with 15 mm hub

Adapter connecting
short flex tubing
to respiratory line

Wide mouth short
flex tubing that slides
over valve

Figure 36-29   *Top,* Passy-Muir speaking valves. *Bottom,* Passy-Muir valve in-line during mechanical ventilation. (Courtesy Passy-Muir, Irvine, Calif.)

cuff is deflated. This type of tube should be considered only for patients with normal upper airway reflexes.

Talking Tracheostomy Tubes

The primary goal of a talking tracheostomy tube is to allow cognitively intact, ventilator-dependent patients to communicate by speaking. If a patient has normally functioning oral and laryngeal structures, the options available are an electrolarynx, a self-activated pneumatic system, or a talking tracheostomy tube. The main drawback of the electrolarynx is its cost, which frequently is beyond reasonable means. Patients also are often frustrated by its unnatural vocal quality and the difficulty some physically impaired patients have in holding the device to the neck while speaking. The pneumatic system also is limited by the dexterity required to operate the tone switch and the inability to speak clearly because of the intraoral catheter.[79] Speaking tracheostomy tubes have been developed that provide communication for ventilator-dependent patients. The most commonly used model is Portex Talk tracheostomy tube (Figure 36-28). It has an opening in the posterior portion above the cuff through which a source of air is provided for speech.

In comparative studies no significant differences were found in the degree of voice intensity produced by the talking tracheostomy tubes. However, on the basis of design differences in posterior air openings and the incidence of plugging by secretions, the Portex Talk was more favorable for longer continuous communication.[80,81] Two deficiencies were cited: the air supply connector is too large, which

causes the oxygen line to the tube to disconnect, and the inner cannula diameter is 2 mm smaller than the outer diameter, which creates increased airway resistance and difficulty breathing with sizes smaller than 8 mm.[81]

Talking tracheostomy tubes provide vital psychologic support. With early speech rehabilitation, patients who are ventilator dependent or who are at risk of aspiration and require a cuffed tracheostomy tube can benefit from a speaking tracheostomy tube.

Passy-Muir Tracheostomy Speaking Valves

The Passy-Muir tracheostomy **speaking valve** (Figure 36-29) is designed to eliminate the need for finger occlusion to communicate by speaking.[82-84] The valve attaches to the 15-mm universal adapter of all tracheostomy tubes and can be used in adult and pediatric patients. The valve opens on inspiration, with air passing through to the lungs, and closes on expiration, with the air directed into the trachea and up past the vocal cords to permit speech. This device can be used in either spontaneously breathing or ventilator-dependent patients. However, it should be used with caution in patients at

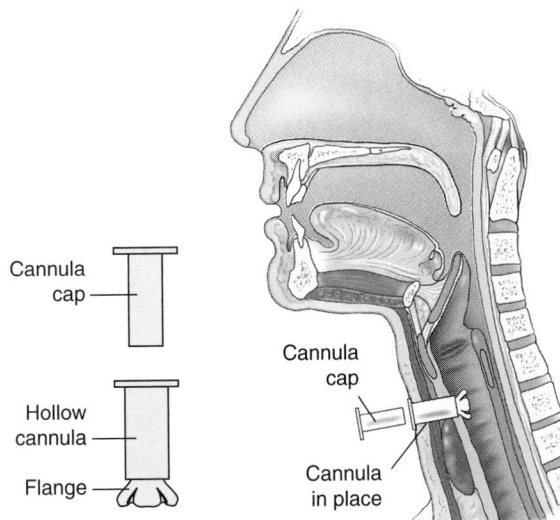

Figure 36-30   Tracheostomy button.

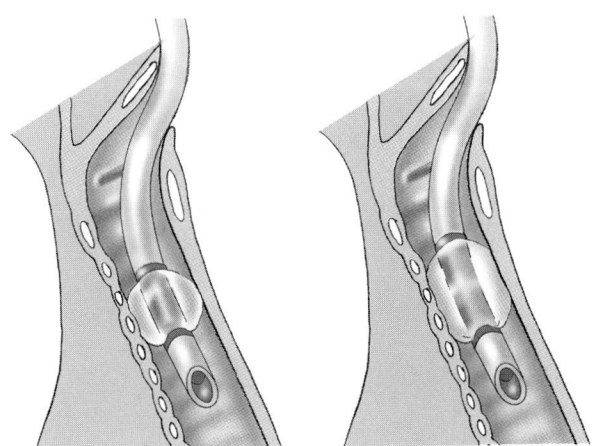

Figure 36-31   The two types of airway cuffs. *Left,* Low-volume, high-pressure cuff. *Right,* High-volume, low-pressure cuff.

risk of aspiration because the cuff of the tracheostomy tube must be deflated to use this device. Increases in ventilator-delivered tidal volume may be needed to compensate for leakage around the tracheostomy tube during mechanical ventilation. After the Passy-Muir valve is removed and the tracheostomy cuff reinflated, overventilation of the patient must be avoided. The Passy-Muir valve may also be used to wean patients from the tracheostomy tube as a means to reorient them to use of the upper airway for breathing.

Tracheal Buttons

Tracheal buttons (Figure 36-30) are used to maintain tracheostomy stomas. They are temporary appliances, generally made of Teflon, consisting of a hollow outer cannula and an inner solid cannula. The device fits from the skin to just inside the anterior wall of the trachea. A tracheal button should be used when the tracheostomy stoma must be maintained, either for replacement of a tracheostomy tube later or for suctioning. A tracheal button does not have a cuff, therefore it is of limited value in cases involving a risk of aspiration or during positive pressure ventilation.

Airway Cuff Concerns

An **airway cuff** is classified as a high-volume, low-pressure cuff or a low-volume, high-pressure cuff (Figure 36-31). Most cuffs used today are high-volume, low-pressure cuffs. The high tracheal wall pressures exerted by the inflated cuff of an endotracheal or a tracheostomy tube can injure the tracheal mucosa.[85-93] The tracheal capillary perfusion pressure normally is 25 to 35 mm Hg. Because the pressure transmitted from the cuff to the tracheal wall usually is less than the pressure in the cuff, it is generally agreed that 25 mm Hg (34 cm H_2O) is the maximum acceptable intracuff pressure. If the cuff pressure is too low, silent aspiration is

more likely.[94,95] Therefore it seems reasonable to maintain cuff pressures at 20 to 25 mm Hg (25 to 35 cm H_2O) to minimize the risks of tracheal wall injury and aspiration.

The cuff typically is inflated with a *minimum occlusion pressure* or *minimum leak* technique. With the minimum occlusion pressure method, the cuff is inflated to a volume that just eliminates an end-inspiratory leak during positive pressure ventilation.[96-99] With the minimum leak technique, the cuff is inflated to a volume that allows a small leak to occur at end-inspiration. With either method, leakage around the cuff is assessed by auscultation over the suprasternal notch or the lateral neck. Although no studies comparing these approaches have been reported, it may be prudent to use the minimum occlusion pressure technique to reduce the risk of silent aspiration of pharyngeal secretions.

Monitoring of the cuff pressure is standard respiratory care practice. The intracuff pressure should be monitored and recorded at least once per shift and more often if the tube position is changed, if the volume of air in the cuff is changed, or if a leak occurs. Cuff pressure is measured with a syringe, stopcock, and manometer (Figure 36-32). With this method, the cuff pressure can be measured simultaneously with adjustment of the cuff volume. Methods in which the manometer is attached directly to the pilot balloon are discouraged, because they cause air to escape from the cuff to pressurize the manometer. Commercially available systems can also be used to measure cuff pressure.

A common cause of high cuff pressure is a tube that is too small, which results in overfilling of the cuff to achieve a seal in the trachea. If the volume of air in the cuff required to achieve a seal exceeds the cuff's *nominal volume,* the tube is too small. The nominal cuff volume is the volume below which the cuff pressure is less than 25 mm Hg ex vivo. Another common cause of high cuff pressure is incorrect positioning of the endotracheal tube, particularly a cephalad position in which the cuff is inflated in the lar-

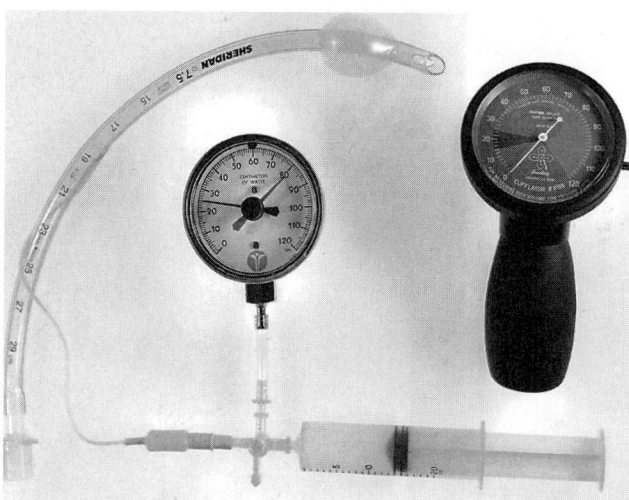

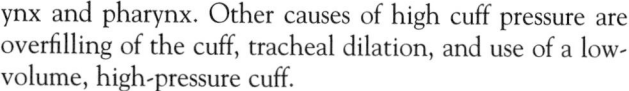

Figure 36-32   Equipment for measuring cuff pressure. (From Bortner PL, May RA. Artificial airways and tubes. In: Eubanks DH, Bone RC, editors. Principles and applications of cardiorespiratory care equipment. St Louis: Mosby; 1994.)

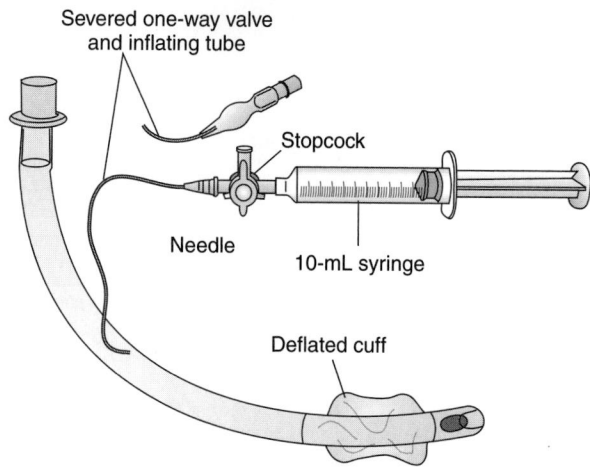

Figure 36-33   Technique for inflating a cuff when the inflating tube has been severed. (Modified from Sills J. An emergency cuff inflation technique. Respir Care 1986;31:199-201.)

ynx and pharynx. Other causes of high cuff pressure are overfilling of the cuff, tracheal dilation, and use of a low-volume, high-pressure cuff.

Occasionally the pilot tube may be severed. To correct this problem, a short, blunt needle can be passed into the pilot tube and a stopcock attached to the needle hub to add and maintain air in the cuff until the tube can be replaced (Figure 36-33).[100] Cuff leaks also can occur, and a continuous flow of gas into the cuff can be used to temporarily maintain cuff inflation until the tube can be changed.[101,102] Interestingly, it has been reported that a large number of endotracheal tubes removed for presumed cuff rupture were flawless, and some researchers have speculated that incorrect tube positioning may be the explanation for this finding.[103]

A simple method can be used to assess cuff rupture. The cuff is inflated with the equipment shown in Figure 36-32. If a leak occurs during this maneuver, there may be a ruptured cuff or an incompetent pilot balloon. This can be further assessed by clamping the pilot tube. If a leak occurs without the clamp, but not with the clamp, the pilot balloon or valve is incompetent. Figure 36-34 presents an algorithm for cuff management. Occasionally an endotracheal tube must be changed, such as when the cuff has ruptured. A tube changer can be used to facilitate this procedure. The tube changer is passed through the endotracheal tube into the trachea, and the endotracheal tube is withdrawn while the tube changer is kept in place. The new endotracheal tube then is passed over the tube changer into the trachea.

Secretion Clearance

Intubated patients should be suctioned whenever a physical examination reveals secretions in the airway. Because

tracheal suctioning is uncomfortable for the patient and carries some risk, it should be performed only when indicated and not at fixed intervals.[104] The upper airway should be suctioned periodically to remove oral secretions.

A suction catheter must be long enough to enter the mainstem bronchi. A thumb port at the proximal end controls suction to the catheter. The catheter must be rigid enough to allow passage through an artificial airway but flexible enough to prevent damage to the airway mucosa. Also to prevent damage to the airway mucosa, the catheter should have smooth, molded ends, one or more side holes near the catheter tip, and minimum frictional resistance when passed through the airway. The catheter should be transparent so that the aspirated secretions can be assessed.

Tracheal suctioning is very irritating and uncomfortable for the patient. The presence of the catheter in the trachea can induce coughing and may stimulate bronchospasm in patients with reactive airways. Airway suctioning has many possible complications.

A number of factors contribute to suction-related hypoxemia,[105-119] including interruption of mechanical ventilation during the suctioning procedure (that is, loss of ventilation, inspired oxygen, and positive end-expiratory pressure [PEEP]), aspiration of gas from the respiratory tract during the application of suction, entrainment of room air into the lungs, the duration of suctioning, and suction-related atelectasis. Hyperoxygenation is the best technique used to prevent suction-related hypoxemia and should be used with all suctioning procedures. This most commonly is accomplished by an increase in the FIO_2 to 1.

Hyperinflation or hyperventilation (or both) to prevent suction-related hypoxemia should be used cautiously because of the hazards of overdistension lung injury.[120-122] In

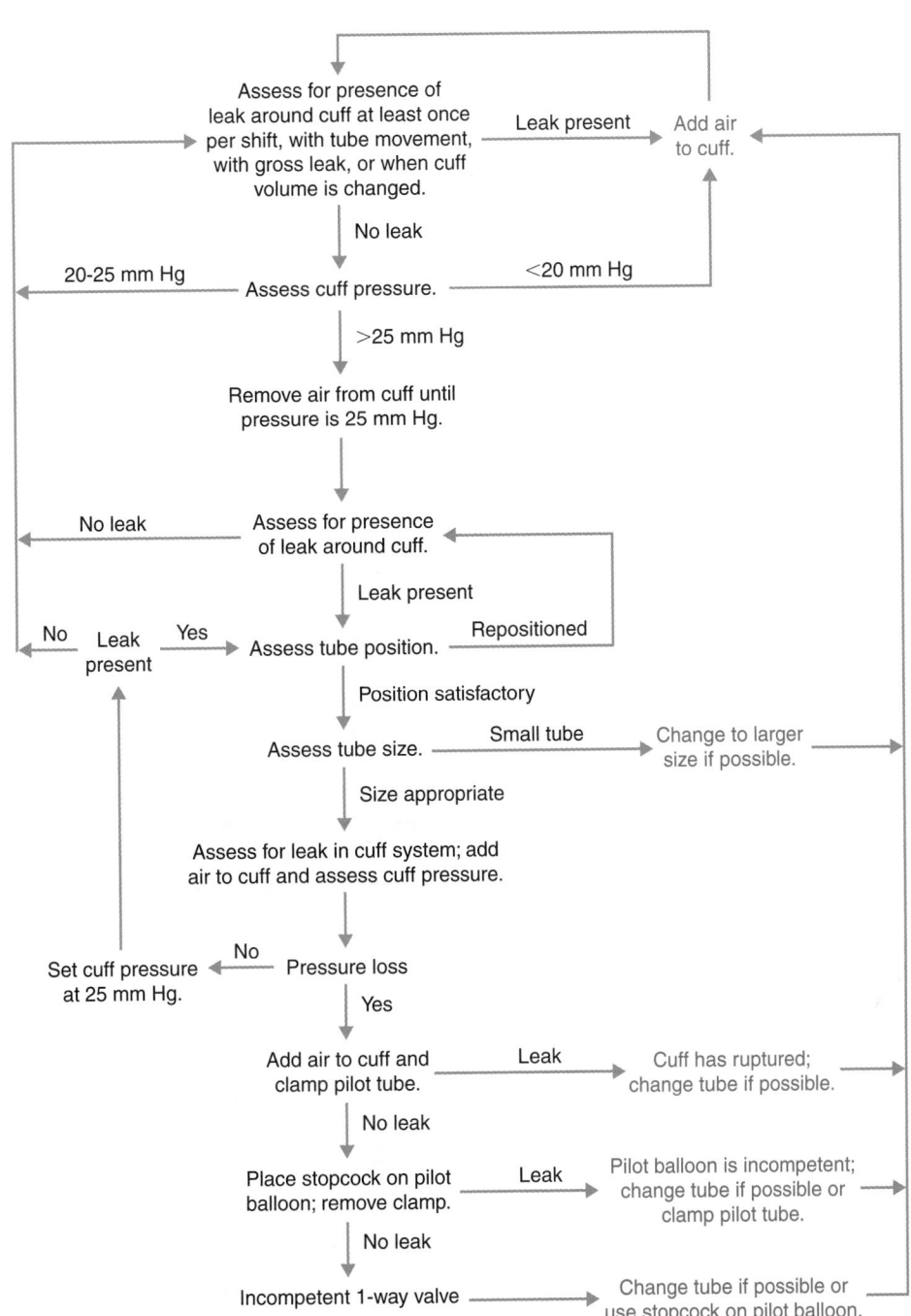

Figure 36-34 Algorithm for the resolution of a cuff leak on an artificial airway. (Modified from Hess DR. Managing the artificial airway. Respir Care 1999;44:759-772.)

some critical care units a manual ventilator (resuscitator) is used for hyperinflation and hyperoxygenation during suctioning procedures. However, this method may not be as effective as hyperinflation and hyperoxygenation provided by the mechanical ventilator. Bedside manual ventilators can be a source of contamination of the lower respiratory tract, and tidal volume delivery and airway pressure are not usually measured. Manual ventilation often does not achieve lung hyperinflation, and adverse hemodynamic se-

quelae may result if hyperinflation is achieved. The duration of suctioning also affects the degree of hypoxemia.[123] A suctioning attempt should be as brief as possible to achieve the desired effect, which is removal of secretions, but should last no longer than 15 seconds.

Atelectasis can occur during suctioning as the result of evacuation of gases from the lower respiratory tract. This is more likely to occur when excessive suction pressures are used and when the size of the suction catheter is large in relation to the size of the endotracheal or tracheostomy tube.[124] The suction pressure should be no greater than that required to remove secretions adequately. It should not exceed 100 mm Hg in infants, 125 mm Hg in children, and 150 mm Hg in adults. Suction catheters are available in a variety of sizes. The catheter size is determined by its OD in French (Fr) units, which refers to the circumference of the tube. Because circumference equals 3.14 (π) $\times$ diameter, the French size is estimated by multiplication of the diameter by 3. The OD of the suction catheter should not exceed one half to two thirds the ID of the artificial airway. A 14 Fr catheter usually is acceptable for adults. A catheter that is too small limits the effectiveness of secretion removal, and a catheter that is too large increases the risk of complications.

Airway edema, hyperemia, mucosal ulceration, hemorrhage, and diminished mucociliary transport have been reported with airway suctioning.[125,126] These effects are related to operator technique and the amount of suction pressure used. Intermittent, rather than continuous, suctioning may be less traumatic to airway mucosa, but little evidence is available on this issue.[127,128] As mentioned previously, the catheter tip should be smooth, molded, and atraumatic,[129-131] and side holes near the tip of the catheter can minimize trauma to the airway mucosa. Pneumothorax that occurs secondary to bronchial perforation by a suction catheter has been reported in infants.[132-136] In infants the suction catheter should not be inserted more than 1 cm beyond the tip of the endotracheal tube. A similar practice should be used for patients who have had a recent tracheal reconstructive surgery or pneumonectomy.

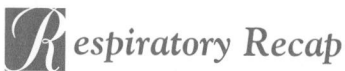espiratory *Recap* ————————

Complications of Suctioning
Hypoxemia
Atelectasis
Airway trauma
Contamination of the lower respiratory tract
Arrhythmias
Increased intracranial pressure
Preferential suctioning of the right bronchus

Contamination of the lower respiratory tract can occur during tracheal suctioning. This complication can be avoided with the use of a sterile technique during the procedure. Care must be taken during suctioning to avoid contamination of the suction catheter, the ventilator circuit or the valve of the manual ventilator, and the clinician performing the procedure.

Arrhythmias may occur during tracheal suctioning as a result of hypoxemia or vagal stimulation.[135-137] This complication often can be avoided by hyperoxygenation of the

> ## Age-Specific Angle
>
> Pneumothorax that occurred secondary to bronchial perforation by a suction catheter has been reported in infants.

patient during suctioning. Aerosolized atropine also has been used to prevent suction-related arrhythmias.

Because the left mainstem bronchus has a smaller diameter than the right bronchus and leaves the trachea at a more acute angle, the suction catheter is more likely to enter the right mainstem bronchus. Secretions therefore are more likely to be suctioned from the right lung than the left. Several techniques can be used for selective endobronchial suctioning, particularly of the left bronchus,[138-145] including use of curved-tip catheters, turning of the head to the side (for example, turning of the head to the right to facilitate suctioning of the left bronchus), and lateral positioning (turning of the patient onto the left side to facilitate passage of the catheter into the left mainstem bronchus). Use of a curved-tip catheter has proved to be the best means to accomplish endobronchial suctioning; when a curved-tip catheter with a guide mark was used for this purpose, successful endobronchial placement was reported in nearly 90% of cases. Factors that affect the success of the selective introduction of a catheter into a mainstem bronchus include the anatomy of the carinal bifurcation, the patient's head and body positions, the route of tracheal tube placement (endotracheal or tracheostomy), the shape and direction of the endotracheal tube's bevel, the configuration and rigidity of the suction catheter, and the location of the tip of the endotracheal tube. Curved-tip catheters may be more effective with tracheostomy tubes than with endotracheal tubes.

An increase in intracranial pressure (ICP) can occur during tracheal suctioning, which may be clinically important in patients with a closed head injury.[146-151] If a patient's ICP is being monitored, it should be watched closely during suctioning. Preoxygenation, hyperventilation, and pharmacologic support may be necessary for suctioning patients with an elevated ICP.

Closed Suction Catheters

With the closed suction system (Figure 36-35), the catheter becomes part of the ventilator circuit.[152-167] Closed suction and conventional suction catheters are equally effective at secretion clearance.[154] However, the closed system may cause significantly fewer physiologic disturbances, such as dysrhythmias and desaturation,[159] and the incidence of both patient and environmental contamination has been reported to be lower with the closed system.[162-164] A problem reported with closed suction catheters involves the catheter remaining in the airway af-

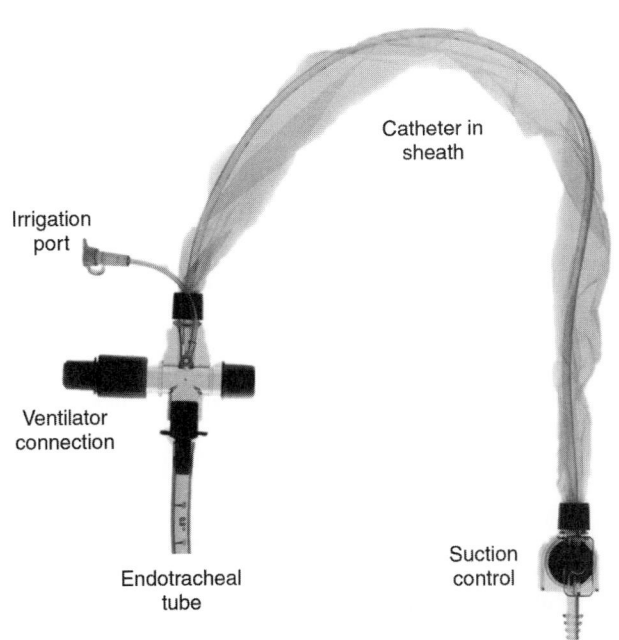

Catheter in sheath

Irrigation port

Ventilator connection

Endotracheal tube

Suction control

Figure 36-35 Closed suction catheter. (From Hess DR. Managing the artificial airway. Respir Care 1999;44:759-772.)

ter suctioning or migrating into the airway between suctioning procedures.[166] This may be of particular concern during pressure ventilation, because the patient's tidal volume may be considerably compromised. Care must also be taken to avoid accidental patient lavage when the catheter is rinsed with saline.

One drawback to the closed suction system is the cost of the catheter. Although the closed system costs many times more than a conventional suction catheter, it also is used many times to suction the patient. One study reported a cost savings of $6,600 in 1 year when closed suctioning was substituted for the open technique,[167] and another study reported that closed suctioning cost $1.88 per patient per day less and required 1 hour less clinician time than open suctioning.[159] Manufacturers recommend changing closed suction catheter systems daily, but the available evidence suggests that these systems need not be changed more often than the ventilator circuit (that is, no more frequently than once a week).[168]

Saline Instillation

Although saline often is instilled into airway as part of the suctioning procedure to facilitate the removal of secretions, this practice is controversial.[169-173] Typically, more saline is instilled than is retrieved by the suctioning, and this may result in an increase in the volume of secretions and worsening of airway obstruction. Saline instillation during suctioning may have an adverse effect on arterial oxygen saturation and may dislodge large numbers of bacteria from the lumen of the endotracheal tube, which may increase the likelihood of organisms being washed from

the endotracheal tube into the lower respiratory tract. In a very few patients, saline instillation may be useful to loosen and remove thick secretions. However, this practice should be used judiciously and should *not* be a routine procedure each time a patient is suctioned.

Extubation and Decannulation

Extubation is the removal of the endotracheal tube (CPG 36-2).[174] A patient generally can be extubated if he or she can keep the upper airway patent, can protect the lower airway from aspiration, can clear secretions from the lower respiratory tract, and can breathe without mechanical ventilation. In other words, the patient may be extubated if none of the indications for endotracheal intubation remain. Before extubation can be performed, the upper airway must be free of swelling and inflammation, which can impede adequate spontaneous ventilation. The absence of these conditions often is assessed qualitatively as the amount of leakage around the endotracheal tube during positive pressure ventilation with the cuff deflated.[175,176]

Before the extubation, secretions are cleared from the lower respiratory tract and pharynx, and oxygen administration equipment is prepared for use after extubation. This often consists of administration of a cool mist, which is believed to reduce the degree of upper airway swelling after extubation. The cuff is deflated, and the endotracheal tube is removed as the patient takes a deep breath. Some prefer to remove the endotracheal tube while applying suction to a catheter placed through the endotracheal tube during extubation to clear upper airway secretions and minimize their aspiration into the lower respiratory tract. After the endotracheal tube has been removed, supplemental oxygen is administered and the patient is encouraged to deep breathe and cough, while the individual is assessed for signs of upper airway obstruction.

Extubation failure, or the need to reintubate, occurs in 5% to 15% of cases for a variety of reasons.[177-179] Most commonly, the patient cannot sustain adequate spontaneous ventilation. Reintubation is not benign and has been associated with increased morbidity and mortality. However, prolonged intubation when successful extubation is possible also is associated with increased morbidity and mortality. Because some risk of extubation failure always exists, it is important that a clinician who can perform reintubation be present at the time of extubation.

*R*espiratory Recap

Extubation and Decannulation
Extubation is the removal of an endotracheal tube. Decannulation is the removal of a tracheostomy tube.

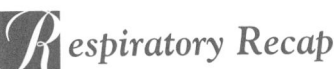

CPG 36-2

Removal of the Endotracheal Tube

Indications

When the airway control afforded by the endotracheal tube is deemed to be no longer necessary for continued care of the patient, the tube should be removed. In general, the patient should be capable of maintaining a patent airway and adequate spontaneous ventilation and should not require high levels of positive airway pressure to maintain normal arterial blood oxygenation.

Patients in whom further medical care is considered (and explicitly declared) futile may have the endotracheal tube removed despite continuing indications for the artificial airway.

Acute obstruction of the artificial airway requires immediate removal of the endotracheal tube if the obstruction cannot be cleared rapidly. Reintubation or other appropriate techniques used to reestablish the airway, such as surgical airway management, must be used to maintain effective gas exchange.

Contraindications

There are no absolute contraindications to extubation; however, some patients will require reintubation, positive pressure ventilation, continuous positive airway pressure, noninvasive ventilation, or a high inspired oxygen fraction (FIO_2) to maintain acceptable gas exchange after extubation. Airway protective reflexes usually are depressed for some time after extubation, therefore measures to prevent aspiration should be considered.

Hazards and Complications

Hypoxemia after extubation may result from but is not limited to failure to deliver adequate FIO_2 through the natural upper airway; acute upper airway obstruction; development of postobstruction pulmonary edema; bronchospasm; development of atelectasis, or lung collapse; pulmonary aspiration; or hypoventilation.

Hypercapnia after extubation may be caused by but is not limited to upper airway obstruction resulting from edema of the trachea, vocal cords, or larynx; respiratory muscle weakness; excessive work of breathing; or bronchospasm.

Death may occur when medical futility is the reason to remove the endotracheal tube.

Modified from AARC Clinical practice guideline: removal of the endotracheal tube. Respir Care 1999;44:85-90. CPG, Clinical Practice Guideline.

Decannulation is the removal of a tracheostomy tube. The considerations for decannulation are similar to those for extubation, but upper airway function can be more completely assessed before this procedure.

Weaning from the tracheostomy tube typically is done through placement of a smaller tracheostomy tube, a fenestrated tracheostomy tube, or a cuffless endotracheal tube. A Passy-Muir valve or a cap can then be placed on the proximal tracheostomy tube to assess the patient's ability to use the upper airway.

Before decannulation the clinician must assess the patient's natural processes to protect the lower respiratory tract from aspiration. Sophisticated evaluation of swallow and airway protection mechanisms requires videofluoroscopy, flexible fiberoptic endoscopy, and scintigraphy.[180] A simple method that can be used at the bedside involves deflating the cuff of the tracheostomy tube and allowing the patient to swallow a small amount of liquid containing a dye, such as food coloring or methylene blue. The tracheal secretions are then suctioned and inspected for coloration from the dye. If the secretions have been colored by the dye, aspiration has occurred. Although a positive result on the colored dye test is useful, the technique has a significant incidence of false-negative results.[180]

$\mathcal{K}$EY $\mathcal{P}$OINTS

- Oropharyngeal airways extend from the lips to the pharynx, following the natural curvature of the tongue, without entering the larynx or esophagus.
- Nasopharyngeal airways follow the anatomy of the nasopharynx so that the tip rests behind the tongue just above the epiglottis.
- Anesthesia personnel have the highest level of intubation skills, but in the hospital setting, the practitioner with the highest level of experience and training outside the operating room is the respiratory therapist.
- Indications for endotracheal intubation include bypassing of an upper airway obstruction, protection of the airway from aspiration, application of positive pressure ventilation, facilitation of secretion clearance, and delivery of high oxygen concentrations.
- Endotracheal intubation is the establishment of an artificial airway by use of a tube passed through the mouth or nose, then through the glottis, and into the trachea.
- The airway consists of five regions: the nose and nasopharynx, oral cavity and oropharynx, hypopharynx, larynx, and tracheobronchial tree.
- Endotracheal intubation is approached calmly; frantic and rushed attempts at intubation often result in failure and worsening of the situation.
- Nasotracheal intubation generally is used for specific indications and has special characteristics compared with orotracheal intubation.
- The shape and design of the laryngeal mask airway allows it to form a seal around the glottic opening that excludes the esophageal opening from the airway.
- The risk of complications associated with endotracheal intubation is reduced by meticulous attention to care of the airway in intubated patients.
- The traditional method used to secure an endotracheal tube is to apply benzoin to the skin and secure the tube with adhesive tape, but commercial holding systems also are available.
- A bite block is placed between the teeth to prevent the patient from biting an orotracheal airway.
- The primary reason to perform a tracheostomy is to maintain a secure airway in patients who require long-term intubation.
- Percutaneous dilational tracheostomy is a comparatively new procedure that is less traumatic than the conventional tracheotomy.
- The fenestrated tracheostomy tube can be useful for assessment of a patient's readiness for decannulation.
- The primary goal of a talking tracheostomy tube is to allow cognitively intact, ventilator-dependent patients to communicate by speaking.
- The Passy-Muir tracheostomy speaking valve is designed to eliminate the need for finger occlusion for oral communication.
- Tracheal buttons are used to maintain tracheostomy stomas.
- Cuff pressure should be kept at 20 to 25 mm Hg to minimize the risks of tracheal wall injury and aspiration.
- Intubated patients should be suctioned whenever a physical examination reveals secretions in the airway.
- Numerous complications are possible with airway suctioning.
- With the closed suction system, the catheter becomes part of the ventilator circuit.
- Saline instillation during suctioning should be used judiciously and should not be performed each time a patient is suctioned.
- The most frequent cause of extubation failure is inability of the patient to sustain adequate spontaneous ventilation.

References

1. Berman RA, Lilienfeld SM. The Berman airway. Anesthesiology 1950;11:136-137.
2. Kupp PJ, Crewe TC. An airway for the edentulous adult. Anesthesia 1974;29:601-602.
3. Greenberg RS, Brimacombe J, Berry A, et al. A randomized trial comparing the cuffed oropharyngeal airway and the laryngeal mask airway in spontaneously breathing anesthetized adults. Anesthesiology 1998;88:970-977.
4. Pollard BJ, O'Leary J. Guedel airway and tooth damage. Anesth Intensive Care 1981;9:395.
5. Wanner A, Zighelboim A, Sacker MA. Nasopharyngeal airway: a facilitated access to the trachea for nasotracheal suction, bedside bronchofiberoscopy, and selective bronchoscopy. Ann Intern Med 1975;75:593-595.
6. Haaf DP, Helms PJ, Diniwiddie R, et al. Nasopharyngeal airways in Pierre Robin syndrome. J Pediatr 1982;100:698-703.
7. Gallagher WI, Pierce AC, Powers SJ. Assessment of a new nasopharyngeal airway. Br J Anaesth 1988;60:112-115.
8. Colice GL. Historical perspective on the development of mechanical ventilation. In: Tobin MJ, editor. Principles and practice of mechanical ventilation. New York: McGraw-Hill; 1994.
9. Stoller JK. The history of intubation, tracheotomy, and airway appliances. Respir Care 1999;44:595-601.
10. Hooke R. [title unknown.] Phil Trans Roy Soc 1667;2:539.
11. MacEwen W. Clinical observations on the introduction of tracheal tubes by the mouth instead of performing tracheostomy or laryngotomy. Br Med J 1880;2:122-124,163-165.
12. O'Dwyer J. Intubation of the larynx. N Y Med J 1885;4:145.
13. Fell GE. Forced respiration in opium poisoning: its possibilities and the apparatus best adapted to produce it. Buffalo Med Surg J 1887;28:145.
14. Murphy FJ. Two improved intratracheal catheters. Anesth Analg 1941;27:102-105.
15. Grillo HC, Cooper JD, Geffin B, et al. A low-pressure cuff for tracheostomy tubes to minimize tracheal injury: a comparative clinical trial. J Thorac Cardiovasc Surg 1971;62:898-907.
16. Kacmarek RM. The role of the respiratory therapist in emergency care. Respir Care 1992;37:523-530.

17. Bishop MJ. Who should perform intubation? Respir Care 1999;44:750-758.

18. Bishop MJ, Michalowski P, Hussey JD, et al. Recertification of respiratory therapists' intubation skills one year after initial training: analysis of skill retention and retraining. Respir Care 2001;46:234-237.

19. Hess DR. Indications for translaryngeal intubation. Respir Care 1999; 44:604-609.

20. Plummer AL, Gracey DR. Consensus conference on artificial airways in patients receiving mechanical ventilation. Chest 1989;96:178-180.

21. Kollef MH, Silver P. Ventilator-associated pneumonia: an update for clinicians. Respir Care 1995;40:1130-1140.

22. AARC. Consensus statement: noninvasive positive pressure ventilation. Respir Care 1997;42:365-369.

23. Pang D, Keenan SP, Cook DJ, et al. The effect of positive pressure airway support on mortality and the need for intubation in cardiogenic pulmonary edema: a systemic review. Chest 1998;114:1185-1192.

24. Keenan SP, Kennerman PD, Cook DJ, et al. Effect of noninvasive positive pressure ventilation on mortality in patients admitted with acute respiratory failure: a metaanalysis. Crit Care Med 1997;25:1685-1692.

25. Keenan SP, Brake D. An evidence-based approach to noninvasive ventilation in acute respiratory failure. Crit Care Clin 1998;14:359-372.

26. Hess D. Noninvasive positive pressure ventilation: predictors of success and failure for adult acute care applications. Respir Care 1997;42:424-431.

27. Branson RD. The nuts and bolts of increasing arterial oxygenation: devices and techniques. Respir Care 1993;38:686.

28. American Society of Anesthesiologists, Task Force on Management of the Difficult Airway. Practice guidelines or management of the difficult airway. Anesthesiology 1993;78:597-602.

29. Williamson JA, Webb RK, Szekely S, et al. The Australian Incident Monitoring Study: difficult intubation: an analysis of 2000 incident reports. Anesth Intensive Care 1993;78:597-602.

30. Wilson ME, Spiegelhalter D, Robertson JA, et al. Predicting difficult intubation. Br J Anaesth 1988;61:211-216.

31. Nath G, Sekar M. Predicting difficult intubation: a comprehensive scoring system. Anesth Intensive Care 1997;25:482-486.

32. Hurford WE. Techniques of endotracheal intubation. Int Anesth Clin 2000;38:1-28.

33. Dunn PF, Goulet RL. Endotracheal tubes and airway appliances. Int Anesth Clin 2000;38:65-94.

34. Jaeger JM, Durbin CG. Special-purpose endotracheal tubes. Respir Care 1999;44:661-683.

35. Rello J, Sonora R, Jubert P, et al. Pneumonia in intubated patients: role of respiratory airway care. Am J Respir Crit Care Med 1996;154:111-115.

36. Valles J, Artigas A, Rello J, et al. Continuous aspiration of subglottic secretions in preventing ventilator-associated pneumonia. Ann Intern Med 1995;122:179-186.

37. Kollef MH, Skubas NJ, Sundt TM. A randomized clinical trial of continuous aspiration of subglottic secretions in cardiac surgery patients. Chest 1999;116:1339-1346.

38. Owen RL, Cheney FW. Endobronchial intubation: a preventable complication. Anesthesiology 1987;67:255-257.

39. Hurford WE. Nasotracheal intubation. Respir Care 1999;44:643-647.

40. Rosen CL, Wolfe RE, Chew SE, et al. Blind nasotracheal intubation in the presence of facial trauma. J Emerg Med 1997;15:141-145.

41. Rouby JJ, Laurent P, Gosnach M, et al. Risk factors and clinical relevance of nosocomial maxillary sinusitis in critically ill patients. Am J Respir Crit Care Med 1994;150:776-783.

42. Asai T, Morris S. The laryngeal mask airway: its features, effects, and roles. Can J Anaesth 1994;41:930-960.

43. Vergnese C, Brimacompe Jr. Survey of laryngeal mask airway usage in 11,910 patients: safety and efficacy for conventional and nonconventional usage. Anesth Analg 1996;82:129-133.

44. Stauffer JL, Silvester RC. Complications of endotracheal intubation, tracheostomy, and artificial airways. Respir Care 1982;27:417-434.

45. Stauffer JL, Olson DE, Petty TL. Complications and consequences of endotracheal intubation and tracheostomy: a prospective study of 150 critical ill adult patients. Am J Med 1981;70:65-76.

46. Tominga GT, Rudzwick H, Scannell G, et al. Decreasing unplanned extubations in the surgical intensive care unit. Am J Surg 1995;170:586-590.

47. Boulain T. Unplanned extubations in the adult intensive care unit: a prospective multicenter study. Am J Respir Crit Care Med 1998;157:1131-1137.

48. Listello D, Sessler CN. Unplanned extubation: clinical predictors for reintubation. Chest 1994;105:1496-1503.

49. Scott PH, Eigen H, Moye LA, et al. Predictability and consequences of spontaneous extubation in a pediatric ICU. Crit Care Med 1985;13:228-232.

50. Christie JM, Dethlefsen M, Cane RD. Unplanned endotracheal extubation in the intensive care unit. J Clin Anesth 1996;8:289-293.

51. Vassal T, Anh NG, Gabillet JM, et al. Prospective evaluation of self-extubations in a medical intensive care unit. Intensive Care Med 1993;19:340-342.

52. Whelan J, Simpson SQ, Levy H. Unplanned extubation: predictors of successful termination of mechanical ventilatory support. Chest 1995;105:1808-1812.

53. Atkins PM, Mion LC, Mendelson W, et al. Characteristics and outcomes of patients who self-extubate from ventilatory support: a case-control study. Chest 1997;112:1317-1323.

54. Betbese A, Perez M, Rialp G, et al. A prospective study of unplanned endotracheal extubation in intensive care unit patients. Crit Care Med 1998;26:1180-1186.

55. Chiang AA, Lee KC, Lee JC, et al. Effectiveness of a continuous quality improvement program aiming to reduce unplanned extubation: a prospective study. Intensive Care Med 1996;22:1269-1271.

56. Sessler CN. Unplanned extubations: making progress using CQI. Intensive Care Med 1997;23:143-145.

57. Kapadia FN, Bajan KB, Raje KV. Airway accidents in intubated intensive care unit patients: an epidemiological study. Crit Care Med 2000;28:659-664.

58. Carrion MI, Ayuso D, Marcos M, et al. Accidental removal of endotracheal and nasotracheal tubes and intravascular catheters. Crit Care Med 2000;28:63-66.

59. Hess DR. Managing the artificial airway. Respir Care 1999;44:759-772.

60. Tasota FJ, Hoffman LA, Zullo TG, et al. Evaluation of two methods used to stabilize oral endotracheal tubes. Heart Lung 1987;16:140-146.

61. Levy H, Griego L. A comparative study of oral endotracheal tube securing methods. Chest 1993;104:1537-1540.

62. Kaplow R, Bookbinder M. A comparison of four endotracheal tube holders. Heart Lung 1994;23:59-66.

63. Conrardy PA, Goodman LR, Lainge F, et al. Alteration of endotracheal tube position: flexion and extension of the neck. Crit Care Med 1976;4:8-12.

64. Schwatz AJ, Dougal RM, Lee WK. Modification of the oral airway as a bite block. Anesth Analg 1980;59:225.

65. Barnson S, Graham J, Wild C, et al. Comparison of two endotracheal tube securement techniques on unplanned extubation, oral mucosa, and facial skin integrity. Heart Lung 1998;27:409-417.

66. Patel N, Smith C, Pinchak A, et al. Taping methods and tape types for securing oral endotracheal tubes. Can J Anaesth 1997;44:330-336.

67. O'Connor DCJ. A new airway-gag. Lancet 1958;1:356-357.

68. Heffner JE. Tracheostomy: indications and timing. Respir Care 1999;44:807-815.

69. Reibel JF. Tracheotomy/tracheostomy. Respir Care 1999;44:820-823.

70. Hill BB, Zweng TN, Maley RH, et al. Percutaneous dilational tracheostomy: report of 356 cases. J Trauma 1996;41:238-243.

71. Cobean R, Beals M, Moss C, et al. Percutaneous dilatational tracheostomy: a safe, cost-effective bedside procedure. Arch Surg 1996;131:265-271.

72. Fernandez L, Norwood S, Roettger R, et al. Bedside percutaneous tracheostomy with bronchoscopic guidance in critically ill patients. Arch Surg 1996;131:129-132.

73. Nates JL, Cooper J, Myles PS, et al. Percutaneous tracheostomy in critically ill patients: a prospective randomized comparison of techniques. Crit Care Med 2000;28:3734-3739.

74. Freeman BD, Isabella K, Lin N, et al. A metaanalysis of prospective trials comparing percutaneous and surgical tracheostomy in critically ill patients. Chest 2000;118:1412-1418.

75. Jackson C. The technique of insertion of intratracheal insufflator tubes. Surg Gynecol Obstet 1913;17:507.

76. Downes JJ, Schreiner MS. Tracheostomy tubes and attachments in infants and children. Int Anesth Clin 1985;23:37-60.

77. Galoof HD, Toledo PS. Comparison of five types of tracheostomy tubes in the intubated trachea. Ann Otol Rhinol Laryngol 1978;87:99-108.

78. Kamen JM, Wilkinson CJ. A new low-pressure cuff for endotracheal tubes. Anesthesiology 1971;34:482.

79. Sparker AW, Robin KT, Newland GN, et al. A prospective evaluation of speaking tracheostomy tubes for ventilator-dependent patients. Laryngoscope 1987;97:89-92.

80. Leder SB, Astrachan DE. Stomal complications and airflow line problems of the Communi-Trach I cuffed talking tracheostomy tube. Laryngoscope 1990;100:1116-1121.

81. Leder SB. Verbal communication for the ventilator-dependent patient: voice intensity with the Portex Talk tracheostomy tubes. Laryngoscope 1990;100:1116-1121.

82. Manzano JL, Lubillo S, Henriquez D, et al. Enhancing communication with the Passy-Muir valve. Crit Care Med 1993;21:512-517.

83. Orringer MK. The effects of tracheostomy tube placement on communication and swallowing. Respir Care 1999;44:845-853.

84. Eibling DE, Gross RD. Subglottic air pressure: a key component of swallowing efficiency. Ann Otol Rhinol Laryngol 1996;105:253-258.

85. Cooper JD, Grillo HC. The evolution of tracheal injury due to ventilatory assistance through cuffed tubes: a pathologic study. Ann Surg 1969;169:334-348.

86. Cooper JD, Grillo HC. Experimental production and prevention of injury due to cuffed tracheal tubes. Surg Gynecol Obstet 1969;129:1235-1241.

87. Cooper JD, Grillo HC. Analysis of problems related to cuffs on intratracheal tubes. Chest 1972;62:21S-27S.

88. Knowlson GTG, Bassett HFM. The pressures exerted on the trachea by endotracheal inflatable cuffs. Br J Anaesth 1970;42:834-837.

89. Dobrin P, Canfield T. Cuffed endotracheal tubes: mucosal and tracheal wall blood flow. Am J Surg 1977;133:562-568.

90. Bernhard WN, Yost L, Joynes D, et al. Intracuff pressures in endotracheal and tracheostomy tubes: related cuff physical characteristics. Chest 1985;87:720-725.

91. Dunn CR, Dunn DL, Moser KM. Determinants of tracheal injury by cuffed tracheostomy tubes. Chest 1974;65:128-135.

92. Seegobin RD, Van Hasselt GL. Endotracheal cuff pressure and tracheal mucosal blood flow: endoscopic study of effects of four large-volume cuffs. Br Med J 1984;288:965-968.

93. Honeybourne D, Costello JC, Barham C. Tracheal damage after endotracheal intubation: comparison of two types of endotracheal tubes. Thorax 1982;37:500-502.

94. Pavlin EG, Van Mimwegan D, Hornbein TF. Failure of a high-compliance low-pressure cuff to prevent aspiration. Anesthesiology 1975;42:216-219.

95. Bernhard WN, Cottrell JE, Sivakumaran C, et al. Adjustment of intracuff pressure to prevent aspiration. Anesthesiology 1979;50:363-366.

96. Guyton DC, Barlow MR, Besselievre TR. Influence of airway pressure on minimum occlusive endotracheal tube cuff pressure. Crit Care Med 1997;25:91-94.

97. Crimlisk JT, Horn MH, Wilson DJ, et al. Artificial airways: a survey of cuff management practices. Heart Lung 1996;25:225-235.

98. Off D, Braun SR, Tompkins B, et al. Efficacy of the minimal leak technique of cuff inflation in maintaining proper intracuff pressures for patients with cuffed artificial airways. Respir Care 1983;28:1115-1120.

99. Cox PM, Schatz ME. Pressure measurements in endotracheal cuffs: a common error. Chest 1974;65:84-87.

100. Sills J. An emergency cuff inflation technique. Respir Care 1986;31:199-201.

101. Ho AM, Contrardi LH. What to do when an endotracheal tube cuff leaks. J Trauma 1990;40:486-487.

102. Tinkoff G, Bakow ED, Smith RW. A continuous flow apparatus for temporary inflation of damaged endotracheal tube cuffs. Respir Care 1990;35:423-426.

103. Kearl RA, Hooper RG. Massive airway leaks: an analysis of the role of endotracheal tubes. Crit Care Med 1993;21:518-521.

104. Tarnow-Mordi W. Is routine endotracheal suction justified? Arch Dis Child 1991;66:374-375.

105. Boutros AR. Arterial blood oxygenation during and after endotracheal suctioning in the apneic patient. Anesthesiology 1978;32:114-118.

106. Ehrhart IC, Hofman WF, Loveland SR. Effects of endotracheal suction versus apnea during interruption of intermittent or continuous positive pressure ventilation. Crit Care Med 1981;9:464-468.

107. Fell T, Cheney FW. Prevention of hypoxia during endotracheal suction. Ann Surg 1971;174:24-28.

108. Karem E, Yatsiv I, Goitein KJ. Effect of endotracheal suctioning on arterial blood gases in children. Intensive Care Med 1990;16:95-99.

109. Berman IR, Stahl WM. Prevention of hypoxic complications during endotracheal suctioning. Surgery 1968;63:586-587.

110. Barnes CA, Kirchhoff KT. Minimizing hypoxemia due to endotracheal suctioning: a review of the literature. Heart Lung 1986;15:164-176.

111. Buchanan LM, Baun MM. The effect of hyperinflation, inspiratory hold, and oxygenation on cardiopulmonary status during suctioning in a lung-injured model. Heart Lung 1986;15:127-134.

112. Skelley BF, Deeren SM, Powaser MM. The effectiveness of two preoxygenation methods to prevent endotracheal suction–induced hypoxemia. Heart Lung 1980;9:316-323.

113. Naigow D, Powaser MM. The effect of different endotracheal suction procedures on arterial blood gases in a controlled experimental model. Heart Lung 1977;6:808-816.

114. Adlkofer RM, Powaser MM. The effect of endotracheal suctioning on arterial blood gases in patients after cardiac surgery. Heart Lung 1978;7:1011-1014.

115. Rogge JA, Bunde L, Baun MM. Effectiveness of oxygen concentrations of less than 100% before and after endotracheal suction in patients with chronic obstructive pulmonary disease. Heart Lung 1989;18:64-71.

116. Goodnough SK. The effects of oxygen and hyperinflation on arterial oxygen tension after endotracheal suctioning. Heart Lung 1985;14:11-17.

117. Preusser BA, Stone KS, Gonyon DS, et al. Effects of two methods of preoxygenation on mean arterial pressure, cardiac output, peak airway pressure, and postsuctioning hypoxemia. Heart Lung 1988;17:290-299.

118. Pierce JB, Piazza DE. Differences in postsuctioning arterial blood oxygen concentration values using two postoxygenation methods. Heart Lung 1987;16:34-38.

119. Baker PO, Baker JP, Koen PA. Endotracheal suctioning techniques in hypoxemic patients. Respir Care 1983;28:1563-1568.

120. Glass C, Grap MJ, Corley MC, et al. Nurses' ability to achieve hyperinflation and hyperoxygenation with a manual resuscitation bag during endotracheal suctioning. Heart Lung 1993;22:158-165.

121. Singer M, Vermaat J, Hall G, et al. Hemodynamic effects of manual hyperventilation in critically ill mechanically ventilated patients. Chest 1994;106:1182-1187.

122. Denehy L. The use of manual hyperinflation in airway clearance. Eur Respir J 1999;14:958-965.

123. George RB. Duration of suctioning: an important variable. Respir Care 1983;28:457-459.

124. Baier H, Begin R, Sackner MA. Effect of airway diameter, suction catheters, and the bronchofiberscope on airflow in endotracheal and tracheostomy tubes. Heart Lung 1976;5:235-238.

125. Amikam B, Landa J, West J, et al. Bronchofiberscopic observations of the tracheobronchial tree during intubation. Am Rev Respir Dis 1972;105:747-755.

126. Landa JF, Chapman GA, Sackner MA. Effects of suctioning on mucociliary transport. Chest 1980;77:202-207.

127. Fluck RR. Suctioning: intermittent or continuous? Respir Care 1985;30:837-838.

128. Czarnik RE, Stone KS, Everhart CC, et al. Differential effects of continuous versus intermittent suction on tracheal tissue. Heart Lung 1991;20:144-151.

129. Link WJ, Spaeth EE, Wahle WM, et al. The influence of suction catheter tip design on tracheobronchial trauma and fluid aspiration efficiency. Anesth Analg 1976;55:290-297.

130. Sackner MA, Landa JF, Greeneltch N, et al. Pathogenesis and prevention of tracheobronchial damage with suction procedures. Chest 1973;64:284-290.

131. Jung RC, Gottlieb LS. Comparison of tracheobronchial suction catheters in humans. Chest 1976;69:179-181.

132. Vaughan RS, Menke JA, Giacoia GP. Pneumothorax: a complication of endotracheal tube suctioning. J Pediatr 1978;92:633-634.

133. Grosfeld JL, Lemons JL, Ballantine TVN, et al. Emergency thoracotomy for acquired bronchopleural fistula in the premature infant with respiratory distress. J Pediatr Surg 1980;15:416-421.

134. Anderson KD, Chandra R. Pneumothorax secondary to perforation of sequential bronchi by suction catheters. J Pediatr Surg 1976;11:687-693.

135. Shim C, Fine N, Fernandez R, et al. Cardiac arrhythmias resulting from tracheal suctioning. Ann Intern Med 1969;71:1149-1153.

136. Winston SJ, Gravelyn TR, Sitrin RG. Prevention of bradycardic responses to endotracheal suctioning by prior administration of nebulized atropine. Crit Care Med 1987;15:1009-1011.

137. Walsh JM, Vanderwarf C, Hoscheit D, et al. Unsuspected hemodynamic alterations during endotracheal suctioning. Chest 1989;95:162-165.

138. Anthony JS, Sieniewicz DJ. Suctioning of the left bronchial tree in critically ill patients. Crit Care Med 1977;5:161-162.

139. Kubota Y, Toyoda Y, Kubota H, et al. Selective left bronchial suctioning in infants and children. Crit Care Med 1986;14:902-903.

140. Kubota Y, Toyoda Y, Kubota H, et al. Treatment of atelectasis with selective bronchial suctioning. Chest 1991;99:510-512.

141. Kubota Y, Magaribuchi T, Toyoda Y, et al. Selective bronchial suctioning in the adult using a curve-tipped catheter with a guide mark. Crit Care Med 1982;10:767-769.

142. Kubota Y, Magaribuchi T, Ohara M, et al. Evaluation of selective bronchial suctioning in the adult. Crit Care Med 1980;8:748-749.

143. Freedman AP, Goodman L. Suctioning the left bronchial tree in the intubated adult. Crit Care Med 1982;10:43-45.

144. Panacek EA, Albertson TE, Rutherford WF, et al. Selective left endobronchial suctioning in the intubated patient. Chest 1989;95:885-887.

145. Salem MR, Wong AY, Mathrubhutham M, et al. Evaluation of selective bronchial suctioning techniques used for infants and children. Anesthesiology 1978;48:379-380.

146. Rudy EB, Baun M, Stone K, et al. The relationship between endotracheal suctioning and changes in intracranial pressure: a review of the literature. Heart Lung 1986;15:488-494.

147. Fisher DM, Frewen T, Swedlow DB. Increase in intracranial pressuring during suctioning: stimulation versus rise in $PaCO_2$. Anesthesiology 1982;57:416-417.

148. Durand M, Sangha B, Cabal LA, et al. Cardiopulmonary and intracranial pressure changes related to endotracheal suctioning in preterm infants. Crit Care Med 1989;17:506-510.

149. Shah AR, Kurth CD, Gwiazdowski SG, et al. Fluctuations in cerebral oxygenation and blood volume during endotracheal suctioning in premature infants. J Pediatr 1991;120:769-774.

150. Brucia J, Rudy E. The effect of suction catheter insertion and tracheal stimulation in adults with severe brain injury. Heart Lung 1996;25:295-303.

151. Wainwright SP, Gould D. Endotracheal suctioning in adults with severe head injury: a literature review. Intensive Crit Care Nurs 1996;12:303-308.

152. Monaco FJ, Meredith KS. A bench test evaluation of a neonatal closed tracheal suction system. Pediatr Pulmonol 1992;13:121-123.

153. Hart TP, Mahutte CK. Evaluation of a closed system, directional-tip suction catheter. Respir Care 1992;37:1260-1265.

154. Witmer MT, Hess D, Simmons M. An evaluation of the effectiveness of secretion removal with the Ballard closed-circuit suction catheter. Respir Care 1991;36:844-848.

155. Craig KC, Benson MS, Pierson DJ. Prevention of arterial oxygen desaturation during closed airway endotracheal suction: effect of ventilator mode. Respir Care 1984;29:1013-1018.

156. Taggart JA, Dorinsky NL, Sheahan JS. Airway pressures during closed system suctioning. Heart Lung 1988;17:536-542.

157. Carlon GC, Fox SJ, Ackerman NJ. Evaluation of a closed tracheal suction system. Crit Care Med 1987;15:522-525.

158. Clark AP, Tyler DO, White KM. Effects of endotracheal suctioning on mixed venous oxygen saturation and heart rate in critically ill adults. Heart Lung 1990;19:552-557.

159. Johnson KL, Kearnery PA, Johnson SB, et al. Closed versus open endotracheal suctioning: costs and physiologic consequences. Crit Care Med 1994;22:654-666.

160. Hrashbarger SA, Hoffman LA, Zullo TG, et al. Effects of a closed tracheal suction system on ventilatory and cardiovascular parameters. Am J Respir Crit Care Med 1992;3:57-61.

161. Deppe SA, Kelly JW, Thoi LL, et al. Incidence of colonization, nosocomial pneumonia, and mortality in critically ill patients using a Trach Care closed suction system versus an open suction system: prospective, randomized study. Crit Care Med 1990;18:1389-1393.

162. Cobley M, Atkins M, Jones PL. Environmental contamination during tracheal suction. Anaesthesia 1991;46:957-961.

163. Ombes P, Fauvage B, Oleyer C. Nosocomial pneumonia in mechanically ventilated patients: a prospective randomized evaluation of the Stericath closed suctioning system. Intensive Care Med 2000;26:878-882.

164. Ritz R, Scott LR, Coyle MB, et al. Contamination of a multiple-use suction catheter in a closed circuit system compared to contamination of a disposable, single-use suction catheter. Respir Care 1986;31:1086-1091.

165. Blackwood B, Webb CH. Closed tracheal suctioning systems and infection control in the intensive care unit. J Hosp Infect 1998,39:315-321.

166. Hamori CA, O'Connell JM. Improperly positioned closed system suction catheter causes elevated peak inspiratory airway pressures. Respir Care 1991;36:1441-1442.

167. DePew CL, Moseley MJ, Clark EG, et al. Open versus closed system endotracheal suctioning: a cost comparison. Crit Care Nurse 1994;14:94-100.

168. Kollef MH, Prentice S, Shapiro SD, et al. Mechanical ventilation with or without daily changes of in-line suction catheters. Am J Respir Crit Care Med 1997;156:466-472.

169. Gray JE, MacIntyre NR, Kronenberger WG. The effects of bolus normal saline instillation in conjunction with endotracheal suctioning. Respir Care 1990;35:785-790.

170. Ackerman MH, Ecklund MM, Abu-Jumah M. A review of normal saline instillation: implications for practice. Dim Crit Care Nurs 1996;15:31-38.

171. Ackerman MH. The effect of saline lavage prior to suctioning. Am J Crit Care 1993;2:326-330.

172. Hagler DA, Traver GA. Endotracheal saline and suction catheters: sources of lower airway contamination. Am J Crit Care 1994;3:444-447.

173. Kinlock D. Instillation of normal saline during endotracheal suctioning: effects on mixed venous oxygen saturation. Am J Crit Care 1999;8:231-242.

174. Campbell RS. Extubation and the consequences of reintubation. Respir Care 1999;44:799-806.

175. Miller RL, Cole RP. Association between reduced cuff leak volume and postextubation stridor. Chest 1996;110:1035-1040.

176. Fisher MM, Raper RF. The "cuff leak" test for extubation. Anaesthesia 1992;47:10-12.

177. Epstein SK, Ciubotaru RL. Independent effects of etiology of failure and time to reintubation on outcome for patients failing extubation. Am J Respir Crit Care Med 1998;158:489-493.

178. Torres A, Gatell JM, Aznar E, et al. Reintubation increases the risk of nosocomial pneumonia in patients needing mechanical ventilation. Am J Respir Crit Care Med 1995;152:137-141.

179. Esteban A, Alia I, Gordo F, et al. Extubation outcome after spontaneous breathing trials with T-tube or pressure support ventilation. Am J Respir Crit Care Med 1997;156:459-465.

180. Peruzzi WT, Logemann JA, Currie D, et al. Assessment of aspiration in patients with tracheostomies: comparison of the bedside colored dye assessment with videofluoroscopic examination. Respir Care 2001;46:243-247.

CHAPTER 37

Cardiopulmonary Resuscitation

Thomas A. Barnes
Dean R. Hess

CHAPTER OUTLINE

OBJECTIVES

1. Describe the components of prudent heart living.
2. Compare basic life support and advanced cardiac life support.
3. Discuss the rationale for rapid response resuscitation teams.
4. Describe the ABCD survey.
5. Describe the techniques of airway opening, emergency ventilation, and external chest compressions for a cardiac-arrested patient.
6. Compare one-rescuer and two-rescuer cardiopulmonary resuscitation.
7. Describe the emergency management of foreign body airway obstruction.
8. Compare the techniques of adult, pediatric, and neonatal resuscitation.
9. Identify electrocardiographic rhythms commonly encountered during cardiopulmonary resuscitation.
10. Compare automated and manual defibrillators.
11. List indications for drugs commonly used during cardiopulmonary resuscitation.
12. Compare defibrillation, cardioversion, and pacing.

KEY TERMS

ABCD Survey	Cardiac Pacing	Face Shield
Advanced Cardiac Life Support (ACLS)	Cardiopulmonary Resuscitation (CPR)	Foreign Body Obstruction
Basic Life Support (BLS)	Cardioversion	Manual Resuscitator
Cardiac Compressions	Defibrillation	Prudent Heart Lifestyle

Cardiopulmonary resuscitation (CPR) includes all care required to treat life-threatening events. Resuscitation of patients in cardiopulmonary arrest requires assessment of the problem and an organized response. Respiratory therapists, nurses, and physicians work together as members of the "code team" providing **basic life support (BLS)** and **advanced cardiac life support (ACLS)** in the hospital. Each institution defines the respiratory therapist's involvement. Expertise in patient assessment,

oxygen therapy, airway management, mechanical ventilation, hemodynamic monitoring, and other critical care procedures by respiratory therapists has led to more responsibility being placed on code teams. Box 37-1 summarizes the CPR responsibilities of respiratory therapists. The American Association for Respiratory Care (AARC) clinical practice guidelines describe the role of respiratory therapists in providing CPR (CPGs 37-1 and 37-2).

Box 37-1

Cardiopulmonary Resuscitation Skills Provided by Respiratory Therapists

Select, Review, Obtain, and Interpret

Electrocardiograms, capnograms, electrolytes, fluid balance, arterial blood gases, hemodynamic data, and vital signs

Assessment of venous distention, capillary refill

Auscultation of heart and lung sounds

Position of endotracheal tube and tracheal tube cuff pressure

Select, Assemble, Check for Proper Function, and Correct Malfunctions of CPR Equipment

Mouth-valve-mask devices, bag-valve-mask devices, mechanical ventilators

Oral and nasopharyngeal airways, oral endotracheal tubes, adjunct airways, and intubation equipment

Automated, semiautomated, and conventional defibrillators

Initiate, Conduct, and Modify Basic and Advanced Life Support Procedures

Evaluation and monitoring of patient response to basic and advanced life support

ECG and hemodynamic monitoring

Emergency ventilation: via mouth-valve-mask, bag-valve-mask, tracheal tube, mechanical ventilators, or transtracheal airways

Airway management: oropharyngeal, nasopharyngeal, endotracheal, and adjunct airways

External cardiac chest compression

Defibrillation

Administration of ACLS drugs and oxygen

Transcutaneous cardiac pacing

ACLS, Advanced cardiac life support.

 ## CPG 37-1

Resuscitation in Acute Care Hospitals

Indications

Cardiac arrest, respiratory arrest, or the presence of conditions that may lead to cardiopulmonary arrest as indicated by rapid deterioration in vital signs, level of consciousness, and blood gas values including airway obstruction (partial or complete)

Acute myocardial infarction with cardiodynamic instability

Life-threatening dysrhythmias

Hypovolemic shock

Severe infections

Spinal cord or head injury

Drug overdose

Pulmonary edema

Anaphylaxis

Pulmonary embolus

Smoke inhalation

High-risk delivery

Contraindications

Resuscitation is contraindicated when the patient's desire not to be resuscitated has been clearly expressed and documented in the medical record.

Resuscitation has been determined to be futile because of the patient's underlying condition or disease.

Monitoring

Patient

1. Clinical assessment: Continuous observation of the patient and repeated clinical assessment by a trained observer provide optimal monitoring of the resuscitation process. Special consideration should be given to the following:
   a. Level of consciousness
   b. Adequacy of airway
   c. Adequacy of ventilation
   d. Peripheral/apical pulse and character
   e. Evidence of chest and head trauma
   f. Pulmonary compliance and airway resistance
   g. Presence of seizure activity
2. Assessment of physiologic parameters: Repeated assessment of physiologic data by trained professionals supplements clinical assessment in management of patients throughout the resuscitation process. Monitoring devices should be available, accessible, functional, and periodically evaluated for function. These data include but are not limited to the following:
   a. Arterial blood gas studies (although investigators have suggested that such values may have a limited role in decision making during CPR)
   b. Hemodynamic data
   c. Cardiac rhythm
   d. Ventilatory frequency, tidal volume, and airway pressure
   e. Exhaled CO_2
   f. Neurologic status

Resuscitation process

Properly performed resuscitation should improve patient outcome. Continuous monitoring of the process will identify areas needing improvement. Among these areas are response time, equipment function, equipment availability, team member performance, team performance, complication rate, and patient survival and functional status.

From AARC Clinical practice guideline: resuscitation in acute care hospitals. Respir Care 1993;38:1179-1188.
CPG, Clinical practice guideline; CPR, cardiopulmonary resuscitation.

CPG 37-2

Defibrillation during Resuscitation

Indications
Cardiac arrest caused by or resulting in ventricular fibrillation
Pulseless ventricular tachycardia

Contraindications
Defibrillation is contraindicated when the patient's desire not to be resuscitated has been clearly expressed and documented in the patient's medical record or other legal document.
Continued resuscitation is determined to be futile by the treating physician.
Immediate danger to the rescuers is present because of the environment, patient's location, or patient's condition.

Assessment of Need
Before arrival of defibrillator: The patient should be assessed for lack of responsiveness, apnea, and pulselessness, and help should be summoned if needed.
After arrival of defibrillator: The patient should be evaluated immediately for the presence of ventricular fibrillation or ventricular tachycardia by the operator (conventional) or the defibrillator (automated or semiautomated). Inappropriate defibrillation can cause harm.

Monitoring
Resuscitation process
Properly performed defibrillation has been shown to improve patient outcome. The most important determinant of survival in adult out-of-hospital ventricular fibrillation is defibrillation. Continuous monitoring of the process identifies components needing improvement. Among these components are response time, witnessed versus unwitnessed arrest, CPR performance, time to first defibrillation attempt, return of spontaneous circulation, complication rate, equipment function, equipment maintenance, and equipment availability.
Equipment
All maintenance should be documented and records preserved. Included in documentation should be routine checks of energy output, condition of batteries, proper functioning of monitor and recorder, and presence of disposables needed for function of defibrillator, including electrodes and defibrillation pads. Defibrillators should be checked each shift for presence, condition, and function of cables and paddles; presence of defibrillating and monitoring electrodes, paper, and spare batteries (as applicable); and charging, message/light indicators, monitors, and ECG recorder (as applicable).
Training
Records should be kept of initial training and continuing education of all personnel who perform defibrillation as part of their professional activities.

From AARC Clinical practice guideline: defibrillation during resuscitation. Respir Care 1995;40:744-748.
CPG, Clinical practice guideline; CPR, cardiopulmonary resuscitation.

Box 37-2

Risk Factors for Coronary Heart Disease

Factors That Cannot Be Changed	Factors That Can Be Changed
Heredity	Cigarette smoking
Gender	Hypertension
Increasing age	Lack of exercise
	Obesity
	Excessive stress
	Diabetes
	Blood cholesterol levels

Risk factors for coronary heart disease (CHD) are listed in Box 37-2. A **prudent heart lifestyle** is an attitude that includes weight control, physical fitness, smart eating habits, and avoidance of stress and cigarette smoking. The most important risk factor is cigarette smoking. The CHD death rate is 70% greater for smokers than nonsmokers, and the risk from smoking increases when combined with other factors (most notably elevated cholesterol and hypertension).[1-3] Sudden death related to CHD is the most prominent medical emergency in the United States.

Indications for CPR are cardiac arrest and/or respiratory arrest. Cardiac arrest usually occurs secondary to ventricular fibrillation (VF) but may be the result of other arrhythmias (for example, asystole). The recognition of VF is particularly important because prompt defibrillation improves the success of CPR. Respiratory problems causing respiratory arrest include an obstructed airway (partial or complete), interference with the respiratory drive mechanism (for example, spinal cord or head injury), or disorders of pulmonary gas transport (for example, pulmonary edema or pulmonary embolus).

Resuscitation Outcomes

Factors affecting resuscitation outcomes include the initial cardiac rhythm, time to initiate CPR, time to defibrillate, duration of CPR, and whether arrest was witnessed.[4-10] Because a longer duration of VF leads to greater myocardial deterioration, late defibrillation is less likely to convert to a spontaneous rhythm.[11-13] The chain of survival illustrates the sequence of actions that improves the rate of survival after cardiac arrest (Figure 37-1): early access, early CPR, early defibrillation, and early ACLS.[3] The highest hospital discharge rate has been achieved in patients for whom

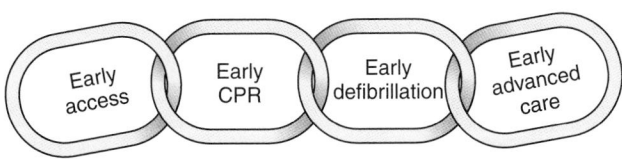

Figure 37-1 The emergency cardiac care systems concept is displayed schematically as the chain of survival. *CPR*, Cardiopulmonary resuscitation. (Modified from Emergency Cardiac Care Committee and Subcommittees, American Heart Association. Guidelines for cardiopulmonary resuscitation and emergency cardiac care. IX. Ensuring effectiveness of community-wide emergency cardiac care. JAMA 1992;268:2289-2295.)

CPR was initiated within 4 minutes of arrest and ACLS initiated within 8 minutes.[14] In the community, early bystander CPR and a rapid emergency medical services response are therefore essential to help improve survival rates with good neurologic recovery. In the hospital, respiratory therapists are often the first responders in the resuscitation effort. Accordingly, respiratory therapists should be trained in ACLS.[15]

ℛ*espiratory Recap*

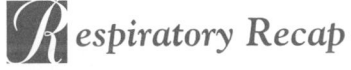

Chain of Survival	
Early access	Early defibrillation
Early CPR	Early ACLS

The ABCD Survey

The approach to resuscitation uses the acronym *ABCD* for *a*irway, *b*reathing, *c*irculation, and *d*efibrillation (Box 37-3).[3,16] Important first actions, such the assessment of unresponsiveness and the call for help, are performed just before the primary **ABCD survey.** In the community, rescuers should immediately activate the emergency medical system (for example, call 911) on recognition of unresponsiveness. Unresponsiveness (that is, clinically comatose) is confirmed by gentle shaking of the patient and shouting of, "Are you okay?" In the hospital, after establishing that the patient is unresponsive, the rescuer should call loudly for help. The person who responds activates the hospital emergency response system, bringing advanced life support in the form of the code team and crash cart to provide early defibrillation, advanced airway management, and intravenous medications. BLS, provided until the code team arrives, includes provision of emergency breathing and cardiac compressions.

In the secondary ABCD survey (see Box 37-3), the code team provides ACLS.[17] ACLS includes use of equipment to maintain the airway, monitoring of the electrocardiogram (ECG) and recognition of dysrhythmias, use of

ℬox 37-3

ABCD Survey

Primary ABCD Survey
(Begin basic life support algorithm.)
Activate emergency response system.
Call for defibrillator.
A *Airway:* open airway; assess breathing (open airway; look, listen, feel)
B *Breathing:* give two slow breaths
C *CPR:* check pulse; if no pulse, proceed to the following step.
C Start chest compressions
D *Defibrillator:* attach AED or monitor/defibrillator when available

Secondary ABCD Survey
A *Intubate* as soon as possible.
B *Confirm* tube placement; use two methods to confirm.
  • Primary physical examination criteria *plus*
  • Secondary confirmation device (qualitative and quantitative measures of end-tidal CO_2)
B *Secure* tracheal tube.
  • Prevent dislodgment; purpose-made tracheal tube holders are recommended over tie-and-tape approaches.
  • If the patient is at risk for transport movement, cervical collar and backboard are recommended.
B *Confirm* initial oxygenation and ventilation.
  • End-tidal CO_2 monitor
  • Oxygen saturation monitor
C *Initiate* oxygen, IV, monitor, and fluids.
  • Rhythm-appropriate medications
C Check *vital signs:* temperature, blood pressure, heart rate, respirations.
D Perform *differential diagnoses.*

From Anonymous. Adult basic life support. Circulation 2000;102:I-22. AED, Automated external defibrillator.

defibrillators, and administration of supplemental oxygen and drugs via parental or endotracheal routes. Endotracheal intubation should be performed before or simultaneously with intravenous (IV) access. Gaining IV access before endotracheal intubation is acceptable if ventilation, oxygenation, and airway protection appear satisfactory. The American Heart Association has published algorithms for emergency cardiac care.

ℛ*espiratory Recap*

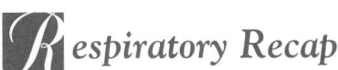

Advanced Cardiac Life Support
Use of airway and ventilation equipment
ECG monitoring
Use of conventional defibrillators
Drug therapy

Airway

Opening the airway is the first step in the primary ABCD survey. The mouth is opened and the upper airway inspected for foreign objects, vomitus, or blood. If present, these items should be removed with a finger sweep, by suctioning, or by placement of the patient in a side-lying position attention is given to the possibility of a cervical spine injury. Posterior displacement of the tongue is the most common cause of airway obstruction in the unconscious person. The loss of control of the submandibular muscles allows the tongue to obstruct the pharynx (Figure 37-2). Because the tongue is attached to the lower jaw, movement of the jaw forward moves the tongue away from the posterior pharynx to open the airway.

The patient's airway is opened via the head-tilt/chin-lift or jaw-thrust maneuver. The head-tilt/chin-lift is performed by placement of the palm of one hand on the victim's forehead and tilting of the head backward. The fingers of the other hand are placed under the bony part of the lower jaw near the chin to lift the chin forward (Figure 37-3). If the head-tilt method is contraindicated because of cervical spine injury, the jaw thrust is accomplished by placement of the fingers behind the angles of the jaw and displacement of the mandible forward (Figure 37-4). If the airway remains obstructed after the jaw-thrust maneuver is performed, the head is tilted gently until the airway opens.

The most effective airway to use during CPR is the endotracheal tube. Early tracheal intubation is an important step in CPR. It has been demonstrated that respiratory therapists can perform emergency tracheal intubation effectively,[18] and their success compares favorably with that of paramedics. The early placement of an endotracheal tube during CPR improves ventilation and oxygenation, prevents gastric insufflation, and provides a route to administer cardiac drugs when IV access cannot be established. In adult patients with depressed levels of consciousness, a Sellick maneuver (Figure 37-5) should be performed during endotracheal intubation.[19] A second person applies pressure to the cricoid cartilage to compress the esophagus and prevent gastric contents from being regurgitated into the hypopharynx and aspirated into the trachea. After endotracheal intubation, it is important to assess the tube position to ensure that the tube is positioned in the trachea (and not in the esophagus or a mainstem bronchus). Tube placement is confirmed by ausculta-

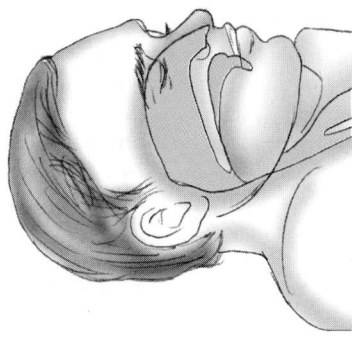

Figure 37-2   Obstruction of the upper airway by the tongue in an unconscious patient.

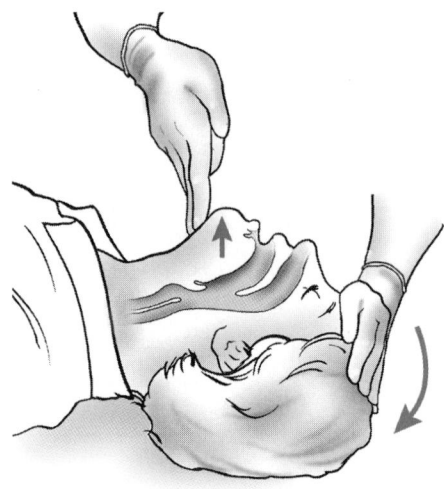

Figure 37-3   Opening the airway.

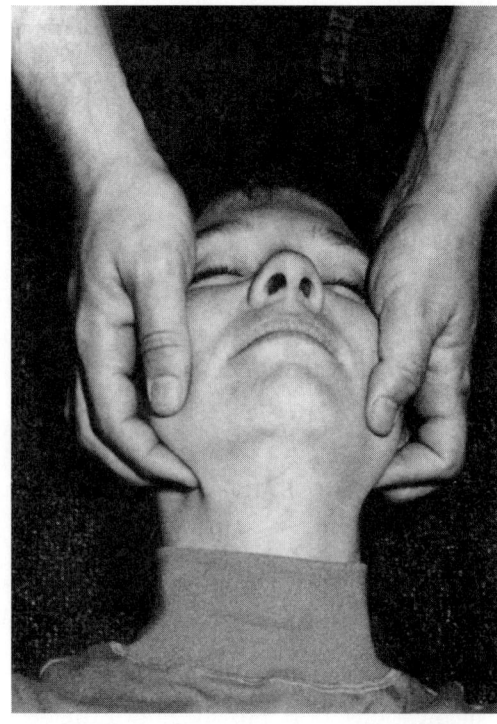

Figure 37-4   Jaw-thrust maneuver for use in cases of suspected cervical spine injury. (From Barnes TA, Boudin KM. Cardiopulmonary resuscitation. In: Burton GG, Hodgkin JE, Ward JJ, editors. Respiratory care practice: a guide to clinical practice. 4th ed. Philadelphia: Lippincott; 1997.)

tion, end-tidal CO_2 detection, esophageal detector devices (Figure 37-6), or direct visualization with a laryngoscope. If the location of the tube is in doubt, the tube should be removed and the patient reintubated.

Oropharyngeal airways facilitate ventilation with a face mask to prevent upper airway obstruction. These are inappropriate for patients who are conscious because stimulation of the gag reflex could cause vomiting and aspiration. Nasopharyngeal airways are used when insertion of an oropharyngeal airway is impossible (for example, when the patient has massive trauma around the mouth) or for patients who do not tolerate an oropharyngeal airway well. Although better tolerated than oral airways, nasopharyngeal airways may precipitate laryngospasm and vomiting.

$\mathcal{R}$espiratory Recap

Equipment for Emergency Airway Management	
Endotracheal tube	Esophageal-Tracheal
Oropharyngeal airway	Combitube
Nasopharyngeal airway	Laryngeal mask airway
Pharyngotracheal lumen airway	

The pharyngotracheal lumen (PTL) airway is a double-lumen tube that is inserted blindly into the trachea or oropharynx (Figure 37-7). After insertion the airway is sealed by inflation of a large proximal balloon that fills the

oropharynx and a smaller cuff on the distal end of the tube. If the long tube is in the trachea, ventilation can be accomplished in a way similar to that with an endotracheal tube. If the long tube is in the esophagus, then the short tube is used to deliver air below the large proximal balloon inflated in the oropharynx. The smaller cuff on

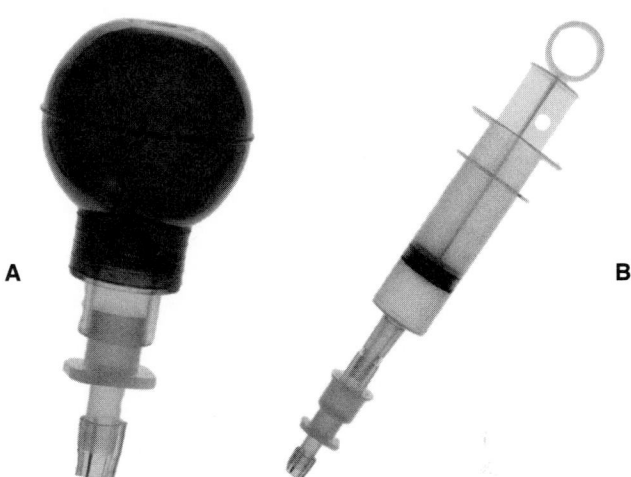

Figure 37-6 **A,** Bulb and **B,** syringe esophageal detector devices. (From Hess DR. Managing the artificial airway. Respir Care 1999; 44:759-772.)

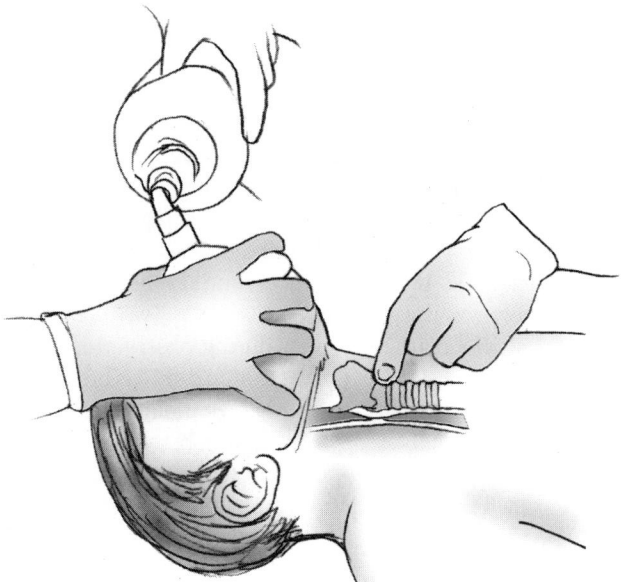

Figure 37-5 The Sellick maneuver.

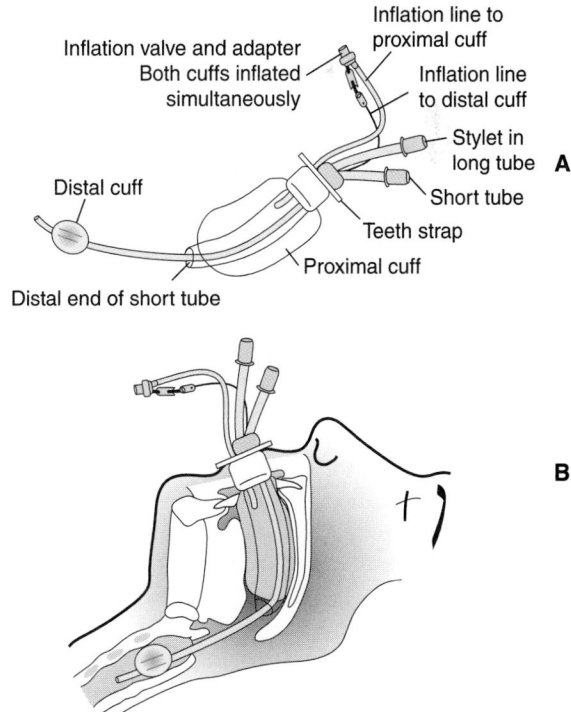

Figure 37-7 **A,** Diagram of the pharyngotracheal lumen (PTL) airway. **B,** Representation of the PTL airway in position. (Modified from Niemann JT, Rosborough JP, Myers R, et al: The pharyngo-tracheal lumen airway: preliminary investigation of a new adjunct. Ann Emerg Med 1984;13:591.)

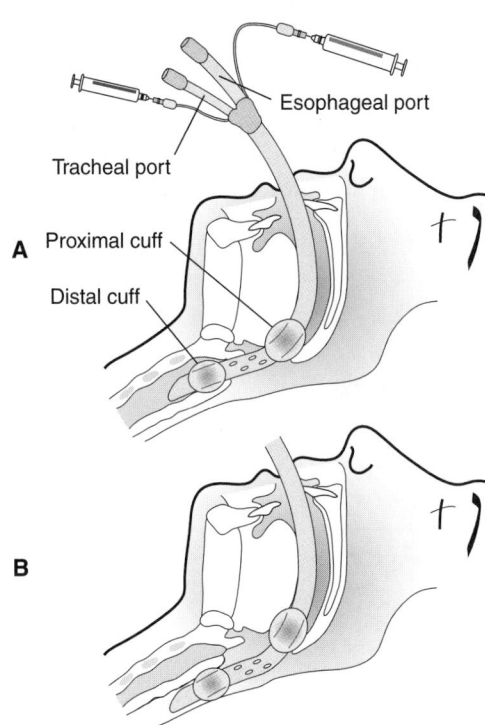

Figure 37-8   **A,** Esophageal-Tracheal Combitube. **B,** Insertion procedure: intubation of either the esophagus or trachea will facilitate ventilation. (Modified from Frass M, Frenzer R, Rausha F, et al: Evaluation of esophageal Combitube in cardiopulmonary resuscitation. Crit Care Med 1986;15:609.)

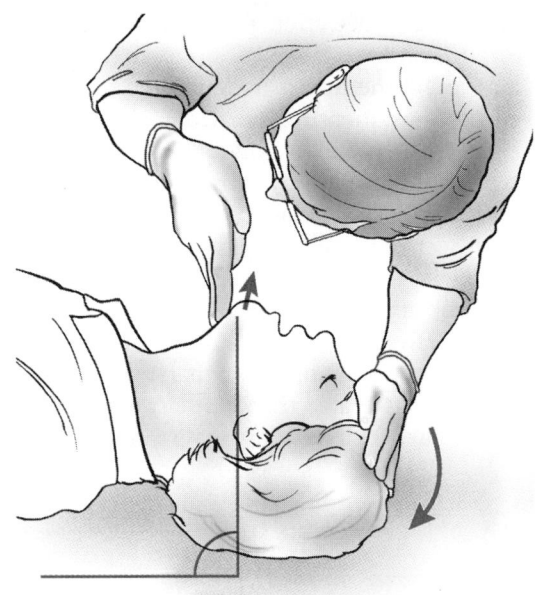

Figure 37-9   Confirming apnea.

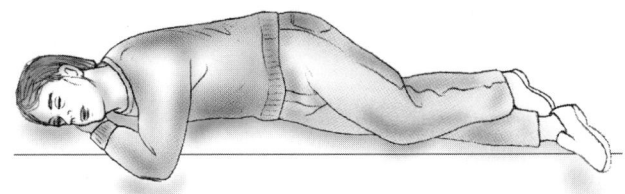

Figure 37-10   Patient in the recovery position.

the long tube prevents air from traveling down the esophagus, and air enters the trachea instead. The cuff on the long tube prevents gastric contents from being aspirated into the lungs.

The Esophageal-Tracheal Combitube (ETC) is similar to the PTL but has two tubes of the same length that are inserted blindly into the laryngopharynx. If the tube is in the trachea, ventilation occurs through the lumen of one of the two tubes in a manner similar to that of an endotracheal tube. If the tube is in the esophagus, air enters the laryngopharynx through side holes from a lumen that has a plug in its distal end. Air enters the trachea because the upper large cuff seals off the upper airway and the smaller lower cuff prevents air from entering the stomach. The lower cuff also prevents gastric contents from moving up the esophagus around the tube (Figure 37-8).

The laryngeal mask airway (LMA) consists of a proximal tube similar to an endotracheal tube, a small mask, and a large inflatable circular cuff intended for placement in the posterior pharynx, sealing the region of the base of the tongue and the glottis. A comparative study of PTL, Combitube, and LMAs during resuscitation reported the effectiveness of the LMA.[20] Despite adequate training, complications may occur with the emergent use of the PTL, ETC, or LMA.

Breathing

Listening over the nose and mouth while the airway is maintained open (Figure 37-9) is the procedure used to assess breathing. In this position, chest movement is observed and airflow is felt and heard during the expiratory phase (for example, "look, listen, and feel" for breathing). If breathing is observed, the patient should be placed in the recovery position (Figure 37-10). Emergency ventilation should begin immediately for the patient with apnea. Two breaths for 2 seconds per breath are given during observation of the chest rise. Ventilation is provided at 10 to 12 breaths per minute. Gastric distention occurs if the tidal volume is too large or flow is delivered too fast, which results in airway pressure exceeding the esophageal opening pressure and allowing air to enter the stomach. Without supplemental oxygen, a tidal volume of 10 mL/kg (700 to 1000 mL) should be provided over 2 seconds. With supplemental oxygen administration, a smaller tidal volume of 6 to 7 mL/kg (400 to 600 mL) is delivered over 1 to 2 seconds.[3]

Mouth-to-mouth breathing is as quick and effective a method of ventilation. The exhaled gas contains about 16% to 18% oxygen, which is adequate to supply emergency needs. To perform mouth-to-mouth breathing, the

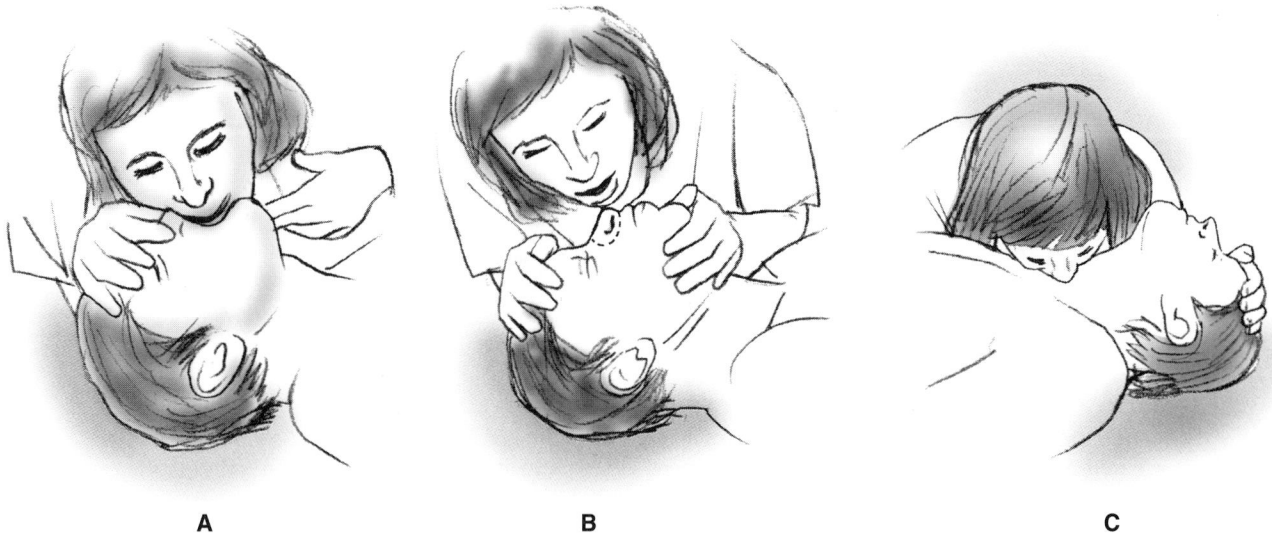

Figure 37-11   **A**, Mouth-to-mouth ventilation. **B,** Mouth-to-nose ventilation. **C**, Mouth-to-stoma ventilation.

patient's mouth is held open and the nose pinched, a deep breath taken, a seal made over the patient's mouth with the rescuer's mouth, and air blown into the patient's mouth while the chest rise is monitored (Figure 37-11). Mouth-to-nose ventilation is used when it is impossible to ventilate through the victim's mouth, the mouth cannot be opened, the mouth is injured, or a tight seal cannot be achieved with mouth-to-mouth ventilation. To perform mouth-to-nose breathing, the mouth is closed with the hand that maintains the jaw thrust. Then the rescuer's mouth is sealed over the nose of the patient and air blown into the nose while the chest rise is monitored. In patients with a tracheal stoma, mouth-to-stoma ventilation is provided with a seal made over the stoma to inflate the lungs. With mouth-to-mouth, mouth-to-nose, or mouth-to-stoma ventilation, the rescuer's mouth is removed from the airway after blowing to allow the patient to exhale.

A barrier device (Figure 37-12) is preferred by most persons to avoid direct contact with the patient and the associated potential for disease transmission.[3] As a general rule a barrier device should be used when emergency ventilation is required outside the home. The two general types of barrier devices are face shields and mouth-to-mask devices. **Face shields** consist of a clear plastic sheet of silicone that separates the patient from the person performing mouth-to-mouth ventilation.[21] Mouth-to-mask devices are more effective than face shields in delivering adequate ventilation.[22] Oxygen enrichment possible with some masks increases the delivered oxygen concentration to greater than 70%.[23] Besides offering oxygen enrichment, other desirable characteristics of mouth-to-mask devices include a nonrebreathing valve to divert the exhaled gas away from the rescuer, a tube extension that lengthens the face-to-face proximity, transparent material that enhances visibility, ease with which they conform to the anatomy of the face, little air resistance, and ease with which a face seal can be achieved.[22] As an extra precaution, in addition to a one-

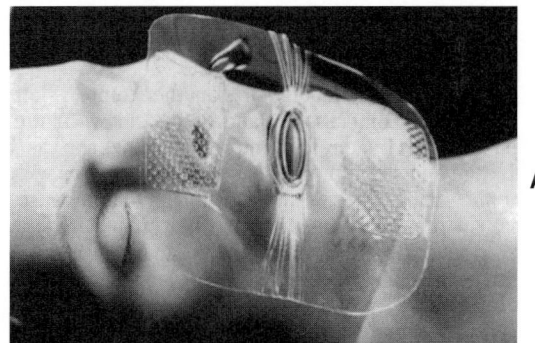

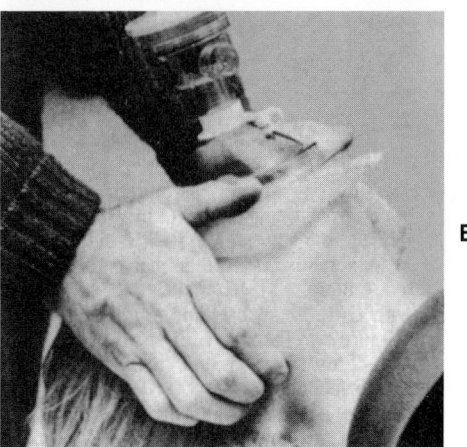

Figure 37-12 Barrier devices. **A**, Microshield face shield with duckbill valve. **B,** Mouth-to-mask ventilation in position using two-hand technique. (From Hess D, Ness C, Oppel A, et al. Evaluation of mask-to-mask ventilation devices. Respir Care 1989;34:1911.)

way valve, a bacterial filter should be placed proximal to the nonrebreathing valve. The mask and the valve should not be affected by the presence of vomitus. Moreover, the mask should work to protect the rescuer from vomitus. The volume of the mask should be as small as possible. The cli-

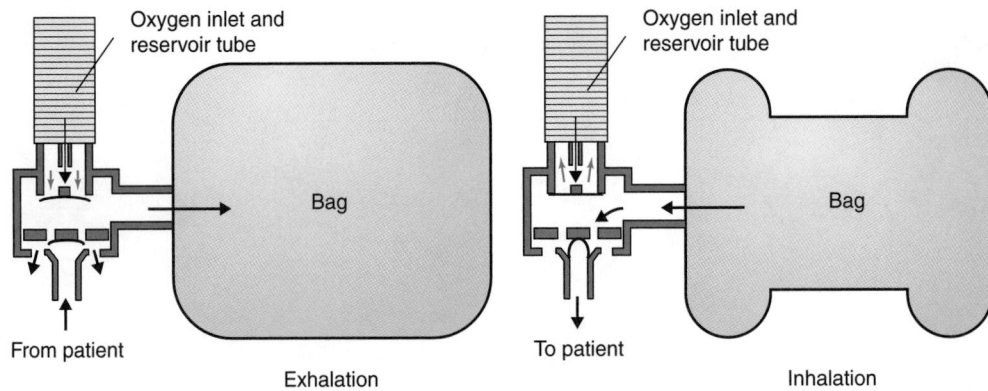

Figure 37-13 Manual resuscitator with gas intake valve located proximal to the patient valve. (Modified from McPherson SP: Respiratory therapy equipment. 4th ed. St Louis: Mosby; 1990.)

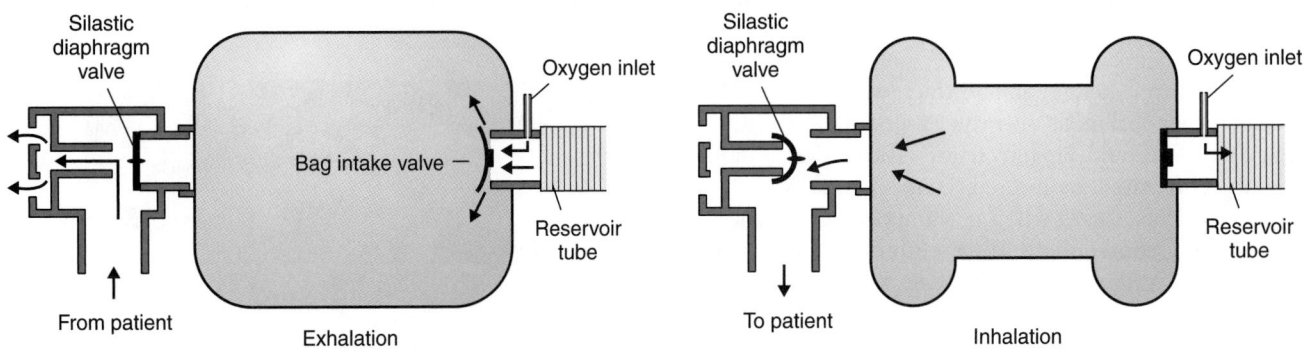

Figure 37-14 Manual resuscitator with gas intake valve located at the bottom of the bag. (Modified from McPherson SP: Respiratory therapy equipment. 4th ed. St Louis: Mosby; 1990.)

nician is positioned at the head of the patient, the mask is placed over the patient's nose and mouth and held in place by the thumbs, the first fingers of each hand are placed under the patient's mandible, and the mandible is lifted as the head is tilted back.

A variety of permanent or disposable manual resuscitators are currently available to ventilate patients during CPR. **Manual resuscitators** (bag-valve devices) consist of a self-inflating bag, an air intake valve, a nonrebreathing valve, an oxygen inlet nipple, and an oxygen reservoir. One end of the nonrebreathing valve connects to the bag; the other end is connected to the patient's tracheal tube or face mask. When the bag is compressed, the nonrebreathing valve directs gas from the bag to the patient. When the bag is released, the exhaled gas is directed through the exhalation port. The bag reinflates through a one-way inlet valve opening directly into the bag. The gas inlet valve is part of the nonrebreathing valve in some units (Figure 37-13) and is part of the valve at the bottom of other units (Figure 37-14). During cardiac arrest, it is important to administer the highest oxygen concentration possible. Manual resuscitators should be able to deliver at least 85% oxygen with a flow of 15 L/min.[24-26] Some manual resuscitators with poorly designed oxygen reservoirs deliver less than 85% oxygen.[27]

*R*espiratory Recap

Manual Resuscitators	
Self-inflating bag	Oxygen inlet
Air intake valve	Oxygen reservoir
Nonrebreathing valve	

Manual ventilation by a bag-valve-mask may not provide adequate tidal volumes,[28] particularly in the hands of an untrained operator. Tidal volume delivery by a bag-valve-mask is improved when used by two persons simultaneously,[29-31] one who opens the airway and holds the mask in place with two hands and the other who squeezes the bag with two hands (Figure 37-15). In the hands of a clinician skilled in its use (for example, a respiratory therapist or an anesthesiologist), manual ventilation may be effective when performed by a single operator. However, it is difficult to deliver an adequate tidal volume with one-hand compression of the bag. Tidal volume delivery during manual ventilation is decreased if lung impedance is high.[29] Persons with small hands deliver 100 to 250 mL

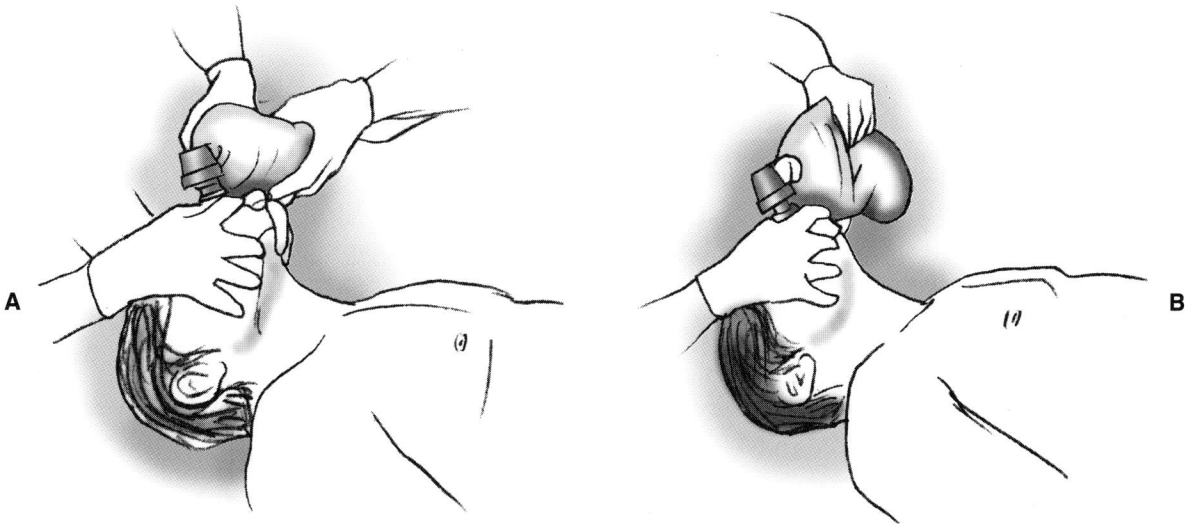

Figure 37-15   **A,** Two-person bag-valve-mask technique. **B,** One-person bag-valve-mask technique.

less volume with a one-hand squeeze of the bag than do those with large hands.[30] It is interesting to note that wearing medical gloves (a universal practice during CPR) does not affect tidal volume delivery during manual ventilation.[32] Intubation ensures the ability to provide adequate ventilation and protects against gastric insufflation and aspiration of gastric material.[33] Use of the bag-valve device to provide oxygen for a spontaneously breathing patient is discouraged because of the increased effort required to breathe through the nonrebreathing valve.[34]

Circulation

The presence of a heartbeat is determined by palpation of the carotid artery (Figure 37-16), which should take no longer than 5 to 10 seconds. Lay rescuers often spend too much time performing the pulse check.[35] Lay rescuers also have difficulty correctly identifying the presence of a pulse. Accordingly, they should not rely on the pulse check to determine the need for chest compressions. However, health care professionals should palpate the carotid artery to determine the presence of a heartbeat. If a pulse is absent, **cardiac compressions** should be initiated. The patient should be placed in the supine position to allow the maximum blood flow to the brain during cardiac compressions. Even when compressions are performed properly, cardiac output is reduced to approximately 25% to 30% of normal. If a patient is in bed, a board is placed under the patient. However, chest compressions should not be delayed while waiting for a board.

External chest compressions are performed on the lower half of the adult sternum, above the notch where the ribs meet the lower sternum (Figure 37-17).[3] The lower margin of the victim's rib cage is located with the middle and index fingers. The fingers are moved along the rib cage to the notch where the ribs meet the sternum, and the middle finger is placed on this notch. The index

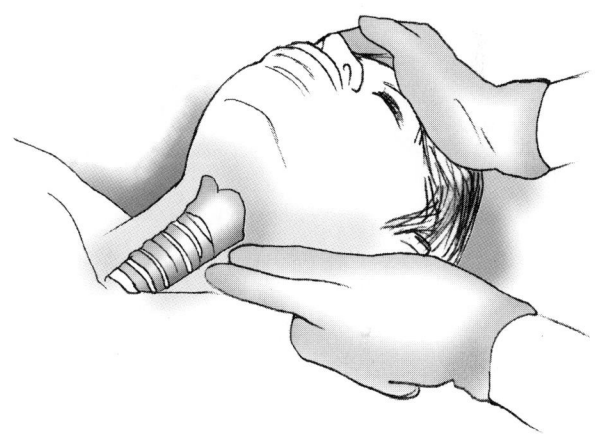

Figure 37-16 Carotid pulse check.

finger is placed next to the middle finger and rests on the lower end of the sternum. The heel of the hand is placed on the lower half of the sternum, close to the index finger, with the long axis of the hand parallel with the sternum. The first hand then is removed from the notch and placed on top of the hand on the sternum. The fingers are extended or interlaced to keep them off the chest. The arms are kept straight, with elbows locked, and the shoulders directly over the sternum (Figure 37-18). Pressure is exerted downward to depress the sternum 1½ to 2 inches (4 to 5 cm) at a rate of 100 per minute. The hands should not be removed from the chest during relaxation. However, pressure must be completely released on the upward stroke of compressions to allow blood to flow into the chest and heart. Arterial blood pressure during chest compression is maximal when the duration of compression is 50% of the compression-release cycle.[3] The effectiveness of chest compressions is evaluated by a second person who palpates the carotid or femoral pulse.

Compressions are usually performed in conjunction with ventilation. The ratio of compressions to ventilations is 15:2, with a pause in chest compression for the ventilations. This compression ratio is used for one-person or two-person CPR until the airway is secured with an endotracheal tube. Once the patient has been intubated, a ratio of compressions to ventilations of 5:1 is used and a pause for ventilation is unnecessary. Because of fear of infectious disease transmission, many persons are reluctant to perform mouth-to-mouth ventilation. Evidence suggests that the outcome of chest compressions without mouth-to-mouth ventilation is significantly better than no CPR.[36] If the rescuer is unwilling or unable to perform mouth-to-mouth ventilation, chest compression-only CPR should be provided rather than no CPR.

Compression of the xiphoid process can cause laceration of the liver that can lead to severe internal bleeding. Rib fractures and costochondral separation can occur if the compressions deviate from midline or if pressure with the fingers is placed on the rib cage. Even when compressions are performed correctly, a possibility still exists that the rescuer may fracture the ribs or sternum. The broken ends of the ribs can, in turn, cause laceration of the lung. Elderly patients and patients on chronic steroids are the most susceptible to such injuries. If cracking of the ribs is felt or heard, the compressor should check the hand position and continue to compress. The formation of fat emboli is another complication of closed chest compressions and may occur without evidence of overt fractures. Compressing bones such as the rib cage and sternum may lead to microfractures within the medulla of the ribs and sternum and an increase in marrow pressure. Fat may enter the venous circulation from the marrow. Cerebral fat emboli may be considered a cause of mental deterioration after CPR. Improperly performed chest compressions may lead to less than optimal cardiac output, causing inadequate blood flow to the brain.

Automatic External Defibrillation

A strong relationship has been established between survival and the speed with which defibrillation is administered.[37-39] The rationale for early defibrillation of VF is that the only effective treatment for VF is electrical defibrillation, the probability of successful defibrillation diminishes rapidly over time, and VF tends to convert to asystole within a few minutes. All health care professionals trained in BLS should be taught to operate a defibrillator if they are expected to respond to people in cardiac arrest.[38] The automated external defibrillator (AED) incorporates a rhythm analysis system. Some are fully automated, whereas others are semiautomated or shock-advisory defibrillators. All AEDs are attached to the patient by two adhesive pads and connecting

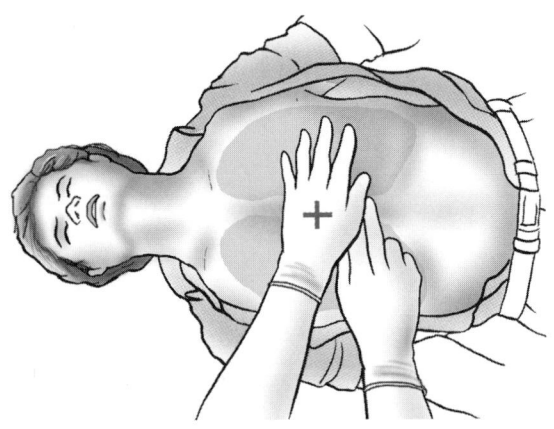

Figure 37-17 Hand position for chest compressions. The fingers should move up the rib cage to the notch where the ribs meet the lower sternum in the center of the lower part of the chest.

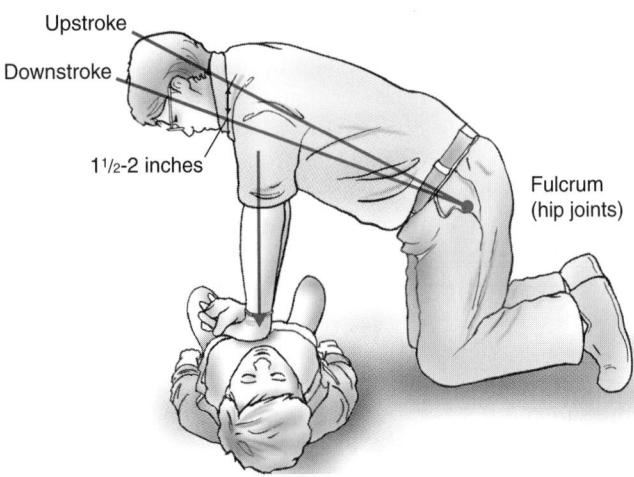

Figure 37-18 Arm position for chest compressions.

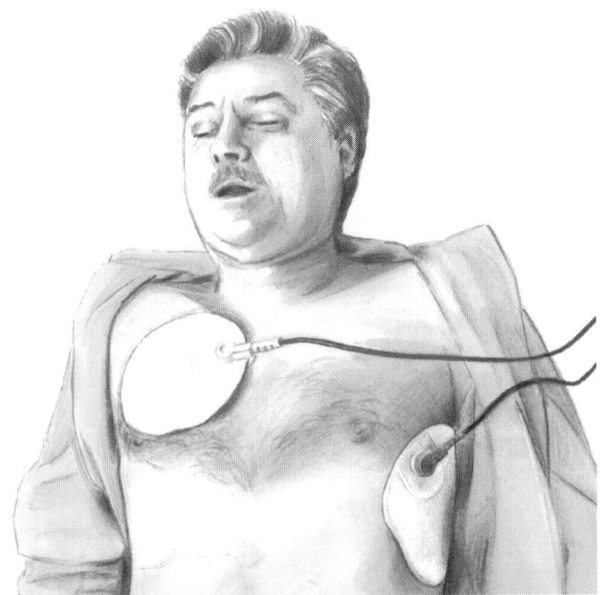

Figure 37-19 Automatic external defibrillator electrode pad placement on the victim. (From The automated external defibrillator: key link in the chain of survival. Circulation 2000;102(Suppl I):I-60–I-76.)

cables (Figure 37-19). To operate an AED the following four steps must be performed: (1) the power turned on, (2) the device attached, (3) the analysis initiated, and (4) the shock delivered if needed. In the hospital setting a defibrillator should be available within 1 to 2 minutes of cardiac arrest.

Adult Foreign Body Airway Obstruction

Most **foreign body obstructions** occur during eating. The universal choking sign is used to alert others of the presence of a complete upper airway obstruction (Figure 37-20). In the case of complete foreign body obstruction, most patients do not lose consciousness immediately but are unable to speak, breathe, or cough. Foreign bodies that cause partial obstruction result in some ability to ventilate. Retraction, agitation, and activity of the accessory muscles are evident. If good air exchange is present, a strong cough may force the foreign body from the airway. A normal cough is superior to any of the artificially induced coughs. If a choking victim can speak or breathe and is coughing with a moderately strong effort, intervention is unnecessary and potentially dangerous.[40] Partial obstruction with poor air exchange requires immediate intervention. Poor air exchange is indicated by a weak, ineffective cough, stridor, and use of accessory muscles. When these signs occur, the management protocol is the same as with a complete airway obstruction.

Emergency maneuvers used to relieve airway obstruction are designed to generate positive intrathoracic pressure to expel a foreign body from the trachea. The abdominal thrust (Heimlich maneuver) is recommended to relieve airway obstruction (Figure 37-21). The rescuer stands behind the victim and puts both arms around the victim's waist. One fist is grasped with the other hand and placed thumb side against the victim's abdomen, in the midline slightly above the navel and well below the tip of the xiphoid process. Each quick thrust should exert force inward and upward. Thrusts are repeated until the object is expelled from the airway or the patient becomes unconscious. If unconsciousness occurs, the victim is placed in a supine position and a call for help is made. A finger sweep of the upper airway is performed.[3] Abdominal thrusts are continued by placement of one hand against the upper abdomen with the second hand on top applying force inward and upward. The abdominal thrusts are more easily applied if the rescuer straddles the victim's legs (Figure 37-22). Complications of abdominal thrusts include pneumoperitoneum, laceration or rupture of the stomach, fractured ribs, regurgitation, and liver laceration.

Another maneuver used to relieve upper airway obstruction is a chest thrust. This maneuver is used for a patient in the late stages of pregnancy or who is extremely obese. To perform a chest thrust, the patient is encircled with the rescuer's arms, placed directly under the patient's armpits, and one fist is placed thumb side on the midsternum, with care to avoid the xiphoid process and the mar-

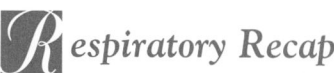

espiratory Recap

Foreign Body Obstruction of the Airway
Abdominal thrusts
Chest thrusts
Finger sweeps

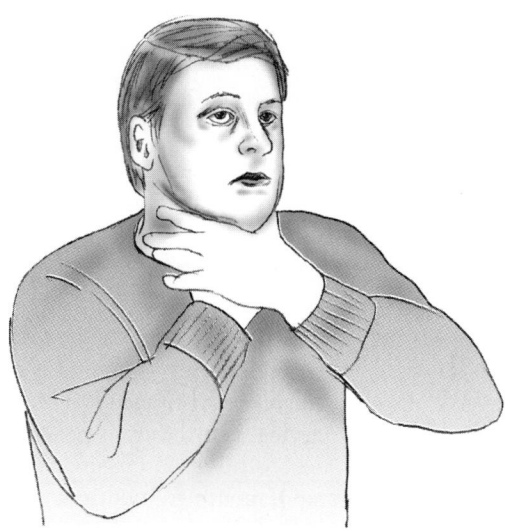

Figure 37-20   Universal choking sign.

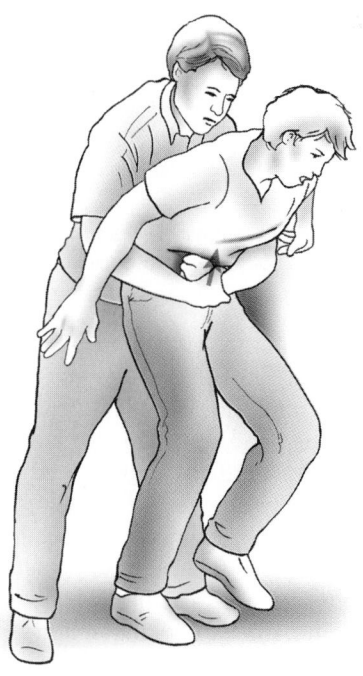

Figure 37-21   Performing the Heimlich maneuver.

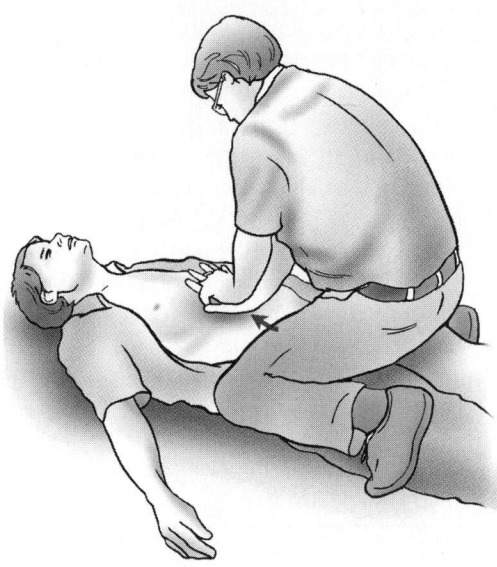

Figure 37-22   Abdominal thrusts administered to an unconscious victim of foreign body airway obstruction.

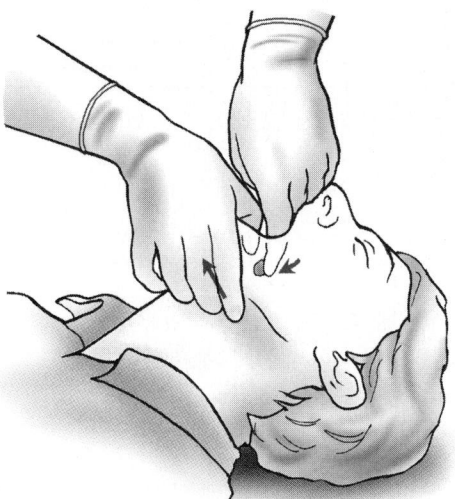

Figure 37-23   Finger sweep maneuver administered to an unconscious victim of foreign body airway obstruction.

gins of the rib cage. The other hand grasps the fist, and as many as five backward thrusts are performed. If the victim is unconscious, the hand position is the same as that used to apply closed chest cardiac compressions.

Finger sweeps may be effective to help remove a foreign body. The mouth is opened by grasping of the lower jaw and tongue between the thumb and fingers and lifting of the mandible (jaw lift). The index finger is inserted to the base of the tongue. A hooking action is used to dislodge the object (Figure 37-23). A Kelly clamp or Magill forceps may be useful if the object is visible. A laryngoscope may help to permit direct visualization of the foreign body. The sequence of abdominal thrusts, finger sweep, and attempt to ventilate should be repeated as long as necessary.

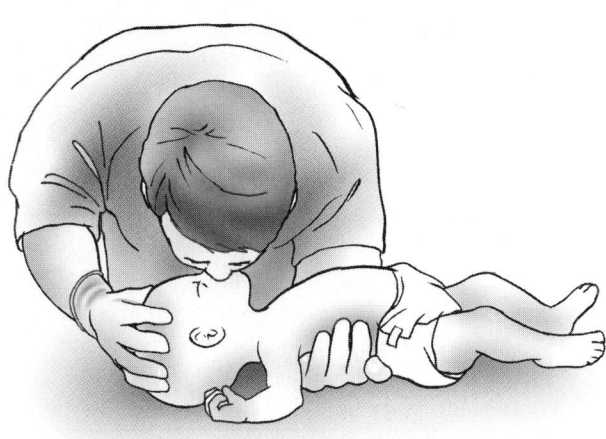

Figure 37-24   Mouth to mouth-and-nose ventilation.

CPR for Infants and Children

Causes of pediatric and neonatal cardiopulmonary arrest often are injury related. Attempts to prevent injury can reduce childhood death and disability, especially when prevention strategies are geared toward the six most common types of severe childhood injuries nationwide: motor vehicle passenger injuries, pedestrian injuries, bicycle injuries, submersion, fire- and burn-related injuries, and firearm injuries.[41] During infancy the most common causes of cardiopulmonary arrest are respiratory emergencies (that is, respiratory diseases and airway obstruction, including foreign body aspiration). Unlike adults, infants rarely suffer a sudden cardiac arrest. It is a progressive deterioration in respiratory function that initiates the cardiopulmonary arrest.

Age-Specific Angle

Pediatric and neonatal cardiopulmonary arrests are most often injury-related. During infancy, cardiopulmonary emergencies are usually the result of respiratory emergencies.

The head-tilt/chin-lift or jaw-thrust maneuver is used to open the airway.[42-44] The presence of breathing is assessed by the look, listen, and feel technique. For the infant (<1 year of age) with apnea, ventilation is provided with mouth-to-mouth-and-nose ventilation (Figure 37-24). For a child (1 to 8 years of age), mouth-to-mouth *or* mouth-to-nose ventilation is provided. Barrier devices and manual resuscitators also can be used.

Two types of manual resuscitators are available—self-inflating and flow-inflating devices (Figure 37-25). Some neonatal resuscitators have a pressure relief valve with an

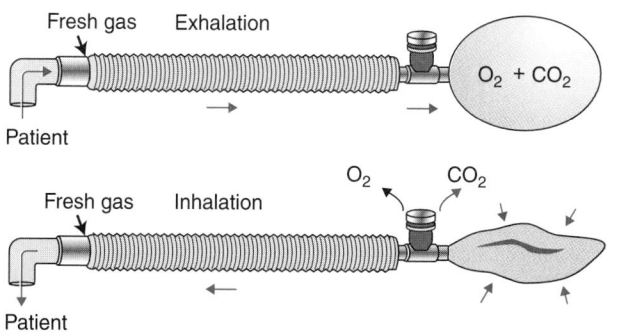

Figure 37-25 Mapleson D system. During expiration, fresh gas (FG) flushes CO_2 and O_2 to the reservoir bag. During inspiration, fresh gas is delivered to the patient and the contents of the reservoir bag exit through a pressure-relief valve. (Modified from Thompson JE, Farrel E, McManus M. Neonatal and pediatric airway emergencies. Respir Care 1992;37:584.)

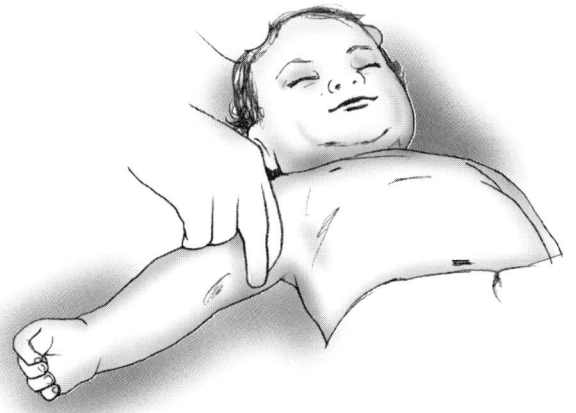

Figure 37-26 Brachial pulse check.

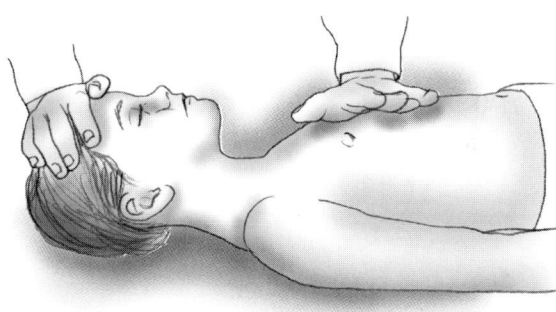

Figure 37-27 One-hand chest compression in the child.

opening pressure of 40 cm H_2O.[25,26] The 40-cm H_2O pressure limit should not be exceeded during normal ventilation conditions, but an override mechanism should be provided for times when lung impedance is high and the patient has a tracheal tube in place. The override mechanism must be designed so that its operating mode is readily apparent to the user.[45] Venting of gas through the pop-off reduces the FIO_2 and lowers the tidal volume.[46] Bag-valve ventilation with an in-line manometer and no pop-off may be safer for neonates, especially for delivery of the first breaths of a neonate's nonaerated lung, during which higher pressures may be needed.[47] Clinicians using pressure manometers to monitor airway pressure must ensure that the manometer is accurate at rates more than 40 per minute.[48] Resuscitation of newborns at birth often involves bag-valve-mask ventilation and the circular face mask.[49-51]

Age-Specific Angle

Bag-valve devices used with infants should have a release valve to limit peak inspiratory pressure.

The size of the neck of an infant under 1 year of age makes palpation of the carotid artery difficult. Thus the brachial artery should be palpated (Figure 37-26). The cardiac compression technique for children is similar to that for adults except that the heel of only one hand is placed over the lower half of the sternum (between the nipple line and the notch), avoiding the xiphoid process. A compression rate of 100 per minute and depression of the sternum of 1 to 1½ inches is used, depending on the size of the child (Figure 37-27). The other hand is used to maintain the child's head position so that it may be possible to ventilate without repositioning the head. A breath is delivered after every fifth compression. With pauses for ventilation the number of compressions is actually about 80 per minute. For infants, two or three fingers are used to compress the

lower half of the sternum ½ to 1 inch (Figure 37-28). The compression rate should be at least 100 per minute, with a breath given after every fifth compression. An alternative technique uses the thumbs to compress the sternum, with the hands encircling the thorax. Table 37-1 compares the BLS maneuvers in infants, children, and adults.

Subdiaphragmatic abdominal thrusts are recommended for relief of airway obstruction in children, just as they are for adults. The sequence of interventions used to treat children with an obstructed airway is identical to that provided to adults. However, blind finger sweeps should not be performed. A finger sweep may be used only when the foreign object is visible. When abdominal thrusts are delivered to a child who is unconscious or who becomes unconscious, the heel of one hand is used rather than two, as for the adult.

The sequence of interventions used to treat infants with an obstructed airway is very different than that provided to adults and children (Table 37-2). In the infant a combination of back blows and chest thrusts is recommended for relief of airway obstruction. The baby is placed between the rescuer's forearms and hands, with the head lower than the trunk. With the infant face down, five forceful back blows should be delivered between the infant's shoulder blades with the heel of one hand (Figure

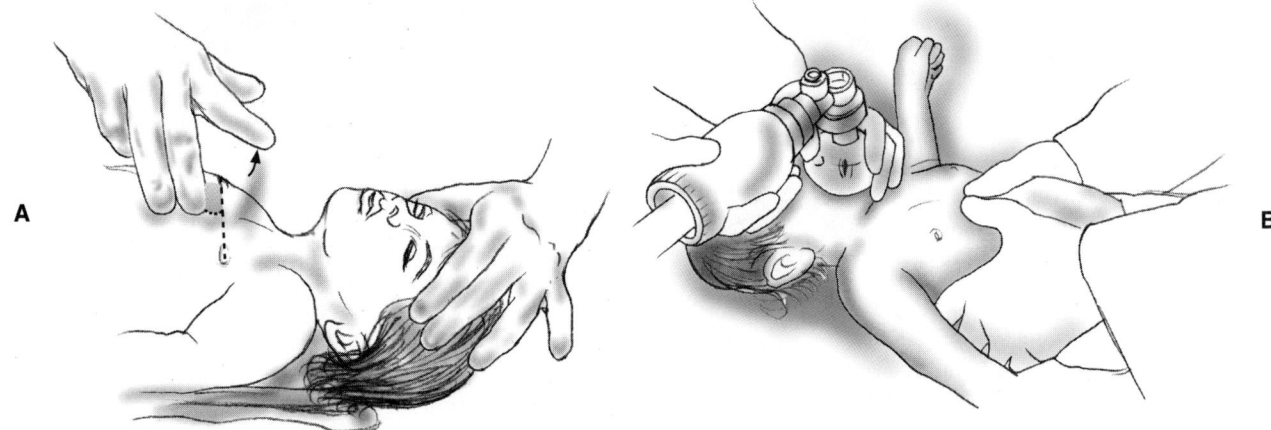

Figure 37-28   A, Two-finger chest compression technique in the infant. **B,** Two-thumb chest compression technique in the infant.

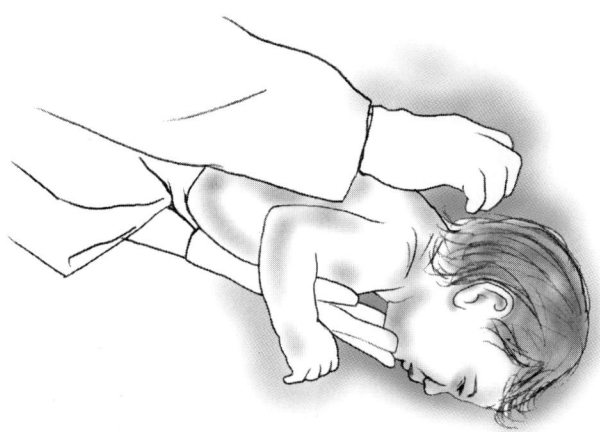

Figure 37-29   Back blows in the infant to clear foreign body obstruction.

37-29). After the baby is turned over to the supine position, with the head lower than the trunk, five quick downward chest thrusts should be delivered in the same location and manner as chest compressions. Rescue breathing is attempted when the infant loses consciousness.

Dysrhythmia Recognition

An important aspect of ACLS is the assessment of the ECG for abnormal cardiac rhythms. Correct identification of the cardiac rhythm dictates the appropriate drug therapy and electrical therapy (for example, defibrillation, cardioversion). Drug therapy is another important aspect of ACLS (Table 37-3). In the cardiac-arrested patient, drugs are administered to improve cardiac output and arterial blood pressure, to control heart rate and rhythm, to promote diuresis, to act as thrombolytic agents, and to treat metabolic acidosis and electrolyte imbalances. To facilitate administration of these drugs, intravenous access should be obtained as soon as possible in the cardiac arrest

situation. Intracardiac injections are not recommended. When intravenous access is delayed, some drugs can be administered through the tracheal tube.[52] Lidocaine, atropine, naloxone, and epinephrine can be administered via the endotracheal tube at 2 to 2½ times the intravenous dose, diluted in 10 mL of normal saline.

Electrical Therapy

The precordial thump is a sharp, quick blow that is delivered with the fleshy part of the fist from a distance of 8 to 12 inches above the chest at the midportion of the sternum. A single precordial thump is recommended for witnessed cardiac arrest when a defibrillator is unavailable. An alternative to the precordial thump in the awake subject is coughing. The subject is asked to cough vigorously and keep coughing at the onset of cardiac arrest. Although how the mechanism works is unclear, coughing converts the rhythm in some cases.

With **defibrillation**, an electrical current is passed through the heart in an attempt to eliminate the chaotic asynchronous activity of VF.[53] If defibrillation is successful, cardiac cells depolarize and then repolarize in a uniform manner with resumption of coordinated cardiac contraction. Defibrillation is indicated for VF, pulseless ventricular tachycardia, and asystole (with the possibility that the rhythm is actually fine VF). The initial defibrillation attempt is applied at 200 joules,

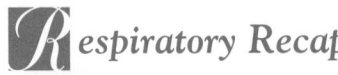

espiratory Recap

Electrical Therapy
Defibrillation
Cardioversion
Pacing

TABLE 37-1

Summary of Basic Life Support Maneuvers for Infants, Children, and Adults

Maneuver	Infant (<1 yr)	Child (1 to 8 yr)	Adult
Assessment of responsiveness	Tapping and speaking loudly	Tapping and speaking loudly	Tapping, shaking, and speaking loudly
Activate EMS	After 1 min CPR, if alone (call fast)	After 1 min CPR, if alone (call fast)	Before opening the airway (phone-first)
Airway	Head-tilt/chin-lift or jaw-thrust	Head-tilt/chin-lift or jaw-thrust	Head-tilt/chin-lift or jaw-thrust
Breathing			
Initial	Two breaths at 1 to $1\frac{1}{2}$ s/breath	Two breaths at 1 to $1\frac{1}{2}$ s/breath	Two breaths at 2 s/breath
Subsequent	20 breaths/min	20 breaths/min	12 breaths/min
Circulation			
Pulse check	Brachial	Carotid	Carotid
Compression area	Lower half of sternum	Lower half of sternum	Lower half of sternum
Compression technique	Two or three fingers, or thumbs	Heel of one hand	Heel of one hand on top of other hand
Compression depth	$\frac{1}{2}$ to 1 in	1 to $1\frac{1}{2}$ in	$1\frac{1}{2}$ to 2 in
Compression rate	At least 100/min	100/min	100/min
Compression: ventilation ratio	5:1 (pause for ventilation)	5:1 (pause for ventilation)	15:2 (pause for ventilation)
Reassessment	After 20 cycles	After 20 cycles	After 4 cycles

EMS, *Emergency medical services;* CPR, *cardiopulmonary resuscitation.*

TABLE 37-2

Summary of Foreign Body Airway Obstruction Maneuvers in Adults, Children, and Infants

Conscious Adult	Conscious Child	Conscious Infant
1. Ask, "Are you choking?" 2. Perform five abdominal thrusts (chest thrusts for pregnant or obese persons). 3. Repeat thrusts until effective or victim becomes unconscious.	1. Ask, "Are you choking?" 2. Perform five abdominal thrusts (chest thrusts for obese persons). 3. Repeat thrusts until effective or victim becomes unconscious.	1. Confirm complete or partial airway obstruction. Check for serious breathing difficulty, ineffective cough, no strong cry. 2. Perform five back blows and five chest thrusts. 3. Repeat step 2 until effective or victim becomes unconscious.

Adult Becomes Unconscious	Child Becomes Unconscious	Infant Becomes Unconscious
1. Activate EMS or code team. 2. Perform tongue-jaw lift followed by blind finger sweep to remove object. 3. Open airway and attempt to ventilate; if still obstructed, reposition and attempt to ventilate again. 4. Give up to five abdominal thrusts. 5. Repeat until effective.	1. If second rescuer available, have that person activate EMS or code team. 2. Perform tongue-jaw lift; if object is visible, perform finger sweep to remove it. 3. Open airway and attempt to ventilate; if still obstructed, reposition and attempt to ventilate again. 4. Give up to five abdominal thrusts. 5. Repeat until effective. 6. If alone and airway obstruction is not relieved after 1 min, activate EMS system or code team.	1. If second rescuer available, have that person activate EMS or code team. 2. Perform tongue-jaw lift; if object is visible, perform finger sweep to remove it. 3. Open airway and attempt to ventilate; if still obstructed, reposition and attempt to ventilate again. 4. Give up to five back blows and five chest thrusts. 5. Repeat until effective. 6. If alone and airway obstruction is not relieved after 1 min, activate EMS system or code team.

EMS, *Emergency medical services.*
Persist in these efforts as long as necessary; do not check pulse or attempt chest compressions until airway is opened. If victim resumes effective breathing, place in recovery position.

TABLE 37-3

Drugs Used During Advanced Cardiac Life Support

Drug	Indication	Dosage/Administration
Drugs to Improve Blood Pressure or Cardiac Output		
Epinephrine (sympathomimetic)	First agent in cardiac arrest VF, VT, PEA, asystole	1 mg of 1:10,000 solution IV push every 3-5 min or infusion titrated at 2-10 μg/min for pulseless VT, VF, or symptomatic bradycardia (not 1st line); side effects: tachydysrhythmias, hypertension
Dopamine (sympathomimetic)	Hypotension Cardiogenic shock	Infusion titrated at 5-20 μg/kg/min; side effects: tachydysrhythmias, hypertension, ischemia
Norepinephrine (sympathomimetic)	Severe hypotension (systolic BP <70 mm Hg) Cardiogenic shock	Infusion titrated at 0.5-30 μg/min; side effect: ischemia
Dobutamine (sympathomimetic)	Refractory congestive heart failure (systolic BP >100 mm Hg and normal diastolic) Cardiogenic shock	Infusion titrated at 2-20 μg/kg/min; side effects: tachydysrhythmias, hypertension, acute myocardial infarction
Amrinone (nonadrenergic non-β-agonist)	Severe CHF that has not responded to diuretics, vasodilators, and conventional inotropes	0-75 mg/kg IV push over 2-3 min followed by an infusion at 5-15 μg/kg/min; side effects: dysrhythmias, hypotension
Vasopressin	Alternative to epinephrine in shock refractory VF; hemodynamic support in vasodilatory shock (e.g., sepsis)	40 units IV, single dose, one time only
Drugs to Control Heart Rate and Rhythm		
Amiodarone (atrial and ventricular arrhythmias)	Rapid atrial arrhythmias, persistent VF or VT, hemodynamically unstable VT	150 mg IV over 10 min, followed by 1 mg/min for 6 hr, and then 0.5 mg/min
Lidocaine (ventricular antidysrhythmic)	VF/pulseless VT, VT with pulse Wide-complex tachycardia of unknown origin Significant ventricular ectopy	1-1.5 mg/kg IV push repeated in 5-10 min to a max dose of 3 mg/kg in VF/pulseless VT; 1-1.5 mg/kg IV push repeated every 5-10 min with 0.5-0.75 mg/kg to a max dose of 3 mg/kg for all others; infusion 2-4 mg/min; side effects: seizure, altered mental status
Procainamide (antidysrhythmic)	Recurrent VT not controlled with lidocaine Refractory pulseless VF/VT Wide-complex tachycardia of unknown origin	20-30 mg/min IV infusion until a max dose 17 mg/kg is given or QRS widens by 50% or hypotension develops or dysrhythmia ceases; infusion (maintenance) 1-4 mg/min; side effects: widening QRS, hypotension, cardiac arrest, seizures
Adenosine (antidysrhythmic)	PSVT Wide-complex tachycardia of unknown origin after lidocaine	6 mg rapid IV push over 1-3 seconds, repeat in 1-2 min with 12 mg, repeat in 1-2 min with another 12 mg (total 30 mg); side effects: transient dysrhythmias, hypotension
Digitalis (antidysrhythmic)	Atrial fibrillation/flutter (chronic) CHF/PSVT (3rd line)	Limited use in emergency cardiac care
Verapamil (Ca^{+2} channel blocker)	Atrial fibrillation/flutter with rapid vent response Narrow PSVT	2.5-5 mg slow IV push over 2 min, repeated with 5-10 mg every 15-30 min to a max dose of 20 mg; side effects: hypotension, bradycardia, asystole, AV block

TABLE 37-3

Drugs Used During Advanced Cardiac Life Support—cont'd

Drug	Indication	Dosage/Administration
Diltiazem (Ca^{+2} channel blocker)	Atrial fibrillation/flutter with rapid ventricular response	0.25 mg/kg IV push over 2 min, repeated with 0.35 mg/kg over 2 min; side effects: hypotension, flushing
Propranolol (β-blocker)	Considered in MI and atrial fibrillation/flutter	Total dose of 0.1 mg/kg slow IV push divided into 3 doses at 2-3 min intervals; side effects: bronchospasm, hypotension, bradycardia
Isoproterenol (β-agonist)	Sympathomimetic bradycardia after all else fails	Infusion titrated at 2-10 μg/min; side effects: increased myocardial oxygen demand, tachycardia
Atropine (anticholinergic, antidysrhythmic, vagolytic)	Bradycardia PEA Asystole	0.4-1.0 mg IV push every 3-5 min to max of 4 mg (starting with I mg for PEA/asystole); side effects: tachycardia, VF, VT
Diuretics		
Furosemide (potent diuretic)	Acute pulmonary edema	0.5-1.0 mg/kg slow IV push; side effects: hypovolemia, hypotension
Vasodilators		
Sodium nitroprusside	Heart failure Hypertension	Infusion titrated at 0.1-5.0 μg/kg/min (max 10 μg/mg/min); side effect: hypotension
Nitroglycerine	Ischemic chest pain Pulmonary edema Unstable angina CHF with MI	Sublingual 0.3-0.4 mg repeated at 5 min intervals times 3 doses; infusion 10-20 μg/min every 5-10 min; side effects: tachycardia, hypotension
Thrombolytic Agents		
Streptokinase, t-PA, Urokinase agent	Chest pain consistent with acute MI	Dosing variable depending on agent and institution; side effect: hemorrhage
Miscellaneous Agents		
Oxygen	All situations	Highest F$_{IO_2}$ possible for cardiac arrests 1-6 L/min nasal cannula or 6-10 L/min simple mask for spontaneously breathing patients
Sodium bicarbonate	Hyperkalemia Long arrest interval	1 mEq/kg IV push, then 0.5 mEq/kg every 10 min; side effect: worsened acidosis from CO_2 and retention
Magnesium sulfate	Torsades de Pointes Pulseless VT/VF AMI Hypomagnesemia	1-2 g IV push over 1-2 min, repeated with infusion (same amount mixed with normal saline over 5-60 min); side effects: depressed respiration, hypotension
Calcium chloride	Hypocalcemia Hyperkalemia Ca^{+2} channel blocker toxicity	2-4 mg/kg IV push over 5 min, repeated every 10 min as needed; side effects: bradycardia, hypotension
Morphine sulphate	Ischemic chest pain CHF	1-3 mg slow IV push every 5 min as needed; side effects: respiratory and CNS depression, hypotension, bradycardia; reversed with naloxone

VF, *Ventricular fibrillation;* VT, *ventricular tachycardia;* PEA, *pulseless electrical activity;* BP, *blood pressure;* CHF, *congestive heart failure;* PSVT, *paroxysmal supraventricular tachycardia;* MI, *myocardial infarction;* AMI, *acute myocardial infarction;* CNS, *central nervous system.*

BOX 37-4

Steps for Defibrillation with a Conventional Manual Defibrillator

1. Turn on defibrillator.
2. Select energy level at 200 joules.
3. Set *lead select* switch on *paddles* (or lead I, II, or III if monitor leads are used).
4. Position conductor pads on patient (or apply gel to paddles).
5. Position paddles on patient (sternum-apex).
6. Visually check the monitor display and assess the rhythm. (Subsequent steps assume VF/pulseless VT is present.)
7. Announce to the team members, "Charging defibrillator—stand clear!"
8. Press *charge* button on apex paddle (right hand) on defibrillator controls.
9. When the defibrillator is fully charged, state firmly in a forceful voice the following chant (or some suitable equivalent) before each shock:
   - "I am going to shock on three. One, I'm clear." (Check and make sure you are clear of contact with the patient or the stretcher and equipment.)
   - "Two, you're clear." (Make a visual check to ensure that no one continues to touch the patient or stretcher. In particular, do not forget about the person doing ventilations. That person should not have hands on the ventilatory adjuncts, including the tracheal tube.)
   - "Three, everybody's clear." (Check yourself one more time before pressing the shock buttons.)
10. Apply 25-lb pressure on both paddles.
11. Press the two *discharge* buttons simultaneously.
12. Check the monitor screen. If unquestionable VF/VT remains, recharge the defibrillator at once. Check a pulse if any question remains about the rhythm display (for example, a lead had been dislodged or the paddles are not displaying the correct signal).
13. Shock at 200 to 300 joules, then at 360 joules, repeating the same verbal statements noted previously.

From Cummins RO, editor. Textbook of advanced cardiac life support. Dallas: American Heart Association; 1994.
VF, Ventricular fibrillation; VT, ventricular tachycardia.

the second at 300 joules, the third at 360 joules, and all subsequent attempts at 360 joules. The procedure for defibrillation is described in Box 37-4.

Synchronized **cardioversion** is an electrical discharge that has been timed to occur at a specific point in the cardiac cycle. The electrical impulse is synchronized to discharge during the nonvulnerable period of the cardiac cycle. The vulnerable period is when the heart is most susceptible to developing VF if excited by an electrical stimulus. Specifically, the vulnerable period just precedes the apex of the T-wave on the ECG. The machine synchronizes the electrical impulse to the R-wave of the ECG (that is, before the vulnerable period). Synchronized cardioversion is initially applied at energy levels lower than what is used for defibrillation (as low as 50 joules).

Cardiac pacing is used for symptomatic bradycardia. Cardiac pacemakers can be transvenous pacemakers, transcutaneous (external) pacemakers, transthoracic pacemakers, or transesophageal pacemakers.

KEY POINTS

- Factors related to resuscitation outcomes after CPR include the initial rhythm, time elapsed before initiation of CPR, time elapsed before defibrillation of ventricular fibrillation or pulseless ventricular tachycardia, duration of CPR, and whether arrest was witnessed.
- The primary ABCD survey consists of airway, breathing, circulation, and defibrillation.
- Masks and face shields can be used for emergency ventilation.
- With two-rescuer CPR, one person performs chest compressions and the other person performs ventilation and assesses cardiopulmonary function.
- The abdominal thrust maneuver is recommended to relieve airway obstruction.
- In airway management, there is no substitute for tracheal intubation.
- Manual ventilation with a bag-valve-mask may not provide adequate tidal volumes.
- During cardiac arrest, it is important to administer the highest oxygen concentration possible.
- Adult and pediatric resuscitators should not have a pressure limiting system.
- An important aspect of ACLS is assessment of the ECG for abnormal cardiac rhythms.
- When intravenous access is delayed, some drugs can be administered through the tracheal tube.
- With defibrillation an electrical current is passed through the heart to eliminate the chaotic asynchronous activity of ventricular fibrillation.
- Synchronized cardioversion is an electrical discharge that has been timed to occur at a specific point in the cardiac cycle.
- Cardiac pacing is used for symptomatic bradycardia.

References

1. Chandra NC, Hazinski MF, editors. Textbook of basic life support for healthcare providers. Dallas: American Heart Association; 1994.
2. Cummins RO, editor. Textbook of advanced cardiac life support. Dallas: American Heart Association; 1994.
3. Anonymous. Adult basic life support. Circulation 2000;102: I-22–I-59.
4. Hess D, Eitel D. Monitoring during resuscitation. Respir Care 1992;37:739-768.

5. Robinson GR, Hess D. Postdischarge survival and functional status following in-hospital cardiopulmonary resuscitation. Chest 1994;105:991-996.

6. Tresch DD, Neahring JM, Duthie EH, et al. Outcomes of cardiopulmonary resuscitation in nursing homes: can we predict who will benefit? Am J Med 1993;95:123-130.

7. Kloeck W, Cummins RO, Chamberlain D, et al. Early defibrillation: an advisory statement from the Advanced Life Support Working Group of the International Liaison Committee on Resuscitation. Circulation 1997;95:2183-2184.

8. Goodlin SJ, Zhong Z, Lynn J, et al. Factors associated with use of cardiopulmonary resuscitation in seriously ill hospitalized patients. JAMA 1999;282:2333-2339.

9. Hossack KF, Hartwig R. Cardiac arrest–associated supervised cardiac rehabilitation. J Cardiac Rehab 1982;2:402-408.

10. Van Camp SP, Peterson RA. Cardiovascular complications of out-patient cardiac rehabilitation programs. JAMA 1986;256:1160-1163.

11. Cummins RO. From concept to standard-of-care? Review of the clinical experience with automated electrical defibrillators. Ann Emerg Med 1989;18:1269-1275.

12. Eisenberg MS, Horwood BT, Cummins RO, et al. Cardiac arrest and resuscitation: a tale of 29 cities. Ann Emerg Med 1990;19:179-186.

13. Eisenberg MS, Cummins RO, Damon S, et al. Survival rates from out-of-hospital cardiac arrest: recommendations for uniform definitions and data to report. Ann Emerg Med 1990;19:1249-1259.

14. Eisenberg MS, Copass MK, Hallstrom AP, et al. Treatment of out of hospital cardiac arrests with rapid defibrillation by emergency medical technicians. N Engl J Med 1980;302:1379-1383.

15. Cummins RO, Sanders A, Mancini E, et al. Inhospital resuscitation: a statement for healthcare professionals from the American Heart Association Emergency Cardiac Care Committee and the Advanced Cardiac Life Support, Basic Life Support, and Pediatric Resuscitation, and Program Administration Subcommittees. Circulation 1997;95:2211-2212.

16. Becker LB, Berg RA, Pepe PE, et al. A reappraisal of mouth-to-mouth ventilation during bystander-initiated cardiopulmonary resuscitation: a statement for healthcare professionals from the Ventilation Working Group of the Basic Life Support and Pediatric Life Support Subcommittees, American Heart Association. Circulation 1997;96:2102-2112.

17. Anonymous. Advanced cardiovascular life support. Circulation 2000;102:I-95.

18. Thalman JJ, Rinaldo-Gallo S, MacIntyre NR. Analysis of an endotracheal intubation service provided by respiratory care practitioners. Respir Care 1993;38:469-473.

19. Selleck BA. Cricoid pressure to control regurgitation of the stomach contents during induction of anesthesia. Lancet 1962;2:404.

20. Rumball C, MacDonald D. The PTL, Combitube, laryngeal mask, and oral airway: a randomized prehospital comparative study of ventilatory device effectiveness and cost-effectiveness in 470 cases of cardiopulmonary arrest. Prehosp Emerg Care 1997;1:1-10.

21. Simmons M, Daeo D, Moon L, et al. Bench evaluation of three face shield CPR devices. Respir Care 1995;40:618-623.

22. Hess D, Ness C, Oppel A, et al. Evaluation of mouth-to-mask devices. Respir Care 1989;34:191-195.

23. Johannigman JA, Branson RD. Oxygen enrichment of expired gas for mouth-to-mask resuscitation. Respir Care 1991;36:99-103.

24. Emergency Cardiac Care Committee and Subcommittees, American Heart Association. Guidelines for cardiopulmonary resuscitation and emergency cardiac care. III. Advanced cardiac life support. JAMA 1992;268:2199.

25. American Society for Testing and Materials. Standard specification for performance and safety requirements for resuscitators intended for use with humans. Designation: F-920-93. Annual Book of ASTM Standards 1995;13.01:266.

26. ISO Technical Committee ISO/TC 121. Anesthetic and respiratory equipment: international standard ISO 8382: resuscitators intended for use with humans. Switzerland: International Organization for Standardization; 1988.

27. Barnes TA. Emergency ventilation techniques and related equipment. Respir Care 1992;37:673.

28. Hess D, Baran C. Ventilatory volumes using mouth-to-mouth, mouth-to-mask, and bag-valve-mask techniques. Am J Emer Med 1985;3:292-296.

29. Hess D, Goff G. The effects of two-hand versus one-hand ventilation on volumes delivered during bag-valve ventilation at various resistances and compliances. Respir Care 1987;32:1025-1028.

30. Hess D, Goff G, Johnson K. The effect of hand size, resuscitator brand, and use of two hands on volumes delivered during adult bag-valve ventilation. Respir Care 1989;34:191-195.

31. Jesudian MC, Harrison RR, Keenan RL, et al. Bag-valve-mask ventilation: two rescuers are better than one: preliminary report. Crit Care Med 1985;13:122-123.

32. Hess D, Spahr C. An evaluation of volumes delivered by selected adult disposable resuscitators: the effects of hand size, number of hands used, and use of disposable medical gloves. Respir Care 1990;35:800-805.

33. Johannigman JA, Branson RD, Davis K, et al. Techniques of emergency ventilation: a model to evaluate tidal volume, airway pressure, gastric insufflation. J Trauma 1991;31:93-98.

34. Hess D, Hirsch C, Marquis-D'Amico C, et al. Imposed work and oxygen delivery during spontaneous breathing with adult disposable manual ventilators. Anesthesiology 1994;81:1256-1263.

35. Eberle B, Dick WF, Schneider T, et al. Checking the carotid pulse: diagnostic accuracy of first responders in patients with and without a carotid pulse. Resuscitation 1996;33:107-116.

36. Hallstrom A, Cobb L, Johnson E, et al. Cardiopulmonary resuscitation by chest compression alone or with mouth-to-mouth ventilation. N Engl J Med 2000;342:1546-1553.

37. Hargarten KM, Stueven HA, Waite EM, et al. Prehospital experience with defibrillation of coarse ventricular fibrillation: a ten-year review. Ann Emerg Med 1990;19:157-162.

38. Kaye W, Mancini JE, Giuliano KK, et al. Strengthening the in-hospital chain of survival with rapid defibrillation by first responders using automated external defibrillators: training and retention issues. Ann Emerg Med 1995;25:163.

39. Anonymous. The automated external defibrillator. Circulation 2000;102:I-60–I-76.

40. Howells TH. Disaster at the dining table. Br Med J 1984;289:510-511.

41. CDC. Fatal injuries to children—US 1986. JAMA 1990;264:952-953.

42. Anonymous. Pediatric basic life support. Circulation 2000;102:I-253–I-290.

43. Anonymous. Pediatric advance life support. Circulation 2000;102:I-291.

44. Anonymous. Neonatal resuscitation. Circulation 2000;102: I-343.

45. Hirschman AM, Kaavath RE. Venting versus ventilating: a danger of manual resuscitation bags. Chest 1982;82:369-370.

46. Finer NN, Barrington KJ, Al-Fadley F, et al. Limitations of self-inflating resuscitators. Pediatrics 1986;77(3):417-420.

47. Goldstein B, Catlin EA, Vetere JM, et al. The role of in-line manometers in minimizing peak and mean airway pressure during the hand-regulated ventilation of newborn infants. Respir Care 1989;34:23-27.

48. Bizzle TL, Kotas RV. Positive pressure hand ventilation: potential errors in estimating inflation pressures. Pediatrics 1983; 72:122-125.

49. Chernick V. Lung rupture in the newborn infant. Respir Care 1986;31:628-635.

50. Field D, Milner AD, Hopkin IE. Efficacy of manual resuscitation at birth. Arch Dis Childhood 1986;61:300-302.

51. Terndrup TE, Kanter RK, Cherry RA. A comparison of infant ventilation methods performed by prehospital personnel, Ann Emerg Med 1989;18:607-611.

52. Hess D, Alagar R. Methods of emergency drug administration. Respir Care 1995;40:498-514.

53. Anonymous. Advanced cardiovascular life support: defibrillation. Circulation 2000;102:I-90.

CHAPTER 38

Pulmonary Rehabilitation

Neil R. MacIntyre*

OBJECTIVES

1. Define pulmonary rehabilitation using the standards established by the American College of Chest Physicians (ACCP) and the American Thoracic Society (ATS).
2. Identify the multidisciplinary team members that comprise a pulmonary rehabilitation program.
3. Describe the two types of pulmonary rehabilitation programs.
4. Identify candidates for a pulmonary rehabilitation program.
5. Describe the components of patient assessment in a comprehensive pulmonary rehabilitation program.
6. Describe the role of education in a pulmonary rehabilitation program.
7. Discuss the benefits of upper and lower extremity exercise training in a pulmonary rehabilitation program.
8. Explain the guidelines used to prescribe an exercise training program.
9. Discuss the roles of the following in a pulmonary rehabilitation program: psychologic therapies, physical therapy, individualized instruction, nutrition counseling, and pharmacologic therapy.

KEY TERMS

Aerobic	Dyspnea Index	Peripheral Deconditioning
Borg Scale	Exercise Assessment	Psychosocial Assessment
Cognitive Function	Exercise Capacity	Pulmonary Rehabilitation
Diaphragmatic Breathing	Exercise Conditioning	Ventilatory Capacity
Dyspnea	Functional Capacity	Ventilatory Reserves

Comprehensive **pulmonary rehabilitation** is a concept that has evolved since the 1960s. Before then, the standard therapy for patients with chronic lung disease was rest and avoidance of physical activity. In the early 1960s, however, studies challenged this standard therapy by

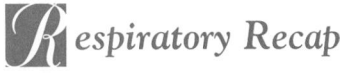

espiratory Recap

> **Role of Exercise in COPD**
>
> Exercise training in patients with COPD increases exercise capacity.
> Exercise training improves the patient's psychologic state.
> Exercise training *does not* improve pulmonary function.

*The author is indebted to the pioneering work of Dr. Nelson Leatherman in establishing the Duke University Pulmonary Rehabilitation Program and providing much of the material on which this chapter is based.

demonstrating that exercise training in individuals with chronic obstructive pulmonary disease (COPD) not only resulted in training effects similar to those observed in normal subjects but also promoted a state of well-being.[1] Numerous subsequent investigations supported these initial findings.[1-3] Almost universally, the early investigations supported three conclusions: (1) Exercise training in individuals with COPD increases **exercise capacity,** (2) exercise training improves the person's psychologic state, and (3) exercise training *does not* improve pulmonary function.

As a consequence of these developments, the American College of Chest Physicians (ACCP) in 1974 and the American Thoracic Society (ATS) in 1981 both formally recognized the effectiveness of pulmonary rehabilitation[4] and offered the following definition:

> Pulmonary rehabilitation may be defined as an art of medical practice wherein an individually tailored multidisciplinary program is formulated, which, through accurate diagnosis, therapy, emotional support, and education, stabilizes or reverses both the physio- and psychopathology of pulmonary diseases and attempts to return the patient to the highest possible functional capacity allowed by his pulmonary handicap and overall life situation.

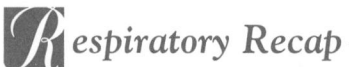
Respiratory Recap

> ### ACCP/ATS *Definition of Pulmonary Rehabilitation*
>
> Pulmonary rehabilitation may be defined as an art of medical practice wherein an individually tailored multidisciplinary program is formulated, which, through accurate diagnosis, therapy, emotional support, and education, stabilizes or reverses both the physiopathology and psychopathology of pulmonary diseases and attempts to return the patient to the highest possible functional capacity allowed by the pulmonary handicap and overall life situation.

Since the 1970s, the number of pulmonary rehabilitation programs has increased dramatically. Indeed, extrapolation of survey data suggests that by the 1980s, several hundred such programs were operational in the United States.[5] These programs have become increasingly multidisciplinary and comprehensive, incorporating psychologic, nutritional, and vocational support; oxygen therapy; bronchial hygiene therapy; education; and exercise.

Mechanisms of Functional Deterioration in Chronic Lung Disease

Without a sudden event to stimulate a change in lifestyle, individuals with chronic pulmonary disease, unlike those with cardiac disease, generally have a long, slow, downhill course. Chronic lung disease progressively damages lung tissue and airways, resulting in a depletion of **ventilatory reserves.** Complicating this damage physiologically are abnormalities in gas exchange and elevations in pulmonary vascular pressures that lead to right ventricular dysfunction. All these factors contribute to the sensation of **dyspnea** and the resultant limitation on physical activity.[6]

As dyspnea and exercise capacity worsen, the need for medical care increases and the individual's ability to self-care decreases; a confusing combination of functional limitations and dependence on others are thrust on the patient. The net effect is a profound sense of loss of control, with a consequent depression and anxiety.

These factors are further worsened by the vicious cycle of inactivity (Figure 38-1). The cycle begins when the individual begins to associate exertional dyspnea with the disease and no longer recognizes dyspnea as a normal response to exertion. In this setting, exertional dyspnea promotes increased levels of anxiety, depression, and fear of exertion, all of which generally lead to an "exertion phobia" and a reduction in physical activity. The lack of exercise in turn leads to both central and **peripheral deconditioning** and ultimately to decreased endurance, weakness, and muscular atrophy. As a result of deconditioning, the individual experiences greater dyspnea, an even greater intolerance to exertion, and further loss of **functional capacity.** As the cycle continues, the individual's exercise capacity spirals progressively downward while the levels of fear, anxiety, and depression increase unabated. As the individual becomes progressively more physically and psychologically incapacitated, the consumption of medical resources increases dramatically. The progressive loss of exercise capacity resulting from the vicious cycle of inactivity is superimposed on the underlying functional reduction caused by the lung disease.

The goal of pulmonary rehabilitation is to improve the quality of life of individuals with chronic lung disease by increasing their functional capacity and sense of well-being. Central to the achievement of this goal is to break this cycle of inactivity with the institution of a lifelong exercise program. The comprehensive nature of pulmonary rehabilitation facilitates this fundamental lifestyle change not only by directing and encouraging formal exercise but also by maximizing all aspects of chronic lung disease management.

Program Structure

The basic elements of pulmonary rehabilitation programs first were outlined by the 1981 ATS Statement on Pulmonary Rehabilitation[4] and later formalized in the American Association of Cardiovascular and Pulmonary Rehabilitation (AACVPR) guidelines and program certification process.[7] Even within these established guidelines, however, the potential exists for diversity in the structure of pulmonary rehabilitation programs. This potential diversity results from consideration of several factors at the time the pulmonary rehabilitation program is under devel-

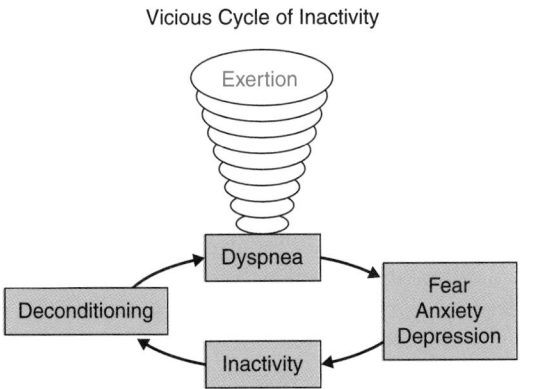

Vicious Cycle of Inactivity

Figure 38-1   The vicious cycle of inactivity. (Modified from Leatherman NA. Pulmonary rehabilitation. In: Dantzker D, MacIntyre N, Bakow E, editors. Comprehensive respiratory care. Philadelphia: WB Saunders; 1995.)

opment, including the patient population, the available physical facilities, and the available pool of allied health professionals.

The pulmonary rehabilitation team is usually a multidisciplinary team that consists of a pulmonary physician and a number of allied health professionals that include respiratory therapists, physical therapists, psychologists, nutritionists, occupational therapists, social workers, a chaplain, and respiratory nurses, among others. Although this description implies the necessity for a large, diverse team, the recommended services for pulmonary rehabilitation may be provided by far fewer personnel if the individuals are appropriately trained in the evaluation and management of pulmonary disease patients. The ultimate provider of the essential services depends on the allied health professionals available to the program and the size of the facility and varies from program to program.

Pulmonary rehabilitation programs often provide two types of programs: (1) a short-term, intensive program that focuses on pulmonary rehabilitation and (2) a long-term maintenance program that is less time intensive.

Intensive Programs

Intensive programs generally provide two to five sessions per week for periods of 4 to 12 weeks. The emphasis of the intensive program is on exercise training, education, medication optimization, bronchial hygiene, and psychosocial support. Much of this program is usually conducted by a respiratory therapist. Other health care specialists who contribute regularly to the program include a physical therapist, an exercise physiologist, a clinical pharmacist, a nutritionist, a pulmonary nurse clinician, and an occupational therapist. Individual consultations with specialists in nutrition, psychology, and smoking cessation are common. The intense focus of this program produces recognized benefits sooner than do less-intensive programs—a factor that serves to enhance patient motivation.

Maintenance Programs

Maintenance programs serve primarily as medically supervised programs for individuals with pulmonary disease who reside locally. Enrollment is usually limited to individuals who have successfully completed the intensive program. Such programs are generally open daily, and participants select their own schedules. Although the primary emphasis is on **exercise conditioning,** all intensive program services are available to the participants as needed. The long-term social interaction with peers and the formation of support groups is a major advantage of this program.

Respiratory Recap

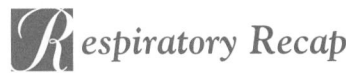

Types of Pulmonary Rehabilitation Programs
Short-term intensive programs
Long-term maintenance programs

Sequence of Pulmonary Rehabilitation

Patient Selection

Any individual with stable chronic respiratory disease who is symptomatic and experiences dyspnea on exertion should be considered a candidate for pulmonary rehabilitation. In addition, candidates must be free of acute illness (including other unstable medical conditions, such as ischemic coronary disease) and must be motivated to lead a more active, healthier life.

The clinical description of persons who potentially may benefit from pulmonary rehabilitation has broadened over the years. In the position statement published by the ATS in 1981 the section on candidate selection mentions only those with COPD, excluding any mention of individuals without COPD. As recently as 1988, 23% of the programs in the United States limited patient selection to those with COPD.[5] Recent evidence has demonstrated that multidisciplinary pulmonary rehabilitation programs are also valuable in the management of patients with restrictive pulmonary diseases and more recently, those undergoing transplantation or lung volume reduction surgery.[7,8] These findings should encourage acceptance of patients with non-COPD pulmonary diseases as well as those with COPD into pulmonary rehabilitation programs.

The observation that individuals with limited **ventilatory capacity** may be unable to exercise with sufficient intensity to receive a training effect has raised concern over whether they can derive benefits from a comprehensive pulmonary rehabilitation program. Although evidence of a true training effect in this group of individuals remains controversial, at a minimum they can benefit from a program designed to improve coordination, muscle strength, suppleness, and state of well-being. Even exercise capacity may be improved in individuals with limited ventilatory capacity because the standard training effect is only one of several ways in which exercise capacity is known to increase.[3,9,10]

Concern that exercise might precipitate respiratory failure by overloading weakened respiratory muscles leads to speculation that exercise training might be contraindicated in hypercapnic COPD patients. However, hypercapnic COPD patients with severe ventilatory impairment and respiratory muscle weakness have been shown to tolerate exercise and benefit significantly from intensive pulmonary rehabilitation.[11] Similarly, exercise hypoxemia has been considered by some clinicians to be a contraindication to an exercise program. The experience of others, however, has been that appropriate supplemental oxygen and proper monitoring (for example, via oximetry) allow such individuals to participate fully in all aspects of the exercise program.

Patient Assessment

A comprehensive patient evaluation is essential to attain the goals of pulmonary rehabilitation and serves as the foundation on which the individually tailored program is constructed. Any condition or attitude that potentially limits the patient's ability to perform desired activities or grasp essential information must be identified by the health care team, assessed, and ultimately addressed. All members of the rehabilitation team are vital participants in the process of gathering and evaluating information from patient questionnaires, interviews, and a variety of clinical evaluations.

The first step in this assessment is to make an accurate diagnosis of the patient's pulmonary problem and any complicating medical problems. The diagnosis should be substantiated by history, physical examination, pulmonary function testing, and as needed, chest roentgenography and other laboratory tests. The importance of this initial step is evidenced by the inability of many patients to report a correct diagnosis. In one study, 64% of the patients entering a pulmonary rehabilitation program reported an incorrect diagnosis of their pulmonary problem. Other diseases or medical problems that have a potential impact on the rehabilitation process also must be identified. As many as 91% of the patients entering a pulmonary rehabilitation program were identified as having other medical problems, such as rhinitis-sinusitis (52%), hypertension (34%), gastrointestinal conditions (30%), and dysrhythmias or coronary artery disease (27%).[12] Other potentially complicating conditions include diabetes, obesity, osteoporosis, and stroke. Once proper diagnoses are made, an appropriate medication regimen can be established.

Exercise assessment is a critical component to be evaluated before participants enter a rehabilitation program. These assessments perform the following two functions:

1. They quantitate the level of disability and provide information used to set initial exercise loads and program expectations.

2. They provide insight into the various cardiorespiratory factors involved in the functional disabilities, permitting focused therapies to be performed.

For instance, the detection of exercise hemoglobin desaturation leads to the initiation of oxygen therapy; the detection of exercise bronchospasm leads to the initiation of improved bronchodilator therapy; and the detection of exercise cardiac dysrhythmias prompts the health care provider to perform a more thorough cardiovascular exam. Moreover, subjects who reach a maximum predicted heart rate without reaching ventilatory or gas exchange limits can be expected to gain particular benefit from the cardiovascular training effects of exercise.

Because psychologic disturbances are common in patients with chronic lung disease,[13,14] an initial **psychosocial assessment** is important to participation in a pulmonary rehabilitation program. The most common emotional consequences of COPD are depression and anxiety, which can further reinforce social isolation and inactivity. **Cognitive function** also has been shown to be impaired in these individuals, perhaps as a consequence of chronic hypoxemia. Medications and psychotherapy can be provided as necessary.

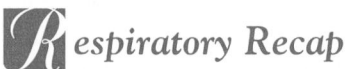
espiratory Recap

Assessment of the Pulmonary Rehabilitation Patient
Accurate diagnosis of patient's pulmonary problem
Exercise evaluation
Psychosocial evaluation
Cognitive function
Physical therapy evaluations
Nutritional evaluations
Occupational therapy evaluations
Educational evaluation

Other assessments necessary before an individual begins pulmonary rehabilitation include physical therapy evaluations, nutritional evaluations, occupational therapy (especially activities of daily living [ADL]) evaluations, and an education assessment focusing on the individual's knowledge and understanding of the disease process and its management. AACVPR guidelines[7] also recommend electrocardiograms, complete blood counts, and serum electrolyte measurements. A particularly important assessment is tobacco usage. Although current smokers reasonably should be able to participate in a rehabilitation program, formal efforts should be made to discontinue smoking.

Program Implementation

Education   A primary purpose of the educational component of pulmonary rehabilitation is to provide the framework for self-care. Through an educational process of instruction, supervision, and practice, patients can acquire an awareness of their disease and its management that allows them to take responsibility for their own care. A spouse, family member, or close friend who participates in the educational activities can provide familial understanding of the disease process and can reinforce the recommended self-care techniques in the home setting.

The educational process usually consists of a combination of lectures, discussions, demonstrations, and practice sessions. During all program activities the patient's knowledge and ability to perform self-management techniques are continually reinforced. Topics typically covered in formal lectures and discussion sessions include the anatomy and physiology of the lung, the pathophysiology of chronic lung disease, pulmonary medications, nutrition, physiologic responses to exercise, sexual concerns, travel concerns, ways to cope with chronic lung disease, early recognition and management of infections and exacerbations, and psychosocial issues.

Respiratory therapy and physical therapy techniques are presented more appropriately in either individual or group demonstrations and in practice sessions. These techniques include cleaning and care of equipment, proper use of metered dose inhalers and spacers, relaxation techniques, clearing of secretions by use of techniques of controlled coughing, postural drainage, percussion and vibration, and supplemental oxygen therapy. Educational material in the form of pamphlets, booklets, and books is available from a multitude of sources, including the American Lung Association. This additional information should be used to support and reinforce the information the patient receives in the lectures, discussions, and demonstrations.

Breathing retraining traditionally has been a key aspect of the educational component of a pulmonary rehabilitation program. Pursed-lip breathing and **diaphragmatic breathing** are commonly used concomitantly to reduce shortness of breath and improve gas exchange. By using pursed-lip breathing, patients may be able to maintain adequate oxygenation without supplemental oxygen.

The success of the program's educational process may be assessed through testing of didactic information before and after instruction and requirements that each patient satisfactorily demonstrate the recommended management techniques.

Exercise Training Prescription
In general the exercise training experience in a pulmonary rehabilitation program should expose the patient to a balance of three types of exercise: stretching and flexibility exercises, strengthening exercises, and endurance exercises.[7,9,10,12] Stretching and flexibility exercises are usually part of a floor exercise routine that develops suppleness, improves range of motion, and helps provide a general warm-up. Strength training may be obtained as part of the floor exercise routine through exercises that require dumbbells, cuff weights, or a stretch band. Pulmonary patients also do well with free weights and weight machines for strength training. Strength exercises require a stimulus of high intensity and low frequency. General endurance training involves exercises that produce a cardiopulmonary stress that results in elevated heart rate and ventilation. Such exercises include walking, rowing, swimming, water aerobics, cycling (arm or leg), stair climbing, and so on, provided that the exercise intensity produces sufficient cardiopulmonary stress. Compared with strength training, endurance training is of lower intensity and higher frequency.

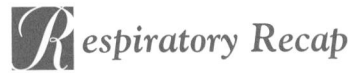

Respiratory Recap

Types of Exercise Used in a Pulmonary Rehabilitation Program
Stretching and flexibility
Strength training
Endurance

The benefits of exercise training are for the most part specific to the muscles and tasks involved in training. For instance, a walking program produces significant improvement in walking performance but not in swimming or biking performance. Therefore considering the particular mode of exercise in conjunction with the needs and goals of the patient is important. If a patient has a stated goal that requires improvement in stair climbing, this activity should be one of the modes of exercise in the prescription. Walking is generally considered an essential exercise because of its prevalence in ADL and most likely for that reason, most exercise training prescriptions use predominantly lower extremity exercises.

Many individuals with chronic airway obstruction experience marked shortness of breath when they use their arms for even simple tasks. Arm exercise may contribute to the dyspnea by contributing to ventilatory muscle fatigue, placing a load on an already stressed system, and placing a nonventilatory demand on shoulder girdle muscles that have been recruited to act as accessory muscles of respiration. Improvement in upper extremity function as a result of specific upper extremity exercises has been demonstrated in individuals with COPD. Improvement in upper extremity function has been observed to carry over to self-care, leisure, and other arm activities. By combining arm and leg exercises in a training program for patients with chronic airway obstruction, other clinicians have shown not only increased exercise performance in both upper and lower extremities but also a significantly improved state of well-being that was greater in the combined training than in either arm or leg training alone. The conclusion is that leg and arm exercise should be combined in exercise programs for patients with chronic airway obstruction.

Upper extremity exercise training may be accomplished through simple games or activities that use the arms above shoulder height (for example, passing an object overhead) or through gravity-resistive exercises (for example, performing arm circles at shoulder height or walking with exaggerated arm movement, possibly with hand weights). Upper extremity strength training may be achieved by performance of exercises with free weights, pulley systems, or weight machines. Arm endurance training may be accomplished with an arm ergometer, rowing machine, combined arm and leg bicycle, or cross-country ski machine.

Well-established guidelines exist to prescribe the intensity of endurance exercise for normal subjects, as well as for cardiac patients. These guidelines are based on target exercise heart rates expressed as a percent of the predicted maximum heart rate. Application of these guidelines, however, may not always be appropriate to pulmonary patients because the ventilatory impairment may prevent the patient from reaching the predicted maximum heart rate.

The initial load prescription should be of sufficiently low intensity that the patient can accomplish it without discomfort. Nothing destroys a patient's motivation faster than failure to complete the initial exercise or experiencing significant discomfort during or after the first exercise session. For example, the initial loads used by the Duke University Pulmonary Rehabilitation Program[12] for the stationary bicycle and arm ergometer are based on the maximum workload reached during the exercise stress test (W_{max}). The initial bicycle workload (W_{bike}) is set at 50% of the maximum workload ($0.5 \times W_{max}$). This value is based on data suggesting that an individual can be expected to work for 8 hours at 50% of maximum work capacity without undue fatigue. The initial load prescription for arm exercise is 30% of W_{max} (or 60% of W_{bike}) and is based on the observation that the aerobic power of the arms ranges from 50% to 70% of the maximum power output of the legs.

Workloads must be reassessed each exercise session and adjusted according to the patient's progress. After the initial settings the appropriate intensity for subsequent target workload (the desired training load) has been an area of controversy. Work from Casaburi suggests that training intensity should be pushed to a training effect if at all possible.[10] Even patients with ventilatory or gas exchange limitations who cannot reach these target heart rates also appear to benefit from higher rather than lower levels of exercise. Thus strategies using target intensities that reach the highest level attained on the initial exercise stress test should be the ultimate goal.

To accomplish the transition from the relatively low initial loads to the higher target loads, the Duke University program relies on the **Borg scale** of perceived exertion as a measure of perceived stress and the exercise heart rate as a measure of cardiopulmonary stress.[15] If the Borg rating of the previous exercise session is less than 15 and the heart rate during exercise is less than the heart rate achieved during the assessment exercise test, consideration is given to an increase in the intensity. Whenever the patient can perform a given load for the duration of the exercise session, the load is increased by 0.25 kilopond for the bicycle ergometer (about 12.5 Watts) and 50 kiloponds per minute for the arm ergometer (about 9 Watts).

After approximately six exercise sessions, most patients will have attained an exercise level representing a high percentage of the target workload.

Whenever the patient experiences significant symptoms of fatigue or dyspnea, instead of a cessation of exercise the load is reduced and the patient encouraged to complete the exercise if possible. When the initial load is already the lowest possible, the patient stops until the symptoms subside and then continues the exercise to completion. The duration of the rest period is considered part of the exercise period. The short-term goal then becomes a reduction in the number of rests during the exercise period.

The recommended minimum duration and frequency of endurance exercise should be no less than 20 minutes, three times per week.[3,10] Increasing the duration and frequency beyond this minimum must take into consideration the motivation and goals of the patient and balance the time spent in training against the benefits derived from a more intense training regimen. The primary benefits of additional time spent training are faster and greater improvement in physical capacity.

All exercise training should be performed under conditions of adequate arterial oxygenation (PaO_2 >55 mm Hg, O_2 saturation >88%). If the initial patient assessment has determined that the resting oxygenation is low or that significant desaturation occurs with exertion, supplemental oxygen must be provided to the patient to maintain adequate oxygen saturation. Usually, oxygen delivered at 2 L/min via nasal cannula is sufficient. In some cases, however, adequate oxygenation during exertion may be difficult to provide with even a partial-rebreathing system. When adequate oxygenation cannot be maintained, either the intensity of the exercise must be reduced or the patient must be instructed to stop exercising until oxygenation is again adequate. Besides reducing the medical risk associated with low oxygenation, supplemental oxygen often allows the patient who needs oxygen to exercise for a longer duration at a higher intensity, thereby enhancing the beneficial effects of the exercise.

Other Interventions   Other focused interventions often depend on the individual patient. Patients with clinically important depression or anxiety may need focused psychologic therapies, whereas those with orthopedic impairments may benefit from physical therapy. Similarly, patients with specific educational needs (for example, medication understanding, equipment operation, chest physical therapy procedures) may need individualized instruction, whereas those with nutritional issues may require nutrition counseling.

Physician review of the medication regimen is particularly important. Chronic medical therapy for COPD and other chronic lung diseases is constantly evolving, and the array of medications (for example, short- and long-acting β-agonists, short- and long-acting anticholinergics, inhaled and oral steroids, and oxygen) can be very confusing to chronically ill patients. The physician should also formulate an action plan for the patient in the event of an acute exacerbation. An undue delay in the initiation of antibiotic and steroid administration (in appropriate patients) can be costly in terms of subsequent health care needs.

Outcomes from a Pulmonary Rehabilitation Program

In 1997 the ACCP/AACVPR published a comprehensive evidence-based review on the effectiveness of pulmonary rehabilitation.[3] In this report, conclusions and recommendations were graded on the strength of the evidence, as follows:

- Grade A conclusions were based on scientific evidence provided by well-designed, well-conducted, controlled trials with statistically significant and consistent findings.
- Grade B conclusions were based on scientific evidence provided by observational studies or by controlled trials with less consistent results.
- Grade C conclusions were based on expert opinions because available scientific evidence did not present consistent results or was lacking.

Table 38-1 summarizes these conclusions.

Evidence supporting the benefits of exercise training in chronic lung disease is compelling and received grade A (lower extremity) and grade B (upper extremity) support in the ACCP/AACVPR review. Lower extremity exercise programs consistently improved walk distance (6% to 33%) and maximum workload (10% to 102%) in all studies reviewed. Proposed mechanisms of improvement include improved **aerobic** capacity (in those who can reach cardiovascular training levels), increased motivation, desensitization to the sensation of dyspnea, improved ventilatory muscle

function, and improved techniques of performance. Data from upper extremity exercise programs were less extensive but did support the concept that upper extremity exercise might improve the thoracic cage muscles of ventilation and improve ADL.

Evidence supporting the effectiveness of pulmonary rehabilitation in reducing dyspnea also received a grade A rating in the ACCP/AACVPR report. This effectiveness was a consistent finding with any number of dyspnea grading scales (for example, visual analog scales, baseline **dyspnea index,** transitional dyspnea index, and other respiratory questionnaires). The mechanisms of reduced dyspnea no doubt depend on many factors but would include better exercise tolerance (and reduced ventilation for a given load), better breathing patterns, better medications, and a better comprehension by the patient of the disease and the ways in which it can be effectively managed.

Many studies have demonstrated that psychosocial function improves as a result of pulmonary rehabilitation.[13,14] Much of this benefit, however, may come from improved exercise tolerance, reduced dyspnea, and a better understanding of the disease process and its management by the patient. Indeed the ACCP/AACVPR report only gave a grade C rating to a pulmonary rehabilitation program for the evidence supporting routine, formal psychosocial components. This rating, however, should not be interpreted as evidence stating that psychosocial support is unimportant or that selected patients would not benefit from focused therapies or medications.

Quality-of-life (QOL) indicators have consistently shown benefit from pulmonary rehabilitation. However, because the instruments used to assess QOL are less rigorous than dyspnea indices for pulmonary patients[16] and because controlled trials

$\mathcal{T}$ABLE 38-1

Summary of Recommendations and Evidence Grades for Pulmonary Rehabilitation Guidelines for Patients with COPD

Component/Outcome	Recommendations	Grade
Lower extremity training	Lower extremity training improves exercise tolerance and is recommended as part of pulmonary rehabilitation.	A
Upper extremity training	Strength and endurance training improve arm function; arm exercises should be included in pulmonary rehabilitation.	B
Ventilatory muscle training	Scientific evidence does not support the routine use of ventilatory muscle training in pulmonary rehabilitation; it may be considered in selected patients with decreased respiratory muscle strength and breathlessness.	B
Psychosocial behavioral, and educational components and outcomes	Evidence does not support the benefits of short-term psychosocial interventions as single therapeutic modalities; longer-term interventions may be beneficial; expert opinion supports inclusion of educational and psychosocial intervention components in pulmonary rehabilitation.	C
Dyspnea	Pulmonary rehabilitation improves the symptom of dyspnea.	A
Quality of life	Pulmonary rehabilitation improves health-related quality of life.	B
Health care use	Pulmonary rehabilitation has reduced the number of hospitalizations and days of hospitalization.	B
Survival	Pulmonary rehabilitation may improve survival.	C

From Pulmonary rehabilitation. Joint ACCP/AACVPR evidence-based guidelines. Chest 1997;112:1363-1396.
COPD, Chronic obstructive pulmonary disease.

are not always consistent, the ACCP/AACVPR report only gave improvements in QOL a grade B rating. Like improvements in dyspnea and psychosocial function, the mechanisms for improved QOL after pulmonary rehabilitation most likely involve many factors.

An important benefit to pulmonary rehabilitation would be a reduction in health care use and costs. The ACCP/AACVPR report identified two randomized trials and two nonrandomized trials assessing health care use after pulmonary rehabilitation, and all demonstrated a reduction. However, because statistical significance was not attained, this evidence received only a grade B rating.

Finally, evidence supporting a survival benefit for pulmonary rehabilitation does not exist. This potential effect thus only received a grade C rating in the ACCP/AACVPR report. However, the rating should not be surprising because the goals of pulmonary rehabilitation are not to reverse the disease process, but rather to improve the patient's functional capabilities within the constraints of the reduced lung function.

𝒦ey 𝒫oints

- Pulmonary rehabilitation programs are comprehensive and multidisciplinary.
- The goal of pulmonary rehabilitation is to improve quality of life and increase functional capacity and sense of well-being.
- Individuals with stable chronic respiratory disease who are asymptomatic, experience dyspnea on exertion, are free from acute illness, and are motivated to lead a more active life are candidates for a pulmonary rehabilitation program.
- Patient education and self-care are critical components of a pulmonary rehabilitation program.
- Exercise training generally entails the enhancement of upper and lower extremity function.
- In the establishment of an exercise training prescription the initial load should be of sufficiently low intensity that the patient can accomplish it without discomfort.
- Both rationale and evidence exist for consideration of physiologic and psychologic mechanisms for the functional benefits derived from pulmonary rehabilitation.

References

1. Casaburi R, Petty TL. Principles and practice of pulmonary rehabilitation. Philadelphia: WB Saunders; 1993.
2. Ries AL. Position paper of the American Association of Cardiovascular and Pulmonary Rehabilitation: scientific basis of pulmonary rehabilitation. J Cardiopulm Rehabil 1990;10: 418-441.
3. ACCP/AACVPR Pulmonary Rehabilitation Guidelines Panel. Pulmonary rehabilitation: evidence based guidelines. Chest 1997;112:1363-1396.
4. American Thoracic Society official statement. Pulmonary rehabilitation. Am Rev Respir Dis 1981;124:663-666.
5. Bickford LS, Hodgkin JE. National pulmonary rehabilitation survey. J Cardiopulm Rehabil 1988;11:473-491.
6. American Thoracic Society. Standards for the diagnosis and care of patients with COPD and asthma. Am J Respir Crit Care Med 1995;152:S77-S121.
7. American Association of Cardiovascular and Pulmonary Rehabilitation. Guidelines for pulmonary rehabilitation programs. 2nd ed. Champaign, Ill: Human Kinetics; 1998.
8. Hilling LR, Connors GL. Pulmonary rehabilitation. Respir Care Clin N Am 1998;4:1-183.
9. Ries AL, Archibald CJ. Endurance exercise training at maximal targets in patients with chronic obstructive pulmonary disease. J Cardiopulm Rehabil 1987;7:594-601.
10. Casaburi R, Petessio A, Ioli F, et al. Reductions in exercise lactic acidosis and ventilation as a result of training in patients with obstructive lung disease. Am Rev Respir Dis 1991;143:9-18.
11. Lacasse Y, Wong E, Guyatt GH, et al. Meta-analysis of respiratory rehabilitation in COPD. Lancet 1996;348:1115-1119.
12. Leatherman NA. Pulmonary rehabilitation. In: Dantzker D, MacIntyre N, Bakow E, editors. Comprehensive respiratory care. Philadelphia: WB Saunders; 1995.
13. Ries AL, Kaplan RM, Linberg TM, et al. Effects of pulmonary rehabilitation on physiological and psychological outcomes in patients with COPD. Ann Int Med 1995;122:823-832.
14. Emery CF, Leatherman NE, Burker EJ, et al. Psychological outcomes of a pulmonary rehabilitation program. Chest 1991; 100:613-617.
15. Borg GA. Psychophysical bases for perceived exertion. Med Sci Sports Exer 1982;14:377-381.
16. Mahler, DA, Wells CK. Evaluation of clinical methods for evaluating dyspnea. Chest 1988;93:580-586.

CHAPTER 39

Mechanical Ventilators: Classification and Principles of Operation

Robert L. Chatburn

OBJECTIVES

1. Write the general outline for classification of ventilators.
2. Describe the major drive mechanisms and output control valves of mechanical ventilators.
3. Describe the Equation of Motion and how it relates to ventilator classification.
4. Compare open- and closed-loop control of mechanical ventilators.
5. Describe dual control.
6. Discuss the differences among pressure, volume, and flow control.
7. Define control variables, phase variables, and conditional variables.
8. Draw the pressure, volume, and flow curves for rectangular pressure output and for rectangular, ramp, and sinusoidal flow output.
9. Describe the major modes of ventilation in terms of the control and phase variables for mandatory and spontaneous breaths.
10. Define *mandatory* and *spontaneous* breaths.
11. Describe the effects of patient circuit compliance and resistance on ventilator output.
12. Compare input power alarms, control circuit alarms, and output alarms.

KEY TERMS

Alarm Event	Cycle	Expiratory Phase
Assisted Ventilation	Cycle Time	Expiratory Time
Closed-Loop Control	Dual Control	External Compressor
Control Circuit	Expiratory Flow Time	Inspiratory Flow Time
Control Variable	Expiratory Pause Time	Inspiratory Pause Time

*K*EY TERMS—cont'd

Inspiratory Phase	Mode of Ventilation	Spontaneous Breath
Inspiratory Time	Open-Loop Control	Time Constant
Internal Compressor	Passive Expiration	Transrespiratory Pressure
Limit	Percent Cycle Time	Trigger
Mandatory Breath	Phase Variable	Ventilatory Period
Mean Airway Pressure	Positive End-Expiratory Pressure (PEEP)	

Among the skills of the respiratory therapist, none is more important or more technically demanding than managing mechanical ventilation. Currently more than 30 critical care ventilators and more than two dozen transport and home care ventilators are being used in the United States. Add to that several dozen modes of ventilation that can be set on these machines and the countless arguments over how they should be used clinically, and the reader has some idea of the magnitude of the educational challenge in this area. Today's ventilators are more than simple life-support machines. They are complex computers with sophisticated software (even artificial intelligence) that can deliver nitric oxide, administer high-frequency ventilation, and monitor lung mechanics. Ventilators have evolved considerably since the simple devices described in Mushin's classic textbook.[1] This chapter presents an updated classification scheme that has been accepted by leading members of the pulmonary and critical care medicine community.[2-4]

Basic Concepts

A ventilator is a machine with a system of related elements designed to alter, transmit, and direct applied energy in a predetermined manner to perform useful work.[5] Energy is put into the ventilator in the form of electricity. That energy is transmitted or transformed by the ventilator's drive mechanism in a predetermined manner (the control circuit) to assist or replace the patient's muscles in performing the work of breathing (referred to as **assisted ventilation**). Therefore to understand mechanical ventilators, the reader first must understand their basic functions of input power, control scheme (including power transmission or conversion), and output (pressure, volume, and flow waveforms).

Input Power

All ventilators require a source of power that can be used to perform the work of ventilating the respiratory system. The most common forms of input power are electric and pneumatic. Input power should not be confused with the power for the control circuit. For example, many ventilators use pneumatic input power to drive inspiration but use electric power for the control circuit.

*R*espiratory Recap

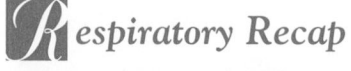

Input Power
Electric
Pneumatic

Electric

Most American ventilators use 110 to 115 volts AC (60 Hz) from common electrical outlets to power the drive mechanism. The AC voltage also is reduced and converted to DC to power electronic control circuits. Some currently used ventilators are designed to use rechargeable batteries as alternative sources of power when the usual AC current is unavailable. This capability makes them useful in the transport of ventilator-dependent patients within the hospital and between hospitals. In the home care setting a battery backup can be lifesaving in the event of a power outage.

Pneumatic

Because compressed air and oxygen are in abundant supply in most hospital intensive care units (ICUs), many ventilators are designed to use the energy stored in pressurized gas. Besides being used to inflate the lungs, the input pressure often is used as the source of power for the control circuit, as in the case of fluidic logic circuits. Ventilators operated by pressurized gas typically have internal reducing regulators so that the normal operating pressure is lower than the source pressure. This feature permits uninterrupted operation from piped gas sources in hospitals, which are usually regulated to 50 pounds per square inch (psi) but are subject to periodic fluctuations. The use of compressed gas as a power source makes a ventilator useful in environments in which no electrical power is available, such as during transport of patients, or in locations where electricity use is undesirable, such as near magnetic resonance imaging (MRI) equipment.

Control Scheme

To understand how a machine can be controlled to replace or assist the natural function of breathing, the reader must understand the mechanics of breathing. Specifically, this knowledge involves the pressure necessary to cause a flow of gas to enter the airway and increase the volume of the lungs. The study of respiratory mechanics relies on simple models. The relatively complex respiratory system can be represented by a simple physical model (for example, a straw connected to a balloon). This simple model is similar to electrical circuits in which compliance is analogous to capacitance, flow resistance is analogous to electrical resistance, and pressure is analogous to voltage. The similarity between the physical and electrical models makes it possible to borrow mathematic models from electrical engineering, substituting pressure, volume, and flow for voltage, charge, and current, respectively (Figure 39-1). The result is known as the *Equation of Motion* for the respiratory system (a simplified version):[6,7]

Muscle pressure + Ventilator pressure = Elastance × Volume + Resistance × Flow   (1)

Muscle pressure + Ventilator pressure = Elastic load + Resistive load   (2)

In this simplified form of the equation, muscle pressure is the imaginary **transrespiratory pressure** (that is, airway pressure minus body surface pressure) generated by the ventilatory muscles to expand the thoracic cage and lungs. Muscle pressure is said to be imaginary because it is not directly measurable. Ventilator pressure is the transrespiratory pressure generated by the ventilator during inspiration. The combination of muscle pressure and ventilator pressure causes volume and flow to be delivered to the patient. Pressure, volume, and flow change with time and hence are *vari-*

ables. Elastance and resistance are assumed to remain constant and are called *parameters*; their combined effect constitutes the load experienced by the ventilator and ventilatory muscles. *Elastance* is defined as the ratio of pressure change to volume change (that is, the reciprocal of compliance), and *resistance* is defined as the ratio of pressure change to flow change. The elastic load is the pressure necessary to overcome the elastance (or compliance) of the respiratory system, and the resistive load is the pressure necessary to overcome the flow resistance of the airways (including endotracheal tube) along with lung and chest wall tissue resistance. The term *parameter* also may refer to a particular aspect of a variable, such as the peak or mean value.

Note that pressure, volume, and flow are all measured relative to their baseline values (that is, their values at end-expiration), which means that the pressure to cause inspiration is measured as the change in airway pressure above **positive end-expiratory pressure (PEEP)**. This is the reason, for example, that pressure-support levels are measured relative to PEEP. Volume is measured as the change in lung volume above functional residual capacity, and the change in lung volume during the inspiratory period is defined as the *tidal volume*. Flow is measured relative to its end-expiratory value (usually zero unless auto-PEEP is present). When pressure, volume, and flow are plotted as functions of time, characteristic waveforms for volume-controlled ventilation and pressure-controlled ventilation are produced (Figure 39-2).

Notice in Figure 39-2 that the expiratory volume and flow waveforms are the same shape (that is, they show exponential decay). This describes **passive expiration** (that is, no muscular effort) in which the respiratory system is

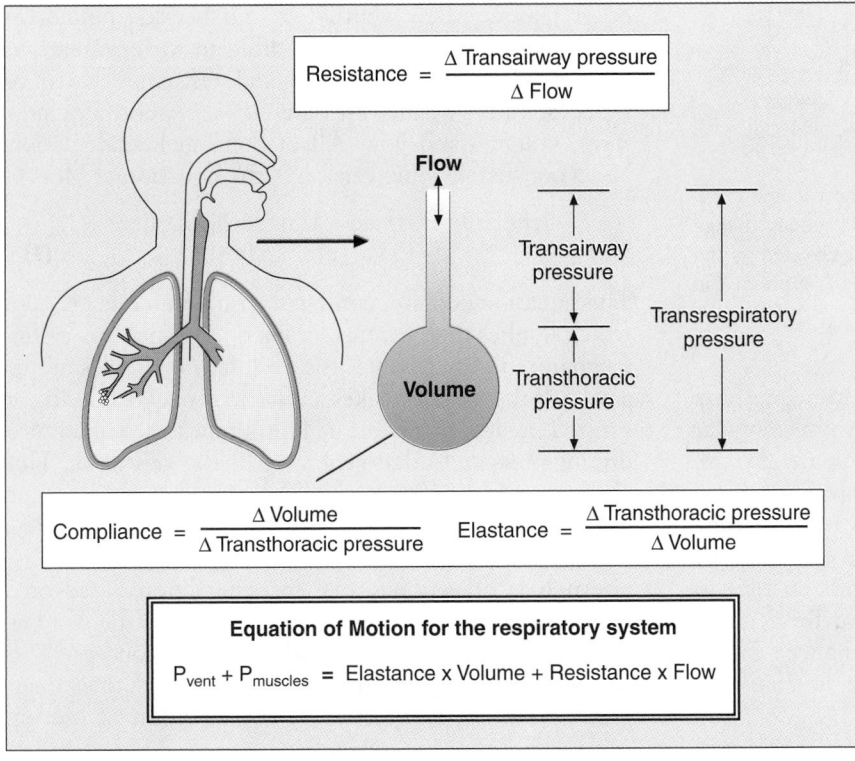

Figure 39-1   The study of respiratory system mechanics is based on graphic and mathematic models. The respiratory system can be modeled as a single-flow conducting tube connected to a single elastic compartment. This physical attribute can be described by a mathematic model called the *Equation of Motion* for the respiratory system. In this model, pressure, volume, and flow are variables (that is, functions of time), whereas resistance and compliance are constants.

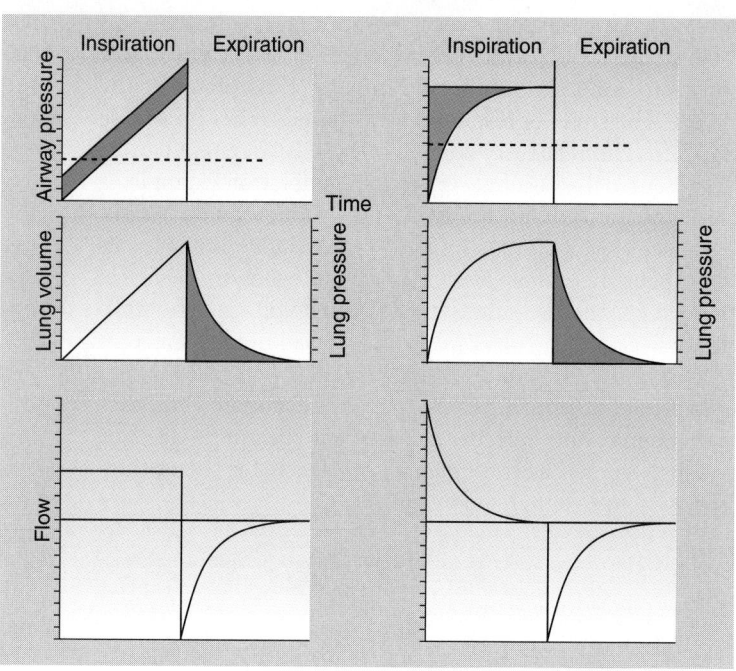

Figure 39-2 This figure illustrates some conventions for the presentation of graphic data. It shows the theoretic output waveforms for flow-controlled inspiration with a rectangular flow waveform on the left compared with pressure-controlled inspiration with a rectangular pressure waveform. The order of presentation is pressure, volume, and flow, according to the order specified by the Equation of Motion. Note that the volume waveform has the same shape as the transthoracic or lung pressure waveform (that is, pressure caused by elastic recoil). The flow waveform has the same shape as the transairway pressure waveform (that is, pressure caused by airway resistance). The origin of the airway pressure waveform is the end-expiratory pressure; the origins of the volume and flow waveforms are both zero. The shaded areas represent pressures resulting from flow resistance; the open areas represent pressure resulting from elastic recoil. The dotted lines represent mean airway pressure.

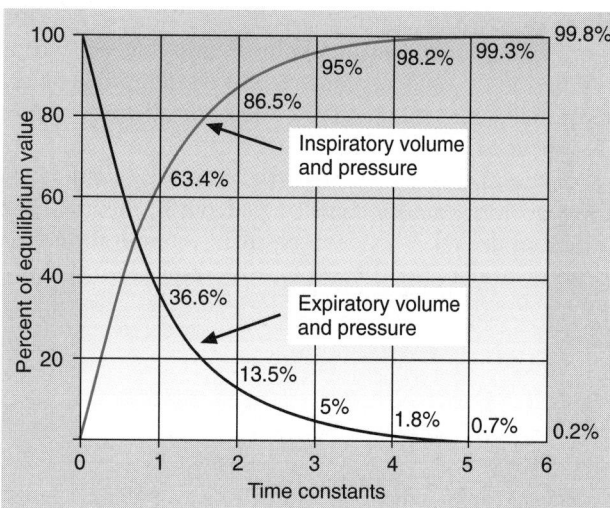

Figure 39-3 The time constant is a measure of how long the respiratory system takes to achieve equilibration with a sudden change in transrespiratory pressure. The time constant is calculated as the product of resistance multiplied by compliance and is expressed in units of time, usually seconds.

responding to a sudden release of inspiratory pressure. Note also that for passive inspiration with a rectangular pressure waveform, inspiratory flow and volume also are exponential. Because the exponential waveform is so common, the convention used to describe it is the **time constant**, which is a measure of the time required for the passive respiratory system to respond to abrupt changes in ventilatory pressure. It has units of time (usually seconds) and is calculated as resistance times compliance.[7] Figure 39-3 shows inspiratory and expiratory time constants marked on exponential curves.

If the patient's ventilatory muscles are not functioning, muscle pressure is zero, and the ventilator must generate all the pressure required to deliver the tidal volume and inspiratory flow. On the other hand, if ventilator pressure equals zero (that is, airway pressure does not rise above baseline during inspiration), no ventilatory support is present. Between these two extremes are an infinite variety of combinations of muscle pressure (that is, patient effort) and ventilator support that are theoretically possible for partial ventilatory support.

The concept of muscle pressure is important for another reason. Many ventilators and bedside pulmonary function monitors provide the clinician with estimates of respiratory system compliance and resistance based on transrespiratory system pressure (that is, ventilator pressure), volume, and flow. All of them make calculations based on the following version of the Equation of Motion:

$$\text{Ventilator pressure} = \text{Elastance} \times \text{Volume} + \text{Resistance} \times \text{Flow} \qquad (3)$$

This equation does not contain a term for muscle pressure, which implies that any measurement of respiratory system mechanics is valid only if the ventilatory muscles are inactive. If the patient makes an inspiratory effort during an assisted breath, this effort adds an unmeasured amount of driving pressure to that generated by the ventilator. Thus elastance and resistance based only on the ventilator's airway pressure sensor measurements underestimate the true values.

Analysis of ventilator-patient interaction based on a mathematic model suggests the proper use of the word *assist*, which is another frequently confused concept. *Webster's Dictionary* defines assist as "to help; to aid; to give support." From the perspective of the Equation of Motion,

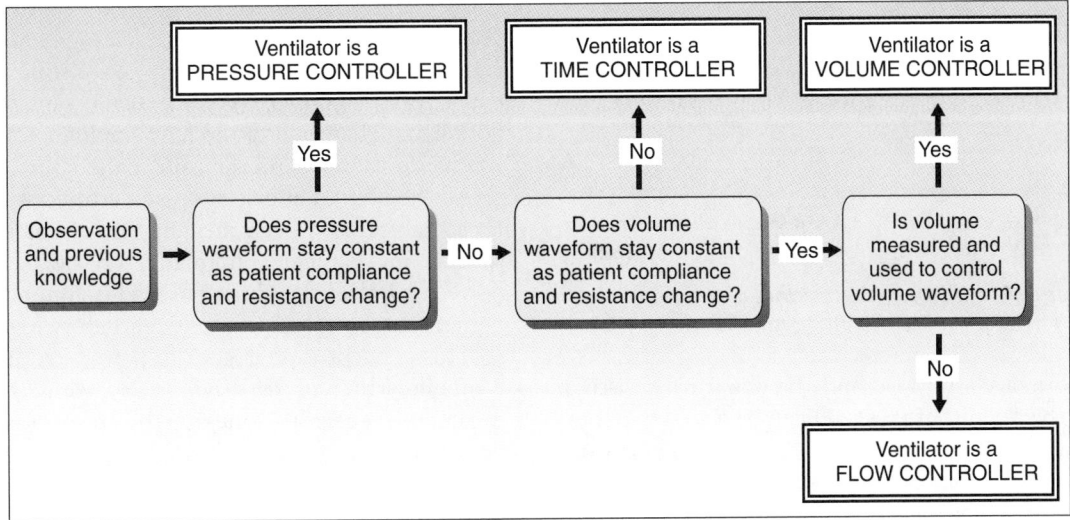

Figure 39-4   Criteria used to determine the control variable during a ventilator-assisted inspiration.

whenever airway pressure (that is, ventilator pressure) rises above baseline during inspiration, the ventilator performs work. Thus the breath is said to be *assisted*, independent of other breath characteristics (that is, whether the breath is classified as spontaneous or mandatory). The reader should not confuse this meaning of the word *assist* with specific names of modes of ventilation (for example, assist/control). Ventilator manufacturers often coin terms for modes without regard to consistency or theoretic relevance.

In the Equation of Motion, the form of any one of the three variables (that is, pressure, volume, or flow) expressed as functions of time can be predetermined, making it the independent variable and making the other two dependent variables. This idea is precisely analogous to the way ventilators operate. During pressure-controlled ventilation, pressure is the independent variable and the shapes of the volume and flow waveforms depend on the shape of the pressure waveform and the resistance and compliance of the respiratory system. On the other hand, during flow-controlled ventilation the ventilator sets the shape of the flow waveform, making flow the independent variable, and

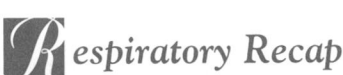espiratory Recap

---

Pressure-Controlled Versus Flow-Controlled Ventilation

During pressure-controlled ventilation, pressure is the independent variable. The shapes of the volume and flow waveforms depend on the shape of the pressure waveform and the characteristics of the patient's lungs.

During flow-controlled ventilation, flow is the independent variable. The shape of the volume and pressure waveforms depends on the shape of the flow waveform and the characteristics of the patient's lungs.

---

the shape of the volume waveform depends on the shape of the flow waveform. During flow-controlled ventilation the shape of the pressure waveform depends on the flow waveform, as well as on resistance and compliance.

This concept provides a theoretic basis for the classification of ventilators as pressure, volume, or flow controllers. The necessary and sufficient criteria used to determine which variable is controlled (that is, which variable is the independent variable) are illustrated in Figure 39-4. Note that if the waveforms for all three variables are not predetermined (that is, none of the variables can be considered independent), then the ventilator is considered to control only the timing of the inspiratory phase and **expiratory phase** and is called a *time controller*.

This theoretic framework is more than just an intellectual exercise. It is essential for the understanding and interpretation of bedside pulmonary mechanics values (for example, resistance, compliance, time constant) calculated by many ventilators. And it is also the basis of a new ventilatory mode known as *proportional assist*.[8] This **mode of ventilation** allows the clinician to support, and essentially cancel, the specific effects of pulmonary pathologic processes. That is, the ventilator can be set to support either the extra elastance or the extra resistance caused by lung disease, or both. To understand this principle, one must begin with the following equation describing spontaneous breathing:

$$\text{Muscle pressure} = \text{Normal elastance} \times \text{Volume} + \text{Normal resistance} \times \text{Flow} \qquad (4)$$

When pathologic processes increase elastance and/or resistance, the result can be expressed by the following equation:

$$\text{Muscle pressure} = (\text{Normal elastance} + \text{Abnormal elastance}) \times \text{Volume} + (\text{Normal resistance} + \text{Abnormal resistance}) \times \text{Flow} \qquad (5)$$

Equation 5 can be rearranged to show the normal and abnormal loads. Load, in this context, is the pressure to overcome either elastance or resistance (that is, Elastance × Volume = Pressure; Resistance × Flow = Pressure), as follows:

> **Muscle pressure = (Normal elastance × Volume) + (Normal resistance × Flow) + (Abnormal elastance × Volume) + (Abnormal resistance × Flow)   (6a)**
>
> **Muscle pressure = (Normal elastance × Volume) + (Normal resistance × Flow) + Abnormal load   (6b)**

The abnormal elastic load and the abnormal resistive load (which have units of pressure) can be added together to obtain the total abnormal load. By comparing Equation 4 with Equation 6b, the reader can see that in the presence of increased load, the muscle pressure must increase to provide the same (that is, normal) tidal volume and flow. To mechanically support the abnormal load(s) and allow muscle pressure to return to normal levels, the ventilator is set to generate a sufficiently large inspiratory pressure, which can be seen by the equating of load to ventilator pressure and the addition of that pressure to the left side of Equation 6b:

> **Muscle pressure + Ventilator pressure = (Normal elastance × Volume) + (Normal resistance × Flow) + Abnormal load   (7)**

In this case, the muscle pressure generates the force necessary to overcome normal elastance and resistance, whereas the ventilator pressure generates the force necessary to overcome abnormal elastance and resistance so that a normal tidal volume and inspiratory flow result. This analysis shows that proportional assist is a form of pressure control. Furthermore, it differs from the pressure-support mode (also a form of pressure control) in that the ventilator pressure does not necessarily generate a preset pressure. On the contrary the ventilator pressure varies continuously throughout inspiration.

To understand this concept requires a review of Equations 6 and 7. The ventilator pressure has two components. One is elastance multiplied by volume and the other is resistance multiplied by flow. Elastance and resistance are assumed to be constant throughout inspiration, whereas volume and flow change with the continuously varying muscle pressure. Because of the requirement for muscle pressure, proportional assist works only with spontaneous breaths. Ventilator pressure is proportional to the volume and flow signals (hence the name *proportional assist*); the constants of proportionality are the abnormal elastance and resistance.

In engineering terms these constants are gain (or amplification) factors set on the volume and flow signals. The ventilator measures airway pressure and flow. The flow signal is integrated into a volume signal. The flow and volume signals are fed through two amplifiers and through a mixer (which combines the amplified signals). The mixed signal is fed to a pressure generator (for example, a piston)

connected to the patient's airway. The ventilator's control circuit is programmed with the Equation of Motion so that each moment of airway pressure is controlled so as to be equal to the amplified volume signal plus the amplified flow signal. The gain of the flow amplifier is set to the abnormal resistance, and the gain of the volume amplifier is set to the abnormal elastance, under the assumption that these values have been measured or estimated. Thus the specific mechanical abnormality of the patient is supported. In effect the abnormal load is eliminated, and the patient perceives only normal ventilatory load.

This concept is analogous to power steering on an automobile, which makes driving easier while still maintaining complete responsiveness to the operator's motions. No ventilator power is wasted to force the patient to breathe in an unnatural pattern, as can happen with pressure support, making proportional assist (at the time of this writing still in the experimental phases) potentially the most comfortable mode of ventilation yet designed. Of course, some practical problems, such as how to continually monitor and reset the abnormal elastance and resistance levels, are inherent, but these issues soon should be resolved.

The Equation of Motion shows that any conceivable ventilator can directly control only one variable at a time: pressure, volume, or flow. Therefore a ventilator can be thought of as simply a machine that controls either the airway pressure waveform, the inspired volume waveform, or the inspiratory flow waveform. Thus pressure, volume, and flow are referred to in this context as **control variables**. Time is a variable that is implicit in the Equation of Motion. As shown in the following paragraphs, in some cases, time is viewed as a control variable. This concept allows the reader to understand any mode of ventilation, no matter how complex, by simply observing how control switches from one variable to the next.

A mechanical system can be controlled in two different ways to achieve the desired output:[9] (1) selection of an input followed by a wait for an output with no interference during the waiting period or (2) selection of an input, observation of the trend in the output, and modification of the input accordingly to get as close as possible to the desired output. For example, when a helmsman steers a boat toward the dock, he may do it in one of the two ways described: (1) point the boat in the direction of the dock and retire to his cabin or (2) continuously steer the boat toward the dock by observing the direction of the dock, observing the direction the boat is moving, and making adjustments as necessary. In this example the system is the boat (motor, propeller, steering mechanism), the input is the position of the boat's steering wheel, and the output is the direction of the boat's motion.

In both cases a change in the input causes a change in the output. But in the first case, no flow of information exists from the output to generate a new input to "close the loop." Hence, this type of control scheme is called **open-loop control**. In the second case the helmsman uses information about the output to modify the input, which in turn improves the output. This control scheme is called **closed-**

loop control, or *feedback control*. Feedback control is also called *servo control*. Figure 39-5 illustrates block diagrams (that is, models) of open- and closed-loop control systems.

To perform closed-loop control the output must be measured and compared with a reference value. In the previous example a human performed the measuring and comparing functions, but in ventilators a transducer and electronic circuitry are necessary to perform automatic closed-loop control. Closed-loop control provides a more consistent output in the presence of unanticipated disturbances. In the previous example, disturbances that affect the direction of the boat might include wind and water currents. In the case of ventilators, disturbances that might affect the delivery of pressure, volume, and flow include pooled condensation or leaks in the patient circuit,

endotracheal tube obstructions, and changes in respiratory system resistance and compliance.

Ventilators use closed-loop control to maintain consistent inspiratory pressure, volume, or flow waveforms in the presence of changing loads. The load presented by the respiratory system changes frequently as a result of pathologic processes of the lung. Ventilator design has evolved from simple mechanical control of pressure to closed-loop electronic control of pressure, volume, and flow within a breath, to dual control. This scheme was developed to obtain the advantages of both pressure-controlled and volume-controlled ventilation while avoiding each of their disadvantages. **Dual control** provides pressure control (that is, limiting peak inspiratory pressure (PIP), at least within a given range, to avoid overdistending the lungs) while

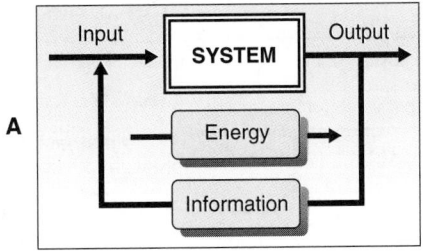

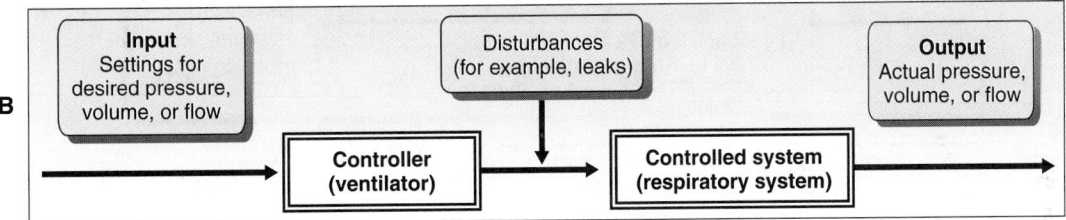

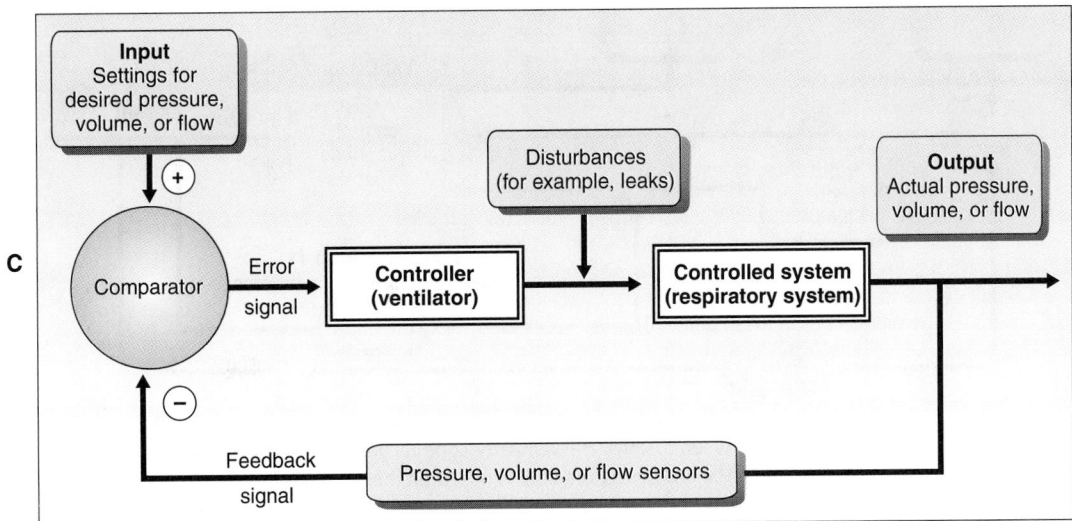

Figure 39-5 A, A simple block diagram of an unspecified system having one input and one output. Energy flows from input to output, and information flows from output to input. **B**, Block diagram for a ventilator using open-loop control. For example, the Newport Breeze ventilator controls airway pressure using open-loop control. **C**, Block diagram for a ventilator using closed-loop control. This also is called *feedback* or *servo control*. For example, the Infant Star ventilator uses closed-loop control of airway pressure.

maintaining the advantage of volume control (that is, delivering a constant tidal volume even if lung mechanics change).

Currently two approaches to dual control are used. The first method is to adjust the pressure waveform between breaths. This scheme was introduced with the volume support mode on the Siemens Servo 300. Inspiration is pressure controlled within a breath, but the pressure limit is automatically adjusted up or down to achieve a preset target tidal volume (Figure 39-6, A). The initial pressure **limit** (that is, change in airway pressure above PEEP) is automatically set based on the calculated value for respiratory system compliance (derived from a test breath): initial pressure limit = set tidal volume / compliance. If the actual tidal volume based on the initial pressure limit is

Respiratory Recap

Approaches to Dual Control

Dual control within breaths
Dual control between breaths

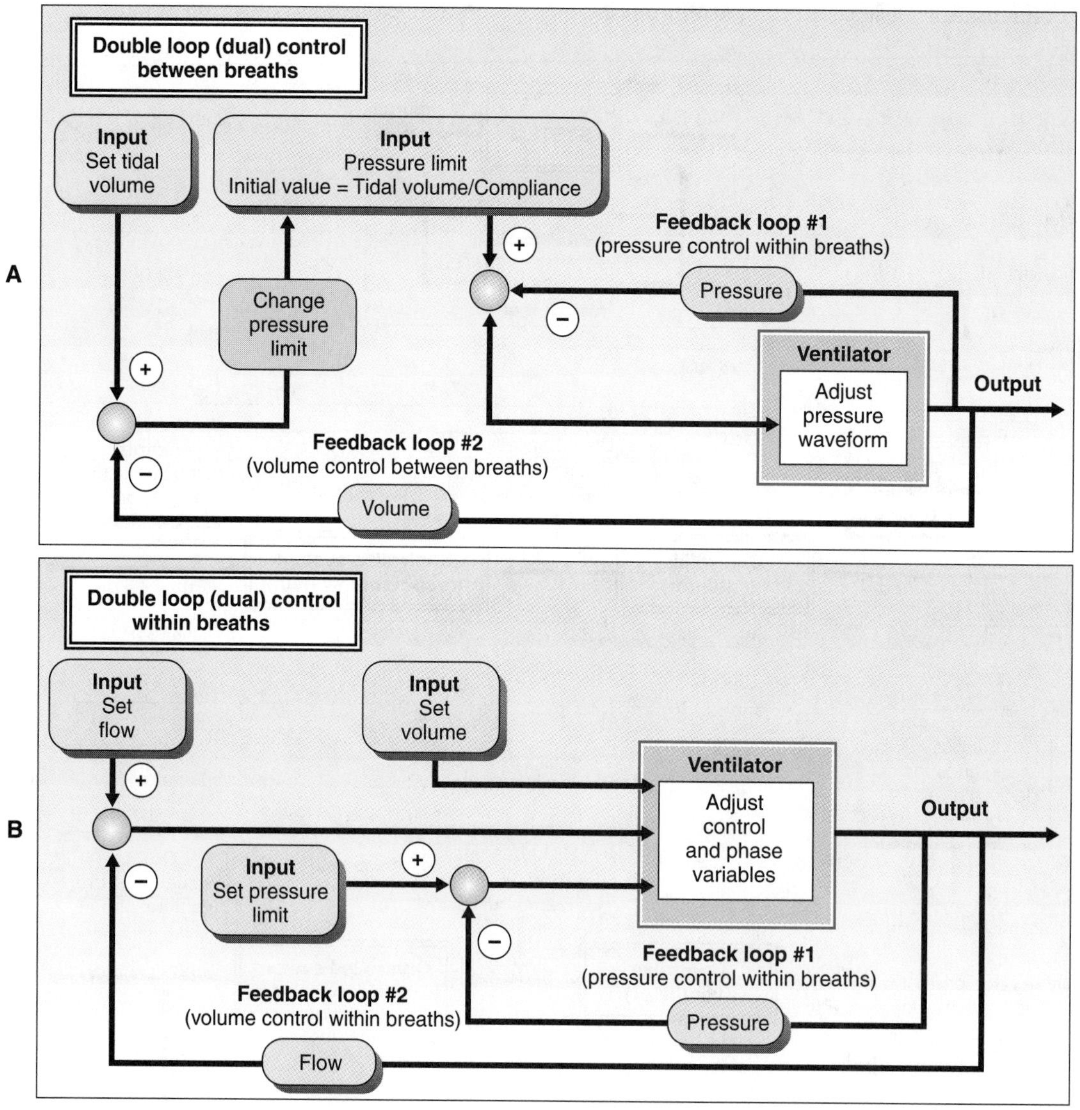

Figure 39-6 **A**, Dual control between breaths. The ventilator controls pressure during inspiration and then checks the resultant tidal volume. The initial pressure limit is based on the set tidal volume and the value for respiratory system compliance the ventilator has calculated from a test breath (for example, volume support on the Siemens 300). If the volume delivered with the initial pressure limit is different from the preset target value, the pressure waveform is changed for the next breath (either higher pressure limit or longer inspiratory flow time). **B**, Dual control within a breath. The ventilator starts inspiration in the pressure-controlled mode. If the set target volume has not been delivered by the time inspiratory flow has decayed to the preset inspiratory flow, the ventilator switches to flow control.

different from the set tidal volume, the pressure limit is adjusted up or down (no more than 3 cm H$_2$O per breath) to get closer to the set tidal volume. This process is repeated over several breaths until the delivered tidal volume equals the set tidal volume.

The other basic approach to dual control is to make adjustments within a breath to achieve the target volume, a process demonstrated in the pressure augment mode on the Bear 1000 and the volume-assured pressure-support (VAPS) mode on the Bird 8400ST (both Thermo Respiratory Group). With this approach the ventilator may switch between pressure control and volume control within a breath, depending on whether a preset tidal volume has been met (Figure 39-6, *B*). Typical pressure and flow waveforms with this form of dual control are illustrated in Figure 39-7.

Another variation of this theme is illustrated by the maximum pressure (P$_{max}$) feature on the Evita 4 (Drager), in which the ventilator begins inspiration in volume control at the set flow limit. When airway pressure reaches the set P$_{max}$ value, the ventilator switches to pressure control at the set pressure limit while tidal volume is monitored. The ventilator attempts to increase the **inspiratory flow time** (that is, the period from the beginning of inspiratory flow to the end of inspiratory flow) until the set tidal volume is delivered, provided that the set inspiratory time (that is, the period from the beginning of inspiratory flow to the beginning of expiratory flow) is long enough. If the set tidal volume is not delivered in the set inspiratory time, an alarm is activated.

Control Variables

A ventilator may be classified as either a pressure, volume, or flow controller. In some cases, classification of a ventilator as a time controller is logical (that is, when it controls only inspiratory and expiratory times).

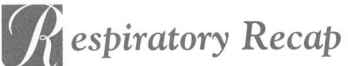
espiratory Recap

Control Variables	
Pressure	Flow
Volume	Time

Ventilators can combine control schemes to create complex modes. For example, the NPB 7200a ventilator can mix flow-controlled breaths with pressure-controlled breaths in the synchronized intermittent mandatory ventilation (SIMV) + pressure-support mode. The Bear 1000 can mix pressure control with flow control within a single breath in its pressure augment mode. The Servo 300 (Siemens) can adjust the level of pressure control automatically to achieve a preset target volume. The great flexibility of today's ventilators is achieved at the expense of added complexity. Thus when ventilator performance is evaluated, simple and unambiguous criteria are vital to any decision about which control variables are in effect.

Pressure

The Equation of Motion states that if the ventilator is an ideal pressure controller, then the left side of the equation (that is, ventilator pressure as a function of time) is determined by the ventilator settings and remains unaffected by changes in parameter values on the right side (that is, compliance and resistance).

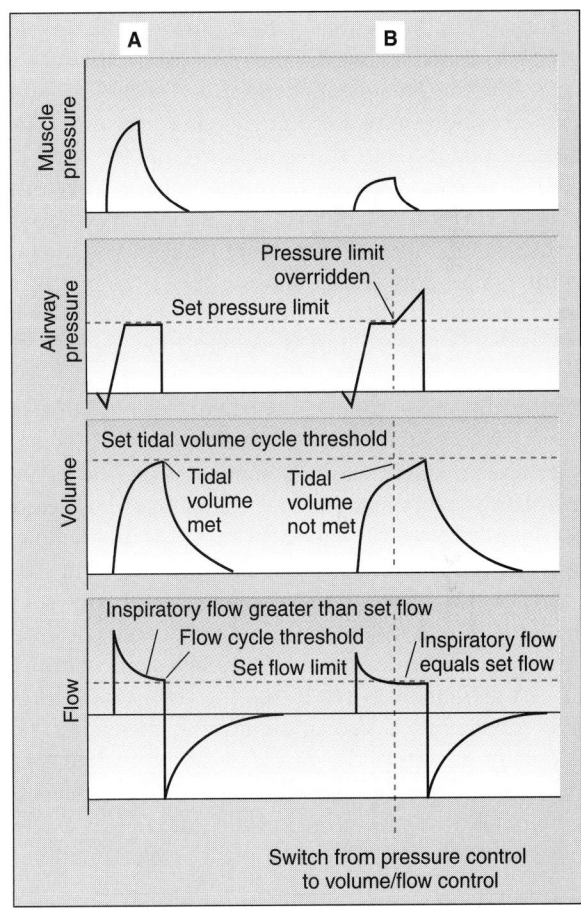

Figure 39-7   Pressure and flow waveforms showing the effects of dual control within breaths. **A,** Pressure-controlled breath with large patient effort (muscle pressure). The set tidal volume has been reached before flow has decayed to the set flow limit, so the breath continues in pressure control until the flow cycle threshold value is reached. This value may be an arbitrary percentage of the peak value for the pressure-controlled portion of the breath (for example, Pressure Augment in the Bear 1000) or the set flow rate (for example, VAPS in the Bird 8400ST). The breath is essentially a pressure-support breath. **B,** Switch from pressure control to flow control because flow decayed to the set flow before the set tidal volume was reached. This result was caused by a smaller patient inspiratory effort. Inspiration continues at the set flow, and pressure rises as expected for a volume/flow controlled breath.

If the control variable is pressure, the ventilator can control either the airway pressure (causing it to rise above body surface pressure for inspiration) or the pressure on the body surface (causing it to fall below airway opening pressure for inspiration). This idea is the basis for classification of ventilators as either positive or negative pressure types. For example, the Newport Wave ventilator would be classified as a positive pressure controller that generates a rectangular pressure waveform, and the Emerson Iron Lung as a negative pressure controller that produces a sinusoidal pressure waveform.

Volume

If the pressure waveform varies as the load imposed by the patient's respiratory system changes, the volume waveform then is examined. However, the observation that the volume waveform remains unchanged is a necessary but not sufficient condition to warrant the classification of a volume controller because the same holds true for a flow controller. The reason is that once the volume waveform is specified, the flow waveform is determined, because they are inverse functions of each other (that is, volume being the integral of flow and flow being the derivative of volume). Therefore if changes in compliance and resistance do not change the volume waveform, they do not affect the flow waveform, and vice versa.

To qualify as a volume controller, a ventilator must maintain a consistent volume waveform in the presence of a varying load and measure volume and use the signal to control the volume waveform. Volume can be measured directly only by the displacement of a piston or bellows or similar device. With a piston or bellows, control of the excursion of the device automatically controls the volume waveform. Alternatively, a volume signal could be derived by integration of a flow signal. Although some ventilators, such as the Siemens Servo 900C, the NPB 7200, the Bear 5, and the Hamilton Veolar, display volume readings, they all actually measure and control flow and calculate volume for displays. Thus they are all flow controllers unless they are operated in a pressure-controlled mode (for example, during pressure-support ventilation). An examination of a ventilator's schematic diagrams and operator's manual should provide the information necessary to decide whether volume or flow is being measured.

Flow

If the volume change (that is, tidal volume) remains consistent when compliance and resistance are varied, and if volume change is not measured and used for control, the ventilator is classified as a flow controller. The simplest example of open-loop flow control in a ventilator consists of a pressure regulator supplying gas to a flowmeter, such as found in infant ventilators. An infant ventilator becomes a flow controller rather than a pressure controller if the airway pressure does not reach the set pressure limit.[10] However, the flowmeter is usually not back-pressure compensated and varies its output slightly in the presence of a changing load. In contrast, the Siemens Servo 900C (so-called because it uses servo control) measures flow and adjusts the output control valve (that is, the inspiratory scissors valve) accordingly. It can maintain a more consistent inspiratory flow waveform as the load changes.

Time

Supposing that both pressure and volume are affected substantially by changes in lung mechanics, then the only form of control is that in which the ventilatory **cycle** is defined, or that involving alternation between inspiration and expiration. Therefore the only variables being controlled are the inspiratory and expiratory times. This situation arises in some forms of high-frequency ventilation when even the designation of an inspiratory and expiratory phase becomes somewhat obscure.

Phase Variables

Once the control variables and the associated waveforms are identified, more detail can be obtained through examination of the events that take place during a ventilatory cycle (that is, the period of time between the beginning of one breath and the beginning of the next). Mushin and colleagues[1] proposed that this time span be divided into four phases: (1) the change from expiration to inspiration, (2) inspiration, (3) the change from inspiration to expiration, and (4) expiration. A particular variable is measured and used to start, sustain, and end the phase. In this context, pressure, volume, flow, and time are referred to as **phase variables**.[11] The criteria used to determine phase variables are defined in Figure 39-8.

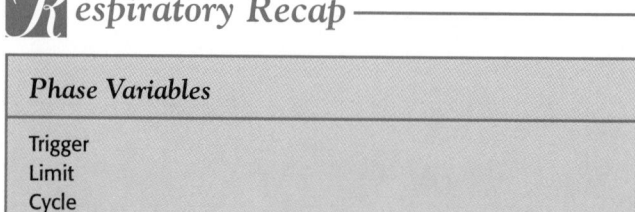

*R*espiratory Recap

Phase Variables
Trigger
Limit
Cycle

Trigger

All ventilators measure one or more of the variables associated with the Equation of Motion (that is, pressure, volume, flow, or time). Inspiration is started when one of these variables reaches a preset value. Thus the variable of interest is the initiating, or **trigger**, variable. The most common trigger variables are time (the ventilator initiating a breath according to a set frequency, independent of the patient's spontaneous efforts), pressure (the ventilator sensing the patient's inspiratory effort in the form of a drop in baseline pressure and starting inspiration independent of the set frequency), and flow (the ventilator sensing the

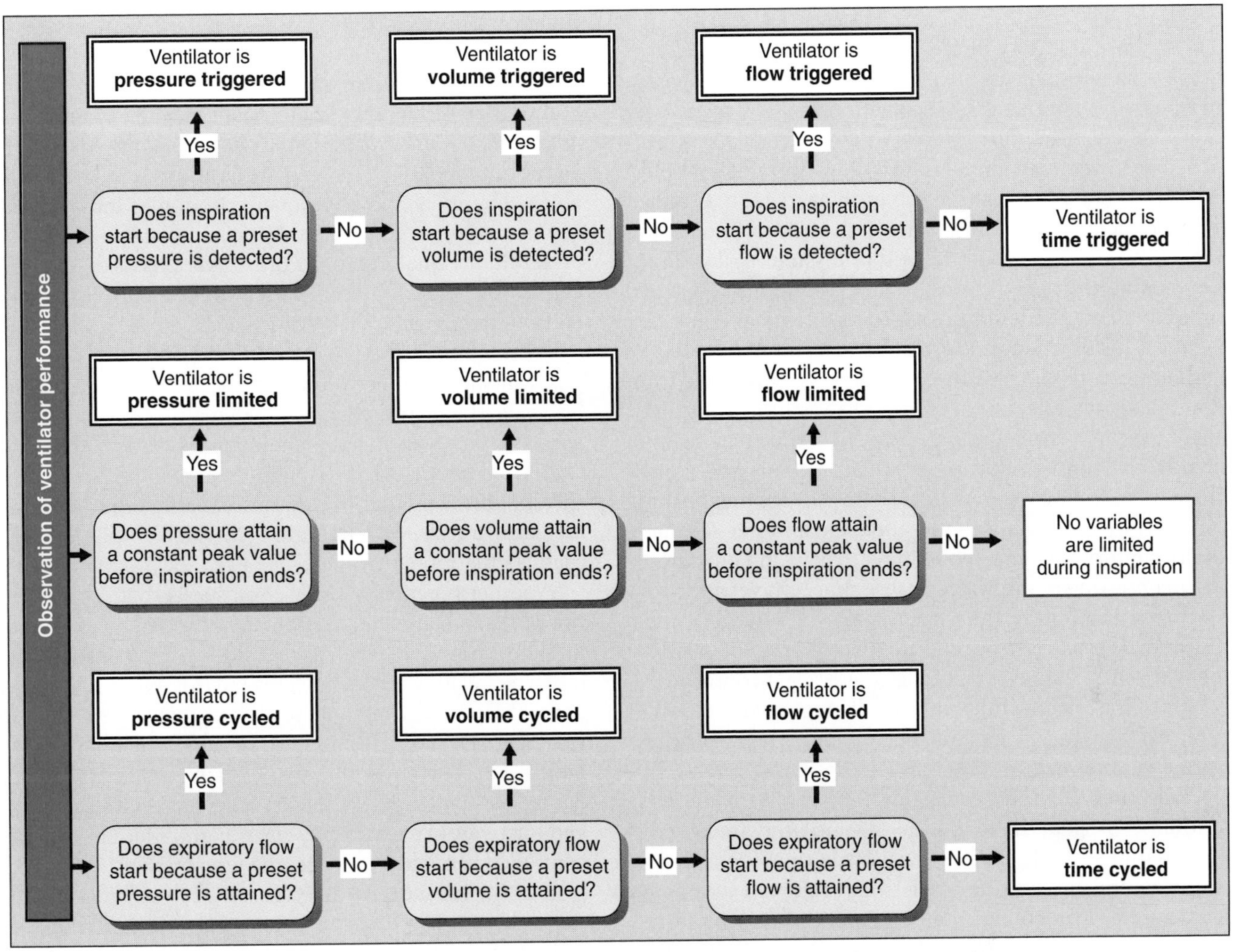

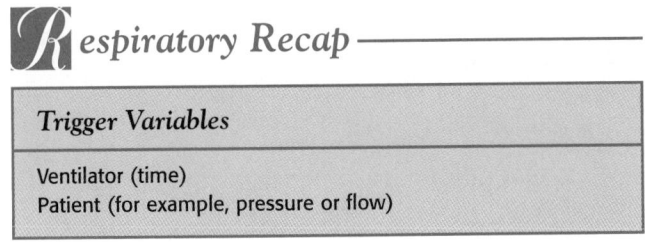

Figure 39-8   Criteria used to determine the phase variables during a ventilator-assisted breath.

patient's inspiratory effort as a drop in the baseline flow through the patient circuit or sensing inspiratory flow directly with a sensor at the patient's airway opening). Any variable that can be measured can potentially be used to trigger inspiration. For example, the Star Sync module allows triggering of the Infant Star ventilator by chest wall movement, whereas the Sechrist SAVI system senses inspiration as a change in chest impedance. Of course, manual triggering of inspiration is relatively simple.

Respiratory Recap

Trigger Variables
Ventilator (time)
Patient (for example, pressure or flow)

Triggering on flow has been shown to reduce the work the patient must perform to trigger inspiration[12] because work is proportional to the volume the patient inspires multiplied by change in baseline pressure necessary for trig-

gering. Pressure triggering obviously requires some pressure change and hence, an irreducible amount of work to trigger. But with flow or volume triggering, baseline pressure need not change and theoretically the patient need not perform work on the ventilator to trigger a response. At least one ventilator, the Drager Babylog, may be volume triggered. The possible advantage of volume triggering over flow triggering is that when the flow signal is integrated to obtain volume, much of the noise in the signal (for example, condensate in the patient circuit) is removed and the likelihood of false triggering reduced. A possible disadvantage of this method is the increased delay from signal processing and the phase lag between flow and volume signals.

The patient effort required to trigger inspiration is determined by the ventilator's sensitivity. The smaller the change in signal (for example, pressure change below baseline) required to trigger, the greater the sensitivity. Many ventilators indicate sensitivity adjustments qualitatively (for example, *min* or *max*). Alternatively, a ventilator may specify a trigger threshold quantitatively. For example, to make a pressure-triggered ventilator more sensitive, the trigger threshold might be adjusted from 2 to 1 cm H_2O below the baseline pressure.

Limit

During the inspiratory phase, pressure, volume, and flow increase above their end-expiratory values. The **inspiratory phase** is quantified by specification of the **inspiratory time**, defined as the time interval from the start of inspiratory flow to the start of expiratory flow. Inspiratory hold (or pause) time is included in the inspiratory time. Distinguishing the inspiratory flow time as the interval from the start of inspiratory flow to the end of inspiratory flow and the **inspiratory pause time** as the interval from the end of inspiratory flow to the start of expiratory flow sometimes is helpful. This distinction is useful because no standardized method exists to set these intervals on ventilators, and the terminology manufacturers use may be confusing. For example, on one ventilator, inspiratory flow time may be indirectly set through setting of tidal volume and flow, whereas pause time may be directly set (in seconds), thus indirectly increasing inspiratory time. On another ventilator, inspiratory time may be set directly with no provision for direct setting of inspiratory pause time. On yet another ventilator, inspiratory time may be set with the *rate* and *percent cycle time* controls and then inspiratory flow time changed via a change in the *percent inspiration* control. Finally, inspiratory flow time must be distinguished from inspiratory time to understand the way P_{max} works on the Evita 4 ventilator.

Cycle time (or total cycle time) is another name for **ventilatory period**, the reciprocal of ventilatory frequency expressed in seconds. The **percent cycle time** is the ratio of inspiratory time to total cycle time expressed as a percentage. The percent inspiratory time is the inspiratory flow time expressed as a percent of total cycle time. The percent pause time is the pause time expressed as a percent of total cycle time. An inspiratory pause is important in estimation of lung pressures and calculation of respiratory system mechanics.

If one (or more) of the inspiratory variables rises no higher than some preset value, the variable is a limit variable. But the limit variable must be distinguished from the variable that is used to end inspiration (the cycle variable). Therefore the additional criterion is imposed that inspiration is not terminated because a variable has met its preset limit value. In other words, a variable is described as *limited* if it increases to a preset value before inspiration ends. The criteria used to distinguish the terms *limit* and *cycle* are illustrated in Figure 39-9.

Clinicians commonly misuse the terms *limit* and *cycle* by using them interchangeably. This practice is encouraged by some ventilator manufacturers who use the term *limit* to describe what happens when a pressure alarm threshold is met (that is, inspiration being terminated and an alarm activated). The term *cycle* is more appropriate in such a situation.

Another potentially confusing issue is that, by convention, PIP, and baseline pressure are measured relative to atmospheric pressure, whereas the pressure limit is sometimes measured relative to baseline pressure (for example, Siemens Servo 900C) and sometimes relative to atmospheric pressure (for example, Bird VIP). On the Bird VIP the high-pressure limit control sets the PIP limit (above ambient pressure) during pressure-controlled ventilation but cycles the breath and activates a high-pressure alarm during volume-controlled ventilation. Hence, the term *pressure limit* in common usage can indicate different clinically significant situations, depending on both the mode of ventilation and the manufacturer. Clearly the lack of standardization among ventilator manufacturers makes the proper use of terminology especially important among clinicians.

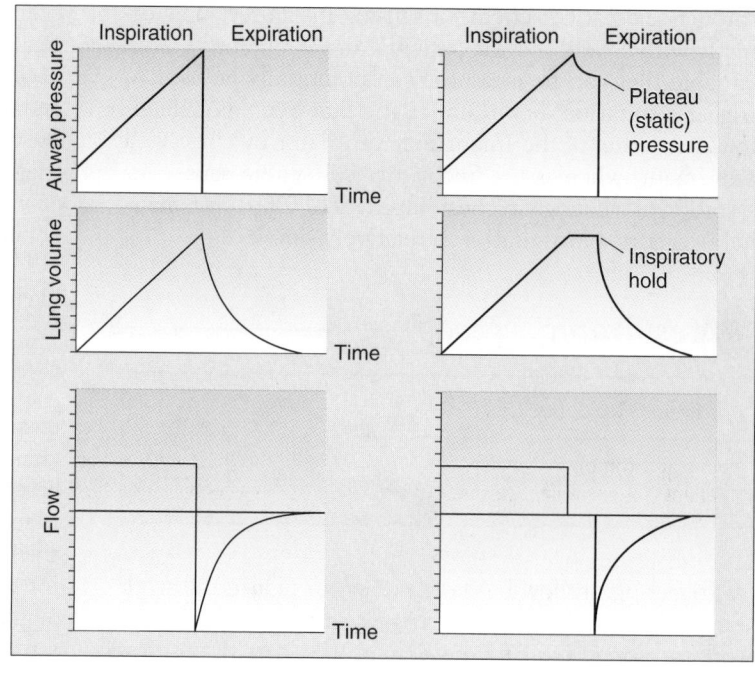

Figure 39-9 This figure illustrates the importance of distinguishing between the terms *limit* and *cycle. Left,* Flow is limited but volume is not, and inspiration is volume cycled. *Right,* Both volume and flow are limited (because they reach preset values before end inspiration), and inspiration is time cycled (after the preset inspiratory pause time).

Cycle

Inspiration always ends (that is, is cycled off) because some variable has reached a preset value. The variable that is measured and used to terminate inspiratory time and begin expiratory time is called the *cycle variable*, which can be pressure, volume, time, or flow. Deciding which variable is used to cycle off inspiration for a given ventilator can be confusing. For a variable to be used as a feedback signal (in this case a cycling signal), it must first be measured. Most current-generation adult ventilators allow the operator to set a tidal volume and inspiratory flow rate, which would lead the reader to believe that the ventilator is volume cycled. However, closer inspection reveals that these ventilators do not measure volume, which is consistent with their all being flow controllers. Rather, they set the inspiratory time necessary to achieve the set tidal volume with the set inspiratory flow rate, making them time cycled. The tidal volume dial can be thought of as an inspiratory time dial calibrated in units of volume rather than time.

As mentioned previously, the term *limit* is often incorrectly substituted for cycle in common usage. But the distinction also is ignored by ventilator designers. An example of the difficulty created by improper terminology is illustrated by the Bear Cub 750vs. This ventilator is designed to be used primarily as a pressure controller for infants. The operator typically sets an inspiratory pressure limit with the knob labeled *inspiratory pressure*. Inspiration is normally time cycled. However, there is a control knob labeled *volume limit*, so inspiration would seem to be both pressure and volume limited at the same time. Not true.

In the first place, the Equation of Motion shows that both volume and pressure cannot be controlled to some preset value at the same time. If the operator sets a pressure limit, the delivered volume depends on lung mechanics, and if the operator sets a volume limit, the pressure varies with lung mechanics. In the second place, the operator's manual describes the volume limit as follows: "When the set threshold is reached, the ventilator will cycle into expiration." So the ventilator does one thing when the *pressure* limit is met (namely, stay at that level until inspiration ends) and another thing when the *volume* limit is met (terminates inspiration). The *volume limit* control is really a *volume cycle threshold*. Calling both functions by the same name is confusing and may obscure the operator's understanding of the ventilator's unique ability to volume cycle in a pressure-controlled mode.

Baseline

The variable controlled during the expiratory time is the baseline variable, which is most commonly PEEP. **Expiratory time** is defined as the time interval from the start of expiratory flow to the start of inspiratory flow. As with inspiratory time, distinguishing the components of expiratory time is helpful: **expiratory flow time**, defined as the interval from the start of expiratory flow to the end of expiratory flow, and **expiratory pause time**, defined as the interval from the end of expiratory flow to the start of inspiratory flow. Expiratory pause time is often initiated to measure auto-PEEP.

Conditional Variables

Figure 39-10 illustrates that for each breath, the ventilator creates a specific pattern of control and phase variables. The ventilator may either keep this pattern constant for each breath or introduce other patterns (for example, one for mandatory breaths and one for spontaneous breaths). In essence, the ventilator must decide which pattern of control and phase variables to implement before each breath, depending on the value of some preset conditional variables. Conditional variables can be thought of as initiating conditional logic in the form of "if-then" statements. That is, if the value of a conditional variable reaches some preset threshold, then some action occurs to change the ventilatory pattern.

A simple example would be a ventilator set to operate in the following way. Each breath is time triggered, flow limited, and volume cycled. The trigger, limit, and cycle variables have preset values (for example, trigger at frequency = 20 cycles/min, limit inspiratory flow at 60 L/min, and cycle at tidal volume = 750 mL). However, every few minutes a sigh breath is introduced that has a different set of phase variable values (for example, trigger at frequency = two sighs every 15 minutes; cycle at tidal volume = 1500 mL). How did the ventilator know to do this? Conceptually, before each breath pattern is selected, the ventilator examines the value of some conditional variable to see whether it has reached a preset threshold value. If the threshold has been met, one pattern is selected; if not, another pattern is selected. In the case of this ventilator example, the conditional variable was time. If a preset time interval has elapsed (that is, the sigh interval), then the ventilator switches to the sigh pattern. Another example is switching from patient-triggered to machine-triggered breaths in the mandatory minute ventilation (MMV) mode.

Spontaneous breaths are those that are both initiated and terminated by the patient. If the ventilator determines either the start or end of inspiration, then the breath is considered mandatory. Figure 39-11 illustrates these definitions with an algorithm. If the ventilator either time-cycles or volume-cycles an inspiration, the breath is considered mandatory because it is terminated by the ventilator. If, however, the ventilator flow-cycles after being patient triggered, as in the pressure-support mode, the breath is considered spontaneous. The rate of decay of inspiratory flow is determined by the patient's lung mechanics and ventilatory muscle activity. Hence, during the pressure-support mode, pressure-limiting inspiration does not constrain inspiratory flow rate, and flow cycling does not necessarily dictate either the inspiratory time or the tidal volume if the ventilatory muscles are active. In other words the ventilator attempts to match the patient's inspi-

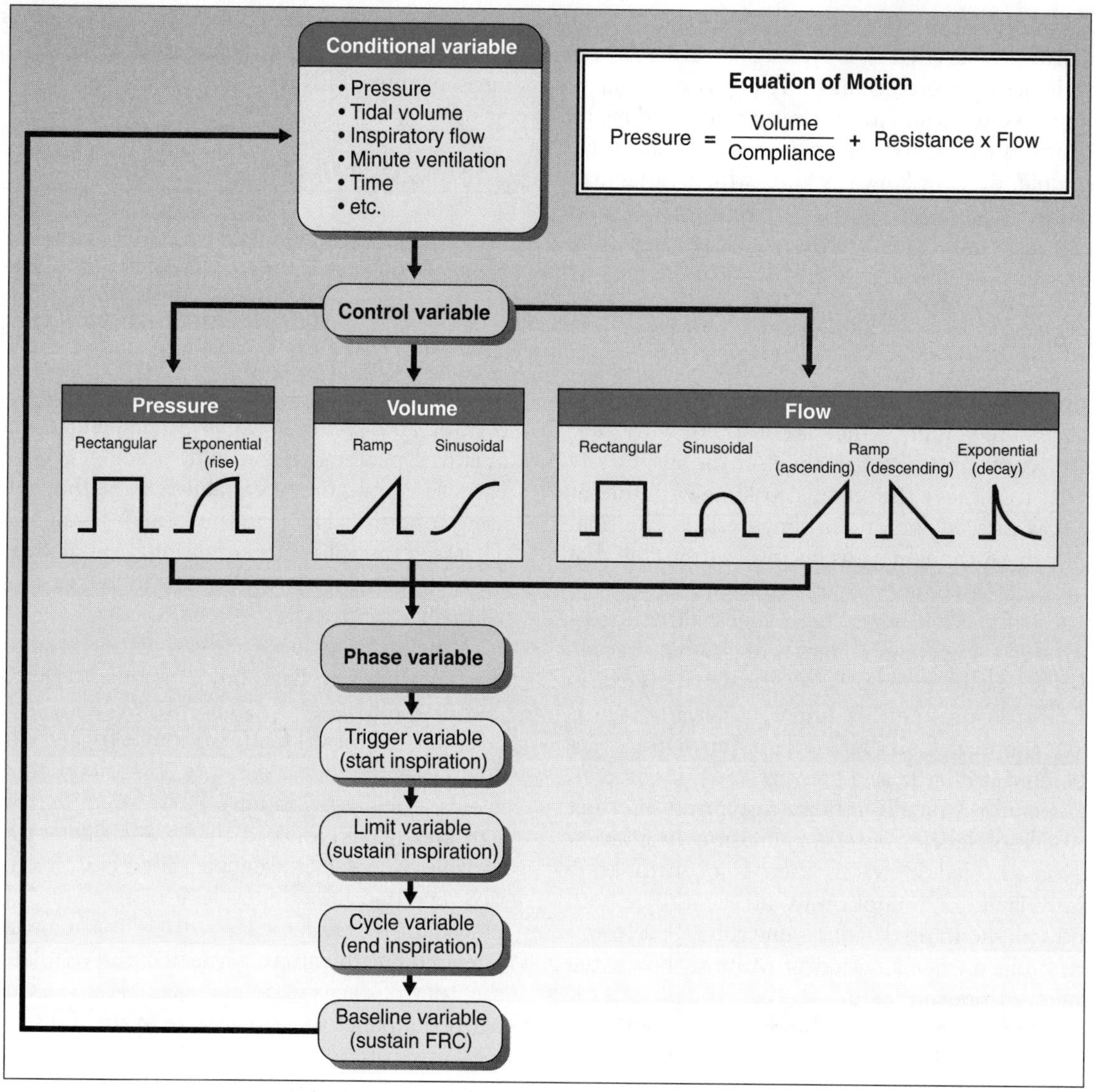

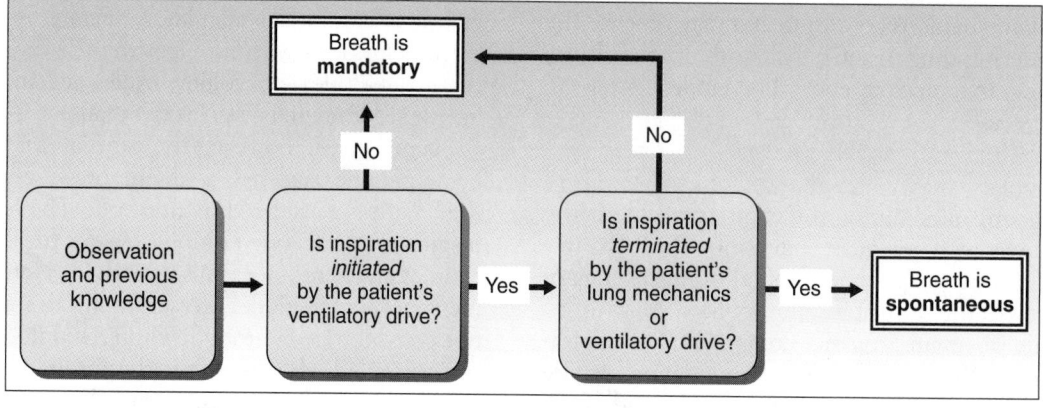

Conditional variable

- Pressure
- Tidal volume
- Inspiratory flow
- Minute ventilation
- Time
- etc.

Equation of Motion

$$\text{Pressure} = \frac{\text{Volume}}{\text{Compliance}} + \text{Resistance} \times \text{Flow}$$

Control variable

Pressure

Rectangular   Exponential (rise)

Volume

Ramp   Sinusoidal

Flow

Rectangular   Sinusoidal   Ramp (ascending)   Ramp (descending)   Exponential (decay)

Phase variable

Trigger variable (start inspiration)

Limit variable (sustain inspiration)

Cycle variable (end inspiration)

Baseline variable (sustain FRC)

Figure 39-10   A ventilator classification scheme based on a mathematic model known as the *Equation of Motion* for the respiratory system. This model indicates that during inspiration the ventilator is able to directly control one and only one variable at a time (that is, pressure, volume, or flow). Some common waveforms provided by current ventilators are shown for each control variable. Pressure, volume, flow, and time also are used as phase variables that determine the parameters of each ventilatory cycle (for example, trigger sensitivity, peak inspiratory flow rate or pressure, inspiratory time, and baseline pressure).

Breath is **mandatory**

No   No

Observation and previous knowledge → Is inspiration *initiated* by the patient's ventilatory drive? — Yes → Is inspiration *terminated* by the patient's lung mechanics or ventilatory drive? — Yes → Breath is **spontaneous**

Figure 39-11   Algorithm defining spontaneous and mandatory breaths.

ratory demand, and the patient actually terminates the breath. If the ventilator is pressure cycled (usually an alarm condition) after being patient triggered, the breath is also spontaneous. Again, the patient's lung mechanics or ventilatory muscle activity has caused airway pressure to rise above the preset threshold (in the absence of ventilator malfunction).

What is confusing to some clinicians is that if a breath is assisted, as in pressure-support ventilation, it somehow seems to them to be mandatory rather than spontaneous. The advantages of separating the definitions of *mandatory* versus *spontaneous* from the definitions of *assisted* versus *unassisted* now should be clear.

Modes of Ventilation

Two general approaches exist in the support of a patient's inspiration: volume/flow control and pressure control. Figure 39-12 is a simplified influence diagram[13-15] that illustrates the important variables for ventilators that are either volume or flow controllers. Figure 39-13 is the influence diagram for ventilators that are pressure controllers. The equations relating these variables are provided in reference textbooks.[16] For pressure-controlled ventilation, with a rectangular pressure waveform, peak inspiratory flow is equal to the set pressure difference (inspiratory pressure limit minus PEEP) divided by the respiratory system resistance. Some ventilators, especially infant ventilators, provide the user with a control knob labeled *flow* (for example, Bear Cub, NPB Infant Star). The meaning of this knob can be confusing. If flow is set relatively low, the set pressure limit is never reached; then the set flow is the peak inspiratory flow. However, if flow is set relatively high, the pressure limit is reached almost immediately; then peak inspiratory flow is determined by the pressure difference and resistance as explained previously. If an intermediate flow is set, then it has the effect of shaping the airway pressure waveform and generally decreasing the peak inspiratory flow.

Beyond these two general approaches to ventilatory support, a variety of breathing patterns, or modes, of ventilation can be created. A *mode of ventilation* represents a set of breath characteristics that are important to the clinician.

Definition of Terms

The following terms represent a minimum set of concepts needed to construct a convenient lexicon of mechanical ventilation modes:

- Mandatory breath: Inspiration is machine triggered and/or machine cycled.
- Spontaneous breath: Inspiration is patient triggered and patient cycled.
- Continuous mandatory ventilation (CMV): Every breath is mandatory.

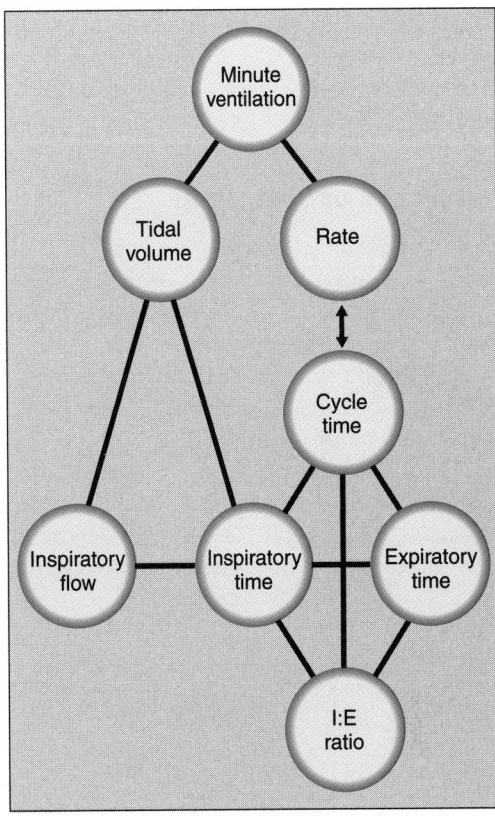

Figure 39-12 Influence diagram for volume-controlled ventilation. Variables are connected by straight lines so that if any two are known, the third can be calculated with standard equations.[16] The *double arrow line* indicates that the ventilatory period is the reciprocal of ventilatory frequency.

- Intermittent mandatory ventilation (IMV): The pattern consists of intermittent (machine-triggered) mandatory breaths, with spontaneous breaths allowed in between.
- SIMV: The pattern consists of synchronized intermittent (patient- or machine-triggered) mandatory breaths, with spontaneous breaths allowed in between.
- Continuous spontaneous ventilation (CSV): Every breath is spontaneous.
- Pressure control: The ventilator attempts to maintain a preset airway pressure waveform during inspiration.
- Volume/flow control: The ventilator attempts to maintain a preset volume or flow waveform during inspiration; direct control of flow implies indirect control of volume, and vise versa.
- Dual control: The ventilatory switches between pressure control and flow control; current examples are (1) inspiration is pressure-controlled within breaths, but the pressure limit is automatically adjusted between breaths to achieve a target tidal volume; and (2) inspiration switches between pressure control and flow control within a breath, depending on the level of patient effort relative to machine settings.

- Assist or assisted inspiration: Externally applied transrespiratory pressure change acts in synchrony with muscle pressure (if present) to increase tidal volume and flow.

General Modes of Ventilation

A mode can be classified simply on the basis of the breathing pattern it produces (Box 39-1), which is identified by the variable manipulated by the system to effect control (that is, the primary breath control variable [for mandatory breaths unless only spontaneous breaths are allowed] and the permissible breath sequence). At the level of detail of the breath control variable, it is only possible to distinguish among pressure-control, volume-control, and dual-control modes. Often this fact is all that is needed to communicate. For example, at the bedside the clinician need only indicate that the patient has been changed from volume control to dual control when it is realized that the condition of the lungs has become unstable. Note that pressure control or volume control can mean either open-loop or closed-loop control, but dual control can be accomplished only with closed-loop (feedback) control. In addition, it is important to be more specific in the discussion of ventilators as opposed to modes. A *ventilator* may be a pressure, volume, or flow controller, whereas a *mode of ventilation* can be classified more simply as either pressure control or volume control.

When the breath sequence is added to the control variable, it is possible to distinguish between, for example, pressure-controlled IMV and pressure-controlled CSV. With the addition of the type of control (see Box 39-1), this description can be used to distinguish among various types of pressure-controlled CSV (for example, that using a set point control [that is, CPAP] and that using servo control [such as proportional assist]).

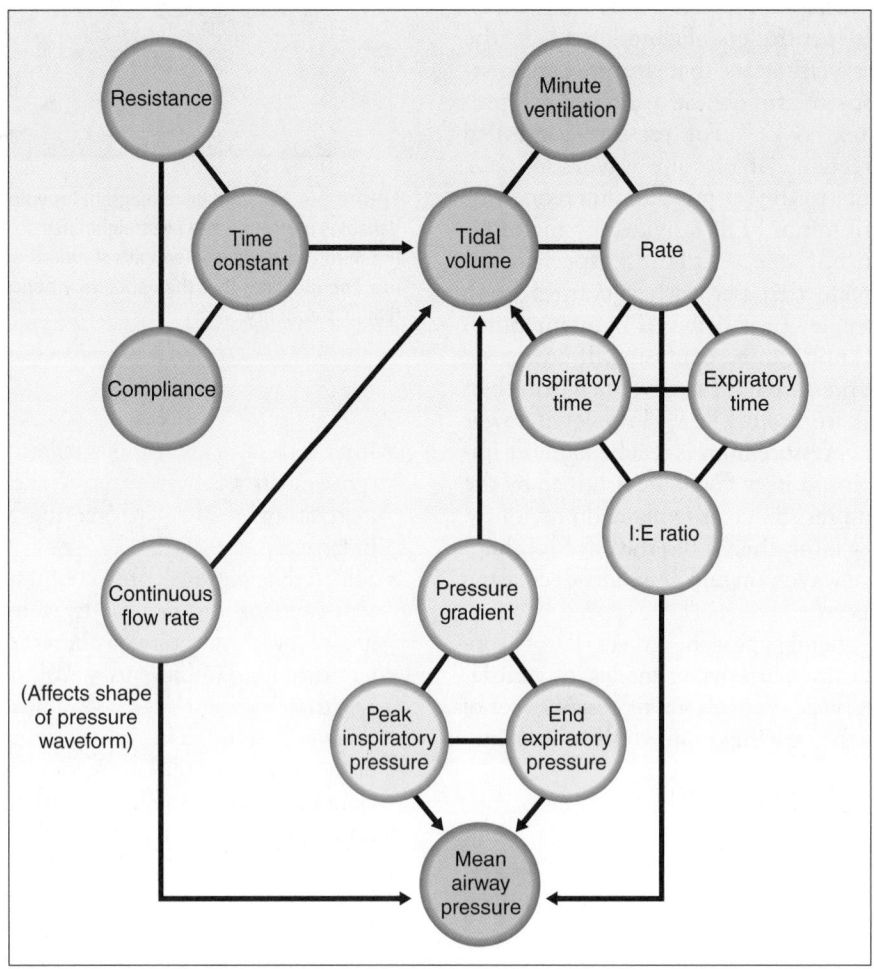

Figure 39-13   Influence diagram for pressure-controlled ventilation. Variables are connected by straight lines so that if any two are known, the third can be calculated with standard equations.[16] *Arrows* represent relations that are either more complex or less predictable. *Open circles* represent variables that can be directly controlled by the ventilator; *shaded circles* are controlled indirectly. (Modified from Chatburn RL, Lough MD. Mechanical ventilation. In: Lough MD, Doershuk CF, Stern RC, editors. Pediatric respiratory therapy. St Louis: Mosby; 1985. pp. 148-191.)

If classification is based solely on the breathing pattern, only 8 possibilities in three groups exist (Table 39-1). The utility of this system is immediately obvious. It is possible to introduce a new mode, such as airway pressure release ventilation (APRV), as simply a form of pressure-controlled IMV. Assuming that the concept of PC-IMV is understood, little effort is necessary to understand the additional nuances of APRV (such as different labels for control settings and alarms). Also possible is the use of PC-IMV and PC-CSV to clarify the meaning of *bilevel positive airway pressure ventilation (BiPAP)*. For example, on the BiPAP S/T-D ventilator (Respironics, Pittsburgh, Pa.), the *timed* BiPAP mode is PC-IMV, whereas the *spontaneous* BiPAP mode is PC-CSV. *BiPAP ventilation* and *bilevel ventilation* are particularly ambiguous terms because any form of assisted ventilation can be thought of as using two levels of pressure.

Not only can a new mode be described in terms of the prototypical breathing pattern it produces, but it is also possible to use this description to group together modes that function the same way but are given different names. For example, both pressure augment (Bear 1000) and volume-assured pressure-support (Bird 8400ST) are dual-control IMV modes. (In addition, they use hierarchical [set-point] control.) Another example is pressure-regulated volume control (Siemens 300) and pressure-controlled assist control + adaptive pressure ventilation (Hamilton Galileo), which are both adaptive dual-control CMV modes. Ventilators also can be grouped in terms of the number of breathing patterns they offer; some offer only one or two, whereas others offer all eight. This grouping might be useful as an initial screening tool in ventilator purchases.

Box 39-1 shows that a more detailed mode description includes the type of control used to manipulate the control variables to produce the permissible breaths. For single-variable, closed-loop control, hierarchical set point and hierarchical servo strategies have been used. Dual-variable, closed-loop control has used hierarchical set point and adaptive set point strategies. Thus ASV and PRVC can be classified as dual adaptive (set-point) control CMV. (The term *set point* could be left out because all dual-control schemes developed by the early twenty-first century are set point.)

Finally, it is possible to fully characterize a mode by the addition of the specific strategy it uses, beginning with the naming of the phase variables and followed by detailing of the operational logic, and, if necessary, provision of the

Box 39-1

Mode Classification Scheme

> The following elements can be used to characterize modes of ventilator operation. If both mandatory and spontaneous breaths are possible in a given mode, the specification of that mode should begin with, and may just be limited to, a description of the mandatory breaths. However, a complete specification would include descriptions of both mandatory and spontaneous breaths.
>
> **Breathing Pattern**
> *Primary breath control variable*
>   Volume
>   Pressure
>   Dual
> *Breath sequence*
>   Continuous mandatory ventilation (CMV)
>   Intermittent mandatory ventilation (IMV)
>   Continuous spontaneous ventilation (CSV)
>
> **Type of Control Strategy (Control Type)**
>   Hierarchical set-point control
>   Hierarchical servo control
>   Adaptive set-point control
>
> **Specific Control Strategy**
> *Phase variables*
>   Trigger
>   Limit
>   Cycle
> *Operational logic*
>   Conditional variables
>   Output variables
>   Performance function (for example, function that is maximized or minimized for adaptive strategies)

Table 39-1

Possible Breathing Patterns

Breath Control Variable	Breath Sequence	Abbreviation
Volume (control)	Continuous mandatory ventilation	VC-CMV
	Intermittent mandatory ventilation	VC-IMV
Pressure (control)	Continuous mandatory ventilation	PC-CMV
	Intermittent mandatory ventilation	PC-IMV
	Continuous spontaneous ventilation	PC-CSV
Dual (control)	Continuous mandatory ventilation	DC-CMV
	Intermittent mandatory ventilation	DC-IMV
	Continuous spontaneous ventilation	DC-CSV

parameter values used in the conditional statements. The specification of the breathing pattern that the mode can produce (that is, breath control variable(s) and breath sequence), and the type of control (hierarchical set point, hierarchical servo, or adaptive set-point control), and the specific strategy (phase variable and operational logic) it uses, for both mandatory and spontaneous breaths, forms a complete classification for any mode of ventilation. A simple example of how a mode can be described with this system is as follows:

- Ventilator name: Bear 1000
- Mode name: SIMV/CPAP (PSV)
- Breathing pattern: Volume-controlled IMV
- Control type: Hierarchical set point
- Control strategy:

Phase variables for mandatory breaths
Trigger: Pressure (sensitivity adjustable from 0.2 to 5.0 cm H_2O)
Time (rate adjustable from 0 to 120 cycles/min)
Limit: Flow (10 to 150 liters/min)
Volume (whenever inspiratory pause time is set >0)
Cycle: Volume (tidal volume adjustable from 100 to 2000 mL)
Time (whenever inspiratory pause time is set >0)
Pressure (when inspiratory pressure violates alarm setting)
Baseline: PEEP/CPAP level adjustable from 0 to 50 cm H_2O

Phase variables for spontaneous breaths
Trigger: Pressure (sensitivity adjustable from 0.2 to 5.0 cm H_2O)
Limit: Pressure (0 to 65 cm H_2O above baseline)
Cycle: Flow (when inspiratory flow decays to 30% of peak flow)
Time (when inspiration exceeds preset threshold)
Baseline: PEEP/CPAP level adjustable from 0 to 50 cm H_2O

Operational logic
If the patient triggers a breath after the start of a ventilatory period (the time equal to the reciprocal of the set ventilatory rate), then a mandatory breath is delivered. If subsequent breathing efforts are detected during the same period, then spontaneous breaths are delivered. If a breathing effort is not detected during a given ventilatory period, then a mandatory breath is time-triggered at the beginning of the next period, and time-triggered mandatory breaths will continue at the set rate until a breathing effort is detected and the sequence repeats.

This system helps to distinguish modes that look the same on graphics monitors and suggests what the operator must do to set the controls. For example, pressure-support mode (for any ventilator) is PC-CSV, for which the operator sets the sensitivity and pressure limit. In contrast, volume-assist mode (Siemens 300) is DC-CSV and looks similar to pressure-support mode on the graphics monitor, but the operator must set a tidal volume in addition to sensitivity and pressure limit.

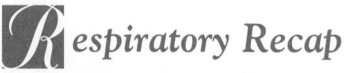

Ventilator Mode Classification Scheme	
Breathing pattern	Specific control strategy
Type of control strategy	Operational logic

Control Subsystems

Control Circuit

The **control circuit** is the subsystem responsible for controlling the drive mechanism and/or the output control valve. A ventilator may have more than one control circuit, which may be one of the following several types:

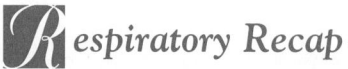

Control Circuits	
Mechanical	Electric
Pneumatic	Electronic
Fluidic	

- *Mechanical control circuits* use levers, pulleys, cams, and so on. These types of circuits were used in the early manually operated ventilators illustrated in history books.[17]
- *Pneumatic control circuits* use gas pressure to operate diaphragms, jet-entrainment devices, pistons, and so on. The original Bird and Bennett PR series ventilators used pneumatic control.
- *Fluidic circuits* are analogs of electronic logic circuits.[18] They use minute gas flows to generate signals that operate timing systems and pressure switches, making them immune to failure from electromagnetic interference (such as that around MRI equipment). Fluidic circuits can be constructed with discrete components, such as comparators and flip-flops, or combined in the form of integrated circuits, analogous to electronic integrated circuits. Examples of ventilators using fluidic logic control circuits are the Sechrist IV-100B and the Bio-Med MVP-10.
- *Electric control circuits* use only simple switches, rheostats (or potentiometers), and magnets to control ventilator operation. One example of a completely electrically controlled ventilator is the Emerson Iron Lung.
- *Electronic control circuits* use devices such as resistors, capacitors, diodes, and transistors, as well as combina-

tions of these components in the form of integrated circuits. Integrated circuits can range in complexity from simple logic gates and operational amplifiers to microprocessors.

Drive Mechanism

The power transmission and conversion system, sometimes referred to as the *drive mechanism*, generates the force necessary to deliver gas to the patient. In general terms this system is composed of either a compressor external to the ventilator in conjunction with a regulator inside the ventilator or an **internal compressor** linked to a motor. A complete description of all possible systems is beyond the scope of this chapter but may be found elsewhere.[19] A brief description of some systems used and their components follows:

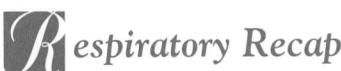espiratory Recap

Drive Mechanisms
Compressor
Motor and linkage
Electric motor with rotating crank and piston rod
Electric motor with rack and pinion
Direct electric motor
Direct compressed gas regulator

- *Compressors:* A compressor is a device, the internal volume of which can be changed to increase the pressure of the gas it contains. Large, water-cooled, piston-type compressors often are used to supply gas under pressure to outlets near patient beds in hospitals. When a ventilator uses compressed gas from wall outlets as its only source of power to drive inspiration, the ventilator is considered to have an **external compressor**. Alternatively, a small compressor designed for use with a single ventilator may be used. The three types of compressors commonly used inside ventilators are (1) piston and cylinder compressors (for example, Emerson IMV), (2) nellows compressors (for example, Servo 900C), and (3) turbine compressors (for example, Bird T-Bird).
- *Motors:* A motor is anything that produces motion. As it relates to a mechanical ventilator, the motor is the device used to drive the compressor. For those ventilators with internal compressors, the characteristics of interest are the type of motor and the linkage between the compressor and motor because these factors influence the waveforms the ventilator can produce.
- *Electric motor/rotating crank and piston rod:* This type of system consists of a piston rod connected to a rotating wheel. The circular motion of the wheel produces a quasi-sinusoidal motion at the distal end of the piston rod (for example, Emerson IMV). A true sinusoidal

motion is generated only by a rotating crank in combination with a Scotch yoke.[20]
- *Electric motor/rack and pinion:* This system produces a linear motion of the rack, driving the piston forward at either a constant or a variable rate, depending on the control circuit.
- *Electric motor/direct:* This system can produce either a rotary motion of the output shaft, such as on a rotating vane air compressor (for example, Bear 2), or a linear motion, as in the case of a linear drive motor. The linear drive motor is particularly versatile because it can produce a wide variety of easily controllable output waveforms.
- *Compressed gas:* When compressed gas is used as the motor, its force is often adjusted by a pressure regulator (pressure reducing valve). The compressed gas either directly inflates the lungs (for example, NPB 7200) or stores energy in a spring (for example, Servo 900C mechanism).

Output Control Valve

The output control valve is used to regulate the flow of gas to the patient. It may be a simple on/off valve (also called an *exhalation valve*) or may be used to shape the output waveform, as in the Siemens ventilators. The following is a list of the most commonly used types:

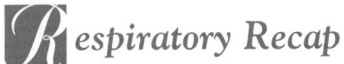espiratory Recap

Output Control Valves	
Electromagnetic poppet valve	Proportional valve
Pneumatic poppet valve	Pneumatic diaphragm

- *Electromagnetic poppet valve:* This type of device (also called a *solenoid valve*) uses magnetic force caused by an electric current to allow a small voltage to control a large pneumatic pressure in an on/off fashion. Examples include the electronic interface valve (for example, Infant Star, which uses a set of valves to approximate various pressure or flow waveforms), the plunger (for example, Bear Cub), and the pinch valve (for example, Bunnell Life Pulse Jet Ventilator).
- *Pneumatic poppet valve:* This type of valve is similar to a solenoid valve except that it uses a small pneumatic pressure (for example, a fluidic signal) to control a larger pneumatic pressure. These valves are particularly useful when electronic signals are inconvenient or hazardous.
- *Proportional valve:* Also known in industrial settings as a *mass flow control valve*, the proportional valve is similar to the solenoid valve in that it is operated by an electromagnet, perhaps in the form of a stepper motor (that is, an electric motor in which rotation can be controlled in discrete arcs or "steps"). The major difference

between the two is that rather than simply turning flow on and off, this type of valve can shape the flow waveform during inspiration by changing the diameter of its outflow port and can be used to create a variety of waveforms. Proportional valves are used in the NPB 7200 and the Hamilton Veolar ventilators and in the form of scissors valves in the Servo 900C or stepper motors in the Bear 5.

- *Pneumatic diaphragm:* Usually operated as an on/off type of valve, the pneumatic diaphragm device uses a flexible diaphragm, or membrane (for example, a "mushroom" valve), to divert gas from one pathway to another. These devices are referred to commonly as *exhalation valves*, which is a misnomer because they are primarily responsible for diverting gas into the patient's lungs during inspiration. However, they also are responsible for slowing exhalation (expiratory retard) and maintaining PEEP. Pneumatic diaphragms are used often in ventilators, such as in the Newport ventilators.

Many ventilators use more than one output control valve. In particular, one valve is often used to direct flow into the patient's airway (for example, a mushroom valve), whereas another may be used to shape the waveform (for example, a proportional valve).

Output

Just as the study of heart physiology involves the study of electrocardiograms and blood pressure waveforms, the study of ventilator operation requires the examination of output waveforms. The waveforms of interest, of course, are the pressure, volume, and flow waveforms used throughout this discussion.

For each control variable, a limited number of waveforms commonly are used by currently available ventilators. These waveforms can be idealized as shown in Figure 39-10 and have been grouped into four basic categories: rectangular (pulse), exponential, ramp, and sinusoidal. A rectangular volume waveform is theoretically impossible because volume cannot change instantaneously from zero to some preset value as can pressure and flow.

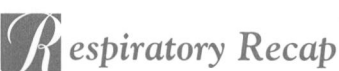 *espiratory Recap*

Ventilator Output Waveforms	
Rectangular	Ramp
Exponential	Sinusoidal

Characteristic idealized ventilator output waveforms shown in Figure 39-10 are precisely defined by mathematic equations and are meant to characterize the operation of the ventilator's control system. As such, they do not show

the minor deviations or "noise" often seen in waveforms recorded during actual ventilator use. These waveform imperfections can be caused by a variety of extraneous variables, such as vibration and turbulence, and the appearance of the waveform is affected by the scaling of the time axis. The waveforms also do not show the effects of the resistance of the expiratory side of the patient circuit because this factor varies depending on the ventilator and type of circuit.

No ventilator is an ideal controller, and ventilators are designed only to approximate a particular waveform. Idealized, or standard, waveforms are nevertheless helpful because they are common in other fields (for example, electrical engineering), which permits the use of mathematic procedures and terminology that have already been developed. For example, a standard mathematic equation is used to describe the most common waveforms for each control variable. This known equation may be substituted into the Equation of Motion, which is then solved to obtain the equations of the other two variables. Once the equations for pressure, volume, and flow are known, they are easily graphed (Figure 39-14).

As mentioned previously, most ventilator waveforms can be classified as one of four general types: rectangular, exponential, ramp, or sinusoidal (including sigmoidal and oscillating). Although many subtypes are possible, only the most common are described in this chapter. Waveforms are listed according to the shape of the control variable waveform. Any new waveforms produced by future ventilators can easily be accommodated by this system.

The ramp waveform is what many respiratory therapists (and ventilator manufacturers) call an *accelerating* or *decelerating* flow waveform. The term *ramp* is borrowed from electronic engineering and is preferred for three reasons. First, the word provides an obvious visual image of the actual shape of the waveform. Second, the term has been described mathematically and used universally for much longer than mechanical ventilators have been in existence. Third, the analogy of something accelerating or decelerating is misapplied. For example, when a car is moving, it is said to have a certain speed (that is, Speed = Change in distance ÷ Change in time). If the speed increases with time, the car is said to accelerate (that is, Acceleration = Change in speed ÷ Change in time), not that the speed accelerates. The speed of moving gas is expressed as a flow (that is, Flow = Area of tube × Change in distance ÷ Change in time). If the flow increases, the gas is said to accelerate (that is, Acceleration = Change in flow rate ÷ Change in time), not that the flow accelerates. In scientific terms, the acceleration of a particle is the rate of change of its velocity with time.[21]

Effects of the Patient Circuit

The pressure, volume, and flow measured inside the ventilator are never the same as pressure, volume, and flow

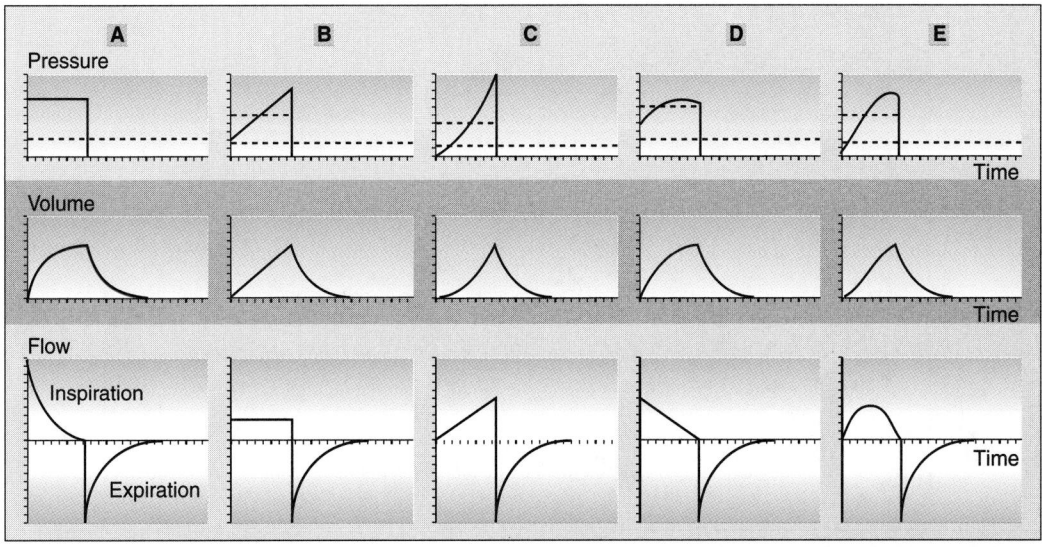

Figure 39-14 Typical pressure, volume, and flow waveforms for pressure-controlled (rectangular pressure waveform) and volume-controlled (various flow waveforms) ventilation. The curves show pressure, volume, and flow as functions of time in accordance with the Equation of Motion (in which muscle pressure is zero). The *upper dotted line* is mean inspiratory pressure. The *lower dotted line* is mean airway pressure measured over one ventilatory period. In **A,** mean inspiratory pressure is equal to peak inspiratory pressure. **A,** Pressure-controlled ventilation with a rectangular pressure waveform. **B,** Volume-controlled ventilation with a rectangular flow waveform. **C,** Volume-controlled ventilation with an ascending ramp flow waveform. **D,** Volume-controlled ventilation with a descending ramp flow waveform. **E,** Flow-controlled ventilation with a sinusoidal flow waveform.

measured at the patient's airway opening. The reason, of course, is because the patient circuit has its own compliance (actually, the compliance of the tubing material plus the compressibility of the inspired gas) and resistance. Therefore the pressure measured inside the ventilator on the inspiratory side (for example, on older ventilators like the Bennett MA-1) is always higher than the pressure at the airway opening because of the elastic and flow resistive pressure drops created by the patient circuit. Volume and flow coming from the ventilator are always more than that delivered to the patient because of the effective compliance of the patient circuit. Patient circuit compliance includes not only the compliance of the material the circuit is made from but also the compressibility of the gas within the circuit. This compliance effect absorbs both volume and flow. Compliance and resistance act together to retard or impede gas delivery to the patient.

Another concept borrowed from electronics is that of *impedance,* a mathematic term that describes the ratio of pressure to flow through a circuit. The higher the impedance, the less flow results from a given pressure. Impedance is directly proportional to resistance and elastance and inversely proportional to compliance. The effects of the patient circuit on rectangular pressure and flow waveforms are illustrated in Figure 39-15.

Via analogy to electrical circuits, compliance of the delivery circuit can be shown to be connected in parallel with the compliance of the respiratory system (that is, both elements sharing the same driving pressure). Pneumatic compliance is analogous to electrical capacitance, and pneumatic resistance is analogous to electrical resistance.[7] Therefore the total compliance of the ventilator-patient system is simply the sum of the two compliances. Similarly the resistance of the delivery circuit is shown to be connected in series with the respiratory system resistance (that is, both elements sharing the same flow) so that the total resistance is the sum of the two. From these assumptions, the relation between the volume input to the patient (at the point of connection to the patient's airway opening) and the volume output from the ventilator (at the point of connection to the patient circuit) can be shown to be described by the following equation:

$$\text{Volume input to patient} = \frac{\text{Volume output from ventilator}}{1 + C_{pc}/C_{rs}} \quad (8)$$

where C_{pc} is the compliance of the patient circuit, and C_{rs} is the total compliance of the patient's respiratory system. The equation shows that the larger the patient circuit compliance compared with the patient's respiratory system, the larger the denominator on the right-hand side of the equation. Hence, the smaller the delivered tidal volume is compared with the volume coming from the ventilator's drive mechanism.

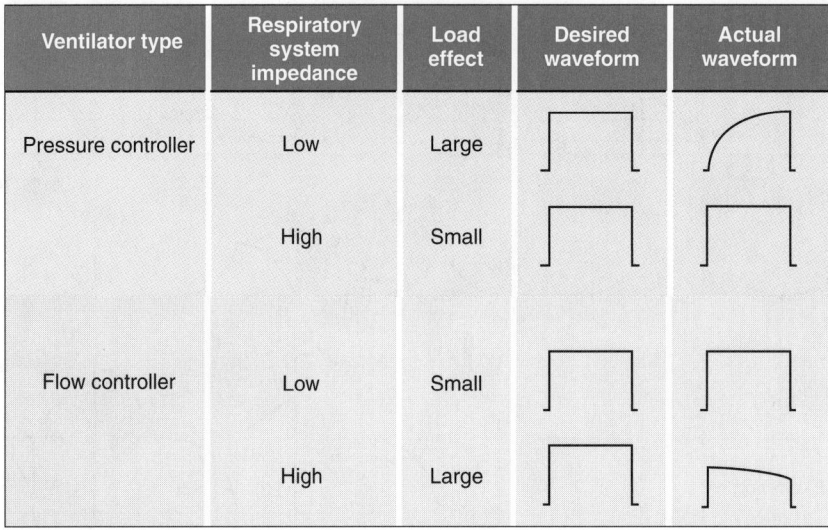

Ventilator type	Respiratory system impedance	Load effect	Desired waveform	Actual waveform
Pressure controller	Low	Large		
	High	Small		
Flow controller	Low	Small		
	High	Large		

Figure 39-15   The effects of loading (by patient circuit and lung mechanics) on ventilator output.

Assuming that the volume exiting the ventilator is the set tidal volume, the patient circuit compliance (C_{pc}) is calculated as follows:

$$C_{PC} = \frac{\text{Set tidal volume}}{P_{plat} - \text{PEEP}} \qquad (9)$$

where P_{plat} is the pressure measured during an inspiratory hold maneuver with the Y-piece of the patient circuit occluded (patient not connected), and PEEP is end-expiratory pressure (that is, baseline pressure). Most authors recommend the use of PIP for P_{plat} in this equation, which is acceptable but may lead to a slight underestimation of patient circuit compliance. P_{plat} is slightly lower than PIP because of the flow-resistive pressure drop of the patient circuit if pressure is not measured at the Y-piece. This difference is greatest in small-bore, corrugated patient circuit tubing but is probably insignificant.

The effects of patient circuit compliance are most troublesome during volume-controlled ventilation. For example, in neonatal ventilation the patient circuit compliance can be as much as three times that of the respiratory system, even with small-bore tubing and a small-volume humidifier. Thus in an attempt to deliver a preset tidal volume, the volume delivered to the patient may be as little as 25% of that exiting the ventilator, whereas 75% is compressed in the patient circuit.

During pressure-controlled ventilation the compliance of the patient circuit has the effect of rounding the leading edge of a rectangular pressure waveform (see Figure 39-15), which could reduce the volume delivered to the patient. This effect is prevented if the pressure limit is maintained for at least five time constants of the respiratory system.

For both pressure- and volume-controlled ventilation the patient circuit compliance and resistance, along with the resistance of the exhalation valve (in series with the patient circuit and respiratory system resistance) increase the expiratory time constant. Thus a large circuit compli-

ance coupled with a short expiratory time can lead to inadvertent auto-PEEP.

In summary, the set values for pressure, volume, and flow may be different from the output (from ventilator) values due to calibration errors and different from the input (to the patient) due to the effects of the patient circuit. Thus two general sources of error cause discrepancies between the desired and actual patient values.

Ventilator Alarm Systems

The ventilator classification scheme described previously centers on the basic functions of input, control, and output. If any of these functions fails, a life-threatening situation may result. Thus ventilators are equipped with various types of alarms, which may be classified in the same manner as the other major ventilator characteristics.

Day and MacIntyre[22,23] have stressed that the goal of ventilator alarms is to warn the operator of events. They define an *event* as any condition or occurrence that requires the clinician's awareness or action. Technical events are those involving an inadvertent change in the ventilator's performance; patient events are those involving a change in the patient's clinical status that can be detected by the ventilator.[18] A ventilator may be equipped with any conceivable vital sign monitor, but the scope in this discussion is limited to include the ventilator's mechanical/electronic operation and those variables associated with the mechanics of breathing (that is, pressure, volume, flow, and time). Because the ventilator is in intimate contact with exhaled gas, the analysis of exhaled oxygen and carbon dioxide concentrations also are included as possible variables to monitor.

Alarms may be audible, visual, or both, depending on the seriousness of the alarm condition. Visual alarms may be as simple as colored lights or as complex as alphanumeric messages to the operator indicating the exact nature of the fault condition. Specifications for an **alarm event** should include (1) conditions that trigger the alarm, (2) the alarm response in the form of audible and/or visual messages, (3) any associated ventilator response, such as termination of inspiration or failure to operate, and (4) whether the alarm must be manually reset or resets itself when the alarm condition is rectified. Alarm categories are based on the ventilator classification scheme and are detailed in the following discussion.

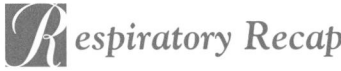

espiratory Recap —————————

Ventilator Alarms	
Input power alarms	Output alarms
Control circuit alarms	

Input Power Alarms

Most ventilators have some sort of battery backup in the case of electrical power failure, even if the batteries only power alarms. Ventilators typically have alarms that are activated if the electrical power is cut off while the machine is still switched on (for example, if the power cord is accidentally pulled from the wall socket). If the ventilator is designed to operate on battery power (for example, transport ventilators), an alarm usually is designed to warn of a low-battery condition.

Ventilators that use pneumatic power have alarms that are activated if either the oxygen or air supply is cut off or reduced below some specified driving pressure. In some cases the alarm is activated by an electronic pressure switch (for example, NPB 7200), but in others the alarm is pneumatically operated as a part of the blender (for example, Siemens Servo 900C).

Control Circuit Alarms

Control circuit alarms are those that either warn the operator that the set control variable parameters are incompatible (for example, inverse inspiration to expiration [I:E] ratio) or indicate that some aspect of a ventilator self-test has failed. In the latter case, something may be wrong with the ventilator control circuitry itself (for example, a microprocessor failure), and the ventilator generally responds with some generic message such as "ventilator inoperative."

Output Alarms

Output alarms are those triggered by an unacceptable state of the ventilator's output. More specifically, an output alarm is activated when the value of a control variable (pressure, volume, flow, or time) falls outside an expected range. Some possibilities include the following:

Pressure Alarms

- *High and low peak airway pressure:* These alarms occur when a possible endotracheal tube obstruction or leak in the patient circuit, respectively, occur.
- *High and low mean airway pressure:* These alarms indicate a possible leak in the patient circuit or a change in ventilatory pattern that might lead to a change in the patient's oxygenation status. That is, within reasonable limits, oxygenation is roughly proportional to **mean airway pressure**.
- *High and low baseline pressure:* These alarms indicate a possible patient circuit or exhalation manifold obstruction (or inadvertent PEEP) and disconnection of the patient from the patient circuit, respectively.
- *Failure to return to baseline:* Failure of airway pressure to return to the baseline level within a specified period indicates a possible patient circuit obstruction or exhalation manifold malfunction.

Volume Alarms

- *High and low expired volume:* These alarms indicate changes in respiratory system time constant during pressure-controlled ventilation, leaks around the endotracheal tube or from the lungs, or possible disconnection of the patient from the patient circuit.

Flow Alarms

- *High and low expired minute ventilation:* These alarms indicate hyperventilation (or possible machine self-triggering) or possible apnea or disconnection of the patient from the patient circuit.

Time Alarms

- *High or low ventilatory frequency:* When these alarms activate, hyperventilation (or possible machine self-triggering) or possibly apnea may be happening.
- *Inappropriate inspiratory time:* A too-long inspiratory time indicates a possible patient circuit obstruction or exhalation manifold malfunction. A too-short inspiratory time indicates that adequate tidal volume may not be delivered (in a pressure-controlled mode) or that gas distribution in the lungs may not be optimal.
- *Inappropriate expiratory time:* A too-long expiratory time may indicate apnea, whereas a too-short expiratory time may warn of alveolar gas trapping. That is, expiratory time should be greater than or equal to five time constants of the respiratory system.

Inspired Gas Alarms

- High/low inspired gas temperature
- High/low F_{IO_2}

Expired Gas Alarms

Because ventilators are designed to control the mechanical results of exhalation, they may be easily adapted to the analysis of exhaled gas composition, and alarms may be set for the following specific parameters:

• *Exhaled carbon dioxide tension:* End-tidal carbon dioxide monitoring may reflect arterial carbon dioxide tension and thus indicate the level of ventilation. Calculation of mean expired carbon dioxide tension along with minute ventilation measurements could provide information about carbon dioxide production and contribute to the calculation of the respiratory exchange ratio and the tidal volume/dead space ratio.

• *Exhaled oxygen tension:*[24] Analysis of end-tidal and mean expired oxygen tension may provide information about gas exchange and could be used along with carbon dioxide data to calculate the respiratory exchange ratio.

KEY POINTS

- The Equation of Motion can be used to describe the pressure required to move a flow of gas into the lungs and produce a tidal volume during mechanical ventilation.
- During pressure-controlled ventilation, pressure is the independent variable, and the shapes of the volume and flow waveforms depend on the shape of the pressure waveform and the resistance and compliance of the respiratory system.
- During flow-controlled ventilation, flow is the independent variable, and the shape of the volume waveform depends on the shape of the flow waveform, with the pressure waveform depending on the flow waveform and the resistance and compliance of the respiratory system.
- A ventilator can directly control only one variable at a time: pressure, volume, or flow.
- Dual-controlled ventilation can be within a breath or between breaths.
- A ventilator can be classified as either a pressure, volume, or flow controller.
- The trigger variable initiates the inspiratory phase, which can be initiated either by the ventilator (that is, time) or by the patient (for example, pressure or flow).
- The ventilator may limit pressure, volume, or flow during the inspiratory phase.

- The variable that is measured and used to terminate the inspiratory phase is the cycle variable.
- Baseline is the variable that is controlled during the expiratory phase.
- Conditional variables determine whether the pattern of control and phase variables for each breath.
- Mandatory breaths are machine triggered and/or machine cycled; spontaneous breaths are patient triggered and patient cycled.
- Every breath is a mandatory breath with continuous mandatory ventilation; every breath is a spontaneous breath with continuous spontaneous ventilation.
- Pressure control occurs when the ventilator attempts to maintain a set airway pressure waveform during inspiration; volume control occurs when the ventilator attempts to maintain a preset volume or flow waveform during inspiration.
- Control subsystems in mechanical ventilators include the control circuit, drive mechanism, and output control valve.
- Output control waveforms on ventilators are rectangular, exponential, ramp, and sinusoidal.
- The compliance, compressibility, and resistance of the ventilator circuit affect gas delivery between the ventilator and the patient.
- Ventilator alarms can be classified as input power alarms, control circuit alarms, and output alarms.

References

1. Mushin M, Rendell-Baker W, Thompson PW, et al. Automatic ventilation of the lungs. Oxford: Blackwell Scientific Publications; 1980. pp. 62-166.
2. Consensus statement on the essentials of mechanical ventilators—1992. Respir Care 1992;37:1000-1008.
3. Chatburn RL. Classification of mechanical ventilators. Respir Care 1992;37:1009-1025.
4. Branson RD, Chatburn RL. Technical description and classification of modes of ventilator operation. Respir Care 1992;37:1026-1044.
5. Morris W. The American heritage dictionary of the English language. Boston: American Heritage Publishing and Houghton Mifflin; 1975. p. 780.
6. Otis AB, McKerrow CB, Bartlett RA, et al. Mechanical factors in distribution of pulmonary ventilation. J Appl Physiol 1956;8:427-443.
7. Chatburn RL, Primiano FP Jr. Mathematical models of respiratory mechanics. In: Chatburn RL, Craig KC, editors. Fundamentals of respiratory care research. Stamford, Conn: Appleton & Lange; 1988.
8. Younes M. Proportional assist ventilation, a new approach to ventilatory support. Am Rev Respir Dis 1992;145:114-120.
9. Rubinstein MF. Patterns of problem solving. Englewood Cliffs, NJ: Prentice-Hall; 1975. pp. 409-473.
10. Hess D, Lind L. Nomograms for the application of the Bourns Model BP200 as a volume-constant ventilator. Respir Care 1980;25:248-250.
11. Desautels DA. Ventilator performance evaluation. In: Kirby RR, Smith RA, Desautels DA, editors. Mechanical ventilation. New York: Churchill Livingstone; 1985. p. 120.
12. Sassoon CSH, Giron AE, Ely EA, et al. Inspiratory work of breathing on flow-by and demand-flow continuous positive airway pressure. Crit Care Med 1989;17:1108-1114.

13. Shachter RD. Evaluating influence diagrams. Operations Res 1986;34:871-882.
14. Seiver A, Holtzman S. Decision analysis: a framework for critical care decision assistance. Int J Clin Monit Comput 1989;6:137-156.
15. Perry DG. A simplified diagram for understanding the operation of volume-preset ventilators. Respir Care 1977;22:42-49.
16. Chatburn RL, Lough MD, Primiano FP Jr. Mechanical ventilation. In: Chatburn RL, Lough MD, editors. Handbook of respiratory care. 2nd ed. St. Louis: Mosby; 1990. pp. 159-223.
17. Morch ET. History of mechanical ventilation. In: Kirby RR, Smith RA, Desautels DA, editors. Mechanical ventilation. New York: Churchill Livingstone; 1985. pp. 1-58.
18. Russell DF, Ross DG, Manson HJ. Fluidic cycling devices for inspiratory and expiratory timing in automatic ventilators. J Biomed Eng 1983;5:227-234.
19. Dupuis YG. Ventilators: theory and application. St. Louis: Mosby; 1986.
20. Beckwith TG, Buck NL, Marangoni RD. Mechanical measurements. 3rd ed. Reading, Mass: Addison-Wesley; 1982. p. 25.
21. Halliday D, Resnick R. Fundamentals of physics. 2nd ed. New York: John Wiley & Sons; 1981. p. 29.
22. Day S, MacIntyre NR. Ventilator alarm systems. Probl Respir Care 1991;4:118-126.
23. MacIntyre NR, Day S. Essentials for ventilator-alarm systems. Respir Care 1992;37:1108-1112.
24. Weingarten M. Respiratory monitoring of carbon dioxide and oxygen: a ten-year perspective. J Clin Monit 1990;6:217-225.

CHAPTER 40

Mechanical Ventilation

Dean R. Hess
Richard D. Branson

CHAPTER OUTLINE

OBJECTIVES

1. List the indications for and complications of mechanical ventilation.
2. Discuss issues related to ventilator-associated lung injury.
3. Discuss issues related to selection of the initial ventilator settings.
4. List parameters that should be monitored during mechanical ventilation.
5. Discuss issues related to weaning from mechanical ventilation.

KEY TERMS

Auto-PEEP
Compressible Volume
Continuous Mandatory Ventilation (CMV)
Continuous Positive Airway Pressure (CPAP)
Dual Control Mode
Flow Triggering
Lung Protection Strategy

Mean Airway Pressure ($\bar{P}_{aw}$)
Oxygen Toxicity
Patient-Ventilator Dyssynchrony
Peak Inspiratory Pressure (PIP)
Permissive Hypercapnia
Plateau Pressure (P_{plat})
Positive End-Expiratory Pressure (PEEP)
Pressure-Control Ventilation (PCV)
Pressure-Support Ventilation (PSV)

Pressure Triggering
Spontaneous Breathing Trial (SBT)
Synchronized Intermittent Mandatory Ventilation (SIMV)
Ventilator-Induced Lung Injury
Volume-Control Ventilation (VCV)
Weaning

Mechanical ventilation is a form of life support. It most often provides a positive pressure to the lungs, but techniques that apply a negative pressure around the thorax can also be used. Mechanical ventilation is a life-saving treatment, but recognition is growing that when used incorrectly, it can increase morbidity and mortality.

Indications for Mechanical Ventilation

Mechanical ventilation is indicated in many situations (Box 40-1).[1-3] Although these conditions are useful in the determination of whether mechanical ventilation is needed, clinical judgment is as important as strict adherence to absolute guidelines. One indication for mechanical ventilation is seemingly imminent acute respiratory failure; in such cases initiating mechanical ventilation may prevent overt respiratory failure and respiratory arrest. Drug overdose and major surgery are indications that may not involve primary respiratory failure. Short-term mechanical ventilation also is commonly used after major surgery, such as open heart surgery, major abdominal surgery, or thoracic surgery.

Complications of Mechanical Ventilation

Mechanical ventilation is not a benign therapy, and it can have major effects on the body's homeostasis (Box 40-2).[4,5] Pulmonary barotrauma (for example, pneumothorax, pneumomediastinum, or subcutaneous emphysema) can result from alveolar overdistention (Figure 40-1).[6,7] Intubated mechanically ventilated patients are at risk for complications associated with the use of artificial airways.[8] Positive pressure ventilation is associated with numerous mechanical complications, the most serious being accidental disconnection.[9] Leaks in the ventilator circuit must be corrected to prevent hypoventilation.

Because positive pressure ventilation increases intrathoracic pressure, it can reduce venous return, which may result in decreased cardiac output and a drop in arterial blood pressure. Fluid administration and drug therapy (such as with vasopressors and inotropes) may be necessary to maintain cardiac output, blood pressure, and urine output. Mechanical ventilation also can cause an increase in plasma antidiuretic hormone (ADH) and a decrease in atrial natriuretic peptide (ANP), which may reduce output and promote fluid retention.[10]

Ventilator-associated pneumonia is a common complication of mechanical ventilation.[11] In the past this was thought to arise from the ventilator circuit, and the circuit and ventilator humidification system were changed every 24 to 48 hours. Evidence now indicates that the ventilator circuit is relatively unimportant in the development of this condition so long as reasonable infection control practices are followed. Ventilator-associated pneumonia usually is caused by aspiration of oropharyngeal secretions (despite the use of a cuffed endotracheal tube) and not by what is breathed through the endotracheal tube. Because the ventilator seldom is the cause

---

Box 40-1

Indications for Mechanical Ventilation

> Apnea
> Acute ventilatory failure (rising partial pressure of arterial carbon dioxide [$Paco_2$] with acidosis, respiratory muscle dysfunction, excessive ventilatory load, altered central ventilatory drive)
> Impending ventilatory failure
> Severe oxygenation deficit

Box 40-2

Complications of Mechanical Ventilation

> **Airway Complications**
>   Laryngeal edema
>   Tracheal mucosal trauma
>   Contamination of the lower respiratory tract
>   Loss of humidifying function of the upper airway
>
> **Mechanical Complications**
>   Accidental disconnection
>   Leaks in the ventilator circuit
>   Loss of electrical power
>   Loss of gas pressure
>
> **Pulmonary Complications**
>   Ventilator-induced lung injury
>   Barotrauma
>   Oxygen toxicity
>   Atelectasis
>   Nosocomial pneumonia
>   Inflammation
>
> **Cardiovascular Complications**
>   Reduced venous return
>   Reduced cardiac output
>   Hypotension
>
> **Gastrointestinal and Nutritional Complications**
>   Gastrointestinal bleeding
>   Malnutrition
>
> **Renal Complications**
>   Reduced urine output
>   Increase in antidiuretic hormone (ADH) and decrease in atrial natriuretic peptide (ANP)
>
> **Neurologic Complications**
>   Increased intracranial pressure
>
> **Acid-Base Complications**
>   Respiratory alkalosis

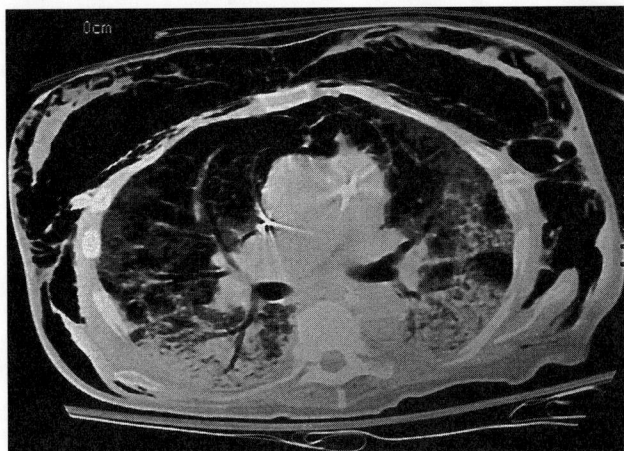

Figure 40-1 Computed tomography (CT) scan of the thorax of a mechanically ventilated patient with severe barotrauma. Note the presence of pneumothorax, pneumomediastinum, and subcutaneous emphysema.

of this type of pneumonia, breathing circuits can be changed weekly or at even longer intervals.[12-16]

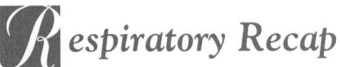espiratory Recap

Indications for and Complications of Mechanical Ventilation
Mechanical ventilation is indicated to support oxygenation and ventilation of patients with acute respiratory failure.
A number of complications are possible with mechanical ventilation, and efforts must be made to minimize these conditions.

Mechanically ventilated patients are at risk for gastrointestinal bleeding and often are given antacids or histamine (H_2) blockers to prevent this complication. Although the evidence is controversial, there is some indication that raising the gastric pH with these medications increases the risk of nosocomial pneumonia.[17] Sucralfate, given orally, may reduce the risk of gastric mucosal bleeding without altering the gastric pH, thereby reducing the risk of ventilator-associated pneumonia.[18] However, aspiration of the stomach contents during sucralfate therapy may increase the risk of lung injury because of the lower pH of the aspirate.[19]

The nutritional needs of mechanically ventilated patients play an important role in preventing or promoting complications.[20] Undernourished patients are at risk for respiratory muscle weakness and pneumonia. An excessive caloric intake, on the other hand, may increase carbon dioxide (CO_2) production, which can markedly increase the patient's ventilatory requirements.

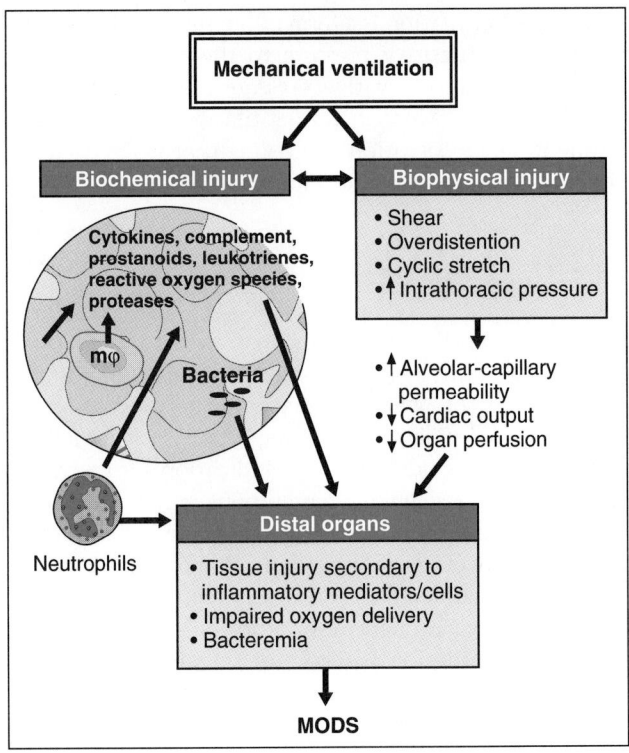

Figure 40-2 Mechanical ventilation can cause biochemical and biophysical injury to the lungs, which may result in multiple organ dysfunction syndrome (MODS). (Modified from Slutsky AS, Trembly L. Am J Respir Crit Care Med 1998; 157:1721-1725.)

Ventilator-Induced Lung Injury

Alveolar overdistention caused by a high peak inflation volume (*volutrauma*) causes acute lung injury.[21] Alveolar overdistention also is associated with high peak alveolar pressures. Because localized overdistention is not easy to monitor, it is inferred from a high peak alveolar pressure. The peak alveolar pressure should be kept below 30 cm H_2O.[22] During mechanical ventilation the peak alveolar pressure is best reflected by the end-inspiratory plateau pressure, which can be easily measured at the bedside. Alveolar overdistention can be minimized during positive pressure ventilation by limiting of the tidal volume (for example, to 6 mL/kg or less in patients with acute respiratory distress syndrome [ARDS]).

Ventilator-induced lung injury also can result from alveolar collapse (*atelectrauma*). The pressure at the junction between an open and a closed alveolus may exceed

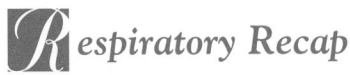espiratory Recap

Types of Ventilator-Induced Lung Injury	
Volutrauma	Biotrauma
Atelectrauma	Oxygen toxicity

TABLE 40-1

Advantages and Disadvantages of Common Modes of Mechanical Ventilation

Mode of Ventilation	Advantages	Disadvantages
Continuous mandatory ventilation (CMV)	Guaranteed volume (or pressure) with each breath Low patient workload if sensitivity and inspiratory flow set correctly	High mean airway pressure Respiratory alkalosis and auto-PEEP if patient triggers at rapid rate Respiratory muscle atrophy
Synchronized intermittent mandatory ventilation (SIMV)	Prevents respiratory alkalosis Lower mean airway pressure Prevents respiratory muscle atrophy	Dyssynchrony if rate set too low High demand valve work of breathing with older ventilators
Pressure-support ventilation (PSV)	Improved patient comfort Overcomes tube resistance Prevents respiratory muscle atrophy Facilitates weaning	Requires spontaneous respiratory effort Fatigue and tachypnea with PSV too low Activation of expiratory muscles with PSV too high

100 cm H_2O,[23] and the cyclic opening of an alveolus during inhalation and closure during exhalation may be injurious to the lungs. This injury is ameliorated by optimal lung recruitment and an expiratory pressure that prevents alveolar derecruitment.

Ventilating the lungs in a manner that promotes alveolar overdistention and derecruitment also increases inflammation in the lungs (*biotrauma*).[24,25] In acute lung injuries, this may slow healing. In addition, inflammatory mediators such as cytokines and chemokines may translocate into the pulmonary circulation, causing systemic inflammation. The way in which the lungs are ventilated therefore may play a role in systemic inflammation (Figure 40-2).

The toxic effects of oxygen (O_2) can cause ARDS-like changes in the lungs.[26] As with overdistention, **oxygen toxicity** primarily affects normal lung units; these areas receive most of the ventilation and therefore are more likely to be injured. To prevent oxygen toxicity, the fractional inspired oxygen concentration (FIO_2) should be set no higher than necessary to maintain adequate arterial oxygenation (over 90% arterial O_2 saturation). Ideally the FIO_2 should be kept below 0.60.

In addition to setting the FIO_2 correctly, the peak alveolar pressure, or **plateau pressure (P_{plat}),** should be kept below 30 cm H_2O, and **positive end-expiratory pressure (PEEP)** should be applied to maintain alveolar recruitment. Such a ventilation technique is known as a **lung protection strategy.** However, this approach may result in respiratory acidosis. Rather than risking damage to the lungs with a high level of ventilation, lung protective strategies permit a high partial pressure of arterial carbon dioxide ($PaCO_2$), known as **permissive hypercapnia.**[27,28] With permissive hypercapnia, the clinical concern generally is related to pH not $PaCO_2$. Most investigators agree that a pH above 7.25 is acceptable, although lower values have been accepted by some clinicians. A pH that allows normal hemodynamic performance, a value that

varies from patient to patient, may be the best target. Complications of permissive hypercapnia include intracellular acidosis, increased intracranial pressure, muscle weakness, and delayed weaning from ventilatory support.

Initial Ventilator Settings

Modes of Ventilation

Options for breath delivery are referred to as *modes of ventilation*.[29,30] Common modes include **continuous mandatory ventilation (CMV), synchronized intermittent mandatory ventilation (SIMV),** and **pressure-support ventilation (PSV).** Dual control modes, which use a feedback loop to enable the ventilator to control pressure or volume, are becoming more widely available on the newest generation of ventilators.[31-33] The choice of mode often is based on institutional policy or the clinician's bias. No one mode is clearly superior; each has its advantages and disadvantages (Table 40-1). When mechanical ventilation is begun, it often is best to use CMV or SIMV to produce nearly complete respiratory muscle rest (that is, full ventilatory support).

CMV delivers a set tidal volume (or pressure) and a minimum respiratory rate (Figure 40-3). The patient can

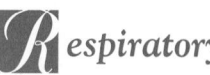
Respiratory Recap

Ventilator Modes
Continuous mandatory ventilation (CMV)
Synchronized intermittent mandatory ventilation (SIMV)
Pressure-support ventilation (PSV)
Continuous positive airway pressure (CPAP)
Dual control modes

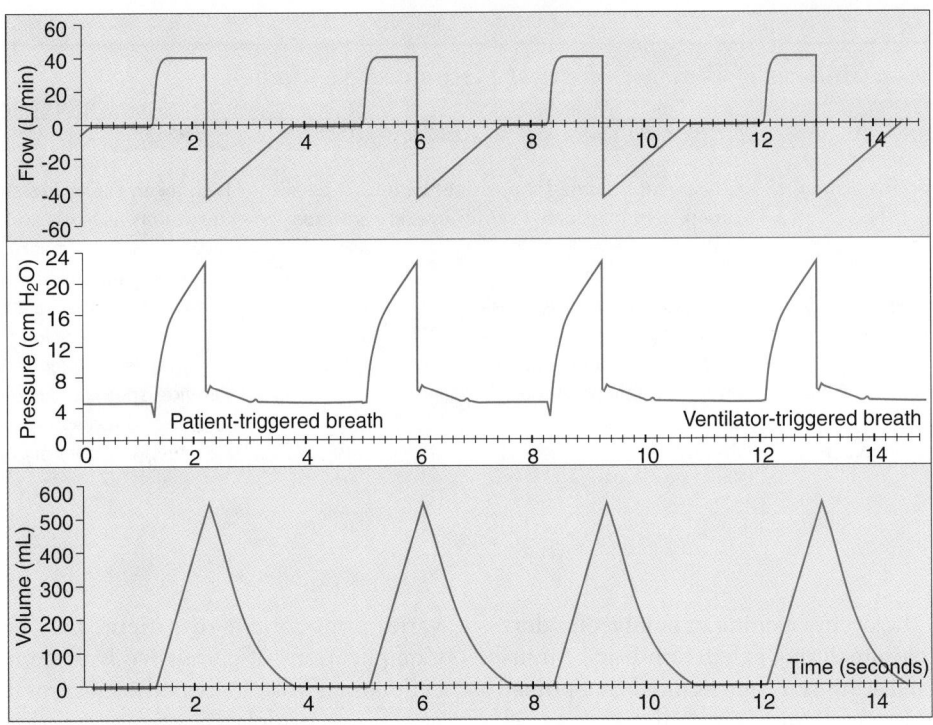

Figure 40-3 Continuous mandatory ventilation (CMV) waveform, showing ventilator triggered and patient-triggered breaths.

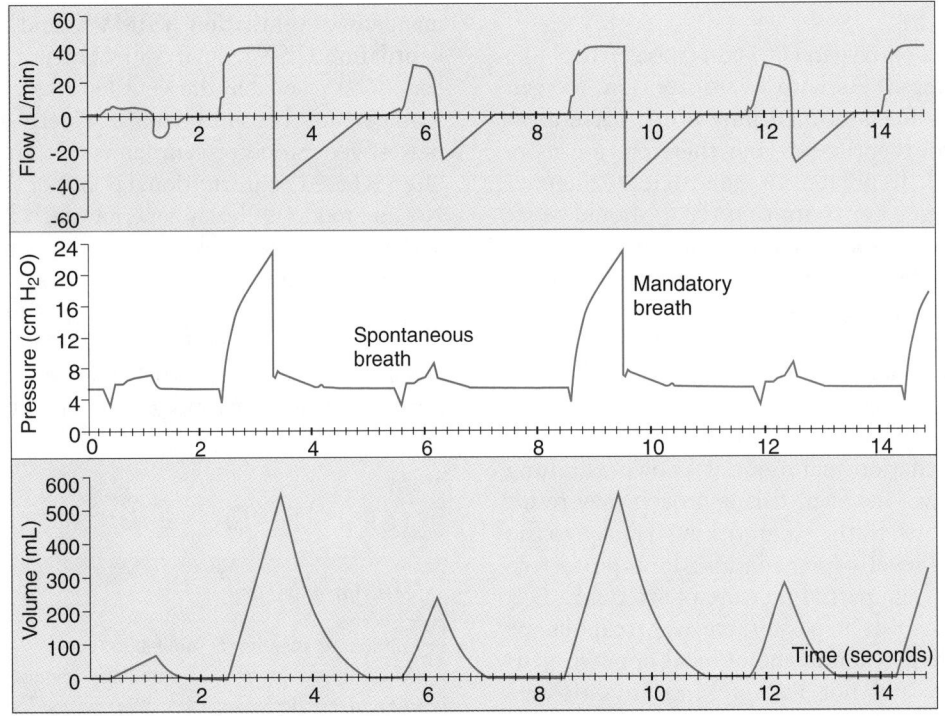

Figure 40-4 Synchronized intermittent mandatory ventilation (SIMV) waveform, showing spontaneous and mandatory breaths.

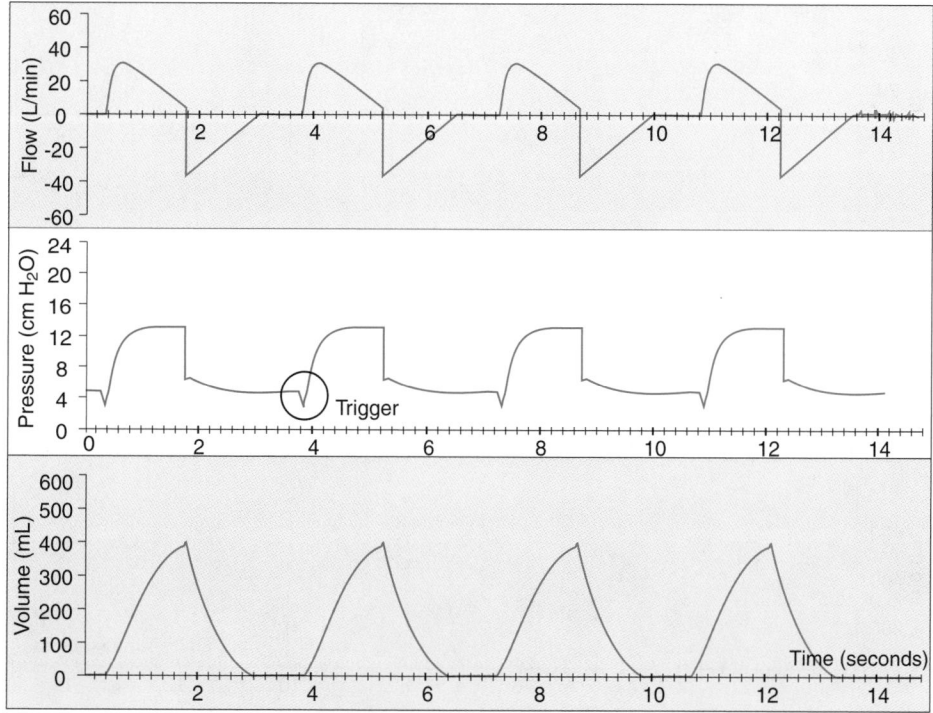

Figure 40-5 Pressure-support ventilation (PSV) waveform.

trigger additional breaths above the minimum rate, but the set volume or pressure remains constant. With SIMV a mandatory breath rate is set, and the patient determines the tidal volume (VT) and the rate of spontaneous breaths between mandatory breaths (Figure 40-4). The mandatory breaths are synchronized with the patient's spontaneous efforts. If the set rate is high enough to satisfy the patient's total ventilatory requirement, SIMV and CMV are similar.

PSV (Figure 40-5) is a spontaneous breathing mode in which patient effort is augmented by a clinician-determined level of pressure during inspiration. Although the clinician sets the level of pressure support, the patient sets the respiratory rate, inspiratory flow, and inspiratory time. The VT is determined by the level of pressure support, the amount of patient effort, and the resistance and compliance of the patient's respiratory system. PSV can be used with SIMV, in which case the spontaneous breaths between mandatory breaths are pressure supported (Figure 40-6). Low-level pressure support can be used to overcome the resistance through the endotracheal tube.

Continuous positive airway pressure (CPAP) is a spontaneous breathing mode (Figure 40-7). The airway pressure is usually but not necessarily greater than atmospheric pressure. CPAP is commonly used to evaluate a patient's ability to breathe spontaneously before extubation.

As was mentioned previously, a **dual control mode** uses a feedback loop to enable the ventilator to control pressure or volume. It is important to remember that the ventilator is controlling only pressure or volume, not both at the same time. Dual control modes are classified as *dual control within a breath* or *dual control breath-to-breath* (Table 40-2). In the dual control within a breath mode, the ventilator switches from pressure control to volume control during the breath. Dual control breath-to-breath is simpler because the ventilator operates in either the pressure-support or pressure-control mode, with the pressure limit increasing or decreasing to maintain a clinician-selected tidal volume.

Regardless of the mode used, the goal is to strike a balance between excessive respiratory muscle rest, which promotes atrophy, and excessive respiratory muscle activity, which promotes fatigue; or, put more simply, to avoid the extremes of too much rest and too much exercise. The highest level of respiratory muscle unloading occurs with CMV. With SIMV the intent is to provide respiratory muscle rest during mandatory breaths and respiratory muscle exercise with the intervening breaths. However, it has been shown that considerable inspiratory effort occurs with both the mandatory breaths and the intervening spontaneous breaths. As the level of SIMV support is reduced, the work of breathing increases for both mandatory and spontaneous breaths (Figure 40-8).[34] This effect can be ameliorated with the addition of pressure support, which results in unloading of both mandatory and spontaneous breaths.[35]

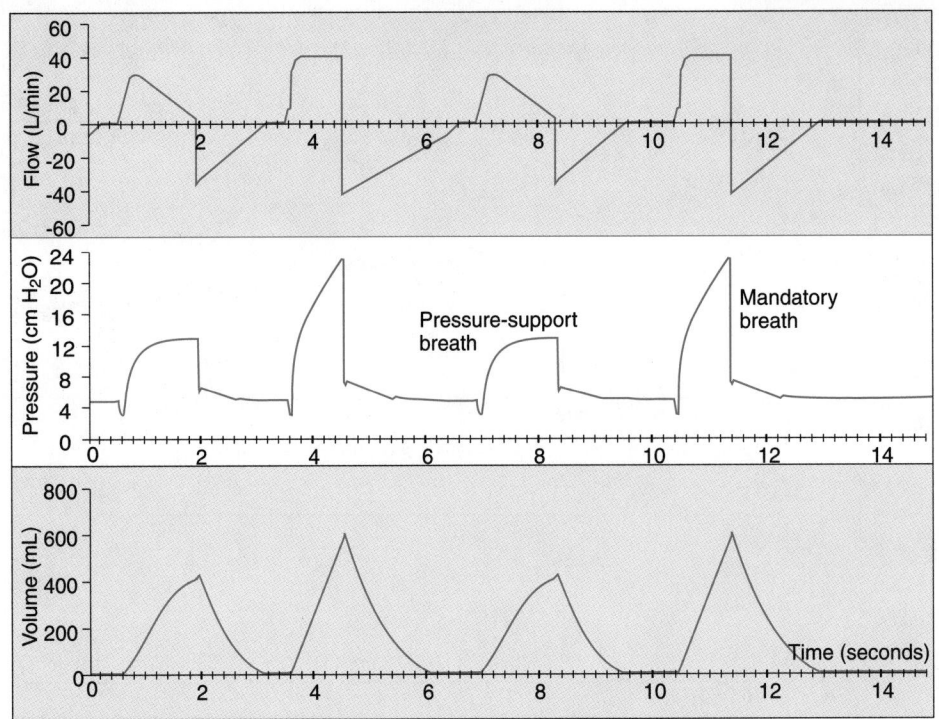

Figure 40-6   Waveform of synchronized intermittent mandatory ventilation (SIMV) with pressure support of spontaneous breaths.

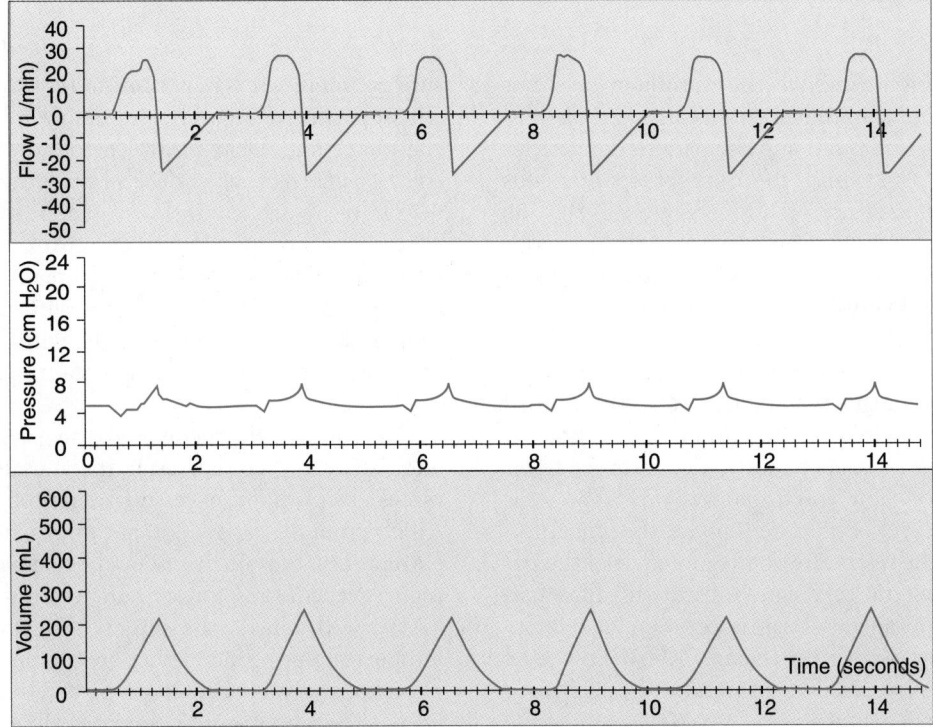

Figure 40-7   Waveform of continuous positive airway pressure (CPAP).

Pressure Triggering Versus Flow Triggering

The effort required to trigger the ventilator is an imposed load for the patient. **Pressure triggering** occurs because of a pressure drop in the system (Figure 40-9). The pressure level at which the ventilator is triggered is set so that the trigger effort is minimal but auto-triggering is unlikely (typically this is 1 to 2 cm H_2O below the PEEP or CPAP).

Flow triggering is an alternative to pressure triggering. With flow triggering the ventilator responds to a change in flow rather than a drop in pressure at the airway (Figure

TABLE 40-2
Dual Control Modes and Ventilators

Mode and Ventilator	Manufacturer's Proprietary Name for Mode
Dual Control within a Breath	
Bird 8400Sti and Tbird (Thermo Respiratory Group)	Volume-assured pressure support
Bear 1000 (Thermo Respiratory Group)	Pressure augmentation
Dual Control Breath-to-Breath	
Pressure-limited, flow-cycled ventilation	
Servo 300 (Siemens)	Volume support
Venturi (Cardiopulmonary Corp.)	Variable pressure support
Pressure-limited, time-cycled ventilation	
Servo 300 (Siemens)	Pressure-regulated volume control
Galileo (Hamilton)	Adaptive pressure ventilation
Evita 4 (Drager)	Autoflow
Venturi (Cardiopulmonary Corp.)	Variable pressure control
Synchronized intermittent mandatory ventilation (SIMV)	
and pressure-support ventilation (PSV)	
Galileo (Hamilton)	Adaptive support ventilation

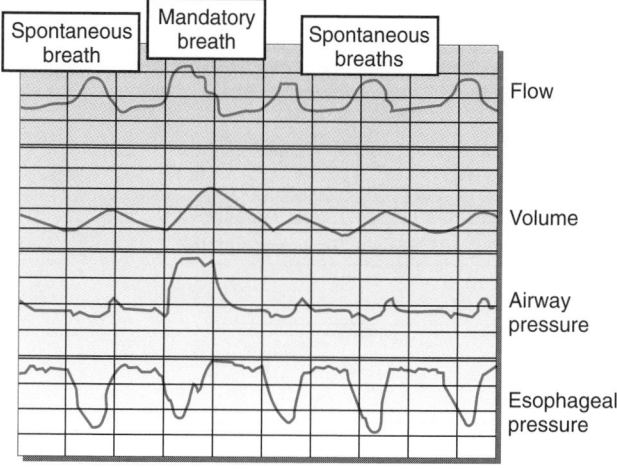

Figure 40-8 Synchronized intermittent mandatory ventilation (SIMV). Note that the esophageal pressure change (that is, the pleural pressure change) for the mandatory breath is nearly as great as that for the spontaneous breaths.

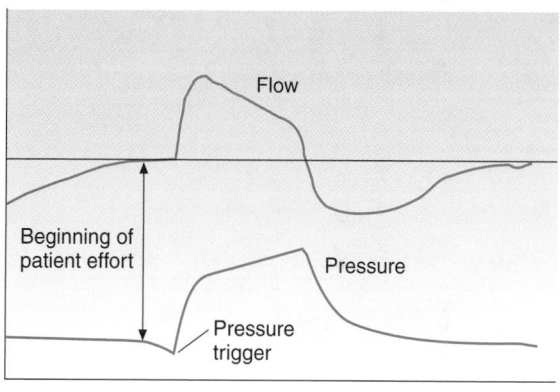

Figure 40-9 Pressure-triggered breath.

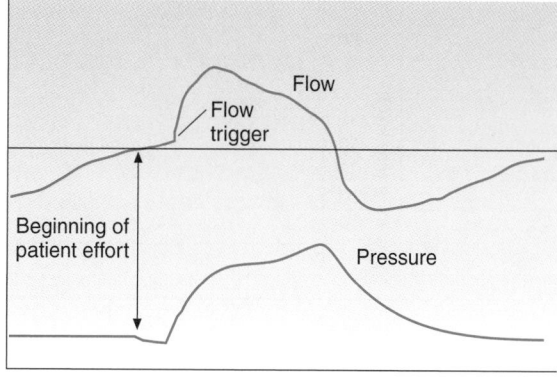

Figure 40-10 Flow-triggered breath.

40-10). With some ventilators, a pneumotachometer is placed between the ventilator circuit and the patient to measure inspiratory flow. In other ventilators, a background or base flow and flow sensitivity are set. When the flow in the expiratory circuit decreases by the amount of the flow sensitivity, the ventilator is triggered. For example, if the base flow is set at 10 L/min and the flow sensitivity is set at 3 L/min, the ventilator triggers when the flow in the expiratory circuit drops to 7 L/min (the assumption is that the patient has inhaled at 3 L/min). Flow triggering has been shown to reduce the work of breathing with CPAP.[36-40] However, it may not be superior to pressure triggering with pressure-supported breaths or mandatory breaths.[41] Neither pressure triggering nor flow trigger-

ing may be effective if **auto-PEEP** is present. Auto-PEEP, which is discussed later in the chapter, is a threshold that must be overcome before the pressure (or flow) decreases at the airway to trigger the ventilator; that is, the patient's inspiratory effort must overcome the level of auto-PEEP

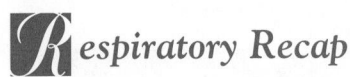espiratory Recap

Types of Ventilator Triggering
Ventilator self-triggers when a set time is reached. Patient triggers the ventilator through changes in pressure or flow.

before either a pressure or flow change is detected at the airway. Regardless of whether pressure triggering or flow triggering is used, the current generation of ventilators is more responsive to patient effort.[42]

Volume Versus Pressure Ventilation

With **volume-control ventilation (VCV),** the ventilator controls the inspiratory flow (Figure 40-11). The tidal vol-

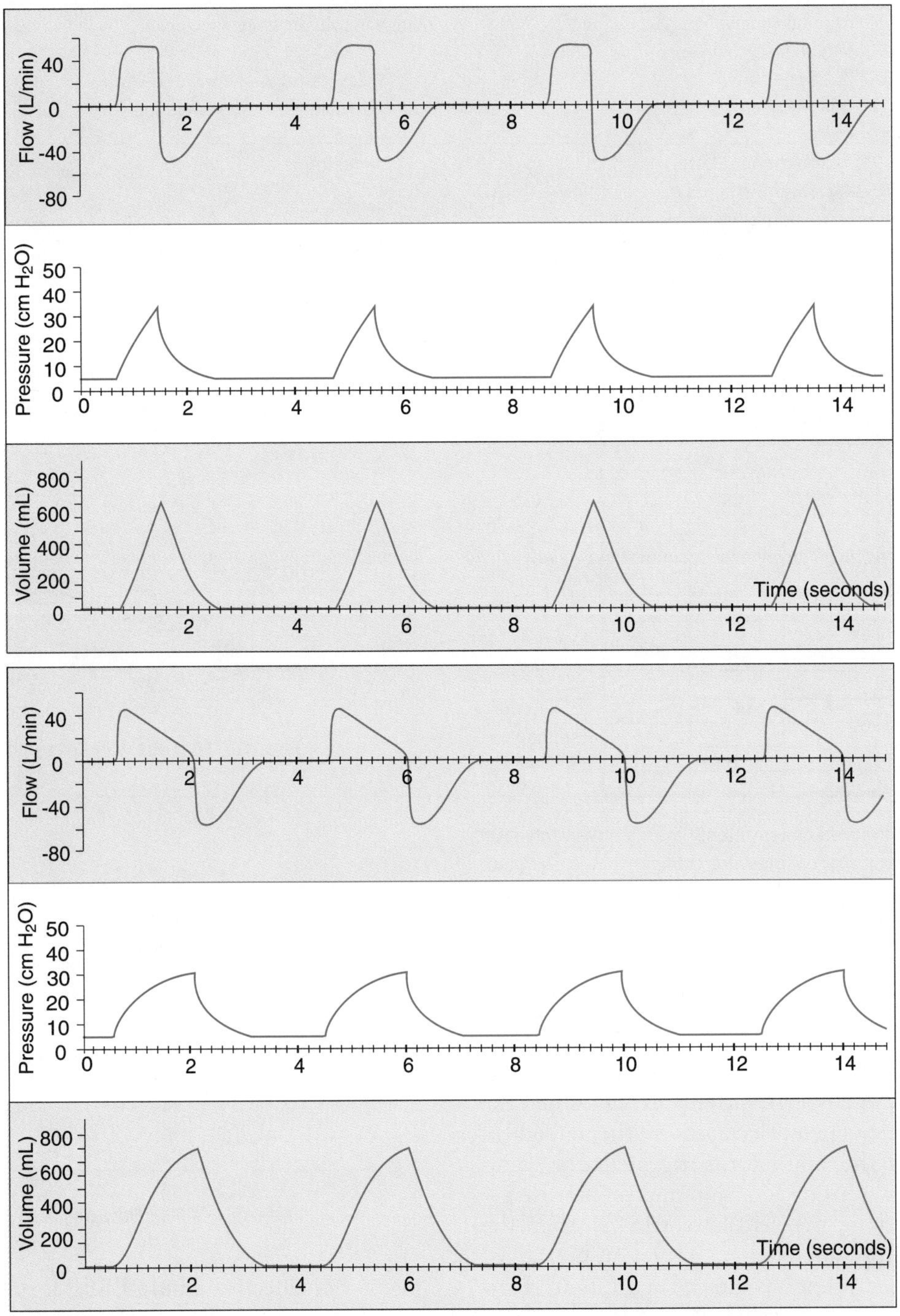

Figure 40-11   Constant flow volume-control ventilation *(top).* Decelerating flow volume-control ventilation *(bottom).*

ume is determined by the flow and the inspiratory time. In practice, however, the flow and tidal volume are set on the ventilator. With VCV the tidal volume is delivered regardless of resistance or compliance, and the peak airway pressure varies (Box 40-3). VCV should be used whenever a constant tidal volume is important in the maintenance of a desired $PaCO_2$, such as with an acute head injury. The principal disadvantage of VCV is that it can produce a high peak alveolar pressure and areas of overdistention in the lungs. Also, because the inspiratory flow is fixed, VCV can cause **patient-ventilator dyssynchrony,** particularly if the inspiratory flow is set too low. With VCV the set flow can be constant or decelerating. A decelerating flow pattern produces a longer inspiratory time unless the peak flow is increased.

With **pressure-control ventilation (PCV),** the airway pressure is set and remains constant despite changes in re-

sistance and compliance (Figure 40-12). Factors that affect the tidal volume with PCV are listed in Box 40-4. The principal advantage of PCV is that it prevents localized alveolar overdistention with changes in resistance and compliance; the peak alveolar pressure cannot be greater than the pressure set on the ventilator. Because the flow can vary with PCV, this mode may improve patient-ventilator synchrony (Figure 40-13).[43,44] The choice of VCV or PCV often is determined by clinician or institutional bias, and both modes have advantages and disadvantages (Table 40-3).

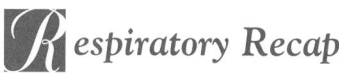

Respiratory Recap

Volume-Control Versus Pressure-Control Ventilation
Volume control: Ventilation remains constant with changes in respiratory mechanics, but airway and plateau pressures can fluctuate.
Pressure control: Ventilation fluctuates with changes in respiratory mechanics, but pressure is limited to the peak pressure set on the ventilator.

PSV is a frequently used mode of mechanical ventilation. However, because it is patient triggered, PSV is not an appropriate mode for patients who do not have an adequate respiratory drive. PSV normally is flow cycled, with secondary cycling mechanisms of pressure and time. Although PSV often is considered a simple mode of ventila-

Box 40-3

Factors that Affect Peak Inspiratory Pressure (PIP) with Volume-Control Ventilation

Peak inspiratory flow setting: A higher flow setting increases the PIP.
Inspiratory flow pattern: PIP is lower with decreasing flow.
Positive end-expiratory pressure (PEEP): An increase in PEEP increases the PIP.
Auto-PEEP: Auto-PEEP increases the PIP.
Tidal volume (V_T): An increase in V_T results in a higher PIP.
Resistance: Greater airways resistance results in a higher PIP.
Compliance: Diminished compliance results in a higher PIP.

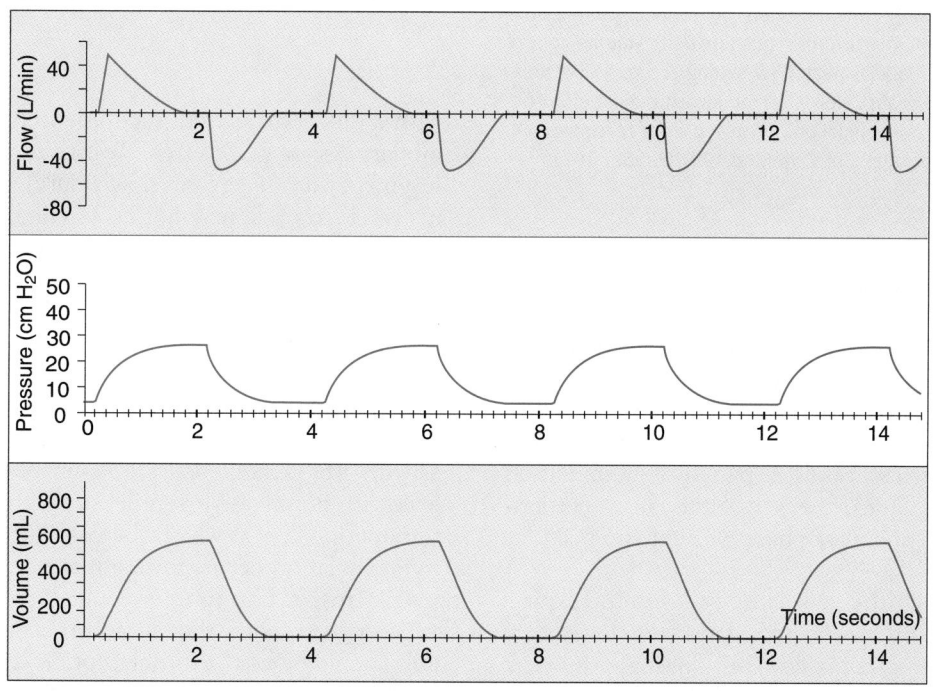

Figure 40-12   Waveform of pressure-control ventilation.

TABLE 40-3

Advantages and Disadvantages of Volume-Control and Pressure-Control Ventilation

Type	Advantages	Disadvantages
Volume ventilation	Constant tidal volume (VT) with changes in resistance and compliance Type of ventilation familiar to most clinicians	Increased plateau pressure (Pplat) with decreasing compliance (alveolar overdistention) Fixed inspiratory flow may cause dyssynchrony
Pressure ventilation	Reduced risk of overdistention with changes in compliance Variable flow improves synchrony	Changes VT with changes in resistance and compliance Clinicians less familiar with pressure-control ventilation

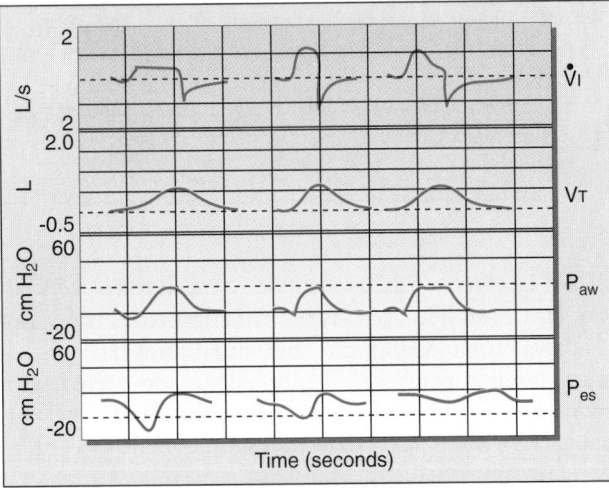

Figure 40-13 Patient effort (reflected by esophageal pressure change) for low-flow, volume-control ventilation *(left)*, volume-control ventilation with an increase in peak flow setting *(center)*, and pressure-control ventilation *(right)*. Note that the lowest patient effort occurs with pressure-control ventilation. (Modified from MacIntyre NR, McConnell R, Cheng KG, et al. Crit Care Med 1997;25:1671-1677.)

BOX 40-4

Factors that Affect Tidal Volume (VT) with Pressure-Control Ventilation

Peak inspiratory pressure: A higher pressure control setting increases the VT.

Auto-PEEP: An increase in auto-PEEP reduces the VT.

Inspiratory time: An increase in inspiratory time increases the VT if inspiratory flow is present; after flow decreases to zero, further increase in the time does not affect the VT.

Compliance: Decreased compliance decreases the VT.

Resistance: Increased resistance decreases the VT if active flow is present; after flow decreases to zero, resistance no longer affects the delivered VT.

Patient effort: Greater inspiratory effort by the patient increases the VT.

tion, it can be quite complex (Figure 40-14). First, the ventilator must recognize the patient's inspiratory effort, which depends on the ventilator's trigger sensitivity and the amount of auto-PEEP. Second, the ventilator must deliver an appropriate flow at the onset of inspiration. A flow that is too high can produce a pressure overshoot, and a flow that is too low can result in patient flow starvation and dyssynchrony. Third, the ventilator must appropriately cycle to the expiratory phase without the need for active exhalation.

The flow at which the ventilator cycles to the expiratory phase during PSV can be a fixed absolute flow, a flow based on the peak inspiratory flow, or a flow based on peak inspiratory flow and elapsed inspiratory time. Several studies have reported dyssynchrony with PSV in individuals with airflow obstruction, such as chronic obstructive pulmonary disease (COPD).[45,46] With airflow obstruction, the inspiratory flow decreases slowly during PSV, and the flow necessary to cycle may not be reached; this course of action stimulates active exhalation to pressure cycle the breath. The problem increases with higher levels of PSV and with higher levels of airflow obstruction. On newer ventilators, the termination flow at which the ventilator cycles can be adjusted to a level appropriate for the patient (Figure 40-15).

Another concern with PSV is leaks in the system, such as with a bronchopleural fistula, uncuffed airway, or mask leak with noninvasive ventilation. If the leak exceeds the termination flow at which the ventilator cycles, either active exhalation occurs to terminate inspiration, or a prolonged inspiratory time is applied. With a leak, either PCV or a ventilator that allows an adjustable termination flow should be used. Another option is to set a maximum inspiratory time during PSV such that the breath can be time cycled at a clinician-determined setting. This sec-

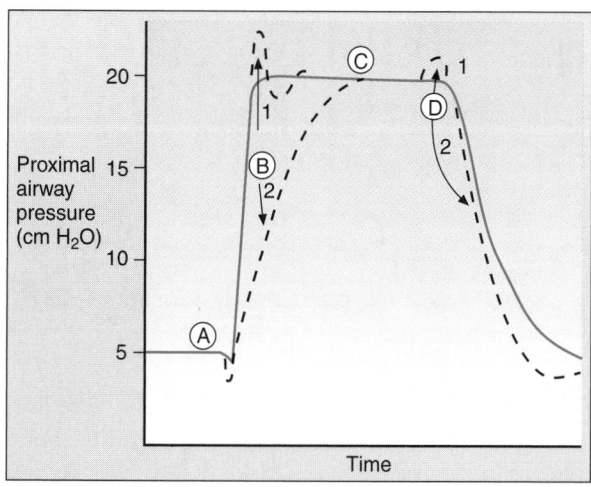

Figure 40-14 Design characteristics of a pressure-supported breath. In this example, the baseline pressure (that is, continuous positive airway pressure [CPAP] is set at 5 cm H_2O (A), and pressure support is set at 15 cm H_2O (a peak inspiratory pressure [PIP] of 20 cm H_2O) (B). The inspiratory pressure is triggered at point A by a patient effort that results in a decrease in airway pressure. Demand valve sensitivity and responsiveness are characterized by the depth and duration of this negative pressure. The rise to pressure (line B) is provided by a fixed high initial flow delivery into the airway. Note that if flows exceed patient demand, the initial pressure exceeds the set level (B1), and if flows fall short of patient demand, a very slow rise to pressure can occur (B2). The plateau of pressure support (line C) is maintained by servo control of flow. A smooth plateau reflects appropriate responsiveness to patient demand, whereas fluctuations reflect less responsiveness of the servo mechanisms. Termination of pressure support occurs at point D and should coincide with the end of the spontaneous inspiratory effort. If termination is delayed, the patient actively exhales (the bump in pressure above the plateau) (D1); if termination occurs prematurely, the patient has continued inspiratory effort (D2). (Modified from MacIntyre N, Nishimura M, Usada Y, et al. The Nagoya Conference on System Design and patient-ventilator interactions during pressure support ventilation. Chest 1990;97:1463-1466.)

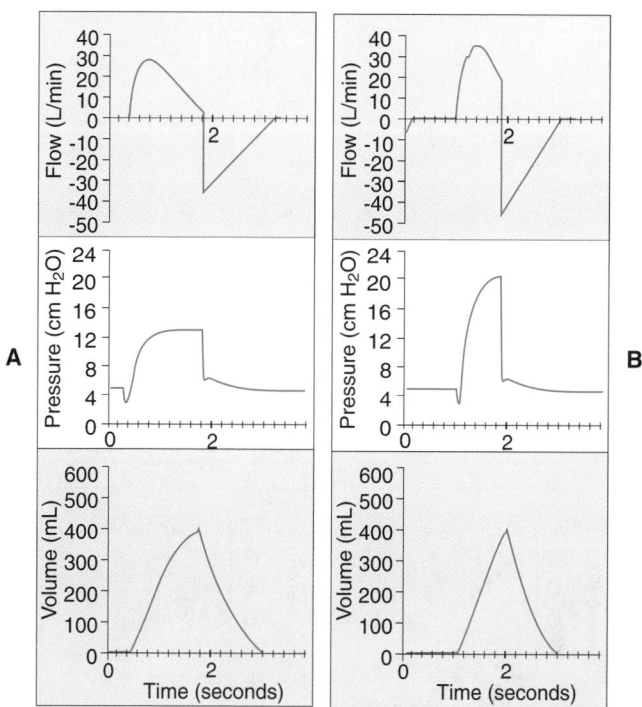

Figure 40-15 The effect of changes in termination flow during pressure-support ventilation. Termination flow is set as a small fraction of peak flow (**A**) and as a greater fraction of peak flow (**B**).

ondary cycle typically has been fixed at a prolonged time to prevent untoward effects of long inspiratory times. Some new ventilators allow both the flow cycle and time cycle to be set.

The flow at the onset of the inspiratory phase may also be important during PCV or PSV. This is called *rise time* and refers to the time required for the ventilator to reach the set pressure at the onset of inspiration. Flows that are too high or too low at the onset of inspiration can cause dyssynchrony. Several of the newer generation of ventilators allow adjustment of the rise time during PSV (Figure 40-16). The rise time should be adjusted to the patient's comfort, and ventilator graphics may be useful as a guide to this setting. However, a high inspiratory flow at the onset of inspiration may not be beneficial.[47] If the flow is higher at the onset of inspiration, the inspiratory phase may be prematurely terminated during PSV if the ventilator cycles to the expiratory phase at a flow that is a fraction of the peak inspiratory flow.

Also, several studies[48,49] have demonstrated the existence of a flow-related inspiratory terminating reflex. Activation of this reflex shortens neural inspiration, which could result in brief, shallow inspiratory efforts, particularly at low pressure-support settings. The clinical effects of this inspiratory flow-terminating reflex have yet to be determined.

Tidal Volume

A tidal volume is selected to provide an adequate $PaCO_2$ but avoid alveolar overdistention, decreased cardiac output, and auto-PEEP. A V_T of 6 mL/kg of ideal body weight (compared with 12 mL/kg of ideal body weight) has been reported to reduce morbidity and mortality in patients with ARDS.[50,51]

For patients with obstructive lung disease, a V_T of 8 to 10 mL/kg is appropriate. In postoperative patients with relatively normal lung function, a V_T of 10 to 12 mL/kg can be used. Ideally a tidal volume should be chosen that maintains the P_{plat} below 30 cm H_2O, provided chest wall compliance is normal.

Respiratory Rate

A respiratory rate is chosen to provide an acceptable minute ventilation, as follows:

$$\dot{V}_E = V_T \times f$$

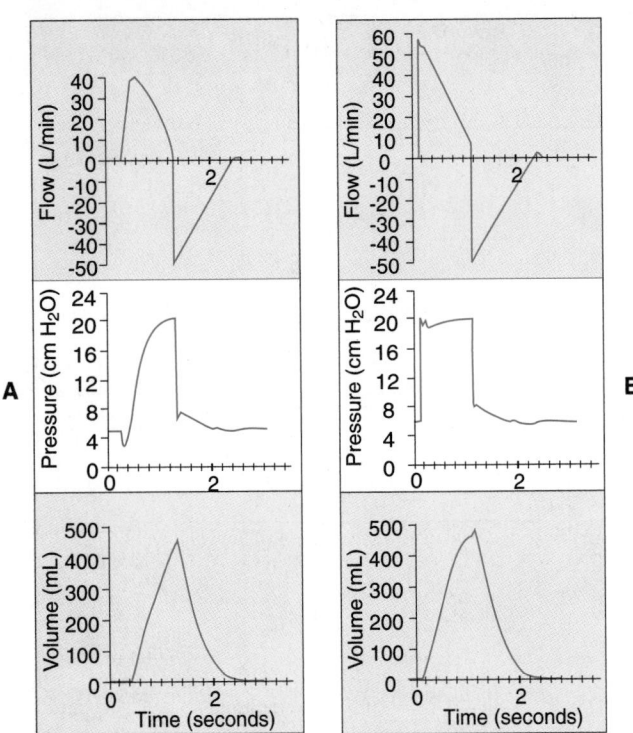

Figure 40-16   Effect of rise time adjustment during pressure-support ventilation. **A,** Slow rise time. **B,** More rapid rise time.

where f is the respiratory rate, $\dot{V}_E$ is the minute ventilation, and V_T is the tidal volume. A rate of 12 to 15 breaths/min is used when mechanical ventilation is initiated. To prevent alveolar overdistention (that is, to keep the P_{plat} <30 cm H_2O), a higher respiratory rate may be required (15 to 30 breaths/min). The respiratory rate is limited by the development of auto-PEEP. The minute ventilation that produces a normal $PaCO_2$ without lung injury may not be possible, and the $PaCO_2$ thus is allowed to increase (permissive hypercapnia).

Inspiratory Time and Inspiration to Expiration Ratio

For patient-triggered mandatory breaths, the inspiratory time should be short (1.5 seconds or less) to improve ventilator-patient synchrony. A shorter inspiratory time requires a higher inspiratory flow, which increases the **peak inspiratory pressure (PIP)** but does not greatly affect the P_{plat}. Increasing the inspiratory time increases the mean airway pressure ($\bar{P}_{aw}$), which may improve oxygenation in some patients with ARDS. When long inspiratory times are used (over 1.5 seconds), paralysis or sedation (or both) often is required. Long inspiratory times also can cause auto-PEEP and may result in hemodynamic instability because of the elevated $\bar{P}_{aw}$ or the auto-PEEP. Although inverse-ratio ventilation has been advocated to improve oxygenation, this extreme (and potentially hazardous) form of ventilation is seldom necessary to achieve adequate oxygenation.

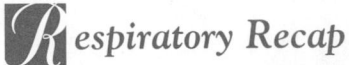

Respiratory Recap

> *Settings for Tidal Volume, Respiratory Rate, and Inspiration to Expiration (I:E) Ratio*
>
> Tidal volume: Set to avoid overdistention
> Respiratory rate: Set for desired partial pressure of arterial carbon dioxide ($PaCO_2$)
> I:E ratio: Set to avoid auto-PEEP and hemodynamic compromise

The inspiration to expiration (I:E) ratio is the relationship between inspiratory time and expiratory time. For example, an inspiratory time of 2 seconds with an expiratory time of 4 seconds produces an I:E ratio of 1:2 and respiratory rate of 10 breaths/min. With VCV the peak inspiratory flow, flow pattern, and tidal volume are the principal determinants of inspiratory time and the I:E ratio. With PCV the inspiratory time, I:E ratio, or percentage inspiratory time are set directly. In both VCV and PCV, the principal determinant of expiratory time is the respiratory rate.

Inspiratory Flow Pattern

For VCV the inspiratory flow pattern can be constant or decelerating. The PIP is greater with constant flow than with decelerating flow; the $\bar{P}_{aw}$ is greater with decelerating flow than with constant flow; and gas distribution is better with a decelerating flow pattern. Because the flow is greater at the beginning of inspiration, patient-ventilator synchrony may be better with a decelerating flow pattern. Although the choice of flow pattern often is based on clinician bias or the capabilities of a specific ventilator, decelerating flow may be desirable compared with other inspiratory flow patterns. An end-inspiratory pause can be set to improve distribution of ventilation, but this prolongs inspiration and may have a deleterious effect on hemodynamics and auto-PEEP.

The inspiratory flow decreases exponentially with PCV. The peak flow and rate of flow decrease depend on the pressure limit, airways resistance, and lung compliance. With high resistance, flow decreases slowly. With a low compliance and long inspiratory time, flow decreases more rapidly, and a period of zero flow may be present at end-inhalation (Figure 40-17).

Positive End-Expiratory Pressure

It is common to use low-level PEEP (3 to 5 cm H_2O) with all mechanically ventilated patients. In patients with ARDS, PEEP should be used to maintain alveolar recruitment. A PEEP level above 15 cm H_2O is seldom necessary but may be needed occasionally. An appropriate PEEP level to maintain alveolar recruitment is part of a lung protection strategy. PEEP should be used cautiously in patients with unilateral disease, because it may overdistend

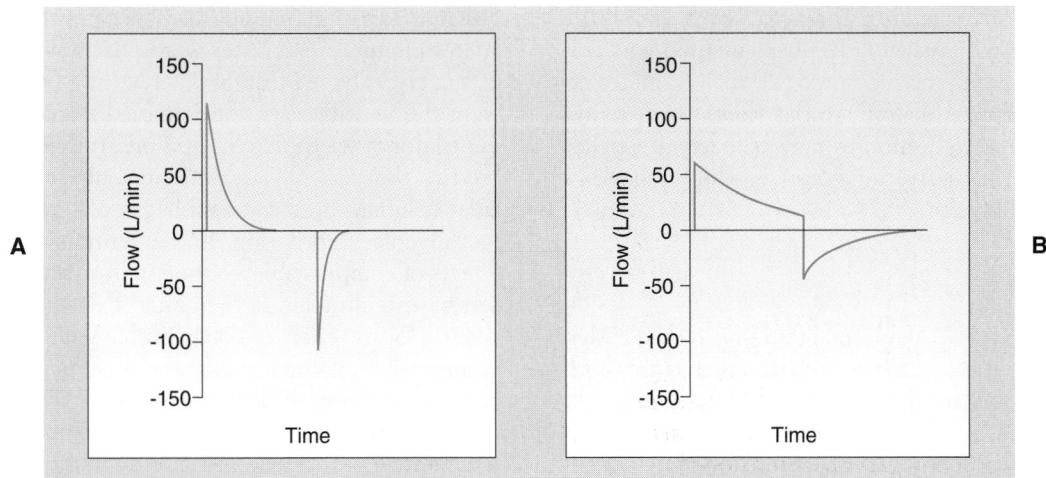

Figure 40-17 Flow waveforms during pressure-control ventilation. **A,** Low resistance and low compliance. **B,** High resistance and high compliance.

the more compliant lung, causing shunting of blood to the less-compliant lung.

PEEP may be useful to improve triggering by patients experiencing auto-PEEP.[52-54] As mentioned earlier, auto-PEEP is a threshold that must be overcome before the pressure (or flow) decreases at the airway to trigger the ventilator. Increasing the set PEEP to a level near the total PEEP (set PEEP + auto-PEEP) may improve the patient's ability to trigger the ventilator (Figure 40-18). Whenever PEEP is used to overcome the effect of auto-PEEP on triggering, the total PEEP level must be monitored to ensure that it does not increase when auto-PEEP is present.

R̲espiratory Recap

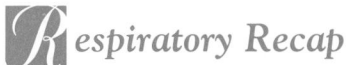

Uses of Positive End-Expiratory Pressure
Maintain alveolar recruitment.
Counterbalance auto-PEEP.

Mean Airway Pressure

Many of the beneficial and deleterious effects of mechanical ventilation are related to the **mean airway pressure ($\bar{P}_{aw}$).** Factors that affect the $\bar{P}_{aw}$ during mechanical ventilation are the PIP, the PEEP (including auto-PEEP), the I:E ratio, the respiratory rate, and the inspiratory flow pattern.[55] A lower $\bar{P}_{aw}$ can help prevent many of the complications of mechanical ventilation. However, a $\bar{P}_{aw}$ over 20 cm H_2O often is necessary for patients with ARDS to maintain adequate arterial oxygenation.

Inspired Oxygen Concentration

An F_{IO_2} of 1 is commonly used when mechanical ventilation is initiated. Pulse oximetry (SpO_2) is useful to guide

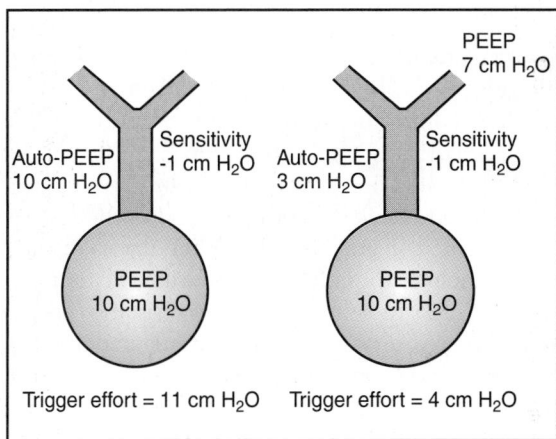

Figure 40-18 Trigger effort is increased with auto-PEEP. To trigger the ventilator, the patient's effort must first overcome the auto-PEEP. Increasing the set PEEP may raise the trigger level closer to the total PEEP, thereby improving the patient's ability to trigger the ventilator. However, this method should not be used if raising the set PEEP increases the total PEEP.

titration of the F_{IO_2}[56] provided periodic blood gas measurements are obtained to confirm the pulse oximetry results. A target SpO_2 of 92% or higher usually provides a partial pressure of arterial oxygen (PaO_2) of 60 mm Hg or

R̲espiratory Recap

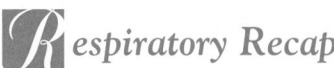

Setting the Fractional Inspired Oxygen Concentration
Initiate mechanical ventilation with 100% oxygen.
Titrate the F_{IO_2} to maintain an acceptable arterial oxygen saturation as measured by pulse oximetry.

higher in Caucasian patients; the target SpO₂ should be 95% or higher in patients with deeply pigmented skin. Although it is common practice to wait 20 to 30 minutes after the FIO₂ is changed before arterial blood gas measurements are obtained, 10 minutes may be adequate unless the patient has obstructive lung disease, which requires a longer equilibration time.[57]

Sigh

Some ventilators are capable of providing periodic sigh volumes.[58] The rationale for use of sighs is that the periodic hyperinflation reduces the risk of atelectasis. For many years the use of sighs during mechanical ventilation was not considered important. However, one study[59] of patients with ARDS showed improved alveolar recruitment with the use of three consecutive sighs per minute at a plateau pressure of 45 cm H₂O.

Alarms

It is particularly important that all alarms are correctly set on the ventilator. The most important alarm is the patient disconnect alarm, which can be a low-pressure alarm or a low exhaled volume alarm. A sensitive alarm should detect not only disconnection but also leaks in the system. The ability to detect a leak depends on the site where the volume is measured (Figure 40-19). Other alarms set on the ventilator include those for high pressure, I:E ratio, FIO₂, and loss of PEEP. To detect changes in resistance and compliance, the peak airway pressure alarm is important with VCV and the low exhaled volume alarm with PCV or PSV.

Circuit

Because of the gas compression in the ventilator circuit and the compliance of the ventilator circuit tubing, as

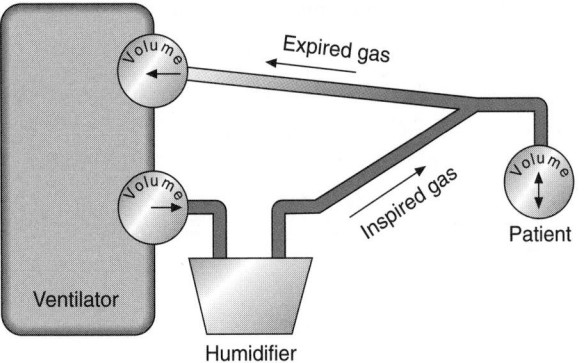

Figure 40-19 The ability to detect a leak depends on where the volume is measured. If the volume on the inspiratory limb is greater than the volume on the expiratory limb, a leak exists in the system (circuit or patient). If the inspired volume at the patient is greater than the expired volume at the patient, a leak exists in the patient (for example, around the cuff of the endotracheal tube or through a bronchopleural fistula).

much as 3 to 5 mL/cm H₂O can be compressed in the ventilator circuit.[60,61] In other words, at an airway pressure of 25 cm H₂O above PEEP, about 100 mL of the gas delivered from the ventilator is not delivered to the patient. If the ventilator is set to deliver 500 mL, only 400 mL is delivered to the patient. For patients ventilated with a small tidal volume, the compressible gas volume can greatly affect alveolar ventilation. Some ventilators adjust for the effects of **compressible volume** such that the volume chosen by the clinician is the actual delivered VT after correction for the effect of compressible volume. The effect of compressible volume on the delivered VT, auto-PEEP, plateau pressure, and mixed exhaled partial pressure of carbon dioxide (P̄ECO₂) is shown in Equation 40-1. The mechanical dead space of the circuit should also be considered. *Mechanical dead space* is that part of the ventilator circuit through which the patient rebreathes and thus becomes an extension of the patient's anatomic dead space. Alveolar ventilation is zero if the sum of the volume loss

*ℰ*QUATION 40-1

Effects of Compressible Volume

The effect of compressible volume on the delivered tidal volume (Vt) can be expressed as follows:

$$V_{T_{pt}} = \frac{1}{1 + (C_{pc}/C_{rs})} \times V_{T_{vent}}$$

where:

$V_{T_{pt}}$ = Tidal volume delivered to the patient
C_{pc} = Compliance of the ventilator circuit
C_{rs} = Compliance of the respiratory system
$V_{T_{vent}}$ = Tidal volume from the ventilator circuit

The effect of compressible volume on auto-PEEP (positive end-expiratory pressure) can be expressed as follows:

$$\text{auto-PEEP} = \frac{C_{rs} + C_{pc}}{C_{rs}} \times \text{Measured auto-PEEP}$$

where *auto-PEEP* is the patient's actual auto-PEEP *(positive end-expiratory pressure)*.

The effect of compressible volume on the plateau pressure (P_plat) can be expressed as follows:

$$P_{plat} = \frac{C_{rs} + C_{pc}}{C_{rs}} \times \text{Measured } P_{plat}$$

where *P_plat* is the patient's actual plateau pressure.

The effect of compressible volume on the mixed exhaled partial pressure of carbon dioxide (P̄ECO₂) can be expressed as follows:

$$P\bar{E}_{CO_2} = P\bar{E}_{CO_2(vent)} \times \frac{V_{T_{vent}}}{V_{T_{pt}}}$$

where:

$P\bar{E}_{CO_2}$ = Patient's actual P̄ECO₂
$P\bar{E}_{CO_2(vent)}$ = P̄ECO₂ from the ventilator circuit
$V_{T_{vent}}$ = Tidal volume from the ventilator circuit
$V_{T_{pt}}$ = Tidal volume delivered to the patient

in the circuit and the mechanical dead space is greater than the VT set on the ventilator.

Humidification

Because the function of the upper airway is bypassed when endotracheal and tracheostomy tubes are used, the inspired gas must be filtered, warmed, and humidified before delivery to the patient. All ventilator circuits include a filter in the inspiratory limb and an active or passive humidifier.[62-64] An *active humidifier* typically humidifies the inspired gas by passing it over or bubbling it through a heated water bath. When an active humidifier is used, the ventilator circuit may be heated to prevent excessive condensation in the circuit. A *passive humidifier* uses an artificial nose (heat and moisture exchanger) to collect heat and humidity from the patient's exhaled gas and returns that to the patient on the next inhalation. Regardless of the humidification technique used, condensation should be seen in the inspiratory ventilator circuit or the proximal endotracheal tube or both, because this indicates that the inspired gas is fully saturated with water vapor.

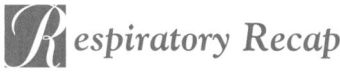espiratory Recap

Methods of Humidification with Mechanical Ventilation
Active humidification: Heated humidifier
Passive humidification: Artificial nose
The presence of condensate in the inspiratory circuit near the patient indicates adequate humidification.

Monitoring the Mechanically Ventilated Patient

It is important to monitor the function of the mechanical ventilator frequently, including checking the ventilator settings and alarm systems, the humidifier and circuitry, and the patient's airway. Flowsheet charting often is used to document monitoring at regular intervals.

Physical Assessment

Asymmetric chest motion may indicate mainstem (endobronchial) intubation, pneumothorax, or atelectasis. Paradoxical chest motion may be seen with flail chest or respiratory muscle dysfunction. Retractions may occur if the inspiratory flow or sensitivity is inappropriately set or if the airway is obstructed. If the patient is not breathing in synchrony with the ventilator (that is, bucking the ventilator), the settings on the ventilator may not be appropriate or the patient may need sedation. A patient respiratory rate greater than the trigger rate on the ventilator indicates the

presence of auto-PEEP. In conjunction with inspection, the chest can be palpated to assess the symmetry of chest movement. Palpation of the tracheal position can help detect pneumothorax. Crepitation indicates subcutaneous emphysema. Percussion can be useful in the detection of unilateral hyperresonance or tympany with a pneumothorax. Unilateral decreased breath sounds may indicate bronchial intubation, pneumothorax, atelectasis, or pleural effusion. An end-inspiratory squeak over the trachea usually indicates insufficient air in the artificial airway cuff.

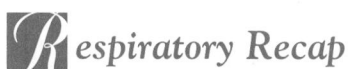espiratory Recap

Monitoring Required during Mechanical Ventilation	
Physical examination	Hemodynamics
Blood gases	Patient-ventilator synchrony
Lung mechanics	Sedation

Blood Gases

The earliest indicators of hypoxemia often are changes in the patient's clinical status (e.g., restlessness and confusion, changes in level of consciousness, tachycardia or bradycardia, changes in blood pressure, tachypnea, bucking the ventilator, and cyanosis). The most commonly used assessment of oxygenation is the partial pressure of arterial oxygen. A low PaO_2 indicates hypoxemia and a dysfunction in the lungs' ability to oxygenate arterial blood. The PaO_2 must always be interpreted in relation to the FIO_2. In mechanically ventilated patients a number of factors can affect the PaO_2, such as a change in the FIO_2, the PEEP level, or the patient's lung function (Figure 40-20). The mixed venous oxygenation ($P\bar{v}O_2$ or $S\bar{v}O_2$) is a better indicator of tissue oxygenation. A $P\bar{v}O_2$ less than 35 mm Hg (or an $S\bar{v}O_2$ less than 70%) indicates tissue hypoxia. The $PaCO_2$ is determined by carbon dioxide production ($\dot{V}CO_2$) and the alveolar ventilation ($\dot{V}_A$). If the $\dot{V}CO_2$ is constant, the $PaCO_2$ varies inversely with the $\dot{V}_A$. The minute ventilation ($\dot{V}_E$) affects the $PaCO_2$ indirectly because of the relationship between the $\dot{V}_E$ and the $\dot{V}_A$. An increase in the $\dot{V}_E$ decreases the $PaCO_2$, and a decrease in the $\dot{V}_E$ increases the $PaCO_2$. This is illustrated by the following relationship:

$$PaCO_2 = \frac{\dot{V}CO_2 \times 0.863}{\dot{V}_E \times [1 - (V_D/V_T)]}$$

where $PaCO_2$ is the partial pressure of arterial carbon dioxide, $\dot{V}CO_2$ is carbon dioxide production, $\dot{V}_E$ is minute ventilation, and V_D/V_T is the ratio of dead space to tidal volume.

The factors that determine the $PaCO_2$ during mechanical ventilation are shown in Figure 40-21.

The use of noninvasive monitors may reduce the need for arterial blood gas determinations, because they allow continuous assessment between blood gas measurements.

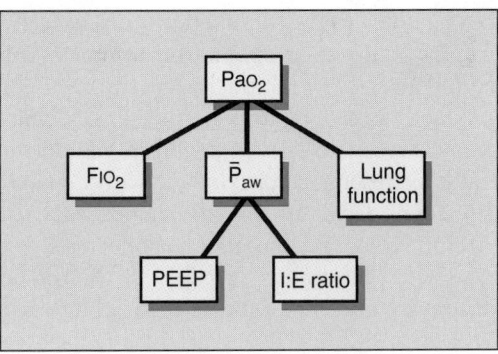

Figure 40-20 Factors that affect the partial pressure of arterial oxygen (Pao_2) during mechanical ventilation. Fio_2, Fractional inspired oxygen concentration; *PEEP*, positive end-expiratory pressure; $\bar{P}_{aw}$, mean airway pressure; *I:E*, inspiration to expiration ratio.

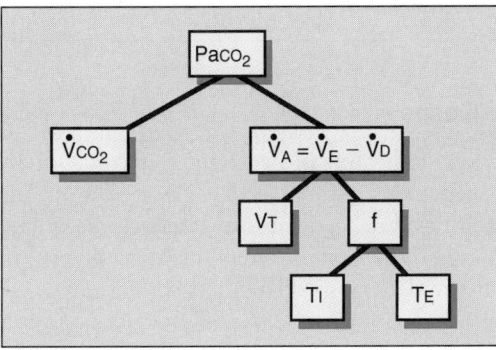

Figure 40-21 Factors that affect the partial pressure of arterial carbon dioxide ($Paco_2$) during mechanical ventilation. $\dot{V}co_2$, Carbon dioxide production; $\dot{V}_A$, alveolar ventilation; $\dot{V}_E$, minute ventilation; $\dot{V}_D$, dead space ventilation; V_T, tidal volume; T_I, inspiratory time; T_E, expiratory time; *f*, respiratory rate.

Pulse oximetry can be used to titrate an appropriate Fio_2. Continuous pulse oximetry has become a standard of care in mechanically ventilated patients. The end-tidal Pco_2 is used to monitor carbon dioxide levels noninvasively.[65,66] In patients with normal lungs, the end-tidal Pco_2 closely approximates the $Paco_2$. However, in patients with an elevated ratio of dead space to tidal volume (V_D/V_T), there can be a large and inconsistent gradient between the $Paco_2$ and the end-tidal Pco_2. For this reason, monitoring of the end-tidal Pco_2 is of limited value for the assessment of the $Paco_2$ during mechanical ventilation. However, the end-tidal Pco_2 is a useful monitor for differentiate tracheal intubation from esophageal intubation.

Lung Mechanics

Breath-by-breath monitoring of airway pressure and V_T is common during mechanical ventilation of adult patients. On current-generation ventilators continuous waveforms of

pressure, flow, and volume are available, as are pressure-volume and flow-volume loops. These are useful in the evaluation of lung mechanics during mechanical ventilation.

Monitoring of the peak pressure, P_{plat}, and auto-PEEP is particularly important (Box 40-5). P_{plat} is measured by application of an end-inspiratory pause of 0.5 to 1.5 seconds, and auto-PEEP is determined by application of an end-expiratory pause of 0.5 to 1.5 seconds (Figure 40-22). Both P_{plat} and auto-PEEP can be accurately measured only when the patient is relaxed and breathing in synchrony with the ventilator. During PCV the inspiratory flow often decelerates to a no-flow period at end-inspiration. In this case, the peak pressure and P_{plat} are equivalent. The P_{plat} is the mean peak alveolar pressure and ideally should be kept below 30 cm H_2O to avoid overdistention and acute lung injury.

Recently interest has arisen in setting the ventilator using the inflation pressure-volume (PV) curve of the respiratory system.[66,67] For patients with ARDS, the PV curve typically is sigmoidal (Figure 40-23). A lower inflection point presumably represents the pressure at which a large number of alveoli are recruited, or opened. An upper inflection point presumably represents the pressure at which a large number of alveoli are overdistended. Therefore it would seem reasonable to set the PEEP above the lower inflection point and the P_{plat} below the upper inflection point.

The PV curve can be measured when a slow, constant flow is set on the ventilator and the ventilator display of the PV curve observed. However, this measurement includes the effect of airways resistance. The PV curve cannot be accurately measured during PCV, and measurement of the PV curve requires heavy sedation or paralysis. The super syringe technique is the traditional method used to

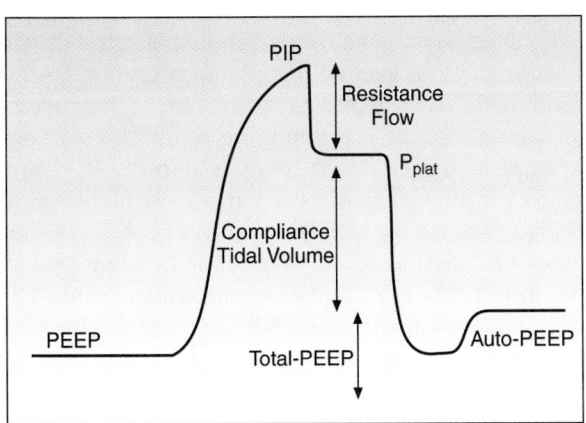

Figure 40-22 Airway pressure waveform during volume-control ventilation. An end-inspiratory and end-expiratory breath-hold is applied to measure the plateau pressure and auto-PEEP. Note that the difference between the peak inspiratory pressure *(PIP)* and the plateau pressure *(P$_{plat}$)* is determined by the flow setting on the ventilator and airways resistance. Note that the difference between the plateau pressure and the total PEEP is determined by the tidal volume setting on the ventilator and the compliance. *PEEP,* Positive end-expiratory pressure; *PIP,* positive inspiratory pressure.

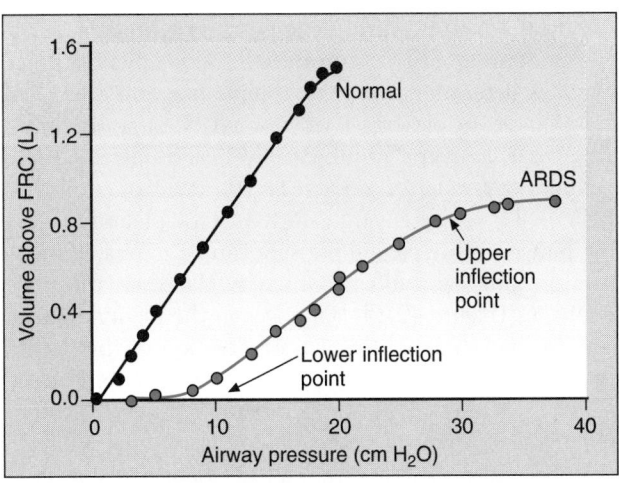

Figure 40-23 Pressure-volume curves for normal lungs and those of individuals with acute respiratory distress syndrome (ARDS). Note the lower and upper inflection points on the pressure-volume curve for ARDS. *FRC,* Functional residual capacity.

measure the PV curve (Figure 40-24). Precise volumes of gas are added to the endotracheal tube, and the pressure at each step change in volume is measured. The PV curve is then plotted as volume as a function of pressure.

The role of the PV curve in setting the ventilator currently is unclear. Although its use is physiologically attractive, more experience is needed with these measurements before the PV curve can be recommended for routine use to set the ventilator.

Hemodynamics

Because positive pressure ventilation can affect cardiac function, it is important to assess hemodynamics during mechanical ventilation. At a minimum, the arterial blood pressure and heart rate should be measured frequently. When the high airway pressures needed to support oxygenation adversely affect cardiac performance, hemodynamics may need to be supported with fluid, inotropes, and pressors. The role of the pulmonary artery catheter in mechanical ventilation is unclear, and its use has declined in recent years.

It is important to appreciate the effect of positive pressure ventilation on hemodynamic assessments. During positive pressure ventilation, pleural pressure increases during inhalation by an amount determined by lung compliance and chest wall compliance:

$$\Delta P_{pl}/\Delta P_{aw} = \frac{C_L}{(C_L + C_{cw})}$$

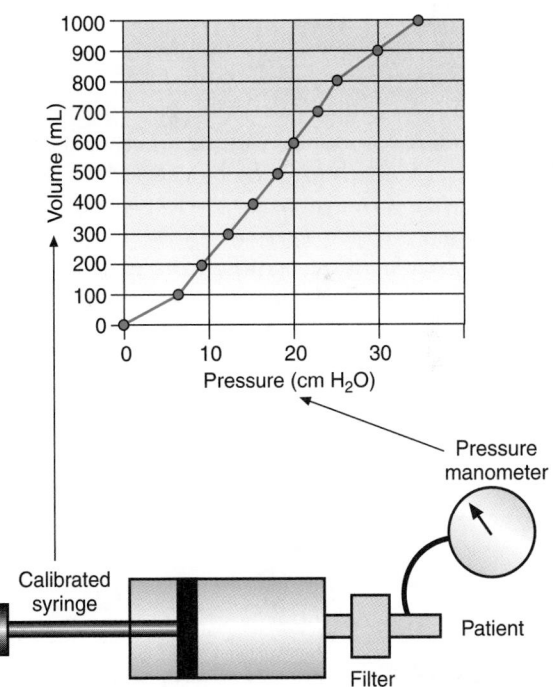

Figure 40-24 Super syringe technique used to measure the pressure-volume curve, with an example of a pressure-volume curve produced with this technique.

where ΔP_{pl} is the change in pleural pressure, ΔP_{aw} is the change in airway (alveolar) pressure, C_L is lung compliance, and C_{cw} is chest wall compliance. By convention hemodynamic measurements are made at end-exhalation to account for the respiratory variation in pleural pressure. At end-exhalation, measurements such as the pulmonary artery occlusion pressure (wedge pressure), pulmonary artery pressure, and central venous pressure are affected by the amount of PEEP transmitted to the pleural space, which is determined by lung compliance and chest wall compliance. In patients with normal chest wall compliance (that is, over 150 mL/cm H₂O) and decreased lung compliance (under 50 mL/cm H₂O), about one fourth of the alveolar pressure is transmitted to the pleural space.

Changes in the pleural pressure can be estimated by use of an esophageal balloon, which is placed in the lower esophagus (Figure 40-25). Changes in the pleural pressure can also be estimated through observation of the respiratory variation in the thoracic vascular catheter pressure measurements (that is, the central venous pressure, pulmonary artery pressure, and pulmonary artery occlusion pressure). With a stiff chest wall, the esophageal pressure or vascular pressure shows greater fluctuation during the respiratory cycle (Figure 40-26), and greater effects of positive pressure ventilation on hemodynamics can be expected.

Patient-Ventilator Synchrony

Dyssynchrony occurs when the patient is not breathing in phase with the ventilator; in its worst form the patient is "bucking" the ventilator. However, dyssynchrony often is much more subtle. Failure of the patient to breathe in synchrony with the ventilator decreases patient comfort and increases both the work of breathing and the oxygen cost of breathing. Dyssynchrony can be categorized as trigger dyssynchrony, flow dyssynchrony, cycle dyssynchrony, and mode dyssynchrony.

Trigger dyssynchrony occurs when the patient has difficulty triggering the ventilator. Trigger dyssynchrony can be caused by an insensitive trigger setting on the ventilator,

which can be corrected by reduction of the pressure or flow required for the patient to trigger the ventilator. The ventilator's trigger point should be as sensitive as possible without causing auto-triggering. If pressure triggering is set on the ventilator, trigger dyssynchrony may be improved by switching to flow triggering and vice versa. The most common cause of trigger dyssynchrony is auto-PEEP. This can be corrected through administration of bronchodilators and clearing of secretions to reduce auto-PEEP or by use of a higher PEEP setting on the ventilator to counterbalance the auto-PEEP. Using PEEP to counterbalance auto-PEEP can be effective for patients with COPD, but this technique is not effective if the auto-PEEP is the result of a high minute ventilation and insufficient expiratory time. Whenever PEEP is used to counterbalance auto-PEEP, care must be taken to avoid hyperinflation with the PEEP. When the attempt is to counterbalance auto-PEEP with PEEP, the clinician should monitor the peak inspiratory pressure as PEEP is increased. If the PIP rises above the desired threshold or increases by a value greater than the increase in PEEP, overdistention should be suspected.

Flow dyssynchrony occurs when the ventilator does not meet the patient's inspiratory flow demand. Lack of synchrony can be detected by evaluating the airway pressure waveform. With dyssynchrony, the pressure waveform with each breath differs from every other, and there is breath-to-breath variability in the peak airway pressure (Figure 40-27). A good way to detect dyssynchrony is to compare patient-triggered breaths with a breath delivered via the manual breath control. Comparing the shape of the mandatory and spontaneous breaths on the pressure-time waveform can

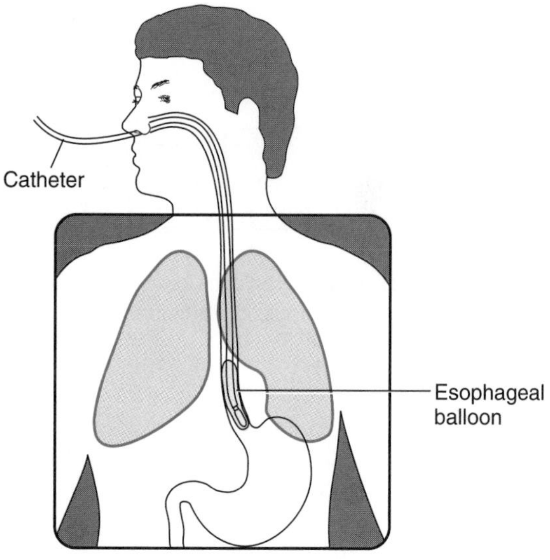

Figure 40-25 Position of esophageal balloon used to measure changes in intrapleural pressure.

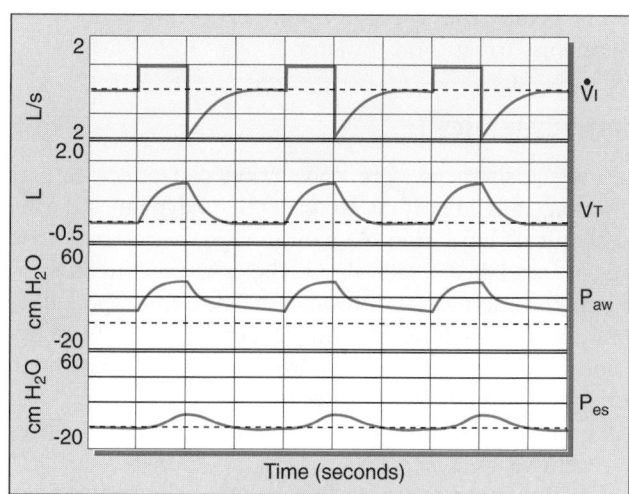

Figure 40-26 Airway flow, volume, and pressure waveforms, along with an esophageal pressure waveform, during positive pressure ventilation. Note the increase in esophageal pressure with each breath; the magnitude of the increase reflects chest wall compliance. (Modified from MacIntyre NR. Respiratory system mechanics. In: MacIntyre NR, Branson RD, editors. Mechanical ventilation. Philadelphia: WB Saunders; 2000.)

demonstrate the effects of patient effort. Clinical signs of dyssynchrony include tachypnea, retractions, and chest-abdominal paradox. Flow dyssynchrony can be corrected by an increase in the flow setting during VCV, by a change in the inspiratory flow pattern, or by an increase in the pressure setting or the rise time setting during PCV or PSV. For patients who have a high respiratory drive because of anxiety or pain, flow dyssynchrony may be improved by appropriate use of sedative agents such as benzodiazepines or narcotics.

Cycle dyssynchrony occurs when the patient begins to exhale before the end of the inspiratory phase set on the ventilator. A common cause of cycle dyssynchrony is due to setting of the inspiratory flow too low during VCV or setting of the inspiratory time too long during PCV. Cycle dyssynchrony can occur during PSV if the patient begins to exhale before the inspiratory flow termination criterion is reached. This occurs most often in patients with obstructive lung disease or when a leak is present. Cycle dyssynchrony during

PSV can be corrected by lowering of the pressure support level, by an increase in the termination flow setting on newer generation ventilators, or by use of pressure control instead of pressure support (pressure control causes inspiration to be time cycled rather than flow cycled). Cycle dyssynchrony is recognized as activation of the expiratory (abdominal) muscles during the inspiratory phase; this can be detected clinically by palpation of the patient's abdomen. Cycle dyssynchrony can also be detected by observation of the ventilator graphics (Figure 40-28).

Mode dyssynchrony occurs when the ventilator delivers different breath types. The best example is SIMV, in which some breath types are mandatory and others are spontaneous. Because the patient's respiratory center cannot adapt to varying breath types, dyssynchrony can develop between the patient and the ventilator.[68]

Sedation

Anxiety is a common cause of failure to breathe in synchrony with the ventilator. In these cases pharmacologic support may be necessary in the form of analgesics (narcotics), sedatives (benzodiazepines), or paralyzing agents. When short-term sedation is necessary to bring a patient into synchrony with the ventilator, propofol may be useful. When ventilation requires long inspiratory times and high airway pressures, pharmacologic control of the patient's breathing is almost always necessary. It must be remembered that all forms of respiratory suppression are associated with adverse side effects. It is most important that disconnect alarms be properly set when the patient's ability to breathe spontaneously is pharmacologically suppressed. Significant problems with pharmacologic suppression of respiration have recently been reported, such as long-term respiratory muscle weakness after use of paralyzing agents during me-

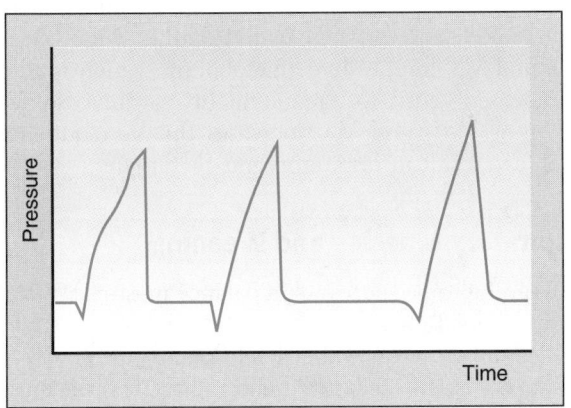

Figure 40-27 Effect of dyssynchrony on airway pressure waveform.

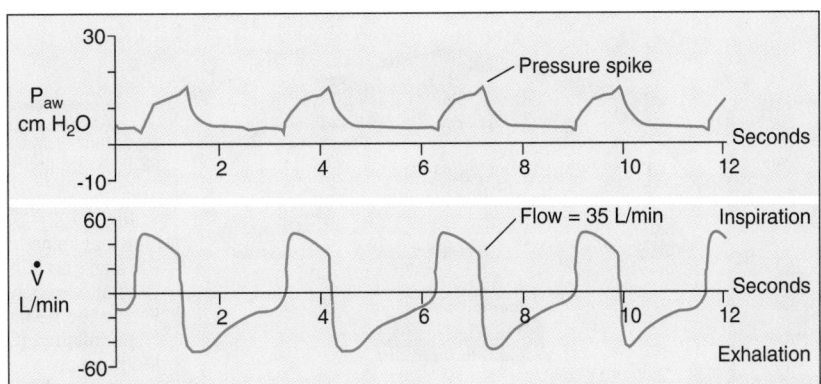

Figure 40-28 Airway pressure *(top)* and flow *(bottom)* waveforms showing active exhalation during pressure-support ventilation. Note that the flow does not decelerate to the flow termination criterion of the ventilator (5 L/min for this ventilator). Also note the pressure spike at the end of each inspiration, which indicates that the ventilator is pressure cycling rather than flow cycling. (Modified from Branson RD. Modes of ventilator operation. In: MacIntyre NR, Branson RD, editors. Mechanical ventilation. Philadelphia: WB Saunders; 2000.)

chanical ventilation.[68-70] It has been shown that assessment of the patient's response to a daily trial of sedation cessation significantly reduces the days of mechanical ventilation.[71] This suggests that many mechanically ventilated patients are excessively sedated and that this excessive sedation prolongs the course of mechanical ventilation.

Weaning from Mechanical Ventilation

Assessing Weaning Readiness

A number of factors should be improved before **weaning** is begun (Box 40-6). Weaning parameters[72] are divided into two categories: parameters affected by lung mechanics and gas exchange parameters. The spontaneous V_T (over 5 mL/kg), respiratory rate (under 30 breaths/min), minute ventilation (under 12 L/min), vital capacity (over 15 mL/kg), and the maximum inspiratory pressure (PI_{max})

$\mathcal{B}$OX 40-6

Criteria to Begin Weaning from Mechanical Ventilation

Resolution of the cause of respiratory failure
Cessation of sedation and paralysis
Absence of sepsis
Stable cardiovascular status
Correction of electrolyte and metabolic disorders
Adequate arterial oxygenation: partial pressure of arterial oxygen (Pao_2) over 60 mm Hg with a fractional inspired oxygen concentration (Fio_2) of 0.5 or less and a positive end-expiratory pressure (PEEP) of 5 cm H_2O or less
Adequate respiratory muscle capability

(under -20 cm H_2O) have been used as predictors of weaning success. However, the best predictor of success or failure of weaning is the rapid shallow breathing index (RSBI),[73,74] which is calculated by division of the spontaneous respiratory rate by the V_T (in liters). An RSBI below 100 is predictive of weaning success, but an RSBI of more than 100 does not necessarily predict failure.

Measurements of the work of breathing may be useful in long-term mechanically ventilated patients who fail to wean from mechanical ventilation. In such patients, a work per minute (W_I/min) of 16 J/min or less and a work per tidal volume (W_I/L) of 1.4 J/min or less are both necessary for successful weaning.[75] Other, more esoteric weaning parameters include measurements of the oxygen cost of breathing and the mouth occlusion pressure 0.1 seconds after the initiation of pressure ($P_{0.1}$).[76] These are not commonly used because they are difficult to measure accurately.

If the Pao_2 is at least 60 mm Hg on an Fio_2 of 0.5 or less, the patient's oxygenation is acceptable to allow satisfactory weaning. The V_D/V_T should be under 0.6 before weaning is begun. Sometimes it is also useful to measure the metabolic rate to assess weaning ability. An increase in $\dot{V}co_2$ and $\dot{V}o_2$ implies hypermetabolism, which results in an increased ventilatory requirement. An increase in the V_D/V_T or $\dot{V}co_2$ and $\dot{V}o_2$ increases the $\dot{V}_E$ requirement, which can result in respiratory muscle fatigue.

Respiratory Muscles and Weaning

For weaning to be successful, a balance must be struck between the load placed on the respiratory muscles and the muscles' ability to meet that load (Figure 40-29). Respiratory muscle fatigue occurs if the load placed on the muscles is excessive, if the muscles are weak, or if the duty cycle (the inspiratory time relative to total cycle time) is too long. Common causes of a high load are high airways re-

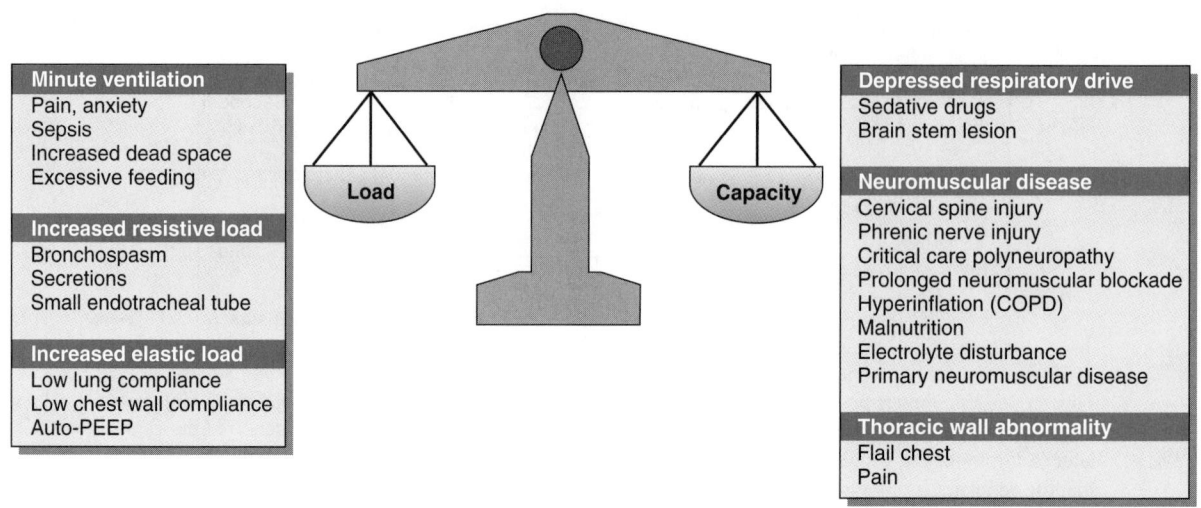

Figure 40-29 Respiratory muscle performance is determined by the balance between the load placed on the respiratory muscles and muscles' capacity to manage that load.

sistance, low lung compliance, and high minute ventilation. Diminished respiratory muscle function may be the result of disease, disuse, malnutrition, hypoxia, or electrolyte imbalance. The clinical signs of respiratory muscle fatigue are tachypnea, abnormal respiratory movements (respiratory alternans and abdominal paradox), and an increase in the $PaCO_2$.[77]

Because the PI_{max} is a good indicator of overall respiratory muscle strength, a low PI_{max} may predict respiratory muscle fatigue. The PI_{max} is measured by attachment of an aneroid manometer to the endotracheal or tracheostomy tube. The patient then forcibly inhales after maximum exhalation. When the PI_{max} is measured, it is recommended that a unidirectional valve be used and that the airway be completely obstructed for 20 to 25 seconds (Figure 40-30).[78-80] A PI_{max} more negative than -20 cm H_2O suggests adequate inspiratory muscle strength. However, if the patient has high airways resistance or low compliance, a PI_{max} of -20 cm H_2O may not prevent fatigue.

The respiratory muscles must be rested if fatigue occurs, and a rest period of 24 hours or longer may be required.[81] Respiratory muscle rest usually is provided by ventilatory support high enough to minimize sponta-neous breathing and provide patient comfort. If respiratory muscle fatigue is the result of an excessive load, the load should be reduced before attempts are made to wean the patient from the ventilator. This is done with provision of therapy that can increase lung compliance or reduce airways resistance.

The tension-time index has been used to predict diaphragmatic fatigue (Figure 40-31).[82] The *tension-time index* is calculated as the product of the contractile force (P_{di}/P_{di-max}) and contraction duration (duty cycle, T_i/T_{tot}). This requires measurement of the mean transdiaphragmatic pressure (P_{di}), the transdiaphragmatic pressure with maximum inhalation (P_{di-max}), the inspiratory time (T_I), and the total respiratory cycle time (T_{tot}). A tension-time index over 0.15 is predictive of respiratory muscle fatigue. Measurement of the transdiaphragmatic pressure requires esophageal and gastric pressure measurements, which are almost never performed in mechanically ventilated patients. A simpler form of tension-time index is the pressure-time index (PTI),[83] which can be determined more readily with equipment available in the critical care unit. It is calculated as follows:

$$PTI = \frac{P_{breath}}{PI_{max}} \times \frac{T_I}{T_{tot}}$$

where P_{breath} is the pressure required to generate a spontaneous breath. The P_{breath} can be determined with esophageal balloon measurements during a short trial of spontaneous breathing. If an esophageal balloon is not available, the P_{breath} can be estimated as follows:

$$P_{breath} = (PIP - PEEP) \times \frac{VT_{sp}}{VT_{mv}}$$

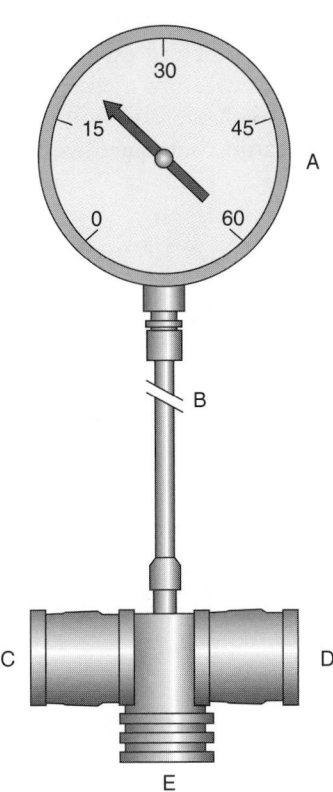

Figure 40-30 The one-way valve system used to measure maximum inspiratory pressure. The patient is connected at *E*, the manometer (*A*) is connected at *B*, the patient exhales through *D*, and the inlet port (*C*) is occluded by the clinician. In this way, maximum inspiratory pressure is measured at the residual volume. (Modified from Kacmarek RM, Cycyk-Chapman MC, Young PJ, et al. Respir Care 1989;34:868-878.)

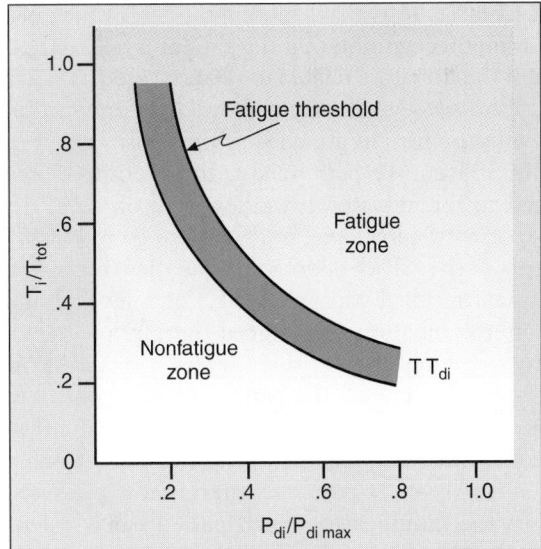

Figure 40-31 Tension-time index. Note that the fatigue threshold is a tension-time index of about 0.15 to 0.18. (Modified from Grassino A, Macklem PT. Annu Rev Med 1984;35:625-647.)

where *PIP* is the peak inspiratory pressure with a ventilator-delivered tidal volume (VT_{mv}), *PEEP* is the total PEEP level (including auto-PEEP), and VT_{sp} is the patient's spontaneous tidal volume.

Weaning Techniques

The **spontaneous breathing trial (SBT)** is the oldest ventilator weaning technique. In the traditional, or T-piece approach, the patient is removed from the ventilator, and humidified supplemental oxygen is provided to the airway. Humidified gas typically is provided as a heated or cool aerosol of water from a large volume nebulizer. For patients with reactive airways, this aerosol may induce bronchospasm. In such cases a humidification system that does not generate an aerosol should be used, such as a heated passover humidifier. Passive humidifiers (that is, artificial noses) should be avoided because of their dead space and resistive workload.

There are two distinctly different applications of the SBT. The first is use of the SBT to identify extubation readiness. Although a 2-hour SBT commonly is used to identify extubation readiness, one study reported similar outcomes with 30-minute and 2-hour SBTs.[84,85] The second application of the SBT is for weaning, in which the length of each SBT is increased, with alternating periods of ventilatory support and SBT. For chronically ventilator-dependent patients, this process may require weeks. For patients with marginal respiratory reserve, nocturnal ventilation may be required, with spontaneous breathing during the waking hours.

The SBT can be conducted without removal of the patient from the ventilator, and this approach has several advantages. No additional equipment is required, and if the patient fails the SBT, ventilatory support can be quickly reestablished. All the monitoring functions and alarms on the ventilator are available during the SBT, which may allow prompt recognition that the patient is failing the SBT. Most of the literature related to weaning used a traditional SBT, although several studies allowed performance of the SBT with the patient attached to the ventilator.[86,87]

The SBT can be performed with no positive pressure applied to the airway, with a low level of CPAP (5 cm H_2O), or with a low level of PSV (5 to 8 cm H_2O). Proponents of the CPAP approach argue that this maintains functional residual capacity (FRC) at a level similar to that after extubation. It is argued that, in a patient with obstructive lung disease, this low level of CPAP maintains airway patency if the patient cannot control exhalation because of the presence of the artificial airway. In patients with marginal left ventricular function, however, a low level of positive intrathoracic pressure may support the failing heart. Such patients may tolerate a CPAP trial but then develop congestive heart failure when extubated.[88]

Proponents of the low level PSV approach argue that this overcomes the resistance to breathing through the artificial airway. However, this argument fails to recognize that the upper airway of an intubated patient typically is swollen and inflamed. One study reported that resistance through the upper airway after extubation was similar to that seen with the endotracheal tube in place.[89] Resistance through the artificial airway is affected by many factors, including the patient's inspiratory flow, the inner diameter of the tube, whether the tube is an endotracheal or tracheostomy tube, and the presence of secretions in the tube. This makes it difficult to choose an appropriate level of pressure support to overcome tube resistance. However, one study reported similar weaning outcomes when the SBT was performed with a T-piece and with 7 cm H_2O PSV.[90] If a passive humidifier is used, a low level of PSV is needed because of the device's imposed resistance and dead space.[91-93]

With pressure-support weaning, the level of pressure support is reduced as tolerated by the patient. When a low level of PSV is successful (for example, 5 to 10 cm H_2O), the patient is considered ready for extubation. With SIMV, weaning is achieved by reduction of the mandatory breath rate, requiring more spontaneous breathing effort to maintain the minute ventilation. Because respiratory center output and respiratory muscle activity are as great during the mandatory breaths of SIMV as with the spontaneous breaths, SIMV may result in a fatiguing load on the respiratory muscles rather than alternating periods of rest and exercise. Although newer generation ventilators feature modes intended to facilitate weaning, no evidence currently shows that these modes improve weaning outcomes over existing modes.

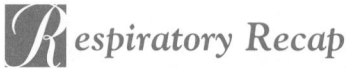

*R*espiratory *Recap* ⎯⎯⎯⎯⎯⎯⎯⎯⎯⎯

Weaning from Mechanical Ventilation
Regularly assess for weaning readiness.
Perform spontaneous breathing trial to assess readiness for extubation.
If spontaneous breathing trial is not tolerated, assess for causes of weaning failure.
Do not use synchronized intermittent mechanical ventilation (SIMV) as a weaning mode.
Use protocols to improve weaning success.

Two prospective, randomized, controlled trials reported that about two thirds of patients are successfully extubated after the first T-piece trial.[94,95] In those who failed the first-day T-piece trial, no difference in outcome (duration of ventilation) was seen between the T-piece and PSV methods. The T-piece and PSV methods were superior to SIMV in both studies.[96] In appropriately selected patients (that is, those recovering from an acute exacerbation of COPD), extubation to noninvasive positive pressure ventilation (NPPV) may reduce the duration of mechanical ventilation.[97,98]

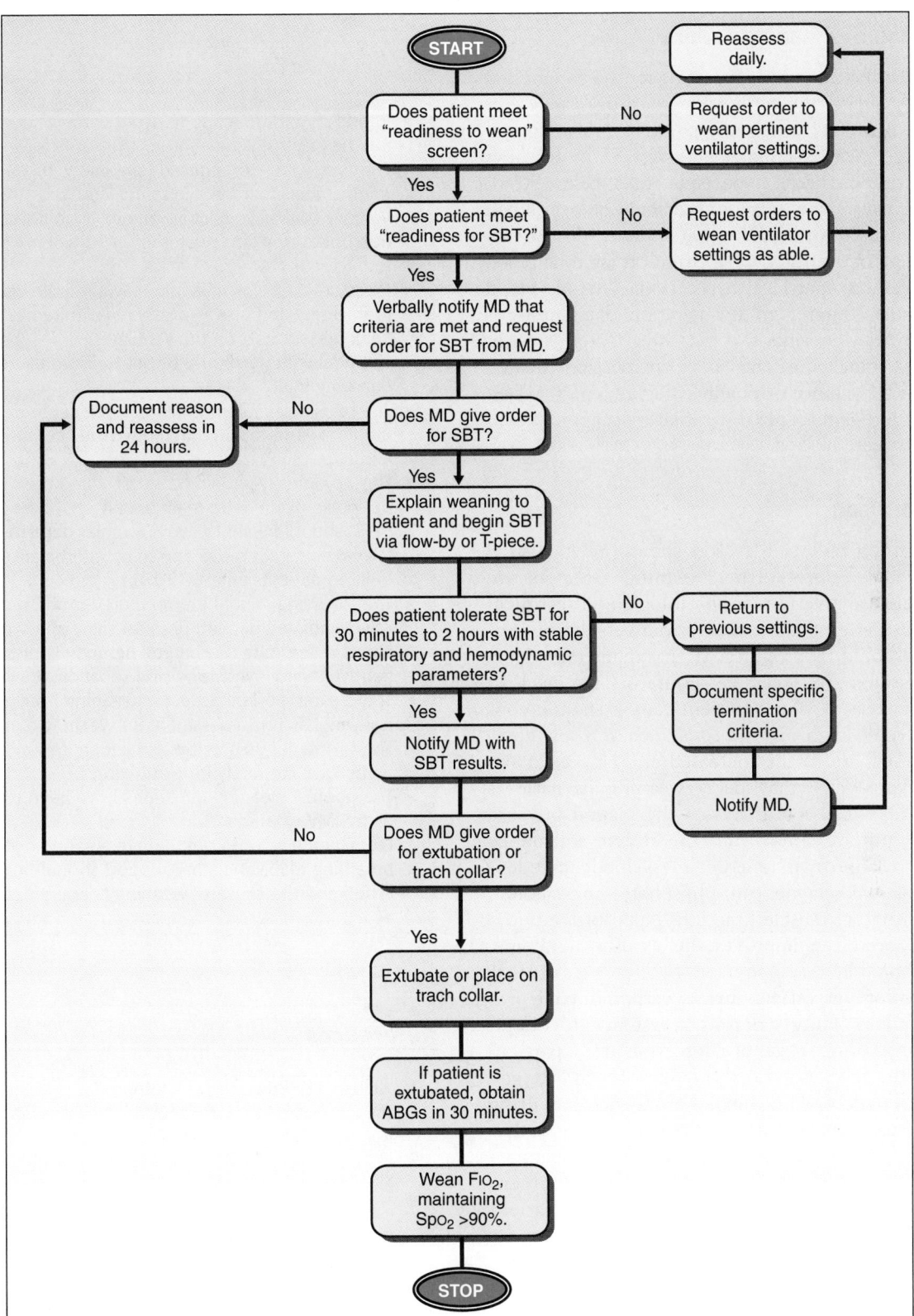

Figure 40-32   Algorithm for weaning from mechanical ventilation. *SBT,* Spontaneous breathing trial. (Modified from Ely EW. Respir Care Clin North Am 2000;6:303-319.)

Recognition of Weaning Failure

A failed weaning trial is discomforting for the patient and may induce significant cardiopulmonary distress. Commonly listed criteria for discontinuation of a weaning trial include tachypnea (respiratory rate over 35 breaths/min for 5 minutes or longer); hypoxemia (SpO_2 below 90%); tachycardia (heart rate over 140 beats/min or a sustained increase above 20%); bradycardia (sustained decrease in the heart rate of over 20%); hypertension (systolic blood pressure over 180 mm Hg); hypotension (systolic blood pressure under 90 mm Hg); and agitation, diaphoresis, or anxiety. In some patients the last three factors are not caused by weaning failure and can be appropriately treated with verbal reassurance or pharmacologic support. When weaning failure is recognized, ventilatory support should be promptly reestablished.

Failure to Wean

When weaning fails, the reason should be identified and corrected before further weaning attempts are made. There are a variety of physiologic and technical reasons why patients fail to wean from ventilatory support. Rest should be provided when exhaustion occurs during weaning. An excessive respiratory muscle load may be the reason why a patient fails a spontaneous breathing trial. High airways resistance and low compliance contribute to the increased effort necessary to breathe. Auto-PEEP may delay weaning in patients with COPD, because it increases the pleural pressure needed to initiate inhalation. Electrolyte imbalance may cause respiratory muscle weakness. Inadequate levels of potassium, magnesium, phosphate, and calcium impair ventilatory muscle function. Appropriate nutritional support often improves the weaning outcome, but care should be taken to avoid overfeeding, because excessive caloric ingestion elevates carbon dioxide production. Failure of any major organ system can precipitate weaning failure. Fever and infection are of particular concern, because they increase both oxygen consumption and carbon dioxide production, resulting in an increased ventilatory requirement. Cardiac dysfunction can delay weaning until appropriate management of cardiovascular status has occurred. A small endotracheal tube or a ventilator unresponsive to patient effort also can delay weaning efforts.

Weaning Protocols

Weaning protocols have become increasingly popular in recent years,[86,87,99,100] and these protocols typically are implemented by respiratory therapists. Studies have reported improved weaning outcomes when weaning protocols are used. Figure 40-32 presents an example of a weaning protocol.

𝒦EY 𝒫OINTS

- Efforts should be made to avoid complications during mechanical ventilation.
- Forms of ventilator-induced lung injury include volutrauma, atelectrauma, biotrauma, and oxygen toxicity.
- Volume-control ventilation maintains minute ventilation but allows airway pressure and plateau pressure to fluctuate.
- Pressure-control ventilation allows minute ventilation to fluctuate, but airway pressure is limited to the peak pressure set on the ventilator.
- The tidal volume should be set to avoid overdistention lung injury.
- The respiratory rate and I:E ratio are set to control the $Paco_2$ and to avoid hemodynamic compromise and auto-PEEP.
- The Fio_2 initially should be set at 1 and then weaned per pulse oximetry to maintain an Spo_2 over 92%.
- PEEP should be set to avoid alveolar derecruitment for patients with ARDS and to counterbalance auto-PEEP in patients with COPD.
- The following should be monitored in the mechanically ventilated patient: physical signs and symptoms, blood gases, lung mechanics, hemodynamics, patient-ventilator synchrony, and sedation.
- The most important aspect of weaning from mechanical ventilation is assessment for weaning readiness.
- The spontaneous breathing trial identifies most patients who are ready for extubation.
- The poorest weaning outcomes have been reported with SIMV weaning.
- For patients who do not tolerate a spontaneous breathing trial, ventilatory support should be reestablished and the cause of weaning failure identified.

References

1. Aldrich TK, Prezant DJ. Indications for mechanical ventilation. In: Tobin MJ, editor. Principles and practice of mechanical ventilation. New York: McGraw-Hill; 1994.
2. Hess DR, Kacmarek RM. Essentials of mechanical ventilation. New York: McGraw-Hill; 1996.
3. Ruiz-Martinez R, Bigatello LM, Hess D. Mechanical ventilation. In: Hurford WE, Bigatello LM, Haspel KL, et al, editors: Critical care handbook of the Massachusetts General Hospital. Philadelphia: Lippincott Williams & Wilkins; 2000.
4. Pingleton SK. Complications associated with mechanical ventilation. In: Tobin MJ, editor. Principles and practice of mechanical ventilation. New York: McGraw-Hill; 1994.
5. Matlu GM, Factor P. Complications of mechanical ventilation. Respir Care Clin North Am 2000;6:213-252.
6. Pierson DJ. Barotrauma and bronchopleural fistula. In: Tobin MJ, editor. Principles and practice of mechanical ventilation. New York: McGraw-Hill; 1994.

7. Pierson DJ. Alveolar rupture during mechanical ventilation: role of PEEP, peak airway pressure, and distending volume. Respir Care 1988;33:472-484.

8. Stauffer JL. Complications of endotracheal intubation and tracheostomy. Respir Care 1999;44:828-843.

9. Hess D, Kacmarek RM. Technical aspects of the patient-ventilator interface. In: Tobin MJ, editor. Principles and practice of mechanical ventilation. New York: McGraw-Hill; 1994.

10. Perreault T, Gutkowska J. Role of atrial natriuretic factor in lung physiology and pathology. Am J Respir Crit Care Med 1995;151:226-242.

11. Morehead RS, Pinto SJ. Ventilator-associated pneumonia. Arch Intern Med 2000;160:1926-1936.

12. Dreyfuss D, Djedanini K, Weber P, et al. Prospective study of nosocomial pneumonia and of patient and circuit colonization during mechanical ventilation with circuit changes every 48 hours versus no change. Am Rev Respir Dis 1991;143:738-743.

13. Hess D, Burns E, Romagnoli D, et al. Weekly ventilator circuit changes: a strategy to reduce costs without affecting pneumonia rates. Anesthesiology 1995;82:903-911.

14. Kollef MH, Shapiro SD, Fraser VJ, et al. Mechanical ventilation with or without 7-day circuit changes: a randomized controlled trial. Ann Intern Med 1995;123:168-174.

15. Fink JB, Krause SA, Barrett L, et al. Extending ventilator circuit change interval beyond 2 days reduces the likelihood of ventilator-associated pneumonia. Chest 1998;113:405-411.

16. Cook D, De Jonghe B, Brochard L, et al. Influence of airway management on ventilator-associated pneumonia: evidence from randomized trials. JAMA 1998;279:781-787.

17. Cook DJ, Laine LA, Guyatt GH, et al. Nosocomial pneumonia and the role of gastric pH: a metaanalysis. Chest 1991;100:7-13.

18. Rijan P, Dawson J, Teres D, et al. Continuous infusion of cimetidine versus sucralfate: incidence of pneumonia and bleeding compared. Crit Care Med 1990;18(Suppl):253.

19. Shepherd KE, Faulkner CS, Thal GD, et al. Acute, subacute, and chronic histologic effects of simulated aspiration of a 0.7% sucralfate suspension in rats. Crit Care Med 1995;23:532-536.

20. Pingleton SK. Nutritional support in the mechanically ventilated patient. Clin Chest Med 1988;9:101-112.

21. Dreyfuss D, Saumon G. Ventilator-induced lung injury. Am J Respir Crit Care Med 1998;157:294-323.

22. Slutsky AS. ACCP [American College of Chest Physicians] consensus conference: mechanical ventilation. Chest 1993;104:1833-1859.

23. Mead J, Takishima T, Leith D. Stress distribution in lungs: a model of pulmonary elasticity. J Appl Physiol 1970;28:596-608.

24. Ranieri VM, Suter PM, Tortorella C, et al. Effect of mechanical ventilation on inflammatory mediators in patients with acute respiratory distress syndrome: a randomized controlled trial. JAMA 1999;282:54-61.

25. Slutsky AS, Trembly L. Multiple system organ failure: Is mechanical ventilation a contributing factor? Am J Respir Crit Care Med 1998;157:1721-1725.

26. Durbin CG, Wallace KK. Oxygen toxicity in the critically ill patient. Respir Care 1993;38:739-753.

27. Laffey JG, Kavanagh BP. Carbon dioxide and the critically ill: Too little of a good thing? Lancet 1999;354:1283-1286.

28. Dries DJ. Permissive hypercapnia. J Trauma 1995;39:984-989.

29. Branson RD, Chatburn RL. Technical description and classification of modes of ventilator operation. Respir Care 1992;37:1026-1044.

30. Chatburn RL. Classification of mechanical ventilators. Respir Care 1992;37:1009-1025.

31. Branson RD, MacIntyre NR. Dual-control modes of mechanical ventilation. Respir Care 1996;41:294-305.

32. Branson RD, Campbell RS, Davis K Jr. New modes of ventilatory support. Int Anesthesiol Clin 1999;37:103-125.

33. Hess D, Branson RD. Ventilators and weaning modes. Respir Care Clin North Am 2000;6:407-435.

34. Marini JJ, Smith TC, Lamb VJ. External work output and force generation during synchronized intermittent mechanical ventilation: effect of machine assistance on breathing effort. Am Rev Respir Dis 1988;138:1169-1179.

35. Leung P, Jubran A, Tobin MJ. Comparison of assisted ventilator modes on triggering, patient effort, and dyspnea. Am J Respir Crit Care Med 1997;155:1940-1948.

36. Sassoon CSH. Mechanical ventilator design and function: the trigger variable. Respir Care 1992;37:1056-1069.

37. Branson RD, Campbell RS, Davis D, et al. Comparison of pressure and flow triggering systems during continuous positive airway pressure. Chest 1994;106:540-544.

38. Sassoon CSH, Gruer SE. Characteristics of the ventilator pressure and flow trigger variables. Intensive Care Med 1995;21:159-168.

39. Sassoon CSH, Rosario ND, Fei R, et al. Influence of pressure- and flow-triggered synchronous intermittent mandatory ventilation on inspiratory muscle work. Crit Care Med 1994;22:1933-1941.

40. Giuliani R, Mascia L, Recchia F, et al. Patient-ventilator interaction during synchronized intermittent mandatory ventilation: effects of flow triggering. Am J Respir Crit Care Med 1995;151:1-9.

41. Goulet RL, Hess D, Kacmarek RM. Flow versus pressure triggering in mechanically ventilated adult patients. Respir Care 1995;40:1205.

42. Aslanian P, El Atrous S, Isabey D, et al. Effects of flow triggering on breathing effort during partial ventilatory support. Am J Respir Crit Care Med 1998;157:135-139.

43. Cinnella G, Conti G, Lofaso F, et al. Effects of assisted ventilation on the work of breathing: volume-controlled versus pressure-controlled ventilation. Am J Respir Crit Care Med 1996;153:1025-1033.

44. MacIntyre NR, McConnell R, Cheng KG, et al. Patient-ventilator flow dyssynchrony: flow-limited versus pressure-limited breaths. Crit Care Med 1997;25:1671-1677.

45. Jubran A, Van de Graaff WB, Tobin MJ. Variability of patient-ventilator interaction with pressure support ventilation in patients with chronic obstructive pulmonary disease. Am J Respir Crit Care Med 1995;152:129-136.

46. Parthasarathy S, Jubran A, Tobin MJ. Cycling of inspiratory and expiratory muscle groups with the ventilator in airflow limitation. Am J Respir Crit Care Med 1998;158:1471-1478.

47. Jubran A. Inspiratory flow: more may not be better. Crit Care Med 1999;27:670-671.

48. Fernandez R, Mendez M, Younes M. Effect of ventilator flow rate on respiratory timing in normal subjects. Am J Respir Crit Care Med 1999;159:710.

49. Manning HL, Molinary EJ, Leiter JC. Effect of inspiratory flow rate on respiratory sensation and pattern of breathing. Am J Respir Crit Care Med 1995;151:751-755.

50. Acute Respiratory Distress Syndrome Network. Ventilation with lower tidal volumes as compared with traditional tidal volumes for acute lung injury and the acute respiratory distress syndrome. N Engl J Med 2000;342:1301-1308.

51. Amato MB, Barbas CS, Medeiros DM, et al. Effect of a protective ventilation strategy on mortality in the acute respiratory distress syndrome. N Engl J Med 1998;338:347-354.

52. Smith TC, Marini JJ. Impact of PEEP on lung mechanics and work of breathing in severe airflow obstruction. J Appl Physiol 1988;65:1488-1499.

53. Petrof BJ, Lagare M, Goldberg P, et al. Continuous positive airway pressure reduces work of breathing and dyspnea during weaning from mechanical ventilation in severe chronic obstructive pulmonary disease. Am Rev Respir Dis 1990;141:281-289.

54. Tobin MJ, Lodato RF. PEEP, auto-PEEP, and waterfalls. Chest 1989;96:449-451.

55. Primiano FP, Chatburn RL, Lough MD. Mean airway pressure: theoretical considerations. Crit Care Med 1982;10:378-383.

56. Jubran A, Tobin MJ. Reliability of pulse oximetry in titrating supplemental oxygen therapy in ventilator-dependent patients. Chest 1990;97:1420-1425.

57. Hess D, Good C, Didyoung R, et al. The validity of assessing arterial blood gases 10 minutes after an FIO_2 change in mechanically ventilated patients without chronic pulmonary disease. Respir Care 1985;30:1037-1041.

58. Branson RD, Campbell RS. Sighs: wasted breath or breath of fresh air? Respir Care 1992;37:462-468.

59. Pelosi P, Cadringher P, Bottino N, et al. Sigh in acute respiratory distress syndrome. Am J Respir Crit Care Med 1999;159:872-880.

60. Hess D, McCurty S, Simmons M. Compression volume in adult mechanical ventilator circuits: a comparison of five disposable circuits and a nondisposable circuit. Respir Care 1991;36:1113-1118.

61. Valeri KL, Hill TV, Taft AA, et al. The effect of time and warming on breathing circuit compliance. Respir Care 1994;39:793-796.

62. Hess D. Prolonged use of heat and moisture exchangers: why do we keep changing things? Crit Care Med 2000;28:1667-1668.

63. Williams R, Rankin N, Smith T, et al. Relationship between the humidity and temperature of inspired gas and the function of the airway mucosa. Crit Care Med 1996;24:1920-1929.

64. Branson RD, Campbell RS. Humidification in the intensive care unit. Respir Care Clin North Am 1998;4:305-320.

65. Hess DR. Capnometry. In: Tobin MJ, editor. Principles and practice of intensive care monitoring. New York: McGraw-Hill; 1998.

66. Hess DR, Medoff BD. Respiratory monitoring. Curr Opin Crit Care 1999;5:52-60.

67. Harris RS, Hess DR, Venegas JG. An objective analysis of the pressure-volume curve in the acute respiratory distress syndrome. Am J Respir Crit Care Med 2000;161:432-439.

68. Kupfer Y, Namba T, Kaldawi E, et al. Prolonged weakness after long-term infusion of vecuronium. Ann Intern Med 1992;117:484-486.

69. Segredo V, Caldwell JE, Matthay MA, et al. Persistent paralysis in critically ill patients after long-term administration of vecuronium. N Engl J Med 1992;327:524-528.

70. Hansen-Flaschen JH, Cowen J, Raps ED. Neuromuscular blockade in the ICU: more than we bargained for. Am Rev Respir Dis 1993;147:234-236.

71. Kress JP, Pohlman AS, O'Connor MF, et al. Daily interruption of sedative infusions in critically ill patients undergoing mechanical ventilation. N Engl J Med 2000;342:1471-1477.

72. Epstein SK. Weaning parameters. Respir Care Clin North Am 2000;6:253-301.

73. Yang KL, Tobin MJ. A prospective study of indices predicting the outcome of trials of weaning from mechanical ventilation. N Engl J Med 1991;324:1445-1450.

74. Tobin MJ, Perez W, Guenther SM, et al. The pattern of breathing during successful and unsuccessful trials of weaning from mechanical ventilation. Am Rev Respir Dis 1986;134:1111-1118.

75. Fiastro JF et al. Comparison of standard weaning parameters and the mechanical work of breathing in mechanically ventilated patients. Chest 1988;94:232-238.

76. Stoller JK. Establishing clinical unweanability. Respir Care 1991;36:186-198.

77. Cohen CA, Zagelbaum G, Gross D, et al. Clinical manifestations of inspiratory muscle fatigue. Am J Med 1982;73:308-316.

78. Branson RD, Hurst JM, Davis K, et al. Measurement of maximal inspiratory pressure: a comparison of three methods. Respir Care 1989;34:789-794.

79. Kacmarek RM, Cycyk-Chapman MC, Young PJ, et al. Determination of maximal inspiratory pressure: a clinical study literature review. Respir Care 1989;34:868-878.

80. Marini JJ, Smith TC, Lamb V. Estimation of inspiratory muscle strength in mechanically ventilated patients: the measurement of maximal inspiratory pressure. J Crit Care 1986;1:32-38.

81. Laghi F, D'Alfonso N, Tobin MJ. Pattern of recovery from diaphragmatic fatigue over 24 hours. J Appl Physiol 1995;79:539-546.

82. Stoller JK. Physiologic rationale for resting the ventilatory muscles. Respir Care 1991;36:290-296.

83. Jabour ER, Rabil DM, Truwitt JD, et al. Evaluation of a new weaning index based on ventilatory endurance and the efficiency of gas exchange. Am Rev Respir Dis 1991;144:531-537.

84. Esteban E, Alia I, Tobin MJ, et al. Effect of spontaneous breathing trial duration on outcome of attempts to discontinue mechanical ventilation. Am J Respir Crit Care Med 1999;159:512-518.

85. Vallverdu I, Calaf N, Subirana M, et al. Clinical characteristics, respiratory functional parameters, and outcome of a 2-hour T-piece trial in patients weaning from mechanical ventilation. Am J Respir Crit Care Med 1998;158:1855-1862.

86. Ely EW, Baker AM, Dunagan DP, et al. Effect of the duration of mechanical ventilation on identifying patients capable of breathing spontaneously. N Engl J Med 1996;335:1864-1869.

87. Ely EW, Bennett PA, Bowton DL, et al. Large-scale implementation of a respiratory therapist–driven protocol for ventilator weaning. Am J Respir Crit Care Med 1999;159:439-446.

88. Lemaire F, Teboul J, Cinotti L, et al. Acute left ventricular dysfunction during unsuccessful weaning from mechanical ventilation. Anesthesiology 1988;69:171-179.

89. Straus C, Louis B, Isabey D, et al. Contribution of the endotracheal tube and the upper airway to breathing workload. Am J Respir Crit Care Med 1998;157:23-30.

90. Esteban A, Alia I, Gordo F, et al. Extubation outcome after spontaneous breathing trials with T-tube or pressure-support ventilation. Am J Respir Crit Care Med 1997;156:459-465.

91. Iotti GA, Olivei MC, Palo A, et al. Unfavorable mechanical effects of heat and moisture exchangers in ventilated patients. Intensive Care Med 1997;23:399-405.

92. LeBourdelles G, Mier L, Fiquet B, et al. Comparison of the effects of heat and moisture exchangers and heated humidifiers on ventilation and gas exchange during weaning trials from mechanical ventilation. Chest 1996;110:1294-1298.

93. Pelosi P, Solca M, Ravagnan I, et al. Effects of heat and moisture exchangers on minute ventilation, ventilatory drive, and work of breathing during pressure support ventilation in acute respiratory failure. Crit Care Med 1996;24:1184-1188.

94. Esteban A, Frutos F, Tobin MJ, et al. A comparison of four methods of weaning patients from mechanical ventilation. N Engl J Med 1995;6:345-350.

95. Brochard L, Rauss A, Benito S, et al. Comparison of three methods of gradual withdrawal from ventilatory support during weaning from mechanical ventilation. Am J Respir Crit Care Med 1994;150:896-903.

96. Cook D, Meade M, Guyatt G, et al. Evidence report on criteria for weaning from mechanical ventilation. Washington, DC: Agency for Health Care Policy and Research, US Department of Health and Human Services; 1999.

97. Girault C, Daudenthun I, Chevron V, et al. Noninvasive ventilation as a systematic extubation and weaning technique in acute on chronic respiratory failure: a prospective, randomized, controlled study. Am J Respir Crit Care Med 1999;160:86-92.

98. Nava S, Ambrosino N, Clini E, et al. Noninvasive mechanical ventilation in the weaning of patients with respiratory failure due to chronic obstructive pulmonary disease: a randomized, controlled trial. Ann Intern Med 1998;128:721-728.

99. Marelich GP, Murin S, Battistella F, et al. Protocol weaning of mechanical ventilation in medical and surgical patients by respiratory care practitioners and nurses: effect on weaning time and incidence of ventilator-associated pneumonia. Chest 2000;118:459-467.

100. Ely EW. The utility of weaning protocols to expedite liberation from mechanical ventilation. Respir Care Clin North Am 2000;6:303-319.

CHAPTER 41

Neonatal Mechanical Ventilation

Patricia English
Steven C. Mason
Dean R. Hess

CHAPTER **OUTLINE**

Manual Ventilation
Nasal Continuous Positive Airway Pressure
Endotracheal Intubation
Conventional Infant Ventilation
   Indications
   Infant Ventilators
   Pressure Limit and Tidal Volume
   Respiratory Rate
   Mode
   Inspiratory Trigger and Expiratory Cycle
   Inspiratory Time
   Positive End-Expiratory Pressure
   Humidification
   Hazards and Complications
   Weaning

High-Frequency Ventilation
   Classification
   Gas Transport Theories
   Patient Selection
   High-Frequency Ventilators
   Management Strategies
   Complications
   High-Frequency Ventilation in Perspective
Airway Care
Adjuncts to Neonatal Mechanical Ventilation
   Surfactant Administration
   Inhaled Nitric Oxide
   Extracorporeal Life Support

OBJECTIVES

1. Compare the use of flow-inflating and self-inflating manual ventilation devices.
2. Describe the use of nasal continuous positive airway pressure (nCPAP) in neonates.
3. Describe the proper position for oral endotracheal tubes in neonates.
4. List indications for mechanical ventilation of neonates.
5. Compare conventional and high-frequency ventilation of neonates.
6. List usual settings for conventional mechanical ventilation of neonates.
7. Discuss the importance of humidification during neonatal mechanical ventilation.
8. List hazards and complications of conventional neonatal mechanical ventilation.
9. Discuss approaches to weaning neonates from mechanical ventilation.
10. Compare the four general types of high-frequency ventilation of neonates.
11. Discuss theories of gas transport during high frequency ventilation.
12. List indications for high-frequency ventilation of neonates.
13. Discuss strategies for implementation of high-frequency ventilation.
14. List complications of high-frequency ventilation of neonates.
15. Discuss issues related to artificial airway care of neonates.
16. Discuss issues related to surfactant administration, inhaled nitric oxide, and extracorporeal life support of neonates.

Neonates may require mechanical ventilation for a variety of reasons. Regardless of the pathologic condition, the goal is to achieve adequate gas exchange while minimizing the risks and complications associated with mechanical ventilation. Many factors influence the respiratory management of a neonate, and no single approach is ideal for all infants. Maintaining adequate support of ventilation and oxygenation by continual reassessment of the infant and adjustment of the ventilator is essential to prevent complications. Mechanical ventilation of the neonate in the intensive care environment is a varied art form. It is practiced differently throughout the world, and the method chosen depends on the strategies adopted by the institution.

Manual Ventilation

Positive pressure ventilation usually begins as manual bag-mask ventilation (BMV), often in the delivery room. Immediately after birth the infant is placed under a warmer, dried, positioned, and provided with tactile stimulation. Positive pressure ventilation is indicated if the infant is apneic or gasping or has a heart rate below 100 beat/min. Appropriate use of positive pressure from the resuscitative efforts can make a significant difference in the infant's course. During the initial resuscitation, administration of 100% oxygen is indicated. Once the infant's condition has been stabilized, with improved color and adequate blood pressure, the oxygen concentration is reduced via pulse oximetry and clinical assessment. Once pulse oximetry is initiated, both the high and low oxygen saturation alarms should be set to reduce the risks of hyperoxia and hypoxia.

Manual resuscitators are classified as self-inflating or flow-inflating bags (Figure 41-1).[1] A **self-inflating bag** inflates automatically and does not need an external gas source to provide positive pressure. These bags usually have a reservoir to deliver 100% oxygen with a flow of 5 to 10 L/min. Most self-inflating bags incorporate a pressure-limiting device (*pop-off valve*) that releases pressure at a preset level. The pop-off valve reduces the risk of exces-

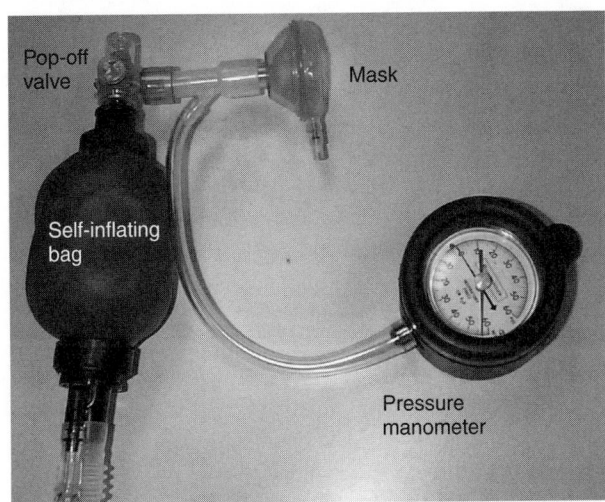

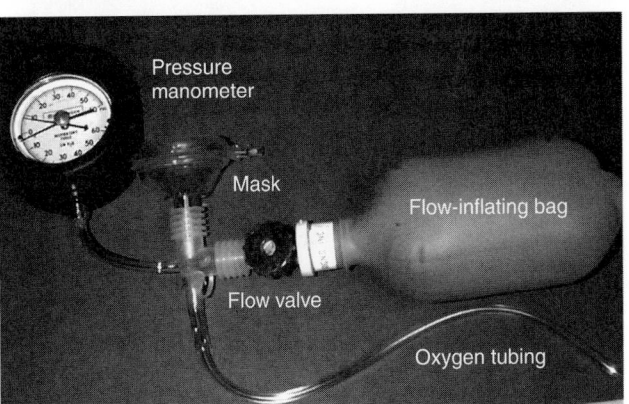

Figure 41-1 **A,** Self-inflating neonatal resuscitation bag. **B,** Flow-inflating neonatal resuscitation bag.

sive pressure being applied, but it can be manually overridden when delivery of high pressures is indicated. Self-inflating bags generally do not allow maintenance of positive end-expiratory pressure (PEEP) unless an external PEEP valve is added.

A **flow-inflating bag** requires a continuous flow from an external gas source. Pressure is determined by the flow and the pressure release valve. Wide ranges of peak inspiratory

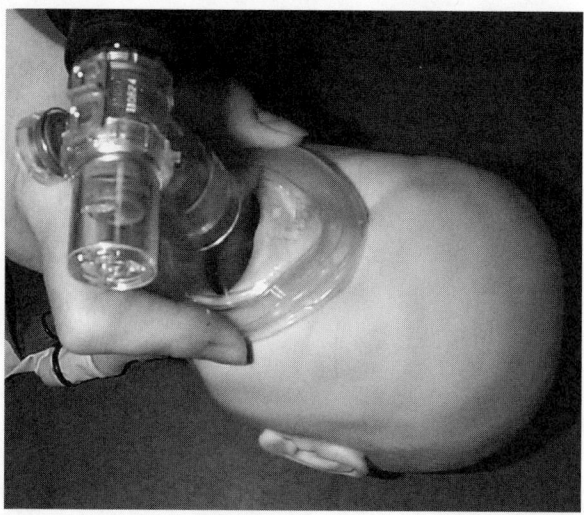

Figure 41-2 Positioning of the mask for neonatal bag-mask ventilation.

pressure (PIP) and PEEP are attainable with flow-inflating bags. Continuous flow at the patient connection makes the device suitable for the delivery of continuous positive airway pressure (CPAP) and a convenient method to deliver oxygen short term to spontaneously breathing infants. Flow-inflating bags are well-suited to the needs of neonates. Clinicians responsible for resuscitating neonates should be familiar with self-inflating and flow-inflating bags and with the specific characteristics of the bags used in their institution.

Respiratory Recap

Neonatal Manual Resuscitators

Self-inflating bags inflate automatically.
Flow-inflating bags require a continuus gas flow.

BMV is ineffective if the mask is not the correct size. A variety of masks are available that fit infants of all sizes. The mask should fit over the infant's nose and mouth, with the edge of the chin resting on the rim of the mask. As the mask is applied to the face, a seal is created by encircling of the mask with the thumb and index finger and application of a gentle downward pressure (Figure 41-2). The ring finger can be used to hold the chin in the mask. Positioning of the infant is critical to achieve effective BMV; slight extension of the neck, often accomplished by placement of a roll under the shoulders, aligns the airway to allow effective ventilation.

Knowledge of the infant's gestational age and prenatal history may be helpful during BMV initiation. Premature infants are likely to need higher ventilating pressures (more than 35 cm H_2O) during the initial breaths

TABLE 41-1

Troubleshooting Bag-Mask Ventilation of the Neonate

Problem	Solution
No seal between mask and face	Reposition mask; consider different mask size.
No chest movement	Check head position; do not overextend neck.
	Check for secretions in airway.
Pressure too low (flow-inflating bag)	Check flow; adjust flowmeter; check manometer connections.
Pressure too low (self-inflating bag)	Ensure pop-off valve is active; consider need to override the valve.

to overcome the surface tension in surfactant-deficient lungs. Depending on lung maturity, successive breaths may require less pressure as lung volume is established. The pressure used to ventilate should be that needed to cause the infant's chest wall to rise. Maintaining PEEP aids in the maintenance of lung volume. Observing chest movement while the bag is being squeezed is essential for correct application of pressure. Common reasons for poor chest movement are an inadequate mask seal, airway obstruction caused by improper head position or secretions in the airway, or inadequate ventilating pressure. Inadequate pressure leads to low lung volume, inability to oxygenate, and hemodynamic compromise. Excessive pressure can result in pneumothorax and further respiratory and hemodynamic compromise. An in-line pressure manometer should be used to monitor the applied peak airway pressure and PEEP levels. Factors to consider to troubleshoot problems with BMV are presented in Table 41-1.

An apneic or distressed infant typically requires a respiratory rate of 40 to 60 breaths/min with an inspiratory time of 0.4 to 0.5 seconds. Administration of 100% oxygen during the initial resuscitative efforts is indicated. Improvement in the skin color, heart rate, and hemodynamics should be apparent after a brief period. If the patient shows no sign of improvement, the adequacy of the delivery system should be reviewed. Oxygen disconnection or inadequacy of the gas source, mask seal, or head position should be considered.

Infants with evidence of meconium below the vocal cords should be intubated and the meconium cleared before they receive positive pressure ventilation. Intubation with the largest possible endotracheal tube is recommended. Clearing of meconium is attempted with a meconium aspirator. The aspirator is attached to the endotracheal tube, suction is applied at 100 mm Hg, and the endotracheal tube is withdrawn. Reintubation is performed with a new tube, and the process is repeated until no particulate meconium is present. After the

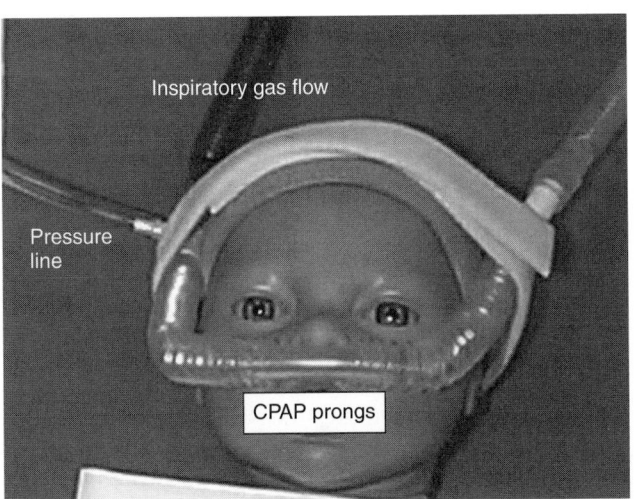

Figure 41-3 Setup for neonatal nasal continuous positive airway pressure (nCPAP) therapy.

Suggested Endotracheal Tube Size Based on Body Weight

Weight (g)	Tube Size*
Less than 1000	2.5
1000 to 2000	3.0
2000 to 3000	3.5
More than 3000	3.5 to 4

Tube size is given as the inside diameter in millimeters.

quately humidified gas can increase the risk of airway obstruction, and inadequately heated gas may result in difficulty in the maintenance of the infant's **neutral thermal environment,** the body temperature at which oxygen concentration is the lowest.

Endotracheal Intubation

After initiating manual ventilation, the clinician reassesses the infant's condition to determine if intubation is necessary. In some cases brief periods of manual ventilation can stabilize the infant's condition, making intubation unnecessary. Improved skin color, spontaneous respiratory efforts, and a stable heart rate are indications for withdrawal of manual ventilation. As the bag and mask are withdrawn, free-flowing oxygen can be placed near the infant's face and the infant reassessed. Infants who do not respond to brief periods of manual ventilation or who require prolonged ventilatory support require intubation.

Oral endotracheal tubes are most commonly used to intubate newborns. Nasal intubation generally requires more time and is reserved for elective settings. The appropriate tube size (Table 41-2) and the distance of insertion can be estimated based on the infant's weight. If the infant's weight is not immediately available, gestational age also is a reliable predictor for tube size (Table 41-3).

Unlike in adults and large children, the narrowest point of an infant's airway is at the cricoid cartilage; this characteristic allows the use of uncuffed airways. Although a complete seal is not always obtained, the cricoid cartilage provides a functional "cuff." Despite some leakage, adequate ventilation can be achieved with an appropriate-sized uncuffed endotracheal tube. Also,

meconium has been cleared, positive pressure ventilation can be provided by BMV or through an endotracheal tube. Insertion of a gastric tube to clear meconium from the stomach may reduce the risk of further meconium aspiration.

Mask positive pressure ventilation also is contraindicated in infants who have or are suspected of having a congenital diaphragmatic hernia. BMV can promote the entry of air into the gastrointestinal tract and further impair gas exchange. These infants should be intubated and ventilated through an endotracheal tube.

Nasal Continuous Positive Airway Pressure

Infants who show adequate spontaneous efforts but whose clinical presentation indicates the potential for low lung volumes and associated hypoxemia may benefit from **nasal continuous positive airway pressure (nCPAP).** nCPAP can be applied via nasal cannula or nasal pharyngeal tubes (Figure 41-3). It can serve as an oxygen delivery source and aid in lung recruitment. nCPAP also is used to minimize airway collapse in patients with tracheomalacia.[2,3] The CPAP level is started at 4 to 5 cm H_2O, and the infant is reevaluated with pulse oximetry or arterial blood gas measurements or both. An appropriately sized nasal cannula is needed to achieve the desired benefit. Cannulas that are too large can cause skin breakdown at the nares, and cannulas that are too small allow the infant to breathe around the device, making continuous airway pressure difficult to maintain. The flow rates must be adequate to meet the infant's inspiratory demand. Insertion of an orogastric tube is advised to minimize air accumulation in the gastrointestinal tract. The circuit used to deliver nCPAP should be heated and humidified, because it becomes the major portion of the infant's inspired air. Inade-

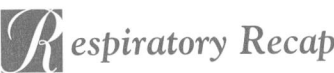*espiratory Recap* —————

Endotracheal Intubation

Oral tubes are most commonly used in neonates.
Neonatal tubes are uncuffed.

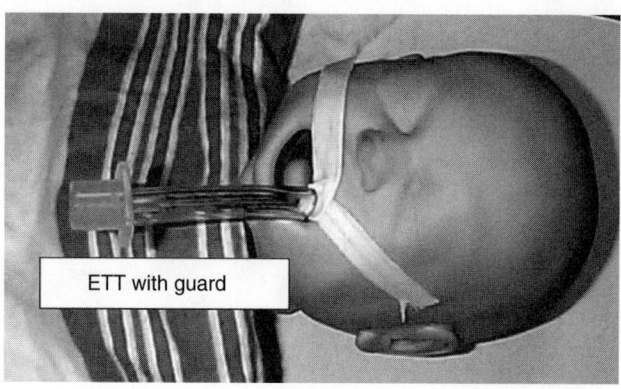

ETT with guard

Figure 41-4   Guard in position over endotracheal tube to prevent kinking.

TABLE 41-3

Suggested Endotracheal Tube Size Based on Gestational Age

Gestational Age (Weeks)	Tube Size*
Less than 30	2.5
30 to 35	3
More than 35	3.5

Tube size is given as the inside diameter in millimeters.

use of an uncuffed tube prevents cuff-related tracheal injury in these patients. For these reasons, cuffed tubes are rarely used in infants.

The approximate distance to insert the endotracheal tube, measured from the infant's lips, can be estimated by the addition of 6 cm to the infant's weight in kilograms. This formula can be used to estimate initial tube placement, but bilateral auscultation of the chest is essential. When bilateral breath sounds are noted, the tube should be secured and its position confirmed by chest radiograph. The tube then can be cut to minimize additional dead space and reduce the risk of inadvertent extubation. A guard to help prevent kinking of the tube can be fashioned from thick-walled tubing, which is wrapped around the outside of the endotracheal tube (Figure 41-4). In addition, a gastric tube should be inserted and suction applied to decompress the stomach of air inadvertently delivered during mask ventilation.

Conventional Infant Ventilation

Indications

Mechanical ventilation is required for a variety of clinical presentations in neonates. Full-term infants who require mechanical ventilation have complex presenting symptoms that often include intrapulmonary and intracardiac shunting. Infants with congenital heart disease have particularly complex circulatory alterations. Some of these patients depend on the fetal blood flow that normally occurs only in utero. Maintaining patency of a ductus arteriosus or septal defect may save a life. During mechanical ventilation, abrupt changes in hemodynamics, normoxia, and hyperoxia can be fatal to these infants. Blood flow through these shunts is sometimes the primary means to maintain blood flow to the systemic circulation. Until corrective procedures can be performed, oxygen concentrations at or below room air can alter intracardiac shunts and ensure the patient's survival. An understanding of various cardiac anomalies is essential to appropriate ventilator management.

Providing adequate oxygenation and ventilation in conditions such as pneumonia, meconium aspiration, and congenital diaphragmatic hernia often is difficult. Nonhomogeneous lung disease increases the risk of barotrauma, because the most compliant alveoli become overdistended. These underlying conditions often cause difficulty in the maintenance of adequate oxygenation and ventilation and lead to pulmonary vasoconstriction and significant pulmonary hypertension. As a result, shunting occurs through a patent ductus arteriosus or patent foramen ovale, making oxygenation more difficult.

Persistent pulmonary hypertension of the neonate (PPHN) can appear as a primary condition and be extremely difficult to manage. In infants with PPHN, either the pulmonary vasculature has increased tone and abnormal responsiveness to vasodilators or the pulmonary arteries are muscularized, with a decreased cross-sectional area. In either condition blood flow is restricted, pulmonary artery pressure increases, and intracardiac shunting occurs. Because limited blood flow reaches the pulmonary vasculature to participate in gas exchange, ventilator adjustments in this population have little effect. Deoxygenated blood is shunted through a patent foramen ovale or a patent ductus arteriosus, making it difficult to achieve an adequate arterial oxygen saturation. The pulmonary vasculature responds to hypoxia with further vasoconstriction, creating the possibility of greater amounts of blood being shunted and worsening oxygenation. Definitive diagnosis of PPHN generally is done by cardiac ultrasound. Clinically, right-to-left shunting is detected when oxygen saturation by pulse oximetry (SpO_2) is monitored at a site receiving preductal blood (generally the right arm) and compared with a simultaneously monitored postductal site (left arm or right or left lower extremity). A difference in the oxygen saturation values from these two sites (preductal value higher than the postductal value) indicates right-to-left shunting, often a result of pulmonary hypertension.

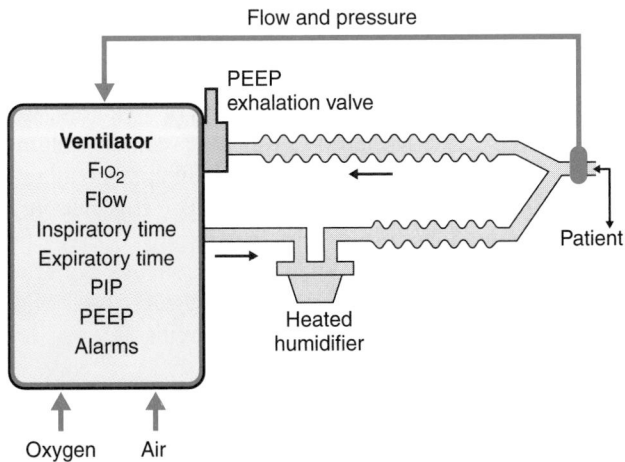

Figure 41-5 Schematic drawing of conventional neonatal ventilator. *F_{IO_2},* Fractional inspired oxygen concentration; *PIP,* peak inspiratory pressure; *PEEP,* positive end-expiratory pressure.

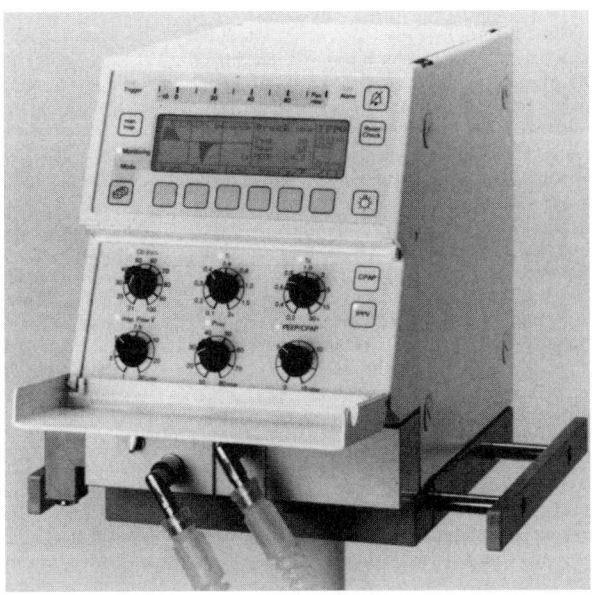

Figure 41-6 Conventional neonatal ventilator. (Courtesy Drager, Inc., Critical Care Systems, Oakdale, Pa.)

Infant Ventilators

Infant ventilators fall into two major categories: conventional ventilators and high-frequency ventilators. A conventional ventilator offers a variety of modes, alarms, and other options.[4-6] Selection of the appropriate mode and other ventilator options is based on the infant's underlying condition and the desired effect of ventilatory support during both spontaneous and ventilator-initiated breaths.

Historically, a conventional neonatal ventilator has been continuous flow, time cycled, and pressure limited (Figure 41-5). These ventilators do not allow for patient triggering. Newer infant ventilators offer volume-limited and pressure-limited options, as well as patient-triggered and non–patient-triggered modes (Figure 41-6). Not all modes and options are appropriate for all neonates. A full understanding of the potential benefits and risks of the available options is essential for proper use of any ventilator. An understanding of the patient-ventilator interaction during both patient-triggered and ventilator-triggered breaths is particularly important.

When initiating infant ventilation, the clinician must select a pressure and/or tidal volume, respiratory rate, ventilator mode, inspiratory time or inspiration to expiration (I:E) ratio, PEEP, and fractional inspired oxygen concentration (F_{IO_2}). Initial ventilator settings for infant ventilation are shown in Table 41-4.

Pressure Limit and Tidal Volume

In neonatal time-cycled, pressure-limited ventilation, the clinician selects a pressure limit and inspiratory time that result in the delivery of a desired tidal volume. The tidal volume varies depending on the PIP, inspiratory time, and lung compliance. For example, if the lungs are less compliant, as in respiratory distress syndrome, a higher PIP is needed to

TABLE 41-4

Initial Ventilator Settings for Conventional Ventilation of the Neonate

Setting	Instructions for Use
Peak inspiratory pressure (PIP)	As needed to provide a tidal volume of 5 to 7 mL/kg
Positive end-expiratory pressure (PEEP)	3 to 5 cm H_2O
Rate	20 to 40/min
Inspiratory time	0.4 to 0.5 seconds
Fractional inspired oxygen concentration (F_{IO_2})	As needed to maintain Sp_{O_2} >90%
Flow	8 to 12 L/min

obtain a desired tidal volume. On the other hand, a lower PIP is needed if the lungs are more compliant. It should also be noted that, unlike most adult ventilators, the pressure limit set on a neonatal ventilator is the PIP—not the pressure above PEEP. Thus the tidal volume is determined by the difference between the pressure limit and PEEP. For this reason, an increase in PEEP may reduce the tidal volume unless the pressure limit is increased by an equivalent amount.

In the volume-limited mode, the delivered tidal volume is preset and the PIP varies. In volume ventilation in neonates the uncuffed endotracheal tube is a concern. The effectiveness of volume ventilation may be limited by leaks around the endotracheal tube, although this mode has been reported useful in neonates with respiratory distress syndrome.[7] Volume preset ventilation can be effective in larger infants with an appropriate-sized endotracheal tube. Careful monitoring of the delivered tidal volume is essential to assess the effect of leaks (Figure 41-7).

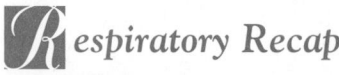espiratory Recap

Neonatal Ventilator Settings
Pressure or tidal volume (or both)
Respiratory rate
Ventilator mode
Inspiratory time or inspiration to expiration (I:E) ratio
Positive end-expiratory pressure (PEEP)
Fractional inspired oxygen concentration (FIO_2)

Pressure-limited ventilation with a target tidal volume is a common approach to neonate ventilation. Whether volume-limited or pressure-limited ventilation is selected,

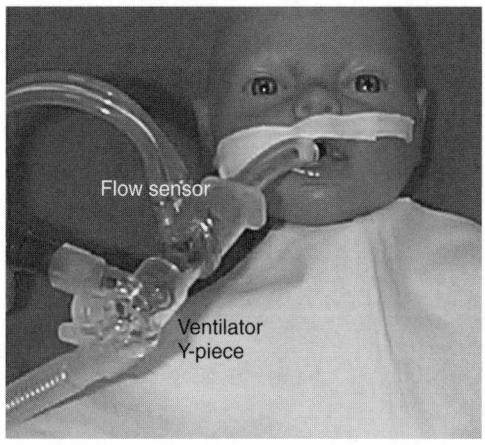

Figure 41-7 Flow sensor at airway to measure delivered tidal volume.

a tidal volume of 5 to 7 mL/kg generally is selected. As changes in tidal volume occur, clinical assessment determines the best intervention (Table 41-5).

A practical issue with the ventilation of neonates is the effect of circuit compliance and compressible volume. These can substantially reduce the tidal volume available, particularly with volume ventilation. For this reason, a noncompliant, low-volume circuit typically is used. Because of the high resistance through this smaller bore tubing, it is important to monitor airway pressure and flow directly at the Y-piece of the ventilator circuit.

Respiratory Rate

After a tidal volume is established, the respiratory rate becomes the primary adjustment for the achievement of a desired minute ventilation. Spontaneously breathing neonates normally breathe 40 to 60 breaths/min to maintain a normal partial pressure of arterial carbon dioxide ($PaCO_2$). During mechanical ventilation, delivery of a larger than normal tidal volume (>5 to 7 mL/kg) at a lower respiratory rate can be more effective at eliminating carbon dioxide because a greater percentage of each tidal volume participates in gas exchange. Higher rates at lower tidal volumes result in a higher percentage of dead space ventilation and may result in less effective ventilation.

The ventilator rate should target a desired $PaCO_2$. The required rate depends on the target $PaCO_2$, the degree of lung disease (that is, the amount of dead space), carbon dioxide production, the ventilator mode, and the amount of spontaneous breathing.

Mode

In the continuous mandatory ventilation (assist/control or CMV) mode, a minimum respiratory rate is set. Each spontaneous respiratory effort triggers a ventilator-assisted breath, and the preset pressure or volume is delivered. The

TABLE 41-5

Troubleshooting Changes in Tidal Volume during Pressure Ventilation of the Neonate

Tidal Volume Change	Possible Causes	Solutions
Increase	Increased compliance, decreased resistance, decreased PEEP, increased inspiratory time, decreased leak	Reduce peak inspiratory pressure.
Decrease	Decreased compliance, increased resistance, decreased peak inspiratory pressure, increased PEEP, decreased inspiratory time, increased leak	Suction airway. Administer surfactant. Increase inspiratory pressure. Perform transillumination to check for pneumothorax. Auscultate to detect pneumothorax or mainstem intubation. Obtain chest radiograph. Check tube position.

PEEP, Positive end-expiratory pressure.

inspiratory time is preset, and the total respiratory rate above the set rate is determined by the infant.

In the synchronized intermittent mandatory ventilation (SIMV) mode, a minimum respiratory rate is set. Between the mandatory breaths the infant can breathe spontaneously. Spontaneous efforts are unassisted and the rate, inspiratory time, and tidal volume are determined by the patient. The patient's inspiratory efforts trigger the mandatory breaths. The mandatory breaths may be pressure or volume limited. If the patient becomes apneic, the SIMV rate is delivered. The intermittent mandatory ventilation (IMV) mode is similar to SIMV except that the mandatory breaths are not synchronized to patient effort. Unlike most adult ventilators, most neonatal ventilators allow spontaneous breathing at both the PIP and PEEP levels.

The use of pressure support in neonates is increasing.[8] With pressure-support ventilation (PSV), all breaths are triggered by the patient. A pressure limit is set to achieve a target tidal volume. The total rate, inspiratory time, expiratory time, and tidal volume are determined by the infant. Because inspiration normally is flow cycled with PSV, leaks around the endotracheal tube are a matter of concern with a prolonged inspiratory time. Some ventilators offer mechanisms to adjust the flow cycle, preventing prolonged inspiratory times with a leak. Pressure support may improve patient-ventilator synchrony in some patients by allowing flow rates and inspiratory times more consistent with the infant's needs. Frequent apnea and periodic breathing are contraindications to this mode.

Inspiratory Trigger and Expiratory Cycle

Patient effort may trigger a breath in two primary ways. Depending on the ventilator, the infant-initiated breaths may be *flow triggered* or *pressure triggered*.[9-11] The signal for neonatal flow triggering typically occurs from a pneumotachometer positioned close to the infant's airway. A change in flow through the pneumotachometer triggers the ventilator. The amount of flow change required to trigger the ventilator is called the *flow-trigger sensitivity*, which is set by the clinician at a level that allows the least trigger effort without auto-triggering. Pressure triggering occurs with a change in the baseline pressure. The amount of pressure change required to trigger the ventilator is the pressure-trigger sensitivity, set in centimeters of water. At a sensitivity of 1 cm H_2O, a patient effort that reduces the baseline system pressure by 1 cm H_2O below PEEP will trigger a breath. The specifics of the trigger mechanism vary from ventilator to ventilator. Some ventilators will flow trigger in one mode and pressure trigger in other modes.

Volume triggering uses the integral of the flow signal for triggering. Because this is an averaging of the flow signal over time, signal noise is reduced. This gives volume triggering a theoretic advantage over flow triggering. Volume triggering is available on the Babylog (Drager, Inc., Critical Care Systems, Oakdale, Pa.), which uses an anemometer at the proximal airway.

Because of the difficulties associated with the measurement of respiratory efforts in neonates and the small endotracheal tubes required, alternative triggers have been explored.[12] On the Sechrist SAVI, (Sechrist Industries, Anaheim, Calif.) the ventilator is triggered by a respiratory impedance signal. Standard electrocardiographic (ECG) electrodes are used, and as the chest wall expands, the change in impedance initiates inspiration. Once inspiratory effort is detected, the control of ventilator limit and cycling variables returns to airway pressure. This method of triggering is not commonly used, and its effectiveness is unclear. The Infant Star (Infrasonics, San Diego, Calif.) uses a motion sensor to trigger the neonatal ventilator. This device (Star Sync) uses an abdominal sensor to detect inspiration. The sensor is a small, air-filled balloon enclosed in a capsule that is taped to the infant's abdomen midway between the umbilicus and the xiphoid. As the abdomen rises, the change in balloon pressure triggers the ventilator.

An adjustable expiratory flow cycle is incorporated into some patient-triggered, pressure-limited modes. The expiratory flow cycle is based on a percentage of the peak flow. This cycle produces a variable inspiratory time, much like pressure support, which may reduce ventilator dyssynchrony. Familiarity with the inspiratory trigger and expiratory cycle mechanisms of the ventilator is essential to determine the appropriate settings for an individual patient.

Inspiratory Time

The inspiratory time is set in conjunction with the respiratory rate. The inspiratory time and the respiratory rate determine the *inspiration to expiration (I:E) ratio*. For example, if the respiratory rate is 30 breaths/min, each breathing cycle takes 2 seconds. If the inspiratory time is 0.5 second, the I:E ratio is 1:3.

An inspiratory time that is too short can compromise both oxygenation and ventilation. The **mean airway pressure** is affected by the inspiratory time. A lower airway pressure may result in a loss of lung volume or inability to establish lung volume, causing a decrease in the partial pressure of arterial oxygen (PaO_2). Decreased ventilation, resulting in less carbon dioxide elimination and a higher $PaCO_2$, occurs if a shortened inspiratory time reduces the delivered tidal volume.

An inspiratory time that is too long may shorten the expiratory time and result in auto-PEEP, which may cause alveolar overdistention, increasing the risk of pneumothorax. Alveolar overdistention may also interfere with pulmonary blood flow, increase dead space ventilation, and reduce carbon dioxide elimination. A typical inspiratory time with conventional positive pressure ventilation for the neonate is 0.3 to 0.5 seconds. Monitoring the expiratory flow with graphics or expiratory flow rate monitors and adjustment of the respiratory rate and inspiratory time can help prevent complications related to the I:E ratio.

Positive End-Expiratory Pressure

PEEP is routinely set in all ventilator modes to prevent alveolar collapse during expiration. PEEP usually is started at 3 to 5 cm H_2O. Lung volumes are assessed by chest radiograph, with the ideal lung volume expansion to 8 or 9 ribs bilaterally. PEEP and PIP are adjusted if the lungs appear underinflated or overinflated. Higher PEEP levels may be indicated for neonates with a persistently low lung volume. Low levels of PEEP are indicated with evidence of pulmonary interstitial emphysema or persistent air leakage after barotrauma. The delivered tidal volumes should be assessed when PEEP levels are adjusted. In pressure-limited ventilation, the change in the PEEP setting may result in a change in the delivered tidal volume. The pressure limit may need to be adjusted to maintain the volume target.

Humidification

Adequate humidification of the inspired gas is critical to the maintenance of airway patency in neonates. A decrease in humidity can lead to dried secretions and may result in partial or complete airway obstruction. This risk is particularly high in neonates because of their small airways. An appropriately humidified circuit shows moisture throughout both the inspiratory and the expiratory limbs. Circuits should be inspected routinely for evidence of humidity. Adequate humidification is also important to maintain the neutral thermal environment of the newborn, particularly the premature newborn. Breathing a cool, dry gas may stress the metabolic demands on the newborn, resulting in increased oxygen consumption.

Heated wire circuits offer some potential advantages over unheated circuits. With unheated wire circuits, the temperature of the gas cools as the gas is exposed to the environmental temperature of the circuit. As a result of this temperature change, a significant amount of condensation accumulates in the circuit. With heated wire circuits the temperature is maintained throughout the circuit, and there is less risk of pooling of condensation in the circuit and reduced risk of accidental aspiration of condensate.

One issue with the neonatal ventilator circuit involves the position of the temperature sensor.[13] Critically ill neonates usually are in an incubator or under a radiant heater. If the temperature sensor in the circuit is placed in the incubator or under the radiant heater, it may be affected by a temperature other than the temperature of the gas in the ventilator circuit. This could result in malfunction of the humidification system. For this reason, the temperature sensor is placed at a point in the circuit outside the incubator or radiant heater, or it is otherwise shielded from the effects of the ambient temperature in these devices.

Hazards and Complications

Complications from mechanical ventilation in the neonate can be significant. Ventilator-associated pneumonia can occur. Tracheal damage from endotracheal tubes can create long-term problems. A neuropathologic consequence of reduced cerebral blood flow known as periventricular leukomalacia (PVL) has been associated with ventilator-induced hypocarbia in preterm infants.

Some neonates who survive the newborn course are left with varying degrees of chronic lung disease, a condition called **bronchopulmonary dysplasia (BPD).** The contribution of mechanical ventilators and oxygen therapy to this condition is not entirely known, but indiscriminate use of high pressure and exposure to high oxygen concentrations over time are thought to be factors. Neonates with BPD have a chronic oxygen requirement, chronic carbon dioxide retention, and pulmonary hypertension. These neonates also have an increased susceptibility to pulmonary infections.

Weaning

Consideration for weaning from ventilatory support should begin as soon as the infant's condition has stabilized from the disorder that required support. The infant's hemodynamic, pulmonary, neurologic, and nutritional status must be assessed. Also, weaning must not be confused with readiness for extubation. Rather, weaning should be an ongoing process of support adjustment to a level that maintains adequate gas exchange without requiring significantly increased work of breathing. No single recipe for weaning can be applied to all infants. The goal is to provide appropriate support by continuous assessment of the infant's total needs and recognizing when weaning is indicated.

Weaning can be done in the SIMV or CMV modes. In the SIMV mode, the set respiratory rate is lowered to assess the infant's ability to breathe spontaneously. The presence of an endotracheal tube reduces the airway size and leaves the infant at risk for increased work of breathing. For this reason, infants generally are not expected to demonstrate the ability to breathe without any assistance before extubation. When weaning in the CMV mode, the tidal volume remains constant and the rate is set lower than the infant's rate to allow all breaths to be triggered by the infant. The pressure or volume limit is adjusted to keep the tidal volume in the range of 5 to 7 mL/kg. The PEEP level usually is maintained at a minimum of 4 to 5 cm H_2O to prevent loss of lung volume.

Work of breathing and the ventilatory pattern are continually assessed during weaning. Periods of apnea are common in premature infants. In infants whose condition otherwise is stable, respiratory stimulants such as caffeine and theophylline may be beneficial in the reduction of apnea during weaning. Pulse oximetry, apnea, respiratory rate, and minute volume monitoring can help alert the clinician to changes in the infant's respiratory status. Infants with persistent tachypnea, retractions, and an increased oxygen requirement during the weaning process use calories needed for normal growth and development. Adequate gas exchange may be achieved, but the expense to the patient can be far greater than the benefit. Continual assessment of the infant's tolerance to weaning from a multisystem perspective is essential throughout the weaning process.

Extubation is considered when no contraindications exist from the neurologic or other nonrespiratory system, when the infant shows the ability to maintain a stable respiratory and heart rate, and when oxygen saturation is acceptable, with an FIO_2 of 0.3 or lower. The ability to feed and the infant's growth pattern also play a role in the decision to extubate. Because of the effects of the endotracheal tube on lung volume and work of breathing, extubation often occurs with ventilator settings of 15 to 20 breaths/min, a PIP of 14 to 18 cm H_2O, and a PEEP of 3 to 5 cm H_2O.

High-Frequency Ventilation

High-frequency ventilation (HFV) is a widely accepted mode of mechanical ventilation in neonatal and pediatric critical care. Although it is categorized as nonconventional ventilation, many neonatal centers now consider it a conventional mode for the treatment of respiratory failure and pulmonary barotrauma. HFV is defined as positive pressure ventilation at a respiratory rate more than 150 breaths/min and tidal volumes approximating anatomic dead space. The advantage of this technique over conventional mechanical ventilation is its ability to deliver an adequate minute volume with a lower airway pressure, often when conventional mechanical ventilation has failed. Treatment with a high mean airway pressure often is better tolerated with HFV than with conventional mechanical ventilation. With conventional mechanical ventilation, the alveolar volume is the difference between tidal volume and the dead space volume. Tidal volumes near the dead space volume produce little alveolar ventilation. The fact that gas exchange occurs with HFV, at times more efficiently than with CMV, is intriguing. HFV is used daily throughout the country, but the exact mechanism by which it accomplishes adequate gas exchange is not completely understood.

Classification

The four general types of high-frequency ventilation are high-frequency positive pressure ventilation, high-frequency jet ventilation, high-frequency flow interrupter ventilation, and high-frequency oscillatory ventilation.

High-frequency positive pressure ventilation (HFPPV) is conventional positive pressure ventilation at a high respiratory rate (more than 150 breaths/min) and small tidal volumes.[14] The inspiratory time is short to facilitate the increased respiratory rate. Exhalation is passive. The use of airway graphics to closely monitor changes in mean airway pressure is essential with HFPPV. Auto-PEEP is much more prevalent in this mode because of the high respiratory rate. Although HFPPV laid the foundation for modern high-frequency ventilation, its use has declined with the availability of other, more effective high-frequency ventilators.

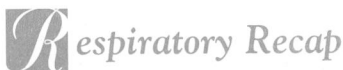 *espiratory Recap*

Categories of High-Frequency Ventilation
High-frequency positive pressure ventilation (HFPPV)
High-frequency jet ventilation (HFJV)
High-frequency flow interrupter ventilation (HFFIV)
High-frequency oscillatory ventilation (HFOV)

High-frequency jet ventilation (HFJV) delivers short pulses of gas directly into the trachea through a narrow-bore cannula or jet injector. Jet ventilators can maintain oxygenation and ventilation over a wide range of patient sizes. These systems have negligible compressible gas volume and operate effectively at rates of 150 to 600 breaths/min. Exhalation is passive. The tidal volume often is equal to or slightly less than the dead space volume. The high-flow jet pulse produces a *jet mixing effect* that creates an area of negative pressure and entrains additional gas into the airway. The high gas velocities and gas mixing effects make pressure monitoring difficult. Jet ventilators are used with a conventional ventilator that provides PEEP, entrained gas, and intermittent sighs.

High-frequency flow interrupter ventilation (HFFIV) delivers inspiratory flow to the patient in short bursts by means of a rotating ball valve or microprocessor-controlled solenoid valve. These ventilators produce breath rates of 2 to 22 Hz (1 Hertz equals 60 breaths/min). HFFIV is similar to high-frequency oscillatory ventilation in that inspiration and exhalation are both active. Active exhalation is defined as a drop in airway pressure during exhalation to accelerate exhaled gas flow.[15] Background mechanical breaths may or may not be used to maintain lung volume.

High-frequency oscillatory ventilation (HFOV) essentially uses airway vibrators, usually with piston pumps or vibrating diaphragms that operate at frequencies ranging from 400 to 2400 breaths/min.[16] During HFOV, inspiration and expiration are both active. Oscillators produce little if any bulk gas delivery. A continuous flow of fresh gas (*bias flow*) provides inspired gas and clears carbon dioxide from the system. Pressure oscillations in the airway produce tiny tidal volumes around a constant

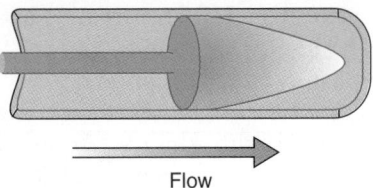

Figure 41-8 Spike formation in the airway during high-frequency ventilation.

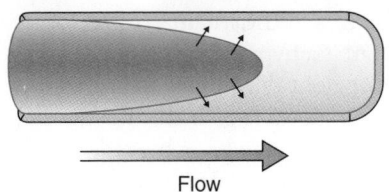

Figure 41-10 Taylor dispersion during high-frequency ventilation.

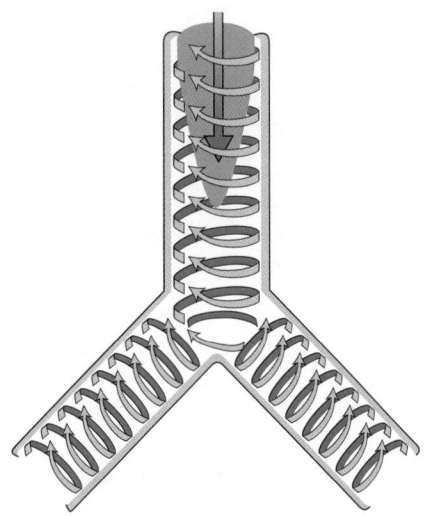

Figure 41-9 Helical diffusion during high-frequency ventilation. (Modified from Karp TB, et al. High frequency ventilation: a neonatal nursing perspective. Neonatal Network 1986; 4(5):43.)

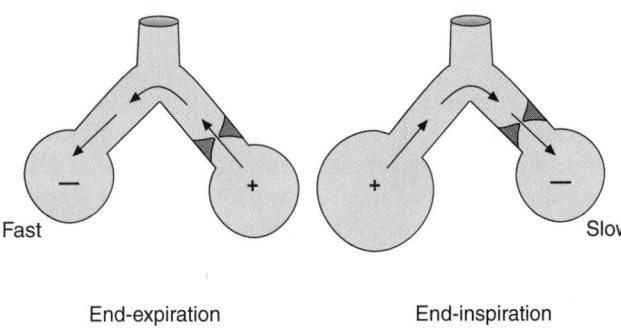

Figure 41-11 Pendelluft during high-frequency ventilation.

mean airway pressure. The tidal volume is determined by the amplitude of airway pressure oscillations, determined by the stroke of the device producing the oscillations.

Gas Transport Theories

Several theories have been proposed to explain gas transport at high respiratory frequencies. The mechanisms of gas exchange during HFV are not completely understood, and several effects interact during HFV.[17]

In **spike formation** (Figure 41-8), a high-energy wave impulse of gas penetrates the center of the airway, enhancing bulk flow of gas in the upper airway and providing a more expansive area of gas mixing in the more distal lung.[18] In the more compliant airway of the premature infant, spike formation is less effective. It is possible that turbulence increases with a more compliant airway, limiting spike effectiveness.

Helical diffusion (Figure 41-9), a variant of the spike theory, may also play a role in HFV. Fresh gas enters the lung through a spike generated in the center of the airway while gas exits the lung circumferentially along the periphery of the airway (*coaxial flow*).[19] This theory assumes that carbon dioxide removal occurs in a spiral fashion, producing a whirlpool effect, whereby fresh gas moves

through the center of the airway while gas simultaneously exits the lung.

Taylor dispersion (Figure 41-10) is the augmented diffusion of gas in situations of parabolic gas flow resulting in high energy spikes.[20] This augmented diffusion can occur wherever two gas streams meet, such as in coaxial flow in larger airways and convective streaming more distal in the lung. This diffusion process is facilitated by the increased surface area between two gas streams during HFV. These high-energy jet spikes probably result in the delivery of more total fresh gas to distal respiratory units before significant contamination of the inflow gas occurs. This preserves the diffusion gradient needed to remove carbon dioxide from the blood.

Pendelluft ventilation (Figure 41-11) is the result of gas mixing between lung regions that have different time constants; this is also called out-of-phase ventilation. When parallel lung units have different time constants, resistance tends to dominate the rate of filling and emptying at rapid respiratory rates.[17] At the end of a rapid inspiration, gas flows from the fast unit, which is beginning to empty, to the slow unit, which is still filling. This motion of gas between two neighboring units during phasic ventilation is called *pendelluft*.[17]

Molecular diffusion is a transport mechanism derived from random thermal oscillation of a molecule. So long as the molecules have a constant temperature, molecular diffusion always occurs. Molecular diffusion is responsible for gas exchange at the level of the alveolar-capillary membrane.[17] Molecular diffusion is altered during HFV. The rapid kinetic motion of oxygen and carbon dioxide molecules during HFV and the process of gas exchange at the alveolar level are speculative at this time.

Patient Selection

Specific strategies for the use of HFV depend on the institution. Therefore the question of when to use HFV in the neonate is not easily answered. Should HFV be implemented early in the treatment of respiratory failure, or should conventional ventilation be used first and HFV applied only if this approach fails? Some centers are very aggressive and institute HFV without trying conventional ventilation, seeking to protect the patient from pulmonary barotrauma at the onset of ventilation. Others try conventional ventilation before HFV. Use of HFV should be considered in the following situations:

- Preterm infants with severe hyaline membrane disease requiring a PIP more than 30 cm H$_2$O
- Infants with severe meconium aspiration syndrome and persistent pulmonary hypertension that does not respond to maximum ventilatory support with a PIP more than 35 cm H$_2$O
- Infants with air leak syndrome, including progressive pulmonary interstitial emphysema, recurring pneumothorax, and pneumopericardium
- Infants with congenital diaphragmatic hernia or pulmonary hypoplasia who have failed conventional ventilation
- Infants with severe parenchymal lung disease, such as group B streptococci pneumonia, who require high levels of ventilatory support
- Any of the above disease states that may preclude the use of conventional ventilation and that indicate the need to institute HFV as an initial point of care

High-Frequency Ventilators

The Infant Star 950 (Nellcor Puritan Bennett, Inc., Pleasanton, Calif.) is a time-cycled, pressure-limited, continuous flow ventilator (Figure 41-12). It is the only ventilator capable of delivering HFV by itself or as an adjunct to IMV. The use of HFV alone or in combination with IMV is determined by institutional preferences. The Infant Star 950 has a bank of 10 computer-controlled proportioning valves that precisely deliver flow from the ventilator. Individual 2-, 4-, 8, and 16-L/min valves provide the cumulative positive pressure pulse. The proportioning valves open and the exhalation valve closes for 18 ms to generate each positive pressure pulse, regardless of the HFV frequency. The

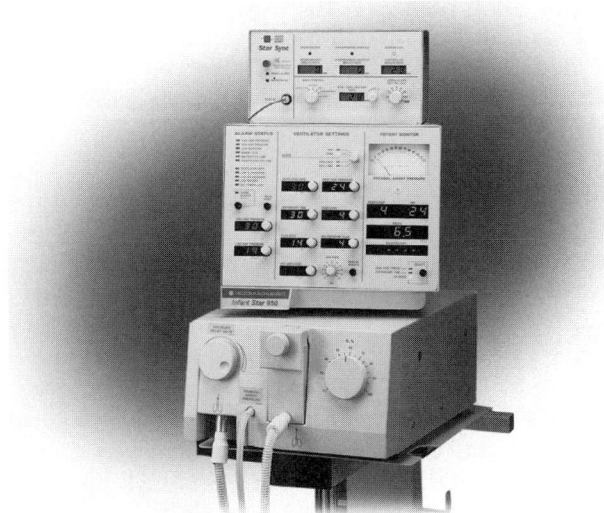

Figure 41-12 Infant Star 950. (Courtesy Nellcor Puritan Bennett, Inc., Pleasanton, Calif.)

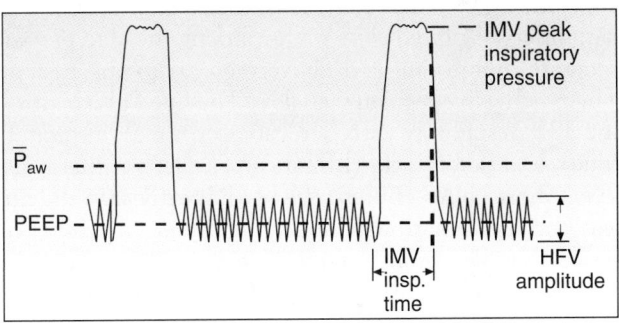

Figure 41-13 Airway pressure pulses with the Infant Star 950. $\bar{P}_{aw}$, Mean airway pressure; *PEEP*, positive end expiratory pressure; *IMV*, intermittent mandatory ventilation, *HFV*, high-frequency ventilation. (Modified from materials courtesy Mallinckrodt, Inc., St. Louis, Mo.)

pulse amplitude is a function of the amount of flow provided by the proportioning valves. The maximum flow is 120 L/min and the minimum flow is 12 L/min during HFV.

An active jet venturi is built into the exhalation valve which, in combination with valve recoil after each positive HFV pulse, produces active exhalation. A typical waveform of the proximal HFV pressure shows that the negative and positive pulse phases are equal above and below the PEEP/CPAP setting (Figure 41-13). The proximal pressure display is derived by sampling of the greatest positive and negative HFV pressures. Change in the amplitude display can occur for many reasons such as a change in water level in the humidifier, kinks or leaks in the patient circuit, changing compliance, mucus plugging, or a change in position of the endotracheal tube.

During an IMV breath, the HFV mode is momentarily shut off. High frequency flow interruption is similar to high frequency jet ventilation without the jet

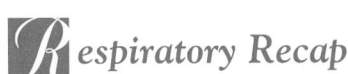
espiratory Recap

<hr>

High-Frequency Ventilators
Infant Star 950
Bunnell Life Pulse Jet Ventilator
SensorMedics 3100A

catheter. The similarities between this ventilator and high frequency oscillation have been argued. However, the negative pressure portion of the cycle is not controlled as in a true oscillator. The target patient size is the 600-2250 gram infant and it has problems ventilating larger infants.

The Bunnell Life Pulse Jet Ventilator (Figure 41-14) is a microprocessor-controlled system capable of delivering and monitoring 240 to 660 breaths/min. It is used in conjunction with a conventional ventilator that provides a source of continuous gas flow, PEEP, and low-rate IMV. The Life Pulse ventilator is approved for clinical use in neonates and infants. It appears to be most effective in disorders in which hypercarbia is the major problem. With HFJV, carbon dioxide removal is achieved at lower airway pressures than with other types of high-frequency ventilators. When managed properly, HFJV can acutely improve oxygenation and the oxygen index in infants with PPHN and other associated pulmonary conditions.

The patient box is an integral component of the Life Pulse ventilator. This box contains the pressure transducer and inhalation pinch valve necessary for operation. The patient box is placed close to the patient's head to provide accurate monitoring and delivery of gas to the patient. The pinch valve regulates gas flow. The Life Pulse controls the PIP, respiratory rate, jet valve on-time (inspiratory time), and on/off ratio (I:E ratio). The jet ventilator delivers short pulses of pressurized gas directly into the airway through a narrow-bore cannula or jet injector. The system has negligible compressible volume, and exhalation is always passive. The tidal volume is difficult to measure but is equal to or slightly greater than the dead space volume. Gas surrounding the injector is entrained into the airway with each jet pulse. Airway pressure must be measured far enough downstream from the jet injector to minimize errors caused by air entrainment effects.

A special triple lumen (Hi-Lo Jet) endotracheal tube has been designed specifically for use during HFJV. In addition to the standard endotracheal tube lumen, this tube has a pressure monitoring port at its distal tip and a jet injector port in the tube wall approximately 7 cm upstream from the pressure monitoring port. A triple lumen endotracheal tube adapter (Figure 41-15) has been designed to allow jet ventilation without the use of the High-Low tube, which eliminates the need to reintubate the infant solely for use of HFJV. This adapter houses the jet injector port and the pressure monitoring port and has been used extensively since 1995.

The Life Pulse ventilator delivers its jet pulse into the endotracheal tube through the injector port. It then servo controls the driving pressure to the jet to maintain a constant predetermined pressure at the endotracheal tube tip. A unique feature of the Life Pulse ventilator is its ability to monitor and display the jet servo pressure. This allows automatic detection of changes in the infant's lung compliance and airway resistance. Servo pressure is proportional to the lung volume being ventilated. For example, as lung compliance or airway resistance (or both) improves, servo pressure increases. This is typically used as an indicator to begin weaning the patient from high-frequency ventilation. Conversely, a decrease in servo pressure indicates that lung compliance or airway resistance has worsened; the endotracheal tube has become obstructed; a tension pneumothorax has devel-

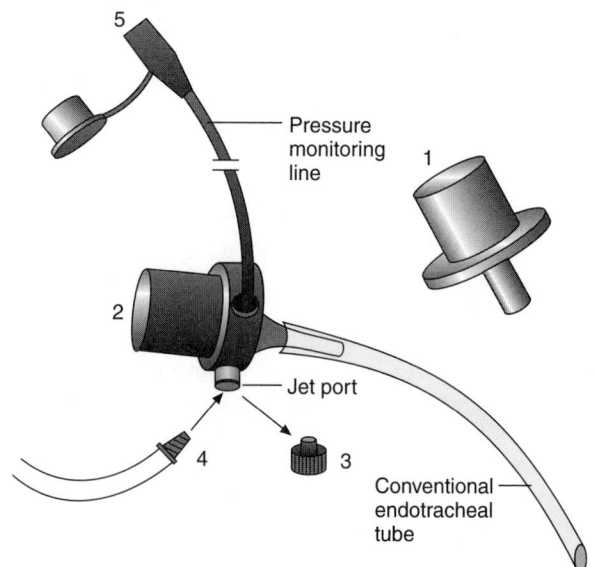

Figure 41-15 Triple lumen endotracheal tube adapter for use with the Bunnell Life Pulse Jet Ventilator. The 15-mm endotracheal tube adapter (1) is replaced with the Life Pulse adapter (2). The cap on the jet port (3) is removed, and the Luer fitting of the Life Pulse circuit (4) is attached to the jet port. The pressure monitoring connector from the jet patient box is attached to the pressure monitoring line (5). The conventional ventilator circuit is attached to the 15-mm port of the Life Pulse adapter. (Modified from Aloan CA, Hill TV. Respiratory care of the neonate and child. 2nd ed. Philadelphia: JB Lippincott; 1997.)

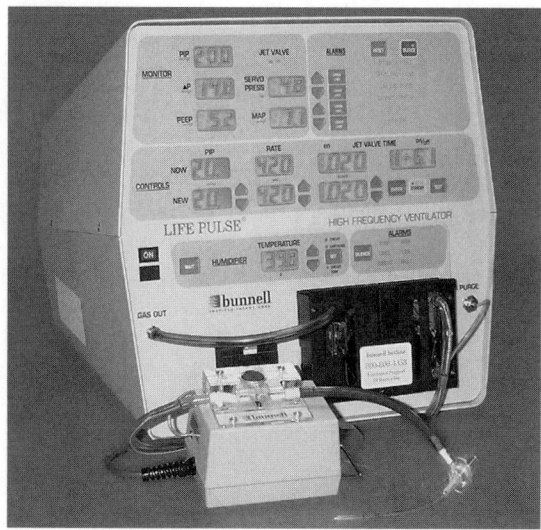

Figure 41-14 Bunnell Life Pulse Jet Ventilator. (Courtesy Bunnell, Inc., Salt Lake City, Utah.)

oped; or the patient requires suctioning. Respiratory therapists and other clinicians find servo pressure helpful for assessing the patient's pulmonary status.

The SensorMedics 3100A (SensorMedics, Inc., Yorba Linda, Calif.) is an electronically controlled oscillatory ventilator (Figure 41-16). Its 365-mL oscillatory driver is a diaphragmatically sealed piston with adjustable displacement, frequency, and I:E ratio. It produces 3- to 15-Hz pressure waves superimposed on an adjustable level of mean airway pressure. The SensorMedics 3100A is distinguished from other types of high-frequency ventilators by its active expiratory phase. It is used for ventilatory support and for treatment of respiratory failure and barotrauma in neonates. The primary therapeutic effects are obtained with just two controls: the oscillatory **pressure amplitude (ΔP)** and the mean airway pressure. In some cases, changing the frequency (Hertz) or the percent inspiratory time or both may provide additional benefits to those infants who do not respond to initial standard settings.

End-expiratory lung volume is determined by the mean airway pressure and remains relatively constant during the respiratory cycle. The SensorMedics 3100A does not require use of a special endotracheal tube. It has fewer control settings than other high-frequency ventilators and once the patient's condition has been stabilized, the ventilator settings are changed infrequently.

The mean airway pressure on the SensorMedics 3100A can be adjusted from 3 to 45 cm H_2O. The mean airway pressure limit can be operated in two modes. In the safety limit mode, the mean airway pressure limit is set to a level higher than the range of normal mean airway pressures to protect the patient from accidental overpressure. In the controlled mode, the mean airway pressure limit is set to a level below that which would otherwise exist through the adjustment of the mean pressure control. In this mode, the mean airway pressure remains constant regardless of changes in bias flow, the percent inspiratory time, or frequency settings. With HFOV the mean airway pressure is the most important determinant of oxygenation. It dictates whether the patient can be weaned from the potentially harmful effects of an elevated FIO_2. The mean airway pressure is maximized initially, with close attention paid to hyperinflation and monitoring of the chest radiograph to maintain lung volume at the level of ribs T8-T9.

Bias flow is necessary to maintain oxygenation, the mean airway pressure, and an oscillatory waveform. The system must be charged with flow to operate effectively. Standardized bias flow settings are 10 to 20 L/min. A common rule-of-thumb is that the smaller the infant, the lower the bias flow. Manipulations of the $PaCO_2$ level are made primarily with the amplitude or power control (ΔP). Increasing the amplitude increases displacement of the bellows, which increases tidal volume delivery. This is measured as an increased pressure amplitude at the airway opening and results in a lower $PaCO_2$. Frequent arterial blood gas measurements or monitoring of the transcutaneous PCO_2 is necessary to titrate the $PaCO_2$.

The respiratory rate on the SensorMedics 3100A is measured in **Hertz (Hz).** The concept of active inspiration and active expiration allows the delivery of very rapid respiratory rates without air trapping. The rate can be set from 3 to 15 Hz. The higher the respiratory rate, the smaller the tidal volume, partly because of the short cycle time at the higher rate. Conversely, the lower the rate, the larger the tidal volume because of the longer cycle time and the ability to move more volume through the circuit. The respiratory therapist must recognize that the delivered tidal volumes are very small and are equal to or less than the dead space volume. As a rule-of-thumb, larger babies (more than 2 kg) fall into the lower rate category (8 to 10 Hz), whereas smaller infants (less than 2 kg) fall into the smaller tidal volume requirement category and hence a higher rate is used (12 to 15 Hz).

The inspiratory time on the SensorMedics 3100A is nearly always set at 33%, which has been determined to be the standard inspiratory time setting for this ventilator. Only in extreme cases (for example, with a large patient with a severely elevated physiologic dead space) is the percent inspiratory time increased to improve carbon dioxide elimination. As with slowing of the respiratory rate, an increase in the percent inspiratory time allows a longer inspiratory phase, thus increasing the delivered tidal volume. The inspiratory time can be adjusted from 33% to 50% in 1% increments.

Management Strategies

Management strategies are divided into two categories, aggressive and nonaggressive. Most patients fall into the aggressive management category. This means that the ventilator parameters are maximized at the clinician's discretion. The only disease that would preclude this ap-

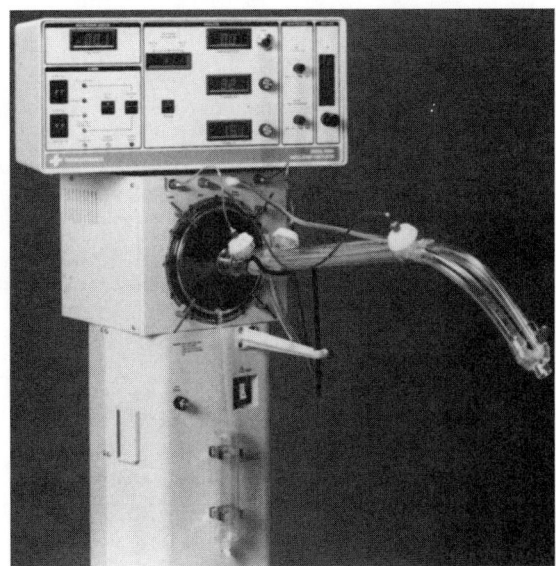

Figure 41-16 SensorMedics 3100A. (Courtesy SensorMedics, Yorba Linda, Calif.)

proach is air leak syndrome. Establishing lung volume and restoring it to an acceptable level is a critical component of HFV. Because the delivered tidal volumes are small, the mean lung volume does not change dramatically during inspiration. PEEP is the primary contributor to mean airway pressure and end-expiratory lung volume during HFV.

The Bunnell Life Pulse HFV (Bunnell, Inc., Salt Lake City, Utah) is used with a conventional ventilator. General management strategies for high-frequency jet ventilation are shown in Table 41-6. The conventional ventilator is responsible for controlling the PEEP level. Hence the mean airway pressure is controlled by the conventional ventilator, and the PIP, respiratory rate, inspiratory time, and I:E ratio are controlled by the HFJV. Once the infant's condition has stabilized, efforts are made to reduce the mean airway pressure. The PIP may be reduced gradually and the respiratory rate dropped to 250 to 300 breaths/min. The PEEP may also be decreased if the PaO_2 is acceptable and the patient tolerates the change.

Management of the infant on HFOV is more straightforward than with HFJV. General management strategies for HFOV are shown in Table 41-7. HFOV *decouples* (separates) ventilation and oxygenation. The mean airway pressure and FIO_2 control oxygenation, whereas amplitude, the percent inspiratory time, and respiratory rate determine ventilation. This simplistic approach to HFOV benefits both clinician and patient. Initially, the mean airway pressure and FIO_2 are maximized. Ventilation may be more difficult to control because the patient's size and disease determine what settings are chosen. The smaller the patient, the higher the rate setting; the percent inspiratory time is set at 33%. Amplitude (ΔP) is a more discretional setting, and the respiratory therapist must be judicious in determining it. Amplitude is what ventilates or moves the chest with HFOV. Although the setting of ΔP is arbitrary, what happens to the patient is not. The higher the amplitude setting, the more vigorously the chest wall moves or wiggles; this is called the *chest wiggle factor*. The clinician

TABLE 41-6

General Guidelines for Use of High-Frequency Jet Ventilation

Setting	Usual	Raise	Lower
HFJV PIP	20 cm H_2O	To lower PcO_2	To raise PcO_2 (raise PEEP simultaneously to keep $\bar{P}_{aw}$ and PO_2 constant)
HFJV respiratory rate	420 breaths/min (neonate)	To increase $\bar{P}_{aw}$ and PO_2 or reduce PcO_2 in *smaller* patients	To lengthen exhalation time and eliminate inadvertent PEEP in larger patients or when weaning, and to increase PcO_2
HFJV inspiratory time	0.02 seconds	To enable jet to reach PIP at low HFJV rates in larger patients	Keep at the minimum of 0.02 seconds in almost all cases.
CV respiratory rate	0 to 3 breaths/min	To reverse atelectasis	Whenever possible, especially when air leaks are a current or potential problem or when hemodynamics may be compromised
CV PIP	15 to 20 cm H_2O	To reverse atelectasis	Whenever air leaks are present or when not attempting to recruit collapsed alveoli
CV inspiratory time	0.4 seconds	To reverse atelectasis	Whenever air leaks are present or when not attempting to recruit collapsed alveoli
PEEP	Neonate: 7 to 8 cm H_2O Pediatric patient: 8 to 15 cm H_2O	To improve oxygenation, optimum PEEP must be determined: raise PEEP until the oxygen saturation (SpO_2) remains constant when the CV is switched from intermittent mandatory ventilation to continuous positive airway pressure ventilation.	Lower PEEP only when air leaks are present and oxygenation is adequate or when lowering PEEP does not reduce PO_2.
FIO_2	0.21 to 1	Raise as needed.	Lower FIO_2 in preference to $\bar{P}_{aw}$ until FIO_2 is below 0.5.

Modified from materials courtesy Bunnell, Inc., Salt Lake City, Utah.

1. *In high-frequency jet ventilation (HFJV), amplitude (ΔP), which is the peak inspiratory pressure minus the positive end-expiratory pressure, is the primary determinant of the partial pressure of carbon dioxide ($PacO_2$). The HFJV rate is secondary.*
2. *The resting lung volume (functional residual capacity [FRC]) and mean airway pressure ($\bar{P}_{aw}$) are crucial determinants of the partial pressure of oxygen (PaO_2).*
3. *Hyperventilation and hypoxemia can be avoided by using the optimum positive end-expiratory pressure (PEEP).*
4. *If increasing the conventional ventilator (CV) rate improves oxygenation, PEEP probably is too low.*
5. *Conventional ventilation should be minimized at all times, especially when air leaks are present.*
6. *The fractional inspired oxygen concentration (FIO_2) should be lowered before the mean airway pressure ($\bar{P}_{aw}$) until the FIO_2 is below 0.5.*

must determine when enough chest wiggle is acceptable for the patient. The patient's compliance determines how aggressive the clinician is with ΔP.

One of the differences between HFOV and HFJV is that higher rather than lower mean airway pressures are required to maintain oxygenation with HFOV. Higher mean airway pressure settings are used early in the ventilatory course and weaned as tolerated when the PaO_2 level is acceptable. In HFOV the mean airway pressure is increased in 1- to 2-cm H_2O increments, provided there is no air leak, until the SpO_2 rises above 95%, which indicates adequate lung recruitment. A chest radiograph must be obtained to ensure that inflation is adequate, to the level of the eighth to the ninth rib. Hyperinflation can adversely affect hemodynamics, and the mean airway pressure should be reduced if hyperinflation occurs. Hyperinflation also poses an increased risk of air leakage. As the patient on HFOV improves, the FiO_2 should be weaned to 0.6 before the mean airway pressure is reduced, unless hyperinflation is noted by chest x-ray. When the mean airway pressure has been reduced 10 to 12 cm H_2O, the clinician should consider transferring the patient back to CMV or continue weaning to extubation on HFOV.

Complications

Complications associated with HFV include tracheal injury, atelectasis, pulmonary overdistention, acute respiratory alkalosis, hypotension, decreased cardiac output, and a displaced or disconnected endotracheal tube.[21] In early uses of HFV tracheal injury was reported in some cases, but improved humidification has eliminated this complication. Atelectasis may occur as a result of mucus plugging or low airway pressures leading to alveolar collapse, which can be prevented through maintenance of an adequate mean airway pressure. The use of in-line suction catheters has made management of the patient on HFV less traumatic.[15] Ventilator disconnects for purposes of pulmonary toilet are now minimized, and loss of lung volume is a less frequent occurrence with these catheters. Pulmonary overdistention and

TABLE 41-7

General Guidelines for Use of High-Frequency Oscillatory Ventilation

Clinical Indicators	Therapeutic Intervention	Treatment Rationale
FiO_2 below 0.70		
High $PaCO_2$ with:		
PaO_2 satisfactory	Increase ΔP.	Increase ΔP to achieve optimum $PaCO_2$.
PaO_2 low	Increase $\bar{P}_{aw}$, ΔP, FiO_2.	Adjust $\bar{P}_{aw}$ and FiO_2 to improve O_2 delivery.
PaO_2 high	Increase ΔP; decrease FiO_2.	Decrease FiO_2 to minimize O_2 exposure.
FiO_2 below 0.70		
Normal $PaCO_2$ with:		
PaO_2 satisfactory	Take no action.	Take no action.
PaO_2 low	Increase $\bar{P}_{aw}$, FiO_2.	Adjust $\bar{P}_{aw}$ and FiO_2 to improve O_2 delivery.
PaO_2 high	Decrease FiO_2.	Decrease FiO_2 to minimize O_2 exposure.
FiO_2 below 0.70		
Low $PaCO_2$ with:		
PaO_2 satisfactory	Decrease ΔP.	Decrease ΔP to achieve optimum $PaCO_2$.
PaO_2 low	Increase $\bar{P}_{aw}$, FiO_2; decrease ΔP.	Adjust $\bar{P}_{aw}$ and FiO_2 to improve O_2 delivery.
PaO_2 high	Decrease FiO_2, ΔP.	Decrease FiO_2 to minimize O_2 exposure.
FiO_2 above 0.70		
High $PaCO_2$ with:		
PaO_2 satisfactory	Increase ΔP.	Increase ΔP to achieve optimum $PaCO_2$.
PaO_2 low	Increase FiO_2, ΔP.	Increase FiO_2 to improve PaO_2.
PaO_2 high	Increase ΔP; decrease $\bar{P}_{aw}$.	Decrease $\bar{P}_{aw}$ to reduce PaO_2.
FiO_2 above 0.70		
Normal $PaCO_2$ with:		
PaO_2 satisfactory	Take no action.	Take no action.
PaO_2 low	Increase FiO_2.	Increase FiO_2 to improve PaO_2.
PaO_2 high	Decrease $\bar{P}_{aw}$, FiO_2.	Decrease $\bar{P}_{aw}$ and FiO_2 to reduce PaO_2.
FiO_2 above 0.70		
Low $PaCO_2$ with:		
PaO_2 satisfactory	Decrease ΔP.	Decrease ΔP to achieve optimum $PaCO_2$.
PaO_2 low	Increase FiO_2; decrease ΔP.	Increase FiO_2 to improve PaO_2.
PaO_2 high	Decrease $\bar{P}_{aw}$, ΔP.	Decrease $\bar{P}_{aw}$, FiO_2 to minimize O_2 exposure.

Courtesy SensorMedics, Yorba Linda, Calif.
FiO_2, Fractional inspired oxygen concentration; $PaCO_2$, partial pressure of arterial carbon dioxide; PaO_2, partial pressure of arterial oxygen; ΔP, pressure amplitude; $\bar{P}_{aw}$, mean airway pressure.

cardiac compromise can result from failure to wean excessive mean airway pressures. Overdistention can cause acute lung injury, pneumothorax, and increased physiologic shunt. Patients must be monitored closely for signs of decreased systemic perfusion when HFV is initiated. A high mean airway pressure may not be tolerated. If myocardial dysfunction occurs, inotropic therapy may be indicated. Minimizing the adverse effects of an increased intrathoracic environment is an essential component of the care of the infant on HFV. An issue related to HFV is the noise caused by the ventilator, which contributes to the noise level in the neonatal intensive care unit.[22,23]

High-Frequency Ventilation in Perspective

HFV is no longer in a stage of infancy. Its use to treat the problem of infant ventilatory insufficiency is well accepted. It produces adequate gas exchange at a higher mean airway pressure than conventional mechanical ventilation. In a very sick infant, it is useful for the safe treatment of severe hypoxemia with an increased mean airway pressure. Still, many questions remain. Should HFV be instituted early in the disease course of the infant? Should the infant be allowed to fail continuous mechanical ventilation before HFV is instituted? What are the recognizable signs and indications for HFV? Should it be used as a lung protection strategy before continuous mechanical ventilation is even tried?

HFV has both positive and negative features. HFJV requires constant monitoring and adjustment of two ventilators. On the other hand, the principles governing the use of the HFOV are straightforward and easy to understand. Does this make one ventilator superior to another? Probably not. Any ventilator is only as good as the respiratory therapist managing its function in relation to the patient. Only with continued use of such technology can clinicians and respiratory therapists develop a better understanding and approach to the specific demands that each disease represents.

Airway Care

Suctioning of an intubated neonate should be performed secondary to clinical assessment and not as a routine procedure. Suctioning can cause hypoxia, atelectasis, infection, tissue damage, and changes in the heart rate, blood pressure, and intracranial pressure. Suctioning needs generally are related to the underlying pathologic condition. Infants intubated because of respiratory distress syndrome, persistent pulmonary hypertension, or apnea require less suctioning than infants with meconium aspiration, sepsis, or pulmonary hemorrhage. Indications for suctioning include evidence of secretions in the endotracheal tube, diminished breath sounds, decreased tidal volume (during pressure ventilation), or increased peak inspiratory pressure (during volume ventilation). An ob-

structed airway or endotracheal tube should always be considered when acute desaturation occurs, particularly in infants with meconium aspiration, pulmonary hemorrhage, or pneumonia. Providing adequate humidity can reduce the risk of tube obstruction, but plugging of artificial airways in infants with thick or abundant secretions is always a concern with the small internal diameter of the tube.

An in-line suction catheter (Figure 41-17) offers several advantages over single-use catheters, and their use has become a routine practice in many neonatal intensive care units. With the in-line catheter, the infant can be suctioned without ventilator disconnection. Maintaining a closed system can reduce the risk of lung volume loss during suctioning. An in-line catheter that connects directly to the endotracheal tube with minimum dead space is ideal.

Selection of the suction catheter size is based on the size of the endotracheal tube. A common rule-of-thumb is to select a catheter with a French size two times the size of the inner diameter (in millimeters) of the endotracheal tube. The distance the catheter is inserted should be determined before the procedure to avoid airway trauma.[24,25] With the endotracheal tube in proper position, the distance is measured from the lips or nares (depending on whether an oral or a nasal tube is present) to the tip of the in-line catheter fully withdrawn. The catheter is then inserted 0.5 cm further than this distance. The recommended suction level is 70 to 100 mm Hg and is applied intermittently during withdrawal of the catheter. In general, an increase in FIO_2 of 0.1 to 0.2 is needed to maintain arterial oxygen saturation. The infant must be assessed throughout the procedure. Decreases in the heart rate or significant arterial oxygen desaturation during suctioning are indications to remove the catheter and support the infant as needed. If further suctioning is indicated, additional oxygen may be required before the procedure continues. After the procedure is completed, reassessment of the heart rate, oxygen

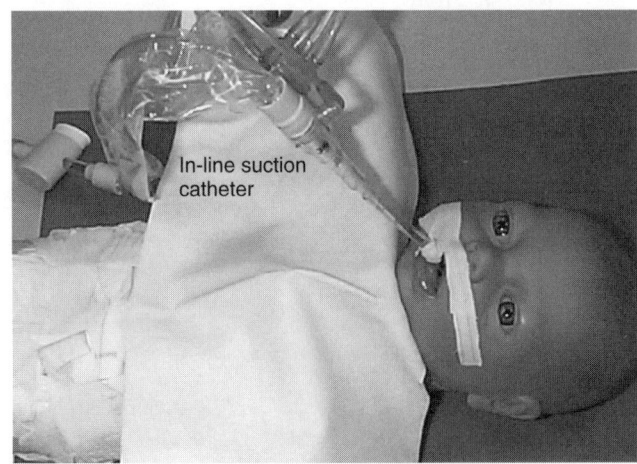

In-line suction catheter

Figure 41-17   Neonatal in-line suction catheter.

saturation, color, chest expansion, and breath sounds are indicated. Ventilator adjustments and changes in the oxygen concentration may be needed to keep the oxygen saturation within the desired range.

Adjuncts to Neonatal Mechanical Ventilation

Surfactant Administration

Preterm infants (those less than 34 weeks of gestational age) have varying degrees of lung maturity, and the respiratory needs of these infants may be significantly different than those of a full-term infant with mature lungs. Infants born at less than 35 weeks' gestation often have a surfactant deficiency. Surfactant production begins about week 23 of gestation, and the fetal lungs reach maturity at week 35. Between weeks 23 and 35, lung maturity may be enhanced in utero by administration of corticosteroids. Corticosteroids often are given to mothers at risk for premature delivery. Infants who receive corticosteroids in utero are likely to have more lung maturity than infants of similar gestational age who were not treated with steroids in utero. However, many infants are born prematurely with either partial treatment or no treatment with steroids and have a surfactant deficiency.

Surfactant is a combination of lipoproteins found in mature alveoli that reduces surface tension at the alveolar air/fluid interface.[26] Alveoli with low surface tension require less pressure to stabilize lung volume and avoid alveolar collapse. Infants with a surfactant deficiency often show signs of respiratory distress syndrome (RDS). The clinical findings associated with RDS are tachypnea, intercostal and sternal retractions, nasal flaring, expiratory grunting, decreased compliance, and an oxygen requirement. The typical chest radiograph of an infant with RDS has a "ground glass" appearance and low lung volumes. Administration of exogenous surfactant has been shown to prevent and treat RDS (Table 41-8).

Surfactant is given endotracheally (Box 41-1). In infants at risk and those with clinical signs of RDS, intubation and early administration of surfactant are recommended. Before the surfactant is administered, the infant's compliance is reduced significantly. It may be necessary to use high pressures to ventilate a surfactant-deficient infant. Reassessment of the infant's ventilatory needs after administration of surfactant is vital. Adjustments to the ventilator are indicated as compliance increases and oxygenation improves. Maintenance of a delivered tidal volume of 5 to 7 mL/kg is achieved by a reduction in the PIP or volume setting. The FIO_2 must be adjusted to keep the arterial oxygen saturation in the desired range. Attention to these details is essential to reduce the risk of ventilator-induced complications.

Inhaled Nitric Oxide

Administration of inhaled nitric oxide (iNO) has been shown to improve oxygenation in neonates with hypoxemia and pulmonary hypertension.[27-29] The primary mechanism is thought to be lowering of pulmonary vascular resistance by vasodilation of the pulmonary vasculature, resulting in decreased right-to-left shunting of blood. Inhaled NO is selective to the pulmonary vasculature and has not been associated with a lowering of systemic blood pressure. Inhaled NO can be administered with either a conventional or high-frequency ventilator. Although the optimum dose of iNO is not entirely clear, 20 ppm or less usually is sufficient. Because administration of iNO can cause methemoglobinemia, this value should be monitored during therapy. NO and oxygen can combine to produce nitrogen dioxide (NO_2). The NO and NO_2 levels should be monitored during therapy, but a high NO_2 level usually can be prevented with proper delivery equipment. The NO concentration is reduced once oxygenation is stable. Continuous monitoring with pulse oximetry as the NO concentration is reduced is essential. Before NO is discontinued, the FIO_2 is increased by 10% to 20% to prevent a rebound effect. To minimize

*T*ABLE 41-8

Commercial Surfactant Preparations

Surfactant	Description	Route of Administration	Dose
Survanta	Bovine lung extract	Endotracheal	4 mL/kg
Curosurf	Isolated from minced pig lungs	Endotracheal	2.5 mL/kg
Exosurf	Synthetic surfactant	Endotracheal	5 mL/kg
Infrasurf	Calf lung surfactant	Endotracheal	3 mL/kg

*B*OX 41-1

Administration of Surfactant

1. Determine the surfactant preparation to be used and the dose.
2. Allow the drug to reach room temperature.
3. Confirm the position of the endotracheal tube.
4. Instill the drug directly into the endotracheal tube.
5. Continuously monitor the heart rate and oxygen saturation as measured by pulse oximetry (SpO_2) during administration; also monitor for endotracheal tube obstruction.
6. Monitor tidal volume and SpO_2 immediately after dose is given.
7. Adjust ventilator support as compliance changes.

the rebound effect, the F_{IO_2} can be increased by 10% to 20% before the iNO is withdrawn. During the administration of NO, the manual resuscitation bag at the bedside should be adapted to provide NO in the event manual ventilation is required to avoid abrupt withdrawal of NO and rebound. NO should not flow into the reservoir of the resuscitation bag until needed to avoid production of NO_2.

Extracorporeal Life Support

Extracorporeal life support (ECLS) helps improve oxygenation and reduce ventilating pressures in some full-term neonates (Table 41-9).[30-32] Approximately 86% of the more than 15,500 neonates treated with ECLS for respiratory failure have survived. ECLS requires cannulation of the right heart. Blood is drained from this cannula into a circuit containing a membrane oxygenator and a pump (Figure 41-18). Oxygen circulates through one side of the membrane, and blood is pumped through the other side. The difference in partial pressures causes oxygen diffusion into the blood and elimination of carbon dioxide from the blood. The oxygenated blood is warmed and returned to the infant. The blood can be reinfused through a separate lumen of the drainage cannula (veno-venous support) or through an additional cannula placed in the carotid artery (veno-arterial support). Both methods of ECLS improve delivery of oxygen to the tissues.

Although ECLS does not specifically treat the underlying condition, it allows time for conditions to improve by reducing the risk of further lung damage from high airway pressures and high oxygen concentrations. While the patient is receiving ECLS, ventilator support generally is minimized with lung rest strategies. PEEP is applied to maintain the functional residual capacity (FRC) with an occasional positive pressure breath (usually 6 to 10 breaths/min), but ventilation and oxygenation are primarily achieved from the extracorporeal support. Additional treatments aimed at the underlying cause of respiratory failure are continued. For example, pulmonary hygiene for an infant with meconium aspiration and antibiotics for a septic infant help improve native gas exchange, and ECLS generally is discontinued after 5 to 7

TABLE 41-9

Extracorporeal Life Support Registry Report

Diagnosis	Number of Patients Who Received ECLS	Percentage of Patients Who Survived
CDH	3422	54
MAS	5509	94
PPHN	2227	79
RDS	1301	84
Sepsis	2107	76
Pneumonia	187	55
Air leak syndrome	78	71
Other	868	67
TOTAL	15,525	86

From Extracorporeal Life Support Organization. International summary. Neonatal respiratory failure. Ann Arbor, Mich: The Organization; 2000. ECLS, Extracorporeal life support; CDH, congenital diaphragmatic hernia; MAS, meconium aspiration syndrome; PPHN, persistent pulmonary hypertension of the newborn; RDS, respiratory distress syndrome.

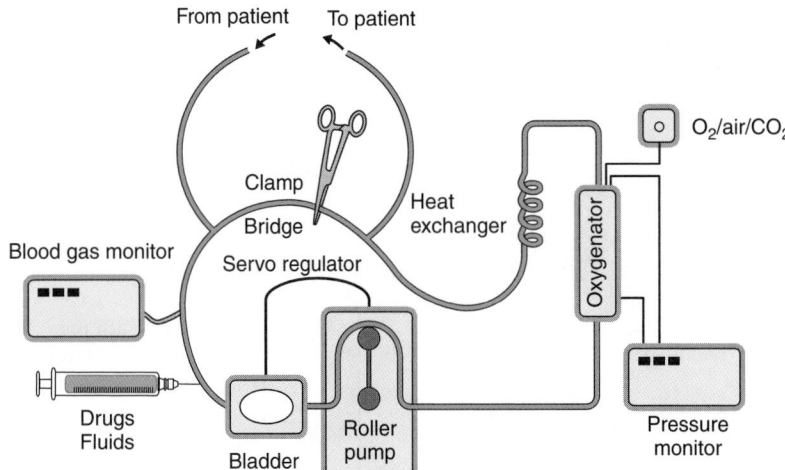

Figure 41-18 Schematic drawing of an extracorporeal membrane oxygenation (ECMO) system. (Modified from English PA, Hess DR. Extracorporeal life support. In: Branson RD, Hess DR, Chatburn RL, editors. Respiratory care equipment. 2nd ed. Philadelphia: JB Lippincott; 1999.)

days. A disadvantage of ECLS is that systemic anticoagulation is required to reduce the risk of clot formation as the blood is circulated through various circuit components. Intracranial, pulmonary, and surgical site bleeding, as well as air embolization and circuit complications, has been associated with ECLS. Because of the need for anticoagulation with the increased risk of intracranial hemorrhage, premature infants generally are not considered candidates for ECLS.

ℋEY 𝒫OINTS

- Positive pressure ventilation usually begins with bag-mask ventilation.
- Nasal CPAP is used to aid lung recruitment and to minimize airway collapse in patients with tracheomalacia.
- Uncuffed oral endotracheal tubes are most commonly used in neonates.
- Infant ventilators are either conventional or high-frequency ventilators.
- Conventional neonatal ventilators are continuous flow, time cycled, and pressure limited.
- Newer generation neonatal ventilators allow patient triggering and modes such as pressure support.
- High-frequency ventilators are classified as high-frequency positive pressure ventilation, high-frequency jet ventilation, high-frequency flow interrupter ventilation, and high-frequency oscillatory ventilation.
- Gas transport during high-frequency ventilation is poorly understood.
- Aggressive and nonaggressive management styles are used for high-frequency ventilation.
- In-line suction catheters allow suctioning of the neonate without disconnection of the ventilator.
- Adjuncts to neonatal mechanical ventilation include surfactant administration, inhaled nitric oxide, and extracorporeal life support.

References

1. Mondolfi AA, Grenier BM, Thompson JE, et al. Comparison of self-inflating bags with anesthesia bags for bag-mask ventilation in the pediatric emergency department. Pediatr Emerg Care 1997;13:312-316.
2. Davis S, Jones M, Kisling J, et al. Effect of continuous positive airway pressure on forced expiratory flows in infants with tracheomalacia. Am J Respir Crit Care Med 1998;158:148-152.
3. Panitch HB, Allen JL, Alpert BE, et al. Effects of CPAP on lung mechanics in infants with acquired tracheobronchomalacia. Am J Respir Crit Care Med 1994;150:1341-1346.
4. MacDonald KD, Johnson SR. Volume and pressure modes of mechanical ventilation in pediatric patients. Respir Care Clin North Am 1996;2:607-618.
5. Hammer GB, Frankel LR. Mechanical ventilation for pediatric patients. Int Anesthesiol Clin 1997;35:139-167.
6. Goldsmith JP, Karotkin EH. Assisted ventilation of the neonate. 3rd ed. Philadelphia: WB Saunders; 1996.
7. Mrozek JD, Bendel-Stenzel EM, Myers PA, et al. Randomized controlled trial of volume-targeted synchronized ventilation and conventional intermittent mandatory ventilation following initial exogenous surfactant therapy. Pediatric Pulmonol 2000;29:11-18.
8. Gullberg N, Winberg P, Sellden H. Pressure support ventilation increases cardiac output in neonates and infants. Paediatr Anaesth 1996;6:311-315.
9. El-Khatib MF, Chatburn RL, Potts DL, et al. Mechanical ventilators optimized for pediatric use decrease work of breathing and oxygen consumption during pressure support ventilation. Crit Care Med 1994;22:1942-1948.
10. Jarreau PH, Moriette G, Mussat P, et al. Patient-triggered ventilation decreases the work of breathing in neonates. Am J Respir Crit Care Med 1996;153:1176-1181.
11. Nishimura M, Hess D, Kacmarek RM. The response of flow-triggered infant ventilators. Am J Respir Crit Care Med 1995;152:1901-1909.
12. John J, Bjorklund LJ, Svenningsen NW, et al. Airway and body surface sensors for triggering in neonatal ventilation. Acta Paediatr 1994;83:903-909.
13. Chatburn RL. Physiologic and methodologic issues regarding humidity therapy. J Pediatr 1989;114:416-420.
14. Sjostrand UH. Review of the physiological rationale for and development of high-frequency positive pressure ventilation. Acta Anaesthesiol Scand 1977;64:7-27.
15. Aloan CA, Hill TV. Respiratory care of the neonate and child. 2nd ed. Philadelphia: JB Lippincott; 1997.
16. Smith R. Ventilation at high respiratory frequencies. Anaesthesia 1982;37:1011.
17. Chunk HK. Mechanisms of gas transport during ventilation by high-frequency oscillation. J Appl Physiol 1984;56:553.
18. Henderson Y, Chillingworth FD, Whitney JL. The respiratory dead space. Am J Physiol 1915;38:1.
19. Fredberg JJ, Glass GM, Boynton BR, et al. Features influencing mechanical performance of neonatal high-frequency ventilators. J Appl Physiol 1987;62:2485-2490.
20. Taylor GI. Dispersion of matter in turbulent flow through a pipe. Proc R Soc Lond B Biol Sci 1954;223:446-448.
21. Boros SJ, Mammel MC, Lewullen PK, et al. Necrotizing tracheobronchitis: a complication of high-frequency ventilation. J Pediatr 1986;109:95.
22. Hoehn T, Busch A, Krause MF. Comparison of noise levels caused by four different high-frequency ventilators. Intensive Care Med 2000;26:84-87.
23. Berens RJ, Weigle CG. Noise measurements during high-frequency oscillatory and conventional mechanical ventilation. Chest 1995;108:1026-1029.
24. Bailey C, Kattwinkel J, Teja K, et al. Shallow versus deep endotracheal suctioning in young rabbits: pathologic effects on the tracheobronchial wall. Pediatrics 1988;82:746-751.
25. Hess DR. Managing the artificial airway. Respir Care 1999;44:759-772.
26. Jobe AH. Which surfactant for treatment of respiratory distress syndrome? Lancet 2000;355:1380-1381.
27. Inhaled nitric oxide in full-term or nearly full-term infants with hypoxic respiratory failure. N Engl J Med 1997;336:597-604.
28. Roberts JD Jr, Fineman JR, Morin FC III, et al. Inhaled nitric oxide and persistent pulmonary hypertension of the newborn:

the Inhaled Nitric Oxide Study Group. N Engl J Med 1997;336:605-610.

29. Clark RH, Kueser TJ, Walker MW, et al. Low-dose nitric oxide therapy for persistent pulmonary hypertension of the newborn: clinical inhaled nitric oxide. N Engl J Med 2000;342:469-474.

30. English PA, Hess DR. Extracorporeal life support. In: Branson RD, Hess DR, Chatburn RL, editors. Respiratory care equipment. 2nd ed. Philadelphia: JB Lippincott; 1999.

31. Bartlett RH, Roloff DW, Custer JR, et al. Extracorporeal life support: the University of Michigan experience. JAMA 2000;283:904-908.

32. Beardsmore C, Dundas I, Poole K, et al. Respiratory function in survivors of the United Kingdom extracorporeal membrane oxygenation trial. Am J Respir Crit Care Med 2000;161:1129-1135.

CHAPTER 42

Mechanical Ventilation in Alternate Care Sites

Peggi Robart

OBJECTIVES

1. List the care settings available for alternate site mechanical ventilation.
2. Describe the demographics of ventilator-assisted individuals.
3. Discuss the general causes of respiratory failure of ventilator-assisted individuals.
4. Discuss the important patient care issues related to triage to the best care site.
5. Compare the ventilator categories used in alternate site mechanical ventilation.
6. Describe the monitoring commonly performed in alternate site mechanical ventilation.
7. Describe elements that can assist in transfers throughout the health care continuum.
8. Discuss the resources necessary for success in alternate site mechanical ventilation.

KEY TERMS

Alternate Site Mechanical Ventilation (ASMV)	Portable Pressure Ventilator	Skilled Nursing Facilities (SNFs)
	Portable Volume Ventilator	Ventilator-Assisted Individuals

Alternate site mechanical ventilation (ASMV) evolved primarily at the end of the twentieth century. Until the early 1980s most chronically ventilated patients were confined to the intensive care unit (ICU). As the number of patients receiving long-term mechanical ventilation grew, long-term ventilator units were developed, most often in the acute care center.[1-3] Protocols and procedures were developed for patients who could be discharged to the home care setting.[4,5] As technology improved, a new emphasis was placed on reduction in the ICU of the number of patients undergoing long-term ventilation, and patients were moved to alternate sites.[6,7] These changes were part of an effort to reduce costs and to improve the quality of life for **ventilator-assisted individuals.** By the end of the twentieth century, many more step-down units and long-term care facilities accepted ventilator-assisted individuals.

The definition of alternate sites has evolved over the years. The two primary alternate site options have been the home and long-term care facilities. With both, the problems originally were similar and daunting. Staffing, reimbursement, appropriate technology, and the necessary expertise to provide the required care all were lacking. However, as technologic advances have been made and the need for alternate site placement has grown, more sites

Sites Available for Alternate Site Mechanical Ventilation Patients

Acute Care
Critical care units
Specialized respiratory care units
Long-term ventilator (weaning) units
Transitional care units
General medical and surgical units

Intermediate Care
Rehabilitation hospitals
Skilled nursing facilities
Transitional care units

Long-Term Care
Home
Assisted-living facility
Congregate-living facility
Foster home care
Skilled nursing facility

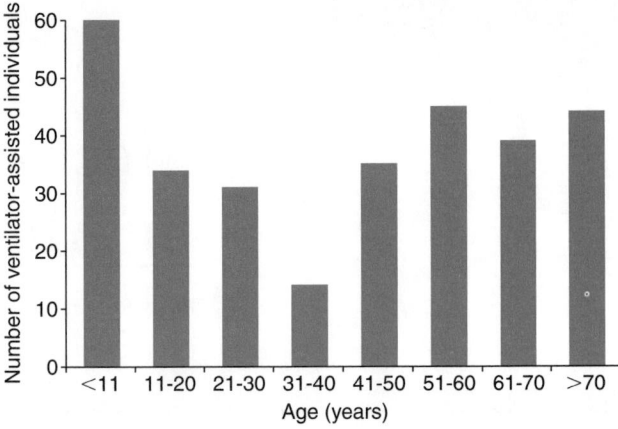

Figure 42-1 Age distribution of ventilator-assisted individuals in Minnesota in 1997. (Modified from Adams AB, Shapiro RS, Marini JJ. Respir Care 1998;43:643-649.)

have become available for ASMV (Box 42-1).[8] This chapter discusses the care settings for ASMV that have developed over the past two decades. The changing technology, personal options, and personnel available for ASMV have dramatically influenced placement of ventilator-assisted individuals,[9] and these changes will continue to affect the options of health care practitioners and patients.

Demographics

Patients with polio have been receiving various forms of ventilatory support since the 1950s; therefore respiratory experts have had decades of experience with individuals receiving positive pressure long-term mechanical ventilation. The number of ventilator-assisted individuals has increased significantly over this period, with a growing proportion receiving noninvasive ventilation.[9-11]

The demographics of ventilator-assisted individuals are different from those of the difficult to wean, chronic obstructive pulmonary disease (COPD) patients often seen

in the ICU. For example, with ventilator-assisted individuals, the age distribution is relatively uniform (Figure 42-1). These patients are young people with congenital abnormalities, middle-aged men with muscular dystrophy and cervical trauma, and elderly individuals with amyotrophic lateral sclerosis (ALS), multiple sclerosis (MS), and COPD.[11]

There are five primary causes of respiratory failure in ventilator-assisted individuals: ventilatory muscle dysfunction, central hypoventilation, obstructive disease, restrictive disease, and miscellaneous causes. The leading diagnoses requiring ventilatory support are polio, COPD, MD, cervical trauma, and ALS.[11] There is a bimodal distribution of patients categorized by their time on mechanical ventilation (Figure 42-2). Patients with parenchymal lung disease are ventilated for a shorter time (1 to 3 years) than patients without lung disease, such as those with cervical trauma, ALS, MD, or polio, who may require mechanical ventilation for many years if not decades.[11,12] Although regional differences can be seen in the placement of ventilator-assisted individuals, nearly two thirds are cared for at home, and the remaining one third receive care in facilities such as those listed in Box 42-1.

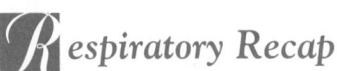*espiratory Recap*

Ventilator-Assisted Individuals

Patients range from children to the elderly.
Two thirds are placed in the home setting.
Leading diagnoses of ventilator-assisted individuals are aftermath of polio, chronic obstructive pulmonary disease (COPD), cervical trauma, multiple sclerosis (MS), amyotrophic lateral sclerosis (ALS), and muscular dystrophy (MD).

espiratory Recap

Categories of Ventilator-Assisted Individuals

Patients with lung diseases who require alternate site mechanical ventilation (ASMV) for 1 to 3 years
Patients with neuromuscular disease or cervical trauma who require ASMV for many years

Patients usually are placed on mechanical ventilation during an acute illness with the expectation that weaning will be possible as the illness resolves. If a need for or dependence on mechanical ventilation persists, economic

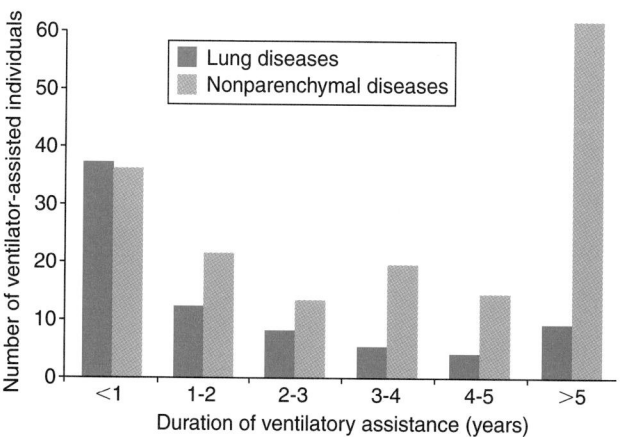

Figure 42-2 Number of ventilator-assisted individuals and the duration of their assistance in Minnesota in 1997. (Modified from Adams AB, Shapiro RS, Marini JJ. Respir Care 1998;43:643-649.)

pressures in the acute care setting work toward a quick transfer out of the ICU.[13,14] Specialized units have developed specifically to continue the weaning process.[15] Of the patients discharged from the ICU, approximately 33% to 55%[15,16] eventually are weaned, about 33% die, and 12% to 33% require continuing ventilatory assistance. Occasionally, for patients with a slowly progressing disease, ASMV can be arranged from an outpatient setting[17] but more often a stay in an acute care hospital precedes ASMV.

Care Issues

The first patients sent home on positive pressure mechanical ventilation in the 1970s were ventilated with acute care ventilators, which required changing of the home care setting into a mini-ICU. The family simply took home a critical care ventilator, with reams of instructions, after gaining experience in caring for the patient in the hospital during months of training. High-pressure (50 psi) oxygen and air systems (with loud, cumbersome air compressors) were set up in the home, and every effort was made to mimic the procedures and care given in the acute care setting. Families often provided all the care until they required respite. On the other end of the spectrum, some agencies provided nurses 24 hours a day, 7 days a week, and the families were called on to practice infrequently used skills on an emergency basis. Coverage for nursing in the home often either would be set for 24 hours a day, 7 days a week, or for very little coverage at all. Either way the family would be taxed to perform care—on the one hand overburdened with care or on the other, not having to provide care at all until the insurance benefit ran out.

It is now well accepted that home care environments do not require practices such as sterile technique for suctioning or frequent ventilator checks. Home care ventilators have many of the options that until recently were available only on critical care ventilators that required

pressurized gases. The resources and systems needed for reliable mechanical ventilation outside the acute care setting are available in a variety of settings. In the past, few long-term care facilities accepted ventilator-assisted individuals. However, during the late 1990s many **skilled nursing facilities (SNFs)** altered their policies to allow admission of mechanically ventilated patients as part of a comprehensive rehabilitation program. Respiratory therapists were added to the staff to monitor and manage these patients. However, when reimbursement for respiratory therapists in SNFs is reduced or eliminated, much of the care of these patients is delegated to nurses or possibly to other nonprofessional staff members.

The history of ASMV can be seen in the list of home care ventilator manufacturers and their products. Recently a new generation of alternate site mechanical ventilators has emerged that expand the options available to the clinician and patient in the alternative site, particularly for patients who require partial ventilatory support or who have serious lung disease. These new models may be optimal for ASMV once more experience has been gained with them. Meanwhile, older generation home care ventilators (for example, piston-driven devices) are still reliable, particularly for patients with neuromuscular disease.

Respiratory therapists must know the individual features of these ventilators and must consider all factors involved in the preparation, discharge, and ongoing care of the patient in the alternate care site. The ventilator chosen, often with the patient's help, must perform effectively for that individual patient.

Triage of the Ventilator-Assisted Individual

The decision on placement of a ventilator-assisted individual is based on a number of variables (Table 42-1). However, a series of events over the past 15 years has curtailed the options of these patients. In the late 1980s and early 1990s, the diagnosis-related group (DRG) reimbursement system for acute care facilities resulted in an increase in the number of patients classified as long-term mechanically ventilated individuals in stable condition; that is, patients who did not require care in the ICU.[11,12] The DRG system increased awareness of the escalating costs of health care, which provided greater motivation for hospitals to find appropriate sites of care for long-term mechanically ventilated patients. As a result, SNFs came under pressure to provide care for ventilator-assisted individuals. As patients were being moved to SNFs for care, respiratory therapists were becoming part of the SNF care system.

The next step in cost containment was the implementation of the prospective-payment system (PPS), which capped payment for SNFs. Because respiratory therapist services had not been reimbursed in SNFs, such services were not incorporated into the planned expenditures for the care of these patients. This fixed payment system effectively eliminated reimbursement for respiratory therapists, whose responsibilities were delegated to nursing per-

TABLE 42-1

Factors in the Placement of a Ventilator-Assisted Individual

Factor	Factor a Consideration?				
	Acute Care	Respiratory Rehabilitation Unit	Long-Term Care Facility	Assisted Living or Group Home	Patient's Home
Level of acuity	Yes	Yes	Yes	Yes	Yes
Availability of bed	Yes	Yes	Yes	Yes	No
Availability of trained staff	No	No	Yes	Yes	Yes
Capable and willing family members	No	No	No	No	Yes
Reimbursement with pre-approval	No	Yes	Yes	Yes	Yes
Patient's ability to care for self	No	No	No	Yes	Yes
Setting appropriate (cleanliness, space, access, distance to acute medical care)	No	No	No	No	Yes

sonnel with little training in respiratory care.[18] Many facilities stopped providing ventilator management altogether. Consequently, because fewer respiratory therapy services are available, fewer facilities offer ASMV to patients. Due in part to these changes, home care has become the more common alternative for discharge from an acute care or a rehabilitation facility. However, not all ventilator-assisted individuals can go home, and not all of them want to go home. Placement of patients in alternative care sites is a complex challenge of coordinating resources.[19,20] Important decisions must be made in the choice of the best site for the patient's needs (Box 42-2).

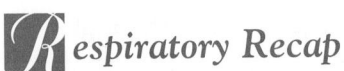

Factors that Increase Demand for Placement of Ventilator-Assisted Individuals in Alternate Sites

Imposition of the diagnosis-related group (DRG) reimbursement system

Awareness of the expense of care in the intensive care unit (ICU)

Awareness of the inappropriateness of ICU care for ventilator-assisted individuals

Realization that patients can live safely on ventilators over extended periods in alternate care settings

Sites of Care

Three care settings are available to ventilator-assisted individuals other than the acute care facility: a SNF, group or assisted living in a group home, and living at home. The SNF offers 24-hour care provided by a professional staff. The group or assisted living setting offers care provided by unlicensed personal care attendants (PCAs) and physicians, nurses, physical therapists, and respiratory therapists, who are consulted as needed but are off-site most of the time. Home care clinical staff support ranges from lit-

tle or no professional monitoring except by the primary care physician and through the equipment management provided by the home care company to nursing coverage 24 hours a day beyond 3 to 4 weeks. Generally, if professional coverage is needed 24 hours a day, the expense may require placement of the patient in a SNF.

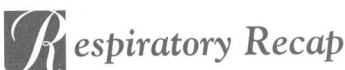

Placement of Ventilator-Assisted Individuals

Skilled nursing facility
Group home arrangement
Individual's home

Placement considerations are as varied as the individuals involved, but there are some common key factors. Placement usually is determined by the patient's finances and the availability of caregivers.[21,22] It is also important to note that the patient's choices may change over the course of the disease. The patient may choose to move to a group home or assisted living facility to gain greater independence. For example, if a pediatric patient, on reaching adulthood, chooses to live away from home, adequate individual monitoring and support in the new care setting must be ensured. With adult patients, a change in the home living situation or the patient's clinical needs may

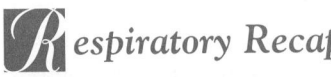

Factors that Affect Placement of Ventilator-Assisted Individuals

Availability of caregivers
Patient's finances

Box 42-2

Choosing the Best Site for a Ventilator-Assisted Individual

Patient and family preference
Patient's physical needs
Resources available
- Family
    Is the family willing and able to take on care
        responsibilities?
    Can the home accommodate the patient and
        equipment?
- Insurance coverage
    Is coverage adequate for needed staff?
    Can the family afford ancillary costs?
    Are community resources available?
- Staffing
    Can a care-giving staff be appropriately trained?
    Will the staff be available when needed?
    Will the staff have the skills to handle contingencies?
- Technology
    Can the patient and environmental supports be well
        matched?

require a move into a skilled nursing or assisted living facility. The options considered change according to the patient's needs and the available care choices. Location options, reimbursement, and technologic advances affect the choices available to the patient at any given time.

Appropriate Technology

Until recently ventilators that could be used without a 50-psi gas source (that is, out-of-hospital ventilators) did not have acute care features even if they were labeled as such. The patient therefore had to adapt to the equipment available. If the patient was unable to adapt and a more sophisticated ventilator was required, the facility's staff or the family had to adapt the environment to that equipment. Caregivers often had to learn to use and to troubleshoot technically complex equipment, to modify the home with high-pressure hoses, to have large tanks and compressors installed adjacent to the care setting, and to care for the patient's physical needs. For example, if a pediatric patient required continuous flow, pressure-controlled ventilation, the first option was to try a volume-controlled ventilator. If the trial succeeded, the patient went home with the volume ventilator, even if it was not the best arrangement. If the patient did not tolerate the volume ventilator, the home could be adapted with large oxygen tanks outside the house, high-pressure hoses, and compressors to provide pressure-controlled ventilation. Occasionally respiratory therapists could alter the ventilators by adding continuous flow with a continuous positive airway pressure (CPAP) machine, but this altered alarms set to detect inadequate ventilation, which was a potential

liability. Options on the latest generation of home care ventilators provide pressure-controlled ventilation, continuous flow, and partial ventilatory support with improved monitoring.

Staffing

Staffing is a common problem in ASMV, especially in the home. The equipment required for a ventilator-assisted individual can be technologically challenging for the caregiver. Nursing support for patients at home is complicated by the logistics in the finding, training, and retention of nurses in ventilator care. Respiratory therapists are not typically employed to provide on-site, continuous care, because there is limited reimbursement for their services except as equipment troubleshooting technicians.

Reimbursement

Before the 1990s, when reimbursement was not available, there was no perceived need for respiratory therapists to manage the respiratory needs of patients in long-term care facilities. This time was before the movement of many chronically ventilated patients residing in acute care facilities into SNFs. These long-term facilities often had to rely on home care equipment companies to supply the equipment and to train staff members to use it. Coverage did not include day-to-day ventilation management, which meant that there was little ongoing evaluation and management of the patient's ventilatory support. The home care companies maintained the equipment and the patient's status quo. Unfortunately, this arrangement can halt any weaning progress in a chronically ventilated patient. Proper equipment function and management of the patient's respiratory needs are best addressed by a respiratory therapist. However, data on the benefits of care provided in ASMV cases by respiratory therapists have not been reported.

Conflicting reports have resulted regarding reimbursement for home mechanical ventilation. Some studies report cost savings in the home setting compared to facility-based care.[21-28] However, one study reports that expenses for professional staffing in home care can be significant and that long-term care requiring highly skilled nursing care should be provided in facilities.[29] The key is the expense borne by the caregivers. Most successful home care arrangements rely on nonprofessional care (usually the family) and regular respite by professionals (usually nurses) to allow the family to sleep, shop, and perform other activities of daily living. The professional care is coordinated by a nursing agency or by the patient or family.

Family Role

Relying on the family for staffing coordination creates a potentially stressful situation that puts the family or patient at risk.[30-32] On the other hand, relying on an agency for such a personal and sensitive task has its own pitfalls. If an agency coordinates nursing care and PCAs for the family, issues may arise regarding the family's comfort level with the background and expertise of the staff. Families sometimes complain that the assigned nursing personnel cannot provide adequate care without previous experience with ventilators. A common reason to delay the discharge of a ventilator-assisted individual is a lack of qualified nursing staff for home care. Also, once the patient has been sent home, a sick call by assigned nursing personnel can place an undue burden on an already stressed family situation. If the family has been providing most of the care (for example, 16 hours/day) and the nurse who was scheduled to relieve them calls in sick, then the family will need to continue attending to the patient for the *next* 24 hours. For example, a parent who is caring for a child on a ventilator from 7 AM to 11 PM ex-

pects the nurse to relieve him or her at 11 so that the parent can sleep. If the nurse calls in sick, the parent cannot sleep, a situation that can turn disastrous. Lack of staffing can devastate the best plans for home mechanical ventilation.

If family members coordinate the nursing and PCA care, they shoulder a tremendous burden that entails advertising, performing background checks, assessing licensure, evaluating expertise, and determining hours of availability. However, if the family is able to manage the personnel involved, they usually can receive reimbursement for staffing services, can reduce staffing costs, and can have greater personal control over the personnel involved. It is important to note that this model is successful only with an involved family that is able and willing to become knowledgeable and operate their own medical staffing agency.

Box 42-3

Choosing the Best Ventilator for a Ventilator-Assisted Individual

Patient's Clinical Needs
Is invasive or noninvasive ventilation required?
Will heated or unheated humidification be used?
Which ventilatory pattern is required?
- Volume or pressure ventilation?
    Pediatric patients often require pressure ventilation. Volume ventilators can achieve higher pressures, which is an important feature for patients with restrictive diseases.
- Is positive end-expiratory pressure (PEEP) required?
    In volume ventilators, the addition of external PEEP compared with the ability to add PEEP internally can make a difference.
- Is continuous flow required?
    Often, the patient may initially appear to require ventilation using continuous flow with the acute care facility's equipment. The individual may be able to adapt to noncontinuous flow ventilation, but the clinician must ask, "At what cost to the patient is the additional work to trigger a non-continuous flow ventilator?"
- How good is the patient's ventilatory demand?
    The patient's ventilatory requirements may determine which ventilator is best. The ventilator must be able to meet the patient's flow and rate demands.

Patient's Personal Preferences
What type of ventilator best suits the patient's lifestyle?
Is the person highly mobile or sedentary?
Will the patient be traveling daily?
    If the patient goes to school or work each day, size and weight considerations are a greater factor than if the patient is primarily bed-bound.
What are the expectations for continued (or increased) mobility?
    On arrival home the prospect of venturing out can seem daunting to the patient, but after taking some time to adjust to the home environment and equipment, many patients want to take regular excursions, which may change their optimal ventilator choice.

How long are the excursions?
    Some ventilators have docking batteries that free the patient for up to 4 hours without having to use an extra external gel cell battery. This allows greater freedom for traveling for shorter distances.
Is travel always done with a wheelchair?
    For most wheelchairs, a special shelf must be made to accommodate the ventilator and an external battery. The amount of extra space available on the wheelchair is a consideration.

Equipment Availability and Cost
Home care company
- Which types of ventilators are available?
- Will appropriate backup service for the equipment be available?
    The patient should not have to change the modality of ventilation if the primary ventilator needs repair.
- Is the staff knowledgeable about the required equipment?
- Is the desired equipment available for use at the patient's location?
    A backup, long-term care facility may be needed in case of caregiver shortages or for regular respite care for the family.
- What sort of ventilators does the company use?
    An effort should be made to allow patients to use their own primary ventilator when admitted, or at the very least patients should not have to change the mode of ventilation because of equipment unavailability.
Is pressurized gas available for use with the ventilator?
    If the long-term care facility uses a significantly different ventilator, can accommodations be made to ensure that the patient is reliably and comfortably ventilated?
Is the facility prepared to manage the patient's equipment needs?
What is the cost of the equipment and is reimbursement available?

Ventilators

Reimbursement

The factors involved in the decision about the best ventilator for a patient are not limited to mechanical features, although such features are a primary concern. A number of issues and concerns must be addressed (Box 42-3). Cost and reimbursement can be the most important factors in the consideration of which ventilator to use. The options for patients receiving Medicare or Medicaid are limited compared to those available in the realm of private pay insurance or plans covered by a health maintenance organization (HMO). This issue is not simply about cost but about what the patient clinically requires. Most insurance companies do not differentiate between ventilators. Unfortunately, this can mean that a ventilator that provides continuous flow, positive end-expiratory pressure (PEEP), and other sophisticated capabilities is reimbursed at the same level as a device with none of these features and covers only a fraction of the more expensive ventilator's cost. The true consideration should be twofold: what patients truly need and what they can afford.

Government-funded insurance does not allow balanced billing. *Balanced billing* is the practice of billing a patient directly for any amount that exceeds the insurance company's payment. For example, if a ventilator rental charge is $800 a month and the insurance coverage is $600 a month, the company is not allowed to bill the difference of $200 a month. This system is intended to prevent home care companies from overcharging patients while receiving adequate reimbursement from the government. A patient who wants a more expensive ventilator with more features or benefits than the basic adequate model is not allowed to pay the amount that exceeds the government reimbursement even if he or she is willing to do so. Therefore if a home care company wants to provide a more expensive ventilator because of clinical requirements or the patient's wishes, it has limited options:

- It can provide the more expensive equipment without adequate reimbursement to cover the additional cost. This results in a fiscal loss for the company every month and has discouraged some home care companies from providing ASMV.
- It can provide a less expensive ventilator that is covered, even if it is not the best ventilator for the patient's growth and development.
- It can bargain with the insurance agency. In some cases an HMO may review the costs and options and allow payment for the needed ventilator. This is why some HMOs provide coverage for a more sophisticated ventilator. Some case managers make allowances for circumstances in which the patient's quality of life will be affected.

If a patient can be safely and effectively ventilated with a less expensive ventilator, most home care companies provide that ventilator rather than one with alleged technologic improvements. This is a matter of business being an integral part of selecting a ventilator under the current system of reimbursement in the United States. However, this system ensures that only those with financial resources substantial enough to pay out of pocket costs, without the use of government-assisted insurance, for improved technology are offered the better option, unless the ventilator-assisted individual cannot be safely and adequately ventilated on a "standard, first-generation ventilator."

First-Generation Portable Volume Ventilators

The first-generation models of the **portable volume ventilator** for ASMV are piston-driven, volume-cycled ventilators (Figure 42-3). Examples include the LP-4, LP-6, and the Bear 33 (no longer manufactured); the PB 2800 and PB 2801 (no longer manufactured or serviced in the United States); and the PLV 100, PLV 102, LP-6 Plus, LP-10, and LP-20 (currently manufactured and serviced in the United States). The LP series, manufactured by Aequitron (Tyco Health Care, Plymouth, Minn.), is the

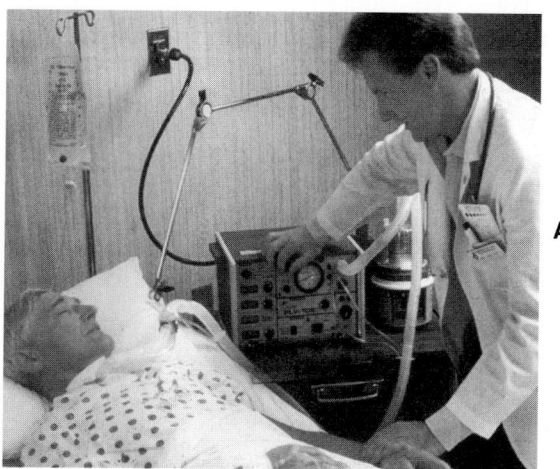

A

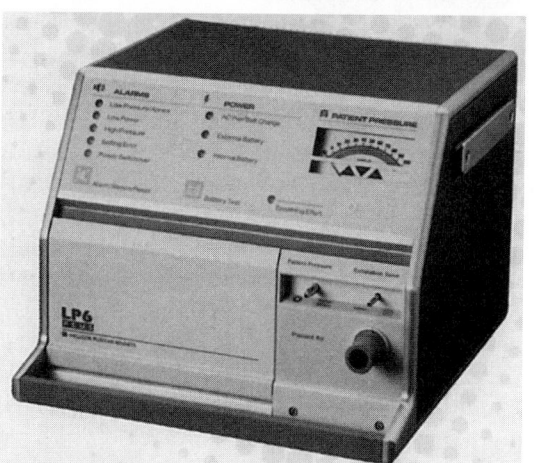

B

Figure 42-3 Portable volume ventilators. **A,** PLV-100. (Courtesy Respironics, Pittsburgh, Pa.) **B,** LP-6 Plus (Courtesy Tyco Health Care, Plymouth, Minn.)

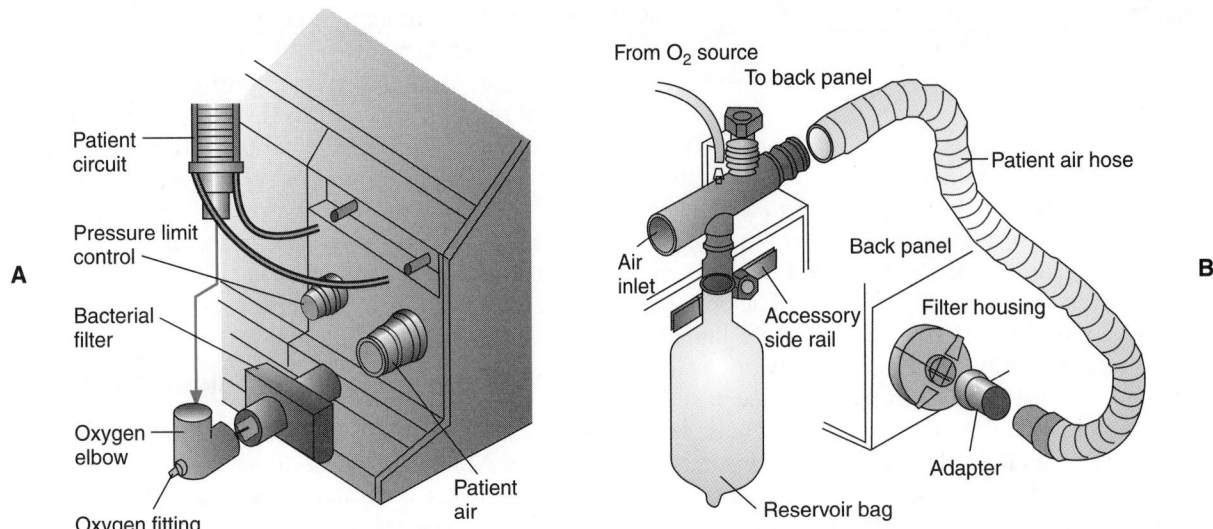

Figure 42-4   Oxygen administration with portable pressure ventilators. **A,** Titration into the inspiratory circuit at the ventilator outlet. **B,** Mixing in a bag before introduction into the piston. (Courtesy Tyco Health Care, Plymouth, Minn.)

first, oldest, and largest family of portable volume ventilators. The ASMV clinician must become familiar with any brand or type of these older ventilators, even those no longer manufactured, because some patients still use them.

First-generation portable ventilators weigh about 13.5 kg (30 pounds). They include basic modes, which provide continuous mandatory ventilation (CMV), intermittent mandatory ventilation (IMV), and monitoring (high and low pressure alarms). Although some of the portable ventilators have a synchronized intermittent mandatory ventilation (SIMV) mode setting, none of them has true SIMV, and the imposed work of breathing is high because of the lack of continuous flow through the circuit or a demand valve. Continuous flow can be added externally, but this can alter the proper functioning of the alarm system. The exhaled tidal volume typically is monitored only during monthly visits by home care equipment personnel. These ventilators use external PEEP valves, which can be bulky and heavy against a patient's chest, and can pull on the tracheostomy tube. In addition, noise can be generated on exhalation through spring-loaded valves when they become wet.

For portability, external batteries are used that can be heavy, bulky, and cumbersome. The batteries weigh approximately 13.5 to 18 kg (30 to 40 pounds) and cannot rest on top of the ventilators, which requires them to have their own space or to be carried separately. The internal battery lasts approximately 15 to 60 minutes and is to be used *only* in emergencies when a power failure occurs, not for short periods of transport. This point must be stressed with family members, who may mistakenly believe that the internal battery can be used for quick errands, such as a brief trip in the car. The result can be an internal failure, because the battery may fail completely after repeated use.

Oxygen must be added after the ventilator outlet to provide an fractional inspired oxygen concentration (FIO_2) of

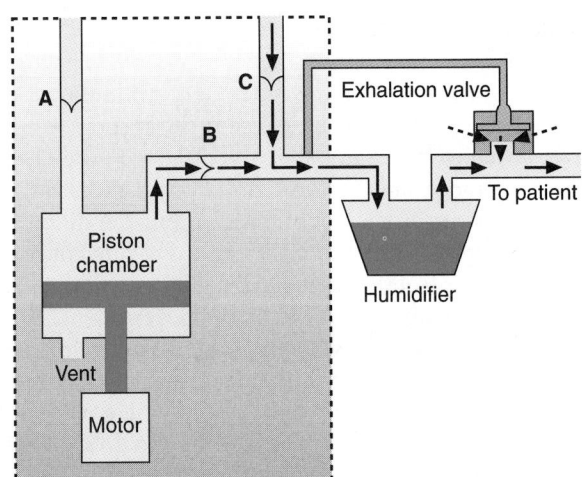

Figure 42-5   Diagram of a piston-driven portable volume ventilator. One-way valve allows gas to enter the piston during the backstroke (*A*). One-way valve prevents retrograde flow into the piston during the backstroke (*B*). Antiasphyxia valve (*C*). (Modified from Kacmarek RM, Stanek KS, McMahon KM, et al. Respir Care 1990;35:405-414.)

0.21 to 0.4 (Figure 42-4). An anesthesia bag or mixing chamber close to the ventilator's air intake can be used for an FIO_2 >0.4. The PLV-102 has an FIO_2 control, but it relies on an external in-line analyzer that responds to changes in the patient's respiratory rate. This feature can be used only in the SIMV mode. As noted previously, the SIMV mode on these first-generation ventilators does not provide the same continuous flow as that provided on acute care ventilators.

First-generation portable volume ventilators deliver a prescribed volume via a piston (Figure 42-5). When a patient is ventilated with an acute care ventilator in SIMV mode, a continuous gas flow or demand valve allows spon-

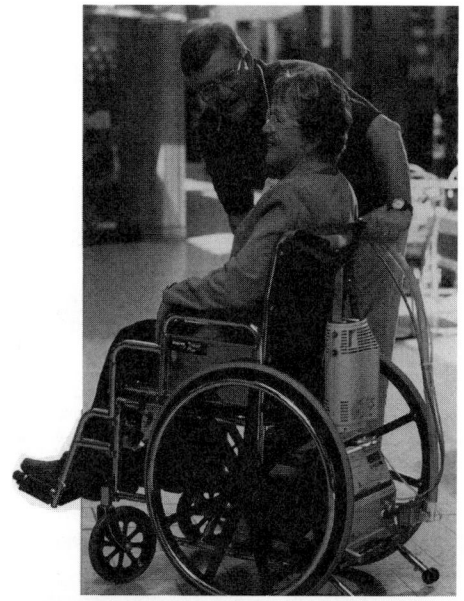

A

taneous breaths with little effort from the patient. However, piston-driven home care ventilators have no demand valve or flow in the circuit when the piston is not in motion.[33] For this reason, patients using SIMV with an acute care ventilator often are given a trial on the home care ventilator to assess how well they tolerate SIMV mode on the piston-driven ventilator. If the clinician switches the patient to the CMV (assist/control) mode, the patient may tolerate the change better.

It should be noted that first-generation ventilators have been used for many years in a wide variety of environments and have proved reliable despite rugged wear and tear. Many ASMV patients become attached to their particular brand, model, and individual ventilator. These ventilators are the workhorses of home care, traveling everywhere with patients and functioning consistently and dependably (Figure 42-6).

Second-Generation Portable Volume Ventilators

The second generation of portable volume ventilators offers more sophisticated features. Examples include the T-Bird Legacy (Bird Products, Palm Springs, Calif.), the Pulmonetic LTV series (LTV 900, 950, and 1000; Pulmonetic Systems, Colton, Calif.), the Achieva (Tyco Health Care, Plymouth, Minn.), and the Ivent (VersaMed, Hackensack, N.J.). Some of the second-generation devices are turbine driven rather than piston driven (Figure 42-7), and many are controlled by a microprocessor. The improved flow delivery of a turbine coupled with microprocessor control gives some of these devices a sophistication that rivals that of critical care ventilators. Furthermore, because a turbine rather than a piston is used for flow delivery, the size of the ventilator can be greatly reduced. The features of second-generation ventilators include continuous flow, FIO_2 control, pressure-support mode, improved patient triggering, internal PEEP control, less weight and smaller size, and built-in batteries for intermediate periods of use (4 hours).

In home care, reliability is the key factor. The need to repair or replace a ventilator model can ruin its potential for long-term use. If the ventilator fails, it does not matter how many otherwise useful features it has. Differences

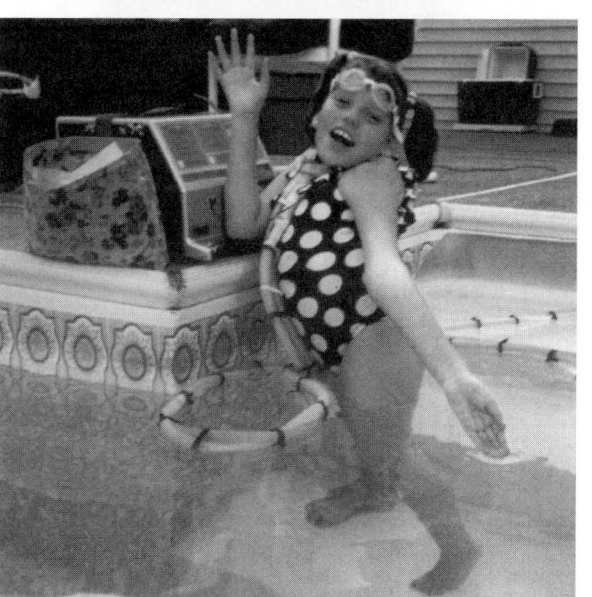

B

Figure 42-6 Examples of the portability of volume ventilators for ventilator-assisted individuals. **A,** Portable volume ventilator on a wheelchair. **B,** Pediatric patient in a pool with a portable volume ventilator.

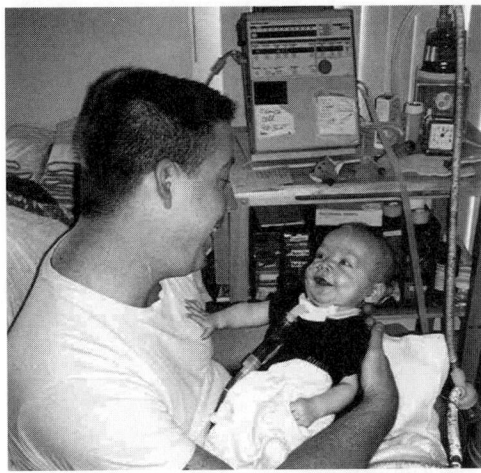 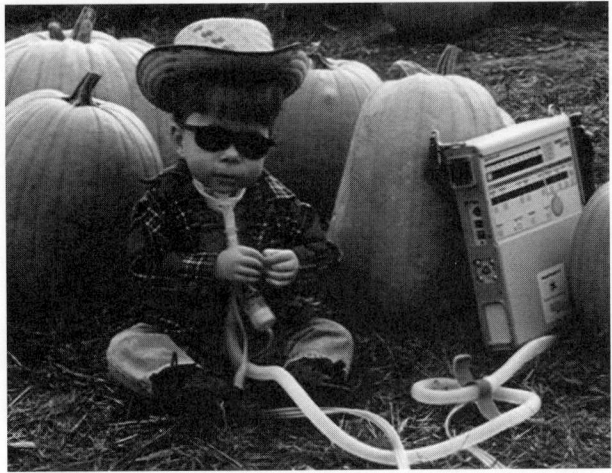

Figure 42-7   Pediatric patients receive ventilatory support with second-generation portable volume ventilators. Note the small size of the turbine-powered ventilator. (Courtesy Pulmonetic Systems, Colton, Calif.)

in performance between first- and second-generation portable volume ventilators are assessed by cost, reliability, and the usefulness of the newer features. Second-generation ventilators demonstrate that there is clearly the potential to greatly reduce size and weight while providing more ventilatory options, even though these new features may not be immediately appreciated. However, there is greater potential for ventilator-patient synchrony with the new features.

Portable Pressure Ventilators

A **portable pressure ventilator** is designed to provide noninvasive positive pressure ventilation (NPPV). Examples include the BiPAP/ST series and the Synchrony BiPAP (Respironics, Pittsburgh, Pa.), the VPAP (Resmed, Poway, Calif.), and the Knightstar 335 (Tyco Health Care, Plymouth, Minn.). Positive features include the simple delivery of pressure-support ventilation, small size and lightweight design, continuous flow, flows that vary according to patient demand, flow compensation for leaks, and responsive triggering. Drawbacks include the lack of sophisticated alarms (with a few exceptions), dependence on leak to clear carbon dioxide, and estimated (calculated) tidal volume monitoring.

NPPV has been used in home care for more than 20 years.[34,35] However, since the advent of the portable pressure ventilators, the number of patients receiving this therapy has increased markedly.[11] Although NPPV can be provided by any ventilator, portable pressure ventilators are simpler and more convenient for ventilator-assisted individuals (Table 42-2). A number of portable pressure ventilators are available, but the BiPAP/ST series is most commonly used. Throughout the early 1990s the BiPAP machine was the only noninvasive ventilator of its type. Many patients now consider portable NPPV a practical option because of

the availability of these smaller, lighter, easy to operate machines.

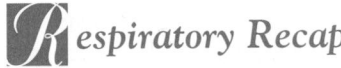

Respiratory Recap

Portable Pressure Ventilators
Types include BiPAP/ST series, Synchrony BiPAP, VPAP, and Knightstar 335. They provide pressure-support ventilation. These machines are used for noninvasive ventilation.

Patients who require airway control or those who have difficulty clearing secretions often do better with a tracheostomy. Pediatric patients also perform better with a tracheostomy, even if only for intermittent ventilator use. The tracheostomy eliminates the need for masks, which are not well accepted or tolerated by young patients. Once these patients are older and better able to cooperate with therapy, a transition to a noninvasive mask may be an appropriate choice.

Age-Specific Angle

Pediatric patients often do better with a tracheostomy than with noninvasive positive pressure ventilation (NPPV).

NPPV ventilators can be used for invasive ventilation with a simple adaptation for connection to a tracheostomy. However, manufacturers and the U.S. Food and Drug Ad-

TABLE 42-2

Features of Portable Pressure and Portable Volume Ventilators

Feature	Portable Pressure Ventilator	Portable Volume Ventilator
Peak inspiratory pressure	20 to 35 cm H_2O	60 to 70 cm H_2O
Leak compensation	Excellent	Poor
Alarms	High and low pressure; disconnect	Several
Monitoring	Varies; estimated tidal volume	More precise; accurate tidal volume
Weight (kg)	4 to 8	12 to 16
Patient comfort	More comfortable than a portable volume ventilator	Less comfortable than a portable pressure ventilator
Internal battery	No	Yes
Cost	Less expensive than a portable volume ventilator	More expensive than a portable pressure ventilator

Modified from Hill NS. Management of long-term noninvasive ventilation: long-term mechanical ventilation. New York: Marcel Dekker; 2001. No. 152. pp. 253-303.

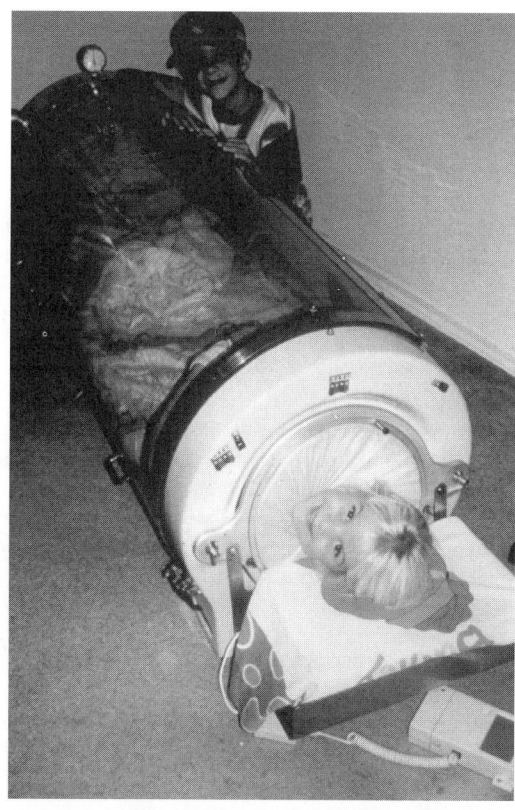

Figure 42-8 Child in a Porta-lung negative pressure ventilator. (Courtesy Respironics, Pittsburgh, Pa.)

ministration (FDA) do not approve of such adaptations. Accordingly, portable pressure ventilators designed for noninvasive ventilation should not be used for invasive ventilatory support.

Negative Pressure Ventilators

Negative pressure ventilators include the NEV-100 (Respironics, Pittsburgh, Pa.) for use with a variety of application devices. The iron lung and the rocking bed (Emerson, Cambridge, Mass.) are still used today but no longer manufactured. For many years the practical application of negative pressure ventilation for ASMV has changed little. These devices apply a negative pressure to the thorax to aid inhalation. Small improvements have been made in alarms and user-friendly mechanisms of the negative pressure devices, but the practical use of these devices today is the same as it has been for more than two decades. In fact, the same principles apply as when the first successful use of the iron lung for ventilation was reported.[36] Although a few negative pressure devices are still in use, they are becoming obsolete with the increased use of portable pressure ventilators.

Negative pressure application systems are powered by a negative pressure device, such as the NEV-100, which can provide negative pressure and active exhalation by the use

of positive pressure to push the air from the patient's lungs. Common application systems include the Porta-lung, the chest shell, and a variety of wraps (Pneumosuit, pneumo jacket, pneumobag; Respironics, Pittsburgh, Pa.). The wraps are made of a material that allows for a seal over the patient's thorax and are used in conjunction with a grid to allow for suspension of the wrap over the thorax without pushing on the patient's chest. The Porta-lung (Respironics, Pittsburgh, Pa.; Figure 42-8) is a lighter, smaller version of the iron lung. These devices can be used with patients for whom secretions and upper airway obstruction are not issues. Negative pressure ventilators may be used in an alternating therapy scheme with positive pressure devices. For example, a patient may use a volume ventilator attached to a mouthpiece while upright in a wheelchair

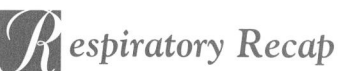 *espiratory Recap* ———

Negative Pressure Ventilators
Types include poncho, chest cuirass, iron lung or Porta-lung, rocking bed. These machines apply a negative pressure to the thorax to initiate or aid inhalation.

CPG 42-1

Long-Term Invasive Mechanical Ventilation in the Home

Goals

The goals of long-term invasive mechanical ventilation in the home are to sustain and extend life, to enhance the quality of life, to reduce morbidity, to provide cost-effective care, to improve or sustain the physical and psychologic function of all ventilator-assisted individuals, and to enhance the growth and development of pediatric ventilator-assisted individuals.

Indications

Patients requiring invasive long-term ventilatory support have demonstrated an inability to be completely weaned from invasive ventilatory support or a progression of disease that requires increasing ventilatory support.

Conditions that meet these criteria may include but are not limited to ventilatory muscle disorders, alveolar hypoventilation syndrome, primary respiratory disorders, obstructive diseases, restrictive diseases, and cardiac disorders, including congenital anomalies.

Contraindications

A physiologically unstable medical condition that requires a higher level of care or resources than are available in the home. Indicators of a medical condition that is too unstable for the home or long-term care setting are a fractional inspired oxygen concentration (FIO_2) above 0.4; a positive end-expiratory pressure (PEEP) more than 10 cm H_2O; a need for continuous invasive monitoring in adult patients; and lack of a mature tracheostomy.

Patient choice not to receive home mechanical ventilation

Lack of an appropriate discharge plan

Unsafe physical environment as determined by the patient's discharge planning team, such as the presence of fire, health, or safety hazards, including unsanitary conditions, and inadequate basic utilities (such as heat, air conditioning, or electricity)

Inadequate resources for care in the home, including inadequate financial resources, personnel, or medical follow-up; inability of the ventilator-assisted individual to care for himself or herself if no caregiver is available; inadequate respite care for caregivers; and an inadequate number of competent caregivers.

Hazards and Complications

Deterioration or an acute change in the clinical status of the ventilator-assisted individual can complicate such therapy. The following factors may result in death or require rehospitalization for acute treatment.

Medical factors: Hypocapnia, respiratory alkalosis, hypercapnia, respiratory acidosis, hypoxemia, barotrauma, seizures, hemodynamic instability, airway complications (stomal or tracheal infection, mucus plugging, tracheal erosion or stenosis), respiratory infection (tracheobronchitis, pneumonia), bronchospasm, exacerbation of underlying disease, or natural course of the disease

Equipment-related factors: Failure of the ventilator, malfunction of equipment, inadequate warming and humidification of the inspired gases, inadvertent changes in ventilator settings, accidental disconnection from the ventilator, or accidental decannulation

Psychosocial factors: Depression, anxiety, loss of resources (caregiver or financial), detrimental change in the family structure or coping capacity

Monitoring

The frequency of monitoring should be determined by the individualized care plan and should be based on the patient's current medical condition. The ventilator settings, proper functioning of equipment, and the patient's physical condition should be monitored and verified with each initiation of invasive ventilation to the patient, including altering the

---

and a Porta-lung for sleep at night.[37] In these instances caregiver training focuses on the ability to secure a good seal, determine the optimal settings (which may change depending on the seal), and monitor the ventilator-assisted individual as needed. The goal of negative pressure devices is to deliver continuous ventilation intermittently without a tracheostomy.

Circuit Components

The seemingly simple issue of ventilator circuitry actually has several aspects. This is a matter not just of the least costly circuit but also of safety, convenience, and environmental effects. The right tubing can make a big difference to the patient. The size and weight of the tubing on the patient's chest or the pull on the tracheostomy can play a role in the patient's quality of life. Many patients prefer soft, silicone-type flex tubes rather than the standard stiff plastic included in disposable circuits. Some tubing, especially the disposable type, can generate a loud noise with every breath, which can diminish the quality of the patient environment. Some long-term patients have modified the tubing so that it is more than 10 m (30 feet) long, allowing them to swim while ventilated. Some patients become reliant on a particular circuit and are not comfortable switching to another model. This can become a problem if the desired tubing is not covered by insurance and the patient cannot afford or is not permitted by insurance regulations to pay for the special circuits. This issue has yet to be addressed in a comprehensive manner by third party payers. When manufacturers stop making a specific circuit, the patient accustomed to that circuit may have difficulty with the transition to a new type of tubing.

Another component of the ventilator circuit is humidification, which is necessary to avoid drying of secretions,

CPG 42-1

Long-Term Invasive Mechanical Ventilation in the Home—cont'd

Monitoring—cont'd

source of ventilation, as from one ventilator or resuscitation bag to another ventilator; with each ventilator setting change; and on a regular basis as specified by individualized plan of care.

All appropriately trained caregivers should follow the care plan and implement the monitoring that has been prescribed. These caregivers may operate, maintain, and monitor all equipment and perform all aspects of care required by the ventilator-assisted individual after having been trained and evaluated as to their level of knowledge about the equipment and the ventilator-assisted individual's clinical response to each intervention.

Lay caregivers should monitor the following regularly:

Patient's physical condition: Respiratory rate, heart rate, color changes, chest excursion, diaphoresis, lethargy, blood pressure, and body temperature

Ventilator settings: Peak pressures, preset tidal volume, frequency of ventilator breaths, verification of oxygen concentration setting, and PEEP level; the frequency of checking these alarms and settings should be specified in the plan of care

Appropriate humidification of inspired gases

Temperature of inspired gases

Heat and moisture exchanger function

Equipment function: Appropriate configuration of the ventilator circuit, alarm function, cleanliness of filters, battery power level (internal and external), overall condition of all equipment

Self-inflating manual resuscitator: Cleanliness and function

A clinician should regularly perform a comprehensive assessment of the patient and the patient ventilator system as prescribed by the plan of care. The clinician should implement, monitor, and assess the results of the following other interventions as indicated by the clinical situation and as anticipated in the care plan:

Pulse oximetry (for patients requiring a change in the prescribed oxygen level or in patients in whom a change in condition is suspected)

Measurement of an end-tidal carbon dioxide level (to establish trends in carbon dioxide levels during weaning

Specimen collection and analysis, as prescribed by physician, including but not limited to sputum and blood work (for example, arterial blood gas analysis and complete blood counts)

Cardiorespiratory monitoring (an electrocardiogram and heart rate trending)

Pulmonary function testing

Ventilator settings

Exhaled tidal volume

F_{IO_2}

Appropriate clinicians are responsible for maintaining interdisciplinary communication concerning the plan of care.

Appropriate clinicians should integrate the respiratory plan of care into the patient's total care plan. The plan of care should include all aspects of the patient's respiratory care and ongoing assessment and education of the caregivers involved.

Modified from AARC Clinical practice guideline: long-term invasive mechanical ventilation in the home. Respir Care 1995;40:1313-1320.
CPG, Clinical practice guideline.

mucus plugging, and lower respiratory tract infection. The two options for humidification are an active heated humidifier or a heat-and-moisture exchanger (artificial nose). For ASMV the use of an artificial nose is convenient and inexpensive. However, the artificial nose may not effectively humidify the inspired gas of some patients. Moreover, many patients prefer an active humidifier. If a leak technique is used with or without a valve (for example, a Passy-Muir valve), an artificial nose should not be used because expiratory gas must pass through it for the device to function properly. The choice of humidification for the ASMV patient usually is a balance of convenience and effectiveness.

Assessment and Monitoring

The frequency and extent of monitoring depend on patient acuity, the care plan, ventilator changes that are to be made, and the patient's overall situation (CPG 42-1 and Box 42-4). Long-term care facilities have policies that determine how often vital signs are checked, including spot checks and emergency monitoring of oxygen saturation, ventilator settings, and circuit integrity.

Arterial blood gas measurements are not easily obtained in most ASMV settings, and blood gas laboratories are not readily available. Also, in the home care setting reimbursement is not available for blood gas determinations. In rare cases patients must be admitted to an acute care facility so that monitoring can be provided during major changes in ventilator settings. Pulse oximetry plays an important role in the monitoring of ASMV patients, but overreliance on oximetry can be misleading and costly. In home care the condition of most patients is quite stable. Oximeter availability may be beneficial for patients with fluctuating oxygen requirements, such as pediatric patients or those with a lung disease that causes intermittent hypoxemia. If an oximeter is available in the home, the caregiver can check the patient's oxygenation if necessary. End-tidal carbon dioxide monitors (capnography) may be useful for monitoring changes in ventilator settings in

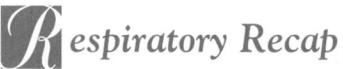

Box 42-4

Monitoring an Alternate Site Mechanical Ventilation Patient

Parameters Monitored Regularly
Vital signs
Ventilator settings
Ancillary alarms
• Primary: High and low pressure, power
• Secondary low pressure: In pediatric ventilators or in circuits with a relatively small tubing diameter, a secondary alarm is added to the built-in high-and low-pressure alarms. A primary low-pressure alarm may not reliably detect a patient disconnect if the tubing diameter is very small.
• Extension of the alarm: This is a simple accessory that allows the caregiver to remain at a distance while monitoring essential alarms.

Parameters Monitored under Certain Circumstances
Oximetry
End-tidal partial pressure of carbon dioxide ($PetCO_2$)
Noninvasive positive pressure ventilation (NPPV)
    A disconnect alarm may sound if (1) the individual cannot replace the mask or interface independently or (2) if the person cannot breathe independently for long and a caregiver must be notified.

ASMV patients. The respiratory therapist measures a baseline end-tidal partial pressure of carbon dioxide ($PetCO_2$), adjusts the ventilator, and compares the baseline value with the end-tidal $PetCO_2$ obtained after the adjustment.

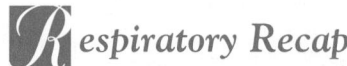

*R*espiratory Recap

Factors Monitored in Alternate Site Mechanical Ventilation Patients*

Vital signs	End-tidal partial pressure of
Ventilator settings	carbon dioxide ($PetCO_2$)
Alarms	in some patients
Oximetry	

*Blood gases need not be monitored routinely.

Interfacility Transport

Transportation of patients who require mechanical ventilation is an added concern because these patients generally are quite cognizant of their ventilatory requirements. For example, patients may have personal preferences for the way in which they prefer to be ventilated, which type of ventilator is most comfortable, and even the specific ventilator that feels right. The mode of transportation must meet the basic clinical requirements for patient ventilation, but it must be reasonably comfortable and available for the transfer. One of the following approaches is used to transport a ventilator-assisted individual between facilities:

• Manual ventilation (this technique generally is not preferred because of inconsistent volumes and provider fatigue, but the patient may prefer it over use of an unknown ventilator)
• A transport ventilator provided by the acute care facility
• The long-term care facility's ventilator
• The patient's own ventilator

*R*espiratory Recap

Interfacility Transport

Keeping the patient on the home ventilator is the best way to accomplish error-free transport.

The preferred arrangement is to maintain patients on their own ventilators throughout the health care spectrum. Optimally, the patient who requires day surgery can continue to be ventilated on the personal ventilator even through the acute care experience. For some patients, this choice is as significant as the choice of anesthesia for surgery. ASMV patients admitted to an acute care facility because of an emergency may need to be ventilated for a brief period on an acute care ventilator to adequately meet their changing respiratory status. However, once the patient's respiratory condition is stable, it is best to return to the usual mode of ventilation. The primary issue involved in this decision is whether the patient has a permanent or an unresolved change in ventilatory status that requires additional mechanical features until discharge to the nonacute facility. Also, the acute or nonacute care facility may have quality control regulations requiring the patient to be on a ventilator that is part of the facility's monitoring and alarm system. This may require some innovation and tolerance on the part of the staff and patience on the part of the patient.

Most portable volume ventilators can use external batteries that operate for up to 24 hours on DC current, depending on the size of the battery and the current draw of the ventilator (depending on the volume and frequency of gas delivered). Portable pressure ventilators can be adapted to DC current to use an external battery, although this is cumbersome. Because portable pressure ventilators are more commonly used with patients who do not require continuous ventilation, the external battery is rarely required.

Factors Affecting Successful Alternate Site Mechanical Ventilation

Patient's Attitude

Attitude makes a difference. Patients with a sense of humor who can adapt and stay optimistic about changing situations tend to do better in home care. Unpredictability is a common factor in the home care setting. Caregivers may not be reliable, equipment may not function properly, and electrical power outages may occur. Some situations can be anticipated, but all problems are better resolved if all those involved cope with a positive attitude.

Family's Capabilities

Every family is unique. Adjustments to the situation are guided by the family members preparing for the patient's discharge to the alternate care site. The family must be included in the process of deciding where the ventilator-assisted individual will live.[38] In most cases the patient will make the choice, or the patient and family decide together. It is important to have a family member who is informed and ready to make the adjustments needed for the transition.[39] This may require a significant amount of training of caregivers. Rooms and sections of the home may require renovation. If the patient is discharged to a long-term care facility, interviews and tours of the facilities must be done. The distance from the family's home to the facility may be an important factor. Generally for the family, preparing to discharge the patient to a long-term care facility is less stressful than preparing to discharge the patient to the home.

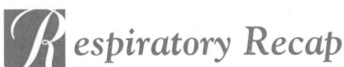espiratory Recap

Factors in Successful Placement of a Ventilator-Assisted Individual at Home
Positive patient attitude Involved and capable family Prepared home Workable financial picture Accessible community resources

The choice to go home involves several steps. Evaluation, training, and adaptation are essential. The level and intensity of training and preparation depend on the resources available as much as the patient's needs. Optimally the patient should be cared for in a manner that is safe and economical and that meets the individual's lifestyle for care. Some ventilator-assisted individuals require complete physical care, whereas others can perform activities of daily living and need only minimal assistance for bathing, transfers, and nighttime monitoring. Care usually is provided by a mix of professionals, PCAs, technicians, trained family members, and the patient. The care can range from 24-hour nursing care, which is very expensive and not often done in the home for extended periods, to intermittent visits by professionals while PCAs and family members provide the bulk of the care. If a ventilator-assisted individual is to be discharged to a SNF, less training and preparation are required than if the patient were going home. Although the facility's staff will require some training regarding the patient's individual needs and a particular ventilator, the family will not need most of the training (that is, airway care, suctioning, and ventilator basics) because this care will be provided by the professionals at the SNF.

Preparation of the Home

Before a decision to go home can be made, the patient's home must be evaluated. Is the home located where a wheelchair van or car can gain access? Is there a ramp into the home? Are the doors wide enough to allow the patient to move about within the home, as well as into and out of it? Are there areas set aside for the storage of supplies, the cleaning of equipment, and good hand washing for those in contact with the patient? If health care professionals will be caring for the patient for extend periods, is there a place where they can write their notes and one where they can stay when not actively caring for the patient? Having an extra family member constantly present can increase the strain on a family. The caregiver cannot be expected to sit in the dark with the sleeping patient during a night shift (nor would most people want someone sitting in the dark and watching them while they sleep).

Electrical requirements also must be considered. How up-to-date is the wiring of the house? Are the circuit breakers for the room easily accessible? Does the room have its own circuit breakers? Do the electrical requirements of the medical equipment exceed the available amperage? What will happen if all the equipment is in use and the vacuum cleaner is turned on in another part of the house? The clinician arranging for the home care transition is responsible for assessing the home for the basic needs of patient access and equipment function. A list showing each piece of equipment, its power requirements, where it can be plugged in, and how it is to be used usually is helpful. Without this advance preparation, a discharge can go quickly awry.

Expense

The care of a ventilator-assisted individual may be financed through private payment, third party payers, and community resources. Private payment comes from the patient's or family's personal resources. The patient is the first party, and the caregiver or home care company is the second party. Third party payers include government programs (Medicare and Medicaid) and private insurance. Funding through nonprofit agencies offsets specific expenses that ASMV patients incur.

Out-of-pocket expenses are almost always a hardship given the long-term nature of ASMV. Even financially secure families can find themselves financially stressed, given the continuous nature of the high-cost services required in ASMV. The financial burden can be a significant pressure that ultimately can lead to an unstable financial situation; this, in turn, can threaten the family's stability and the provision of a suitable home care situation for some patients. Waiting for funding approval can present a significant obstacle to discharge of a ventilator-assisted individual.[38]

Insurance companies' policies vary radically in the way in which services and equipment may be reimbursed. A multitude of considerations can influence how care will be administered based on reimbursement issues.[19] This may alter the clinical outcome and remains a critical factor in the respiratory therapist's ability to fully care for the patient.

The options for home care versus facility-based care are tied to caregiver availability. Caregiver availability depends on two things: time and money. If family members are able and willing to provide care, the expense of a caregiver is reduced or possibly eliminated. If a caregiver must be paid, the expense depends on how much time is needed and whether the caregiver is a PCA or must be a licensed health care practitioner (traditionally a registered nurse). The training, monitoring, and follow-up for a given family depend very much on who is operating and troubleshooting the ventilator. The likelihood of keeping a patient at home rather than in a facility-based location can be tied to the success of the caregivers' management of ventilator alarms and airway care.

Community Resources

Community resources vary widely. Some large national not-for-profit organizations, such as the Muscular Dystrophy Association, can provide funds to certain families, but other resources also can be investigated for families learning to manage the expense of ASMV in the home. Large cities may have more established mechanisms to find and distribute funds to help those with medical needs. On the other hand, in some instances making a need known can rally a small town and result in meaningful assistance for those having difficulty paying for essential services. Supportive resources may include church groups, Lions and Rotary clubs, and other such private organizations that may be motivated to help with fund-raising for specific needs. Social services may be available through government-funded organizations to help locate and use the agencies available to patients requiring ASMV.

KEY POINTS

- Significant changes in ASMV have occurred, both in the options available to the patient and the technology to support the patient's lifestyle choices.
- The number of ventilator-assisted individuals has increased markedly, as has the use of noninvasive ventilation and second-generation portable volume ventilators, which have improved the flexibility of ASMV.
- Changes in reimbursement have dramatically affected the placement of ventilator-assisted individuals, placing greater dependence on the availability and financial resources of caregivers.
- Obtaining and coordinating the care required for ventilator-assisted individuals puts a burden on the patients' families and the health care system.
- Ventilator-assisted patients need the respiratory therapist's expertise and training in mechanical ventilation; however, reimbursement controls have placed the respiratory therapist in the position of marginally assisting in the optimal care of these individuals.
- Second-generation portable ventilators have improved the clinical management, comfort, and convenience for ventilator-assisted individuals.

References

1. Indihar FJ, Walker NE. Experience with a prolonged respiratory care unit revisited. Chest 1984;86:616-620.
2. Gilmartin M. Transition from the intensive care unit to home: patient selection and discharge planning. Respir Care 1994; 39:456-477.
3. Gracey DR, Viggiano RW, Naessens JM, et al. Outcomes of patients admitted to a chronic ventilator-dependent unit in an acute care hospital. Mayo Clin Proc 1992;67:131-136.
4. Gilmartin M, Make B. Home care of the ventilator-dependent person. Respir Care 1983;28:1490-1497.
5. O'Donohue WJ, Giovannoni RM, Goldberg AI, et al. Long-term mechanical ventilation: guidelines for management in the home and at alternate community sites. Chest 1986;90;1S-35S.
6. Plummer AL, O'Donohue WJ, Petty TL. Consensus conference on problems in home mechanical ventilation. Am Rev Respir Dis 1989;140:555-560.
7. Bone RC. Long-term ventilator care: a Chicago problem and a national problem. Chest 1987;92:536-539.
8. Make BJ. Epidemiology of long-term ventilatory assistance. In: Hill N, editor. Long-term mechanical ventilation. New York: Marcel Dekker; 2001.
9. Goldberg AI. The ventilator-assisted individuals study. Chest 1990;98:428-433.
10. Make B, Dayno S, Gertment P. Prevalence of chronic ventilator dependency. Am Rev Respir Dis 1986;132:A167.
11. Adams AB, Whitman J, Marcy T. Surveys of long-term ventilatory support in Minnesota: 1986 and 1992. Chest 1993;103: 1463-1469.

12. Adams AB, Shapiro RS, Marini JJ. Changing prevalence of chronically ventilator-assisted individuals in Minnesota: increases, characteristics, and the use of noninvasive ventilation. Respir Care 1998;43:643-649.

13. Nochomovitz ML, Montenegro HD, Parran S, et al. Placement alternatives for ventilator-dependent patients outside the intensive care unit. Respir Care 1991;36:199-204.

14. Wagner D. Economics of prolonged mechanical ventilation. Am Rev Respir Dis 1989;140:S14-S18.

15. Sheinhorn DJ, Chao DC, Stearn-Hassenpflug, et al. Post-ICU mechanical ventilation: treatment of 1123 patients in a regional weaning center. Chest 1997;111:1654-1659.

16. Indihar FJ. A report of patients in a prolonged respiratory care unit. Minn Med 1991;74:23-27.

17. Goldstein RS, Avendano MA. Long-term mechanical ventilation as elective therapy: clinical status and future prospects. Respir Care 1991;36:297-304.

18. Czachowski R. Study finds respiratory care instruction very limited in nursing schools. AARC Times 1994;8:99-108.

19. DeWitt PK, Jansen MT, Ward SL, et al. Obstacles to discharge of ventilator-assisted children from the hospital to home. Chest 1993;103:1560-1565.

20. Fischer DA, Prentice WS. Feasibility of home care for certain respiratory-dependent restrictive or obstructive lung disease patients. Chest 1982;82:739-743.

21. Moss AH, Casey P, Stocking CB, et al. Home ventilation for amyotrophic lateral sclerosis patients: outcomes, costs, and patient, family, and physician attitudes. Neurology 1993;43:438-443.

22. Fields AI. Home care cost-effectiveness for respiratory technology–dependent children. Am J Dis Child 1991;145:729-733.

23. Splaingard ML, Frates RC, Harrison GM, et al. Home positive pressure ventilation: twenty years' experience. Chest 1983;84:376-382.

24. Frates RC, Splaingard ML, Smith EO, et al. Outcome of home mechanical ventilation in children. J Pediatr 1985;106:850-856.

25. Creese AL, Fielden R. Hospital or home care for the severely disabled: a cost comparison. Br J Prevent Soc Med 1977;31:116-121.

26. Indihar FJ, Forsberg D. Experience with a prolonged respiratory care unit. Chest 1982;81:89-92.

27. Sivak ED, Cordasco EM, Gipson WT. Pulmonary mechanical ventilation at home: a reasonable and less expensive alternative. Respir Care 1983;28:42-49.

28. Bach J. The ventilator-assisted individual: cost analysis of institutionalization versus rehabilitation and in-home management. Chest 1992;101:S26-S30.

29. Prentice WS. Placement for long-term ventilator care. Respir Care 1986;31:288-293.

30. Quint RD, Chesterman E, Crain LS, et al. Home care for ventilator-dependent children. Am J Dis Child 1990;144:1238-1241.

31. Thomas VM, Ellison K, Howell EV, et al. Caring for the person receiving ventilatory support at home: caregivers' needs and involvement. Heart Lung 1992;21:180-186.

32. Miller JR, Colbert AP, Schock NC. Ventilator use in progressive neuromuscular disease: impact on patients and their families. Dev Med Child Neurol 1988;30:200-207.

33. Kacmarek RM, Stanek KS, McMahon KM, et al. Imposed work of breathing during synchronized intermittent mandatory ventilation provided by five home care ventilators. Respir Care 1990;35:405-414.

34. Hill NS. Management of long-term noninvasive ventilation. In: Hill N, editor. Long-term mechanical ventilation. New York: Marcel Dekker; 2001.

35. Bach JR, Alba AS, Shin D. Management alternatives for post-polio respiratory insufficiency: assisted ventilation by nasal or oral-nasal interface. Am J Phys Med Rehabil 1989;68:264-271.

36. Drinker PD, McKhann CF. The use of a new apparatus for the prolonged administration of artificial respiration. JAMA 1929;92:1658-1660.

37. Bach JR. Ventilator use by Muscular Dystrophy Association patients. Arch Phys Med Rehabil 1992;73:179-183.

38. Smith CE, Mayer LS, Parkhurst C, et al. Adaptation in families with a member requiring mechanical ventilation at home. Heart Lung 1991;20:349-356.

39. Thompson CL, Richmond MR. Teaching home care for ventilator-dependent patients: the patient's perception. Heart Lung 1990;19:79-83.

CHAPTER 43

Noninvasive Ventilation and Continuous Positive Airway Pressure

Dean R. Hess
Allan B. Saposnick

CHAPTER OUTLINE

Noninvasive Positive Pressure Ventilation
Acute Care Applications
Chronic Applications
Patient Interface
Ventilators for Noninvasive Positive Pressure Ventilation
Caregiver Issues
Clinical Application

Negative Pressure Ventilation, Rocking Beds, and Pneumobelts
Continuous Positive Airway Pressure
Acute Care Applications
Chronic Applications

OBJECTIVES

1. Compare noninvasive positive pressure ventilation (NPPV), negative pressure ventilation, and continuous positive airway pressure (CPAP).
2. List selection criteria for noninvasive positive pressure ventilation (inclusion and exclusion).
3. Describe interfaces and ventilators for NPPV and CPAP.
4. Describe the principles of negative pressure ventilation, rocking beds, and pneumobelts.
5. Discuss acute care applications of CPAP.
6. Discuss the use of CPAP to treat obstructive sleep apnea.
7. Discuss the role of humidification in the application of NPPV and CPAP.
8. Discuss issues of compliance with CPAP for treatment of obstructive sleep apnea.
9. Describe the operation and use of auto-positive airway pressure devices.

KEY TERMS

Auto-Positive Airway Pressure (APAP)	Expiratory Positive Airway Pressure (EPAP)	Noninvasive Positive Pressure Ventilation (NPPV)
Bilevel Positive Airway Pressure	Inspiratory Positive Airway Pressure (IPAP)	Pneumobelt
Continuous Positive Airway Pressure (CPAP)	Iron Lung	Rocking Bed
Cuirass	Negative Pressure Ventilation (NPV)	

Noninvasive ventilation provides ventilatory support without an endotracheal tube or tracheostomy tube. Both positive pressure and negative pressure approaches can be used to provide noninvasive ventilation. With noninvasive ventilation the minute ventilation of the patient is partially or fully provided by the ventilator. With **continuous positive airway pressure (CPAP),** a pressure greater-than-atmospheric pressure is applied to the airway throughout the respiratory cycle. Although CPAP can be provided either invasively (that is, through an artificial airway) or noninvasively (that is, with a nasal or oronasal mask), only noninvasive approaches to CPAP are dis-

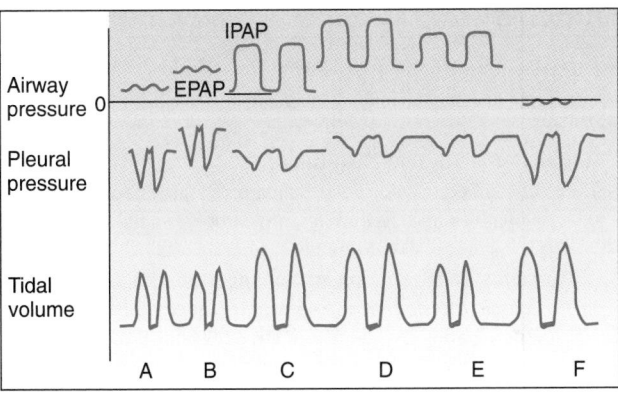

Figure 43-1   *A,* Continuous positive airway pressure (CPAP). Note negative pleural pressure swings in the negative direction (resulting from respiratory muscle contraction) to produce the delivered tidal volume. *B,* An increase in CPAP shifts the pleural pressure in a positive direction, but respiratory muscle effort and tidal volume are unchanged. *C,* Noninvasive positive pressure ventilation. Note that pleural pressure swings are smaller (respiratory muscle unloading) and tidal volume is increased. *D,* An increase in expiratory positive airway pressure (EPAP) increases the pleural pressure. Because the inspiratory positive airway pressure (IPAP) is increased by the same magnitude as the EPAP, respiratory muscle unloading and tidal volume are unchanged. *E,* A decrease in IPAP results in a decrease in tidal volume. *F,* Negative pressure ventilation. Pleural pressure swings and tidal volume are increased because of the negative pressure applied to the chest wall.

cussed in this chapter. **Noninvasive positive pressure ventilation (NPPV), negative pressure ventilation (NPV),** and CPAP are compared in Figure 43-1.

Noninvasive Positive Pressure Ventilation

Acute Care Applications

Recently clinical interest has intensified on the provision of mechanical ventilation by noninvasive means to selected patients with acute respiratory failure.[1,2] Many controlled and uncontrolled clinical trials of NPPV for acute respiratory failure have been published.[3] In the controlled studies the predominant diagnosis was chronic obstructive pulmonary disease (COPD), although NPPV has been used successfully in patients with other diagnoses. A primary outcome variable in controlled studies of NPPV is the requirement for intubation, with a lower intubation rate for patients receiving NPPV. In a meta-analysis, NPPV was associated with a lower need for endotracheal intubation and decreased mortality.[4] Improved long-term survival has been reported for patients receiving NPPV during acute respiratory failure at 6 months and at 12 months for patients who received NPPV.[5,6] The incidence of ventilator-associated pneumonia (VAP) also has been shown to be lower in patients receiving NPPV compared with invasive ventilatory support.[7,8] In a prospective epi-

demiologic survey of VAP in patients receiving invasive and noninvasive ventilatory support, one study reported a fourfold greater risk of VAP in patients receiving invasive ventilatory support, even when corrected for severity of illness.[7] In addition to avoidance of intubation, the use of NPPV is reportedly beneficial in the weaning of patients with COPD from invasive ventilatory support.[9,10] In such studies, selected patients were extubated to NPPV instead of being maintained on invasive ventilatory support until the time of extubation.

Respiratory Recap

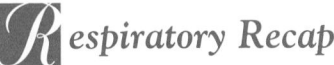

Benefits of NPPV for Acute Respiratory Failure
Decreased intubation rate
Improved survival
Decreased pneumonia rates

Appropriate patient selection is an important predictor of success. Common selection criteria include acute respiratory distress (moderate to severe dyspnea, accessory muscle use, tachypnea) and acute hypercapnia (pH <7.35 and $PaCO_2$ >45 mm Hg). Patients with a rapidly reversible process (for example, within 48 hours) may derive the greatest benefit from NPPV for acute respiratory failure. The routine use of NPPV, without careful patient selection, provides no benefit to patients with COPD.[11] Common exclusion criteria include the need for airway protection (for example, impaired neurologic state, upper airway obstruction, inability to clear secretions), inability to fit the mask or other interface, and lack of cooperation with the technique.

Respiratory Recap

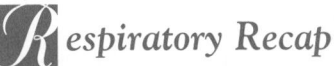

Exclusions for NPPV
Need for airway protection
Inability to fit mask or other interface
Uncooperative patient

The strongest evidence of the effectiveness of NPPV for acute respiratory failure comes from patients with acute decompensation of COPD.[3,12] Although the strongest evidence (that is, controlled clinical trials) suggests that NPPV is more likely to be successful for patients with COPD and/or hypercapnic respiratory failure, NPPV has been used successfully in the treatment of hypoxemic respiratory failure. The role of NPPV in patients with acute cardiogenic pulmonary edema is unclear. One study reported a higher rate of myocardial infarction (MI) in patients with acute cardiogenic pulmonary edema randomized to receive NPPV, compared with those who received mask CPAP.[13] In a study of patients with acute cardiogenic pulmonary edema, a high rate of NPPV failure was reported in patients with acute MI.[14] Based on the available evidence, NPPV should be avoided in patients with cardiogenic pulmonary edema secondary to acute MI.

The initial response to NPPV may predict success or failure. A more rapid decrease in $PaCO_2$ occurs in patients in which NPPV is successful. Unsuccessful nasal NPPV has been associated with greater severity of illness, greater mouth leak, and increased difficulty acclimating to NPPV.[15] The greater mouth leak was associated with patients who were edentulous, had excess secretions, and used pursed-lip breathing. Success of NPPV also has been reported to be greater for patients with higher baseline pH levels, perhaps because low pH was considered a marker of more severe illness.[16] A good level of consciousness also has been associated with successful responses to NPPV for patients with COPD and acute hypercapnic respiratory failure.[17]

Chronic Applications

Another trend is the use of NPPV for chronic respiratory failure resulting from restrictive lung disease, COPD, and nocturnal hypoventilation. In some patients with severe neuromuscular disease, NPPV may be used to provide full ventilatory support.[18,19] In many patients receiving chronic NPPV, however, the therapy is administered only at night. Common goals of this therapy are to improve symptoms (for example, fatigue, morning headache), to decrease $PaCO_2$, and to decrease the degree of nocturnal arterial oxygen desaturation. A major concern regarding chronic use of NPPV is the cost of this therapy, particularly if patient selection is inappropriate. A recent consensus statement recommended clinical indications for the use of NPPV in chronic applications (Box 43-1).[20] A recent randomized controlled trial reported that domiciliary use of NPPV (average inspiratory pressure of 16 cm H_2O) resulted in improvements in exercise tolerance and quality of life.[21] These results are of particular interest because the benefit was reported after only 12 weeks of treatment, and the patients used the ventilator only about 2 hours per day on average (although they were instructed to use it 8 hours per day). This finding suggests a potential benefit of daily short-

term use of NPPV in patients with COPD. However, a 1-year controlled trial of NPPV in patients with severe COPD reported no effect on the natural course of the disease and marginal benefit for stable COPD.[22]

Patient Interface

Patient interfaces for NPPV include basic plastic masks, masks with bubble cushions, masks with gel cushions, masks that engulf the entire nose, and those that cover only the nares. Some patients, especially mouth breathers, may do better with an oronasal mask, whereas others prefer a mask that covers the entire face from forehead to under the chin. The use of nasal prongs, also referred to as *nasal pillows*, offers another option. Most brands of masks are available in two or more sizes to accommodate and comfortably fit the many sizes and shapes

---

$\mathcal{B}$OX 43-1

Clinical Indications for Noninvasive Positive Pressure Ventilation in Chronic Respiratory Failure

> **Restrictive Thoracic Disorders**
> *Examples:* Sequelae of polio, spinal cord injury, neuropathies, myopathies and dystrophies, amyotrophic lateral sclerosis (ALS), chest wall deformities, kyphoscoliosis
> *Symptoms:* Fatigue, dyspnea, morning headache
> *Physiologic criteria:* $PaCO_2 \geq 45$ mm Hg, nocturnal oximetry demonstrating oxygen saturation $\leq 88\%$ for 5 consecutive minutes, maximal inspiratory pressures < -60 cm H_2O or forced vital capacity $<50\%$ of predicted
>
> **Chronic Obstructive Pulmonary Disease**
> *Examples:* Chronic bronchitis, emphysema, bronchiectasis, cystic fibrosis
> *Symptoms:* Fatigue, dyspnea, morning headache
> *Physiologic criteria:* $PaCO_2 \geq 55$ mm Hg, $PaCO_2$ of 50 to 54 mm Hg and nocturnal oximetry demonstrating oxygen saturation $\leq 88\%$ for 5 consecutive minutes while receiving oxygen therapy ≥ 2 L/min, $PaCO_2$ of 50 to 54 mm Hg and hospitalization related to recurrent episodes of hypercapnic respiratory failure

Modified from Clinical indications for noninvasive positive pressure ventilation in chronic respiratory failure due to restrictive lung disease, COPD, and nocturnal hypoventilation—a consensus conference report. Chest 1999;16:521-534.

$\mathcal{R}$*espiratory Recap* ————

Goals of Chronic Use of NPPV

Improve symptoms.
Decrease $PaCO_2$.
Decrease degree of nocturnal oxygen desaturation.

$\mathcal{R}$*espiratory Recap* ————

NPPV Interfaces

Nasal mask	Nasal prongs
Oronasal mask	Mouthpieces
Full face mask	

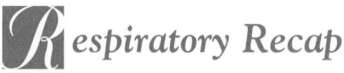

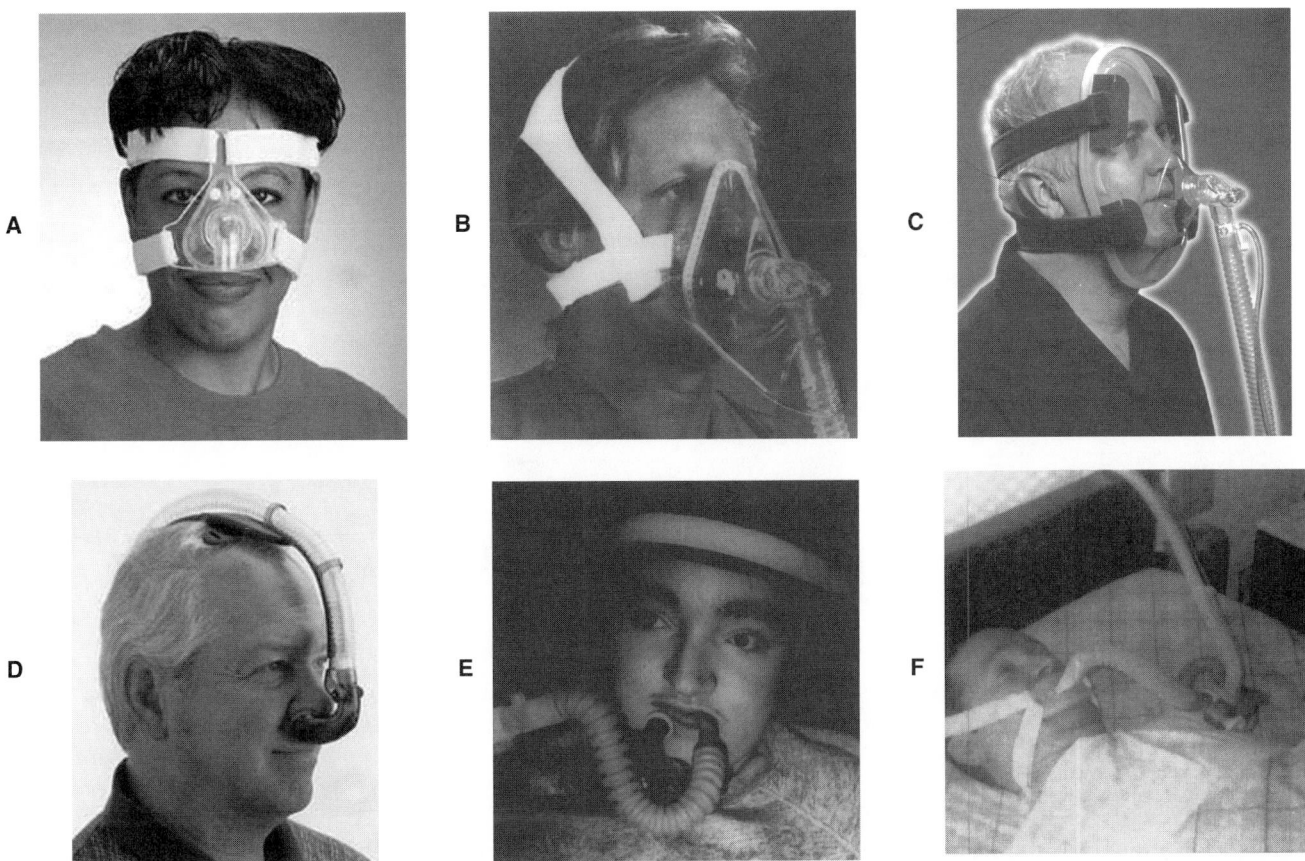

Figure 43-2 Examples of noninvasive positive pressure ventilation (NPPV), or continuous positive airway pressure (CPAP) interfaces. **A,** Nasal mask. **B,** Oronasal mask **C,** Full face mask. **D,** Nasal pillows (prongs). **E,** Mouthpiece. **F,** Mouthpiece with lipseal. (*B,* From Hill NS. Complications of noninvasive positive pressure ventilation. Respir Care 1997;42:432-442. *C,* Courtesy Respironics, Pittsburgh, Pa. *D,* Courtesy Mallinckrodt, Carlsbad, Calif. *E,* From Bach JR, Alba AS, Saporito LR. Intermittent positive pressure ventilation via the mouth as an alternative to tracheostomy for 257 ventilator users. Chest 1993;103:174-182. *F,* From Bach JR. A historical perspective on the use of noninvasive ventilatory support alternatives. Respir Care Clin NA 1996;2:161-181.)

of faces and noses (Figure 43-2). Mouthpieces also can be used to provide NPPV. Having several interfaces available (for example, mouthpiece during the day, mask or nasal pillows at night) may be preferable for patients who use chronic NPPV.

The patient interface has a major impact on patient comfort and compliance during noninvasive ventilation. A poorly fitting interface decreases both the clinical effectiveness and the patient compliance of this therapy. The most commonly used interfaces for NPPV with acute respiratory failure are nasal masks or oronasal masks; each has advantages and disadvantages (Table 43-1). They can be custom-molded, but this feature is generally unnecessary because of the variety of sizes and designs commercially available. Desirable features of a mask for noninvasive ventilation include a low dead space, a transparent design, and an adequate seal with low facial pressure; the mask should be lightweight, easy to secure, disposable or easy to clean, nonirritating to the skin (nonallergenic), and inexpensive.

The mask cushion comes into contact with the face and produces the seal between the mask and the patient. Although the cushion should minimize air leak during noninvasive ventilation, leaks are common and may not necessarily compromise the effectiveness of noninvasive ventilation. The cushion should be soft and malleable to the facial anatomy. The traditional cushion available on anesthesia and resuscitation oronasal masks was a hard plastic or air-filled cushion. These masks are not desirable for noninvasive ventilation because they seal poorly and apply high pressure to the face, which is uncomfortable and increases the likelihood of facial pressure sores. Many commercially available oronasal masks now have a soft air-filled cushion or a soft foam-filled cushion. Some oronasal masks have an inflatable cushion, allowing air to be added or removed from the mask after it is fitted to the patient for improved mask fit. Most nasal or oronasal masks designed specifically for noninvasive ventilation use an open cushion with an inner lip. With this design the cushion pushes against the face as pressure increases

*T*ABLE 43-1

Comparison of Advantages and Disadvantages of Nasal Versus Oronasal Masks

Mask	Advantages	Disadvantages
Nasal	Less risk of aspiration	Mouth leak
	Easier secretion clearance	Less effectiveness with nasal obstruction
	Less claustrophobia	Nasal irritation and rhinorrhea
	Easier speech	Mouth dryness
	Less dead space	
Oronasal	More effective for dyspneic patients	Increased dead space
		Difficulty in maintenance of adequate seal
		Increased risk of facial pressure sores
		Claustrophobia
		Increased aspiration risk
		More difficulty with speech
		Inability to eat
		More difficulty with secretion clearance
		Asphyxiation with ventilator malfunction

inside the mask. With a correctly sized mask, this design should minimize leak and improve comfort with noninvasive ventilation.

Selecting the correct mask size is critical.[23] The nasal mask should fit just above the junction of the nasal bone and cartilage, directly at the sides of both nares, and just below the nose above the upper lip. The oronasal mask should fit from just above the junction of the nasal bone and cartilage to just below the lower lip. Sizing gauges are available to properly fit masks. These sizing gauges are mask specific and cannot be interchanged between manufacturers or different mask styles of the same manufacturer. A common mistake is to choose a mask that is too large, which results in leaks, decreased effectiveness, and patient discomfort. An assortment of various mask styles and sizes should be available. The patient may have to try several masks before finding the best fit.

Leaks through the mouth are not uncommon with the nasal mask. Typically, leaks are more problematic during acute respiratory failure than during chronic applications. When mouth leak interferes with the effectiveness of ventilation, a chin strap or an oronasal mask can be used. Upper airway dryness may occur with the use of a nasal mask and mouth leak. Heated humidification or an oronasal mask may reduce discomfort.[24,25] The greatest concerns with an oronasal mask are aspiration in case of regurgitation and asphyxiation in the event of a ventilator mal-

function. Commercial oronasal masks now are available with antiasphyxia valves and quick-release features. Even with this design, close patient monitoring is prudent whenever an oronasal mask is used for noninvasive ventilation.

The choice of interface for NPPV often is based on patient or clinician preference. The nasal mask is better tolerated by patients than the oronasal mask or nasal pillows.[26] However, minute ventilation and $PaCO_2$ are better with an oronasal mask or nasal pillows than with a nasal mask. For acute respiratory failure, NPPV often is initiated with an oronasal mask. As the patient's respiratory failure improves, the transition is made to a nasal interface (nasal mask or nasal pillows). For chronic applications a nasal mask is most commonly used because of improved patient comfort.

An appropriate headgear or harness is needed to maintain the correct position of the mask. Elastic straps with holes that attach to hooks are commonly used with oronasal masks. The hooks on oronasal masks can be either on the outer edge of the mask or more commonly, near the center of the mask. Attachment of the headgear to the outer edge of the mask may better distribute the pressure of the mask and facilitate a seal. Most masks designed specifically for noninvasive ventilation use cloth straps and Velcro to secure the mask. The cloth straps fit through slots at the sides and top of the mask. Use of Velcro to secure the mask allows nearly infinite headgear adjustments.

A common mistake is to fit the headgear too tightly. The clinician or patient should be able to pass one or two fingers between the headgear and the face. Fitting the headgear too tightly usually does not improve the fit and always decreases patient comfort and compliance. The design of most masks for noninvasive ventilation is such that the top of the mask is secured on the forehead rather than at the bridge of the nose. Forehead spacers are an important feature of this design. These cushions fill the gap be-

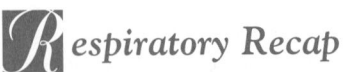

*R*espiratory Recap

Choosing an Interface
Use the proper interface for the patient.
Avoid an interface that is too large.

tween the forehead and the mask, thus reducing pressure on the bridge of the nose, improving comfort and decreasing the likelihood of pressure sores.

Aerophagia commonly occurs with noninvasive mask ventilation, but this occurrence is usually benign because the airway pressure is less than the esophageal opening pressure. Therefore a gastric tube is not routinely necessary for mask ventilation. In fact, a gastric tube may interfere with the effectiveness of mask ventilation in several ways. Achieving a mask seal may be more difficult if a gastric tube is present. Compression of the gastric tube against the face by the mask cushion may increase the likelihood of facial skin breakdown. A nasogastric tube increases resistance to nasal gas flow, which may decrease the effectiveness of mask ventilation (particularly nasal mask ventilation).

Pressure sores on the bridge of the nose are a common complaint during noninvasive ventilation. Fortunately, ulceration and skin breakdown are prevented in many patients. Signs of soreness at the bridge of the nose should alert the clinician to reduce pressure injury using the following strategies:

- Reassess correct mask fit and size.
- Reduce the tension of the headgear.
- Try a different mask style.
- Apply a wound care dressing over the bridge of the nose.

Ventilators for Noninvasive Positive Pressure Ventilation

Critical care ventilators are commonly available in most hospitals to provide noninvasive ventilation. Theoretically any ventilator can attach to a mask rather than to an artificial airway to provide noninvasive ventilation. This approach has the advantages of precise control of F_{IO_2}, various modes and inspiratory flow patterns, and separation of inspiratory and expiratory gases to limit rebreathing. Critical care ventilators have extensive monitoring devices and alarms, which are desirable during invasive ventilation but can be distracting and annoying (for patients and clinicians) during noninvasive ventilation. Although critical care ventilators are more expensive than noninvasive ventilators, this is not important unless the hospital inventory of critical care ventilators can be reduced in favor of noninvasive ventilators. The greatest disadvantage of critical care ventilators is their difficulty

in dealing with leaks that invariably occur during noninvasive ventilation.

Pressure-limited ventilation commonly is used for NPPV. A theoretic advantage of pressure ventilation is that it varies the inspiratory flow as needed to meet the demands of the patient, a feature which should improve patient comfort during NPPV. One study reported that both pressure-support and volume-control modes similarly improved breathing pattern and gas exchange.[27] In that study the inspiratory workload was less with volume control, but patient comfort was greater with pressure support. Another study reported no physiologic differences during NPPV with volume-control or pressure-support ventilation.[26]

Pressure support can be problematic when noninvasive ventilation is provided with a critical care ventilator. Critical care ventilators cycle to the expiratory phase during pressure support when the flow decreases to ventilator preset level (for example, 5 L/min or 25% of peak inspiratory flow). If the leak is greater than the flow at which the ventilator cycles, then inspiration is prolonged and patient compliance reduced.[28] For some ventilators the inspiratory termination flow during pressure support can be adjusted. Alternatively, pressure control with a short inspiratory time (≤ 1 second) can be used rather than pressure support. One study reported increased patient comfort during time-cycled pressure ventilation (that is, pressure control) compared with flow-cycled ventilation (that is, pressure support).[29] Even without a leak, patients with COPD may have a prolonged inspiratory time with pressure support using a critical care ventilator[30,31] and may benefit from pressure control or pressure support using a ventilator in which the termination flow can be adjusted. During NPPV a relatively narrow range for inspiratory termination flow may provide adequate ventilation without causing hyperinflation.[32]

Conventional home care ventilators have been used to provide noninvasive ventilation, particularly for patients with neuromuscular diseases. These ventilators function well when little patient-ventilator interaction occurs, such as with neuromuscular disease. Generally the trigger on these ventilators is poor, and inspiratory flow is fixed, which limits their use for noninvasive ventilation during acute respiratory failure. Similar to critical care ventilators, these machines generally do not tolerate large leaks, although an increase in the delivered tidal volume somewhat compensates for leaks. These ventilators have a limited number of alarms and operate from internal or external batteries during external power failure, both of which are benefits for home use. They perform best for patients with neuromuscular disease who require volume-controlled noninvasive ventilation. These ventilators have a true exhalation valve, so carbon dioxide rebreathing is not a problem.

Portable pressure ventilators are available from several manufacturers specifically to provide NPPV (Figure 43-3).

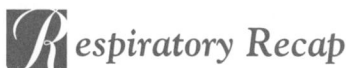

Respiratory Recap

Ventilators for NPPV
Critical care ventilators
Home care ventilators
Portable pressure ventilators

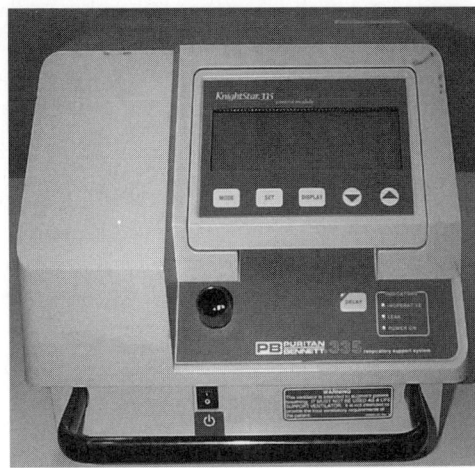
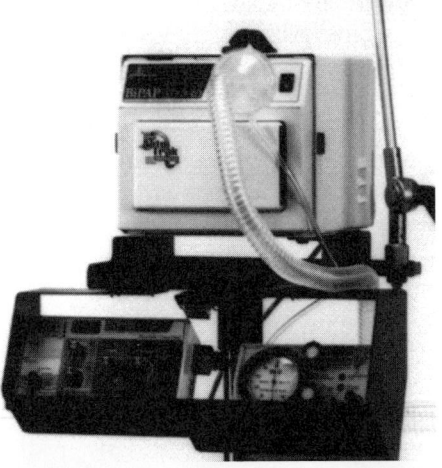
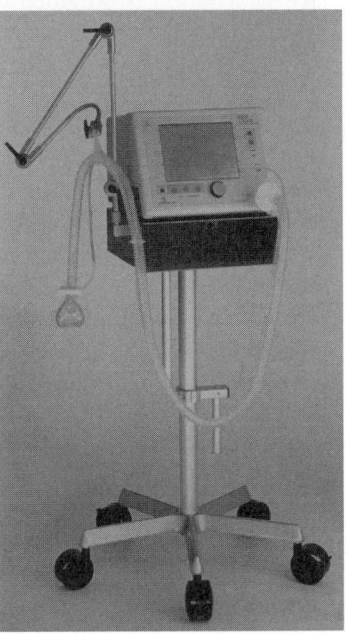
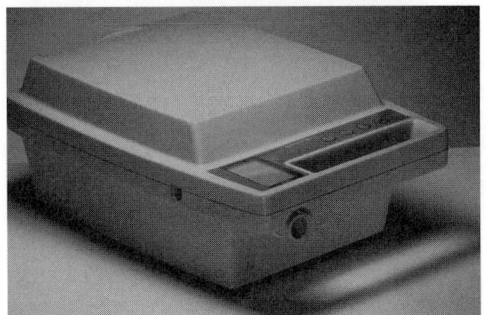

Figure 43-3 Portable pressure ventilators for noninvasive positive pressure ventilation. (*Bottom right,* Courtesy ResMed, Poway, Calif.)

Their major advantage is their ability to function correctly in the presence of leaks. In fact, they require a leak to function correctly. They are blower devices that vary inspiratory and expiratory pressures in response to patient demand. These ventilators provide pressure ventilation; none provides volume ventilation. Although they can be used to provide pressure-controlled ventilation in the absence of patient effort, they are usually used to provide pressure-support ventilation. These ventilators typically

provide modest inspiratory (≤ 30 cm H_2O) and expiratory (≤ 15 cm H_2O) pressures.

For ventilators designed specifically to provide NPPV, inspiratory pressure is called **inspiratory positive airway pressure (IPAP)** and expiratory pressure is called **expiratory positive airway pressure (EPAP).** IPAP is usually the absolute inspiratory pressure and includes the expiratory pressure, which differs from most critical care ventilators, in which the inspiratory pressure setting is above the level of expiratory pressure. EPAP is synonymous with CPAP. The difference between IPAP and EPAP is the level of pressure support. The IPAP level must be changed if the EPAP level is changed to maintain a constant pressure-support level.

Two important issues relate to how well these ventilators trigger the inspiratory phase and cycle to the expiratory phase. Some noninvasive ventilators automatically adjust the inspiratory trigger and expiratory cycle by tracking the patient's inspiratory and expiratory flows. Others allow the clinician to adjust the trigger and/or cy-

$\mathcal{R}$*espiratory Recap*

Portable Pressure Ventilators for NPPV

Use blower devices
Allow adjustment of IPAP and EPAP
Associated with CO_2 rebreathing, which can be problematic
Adjust F_{IO_2} by titration

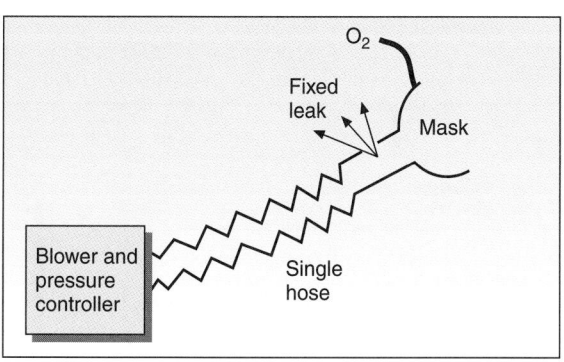

Figure 43-4   Schematic drawing of a portable pressure ventilator to provide noninvasive positive pressure ventilation.

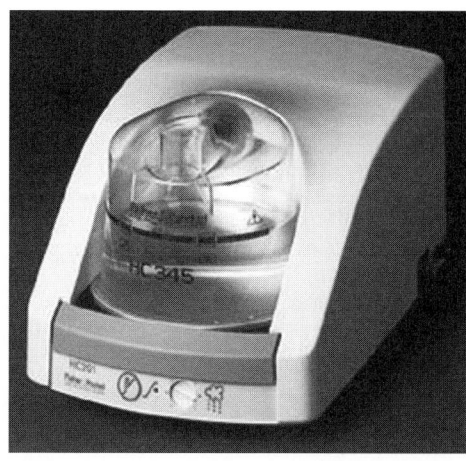

Figure 43-5   An in-line heated humidifier consisting of a temperature-adjustable heating plate and a removable/replaceable water chamber. (Courtesy Fisher & Paykel, Laguna Hills, Calif.)

cle. The ability to adjust the trigger sensitivity allows the clinician to balance the ability of the patient to initiate the inspiratory phase and the tendency of the ventilator to auto-trigger. The ability to adjust the cycle sensitivity is a balance between premature termination of the inspiratory phase and active expiratory muscle activity to terminate the inspiratory phase. Studies of the performance of NPPV ventilators report them to be satisfactory for many commercially available devices.[32-37]

A concern with portable pressure ventilators, particularly for patients with hypercapnic respiratory failure, is the potential for CO_2 rebreathing.[38,39] Most of these ventilators use a single hose without a true exhalation valve (Figure 43-4). Expired gas passes through a fixed leak established in the device. Particularly with low flow from the ventilator, as may occur with low EPAP levels, inadequate flushing of CO_2 and subsequent rebreathing may occur. This problem can be resolved by the use of higher EPAP levels (≥ 6 cm H_2O) or a valve that prevents rebreathing. Increasing the leak flow also flushes CO_2 from the system. Theoretically a fixed leak in the mask should produce less rebreathing than a fixed leak in the hose.

Precise and constant oxygen administration is nearly impossible with portable pressure ventilators.[40] Typically supplemental oxygen is titrated into the inspiratory circuit at the ventilator outlet or directly into the mask. In each case, the FIO_2 is determined by the oxygen flow and ventilatory pattern. Thus the FIO_2 varies as the ventilatory pattern changes. Because of the high flow from the ventilator, achievement of an FIO_2 greater than 0.50 is generally difficult. Newer-generation noninvasive ventilators allow the user to precisely set the FIO_2.

The appropriate role of alarms and monitoring for noninvasive ventilators is controversial. Many patients receiving this therapy can sustain adequate spontaneous breathing for short periods of time without ventilatory support. Nonetheless, disconnect and power-loss alarms are recommended.[1] Airway pressure and volume monitors are desirable but not mandatory for acutely ill patients in whom noninvasive ventilation is used. Newer-generation noninvasive ventilators provide sophisticated monitoring (including graphics), alarms, and backup ventilatory support in the event of apnea.

Humidity is added by placement of a humidifier between the ventilator and the patient interface. A cool, ambient-temperature, passover humidifier chamber adds a small amount of water vapor to the air flowing to the patient. However, because of the velocity and volume of airflow, the limited surface area of the water chamber, and the evaporative cooling effect, the water content of the air being delivered to the patient increases only slightly. For some patients this may be enough to minimize nasal mucous membrane drying. For others a heated humidifier may be necessary. Heating the water in the reservoir counters the effects of evaporative cooling and raises the temperature of the air passing through the humidifier, allowing it to carry more water content (Figure 43-5).

In-line nebulizer therapy also can be provided during NPPV. To improve drug delivery, the nebulizer should be placed near the mask rather than at the outlet of the ventilator during NPPV. Although the amount of aerosol that penetrates the upper airway may be reduced during NPPV, a sufficient quantity is delivered to the lungs to produce a physiologic response.[41,42]

Caregiver Issues

Successful NPPV requires commitment by those caring for the patient (physicians, nurses, respiratory therapists).[43,44] Some clinicians are reluctant to initiate NPPV because they are concerned about time requirements and potential difficulties. Fitting the mask, selecting appropriate ventilator settings, and coaching the patient may be labor intensive for the first hours of NPPV. During the first 8 hours the time requirement for respiratory therapists has been reported as greater for patients treated with

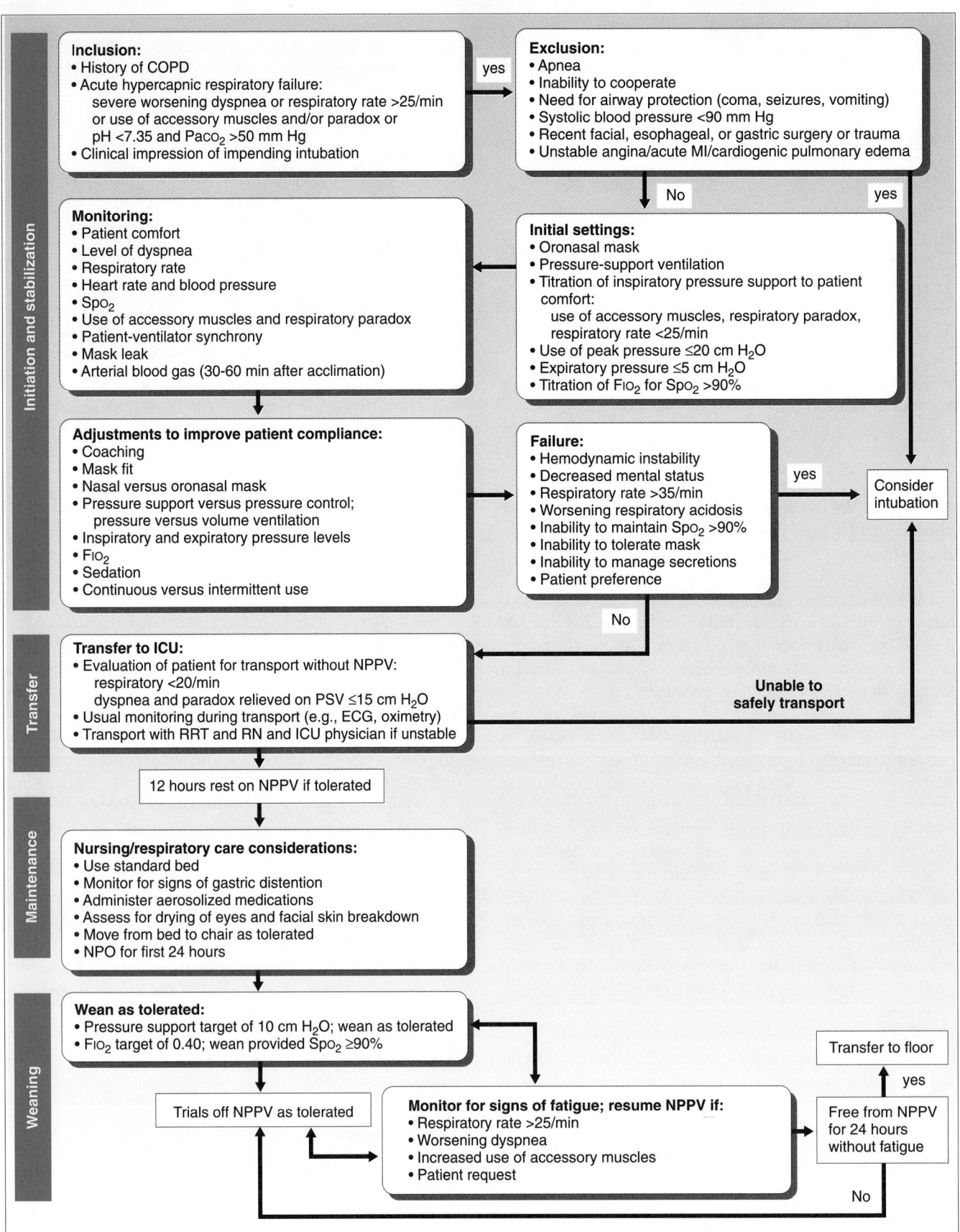

Figure 43-6 An algorithm for noninvasive positive pressure ventilation (NPPV) to treat acute respiratory failure. *COPD*, Chronic obstructive pulmonary disease; *Spo₂*, oxygen saturation measured by pulse oximetry; *PSV*, pressure-support ventilation; *RRT*, registered respiratory therapist; *RN*, registered nurse; *ICU*, intensive care unit; *ECG*, electrocardiography; *NPO*, nothing by mouth; *Paco₂*, partial pressure of arterial carbon dioxide; *MI*, myocardial infarction.

*Monitoring the Effect of Noninvasive Positive
Pressure Ventilation (NPPV)*

Response to NPPV
Physiologic: ABG, oximetry
Objective: Respiratory rate, hemodynamics
Subjective: Dyspnea, comfort, neurologic status

Mask
Fit
Comfort
Leak
Skin breakdown

Respiratory Muscle Unloading
Accessory muscle use
Thoracoabdominal paradox

Abdomen
Gastric distention
Activation during inspiration

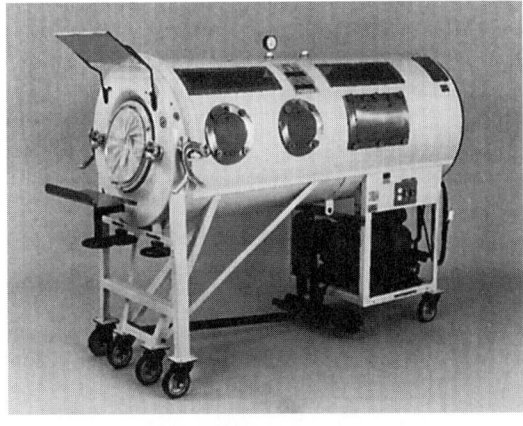

Figure 43-7   Iron lung. (From Gilmartin ME. Body ventilators. Equipment and techniques. Respir Care Clin N Am 1996;2:195-222.)

- Silence alarms and choose low settings.
- Initiate NPPV while holding mask in place.
- Secure mask, avoiding a tight fit.
- Titrate inspiratory pressure to patient comfort.
- Titrate FIO_2 to SpO_2 >90%.
- Avoid peak pressure >20 cm H_2O.
- Titrate expiratory pressure per trigger effort and SpO_2.
- Continue to coach and reassure patient; make adjustments to improve patient compliance.

Figure 43-6 is an algorithm for the initiation of NPPV for patients suffering acute respiratory failure.

Complications of NPPV are usually minor and include leaks, mask discomfort, eye irritation, facial skin breakdown, sinus congestion, oropharyngeal drying, patient-ventilator dyssynchrony, gastric insufflation, and hemodynamic compromise.[49] Parameters that should be monitored during NPPV are listed in Box 43-2.[50] The best approach to weaning from NPPV is unclear. In many cases the patient requests removal of the mask after several hours of therapy. If the patient's condition deteriorates after removal of the mask, then the therapy should be resumed.

Negative Pressure Ventilation, Rocking Beds, and Pneumobelts

Negative pressure ventilators (body ventilators) provide intermittent subatmospheric pressure around the thorax and abdomen.[51,52] Typically the patient is partially enclosed in a chamber, with the ventilator providing negative pressure to the area between the chamber and the chest wall. This subatmospheric pressure is transmitted to the pleural space, which promotes gas flow into the lungs. The prototype negative pressure ventilator was the **iron lung** (or tank ventilator), which was popular during the polio epidemic 50 years ago and remains in limited use today (Figure 43-7). The **cuirass** (also called the *chest shell*

NPPV than those intubated.[45] Respiratory therapy time decreased significantly for the second 8 hours and was less for patients treated with NPPV than those who received conventional therapy.

Another study also has reported a greater time requirement by respiratory therapists for NPPV than for invasive mechanical ventilation.[46] However, the total time required of physicians and nurses may not differ for invasive and noninvasive ventilation.[46,47] Although the first hour of NPPV is labor intensive, this time is well worth the benefit of avoiding intubation and a long course of invasive mechanical ventilation. NPPV for the treatment of acute exacerbation of COPD has been shown to be cost effective.[48]

Clinical Application

The application of NPPV requires caregiver patience and skills with both the technical aspects of mechanical ventilation and patient coaching to adapt to the mask and ventilator. In many cases the appropriate settings for NPPV are determined largely by trial-and-error, with appropriate feedback from the patient. The primary goal in the initiation of NPPV is patient comfort and not an improvement in arterial blood gases per se. (An improvement in blood gases usually follows if patient comfort and respiratory muscle unloading are achieved.) Important steps in the clinical application of NPPV are as follows:

- Choose a ventilator capable of meeting patient needs (usually pressure ventilation).
- Choose the correct interface; avoid a mask that is too large.
- Explain therapy to the patient.

or *turtle shell*) consists of a lightweight rigid dome that fits over the anterior chest wall (Figure 43-8) and connects to a negative pressure generator. Other versions of negative pressure ventilators include the wrap devices (ponchos, body suits, and pneumosuits) that fit over the patient, sur-

round a semicylindric grid, and attach to a negative pressure generator (Figure 43-9).

With the increased popularity of NPPV, negative pressure devices are no longer in common use. However, they provide a treatment option for patients who cannot use NPPV. Negative pressure devices are more complex and bulky than NPPV devices. In addition, negative pressure devices can produce upper airway obstruction and thus are contraindicated in patients with obstructive sleep apnea (OSA). Selection criteria for body ventilators are outlined in Table 43-2, and typical settings for these devices are provided in Table 43-3.

An unconventional ventilation device is the **rocking bed** (Figure 43-10). The action of the rocking bed has been compared with a piston in a cylinder. As the patient's head moves down, the piston-like viscera and diaphragm slide cephalad within the cylinder-like chest wall, assisting exhalation. In the foot-down position the abdominal contents and diaphragm slide caudad, assisting inhalation. Another unconventional ventilation device is the **pneumobelt** (Figure 43-11). It consists of an inflatable rubber bladder held over the abdomen by an adjustable corset and assists diaphragmatic motion by causing piston-like motions of the abdominal viscera.

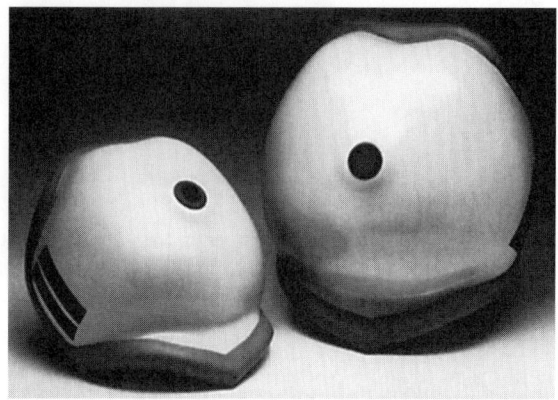

Figure 43-8   Chest shells (cuirass) to provide negative pressure ventilation. (From Gilmartin ME. Body ventilators. Equipment and techniques. Respir Care Clin N Am 1996;2:195-222.)

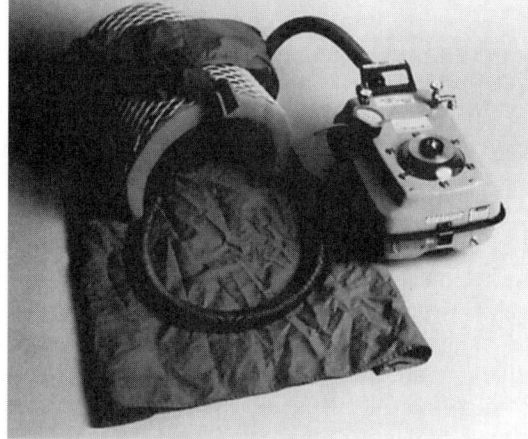

A

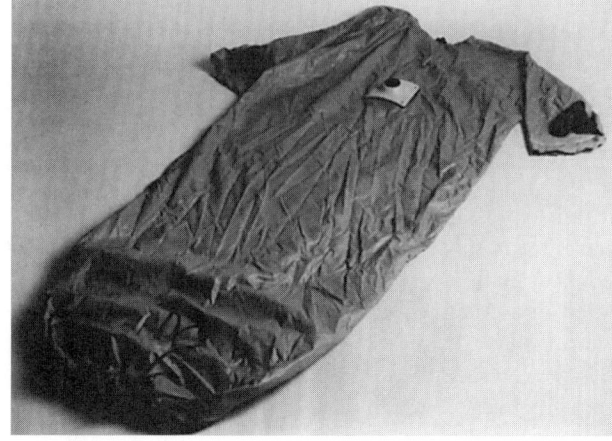

B

Figure 43-9   **A,** Poncho wrap. **B,** Pneumosuit. (From Gilmartin ME. Body ventilators. Equipment and techniques. Respir Care Clin N Am 1996;2:195-222.)

TABLE 43-2

Selection Criteria for Body Ventilators

Considerations	Possible Solutions
Patient preference	
Portability	Wrap, cuirass, pneumobelt
Convenience	Rocking bed, cuirass
Freedom of hands and face	Rocking bed, pneumobelt
Efficiency and reliability	Iron lung
Diagnosis	
Bilateral diaphragm paralysis	Rocking bed, pneumobelt
High spinal cord lesion	Pneumobelt
Obstructive sleep apnea	Noninvasive positive pressure ventilation
Body habitus	
Marked kyphoscoliosis or obesity	Noninvasive positive pressure ventilation, iron lung

TABLE 43-3

Typical Settings for Body Ventilators

Ventilator	Rate (breaths/min)	Pressure (cm H₂O)
Iron lung	12 to 24	−10 to −35
Porta lung	12 to 24	−10 to −35
Wrap	14 to 28	−15 to −45
Shell	14 to 28	−15 to −45
Pneumobelt	12 to 24	+15 to +50
Rocking bed	12 to 24	40°

Continuous Positive Airway Pressure

CPAP has applications in both the acute care and chronic care of patients. In acute care, noninvasive (mask) CPAP is used to administer intermittent lung expansion therapy, to treat acute hypoxemic respiratory failure, and to treat acute cardiogenic pulmonary edema. In chronic care, CPAP is used to treat OSA.

Acute Care Applications

Intermittent mask CPAP with 5 to 10 cm H_2O has been used for a prophylactic postoperative respiratory therapy.[53-59]

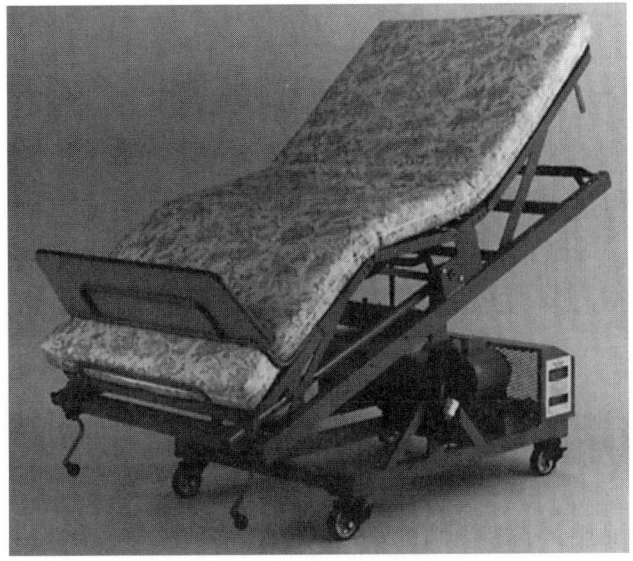

Figure 43-10 Rocking bed. (From Gilmartin ME. Body ventilators. Equipment and techniques. Respir Care Clin N Am 1996;2:195-222.)

Mask CPAP may be an effortless, painless type of postoperative respiratory care. Nasal mask CPAP at 8 to 10 cm H_2O has been reported as a beneficial method to avoid endotracheal reintubation in postoperative high-risk patients with nonhypercapnic oxygenation failure.[60] Mask CPAP also reportedly improves the safety of bronchoscopy in hypoxemic patients.[61]

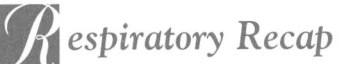

espiratory Recap

Acute Care Applications of Mask CPAP
Postoperative pulmonary complications
Hypoxemic respiratory failure
Cardiogenic pulmonary edema

Mask CPAP (5 to 10 cm H_2O by nasal or oronasal mask) has been used in patients with acute hypoxemic respiratory failure to recruit collapsed alveoli, increase functional residual capacity (FRC), decrease shunt, and increase PaO_2. Its use in this setting is supported by several uncontrolled reports.[62-65] However, the results of a prospective randomized controlled trial comparing mask CPAP with oxygen therapy are less optimistic.[66] Although mask CPAP produced an initial improvement in PaO_2, it did not improve important outcomes such as intubation rate or hospital mortality. Furthermore, a higher number of adverse events occurred with mask CPAP.

The strongest evidence for the use of mask CPAP is for patients with acute cardiogenic pulmonary edema. In these patients the increase in intrathoracic pressure decreases preload, decreases afterload, improves lung compliance, decreases intrapulmonary shunt, and increases PaO_2.

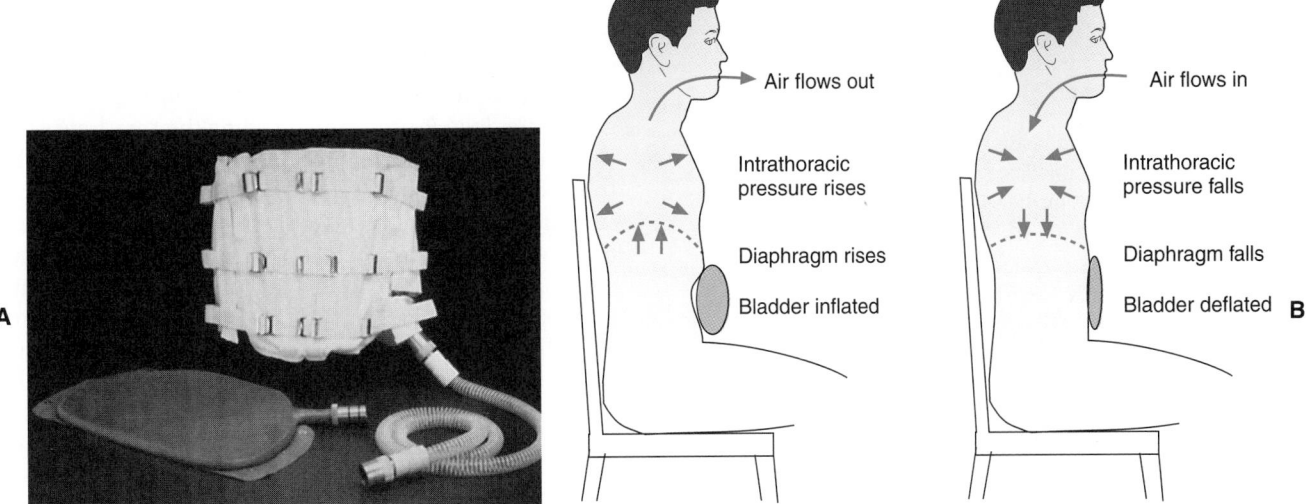

Figure 43-11 **A,** Pneumobelt. **B,** Mode of action of pneumobelt. (Modified from Gilmartin ME. Body ventilators. Equipment and techniques. Respir Care Clin N Am 1996;2:195-222.)

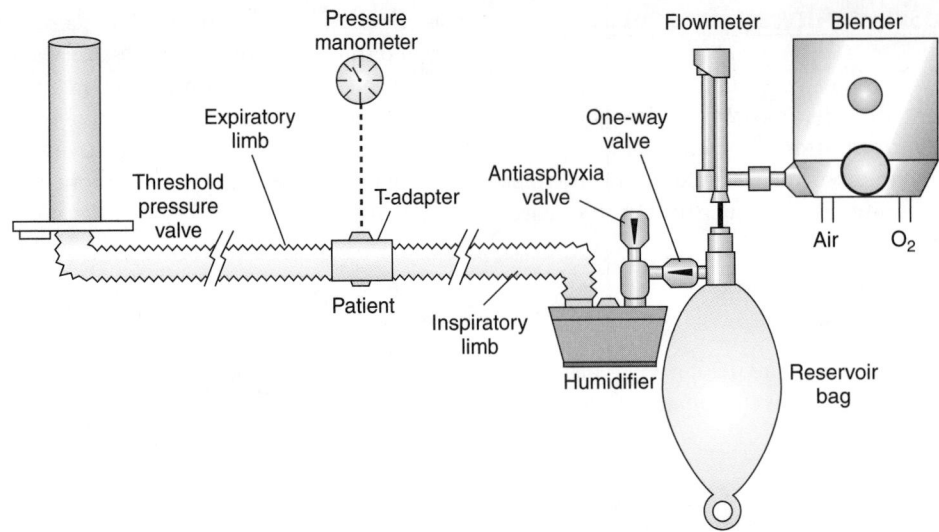

Figure 43-12 Continuous positive airway pressure circuit for acute respiratory failure. (Modified from Branson RD. Spontaneous breathing systems: IMV and CPAP. In: Branson RD, Hess DR, Chatburn RL. Respiratory Care Equipment. 2nd ed. Philadelphia: JB Lippincott; 1999.)

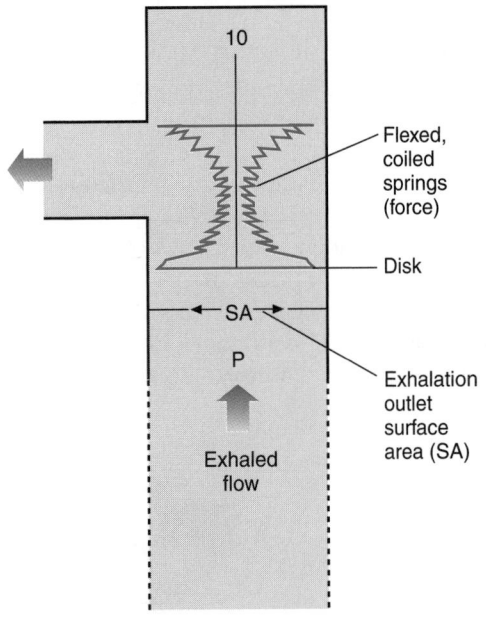

Figure 43-13 Threshold resistor continuous positive airway pressure valve. *P,* Pressure. (Modified from Banner MJ, Lampotang S. Expiratory pressure valves. In: Branson RD, Hess DR, Chatburn RL. Respiratory Care Equipment. 2nd ed. Philadelphia: JB Lippincott, 1999.)

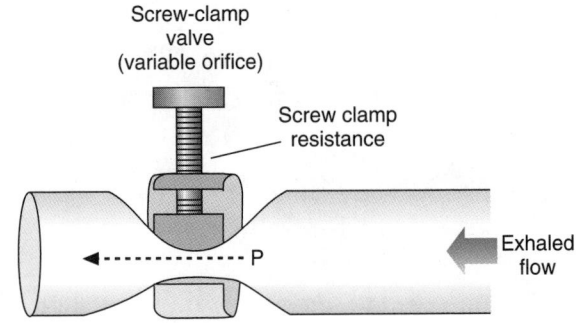

Figure 43-14 Fixed-orifice continuous positive airway pressure valve. (Modified from Banner MJ, Lampotang S. Expiratory pressure valves. In: Branson RD, Hess DR, Chatburn RL. Respiratory Care Equipment. 2nd ed. Philadelphia: JB Lippincott, 1999.)

A typical CPAP level of 5 to 10 cm H_2O is used. A systematic review reported that mask CPAP in these patients decreases the intubation rate and improves survival rate.[67]

The CPAP circuit (Figure 43-12) consists of a high-flow gas source and an expiratory valve that maintains pressure in the circuit at the desired level (5 to 20 cm H_2O).[68] CPAP requires a relatively high gas flow to maintain the desired positive airway pressure. CPAP valves are classified as *threshold resistors* or *fixed orifices*. Threshold resistors maintain a constant pressure in the circuit, regardless of flow. A pressure exceeding the threshold opens the valve and allows expiration, whereas pressures below threshold allow the valve to close, sealing the circuit and stopping the flow of gas. Commonly used threshold resistor devices use spring tension to produce CPAP (Figure 43-13). With the fixed-orifice device a restricted opening of a fixed size is placed at the end of the expiratory limb of a breathing circuit (Figure 43-14). The resistance through the fixed orifice produces back-pressure, which is CPAP pressure produced in the circuit. For a given flow a higher pressure is generated with a smaller orifice. Expiratory pressure is flow dependent, so pressure decreases as flow decreases. The fixed-orifice resistor has been abandoned in adult respiratory care but remains in use in neonatal care.

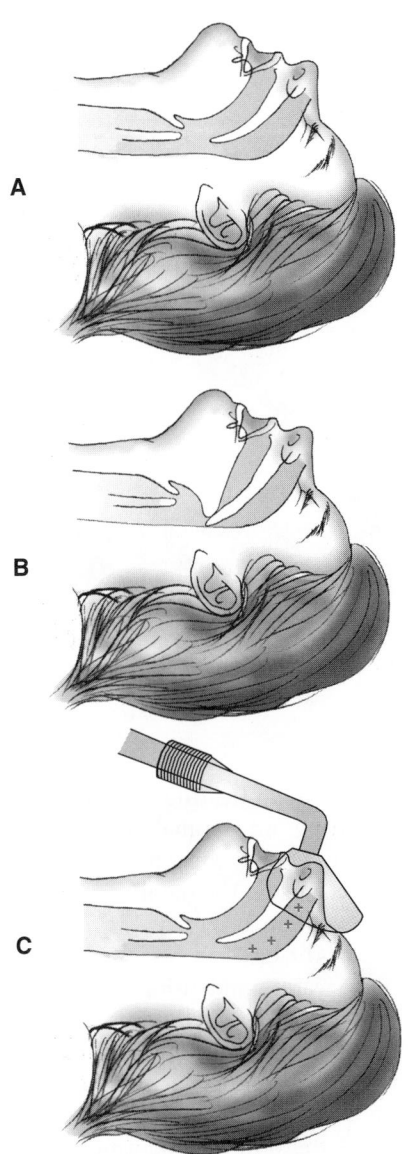

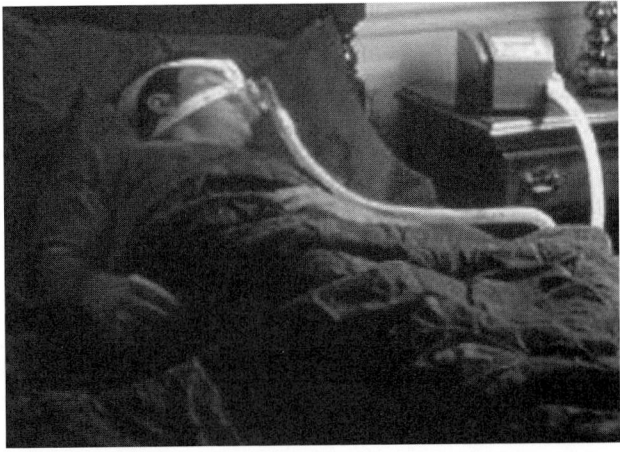

Figure 43-16   Nasal continuous positive airway pressure system in use. (Courtesy Respironics, Pittsburgh, Pa.)

Figure 43-15   A, Normal upper airway. **B,** Upper airway obstruction. **C,** Upper airway obstruction relieved with the addition of continuous positive airway pressure. (Modified from Branson RD. Spontaneous breathing systems: IMV and CPAP. In: Branson RD, Hess DR, Chatburn RL. Respiratory Care Equipment. 2nd ed. Philadelphia: JB Lippincott; 1999.)

Chronic Applications

OSA is a serious, potentially life-threatening condition characterized by repeated collapse of the upper airway during sleep, with subsequent cessation of breathing.[69] The most effective and most widely prescribed noninvasive treatment for OSA is CPAP therapy. When applied at the appropriate pressure setting, CPAP eliminates the soft tissue obstruction of the upper airway. With the mechanical cause of obstruction alleviated the symptoms and effects of OSA quickly vanish (Figure 43-15). With CPAP, air flows through the nasopharynx and oropharynx at a preset pressure to maintain a constant positive pressure within the upper airway. This action has the effect of splinting the soft tissue, preventing its collapse into the airway during sleep and the subsequent obstruction. The CPAP pressure is prescribed after a sleep study during which the pressure is slowly increased (titrated) until the pressure necessary to significantly eliminate the apneas and hypopneas has been achieved.

CPAP was described by Sullivan[70] and Sanders and colleagues[71] as a treatment for OSA. In 1984 the FDA approved CPAP for the treatment of OSA in the home. These first units were large, heavy, and noisy and operated on purely mechanical principles. They have evolved to small (about 10 inches × 5 inches × 6 inches), light (4 to 6 pounds), quiet devices with miniaturized electronics and microprocessors (Figure 43-16).

Numerous brands and models of CPAP machines are commercially available. The basic models are relatively simple devices consisting of an electrically operated flow generator (fan or turbine) that draws in room air through a particulate filter (a gross particulate filter to remove dust, lint and other large airborne matter) and a secondary filter (to capture smaller particles, such as pollen and spores). The prescribed pressure is entered, usually through digital electronics, into the unit's microprocessor, which causes the flow generator to deliver the flow of air necessary to maintain the prescribed pressure. CPAP systems, similar to ventilators for NPPV, are designed to operate with a built-in leak in the circuit. This leak port usually is found in the mask or between the tubing and mask. Because the system is designed to automatically compensate for this leak and to maintain the designated pressure, it also accommodates other small to moderate leaks that occur at the various patient interfaces.

The pressure settings on most CPAP units are in the range of 3 to 20 cm H_2O. Most units also have an adjustable setting referred to as *ramp* or *delay*. When the prescribed pressure is greater than 10 cm H_2O, some CPAP users find it difficult to fall asleep, bothered by the high air flow. Because obstructive episodes do not occur until the patient has been asleep for a period of time, the patient, after putting on the interface and adjusting for any leaks, can activate the ramp/delay feature. This activation causes the pressure to drop to 2 to 4 cm H_2O, a more tolerable level, while the patient falls asleep. The ramp feature can be preset to from 5 to 45 minutes. The unit's microprocessor divides the set prescribed pressure by the number of ramp minutes and, beginning at 2 to 4 cm H_2O, delivers an increasing pressure until the prescribed level is reached, by which time the patient has been able to fall asleep.

The patient interface used for nocturnal CPAP therapy is the same as that used for NPPV. The interface tends to be the most troublesome point in the achievement and maintenance of long-term compliance. Selecting the most appropriate interface and the correct size for each individual patient is one of the most important aspects determining whether a patient will be successful in long-term use of CPAP therapy. Inappropriate selection of the interface and its size, or incorrect selection, fitting, or adjustment of the headgear results in air leaks around the mask (especially around the bridge of the nose at the corners of the eyes) and skin irritation, which can lead to tissue breakdown and ulceration. Care by the sleep laboratory personnel and the home medical equipment provider in selecting, fitting, and adjusting the interface and taking adequate time to fully train the patient and family members in the proper techniques used to apply, adjust, maintain, and clean the interface significantly enhances patient compliance.

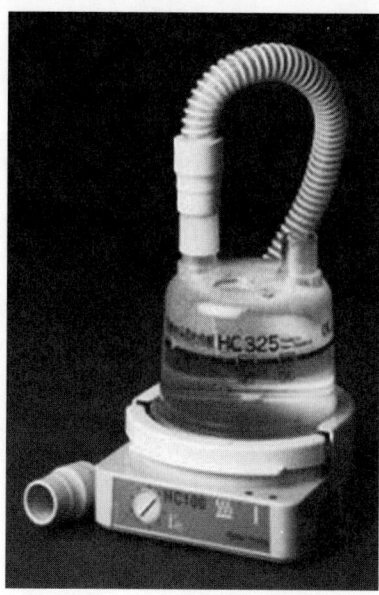

Figure 43-17 A nasal continuous positive airway pressure unit combined with a built-in heated humidifier. (Courtesy Fisher & Paykel, Laguna Hills, Calif.)

ℛ*espiratory Recap*

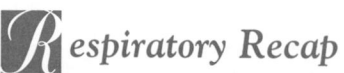

Factors Affecting CPAP Compliance
Poor patient education and understanding
Improper interface size, selection, and fit
Drying of nose and mouth
High inward flow during expiration

Upper airway discomforts of dryness of the nasal passages and/or the mouth, epistaxis, nasal congestion, and rhinitis are frequent complaints of CPAP users, often leading to decreased use of CPAP therapy.[72] The unidirectional flow of air through the nasal passages during CPAP therapy, especially when high pressures are required, leads to drying and inflammation of the mucous membranes. The inflamed nasal mucosa restricts airflow, increasing nasal airway resistance, which is especially true in patients who sleep with their mouths open. The use of a chin strap to help keep the mouth closed may be helpful to lessen this problem in some patients. Humidification of the air being delivered by the CPAP device often is necessary to improve the patient's comfort level and subsequent compliance to therapy. Humidification may be achieved by the addition of an in-line ambient temperature passover hu-

midifier or one having a heating element. By adjustment of the heater setting, an optimal point can be found at which the patient receives enough humidification to alleviate the drying effects on the nasal mucosa, leading to increased CPAP compliance (Figure 43-17).[73] Water should not accumulate in the circuit when the humidifier is used. Accumulation of water condensing in the circuit may result in below-therapeutic CPAP levels.[74]

Most CPAP units have an hour meter that displays the cumulative hours of operation. This reading does not reflect the hours of therapeutic use. If the mask comes off during the night, the unit may continue to operate with no patient benefit. Measuring time in use at the CPAP pressure setting is a reflection of the therapeutic use. Most units now have compliance meters that record hours of use at the CPAP therapeutic pressure setting and a separate meter for hours of operation. Many insurers seek compliance information to make determinations about continuing rental payments or purchasing the unit for the long-term use of the beneficiary.

One manufacturer has included in one of its basic CPAP units the Functional Outcomes of Sleep Questionnaire (FOSQ),[75] which the patient can access through a small digital screen. From time to time, usually at the initiation of therapy and at regular 30- to 90-day intervals thereafter, the patient is instructed to answer the 30 questions through the unit's keypad. The patient is asked to rate the level of difficulty in performing certain activities because of being tired or sleepy. If the CPAP therapy is effective, the FOSQ score should show improvement with continued use.

A number of manufacturers have incorporated into their units the capability to record and hold in memory

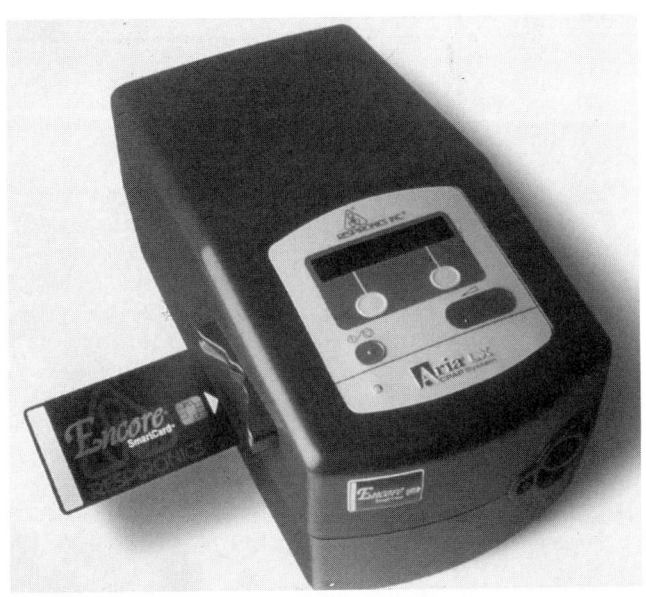

Figure 43-18   Nasal continuous positive airway pressure unit showing the removable data storage card on which patient usage and compliance information is stored and can be downloaded onto a personal computer where, with compatible software, a report is generated. (Courtesy Respironics, Pittsburgh, Pa.)

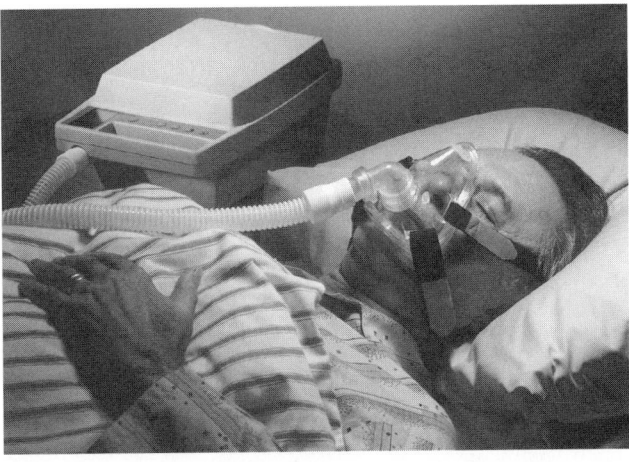

Figure 43-19   A bilevel device being used with an oronasal mask. (Courtesy ResMed, Poway, Calif.)

weeks to months of data, such as the date, time on and off, time at pressure, leak, and use of a ramp. The stored data can be retrieved as needed by downloading to a laptop computer or similar device in the field, directly by modem from a central location, or from a removable/exchangeable data storage device (Figure 43-18). The data is uploaded to a computer program that displays the data in various graphic and tabular formats. This information is valuable to the equipment provider, referring physician, sleep laboratory, and insurer because it provides details of ongoing patient compliance and helps identify problems requiring intervention.

CPAP is an effective therapeutic means to maintain upper airway patency. However, because the airflow is continuous throughout the respiratory cycle, some patients find exhaling against this pressure difficult, creating a feeling of discomfort and anxiety. For patients on high CPAP pressure, this difficulty is often a major factor in poor compliance. **Bilevel positive airway pressure** systems are an alternative for individuals unable to tolerate CPAP therapy. These units are functionally the same machines as those used for NPPV. Treatment of OSA with bilevel devices has been shown to be as effective as treatment with CPAP.[76] With a bilevel device the IPAP and EPAP are adjusted independently. The IPAP level is set at a point that eliminates the sleep-disordered breathing (apneas, hypopneas, snoring). The EPAP is set at a lower pressure to allow the patient to exhale against less resistance yet maintain airway splinting and patency. The use of bilevel therapy causes the mean airway pressure to be lower, generally increasing comfort and ther-

apy tolerance and leading to increased acceptance and compliance. Some insurers, including Medicare, cover bilevel devices only after the patient has been treated with CPAP that proved ineffectual and/or intolerable (Figure 43-19).

The pressure required to prevent airway collapse varies in most patients from night to night and from hour to hour throughout any night because of changes in body position, level and stage of sleep, ingestion of alcohol or caffeine, and airway congestion.[77] Several available CPAP devices actively monitor one or more airway variables during sleep and respond to upper airway changes by automatically adjusting the pressure within a range of 4 to 20 cm H_2O. These devices are referred to as *auto-CPAP* or **auto-positive airway pressure (APAP)**, or auto-titrating, devices. One or more of the following parameters are monitored: pharyngeal wall vibration (snoring), inspiratory flow limitations, hypopneas, and apneas. The system responds automatically when it senses an impending respiratory event by slowly increasing the CPAP pressure in a steplike pattern until airway patency is reestablished. After a few minutes the pressure slowly decreases to the lowest pressure possible to maintain airway stability (Figure 43-20).

The use of APAP is as effective as CPAP in reducing the apnea-hypopnea index (AHI) and improving sleep. The auto-adjustment of pressure during the night does not disrupt sleep, and mean airway pressure is significantly reduced.[78,79] APAP units can be used in the home setting to effectuate OSA therapy before or in place of a sleep laboratory titration.[80] After an APAP unit is used for 1 to 4 or more weeks, the accumulated data are reviewed and a

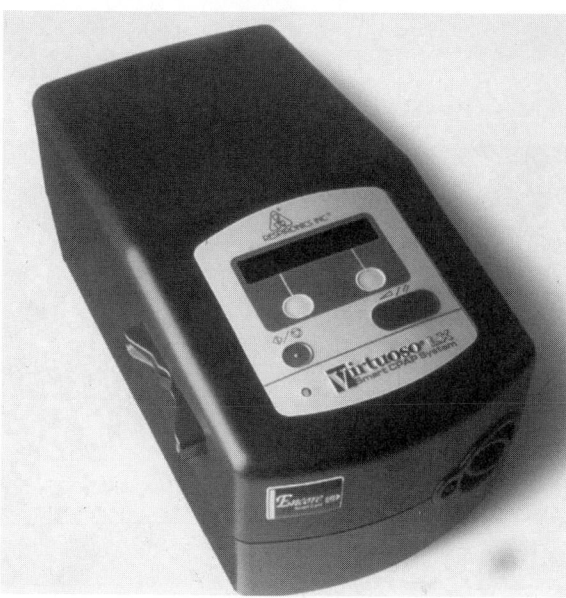

Figure 43-20 Example of an auto-CPAP (continuous positive airway pressure) unit, which adjusts pressure automatically in response to the user's needs to maintain airway patency. (Courtesy Respironics, Pittsburgh, Pa.)

traditional CPAP or bilevel system ordered, with pressure settings based on the APAP data. This change of equipment is necessitated because most insurers reimburse only for standard CPAP and do not pay higher rates for CPAP units that cost considerably more because of additional options or features.

KEY POINTS

- NPPV for acute respiratory failure has been demonstrated to decrease intubation rate, decrease pneumonia rate, and increase survival rates.
- Some patients—particularly those with neuromuscular disease—may benefit from chronic nocturnal NPPV.
- Nasal and oronasal interfaces are available for NPPV.
- Any ventilator can be used to provide NPPV.
- The choice of interface, ventilator, and ventilator mode for NPPV is determined primarily by clinician and patient preference.
- Mask CPAP can be used in acute care applications to prevent postoperative pulmonary complications, to improve oxygenation in patients with hypoxemic respiratory failure, and to treat cardiogenic pulmonary edema.
- Nocturnal nasal CPAP is used to treat OSA.
- CPAP compliance can be improved by the use of an appropriate interface, by humidification of the gas flow, by use of the ramp/delay function, and by use of bilevel therapy.
- Auto-CPAP units vary pressure by monitoring changes in upper airway obstruction.

References

1. Bach JR, Brougher P, Hess DR, et al. Consensus statement: Noninvasive positive pressure ventilation. Respir Care 1997;42:365-369.
2. Evans TW. International consensus conference in intensive care medicine: non-invasive positive pressure ventilation in acute respiratory failure. Intensive Care Med 2001;27: 166-178.
3. Hess D, Chatmongkolchart S. Techniques to avoid intubation: noninvasive positive pressure ventilation and heliox therapy. International Anesthesiology Clinics 2000;38:161-187.
4. Keenan SP, Kernerman PD, Cook DJ, et al. Effect of noninvasive positive pressure ventilation on mortality in patients admitted with acute respiratory failure: a meta-analysis. Crit Care Med 1997;25:1685-1692.
5. Confalonieri M, Parigi P, Scartabellati A, et al. Noninvasive mechanical ventilation improves the immediate and long-term outcome of COPD patients with acute respiratory failure. Eur Respir J 1996;9:422-430.
6. Vitacca M, Clini E, Rubini F, et al. Non-invasive mechanical ventilation in severe chronic obstructive lung disease and acute respiratory failure: short- and long-term prognosis. Intensive Care Med 1996;22:94-100.
7. Nourdine K, Combes P, Carton MJ, et al. Does noninvasive ventilation reduce the ICU nosocomial pneumonia risk? A prospective clinical survey. Intensive Care Med 1999;25: 567-573.
8. Girou E, Schortgen F, Delclaux C, et al. Association of noninvasive ventilation with noscomial infections and survival in critically ill patients. J Am Med Assoc 2000;284:2361-2367.
9. Nava S, Ambrosino N, Clini E, et al. Noninvasive mechanical ventilation in the weaning of patients with respiratory failure due to chronic obstructive pulmonary disease. A randomized, controlled trial. Ann Intern Med 1998;128:721-728.
10. Girault C, Daudenthun I, Chevron V, et al. Noninvasive ventilation as a systematic extubation and weaning technique in acute-on-chronic respiratory failure. A prospective, randomized controlled study. Am J Respir Crit Care Med 1999;160: 86-92.
11. Barbe F, Togores B, Rubi M, et al. Noninvasive ventilatory support does not facilitate recovery from acute respiratory failure in chronic obstructive pulmonary disease. Eur Respir J 1996; 9:1240-1245.
12. Hess D. Noninvasive positive pressure ventilation: Predictors of success and failure for adult acute care applications. Respir Care 1997;42:424-431.
13. Mehta S, Jay GD, Woolard RH, et al. Randomized, prospective trial of bilevel versus continuous positive airway pressure in acute pulmonary edema. Crit Care Med 1997;25: 620-628.
14. Rusterholtz T, Kempt J, Berton C, et al. Noninvasive pressure support ventilation (NIPSV) with face mask in patients with acute cardiogenic pulmonary edema (ACPE). Intensive Care Med 1999;25:21-28.
15. Soo Hoo GW, Santiago S, Williams AJ. Nasal mechanical ventilation for hypercapnic respiratory failure in chronic obstructive pulmonary disease: determinants of success. Crit Care Med 1994;22:1253-1261.
16. Ambrosino N, Folgio K, Rubini F, et al. Non-invasive mechanical ventilation in acute respiratory failure due to chronic obstructive pulmonary disease: correlates for success. Thorax 1995;50:755-757.

17. Anton A, Guell R, Gomez J, et al. Predicting the result of non-invasive ventilation in severe acute exacerbations of chronic airflow limitation. Chest 2000; 117:828-833.

18. Bach JR, Niranjan V, Weaver B. Spinal muscular atrophy Type 1. A noninvasive respiratory management approach. Chest 2000;117:1100-1105.

19. Tang AC, Back JR. Prevention of pulmonary morbidity for patients with neuromuscular disease. Chest 2000;118:1390-1396.

20. Clinical indications for noninvasive positive pressure ventilation in chronic respiratory failure due to restrictive lung disease, COPD, and nocturnal hypoventilation—a consensus conference report. Chest 1999;116:521-534.

21. Garrod R, Mikelsons C, Paul EA, et al. Randomized trial of domiciliary noninvasive positive pressure ventilation and physical training in severe chronic obstructive lung disease. Am J Respir Crit Care Med 2000;162:1335-1341.

22. Casanova C, Celli BR, Tost L, et al. Long-term controlled trial of nocturnal nasal positive pressure ventilation in patients with severe COPD. Chest 2000;118:1582-1590.

23. Turner RE. Patient-interface issues in noninvasive positive pressure ventilation. Respir Care 1997;42:389-393.

24. Richards GN, Cistulli PA, Ungar G, et al. Mouth leak with nasal continuous positive airway pressure increases nasal airway resistance. Am J Respir Crit Care Med 1996;154:182-186.

25. de Araujo MTM, Vieira SB, Vasquez EC, et al. Heated humidification or face mask to prevent upper airway dryness during continuous positive airway pressure therapy. Chest 2000;117:142-147.

26. Navalesi, P, Fanfulla F, Frigerio P, et al. Physiologic evaluation of noninvasive mechanical ventilation delivered with three types of masks in patients with chronic hypercapneic respiratory failure. Crit Care Med 2000;28:1785-1790.

27. Girault C, Richard JC, Chevron V, et al. Comparative physiologic effects of noninvasive assist-control and pressure support ventilation in acute hypercapnic respiratory failure. Chest 1997;111:1639-1648.

28. Black JW, Grover BS. A hazard of pressure support ventilation. Chest 1988;93:333-335.

29. Calderini E, Confalonieri M, Puccio PG, et al. Patient-ventilator asynchrony during noninvasive ventilation: the role of expiratory trigger. Intensive Care Med 1999;25:662-667.

30. Jubran A, van de Graaff WB, Tobin MJ. Variability of patient-ventilator interaction with pressure support ventilation in patients with chronic obstructive pulmonary disease. Am J Respir Crit Care Med 1995;152:129-136.

31. Parthasarathy S, Jubran A, Tobin MJ. Cycling of inspiratory and expiratory muscle groups with the ventilator in airflow limitation. Am J Respir Crit Care Med 1998;158:1471-1478.

32. Adams AB, Bliss P, Hotchkiss J. Effects of respiratory impedance on the performance of bi-level pressure ventilators. Respir Care 2000;45:390-400.

33. Strumpf DA, Carlisle CC, Millman RP, et al. An evaluation of the Respironics BiPAP bi-level CPAP device for delivery of assisted ventilation. Respir Care 1990;35:415-422.

34. Hill NS, Mehta S, Carlisle CC, McCool FD. Evaluation of the Puritan-Bennett 335 portable pressure support ventilator: comparison with the Respironics BiPAP S/T. Respir Care 1996;41:885-894.

35. Kacmarek RM. Performance characteristics of portable ventilators used for noninvasive positive pressure ventilation. Respir Care 1997;42:380-388.

36. Bunburaphong T, Imanaka H, Nishimura M, et al. Performance characteristics of bilevel pressure ventilators: a lung model study. Chest 1997;111:1050-1060.

37. Lofaso F, Brochard L, Hang T, et al. Home versus intensive care pressure support devices. Experimental and clinical comparison. Am J Respir Crit Care Med 1996;153:1591-1599.

38. Lofaso F, Brochard L, Touchard D, et al. Evaluation of carbon dioxide rebreathing during pressure support ventilation with airway management system (BiPAP) devices. Chest 1995;108:772-778.

39. Ferguson GT, Gilmartin M. CO_2 rebreathing during BiPAP ventilatory assistance. Am J Respir Crit Care Med 1995;151:1126-1135.

40. Waugh JB, de Kler RM. Inspiratory time, pressure settings, and site of supplemental oxygen insertion on delivered oxygen fraction with the Quantum PSV noninvasive positive pressure ventilator. Respir Care 1999;44:520-523.

41. Pollack CV, Fleisch KB, Dowsey K. Treatment of acute bronchospasm with beta-adrenergic agonist aerosols delivered by a nasal bilevel positive airway pressure circuit. Ann Emerg Med 1995;26:552-557.

42. Parkes SN, Bersten AD. Aerosol kinetics and bronchodilator efficacy during continuous positive airway pressure delivered by a face mask. Thorax 1997;52:171-175.

43. Meduri GU, Turner RE, Abou-Shala N, et al. Noninvasive positive pressure ventilation via face mask. First-line intervention in patients with acute hypercapnic and hypoxemic respiratory failure. Chest 1996;109:179-193.

44. Sinuff T, Cook D, Randall J, Allen C. Noninvasive positive-pressure ventilation: a utilization review of use in a teaching hospital. CMAJ 2000;163:969-973.

45. Kramer N, Meyer TJ, Meharg J, et al. Randomized, prospective trial of noninvasive positive pressure ventilation in acute respiratory failure. Am J Respir Crit Care Med 1995;151:1799-1806.

46. Nava S, Evangelisti I, Rampulla C. Human and financial costs of noninvasive mechanical ventilation in patients affected by COPD and acute respiratory failure. Chest 1997;111:1631-1638.

47. Hilbert G, Gruson D, Vargas F, et al. Noninvasive ventilation for acute respiratory failure. Quite low time consumption for nurses. Eur Respir J 2000;16:710-716.

48. Keenan S, Gregor J, Sibbald WJ, et al. Noninvasive positive pressure ventilation in the setting of severe, acute exacerbations of chronic obstructive lung disease: more effective and less expensive. Crit Care Med 2000;28:2094-2102.

49. Hill NS. Complications of noninvasive positive pressure ventilation. Respir Care 1997; 42:432-442.

50. Meduri GU. Noninvasive positive-pressure ventilation in patients with acute respiratory failure. Clin Chest Med 1996;17:513-553.

51. Hill NS. Use of negative pressure ventilation, rocking beds, and pneumobelts. Respir Care 1994;39:532-549.

52. Gilmartin ME. Body ventilators. Equipment and techniques. Respir Care Clin N Am 1996;2:195-222.

53. Andersen JB, Olesen KP, Eikard E, et al. Periodic continuous positive airway pressure, CPAP, by mask in the treatment of atelectasis: A sequential analysis. Eur J Respir Dis 1980;61:20-25.

54. Pontoppidan H. Mechanical aids to lung expansion in nonintubated surgical patients. Am Rev Respir Dis 1980;122:109-119.

55. Carlsson C, Sonden B, Thylen U. Can postoperative continuous positive airway pressure (CPAP) prevent pulmonary complications after abdominal surgery? Intensive Care Med 1981;7:225-229.

56. Stock MC, Downs JB, Corkran ML. Pulmonary function before and after prolonged positive airway pressure by mask. Crit Care Med 1984;12:973-974.

57. Stock MC, Downs JB, Cooper RB, et al. Comparison of continuous positive airway pressure, incentive spirometry, and conservative therapy after cardiac operations. Crit Care Med 1984;12:969-972.

58. Stock MC, Downs JB, Gauer PK, et al. Prevention of postoperative pulmonary complication with CPAP, incentive spirometry and conservative therapy. Chest 1985;87:151-157.

59. Lindner KH, Lotz P, Ahnefeld FW. Continuous positive airway pressure effect on functional residual capacity, vital capacity and its subdivisions. Chest 1987;92(1):66-70.

60. Kindgen-Milles D, Buhl R, Gabriel A, et al. Nasal continuous positive airway pressure. A method to avoid endotracheal reintubation in postoperative high-risk patients with severe nonhypercapnic oxygenation failure. Chest 2000;117:1106-1111.

61. Maitre B, Jaber S, Maggiore SM, et al. Continuous positive airway pressure during fiberoptic bronchoscopy in hypoxemic patients. A randomized double-blind study using a new device. Am J Respir Crit Care Med 2000;162:1063-1067.

62. Greenbaum DM, Millen JE, Eross B, et al. Continuous positive airway pressure without intubation in spontaneously breathing patients. Chest 1976;69:615-620.

63. Smith RA, Kirby RR, Gooding JM, et al. Continuous positive airway pressure (CPAP) by face mask. Crit Care Med 1980;8:483-485.

64. Covelli HD, Weled BJ, Beekman JF. Efficacy of continuous positive airway pressure administered by face mask. Chest 1982;81:147-150.

65. Hurst JM, DeHaven CB, Branson RD. Use of CPAP mask as the sole mode of ventilatory support in trauma patients with mild to moderate respiratory insufficiency. J Trauma 1985;25:1065-1068.

66. Delclaux C, L'Her E, Alberti C, et al. Treatment of acute hypoxemic nonhypercapnic respiratory insufficiency with continuous positive airway pressure delivered by a face mask. A randomized controlled trial. J Am Med Assoc 2000;284:2352-2360.

67. Pang D, Keenan SP, Cook DJ, et al. The effect of positive pressure airway support on mortality and the need for intubation in cardiogenic pulmonary edema. A systematic review. Chest 1998;114:1185-1192.

68. Banner MJ, Lampotang S. Expiratory pressure valves. IN: Branson RD, Hess DR, Chatburn RL. Respiratory care equipment, 2nd ed. Philadelphia: JB Lippincott; 1999.

69. National Heart, Lung, and Blood Institute, National Institutes for Health. Sleep apnea: is your patient at risk? Bethesda, Md: NIH Publication 95-3803, 1995. Reprinted in Respir Care 1995;40:1287-1298.

70. Sullivan CE, Issa FG, Berthon-Jones M, et al. Reversal of obstructive sleep apnoea by continuous positive airway pressure applied through the nares. Lancet 1981;1:862-865.

71. Sanders MH, Moore SE, Eveslage J. CPAP via nasal mask: a treatment for occlusive sleep apnea. Chest 1983;83:144-145.

72. Pepin JL, Leger P, Veale D, et al. Side effects of nasal continuous positive airway pressure in sleep apnea syndrome. Chest 1995;107:375-381.

73. Massie CA, Hart RW, Peralez K, et al. Effects of humidification on nasal symptoms and compliance in sleep apnea patients using continuous positive airway pressure. Chest 1999;116:403-408.

74. Bacon JP, Farney RJ, Jensen RL, et al. Nasal continuous positive airway pressure devices do not maintain set pressure dynamically when tested under simulated clinical conditions. Chest 2000;118:1441-1449.

75. Weaver TE, Laizner AM, Evans LK, et al. An instrument to measure functional status outcomes for disorders of excessive sleepiness. Sleep 1997;20:835-843.

76. Sanders MH, Kern N. Obstructive sleep apnea treated by independently adjusting inspiratory and expiratory positive airway pressure via nasal mask. Chest 1990;98:317-324.

77. Berthon-Jones M. Feasibility of a self-setting CPAP machine. Sleep 1993;16:S120-S123.

78. Behbehani K, Yen F-C, Lucas EA, et al. A sleep laboratory evaluation of an automatic positive airway pressure system for treatment of obstructive sleep apnea. Sleep 1998;21:485-491.

79. d'Ortho M, Grillier-Lanoir V, Levy P, et al. Constant vs automatic continuous positive airway pressure. Home evaluation. Chest 2000;118:1010-1017.

80. Series F. Accuracy of an unattended home CPAP titration in the treatment of obstructive sleep apnea. Am J Respir Crit Care Med 2000;162:94-97.

CHAPTER 44

Nonconventional Respiratory Therapeutics

Dean R. Hess

OBJECTIVES

1. Discuss the biology of nitric oxide.
2. Describe selective pulmonary vasodilation.
3. Compare FDA-approved and off-label use of inhaled nitric oxide.
4. List potential toxicities and adverse effects of inhaled nitric oxide.
5. Describe the delivery systems for administration of inhaled nitric oxide.
6. Describe the physical basis for the use of heliox therapy.
7. List patient types likely to benefit from heliox therapy.
8. Describe the effects of heliox on the operation of respiratory care equipment.
9. Discuss the physiologic basis for tracheal gas insufflation.
10. Describe mechanisms whereby prone position improves oxygenation.
11. Describe the goal of lung recruitment maneuvers.
12. Discuss the potential benefit of partial liquid ventilation.

KEY TERMS

Heliox	Nitric Oxide Synthase (NOS)	Recruitment Maneuver
Kinetic Therapy	Nitrogen Dioxide (NO_2)	Tracheal Gas Insufflation (TGI)
Methemoglobin (metHb)	Partial Liquid Ventilation (PLV)	
Nitric Oxide (NO)	Prone Position	

A variety of nonconventional respiratory therapeutics are now available. These therapies range from pharmacologic (for example, inhaled nitric oxide) to physical (for example, heliox) to positional (for example, prone positioning). Some have been available for many years, whereas others are in experimental stages (for example, partial liquid ventilation).

Inhaled Nitric Oxide

Nitric oxide (NO) is a ubiquitous, highly reactive, gaseous, diatomic radical[1] that is important physiologically at low concentrations (Box 44-1). Atmospheric concentrations of NO usually range from 10 to 100 ppb. Concentrations of 400 to 1000 ppm are routinely inhaled by people who smoke cigarettes.[2] NO is present in low

Typical Expression of Concentration of Nitric Oxide and Nitrogen Dioxide

Concentrations are usually expressed in concentrations of parts per million (ppm) or parts per billion (ppb) as follows:

$$\% = \frac{1}{100}$$
$$ppm = \frac{1}{1,000,000}$$
$$10,000 \ ppm = 1\%$$
$$1000 \ ppb = 1 \ ppm$$

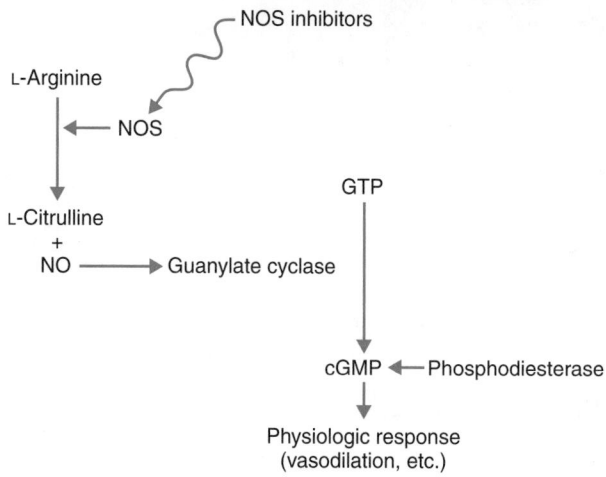

Figure 44-1 Biologic pathway for nitric oxide production and its biologic effect of increasing the production of cGMP.

concentration in the hospital compressed gas supply, which may have physiologic effects on patients.[3,4] Because it is considered an occupational and environmental pollutant, the Occupational Safety and Health Administration (OSHA) developed exposure limits for NO in the workplace.[5] NO is an important messenger molecule and many cell types have shown the capacity to produce NO.

The action of common nitrosovasodilators (for example, sodium nitroprusside and nitroglycerin) is due to their release of NO. Since the early 1990s, clinical and academic interest in NO shifted from environmental and public health to cellular biology and physiology.

Biology of Nitric Oxide

L-Arginine is the substrate for NO synthesis in biologic systems (Figure 44-1).[1,6] NO is produced in the presence of **nitric oxide synthase (NOS).** NO is lipophilic and readily diffuses across cell membranes to adjacent cells, thus serving as a local messenger molecule. It typically diffuses from its cell of origin to a neighboring cell, where it binds with guanylate cyclase. Activation of guanylate cyclase results in the production of cyclic guanosine 3′,5′-monophosphate (cGMP) from guanosine triphosphate (GTP), which produces a biologic effect within the cell (for example, smooth muscle relaxation). The time between NO production and guanylate cyclase activation is minimal because NO in physiologic systems has a half-life of less than 5 seconds. Inhibitors of guanylate cyclase (for example, methylene blue) and inhibitors of NOS decrease cGMP levels, whereas inhibitors of phosphodiesterase (for example, sildenafil and dypyridamole) increase cGMP levels.[7,8]

NO also has cGMP-independent effects. Inhaled NO may have important effects in reducing some forms of lung and tissue injury, including the ability to scavenge oxygen free radicals, reduce oxygen toxicity, and inhibit platelet and leukocyte aggregation.[1] The cGMP-independent effect of inhaled NO on hemoglobin function may be important in individuals with sickle cell disease.[9]

NO is present in the exhaled gas.[10,11] Measurable levels of NO (7 to 130 ppb) are present in the nasopharynx. In the paranasal sinuses, NO levels are much higher (ap-

proximately 10 ppm), and the bacteriostatic effects of NO may be responsible for maintaining the sterility of the sinuses.[12] NO in the nasopharynx is inhaled and much of that is absorbed. When the trachea is intubated, NO levels are reduced in inhaled and exhaled gas.[13,14] Exhaled NO has been reported to be increased in asthma,[15-18] the hepatopulmonary syndrome,[19] and bronchiectasis.[20] The analysis of exhaled NO concentration is complicated because exhaled levels may vary with changes of ventilatory pattern, pulmonary blood flow, and diffusing capacity.[21,22]

Selective Pulmonary Vasodilation

The term *selective pulmonary vasodilation* is used to indicate two physiologic phenomena (Figure 44-2). First, selective pulmonary vasodilators reduce pulmonary vascular resistance without affecting systemic vascular resistance. Second, a selective pulmonary vasodilator affects vascular resistance only near ventilated alveoli. Inspired vasodilators are delivered to those lung units that are ventilated. NO is not a selective pulmonary vasodilator but becomes one when inhaled. Inhaled NO selectively improves blood flow to ventilated alveoli and produces a reduction in intrapulmonary shunt and improved arterial oxygenation. The selective pulmonary vasodilation demonstrated by inhaled NO is due to the high affinity of hemoglobin for NO, which is about 10^6 times as great as the affinity of hemoglobin for O_2. In contrast to inhaled NO, intravenous vasodilators (for example, sodium nitroprusside, nitroglycerin, prostacyclin) are not selective. Although intravenous vasodilators lower pulmonary artery pressure, they also lower systemic blood pressure. These agents increase blood flow to both ventilated and unventilated lung units, resulting in an increased intrapulmonary shunt and a lower PaO_2.

Clinical Applications

Multicenter, randomized, double-blind placebo-controlled studies of inhaled NO for persistent pulmonary hypertension of the newborn (PPHN) have reported improvements in PaO_2 and a reduction in the requirement for extracorporeal life support (ECLS) with the use of inhaled NO.[23-29] These studies established a role for inhaled NO in term infants with PPHN. This led to approval by the FDA for use of inhaled NO (INOmax, INO Therapeutics, Clinton, N.J.):

> INOmax, in conjunction with ventilatory support and other appropriate agents, is indicated for the treatment of term and near-term (>34 weeks) neonates with hypoxic respiratory failure associated with clinical or echocardiographic evidence of pulmonary hypertension, where it improves oxygenation and reduces the need for extracorporeal membrane oxygenation.

This is the only FDA-approved indication for inhaled NO, and all other uses are off-label. NO should not be used for hypoxemic newborns with congenital cardiac defects who are dependent upon right-to-left shunt. The usual starting dose of inhaled NO is 20 ppm. This dose is then weaned to the lowest effective dose (for example, 5 ppm) and continued until the condition of the baby is improved.

Acute respiratory distress syndrome (ARDS) is characterized by hypoxemia and pulmonary hypertension. Case series[30,31] reporting improvements in PaO_2 and pulmonary hypertension with the use of inhaled NO resulted in considerable enthusiasm for the use of NO in this patient population.[32,33] Unfortunately, however, randomized multicentered trials failed to report improvements in important patient outcomes (for example, ventilator days and mortality) with the use of NO.[34,35] Inhaled NO produced an initial improvement in PaO_2, but this was short-lived; after

several days of therapy patients receiving NO and those receiving placebo were indistinguishable. Although it remains attractive to use inhaled NO for hypoxemic patients with ARDS, limited evidence supports its use in this patient population.

Age-Specific Angle

The only FDA-approved indication for inhaled nitric oxide is hypoxic respiratory failure of the newborn.

Inhaled NO is being investigated for primary pulmonary hypertension,[36-38] bronchospasm,[39,40] sickle cell disease,[9,41] cardiothoracic surgery,[42,43] heart or lung transplantation,[44,45] and for diagnostic testing of pulmonary vascular reactivity.[36] However, these applications remain investigational until completion of appropriately designed clinical trials.

Toxicity and Complications

The toxicity of inhaled NO appears to be low when administered by clinicians familiar with its use. However, a number of potential toxicities and complications exist.[46,47] In high concentrations, inhaled NO may have direct toxic effects on the lungs. Farmers exposed to high levels of the oxides of nitrogen develop silo-filler's disease, characterized by dyspnea, hypoxemia, and pulmonary edema. However, the NO concentrations in these instances are extremely high—much greater than those used therapeutically or stored in NO cylinders.

Nitrogen dioxide (NO_2) is produced spontaneously from NO and O_2. The conversion rate of NO to NO_2 is determined by the O_2 concentration, the square of the NO concentration, and the residence time of NO with O_2.[48] The Occupational Safety and Health Administration (OSHA) has set safety limits for NO_2 at 5 ppm,[5] but airway reactivity and parenchymal lung injury have been reported with inhalation of 2 ppm NO_2 or less.

Methemoglobin (metHb) is produced when the iron in heme is oxidized from Fe^{+2} to Fe^{+3}. In the oxidized form, iron cannot bind O_2 and the affinity of the other heme groups for O_2 increases (that is, shifts the oxyhemoglobin dissociation curve to the left). Normal metHb is less than 2% and levels less than 5% do not require treatment. The normal metHb blood level may be due to metabolism of endogenous NO. Methemoglobin reductase within erythrocytes converts endogenously produced metHb to normal hemoglobin. Methemoglobin production after NO exposure is uncommon at the NO doses used for therapeutic inhalation (20 ppm or less). A few cases of methemoglobinemia were reported in association with inhaled NO therapy, generally with high does of inhaled NO (for example, 80 ppm). In patients with decreased metHb reductase (for example, newborns and those with an hereditary deficiency), methemoglobinemia may be more likely.

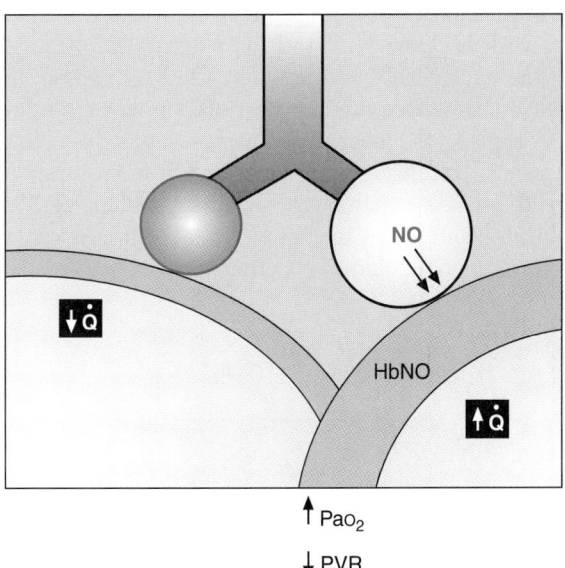

Figure 44-2   The mechanism by which inhaled nitric oxide acts as a selective pulmonary vasodilator.

In biologic systems NO reacts with O_2^- to produce peroxynitrite ($ONOO^-$), which is unstable at physiologic pH because it protonates to peroxynitrous acid, which decomposes with a half-life less than 1 second to NO_2 and the hydroxyl radical. The toxicity of O_2^- may be related to its reactivity with NO to produce $ONOO^-$. Superoxide dismutase may prevent the production of $ONOO^-$ by decreasing the availability of O_2^- to react with NO. Virtually nothing is known about the potential intracellular toxicity of inhaled NO resulting from peroxynitrite at the doses used therapeutically.

Some patients do not respond to inhaled NO. About 40% of patients with ARDS will fail to have an initial improvement in PaO_2/FIO_2 or pulmonary vascular resistance of at least 20%.[49] Worsening of hypoxemia in patients with COPD who received inhaled NO also has been reported and attributed to impaired matching of ventilation to perfusion.[50,51] To improve the responsiveness to inhaled NO, it has been combined with other therapies such as phosphodiesterase inhibitors, vasoconstrictors, prone positioning, and lung recruitment.[52]

Inhibition of platelet adhesion, aggregation and agglutination have been reported with inhaled NO.[53] Although consideration of coagulopathy is prudent in a decision to use inhaled NO, the clinical importance of this effect remains unclear. An increased incidence of bleeding diathesis has not been noted in prospective randomized trials of NO inhalation.

At high doses (40 to 80 ppm), inhaled NO reportedly decreases pulmonary vascular resistance and increases pulmonary capillary wedge pressure in some patients with severe left ventricular dysfunction.[54,55] The acute reduction of right ventricular afterload may produce an increase in pulmonary venous return to the left heart. This increases left ventricular filling pressure and might worsen pulmonary edema. Although this effect may be dose related, inhaled NO should be avoided in patients with severe left ventricular dysfunction (pulmonary capillary wedge pressure of at least 25 mm Hg). Treatment of the left ventricular dysfunction (for example, diuretics, inotropes) often corrects the associated pulmonary dysfunction so that a selective pulmonary vasodilator is not necessary.

Withdrawal of inhaled NO is problematic for some patients.[56-60] In some cases, the degree of hypoxemia and pulmonary hypertension is greater after discontinuation of NO than at baseline, leading to hemodynamic instability. Reinstitution of NO inhalation promptly corrects the hemodynamic instability and NO withdrawal is postponed until the patient is less severely ill. The reasons for rebound are not known but may relate to feedback inhibition of NOS activity. The following guidelines may prevent the deleterious effects of rebound during withdrawal of inhaled NO:

1. Use the lowest effective NO dose (5 ppm or less).
2. Do not withdraw inhaled NO until the patient's clinical status has improved sufficiently.

3. Set the NO dose at 1 ppm for a short time (30 minutes to 1 hour) before discontinuing NO.
4. Increase the FIO_2 before withdrawal of inhaled NO and prepare to support the patient's hemodynamics if necessary.

Delivery Systems for Inhaled Nitric Oxide

In the United States the INOvent Delivery System (Ohmeda, Madison, Wis.) is a universal NO delivery system.[61,62] It can be used with neonatal ventilators,[63] adult ventilators,[64] anesthesia machines,[65] and with spontaneously breathing patients (Figure 44-3). The system is configured for 0 to 80 ppm with an 800 ppm NO source cylinder. These cylinders are either D-size or size 88 (1963 L at 2000 psig), are constructed of aluminum alloy, and have threaded connections specific for NO (CGA 626).

NO is stored in nitrogen gas. The injection module of the INOvent is inserted into the inspiratory circuit at the outlet of the ventilator. The injection module consists of a hot film flow sensor and a gas injection tube. Flow in the ventilator circuit is precisely measured and NO is injected proportional to that flow to provide the desired NO dose. This design allows a precise and constant NO concentration in the inspired gas for any ventilatory pattern. The INOvent Delivery System includes gas monitoring of O_2, NO, and NO_2. Gas is sampled downstream from the point of injection near the Y-piece in the inspiratory circuit with electrochemical cells. A number of alarms can be set by the user.

A manual NO delivery system is provided by the INOvent Delivery System. With an oxygen flow to the manual ventilator set at 15 L/min, INOvent injects gas to provide an NO concentration of 20 ppm. Squeezing the bag three to five times to clear residual NO_2 is prerequisite for the use of a manual ventilator system for NO.

Concern exists regarding contamination of the environment with NO and NO_2 and the potential for adverse effects on health care providers. The OSHA exposure limits for NO (a time-weighted average of 25 ppm for 8 hours in the workplace) is higher than the typical NO dose (20 ppm or less). In intensive care unit environments that have more than six air exchanges per hour, ambient NO levels remain low without scavenging.[66] Scavenging is generally not recommended during NO therapy.

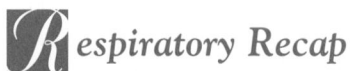

espiratory Recap

Inhaled Nitric Oxide
A selective pulmonary vasodilator
FDA-approved for the treatment of hypoxic respiratory failure of the newborn
Toxicity low at usual clinical doses
Administered via the INOvent Nitric Oxide Delivery System

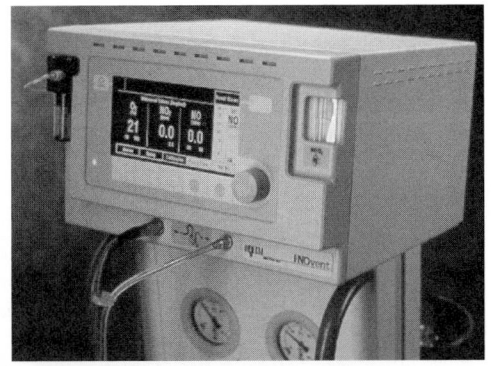

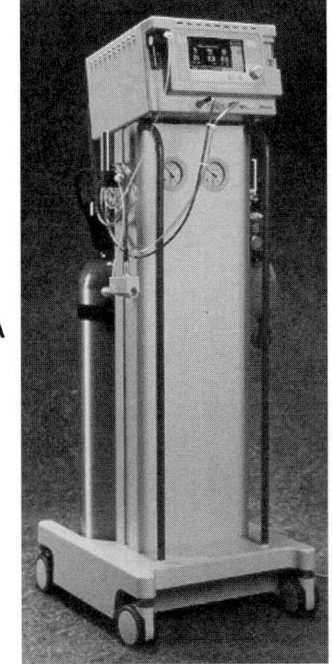

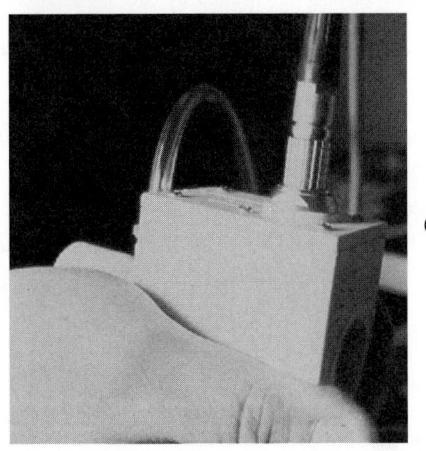

Figure 44-3 A, INOvent Nitric Oxide Delivery System. **B,** Monitoring panel of INOvent. **C,** Nitric oxide injector port that fits into the inspiratory limb of the ventilator circuit.

During NO therapy, analysis is mandatory to avoid complications from inaccurate dosing. Measuring NO_2 is also important because it may be generated in NO delivery systems. Chemiluminescence techniques measure gas concentrations by stimulated photoemission.[67-69] The sample gas reacts with ozone (O_3) to produce NO_2 with an electron in an excited state (NO_2^*). A photon is released when the excited electron of NO_2^* decays to its basal energy level. This is measured by a photomultiplier tube that proportionately converts the intensity of luminescence into an electrical signal for display. Electrochemical techniques for detection of NO and NO_2 are based on the principle that these gases react with electrolyte solutions.[67,68] Electrons are liberated or consumed, generating a current between two polarized electrodes in proportion to the concentration of NO or NO_2 in the sample gas. The accuracy of electrochemical analyzers has been found acceptable in the range used clinically.[70]

Heliox

Heliox is a gas mixture of helium and oxygen. Heliox is used clinically because of its low density. The only gas with a density less than helium is hydrogen. Unlike hydrogen, helium is an inert gas and is thus nonreactive. He-

TABLE 44-1

Physical Properties of Oxygen, Air, and Helium

Gas	Density (g/L)	Viscosity (µpoise)	Thermoconductivity (µcal × cm × s × °K)
Air	1.293	170.8	58.0
Oxygen	1.429	192.6	58.5
Helium	0.179	188.7	352.0

lium is relatively insoluble in body fluids. Because helium does not support life, for clinical applications it must always be delivered in a gas mixture containing at least 20% oxygen. In addition to its use for diagnostic purposes such as measurement of lung volumes (for example, functional residual capacity), it may be of therapeutic use in patients with obstructive lung diseases.

Physics and Physiology

The physical properties of helium are different from those of air or oxygen (Table 44-1). These physical properties of helium affect its flow through airways of the lungs (Equation 44-1). Because turbulent flow is

EQUATION 44-1

Physical Principles that Explain the Benefits of Heliox Therapy

For turbulent flow, the Hagen-Poiseuille equation predicts that flow is affected by the radius of the conducting tube, the pressure gradient, the density of the gas (ρ), and the length of the conducting tube (l) as follows:

$$\dot{V}^2 \approx \frac{4\pi r^5 \Delta P}{\rho l}$$

where $\dot{V}$ is flow and ΔP is the pressure gradient.

Whether flow is laminar or turbulent is determined by the Reynolds number (Re) as follows:

$$Re \approx \frac{\text{Inertial forces}}{\text{Viscous forces}} \approx \frac{vr\rho}{\eta}$$

where v is the velocity of gas movement, r is the radius, and η is viscosity. A low Reynolds number causes flow to be laminar.

For gas flow through an orifice (for example, axial acceleration), flow has only a weak dependence on the Reynolds number and is affected by density as follows:

$$\dot{V}^2 \approx \frac{\Delta P}{\rho}$$

In other words, flow through an orifice (for example, constricted airway) will increase if the density of the gas decreases (for example, heliox).

The Bernoulli principle states that the pressure required to produce flow is affected by the mass of the gas as follows:

$$(P_1 - P_2) = \frac{1}{2} \times m \times (v_2^2 - v_1^2)$$

where:

$(P_1 - P_2)$ = Pressure required to produce flow
$(v_2^2 - v_1^2)$ = Difference in velocity between P_1 and P_2
$\qquad m$ = Mass of the gas

In other words, less pressure is required to produce flow with heliox than with air or oxygen.

Graham's law states that the rate of diffusion is inversely related to the square root of gas density. Thus heliox (80% He/20% O_2) will diffuse at a rate 1.8 times faster than oxygen, which explains why the flow of heliox through an oxygen flowmeter is 1.8 times faster than the indicated flow.

According to wave speed theory, flow through an airway cannot be greater than the flow at which gas velocity equals wave speed. Wave speed is the speed at which a small disturbance travels in a compliant tube filled with a fluid. The wave speed (c) in an airway depends on the cross-sectional area of the airway (A), the density of the fluid, and the slope of the pressure-area curve of the airway (dP/dA) as follows:

$$c^2 = \frac{A}{\rho} \times \frac{dP}{dA}$$

Note that maximal flow ($\dot{V}_{max}$) is the product of the fluid velocity at wave speed and the airway area (cA). If $\dot{V}_{max} = cA$, then the following occurs:

$$\dot{V}_{max} = A \left(\frac{A}{\rho} \times \frac{dP}{dA} \right)^{1/2}$$

According to wave speed theory, $\dot{V}_{max}$ increases as gas density decreases. However, wave speed theory is useful only when gas flow is density dependent. In small airways, and particularly at low lung volumes, gas flow is density independent and viscous flow limitation becomes more important than wave speed.

---

density dependent, whereas laminar flow is density independent, use of heliox is expected to have a greater effect on turbulent flow. Because of its lower density and higher viscosity, heliox produces a lower Reynolds number and a greater tendency for laminar flow. Laminar flow is desirable because it is more energy efficient than turbulent flow. According to the Reynolds number, gas flow tends to be laminar in small peripheral airways of the lungs and turbulent in larger central airways. Therefore heliox may have limited benefit for diseases affecting small airways (for example, emphysema), whereas it may be useful for diseases affecting larger airways (for example, asthma or postextubation stridor). For gas flow through an orifice (that is, axial acceleration), flow through the orifice (for example, constricted airway) will increase if the density of the gas decreases (for example, heliox). Because of the Bernoulli principle, less pressure is required to produce flow with heliox than air or oxygen. According to Graham's law, heliox (80% helium/20% oxygen) diffuses at a rate 1.8 times greater than oxygen.

Clinical Applications

A common use of heliox is to reduce resistance with partial upper airway obstruction.[71-82] An example of this application is postextubation stridor, most of the evidence for which comes from anecdotal reports. In a study of children with postextubation stridor, heliox breathing reduced respiratory distress 38%, but no significant effect with oxygen-enriched air.[75]

Heliox has potential use in case of acute asthma.[83-94] In spontaneously breathing asthmatic patients, heliox has been reported to decrease $PaCO_2$, increase peak flow, and decrease pulsus paradoxus. The reduction in pulsus paradoxus may be particularly important because it reflects a reduction in inspiratory muscle work.[87] Heliox has been used also with intubated and mechanically ventilated asthmatic patients, in whom it reportedly produces a reduction in $PaCO_2$ with a lower peak airway pressure[86] and an improvement in oxygenation.[94]

Several studies have reported no benefit of heliox in acute asthma patients.[90-92] In one of those,[92] heliox was administered for only 5 minutes, which might not be long

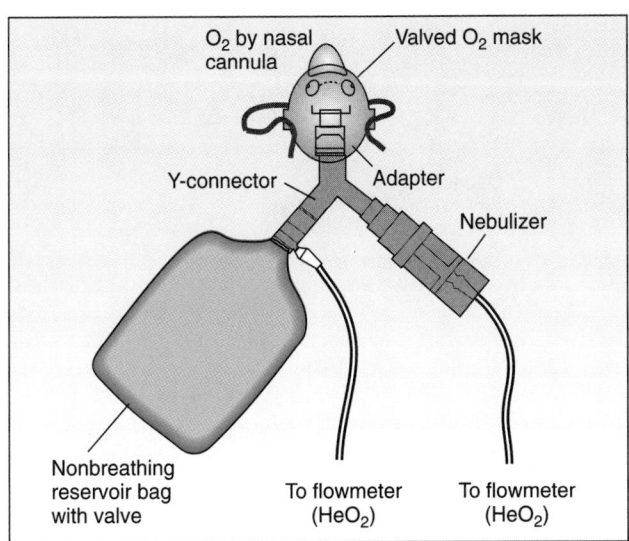

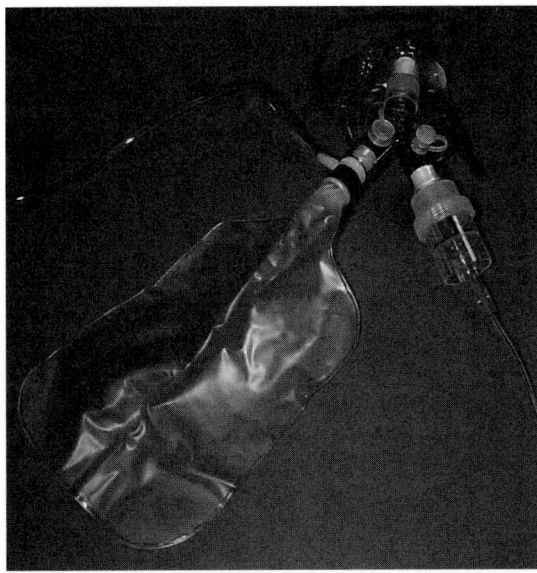

Figure 44-4 Equipment for administration of heliox.

enough to detect a benefit. A prospective, randomized, double-blind, crossover study[90] reported that heliox did not improve spirometry, clinical signs of asthma severity, or dyspnea. However, patients were enrolled after at least 6 hours of treatment for the acute asthma. Perhaps heliox is most useful during acute asthma with a short duration of symptoms.

The role of heliox in the treatment of COPD is unclear. COPD is a disease of small airways, a region of the lungs in which flow is density independent. In fact, failure of forced expiratory flow to increase after breathing heliox has been used as a diagnostic test for small airway disease.[95] However, several reports exist of benefit with heliox in patients with COPD.[96-99]

In two case series, an improvement in oxygenation and dynamic compliance was reported with heliox breathing after cardiac surgery.[100,101] These reports were uncontrolled and the mechanism is unclear, particularly because relatively low concentrations of helium were used.

Monitoring the Effect

Because of the expense of this therapy and the difficulties of its administration, heliox therapy should not be continued unless a clinical benefit is demonstrated. A decreased work of breathing with heliox should reduce the respiratory rate, decrease use of accessory muscles of breathing, decrease pulsus paradoxus, decrease the $PaCO_2$, improve air entry as assessed by auscultation, and improve the subjective breathing effort. Peak flowmeters and pulmonary function monitors may be inaccurate unless they are calibrated for the effects of heliox. Monitoring oxygenation (for example, pulse oximetry) during this therapy is important to ensure delivery of an adequate FIO_2.

Delivery Systems for Heliox

Administering heliox in a safe and effective manner requires caution. To avoid administration of a hypoxic gas mixture, 20% O_2/80% He should be mixed with oxygen to provide the desired helium concentration and FIO_2. The FIO_2 requirement limits the helium concentration that can be administered. If an FIO_2 greater than 0.40 is required, the limited concentration of helium is unlikely to produce clinical benefit. However, the FIO_2 requirement may decrease if heliox therapy is effective.[94]

For spontaneously breathing patients, heliox is administered by face mask with a reservoir bag (Figure 44-4). A Y-piece attached to the mask allows concurrent delivery of aerosolized medications. Sufficient flow is required to keep the reservoir bag inflated. This is often 12 to 15 L/min and requires three to six H-size cylinders per day. Using an oxygen-calibrated flowmeter for heliox therapy causes the flow of heliox (80% helium, 20% oxygen) to be 1.8 times greater than the indicated flow.

Heliox administration during mechanical ventilation can be problematic.[102,103] Ventilators are designed to deliver a mixture of air and oxygen. The density, viscosity, and thermal conductivity of helium can affect the delivered tidal volume and the measurement of exhaled tidal volume. With some ventilators (for example, Nellcor-Puritan-Bennett 7200), no reliable tidal volume is delivered with heliox. Use of other ventilators may result in a much higher delivered tidal volume than desired. This problem can be partially circumvented through the use of pressure ventilation rather than volume ventilation. Unlike flow sensors, pressure sensors are not affected by gas composition. Volume correction factors are necessary for critical care ventilators when heliox is used.[102]

The effect of heliox on the ability of the ventilator to correctly monitor flow and tidal volume depends on the method used for this measurement. Monitoring devices that are density dependent or that use thermal conductivity will be inaccurate in the presence of helium. Devices affected by gas viscosity will be affected to a lesser degree because the viscosity of helium is only slightly greater than that of air or oxygen. Screen pneumotachometers, such as those used in the Servo 900C and 300 ventilators, are affected by viscosity rather than density. Thus these ventilators are affected to a lesser degree than other ventilators. The accuracy of commonly used bedside respirometers are also affected by heliox. Regardless of the ventilator, clinicians must exercise extreme caution with the delivery of heliox, providing this therapy only when familiar with the performance of the ventilator with heliox. Unless a volume displacement spirometer is used, exhaled tidal volumes are likely incorrect. Some ventilators waste gas as part of the normal pneumatic function of the device, resulting in gas loss and frequent cylinder changes.

Effect of Heliox on Aerosol Delivery

Several studies reported improved aerosol penetration and deposition in the lungs with the nebulizer powered with heliox rather than air.[104-107] However, several studies reported no benefit with the use of heliox-driven nebulizer therapy.[108,109] Heliox can affect nebulizer function, resulting in a smaller particle size, reduced output, and longer nebulization time.[110] When heliox (rather than air or oxygen) is used to power the nebulizer, the flow should be increased by 50% to 100% to ensure adequate output from the nebulizer. Heliox has been shown also to improve aerosol delivery during mechanical ventilation.

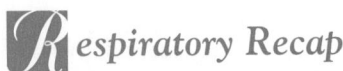*espiratory Recap*

Heliox
Therapeutic benefit related to its low density
Beneficial in some patients with partial upper airway obstruction or asthma
Adversely affects the function of equipment such as flowmeters, nebulizers, and ventilators

Combined Noninvasive Positive Pressure Ventilation and Heliox Therapy

Some clinicians are interested in combining the beneficial effects of NPPV and heliox therapy. In COPD patients, several studies[111,112] reported that heliox reduced PaCO2, dyspnea, and work of breathing to a greater extent than oxygen alone without heliox. Because of the technical complexity involved in the combination of these therapies, further research is needed before this can be recommended in clinical practice. Some interest also exists in the use of heliox with portable pressure ventilators. However, delivering high helium concentrations is difficult with these blower devices—even when high heliox flows are titrated into the system.[113]

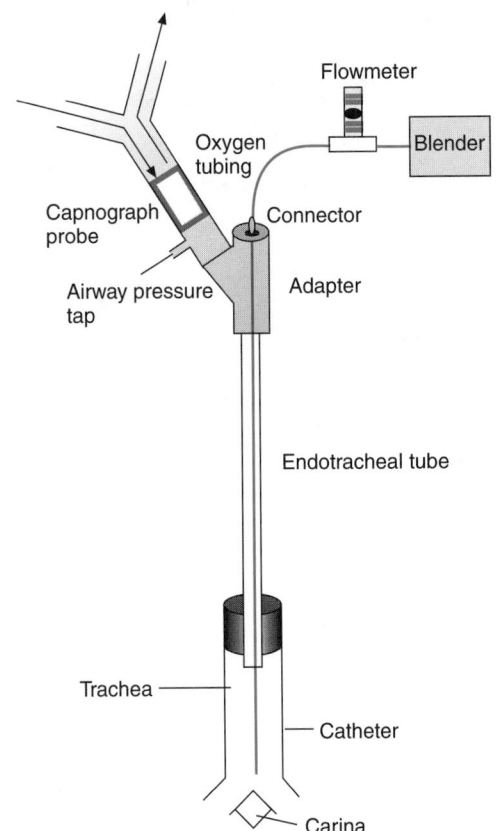

Figure 44-5   System for tracheal gas insufflation, with catheter placed through the endotracheal tube into the trachea. (Modified from Adams AB. Tracheal gas insufflation [TGI]. Respir Care 1996;41:285-293.)

Tracheal Gas Insufflation

Tracheal gas insufflation (TGI) is the injection of fresh gas into the central airways to improve the efficiency of alveolar ventilation and/or minimize the ventilatory requirement.[114-116] It is used as an adjunct to mechanical ventilation. A catheter is placed into the central airway proximal to the carina (Figure 44-5). Flow is introduced through the catheter to flush the proximal airways of CO2-laden gas (Figure 44-6). The result is less CO2 rebreathing on the subsequent inspiration, which effectively lowers the dead space. TGI has been studied extensively in lung models and animals.[117] In recent years, the number of reports of the use of TGI is increasing for patients with acute respiratory failure.[118] As it has become more widely recognized that alveolar overdistention during mechanical ventilation may result in increased morbidity and mortality, TGI may be useful as a technique to reduce the ventilatory requirement of patients with acute respiratory failure.

Approaches to TGI vary. The catheter can be introduced into the trachea either beside the endotracheal tube or through the endotracheal tube, or it can be incorporated into endotracheal tube design. Catheters can introduce flow either toward the carina or away from the carina (retrograde or reverse-thrust catheters).[119] The flow can be

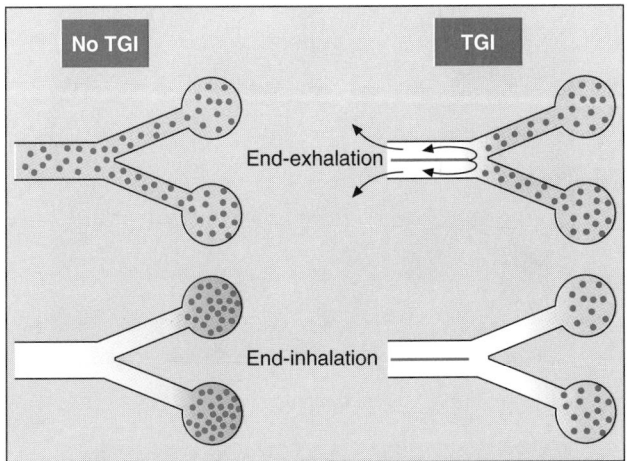

Figure 44-6 With no TGI, CO_2 in the central airway is delivered to the alveoli on the subsequent breath. With TGI, the central airway is cleared of CO_2 during the expiratory phase. (Modified from Ravenscraft SA. Tracheal gas insufflation: adjunct to conventional mechanical ventilation. Respir Care 1996;41:105-111.)

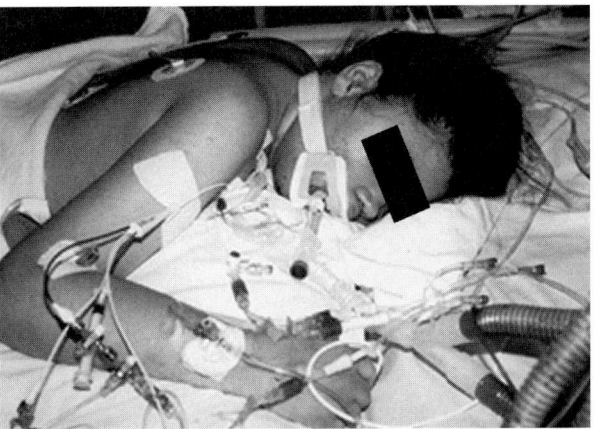

Figure 44-7 Patient in prone position.

continuous throughout the respiratory cycle, restricted to the expiratory phase, or constrained to a specific portion of the expiratory phase. Regardless of the approach, a concern with the use of TGI is the interaction between the TGI flow and the ventilator.[120]

Respiratory Recap

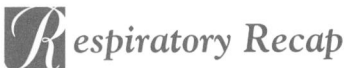

> **Tracheal Gas Insufflation**
>
> Flushes CO_2 from the anatomic dead space during exhalation
> May improve the efficiency of alveolar ventilation
> May adversely affect ventilator function

An alternative to TGI is aspiration of airway dead space-tracheal gas exsufflation (TGE).[121,122] With this technique, airway dead space gas is aspirated from the distal endotracheal tube and replaced by fresh gas from the ventilator circuit. A potential advantage of this approach is elimination of TGI-related problems such as airway injury resulting from jet streams from the catheter and difficulties with humidification of the TGI gas flow.

Prone Position

Critically ill patients, such as those with ARDS, are traditionally cared for in a supine position. Changing such patients to a **prone position** (Figure 44-7) may result in a significant improvement in oxygenation.[123] Lung consolidation and collapse occur primarily in the dependent lung zones in patients with ARDS.[124] The dorsal to ventral distribution of blood flow changes little when these patients are turned prone.[125] However, ventilation of the dorsal lung regions is increased when

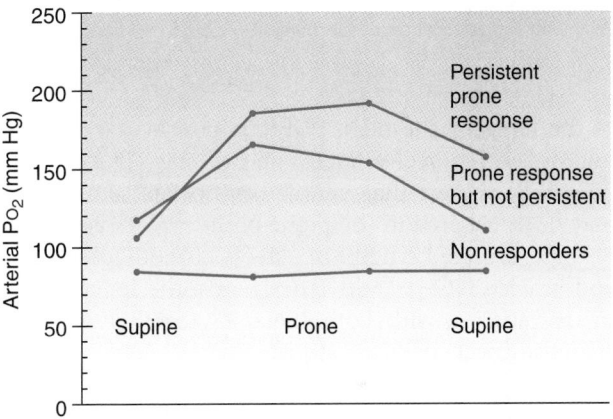

Figure 44-8 Three patterns of response to prone position. Some patients respond with an increase in Pao_2; this response persists when the patient is returned to supine. Some patients increase their Pao_2 when turned prone, but the response does not persist when they are returned to supine. Other patients do not respond to prone positioning. (Modified from Chatte G, Sab JM, Dubois JM, et al. Prone position in mechanically ventilated patients with severe acute respiratory failure. Am J Respir Crit Care Med 1997;155:473-478.)

prone, resulting in recruitment of these lung zones. The result is an improvement is shunt and arterial oxygenation when patients with ARDS are turned to a prone position. An improvement in oxygenation is seen in about two thirds of patients when they are turned prone (Figure 44-8).[126,127]

Several mechanisms have been used to describe the improvement in arterial oxygenation with prone position.[128] A more uniform pleural pressure in the prone position results in improved ventilation of dorsal lung regions. Prone positioning may result in a decrease in ventral thoracic chest wall compliance, promoting redistribution of ventilation to dorsal lung regions. Interestingly, some patients demonstrate an improvement in arterial oxygenation when sandbags are placed on the anterior chest wall with the patient in a supine position (Figure 44-9). The prone position eliminates compression

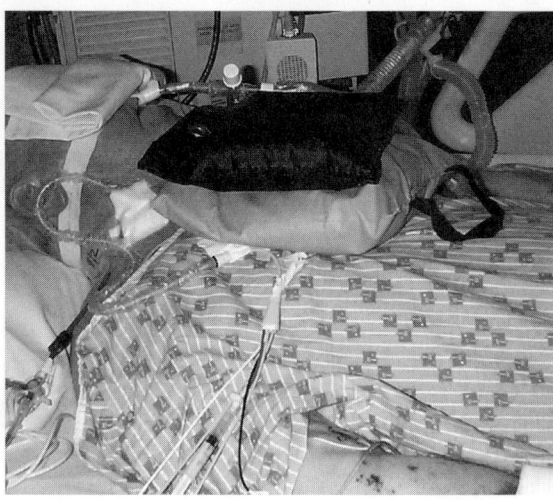

Figure 44-9 A patient with acute respiratory distress syndrome has sandbags placed on the anterior chest to decrease chest wall compliance. In this patient, there was a dramatic improvement in Pao₂ with the application of sandbags.

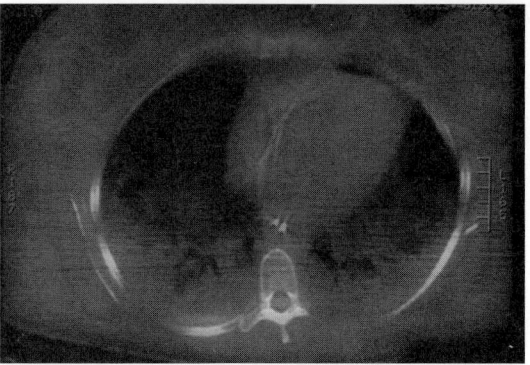

Before recruitment

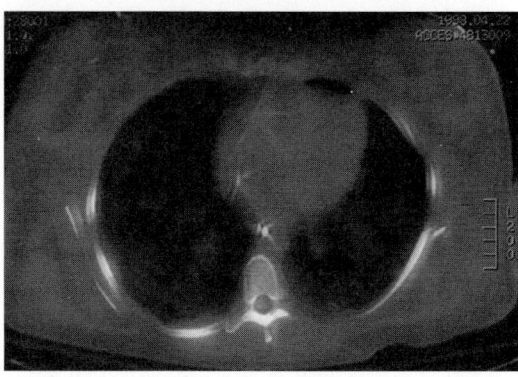

After recruitment

Figure 44-10 Computed tomography of the chest of a patient with acute respiratory distress syndrome before and after application of a recruitment maneuver.

of the lungs by the heart.[129] Prone positioning also may improve secretion clearance from the lungs. The results of one study suggest that ventilator-associated lung injury may be attenuated in the prone position.[130] Several studies have reported synergistic effects of prone positioning and inhaled NO.[131,132] In other words, the improvement in oxygenation with both therapies together is greater than the effects of either alone.

ℛespiratory Recap

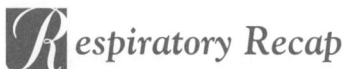

Prone Position
Improves oxygenation of some patients with ARDS
Requires caution during positioning of patients prone to prevent airway or vascular line dislodgement

Turning the patient prone requires at least four persons. One person, usually a respiratory therapist, is responsible for maintaining the airway. Another person is responsible for maintaining vascular lines, chest tubes, and the foley catheter. At least two others then log roll the patient to a prone position. The amount of time that the patient should remain prone is unclear. Generally, a set schedule of prone and supine is not necessary. The patient should remain prone as long as this strategy is beneficial. Periodically, the patient is turned supine for nursing care. At that time, patient response is assessed and the patient is returned to a prone position if deterioration is noted when supine. Prone positioning can be achieved effectively with an ordinary hospital bed (in other words, a special bed is not required). Some investigators have recommended elevation of the hips during prone position to allow the ab-

domen to hang free, but the necessity of this practice is unclear.[128]

Complications of prone positioning are relatively few and infrequent.[128,133] Occasionally, a vascular line or airway is removed if caregivers are not vigilant during the position change. Many patients develop some degree of facial edema while in the prone position. Occasionally, pressure sores on the face, ventral chest wall, or penis can occur. Periodic repositioning of the patient while he or she is in the prone position eliminates these effects. Some clinicians advocate the use of a swimmer's position, with the position changed from right to left on a regular basis while the patient is prone. The only absolute contraindication of prone positioning is a spinal cord injury.

In patients with unilateral lung disease, an improvement in oxygenation may occur with positioning of the patient in a lateral position with the good lung down. Presumably, this improves blood flow to the ventilated lung. **Kinetic therapy** uses a special bed that rotates the patient continuously from one lateral position to another, reaching a 124-degree angle, every 4 minutes. Although kinetic therapy may improve oxygenation and decrease the risk of pneumonia in selected mechanically

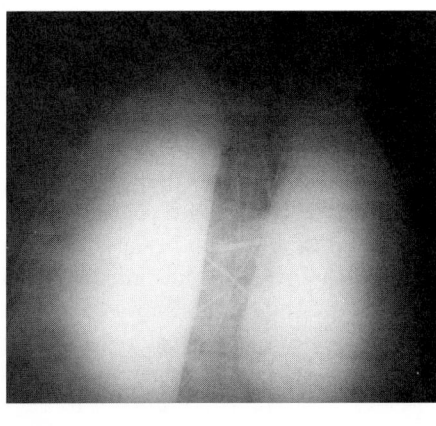

Gas ventilator

Liqui Vent

Endotracheal tube

A

Inhalation   Exhalation

Gas →

PFC   PFC

Alveoli filled
with *Liqui Vent*

B

Figure 44-11   **A,** Administration of partial liquid ventilation. **B,** Chest x-ray of a patient receiving partial liquid ventilation resulting from the radiopaque property of perflubron. (**A,** Modified courtesy Alliance Pharmaceutical, San Diego.)

TABLE 44-2

Physical Properties of Perflubron and Saline

Property	Perflubron	Saline
Oxygen solubility	53 mL/100 mL	2 mL/100 mL
Carbon dioxide solubility	210 mL/100 mL	70 mL/100 mL
Surface tension	18 dynes/cm	75 dynes/cm
Density	1.92 g/mL	1 g/mL
Spreading coefficient	2.7 dynes/cm	
Vapor pressure	11 mm Hg	

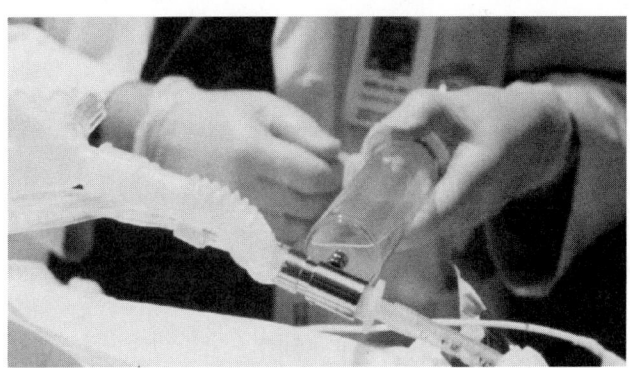

Figure 44-12   Instillation of perflubron into the proximal endotracheal tube.

ventilated patients, it has not been shown to decrease mortality.[134,135]

Recruitment Maneuvers

A characteristic of the lungs of the patient with ARDS is dependent atelectasis. These atelectatic alveoli may have high opening pressure. A **recruitment maneuver** is a sustained inflation at high airway pressure, which has been advocated as an adjunct to mechanical ventilation in patients with ARDS.[128] The result of a recruitment maneuver is decreased dependent atelectasis (Figure 44-10).

A common procedure used to perform a recruitment maneuver is to apply a sustained inflation (with CPAP mode on the ventilator) with a pressure of 30 to 45 cm H_2O for 30 to 45 seconds.[128,136] Other approaches used to perform recruitment maneuvers consist of an increase in PEEP for several breaths each minute[137] or the provision of several sigh breaths each minute at a plateau pressure of 45 cm H_2O.[138] An important aspect of lung recruit-

ment is the application of an adequate level of PEEP.[139] Although recruitment maneuvers are apparently safe, relative contraindications include hemodynamic instability, barotrauma, localized atelectasis (for example, unilateral lung disease), and bullous lung disease.

Partial Liquid Ventilation

Liquid ventilation uses fluorinated organic liquids (perfluorocarbons) as a respiratory medium.[140] These liquids have several properties that make them attractive for gas exchange (Table 44-2). Total liquid ventilation uses a special ventilator to deliver perfluorocarbon tidal volumes to the lungs. More commonly studied has been **partial liquid ventilation (PLV).** With PLV, the lungs are partially filled with perfluorocarbon and a conventional ventilator provides gas ventilation (Figure 44-11). The perfluorocarbon is administered by direct instillation into the endotracheal tube (Figure 44-12). The most commonly used perfluorocarbon for PLV has been perflubron. Perflubron is an eight-carbon molecule that is fluorinated in every position except for a terminal bromine ($C_8F_{17}Br$). This terminal bromine makes the molecule radiopaque (see Figure 44-11). Proposed mechanisms for benefit of PLV include recruitment of dependent lung regions because of the density of perflubron, improved compliance because of the low surface tension of perflubron, and lung lavage because perflubron is a poor solvent of water-based solutions. Because it has a low vapor pressure, perflubron is eliminated from the lungs by evaporation. Clinical trials of the use of perflubron are in their infancy. PLV is apparently safe, but its benefit in diseases such as ARDS remains to be determined.

$\mathcal{K}$EY $\mathcal{P}$OINTS

- Inhaled nitric oxide is a selective pulmonary vasodilator.
- The only FDA-approved indication for inhaled nitric oxide is hypoxic respiratory failure of the newborn.
- When administered by inhalation at low doses, inhaled nitric oxide is relatively risk free.
- The usual dose of inhaled nitric oxide is 20 ppm or less.
- Heliox is a mixture of oxygen and helium.
- Heliox may improve gas flow through a partially obstructed airway because of its low density.
- Because respiratory care equipment is designed to operate with air or oxygen, use of heliox frequently adversely affects its performance.
- Tracheal gas insufflation flushes carbon dioxide from the central airways during exhalation and thus improves the efficacy of alveolar ventilation.
- Many patients with ARDS have an improvement in oxygenation when turned to a prone position.
- Recruitment maneuvers are used to open atelectatic lung regions in patients with ARDS.
- Liquid ventilation uses fluorinated organic liquids (perfluorocarbons) as a respiratory medium.

References

1. Hurford WE. The biological basis for inhaled nitric oxide. Respir Care Clin N Am 1997;3:357-369.
2. Dupuy PM, Lancon JP, Francoise M, et al. Inhaled cigarette smoke selectively reverses human hypoxic vasoconstriction. Intensive Care Med 1995;21:941-944.
3. Lee KH, Tan PS, Rico P, et al. Low levels of nitric oxide as contaminant in hospital compressed air: physiologic significance? Crit Care Med 1997;25:1143-1146.
4. Pinsky MR, Genc F, Lee KH, et al. Contamination of hospital compressed air with nitric oxide: unwitting replacement therapy. Chest 1997;111:1759-1763.
5. NIOSH recommendations for occupational safety and health standards, 1988. MMWR 1988;37:1-29.
6. Aranda M, Pearl RG. The biology of nitric oxide. Respir Care 1999;44:156-168.
7. al-Alaiyan S, al-Omran A, Dyer D. The use of phosphodiesterase inhibitor (dipyridamole) to wean from inhaled nitric oxide. Intensive Care Med 1996;22:1093-1095.
8. Bigatello LM, Hess D, Dennehy KC, et al. Sildenafil can increase the response to inhaled nitric oxide. Anesthesiology 2000;92:1827-1829.
9. Head CA, Brugnara C, Martinez-Ruiz R, et al. Low concentrations of nitric oxide increase oxygen affinity of sickle erythrocytes in vitro and in vivo. J Clin Invest 1997;100:1193-1198.
10. Lundberg JO, Weitzberg E, Lundberg JM, et al. Nitric oxide in exhaled air. Eur Respir J 1996;9:2671-2680.
11. Hess D, Bigatello L, Kacmarek RM, et al. Use of inhaled nitric oxide in patients with acute respiratory distress syndrome. Respir Care 1996;41:424-446.
12. Lundberg JO, Farkas-Szallasi T, Weitzberg E, et al. High nitric oxide production in human paranasal sinuses. Nat Med 1995;1:370-373.
13. Gerlach H, Rossaint R, Pappert D, et al. Autoinhalation of nitric oxide after endogenous synthesis in nasopharynx. Lancet 1994;343:518-519.
14. Gerlach M, Gerlach H. Exhaled nitric oxide. Respir Care 1999;44:349-359.
15. Kharitonov SA, Yates D, Robbins RA, et al. Increased nitric oxide in exhaled air of asthmatic patients. Lancet 1994;343:133-135.
16. Alving K, Weitzberg E, Lundberg JM. Increased amount of nitric oxide in exhaled air of asthmatics. Eur Respir J 1993;6:1368-1370.
17. Massaro AF, Mehta S, Lilly CM, et al. Elevated nitric oxide concentrations in isolated lower airway gas of asthmatic subjects. Am J Respir Crit Care Med 1996;153:1510-1514.
18. Kharitonov SA, Chung KF, Evans D, et al. Increased exhaled nitric oxide in asthma is mainly derived from the lower respiratory tract. Am J Respir Crit Care Med 1996;153:1773-1780.
19. Cremona G, Higenbottam TW, Mayoral V, et al. Elevated exhaled nitric oxide in patients with hepatopulmonary syndrome. Eur Respir J 1995;8:1883-1885.
20. Kharitonov SA, Wells AU, O'Connor BJ, et al. Elevated levels of exhaled nitric oxide in bronchiectasis. Am J Respir Crit Care Med 1995;151:1889-1893.
21. Hyde RW, Geigel EJ, Olszowka AJ, et al. Determination of production of nitric oxide by lower airways of humans—theory. J Appl Physiol 1997;82:1290-1296.
22. Recommendations for standardized procedures for the on-line and off-line measurement of exhaled lower respiratory nitric oxide and nasal nitric oxide in adults and children—1999. Am J Respir Crit Care Med 1999;160:2104-2117.
23. Roberts JD, Fineman JR, Morin FC, et al. Inhaled nitric oxide and persistent pulmonary hypertension of the newborn. New Engl J Med 1997;336:605-610.
24. Inhaled nitric oxide in full-term and nearly full-term infants with hypoxic respiratory failure. N Engl J Med 1997;336:597-604.
25. Kinsella JP, Truog WE, Walsh WF, et al. Randomized, multicenter trial of inhaled nitric oxide and high-frequency oscillatory ventilation in severe, persistent pulmonary hypertension of the newborn. J Pediatr 1997;131:55-62.
26. Clark RH, Kueser TJ, Walker MW, et al. Low-dose inhaled nitric oxide treatment of persistent pulmonary hypertension in the newborn. N Engl J Med 2000;342:469-474.
27. Davidson D, Barefield ES, Kattwinkel J, et al. Inhaled nitric oxide for the early treatment of persistent pulmonary hyper-

tension of the term newborn: a randomized, double-masked, placebo-controlled, dose-response, multicenter study. Pediatrics 1998;101:325-334.

28. Kinsella JP, Abman SH. Clinical approach to inhaled nitric oxide therapy in the newborn with hypoxemia. J Pediatr 2000;136:717-726.

29. Jacobs P, Finer NN, Robertson CMT, et al. A cost effectiveness analysis of the application of nitric oxide versus oxygen gas for near-term newborns with respiratory failure: results of a Canadian randomized clinical trial. Crit Care Med 2000;28:872-878.

30. Rossaint R, Falke KJ, Lopez F, et al. Inhaled nitric oxide for the adult respiratory distress syndrome. N Engl J Med 1993;328:399-405.

31. Bigatello LM, Hurford WE, Kacmarek RM, et al. Prolonged inhalation of low concentrations of nitric oxide in patients with severe adult respiratory distress syndrome. Effects on pulmonary hemodynamics and oxygenation. Anesthesiology 1994;80:761-770.

32. Bigatello LM, Hurford WE, Hess D. Use of inhaled nitric oxide for ARDS. Respir Care Clin NA 1997;3:437-458.

33. Gerlach M, Keh D, Gerlach H. Inhaled nitric oxide for acute respiratory distress syndrome. Respir Care 1999;44:1184-1195.

34. Dellinger RP, Zimmerman JL, Taylor RW, et al. Effects of inhaled nitric oxide in patients with acute respiratory distress syndrome: results of a randomized phase II trial. Crit Care Med 1996;26:15-24.

35. Lundin S, Mang H, Smithies M, et al. Inhalation of nitric oxide in acute lung injury: results of a European multicenter study. Intensive Care Med 1999;25:911-919.

36. Sitbon O, Brenot F, Denjean A, et al. Inhaled nitric oxide as a screening vasodilator agent in primary pulmonary hypertension. A dose-response study and comparison with prostacyclin. Am J Respir Crit Care Med 1995;151:384-389.

37. Channick RN, Newhart JW, Johnson FW, et al. Pulsed delivery of inhaled nitric oxide to patients with primary pulmonary hypertension: an ambulatory delivery system and initial clinical tests. Chest 1996;109:1545-1549.

38. Channick RN, Yung GL. Long-term use of inhaled nitric oxide for pulmonary hypertension. Respir Care 1999;44:212-221.

39. Kacmarek RM, Ripple R, Cockrill BA, et al. Inhaled nitric oxide. A bronchodilator in mild asthmatics with methacholine-induced bronchospasm. Am J Respir Crit Care Med 1996;153:128-135.

40. Nakagawa TA, Johnston SJ, Falkos SA, et al. Life-threatening status asthmaticus treated with inhaled nitric oxide. J Pediatr 2000;137:119-122.

41. Gladwin MT, Schechter AN, Shelhamer JH. Inhaled nitric oxide augments nitric oxide transport on sickle cell hemoglobin without affecting oxygen affinity. J Clin Invest 1999;104:937-945.

42. Fullerton DA, McIntyre RC. Inhaled nitric oxide: therapeutic applications in cardiothoracic surgery. Ann Thorac Surg 1996;61:1856-1864.

43. Mathisen DJ, Kuo EY, Hahn C, et al. Inhaled nitric oxide for adult respiratory distress syndrome after pulmonary resection. Ann Thorac Surg 1998;66:1894-1902.

44. Bacha EA, Herve P, Murakami S, et al. Lasting beneficial effect of short-term inhaled nitric oxide on graft function after lung transplantation. J Thorac Cardiovasc Surg 1996;112:590-598.

45. Bacha EA, Sellak H, Murakami S, et al. Inhaled nitric oxide attenuates reperfusion injury in non-heartbeating-donor lung transplantation. Transplantation 1997;63:1380-1386.

46. Hess D, Bigatello L, Hurford WE. Toxicity and complications of inhaled nitric oxide. Respir Care Clin NA 1997;3:487-503.

47. Hess DR. Adverse effects and toxicity of inhaled nitric oxide. Respir Care 1999;44:315-330.

48. Nishimura M, Hess D, Kacmarek RM, et al. Nitrogen dioxide production during mechanical ventilation with nitric oxide in adults. Effects of ventilator internal volume, air versus nitrogen dilution, minute ventilation, and inspired oxygen fraction. Anesthesiology 1995;82:1246-1254.

49. Manktelow C, Bigatello LM, Hess D, et al. Physiologic determinants of the response to inhaled nitric oxide in patients with acute respiratory distress syndrome. Anesthesiology 1997;87:297-307.

50. Barbera JA, Roger N, Roca J, et al. Worsening of pulmonary gas exchange with nitric oxide inhalation in chronic obstructive pulmonary disease. Lancet 1996;347:436-440.

51. Katayama Y, Higenbottam TW, Diaz dAMJ, et al. Inhaled nitric oxide and arterial oxygen tension in patients with chronic obstructive pulmonary disease and severe pulmonary hypertension. Thorax 1997;52:120-124.

52. Bigatello LM. Strategies to enhance the efficacy of nitric oxide therapy. Respir Care 1999;44:331-339.

53. Samama CM, Diaby M, Fellahi JL, et al. Inhibition of platelet aggregation by inhaled nitric oxide in patients with acute respiratory distress syndrome. Anesthesiology 1995;83:56-65.

54. Loh E, Stamler JS, Hare JM, et al. Cardiovascular effects of inhaled nitric oxide in patients with left ventricular dysfunction. Circulation 1994;90:2780-2785.

55. Semigran MJ, Cockrill BA, Kacmarek R, et al. Hemodynamic effects of inhaled nitric oxide in heart failure. J Am Coll Cardiol 1994;24:982-988.

56. Lavoie A, Hall JB, Olson DM, et al. Life-threatening effects of discontinuing inhaled nitric oxide in severe respiratory failure. Am J Respir Crit Care Med 1996;153:1985-1987.

57. Miller OI, Tang SF, Keech A, et al. Rebound pulmonary hypertension on withdrawal from inhaled nitric oxide. Lancet 1995;346:51-52.

58. Atz AM, Adatia I, Wessel DL. Rebound pulmonary hypertension after inhalation of nitric oxide. Ann Thorac Surg 1996;62:1759-1764.

59. Davidson D, Barefield ES, Kattwinkel J, et al. Safety of withdrawing inhaled nitric oxide therapy in persistent pulmonary hypertension of the newborn. Pediatrics 1999;104:231-236.

60. Aly H, Sahni R, Wung JT. Weaning strategy with inhaled nitric oxide treatment in persistent pulmonary hypertension of the newborn. Arch Dis Child 1997;76:F118-F122.

61. Hess D, Ritz R, Branson RD. Delivery systems for inhaled nitric oxide. Respir Care Clin N Am 1997;3:371-410.

62. Branson RD, Hess DR, Campbell RS, et al. Inhaled nitric oxide: delivery systems and monitoring. Respir Care 1999;44:281-307.

63. Fujino Y, Kacmarek RM, Hess DR. Nitric oxide delivery during high-frequency oscillatory ventilation. Respir Care 2000;45:1097-1104.

64. Kirmse M, Hess D, Fujino Y, et al. Delivery of inhaled nitric oxide using the Ohmeda INOvent Delivery System. Chest 1998;113:1650-1657.

65. Ceccarelli P, Bigatello LM, Hess D, et al. Inhaled nitric oxide delivery by anesthesia machines. Anesth Analg 2000;90:482-488.

66. Phillips ML, Hall TA, Sekar K, et al. Assessment of medical personnel exposure to nitrogen oxides during inhaled nitric oxide treatment of neonatal and pediatric patients. Pediatrics 1999;104:1095-1100.

67. Body SC, Hartigan PM, Shernan SK, et al. Nitric oxide delivery, measurement and clinical application. J Cardiothor Vasc Anesth 1995;9:748-763.

68. Body SC, Hartigan PM. Manufacture and measurement of nitrogen oxides. Respir Care Clin N Am 1997;3:411-434.

69. Nishimura M, Imanaka H, Uchiyama A, et al. Nitric oxide (NO) measurement accuracy. J Clin Monit 1977;13:241-248.

70. Purtz EP, Hess D, Kacmarek RM. Evaluation of electrochemical nitric oxide and nitrogen dioxide analyzers suitable for use during mechanical ventilation. J Clin Monit 1997;13:25-34.

71. Skrinskas GJ, Hyland RH, Hutcheon MA. Using helium-oxygen mixtures in the management of acute upper airway obstruction. Can Med Assoc J 1983;128:555-558.

72. Lu TS, Ohmura A, Wong KC, Hodges MR. Helium-oxygen in treatment of upper airway obstruction. Anesthesiology 1976; 45:678-680.

73. Curtis JL, Mahlmeister M, Fink JB, et al. Helium-oxygen gas therapy. Use and availability for the emergency treatment of inoperable airway obstruction. Chest 1986;90:455-457.

74. Boorstein JM, Boorstein SM, Humphries GN, et al. Using helium-oxygen mixtures in the emergency management of acute upper airway obstruction. Ann Emerg Med 1989;18:688-690.

75. Kemper KJ, Ritz RH, Benson MS, et al. Helium-oxygen mixture in the treatment of postextubation stridor in pediatric trauma patients. Crit Care Med 1991;19:356-359.

76. Kemper KJ, Izenberg S, Marvin JA, et al. Treatment of postextubation stridor in a pediatric patient with burns: the role of heliox. J Burn Care Rehab 1990;11:337-339.

77. TenEyck LG, Colgan FJ. Methods and guidelines for mechanical ventilation with helium-oxygen for severe upper-airway obstruction. Respir Care 1984;29:155-159.

78. Mizrahi S, Yaari Y, Lugassy G, et al. Major airway obstruction relieved by helium/oxygen breathing. Crit Care Med 1986; 14:986-987.

79. Rudow M, Hill AB, Thompson NW, et al. Helium-oxygen mixtures in airway obstruction due to thyroid carcinoma. Can Anaesth Soc J 1986;33:498-501.

80. Sauder RA, Rafferty JF, Bilenki AL, et al. Helium-oxygen and conventional mechanical ventilation in the treatment of large airway obstruction and respiratory failure in an infant. Southern Med J 1991;84:646-648.

81. Rodeberg DA, Easter AJ, Washam MA, et al. Use of a helium-oxygen mixture in the treatment of postextubation stridor in pediatric patients with burns. J Burn Care Rehab 1995;16: 476-480.

82. Jordan WS, Graves CL, Elwyn RA. New therapy for postintubation laryngeal edema and tracheitis in children. JAMA 1970;212:585-588.

83. Tobias JD. Heliox in children with airway obstruction. Pediatr Emerg Care 1997;13:29-32.

84. Smith SW, Biros M. Relief of imminent respiratory failure from upper airway obstruction by use of helium-oxgyen: a case series and brief review. Acad Emerg Med 1999;6:953-956.

85. Shiue ST, Gluck EH. The use of helium-oxygen mixtures in the support of patients with status asthmaticus and respiratory acidosis. J Asthma 1989;26:177-180.

86. Gluck EH, Onorato DJ, Castriotta R. Helium-oxygen mixtures in intubated patients with status asthmaticus and respiratory acidosis. Chest 1990;98:693-698.

87. Manthous CA, Hall JB, Caputo MA, et al. Heliox improves pulsus paradoxus and peak expiratory flow in nonintubated patients with severe asthma. Am J Respir Crit Care Med 1995; 151:310-314.

88. Kass JE, Castriotta RJ. Heliox therapy in acute severe asthma. Chest 1995;107:757-760.

89. Austan F. Heliox inhalation in status asthmaticus and respiratory acidemia: a brief report. Heart Lung 1996;25:155-157.

90. Carter ER, Webb CR, Moffitt DR. Evaluation of heliox in children hospitalized with acute severe asthma. A randomized crossover study. Chest 1996;109:1256-1261.

91. Kudukis TM, Manthous CA, Schmidt GA, et al. Inhaled helium-oxygen revisited: effect of inhaled helium-oxygen during the treatment of status asthmaticus in children. J Pediatr 1997;130:217-224.

92. Verbeek PR, Chopra A. Heliox does not improve FEV_1 in acute asthma patients. J Emerg Med 1998;16:545-548.

93. Kass JE, Terregion CA. The effect of heliox in acute severe asthma. Chest 1999;116:296-300.

94. Schaeffer EM, Pohlman A, Morgan S, et al. Oxygenation in status asthmaticus improves during ventilation with helium-oxygen. Crit Care Med 1999;27:2666-2670.

95. Despas PJ, Leroux M, Macklem PT. Site of airway obstruction in asthma as determined by measuring maximal expiratory flow breathing air and a helium-oxygen mixture. J Clin Invest 1972;51:3235-3243.

96. Grape B, Channin E, Tyler JM. The effect of helium and oxygen mixtures on pulmonary resistance in emphysema. Am Rev Respir Dis 1960;81:823-829.

97. Swidwa DM, Montenegro HD, Goldman MD, et al. Helium-oxygen breathing in severe chronic obstructive pulmonary disease. Chest 1985;87:790-795.

98. Polito A, Fessler H. Heliox in respiratory failure from obstructive lung disease. N Engl J Med 1995;332:192-193.

99. Tassaux D, Jolliet P, Roeseler J, et al. Effects of helium-oxygen on intrinsic positive end-expiratory pressure in intubated and mechanically ventilated patients with severe chronic obstructive pulmonary disease. Crit Care Med 2000; 28:2721-2728.

100. Yahagi N, Kumon K, Tanigami H, et al. Helium/oxygen breathing improved hypoxemia after cardiac surgery: case reports. Anesth Analg 1995;80:1042-1045.

101. Yahagi N, Kumon K, Haruna M, et al. Helium/oxygen breathing improves hypoxemia after cardiac surgery. Artificial Organs 1997;21:24-27.

102. Tassaux D, Jolliet P, Thouret J, et al. Calibration of seven ICU ventilators for mechanical ventilation with helium-oxygen mixtures. Am J Respir Crit Care Med 1999;160:22-32.

103. Devabhaktuni VG, Torres A, Wison S, et al. Effect of nitric oxide, perfluorocarbon, and heliox on minute volume measurement and ventilator volumes delivered. Crit Care Med 1999;27(8):1603-1607.

104. Anderson M, Svartengren M, Bylin G, et al. Deposition in asthmatics of particles inhaled in air or in helium-oxygen. Am Rev Respir Dis 1993;147:524-528.

105. Svartengren M, Anderson M, Philipson K, et al. Human lung deposition of particles suspended in air or in helium/oxygen mixture. Exper Lung Res 1989;15:575-585.

106. Habib DM, Garner SS, Brandeburg S. Effect of helium-oxygen on delivery of albuterol in a pediatric, volume-cycled, ventilated lung model. Pharmacotherapy 1999;19:143-149.

107. Goode ML, Fink JB, Dhand R, et al. Improvement in aerosol delivery with helium-oxygen mixtures during mechanical ventilation. Am J Respir Crit Care Med 2001;163:109-114.

108. Henderson SO, Acharya P, Kilaghbian T, et al. Use of heliox-driven nebulizer therapy in the treatment of acute asthma. Ann Emerg Med 1999;33:141-146.

109. deBoisblanc BP, DeBleiux P, Resweber S, et al. Randomized trial of the use of heliox as a driving gas for updraft nebulization of bronchodilators in the emergent treatment of acute exacerbations of chronic obstructive pulmonary disease. Crit Care Med 2000;28:3177-3180.

110. Hess DR, Acosta FL, Ritz RH, et al. The effect of heliox on nebulizer function using a beta-agonist bronchodilator. Chest 1999;115:184-189.

111. Jolliett P, Tassauz D, Thouret J, et al. Beneficial effects of helium:oxygen versus air:oxygen noninvasive pressure support in patients with decompensated chronic obstructive lung disease. Crit Care Med 1999;27:2422-2429.

112. Jaber S, Fodil R, Carlucci A, et al. Noninvasive ventilation with helium-oxygen in acute exacerbations of chronic obstructive pulmonary disease. Am J Respir Crit Care Med 2000;161:1191-1200.

113. Chatmongkolchart S, Kacmarek RM, Hess DR. Heliox delivery by ventilators designed for noninvasive ventilation. Respir Care 2001;46:248-254.

114. Adams AB. Tracheal gas insufflation (TGI). Respir Care 1996; 41:285-293.

115. Ravenscraft SA. Tracheal gas insufflation: adjunct to conventional mechanical ventilation. Respir Care 1996;41:105-111.

116. Hess DR, Gillette MA. Tracheal gas insufflation and related techniques to introduce gas flow into the trachea. Respir Care 2001;46:119-129.

117. Nahum A. Animal and lung model studies of tracheal gas insufflation. Respir Care 2001;46:149-157.

118. Blanch LL. Clinical studies of tracheal gas insufflation. Respir Care 2001;46:158-166.

119. Adams AB. Catheters for tracheal gas insufflation. Respir Care 2001;46:177-184.

120. Kacmarek RM. Complications of tracheal gas insufflation. Respir Care 2001;46:167-176.

121. De Robertis E, Sigurdsson SE, Drefeldt B, Jonson B. Aspiration of airway dead space. A new method to enhance CO_2 elimination. Am J Respir Crit Care Med 1999;159:728-732.

122. Takahashi T, Bugedo G, Adams AB, et al. Effects of tracheal gas insufflation and tracheal gas exsufflation on intrinsic positive end-expiratory pressure and carbon dioxide elimination. Respir Care 1999;44:918-924.

123. Curley MA. Prone positioning of patients with acute respiratory distress syndrome: a systematic review. Am J Crit Care 1999;8:397-405.

124. Gattinoni L, Mascheroni D, Torresin A, et al. Morphological response to positive end expiratory pressure in acute respiratory failure. Computerized tomography study. Intensive Care Med 1986;12:137-142.

125. Lamm SJ, Graham MM, Albert RK. Mechanism by which the prone position improves oxygenation in acute lung injury. Am J Respir Crit Care Med 1994;150:184-193.

126. Chatte G, Sab JM, Dubois JM, et al. Prone position in mechanically ventilated patients with severe acute respiratory failure. Am J Respir Crit Care Med 1997;155:473-478.

127. Curley MA, Thompson JE, Arnold JH. The effects of early and repeated prone positioning in pediatric patients with acute lung injury. Chest 2000;118:156-163.

128. Kacmarek RM, Schwartz DR. Lung recruitment. Respir Care Clin N Am 2000;6:597-623.

129. Albert RK, Hubmayr RD. The prone position eliminates compression of the lungs by the heart. Am J Respir Crit Care Med 2000;161:1660-1665.

130. Broccard A, Shapiro RS, Schmitz LL, et al. Prone positioning attenuates and redistributes ventilator-induced lung injury in dogs. Crit Care Med 2000;28:295-303.

131. Papazian L, Bregeon F, Gaillet F, et al. Respective and combined effects of prone position and inhaled nitric oxide in patients with acute respiratory distress syndrome. Am J Respir Crit Care Med 1998;157:580-585.

132. Borelli M, Lampati L, Vascotto E, et al. Hemodynamic and gas exchange response to inhaled nitric oxide and prone positioning in acute respiratory distress syndrome patients. Crit Care Med 2000;28:2707-2712.

133. Offner PJ, Haenel JB, Moore EE, et al. Complications of prone ventilation in patients with multisystem trauma with fulminant acute respiratory distress syndrome. J Trauma 2000; 48:224-228.

134. Staudinger T, Kofler J, Mullner M, et al. Comparison of prone positioning and continuous rotation of patients with adult respiratory distress syndrome: results of a pilot study. Crit Care Med 2001;29:51-56.

135. Hess D, Agarwal NN, Myers CL. Positioning, lung function, and kinetic bed therapy. Respir Care 1992;37:181-197.

136. Medoff BD, Harris RS, Kesselman H, et al. Use of recruitment maneuvers and high positive end-expiratory pressure in a patient with acute respiratory distress syndrome. Crit Care Med 2000;28:1210-1216.

137. Foti G, Cereda M, Sparacino ME, et al. Effects of periodic lung recruitment maneuvers on gas exchange and respiratory mechanics in mechanically ventilated acute respiratory distress syndrome (ARDS) patients. Intensive Care Med 2000;26: 501-507.

138. Pelosi P, Cadringher P, Bottino N, et al. Sigh in acute respiratory distress syndrome. Am J Respir Crit Care Med 1999; 159:872-880.

139. Lapinsky SE, Aubin M, Mehta S, et al. Safety and efficacy of a sustained inflation for alveolar recruitment in adults with respiratory failure. Intensive Care Med 1999;25:1297-1301.

140. Multz AS. Liquid ventilation. Respir Care Clin N Am 2000; 6:645-657.

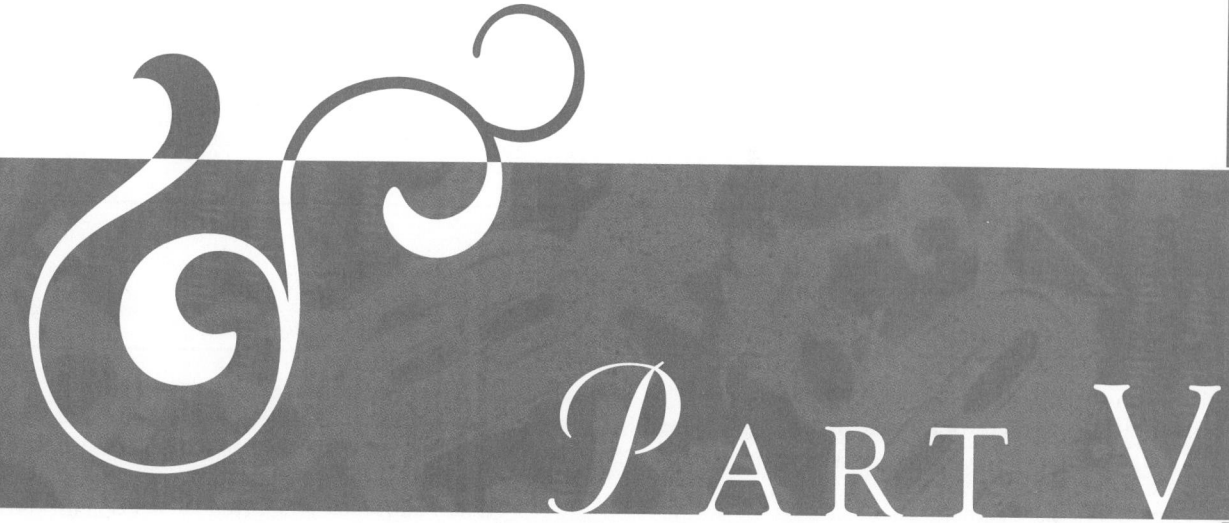

PART V

Respiratory Disease Management

CHAPTER 45

Principles of Disease Management

William F. Galvin

OBJECTIVES

1. Identify the forces driving disease management and the new mindset in managing disease.
2. Explain the history and evolution of disease management.
3. Define disease management and terms associated with care management.
4. Explain the difference between case management and disease management.
5. List the factors associated with the disease management movement.
6. Identify the core components of disease management.
7. Describe the concept of health value as it pertains to disease management.
8. List and explain the basic principles of disease management.
9. Identify the diseases best suited for disease management programs.
10. Identify and explain the steps used to develop a disease management program.
11. List and explain the barriers and opportunities of disease management.
12. Explain the roles of respiratory therapists with regard to disease management.

KEY TERMS

Care Management	Demand Management	Pathways
Case Management	Disease Management	Protocols
Component Management	Evidence-Based Medicine	

The primary forces driving disease management are cost and the changing pattern of disease (Figure 45-1 and Box 45-1). The health care cost component of the gross domestic product (GDP) shifted from 5% in 1960 to almost 14% by the end of the twentieth century. This escalating increase in the health care component of the GDP is at the heart of efforts to reform and restructure the health care system.

The infectious diseases prevalent in 1900 have given way to chronic, lifestyle diseases by the year 2000. This issue of chronicity is especially important because more than 90 million Americans have chronic conditions and they account for approximately $660 billion in health care costs.[1] Lifestyle, which is reflected in an individual's health behaviors, is also an important consideration be-

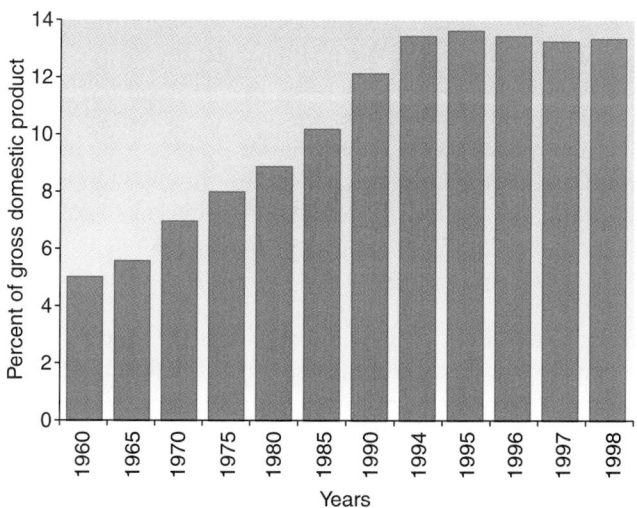

Figure 45-1 Health care expenditures as a percent of gross domestic product (1960-1995). (Data from Centers for Disease Control and Prevention, National Center for Health Statistics. Health care expenditures. Hyattsville, Md: The CDC; 2000. [http://www.cdc.gov/nchs/data/hus99ncb.pdf])

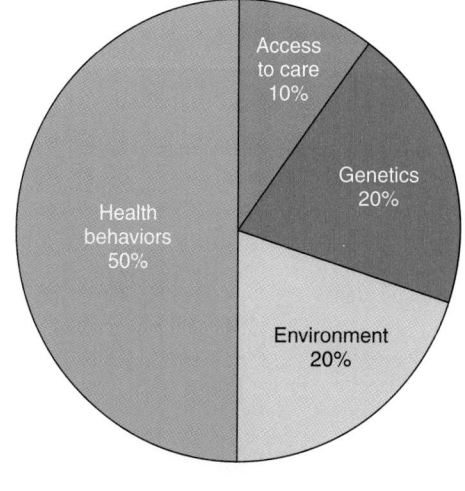

Figure 45-2 Determinants of health. (Data from Centers for Disease Control and Prevention. Ten leading causes of death in the United States, 1975. Atlanta: The CDC; 2000. [http://www.cdc.gov/nchs/data/hus99ncb.pdf])

Box 45-1

Changing Patterns of Disease (1900-1999)

1900*	1999*
Pneumonia	Heart disease
Tuberculosis	Cancer
Diarrhea and enteritis	Stroke
Heart disease	Chronic lung disease
Stroke	Unintentional injury
Liver disease	Pneumonia and influenza
Injuries	Diabetes
Cancer	HIV infection
Senility	Suicide
Diphtheria	Chronic liver disease

From Center for Disease Control and Prevention. Control of Infectious Diseases, 1900-1999. Morbidity and Mortality Weekly Report 1999;48:621-629.
*Diseases listed are in order of prevalence, from most prevalent to least prevalent for the time spans stated.

Table 45-1

Behavioral Causes of Death in the United States in 1990

Cause	Percentage of Total Deaths
Tobacco	19
Diet/activity patterns	14
Alcohol	5
Microbial agents	4
Toxic agents	3
Firearms	2
Sexual behavior	1
Motor vehicles	1
Illicit use of drugs	<1
TOTAL	50

From McGinnis J, Foege WH. Actual causes of death in the United States. JAMA 1993;270:2207-2212.

cause it accounts for about 50% of an individual's health status (Figure 45-2) and is associated with every leading cause of death in the United States.[2] Its impact is even more pronounced when one views the leading causes of death from the perspective of the behavioral causes of death (Table 45-1). These forces have given rise to the adoption of a new mindset in the way we perceive health (Table 45-2).[3] These new mindsets are the impetus behind the disease management movement and are the themes of this chapter. This chapter addresses specifically the history and evolution of the disease management movement. It defines the terms associated with disease management and addresses the goals, principles, and specific cardiopul-

monary diseases targeted for disease management programs. It identifies the steps in development of a disease management program and barriers and future opportunities and concludes with an explanation of the role of the respiratory therapist as a disease manager.

History and Evolution of Disease Management

The origin and evolution of **disease management** is rooted in the desire to improve health care quality and contain health care costs. Disease management first became popu-

TABLE 45-2

Adopting New Mindsets

Previous Focus	Current Focus
Disease orientation	Health orientation
Fragmentation	Integration
Competing institutions	Shared power and collaboration
Physicians as adversaries	Physicians as partners
Limited financial risk	Broad financial risk
Providers as independent agents	Providers of a community of social agents
Accountability to governing bodies	Accountability to the community
Focus on the individual	Focus on the broader population
Hospitals and health care systems	Organizers and joiners of community care networks

Modified from American Hospital Association. American Hospital Association Booklet, Chicago: The Association; 1996.

TABLE 45-3

Selected List of Participants in the Disease Management Movement

Parent Group	Specific Organizations
Managed care organizations	Aetna U.S. Healthcare, Group Health Care of Puget Sound
Pharmaceutical firms	Merck, SmithKline Beecham, Glaxo Wellcome
Integrated delivery systems	Lovelace Health System, Henry Ford Health System, Mayo Clinic
Specialty centers	National Jewish Center for Immunology and Respiratory Diseases, Memorial Sloan Kettering
Academic health centers/systems	University of Pennsylvania Health System, Johns Hopkins Health System
Multihospital chains	Columbia HCA, Tenet, Intermountain Health Care
Employers and coalitions	Xerox, GTE, Digital, Business Health Care Action Group
Pharmaceutical benefit companies	Medco, PCS, DPS, Caremark, Value Rx
"Independent" disease management companies	Greenstone Health Care, Stuart Disease Management, AirLogix

From Couch JB. The physician's guide to disease management. Gaithersburg, Md: Aspen; 1997. p. 2.

lar in 1993 when the Boston Consulting Group introduced the term in its study of the pharmaceutical industry.[4] Since that time, every health care–related group or entity is involved in some way with the evolution, development, and implementation of disease management (Table 45-3). Two groups in particular are considered responsible for spearheading the popularity of disease management—managed care organizations and the pharmaceutical industry. Their goals are to optimize profits, contain health care costs, and provide quality patient care.

Large pharmaceutical corporations purchased pharmaceutical benefits companies with the initial intention of capturing market distribution channels into managed care organizations and leveraging resources and contacts to develop state-of-the-art programs to manage the various diseases of these large populations.[5] Although pharmaceutical companies do not provide direct treatment, they do have extensive data-bases and can use them to influence the industry. Local pharmacies have a distinct advantage: they are strategically placed in the community and have access to the databases of both physicians and patients. This allows them to provide advice, guidance and support, identify adverse drug interactions, adjust dosages and schedules, employ utilization review, and document compliance through knowledge of refill and usage patterns of their customers.[6] Disease management provides them with an opportunity to demonstrate how appropriately selected and administered drug and device interventions may result in improved outcomes, patient satisfaction, and financial rewards.

The impetus for utilization of disease management programs by managed care organizations comes from two sources: the employment benefits consultant community and the employer coalition community. The people who write the request for proposals (employee benefits managers) are the ones that drive the market. The employer coalition community is bringing enormous numbers of employees to managed care. Accordingly, this fact serves to shape thought and acceptable standards.[7] Managed care organizations have strong motivation and strong financial incentives to cut resource consumption in all provider sites and they tend to move aggressively to this end. They are at the forefront of adopting this approach because the shift from discounted fees to a prepaid per-member formula for enrollees drives the demand to increase efficiencies, ensuring that providers are uniformly using the most effective procedures, drugs, and supplies.[8]

Disease management has become a way for pharmaceutical firms to sell more products, for managed care organizations to contain costs, and for health care professionals (for example, respiratory therapists) to improve patient outcomes.[6] For disease management to be effective, a partnership must exist between the patient, health plan, and provider.

Terms, Factors, and Concepts Associated with Disease Management

Care Management

Care management is a general term for the coordination of patient interventions. It is an umbrella term under which many loosely related terms flow. The more popular terms associated with care management are **component**

management, demand management, case management, and disease management. Respiratory therapists must have an understanding of these terms, because efforts are continuously underway to institute measures aimed at coordination of the care and management of respiratory diseases.

Component Management

Component management, is the opposite of disease management.[9] Component management is the predominant method used to control health care costs since the 1980s. Its focus is cost control through limitation of the use of resources or services such as therapeutic procedures, diagnostic tests, medications, or hospital lengths of stay. Unfortunately, component management often results in lower quality of care and poorer clinical outcomes and is an ineffective way to truly control costs.

The problem with component management is that each aspect of care is managed separately—emergency room visits, physician services, medications—and services are not integrated. In the case of the patient with asthma, all health plans cover emergency room visits, inpatient hospital stays, and physician services. Medications may or may not be covered. However, few provide coverage for patient education and counseling. Consequently, the limited coverage for medications and patient education converts into significantly higher costs in the form of emergency room visits, inpatient hospitalizations, and physician office visits. When respiratory therapy departments were revenue generators, component care approaches allowed them to flourish. However, component management is flawed: it is episodic, uncoordinated, emphasizes treatment instead of prevention, and provides little incentive to treat the entire disease. Shortcomings of component management are identified in Box 45-2.[9]

Demand Management

Demand management entails any organized effort or program designed to guide health care consumers into the most appropriate level of health care service by involving them in their own care.[10] It reduces the need for and use of costly, often unnecessary, medical services, and arbitrary managed care interventions. The tools of demand management consist of patient **protocols,** clinical **pathways,** case management, and disease management. These tools were developed to enable the clinician to achieve better outcomes by making it easier to give patients what they need when they need it. The intention was to weed out inappropriate and unnecessary care.[11]

Case Management

Case management is defined as a collaborative process that assesses, plans, implements, coordinates, monitors, and evaluates the options and services required to meet an individual's health needs, using communication and available resources to promote quality, cost, and effective

Box 45-2

Shortcomings of Component Management

- Often pays for only the most expensive services (hospitalizations, physician visits) leading to increases in high-cost treatments
- Provides powerful incentives for fragmentation of the health care system
- Does not recognize the relationship between health care services and total health care costs
- Frequently puts providers in opposition with financial managers and each other
- Emphasizes treatment over prevention

From Patterson R. Disease management. Case Review 1995 (Fall).

outcomes.[12] It is generally employed for the high-risk, high-cost patient who suffers repeated admissions, encounters significant variances, is unpredictable and may be socioeconomically disadvantaged.[11] Case management was built on the notion that 20% of the patients were responsible for 80% of the costs. The rationale was a focus on the care of the 20%, would reduce this 80% cost. Traditional case management is one-on-one care and expensive.[13] Case managers focus on an individual patient and assist in acquiring equipment and services, work with schools and other community-based organizations, provide technical support, conduct patient education, and identify and remove barriers to effective implementation of the care plan.[11]

Disease Management

Disease management is one of the most innovative and exciting concepts facing the health care delivery system. Numerous synonyms are associated with the concept, and some of the more popular are *disease state management, system-based disease management, total health management, medical management, population-based management, best practices, care-mapping,* and *outcomes management.* The different terminology attempts to capture or highlight one or more of the numerous principles that drive the disease management movement.

The following definitions for disease management are numerous and diverse:

- A clinical management process of care that spans the continuum of care from primary prevention to ongoing long-term health maintenance for individuals with chronic health conditions or diagnoses[7]
- An approach to identify a specific subpopulation of patients at high risk for undesirable outcomes and intervene to modify that risk[14]
- The cure to high-cost conditions[7]
- An ongoing, comprehensive case management program for specific chronic diseases that is based on clearly defined, well-established best practices of care[11]

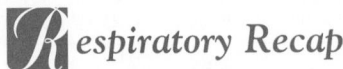

Key elements are repeated throughout the various definitions—a coordinated effort, comprehensive care across the continuum, and integration within the health system. For purposes of this chapter, the following definition is used: Disease management is an approach to patient care that emphasizes coordinated, comprehensive care along the continuum of disease and across health care delivery systems.[15]

Often the difference between case management and disease management is not apparent. However, the goal, emphasis, scope, timing, guidelines, caregivers involved, and data sources are strikingly unique and different for each management approach (Table 45-4).

Factors Associated with Disease Management

Some of the factors associated with the concept of disease management are as follows:

- An emphasis on primary and secondary prevention, featuring both patient and provider education and extensive self-care
- The use of clinical guidelines and practice protocols, and other tools that direct practitioners toward rigorously defined best practices that cross practice setting boundaries
- The application of quality improvement principles to the entire spectrum of care, focusing on disease states

Table 45-4

Comparison of Conventional Case Management and Disease Management

Case Management	Disease Management

Goal
   Streamlining components
   Critical path component cost control
	Integrating components
	Improvement in long-term outcome

Emphasis
   Treatment of sickness, especially in a complex patient
	Prevention and education
	   For patients, families, and physicians
	   For common outpatient conditions
	   Low technology and nonsurgical procedures
	   Prescription drug managed

Scope Patient often has multiple diseases	Patient often is evaluated for a single disease
Timing Periodic inspection	Prospective and concurrent

Guidelines
   Generic
   Externally imposed
	Customized to diagnosis
	Internally designed

Caregivers
   Generalists
   Nurses (primarily)
	Specialists
	Multidisciplinary team

Data Sources
   Primarily inpatient (tracking length of stay, profit margin per
     stay, mortality)
   Not integrated
	All points of service (tracking annual episodes of care cost,
	     medication compliance, functional status)
	Integrated

Financial Risk Lacks ability to bear financial risk	Demonstrates increased ability to bear financial risk

From Kongstvedt P. Essentials of managed health care. 2nd ed. Gaithersburg, Md: Aspen; 1997.

rather than on acute episodes of care and including inpatient, outpatient, and ancillary services

- An integrated, systems-based approach that features strong communication among providers and measurable, high-quality standards
- The collection and evaluation of outcomes information[6]

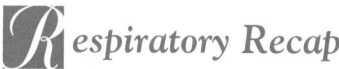

Respiratory Recap

Factors Associated with Disease Management
Emphasis on prevention
Use of clinical guidelines and practice protocols
Application of quality improvement principles to the entire spectrum of care
Integrated, systems-based approach
Collection and evaluation of outcomes information

Core Components of Disease Management

In a study conducted by Migliara and Kaplan for the National Managed Health Care Congress,[16] 16 components of disease state management were presented in three segments

TABLE 45-5

Core Components of a Disease Management Program

Components	Percentage of Respondents Who Selected Component
Core Components	
Clinical guidelines	87
Clinical outcomes management	83
Outcomes studies	82
Computer data collection/ management/tracking	81
Provider education	78
Patient satisfaction	77
Additional Components	
Benchmarking	66
Patient compliance monitoring	65
Patient education	63
Provider compliance monitoring	59
Treatment algorithms	56
Wellness programs	48
Noncomputerized data collection/ management/tracking	47
Pharmacoeconomic analysis	32
Demand management	22
Formulary compliance	15

From Johnson SK. The state of disease state management. Case Review 1996; (Fall):53-57.

of health care: managed care organizations, employers, and ancillary vendors and providers. The surveyed organizations were asked to rate components in terms of their significance to an effective program. More than 70% of respondents selected the same core components (Table 45-5).[7] A second string of core components were also identified (see Table 45-5). Although these core components are considered key components of a disease management program, others have streamlined the list to five cornerstones of disease management. The five cornerstones are as follows:

1. Expert guidance on clinical decisions
2. A new team approach to peer consulting
3. Changes in the way the cooperative operates
4. Savvy ways to educate patients to cope with their illnesses (need to know how human behavior works and help people set clear, achievable goals)
5. Better, faster information when and where the doctors need it[8]

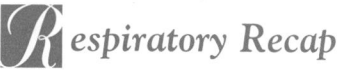

Respiratory Recap

Cornerstones of Disease Management
Expert guidance on clinical decisions
A new team approach to peer consulting
Changes in the way the cooperative operates
Savvy ways to educate patients to cope with their illnesses
Better, faster information when and where the doctors need it

Goals of Disease Management

The purpose of disease management is to take what was learned in epidemiology and research and incorporate that knowledge into everyday practice, while the results are measured and improvements attempted. The plan is never really finished but rather under continuous quality improvement.[8] The challenge is to apply a gradation of resources to members of the population in question so that each does not get too little (low quality) or too much (poor cost-containment), but just the right amount of resources (high value).[13] In short, disease management attempts to achieve better control of episode cost of care, reduce mortality, improve functional status, improve patient and physician satisfaction, acquire meaningful outcome data (for example, medication compliance), and develop an improved ability to bear financial risk for service.[12]

Health Value

Although the goal of disease management is reduction of cost and improvement in quality, the overriding goal of health care is value.[5,13] Value (Equation 45-1) is defined as

Equation 45-1
Health Care Value

$$\text{Health care value} = \frac{\text{Quality of clinical, economic, service, humanistic outcomes}}{\text{Overall costs, time, resources, and ``hassles'' to all stakeholders}}$$

quality of outcomes per unit of cost to the stakeholders.[5] Outcomes can be of a clinical, economic, service, and/or humanistic nature. Clinical outcomes can entail rates of mortality, morbidity, complications, and/or infection. Economic outcomes can be measured in terms of overall costs for hospitalization, emergency room visits, outpatient-, physician- and pharmaceutical-related services, and member/month costs. Service outcomes are generally subjective and include patient perception of care, patient and provider satisfaction, and health plan enrollment rates. Humanistic outcomes can include overall perception of health status, physical, role and social functioning, and levels of pain.

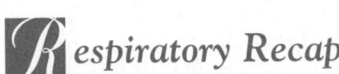 *espiratory Recap*

Goals of Disease Management
Achieve control of episode cost of care
Reduce morbidity
Improve functional status
Improve patient and physician satisfaction
Acquire more meaningful outcome data
Develop an improved ability to bear financial risk for the service

Costs include the total of all costs involved in health care delivery and include time, resources, and hassles. This entails appropriate choice of equipment, personnel, and services and utilization of all three of these in a timely fashion. Efficiency and effectiveness minimize absenteeism and losses in productivity. All stakeholders (purchasers, payers, providers, and patients) experience hassles, such as providers submitting claims and patients securing referrals. Stakeholder concerns with hassles are real and should not be taken lightly.[5]

Basic Principles of Disease Management

Natural Course, Causes, and Cost Drivers of Disease

One of the more important principles of disease management (Box 45-3)[17] is to understand the natural course of the disease, the causes of the disease, and the factors that typically drive costs. The course and causes of most car-

Box 45-3
Principles Characterizing Disease Management

- Understanding of the disease's natural course, causes, and cost drivers
- Diagnosis and treatment based on the disease process rather than on reimbursement patterns
- Patient education and compliance programs for chronic disease management
- Management of treatment that cuts across care settings and provides full continuity of care
- Direct resources toward the best and most cost-effective treatments and compare outcomes among plans and treatments

Modified from Zitter M. Disease management: a new approach to health care. Medical Interface 1994; (August):70-76.

diopulmonary disease are fairly predictable and straightforward. However, what are not obvious are the factors that drive the cost of disease. Cost drivers of disease are compliance, prevention, rapid resolution, acute flare-ups, and the 80/20 rule.[17]

espiratory Recap

Cost Drivers of Disease	
Compliance	Acute flare-ups
Prevention	The 80/20 Rule
Rapid resolution	

Tuberculosis is an example of a respiratory disease in which noncompliance to long-term pharmacologic management results in ineffective treatment, lack of resolution of the disease process, and risk of exposure and transmission to the public. Patients with tuberculosis typically require a regimen of multiple medications for a prolonged period of time (6 to 12 months). However, patients often feel better shortly after initial treatment and stop taking their medications. The result is a lack of eradication of the disease and potentially serious health consequences to the individual and to the public. In short, compliance to the care plan results in a significant impact on cost containment.

With regard to prevention, many patients with acquired immune deficiency syndrome (AIDS) could be spared disease by practicing safe sex. In other words, the high cost of treatment could have been prevented if the individuals engaged in a healthy lifestyle practice. About 85% of managed care organization's disease management efforts are focused on treatment rather than prevention. In the future this is likely to shift: efforts will be directed at prevention rather than treatment.[7]

Rapidly resolving the disease or condition curtails health care costs. For example, a patient who develops a serious case of pneumonia should receive immediate treatment with antibiotics. Ideally, the invading organism is identified, the appropriate antibiotic ordered, and the patient adheres to the therapeutic care plan. Often delays in a patient's seeking medical attention or inaccurate assessment and diagnosis will result in a more serious affliction and a condition that is protracted or sustained. A prolonged illness can result in an increase in the number and intensity of additional services, an increased length of stay, and ultimately increased health care costs. Efforts should always be directed at rapidly resolving the disease or condition.

Asthma is often characterized by acute exacerbation of the disease. These acute flare-ups are preventable by identification of triggers, education on the action and use of medications, and instruction in the proper use of medication delivery devices. Hospitalization and frequent emergency room visits are extremely costly. Efforts directed at curtailing these acute flare-ups result in significant reduction of health care costs.

The 80/20 rule indicates that a high percentage of health care costs are represented by a relatively small number of conditions. A report states that in a typical employee group, 10% of employees make up 70% of the group's health care costs, whereas just 1% consume 30% of total expenditures.[18] With regard to specific diseases, more than 10 million people have asthma and less than 4% of that population accounts for more than 50% of the total costs associated with this chronic disease.[19] Using the 80/20 rule and targeting the at-risk for prevention and treatment is an effective and efficient means to control cost drivers.[17]

Diagnosis and Treatment Based on Disease Rather than Reimbursement Patterns

Fragmentation is a major problem within the health care system. The critically important functions of the provision of care and reimbursement for services rendered are fragmented and disharmonious. The provider network made up of physicians and other care providers is interested primarily in quality of care issues, whereas the payer network is concerned almost exclusively with the costs of services and method and amount of reimbursement. The two seem to be going in different directions. Under a disease management program, the system is integrated and the primary focus is to diagnose and treat the disease process with emphasis on preventive measures.

Patient Education and Compliance Programs for Chronic Disease Management

With regard to disease management, strong patient education skills and abilities takes on new meaning. Failure to achieve desired results from noncompliance reportedly averages 40%, depending on the condition being treated. The rate for asthma is approximately 20%, whereas the rate for arthritis is 71% and hypertension is approximately 40%.[20] About 10% of all hospitalizations and 23% of all nursing home admissions are attributed to nonadherence.[21] The cost of nonadherence in the United States has been estimated at more than $100 billion dollars each year.[22] The problem of noncompliance is monumental and the critical need for patient education through scheduled inpatient sessions at the bedside, counseling, telephone and mail prompts, and/or home visits is crucial. Disease management programs emphasize and employ many of these measures on a more concerted basis.

Empowering the patient and stressing the importance of self-management of the disease process are emphasized. The patient needs to be more knowledgeable and better informed. In addition, patients must be held accountable for their actions. This is often difficult; however, patient involvement is key because one of the major measures of quality is patient satisfaction.

Management of Treatment across Full Continuum of Care

Disease management programs have the ability to coordinate all aspects of care across all elements of the health care delivery system and to individualize that care to the specific needs of the patient. Coordinating care across the continuum implies that health care settings are no longer confined to the hospital or the physician's office. Delivery settings have proliferated in response to the changing configuration of economic incentives and disease management programs treat disease across a broader array of settings that include extended care (skilled nursing homes), acute care (hospitals), ambulatory care (physician offices and outpatient clinics), home care (hospice, durable medical equipment, home health visits), outreach (screening, information and referrals, telephone contact), wellness and health promotion (educational and exercise programs, support groups), and housing (assisted living, retirement communities). Acute care is clearly the most expensive form of care, whereas home care and self-care is significantly cheaper. This is especially true in the critical care areas in which significant human and technologic resources are expended. In addition, most patients prefer the home care setting, because it offers the added advantages of comfort, familiarity, and proximity to the family.

Funding for the Most Powerful Interventions

Disease management entails funding of the most powerful and successful interventions. It calls for physicians to discard their old, autonomous way of making decisions and substitute new group-tested approaches for the treatment of common conditions. It swaps medicine's tradition of independence for "group think."[8] The notion of group think has given rise to the term **evidence-based medicine,** an approach to practice and teaching that integrates pathophysiologic rationale, caregiver experience, and patient preferences with valid and current clinical research evidence.[23] It entails precise definition of the patient problem, proficient searching and critical appraisal of relevant information from the literature, and subsequent incorporation of the information into medical practice.[24] This prevents common conditions from spiraling out of control and creates a clinical road map for each targeted condition.[8]

Diseases Targeted for Disease Management Programs

A number of cardiorespiratory diseases are ideally suited for a disease management program and include asthma, congestive heart failure (CHF), acquired immunodeficiency syndrome (AIDS), cancer, COPD, and pneumonia. Many of the cardiorespiratory diseases are considered ideal illnesses for implementation of a disease management intervention.[25] A short list of characteristics of the ideal illness is provided in Box 45-4. However, what makes specific diseases especially well suited for a disease management intervention are the following:

- A high rate of preventable complications (with the goal of a reduction in emergency department visits and hospital readmissions)
- Short time frame during which alterations in natural history can show a measurable impact (for example, 1 to 3 years)
- Chronic, outpatient-focused conditions that are common, low technology, and nonsurgical
- High rate of variability in patterns of therapeutics from patient to patient and from physician to physician
- High rates of patient noncompliance with the therapeutic regime (amenable to change by education directed at patients, family members, and physicians)
- Existence of or development of practice guidelines on optimal treatment
- Achievable consensus on what constitutes good quality, which outcomes to measure, and how to improve them[12]

Box 45-4

Characteristics of the Ideal Illness

> High incidence of preventable complications
> Improper prescribing that can be addressed through physician education
> A chronic nature that lends itself to management
> A large patient population
> Highly visible costs
> The ability to lower costs through patient education
> The ability to measure outcomes

From Dubbs WH. Disease management: a proven strategy for reducing costs, enhancing care. AARC Times 1996;20(12):30-32.

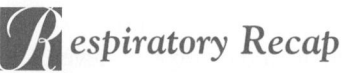 *espiratory Recap*

Cardiopulmonary Conditions Targeted for Disease Management	
Asthma	Cancer
CHF	COPD
AIDS	Pneumonia

Steps to Develop a Disease Management Program

Numerous approaches exist to the development of a disease management program.[5,26] An approach suggested by Ellrodt and colleagues[23] will be employed here, because it is evidence-based and well-suited for respiratory care. The Ellrodt model includes the following characteristics (Box 45-5): a multidisciplinary team of health care workers to define the problem; a process to search, select, appraise, and summarize the relevant literature to develop practice guidelines, pathways, and algorithms; implementation of the guidelines, pathways, and algorithms; and development of a method to measure and report process and outcome measures that inform the quality improvement exercise.[23]

The first step taken to create a disease management program is to define clearly the clinical and economic scope of the condition. What is the economic cost to society? How large a population is affected? Which patients should be included in the program? What critical interventions are likely to improve clinical and economic outcomes? What is the problem and what are the realistic goals or desired outcomes of the disease man-

Box 45-5

Steps in the Development of a Disease Management Program

> 1. Formulate a clear definition of the disease, its scope, and its impact over time using a multidisciplinary team.
> 2. Develop comprehensive baseline information to understand current health care delivery and resource utilization.
> 3. Generate specific clinical and economic questions and search the literature.
> 4. Critically appraise and synthesize the evidence.
> 5. Evaluate the benefits, harms, and costs.
> 6. Develop evidence-based practice guidelines, clinical pathways, and algorithms.
> 7. Create a system for process and outcome measurement and reporting.
> 8. Implement the evidence-based guidelines, pathways, and algorithms.
> 9. Complete the quality improvement cycle.

agement process? Additionally, team composition is crucial and involvement of all relevant caregivers should be ensured. Typically, the team includes a physician, a nurse, a respiratory therapist, a financial and actuarial professional, and individuals with marketing and communications expertise.

After the scope is defined and the team assembled, data must be garnered on current practice patterns, patient outcomes, and resource utilization. Ascertaining prevailing practices and measuring accurately the impact of the program is important. At this point in the process, the team needs to develop questions regarding clinical and economic measures related to the condition. In the case of asthma, what medications are appropriate? What mode of medication delivery is most effective? Which medications are most cost effective? Critical and insightful questions must be asked.

The next step is literature reviews that are systematic, comprehensive, and rigorous. The results of the search require critical appraisal and finally a summary of the findings. The summary should include a description of the design, population, intervention, and outcomes of each article. The conclusions and recommendations are graded to indicate the quality of the evidence. After the summary, the team considers the anticipated benefits, harm, and costs in light of local practice and administrative constraints. In the absence of high-quality research, patient values are considered.

The team then attempts to gain consensus on the results of the effort and to format the findings into practice guidelines. The guidelines should reflect the best scientific evidence (from controlled clinical trials, the medical literature, and outcome-validated databases) concerning which clinical processes have achieved the best results for the best expenditure of resources. The guidelines and protocols should be user friendly and widely disseminated. The practice guidelines are converted to pathways that become timed and sequenced events. Algorithms entail conditional responses and are generally if–then statements.

The impact of the effort should be measured and a system of reporting the results determined. Key questions must be addressed. What will be measured? Who will do the measuring? Who will report the findings? How will it be reported? The intention is to compare the post-intervention actual outcomes measured with the original goals.

Another step in the development of a disease management program entails facilitation of the implementation of the guidelines, pathways, and algorithms into clinical practice. The intention is to communicate the intervention (guidelines, pathways, and algorithms) in a manner most likely to change clinical decision-making. This step is often underrated. The most important variables are message content, the media for delivery, and the feedback. Even the most rigorously validated evidence-based guidelines must be recast into an appropri-

ate format to influence the clinical decision-making behavior of clinicians and patients.

Clinicians prefer to receive short manuals, executive summaries of guideline recommendations, or a synopsis of the supporting evidence and quantification of the expected benefits. Involving respected peers and opinion leaders is an important consideration used to gain acceptance and compliance; this has proven to be an effective way to change practice patterns.

Steps are essential to ensure compliance with the evidence-based practice guidelines. Compliance can be undermined for a number of reasons. Clinicians may be unaware of the guidelines, they may lack confidence in the recommendations because of controversy or divergence in the literature, or inefficiencies or barriers in the system may preclude their use. Updated literature searches and feedback on outcome measures should be periodically provided.

Obstacles and Future Opportunities

The major obstacles to the success of the disease management movement are listed in Box 45-6[23] and speculation about the future is provided in Box 45-7.[12] Two main issues confront the broad topic of medical management. The first is the debate over which care processes are used and the second deals with clinician variation in the care and management of patients.[27]

Although considerable effort has been given to the development of guidelines, protocols, and algorithms, little agreement exists regarding how, where, or when to use them. A major stumbling block in the resolution of this dilemma is the lack of a standardized computerized patient record. The medical record continues to serve as the best primary source used to evaluate the patient's disease, severity of illness, diagnostic and therapeutic interventions, results, and progress. Little hope exists for disease management to reach its true potential, however, until this information can be recorded, captured,

---

Box 45-6

Obstacles to the Implementation of Disease Management

> Limited resources to develop the program
> Information systems that are inadequate to identify patients for disease management program and to measure process and outcome
> Physician buy-in
> Disruption of continuity of care if managed by other providers
> Perception of cookbook approach
> Difficulty changing practice patterns

Ellrodt G, Cook D, Lee J, et al. Evidence-based disease management. JAMA 1997;278;1690.

Box 45-7

Speculation on the Future of Disease Management

> Information technology advances hold the greatest promise for improvement, starting with the electronic longitudinal patient medical record and including on-line educational services for patients.
>
> Continuous updates in optimal treatment guidelines will drive improvements in care.
>
> Customized programs for Medicare and Medicaid populations will be necessary and rely heavily on outreach programs.
>
> Interventions must include attention to the patient's psychosocial needs rather than focus only on clinical morbidity because care-seeking behavior is often not directly related to burden of illness.
>
> Treatment decision support systems will need to rediscover the role of patient choice in the equation for controversial circumstances.
>
> Progression is necessary from concentrated efforts on the single disease toward better coordination of care for patients with two or more diseases.
>
> Health risk appraisals need to become better risk predictors.
>
> Population health management will require use of both disease-specific functional status measures and health status measures.

aggregated in a single depository, and analyzed in a systematic manner.[5]

With regard to a reduction in clinician variation in the care and management of patients, physicians and practitioners are disturbed by the notion that anybody or anything might be engaged in patient management other than themselves. Consequently, they have regarded disease management as an intrusion into the sacrosanct physician-patient relationship and until they embrace the issues of evidenced-based disease management little progress is likely to occur.[5]

The roles of the payer and the provider will continue to conflict as payers will strive for decreases in per-member-per-month costs; strive to stay within capitation allowances; attempt to improve members health status and plan satisfaction; maintain and increase plan enrollment and reenrollment; keep premiums at a competitive level; and demonstrate superior value to purchasers. Providers will advocate for their patients; strive for improved patient outcomes; attempt to demonstrate superior value to purchasers, payers, and patients; and rationalize and standardize diagnosis and treatment.[5]

With regard to standardization of treatments and development of guidelines and protocols, in the next decade the focus will shift from guideline design to enforcement in guideline use. This latter point is especially important, because it will provide opportunities for professionals involved in disease management and care coordination. This highlights the urgent and critical nature of this issue for the respiratory therapist.

Respiratory Therapists as Disease Managers

Respiratory therapists are bedside specialists in the care and treatment of the patient with cardiopulmonary disease. Their experience and expertise make them the ideal professionals to engage in cardiopulmonary disease management and care coordination. An opportunity exists for them to position themselves for such a role and they would be wise to embrace the merits of the disease management movement.

Key Points

- The two major forces driving disease management are escalating health care costs and the changing patterns of cardiopulmonary diseases.
- The origin and evolution of the disease management movement are rooted in the pharmaceutical industry and managed care organizations.
- Care management is an umbrella term for component management, demand management, case management, and disease management.
- Component management is episodic, uncoordinated, and focuses on treatment versus prevention.
- The tools of demand management are patient-driven protocols, clinical pathways, case management, and disease management.
- Case management focuses on an individual patient and is expensive.
- Disease management focuses on subpopulations of patients and emphasizes coordinated comprehensive care along the continuum of disease and across health care delivery systems.
- The challenge of disease management is to apply a gradation of resources to members of the population so that each does not get too little (low quality) or too much (high cost), but just the right (high quality) amount of care.
- The goal of health care is to provide value, defined as quality outcomes per unit of cost.
- The principles of disease management include an understanding and treatment of the course, cause, and cost drivers of a disease, diagnoses and treatment based on the disease process, emphasis on patient education and compliance for chronic disease management, management across care settings with full continuity of care, and direction of resources to proven methodologies.
- The cost drivers of a disease are compliance, prevention, rapid resolution, acute flare-ups, and that 80% of the costs are produced by 20% of the diseases.
- Disease management program entails assembly of a multidisciplinary team to define the problem, an extensive search of the literature, development of guidelines and protocols, implementation of the guidelines and protocols, and assessment of the process and outcomes measures.

References

1. Hoffman C. Persons with chronic conditions: their prevalence and costs. JAMA 1996;276:1473.

2. McGinnis JM, Foege WH. Actual causes of death in the United States. JAMA 1993;270:2208.

3. American Hospital Association. American Hospital Association booklet. Chicago: The Association; 1996.

4. The Boston Consulting Group. The changing environment for pharmaceuticals. Boston: Boston Consulting Group; 1993.

5. Couch JB. The physician's guide to disease management. Gaithersburg, Md: Aspen; 1997.

6. Phillips L. Disease management: the next step in managed care depends on information sharing. AHIMA 1996;67:44-46.

7. Johnson SK. The state of disease state management. Case Review 1996; (Fall):53-55.

8. Lumsdon K. Disease management: the heat and heartaches of retooling patient care create hard labor. Hospitals and Health Networks 1995; (April 5):34-42.

9. Patterson R. Disease management. Case Review 1995 (Fall).

10. Ward M, Rieve J. Disease management: case management's return to patient-centered care. Care Management 1995;1:8.

11. Bunch D. Demand management tools help providers lower costs of care. AARC Times 1996;20(12):24-27.

12. Kongstvedt P. Essentials of managed health care. 2nd ed. Gaithersburg, Md: Aspen; 1997.

13. O'Brien K. Asthma management: a new paradigm. Case Review 1998; (March/April):16,18,59,60.

14. Durbin CG. The role of the respiratory care practitioner in the continuum of disease management. Respir Care 1997;42:159-165.

15. The Boston Consulting Group. The promise of disease management. Boston: Boston Consulting Group; 1995.

16. National Managed Health Care Congress. The disease management strategic research and resource guide. Case Review 1996:54.

17. Zitter M. Disease management: a new approach to health care. Medical Interface 1994; (August):70-76.

18. Meyer LC, Rohl B. An innovative approach to treating chronic disabling asthma. The Case Manager 1993;4:54-69.

19. National Jewish Medical and Research Center [http://www.njc.org/dmp/dmp.html].

20. Greenberg RN. Overview of patient compliance with medication dosing: a literature review. Clin Ther 1984;6:592-599.

21. McKenny JM, Harrison TL. Drug-related hospital admissions. Am J Hosp Pharm 1976;33:792-795.

22. Muma R, et al. Patient education: a practical approach. Stamford, Conn: Appleton & Lange; 1996.

23. Ellrodt G, Cook D, Lee J, et al. Evidence-based disease management. JAMA 1997;278:1687.

24. Evidence-Based Working Group. Evidence-based medicine: a new approach to teaching the practice of medicine. JAMA 1992;268:2420-2425.

25. Dubbs WH. Disease management: a proven strategy for reducing costs, enhancing care. AARC Times 1996; (December):31.

26. Mayo Clinic uses clinical data to develop aggressive disease management strategy. Clinical Data Management 1995;2:2.

27. Institute for the Future. Health and healthcare 2010: the forecast, the challenge. San Francisco: Jossey-Bass; 2000.

CHAPTER 46

Asthma

Timothy R. Myers
Robert L. Chatburn

CHAPTER OUTLINE

OBJECTIVES

1. Define asthma.
2. Discuss the epidemiology of asthma.
3. Discuss the pathophysiology of asthma.
4. List the risk factors for asthma.
5. Describe the clinical features of nocturnal asthma, exercise-induced asthma, and occupational asthma.
6. Describe the disease severity classification proposed by the National Asthma Education and Prevention Program.
7. Discuss the role of peak flow monitoring in the management of asthma.
8. Compare the role of controller medication and quick-relief medications in the management of asthma.

OBJECTIVES—cont'd

9. Compare the use of nebulizers, metered dose inhalers, and dry powder inhalers in the delivery of aerosols to the patient with asthma.
10. Discuss the role of alternative treatment modalities in the management of asthma.
11. List the goals of mechanical ventilation of the patient with asthma.
12. Discuss the role of education in the disease management of asthma.

KEY TERMS

Airway Hyperresponsiveness	Exercise-Induced Asthma (EIA)	National Asthma Education and
Airway Inflammation	Exhaled Nitric Oxide	Prevention Program (NAEPP)
Allergen	Extrinsic Asthma	Nocturnal Asthma
Asthma	Heliox	Peak Flowmeter
Asthma Education Program	Intrinsic Asthma	Quick-Relief Medication
Asthma Trigger	Mild Intermittent Asthma	Severe Persistent Asthma
Bronchial Challenge Testing	Mild Persistent Asthma	
Controller Medication	Moderate Persistent Asthma	

Asthma is one of the most common chronic diseases of the pulmonary system. An expert panel report from the **National Asthma Education and Prevention Program (NAEPP)** of the National Institutes of Health issued this working definition of asthma[1]:

Asthma is a chronic inflammatory disorder of the airways in which many cells and cellular elements play a role, in particular, mast cells, eosinophils, T lymphocytes, macrophages, neutrophils, and epithelial cells. In susceptible individuals, this inflammation causes recurrent episodes of wheezing, breathlessness, chest tightness, and coughing, particular at night or in the early morning. These episodes are usually associated with widespread but variable airflow obstruction that is often reversible either spontaneously or with treatment. The inflammation also causes an associated increase in the existing bronchial hyperresponsiveness to a variety of stimuli.

In this chapter, issues related to the respiratory care of patients with asthma are presented.

Epidemiology

Asthma is a common chronic disease that is increasing in prevalence and severity. The asthma literature frequently mentions epidemiology, prevalence, and incidence. Webster's Ninth *New Collegiate Dictionary* defines *epidemiology* as a branch of medical science that deals with the incidence, distribution and control of disease in a population.[2] *Prevalence* refers to the number of individuals with a diagnosis at any given time (for example, 1990), whereas *incidence* refers specifically to the number of newly diagnosed cases that occur within a specific period of time (for example, the past century).

Estimation of the prevalence and incidence of asthma is difficult to assess because of the inherent problems with surveys and varying definitions for asthma. Asthma is prevalent in approximately 10% of the world's population. Despite recent advances in both pharmacologic and management strategies, both the prevalence and incidence of asthma is rapidly increasing. Between 1980 and 1987, the prevalence of asthma increased an estimated 25% to 30%.

All segments of the population are experiencing rapid growth in the prevalence of asthma. Although prevalence, acute care visits, and deaths resulting from asthma have increased nationwide, these increased rates are not evenly distributed across the nation.[3] The fastest growing segment is in children younger than 5 years of age.[4] Although asthma is more prevalent in males, it tends to be more severe in women. African Americans, especially those residing in urban areas, are three times more likely to be diagnosed with asthma. In the United States, asthma is the third leading cause of preventable hospitalization and results in approximately 2000 deaths each year.[5]

Age-Specific Angle

Asthma is increasing at the fastest rate in children less than 5 years of age.

The mortality rates for asthma have remained stable or experienced slight increases in the past decade. Death rates are most prominent in people with asthma who are under the age of 35 years. African Americans have death rates that are five times higher than those of Caucasians. Patients who have frequent hospital admissions or previous life-threatening asthma are the most susceptible to asthma mortality. Patients classified as having life-threatening asthma have been subgrouped into the following three separate classes:

1. The typical case, a patient who presents with a gradual deterioration over time and experiences a life-threatening episode[6]
2. The patient with relatively mild, asymptomatic chronic asthma and suffers an acute episode in a relatively short time frame (referred to as *acute asphyxia asthma*)[7]
3. The patient who is a combination of the previous two classes

Misdiagnosis and inadequate treatment by disease severity are significant factors contributing to the increased incidence and prevalence of asthma.

Age-Specific Angle

Death rates are greatest for people with asthma younger than 35 years of age.

The spread of this chronic inflammatory disease is alarming enough, but disease severity and frequency of acute care visits for treatment are also increasing. The severity of acute episodes may vary from mild to life threatening within a given patient over the course of the disease or within a given year. People with asthma suffer more than 1,000,000 days of restricted activity of daily living per year and experience more than 470,000 hospitalizations annually.[1]

Along with the increasing prevalence of asthma is the economic burden that comes with this chronic condition. In the early 1990s, the cost to treat asthma was estimated to be approximately $6 billion per year with 43% of the cost associated with hospitalizations, emergency room visits, and death.[8] The cost of emergency department therapy for asthma in the same year was $270 million, which represented 8% of the total direct cost of caring for asthma.[4] The fastest growing age segment with asthma is children, which has been reported to have a staggering impact on the cost to treat asthma. A recent study suggests that the cost for children under the age of 5 years hospitalized with asthma reaches approximately 74% of their total health care costs.[9] The same study reported that the highest sector in the adult population for cost also is associated with hospitalizations (54%). Medications resulted in 16.5% of the total cost to treat asthma in adults compared with 5.4% in children under the age of 5 years.

The high cost associated with acute care treatment of asthma has led to implementation of disease management programs.[10-12] Because of the high volume of asthma visits and/or admissions in most urban areas, disease manage-

ment programs or clinical practice guidelines can reduce cost by eliminating practice variation in the emergency room or hospital in the treatment of asthma. Eliminating acute treatment that adds cost but does not degrade the overall quality of care can be an effective tool in the management of asthma.[13-15]

Although asthma is not a curable disease, it can be managed effectively. Asthma mortality, and to a lesser degree morbidity, is largely preventable. Appropriate medications based on disease severity, and patient compliance with medication can result in highly effective disease management. Patient education and awareness of environmental triggers also play a significant role in the overall management of the disease. Even with the overall effective management from an education, medical, and compliance standpoint, some patients develop severe persistent asthma with frequent exacerbations that may result in emergency department visits or hospitalizations.

Pathophysiology

The exact underlying cause of asthma is still unknown. Asthma is a multifactorial disease that has been associated with allergenic, hereditary, psychosocial, socioeconomic, environmental, and infectious causes.[16] Asthma is not the only cause of wheezing. Box 46-1 lists other potential causes or diagnoses associated with wheezing.

Even if the underlying cause of asthma is known in an individual, the trigger stimuli of an exacerbation may change over time. The pathophysiology of the disease is largely related to inflammation, hyperresponsiveness,

---

Box 46-1

Differential Diagnosis of Wheezing

Small and Large Airway Obstruction
Asthma
Airway tumors
Bronchiolitis (in children)
Cardiogenic pulmonary edema
Cystic fibrosis
Pneumonias; aspiration
Bronchopulmonary dysplasia

Large Airway Obstruction
Airway and esophageal foreign bodies
Pulmonary emboli
Tumors
Vascular rings
Focal pneumonia
Laryngeal webs or malacia
Tracheal stenosis
Lymphadenopathies
Vocal cord dysfunction

and obstruction. Figure 46-1 demonstrates the interrelationship of these three factors in the underlying mechanism of the disease.

Airway Inflammation

Regardless of the trigger mechanism or the underlying cause of asthma, **airway inflammation** plays an important role. The mediators that appear to be the most significant are mast cells, eosinophils, macrophages, epithelial cells, and T lymphocytes. Many cell types can influence newly synthesized mediators that either act alone or in conjunction with other mediators.[17] The release of inflammatory mediators results in recurrent exacerbations that manifest as wheezing, progressive shortness of breath, chest tightness, and coughing that may be more persistent nocturnally or in the early mornings.[18] In most patients, these exacerbations are usually self-limiting or resolve rapidly to appropriate asthma treatment.

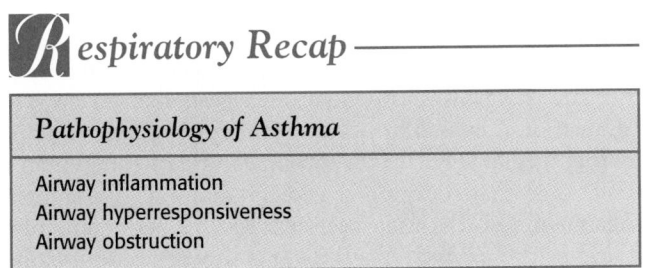

Pathophysiology of Asthma

Airway inflammation
Airway hyperresponsiveness
Airway obstruction

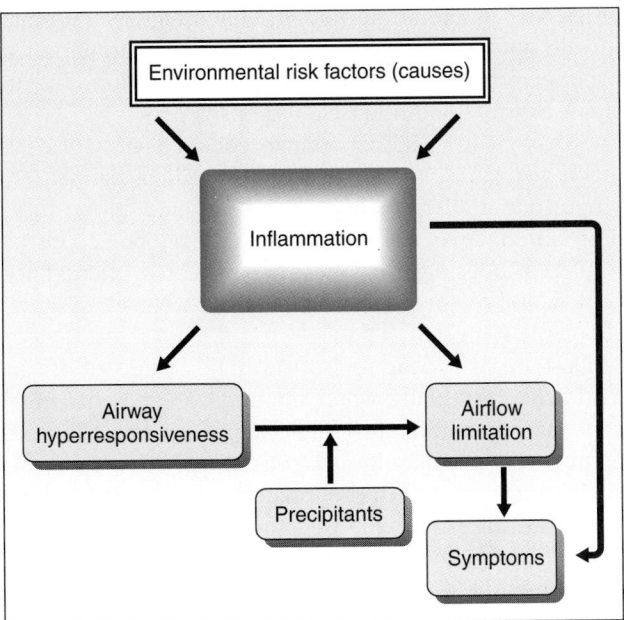

Figure 46-1 Mechanisms underlying the definition of asthma. (Modified from National Asthma Education Program, National Heart, Lung, and Blood Institute. Expert panel report 2: guidelines for the diagnosis and management of asthma. Publication No. 97-4051. Bethesda, Md: National Institutes of Health; 1997.)

Airway inflammation may be classified as acute, subacute, or chronic. The acute inflammatory response is represented by the early recruitment of cells to the airway. In the subacute phase, recruited and resident cells are activated to cause a more persistent pattern of inflammation. Chronic inflammation is characterized by a persistent level of cell damage and an ongoing repair process, changes that may cause permanent damage in the airway.[1]

Over time, recurrent episodes of airway inflammation result in an increase hyperresponsiveness of the airways. Inflammation can also play an important role in the development of acute and severe airflow limitation through bronchoconstriction, epithelial wall remodeling, pulmonary edema, and mucus plug formation from cellular debris or breakdown. The new hypothesis is that inflammation is present in the acute and chronic phases of asthma and therapy directed at the inflammation must be continuous and long term.

Airway Hyperresponsiveness

A marker associated with asthma is the increased sensitivity or **airway hyperresponsiveness** to both specific and nonspecific factors. These factors have little or no effect on people with normal airways. The Lung Health Study showed that the majority of women and half the men diagnosed with COPD also have a component of hyperresponsiveness.[19]

Airway hyperresponsiveness is a mechanism in which the airways constrict too easily and frequently. Factors associated with hyperresponsive airways include environmental factors (both indoor and outdoor), exercise, **allergens,** and viral infections. The degree or level of airway hyperresponsiveness usually correlates with the clinical severity of the disease.[1]

Bronchial challenge testing with either methacholine or histamine serves as a measure of responsiveness to general stimuli. Asthma is characterized by the disease's ability to have reversible airflow obstruction. These challenge tests are administered usually in a pulmonary function lab and followed (usually within 15 minutes) with a short-acting, β_2-agonist that results in a 12% to 15% increase in a patient's forced expiratory volume in 1 second (FEV_1). A recent study of FEV_1 demonstrated that the reversibility of asthma was associated with a 16% increase and the reversibility of COPD was associated with a 10% change.

Airway Obstruction

The final component in the definition of asthma is airway obstruction or the limitation of airflow through the airways. Airflow limitation is most commonly caused by IgE mediators released into the airways and coming into contact with airway smooth muscles. More specifically, the mediators usually associated with an IgE response include histamine, tryptase, prostaglandin, and leukotrienes. However, when the airways do have some degree of hyperresponsiveness, several stimuli can exac-

$\mathcal{B}$OX 46-2

Changes that Lead to Airway Obstruction

> Acute bronchoconstriction
> Chronic mucus plug formation
> Airway edema
> Airway remodeling

erbate bronchoconstriction (Box 46-2). In most patients, this airflow limitation or bronchoconstriction will spontaneously resolve or with the administration of a short-acting β_2-agonist. Patients who have severe disease or who have had asthma for a number of years may develop an incomplete response. These patients are difficult to separate from the COPD population. Patients who continue to have airway obstruction after initiation of therapy are considered to be in status asthmaticus.

Risk Factors

The strongest identifiable predisposing factor for the development of asthma is atopy.[20] Atopy is the familial or genetic predisposition to develop an IgE-mediated response to common allergens in the environment. Asthma in childhood is normally linked to atopic factors. This is called *pediatric asthma*, or *allergic asthma*. A study of 6- to 34-year olds in Tucson, Arizona, found a strong, direct correlation between serum IgE levels and the development or presence of asthma and a weaker correlation between positive skin test reactions and the development or presence of asthma.[21]

The easiest diagnosis of atopic asthma is through skin-prick testing, in which a multitude of known allergens are introduced to the patient system through small pricks in the arms of suspected patients. The most common method of skin testing is a radioallergosorbent test (RAST) that measures antigen-specific IgE. A recent study of children in eight metropolitan areas indicated that the highest risk factors of atopic asthma in inner-city children were cockroach antigen, animal dander, and dust mites.[22]

Factors that may contribute or enhance the development of asthma on exposure or increase the susceptibility include environmental pollution, low birth weight, tobacco smoke, diet, or viral infections.[16] Asthma has also been associated with sinusitis and gastrointestinal reflux.

Allergens

The majority of asthmatics suffer attacks exacerbated from inhalation of an allergen. Many allergens, both indoor (that is, mold, animal dander, cleaning chemicals, cockroach antigen, dust mites) and outdoor (that is, cold air, noxious fumes, grass and tree pollens), may trigger an exacerbation. Allergenic asthma usually manifests in two

distinct components. The first component is an acute triggering phase. The presence of an **asthma trigger** on a hypersensitive airway causes a rupture and degranulation of the mast cell. The mast cells of the airways release several chemical mediators into the tracheobronchial tree. These mediators include leukotrienes, eosinophils chemotactic factor of anaphylaxis (ECF-A), prostaglandins, and histamine. These mediators all interact with the airway smooth muscle, resulting in bronchoconstriction, edema, vasodilation, eosinophil release, and may include increased secretion production.[23]

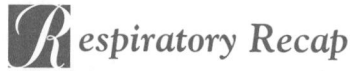

$\mathcal{R}$espiratory Recap

> ### *Risk Factors for Asthma*
>
> | Allergens | Food and drug additives |
> | --- | --- |
> | Pollution | Viral agents |

The second component of an asthma attack is the inflammatory response. Inflammatory mediators are released into the airway. Recent evidence suggests that airway inflammation is caused by not one particular type of inflammatory mediator but by an intricate cycle of complex interactions that develop between multiple mediators, inflammatory cells, and other cells and tissues commonly found in the airways. The inflammatory response usually results in the migration of these various inflammatory cells and mediators into the airways where they cause direct injuries, such as alterations in epithelial integrity, abnormalities in autonomic neural control of airway tone, mucus hypersecretion, change in mucociliary function, and increase airway smooth muscle responsiveness.[1]

Allergens from indoor sources consist mainly of cockroach antigen, domestic dust mites, animal dander, and fungi. Indoor allergens appear to be a main trigger in industrialized, developed countries. In developed countries, insulated housing that has been heated, humidified, cooled, and carpeted is prone to increased levels of indoor allergenic sources.

Dust mites appear to be the major cause of asthma worldwide, especially when infants are exposed to high concentrations in the first 3 to 6 months of life.[24] The predominant domestic mite is *Dermatophagoides* species. The allergens are located in the inhaled microscopic fecal pellets. Dust mites are found in common household products but are especially prominent in bedding, carpet, and soft furnishings. Dust mites grow best in humid, room air (22° to 26° C) temperatures. The best method for eradicating mites is to wash potential breeding material in hot water.

A recent study indicated cockroach antigen as the leading allergenic cause of inner-city asthma.[25] Cockroach antigen is found in the microscopic excrement and is inhaled by the sensitized patient.

Cats are highly allergenic. The principal source of allergen is again found in cat excrement. Cat saliva has also been associated as a source of cat antigen. Dog sensitivity is not as well documented as a leading cause but has been found to contribute to allergenic sources.

Fungi and molds have also been identified as allergenic risks in specific individuals with moderate to severe asthma. Fungi are most commonly found to grow extremely well in areas used for heating, cooling, or humidification. Home humidifiers provide a special risk for indoor fungal growth and air contamination.[26]

Outdoor allergen sources are primarily pollens. The sources of these pollens include grasses, trees, flowers, weeds, and fungi. Each season particular outdoor allergen sources appear as major contributing factors to initiating asthma exacerbations. In the early spring, trees are the prominent trigger in pollen-associated asthma attacks. As the temperatures warm in the late spring and early summer, grasses and flowers reign as the initiators. In early fall, weeds play an important role in eliciting asthma exacerbations. The fall season also initiates the mold-induced exacerbations, predominately from *Alternaria* and *Cladosporium* species. Temperature changes have often been associated with eliciting asthma exacerbations. Although this appears to be largely unfounded, the roles of humidity in the summer months and cold air during winter months are still a mystery.

Pollution

The role of indoor and outdoor air pollution in the development or initiation of an asthma attack remains unproved and controversial. Air pollution has often been accused of being a viable source for the increase prevalence of asthma, but research has failed to produce a direct link to air pollution and asthma.[27] Outdoor types of pollution are mainly associated in industrialized nations that have a large amount of industrial or photochemical smog.

Indoor air pollutants have had a higher association with the development of respiratory symptoms. Although active smoking has not been indicated as a general risk factor for the development of asthma, it does seem to play a role in eliciting exacerbations to asthmatics that are exposed. The main source of indoor air pollution is tobacco smoke, which correlates to an increased risk of asthma development or exacerbation in children. Other potential sources of indoor air pollution include nitric oxide, carbon dioxide, carbon monoxides, nitrogen oxides, sulfur dioxides, formaldehydes, and biologic sources such as endotoxins.[16]

Food and Drug Additives

Many patients with asthma who have allergies to specific foods increase their potential to develop exacerbations from intake of these foods. Foods that contain salicylates, some food-coloring agents, food preservatives (for example, sulfites), and monosodium glutamate are substances known to be associated with asthma exacerbations.[24]

Many drugs may or may not be associated with the increased likelihood exacerbation. The primary risk is with nonsteroidal antiinflammatory agents and aspirin. Patients that have sensitivity to aspirin have an increased risk of developing asthma later in life. Patients with asthma are also sensitive to β-blockers.

Viral Agents

Viral illness seasons (October through December and February through April) coincide with the most prevalent hospitalization periods for asthma in both children and adults. A study published in 1997 by Teichtahl and colleagues reported that 37% of adult patients with acute asthma admitted over a 12-month period had evidence of recent respiratory tract infection.[28] This has been called **intrinsic asthma,** in contrast to **extrinsic asthma.** The inflammatory responses to viral infections (especially lower respiratory tract) may start the cascade of symptomatic wheezing from inflammatory debris or excessive mucous production in the airways.

Pizzichini and colleagues studied induced sputum as a useful marker on the effects of natural colds and influenza on the airways of the lungs. The results suggested that natural colds (by day 4) cause neutrophilic lower airway inflammation that is greater in people with asthma than in healthy subjects. These researchers hypothesized that the greater inflammatory response in people with asthma may be due to the changes associated with trivial eosinophilia or to the different viruses involved.[29]

Recent publications suggest a relationship between respiratory viral infections early in childhood and the development of asthma. Martinez and colleagues[30] found that in children exposed to lower respiratory tract infections early in life, alterations in acute immune existed in response to the viral infection. These immune response alterations may be detected at the time of the first wheezing episode in subjects who eventually have persistent wheezing symptoms.

The most prominent of these viral infections is respiratory syncytial virus (RSV). The population at highest risk for severe cases of RSV and other lower respiratory tract infections, indigent inner-city populations, is also at high risk for asthma. A study by Welliver and colleagues[31] reported that infants with RSV early in life and developed high titers of RSV IgE were three times more likely to have recurrent wheezing after 48 months.

The exact role that early childhood respiratory tract infections play on the development of asthma is yet unclear. However, respiratory tract infections are a significant risk factor for the initiation of an asthma exacerbation that may or may not result in an individual seeking acute care. Infections should be identified to the patient with asthma as a trigger. Furthermore, written asthma treatment plans should include a component for increasing or stepping up therapy at the onset of symptoms. Lieu and colleagues[32] demonstrated the advantage of hospitalization prevention when families of children with asthma had a written treatment plan that could initiate more aggressive outpatient management with the onset of cold-like symptoms.

Nocturnal Asthma, Exercise-Induced Asthma, and Occupational Asthma

Nocturnal Asthma

Nocturnal symptoms are quite common in people of all ages with asthma and even in patients who have mild intermittent or mild persistent asthma. Although **nocturnal asthma** is prevalent in up to 75% of all patients with asthma,[33] many do not correlate these nighttime symptoms with asthma. The presence of nocturnal asthma is a marker for uncontrolled or more severe asthma.[34-36]

A variety of mechanisms are interactive when nocturnal asthma is present.[7,37,38] The mechanisms seem to revolve around circadian alterations of body temperature, vagal tone, mediators, inflammation, epinephrine, and β_2-receptor function.[39,40] Other variables considered to be potential causes include gastroesophageal reflux, aspiration, sinusitis, increased mucus production, sleep apnea, and the normal decrease in lung function of patients sleeping.

An extensive amount of research has been undertaken in an attempt to optimize the treatment of nocturnal asthma. Martin[37] emphasizes that treatment of nocturnal asthma requires therapy that uses a chronopharmacologic approach. An optimal therapeutic regimen should include some or multiple components of sustained-release theophylline, sustained-release β-adrenergics, long-acting β-adrenergics, and/or inhaled corticosteroids.

Exercise-Induced Asthma

Exercise-induced asthma (EIA) is characterized by transient airway obstruction, typically occurring 5 to 15 minutes after strenuous exertion. EIA is prevalent in 90% of individuals with asthma. The prevalence of EIA among athletes is estimated to range between 3% and 11%.

Studies have reported undiagnosed asthma that suddenly appears in competitive high school athletes.[41] Diag-

Box 46-3

Etiology Theories for Exercise-Induced Asthma

Respiratory heat or water loss (or both) from the bronchial mucosa
Mucosal drying and increased osmolarity stimulating mast cell degranulation
Rapid airway rewarming after exercise, causing vascular congestion, increased permeability, and edema leading to obstruction
Hyperventilation, causing discharge of bronchospastic chemical mediators

nosis of EIA may be made based on a history of symptoms (cough, wheeze, and chest tightness with exercise). More traditionally or for definitive diagnosis, a fall of 10% or more in the FEV_1 or in peak expiratory flow (PEF) rate after exercise is diagnostic.

The exact etiology of EIA is unclear. Theories range from temperature-related causes to inflammatory mediator release (Box 46-3). EIA symptoms typically appear after exercise and peak at 8 to 15 minutes and eventually spontaneously resolve in about 60 minutes. Frequently, a refractory period (of up to 3 hours) occurs after initial recovery, during which repeat exercise causes less bronchospasm.

Although β_2-agonists continue to be the cornerstone of therapy for EIA, treatment can be by either pharmacologic or nonpharmacologic means. From a pharmacologic standpoint, cromolyn sodium and nedocromil sodium are alternatives to the β_2-agonists. Medications that can be added if inhaled β_2-agonists, cromolyn, or nedocromil is not adequate include anticholinergic agents (such as ipratropium bromide), oral β-agonists, α-agonists, theophylline, calcium channel blockers, and antihistamines. Some newer asthma medications (anti-leukotriene modifiers), and some non-asthma medications (inhaled heparin and inhaled furosemide) have been reported as treatment of EIA. Combination therapy of two classes of medications can provide additive benefits.[42]

Although aerobic fitness and good control of baseline airway hyperreactivity diminish the effects of EIA, a number of nonpharmacologic measures can be utilized. Nonpharmacologic measures include warming up before vigorous exertion, covering the mouth and nose in cold weather, exercising in warm, humidified environments if possible, and cooling down after exercise.

Although prevention is the main objective in managing EIA, education regarding the nature and management is important. Most patients respond well to preexercise treatment with an inhaled quick-acting β-agonist and nonpharmacologic measures. Some times a patient presents with the symptoms of EIA but responds poorly to treatment. Further investigation may lead to a totally different diagnosis, such as vocal cord dysfunction.

Occupational Asthma

Occupational asthma is characterized by variable airway hyperresponsiveness in the workplace. The patient typically reports increased symptoms while at work or within several hours of the completion of a shift, with improvement on weekends or during vacations. The diagnosis can be made by monitoring peak flows in the workplace. Both new onset asthma and exacerbations of preexistent asthma may occur as a result of occupational exposures. Occupational asthma is the most common occupational lung disease in developed countries. Isocyanates are the most common etiologic agents. Inciting agents are divided into two broad categories: low molecular weight chemicals (for example, trimellitic anhydride, formaldehyde), which require combination of the chemical, which is an incomplete antigen (that is, a hapten), with a protein conjugate to produce a sensitizing neoantigen; high molecular weight organic materials (for example, grain dust, avian proteins), which may serve as complete antigens. Cigarette smoking is also an important risk factor for occupational asthma.

Disease Severity Classification

An important initiative in the management of asthma promoted in recent years is linking asthma treatment to chronic disease severity. Multitudes of factors influence the classification of disease severity in asthma. Determining a patient's true degree of chronic severity from that of noncompliant, uncontrolled asthma is often difficult. Researchers and clinicians have developed a large conglomeration of tools to assess chronic disease severity. Some potential tools include asthma-specific histories, physical examination, questionnaires, and pulmonary function studies.

The NAEPP Expert Panel[1] has developed a four-tiered level to classify chronic disease severity. These four categories are mild intermittent, mild persistent, moderate persistent, and severe persistent asthma. Each category or classification has specific symptomatic or utilization components that separate it from the others.

Mild Intermittent

Mild intermittent asthma is the least severe of the four classes of disease severity. People with asthma in this category experience symptoms of coughing or wheezing no more than two times per week. These patients have asymptomatic or normal PEFs between exacerbations, although their exacerbations are generally brief (from a few hours to a few days). These patients generally are expected to experience nocturnal symptoms of coughing, wheezing, or breathlessness no more than two times per month. The measured FEV_1 or PEF should fall consistently in the green zone of at least 80% of predicted, while maintaining less than 20% variability in PEF routinely.

Routine management of these patients generally consists of as needed short-acting β-agonist. Although these patients may have the chronic component of their disease classified as mild intermittent, the periodic exacerbations that occur may vary in their intensity. Sometimes, although rarely, these exacerbations result in this class of patients needing to seek emergency room treatment or occasionally result in hospitalization.

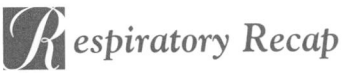
espiratory Recap

Asthma Disease Severity Classification	
Mild intermittent	Moderate persistent
Mild persistent	Severe persistent

Mild Persistent

People with **mild persistent asthma** experience symptoms of coughing or wheezing more than two times per week but less than once per day. These patients have symptoms that affect normal daily activities of living or normal nighttime sleep patterns. These patients generally experience nocturnal symptoms of coughing, wheezing, or breathlessness more than two times per month. The measured FEV_1 or PEF should fall consistent in the green zone of at least 80% of predicted or personal best, while maintaining approximately 20% to 30% variability in PEF rates. Routine management of these patients generally consists of as needed short-acting β-agonist with the addition of a controller medication. In adults this controller medication is an inhaled corticosteroid, whereas in children the options of cromolyn sodium or nedocromil are indicated as a potential substitute for inhaled corticosteroids. Dependent on the nocturnal symptoms these patients are experiencing, a long-acting, inhaled β-agonist or an oral sustained released theophylline or long-acting oral β-agonist may be prescribed. Although these patients may have the chronic component of their disease classified as mild persistent, the periodic exacerbations that occur also vary in their intensity. These exacerbations periodically result in this class of patients needing to seek emergency room treatment or occasionally result in hospitalization.

Moderate Persistent

People with **moderate persistent asthma** experience symptoms of coughing or wheezing on a near-daily basis. Exacerbations are experienced at least two times per week and often persist for multiple days. These patients have symptoms that routinely interfere with normal daily activities of living or normal nighttime sleep patterns. Moderate persistent asthma patients generally experience nocturnal symptoms of coughing, wheezing, or breathlessness more than once per week. The measured FEV$_1$ or PEF routinely falls in the yellow zone of 60% to 80% of predicted or personal best, while consistently maintaining at least 30% variability in PEF rates. Management of these patients consists of short-acting β-agonist for exacerbations and an inhaled corticosteroid on a routine frequency of two to three times per day. Most children that fall in this category are also indicated for inhaled corticosteroids either perennially or during seasons of high probability. These patients are routinely prescribed a long-acting, inhaled bronchodilator to manage their nocturnal symptoms. These patients routinely need to seek emergency room treatment or require hospitalization secondary to the chronic inflammatory component of their asthma.

Severe Persistent

This category is the highest level of the four classes of disease severity. Patients with asthma in this category experience symptoms of coughing or wheezing almost continually. Exacerbations are experienced frequently and often persist for multiple days or sometimes weeks. These patients have symptoms that limit normal daily activities of living or normal nighttime sleep patterns. **Severe persistent asthma** patients experience nocturnal symptoms of coughing, wheezing, or breathlessness almost every night. The measured FEV$_1$ or PEF routinely falls in the red zone of 60% or less of predicted or personal best, while consistently maintaining at least 30% variability in PEF rates. Management of these patients consists of short-acting β-agonist for exacerbations and an inhaled corticosteroid on a scheduled frequency of two to three times per day. Most children that fall in this category are also indicated for an inhaled steroid. These patients are routinely prescribed a long-acting, inhaled bronchodilator to manage their nocturnal symptoms. These patients also are indicated for chronic oral corticosteroid use for a period of time to aid in the control of their symptoms. These patients frequently seek emergency room treatment and require hospitalization secondary to the chronic inflammatory component of their asthma.

Although patients may be classified in any of the four categories, periodic review of chronic symptoms and medication usage is necessary. Quite often asthma is controlled with appropriate medications and compliance and treatment can be decreased to a lower severity class with a decrease in symptoms. From the opposite perspective, with increasing symptomatic data and medication compliance, it may be necessary to intensify the treatment regimen to address the increase in symptoms.

Status Asthmaticus

Severe attacks of asthma poorly responsive to adrenergic agents and associated with signs or symptoms of potential respiratory failure are often referred to as *status asthmaticus*. The mechanisms of airflow obstruction and the principles

of treatment for status asthmaticus are similar to those in which the asthma responds promptly to treatment.

Objective Measurements

One of the primary goals of asthma management and control is to maintain normal (or near normal) lung function. Objective assessment of the degree of variable airflow obstruction, hyperresponsiveness, and/or airflow reversibility is a fundamental component in the diagnosis of asthma. The precise measurement of airflow changes is important to evaluate the effectiveness of therapeutic maintenance or interventions.

The most familiar ways to diagnose and monitor airflow rates are pulmonary function testing (spirometry) and **peak flowmeters.** In 1994 the American Thoracic Society (ATS) differentiated between diagnostic and monitoring devices.[43] Diagnostic evaluation by pulmonary function testing includes bronchial challenge, spirometry, lung volumes, and airway resistance. A relatively diagnostic tool for the inflammatory component of asthma is measurement of exhaled nitric oxide levels.

Spirometry

Studies have demonstrated that children as young as three years of age can perform spirometry approximately 20% of the time.[44] The NAEPP recommends diagnostic spirometry at initial diagnosis and at least yearly after initial diagnosis. The airflow obstructive component of asthma is caused primarily by a decrease in expiratory flows and/or a high airway resistance. The general spirometry data of an asthmatic with airflow obstruction show a normal or slightly decreased forced vital capacity (FVC), a decreased or normal FEV$_1$, a decreased or normal PEF, and a decreased percentage of FEV$_1$/FVC. The ATS[43] has recommended a diagnosis of asthma when airflow reversibility achieves 12% to 15% reversibility. Pre- and post-bronchodilator testing is the hallmark intervention to decipher airflow reversibility. Normal spirometry with a suspected history of asthma symptoms may be an indication for more advanced diagnostic testing. During periods of acute exacerbations, people with asthma may have significant amounts of hyperinflation and air-trapping that will suggest a restrictive disease and require the measurement of lung volumes for accurate diagnosis.

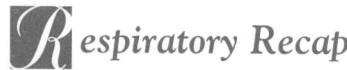

*R*espiratory Recap

Objective Measurements in Asthma
Spirometry Lung volumes and airway resistance Peak flowmeters Exhaled nitric oxide

Lung Volumes and Airway Resistance

Body plethysmography is the diagnostic tool that is utilized to achieve measurements of airway resistance (R_{aw}), airway conductance (G_{aw}), and static lung volumes. Static lung volumes are the primary test that differentiates restrictive diseases from obstructive diseases. Static lung volumes are useful also to detect the presence of hyperinflation. R_{aw} may be normal in asymptomatic asthma, although G_{aw} may be decreased. Normally during acute exacerbations, R_{aw} is increased. Bronchodilator effectiveness is accurately evaluated with measurements of R_{aw} during acute exacerbations.

Peak Flowmeters

Peak flowmeters (Figure 46-2) have been classified by the ATS as a monitoring device[43] for the management of asthma. The NAEPP published guidelines that recommended daily peak flow monitoring in all people with asthma.[1] This started a deluge of studies to determine the overall effectiveness of this type of asthma monitoring. The application and use of peak flowmeters was found to be beneficial in selected patient populations. In the second release of guidelines by the NAEPP in 1997, the recommendation of peak flow monitoring was modified based on the results of many of these studies. The current recommendations are for patients that have moderate to severe asthma, 5 years of age and older.[1]

The accuracy and reliability of different peak flowmeters have been questioned. Variation occurs even within a manufactured brand of peak flowmeters. For this reason, a patient should use a specific device for consistent readings. When analyzing peak flow data, one must realize the limitations of the measurements. Peak flow readings are extremely effort dependent and are an indicator of large airway obstruction. Often the mistake is made to attribute all low measurements to poor effort or lack of cooperation when there is airway obstruction present. Sometimes the clinician cannot differentiate between poor data or airway obstruction. PEF readings are often incorporated into care path protocols or home management plans as an objective measurement on which to base therapy. Consensus opinion from the NAEPP committee established a traditional three-zone approach to the management of acute asthma exacerbations: green, yellow, and red (Box 46-4). Some new treatment plans are separating the yellow zone into a high and low categories that each has different management strategies based on severity. Most of the predicted normal values or nomograms for peak flow values are based on sex and height in healthy subjects. Most people with moderate to severe asthma could not achieve these predicted values on their best days. This is the rationale to develop a personal best reading for peak flows on an individual-by-individual basis.

Exhaled Nitric Oxide

In 1993, Jorgens and colleagues[45] described the potential significance of measuring **exhaled nitric oxide** in disorders of the pulmonary system. Exhaled nitric oxide (NO) has been indicated as a useful marker of airway inflammation in patients with asthma. The use of exhaled nitric oxide as a potential marker of macrophage or neutrophil production in the lower airways was hypothesized and documented by Alving and colleagues.[46] Unfortunately, varied protocols make it difficult to compare and compile information from early studies on exhaled nitric oxide and asthma.

An important issue is standardization of measurement techniques for exhaled nitric oxide analysis. Measurement of exhaled nitric oxide can be complicated by two factors: contamination by nasal nitric oxide and variable expiratory flow rates. Exhaled nitric oxide concentration can be up to 1000 times higher in the nasal cavity and paranasal sinuses than concentrations found in the lower airways. Turbulent gas mixing during exhalation allows nitric oxide contamination from the nasal cavity. Nitric oxide concentration is also highly flow dependent allowing for measurement difficulty with variable flow rates.

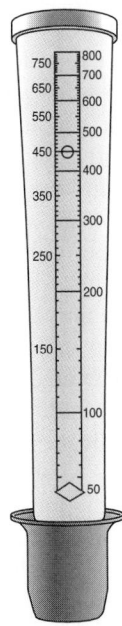

Figure 46-2   Peak flowmeter. (Modified from materials courtesy Monaghan Medical, Plattsburg, NY.)

$\mathcal{B}$OX 46-4
_____

Traditional Peak Flow Zones

Green Zone: Normal Zone
Predicted or personal best in the range of 80% to 100%

Yellow Zone: Caution Zone
Predicted or personal best in the range of 50% to 80%

Red Zone: Danger Zone
Predicted or personal best less than 50%

With high expiratory flow rates, nitric oxide levels will be lower than with a constant and slow expiratory maneuver. Silkoff and colleagues[47] have developed a technique for measuring exhaled nitric oxide that potentially overcomes these factors.

Exhaled nitric oxide is an important measurement of the inflammatory component to both acute and chronic asthma in both children and adults. People with asthma who suffer from nocturnal asthma have higher exhaled nitric oxide levels during the day and night than those who do not suffer from nocturnal symptoms.[48] With recent efforts to standardize measurement techniques, information concerning the role and degree of inflammation in both acute and chronic asthma will be available. Also the role of corticosteroid impact on decreasing or suppressing inflammation will be readily at hand for clinicians.

Pharmacologic Therapy

The purpose of pharmacologic therapy in the treatment of asthma is to prevent and/or control asthma symptoms or at least to attempt to reduce the frequency or severity of acute exacerbations. Medications for asthma are classified into two categories in the new guidelines released by the expert panel[1]—as either long-term controllers or quick relievers. The long-term controller classes of medications are taken daily in an attempt to primarily control or maintain the degree of inflammatory mediator release in the airways. The class of medications known as **controller medications** includes antiinflammatory agents, long-acting bronchodilators, and leukotriene modifiers.

Quick-relief medications are primarily short-acting, β-agonists that are used to combat acute exacerbations of bronchoconstriction or provide quick, complete resolution of airflow obstruction and its accompanying symptoms of cough, wheezing, and chest tightness. This class of quick-relief medications includes short-acting β_2-agonist and anticholinergics. All severity classes of asthma should be prescribed quick-relief medications for use during acute exacerbations.

Because the new asthma guidelines stress the importance of inflammatory component in asthma, the following medication sections start with a description of the controller medications.

Controller Medications

Inhaled Corticosteroids

This class of medications is considered the most potent and consistent antiinflammatory agent currently available by inhaled therapy in the long-term management of the inflammatory component of asthma. Antiinflammatory medications are now stressed as the first line of treatment in the management of the asthma. All asthma severity classes that have a persistent component are most effectively controlled with daily antiinflammatory therapy.

Corticosteroids have been shown to suppress the release of certain inflammatory mediators.[49] The use of corticosteroids in the management of asthma has been correlated with an overall reduction in asthma symptoms, an increase in lung function (as well as a decrease in the decline of FEV_1 over years of the disease), a decrease in airway hyperresponsiveness, a decrease in the frequency of acute exacerbations and possibly a decrease in the amount of airway remodeling in both adults and children.[50]

The exact mechanism of action involved with corticosteroids and inflammation is not well understood. Several mechanisms appear to be actively and intimately involved. Corticosteroid therapy has provided evidence of an interference of production or suppression of cytokine-release,[51] a depression in the production of leukotrienes, and active recruitment of eosinophils.[52] Clinical effects may take 2 to 3 weeks or more, but some newer agents such as fluticasone have demonstrated improvement in a day.

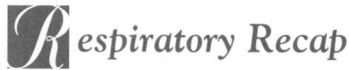

Respiratory Recap

Asthma Controller Medications
Inhaled corticosteroids
Nonsteroidal antiinflammatories
Long acting β_2-agonists
Methylxanthines
Leukotriene modifiers

Dosage and frequency of corticosteroids can vary, depending on the specific type of product or delivery device. However, dosing to effect is patient- and time-dependent. The ability to eventually wean patients off corticosteroids also depends on patient physiology. Patients who have moderate to severe persistent asthma often have persistent symptoms and a decline in lung function with attempts to wean or decrease the dose or use of corticosteroids.

The most frequent type of corticosteroid dose and frequency appears to be two to four puffs given two to three times per day. In cases of uncontrolled asthma or increasing disease severity, the dosage and frequency can be increased. Some studies have demonstrated that once-daily dosing can be effective in people with mild persistent asthma.[53,54]

Some common complications are associated with the use of corticosteroids. The most common are persistent reflex cough, occasional dysphonia, and oral pharyngeal candidiasis. The majority of these short-term complications can be eliminated or greatly reduced with the use of spacer devices and a rinsing of the mouth after inhalation. Systemic toxic effects are a rare occurrence with inhaled corticosteroids.[55] The effect of corticosteroids on the linear growth of preadolescents who are taking this class of medications long term is controversial.[56,57]

Nonsteroidal Antiinflammatory Medications

This class of long-term controller medications is predominantly utilized in adolescents and children. These medications appear to be clinically useful with patients that have mild intermittent or mild persistent asthma. In patients with moderate or severe persistent asthma, these medications are less effective as a prime method of treatment. If stepping down in therapy to a mild category, these agents can again be effective. Primarily two drugs are found in this category: cromolyn sodium and nedocromil (Table 46-1).

Both medications have distinct properties but appear to have similar antiinflammatory actions.[58] The mechanism

*T*ABLE 46-1

Long-Term Controller Medications

Medication	Dose Strength	Frequency
Corticosteroids		
Metered dose inhalers		
Beclomethasone dipropionate (Beclovent, Vanceril)	42 and 84 µg/puff	bid-qid
Budesonide	250 µg/puff	bid
Flunisolide (AeroBid, AeroBid M)	44, 110, and 220 µg/puff	bid
Fluticasone propionate (Flovent)	200 µg/puff (100 µg to patient)	bid-qid
Triamcinolone (Asthmacort)		
Systemic liquids		
Prednisone	5 mg/ 5 mL	qd
Prednisolone	5 mg/ 5 mL; 15 mg/ 5 mL	qd
Tablets		
Prednisone	1, 2.5, 5, 10, 20, 25, and 50 mg	qd
Prednisolone	5 mg	qd
Methylprednisolone	2, 4, 8, 16, 24, and 32 mg	qd
Nonsteroidal Antiinflammatories		
Metered dose inhalers		
Cromolyn sodium (Intal)	1 mg/puff	bid-qid
Nedocromil sodium (Tilade)	1.75 mg/puff	bid-qid
Nebulization		
Cromolyn sodium (Intal)	20 mg/2-mL ampule	bid-qid
Nedocromil sodium (Tilade)		
Dry powder inhaler		
Cromolyn sodium (Intal)	20-mg capsule	bid-qid
Long-Acting β₂-Agonists		
Metered dose inhalers		
Salmeterol (Serevent)	25 µg/puff	bid
Dry powder inhaler		
Salmeterol (Serevent)	25 µg/puff	bid
Oral		
Sustained-release albuterol	4 and 8 mg	bid
Methylxanthines (Oral)		
Theophylline (Slo-bid, Theo-24, Theo-Dur, Uniphyl)	Various, depending on formulation	
Leukotriene Modifiers (Oral)		
Receptor antagonists		
Zafirlukast (Accolate)	20-mg tablets	bid
Montelukast (Singulair)	5-mg tablets	qd
Receptor inhibitor		
Zileuton	600-mg tablets	qid

bid, *Twice a day;* qid, *four times a day;* qd, *daily.*

of action with these medications appears a chloride channel blockade and they modulate mast cell mediator release and promote eosinophil release.[59,60]

These antiinflammatories appear to reduce the need for quick-relievers, reduce bronchial hyperresponsiveness, improve morning peak flows, and decrease the symptoms of nocturnal asthma.[61,62] Nedocromil may have a broader range of activity in protection of EIA,[63] cough-variant asthma,[64] and cold air–induced bronchospasm.[65]

The side effects of these drugs are practically nonexistent. Both drugs have a strong safety profile with a low adverse event profile. Cromolyn is available as a unit dose, nebulized medication, and in a metered dose inhaler (MDI). Nedocromil is available at this time only in the MDI form. General MDI dosing recommendations are two puffs given four times per day. The onset of action for both drugs is about 4 to 6 weeks.

Long-Acting β2-Agonist

This class of long-term controller medications is predominantly utilized to provide a longer duration of airway smooth muscle protection. This class of medication is not intended for acute bronchospasm relief. Long-acting β2-agonists have a bronchodilation duration of approximately 12 hours but a longer onset of action than short-acting β2-agonists. Two medications are in this class of controllers: salmeterol and formoterol (see Table 46-1).

The mechanism of action for this long-acting β2-agonist is more β selective than short-acting β2-agonist. This class of medications acts as a stimulation to increase cyclic AMP and produce antagonistic reactions to bronchoconstriction by relaxing airway smooth muscle and releasing mass cell mediators. These medications have proven to work well as adjunct therapy to antiinflammatory medications in the long-term control of symptoms.[66,67] Long-acting β2-agonist appear to work exceptionally well at controlling symptoms that occur at night[68] and to prevent exercise-induced exacerbations.[69]

The complications of long-acting β2-agonist are still somewhat controversial. Case reports exist of sudden severe asthma attacks that could have been worsened or initiated with the use of salmeterol.[70] Two studies that looked closely at this issue in a large cohort of patients found more deaths in patients that were taking salmeterol compared with those that were not taking salmeterol. However, this higher mortality rate did not reach statistical significance.[71,72] Based on this data, clinicians need to pay close attention to properly educating patients who are using salmeterol. Salmeterol should be used only as a supplement to inhaled corticosteroids and never as a quick-relief medication.

Methylxanthines

This class of long-term controller medications is utilized predominantly to provide mild to moderate bronchodilation. The principal medication in this class is theophylline.

Slow-release theophylline is used primarily as adjuvant therapy for nocturnal asthma (see Table 46-1). It has been relegated for patients in the moderate to severe persistent class that are not well controlled on corticosteroids.

The exact mechanism of action of methylxanthines in asthma is not well established.[73,74] Theophylline acts as a nonselective phosphodiesterase inhibitor. This results in an increase in cyclic guanosine monophosphate levels and cyclic adenosine monophosphate levels that inhibit inflammation cells and produce bronchodilation. Recent clinical studies have indicated that low serum concentrations of theophylline may act as mild antiinflammatory medication.[75-77] This is possible most likely because of the decreased mediator release from mast cells and reactive oxygen species, and inhibition of neutrophil activity.

Theophylline is relatively safe. Its use requires frequent monitoring of serum drug levels so that therapeutic, but not toxic, levels are achieved. Potential toxic side effects include tachycardia, nausea and vomiting, central nervous system stimulation, arrhythmias, headache, seizures, hyperglycemia, and hypokalemia. The therapeutic serum range has recently been decreased from 10 to 20 mg/L to 5 to 15 mg/L to limit potential toxic effects. Clinicians must pay close attention to other medications patients receiving theophylline are receiving (antibiotics, β2-blockers, and quinolones).

Leukotriene Modifiers

This is the first new class of asthma medications introduced to clinicians in more than 20 years. These medications also fall into the class of controller medications. This class of medications acts on the inflammatory cells known as leukotrienes. Leukotrienes are mediators responsible for the release of inflammatory cells such as mast cells, eosinophils, and basophils. These inflammatory cells are responsible for airway bronchoconstriction, inflammatory cell recruitment, increase vascular permeability, and secretion production.

The mechanism of action of leukotriene modifiers is through two routes. One form of leukotriene modifiers (zafirlukast and montelukast) acts as leukotriene receptor antagonist. These medications block the receptor sites of leukotrienes. The other form of leukotriene modifiers (zileuton) acts as an inhibitor to the release of leukotrienes (see Table 46-1).

Leukotriene modifiers appear to work best in patients that have mild to moderate chronic asthma. Leukotriene modifiers are being promoted as an oral alternative therapy to low-dose inhaled corticosteroids. It appears that leukotriene modifiers improve lung function, diminish asthma symptoms, and decrease the need for short-acting β2-agonists.[78-80] Leukotriene modifiers are so new that the complication and risk profiles are still under investigation. Zileuton has been documented as potentially increasing the half-life of the drug warfarin, resulting in the need to monitor prothrombin times of warfarin and to adjust its dose accordingly.[1] The drug zileuton has received much more scrutiny from its potential to induce liver toxicity.

Because zileuton is a microsomal CYP3A4 enzyme inhibitor, it can interfere with the metabolism of terfenadine, warfarin, and theophylline. Because of this potential toxicity, patients on zileuton should have hepatic enzymes (ALT) monitored on a frequent basis.

Quick-Relief Medications

Short-Acting β₂-Agonist

This class of quick-relief medications is utilized predominantly to relieve airway bronchoconstriction and symptoms of cough, chest tightness, and wheezing. Short-acting β₂-agonists are the first-line medications used to treat an acute asthma exacerbation and for preventing exercise-induced bronchoconstriction. Before the 1990s, this was the first line of medications prescribed to result in overall control of asthma symptoms. With the new impetus of the role airway inflammation plays in the chronic management of asthma, short-acting β₂-agonist have become rescue medications. This class of medications includes albuterol, metaproterenol, bitolterol, pirbuterol, terbutaline, and isoetharine (Table 46-2).

The mechanism of action is to relax smooth airway muscle and cause quick (15- to 30-minute) resolution to airway obstruction. Bronchodilation occurs primarily through β₂-adrenergic receptor stimulation in bronchial

TABLE 46-2

Quick-Relief Medications

Medication	Dose Strength	Frequency
Short-Acting β₂-Agonists		
Metered dose inhalers		
Albuterol (Ventolin, Proventil, generic)	90 μg/puff	prn; q4h-q6h
Bitolterol (Tornalate)	370 μg/puff	
Isoetharine (Bronkometer)	340 μg/puff	
Metaproterenol (Alupent, Metaprel)	650 μg/puff	
Pirbuterol (Maxair)	200 μg/puff	
Terbutaline (Brethine, Bricanyl)	200 μg/puff	
Nebulization		
Albuterol (Ventolin, Proventil, generic)	2.5 mg (0.5% solution)	prn; q4h-q6h
Albuterol (Xopenex)	0.31 mg and 0.63 mg	
Bitolterol	0.2% solution	
Isoetharine	1% solution	
Metaproterenol	5% solution	
Dry powder inhaler		
Albuterol	200-μg capsule	prn; q4h-q6h
Oral tablet		
Albuterol (Repetabs, Volmax)	2 and 4 mg	prn; q4h-q6h
Metaproterenol	10 and 20 mg	
Terbutaline (Brethaire)	2.5 and 5 mg	
Syrup		
Albuterol	2 mg/5 mL	
Metaproterenol	10 mg/5 mL	prn; q4h-q6h
Subcutaneous injection		
Terbutaline	1 mg/mL injection	prn; q4h-q6h
Anticholinergics		
Metered dose inhalers		
Ipratropium bromide (Atrovent)	18 μg/puff	bid-qid
Nebulization		
Ipratropium bromide (Atrovent)	500-μg solution	bid-qid
Methylxanthines		
Intravenous		
Aminophylline	Various, depending on formulation	

prn, *As needed;* bid, *twice a day;* qid, *four times a day;* q4h, *every 4 hours;* q6h, *every 6 hours.*

smooth muscle. These receptors are also present in airway epithelium, airway smooth muscle, mucus glands, and mast cells. The onset of action for short-acting β_2-agonist is approximately 5 to 15 minutes under most circumstances of mild to moderate acute exacerbations.

Complications from short-acting β_2-agonist are usually mild and self-limiting upon stopping the medication. Potential side effects include tachycardia, nausea, vomiting, tremors, headache, palpitation, paradoxical bronchospasm, and hypokalemia. Some potential complications from high use or prolonged use over time include subsensitivity (reduction in bronchodilation affect), increased airways hyperreactivity, and life-threatening episodes with overuse. The frequency of short-acting β_2-agonist use or prescription refills can be used as a marker of disease worsening or indicating an increased risk for death or near death.[81]

Anticholinergics

This class of quick-relief medications is used predominantly as an adjunct to short-acting β_2-agonists in acute severe exacerbations of airway bronchoconstriction. The mechanism of action of this class of medications is airway smooth muscle tone relaxation through cholinergic innervation. Ipratropium bromide is the primary asthma medication in the anticholinergic class. Ipratropium bromide is a derivative of atropine without the common side effects of atropine (see Table 46-2).

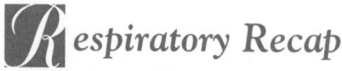

Respiratory Recap

Asthma Quick-Relief Medications
Short-acting β_2-agonists Anticholinergics Systemic corticosteroids

The overall effectiveness of ipratropium bromide in the management of asthma remains controversial.[82-86] Its effectiveness for long-term asthma management has not been demonstrated.[87,88] Adult patients who have asthma and a component of chronic obstructive pulmonary disease apparently experience some beneficial outcomes.[89]

Recent studies in pediatrics have demonstrated the use of ipratropium bromide in combination with β_2-agonists in patients with acute exacerbations or severe airway obstruction may be beneficial. However, routine administration of this combination therapy does not appear to be beneficial.[90, 91]

Systemic Corticosteroids

This class of quick-relief medications is usually combined with a short-acting β_2-agonist for a quick resolution of air-

way obstruction in an emergency room or hospital setting.[92-94] These drugs may be given either orally or intravenously. Normal dosage in this setting is 2 mg/kg (given every 6 hours, up to a maximum dose of 120 mg). The mechanism of action for systemic corticosteroids is the same as inhaled corticosteroids. For outpatient use, systemic corticosteroids are prescribed for "short-term" burst therapy (once a day for 3 to 10 days). Normal dosing is prescribed at the lowest possible dose (0.5 to 2 mg/kg/day). Maximum dose is normally restricted to 60 mg for outpatient use. If chronic utilization of systemic corticosteroids is needed, a study has documented that improved efficacy if given at 3 PM instead of in the morning.[95]

Aerosol Therapy

The main routes of delivery for asthma medications are systemic or inhaled. The main routes of systemic delivery are oral (ingested) or parenteral (subcutaneous, intramuscular, or intravenous).[1] Oral medications are mainly in either pill or liquid form. Parenteral medications are limited to predominantly patients who are in either the emergency room or the hospital.

The inhaled route is more convenient and common because of fewer side effects and quicker onset of action. The disadvantages of the inhaled route are associated with the delivery device and the factors that affect drug penetration and deposition in the lungs. The main factors involved in penetration and deposition consist of physical (sedimentation, inertial impaction, and diffusion) and clinical (particle size, ventilatory pattern, and lung function).[96]

Inhaled medications consist basically of nebulization, MDIs, and dry powder inhalers (DPIs). Numerous studies have been performed over the past 15 years to discern the best and most efficient aerosol delivery method by inhalation. Opinions and research has varied from time to time on the best and most efficient method, but recent trial demonstrated that all three (nebulized, MDIs, and DPIs) appear to be adequate in treating an acute exacerbation.[97]

Nebulizers

The small-volume nebulizer (SVN) is the most common device used to deliver medications to small children and patients requiring hospitalization. These devices utilize the Bernoulli principle, in which a compressed gas (oxygen or air) is passed through a jet to create a source of low pressure. The area of low pressure siphons medication from a reservoir chamber through a liquid feed and baffles the medication into particles that are distributed by the gas stream. Baffling of the medication allows for the larger particles to remain in the reservoir for rebaffling and the smallest (and optimal) size particles to be delivered to the patient's airways. Although theoretically aerosol delivery and deposition in an asthmatic airway may be improved with a less dense gas (helium), published research has not proved this to be true and has documented other potential problems with the use of nebulizers powered by heliox.[77,98]

A number of factors can affect an SVN's performance. These include the drug being delivered,[99] flow of the source gas,[100] type of gas source to power the nebulizer,[101] temperature and humidity of the gas source,[102] dead volume of the nebulizer,[103] the presence of a reservoir or extension,[104,105] and nebulizer brand.[106,107] Even with optimal technique and SVN performance, as little as 20% of the medication placed in a nebulizer reaches the mouthpiece, and less than 10% is deposited in the lower respiratory tract.[108-110] The clinical application of nebulizers relies on proper technique. Deposition of appropriate particle size in the lower respiratory tract depends on ventilatory pattern. To ensure optimal particle deposition, a slow breath (through the mouth) to total lung capacity with an end-inspiratory breath hold is ideal. With proper breathing technique, aerosol delivery with an SVN is equally effective with a mask or mouthpiece.[111]

Continuous Aerosols

For people with asthma who are in status, even aggressive intensive care aerosol therapy may fail. SVNs present a unique characteristic that is not available with other delivery systems—continuous nebulizer therapy. Compared with most methods and forms of acute asthma management, continuous aerosol therapy is a relatively new modality. In the late 1980s, two studies documented the benefits of continuous nebulization of terbutaline in the hospital management of children with acute asthma exacerbations.[112,113]

Although an early study in an adult emergency department demonstrated the positives (an increase FEV_1) and the negatives (β_1 side-effects) of continuous therapy,[114] studies in a pediatric population showed continuous therapy to be relatively safe.[115] Eventually, many randomized studies demonstrated that continuous therapy was as effective or more effective than intermittent therapy.[116-119]

Recent studies have investigated the ability to safely deliver continuous aerosol therapy, and to do so at higher doses or at least identify the amount of drug being delivered.[120-122] Continuous aerosol therapy has become a medically accepted alternative to intermittent therapy in emergency rooms for patients who are failing to respond or developing increased respiratory distress. Continuous therapy also appears to have become a routine practice for newly admitted people with asthma to both adult and pediatric intensive care settings. Continuous nebulization may be more effective in patients with low peak flows (less than 200 L/min) or FEV_1 (less than 50% predicted).

Metered Dose Inhalers

The MDI is the most common device used to deliver medications in an ambulatory setting and is rapidly increasing in use in hospitalized and emergency room treatment.

Medications delivered by MDIs are micronized crystals suspended in a mixture of surfactant and propellant.[123] This mixture is contained in a canister activated by compressing it into a mouthpiece. This results in a metered dose of the drug being delivered for inhalation. Because the MDI canister is pressurized, the medication is dispensed quickly and directionally. This often results in the majority of the medication being deposited in the mouth and oropharynx.[124,125] Because of the potential for ineffective drug delivery with this device, use of an accessory device (spacer, holding chamber) is recommended for all MDIs.

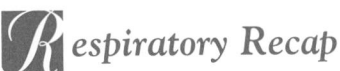 *espiratory Recap*

Aerosol Delivery Devices for the Patient with Asthma
Metered dose inhaler
Metered dose inhaler with accessory device
Dry powder inhaler

A number of factors can affect an MDI's performance and drug delivery. A potential factor that can interfere with appropriate metered dose delivery is in utilizing medications from one manufacturer with an actuator or accessory device of another manufacturer. Most of the factors that affect optimal delivery are in patient delivery technique; this is especially prominent in the very young or elderly. Factors critical in the effectiveness of MDI performance include timing of actuation, lung volume, MDI position to the mouth (without spacer), inspiratory flow rate, and the ability to perform a breath hold.[86]

Accessory Spacing Devices

To enhance optimal drug delivery with MDIs, patients should utilize an accessory spacing device. With optimal MDI delivery technique, evidence exists (even with children) of no difference in deposition with or without a spacing device.[126] For patients that are unable to coordinate and demonstrate appropriate MDI delivery technique and patients receiving inhaled corticosteroids, a spacing device is required.

With an accessory spacing device, an MDI is actuated into a holding chamber and the patient breathes the medication from a mouthpiece or mask attached to the spacer. For optimal medication availability, a spacing device that has a one-way value on inspiration is preferred. This decreases the potential of medication being lost through the device on exhalation. Different spacing devices affect drug delivery[127] and more studies are indicated with the rapid development of new medications and spacing devices. Another potential factor that may impact the amount of drug delivered with a spacing device is a static charge that occurs from rinsing spacers after use. Manufacturer instructions should be carefully read regarding appropriate spacer cleansing methodology.

An alternative to a spacer is the breath-actuated MDI. With such a device, the MDI fires automatically as the patient begins to inhale, thus appropriately timing drug delivery with inspiration.

Dry Powder Inhalers

DPIs have been commonly used in European countries for many years. Their use in the United States has not been as common but has increased with the introduction of new medications into the market. Two types of DPIs exist: single dose devices (that is, Spinhaler, Rotahaler), and multi-dose devices (that is, budesonide, fluticasone, salmeterol). DPIs are breath-activated with a high-inspiratory flow generated from a mouthpiece. In the past, many DPIs required the patient to load doses for delivery. This is no longer necessary with some of the newer DPIs on the market (for example, Turbuhaler). Because of the requirement of a high-inspiratory flow for actuation, DPIs are not indicated for use in children under 12 years of age.

Alternative Treatment Modalities

Oxygen, inhaled β_2-adrenergic agonists, and corticosteroids remain the cornerstones of therapy for asthma. This section discusses four alternative therapies to aerosolized medications in the treatment of status asthmaticus: helium–oxygen gas mixtures (heliox), magnesium sulfate, noninvasive ventilation, and mechanical ventilation. Because of the risk of immediate respiratory decompensation, these therapies are normally administered in the confines of an intensive care unit or emergency room.

Heliox

Helium is a gas that is less dense than air, which may be beneficial in the treatment of asthma.[128] **Heliox** is not a stand-alone therapy to treat status asthmaticus, but supportive therapy before intubation to allow time for bronchodilators and corticosteroids to take effect.[129] A difficulty in the provision of heliox in nonintubated patients is that the available gas mixtures in concentrations may not provide adequate supplemental oxygen to achieve acceptable oxyhemoglobin saturations (80% helium:20% oxygen or 70% helium:30% oxygen).

Therapeutic benefits of heliox are controversial. Reports of the therapeutic benefits of heliox are isolated primarily to the management of pediatric asthma[130] or in the management of adult patients who present to the emergency department with a respiratory acidosis and/or a short duration of symptoms.[131] Some studies have shown that the use of heliox has no effect on FEV_1.[132,133] Given

the safety profile of heliox and the short time to achieve a positive response, a brief trial of heliox may serve as a therapeutic bridge until corticosteroid therapy has taken effect. One study documented a rapid resolution (less than 60 minutes) to respiratory acidosis by using heliox, especially in patients that had brief duration of symptoms (less than 24 hours) and a severely acidotic pH (7.20 or less) at presentation.[134] A randomized trial in patients with asthma has also reported benefit with the use of heliox.[135]

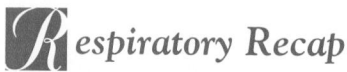

*R*espiratory Recap

Alternative Treatments for Asthma
Heliox
Magnesium sulfate
Noninvasive ventilation

Magnesium Sulfate

Administration of magnesium sulfate is an alternative treatment for status asthmaticus.[136,137] Magnesium is proven to be beneficial in the management of status asthmaticus. The mechanisms of action include calcium-channel blockade in the airway smooth muscle and inhibitor of acetylcholine and histamine release. Magnesium may promote bronchodilation that would improve β_2-agonist delivery.[138] A recent study comparing nebulized magnesium to salbutamol demonstrated a similar response,[139] but nebulized magnesium does not consistently have this bronchodilator effect. Other studies have documented no improvement in FEV_1 in patients who were treated with magnesium intravenously.[140-143]

The dose for intravenous magnesium is 30 to 70 mg/kg (maximum 2 to 3) administered over a half hour. The onset of action for magnesium can occur within minutes of administration. Potential side effects are usually minor (facial warmth and flushing). However, magnesium can be toxic with high serum levels. Signs of magnesium toxicity include hypotension, dysrthymias, areflexia, and muscle weakness. The use of magnesium sulfate in the treatment of status asthmaticus remains controversial as a first-line therapy. In moderate to severe asthma exacerbations that are unresponsive to β_2-agonists, magnesium may be beneficial as an adjunctive therapy.[144,145]

Noninvasive Ventilation

The use of noninvasive positive pressure ventilation (NPPV) has taken a role in the management of patients that are at high risk for intubation and mechanical ventilation. NPPV offers a viable means of overcoming increased work of breathing without an endotracheal tube and ventilator. Uncontrolled studies have documented the use of noninvasive ventilation as a viable alternative to mechanical ventilation.[146,147] The key factor in the use of NPPV is the early initiation of the therapy in conjunction with bronchodilators and corticosteroids. Appropriate inspiratory flow is important to ensure patient comfort and to decrease the work of breathing. Avoiding delivery of excessive minute ventilation is important, because it could lead to hyperinflation and air trapping. The use of aerosolized medications with NPPV is feasible but remains controversial in its overall effectiveness.[148] The use of NPPV in an asthmatic population is supportive and meant to be utilized in conjunction with established therapies.

Mechanical Ventilation

Mechanical ventilation of patients with asthma is a treatment of last resort for patients experiencing respiratory failure.[149] Respiratory failure that leads to mechanical ventilation of the patient with asthma because of severe airflow obstruction, increased mucous production, and/or severe airway inflammation. Asthma resulting in intubation and mechanical ventilation is not a common event, consisting of less than 5% of patients treated.[150] The general indications for mechanical ventilation in the patient with asthma are listed in Box 46-5. The obstructive nature of a severe exacerbation of asthma produces a ventilation-perfusion mismatch and an increased work of breathing, but this rarely produces severe hypoxemia.[151] The more difficult issue in the acute asthmatic patient is optimizing the pH and $PaCO_2$ because of air trapping, bronchoconstriction, and increased dead space.[152]

Goals of Mechanical Ventilation

On intubation of an acute asthmatic, full ventilatory support is usually provided (that is, no spontaneous breathing by the patient). This allows optimization of the patient-ventilator interface under the best possible conditions. The principal goal of mechanical ventilation of the patient with asthma is to provide acceptable gas exchange while avoiding air trapping (auto-PEEP [positive end-expiratory pressure]). With auto-PEEP, alveolar

---

Box 46-5

Indications for Mechanical Ventilation of the Patient with Asthma

> $PaCO_2$ >40 mm Hg (especially if increasing)
> Refractory hypoxemia (PaO_2 <60 mm Hg on FIO_2 ≥50%)
> Mental status deterioration
> Decrease or loss of breath sounds
> Apneic episodes

---

overdistention may occur with concomitant hypotension and barotrauma.

Mode of Ventilation

The choice of ventilator mode is often based on clinical preference or institutional bias. Either volume or pressure modes can be used, and advantages and disadvantages exist for both. With volume controlled ventilation, auto-PEEP results in increased plateau pressures and alveolar overdistention. With pressure-controlled ventilation, auto-PEEP results in decreased tidal volumes and respiratory acidosis. In patients with asthma with severe airflow obstruction, it may be difficult to deliver an adequate tidal volume with pressure-controlled ventilation. Regardless of the mode chosen, auto-PEEP and plateau pressures must be monitored closely.

Tidal Volume

The ultimate goal of a delivered tidal volume in status asthmaticus is to avoid overdistention of the alveoli. Generally, tidal volumes are set in the 5 to 8 mL/kg range and adjusted to minimize over distention (that is, to avoid a plateau pressure of more than 35 cm H_2O). This often results in a ventilator strategy of permissive hypercapnia. With permissive hypercapnia, $PaCO_2$ is allowed to rise and an acidic pH is tolerated. The limits of safe $PaCO_2$ and pH are debated, but general consensus suggests that $PaCO_2$ levels of 80 to 100 mm Hg and pH levels of 7.15 to 7.20 are acceptable.[152-157]

Positive End-Expiratory Pressure

The use of positive end-expiratory pressure (PEEP) when ventilating the patient with asthma is controversial. PEEP as a means to prevent atelectasis or collapse is not necessary. PEEP has been used to combat auto-PEEP. The intent is to counterbalance auto-PEEP by applying PEEP so that the patient will be better able to trigger the ventilator. However, care must be taken to avoid increased over distention with the application of PEEP. PEEP has no role in counterbalancing auto-PEEP in the patient who is not attempting to trigger the ventilator.[158-162] Generally, no more than 10 cm H_2O PEEP is used to counterbalance auto-PEEP. Some auto-PEEP that occurs during mechanical ventilation of the patient with asthma may not be measurable in the usual manner because of complete airway closure during the expiratory phase.[163]

Inspiratory to Expiratory Ratio

The inspiratory to expiratory ratio (I:E) in a patient with airflow obstruction is important to avoid air trapping. The I:E ratio is determined by the inspiratory time (flow and tidal volume for volume-controlled ventilation) and respiratory rate. The goal when setting the I:E ratio in patients with asthma is to allow adequate expiratory time to minimize auto-PEEP. Use of prolonged expiratory times require a low respiratory rate and a shortened inspiratory time. Typically, a respiratory rate of 12/minute or less with an inspiratory time of 1 second is used.

Aerosol Therapy with Mechanical Ventilation

When aggressive therapy fails to stabilize a patient's asthma and intubation occurs, the need to provide aerosol therapy remains important in the resolution of the acute exacerbation. Aerosol therapy of the intubated patient has been an area of debate.[164] Some support either nebulization or MDI as the most effective and efficient method from a clinical and financial standpoint. Aerosol delivery to intubated patients with either nebulization or MDI is less effective than when delivered to a spontaneously breathing patient. Many factors in intubated patients affect optimal aerosol delivery and deposition. Higher-than-standard doses may be necessary to elicit a desired response because of potential barriers involved with mechanically ventilated patients. Aerosol administration by both nebulizers and MDIs is an effective means of delivering medication to ventilated patients. Studies utilizing both devices have demonstrated lung deposition efficiency of 5% to 15%.[164] Sufficient attention to detail, including the use of an efficient nebulizer and/or adapter and proper placement and operating method, is required to provide optimal delivery.

Heliox with Mechanical Ventilation

The use of heliox with mechanical ventilation may be beneficial when a patient with asthma is difficult to manage with traditional mechanical ventilator manipulations.[128] However, caution is warranted because the addition of heliox may result in ventilator malfunction.[165]

Complications

Mechanical ventilation of the patient with asthma may be a lifesaving measure, but it can also be associated with significant morbidity and mortality.[152,166-169] The major complications of mechanical ventilation of the patient with asthma include over distention, pneumothorax, hypotension, air trapping, patient-ventilator dyssynchrony, and neuromuscular blocking agent-related myopathies.

Education

Asthma education begins at diagnosis and is reinforced with each visit. The ability to modify morbidity and re-

---

Box 46-6

Educational Recommendations of the NAEPP

Teach basic facts about asthma.
Teach the necessary medication skills (techniques, delivery devices, and dosing regimens).
Teach self-monitoring skills: symptom-based, peak flow monitoring.
Teach relevant environmental control/avoidance strategies.
Provide a written asthma exacerbation treatment plan.

From National Asthma Education and Prevention Program, National Heart, Lung, and Blood Institute. Expert panel report 2: guidelines for the diagnosis and management of asthma. Publication No. 97-4051. Bethesda, Md: National Institutes of Health; 1997.

Table 46-3

Theoretic Look at Regression Toward the Mean

| | Percentage of Resource Cost Consumption | | | |
	Original Percentage of Patients	Year 1	Year 2	Year 3
High-resource consumers	10	80	10	4
Low-resource consumers	90	20	90	96

---

source consumption through education has also been well-documented in asthma.[170,171] Over the past 20 years, many programs and formats have been designed and implemented to demonstrate that asthma education is a main component to the overall successful management of the disease. The items in Box 46-6 should be included in all **asthma education programs.**[1]

Many studies of educational interventions are available in the literature, covering many different care settings. These include ambulatory clinics, allergy or pulmonary specialty clinics, emergency departments, hospitals, patient homes, and asthma camps. Educational interventions have evaluated the impact on readmission rates, hospitalizations, compliance, emergency room visits, clinic follow-up rates, test scores, and behavior changes.

The rapid expansion of managed health care in the 1990s, led to the study of the financial aspects of providing asthma education. Some of the earlier managed care education interventions assessed patients with asthma determined to be high risk. Although these programs still exist, asthma educators are looking at ways to target a variety of patients with asthma, because of a regression-to-the-mean concept. The theory of regression-toward-the-mean implies that patients with chronic conditions do not have steady-state health-care resource consumption year after year. One year's high-resource consumers do not necessarily translate into the next year's high-resource consumers. Therefore these earliest managed care programs and interventions resulted in a shifting of the costs from group to group or from year to year (Table 46-3).

The asthma education program needs to take a proactive approach. An asthma education program should provide education to the patient with asthma and include all potential caregivers (spouses, parents, older children, day-care providers, teachers, coaches, group leaders, and counselors). The National Cooperative Inner City Asthma Study (NCICAS) reported that often a child has several care providers in the home.[172] This pediatric study demonstrated the importance of involving as many caregivers as possible in the asthma education to ensure consistent management. This study also identified that pediatric asthma has additional educational barriers. Often education providers overlook the child to concentrate their educational efforts on the caregivers. However, children as young as 2 years can begin learning about their asthma and its management. As children age, the scope and the depth of the information will need to continue to grow. As children grow into adolescents, they should receive all asthma information themselves.[173]

Age-Specific Angle

Children as young as 2 years of age can begin learning about asthma and its management.

Asthma education information should be repeated several times for maximum effect, and educational objectives should be reinforced with written materials targeted for age appropriateness. Asthma self-management education should be modified to the needs of each individual patient. Cultural beliefs and unharmful practices should be approached and discussed with sensitivity and understanding. The education provider should be attentive and document concerns of the patient and the family regarding medications and asthma management. Addressing concerns and explaining the rationale may be the overriding factor to patient compliance with chronic asthma management. The asthma educator also must be prepared to intervene and problem-solving areas of medications, level of treatment, trigger avoidance, compliance, and self-management skills.

One of the indicators of a chronic condition is the ability to modify or reduce morbidity and mortality risks through patient education. Asthma is a chronic disease condition that has demonstrated this ability. An unlimited number of approaches or interventions are readily available to provide effective and efficient asthma education to health care providers. Perhaps one method is not truly better than another. The important features are to provide the resources and information at diagnosis and consistently thereafter to each patient with asthma individually.

CASE STUDIES

Case One
Ambulatory Asthma Management

A 43-year-old woman with asthma presents to an inner-city emergency room with coughing, wheezing, and shortness of breath. She reports a respiratory viral infection within the last week that resolved with over-the-counter medicines in 3 or 4 days. Her initial physical examination reveals the following: respiratory rate of 36 breaths per minute, and labored; heart rate of 120/min; blood pressure 120/80 mm Hg; pulse oximetry of 93% in room air; inspiratory and expiratory wheezing upon auscultation; equal air exchange bilaterally; moderate intercostal retractions; and PEF of 290 L/min (60% of predicted). The initial treatment consists of six puffs of albuterol, administered via an MDI with a holding chamber. Each puff is given with the appropriate technique. Posttreatment PEF is 300 L/min (62% of predicted).

The woman reports that she stopped taking her beclomethasone about 2 months before this visit. The following additional information is acquired:

- *Reported medications:* Beclomethasone 2 puffs bid and albuterol 2 puffs as needed and before exercise
- *Treatment before arrival:* None
- *Peak flowmeter diary:* None
- *Unscheduled ED/MD visits in the past month:* 0
- *Unscheduled ED/MD visits in the past year:* 3
- *Hospital admissions in the past year:* 1
- *Prior intensive care unit (ICU) admissions:* 0
- *Cough or wheeze frequency:* Two times per week
- *Activity limitations:* Occasionally
- *Nocturnal cough or wheeze:* Two to three times per week
- *Work absenteeism:* 6 days per year

Approximately 20 minutes after the initial treatment, a second treatment is administered with six puffs of albuterol via MDI and holding chamber as before. The patient is also given 60 mg of prednisolone. Posttreatment assessment reveals a respiratory rate of 24 breaths per minute; heart rate of 100 beats per minute; oxygen saturation of 95% breathing room air; inspiratory and expiratory wheezing upon auscultation; equal air exchange bilaterally; mild intercostal retractions; and PEF of 315 L/min (65% predicted).

Approximately 20 minutes after the second treatment, a third treatment of albuterol (six puffs) is administered, along with 2 puffs of Atrovent. Posttreatment assessment reveals a respiratory rate of 16 breaths per minute; heart rate of 80 beats per minute; oxygen saturation of 95% breathing room air; faint end-expiratory wheezes with auscultation and bilateral equal air exchange; no intercostal retractions; and PEF of 365 L/min (75% predicted).

The woman's next β_2-agonist treatment is withheld and she is reassessed in 60 minutes. The prior assessment response is sustained upon physical examination and the woman is readied for discharge. Based on the self-reported asthma history, the woman's chronic asthma is determined to be moderate persistent asthma. She is instructed to continue her albuterol treatments with two puffs every 4 to 6 hours for the next several days. She is also told to resume her beclomethasone therapy of two puffs bid for chronic inflammatory control. She is given a peak flowmeter and instructed in its proper use. She is also instructed in the use of an asthma action plan with a peak flow diary that illustrates meter readings in three color-coded zones to assist her in self-management. She is also instructed to call her primary care physician and to schedule a follow-up visit in the next week to 10 days.

Case Two
Life-Threatening Asthma Management

A 10-year-old boy with asthma presents to an inner-city emergency room with dyspnea at rest, talking in phrases, agitated, and dusky in color. The boy's mother reports having administered three nebulizer treatments before arrival in the emergency room. The child's initial physical examination reveals the following: respiratory rate of 48 breaths per minute, and labored; heart rate of 170 beats per minute; blood pressure 160/100 mm Hg; oxygen saturation of 89% breathing room air; breath sounds muffled to inaudible; severe intercostal and substernal retractions; and inability to perform a PEF.

The initial treatment consists of 0.5 mg of epinephrine given subcutaneously. The patient is then started on undiluted albuterol that was nebulized with 100% oxygen. An IV is placed and he is given 60 mg methylprednisone. During the aerosol treatment, an asthma history is taken from the boy's mother. She reports that her child had been outside playing basketball with his friends for most of the afternoon. Before this episode, he was in good health. The following information is acquired:

- *Reported medications:* Serevent two puffs bid and albuterol two puffs as needed before exercise
- *Treatment before arrival:* Three nebulized treatments with albuterol
- *Peak flowmeter diary:* None

- *Unscheduled ED/MD visits in the past month:* 0
- *Unscheduled ED/MD visits in the past year:* 1
- *Hospital admissions in the past year:* 1
- *Prior ICU admissions:* 1 (3 years ago)
- *Cough or wheeze frequency:* With respiratory infections
- *Activity or play limitations:* Always
- *Nocturnal cough or wheeze:* One to two times per week
- *School absenteeism:* Three to four days per year

While receiving continuous albuterol treatments, the child is assessed every 20 minutes. ECG and pulse oximetry is monitored continuously. After the initial 20 minutes, 0.5 mg of ipratropium is added to the aerosol. Thirty-five minutes after treatment was started, the boy's status is respiratory rate of 20 breaths per minute, and labored; heart rate of 80 beats/ per minute; blood pressure 200/100 mm Hg; oxygen saturation of 88% on continuous nebulizer; inaudible breath sounds; severe intercostal and substernal retractions; inability to perform PEF; lethargy and drowsiness. Arterial blood gas results are pH 7.29, PaCO$_2$ 52 mm Hg, PaO$_2$ 60 mm Hg, HCO$_3^-$ 26 mmol/L, and oxygen saturation of 87%.

The decision is made to intubate the child. After atropine, ketamine, and succinylcholine are administered, he is intubated with 6.0 mm cuffed endotracheal tube. Upon arrival in the pediatric intensive care unit, the child is placed on the following settings: SIMV with pressure support, tidal volume 350 mL (7 mL/kg), PEEP 4 cm H$_2$O, mandatory breath rate 10 breaths/min, I:E ratio of 1:5, FIO$_2$ 0.50, and pressure support 5 cm H$_2$O. After 1 hour on the ventilator, the arterial blood gas results are pH 7.32, PaCO$_2$ 46 mm Hg, PaO$_2$ 120 mm Hg, HCO$_3^-$ 22 mmol/L, and oxygen saturation 99%. The FIO$_2$ is weaned by 10%. The patient is ventilated with permissive hypercapnia to protect auto-PEEP and overdistention. Continuous ventilator waveform analysis is used to detect auto-PEEP and a long expiratory time is set. The patient is kept moderately sedated and paralytics is not necessary at this time. The child is given albuterol via MDI through the ventilator circuit with 10 puffs every 30 minutes and two puffs of Atrovent every 6 hours. The patient remains on IV methylprednisone.

After 6 hours of this therapy, the albuterol treatments are changed to a frequency of every hour. After 12 hours of mechanical ventilation and pharmacologic therapy, blood gas results are pH 7.42, PaCO$_2$ 33 mm Hg, PaO$_2$ 95 mm Hg (on FIO$_2$ of 0.25), HCO$_3^-$ 24 mmol/L, and oxygen saturation of 99%. He is awake and spontaneously breathing at a rate of 6 to 10/min above the mandatory rate with spontaneous tidal volumes of 4 to 5 mL/kg. He is extubated to a 2 L/min nasal cannula and receives 5.0 mg nebulized albuterol every hour with IV methylprednisone and ipratropium 0.5 mg every 6 hours.

$\mathcal{K}$EY $\mathcal{P}$OINTS

- Asthma is a common chronic disease that is increasing in prevalence and severity.
- The pathophysiology of asthma is largely related to inflammation, hyperresponsiveness, and airway obstruction.
- The most identifiable predisposing factor for the development of asthma is atopy.
- Nocturnal symptoms of asthma are common.
- Exercise-induced asthma is characterized by transient airway obstruction after strenuous exercise.
- Occupational asthma is characterized by variable airway hyperresponsiveness in the workplace.
- The NAEPP has developed a four-tiered level to classify asthma disease severity.
- The most common ways to diagnose and monitor airflow obstruction in asthma are spirometry and peak flowmeters.
- Asthma medications are classified as either long-term controllers or quick-relievers.
- Inhaled medications are delivered by nebulizer, metered dose inhaler, or dry powder inhalers.
- Oxygen, inhaled β-agonists, and corticosteroids are the cornerstones of therapy for asthma.
- Mechanical ventilation is the treatment of last resort for patients with asthma and respiratory failure.
- Asthma education begins with diagnosis and is reinforced with each visit.

References

1. Expert Panel Report 2: Guidelines for the Diagnosis and Management of Asthma. National Asthma Education Program, National Heart, Lung, and Blood Institute, National Institutes of Health. Bethesda, Maryland: Publication No. 97-4051, April 1997.
2. Webster's Ninth New Collegiate Dictionary. Merriam-Webster Inc, Springfield, Mass, 1984.
3. Weiss KB, Wagoner DK. Changing patterns of asthma mortality. Identifying target populations at high risk. JAMA 1990;264:1683-1687.
4. Schaubel D, Johansen H, Mao Y, et al. Risk of preschool asthma; incidence, hospitalization, recurrence, and readmission probability. J Asthma 1996;33:97-103.
5. Pappas G, Hadden WC, Kozak LJ, et al. Potentially avoidable hospitalizations: inequalities in rates between US socioeconomic groups. Am J Public Health 1997;87:811-816.
6. Kussin PS, McIntyre N. Adult asthma. Respir Care Clin N Am 1995;1:178.
7. Wasserfallen JB, Schaller MD, Feihl F, et al. Sudden asphyxia asthma: A distinct entity? Am Rev Respir Dis 1990;142:108-111.
8. Weiss KB, Gergan PJ, Hodgson TA. An economical evaluation of asthma in the US. N Engl J Med 1992;326:862-866.
9. Smith D, Malone D, Lawson K et al. A national estimate of the economic costs of asthma. Am J Respir Crit Care Med 1997;156:787-793.
10. McFadden, ER, Elsanadi N, Dixon L, et al. Protocol therapy for acute asthma: therapeutic benefits and cost savings. Am J Med 1995;99:651-660.
11. Myers TR, Chatburn RL, Kercsmar CM. A pediatric asthma unit staff by respiratory therapists demonstrates positive clinical and financial outcomes. Respir Care 1998;43:22-29.
12. McDowell KM, Chatburn RL, Myers TR, et al. A cost-saving algorithm for children hospitalized for status asthmaticus. Arch Pediatr Adolesc Med 1998;152:977-984.
13. Mayo PH, Weinberg BJ, Kramer B, et al. Results of a program to improve the process of inpatient care of adult asthmatics. Chest 1996;110:48-52.
14. Kwann-Ghett TS, Lozano P, Mullin K, et al. One-year experience with an inpatient asthma clinical pathway. Arch Pediatr Adolesc Med 1997;151:684-689.
15. Headrick L, Katcher W, Neuhauser D, et al. Continuous quality improvement and knowledge for improvement applied to asthma care. J Joint Commission Qual Improvement 1994; 562-568.
16. Weiss KB, Gergen PJ, Wagener DK. Breathing better or wheezing worse? The changing epidemiology of asthma morbidity and mortality. Annu Rev Public Health 1993;14:491-513.
17. Emanuel MB, Howarth PH. Asthma and anaphylaxis: a relevant model for chronic disease? An historical analysis of directions in asthma research. Clin Exp Allergy 1994;25:15-26.
18. Global Initiative for Asthma: Global Strategy for Asthma Management or Prevention. NHLBI/WHO Workshop Report. Bethesda, Md. National Institutes of Health, Publication no. 95-3659, 1995, 78-79.
19. Anthonisen NR, Connett JE, Kiley JP, et al. Effects of smoking intervention and the use of an inhaled anticholinergic bronchodilator on the rate of decline of FEV_1. JAMA 1994;272:1497-1505.
20. Sporik R, Holgate ST, Platts-Mills TA, et al. Exposure to house-dust mite allergen (Der pI) and the development of asthma in childhood. A prospective study. N Engl J Med 1990;323:502-507.
21. Burrows B, Martinez FD, Halonen M, et al. Association of asthma with serum IgE levels and skin test reactivity to allergens. N Engl J Med 1989;320:271.
22. Eggleston PA, Rosenstreich D, Lynn H, et al. Relationship of indoor allergen exposure to skin test sensitivity in inner-city children with asthma. J Allergy Clin Immunol 1998;102:563-570.
23. Whitaker K. Pediatric diseases requiring respiratory care. In: Comprehensive perinatal & pediatric respiratory care, 2nd ed. Albany: Delmar Publishers; 1997. pp. 425-431.
24. Feather IH, Warner JA, Holgate ST. Cohabitating with domestic mites. Thorax 1993;48:5-9.
25. Rosenstreich DL, Eggleston P, Kattan M, et al. The role of cockroach allergy and exposure to cockroach allergen in causing morbidity among inner-city children with asthma. N Engl J Med 1997;336:1356-1363.
26. Donahue J. Ambulatory care of the adult asthma patient. Respir Care Clin N Am 1995;1:193-213.
27. Rossi OVJ, Kinnula VL, Tiermari J, et al. Association of severe asthma attacks with weather, pollen, and air pollutants. Thorax 1994;49:1185-1188.

28. Teichtahl H, Buckmaster N, Pertnikovs E. The incidence of respiratory tract infection in adults requiring hospitalization for asthma. Chest 1997;112:591-596.

29. Pizzichini MM, Pizzichini E, Efthimiadis A, et al. Asthma and natural colds. Inflammatory indices in induced sputum: a feasibility study. Am J Respir Crit Care Med 1998;158:1178-1184.

30. Martinez FD, Stern DA, Wright AL, et al. Differential immune responses to acute lower respiratory illness in early life and subsequent development of persistent wheezing and asthma. J Allergy Clin Immunol 1998;102(6 Pt 1):915-920.

31. Welliver RC, Sun M, Rinaldo D, et al. Predictive value of respiratory syncytial virus-specific IgE responses for recurrent wheezing following bronchiolitis. J Pediatr 1986;109:776-780.

32. Lieu TA, Quesenberry CP Jr, Capra AM, et al. Outpatient management practices associated with reduced risk of pediatric asthma hospitalization and emergency department visits. Pediatrics 1997;100:334-341.

33. Martin RJ. Nocturnal asthma and the use of theophylline. Clin Exp Allergy 1998;28:64-70.

34. Meijer GG, Postma DS, Wempe JB, et al. Frequency of nocturnal symptoms in asthmatic children attending a hospital out-patient clinic. Eur Respir J 1995;8:2076-2080.

35. Di Stefano A, Lusuardi M, Braghiroli A, et al. Nocturnal asthma: mechanisms and therapy. Lung 1997;175:53-61.

36. Fix A, Sexton M, Langenberg P, et al. The association of nocturnal asthma with asthma severity. J Asthma 1997;34:329-336.

37. Martin RJ. Nocturnal asthma. Mount Kisco, NY: Futura Publishing Company; 1993.

38. Douglas NJ. Nocturnal asthma. Thorax 1993;48:100-102.

39. Silkoff PE, Martin RJ. Pathophysiology of nocturnal asthma. Ann Allergy Asthma Immunol 1998;81:378-383.

40. Syabbalo N. Chronobiology and chronopathophysiology of nocturnal asthma. Int J Clin Pract 1997;51:455-462.

41. Kukafka DS, Lang DM, Porter S, et al. Exercise-induced bronchospasm in high school athletes via a free running test: incidence and epidemiology. Chest 1998;114:1613-1622.

42. de Benedictis FM, Tuteri G, Pazzelli P, et al. Combination drug therapy for the prevention of exercise-induced bronchoconstriction in children. Ann Allergy Asthma Immunol 1998;80:352-356.

43. American Thoracic Society. Standardization of spirometry: 1994 update. Am J Respir Care Med 1995;152:1107-1136.

44. Le Souf PN, La Fortune BC, Landau LI. Spirometric assessments of asthmatic children aged two to six years. Aust NZ J Med 1986;16:625.

45. Jorgens PG, Vermeire PA, Herman AG. L-Arginine-dependent nitric oxide synthase: a new metabolic pathway in the lung and airways. Eur Respir J 1993;6:258-266.

46. Alving K, Weitzberg E, Lundberg JM. Increased amount of nitric oxide in exhaled air of asthmatics. Eur Respir J 1993;6:1368-1370.

47. Silkoff PE, McClean PA, Slutsky AS, et al. Marked flow-dependence of exhaled nitric oxide using a new technique to exclude nasal nitric oxide. Am J Respir Crit Care Med 1997;155:260-267.

48. ten Hacken NH, van der Vaart H, van der Mark TW, et al. Exhaled nitric oxide is higher both at day and night in subjects with nocturnal asthma. Am J Respir Crit Care Med 1998;158:902-907.

49. Mathewson HS. Asthma and bronchitis: a shift of therapeutic emphasis. Respir Care 1990;35:273-277.

50. Barnes PJ, Pederson S. Efficacy and safety of inhaled corticosteroids in asthma. Am Rev Respir Dis 1993;146:1524-1530.

51. Barnes P. Inhaled glucocorticoids for asthma. N Engl J Med 1995;332:866-867.

52. Busse WW. What role for inhaled steroids in chronic asthma. Chest 1993;104:1565-1571.

53. Jones AH, Langdon CG, Lee PS, et al. Pulmicort Turbuhaler once daily as initial prophylactic therapy for asthma. Respir Med 1994;88:293-299.

54. Pincus DJ, Szefler SJ, Ackerson LM, et al. Chronotherapy of asthma with inhaled steroids: the effect of dosage timing on drug efficacy. J Allergy Clin Immunol 1995;95:1172-1178.

55. Monson JP. Systemic effects of inhaled corticosteroids. Thorax 1993;48:955-956.

56. Russell G. Inhaled corticosteroid therapy in children: an assessment of the potential for side-effects. Thorax 1994;49:1185-1188.

57. Wolthers OD, Pederson S. Short-term growth during treatment with inhaled fluticasone propionate and beclomethasone dipropionate. Arch Dis Child 1993;68:673-676.

58. Clark B. General pharmacology, pharmacokinetics, and clinical toxicology of nedocromil sodium. J Allergy Clin Immunol 1993;92:200-202.

59. Alton E, Norris AA. Chloride transport and the actions of nedocromil sodium and cromolyn sodium in asthma. J Allergy Clin Immunol 1994;98:S102-S106.

60. Eady RP. The pharmacology of nedocromil sodium. Eur J Respir Dis 1986;147:S112-119.

61. Wasserman SI. Nedocromil sodium: a pyranoquinoline antiinflammatory agent for the treatment of asthma. J Allergy Clin Immunol 1993;92:143-216.

62. Schwartz HJ, Blumenthal M, Brady R, et al. A comparative study of the clinical efficacy of nedocromil sodium and placebo. Chest 1996;109:945-952.

63. Novembre G, Frongia GF, Veneruso G, et al. Inhibition of exercise-induced asthma (EIA) by nedocromil sodium and sodium cromoglycate in children. Pediatr Allergy Immunol 1994;5:107-110.

64. Lal S, Dorow PD, Venho KK, et al. Nedocromil sodium is more effective than cromolyn sodium for the treatment of chronic reversible obstructive airway disease. Chest 1993;104:438-447.

65. Juniper EF, Kline PA, Morris MM, et al. Airway constriction by isocapnic hyperventilation of cold, dry air: comparison of magnitude and duration of protection by nedocromil sodium and sodium cromoglycate. Clin Allergy 1987;17:523-528.

66. Greening AP, Wind P, Northfield M, et al. Added salmeterol versus higher-dose corticosteroids in asthma patients with symptoms on existing corticosteroids. Lancet 1994;344:219-224.

67. Woolcock A, Lundback B, Ringdal N, et al. Comparison of addition of salmeterol to inhaled steroids with doubling of the dose of inhaled steroid. Am J Respir Crit Care Med 1996;153:1481-1488.

68. Yates DH, Sussman HS, Shaw MJ, et al. Regular formoterol treatment in mild asthma. Effect of bronchial responsiveness during and after treatment. Am J Respir Crit Care Med 1995;152:1170-1174.

69. Green CP, Price JF. Prevention of exercise-induced asthma by inhaled salmeterol xinzfoate. Arch Dis Child 1992;67:1014-1017.

70. Clark CE, Ferguson AD, Siddorn JA. Respiratory arrests in young asthmatics on salmeterol. Respir Med 1993;87:227-228.

71. Castle W, Fuller R, Hall J, et al. Serevent nationwide surveillance study: comparison of salmeterol with salbutamol in asthmatic patients who require bronchodilator treatment. BMJ 1993;306:1034-1037.

72. Mann RD, Kubota K, Pearce G, et al. Salmeterol: a study by prescription-event monitoring in a UK cohort of 15,407 patients. J Clin Epidemiol 1996;49:247-250.

73. Weinberger M, Hendeles L. Theophylline in asthma. N Engl J Med 1996;334:1380-1388.

74. Hendeles L, Harman E, Huang D, et al. Theophylline attenuation of airway responses to allergen: comparison with cromolyn metered-dose inhaler. J Allergy Clin Immunol 1995;95:505-514.

75. Sullivan P, Bekir S, Jaffar Z, et al. Anti-inflammatory effects of low-dose oral theophylline in atopic asthma. Lancet 1994;343:1006-1008.

76. Kidney J, Dominguez M, Taylor PM, et al. Immunodilation by theophylline in asthma. Am J Respir Crit Care Med 1995;151:1907-1914.

77. Pauwels RA. New aspects of the therapeutic potential of theophylline in asthma. J Allergy Clin Immunol 1989;83:548-553.

78. Gaddy JN, Margolskee DJ, Bush RK, et al. Bronchodilation with potent and selective leukotriene D4 (LTD4) receptor antagonist (MK-571) in patients with asthma. Am Rev Respir Dis 1992;146:358-363.

79. Spector Sl, Smith Lj, Glass M. Effects of 6 weeks of therapy with oral doses of ICI 204,219, a leukotriene D4 receptor antagonist, in subjects with bronchial asthma. Am J Respir Crit Care Med 1994;150:618-623.

80. Israel E, Chn J, Dube L, et al. Effects of treatment with zileuton, a 5-lipoxygenase inhibitor, in patients with asthma. JAMA 1996;275:931-936.

81. Spitzer WO, Suissa S, Ernst P, et al. The use of beta-agonist and the risk of death and near death from asthma. N Engl J Med 1992;326:501-501.

82. Chapman KR. An international perspective on anticholinergic therapy. Am J Med 1996;29;100:2S-4S.

83. Karpel JP, Schacter EN, Fanta C, et al. A comparison of ipratropium and albuterol vs albuterol alone for the treatment of acute asthma. Chest 1996;110:611-616.

84. FitzGerald JM, Grunfeld A, Pare PD, et al. The clinical efficacy of combination nebulized anticholinergic and adrenergic bronchodilators vs nebulized adrenergic bronchodilator alone in acute asthma. Canadian Combivent Study Group. Chest 1997;111:311-315.

85. McFadden ER Jr, el Sanadi N, Strauss L, et al. The influence of parasympatholytics on the resolution of acute attacks of asthma. Am J Med 1997;102:7-13.

86. Lanes SF, Garrett JE, Wentworth CE, et al. The effect of adding ipratropium bromide to salbutamol in the treatment of acute asthma: a pooled analysis of three trials. Chest 1998;114:365-372.

87. Kerstjens HA, Brand PI, Hughes MD, et al. A comparison of bronchodilator therapy with or without inhaled corticosteroid therapy for obstructive airways disease. N Engl J Med 1992;327:1413-1419.

88. Gross NJ. Ipratropium bromide. N Engl J Med 1988;319:486-494.

89. Levin DC, Little KS, Laughlin KR, et al. Addition of anticholinergic solution prolongs bronchodilator effect of beta-2 agonists in patients with chronic obstructive pulmonary disease. Am J Med 1996;100:40S-48S.

90. Ducharme FM, Davis GM. Randomized controlled trial of ipratropium bromide and frequent low doses of salbutamol in the management of mild and moderate acute pediatric asthma. J Pediatr 1998;133:479-485.

91. Qureshi F, Pestian J, Davis P, et al. Effect of nebulized ipratropium on the hospitalization rates of children with asthma. N Engl J Med 1998;339:1030-1035.

92. Scarfone RJ, Fuchs SM, Nager AL, et al. Controlled trial of oral prednisone in the emergency department treatment of children with acute asthma. Pediatrics 1993;70:513-518.

93. Connett GJ, Warde C, Wooler E, et al. Prednisolone and salbutamol in the hospital treatment of acute asthma. Arch Dis Child 1993;70:170-173.

94. Fanta CH, Rossig TH, McFadden ER. Glucocorticoids in acute asthma. A critical controlled trial. Am J Med 1983;74:845-851.

95. Beam WR, Weiner DE, Martin RJ. Timing of prednisone and alterations of airways inflammation in nocturnal asthma. Am Rev Respir Dis 1992;146:1524-1530.

96. Dolovich M. Clinical aspects of aerosol physics. Respir Care 1991;36:931.

97. Raimondi AC, Schottlender J, Lombardi D, et al. Treatment of acute asthma with inhaled albuterol delivered via jet nebulizer, metered dose inhaler with spacer, or dry powder. Chest 1997;112:24-28.

98. Henderson SO, Acharya P, Kilaghbian T, et al. Use of a heliox-driven therapy in the treatment of acute asthma. Ann Emerg Med 1999;33:141-146.

99. Clay MM, Pavia D, Newman SP, et al. Factors influencing the size distribution of aerosols from jet nebulizers. Thorax 1983;38:755.

100. Handfiel JW, Windebank WJ, Bateman RM. Is driving gas flow rate clinically important for nebulizer therapy? Br J Dis Chest 1986;80:50.

101. Hess DR, Acosta FL, Ritz RH, et al. The effect of heliox on nebulizer function using a beta-agonist bronchodilator. Chest 1999;115:184-189.

102. Phipps PR, Gonda I. Droplets produced by medical nebulizers: some factors affecting their size and solute concentration. Chest 1990;97:1327.

103. Hess DR, Horney D, Snyder T. Medication-delivery performance of eight small-volume, hand-held nebulizers: effects of diluent volume, gas flowrate, and nebulizer model. Respir Care 1989;34:717.

104. Hoffman L, Smithline H. Comparison of Circulaire to conventional small volume nebulizer for the treatment of bronchospasm in the emergency department. Respir Care 1997;42:1170-1174.

105. Mason JW, Miller WE, Small S. Comparison of aerosol delivery via Circulaire system vs conventional small volume nebulizer. Respir Care 1993;39:1157-1161.

106. Loffert DT, Ikle D, Nelson HS. A comparison of commercial jet nebulizers. Chest 1994;106:1788.

107. Alvine GF, Rodgers P, Fitzsimmons KM, et al. Disposable jet nebulizers. How reliable are they? Chest 1992;101:306.

108. Pooler S, Hess D, Williams P, et al. Drug delivery by medication nebulizers: aerosol inhaled. Resp Care 1994;39:1086.

109. O'Callaghan CO, Barry PW. The science of nebulised drug delivery. Thorax 1997;52:S31-S44.

110. Kacmarek RM, Hess DR. The interface between patient and aerosol generator. Respir Care 1991;36:952-976.

111. Hess DR. Aerosol therapy. Respir Care Clin N Am 1995;1:239.

112. Portnoy J, Aggarwal J. Continuous terbutaline nebulization for the treatment of severe exacerbations of asthma in children. Ann Allergy 1988;60:368-371.

113. Moler FW, Hurwitz ME, Custer JR. Improvement in clinical asthma score and PaCO₂ in children with severe asthma treated with continuously nebulized terbutaline. J Allergy Clin Immunol 1988;81:1101-1109.

114. Lin RY, Smith AJ, Hergenroeder P. High serum albuterol levels and tachycardia in adult asthmatics treated with high-dose conitinuously aerosolized albuterol. Chest 1993;103:221-225.

115. Katz RW, Kelly HW, Crowley MR, et al. Safety of continuous nebulized albuterol for bronchospasm in infants and children. Pediatrics 1993;92:666-669.

116. Papo MC, Frank J, Thompson AE. A prospective, randomized study of continuous versus intermittent nebulized albuterol for severe status asthmaticus in children. Crit Care Med 1993;21:1479-1486.

117. Rudnitsky GS, Eberlein RS, Schoffstall JM, et al. Comparison of intermittent and continuously nebulized albuterol for treatment of asthma in an urban emergency department. Ann Emerg Med 1993;22:1842-1846.

118. Lin RY, Sauter D, Newman T, et al. Continuous versus intermittent albuterol nebulization in the treatment of acute asthma. Ann Emerg Med 1993;22:1847-1853.

119. Reisner C, Kotch A, Dworkin G. Continuous versus frequent intermittent nebulization of albuterol in acute asthma: a randomized, prospective study. Ann Allergy Asthma Immunol 1995;75:41-47.

120. Shretha M, Bidadi K, Gourlay S, et al. Continuous vs intermittent albuterol, at high and low doses, in the treatment of severe acute asthma in adults. Chest 1996;110:42-47.

121. Raabe OG, Wong TM, Wong GB, et al. Continuous nebulization therapy for asthma with aerosols of beta₂ agonists. Ann Allergy Asthma Immunol 1998;80:499-508.

122. McPeck M, Tandon R, Hughes K et al. Aerosol delivery during continuous nebulization. Chest 1997;111:1200-1205.

123. Newman SP. Aerosol generators and delivery systems. Respir Care 1991;36:939-951.

124. Newman SP, Pavia D Moren F, et al. Deposition of pressurized aerosols in the human respiratory tract. Thorax 1981;36:52-55.

125. Vidgren MT, Karkkainen A, Karjalainen P, et al. A novel labelling method for measuring the deposition of drug particles in the respiratory tract. Int J Pharm 1987;37:239-244.

126. Lee H, Evans HE. Evaluation of inhalation aids of metered dose inhalers in asthmatic children. Chest 1987;91:366-369.

127. Barry PW, O'Callaghan C. Inhalational drug delivery from seven different spacer devices. Thorax 1996;51:835-840.

128. Gluck EH, Onorato DJ, Castriotta R. Helium-oxygen mixtures in intubated patients with status asthmaticus and respiratory acidosis. Chest 1990;98:693-698.

129. Tobias JD. Heliox in children with airway obstruction. Pediatr Emerg Care 1997;13:29-32.

130. Kudukis TM, Manthous CA, Schmidt GA, et al. Inhaled helium-oxygen revisited: effect of inhaled helium-oxygen during the treatment of status asthmaticus in children. J Pediatr 1997;130:217-224.

131. Kass JE, Castriotta RJ. Heliox therapy in acute severe asthma. Chest 1995;107:757-760.

132. Carter ER, Webb CR, Moffitt DR. Evaluation of heliox in children hospitalized with acute severe asthma. A randomized crossover trial. Chest 1996;109:1256-1261.

133. Verbeek PR, Chopra A. Heliox does not improve FEV₁ in acute asthma patients. J Emerg Med 1998;16:545-548.

134. Kass JE, Castratta RJ. Heliox therapy in acute severe asthma. Chest 1995;107:757.

135. Kass JE, Terregino CA. The effect of heliox in acute severe asthma: a randomized controlled trial. Chest 1999;116:296-300.

136. Ciarallo L, Sauer AH, Shannon MW. Intravenous magnesium therapy for moderate to severe pediatric asthma: results of a randomized placebo-controlled trial. J Pediatr 1996;129:809-814.

137. Bloch H, Silverman R, Mancherje N, et al. Intravenous magnesium sulfate as an adjunct in the treatment of acute asthma. Chest 1995;107:1576-1581.

138. Noppen M, Vanmaele L, Impens N, et al. Bronchodilating effect of intravenous magnesium sulfate in acute severe bronchial asthma. Chest 1990;97:373-376.

139. Mangat HS, D'Souza GA, Jacob MS. Nebulized magnesium sulphate versus nebulized salbutamol in acute bronchial asthma: a clinical trial. Eur Respir J 1998;12:341-344.

140. Hill J, Britton J. Dose-response relationship and time-course of the effect of inhaled magnesium sulphate on airflow in normal and asthmatic subjects. Br J Clin Pharmacol 1995;40:539-544.

141. Bernstein WK, Khastgir T, Khastgir A, et al. Lack of effectiveness of magnesium in chronic stable asthma. A prospective, randomized, double-blind, placebo-controlled, crossover trial in normal subjects and in patients with chronic stable asthma. Arch Intern Med 1995;155:271-276.

142. Tiffany BR, Berk WA, Todd IK, et al. Magnesium bolus or infusion fails to improve expiratory flow in acute asthma exacerbations. Chest 1993;104:831-834.

143. Green SM, Rothrock SG. Intravenous magnesium sulfate for acute asthma. Failure to decrease emergency treatment duration or need for hospitalization. Am Emerg Med 1992; 21:260.

144. Nopper M, Vanmaele L, Impens N et al. Bronchodilating effect of intravenous magnesium sulfate in acute severe bronchial asthma. Chest 1990;97:373.

145. Skobeloff EM, Spivey WH, McNamara RM, et al. Intravenous magnesium sulfate for the treatment of acute asthma in the emergency department. JAMA 1989;262:1210-1213.

146. Meduir GU, et al. Noninvasive positive pressure ventilation in status asthmaticus. Chest 1996;110:767-774.

147. Teague GW, Fortenberry JD. Noninvasive ventilator support in pediatric respiratory failure. Respir Care 1995;40:86-95.

148. Pollack C, Fleisch K, Dowsey K. Treatment of acute bronchospasm with beta-adrenergic agonist aerosols delivered by a nasal bilevel positive airway pressure circuit. Ann Emerg Med 1995;26:552-557.

149. Marquette CH, Saulnier F, Leroy O, et al. Long-term prognosis of new fatal asthma. A 6 year follow-up of 145 asthmatic patients who underwent mechanical ventilation. Am Rev Respir Dis 1992;146:76-81.

150. Mansel JK, Stogner SW, Patrini MF, et al. Mechanical ventilation in patients with acute severe asthma. Am J Med 1990;87:42-48.

151. Rodriguez-Roison R, Ballestar E, Roca J, et al. Mechanisms of hypoxemia in patients with status asthmaticus requiring mechanical ventilation. Am Rev Respir Dis 1989;139:732-739.

152. Leatherman J. Life-threatening asthma. Clin Chest Med 1994;15:453-479.

153. Mansel JK, Stogner SW, Patrini MF, et al. Mechanical ventilation in patients with acute severe asthma. Am J Med 1990;87:42-48.

154. Hickling KC, Henderson SJ, Jackson R. Low mortality associated with low volume pressure limited ventilation and permissive hypercapnia in severe adult respiratory distress syndrome. Intensive Care Med 1990;16:372-377.

155. ACCP Mechanical Ventilation Consensus Group: Mechanical ventilation. Chest 1993;104:1833-1859.

156. Feihl F, Perret C. Permissive hypercapnia: How permissive should we be? Am J Respir Crit Care Med 1994;150: 1722-1737.

157. Darioli R, Perret C. Mechanical controlled hypoventilation in status asthmaticus. Am Rev Respir Dis 1984;129: 385-387.

158. Ranieri VM, Grasso S, Fiore T, et al. Auto-positive end-expiratory pressure and dynamic hyperinflation. Clin Chest Med 1996;17:379-394.

159. Marini JJ. Should PEEP be used in airflow obstruction? Am Rev Respir Dis 1989; 140:1-3.

160. Tuxen DV. Detrimental effects of PEEP during controlled mechanical ventilation of patients with severe airflow obstruction. Am Rev Respir Dis 1989;140:5-9.

161. Tuxen DV, Williams TJ, Scheinkestel CD, et al. Use of a measurement of pulmonary hyperinflation to control the level of mechanical ventilation in patient with acute severe asthma. Am Rev Resp Dis 1992;146:1136-1142.

162. Tuxen DV, Lane S. The effect of ventilatory pattern on hyperinflation, airway pressures and circulation in mechanical ventilation of patients with severe airflow obstruction. Am Rev Respir Dis 1987;136:872-879.

163. Leatherman JW, Ravenscraft SA. Low measured auto-positive end-expiratory pressure during mechanical ventilation of patients with severe asthma: hidden auto-positive end-expiratory pressure. Crit Care Med 1996;24:541-546.

164. Dhand R, Tobin MJ. Inhaled bronchodilator therapy in mechanically ventilated patients. Am J Respir Crit Care Med 1997;156:3-10.

165. Tassaux D, Jolliet P, Thouret JM, et al. Calibration of seven ICU ventilators for mechanical ventilation with helium-oxygen mixtures. Am J Respir Crit Care Med 1999;160:22-32.

166. Douglass JA, Tuxen DV, Horne M, et al. Myopathy in severe asthma. Am Rev Respir Dis 1992;146:517-519.

167. Picado C, Montserrat J, Agusti-Vidal A. Muscle atrophy in severe exacerbation of asthma requiring mechanical ventilation. Respiration 1988;53:201-203.

168. Levy BD, Kitch B, Fanta CH. Medical and ventilatory management of status asthmaticus. Intensive Care Med 1998;24: 105-117.

169. Jain S, Hanania NA, Guntupalli KK. Ventilation of patients with asthma and obstructive lung disease. Crit Care Clin 1998;14:685-705.

170. Trautner C, Richter B, Berger M. Cost-effectiveness of structured treatment and teaching programme on asthma. Eur Respir J 1993;6:1485-1491.

171. Clark NM, Feldman CH, Evans D, et al. The impact of health education on frequency and cost of health care use by low income children with asthma. J Allergy Clin Immunol 1986; 78:108-115.

172. Wade S, Weil C, Holden G, et al. Psychosocial characteristics of inner-city children with asthma: a description of the NCICAS psychosocial protocol. National Cooperative Inner-City Asthma Study. Pediatr Pulmonol 1997;24:263-276.

173. Wade SL, Islam S, Holden G, et al. Division of responsibility for asthma management tasks between caregivers and children in the inner city. Dev Behav Pediatr 1999;20:93-98.

CHAPTER 47

Chronic Obstructive Pulmonary Disease

John E. Heffner
Michael Duane Frye

CHAPTER OUTLINE

OBJECTIVES

1. Define chronic obstructive pulmonary disease (COPD), asthma, bronchitis, and asthmatic bronchitis.
2. Describe the epidemiology, pathogenesis, and pathophysiology of COPD.
3. Compare therapeutic strategies for stable patients and patients experiencing an acute exacerbation in the ambulatory or inpatient setting.
4. Discuss the surgical approaches to improve lung function in COPD.
5. Identify important aspects of end-of-life care for patients with COPD.

KEY TERMS

Acute Exacerbation	Chronic Obstructive Pulmonary Disease	Lung Volume Reduction Surgery (LVRS)
Air Trapping	(COPD)	Methylxanthines
α_1-Antitrypsin (AAT) Deficiency	Corticosteroids	Mucokinetic Agents
Antibiotics	Dynamic Airway Compression	Negative Pressure Ventilation (NPV)
Anticholinergic Agent	Dyspnea	Noninvasive Positive Pressure
Asthmatic Bronchitis	Emphysema	Ventilation (NPPV)
Bullae	Hyperinflation	Pulmonary Cachexia
Bullectomy	Long-Term Oxygen Therapy (LTOT)	Pulmonary Rehabilitation
Chronic Bronchitis	Lung Transplantation	Smoking Cessation

Chronic obstructive pulmonary disease (COPD) has emerged as a major health condition worldwide. In the United States, more than 14 million people are affected by COPD, which is now the fourth most common cause of death. The prevalence of chronic bronchitis is 3% to 17% in most developed countries and 13% to 27% in less developed regions of the world.[1] The prevalence of COPD is increasing worldwide. It is currently the twelfth leading condition contributing to the global burden of disease and is predicted to be ranked as the fifth within the next 20 years.[2] All stages of the disease impact patients' lives to varying degrees. Early symptomatic disease decreases exercise capacity, causes work absenteeism, and interferes with vigorous life-style pursuits. More advanced COPD increases the risk of pneumonia and lung cancer[3] and causes respiratory failure related to acute exacerbations of airway disease. Severely affected patients experience major limitations in activities of daily living and assume dependent roles in their family units. At a time when the number of deaths caused by heart disease and strokes has decreased substantially,[4] the mortality from COPD has increased by 33% during the last decade.[5] Because of the chronic nature of COPD and its typically relentless symptomatic progression, few conditions present such long-term and disabling burdens for personal health and well-being.

This chapter provides a general discussion of the diagnosis and care of patients with COPD with an emphasis on practical elements of management. It centers on the premise that respiratory therapists have the needed expertise to intercede at all stages of COPD to improve patients' functional status, quality of life, and the outcome of their disease.

Definitions and Staging of Disease

The term **chronic obstructive pulmonary disease (COPD)** refers to a group of disorders characterized by progressive limitations in predominantly expiratory airflow that are at best only partially reversible by bronchodilator or antiinflammatory therapy. Emphysema, chronic bronchitis, and asthmatic bronchitis are the three disorders categorized as COPD. Isolated asthma was previously considered to be a form of COPD but is no longer classified as such because of its unique pathophysiology, etiology, and clinical course. Several specific causes of chronic airflow limitation, such as cystic fibrosis, bronchiolitis obliterans, and bronchiectasis, are not considered to be COPD.[6]

Chronic bronchitis is defined by the presence of cough and sputum production for 3 or more months in 2 successive years in patients who do not have other causes of cough. This definition may be less than ideal considering that mucus hypersecretion occurs in the proximal airways but the site of increased airway resistance in COPD is in the peripheral, small airways, where inflammation results in fibrosis and distortion of terminal airways.[6] Patients with chronic bronchitis and limitation of expiratory airflow are considered to have COPD; patients with cough without measurable airflow obstruction have a relatively good prognosis and are classified as simple chronic bronchitis without COPD. The airflow limitation in chronic bronchitis does not demonstrate significant reversibility with bronchodilator therapy. The chest radiograph and measured lung diffusion are normal because the disease does not affect the lung parenchyma and the pathologic changes are confined to the airways. These changes include hyperplasia of surface mucous glands, ciliary dyskinesia and loss of cilia, enlargement of tracheobronchial submucosal glands, excess mucus, and the presence of inflammatory cells (Figure 47-1).

Emphysema occurs in patients who experience damage to the lung parenchyma that results in histopathologic evidence of alveolar wall destruction without fibrosis and who have physiologic evidence of decreased lung elastic recoil.[7] Air spaces are permanently enlarged distal to the terminal bronchioles (see Figure 47-1). Air space enlargements greater than 1 cm are termed **bullae** (Figure 47-2). Bullae can progressively enlarge and compress adjacent lung tissue, thereby impairing respiratory function. Patients with pure emphysema uncomplicated by bronchitis have irreversible airflow limitation. Decreased lung elasticity results in increased expiratory airway resistance because of **dynamic airway compression**, which results in air trapping and hyperinflation (Figure 47-3). **Hyperinflation** with increased lung volumes may be apparent on chest radiographs (Figure 47-4) and chest computed tomography (CT) scans. Structural abnormalities in the alveolar–capillary units impair gas exchange causing hypoxemia, hypercapnia, and decreased lung diffusion as measured by the diffusing capacity for carbon monoxide (DLCO).

Asthmatic bronchitis produces cough, dyspnea, and wheezing with expiratory airflow limitation that improves to a degree when treated with bronchodilators and corticosteroids. Complete reversibility is not observed and would suggest the alternative diagnosis of asthma. Patients with asthmatic bronchitis develop progressive symptoms, and airflow limitation becomes less reversible over time.

Most patients with COPD have a mixture of emphysema, chronic bronchitis, and asthmatic bronchitis to varying degrees. Because the clinical manifestations and therapy of these three conditions merge as the severity of COPD progresses, the general term *COPD* is most often used for patients with advanced airflow limitation. Measurement of the forced expiratory volume at 1 second (FEV_1) is the best measure of the severity of COPD.[7] Mild (stage I disease) COPD, is defined as an FEV_1 greater than or equal to 50% of predicted; moderate (stage II) COPD has an FEV_1 35% to 49% of predicted; and severe (stage III) COPD has an FEV_1 less than 35% of predicted.[8]

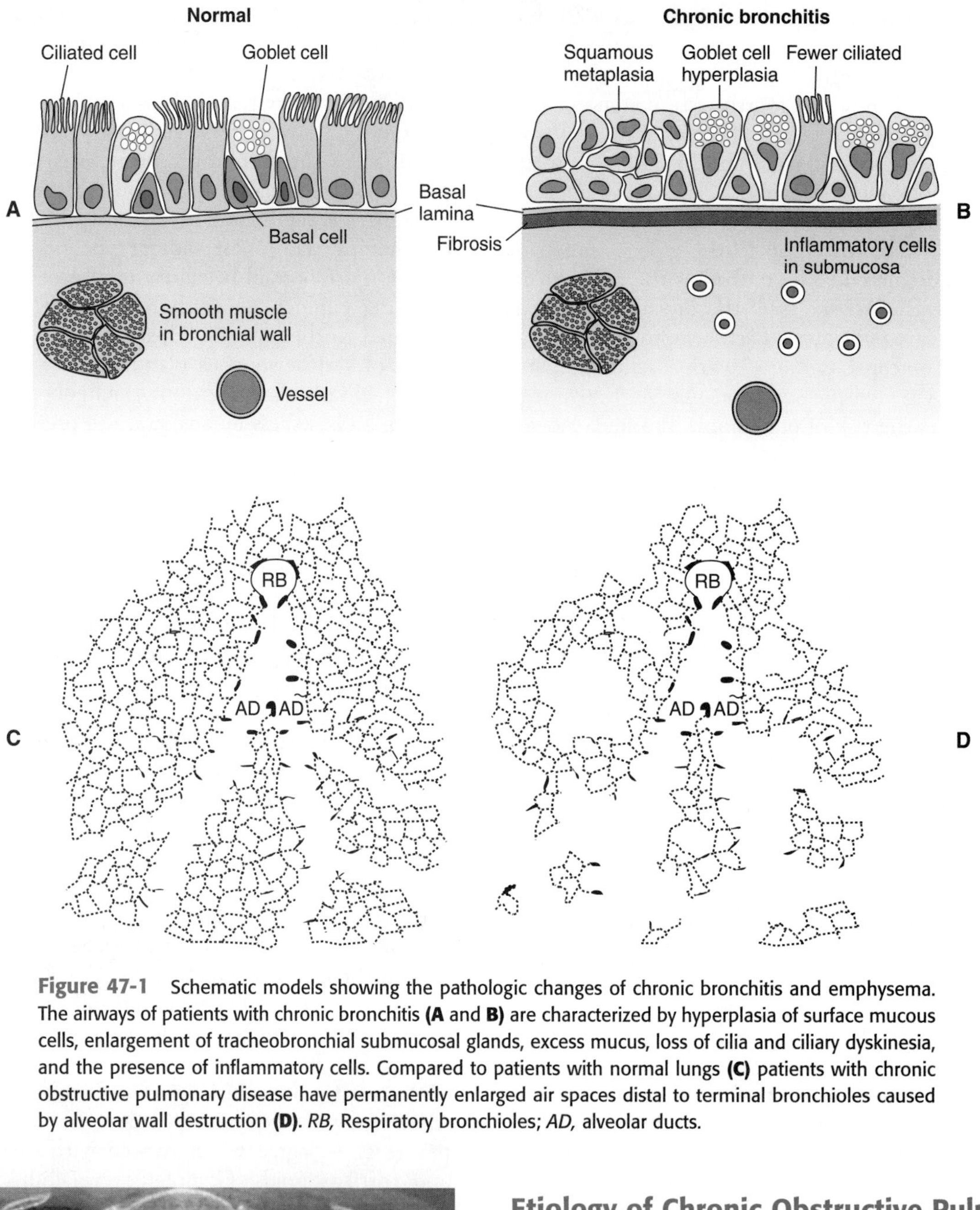

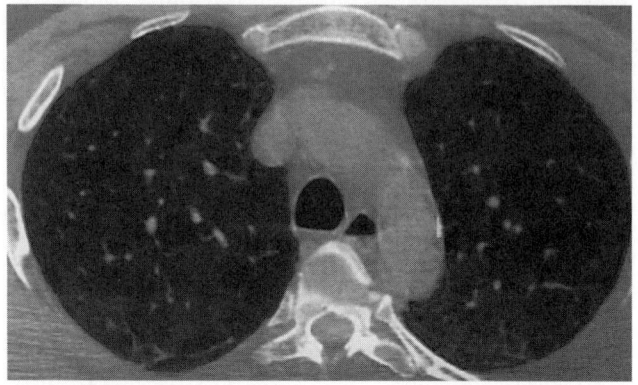

Normal

Ciliated cell   Goblet cell

A

Basal cell

Smooth muscle
in bronchial wall

Vessel

Chronic bronchitis

Squamous
metaplasia   Goblet cell
hyperplasia   Fewer ciliated

Basal
lamina

Fibrosis

B

Inflammatory cells
in submucosa

C   RB

AD AD

D   RB

AD AD

Figure 47-1   Schematic models showing the pathologic changes of chronic bronchitis and emphysema. The airways of patients with chronic bronchitis **(A** and **B)** are characterized by hyperplasia of surface mucous cells, enlargement of tracheobronchial submucosal glands, excess mucus, loss of cilia and ciliary dyskinesia, and the presence of inflammatory cells. Compared to patients with normal lungs **(C)** patients with chronic obstructive pulmonary disease have permanently enlarged air spaces distal to terminal bronchioles caused by alveolar wall destruction **(D)**. *RB,* Respiratory bronchioles; *AD,* alveolar ducts.

Figure 47-2   Computed tomography (CT) scan of a patient with severe emphysema. Note the multiple bullae throughout the lung parenchyma, which appears hyperlucent, indicating generalized loss of lung tissue and hyperinflation.

Etiology of Chronic Obstructive Pulmonary Disease

Overwhelming epidemiologic and experimental evidence demonstrates that smoking is the major cause of COPD.[9-15] It is notable that only 15% of smokers develop measurable airflow limitation, indicating that host factors contribute to the pathophysiology of the disease. With α_1-**antitrypsin (AAT) deficiency,** it is not possible to identify smokers who are at risk of developing COPD, although one recent study indicates that middle-aged male smokers who have both a reduced FEV_1 as a proportion of forced vital capacity (FVC) and an abnormal nitrogen washout are at greatest risk of developing COPD over a 13-year period.[16]

The best characterized risk factor for COPD is AAT deficiency, which is a hereditary defect occurring almost en-

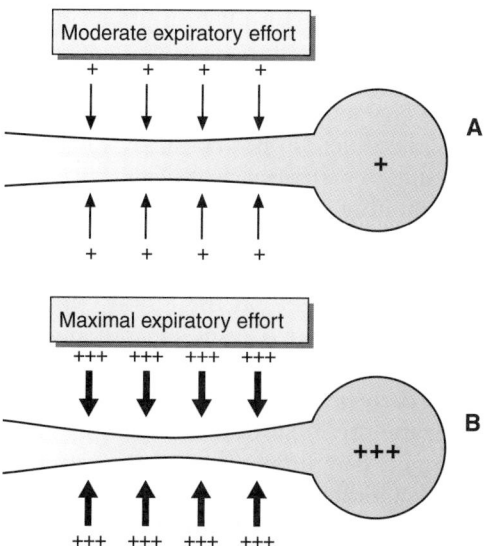

Figure 47-3 Schematic model demonstrating the morphologic changes associated with dynamic airway compression in patients with emphysema. The loss of parenchymal tethering external to airways causes airway collapse during forced expiration and increased expiratory airway resistance. Maximal expiratory effort **(A)** creates greater compressing pressure around airways and produces more dynamic compression compared to moderate expiratory effort **(B)**.

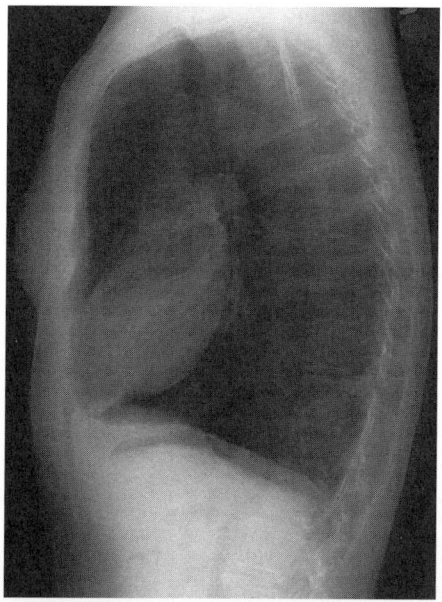

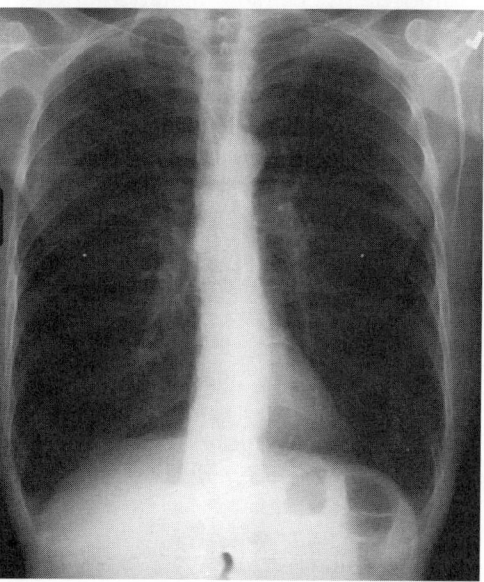

Figure 47-4 Chest radiograph of a patient with emphysema showing hyperinflation as evidenced by the flat diaphragms and hyperlucent lung fields.

tirely in whites that results in abnormally functioning or insufficient production of AAT.[17] These patients do not demonstrate a normal antiprotease response to the proinflammatory effects of tobacco smoke. The resulting activation of proteases and toxic oxygen metabolites with smoking results in accelerated lung destruction and emphysema in early life. Even nonsmokers with AAT deficiency may develop COPD, but symptoms usually occur late in life. The discovery of the importance of AAT deficiency of antiprotease defenses in protecting the lung from the effects of collagenase and elastase release by inflammatory cells activated by smoking has led to the protease-antiprotease theory of the pathophysiology of COPD in general.

Other host factors are suspected to contribute to COPD caused by smoking as evidenced by family clusterings of obstructive lung disease independent of the presence of AAT deficiency.[18] This observation suggests that genetic risk factor(s) for COPD are expressed in response to cigarette smoking. In addition, not all patients with AAT deficiency who smoke develop COPD,[18] and women appear to be at higher risk than men for smoking-related COPD.[19] In addition to undefined genetic factors, underlying bronchial hyperreactivity may amplify the damaging effects of cigarette smoking and promote the development of COPD.[20]

Various occupational dusts, including coal and grain dusts, air pollution, indoor air pollution caused by cooking fuels or cigarette smoke, and childhood respiratory infections are additional risk factors for the development of COPD.[21-25] Low socioeconomic class, excessive alcohol consumption, and diet deficient in antioxidants have been considered potential risk factors for the disease.[15]

Pathophysiology of Chronic Obstructive Pulmonary Disease

The major structural abnormalities in COPD occur in the central airways, the small peripheral bronchi and bronchioles, and the lung parenchyma. The central airways are the site of most of the excess mucus production in chronic bronchitis. Histologic studies of large airways detect enlargement of tracheobronchial submucosal glands and hyperplasia of tracheobronchial surface mucous cells.[26] Inflammation is present in the form of mononuclear cells in the airway mucosa and neutrophils in addition to eosinophils in airway secretions.[27] Abnormalities in the peripheral bronchi and bronchioles produce the majority of the increased airflow resistance that is observed in COPD.[28]

Histologic features are characterized by hyperplasia and alterations in morphology of mucous cells, increased airway mucus, increased peribronchiolar muscle mass, inflammation, fibrosis, obliteration and narrowing of airways, and loss of alveolar attachments to bronchioles.[29-31] In the lung parenchyma, permanent destructive enlargement of air spaces distal to the terminal bronchioles occurs without obvious fibrosis.[7] The loss of alveolar attachments to airways results in stenosis and tortuosity of bronchioles. Additional structural abnormalities can be detected in the pulmonary vasculature (intimal thickening, muscularization of arterioles, and diminution of the vascular bed), heart (right ventricular enlargement), and respiratory muscles (atrophy of the diaphragm) of patients with severe COPD.[32-34]

The pathogenesis of airflow limitation in COPD is not entirely understood. Multiple factors, such as the loss of airway tethering caused by decreased elastic recoil of the lung parenchyma, airway secretions, changes in the properties of lining fluid, smooth muscle contraction, mucous gland hypertrophy, and airway inflammation interact in complex ways to obliterate peripheral airways or narrow the caliber of conducting airways and limit airflow.[35-37] Any one of these factors, however, does not appear to be predominant in determining the severity of airflow limitation. In severe COPD, however, most experts consider that emphysematous changes represent the major factors in the production of airflow limitation. Changes in the peripheral airways contribute to airflow limitation more predominantly in mild to moderate COPD.[38] Radiographic or histologic measures of the severity of emphysema or bronchitis do not correlate with the degree of measured airflow

limitation. Functional measures of airflow limitation, such as FEV_1 and blood gas abnormalities, provide the best correlates with prognosis and survival and are used in clinical practice to characterize the severity of COPD.[7] Spirometric values, however, do not correlate with health-related quality of life in patients with COPD.[39]

The expiratory airflow limitation that occurs in COPD is most prominent during maximal, forced expiratory efforts. During inspiration, airflow is linearly proportional to the applied pressure on the airway, which correlates with inspiratory effort. During expiration, however, airflow is linearly related to pressure (expiratory effort) only during the early phases of expiration, after which time increases in the driving pressure (expiratory effort) do not result in increased airflow (Figures 47-3 and 47-5). This limitation of airflow results from the airway compression that occurs from increased intrathoracic pressure during forced expiration. This dynamic airway compression results in greater increases in airway resistance with greater expiratory effort.

Expiratory flow-volume curves present a visual image of these relationships (Figure 47-6). Individuals with normal lung function increase their expiratory airflow during forced expiratory maneuvers until dynamic airway compression occurs, at which point airflow does not increase with increased effort. During tidal breathing, expiratory airflow is much lower than during a maximal, forced expiration indicating that patients in good health have considerable ventilatory reserve available for increasing $\dot{V}_E$.

In patients with COPD, decreased diameter of conducting airways lowers the maximal expiratory airflow and airflow at all other lung volumes compared to normal individuals. Because of the loss of lung elasticity and the collapsibility of airways in patients with emphysema, dynamic airway compression occurs at lower intrathoracic pressures. In patients with progressive COPD, maximal airflow may be reached during exercise and eventually at resting tidal breathing (see Figure 47-6). In severe COPD when maximal airflow is reached during tidal breathing, patients faced with increased ventilatory demands from

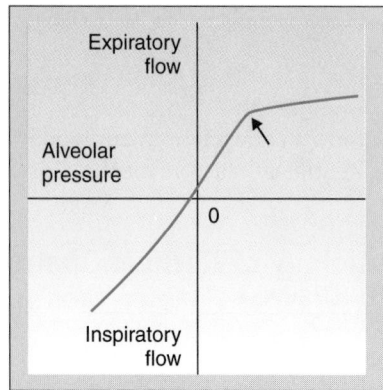

Figure 47-5 Relationship of flow to pressure during inspiration and expiration at a given lung volume. This relationship is linear during inspiration, but dynamic airway compression (*arrow*) causes expiratory flow to reach an early maximal value that does not increase with further increases in alveolar pressure.

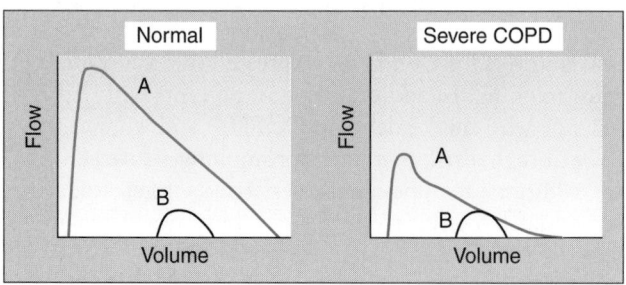

Figure 47-6 Expiratory flow-volume curves of a patient with severe chronic obstructive pulmonary disease (COPD) (*right*) compared to an individual with normal lungs (*left*). The patient with COPD reaches maximal expiratory airflow during tidal breathing. *A*, Forced vital capacity; *B*, tidal breathing.

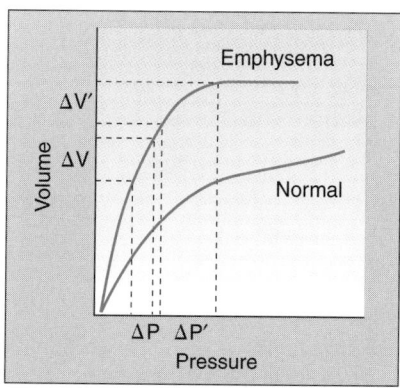

Figure 47-7 Volume-pressure relationships of individuals with normal lungs and patients with emphysema. Patients with emphysema experience a small increase in pressure (ΔP) with an increase in volume (ΔV) while breathing at low lung volumes. In contrast, patients with emphysema have large increases in pressure (ΔP′) for a similar change in volume (ΔV′) when breathing at high lung volumes, at which point their lungs become hyperinflated and "stiff." Patients with emphysema have heterogeneous distribution of emphysema so that normal regions of lung follow the "normal" volume-pressure curve and emphysematous regions follow the "emphysema" curve.

exercise or increased airway resistance cannot increase airflow to recruit larger tidal volumes so they raise minute ventilation by generating higher respiratory rates. An increased respiratory rate decreases expiratory time, which promotes air trapping and further dynamic airway compression.[40] Positive end-expiratory recoil pressure of the total respiratory system develops because of this hyperinflation and is termed *intrinsic positive end-expiratory pressure (PEEPi)*.[41,42] PEEPi places an inspiratory threshold load that increases the work of breathing because patients must contract inspiratory muscles to create negative alveolar pressure to initiate inspiration. These changes result in patients breathing with decreased tidal volumes and increased respiratory rates at higher lung volumes. In addition to expiratory limitation, inspiratory limitation also occurs in COPD, which further limits ventilatory capacity leading to hyperinflation.

The loss of lung elastic recoil in emphysema is an important factor in causing increased airway resistance and hyperinflation at resting lung volumes.[43] Abnormalities in elastic recoil are distributed throughout the lungs in a heterogeneous pattern. An admixture of regions with normal elastic recoil and regions of low elasticity produces varying volume and pressure relationships. Regions of relatively normal elastic recoil respond to airway pressure changes with volume changes that follow a normal volume-pressure relationship (Figure 47-7). In contrast, the volume-pressure curve for emphysematous regions of the lung have curves shifted upward and to the left. This heterogeneous distribution of decreased elastic recoil suggests that lung function may improve if more severely affected lung regions are resected, thereby improving the overall elastic recoil of the lung (see following discussion).

The severity of airflow limitation also varies between regions of the lung. Combined with the heterogeneous distribution of elastic recoil abnormalities, varying degrees of mismatching of ventilation and perfusion occur throughout the lung in patients with emphysema.[44] Although emphysematous regions of the lung are underventilated, perfusion is more severely decreased so that ventilation-perfusion ratios ($\dot{V}/\dot{Q}$) increase. Consequently, emphysematous lung regions have increased dead space and contribute to hypoxemia and hypercapnia. In other regions of the lung, increased resistance or partial obstruction of airways that ventilate relatively normal alveolar-capillary units generates decreased $\dot{V}/\dot{Q}$ ratios that cause venous admixture and hypoxemia. The combination of lung regions with high and low $\dot{V}/\dot{Q}$ alter gas exchange and place demands on the ventilatory capacity of patients, thereby increasing respiratory work.[45,46] Worsening $\dot{V}/\dot{Q}$ abnormalities eventually result in hypoxemia and, if ventilation is markedly impaired, hypercapnia, both of which are associated with a poor prognosis in patients with COPD.[47] Shunts are notably absent in stable patients with COPD, indicating the efficiency of collateral ventilation and hypoxic pulmonary vasoconstriction and the absence of complete airway obstruction.[6]

Patients with COPD also experience abnormalities in the coordination of respiratory muscle function. During exercise and voluntary hyperventilation, patients demonstrate early fatigue of the exercising muscle groups combined with dyssynchrony of respiratory muscles with poor coordination of rib cage and diaphragm-abdominal muscles.[48,49]

As the severity of COPD progresses, patients become aware of the effort to breathe. When this effort is perceived as work, patients experience *dyspnea*. **Dyspnea** related to COPD derives from alterations in ventilatory mechanics. Patients with airflow limitation initially respond to abnormalities in gas exchange by increasing their respiratory drive and $\dot{V}_E$ by recruiting a larger V_T to normalize P_{CO_2} and P_{O_2}.[50-52] With more severe disease, increasing V_T causes too much work of breathing so $\dot{V}_E$ is maintained through an increase in respiratory rate in a linear manner with increasing airway resistance.[53]

To increase respiratory rate, patients shorten their inspiratory time (T_i) resulting in a decreased fractional duration of inspiration (T_i/T_{tot}) and an increased mean inspiratory flow rate (V_T/T_i). The heightened central respiratory drive underlying these accommodations can be noninvasively quantified by measurement of mouth occlusion pressure, which is measured 0.1 seconds after the initiation of inspiratory effort ($P_{0.1}$).[54] $P_{0.1}$ increases in COPD as the degree of airflow limitation progresses.

An increased respiratory rate eventually decreases expiratory time to such a degree that air space emptying cannot occur and further hyperinflation develops. Worsening hyperinflation shifts the pressure-volume curve of emphysematous lung units further upward and to the left, adding a restrictive pulmonary defect to the underlying airflow limitation. This produces the rapid and shallow respiratory pattern commonly observed in patients with severe COPD.[55]

Rapid and shallow breathing places greater demands on respiratory muscles both in terms of the amount of pressure they need to generate for breathing (P_{breath}) and the proportion of the respiratory cycle during which muscle contraction is required to occur (T_i/T_{tot}). Progressive dyspnea correlates both with increasing P_{breath} and T_i/T_{tot}.[56,57] As P_{breath} approaches the maximal pressure that respiratory muscles can generate (PI_{max}), patients begin to function near their limits of ventilatory reserve and fatigue threshold. Further demands on respiratory muscles, such as an acute exacerbation with increased airway resistance, can overburden compensatory mechanisms and cause acute respiratory failure.

Clinical Course and Prognosis

Patients with COPD follow a variable clinical course. Those with features of chronic bronchitis or asthmatic bronchitis and a relatively low smoking intensity, a positive bronchodilator response, evidence of atopy, normal lung volumes, and no gas exchange abnormalities have a better prognosis than patients who are heavy smokers with lung diffusion abnormalities and hyperinflation. The latter patients have emphysema predominantly. Most studies of COPD indicate that patients who continue to smoke experience a decline in FEV_1 of 48 to 1 mL/year.[37,58]

The clinical course of COPD is improved by **smoking cessation.** The rate of decline in FEV_1 in ex-smokers who quit smoking at age 45 decreases and begins to parallel never-smokers.[59,60] Patients over the age of 60 years also slow their decline in lung function after smoking cessation.[14] No evidence indicates that acute exacerbations of COPD accelerate the decline in FEV_1,[61] although acute exacerbations become more frequent with progressive disease. Increasing severity of COPD also is associated with an increased risk of lung cancer.[62]

To date, no pharmacologic intervention has been validated in large scale studies to alter baseline lung function.[63-67] Some studies suggest that inhaled ipratropium[65] and inhaled corticosteroids[66] improve long-term lung function, but final conclusions of benefit await the results of ongoing, large scale studies.[67,68]

Outpatient Care

An integrated outpatient approach to the management of COPD provides opportunities to reduce symptoms and improve quality of life, reducing decline in lung function, preventing complications, preventing or minimizing adverse effects of therapy, and prolonging survival.[6] These approaches incorporate drug therapy, surgical interventions, rehabilitation services, education, prophylactic measures, and supplemental oxygen support (Figure 47-8).

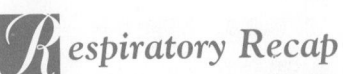

Respiratory Recap

Outpatient Care of the Patient with COPD

Smoking cessation is indicated for all smokers.
Drug therapy is prescribed for all symptomatic patients.
   First line: anticholinergics
   Second line: β-agonists
   Third line: methylxanthines
   Use of steroids: controversial
   Antibiotics: limited role
   Mucokinetics: possible use if the patient has difficulty with secretion clearance
Long-term oxygen therapy improves survival.
Vaccinations have an important preventive role.
Noninvasive ventilation is controversial.
Sleep-disordered breathing should be considered.
Pulmonary rehabilitation benefits patients with COPD.

Smoking Cessation

Smoking cessation is the most effective intervention to prevent complications from COPD.[59,69,70] Although 70% of smokers state a desire to stop smoking,[71] approximately 80% of individuals who quit smoking relapse within 6 months, and only 10% remain abstinent after 1 year.[72] Patients who are successful in the long-term, however, have one or more previous failures at smoking cessation, emphasizing the importance of ongoing encouragement to stop smoking. Recent advances in the understanding of the psychodynamics of smoking cessation assist clinicians in managing patients with COPD (Box 47-1).[73]

Pharmacologic approaches exist to assist motivated patients in their smoking-cessation efforts (Box 47-2). Nicotine replacement therapy reduces symptoms related to nicotine withdrawal and improves abstinence rates at 1 year.[74] Clonidine, naloxone, and buspirone demonstrate short-term benefits in the relief of withdrawal symptoms, but long-term benefits are not well documented.[75] Bupropion HCl, an antidepressant, has recently been shown to improve abstinence compared to placebo.[76]

Drug Therapy

Most symptomatic patients with COPD require pharmacologic therapy. Oral and inhaled medications are directed toward relieving bronchospasm, reducing airway inflammation, promoting expectoration of airway secretions, and preventing or reversing acute exacerbations of bronchitis and worsening of lung function. The modern approach to pharmacotherapy in COPD management initiates drug therapy in a stepwise fashion and accelerates the therapeutic regimen at the onset of an acute exacerbation.[7,77] The following discussion considers pharmacologic therapy in terms of the management of the stable patient and also patients experiencing an acute exacerbation.

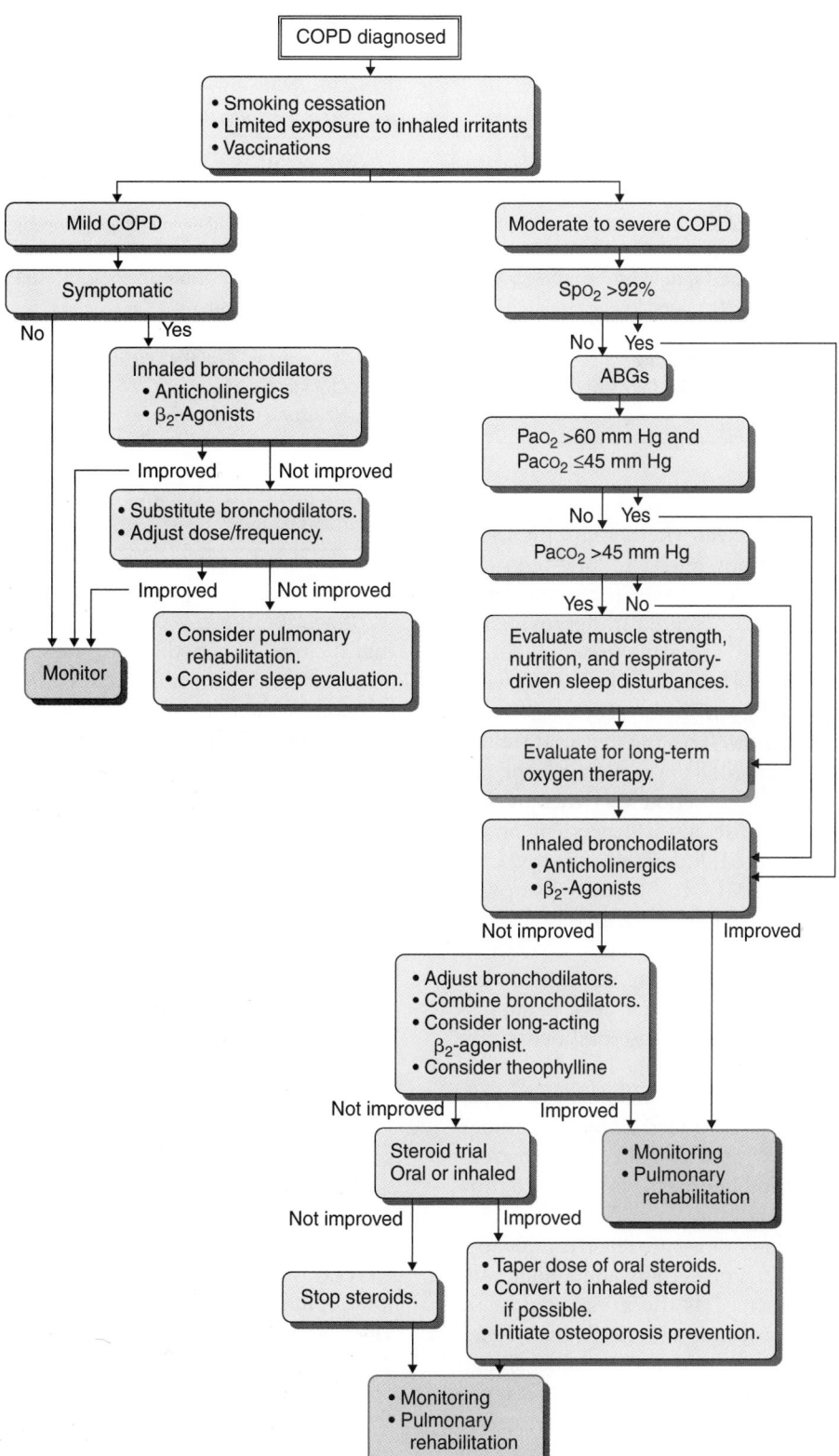

Figure 47-8   Algorithm for management of patients with chronic obstructive pulmonary disease (COPD) based on recently published clinical practice guidelines.

Box 47-1

*Stages in Transition from Smoking
to Nonsmoking Status*

> *Precontemplation.* Smokers who have not thought about quitting, do not appreciate the health risks of smoking, and have little information on smoking cessation.
> *Contemplation.* Smokers who are seriously thinking about stopping smoking within the next 6 months.
> *Preparation.* Smokers who are determined to quit within the next month.
> *Action.* Smokers who have stopped smoking.
> *Maintenance.* Smokers who have successfully stopped smoking for 6 or more months.

Box 47-2

*Pharmacologic Interventions to Assist
Smoking Cessation*

> **Nicotine Replacement Therapy**
> Gum: 2 and 4 mg per piece at 1- to 2-hour intervals; one 2-mg piece of gum replacing two cigarettes
> Patch: 5 to 21 mg per patch
> Nasal inhalers: two sprays each nostril once or twice an hour to 40 sprays a day
>
> **Reduction of Opiate Withdrawal Symptoms**
> Clonidine
> Naloxone
> Buspirone
>
> **Antidepressant Therapy**
> Buproprion

In stable patients, it is unclear whether chronic use of inhaled bronchodilator therapy improves long-term outcome in COPD.[65,69,78] It is clear, however, that some degree of improvement in airflow is observed in approximately 80% of patients treated with inhaled bronchodilators[79] and a larger proportion of patients have improved symptoms and exercise capacity even in the absence of measured improvements in airflow. The inhaled route either with a metered dose inhaler (MDI) or nebulizer is the preferred mode used to provide bronchodilator therapy. Unfortunately, effectiveness of therapy is dependent on the ability of patients to use the MDI devices correctly. Only 60% of patients have good MDI technique.[80] Even with good technique, only 15% of the drug is delivered into the lung; the remainder is deposited in the mouth. To limit absorption from oral mucosa, patients are advised to rinse their mouths after an inhalation. Spacer devices improve drug delivery into the lung and decrease oral deposition. Some patients with poor MDI technique benefit from dry powder preparations or automatic discharge devices. Nebulizers are recommended for the first several treatments with bronchodilator drugs during acute exacerbations. Nebulizers provide bronchodilatory effects similar to those of MDI devices with spacers.[81]

Among the bronchodilator drugs used by the inhalation route, ipratropium bromide, a quaternary ammonium **anticholinergic agent,** has emerged as the initial step in the management of COPD. Associated with negligible systemic adverse reactions,[82] it promotes bronchodilation by antagonizing vagal nerve stimulation. Patients with COPD appear to have increased cholinergic muscle tone and decreased responses to adrenergic drugs supplied to the airways compared with patients who have asthma.[83] Ipratropium has a longer duration of action and delayed onset compared to β_2-agonists, so it is used for maintenance rather than rescue therapy.[84] At conventional doses, ipratropium provides greater bronchodilatory potency compared to β_2-agonists, although bioactivity is similar at maximal doses.[85] Long-term use does not promote tolerance. Usual doses with an MDI are two to four puffs every 6 or 8 hours.

β_2-agonist therapy provides several benefits in COPD that include bronchodilation, improved mucociliary clearance, inhibition of cholinergic neurotransmission, and inhibition of inflammatory mediator release from mast cells and basophils.[86] Their primary role, however, is to promote smooth muscle relaxation by stimulating β_2-adrenergic receptors in the airways.

Inhalation of short- and long-acting β_2-agonists in MDI or dry powder formulations is the primary mode used to administer these agents in COPD. Short-acting agents have a more rapid onset of action compared to ipratropium and are consequently appropriate for rescue therapy and management of acute symptoms. Long-acting β_2-agonists provide bronchodilation that lasts up to 12 hours with an onset of action that requires 10 to 20 minutes.[86] Because of their slow onset to effect, these long-acting agents are appropriate for maintenance rather than rescue therapy.

Ongoing studies are examining the role of long-acting β_2-agonists in COPD. At present, they are recommended to decrease dose requirements for patients who require multiple daily treatments with short-acting agents, provide management of nocturnal symptoms, and supplement other interventions when symptoms persist. The combination of ipratropium and β_2-agonists, both at submaximal doses, provides additive bronchodilatory effects without causing increased adverse reactions.[79,87] β_2-agonists are therefore added as the second step of management in patients who show incomplete resolution of symptoms with ipratropium alone. Combination MDI formulations of ipratropium with albuterol are now available to simplify therapy. Patients with severe COPD, however, benefit from therapy with individual canisters to allow tailoring of drug dosages.

Long-term therapy with inhaled β_2-agonists may promote tolerance and increased sensitivity to nonspecific bronchoconstrictor stimuli that can promote mild and transient bronchial hyperreactivity with the abrupt discontinuation of these agents. Rarely, paradoxic bronchoconstriction with the use of β_2-agonists has been reported. Side effects are common but rarely serious.[88] Reported complications include tachycardia, dysrhythmias, hypertension, hypokalemia, hyperglycemia, tremor, insomnia, and anxiety.

The **methylxanthines** are traditional agents in the care of patients with COPD. Their narrow therapeutic index compared to other available agents has decreased the popularity of their use for long-term care. Methylxanthines, however, provide significant bronchodilator effects in patients with COPD, although less than that observed with anticholinergic and β_2-agonist agents.[89,90] They also decrease the sensation of dyspnea and enhance perceptions of health-related quality of life that do not depend on measurable improvement of airflow in patients with COPD.[91,92] Other pulmonary effects of these agents include enhanced diaphragmatic muscle strength, prevention of respiratory muscle fatigue, and improved mucociliary clearance.[93,94] Nonpulmonary effects that present a potential to benefit patients with COPD include an anti-inflammatory effect, improved cardiac output, and reduced pulmonary vascular resistance.[95]

Methylxanthines, most often in the form of anhydrous theophylline, serve as third-line therapy and are introduced when ipratropium and β_2-agonist do not optimize lung function. Sustained-release formulations allow once- or twice-daily dosing. Because of the multiple drug-drug interactions and health conditions that alter theophylline elimination kinetics and inter-individual variation in pharmacokinetics, careful dosing of theophylline with periodic serum drug assays is required. Traditional recommended serum drug levels of 10 to 20 mg/dL have been modified to 5 to 15 mg/dL to decrease drug toxicity and maintain clinical benefit.[96] Patients with severe COPD and incomplete responses to theophylline at these serum levels may obtain benefit at serum levels of 17 mg/dL.[92] Adverse reactions caused by methylxanthines include nausea, vomiting, abdominal pain, diarrhea, tremor, irritability, sleep disorders, headache, seizures, and cardiac dysrhythmias.

Corticosteroids are often introduced in the care of patients with COPD when they do not experience optimal symptom control despite maximum bronchodilator therapy. The efficacy of corticosteroids in long-term management of COPD remains controversial. Although some studies suggest that inhaled corticosteroids slow the progression of airflow limitation, large-scale studies examining this potential benefit have not been completed.[63,66] It is estimated, however, that 10% to 30% of patients with COPD will demonstrate short-term improvement of FEV_1 after initiation of steroid therapy.[97]

Common clinical practice is to perform baseline spirometry and initiate oral prednisone at a dose of 0.5 mg/kg/day for a therapeutic trial of 2 weeks, after which spirometry is repeated. Patients who improve their FEV_1 by 10% or by an absolute value of 200 mL can be considered for long-term corticosteroid therapy.[97] Corticosteroids are tapered to the minimally effective dose. Recent placebo-controlled studies indicate that inhaled fluticasone provides modest benefit in terms of spirometric values, frequency of acute exacerbations, sputum production, functional status, and symptom scores over a 6-month period.[98] The role of inhaled corticosteroids in COPD, however, awaits further controlled trials.[67] Clinicians have to carefully consider the ongoing use of corticosteroids in patients who experience a subjective response but fail to have objective evidence of benefit. No studies have examined health-related quality of life indices to monitor the effectiveness of prednisone therapy. Also, insufficient data exist to recommend the substitution of inhaled corticosteroids for patients with COPD who respond to oral prednisone.

Side effects of long-term corticosteroid therapy include osteoporosis, diabetes, fluid retention, hypertension, cataracts, immunosuppression with risk of infection, integument changes, and redistribution of fat. Clinical practice guidelines recommend measurement of bone density and initiation of vitamin D and calcium in patients initiating long-term corticosteroid therapy.[99]

Antibiotics have a limited role in stable patients with COPD. Chronic use of antibiotics has not been shown to preserve lung function or prevent acute exacerbations. Although ongoing use of antibiotics may benefit only subgroups of patients who have more than four exacerbations per year,[61] the role of antibiotics is still important during acute exacerbations for hospitalized patients with deterioration of lung function.

Multiple agents with stimulatory effects on central respiratory centers, peripheral chemoreceptors, and $\dot{V}/\dot{Q}$ matching have been evaluated in patients with COPD. Ethamivan, almitrine, and doxapram increase minute ventilation through central and peripheral chemoreceptor effects, thereby lowering P_{CO_2} and increasing P_{O_2}.[100-105] Almitrine also improves $\dot{V}/\dot{Q}$ matching and intrapulmonary shunt.[102] These agents are not used in COPD, however, because of troublesome side effects. Theophylline is a mild respiratory stimulant, although the clinical importance of this effect is unknown.[106] Inhaled nitric oxide has been shown to improve oxygenation in patients with COPD in initial studies by vasodilating pulmonary vascular beds.[107]

Mucokinetic agents are intended to reduce mucus viscosity and assist with the mobilization of airway secretions. Iodinated glycerol has been demonstrated in a placebo-controlled trial to improve cough symptoms and sense of well-being although objective markers of airflow limitation did not improve.[108] Acetylcysteine breaks sulfhydryl bonds and has antioxidant properties. Some,[109-114] but not all,[115] studies suggest that it may have utility when administered orally to help prevent acute exacerbations of COPD, improve general health, and diminish airway secretions. It is presently undergoing more extensive trials. The efficacy of dornase in COPD is presently unproved, and its use is not recommended.[116] Aerosolized surfactant has recently been shown to improve pulmonary function and ciliary sputum transport in patients with stable chronic bronchitis.[117] Presently mucokinetic agents are used empirically in patients who have marked difficulty expectorating secretions despite maximal therapy.

Patients with severe COPD occasionally experience dyspnea at rest despite maximal medical therapy and oxygen supplementation. Oral opiates in such patients may relieve dyspnea symptoms. Some studies indicate that opiates through the inhaled route similarly improve dyspnea with less systemic toxicity.[118] Benzodiazepines have not been shown to improve dyspnea, and their use increases the risk for falls.[119]

Patients with severe COPD frequently experience debilitating muscle and weight loss, which has a negative effect on survival.[120] Although the cause of **pulmonary cachexia** is uncertain, it appears to be related to altered energy balance that increases energy expenditure. Resting energy expenditure[121] and total free living energy expenditure[122] are increased in patients with COPD compared to normal individuals, and patients with COPD are hypermetabolic compared to patients without COPD who are matched by severity of malnutrition.[123] Recent interest has focused on anabolic agents being used to reverse muscle loss in COPD. Several studies have demonstrated increased muscle mass in patients treated with anabolic steroids but no improvement in exercise tolerance or endurance and no enhancement of health-related quality of life.[124-126] To date, anabolic steroids remain investigational in the care of pulmonary cachexia.

The onset of cor pulmonale in patients with COPD is associated with a poor clinical prognosis.[127] Unfortunately, cardiovascular pharmacologic therapy directed at the improvement of right ventricular function or the reduction of pulmonary vascular resistance has not been associated with an improved clinical outcome. Vasodilator therapy can reduce pulmonary artery pressure acutely, but long-term benefits have not been shown. Also, vasodilators may aggravate hypoxemia by inhibiting adaptive hypoxic vasoconstriction[128,129] and worsen $\dot{V}/\dot{Q}$ mismatching. Some clinicians use digoxin for the management of right ventricular failure with marked peripheral edema in patients with cor pulmonale. No clinical evidence demonstrates improved outcome, however, and most experts reserve digoxin for patients with left ventricular systolic dysfunction or supraventricular dysrhythmias. Diuretic therapy can promote patient well-being by mobilizing lower extremity edema and improving ambulation, in addition to decreasing circulating blood volume and enhancing right-sided cardiac function. Methylxanthines and β_2-agonists enhance cardiac contractility,[95] although limited clinical benefits related to manifestations of cor pulmonale are noted with these agents.[128] Phlebotomy can improve right ventricular function in patients with marked secondary polycythemia.

Long-Term Oxygen Therapy

Long-term oxygen therapy (LTOT) is the only pharmacologic intervention available for hypoxemic patients with COPD that has been shown to prolong survival.[130,131] The mechanisms of benefit are unclear, although patients treated with LTOT for an average of 19 hours/day have a slower progression of pulmonary hypertension compared to those treated with 12 hours/day or less, suggesting a positive effect on pulmonary vasculature as the basis for improved survival.[131] LTOT also decreases dyspnea awareness,[132] oxygen cost of breathing,[133] pulmonary hypertension,[131] disordered sleep, and nocturnal dysrhythmias.[134] Oxygen therapy improves exercise endurance,[132] strength,[135] and mental alertness.[135]

Because of the expense of home oxygen, patients are selected for therapy on the basis of specific indications derived from clinical evidence (Box 47-3).[136,137] Demonstration of hypoxia should occur after a 4-week stable period when patients are receiving full medical therapy and not smoking. Subsequent monitoring of oxygenation is performed on an individual basis. Up to 40% of patients initiated on LTOT experience improved oxygenation after 1 month of therapy and no longer fulfill the indications for supplemental oxygen.[137]

Patients receiving continuous LTOT should be counseled to use oxygen 24 hours/day. Some clinicians increase flow rates empirically by 1 L/min during sleep.[136] Patients should be carefully matched with the three types of oxygen delivery systems available, which are oxygen concentrators, compressed gas cylinders, and liquid oxygen. The relative benefits of these three systems are listed in Table 47-1.[138] Most patients need a stationary unit (usually an oxygen concentrator) and a portable unit (usually gas cylinders) unless they are homebound. Liquid oxygen systems benefit active patients who require greater portability than that provided by gas cylinders.[138]

Multiple oxygen cannula systems are available. Most patients use nasal prongs, which supply variable concentrations of oxygen to the lungs depending on the selected flow rate and patients' breathing patterns. On average, delivered F_{IO_2} values are 24% at 1 L/min, 28% at 2 L/min, and 32% at 3 L/min. Humidification systems are not required with oxygen flow rates less than 5 L/min. Flow rates

Box 47-3

Indications for Long-Term Oxygen Therapy

Continuous Oxygen Therapy
Pa_{O_2} ≤55 mm Hg or oxygen saturation ≤88% at rest during breathing of room air
Pa_{O_2} between 56 to 59 mm Hg or oxygen saturation of 89% at any time during breathing of room air with one or more of the following:
  Cor pulmonale
  Polycythemia (Hct >56%)
  Pulmonary hypertension

Noncontinuous Oxygen Therapy
Pa_{O_2} ≤55 mm Hg or oxygen saturation ≤88% during exertion or sleep during breathing of room air

Pa_{O_2}, *Partial pressure of arterial oxygen*; *Hct, hematocrit*.

above 5 L/min are poorly tolerated and indicate a need for a different oxygen supplementation system, such as a face mask or transtracheal oxygen.

To conserve oxygen, several devices have been developed to limit the loss of oxygen observed with continuous flow nasal cannulae.[7,137] Mechanical reservoirs store 15 to 20 mL of 100% oxygen in a space that is delivered during the initial phase of inspiration. Electronic demand devices sense the pressure or flow changes with early inspiration and deliver an oxygen pulse. Transtracheal oxygen systems can be used in highly motivated patients who have difficulty using nasal prongs or who require more than 3 L/min of oxygen flow.[139] Transtracheal catheters are inserted into the trachea between the second and third tracheal rings under local anesthesia. Humidification of delivered oxygen is required to prevent inspiration of secretions. The relative features and complications of these systems are shown in Table 47-2.

LTOT is directed toward maintenance of PaO_2 above 60 mm Hg or oxygen saturation above 90% without an induction of marked hypercarbia. Oxygen therapy increases $PaCO_2$ by altering $\dot{V}/\dot{Q}$ matching and increasing dead space ventilation in addition to blunting respiratory drive.[140] Consequently, oxygen is initiated at low flow rates of 0.5 to 2 L/min with monitoring of arterial blood gases within the first 1 or 2 hours with gradual increases in subsequent flow rates as needed.[7,137,138,141] Patients should be warned of oxygen's capacity to support combustion and the risks of smoking while using oxygen.

Patients dependent on oxygen can travel by air plane, but advance arrangements are necessary to obtain oxygen units during flight and provide units on arrival.[142,143] Because airline cabins are pressurized to 6000 to 8000 feet, patients should increase their usual oxygen flow rates by 1 to 2 L/min. A high altitude simulation test (HAST) can be performed when the patients breathe 16% oxygen at sea level and administered oxygen is titrated to achieve adequate oxygenation.[142]

TABLE 47-1

Relative Features of Different Types of Oxygen Delivery Systems

Feature	Oxygen Concentrator	Compressed Gas	Liquid Oxygen
Availability	Good	Good	Limited
Oxygen supply	½-5 L/min continuously	Large cylinders: 2 L/min for 2-3 days	Stationary unit: 2 L/min for 7 days
		Smaller cylinders: 2 L/min for 5.2, 2, or 1.2 hr	Portable unit: 2 L/min 4 to 8 hours
		Time enhanced with use of conserving device by 2-4 times	Time enhanced with use of conserving device by 2-4 times
Power	AC	Not needed	Not needed
Weight	Heavy (about 50 lb)	Heavy	Portables: light to moderate; stationary units: heavy
Portability	Limited	Good	Good to excellent
Cost	Low	Moderate	High

TABLE 47-2

Relative Features of Oxygen-Conserving Devices

Feature	Mechanical Reservoir	Electronic Demand	Transtracheal Oxygen
Cost	Low	Moderate	High
Appearance	Poor	Good	Excellent
Complications		Mechanical failures	Inspirated mucous plugs
		Not recommended for use while asleep	Cough
			Bronchospasm
			Subcutaneous emphysema
			Stomal infection
			Hemorrhage
			Catheter misplacement

Vaccinations

Vaccinations are a central preventive measure in the management of patients with COPD. All caregivers interacting with patients should counsel them regarding their annual vaccination with trivalent influenza vaccine, which is 70% effective in decreasing morbidity during influenza epidemics. Pneumococcal vaccination is recommended for patients with COPD.[7]

Ancillary Measures

Ancillary measures in the care of patients with COPD include breathing exercises, physical therapy to mobilize secretions, and assisted ventilation. Pursed-lip and diaphragmatic breathing is encouraged for patients with moderate to severe COPD when they experience increased dyspnea with exercise or increased anxiety. Although little objective data support their use, many patients have an enhanced sense of well-being with these breathing exercises. Physical therapy to assist the mobilization of secretions is directed primarily at the improvement of symptoms, although some data suggest that mucus hypersecretion correlates with increased rates of hospitalization.[144]

Outcome data support the benefit of these interventions in patients with cystic fibrosis, but little evidence supports their efficacy in COPD. Subgroups of patients with COPD who have more than 30 mL of expectorated secretions per day or severe debilitation that appears aggravated by the inability to raise airway secretions are selected for physical therapy.[7] Physical therapy interventions include postural drainage, chest percussion and vibration, directed coughing, and positive expiratory pressure techniques. Patients are selected for one or more of these interventions empirically with careful monitoring of benefit. Increasing fluid intake does not thin airway secretions in adequately hydrated patients. Aerosolized water or saline provides no benefit and can trigger bronchospasm and promote infection.[7]

Ventilatory Support

The benefits of mechanical ventilation in the outpatient management of patients with COPD is yet to be defined. The theory behind intermittent ventilator support is to unload respiratory muscles and treat or prevent muscle fatigue. Such therapy has been shown to benefit patients with chronic respiratory failure caused by restrictive lung diseases.[145] Negative pressure ventilator devices, such as poncho wrap ventilators or tank ventilators, have not shown benefit in long-term use.[146] **Negative pressure ventilation (NPV)** also may induce a pressure-related collapse of upper airways during sleep and symptoms related to obstructive sleep apnea.

Intermittent **noninvasive positive pressure ventilation (NPPV)** by way of a mouthpiece or a nasal or face mask has been examined in several controlled trials. Results from these studies have conflicted with some studies detecting no benefit[147,148] and others showing improvement in total sleep time, quality of life, gas exchange, and respiratory symptoms.[149] One recent study demonstrates a trend toward improved survival in patients treated with NPPV.[150] Presently the indications for NPPV in patients with stable COPD are unclear. Highly motivated patients with daytime hypercapnia (more than 50 mm Hg) or nocturnal oxygen desaturation recalcitrant to supplemental oxygen may be considered for a 1- to 2-month trial.[151]

Management of Sleep-Related Abnormalities

Patients with COPD are at risk for sleep-related disorders characterized primarily by worsening hypoxia at night.[152,153] The prevalence of sleep-related disorders in COPD is unknown although recent studies indicate that sleep complaints are found in 40% to 50% of patients with chronic respiratory symptoms.[154] Bronchitic symptoms, but not spirometric results, correlate with the occurrence of sleep complaints.[155] It is uncertain whether daytime severity of hypoxemia does[153] or does not[156] correlate with nocturnal oxygen desaturation. Daytime hypercapnia increases the risk of nocturnal desaturation.[157] No clinical predictors, however, identify patients with COPD at risk for nocturnal oxygen desaturation with sufficient accuracy to be used in clinical practice.[158,159]

Causative factors in sleep-related disorders in COPD include nocturnal hypoventilation with decreased ventilation most apparent during rapid eye motion (REM) sleep,[160,161] worsening lung mechanics with decreased tone in accessory respiratory muscles[162] and increased upper airway resistance,[163] and impairment of gas exchange with worsening $\dot{V}/\dot{Q}$ mismatch during sleep because of decreased functional residual capacity[164] and small airways disease.[165]

The coexistence of COPD with obstructive sleep apnea (OSA) is a relatively common condition and is termed the *overlap syndrome*.[166] It remains unresolved whether the overlap syndrome results from the coincidental occurrence of these two relatively common conditions in the same individual or if COPD predisposes patients to OSA.[152] Affected patients present with daytime sleepiness, rapidly worsening pulmonary hypertension, or respiratory failure.

Multiple complications of sleep-disordered breathing with recurrent nocturnal oxygen desaturation have been evaluated in patients with COPD. Ventricular ectopy increases during sleep in patients with COPD and nocturnal hypoxemia.[167,168] Acute worsening of pulmonary hypertension can occur during REM sleep. Some evidence suggests that nocturnal oxygen desaturation can contribute to the long-term progression of chronic pulmonary hypertension,[169] but a causative relationship has not yet been confirmed. Among patients with the overlap syndrome, however, 42% have daytime pulmonary hypertension.[170] It is suspected but not established that patients with COPD with sleep hypoxemia are at increased risk for secondary polycythemia.[152] Patients with the overlap syndrome demonstrate diurnal hypercapnia more often than patients with COPD alone[171] and may be at increased risk for acute respiratory failure.[172]

The presence of COPD is not an indication for routine polysomnography. Patients with COPD who demonstrate symptoms suggestive of sleep apnea/hypopnea syndrome should be considered for study.[153] The American Thoracic Society (ATS) further recommends that any patient with COPD who has a diurnal PaO_2 greater than 55 mm Hg with evidence of pulmonary hypertension, cor pulmonale, or polycythemia should be evaluated with polysomnography.[173] It remains unclear whether the demonstration of isolated nocturnal desaturation warrants a consideration of nocturnal oxygen therapy. Studies to date have not demonstrated a survival benefit from isolated nocturnal oxygen therapy in patients with COPD who experience hypoxemia only during sleep.[172] Studies examining sleep quality with and without nocturnal supplemental oxygen have been conflicting.[174,175] At present, the data are insufficient to recommend isolated nocturnal O_2 therapy for patients with nocturnal desaturation who do not qualify for conventional O_2 therapy.[176]

It also is not established that pharmacologic agents improve sleep architecture or reduce nocturnal oxygen desaturation in patients with COPD.[152] Nasal continuous positive airway pressure (CPAP) remains the mainstay of therapy for patients with overlap syndrome, although little data exist demonstrating the outcome of this therapy in patients with COPD.[152]

Pulmonary Rehabilitation

Enrollment of patients with moderate to severe COPD in outpatient **pulmonary rehabilitation** programs provides opportunities to restore patients to the highest possible level of independence and functioning in the community.[177-179] Components of an effective, multidisciplinary rehabilitation program include exercise training, education for patients and family, instruction in respiratory and chest physiotherapy, and psychologic support. The effectiveness of pulmonary rehabilitation has long been debated because of the limited outcomes data that demonstrate measurable improvements in post-rehabilitation endpoints.

A recent systematic review and a clinical practice guideline sponsored by the American College of Chest Physicians and the American Association of Cardiovascular and Pulmonary Rehabilitation have examined the existing evidence for benefit.[179,180] Both reports indicate that varying levels of evidence support the effectiveness of different elements of pulmonary rehabilitation and that pulmonary rehabilitation represents a cost-effective intervention by decreasing the frequency of hospitalizations. Consensus is developing that pulmonary rehabilitation benefits patients with COPD.[181] Future efforts are needed to design programs that maintain long-term and short-term benefits of pulmonary rehabilitation on functional status improvement, which often diminish over time.[182,183] Pulmonary rehabilitation has provided a framework for the development of disease management programs to promote self-care and integrate regular exercise into lifestyle changes in patients with COPD.[184]

Surgery

Multiple surgical approaches have been attempted in patients with COPD over the last 50 years to improve baseline lung function.[185-187] Unfortunately, most of these interventions did not result in lasting functional improvement.[188] Presently, bullectomy, lung volume reduction surgery (LVRS), and lung transplantation have clinical utility for selected patients with COPD.

Bullectomy

Bullectomy is performed for patients with emphysema who develop giant bullae, which are air space enlargements that occupy one third of a hemithorax (Figure 47-9). Giant bullae are an unusual complication of emphysema but represent a reversible cause of pulmonary decompensation, which results from compression of an adjacent lung by expanding bullae.[189] Patients are selected for bullectomy on the basis of the degree of lung compression and the functional status of the compressed lung to determine the amount of improvement that can be anticipated by removal of bullae. Patients with giant bullae and reduced lung function attributable to the bullae rather than underlying diffuse emphysema are the best surgical candidates.[188] Patients with giant bullae without compressed lung tissue, which is termed "vanishing lung syndrome," gain no benefit from bullectomy.[190] Patients with giant bullae, compressed lung tissue, and diffuse emphysema with moderate to severe functional impairment require careful individualization of the decision to perform bullectomy.

CT scans have supplanted pulmonary angiography as the standard imaging approach to provide an accurate assessment of the size of bullae, the amount of compressed lung, and the severity of diffuse emphysema.[191,192] Pulmonary function tests assess the degree of diffuse emphysema. Patients with isolated giant bullae without diffuse emphysema have a restrictive pattern on spirometric evaluation.[188] Evidence of airway obstruction, therefore, quantifies the degree of generalized COPD. The volume of a giant bullae can be calculated by subtraction of the total lung volume (TLC) determined by helium dilution (which does not measure the volume of bullae) from the TLC measured by plethysmography (which includes the volume of bullae in the determination of TLC).

Bullectomy is performed by the excision of bullae and placement of a suture or staple line across the base of the lesion by way of a sternotomy or thoracotomy incision or by thoracoscopy. Postoperative air leaks are the major complication of bullectomy and can be prevented to a degree by placement of staple or suture lines across strips of bovine pericardium or the folded back edges of the base of the bullae to reinforce the tissue. Overall mortality rates are 8% in carefully selected patients.[189]

Lung Volume Reduction Surgery

Lung volume reduction surgery (LVRS) is undergoing evaluation in a multicenter study as a surgical intervention

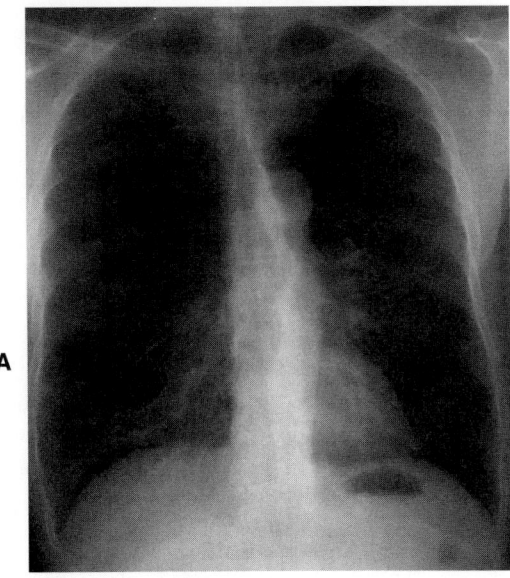

Preoperative spirometry

FEV$_1$ (L)	1.42
FVC (L)	2.60
FEV$_1$/FVC (%)	55

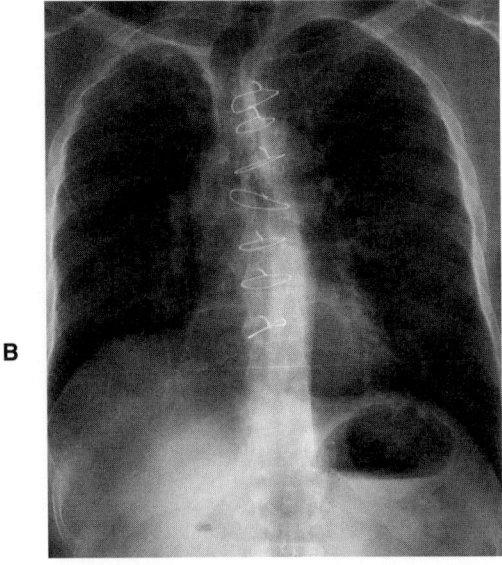

Postoperative spirometry

FEV$_1$ (L)	2.50
FVC (L)	2.96
FEV$_1$/FVC (%)	84

Figure 47-9 Chest radiographs and spirometric values in a patient who underwent bilateral bullectomy through a sternotomy incision. **A,** This chest radiograph shows the bilateral upper lobe bullae with increased density in the mid lung fields consistent with lung crowding. **B,** This chest radiograph was obtained after bullectomy and demonstrated decreased lung volumes and the absence of lung crowding. The preoperative spirometric values improved postoperatively.

that may have application for large numbers of patients with advanced emphysema. The procedure removes 20% to 30% of the lung tissue that is most severely affected by emphysema. The remaining lung gains recoil elasticity and

improves lung, chest wall, and diaphragmatic mechanics in addition to right ventricular performance.[193-195] Increased lung elasticity improves airway tethering, thereby preventing early expiratory airway closure and reversing to a degree the overexpanded configuration of the chest and diaphragm, which improves inspiratory muscle efficiency.[196]

Criteria used to select patients for LVRS have not yet been established. Many centers require patients to demonstrate moderate to severe hyperinflation and airflow limitation with CT quantification measurements of emphysema and evidence of heterogeneous distribution of emphysematous changes.[186,197,198] Exclusion criteria include continued smoking, severe abnormalities in gas exchange, copious airway secretions, physical deconditioning, hyperreactive airways, and serious comorbid conditions such as cardiac disease, morbid obesity, or cachexia. Most centers report that only 20% to 40% of evaluated patients are appropriate candidates for LVRS.[199]

Surgical approaches used to perform LVRS include unilateral and bilateral thoracoscopy,[200] anterior thoracotomy, bilateral thoracosternotomy, and median sternotomy. Most centers perform LVRS on both lungs during the same procedure. The surgeon removes the most emphysematous regions of the lung as guided by direct inspection and the results of preoperative V̇/Q̇ lung scans. Lung tissue is stapled and exised,[201] laser ablated,[202] or plicated and stapled without excision.[203]

Postoperative pain control is an important aspect of care to reduce the risk of atelectasis and pneumonia. Patients are managed with epidural catheters for the infusion of bupivacaine. Postoperative hypercapnia is common and may require temporary management with NPPV.[204] Minitracheostomy may improve postoperative clearance of airway secretions.[201] Respiratory therapy plays an important role in the postoperative period in the administration of bronchodilators, chest physical therapy, and incentive spirometry.[186]

Studies report that LVRS results in short-term improvement in pulmonary function, gas exchange, and exercise tolerance with reduced dependency on LTOT.[201,205] The degree of subjective improvement in dyspnea does not always correlate with changes in pulmonary function test results.[206] Recent data suggest that symptomatic improvement correlate with increments in postoperative elastic recoil.[207] Maximal functional and physiologic improvement occurs within 3 to 6 months of surgery.

The long-term results of LVRS are not completely defined. Reported patient series differ regarding the proportion of patients who maintain improved functional capacity and spirometric values during the first 1 to 3 years after surgery.[201,208,209] Some studies report improved lung function and gas exchange after 12 months,[201,208] and other studies indicate that benefits from LVRS may persist in only 31% of patients after 3 years.[209] The effect of LVRS on COPD-related mortality remains unknown, although a recent nonrandomized study observed a higher mortality in patients who were selected for LVRS but denied the procedure because of funding issues compared with comparable patients who underwent the procedure.[210] Complications of LVRS include prolonged air leak, pneumonia, respiratory failure, postoperative ileus and colonic or cecal perforation, and cardiac ischemia.[186]

Lung Transplantation

Lung transplantation is a therapeutic option for patients with severe COPD who do not have serious comorbid conditions. Patient selection criteria include age less than 65 years, abstinence from smoking, ambulatory status, an ability to participate in pulmonary rehabilitation, an absence of malignancy or nonpulmonary organ dysfunction, and no serious chronic disorders such as morbid obesity, severe hypertension, heart failure, or cachexia. Most patients have an FEV_1 less than 25% of predicted at the time they are listed on a transplant list and considerably less than that value when an allograft becomes available, which usually takes 2 years.

Multiple surgical approaches exist for lung transplantation.[211] Single lung transplantation is usually performed through a median sternotomy or anterior thoracotomy incision. Bilateral lung transplantation is done most often through a transverse thoracosternotomy incision.[212] Postoperative pain is managed with epidural anesthesia. Careful fluid management is required because of increased permeability in the transplanted lung and the absence of lymphatic drainage.[213] Respiratory therapy is directed toward assisting patients with airway secretion, administering inhaled bronchodilators, and assisting with deep breathing.

Perioperative mortality for single and bilateral lung transplantation approaches 10% and 1-year survival is 70% to 80%. Recent studies suggest that patients with COPD have better 1-year survival after bilateral compared to single lung transplantation.[201,214] Although lung transplantation in COPD has not been subjected to randomized trials to determine its effect on survival, analysis of retrospective data controlled for independent risk factors of death indicate improved survival compared to patients with severe COPD who have not been transplanted.[215] Both single and bilateral lung transplantation is associated with marked improvements in FEV_1 and exercise capacity.[214] After trans-

plantation, patients with COPD have exercise limitations based on peripheral muscle weakness and chronic deconditioning rather than ventilatory capacity.[216]

Complications of lung transplantation include infection, early allograft dysfunction that may progress to acute lung injury, hemorrhage, dehiscence of the bronchial anastomoses, and acute and chronic lung rejection.[201,217] The development of acute postoperative allograft edema that requires mechanical ventilation in patients who have undergone single lung transplantation complicates ventilator management. The overexpansion of the highly compliant native lung compared to the low-compliant allograft may necessitate independent lung ventilation with a double-lumen endotracheal tube.[218]

Managing Acute Exacerbations

Despite comprehensive outpatient care, patients with COPD are at risk of developing an acute exacerbation of their airways disease that requires inpatient care. On average, patients with symptomatic COPD experience one to four acute exacerbations per year.[219] An **acute exacerbation** is defined as a sudden worsening of respiratory symptoms accompanied by deteriorating lung function.[136] Most often, patients will present with increased dyspnea, cough, and changes in the quality or quantity of sputum. A patient with an acute exacerbation often may be managed successfully as an outpatient with an increased intensity of bronchodilator therapy and corticosteroid agents with oral antibiotics. Each exacerbation, however, has the potential to progress in severity and require hospitalization to prevent the onset of respiratory failure and a need for mechanical ventilation. Multiple clinical conditions can precipitate an acute exacerbation (Box 47-4).[136,220]

Box 47-4

Precipitating Causes of an Acute Exacerbation of COPD

Bronchial infections (usually viral)
Pneumonia
Pulmonary emboli
Myocardial infarction, congestive heart failure, or dysrhythmias
Pneumothorax
Aspiration
Neuromuscular weakness or end-stage COPD with muscle fatigue
Rib or vertebral body fractures
Postsurgical thoracoabdominal pain
Metabolic acidosis or other electrolyte disturbance
Pleural effusion
Sedating drugs or β-blocking agents
Environmental respiratory irritants
Inappropriate use of oxygen
Other organ dysfunction (gastrointestinal hemorrhage)

COPD, *Chronic obstructive pulmonary disease.*

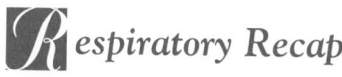

Respiratory Recap

Acute Exacerbation of the Patient with COPD

Mild exacerbations can be managed at home.
Inhaled β-agonists and anticholinergics are the first line therapy.
The use of steroids for severe exacerbations is standard practice.
Antibiotics are used for exacerbations severe enough to warrant hospitalization.
Oxygen therapy is titrated to maintain an adequate Pao_2 without CO_2 retention.
Many studies have confirmed the value of noninvasive ventilation for acute exacerbation of COPD.
Life-threatening respiratory failure requires intubation and mechanical ventilation (particularly if noninvasive ventilation is failing).

Mild acute exacerbations can be managed with home therapy (Figure 47-10). Patients should be encouraged to maintain adequate fluid intake to avoid dehydration. If they cannot cough and raise secretions, home physiotherapy should be offered. Patients benefit from a written action plan to manage their medications and alert them to when they should contact their physician or go to the emergency department. Inhaled bronchodilators should be increased to their maximum dosages. β_2-Agonists have greater efficacy than ipratropium for acute symptoms.

The role of antibiotics in acute exacerbations is controversial. At least a third of respiratory infections that underlie acute exacerbations are viral in etiology[221] and would not be expected to respond to antibiotics. A recent meta-analysis concluded that antibiotics provide only a small but statistically significant benefit for patients with COPD experiencing an acute exacerbation.[222] Nevertheless, recent consensus statements[136,220] recommend the initiation of antibiotics for acute exacerbations if any two of the following three features are present: increased dyspnea, sputum volume, or sputum purulence.[61,223] An oral antibiotic is selected with activity against the common pathogens in COPD exacerbations, which are *Streptococ-*

cus pneumoniae, Haemophilus influenzae, and *Moraxella catarrhalis.*[61] Recent data suggest that *Mycoplasma pneumoniae* and *Chlamydia pneumoniae* may be common pathogens in acute exacerbations and may require antibiotic therapy in some patients.[224,225] Amoxicillin, tetracycline, a second-generation cephalosporin, a macrolide, or trimethoprim-sulfamethoxazole are usually continued for 7 to 10 days. Newer azalide antibiotics allow shorter durations of therapy. Patients with FEV_1 values less than 35% of predicted may have gram-negative bacteria, especially *Enterobacteriaceae* and *Pseudomonas* species, as a cause of acute exacerbations.[226] These patients may benefit from antibiotic therapy with broad-spectrum activity.[227]

The addition of corticosteroids to the therapy for patients with severe acute exacerbations or exacerbations with wheezing or a history of airway hyperreactivity has become standard practice despite the relatively limited data that support their use. A recent study, however, indicated that a brief course of outpatient prednisone accelerated improvement in hypoxemia, FEV_1, and peak flow with decreased treatment failures in patients with COPD experiencing acute exacerbations.[228] Most physicians initiate prednisone for outpatients at a dose of 0.5 to 1 mg/kg/day for 7 to 10 days.

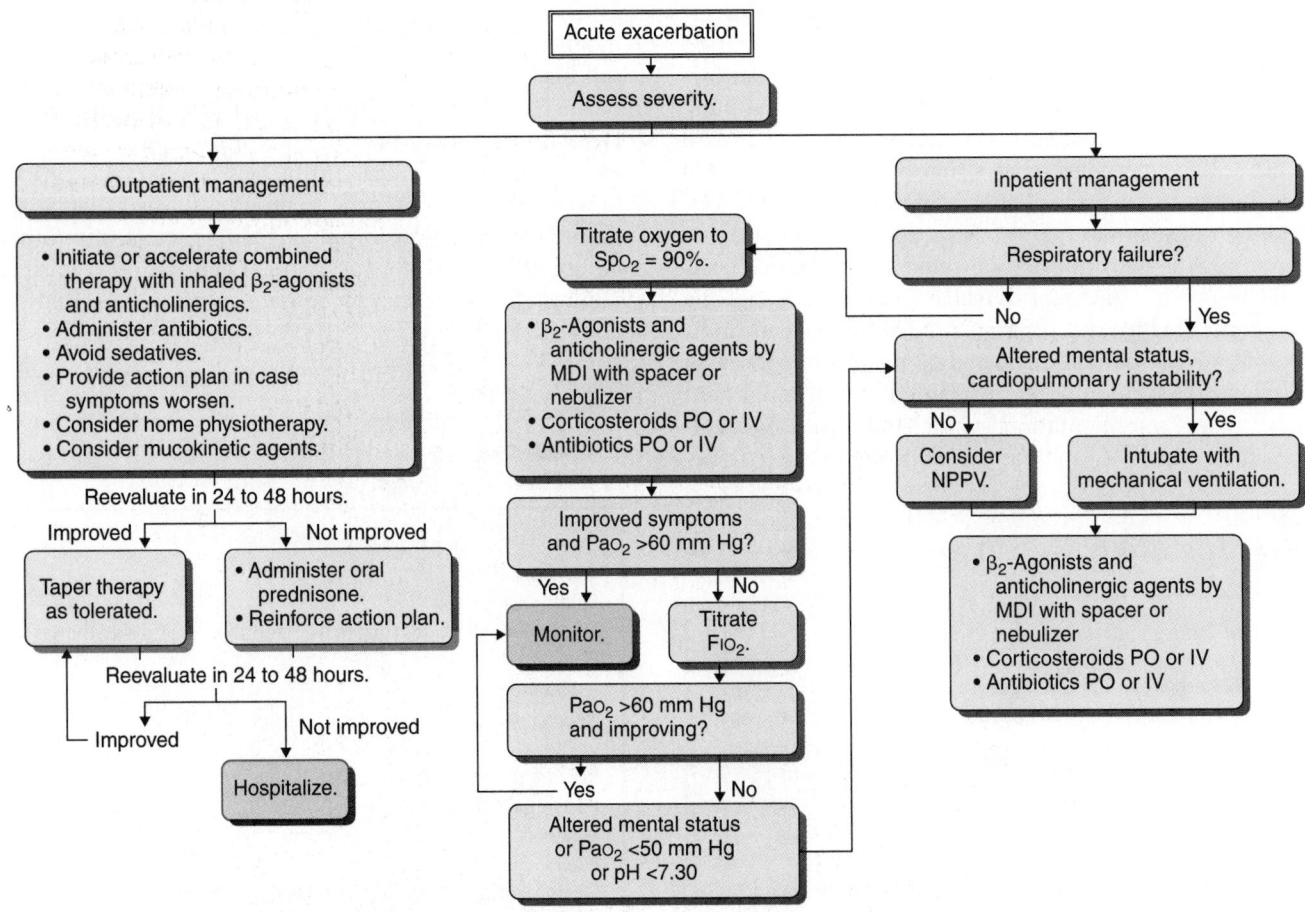

Figure 47-10 Algorithm for management of patients with an acute exacerbation of chronic obstructive pulmonary disease (COPD) based on recently published clinical practice guidelines. *SpO₂,* Arterial oxygen saturation by pulse oximetry; *MDI,* metered dose inhaler; *NPPV,* noninvasive positive pressure ventilation; *FIO₂,* fractional inspired oxygen concentration; *po,* by mouth.

Box 47-5

Criteria for Hospitalization of Patients with Acute Exacerbations of COPD

Increased respiratory symptoms with any one of the following:
    Failure of outpatient management
    Inability to ambulate (for example, walk between rooms) in a previously mobile patient
    Inability to sleep or eat because of increased dyspnea or cough
    Inadequate home resources for care
    Prolonged deterioration before emergency evaluation
    Altered mentation
    Worsening hypoxemia
    New or worsening hypercarbia
    Emergency department visit within previous 1 week
    Failure to improve with maximal therapy during an emergency department evaluation
New or worsening cor pulmonale unresponsive to outpatient care
Comorbid condition (for example, acute vertebral compression fracture, severe steroid myopathy) that is not immediately reversible and compromises respiratory function

From Celli BR, et al. Standards for the diagnosis and care of patients with chronic obstructive pulmonary disease (COPD) and asthma. Am J Respir Crit Care Med 1995;154:120.
COPD, Chronic obstructive pulmonary disease.

Severe exacerbations of COPD are characterized by deterioration in arterial blood gas tensions with varying degrees of hypoxia and hypercapnia. Abnormalities in $\dot{V}/\dot{Q}$ worsen and intrapulmonary shunts develop, indicating the presence of complete obstruction of some airways.[229] PEEPi develops or increases from baseline values.[230] These changes require evaluation of patients for hospitalization and inpatient care (see Figure 47-10). Despite advances in respiratory care, the inpatient mortality of patients hospitalized for an acute exacerbation of COPD remains substantial, ranging from 6% to 30%.[231-233] Markers of increased mortality include advanced age, need for mechanical ventilation, ventricular dysrhythmia, atrial fibrillation, acute or chronic cardiac disease, associated nonpulmonary organ failure, high APACHE (Acute Physiology and Chronic Health Evaluation) III score, poor nutritional status, poor baseline health status, and an alveolar-arterial oxygen gradient on room air greater than 40 mm Hg or a low PaO_2/FIO_2.[231-233] No scoring system, however, predicts survival in patients with acute exacerbations of COPD with sufficient accuracy for clinical practice.[234]

Few clinical studies have examined the indications for hospitalization.[235] In contrast to patients with asthma, spirometric or peak flow measurements do not predict with sufficient accuracy the need for hospitalization.[235] In the absence of extensive outcome data, the ATS has devised general indications for hospitalization of patients with COPD (Box 47-5).[7] The availability of daily home visits by respiratory nurses during an acute exacerbation can limit the need for hospitalization.[236]

Box 47-6

American Thoracic Society Criteria to Determine Readiness for Hospital Discharge of Patients with Acute Exacerbations

Inhaled bronchodilator use no more frequently than every 4 hours
Previously ambulatory patients can walk across the room
Degree of dyspnea does not interfere with eating or sleeping
Airway reactivity is stable and controlled
Stable respiratory status when off of parenteral therapy for 12 to 24 hours
Patient or home caregivers understand therapeutic plan
Home care and follow-up plan are completed
Patient, family, and physician are confident of discharge success

Limited data exist to accurately identify patients who would benefit from admission to an intensive care unit (ICU). The ATS consensus statement[7] recommends ICU admission for patients with severe dyspnea who fail to improve adequately with emergency department therapy, have acute mental status changes, impending respiratory muscle fatigue, hypoxemia or respiratory acidemia that progresses despite emergency department therapy, or cardiorespiratory instability that signifies a need or potential need for ventilator support. Unfortunately, scoring systems have not been developed that identify patients who can benefit from ICU care. A recent study indicates that the presence of atrial fibrillation, ventricular dysrhythmias, an alveolar-arterial oxygen gradient greater than 41 mm Hg, and advanced age identify patients with an increased risk of death.[232] Most patients treated with NPPV for acute respiratory failure should be cared for in an ICU environment.[237]

Evidence-based guidelines do not exist to guide decisions regarding duration of hospitalization. Mushlin and colleagues[238] demonstrated that most complications of acute exacerbations, such as need for mechanical ventilation, occur in the first 6 days of hospitalization in 90% of patients. In their reported patient population, the average duration of hospitalization was 7 to 9 days, although hospitalization ranged between 1 to 57 days. Predictors of prolonged hospitalization included admission $PaCO_2$ greater than 45 mm Hg, preadmission duration of symptoms greater than 1 day, and need for antibiotics on admission.[238] The ATS has recommended guidelines used to determine a patient's readiness for discharge (Box 47-6). Although recommended by some guidelines,[239] no evidence supports the measurement of airflow to determine readiness for discharge.

An acceleration of outpatient pharmacologic therapy is the keystone to manage an acute exacerbation of COPD that requires inpatient care. Goals of pharmacologic therapy center on assistance in the mobilization of airway secretions, treatment of the airway infection, and relief of bronchospasm to prevent the need for intubation. The pharmacologic approach requires individualization of care based on the chronic outpatient drug regimen, recent drug doses during the early phases of the exacerbation, degree of bronchospasm reversibility, history of toxicity to medications, comorbid conditions to increase drug toxicity, and the need for specific therapy for underlying precipitants of the exacerbation.

Inhaled β_2-adrenergic agents and anticholinergic bronchodilators are first-line therapy for COPD exacerbations. Among the available β_2-adrenergic agents, short-acting drugs are used to allow a rapid onset of effect and repeated doses at short intervals.[7] Oral formulations of the drugs are avoided because of delayed onset; parenteral routes are used only if patients cannot be managed with inhaled agents. Parenteral administration increases the risk of cardiac complications in patients with coexisting coronary artery disease. β_2-Agonists, but not anticholinergic agents, may transiently worsen hypoxia through pulmonary vascular effects.[240,241]

Consensus statements recommend administration of inhaled β_2-agonists with an MDI rather than a nebulizer unit,[7,220] although consensus does not exist regarding equivalency of these two routes of drug administration.[242] With the MDI mode of administration, patients are given three to four puffs at hourly intervals as tolerated depending on the course of the bronchospasm. Patients need to be closely monitored for signs of toxicity, such as tachycardia, tremulousness, and dysrhythmias.

Inhaled anticholinergic bronchodilators, such as ipratropium bromide, can be added to inhaled β_2-agonists in an effort to maximize bronchodilator response. The available data, however, do not clearly demonstrate added benefit of combined therapy during acute exacerbations.[6,7,243] Several studies suggest that ipratropium as compared with β_2-agonists has a delayed onset of maximal bronchodilation effect, an equivalent bronchodilator efficacy, and a greater effect on the improvement of oxygenation.[243,244] Based on these observations and the low toxicity of ipratropium, combined therapy is usually recommended.[7]

Randomized studies have not demonstrated benefit in terms of bronchodilator response in the addition of intravenous aminophylline to inhaled β_2-agonists during acute exacerbations.[244] Because of the toxicity of methylxanthines and their unpredictable pharmacokinetics and potential for drug-drug interactions during acute exacerbations, some expert panels discourage their use.[220,245] The ATS recommends considering methylxanthines for patients who cannot receive inhaled bronchodilators and for patients who demonstrate an inadequate response to bronchodilator therapy because of the possibility of a small added benefit from methylxanthines.[136]

If used during acute exacerbations, the narrow therapeutic window of methylxanthines requires careful dosing. Patients who are taking outpatient methylxanthine drugs should not receive intravenous therapy with these agents until toxic serum concentrations are excluded. Target serum levels are 10 to 12 μg/ml, which provides physiologic benefit and avoids adverse reactions. Drug doses require careful monitoring in the presence of clinical conditions and coexisting drugs that alter the elimination rate of methylxanthines. The initial clinical manifestation of an adverse reaction may be a life-threatening seizure or cardiac dysrhythmia.

Most clinicians prescribe corticosteroids for hospitalized patients with acute exacerbations of COPD, although reports supporting evidence of clinical benefit are few. Albert and colleagues demonstrated that intravenous methylprednisolone (Solu-Medrol) produced a greater percentage improvement in FEV_1 as compared with placebo.[246] No significant difference was noted, however, when these data were reanalyzed as changes in absolute values of FEV_1.[247] Other endpoints in the study, such as duration of hospitalization, survival, and need for intubation were not affected by corticosteroid therapy. In a short-term study of patients with acute exacerbations of COPD treated in an emergency department, no benefit from corticosteroids were noted during a 4.5-hour period in one study,[248] but another study indicated that corticosteroids administered in the emergency department decreased the 48-hour relapse rate.[249] A small study of eight tracheotomized patients with acute exacerbations of COPD demonstrated decreased airways resistance and intrinsic PEEP after 90 minutes of corticosteroid therapy.[250] Recent data from the Systemic Corticosteroids in COPD Exacerbations clinical trial indicate that hospitalized patients treated with corticosteroids had fewer treatment failures, shorter hospitalization, and more rapid normalization of spirometric values.[251] The dose and duration of corticosteroids are controversial, but many physicians initiate therapy with 0.5 to 1.0 mg/kg/day of Solu-Medrol with conversion to oral prednisone within 2 to 3 days and a rapid taper if objective measures of a corticosteroid response occur or a discontinuance in therapy after 2 to 3 days if the patient does not respond. A response to corticosteroids during an acute hospitalization should not be interpreted as an indication for chronic corticosteroid therapy.

Consensus statements recommend starting antibiotics for acute exacerbations that are sufficiently severe to warrant hospitalization.[6,136,220] This recommendation receives support from the previously discussed data that demonstrates benefit in outpatients treated with antibiotics for acute exacerbations of bronchitis.[222] Sputum cultures may guide therapy for appropriate second choices of antibiotics for patients who fail initial therapy.[6] Because gram-negative pathogens may contribute to acute exacerbations in patients with severe COPD[226] and are found commonly in the airways of patients intubated for COPD-related respiratory failure,[252] patients at high risk for treatment failure or with respiratory failure may benefit from broad-spectrum antibiotics.[252-254]

Oxygen is administered to all patients hospitalized for acute exacerbations. Patients with hypercapnia are at risk for developing increasing respiratory acidosis on the basis of oxygen-induced alterations in $\dot{V}/\dot{Q}$ and depressed respiratory drive. Oxygen is titrated to minimize its effects on $PaCO_2$ without a sacrifice in the oxygenation goal of therapy, which is to maintain a PaO_2 of 60 mm Hg (Figure 47-11).[136]

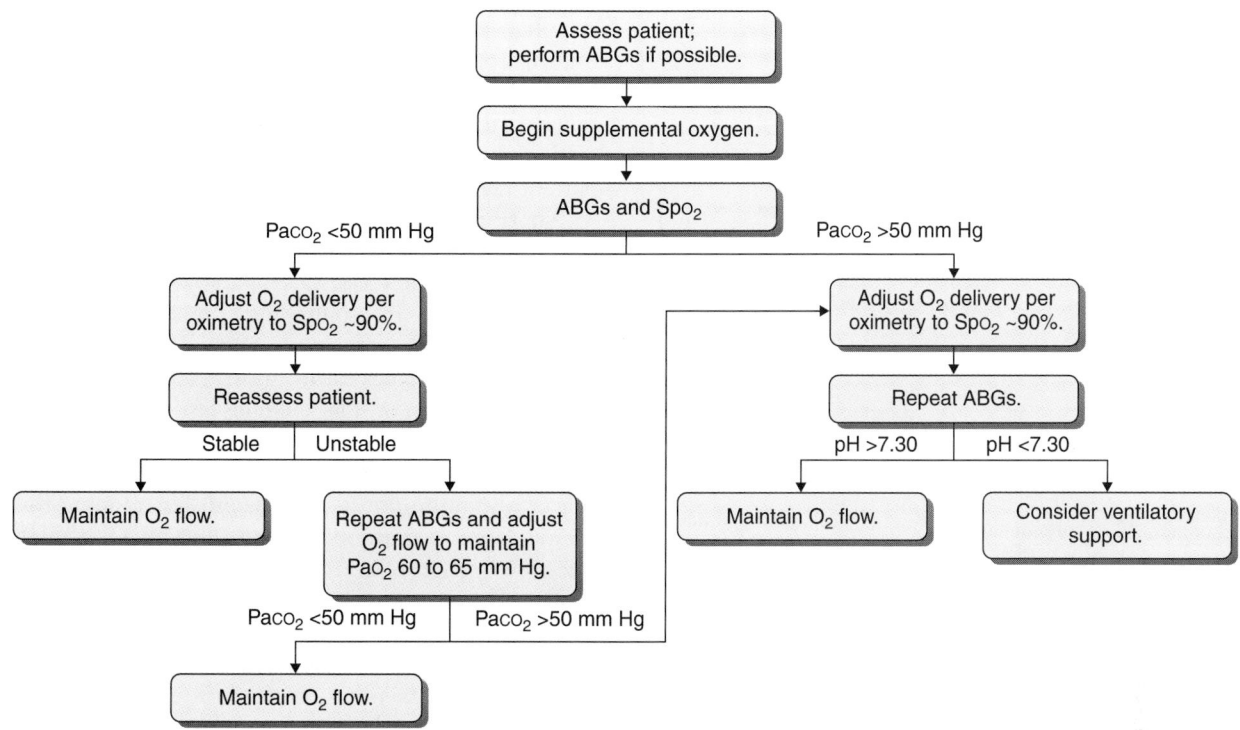

Figure 47-11 Algorithm for the management of supplemental oxygen in patients hospitalized for an acute exacerbation. *ABGs,* Arterial blood gases; *Spo₂,* arterial oxygen saturation by pulse oximetry; *Paco₂,* partial pressure of arterial carbon dioxide.

Multiple clinical trials have examined the utility of NPPV for the management of respiratory failure related to acute exacerbations of COPD.[255-260] Most,[256-260] but not all,[255] studies have demonstrated benefit from the use of NPPV for various endpoints that include hospital survival, 6-month survival, and avoidance of intubation. A meta-analysis of existing studies concluded that patients with COPD treated with NPPV had a lower mortality rate and incidence of progressing to the need of intubation and mechanical ventilation.[261] Specific indications for the use of NPPV for acute respiratory failure related to COPD have not been established.[262] Some experts recommend the initiation of noninvasive support when the respiratory rate is greater than 30 breaths/min and the pH is below 7.35.[263]

Patients with respiratory failure that appears immediately life-threatening as characterized by severe hypoxemia, hypercapnia, hemodynamic instability, altered mental status, or increased work of breathing with impending apnea require intubation and mechanical ventilation. Also, patients who fail to improve with NPPV are identified early and semi-urgently intubated. Either nasotracheal or orotracheal routes of intubation are appropriate although increasing consensus favors the orotracheal route so as to avoid nasal obstruction and nosocomial sinusitis.[264,265] The nasotracheal route also requires a smaller caliber endotracheal tube as compared with the oral route, which may impede weaning efforts by an increase in airway resistance[266] and a decrease in the efficiency of aerosol delivery.[267] For these reasons, patients intubated through the nasotracheal route are often converted to oral intubation after 24 hours of stabilization. The early complications of intubation (Box 47-7) depend on operator experience.[268]

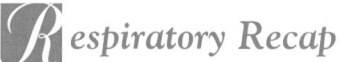

espiratory Recap

Goals of Mechanical Ventilation in the Patient with COPD

Avoid auto-PEEP.
Prevent overdistention.
Prevent overventilation and respiratory alkalosis.
Prevent patient-ventilator dyssynchrony.
Assess for continued need for mechanical ventilation; wean and extubate when respiratory failure has resolved.

Figure 47-12 presents an algorithmic approach to the initiation of mechanical ventilation for patients with COPD. Because of their increased airway resistance and lung compliance, intubated patients with COPD are at risk for air trapping, which produces discomfort and patient-ventilator dyssynchrony. Pressure ventilation, in contrast to volume ventilation, appears to prevent dyssynchrony, lowers peak airway and alveolar pressures, and decreases the likelihood of alveolar overdistention.[269,270] This benefit results from the variable inspiratory flow provided

Major Immediate Complications of Orotracheal and Nasotracheal Intubation

Both Intubation Routes	Orotracheal Intubation	Nasotracheal Intubation
Esophageal intubation	Oral trauma	Epistaxis
Failure to intubate	Soft tissues	Bacteremia
Emesis-aspiration	Dental	Dislodged adenoids; glottic injury to tonsils
Perforated esophagus		Tube kinking
Perforated pharynx		Turbinate trauma
Hypoxemia		
Cardiac dysrhythmias		

From Heffner JE. Tracheal intubation in mechanically ventilated patients. Clin Chest Med 1988;9:23-35.

by pressure ventilation that matches the patient's inspiratory efforts.[271] Pressure ventilation is available as either pressure support or pressure control. Special caution is required in the use of pressure support ventilation in patients with COPD and extreme airway obstruction because airway flow is used by most pressure support ventilators to cycle from inspiration to expiration. Because flow deceleration may be extremely slow near end-inspiration in these patients, inspiratory time may be prolonged, requiring patients to actively exhale to cycle the ventilator.[272] This problem can be circumvented with pressure control ventilation that is set to maintain the inspiratory time between 0.8 to 1.2 seconds and allow patient triggering (set rate less than 6 breaths/min) so as to terminate the inspiratory cycle early.[271]

The goals in the selection of a mode of ventilation for patients with COPD center on the provision of sufficient unloading of respiratory muscles to prevent or reverse fatigue but not to maintain a degree of ventilatory work so as to avoid respiratory muscle atrophy.[271] The assist-control mode of ventilation provides the greatest degree of respiratory muscle unloading[273] and may be appropriate as pressure-control ventilation for extremely fatigued patients during the first 24 hours of ventilatory support when respiratory muscle fatigue is at its worst.[274] Synchronized intermittent mandatory ventilation (SIMV) is intended to alternate mandatory breaths that provide muscle rest with spontaneous breaths that require patient effort. It has been demonstrated, however, that significant work is required during both the mandatory and spontaneous breaths in SIMV modes of ventilation.[275] This work can be diminished with the addition of pressure support.[273] Patients with COPD, therefore, are managed with pressure support when the SIMV mode of ventilation is used.

Regardless of the mode of ventilation selected, it is important to provide short inspiratory times to prevent air trapping in patients with COPD. Short inspiratory times improve pulmonary mechanics and gas exchange by decreasing measured dead space and shunt through enhanced alveolar emptying.[276] Shorter inspiratory times may result in increased respiratory rates[277] that may require patient sedation to control.

Air trapping is prevented by the prevention of excessive tidal volumes and the maintenance of transpulmonary pressures below 30 cm H_2O. In patients with normal chest wall compliance, transpulmonary pressures of 30 cm H_2O occur with plateau airway pressures of 35 cm H_2O. These goals can be achieved in most patients with COPD through selection of tidal volumes less than 8 mL/kg. The detection of high plateau pressures or auto-PEEP may require adjustment of the ventilator to lower tidal volumes. Lower respiratory rates also prevent air trapping through an increase in expiratory time to allow alveolar emptying. Excessively high respiratory rates, in addition to promoting alveolar overdistention, may lower $PaCO_2$ below baseline levels in patients with chronic respiratory failure, delaying weaning from mechanical ventilation if renal compensation lowers base buffer stores. During the first 24 hours of mechanical ventilation, patients may benefit from controlled ventilation with higher respiratory rates to provide respiratory muscle rest, but auto-PEEP and high transpulmonary pressures must be avoided.

Inspired oxygen concentrations in ventilated patients with COPD are administered with the goal to maintain oxygen saturation above 90% and PaO_2 above 55 mm Hg. Increasing FIO_2 to needed levels to maintain oxygenation does not alter dead space, respiratory drive, or $PaCO_2$.[278]

Applied PEEP may benefit some ventilated patients with COPD who are experiencing auto-PEEP. The application of PEEP at a level less than or equal to 85% of auto-PEEP may decrease auto-PEEP, expiratory resistance, and the amount of patient effort to trigger the ventilator without increasing peak alveolar pressure.[279,280] To achieve these benefits, PEEP is adjusted to improve patient comfort and decrease auto-PEEP, but applied PEEP is kept less than or equal to 85% of auto-PEEP, or 10 cm H_2O. Patients are carefully monitored to be certain that applied PEEP does not increase the level of measured auto-PEEP, which would indicate the presence of worsening hyperinflation.

In preparation for weaning of patients with COPD, completion of a "weaning checklist" is required to determine readiness for weaning (Box 47-8). Appropriate weaning candidates are then evaluated with weaning parameters to measure pulmonary mechanics and respiratory muscle strength. Multiple weaning parameters are available that have different clinical applications and relative diagnostic accuracies.[281] The rapid shallow breathing index (RSBI = respiratory rate ÷ VT in liters) is the most accurate predictor of successful weaning in general populations of patients with respiratory failure.[281,282] A value for RSBI below 105 increases the probability of a successful wean.

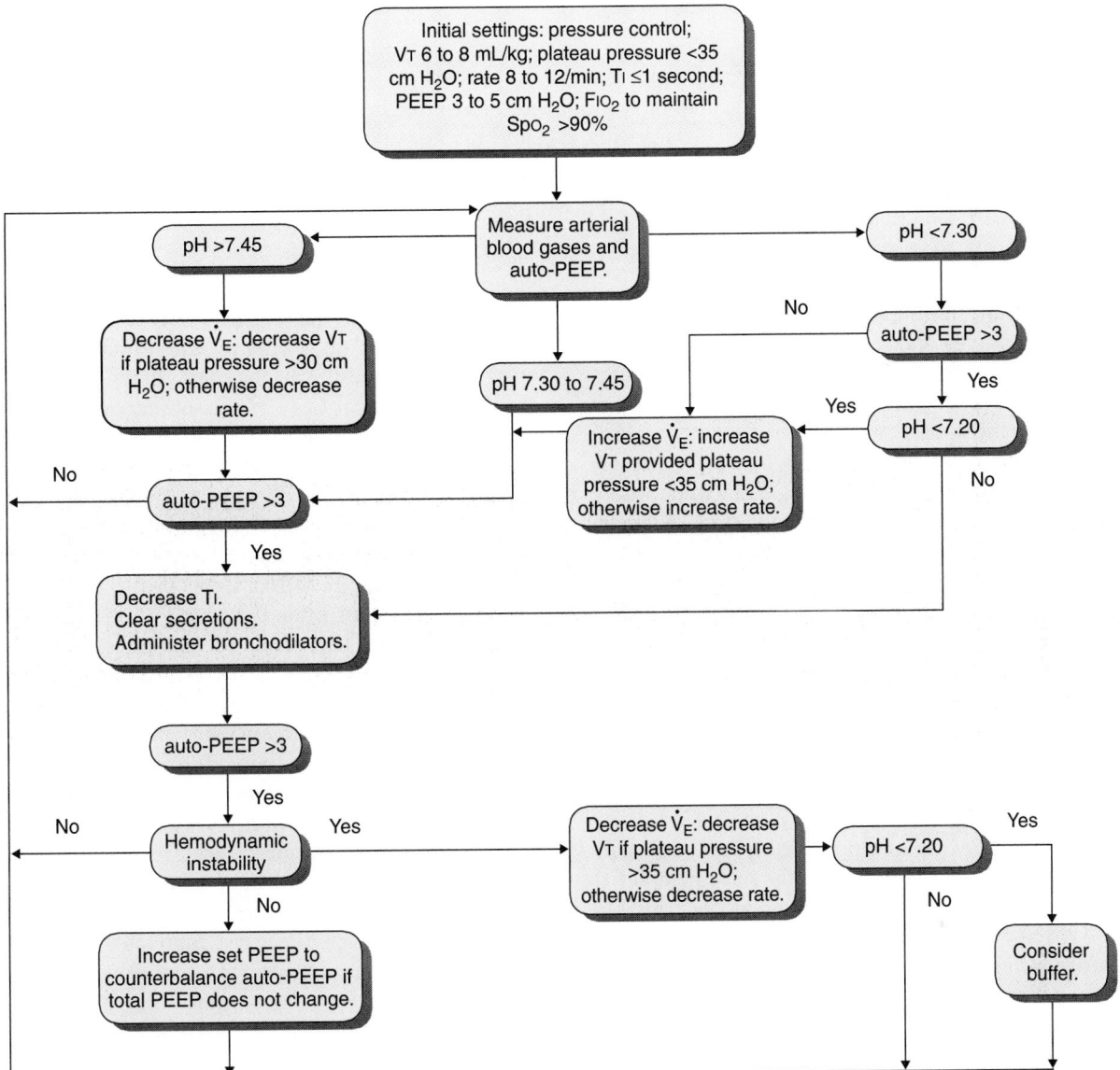

Figure 47-12 Algorithm for the initiation of mechanical ventilation for patients with chronic obstructive pulmonary disease (COPD). (Modified from Hess DR, Medoff BD. Mechanical ventilation of the patient with chronic obstructive pulmonary disease. Respir Care Clin N Am 1998;4:439-473.)

Large-scale studies have not examined the comparative benefit of different weaning techniques in ventilator-dependent patients with COPD. Recent prospective randomized studies in general populations of ventilator-dependent patients, however, reported the highest rates of success with trials of spontaneous breathing[283] or pressure support weaning.[284]

There are several causes for failure to wean from mechanical ventilation (Box 47-9). Identification of these factors and delaying weaning until the patient improves prevents an aggravation in respiratory muscle fatigue. Prolonged weaning failure presents considerations of a tracheostomy. Conversion of a translaryngeal endotracheal tube to a tracheostomy increases patient comfort, provides easier access for suctioning, enhances patient mobility, and may allow a more aggressive weaning approach.[285,286] Pa-

tients also may have an improved sense of well-being because of the ability to speak with a tracheostomy in place.[287,288] No data indicate that a tracheostomy must be performed after any specific duration of translaryngeal intubation. Patients with COPD are selected for tracheostomy after an initial 7 days of mechanical ventilation if successful weaning is not imminent.[285] Earlier tracheostomy can be considered if the seriousness of the illness makes extubation unlikely within a reasonable time. Considering that most of the benefits of tracheostomy are comfort related, it is less compelling to perform an early tracheostomy in patients with depressed mental status who are otherwise tolerating translaryngeal intubation well. The decision for tracheostomy should be based on the individual needs of a specific patient rather than general guidelines that direct routine tracheotomy only after 21 days of intubation.[289]

Ethical Considerations and End-of-Life Care

The progressive nature of COPD, which affects older age groups and often ends with a terminal episode of respiratory failure and ventilator dependency, presents clinicians with challenging ethical dilemmas.[234,290] Most patients hospitalized for acute exacerbations of COPD survive to hospital discharge irrespective of the occurrence of respiratory failure.[291,292] A subgroup of patients, however, presents with acute respiratory failure as the terminal event in their disease. Intubation and life-support are burdensome for this latter group of patients and may only prolong their dying process. Unfortunately, clinical and laboratory findings available at the time of admission are poor discriminators between those patients who will survive their hospitalization and those who will not recover.[234] In such circumstances, decisions about the withholding and withdrawal of life support are aided by clinicians having a clear understanding of their patients' end-of-life wishes. Patients can formulate their own decisions about the acceptability of life support by blending their life goals and values with their physicians' estimates of anticipated outcome from life support interventions. This process centers on a patient's ability to provide informed decision-making and requires an ongoing dialogue between patients, families, and caregivers.

Less than 20% of patients with moderate to severe COPD enrolled in pulmonary rehabilitation programs have discussed end-of-life advance planning or their wishes regarding the acceptability of life support with their physicians.[293] Also, only 42% of patients have completed written advance directives, such as living wills or durable powers of attorney for health care, even though 89% of patients desire information on end-of-life planning.[293] Consequently, less than 15% of patients with moderate to severe COPD have confidence that their longtime physicians understand their end-of-life wishes.[293]

Nonphysician educators can supplement physician discussions on end-of-life issues to promote patients' abilities to provide informed decisions.[290] Nurses, for instance, often have heightened sensitivities to their patients' needs and greater opportunities than physicians for discussing emotionally charged issues, such as advance planning.[294] Although not yet studied, end-of-life discussions initiated by respiratory therapists may effectively introduce patients with COPD to topics of life support and advance planning during hospitalizations, home visits, and enrollment in pulmonary rehabilitation. Patients have demonstrated that they are willing to learn about advance planning from a wide range of nonphysician sources.[295] The Society of Critical Care Medicine encourages all members of the health care team, physicians and nonphysicians alike, to initiate discussions with their patients about end-of-life issues.[296]

Patients indicate that they are more interested in receiving information on advance planning in the outpatient clinic during periods of stable health rather than during hospitalizations when the need for life support appears imminent.[293,295] The ATS[297] recommends that education about end-of-life issues occur during periods of stable health. An ideal opportunity for such educational programs exists in conjunction with pulmonary rehabilitation. Unfortunately, less than 8% of pulmonary rehabilitation programs provide information on advance planning even though 72% of nonphysician program directors would favor adding end-of-life education into their curricula.[295] A recent study indicates that a brief self-education program supplemented with videotapes promotes the adoption of advance directives, motivates patients to initiate end-of-life discussions with their physicians, and increases the proportion of patients who have confidence that their primary physicians understand their wishes regarding the acceptability of life support.[298]

Box 47-8

Weaning Checklist to Determine Patient's Readiness for Weaning

> The underlying cause of respiratory failure is corrected
> Respiratory muscle fatigue has resolved
> Respiratory depressant drugs are no longer needed
> Mental status has improved to baseline status
> Patient education and reassurance regarding weaning has controlled "weaning anxiety"
> Major organ failure is not present
> Nutritional support is tailored to the patient's caloric needs
> Electrolyte balance is achieved
> Adequate gas exchange is achieved ($FIO_2 \geq 0.50$; PEEP ≤ 5 cm H_2O; $\dot{V}_E \leq 12$ L/min; pH ≥ 7.35 at baseline $PaCO_2$)

FIO_2, Fractional inspired oxygen concentration; PEEP, positive end-expiratory pressure; $\dot{V}_E$, minute ventilation; $PaCO_2$, partial pressure of arterial carbon dioxide.

Box 47-9

Common Reasons for Failure to Wean from Mechanical Ventilation

> Patient was not ready to wean for following reason(s):
>   Electrolyte disturbances
>   Organ failures
>   Depressed mental status
>   Infection, fever, or sepsis
>   Bronchospasm
>   Copious airway secretions
> Auto-PEEP increases work of breathing
> Respiratory fatigue develops from overly aggressive weaning or excessive resistance of the ventilatory circuit including artificial airway
> Respiratory muscle weakness resulting from corticosteroid, paralytic agent, or aminoglycoside therapy
> Overfeeding or underfeeding
> Left ventricular failure or myocardial ischemia during weaning

PEEP, Positive end-expiratory pressure.

In preparing to discuss end-of-life issues, caregivers should recognize that most patients want explicit information about the probability of benefiting from life support related to the severity of their lung disease and their specific clinical circumstances. Without this information, patients tend to have overly optimistic impressions of the probability of surviving life support and resuming their pretreatment quality of life.[293,299] When patients receive information regarding anticipated survival and posttreatment quality of life, they often alter their wishes and choose less aggressive terminal care (Figure 47-13).[293] Appropriately informed patients are more capable of preparing detailed advance directives, which are more compelling and more likely to be followed by their physicians.[300]

The manner by which patients can best be informed and educated regarding end-of-life care has not been extensively studied.[301] Self-directed questionnaires can effectively assess patients' life values and interests for life support in various clinical settings and prepare them for informed discussion with their physicians.[299,302] Better caregiver training is required to prevent the presentation of biased end-of-life therapeutic recommendations that influence patients' decisions.[303] Physicians tend to use medical jargon, fail to present quantitative information about likely outcomes, and often fail to explore patients' life goals and values when they discuss the value of life support and terminal care.[304,305]

Patients with severe COPD who choose to forego life supportive care in the terminal phases of their disease must be continuously reassured by all caregivers that they will not be medically or emotionally abandoned.[294] Intensive comfort care and close monitoring to detect a need for aggressive pain, anxiety, and dyspnea relief are fundamentally important. In such settings, the principle of "double-effect" ethically, morally, and legally allows the administration of sufficient sedatives and analgesics to relieve pain and suffering even if drug therapy accelerates the patient's death.[306] Alternatives to acute care hospitalization do exist for patients with terminal COPD. COPD is recognized as a condition warranting hospice services by the National Hospice Organization, which has published guidelines to identify patients who qualify for hospice care (Box 47-10).[307]

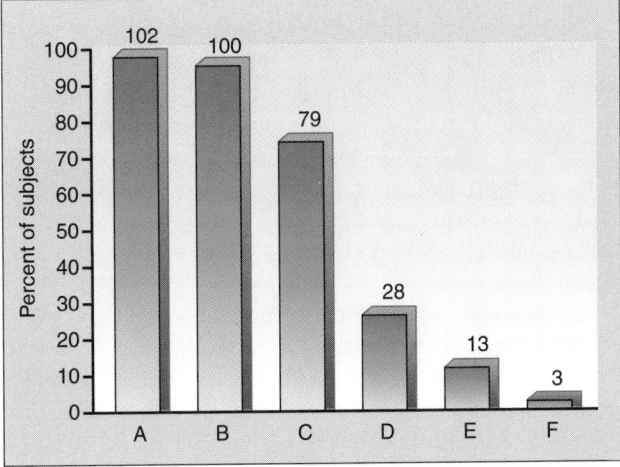

Figure 47-13 Willingness of patients with chronic obstructive pulmonary disease (COPD) to accept intubation and mechanical ventilation based on likely survival outcome. Numbers above each bar indicate the number of subjects who desired life-support at each likelihood of survival. The hypothetical survival likelihoods were as follows: *A* = a very good likelihood of survival, *B* = a quite reasonable likelihood, *C* = a fair likelihood, *D* = a poor likelihood, *E* = a very poor likelihood, *F* = subjects who would not accept life support regardless of the likelihood of survival. (Modified from Heffner JE, Fahy B, Hilling L, et al. Attitudes regarding advance directives among patients in pulmonary rehabilitation. Am J Respir Crit Care Med 1996; 154:1735.)

$\mathcal{B}$OX 47-10

Parameters to Identify Patients Who Qualify for Hospice Services

1. Severity of chronic lung disease documented by the following:
   a. Disabling dyspnea at rest, poorly responsive or unresponsive to bronchodilators, resulting in decreased functional activity, for example, bed-to-chair existence, often exacerbated by other debilitating symptoms such as fatigue and cough FEV_1 after bronchodilator, less than 30% of predicted, is helpful supplemental objective evidence but should not be required if not already available
   b. Progressive pulmonary disease
      (1) Increasing visits to the emergency department or hospitalizations for pulmonary infections and/or respiratory failure
      (2) Decrease in FEV_1 on serial testing of greater than 40 ml per year is helpful supplemental objective evidence but should not be required if not already available
2. Presence of cor pulmonale or right heart failure
   a. These should be the result of advanced pulmonary disease, not primary or secondary to left heart disease or valvulopathy
   b. Cor pulmonale may be documented by the following:
      (1) Echocardiography
      (2) Electrocardiogram
      (3) Chest x-ray film
      (4) Physical signs of right heart failure
3. Hypoxemia at rest on supplemental oxygen
   a. Pao_2 ≤55 mm Hg on supplemental oxygen
   b. Oxygen saturation ≤88% on supplemental oxygen
4. Hypercapnia ($Paco_2$ ≥50 mm Hg)
5. Unintentional progressive weight loss of greater than 10% of body weight over the preceding 6 months
6. Resting tachycardia greater than 100/minute in a patient with known severe chronic obstructive pulmonary disease

From Stuart B, Alexander C, Arenella C, et al. Medical guidelines for determining prognosis in selected non-cancer diseases. 2nd ed. Arlington, Va: The National Hospice Organization; 1996. pp. 10-11.

CASE STUDIES

Case One
Initial Presentation of Chronic Obstructive Pulmonary Disease

During a routine physical examination, a 62-year-old woman complains of increasing shortness of breath with exertion. She has a 40-year smoking history and presently smokes one pack of filtered cigarettes per day. She reports occasional nonproductive cough. Physical examination reveals bilateral breath sounds with no adventitious sounds. Respiratory rate and pattern are normal at rest. No cyanosis or edema is present, and the remainder of the history and physical examination are unremarkable. She is referred to the pulmonary clinic for consultation, pulmonary function testing, and arterial blood gas analysis.

Results of pulmonary function testing are a FVC of 2.10 L (80% predicted), FEV_1 1.20 L (65% predicted), and FEV_1/FVC 58%. After administration of inhaled β-agonist, the FEV_1 increases to 1.35 L. Lung volumes (residual volume [RV], functional residual capacity [FRC], and total lung capacity [TLC]) reveal mild hyperinflation. Single-breath $D_{L}CO$ is 70% of predicted. Arterial blood gases on the breathing of room air are pH 7.42, $PaCO_2$ 39 mm Hg, and PaO_2 72 mm Hg. A chest x-ray film is unremarkable other than giving the suggestion of mild hyperinflation.

The patient is referred to a smoking-cessation program. She receives influenza and pneumococcal vaccinations. Ipratropium bromide (Atrovent) is prescribed, 2 puffs qid. Albuterol (Proventil) is also prescribed, 2 puffs prn. She is instructed in the proper use of the inhalers with a valved spacer (Aerochamber). Pulmonary rehabilitation is deferred at this time. She is scheduled for a follow-up at 6 months in the pulmonary clinic.

Case Two
Acute Exacerbation of Chronic Obstructive Pulmonary Disease

A 72-year-old male with a history of COPD is admitted to the emergency department with progressively increasing dyspnea over the past 48 hours. He uses continuous home oxygen at 2 L/min. He also uses inhaled ipratropium and albuterol by MDI. His sputum became purulent 3 days ago,

and his primary care physician prescribed antibiotic therapy (tetracycline). The patient has a respiratory rate of 30/min with use of accessory muscles and pursed lip exhalation. Breath sounds are distant, but no adventitious sounds are present. The chest is hyperinflated. Mild neck vein distention and ankle edema are present. The ECG is normal with the exception of a mild tachycardia (110/min). The patient appears dyspneic, but he cooperates with the physical examination. An arterial blood gas is obtained with the patient breathing oxygen at 2 L/min: pH 7.28, $PaCO_2$ 78 mm Hg, and PaO_2 52 mm Hg.

Noninvasive ventilation is initiated. An oronasal mask is necessary because of the patient's dyspnea and inability to maintain a closed mouth. Pressure ventilation is used and the inspiratory pressure is titrated to 16 cm H_2O, which results in decreased accessory muscle use, a decrease in the respiratory rate, and improvement in dyspnea reported by the patient. Missed trigger efforts are noted and attributed to the presence of auto-PEEP. The expiratory pressure (PEEP) is titrated up to 6 cm H_2O, at which every inspiratory effort of the patient triggers the ventilator. Inspired oxygen is titrated to maintain a SpO_2 of 88% to 90%. Preparations are made to admit him to the ICU.

Two hours later, the patient is in the ICU. He continues on noninvasive ventilation, but appears more comfortable. A nebulizer treatment has been administered with albuterol and ipratropium. Arterial blood gases at this time are pH 7.36, $PaCO_2$ 65 mm Hg, PaO_2 66 mm Hg. Four hours later, the patient asks to have the mask removed. He initially appears comfortable, but after 1 hour he has increasing dyspnea and accessory muscle use. Noninvasive ventilation is resumed at the previous settings, but with the use of a nasal mask instead of the oronasal mask. This pattern of failed attempts to discontinue noninvasive ventilation continues for the next 36 hours, at which time he remains comfortable after removal of the mask. Six hours after discontinuation of noninvasive ventilation, his arterial blood gases breathing 2 L/min of oxygen by nasal cannula are pH 7.37, $PaCO_2$ 60 mm Hg, and PaO_2 62 mm Hg. The patient is transferred from the ICU to a general ward.

The following day, he continues to do well and plans are made for discharge home. Options related to future exacerbations are discussed with the patient and his wife. He decides that noninvasive ventilation may be used for future exacerbations, but that he will not be intubated or receive other resuscitative measures.

KEY POINTS

- Chronic obstructive pulmonary disease is the fourth most common cause of death in the United States, and its prevalence is increasing worldwide.
- Chronic bronchitis, asthmatic bronchitis, and emphysema are the lung conditions categorized as COPD. The clinical expressions of these disorders tend to merge with increasing severity of disease, so patients are usually described as having COPD rather than any one of these three more specific conditions.
- Smoking is the overwhelmingly predominant cause of COPD. The prognosis of this progressive disorder is improved at any age with smoking cessation.
- Airflow limitation with decreased ventilatory reserve is the major pathophysiologic consequence of COPD. The multiple factors that contribute to airflow limitation include loss of airway tethering because of decreased elastic recoil of the lung parenchyma, airway secretions, changes in the properties of lining fluid, smooth muscle contraction, mucous gland hypertrophy, and airway inflammation.
- The management of patients with COPD is directed toward a reduction in symptoms and an improvement in quality of life, reducing decline in lung function, preventing complications, preventing or minimizing adverse effects of therapy, and prolonging survival.
- End-of-life planning is an important component in the management of patients with all stages of COPD.

References

1. Ball P, Make B. Acute exacerbations of chronic bronchitis: an international comparison. Chest 1998;113:199S-204S.
2. Murray CLJ, Lopez A. Evidence-based health policy: lessons from the global burden of diseases study. Science 1996;274:740-743.
3. Petty TL. Lung cancer and chronic obstructive pulmonary disease. Med Clin North Am 1996;80:645-655.
4. Rosamond ED, Chambless DE, Folsom AR, et al. Trends in the incidence of myocardial infarction and in mortality due to coronary heart disease, 1987 to 1994. N Engl J Med 1998;339:861-867.
5. Speizer FE. The rise in chronic obstructive pulmonary disease mortality: overview and summary. Am Rev Respir Dis 1989;140:S106-S107.
6. Siafakas NM, Vermeire P, Pride NB, et al. Optimal assessment and management of chronic obstructive pulmonary disease (COPD). Eur Respir J 1995;8:1398-1420.
7. Celli BR, et al. Standards for the diagnosis and care of patients with chronic obstructive pulmonary disease (COPD) and asthma. Am J Respir Crit Care Med 1995;154:1-20.
8. American Thoracic Society. Lung function testing: selection of reference values and interpretative strategies. Am Rev Respir Dis 1991;144:1201-1218.
9. US Department of Health and Human Services. The health consequences of smoking: chronic obstructive pulmonary disease. DHHS publication no: (PHS) 84-50205. Rockville, Md: US Department of Health and Human Services, Public Health Service, Office of Smoking; 1984.
10. Buist AS, Vollmer WM, Wu Y, et al. Effects of cigarette smoking on lung function in four population samples in the People's Republic of China: The PRC-US Cardiovascular and Cardiopulmonary Epidemiology Research Group. Am J Respir Crit Care Med 1995;151:1393-1400.
11. Burrows B, Bloom JW, Traver GA, et al. The course and prognosis of different forms of chronic airways obstruction in a sample from the general population. N Engl J Med 1987;317:1309-1314.
12. Burrows B. The course and prognosis of different types of chronic airflow limitation in a general population sample from Arizona: comparison with the Chicago "COPD" series. Am Rev Respir Dis 1989;140:S92-S94.
13. Burrows B, Lebowitz MD, Barbee RA, et al. Interactions of smoking and immunologic factors in relation to airways obstruction. Chest 1983;84:657-661.
14. Higgins MW, Enright PL, Kronmal RA, et al. Smoking and lung function in elderly men and women. The Cardiovascular Health Study. JAMA 1993;269:2741-2748.
15. Higgins M. Risk factors associated with chronic obstructive lung disease. Ann NY Acad Sci 1991;624:7-17.
16. Stanescu D, Sanna A, Veriter C, et al. Identification of smokers susceptible to development of chronic airflow limitation: a 13-year follow-up. Chest 1998;114:416-425.
17. Wiedemann HP, Stoller JK. Lung disease due to alpha-1-antitrypsin deficiency. Curr Opin Pulm Med 1996;2:155-160.
18. Silverman EK, Chapman HA, Drazen JM, et al. Genetic epidemiology of severe, early-onset chronic obstructive pulmonary disease: risk to relatives for airflow obstruction and chronic bronchitis. Am J Respir Crit Care Med 1998;157:1770-1778.
19. Silverman EK, Pierce JA, Province MA, et al. Variability of pulmonary function in alpha-1-antitrypsin deficiency: clinical correlates. Ann Intern Med 1989;111:982-991.
20. O'Connor GT, Sparrow P, Weiss ST. The role of allergy and nonspecific airway hyperresponsiveness in the pathogenesis of chronic obstructive pulmonary disease. Am Rev Respir Dis 1989;140:225-232.
21. Coultas DB. Passive smoking and risk of adult asthma and COPD: an update. Thorax 1998;1998:381-387.
22. Burrows B, Knudson RJ, Lebowitz MD. The relationship of childhood respiratory illness to adult obstructive airway disease. Am Rev Respir Dis 1977;115:751-760.
23. Behera D, Jindal SK. Respiratory symptoms in Indian women using domestic cooking fuels. Chest 1991;100:385-388.
24. Tager IB, Segal MR, Munoz A, et al. The effect of maternal cigarette smoking on the pulmonary function of children and adolescents: analysis of data from two populations. Am Rev Respir Dis 1987;136:1366-1370.
25. Bates DV. Detection of chronic respiratory bronchiolitis in oxidant-exposed populations: analogy to tobacco smoke exposure. Environ Health Perspect 1993;101(Suppl 4):217-218.
26. Jeffery PK. Comparative morphology of the airways in asthma and chronic obstructive pulmonary disease. Am J Respir Crit Care Med 1994;150:S6-S13.
27. Lacoste J-Y, Bousquet J, Chanez P, et al. Eosinophilic and neutrophilic inflammation in asthma, chronic bronchitis, and chronic obstructive pulmonary disease. J Allergy Clin Immunol 1993;92:537-548.

28. Hogg JC, Wright JL, Wiggs BR, et al. Lung structure and function in cigarette smokers. Thorax 1994;49:473-478.

29. Cosio MG, Hale KA, Niewoehner DE. Morphologic and morphometric effects of prolonged cigarette smoking on the small airways. Am Rev Respir Dis 1980;122:265-271.

30. Wright JL, Hobson JE, Wiggs B, et al. Airway inflammation and peribronchiolar attachments in the lungs of nonsmokers, current and ex-smokers. Lung 1988;166:277-286.

31. Saetta M, Shiner RJ, Angus GE, et al. Destructive index: a measurement of lung parenchymal destruction in smokers. Am Rev Respir Dis 1985;131:764-769.

32. Arora NS, Rochester DF. COPD and human diaphragm muscle dimensions. Chest 1987;91:719-724.

33. Wright JL, Churg A. Effect of long-term cigarette smoke exposure on pulmonary vascular structure and function in the guinea pig. Exp Lung Res 1991;17:997-1009.

34. Musk AW. Relation of pulmonary vessel size to transfer factor in subjects with airflow obstruction. AJR Am J Roentgenol 1983;141:915-918.

35. Di Stefano A, Capelli A, Lusuardi M, et al. Severity of airflow limitation is associated with severity of airway inflammation in smokers. Am J Respir Crit Care Med 1998;158:1277-1285.

36. Nagai A, Yamawaki I, Takizawa T, et al. Alveolar attachments in emphysema of human lungs. Am Rev Respir Dis 1991;144:888-891.

37. Postma DS, Slinter HJ. Prognosis of chronic obstructive pulmonary disease: the Dutch experience. Am Rev Respir Dis 1989;1989:100-105.

38. Snider GL. Chronic obstructive pulmonary disease: a definition and implications of structural determinants of airflow obstruction for epidemiology. Am Rev Respir Dis 1989;140:S3-S8.

39. Mahler DA, Faryniarx K, Tomlinson D, et al. Impact of dyspnea and physiologic function on general health status in patients with chronic obstructive pulmonary disease. Chest 1992;102:395-401.

40. O'Donnell SE, Sanil R, Anthonisen NR, et al. Effect of dynamic airway compression on breathing pattern and respiratory sensation in severe chronic obstructive pulmonary disease. Am Rev Respir Dis 1987;135:912-918.

41. Del Vecchio L, Polese G, Poggi R, et al. "Intrinsic" positive end-expiratory pressure in stable patients with chronic obstructive pulmonary disease. Eur Respir J 1990;3:74-80.

42. Ninane V, Yernault JC, De Troyer A. Intrinsic PEEP in patients with chronic obstructive pulmonary disease. Am Rev Respir Dis 1993;148:1037-1042.

43. Greaves IA, Colebatch HJ. Elastic behavior and structure of normal and emphysematous lungs post mortem. Am Rev Respir Dis 1980;121:127-136.

44. Buist AS, Van Fleet DL, Ross BB. A comparison of conventional spirometric tests and the tests of closing volume in one emphysema screening center. Am Rev Respir Dis 1973;107:735-740.

45. Javaheri S, Blum J, Kazemi H. Pattern of breathing and carbon dioxide retention in chronic obstructive lung disease. Am J Med 1981;71:228-234.

46. Parot S, Miara B, Milic-Emili J, et al. Hypoxemia, hypercapnia, and breathing patterns in patients with chronic obstructive pulmonary disease. Am Rev Respir Dis 1982;126:882-886.

47. Anthonisen NR. Prognosis in chronic obstructive pulmonary disease. Results from multicenter clinical trials. Am Rev Respir Dis 1989;133:95-99.

48. Sharp JT. The respiratory muscles in emphysema. Clin Chest Med 1983;4:421-432.

49. Sharp JT, Beard GA, Sunga M, et al. The rib cage in normal and emphysematous subjects: a roentgenographic approach. J Appl Physiol 1986;61:2050-2059.

50. Rochester DF. The diaphragm contractile properties and fatigue. J Clin Invest 1985;75:1397-1402.

51. Sassoon CS, Te TT, Mahutte CR, et al. Airway occlusion pressure: an important indicator for successful weaning in patients with chronic obstructive pulmonary disease. Am Rev Respir Dis 1987;135:107-113.

52. Sears TA. Central rhythm and pattern generation. Chest 1990;97:455-515.

53. Martinez FJ, Couser JI, Celli BR. Factors influencing ventilatory muscle recruitment in patients with chronic airflow obstruction. Am Rev Respir Dis 1990;142:276-282.

54. Murciano D, Broczkowski J, Lecocguic M, et al. Tracheal occlusion pressure: a simple index to monitor respiratory muscle fatigue during acute respiratory failure in patients with chronic obstructive pulmonary disease. Ann Intern Med 1988;108:800-805.

55. Loveridge B, West P, Anthonisen NR, et al. Breathing patterns in patients with chronic obstructive pulmonary disease. Am Rev Respir Dis 1984;130:730-733.

56. Killian K, Jones N. Respiratory muscles and dyspnea. Clin Chest Med 1988;9:237-248.

57. Bellemare F, Grassino A. Force reserve of the diaphragm in patients with chronic obstructive pulmonary disease. J Appl Physiol 1983;55:8-15.

58. Burrows B. Course and prognosis of patients with chronic airways obstruction. Chest 1980;77:250-251.

59. Anthonisen NR, Connett JE, Kiley JP, et al. Effects of smoking intervention and the use of an inhaled anticholinergic bronchodilator on the rate of decline of FEV_1. The Lung Health Study. JAMA 1994;272:1497-1505.

60. Peto R, Speizer FE, Cochrane AL, et al. The relevance in adults of airflow obstruction, but not of mucus hypersecretion to mortality from chronic lung disease. Am Rev Respir Dis 1983;128:491-500.

61. Murphy TF, Sethi S. Bacterial infection in chronic obstructive pulmonary disease. Am Rev Respir Dis 1992;146:1067-1083.

62. Skillrund DM, Offord KP, Miller RD. Higher risk of lung cancer in chronic obstructive pulmonary disease: a prospective, matched controlled study. Ann Intern Med 1986;105:503-507.

63. Postma DS, Steenhuis EJ, van der Weele LT, et al. Severe chronic airflow obstruction: can corticosteroids slow down progression? Eur J Respir Dis 1985;67:56-64.

64. Tashkin DP, Altose MD, Bleecker ER, et al. The lung health study: airway responsiveness to inhaled methacholine in smokers with mild to moderate airflow limitation. The Lung Health Study Research Group. Am Rev Respir Dis 1992;145:301-310.

65. Rennard SI, Serby CW, Ghafouri M, et al. Extended therapy with ipratropium is associated with improved lung function in patients with COPD. Chest 1996;110:62-70.

66. Dompeling E, van Schayck C, van Grunsven P, et al. Slowing the deterioration of asthma and chronic obstructive pulmonary disease observed during bronchodilator therapy by adding inhaled corticosteroids: a 4-year prospective study. Ann Intern Med 1993;188:770-778.

67. Wedzicha JA. Inhaled corticosteroids in COPD: awaiting controlled trials. Thorax 1993;48:305-307.

68. Owens GR. The Lung Health Study. Curr Opin Pulm Med 1996;2:81-83.

69. Kerstkens HAM, Brand PLP, Pstma DS. Risk factors for accelerated decline among patients with chronic obstructive pulmonary disease. Am J Respir Crit Care Med 1996;154:S266-S272.

70. Fiore MC. How to prevent the progression of chronic bronchitis: the role of smoking cessation prevention. Monaldi Arch Chest Dis 1994;49:13-16.

71. US Department of Health and Human Services. Preventing tobacco use among young people: a report of the Surgeon General. Atlanta, Ga: US Department of Health and Human Services, Public Health Service, Centers for Disease Control and Prevention, Center for Chronic Disease Prevention and Health Promotion, Office on Smoking and Health; 1994.

72. Fiore MC. Trends in cigarette smoking in the United States: The epidemiology of tobacco use. Med Clin North Am 1992;76:289-303.

73. Prochaska JO, Goldstein MG. Process of smoking cessation. Clin Chest Med 1991;12:727-735.

74. Henningfield JE. Nicotine medications for smoking cessation. N Engl J Med 1995;333:1196-1203.

75. Law M, Tang J. An analysis of the effectiveness of interventions intended to help people stop smoking. Arch Intern Med 1995;155:1933-1941.

76. Hurt RD, Sachs DPL, Glover ED, et al. A comparison of sustained-release bupropion and placebo for smoking cessation. N Engl J Med 1997;337:1195-1202.

77. Friedman M. Changing practices in COPD. A new pharmacologic treatment algorithm. Chest 1995;107(Suppl):194S-197S.

78. Buist AS. The US Lung Health Study. Respirology 1997;2:303-307.

79. COMBIVENT Inhalation Aerosol Study Group. In chronic obstructive pulmonary disease, a combination of ipratropium bromide and albuterol is more effective than either agent alone: an 85-day multicenter trial. Chest 1994;105:1411-1419.

80. Shim C, Williams MH. The adequacy of inhalation of aerosol from canister nebulizers. Am J Med 1980;69:891-894.

81. Jenkins SC, Heaton RW, Fulton TJ, et al. Comparison of domiciliary nebulized salbutamol and salbutamol from a metered dose inhaler in stable chronic airflow limitation. Chest 1987;91:804-807.

82. Gross NJ. The influence of anticholinergic agents on treatment for bronchitis and emphysema. Am J Med 1991;91:11S-12S.

83. Gross NJ. Ipratropium bromide. N Engl J Med 1988;319:486-494.

84. Mann KV, Leon AL, Tietze KJ. Use of ipratropium bromide in obstructive lung disease. Clin Pharm 1988;7:670-680.

85. Easton PA, Jadue C, Dhingra S, et al. A comparison of the bronchodilating effects of a beta-2 adrenergic agent (albuterol) and an anticholinergic agent (ipratropium bromide), given by aerosol alone or in sequence. N Engl J Med 1986;315:735-739.

86. Nelson HS. Beta-adrenergic bronchodilators. N Engl J Med 1995;333:499-506.

87. Ikeda A, Nishimura K, Koyama H, et al. Bronchodilating effects of combined therapy with clinical dosages of ipratropium bromide and salbutamol for stable COPD: comparison with ipratropium bromide alone. Chest 1995;107:401-405.

88. Skorodin MS. Pharmacotherapy for asthma and chronic obstructive pulmonary disease. Current thinking, practices and controversies. Arch Intern Med 1993;153:814-828.

89. Murciano D, Auclair MH, Pariente R, et al. A randomized, controlled trial of theophylline in patients with severe chronic obstructive pulmonary disease. N Engl J Med 1989;320:1521-1525.

90. Ramsdell J. Use of theophylline in the treatment of COPD. Chest 1995;107:206S-209S.

91. Mahler DA, Matthay RA, Snyder PE, et al. Sustained-release theophylline reduces dyspnea in non-reversible obstructive airway disease. Am Rev Respir Dis 1985;131:22-25.

92. McKay SE, Howie CA, Thompson AH, et al. Value of theophylline treatment in patients handicapped by chronic obstructive lung disease. Thorax 1993;48:227-232.

93. Murciano D, Aubier MH, Lecocquic Y, et al. Effects of theophylline on diaphragmatic strength and fatigue in patients with chronic obstructive pulmonary disease. N Engl J Med 1984;311:349-353.

94. Sutton PP, Pavia D, Bateman JR, et al. The effect of oral aminophylline on lung mucociliary clearance in man. Chest 1981;80:889-892.

95. Matthay RA, Berger HJ, Davies R, et al. Improvement in cardiac performance by oral long-acting theophylline in chronic obstructive pulmonary disease. Am Heart J 1982;104:1022-1026.

96. Rogers RM, Owen GR, Penncock BE. The pendulum swings again: towards a rational use of theophylline. Chest 1985;87:280-282.

97. Callahan C, Dittus RC, Katz BP. Oral corticosteroid therapy for patients with chronic obstructive pulmonary disease: a meta-analysis. Ann Intern Med 1991;114:216-223.

98. Paggiaro PL, Dahle R, Bakran I, et al. Multicentre randomised placebo-controlled trial of inhaled fluticasone propionate in patients with chronic obstructive pulmonary disease. International COPD Study Group. Lancet 1998;351:773-780.

99. Hochberg MC, Prashker MJ, Greenwald M, et al. Recommendations for the prevention and treatment of glucocorticoid-induced osteoporosis. Arthritis Rheum 1996;39:1791-1801.

100. Stradling JR, Nicholl CG, Cover D, et al. The effects of oral almitrine on pattern of breathing and gas exchange in patients with chronic obstructive pulmonary disease. Clin Sci 1984;66:435-442.

101. Magnussen H, Radenbach D, Kiwull-Schone H. The acute effect of a single oral dose of 200 mg almitrine on gas exchange in patients with chronic obstructive bronchitis and emphysema, bronchial asthma and lung fibrosis. Bull Eur Physiopathol Respir 1987;23(Suppl 11):211S-214S.

102. Winkelmann BR, Leinberger H, Hertrich FF, et al. Acute and chronic effects of low dose almitrine bismesylate in the treatment of chronic bronchitis and emphysema. Eur J Med 1992;1:469-481.

103. Stanley NN. Effects of almitrine bismesylate 100 mg daily for four weeks on respiratory regulation in patients with chronic bronchitis. Eur J Respir Dis Suppl 1986;146:635-639.

104. Yoshikawa T, Yamamoto H, Nishimura M, et al. Doxapram on blunted respiratory chemosensitivity to hypoxia in hypoxemic, chronic obstructive pulmonary disease. Jpn J Med 1987;26:194-202.

105. Rodman T, Fennelly JF, Kraft AJ. Effect of ethamivan on alveolar ventilation in patients with chronic lung disease. N Engl J Med 1962;267:1279-1285.

106. Sanders JS, Berman TM, Bartlett MM, et al. Increased hypoxic ventilatory drive due to administration of aminophylline in normal men. Chest 1980;78:279-282.

107. Germann P, Ziesche R, Leitner C, et al. Addition of nitric oxide to oxygen improves cardiopulmonary function in patients with severe COPD. Chest 1998;114:29-35.

108. Petty TL. The National Mucolytic Study. Results of a randomized, double-blind, placebo-controlled study of iodinated glycerol in chronic obstructive bronchitis. Chest 1990;97:75-83.

109. Oral N-acetylcysteine and exacerbation rates in patients with chronic bronchitis and severe airways obstruction. British Thoracic Society Research Committee. Thorax 1985;40:832-835.

110. Boman G, Backer U, Larsson S, et al. Oral acetylcysteine reduces exacerbation rate in chronic bronchitis: report of a trial organized by the Swedish Society for Pulmonary Diseases. Eur J Respir Dis 1983;64:405-415.

111. Hansen NC, Skriver A, Brorsen-Riis L, et al. Orally administered N-acetylcysteine may improve general well-being in patients with mild chronic bronchitis. Respir Med 1994;88:531-535.

112. Jackson IM, Barnes J, Cooksey P. Efficacy and tolerability of oral acetylcysteine (Fabrol) in chronic bronchitis: a double-blind placebo controlled study. J Int Med Res 1984;12:198-206.

113. Rasmussen JB, Glennow C. Reduction in days of illness after long-term treatment with N-acetylcysteine controlled-release tablets in patients with chronic bronchitis. Eur Respir J 1988;1:351-355.

114. Allegra L, Cordaro CI, Grassi C. Prevention of acute exacerbations of chronic obstructive bronchitis with carbocysteine lysine salt monohydrate: a multicenter, double-blind, placebo-controlled trial. Respiration 1996;63:174-180.

115. Millar AB, Pavia D, Agnew JE, et al. Effect of oral N-acetylcysteine on mucus clearance. Br J Dis Chest 1985;79:262-266.

116. Hudson TJ. Dornase in treatment of chronic bronchitis. Ann Pharmacother 1996;30:674-675.

117. Anzueto A, Jubran A, Ohar JA, et al. Effects of aerosolized surfactant in patients with stable chronic bronchitis: a prospective randomized controlled trial. JAMA 1997; 278:1426-1431.

118. Farncombe M, Chater S, Gillin A. The use of nebulized opioid for breathlessness: a chart review. Palliative Med 1994; 8:306-312.

119. O'Donnell DE. Breathlessness in patients with chronic airflow limitation: mechanisms and management. Chest 1994;106:904-912.

120. Schols AMWI, Slangen J, Volovics L, et al. Weight loss is a reversible factor in the prognosis of chronic obstructive pulmonary disease. Am J Respir Crit Care Med 1998;157:1791-1797.

121. Goldstein S, Askanazi J, Weissman C, et al. Energy expenditure in patients with chronic obstructive pulmonary disease. Chest 1987;91:222-224.

122. Barends EM, Schols AMWJ, Pannemans DLE, et al. Total free living energy expenditure in patients with severe chronic obstructive pulmonary disease. Am J Respir Crit Care Med 1997;155:549-554.

123. Goldstein SA, Thomashow BM, Kvetan V, et al. Nitrogen and energy relationships in malnourished patients with emphysema. Am Rev Respir Dis 1988;138:636-644.

124. Casaburi R, Carithers E, Tosolini J, et al. Randomized placebo controlled trial of growth hormone in severe COPD patients undergoing endurance exercise training. Am J Respir Crit Care Med 1997;155:A498.

125. Schols AMWJ, Soeters PB, Mostert R, et al. Physiologic effects of nutritional support and anabolic steroids in patients with chronic obstructive pulmonary disease. Am J Respir Crit Care Med 1995;152:1268-1274.

126. Ferreira IM, Verreschi IT, Nery LE, et al. The influence of 6 months of oral anabolic steroids on body mass and respiratory muscles in undernourished patients. Chest 1998;114:19-28.

127. Weitzenblum E, Mammosser M, Ehrhart M. Evolution of pulmonary hypertension in chronic obstructive pulmonary diseases. G Ital Cardiol 1984;14:33-38.

128. Klinger JR, Hill NS. Right ventricular dysfunction in chronic obstructive pulmonary disease. Evaluation and management. Chest 1991;99:715-723.

129. Weitzenblum E, Kessler R, Oswald M, et al. Medical treatment of pulmonary hypertension in chronic lung disease. Eur Respir J 1994;7:148-152.

130. Long term domiciliary oxygen therapy in chronic hypoxic cor pulmonale complicating chronic bronchitis and emphysema. Report of the Medical Research Council Working Party. Lancet 1981;1:681-686.

131. Nocturnal Oxygen Therapy Trial Group. Continuous or nocturnal oxygen therapy in hypoxemic chronic obstructive lung disease: a clinical trial. Ann Intern Med 1980;93:391-398.

132. Dean NC, Brown JK, Himelman RB, et al. Oxygen may improve dyspnea and endurance in patients with chronic obstructive pulmonary disease and only mild hypoxemia. Am Rev Respir Dis 1992;146:941-945.

133. Couser JI, Make BJ. Transtracheal oxygen decreases inspired minute ventilation. Am Rev Respir Dis 1989;139:627-663.

134. Tirlapur VG, Mir MA. Nocturnal hypoxemia and associated electrocardiographic changes in patients with chronic obstructive pulmonary disease. N Engl J Med 1982;306:125-130.

135. Heaton RK, Grant I, McSweeny AJ, et al. Psychologic effects of continuous and nocturnal oxygen therapy in hypoxemic chronic obstructive pulmonary disease. Arch Intern Med 1983;333:1196-1203.

136. Standards for the diagnosis and care of patients with chronic obstructive pulmonary disease. Am J Respir Crit Care Med 1995;152:S77-S120.

137. Tarpy SP, Celli BR. Long-term oxygen therapy. N Engl J Med 1995;333:710-714.

138. Tiep BL. Long-term oxygen therapy. Clin Chest Med 1990;11:505-521.

139. Orvidas LJ, Kasperbauer JL, Staats BA, et al. Long-term clinical experience with transtracheal oxygen catheters. Mayo Clin Proc 1998;73:739-744.

140. Aubier M, Murciano D, Fournier M, et al. Central respiratory drive in acute respiratory failure of patients with chronic obstructive pulmonary disease. Am Rev Respir Dis 1980;122:191-199.

141. O'Donahue WJ. Home oxygen therapy. Med Clin North Am 1996;80:611-622.

142. Gong H. Air travel and oxygen therapy in cardiopulmonary patients. Chest 1992;101:1104-1113.

143. Schwartz JS, Bencowitz HZ, Moser KM. Air travel hypoxemia with chronic obstructive pulmonary disease. Ann Intern Med 1984;100:473-477.

144. Vestbo J, Knudsen KM, Rasmussen FV. The value of mucus hypersecretion as a predictor of mortality and hospitalization: an 11-year register based follow-up study of a random population sample of 876 men. Respir Med 1988;83:207-211.

145. Simonds AK, Elliott MW. Outcome of domiciliary nasal intermittent positive pressure ventilation in restrictive and obstructive disorders. Thorax 1995;50:604-609.

146. Shapiro SH, Ernst P, Gray-Donald K, et al. Effect of negative pressure ventilation in severe chronic obstructive pulmonary disease. Lancet 1992;340:1425-1429.

147. Strumpf DA, Millman RP, Carlisle CC, et al. Nocturnal positive-pressure ventilation via nasal mask in patients with severe chronic obstructive pulmonary disease. Am Rev Respir Dis 1991; 144:1234-1239.

148. Lin CC. Comparison between nocturnal nasal positive pressure ventilation combined with oxygen therapy and oxygen montherapy in patients with severe COPD. Am J Respir Crit Care Med 1996;154:353-358.

149. Meecham Jones DJ, Paul EA, Jones PW, et al. Nasal pressure support ventilation plus oxygen compared with oxygen therapy alone in hypercapnic COPD. Am J Respir Crit Care Med 1995;152:538-544.

150. Muir JF, Cuvelier A, Tengang B, et al. Long-term home nasal intermittent positive ventilation (NIPPV) + oxygen therapy (LTOT) versus LTOT alone in severe hypercapnic COPD. Am J Respir Crit Care Med 1997;155:A408.

151. Wedzicha JA, Meecham Jones DJ. Domiciliary ventilation in chronic obstructive pulmonary disease: where are we? Thorax 1996;51:455-457.

152. Brown LK. Sleep-related disorders and chronic obstructive pulmonary disease. Respir Care Clin North Am 1998;4: 493-512.

153. Douglas NJ. Sleep in patients with chronic obstructive pulmonary disease. Clin Chest Med 1998;19:115-125.

154. Klink ME, Dodge R, Quan SF. The relation of sleep complaints to respiratory symptoms in a general population. Chest 1994;105:151-154.

155. Larsson LG, Lundback B, Jonsson E, et al. Are symptoms of obstructive sleep apnoea syndrome related to bronchitic symptoms or lung function impairment? Report from the Obstructive Lung Disease in Northern Sweden Study. Respir Med 1998;92:283-288.

156. Mohsenin V, Guffanti EE, Hilbert J, et al. Daytime oxygen saturation does not predict nocturnal oxygen desaturation in patients with chronic obstructive pulmonary disease. Arch Phys Med Rehabil 1994;75:285-289.

157. Laks L, Lehrhaft B, Grunstein RR, et al. Pulmonary hypertension in obstructive sleep apnoea. Eur Respir J 1995;8:537-541.

158. McKeon JL, Murree-Allen K, Saunders NA. Prediction of oxygenation during sleep in patients with chronic obstructive lung disease. Thorax 1988;43:312-317.

159. Mulloy E, Fitzpatrick M, Bourke S, et al. Oxygen desaturation during sleep and exercise in patients with severe chronic obstructive pulmonary disease. Respir Med 1995; 89:193-198.

160. Catterall JR, Calverley PM, MacNee W, et al. Mechanism of transient nocturnal hypoxemia in hypoxic chronic bronchitis and emphysema. J Appl Physiol 1985;59:1698-703.

161. Douglas NJ. Control of ventilation during sleep. Clin Chest Med 1985;6:653-675.

162. Millman RP, Knight H, Kline LR, et al. Changes in compartmental ventilation in association with eye movements during REM sleep. J Appl Physiol 1988;65:1196-1202.

163. White JES, Drinnen MJ, Smithson AJ, et al. Respiratory muscle activity during rapid eye movement (REM) sleep in patients with chronic obstructive pulmonary disease. Thorax 1995;50:376-382.

164. Hudgel DW, Martin RJ, Capehart M, et al. Contribution of hypoventilation to sleep oxygen desaturation in chronic obstructive pulmonary disease. J Appl Physiol 1983;55:669-677.

165. Sandek K, Andersson T, Bratel T, et al. Ventilation-perfusion inequality in nocturnal hypoxaemia due to chronic obstructive lung disease (COLD). Clin Physiol 1995;15:499-513.

166. Flenley DC. Sleep in chronic obstructive lung disease. Clin Chest Med 1985;6:651-661.

167. Glick MR, Block AJ. Nocturnal versus diurnal cardiac arrhythmias in patients with chronic obstructive pulmonary disease. Chest 1979;75:8-11.

168. Shepard JW, Garrison MW, Grither DA, et al. Relationship of ventricular ectopy to nocturnal oxygen desaturation in patients with chronic obstructive pulmonary disease. Am J Med 1985;78:28-34.

169. Levi-Valensi P, Weitzenblum E, Rida Z, et al. Sleep-related oxygen desaturation and daytime pulmonary haemodynamics in COPD patients. Eur Respir J 1992;5:301-307.

170. Chaouat A, Weitxenblum E, Krieger J, et al. Association of chronic obstructive pulmonary disease and sleep apnea syndrome. Am J Respir Crit Care Med 1995;151:82-86.

171. Bradley TD, Rutherford R, Lue F, et al. Role of diffuse airway obstruction in the hypercapnia of obstructive sleep apnea. Am Rev Respir Dis 1986;134:920-924.

172. Fletcher EC, Luckett RA, Goodnight-White S, et al. A double-blind trial of nocturnal supplemental oxygen for sleep desaturation in patients with chronic obstructive pulmonary disease and a daytime PaO_2 above 60 mm Hg. Am Rev Respir Dis 1992;145: 1070-1076.

173. American Thoracic Society. Indications and standards for cardiopulmonary sleep studies. Am Rev Respir Dis 1989;139: 559-568.

174. Calverley PM, Brezinova V, Douglas NJ, et al. The effect of oxygenation on sleep quality in chronic bronchitis and emphysema. Am Rev Respir Dis 1982;126:206-210.

175. McKeon JL, Murree-Allen K, Saunders NA. Supplemental oxygen and quality of sleep in patients with chronic obstructive lung disease. Thorax 1989;44:184-188.

176. Weitzenblum E, Chaouat A, Charpentier C, et al. Sleep-related hypoxaemia in chronic obstructive pulmonary disease: causes, consequences and treatment. Respiration 1997;64:187-193.

177. Resnikoff PM, Ries AL. Maximizing functional capacity: pulmonary rehabilitation and adjunctive measures. Respir Care Clin North Am 1998;4:475-492.

178. Fishman AP. Pulmonary rehabilitation research. NIH workshop summary. Am J Respir Crit Care Med 1994;149: 825-833.

179. Pulmonary rehabilitation: Joint ACCP/AACVPR evidence-based guidelines. ACCP/AACVPR Pulmonary Rehabilitation Guidelines Panel. American College of Chest Physicians. American Association of Cardiovascular and Pulmonary Rehabilitation. Chest 1997;112:1363-1396.

180. Lacasse Y, Guyatt GH, Goldstein RS. The components of a respiratory rehabilitation program. A systemic overview. Chest 1997;111:1077-1088.

181. Lacasse Y, Guyatt GH, Goldstein RS. Is there really a controversy surrounding the effectiveness of respiratory rehabilitation in COPD? Chest 1998;114:1-4.

182. Ketelaars CA, Abu-Saad HH, Schlosser MA, et al. Long-term outcome of pulmonary rehabilitation in patients with COPD. Chest 1997;112:363-369.

183. Mahler DA. Pulmonary rehabilitation. Chest 1998;113:263S-268S.

184. Tiep BL. Disease management of COPD with pulmonary rehabilitation. Chest 1997;112:1630-1656.

185. Benditt JO, Albert RK. Surgical options for patients with advanced emphysema. Clin Chest Med 1997;18:577-593.

186. Edelman JD, Kotloff RM. Surgical approaches to advanced emphysema. Respir Care Clin North Am 1998;4:513-539.

187. Cooper JD. The history of surgical procedures for emphysema. Ann Thorac Surg 1997;63:312-319.

188. Gaensler EA, Cugell DW, Knudson RJ, et al. Surgical management of emphysema. Clin Chest Med 1983;4:443-463.

189. Snider GL. Reduction pneumoplasty for giant bullous emphysema. Implications for surgical treatment of nonbullous emphysema. Chest 1996;109:540-548.

190. Laros CD, Gelissen HJ, Bergstein PG, et al. Bullectomy for giant bullae in emphysema. J Thorac Cardiovasc Surg 1986;91:63-70.

191. Morgan MD, Denison DM, Strickland B. Value of computed tomography for selecting patients with bullous lung disease for surgery. Thorax 1986;41:855-862.

192. Nickoladze GD. Functional results of surgery for bullous emphysema. Chest 1992;101:119-122.

193. Sciurba FC, Rogers RM, Keenan RJ, et al. Improvement in pulmonary function and elastic recoil after lung-reduction surgery for diffuse emphysema. N Engl J Med 1996;334:1095-1099.

194. Sciurba FC. Early and long-term functional outcomes following lung volume reduction surgury. Clin Chest Med 1997;18:259-276.

195. Gelb AF, McKenna RJ Jr, Brenner M, et al. Contribution of lung and chest wall mechanics following emphysema resection. Chest 1996;110:11-17.

196. Rochester DF, Arora NS, Braun NMT, et al. The respiratory muscles in chronic obstructive pulmonary disease (COPD). Eur Physiopathol Respir 1979;15:971-975.

197. Gierada DS, Slone RM, Bae KT, et al. Pulmonary emphysema: comparison of preoperative quantitative CT and physiologic index values with clinical outcome after lung-volume reduction surgery. Radiology 1997;205:235-242.

198. Slone RM, Pilgram TK, Gierada DS, et al. Lung volume reduction surgery: comparison of preoperative radiologic features and clinical outcome. Radiology 1997;204:685-693.

199. Kotloff RM, Tino G, Bavaria JE, et al. Bilateral lung volume reduction surgery for advanced emphysema. A comparison of median sternotomy and thoracoscopic approaches. Chest 1996;110:1399-1406.

200. Keller CA, Ruppel G, Hibbett A, et al. Thoracoscopic lung volume reduction surgery reduces dyspnea and improves exercise capacity in patients with emphysema. Am J Respir Crit Care Med 1997;156:60-67.

201. Cooper JD, Patterson GA, Sundaresan RS, et al. Results of 150 consecutive bilateral lung volume reduction procedures in patients with severe emphysema. J Thorac Cardiovasc Surg 1996;112:1319-1329; discussion 1329-1330.

202. Wakabayashi A. Thoracoscopic laser pneumoplasty in the treatment of diffuse bullous emphysema. Ann Thorac Surg 1995;60:936-942.

203. Swanson SJ, Mentzer SJ, DeCamp MM Jr, et al. No-cut thoracoscopic lung plication: a new technique for lung volume reduction surgery. J Am Coll Surg 1997;185:25-32.

204. Keller CA, Naunheim KS. Perioperative management of lung volume reduction patients. Clin Chest Med 1997;18:285-300.

205. Kotloff RM, Tino G, Palevsky HI, et al. Comparison of short-term functional outcomes following unilateral and bilateral lung volume reduction surgery. Chest 1998;113:890-895.

206. Brenner M, McKenna RJ, Gelb AF, et al. Dyspnea response following bilateral thoracoscopic staple lung volume reduction surgery. Chest 1997;112:916-923.

207. Scharf SM, Rossoff L, McKeon K, et al. Changes in pulmonary mechanics after lung volume reduction surgery. Lung 1998;176:191-204.

208. Cordova F, O'Brien G, Furukawa S, et al. Stability of improvements in exercise performance and quality of life following bilateral lung volume reduction surgery in severe COPD. Chest 1997;112:907-915.

209. Roue C, Mal H, Sleiman C, et al. Lung volume reduction in patients with severe diffuse emphysema: a retrospective study. Chest 1996;110:28-34.

210. Meyers BF, Yusen RD, Lefrak SS, et al. Outcome of Medicare patients with emphysema selected for, but denied, a lung volume reduction operation. Ann Thorac Surg 1998;66:331-336.

211. Trulock EP, III. Lung transplantation for COPD. Chest 1998;113:269S-276S.

212. Patterson GA, Cooper JD. Lung transplantation for emphysema. Chest Surg Clin N Am 1995;5:851-868.

213. Kaplan JD, Trulock EP, Cooper JD, et al. Pulmonary vascular permeability after lung transplantation: a positron emission tomographic study. Am Rev Respir Dis 1992;145:954-957.

214. Bavaria JE, Kotloff R, Palevsky H, et al. Bilateral versus single lung transplantation for chronic obstructive pulmonary disease. J Thorac Cardiovasc Surg 1997;113:520-528.

215. Geertsma A, Ten Vergert EM, Bonsel GJ, et al. Does lung transplantation prolong life? A comparison of survival with and without transplantation. J Heart Lung Transplant 1998;17:511-516.

216. Hokanson JF, Mercier JG, Brooks GA. Cyclosporine A decreases rat skeletal muscle mitochondrial respiration in vitro. Am J Respir Crit Care Med 1991;151:1848-1851.

217. Badesch DB, Zamora M, Fullerton D, et al. Pulmonary capillaritis: a possible histologic form of acute pulmonary allograft rejection. J Heart Lung Transplant 1998;17:415-422.

218. Gavazzeni V, Iapichino G, Mascheroni D, et al. Prolonged independent lung respiratory treatment after single lung transplantation in pulmonary emphysema. Chest 1993;103:96-100.

219. Cherniak NS. Chronic obstructive pulmonary disease. Philadelphia: Saunders; 1991.

220. Canadian Thoracic Society Workshop Group. Guidelines for the assessment and management of chronic obstructive pulmonary disease. Can Med Assoc J 1992;147:420-426.

221. Smith CB, Golden CA, Kanner RE, et al. Association of viral and *Mycoplasma pneumoniae* infections with acute respiratory illness in patients with chronic obstructive pulmonary diseases. Am Rev Respir Dis 1980;121:225-232.

222. Saint S, Bent S, Vittinghoff E, et al. Antibiotics in chronic obstructive pulmonary disease exacerbations: a meta-analysis. JAMA 1995;273:957-960.

223. Anthonisen NR, Manfreda J, Warren CP, et al. Antibiotic therapy in exacerbations of chronic obstructive pulmonary disease. Ann Intern Med 1987;106:196-204.

224. Monso E, Ruiz J, Rosell A, et al. Bacterial infection in chronic obstructive pulmonary disease. Am J Respir Crit Care Med 1995;152:1316-1320.

225. Blasi F, Legnani D, Lombado VM, et al. *Chlamydia pneumoniae* infection in acute exacerbations of COPD. Eur Respir J 1993;6:19-22.

226. Eller J, Ede A, Schaberg T, et al. Infective exacerbations of chronic bronchitis: relation between bacteriologic etiology and lung function. Chest 1998;113:1542-1548.

227. Grossman R, Mukherjee J, Vaughan D, et al. A 1-year community-based health economic study of ciprofloxacin vs usual antibiotic treatment in acute exacerbations of chronic bronchitis: the Canadian Ciprofloxacin Health Economic Study Group. Chest 1998;113:131-141.

228. Thompson WH, Nielson CP, Carvalho P, et al. Controlled trial of oral prednisone in out-patients with acute COPD exacerbation. Am J Respir Crit Care Med 1996;154:407-412.

229. Rodriguez-Roisin R, Barbera JA. Chronic obstructive pulmonary disease: mechanism of hypoxaemia (structure and gas exchange relationships). Monaldi Arch Chest Dis 1993;48:415-417.

230. Rossi A, Polese G, De Sandre G. Respiratory failure in chronic airflow obstruction: recent advances and therapeutic implications in the critically ill patient. Eur J Med 1992;1:349-357.

231. Connors AFJ, Dawson NV, Thomas C, et al. Outcomes following acute exacerbation of severe chronic obstructive lung disease. J Respir Crit Care Med 1996;154:959-967.

232. Fuso L, Incalzi RA, Pistelli R, et al. Predicting mortality of patients hospitalized for acutely exacerbated chronic obstructive pulmonary disease. Am J Respir Crit Care Med 1995;98:272-277.

233. Seneff MG, Wagner DP, Wagner RP. Hospital and 1-year survival of patients admitted to intensive care units with acute exacerbation of chronic obstructive pulmonary disease. JAMA 1995;20:1852-1857.

234. Heffner JE. Chronic obstructive pulmonary disease: ethical considerations of care. Clin Pulm Med 1996;3:1-8.

235. Murata GH, Gorby MS, Kapsner CO, et al. A multivariate model for the prediction of relapse after outpatient treatment of decompensated chronic obstructive pulmonary disease. Arch Intern Med 1992;152:73-77.

236. Gravil JH, Al-Rawas OA, Cotton MM, et al. Home treatment of exacerbations of chronic obstructive pulmonary disease by an acute respiratory assessment service. Lancet 1998;351:1853-1855.

237. Bach JR, Brougher P, Hess DR, et al. Consensus conference: non-invasive positive pressure ventilation. Respir Care 1997;42:361-369.

238. Mushlin AI, Black ER, Connolly CA, et al. The necessary length of hospital stay for chronic pulmonary disease. JAMA 1991;266:80-83.

239. Pearson MG, Alderslade R, Allen SC, et al. BTS guidelines for the management of chronic obstructive pulmonary disease. Thorax 1997;52(Suppl 5):S1-S28.

240. Cazzola M, Spina D, Matera MG. The use of bronchodilators in stable chronic obstructive pulmonary disease. Pulm Pharmacol Ther 1997;10:128-144.

241. Gross NJ, Bankwala Z. Effects of an anticholinergic bronchodilator on arterial blood gases of hypoxemic patients with chronic obstructive pulmonary disease: comparison with a beta-adrenergic agent. Am Rev Respir Dis 1987;136:1091-1094.

242. Turner JR, Corkery KJ, Eckman D, et al. Equivalence of continuous flow nebulizer and metered dose inhaler with reservoir bag for treatment of acute airflow obstruction. Chest 1988;93:476-481.

243. Karpel JP, Pesin J, Greenberg D, et al. A comparison of the effects of ipratropium bromide and metaproterenol sulfate in acute exacerbations of COPD. Chest 1990;98:835-839.

244. Rebuck AS, Chapman KR, Abboud R, et al. Nebulized anticholinergic and sympathomimetic treatment of asthma and chronic obstructive airways disease in the emergency room. Am J Med 1987;82:59-64.

245. Leuenberger P, Anderhub HP, Brandi O, et al. Management 1997 of chronic obstructive pulmonary disease. Working Group of the Swiss Society of Pneumology. Schweiz Med Wochenschr 1997;127:766-782.

246. Albert R, Martin T, Lewis S. Methylprednisolone improves chronic bronchitics with acute respiratory insufficiency. Chest 1980;77:314-315.

247. Glenny RW. Steroids in COPD. The scripture according to Albert. Chest 1987;91:289-290.

248. Emerman CL, Connors AF, Lukens TW, et al. A randomized controlled trial of methylprednisolone in the emergency treatment of acute exacerbations of COPD. Chest 1989;95:563-567.

249. Murata GH, Gorby MS, Chick TW, et al. Intravenous and oral corticosteroids for the prevention of relapse after treatment of decompensated COPD. Chest 1990;98:845-849.

250. Rubini F, Rampulia C, Nava S. Acute effect of corticosteroids on respiratory mechanics in mechanically ventilated patients with chronic airflow obstruction and acute respiratory failure. Am J Respir Crit Care Med 1994;149:306-310.

251. Erbland ML, Niewoehner D. Results from SCCOP: systemic corticosteroids for the prevention of relapse after treatment of decompensated COPD. Presented at the International Conference for the American Lung Association/American Thoracic Society; 1998 April 24-29; Chicago, Ill.

252. Soler N, Torres A, Ewig S, et al. Bronchial microbial patterns in severe exacerbations of chronic obstructive pulmonary disease (COPD) requiring mechanical ventilation. Am J Respir Crit Care Med 1998;157:1498-1505.

253. Grossman RF. Guidelines for the treatment of acute exacerbations of chronic bronchitis. Chest 1997;112:310S-313S.

254. Grossman RF. The value of antibiotics and the outcomes of antibiotic therapy in exacerbations of COPD. Chest 1998; 113:249S-255S.

255. Barbé F, Togores B, Rubi M, et al. Noninvasive ventilatory support does not facilitate recovery from acute respiratory failure in chronic obstructive pulmonary disease. Eur Respir J 1996;9:1240-1245.

256. Bott J, Carroll MP, Conway JH, et al. Randomised controlled trial of nasal ventilation in acute ventilatory failure due to chronic obstructive airways disease. Lancet 1993;341:1555-1557.

257. Brochard L, Isabey D, Piquet J, et al. Reversal of acute exacerbations of chronic obstructive lung disease by inspiratory assistance with a face mask. N Engl J Med 1990;323: 1523-1530.

258. Brochard L, Mancebo J, Wysocki M, et al. Noninvasive ventilation for acute exacerbations of chronic obstructive pulmonary disease. N Engl J Med 1995;333:817-822.

259. Kramer N, Meyer TJ, Meharg J, et al. Randomized, prospective trial of noninvasive positive pressure ventilation in acute respiratory failure. Am J Respir Crit Care Med 1995;151:1799-1806.

260. Vitacca M, Clini E, Rubini F, et al. Non-invasive mechanical ventilation in severe chronic obstructive lung disease and acute respiratory failure: short- and long-term prognosis. Intensive Care Med 1996;22:94-100.

261. Keenan SP, Kernerman PD, Cook DJ, et al. Effect of noninvasive positive pressure ventilation on mortality in patients admitted with acute respiratory failure: a meta-analysis. Crit Care Med 1997;25:1685-1692.

262. Make BJ, Hill NS, Goldberg AI, et al. Mechanical ventilation beyond the intensive care unit. Report of a consensus conference of the American College of Chest Physicians. Chest 1998;113:289S-344S.

263. Elliott MW. Noninvasive ventilation in chronic obstructive pulmonary disease. N Engl J Med 1995;333:870-871.

264. Rouby JJ, Laurent P, Gosnach M, et al. Risk factors and clinical relevance of nosocomial maxillary sinusitis in the critically ill. Am J Respir Crit Care Med 1994;150:776-783.

265. Heffner JE. Nosocomial sinusitis. Den of multiresistant thieves? Am J Respir Crit Care Med 1994;150:608-609.

266. Heffner JE. Tracheal intubation in mechanically ventilated patients. Clin Chest Med 1988;9:23-35.

267. Crogan SJ, Bishop MJ. Delivery efficiency of metered dose aerosols given via endotracheal tubes. Anesthesiology 1989;70:1008-1010.

268. Salem MR, Mathrubhutham M, Bennett EJ. Difficult intubation. N Engl J Med 1976;295:879-881.

269. Cinnella G, Conti G, Lofaso F, et al. Effects of assisted ventilation on the work of breathing: volume-controlled versus pressure-controlled ventilation. Am J Respir Crit Care Med 1996;153:1025-1033.

270. MacIntyre NR, McConnell R, Cheng KG, et al. Patient-ventilator flow dyssynchrony: flow-limited versus pressure-limited breaths. Crit Care Med 1997;25:1671-1677.

271. Hess D, Medoff B. Mechanical ventilation of the patient with chronic obstructive pulmonary disease. Respir Care Clin North Am 1998;4:439-473.

272. Jubran A, van de Graff WB, Tobin MJ. Variability of patient-ventilator interaction with pressure support ventilation in patients with chronic obstructive pulmonary disease. Am J Respir Crit Care Med 1995;152:129-136.

273. Leung P, Jubran A, Tobin MJ. Comparison of assisted ventilator modes on triggering patient effort and dyspnea. Am J Respir Crit Care Med 1997;155:1940-1948.

274. Laghi F, D'Alfonso N, Tobin MJ. Pattern of recovery from diaphragmatic fatigue over 24 hours. J Appl Physiol 1995;79:539-546.

275. Marini JJ, Smith TC, Lamb VJ. External work output and force generation during synchronized intermittent mechanical ventilation. Effect of machine assistance on breathing effort. Am Rev Respir Dis 1988;138:1169-1179.

276. Connors AF, McCaffree DR, Gray BA, et al. Effect of inspiratory flow rate on gas exchange during mechanical ventilation. Am Rev Respir Dis 1981;124:537-543.

277. Corne S, Gillespie D, Roberts D, et al. Effect of inspiratory flow rate on respiratory rate in intubated ventilated patients. Am J Respir Crit Care Med 1997;156:304-308.

278. Crossley DJ, McGuire GP, Barrow PM, et al. Influence of inspired oxygen concentration on dead space, respiratory drive, and $PaCO_2$ in intubated patients. Crit Care Med 1997;25:1522-1526.

279. Smith TC, Marini JJ. Impact of PEEP on lung mechanics and work of breathing in severe airflow obstruction. J Appl Physiol 1988;65:1488-1499.

280. MacIntyre NR, Cheng KC, McConnell R. Applied PEEP during pressure support reduces the inspiratory threshold load of intrinsic PEEP. Chest 1997;111:188-193.

281. Lessard MR, Brochard LJ. Weaning from ventilatory support. Clin Chest Med 1996;17:475-489.

282. Yang KL, Tobin MJ. A prospective study of indexes predicting the outcome of trials of weaning from mechanical ventilation. N Engl J Med 1991;324:1445-1450.

283. Esteban A, Frutos F, Tobin MJ, et al. A comparison of four methods of weaning patients from mechanical ventilation. N Engl J Med 1995;332:345-350.

284. Brochard L, Rauss A, Benito S, et al. Comparison of three methods of gradual withdrawal from ventilatory support during weaning from mechanical ventilation. Am J Respir Crit Care Med 1994;150:896-903.

285. Heffner JE. Timing of tracheotomy in mechanically ventilated patients. Am Rev Respir Dis 1993;147:768-771.

286. Heffner JE. Timing of tracheotomy in ventilator-dependent patients. Clin Chest Med 1991;12:611-625.

287. Heffner JE, Casey K, Hoffman C. Care of the mechanically ventilated patient with a tracheotomy. In: Tobin MJ, editor. Principles and practice of mechanical ventilation. New York: McGraw Hill; 1994. pp. 749-774.

288. Godwin JE, Heffner JE. Special critical care considerations in tracheostomy management. Clin Chest Med 1992;12:573-583.

289. Heffner JE. Timing tracheotomy: calendar watching or individualization of care. Chest 1998;114:361-363.

290. Heffner JE. End-of-life issues. Respir Care Clin North Am 1998;4:541-559.

291. Martin TR, Lewis SW, Albert RK. The prognosis of patients with chronic obstructive pulmonary disease after hospitalization for acute respiratory failure. Chest 1982;82:310-314.

292. Rieves RD, Bass D, Carter RR, et al. Severe COPD and acute respiratory failure: correlates for survival at the time of tracheal intubation. Chest 1993;104:854-860.

293. Heffner JE, Fahy B, Hilling L, et al. Attitudes regarding advance directives among patients in pulmonary rehabilitation. Am J Respir Crit Care Med 1996;154:1735-1740.

294. Youngner SJ. Do-not-resuscitate orders: no longer a secret but still a problem. Hastings Center Report 1987;17:24-33.

295. Heffner JE, Fahy B, Barbieri C. Advance directive education during pulmonary rehabilitation. Chest 1996;109:373-379.

296. Task Force on Ethics of the Society of Critical Care Medicine. Consensus report on the ethics of foregoing life-sustaining treatments in the critically ill. Critical Care Medicine 1990;18:1435-1439.

297. American Thoracic Society Bioethics Task Force. Withholding and withdrawing life-sustaining therapy. Am Rev Respir Dis 1991;144:726-731.

298. Heffner JE, Fahy B, Hilling L, et al. Outcomes of advance directive education of pulmonary rehabilitation patients. Am J Respir Crit Care Med 1997;155:1055-1059.

299. Murphy DJ, Burrows D, Santilli S, et al. The influence of the probability of survival on patients' preferences regarding cardiopulmonary resuscitation. N Engl J Med 1994;330:545-549.

300. Mower MR, Baraff LJ. Advance directives: effect of type of directive on physicians' therapeutic decisions. Arch Intern Med 1993;153:375-381.

301. Markson LJ, Fanale J, Steel K, et al. Implementing advance directives in the primary care setting. Arch Intern Med 1994;154:2321-2327.

302. Sachs G, Stocking C, Miles S. Empowerment of the older patient? A randomized, controlled trial to increase discussion and use of advance directives. J Am Geriatrics Soc 1992;40:269-273.

303. Tulsky JA, Fischer GS, Rose MR, et al. Opening the black box: how do physicians communicate about advance directives? Ann Intern Med 1998;129:441-449.

304. Tulsky JA, Chesney MA, Lo B. How do medical residents discuss resuscitation with patients? J Gen Intern Med 1995;10:436-442.

305. Tulsky JA, Chesney MA, Lo B. See one, do one, teach one? House staff experience discussing do-not-resuscitate orders. Arch Intern Med 1996;156:1285-1289.

306. Fried TR, Stein MD, O'Sullivan PS, et al. Limits of patient autonomy–physician attitudes and practices regarding life-sustaining treatments and euthanasia. Arch Intern Med 1993;153:722-728.

307. Stuart B, Alexander C, Arenella C, et al. Medical guidelines for determining prognosis in selected non-cancer diseases. Arlington, Va: The National Hospice Organization; 1996.

CHAPTER 48

Interstitial Lung Disease

Andrew J. Ghio

CHAPTER OUTLINE

OBJECTIVES

1. Describe the precipitating causes, clinical manifestations, and radiographic, laboratory, and pathophysiologic findings of interstitial lung disease.
2. Describe the diseases associated with idiopathic pulmonary fibrosis.
3. Describe the management and therapy of interstitial lung disease.
4. Discuss the prognosis of interstitial lung disease.

KEY TERMS

Bronchiolitis Obliterans with Organizing Pneumonia (BOOP)
Collagen Vascular Disease

Eosinophilic Granuloma
Idiopathic Pulmonary Fibrosis (IPF)
Interstitial Lung Disease (ILD)

Pulmonary Alveolar Proteinosis (PAP)
Respiratory Bronchiolitis
Sarcoidosis

Interstitial Lung Disease

The term **interstitial lung disease (ILD)** encompasses approximately 200 distinct diseases in which the interstitium is altered by inflammation or fibrosis or both. The interstitium comprises the alveolar walls (and lumens), pulmonary microvasculature, interstitial macrophages, fibroblasts, myofibroblasts, and matrix components of the lungs (Figure 48-1). The inflammatory and fibrotic disorders of ILD can affect any of these components. The resulting infiltration of the acinar region by cellular and extracellular elements either distorts or destroys the alveolar and bronchiolar architecture, or it may cause little associated damage (Figure 48-2).

ILD is an extremely diverse group of both acute and chronic disorders. Common clinical, radiographic, and patho-physiologic features form the basis for collective reference to this complex group of disorders as interstitial lung disease (Box 48-1). Most often the patient complains of dyspnea; a chest radiograph shows abnormal markings; and lung function tests demonstrate a loss of function, including decreased volumes and reduced diffusing capacity. To make the diagnosis, the clinical presentation, radiographic findings, pulmonary function test results, laboratory values, and lung biopsy findings all must be correlated. In most cases a definitive diagnosis cannot be made without a biopsy.

Pathophysiology

A common sequence of events that results in ILD begins when either a recognized or an unidentified agent induces

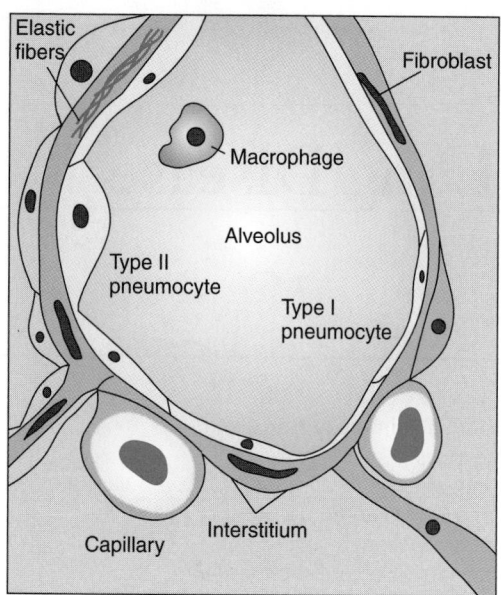

Figure 48-1 Schematic drawing of the lung showing the components of the interstitium.

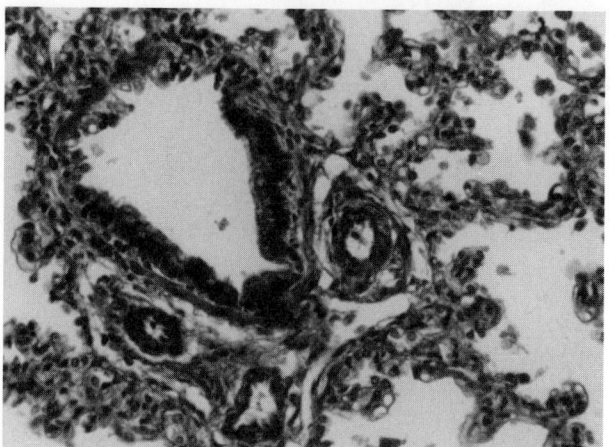

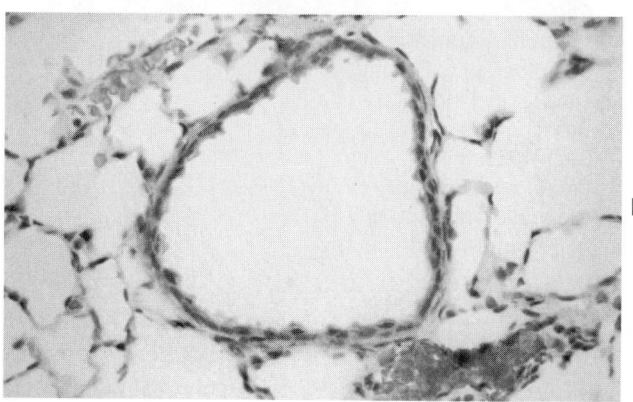

Figure 48-2 **A,** Micrograph of a newborn with bronchopulmonary dysplasia, an interstitial lung disease. **B,** Hematoxylin-eosin staining shows an accumulation of inflammatory cells and subsequent widening in the interstitium.

$\mathcal{B}$OX 48-1

Key Diagnostic Features of Interstitial Lung Disease

> Dyspnea at rest or with exertion (or in both cases)
> Bilateral diffuse interstitial infiltrates on chest radiograph
> Physiologic abnormalities of a restrictive lung defect: decreased lung volumes, decreased diffusing capacity for carbon monoxide (DLCO), and abnormal difference between the alveolar and arterial partial pressures of oxygen (P[A − a]o₂) at rest and/or with exertion
> Histopathologic features of inflammation or fibrosis (or both) of the pulmonary parenchyma

---

$\mathcal{B}$OX 48-2

Pathophysiology of Interstitial Lung Disease

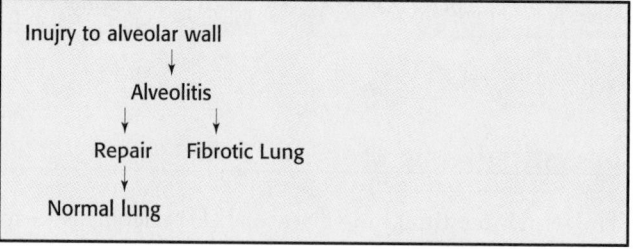

---

alveolitis and vasculitis (Box 48-2). Persistence of this inflammatory lesion results in alveolar, capillary, and parenchymal cell injury. Abnormal repair leads to proliferation of mesenchymal cells, with the production of excess collagen and other extracellular matrix connective tissue elements. In the later stages of ILD, the normal architecture of the lung is replaced by cystic spaces separated by thick bands of fibrous tissue, a condition called *honeycomb lung.*

Although the end stage of the lung is histologically similar in all types of ILD, the alveolitis stage often is distinctive because of the number and influence of various inflammatory and immune effector cells present, such as neutrophils, eosinophils, and lymphocytes. Elaboration of neutrophil proteases, such as elastase, collagenase, and cathepsins, and endogenous oxidant production is assumed to mediate some portion of tissue injury in many of these disorders. The alveolar macrophage previously was considered to be central to the perpetuation of this injury because of its release of reactive oxygen species, chemoattractants for neutrophils, and growth factors for mesenchymal cells, including fibronectin, platelet-derived growth factor, and insulin-like factor 1, which probably are important in the progression to fibrosis. However, it has been demonstrated that respiratory epithelial cells have a similar capacity to elaborate these same mediators and coordinate an inflammatory and fibrotic response to numerous agents.

Box 48-3

Classification of Interstitial Lung Disease

Known Cause
Infection
 Bacteria (*Legionella pneumophila, Bordetella pertussis*)
 Viruses (cytomegalovirus, human immunodeficiency virus, respiratory syncytial virus, adenovirus, influenza, parainfluenza, measles)
 Mycoplasma species
 Mycobacterium species
 Fungi (*Aspergillus* species)
 Parasites
 Pneumocystis carinii pneumonia
Occupational exposure
 Inorganic dusts (silicosis, asbestosis, talcosis, berylliosis, coal workers' pneumoconiosis, siderosis, baritosis)
 Microbial antigens (farmer's lung, humidifier lung, bird fancier's lung)
 Fumes (lung injury from exposure to chlorine gas, sulfuric acid, hydrochloric acid, nitrogen dioxide, or ammonia)
Neoplasm
 Bronchoalveolar carcinoma
 Leukemia
 Hodgkin's disease
 Non-Hodgkin's lymphoma
Congenital and metabolic causes
 Lipoidoses (Gaucher's disease, Niemann-Pick disease)
 Storage disorders (Hermansky-Pudlak syndrome)
 Cystic fibrosis
 Radiation
Drug reactions
 Nitrofurantoin, Furatoin, gold, sulfasalazine, thiazides, cytarabine, bleomycin, methotrexate, cyclophosphamide, carmustine, busulfan, procarbazine, azathioprine, 6-MP, vinblastine, mitomycin, chlorambucil, amiodarone, adrenergic antagonists, tocainide, salicylates, nonsteroidal antiinflammatory drugs (NSAIDs), narcotics, methadone, codeine, buprenorphine, naloxone, terbutaline, ritodrine, Dilantin, carbamazepine, angiotensin-converting enzyme inhibitors, contrast media, paraquat, oxygen
Recurrent aspiration
Lipoid pneumonia
Amyloidosis
Microlithiasis

Heart disease (congestive heart failure)
Liver disease (chronic active hepatitis, primary biliary cirrhosis)
Renal disease (renal failure)
Bowel disease (ulcerative colitis, Crohn's disease)
Graft-versus-host disease
Pulmonary venoocclusive disease
Acute respiratory distress syndrome (ARDS)
Acute eosinophilic pneumonia (parasitic infections, such as with *Strongyloides, Ascaris,* and *Ancylostoma* subspecies)

Unknown Cause
Idiopathic pulmonary fibrosis
Sarcoidosis
Vasculitides
 Wegener's granulomatosis, Churg-Strauss angiitis, lymphomatoid granulomatosis, alveolar hemorrhage syndromes accompanied by capillaritis, microscopic polyangiitis, Behçet's syndrome, Takayasu's disease, Henoch-Schönlein purpura.
Collagen vascular diseases
 Rheumatoid arthritis, systemic sclerosis, systemic lupus erythematosus (SLE), polymyositis, dermatomyositis, Sjögren's syndrome, mixed connective tissue disease, ankylosing spondylitis
Diffuse alveolar hemorrhage syndromes
 Antiglomerular basement membrane antibody disease (Goodpasture's syndrome), bleeding in patients with systemic necrotizing vasculitis (Wegener's granulomatosis and microscopic polyangiitis) and collagen vascular diseases, hemorrhage in immunocompromised hosts and after administration of exogenous agents (trimellitic anhydride, cocaine, and penicillamine), idiopathic pulmonary hemosiderosis
Eosinophilic granuloma
Chronic eosinophilic pneumonia
Bronchiolitis obliterans with organizing pneumonia
Respiratory bronchiolitis
Pulmonary alveolar proteinosis
Lymphangioleiomyomatosis, tuberous sclerosis, and ataxia-telangiectasia
Lymphoid interstitial pneumonitis
Acute interstitial pneumonitis

Classification

A satisfactory classification system for ILD is not yet available. For practical purposes it is useful to categorize the disorders by whether the cause is known or unknown (Box 48-3). An alternative criterion is the presence or absence of granuloma as a feature of the inflammatory process. Hypersensitivity pneumonitis, sarcoidosis, eosinophilic granuloma, Wegener's granulomatosis, Churg-Strauss syndrome, and silicosis all are associated with the formation of granulomas. Idiopathic pulmonary fibrosis (IPF), connective tissue disorders, asbestosis, and disease caused by

drugs, radiation, and toxic gas exposure are not associated with granulomas.

Clinical Manifestations

The most common presentation of ILD is a slowly progressive onset of dyspnea and a nonproductive cough. The dyspnea may occur on exertion at first but progresses to dyspnea at rest. The history is the most important tool in the identification of the etiology of ILD. A thorough history limits the differential diagnosis and may preclude the need for biopsy. However, even with a detailed history, the causative agent is identified in fewer than 20% to 30% of patients with ILD.[1]

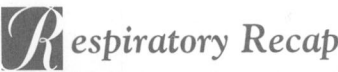
espiratory Recap

Clinical History of Interstitial Lung Disease
Dyspnea on exertion or at rest
Cough
Fevers, chills, night sweats
Medications taken
Detailed work history
Hobbies
Environmental exposures
Risk factors for infection with the human immunodeficiency virus (HIV)
Past medical history of pneumothoraces
Family medical history of interstitial lung disease
Cigarette smoking

In attempting to determine the causative agent, the clinician must ask specific questions and note specific symptoms. A list of all medications the patient has been taking should be compiled to detect drug-related causes of ILD. It should be remembered that patients are notoriously vague about medications they are currently taking or may have taken in the past. A detailed job history can help define occupational exposures and possible dusts, fumes, and antigens associated with ILD. Hobbies and environmental exposures (for example, pigeon breeding, home saunas, and heating and air conditioning units) should also be noted. Knowledge of the agents that can cause ILD can serve as a guide to the areas that should be emphasized in the occupational and environmental history. Risk factors for infection with the human immunodeficiency virus (HIV) must be explored. A review of systems must include attention to fevers, chills, night sweats (hypersensitivity pneumonitis and vasculitis), arthralgia and myalgia (ILD with connective tissue disorders), sinusitis, hemoptysis

(alveolar hemorrhage syndromes), and chest pain (ILD resulting from toxic gas exposure). A past medical history should inquire into episodes of pneumothoraces. The family medical history should be reviewed closely to rule out a number of inherited disorders known to cause interstitial lung disease, such as IPF, tuberous sclerosis, and neurofibromatosis. A history of cigarette smoking is important in the pathogenesis of some ILD diseases, including eosinophilic granuloma, respiratory bronchiolitis, and alveolar hemorrhage syndromes.

The physical examination may be less helpful than the history in the determination of a specific diagnosis in ILD (Table 48-1). Bilateral, end-inspiratory, basilar crackles are a feature in several ILD diseases, including IPF, ILD with collagen vascular diseases, and asbestosis. Wheezes are rare except in Churg-Strauss syndrome. Other findings on the physical examination can assist in the differential diagnosis. Patients who have had severe disease for a protracted period may show evidence of pulmonary hypertension on the physical examination.

Pulmonary Function

The initial evaluation of pulmonary function in the patient with ILD should include spirometry, measurement of lung volumes and diffusing capacity (D_LCO), inspiratory effort, maximum voluntary ventilation, arterial blood gas measurements, and exercise oxygen saturation. These studies characteristically reveal restriction with a decreased forced vital capacity (FVC), a decreased forced expiratory volume in 1 second (FEV_1), and a normal or increased FEV_1 to FVC ratio. Total lung capacity (TLC) and the D_LCO are decreased. The D_LCO can be the most sensitive of the pulmonary function measures and may be abnormal even when lung volumes are preserved.[2]

A mild resting hypoxemia with significant arterial oxygen desaturation after exercise often is seen. The resting hypoxemia is the result both of ventilation-perfusion mismatch and shunt; the worsening of the condition with exercise may reflect diffusion restrictions in addition to mismatch and shunt. In patients with normal lung volumes or spirometry results, desaturation with ambulation may be a

TABLE 48-1
Physical Examination Findings with Interstitial Lung Disease

Finding	Associated Disease
Digital clubbing	Idiopathic pulmonary fibrosis
Cutaneous lesions	Sarcoidosis, tuberous sclerosis, necrotizing vasculitis, dermatomyositis, collagen vascular diseases
Ocular signs	Sarcoidosis, ILD in systemic vasculitis, ILD with Sjögren's syndrome or other connective tissue disorders
Polyarthritis	Sarcoidosis, ILD in systemic vasculitis, ILD with Sjögren's syndrome or other connective tissue disorders
Peripheral lymphadenopathy	Sarcoidosis, lymphoid interstitial pneumonitis, ILD with connective tissue disorders
Hepatosplenomegaly	Sarcoidosis, amyloidosis, eosinophilic granuloma, chronic cor pulmonale
Neurologic manifestations	Tuberous sclerosis, systemic vasculitis, sarcoidosis, eosinophilic granuloma

ILD, Interstitial lung disease.

clue to the presence of pulmonary fibrosis.[2] A 6-minute walk test with a finger oximeter in place is well tolerated, provides a measure of oxygen requirements, and can be a quantifiable index of disease progression.

Pulmonary function test results reflecting airway obstruction sometimes are seen in sarcoidosis, hypersensitivity pneumonitis, eosinophilic granuloma, Wegener's granulomatosis, and lymphangioleiomyomatosis.

Radiographic Findings

The classic findings of ILD on a chest radiograph are those of a reticular, nodular, or reticulonodular pattern and reduced lung volume (Figure 48-3). Upper lobe predominance is seen in sarcoidosis, eosinophilic granuloma, silicosis, coal workers' pneumoconiosis, eosinophilic pneumonia, and ILD with ankylosing spondylitis. Lower lobe predominance is found in IPF, ILD with collagen vascular diseases,

and asbestosis. The presentation usually is bilateral and symmetric but may be asymmetric and even unilateral, and alveolar infiltrates may be seen rather than small opacities. If the disorder has been long-standing, pulmonary hypertension may have developed and sometimes can be documented by chest radiograph. An array of abnormalities can be seen on the chest radiographs of patients with ILD, which sometimes can be helpful in the determination of the differential diagnosis (Table 48-2).

High-resolution computed tomography (HRCT) is an important advance in the diagnosis and staging of ILD. Thin sections (1 to 2 mm) are used to portray two distinct patterns of disease: a ground glass increase in attenuation and a reticular pattern. The ground glass appearance is associated with a cellular histologic appearance of that area of lung, whereas the reticular pattern is found in patients whose subsequent lung biopsy confirms fibrosis. HRCT is significantly more sensitive and specific than a chest radi-

TABLE 48-2

Radiographic Findings with Interstitial Lung Disease

Finding	Associated Disease
Normal radiograph (10% of ILD cases)	Early IPF, sarcoidosis, and hypersensitivity pneumonitis
Spontaneous pneumothorax	Eosinophilic granuloma and lymphangioleiomyomatosis
Hilar or mediastinal lymphadenopathy	Sarcoidosis, berylliosis, and silicosis
Eggshell calcification	Silicosis
Pleural disease	Asbestos-related ILD, tuberculosis, ILD with collagen vascular disease, malignancies, and lymphangioleiomyomatosis
Honeycombing	IPF, eosinophilic granuloma, collagen vascular diseases, pneumoconioses, sarcoid

ILD, *Interstitial lung disease;* IPF, *idiopathic pulmonary fibrosis.*

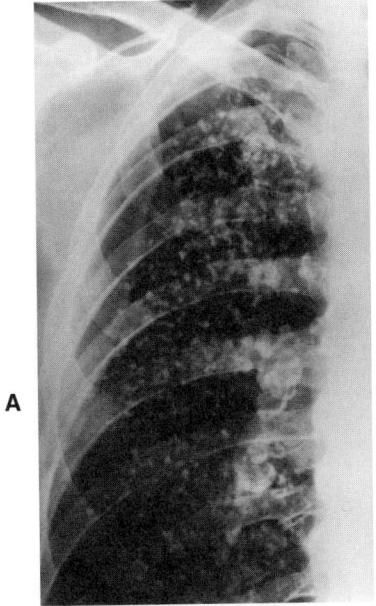
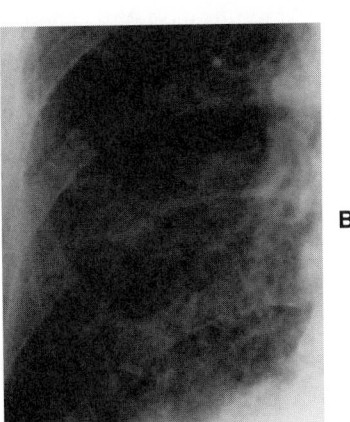

Figure 48-3 A, Chest radiograph showing predominantly rounded opacities in the upper lung fields; this finding is consistent with silicosis or coal workers' pneumoconiosis. **B,** Asbestosis is characterized by linear markings, most commonly seen in the lower lung fields.

ograph in the diagnosis of ILD and in the assessment of both the extent and severity of the disease.[3] It can identify disease before any abnormality is apparent on a chest radiograph. The distribution patterns and anatomic variability of ILD are more evident with HRCT. Although they can be virtually pathognomonic for several forms of ILD, such as eosinophilic granuloma, IPF, lymphangioleiomyomatosis, lymphangitis carcinomatosa, sarcoidosis, and hypersensitivity pneumonitis, dissimilar patterns can be present in patients with different causes of ILD.[4] HRCT also has prognostic value in that a demonstration of honeycomb cysts indicates end-stage, irreversible fibrosis and loss of alveolar walls. HRCT can guide parenchymal biopsy sites or direct the surgeon to lymph nodes for biopsy by mediastinoscopy.[4]

*R*espiratory Recap

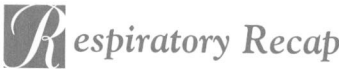

High-Resolution Computed Tomography

High-resolution computed tomography (HRCT) can aid in the diagnosis of idiopathic pulmonary fibrosis, eosinophilic granuloma, lymphangioleiomyomatosis, sarcoidosis, and hypersensitivity pneumonitis.

Nuclear scintigraphy with gallium-67 citrate has been proposed as a diagnostic and staging tool in the assessment of patients with ILD, particularly sarcoidosis and IPF. However, gallium uptake is nonspecific, and there is no clinical utility either in the monitoring or prediction of the clinical course of patients with ILD. Similarly, technetium-99 radionuclide scans and positron-emission tomography (PET) scans currently have no clinical role in either the diagnosis or staging of ILD.

Laboratory Findings

Routine blood and serologic test results most often are unremarkable for patients with ILD. Many patients have a mild anemia and elevated erythrocyte sedimentation rate, reflecting inflammation. Sputum cultures and cytologic studies rarely are diagnostic. Serologic tests, including angiotensin-converting enzyme, antinuclear antibody, and antineutrophil cytoplasmic antibody determinations; hypersensitivity pneumonitis screening (serum precipitins); and complement fixation for fungi can be helpful in some patients.

Although nonspecific, laboratory results can support diagnoses and narrow the differential diagnosis in ILD. Evidence of renal insufficiency or hematuria raises the possibility of renal-pulmonary syndromes (for example, Wegener's granulomatosis, Goodpasture's syndrome, systemic lupus erythematosus, systematic necrotizing vasculitis), whereas abnormal results on liver function tests and high serum cal-

cium levels are clues to the diagnosis of either sarcoidosis or metastatic malignancy.

Bronchoscopy

With ILD it is unusual to reach a specific diagnosis on the basis of the history, physical examination, pulmonary function test results, chest radiograph, and laboratory studies. The next step is to obtain an HRCT scan, and bronchoscopy with lavage and transbronchial lung biopsy usually follows. The exception to this order of investigation is the patient for whom bronchoscopy is thought to be more diagnostic; in such cases this procedure is done before HRCT (Figure 48-4).

In the United States more than 60% of all patients with ILD undergo bronchoscopy.[1] In the evaluation of ILD, bronchoalveolar lavage samples cells and noncellular material from the lower respiratory tract.[5] Currently the clinical application of lavage in ILD is limited. Although the technique can be diagnostic (for example, in cases of pulmonary alveolar proteinosis and pneumoconiosis), especially when particular cytologic or immunohistologic stains are applied (such as in cases of eosinophilic granuloma and alveolar hemorrhage syndromes), precise information is not obtained for most ILD disorders. However, lavage can be extremely useful in the exclusion of specific etiologies and the provision of supportive data to determine the differential diagnosis. The processing of lavage fluid should include cytologic studies and smears or cultures for acid-fast bacilli, fungi, *Pneumocystis carinii*, or viruses. This allows the clinician to exclude certain malignancies and specific infectious agents.

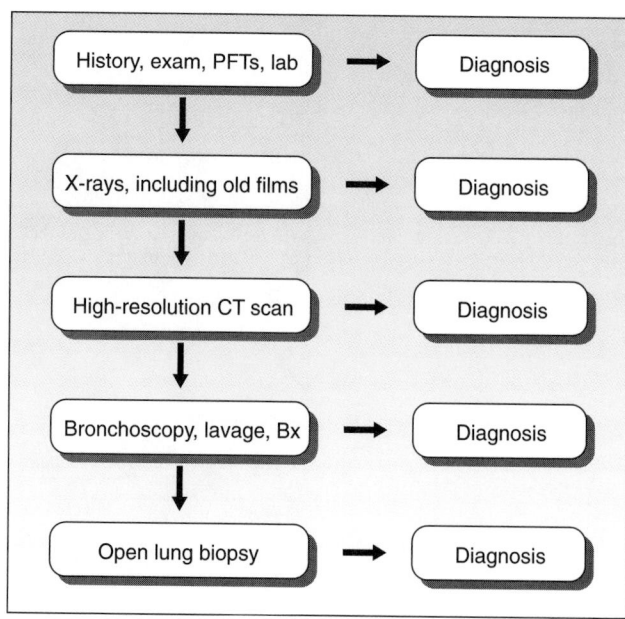

Figure 48-4 Approach to the evaluation of a patient with interstitial lung disease.

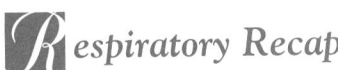espiratory Recap

The cellular profiles obtained through analysis of the lavage fluid may indicate the underlying nature of the ILD. A lymphocytosis can be seen in sarcoidosis, berylliosis, and hypersensitivity pneumonitis. The CD_4 (T-helper) cells increase in sarcoid, with a ratio of CD_4 to CD_8 (T-suppressor) cells more than 3.5, whereas CD_8 cells predominate with hypersensitivity pneumonitis. A lavage sample yielding more than 30% eosinophils supports a diagnosis of chronic or acute eosinophilic pneumonia. Neutrophils abound in several forms of ILD, including IPF and asbestosis.

Transbronchial biopsies (TBBs) are particularly helpful if a primary lung neoplasm, infectious pneumonitis, or sarcoidosis is high in the differential diagnosis. TBBs also can sometimes diagnose Wegener's granulomatosis, rheumatoid lung disease, lymphangioleiomyomatosis, eosinophilic granuloma, eosinophilic pneumonitis, pulmonary alveolar proteinosis, silicosis, hypersensitivity pneumonitis, lymphangitic spread of carcinoma, and Goodpasture's syndrome. Several specimens (up to six) should be obtained from both the upper and lower lobes of either the right or the left lung. If lavage and TBB are not diagnostic, surgical lung biopsies should be done unless specific contraindications exist.

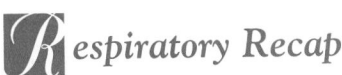espiratory Recap

Surgical Lung Biopsy

Lung biopsy is conventionally regarded as the gold standard used to determine a specific diagnosis for patients with ILD. In the United States 42% of patients with ILD have a lung biopsy of some type for diagnostic purposes,[6] although the decision to obtain a surgical lung biopsy must be individualized. There are several indications for surgical lung biopsy (Box 48-4). Examination of tissue allows confirmation of a specific diagnosis, development of a plan of treatment, prediction of response to therapy,

prognostic information, arguments for long-term therapy with drugs that have significant adverse effects, promotion of transplantation, and insight into the pathogenesis of the ILD. Morbidity and mortality rates are low with open biopsy and even lower with minithoracotomy or thoracoscopic biopsy.[7] Thoracoscopic biopsy is tolerated extremely well and results in less pain and fewer complications than the open approach. Thoracoscopy-guided lung biopsy (TGLB) is rapidly substituting for open lung biopsy because of its reduced perioperative morbidity and the shorter hospital stay for the patient. Lung specimens obtained through TGLB provide equivalent specimen volume and diagnostic accuracy.

Biopsy specimens must be obtained from several sites, including apparently normal lung tissue adjacent to and remote from obviously involved tissue. HCRT can help determine the needed biopsy sites. Alveolar tissue is preferred. Tissue processing requirements include untreated samples for bacteriologic and virologic studies; samples fixed in 10% formalin; samples fixed in methacarnoys solution for immunofluorescence; samples fixed in glutaraldehyde for electron microscopy; and samples cryopreserved for immunologic and molecular studies.

Pathologic Findings

The pathologic findings in ILD are remarkably similar. An alveolitis (granulomatous or nongranulomatous) is initially observed, which may continue for a prolonged period. Eventually collagen is deposited in the interstitium, and fibrosis results. Airways, blood vessels, and pleura may be involved. Different clinical entities may have similar underlying histologic pictures, and several histologic patterns may evolve for one clinical entity (Table 48-3).

Prognosis and Mortality

The prognosis of ILD depends on the specific diagnosis, and most of the current information results from studies of

TABLE 48-3

Histologic Patterns with Interstitial Lung Disease

Pattern	Associated Disease
Common interstitial pneumonitis	IPF, ILD with collagen vascular disease, asbestosis, sarcoidosis, hypersensitivity pneumonitis, drug reactions, organizing pneumonia
Cellular interstitial pneumonitis	IPF, ILD with collagen vascular disease, idiopathic BOOP, drug reactions, hypersensitivity pneumonitis, lymphocytic interstitial pneumonitis
Desquamative interstitial pneumonitis	IPF, respiratory bronchiolitis, eosinophilic granuloma, drug reactions, lipoid pneumonia
Diffuse alveolar damage	Acute respiratory distress syndrome, cytotoxic drugs, ILD with collagen vascular disease, Hamman-Rich syndrome
Bronchiolitis obliterans with organizing pneumonia	IPF, ILD with collagen vascular disease, drug reactions, radiation, alveolar hemorrhage, eosinophilic pneumonia, hypersensitivity pneumonitis
Diffuse alveolar hemorrhage	Vasculitis, ILD with collagen vascular disease, Goodpasture's syndrome, idiopathic pulmonary hemosiderosis
Eosinophilic pneumonia	IPF, drug reactions, allergic granulomatosis of Churg-Strauss, tropical eosinophilia, hypereosinophilic syndrome

ILD, *Interstitial lung disease;* IPF, *idiopathic pulmonary disease;* BOOP, *bronchiolitis obliterans with organizing pneumonia.*

IPF. Findings in the history, the chest radiograph, the pathology of the disease, and the response to therapy can provide prognostic information. In IPF, factors that predicted a better chance of survival in an untreated group were female gender and a younger age at presentation or at the onset of symptoms; the median survival among these patients was 4½ years. In a treated group, factors associated with a better chance of survival were a younger age at presentation or onset of symptoms, less dyspnea, less impairment of carbon monoxide transfer factor, less radiographic abnormality, a more cellular histologic appearance on biopsy, and an early response to corticosteroids. The response to steroids was closely linked with a more cellular appearance on biopsy. The median survival in patients who responded to corticosteroid treatment approached 9 years.

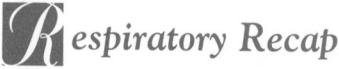

Respiratory Recap

> **Factors Indicating an Improved Prognosis in Idiopathic Pulmonary Fibrosis**
>
> Female patient
> Younger age
> Less dyspnea
> Greater cellular response in lavage

HRCT has been used to predict response to treatment and outcome and is deemed more accurate than a chest radiograph.[8,9] A ground glass appearance was associated with 100% survival rate at 50 months after diagnosis of IPF, compared with a 50% survival rate for patients with disease that appeared with a more reticular pattern. Bronchoscopy with lavage also can provide prognostic information. An increased number of lymphocytes can be associated with a good response to corticosteroids and a better overall prognosis, compared with an elevated number of eosinophils and neutrophils, which predicts a poorer response to corticosteroids in IPF but a better response to cyclophosphamide.

Management and Therapy

Left untreated, most of the disorders included in ILD are progressive and result in death that occurs secondary to respiratory insufficiency and cor pulmonale. The most important tenet of therapy is to remove the agent of injury to the lung if possible, which may mean an exhaustive search for a causative agent.

If no agent is found, therapy can be directed toward suppression of inflammatory and cellular immune responses.[10] Agreement has never been reached on guidelines for standards of care and the time of treatment for patients with ILD. The natural history of many with ILD is a steady progression and functional deterioration to the point where treatment is warranted. An important and challenging issue is when to start treatment. Most of the drugs used to treat ILD have the potential for serious side effects, which often is a disincentive to their use until no choice remains. By this time the patient has developed unequivocal breathlessness, and a considerable proportion of functional lung capacity has already been lost. It therefore is not surprising that meaningful improvements in lung function are uncommon and that often the best that can be achieved is stabilization of the disease to prevent further deterioration.

In ILD few diseases are amenable to specific treatments, although lavage in pulmonary alveolar proteinosis is an exception. Effective therapy is not available because the etiology or mechanism of disease is not recognized. The alveolitis may be suppressed with either corticosteroids or immunosuppressive agents, but these medications do not cure the disease. Corticosteroids almost always are the initial therapy, but they are associated with many adverse side effects. A few adequately controlled trials have assessed corticosteroid use in ILD. Among IPF patients, half experienced subjective improvement with steroids, yet only 15% to 20% improved by objective measures. The specific steroid regimen varies. Most commonly therapy is initiated with prednisone, 1 mg/kg, which is given for 3 to 6 months and then tapered over 4 to 6 months to 0.25 mg/kg. The efficacy of alternate-day regimens is not known.

Immunosuppressive or cytotoxic agents may be considered for patients for whom corticosteroids appear to have failed or for those who experience adverse side effects or have contraindications to corticosteroids, such as age, morbid obesity, insulin-dependent diabetes mellitus, or severe osteoporosis. Cyclophosphamide and methotrexate have been used in a number of disorders included in ILD. Methotrexate has been used infrequently because pulmonary toxicity can occur in a significant number of patients. Azathioprine also has been used as a corticosteroid-sparing agent in diverse autoimmune disease and as therapy for sarcoidosis, IPF, and ILD with collagen vascular disease. This medication is given orally and is associated with fewer adverse side effects than methotrexate, cyclophosphamide, or alkylating agents.

Meticulous supportive care can improve the quality of life of patients with ILD. Supportive therapy includes vaccines, antibiotics for episodes of purulent sputum, bronchodilators for wheezing, supplemental oxygen when the partial pressure of arterial oxygen (PaO_2) drops below 55 mm Hg, psychosocial therapy, and pulmonary rehabilitation.

Associated Diseases

Idiopathic Pulmonary Fibrosis

Idiopathic pulmonary fibrosis (IPF) predominantly affects males in the fifth to seventh decade of life.[11] No genetic basis has been found. The pathogenesis is not known but is likely to reflect an aberrant host response to injury of the alveolar epithelium and endothelium or a protracted response to the same. A history of a gradual onset of dyspnea with exercise is typical. More than 30% of patients experience constitutional symptoms such as weight loss, malaise, and easy fatigability. With progression of the disease, clubbing of the fingers and toes, crackles in lung bases, dyspnea at rest, and evidence of cor pulmonale become more prominent. The chest radiograph correlates poorly with clinical findings. In 10% of patients the radiograph is normal, but a reticulonodular pattern in the lung bases is characteristic in IPF. The distribution and pattern of the lesions are highly distinctive on HRCT scans, which show patchy subpleural and basilar lesions.

Pulmonary function tests show reduced lung volumes, reduced compliance, and a decrease in diffusing capac-

ity. Laboratory values are nonspecific. TBB usually is not diagnostic. Most but not all patients with IPF ultimately require a surgical lung biopsy. Biopsies reveal a mixture of fibrosis and inflammatory cell infiltration with the pulmonary interstitium and alveolar walls. IPF has no pathognomonic clinical, biochemical, or pathologic finding and therefore is currently diagnosed by histologic exclusion of other specific entities. As the lesions progress, the lung architecture is distorted, and respiratory failure ensues within 5 years. The mortality rate approximates 50% at 5 years. The prognosis is worse in men and for patients with honeycombing, severely depressed pulmonary function, and absence of lymphocytes on lavage.

The decision as to which patients should be treated with steroids or cytotoxic agents is difficult. Most would agree in the treatment of patients who have significant gas exchange abnormalities with ILD symptoms. Corticosteroids have been associated with a favorable response in 10% to 30% of these patients. An initial trial of 40 to 60 mg given orally daily for 3 months is reasonable. Continuation of therapy should depend on an objective response to these agents. Criteria and end points used to document a response are controversial. A 10% or greater increase in the FVC and FEV_1 or a 20% or greater increase in the D_{LCO} is considered a favorable response. Responders should be tapered to 10 to 20 mg given orally daily within 6 months. The optimum duration of therapy has not been determined. In nonresponders the corticosteroid should be tapered and stopped. Immunosuppressive or cytotoxic agents (cyclophosphamide and azathioprine) should be considered for patients in whom corticosteroids appear to be ineffective or who are at risk of adverse effects from corticosteroids. However, data show a low rate of response to alternative therapies in patients whose condition is resistant to steroids. Single-lung transplantation is an option for younger patients whose condition fails to respond to medical therapy.

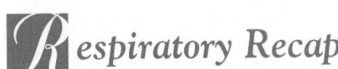

espiratory Recap

Characteristics of Idiopathic Pulmonary Fibrosis

Disease predominantly affects men in the fifth to seventh decades of life.

History of exertional dyspnea is typical.

Chest radiograph correlates poorly with clinical findings.

High-resolution computed tomography shows the disease's highly distinctive distribution and pattern of lesions.

Transbronchial biopsy usually is not diagnostic.

Most patients require a surgical lung biopsy.

Disease currently is diagnosed by histologic exclusion of other specific entities.

Mortality rate is approximately 50% at 5 years.

Initial trial of prednisone (40 to 60 mg given orally once a day for 3 months) is a reasonable treatment choice; continuation of therapy depends on an objective response.

Sarcoidosis

Sarcoidosis is a disorder in which multiple organ systems usually develop noncaseating granulomas.[12] It is a common disorder and is the most prevalent ILD of unknown etiology. The prevalence of sarcoidosis in North America is 10 to 20 cases per 100,000 people, and the rate in Scandinavia is approximately 80 per 100,000. The disorder is rare in Africa, South America, and Central America. Most cases occur between 20 and 45 years of age, and the disease is rare in children and the elderly. Sarcoidosis is common in African Americans.

Respiratory Recap

Characteristics of Sarcoidosis

Disease causes noncaseating granulomas in several organ systems.

Sarcoidosis is the most common interstitial lung disease (ILD) of unknown etiology.

Most cases are seen in patient 20 to 45 years old.

Disease is common in African Americans.

Lung is the organ most frequently involved.

Chest radiograph shows bilateral hilar lymph node enlargement (stage I), ILD with lymph node enlargement (stage II), and ILD alone (stage III).

Adenopathy and ILD frequently regress spontaneously.

Extrapulmonary involvement is common.

Transbronchial biopsy demonstrates noncaseating granulomas.

Thoracoscopic or open lung biopsy is rarely needed for diagnosis.

Steroids are given with functional impairment of one or more organs.

In sarcoidosis the lung is the organ most frequently involved. This high frequency of respiratory tract involvement may represent a response to an inhaled antigen. A significant proportion of individuals with sarcoidosis are asymptomatic (40% to 60%), but the chest radiograph is abnormal in more than 90%. The chest radiograph in sarcoidosis shows one of the following patterns: lymph node enlargement, which most frequently is bilateral and hilar (stage I disease); ILD with lymph node enlargement (stage II); or ILD alone (stage III). HRCT has no routine role in the diagnosis or staging of sarcoidosis. Most patients with stage II or stage III disease demonstrate restrictive results on pulmonary function tests. Some of these individuals may also show a pattern of airway obstruction. Laboratories can demonstrate an increased serum concentration of angiotensin-converting enzyme (ACE) and hypercalcemia. The level of ACE may correspond to disease activity and has been used as a measure of granuloma burden.

Over time both the adenopathy and the ILD may regress spontaneously in approximately 60% of all patients (this occurs in 80% of patients in stage I, 40% in stage II, and 10% in stage III). However, at the other extreme, the interstitial disease may progress to extensive scarring and end-stage lung disease, at which point the patient may have severe respiratory compromise. The course of the disease usually is dictated in the first 24 months, with almost all spontaneous remissions occurring during this time.

Extrapulmonary involvement is common. Eye and skin involvement are particularly common manifestations of sarcoidosis, but the disease may also have cardiac, neuromuscular, hematologic, hepatic, endocrine, and peripheral lymph node effects. Mortality from sarcoidosis most often is the result of cardiac involvement.

The diagnosis can be made in several ways. The history, a physical examination, and chest radiography may provide the diagnosis in a young African-American woman with bilateral hilar adenopathy. Bronchoscopy with lavage can assist in the diagnosis with lavage cells displaying a predominance of lymphocytes with an abnormally elevated CD_4 to CD_8 ratio. TBB demonstrates noncaseating granulomas (which have a central core of histiocytes, epithelioid cells, and multinucleated giant cells) in as many as 90% of patients, because this process involves peribronchial and bronchiolar tissue. If bronchoscopy is not diagnostic, mediastinoscopy may be done to sample hilar and mediastinal lymph nodes. Biopsies of other involved tissues (skin, conjunctiva, salivary glands, or liver) can also provide a diagnosis. Thoracoscopic or open lung biopsy is rarely needed for diagnosis.

Treatment of sarcoidosis consists of steroid administration when evidence of progressive functional impairment of one or more vital organs is seen. Treatment of patients with mild symptoms or nonprogressive disease is inappropriate. Severe pulmonary dysfunction, hypercalcemia, and myocardial, nervous system, and eye involvement and disfiguring skin lesions necessitate corticosteroid treatment. The appropriate dose, duration, and tapering of the corticosteroid has not been defined. Response to the treatment is evident within 12 weeks, but the corticosteroid should be continued for at least 12 months at a minimally effective dose, because relapses of sarcoidosis occur often as the corticosteroid is tapered. Immunosuppressive agents (methotrexate and azathioprine) have been used for steroid-resistant cases, for steroid sparing, and for individuals who have contraindications to or who have had adverse effects from steroids. Transplantation has been used in end-stage lung disease with sarcoidosis.

Interstitial Lung Disease with Collagen Vascular Disease

Patients with a **collagen vascular disease** can develop ILD.[13] The collagen vascular diseases include progressive systemic sclerosis, systemic lupus erythematosus (SLE), polymyositis and dermatomyositis, Sjögren's syndrome, and mixed connective tissue disease. Although progression of ILD with collagen vascular diseases is slower, the clinical presentation is comparable to that of IPF. The histopathologic features of ILD in this setting also correspond to those of IPF, with the additional features of lymphoid hyperplasia, cellular interstitial pneumonitis, lymphoid interstitial pneumonitis, diffuse alveolar damage, and bronchiolitis obliterans with organizing pneumonia. The diagnosis is assumed in patients with a known, underlying collagen vascular disease and classic clinical features of ILD (rales, dyspnea, interstitial infiltrates, and restrictive results on pulmonary function tests). Before aggressive immunosuppressive therapy is begun, bronchoscopy with lavage and TBB should be performed to exclude alternative etiologies such as malignancy and infection. For patients with a deteriorating course, treatment involves administration of corticosteroids or immunosuppressive agents or both.

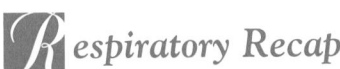

Respiratory Recap

> **Interstitial Lung Disease with Collagen Vascular Disease**
>
> Progression of interstitial lung disease (ILD) with collagen vascular diseases is slow, but the clinical presentation is comparable to that of idiopathic pulmonary fibrosis (IPF), as is the histopathology.
> Diagnosis is assumed in patients with a known underlying collagen vascular disease and classic clinical features of ILD.
> Treatment involves administration of corticosteroids or immunosuppressive agents or both.

ILD shows a high association with progressive systemic sclerosis, and most patients with this disorder have ILD at some time during the course of their illness. There is an even greater prevalence of pulmonary hypertension (80% to 95%).

Eosinophilic Granuloma

Eosinophilic granuloma, also called *Langerhans' cell granulomatosis,* was first described in 1953 as a bone disease having characteristics similar to those of Letterer-Siwe disease and Hand-Schüller-Christian disease.[13] Since then, it has been shown to be predominantly a pulmonary disorder. Eosinophilic granuloma is a rare disease that occurs almost exclusively in smokers or former smokers 10 to 40 years of age. Although the etiology remains unknown, eosinophilic granuloma probably is an inflammatory response by Langerhans' cells to a component of tobacco smoke.[14] Common presenting symptoms are a nonproductive cough, chest pain, and dyspnea on exertion. Weight loss, fever, and hemoptysis occasionally occur. Extrapulmonary features, including involvement of the posterior pituitary gland with the development of diabetes insipidus and lytic bony lesions, have frequently been described (20% of patients).

The physical examination often is unremarkable, but occasional wheezing may be heard. Pulmonary function tests show a decrease in lung volumes and diffusing capacity with normal or reduced expiratory flow rates. Radiographic findings of nodular densities in the upper and midlung fields with sparing of the lung bases are characteristic, but reticular, reticulonodular, and cystic lesions can be observed. Pleural effusions are uncommon. Pneumothoraces occur in approximately 10% of patients. The HRCT scans are highly distinctive, revealing numerous peribronchiolar nodular and cystic lesions.

As the disease progresses, the nodules are replaced by cysts that become confluent. Biopsy shows a mixture of inflammatory, cystic, nodular, and fibrotic lesions centered at or adjacent to bronchioles. Light microscopy shows the cleft nuclei of the Langerhans' cells and the stellate pattern of fibrosis in 80% of patients. Aggregates of Langerhans' cells (HX cells) can be demonstrated by immunostaining for S-100 protein or OKT6 antigen. Electron microscopy reveals Birbeck granules (X bodies) within these large, mononuclear phagocytes. As the inflammation progresses, alveolar architecture is destroyed and replaced by cysts and fibrosis.

In some cases TBB can provide the diagnosis. Spontaneous remissions are the rule, and no therapy beyond symptomatic and supportive care has been shown to be effective. Cigarette smoking must be stopped. There is progressive loss of pulmonary function in up to one quarter of these individuals, who can die of respiratory failure. Corticosteroids often are used in severe and progressive disease, but no data are available on their efficacy.

Respiratory Recap

> **Characteristics of Eosinophilic Granuloma**
>
> Disease is also called Langerhans' cell granulomatosis.
> Eosinophilic granuloma was first described as a bone disease but is now recognized as a predominantly pulmonary disorder.
> Disease occurs almost exclusively in smokers or former smokers 10 to 40 years old.
> Etiology is unknown.
> Common presenting symptoms are a nonproductive cough, chest pain, and dyspnea on exertion.
> Extrapulmonary features include diabetes insipidus and lytic bony lesions.
> High-resolution computed tomography scans are highly distinctive.
> Light microscopy shows the cleft nuclei of the Langerhans' cells and stellate pattern of fibrosis in 80% of patients.
> Spontaneous remissions are the rule.
> Patient must stop smoking if the disease is to resolve.

Respiratory Bronchiolitis

Respiratory bronchiolitis is a rare disorder that occurs exclusively in cigarette smokers.[15] Most of these individuals are asymptomatic, but they may have a mild cough, dyspnea, and sputum production. Crackles can be detected in some of these patients in the physical examination. The chest radiograph may demonstrate reticulonodular infiltrates at the bases, but it also may be normal. Pathologic studies reveal intracytoplasmic, golden-brown, granular pigment in alveolar macrophages in the respiratory and terminal bronchioles. The disease resolves in almost all patients after the person stops smoking.

Pulmonary Alveolar Proteinosis

Pathologically **pulmonary alveolar proteinosis (PAP)** is characterized by filling of alveolar spaces with a lipoproteinaceous exudate and interstitial fibrosis.[16] The intraalveolar phospholipid stains bright pink with periodic–acid Schiff (PAS) reagent. Although some patients are asymptomatic, most have dyspnea and cough, and alveolar infiltrates are seen on the chest radiograph. Laboratory values can verify hypoxemia. The disease spontaneously remits in one third of patients. Although the mortality rate formerly was high, death is now rare. Treatment involves whole lung lavage, performed under general anesthesia, with 20 to 40 L of saline. The etiology remains unknown, but some patients have a history of exposure to silica and hydrocarbons.

Drug-Induced Interstitial Lung Disease

A number of different drugs can result in ILD.[17] The clinical and radiographic features differ depending on the implicated agent. Clinical presentations are specified as syndromes of acute pneumonitis, chronic interstitial pneumonitis, acute alveolar hemorrhage, or noncardiac pulmonary edema. A dose-related toxicity (for example, as with antineoplastic agents) may be seen but often is not (such as with bleomycin), and the presentation may be that of an idiosyncratic reaction. Agents may be synergistic with each other, with radiation, or with oxygen exposure in the resultant lung toxicity.

A number of mechanisms are involved in drug-induced ILD, including cytotoxicity, hypersensitivity pneumonitis, and noncardiogenic pulmonary edema. Cytotoxic drug injury may occur with bleomycin, alkylating agents, and nitrosoureas. Previous chemotherapy or radiation therapy can amplify the risk of ILD with use of these drugs. The histopathologic features include type II pneumocyte proliferation with cellular atypia (large nuclei, prominent nucleoli, and bizarre chromatin patterns), inflammatory cell incursion, and fibrosis. Cytotoxic lung injury has a significant mortality rate (10% to 50% of patients, depending on the drug). Corticosteroids are most effective if given early, when a cellular rather than a fibrotic histology is present; the response is extremely variable and often negative with established disease. Methotrexate, nitrofurantoin, gold, and sulfasalazine are associated with hypersensitivity pneumonitis. Both acute and subacute forms manifest with fever, chest pain, and interstitial or alveolar infiltrates on the radiograph. The prognosis is good when the medication is stopped. Corticosteroids may hasten resolu-

tion. Salicylates, thiazides, narcotics, and cytarabine all can induce a noncardiac pulmonary edema.

Acute Interstitial Lung Disease

A number of interstitial lung diseases manifest in a more acute fashion. They include acute interstitial pneumonitis (Hamman-Rich syndrome), acute **bronchiolitis obliterans with organizing pneumonia (BOOP),** acute eosinophilic pneumonia, and lymphoid interstitial pneumonitis.[18] The presentation of these diseases mimics an atypical pneumonia, with the patient reporting an unproductive cough, dyspnea, fever, and malaise. It is not unusual for these patients to develop acute respiratory failure that requires mechanical ventilation.

Acute interstitial pneumonitis is a rapidly progressive form of interstitial pneumonitis thought either to exemplify an accelerated phase of IPF or to be a distinct entity of unknown etiology. It has been described as an acute respiratory distress syndrome without an underlying precipitating injury. Acute interstitial pneumonitis is characterized by an epithelial cell injury that results in denudation of the epithelial lining of the alveolus and edema of the alveolar walls (that is, diffuse alveolar damage). Intraalveolar fibrin, edema accumulation, mild acute and chronic interstitial inflammation, and formation of intraalveolar hyaline membranes also are frequently described. Collagen deposition by fibroblasts and honeycomb lung can follow. Hypoxemic respiratory failure is common, and the mortality rate is high. Patients are treated with corticosteroids, but the drugs' effectiveness is not known.

Acute BOOP appears to be a response of the lung to a variety of injuries that affect the smaller airways and alveoli as a unit. These injuries include infections, exposure to toxic gases, radiation therapy, drug toxicity, eosinophilic pneumonia, Wegener's granulomatosis, and hypersensitivity pneumonitis. Acute BOOP manifests as an upper respiratory infection with a persistent cough and then dyspnea. Focal alveolar infiltrates are seen on the chest radiograph. Histologically, proliferating fibroblasts are noted in alveolar spaces, and polyps (inflammatory cells and fibrosis) project into the lumina of distal bronchioles. Extrapulmonary involvement does not occur. Treatment is administration of corticosteroids, with most individuals demonstrating good response.

Acute eosinophilic pneumonia is distinguished by fleeting pulmonary infiltrates and peripheral eosinophilia. Simple pulmonary eosinophilia (Löffler's syndrome) is most commonly the result of infection with parasites such as *Strongyloides, Ascaris,* and *Ancylostoma* species but also can be caused by a drug reaction. The most common symptom is a dry cough. The infiltrates resolve within 2 weeks, and the peripheral eosinophilia is transitory. Treatment is directed at an identifiable underlying cause. Tropical eosinophilia can manifest as an acute eosinophilic pneumonia and is believed to be part of a hypersensitivity reaction to the filarial worm. Cough, fever, myalgia, and dyspnea are common. The histologic appearance is that of a cellular interstitial pneumonia with both infiltration of the interstitium and alveolar spaces by mononuclear cells and eosinophils and areas of BOOP. This can lead to respiratory failure requiring mechanical ventilation.

Various drugs have also been reported to produce acute eosinophilic pneumonia. In these cases the bronchoalveolar lavage shows a predominance of eosinophils. Treatment with corticosteroids cures the disease, and recurrences are unusual.

Allergic bronchopulmonary aspergillosis manifests as an acute eosinophilic pneumonia and is seen in asthmatics. Patients have a productive cough, eosinophilia, and a patchy infiltrate. Treatment is administration of corticosteroids.

Lymphoid interstitial pneumonitis is distinguished by dense lymphocytic infiltrates in the alveolar interstitium and lymphatics. The patient complains of cough and dyspnea. On the radiograph, bilateral reticular and reticulonodular infiltrates, dense alveolar infiltrates, or focal nodules are observed. The disease is considered a lymphoproliferative disorder. Lymphoid interstitial pneumonitis is associated most commonly with HIV infection (especially in children) but also with dysproteinemias, hypogammaglobulinemia, common variable immunodeficiency syndrome, monoclonal gammopathy, SLE, Sjögren's syndrome, chronic active hepatitis, primary biliary cirrhosis, and bone marrow transplantation. Treatment is administration of corticosteroids, but no data are available on their effectiveness. The mortality rate for lymphoid interstitial pneumonitis is high.

KEY POINTS

- Interstitial lung disease is a heterogenous group of disorders classified together because of similarities in their clinical and pathologic presentation.
- The most common identifiable causes of interstitial lung disease are related to occupational or environmental exposure.
- A large number of ILD patients have interstitial lung disease of unknown etiology, including idiopathic pulmonary fibrosis and sarcoidosis.
- Treatment of interstitial lung disease most often is supportive.

References

1. Du Bois RM. Diffuse lung disease: an approach to management. Br Med J 1994;309:175-179.
2. Robertson HT. Clinical application of pulmonary function and exercise tests in the management of patients with interstitial lung disease. Semin Respir Crit Care Med 1994;15:1-16.
3. Muller NL. Clinical value of high-resolution CT in chronic diffuse lung disease. Am J Radiol 1991;157:1163-1170.
4. Raghu G. Interstitial lung disease: a diagnostic approach: are CT scan and lung biopsy indicated in every patient? Am J Respir Crit Care Med 1995;151:909-914.
5. Reynolds HY, Fulmer JD, Kazmierowski JA, et al. Analysis of cellular and protein content of bronchoalveolar lavage fluid from patients with idiopathic pulmonary fibrosis and chronic hypersensitivity pneumonitis. J Clin Invest 1977;59:165-175.
6. Smith CM, Holbrook T. Utilization of the transbronchial biopsy and open lung biopsy for tissue to establish the diagnosis of idiopathic pulmonary fibrosis. Am Rev Respir Dis 1990; 141:A62.
7. Venn GE, Kay PH, Midwood CJ, et al. Open biopsy in patients with diffuse pulmonary shadowing. Thorax 1985;40:931-935.
8. Lee JS, Im JG, Ahn JM, et al. Fibrosing alveolitis: prognostic implication of ground glass attenuation at high-resolution CT. Radiology 1992;184:451-454.
9. Wells AU, Hansell DM, Corrin B, et al. High-resolution computed tomography as a predictor of lung histology in systemic sclerosis. Thorax 1992;47:738-742.
10. Hunninghake GW, Kalica AR. Approaches to treatment of pulmonary fibrosis. Am J Respir Crit Care Med 1995;15:915-918.
11. Ryu JH, Colby TV, Hartman TE. Idiopathic pulmonary fibrosis: current concepts. Mayo Clin Proc 1998;73:1085-1101.
12. Belfer MH, Stevens RW. Sarcoidosis: a primary care review. Am Family Physician 1998;58:2041-2050, 2055-2056.
13. Lynch JP III, Hunninghake GW. Pulmonary complications of collagen vascular disease. Annu Rev Med 1992;43:17-35.
14. Colby TV, Lombard C. Histiocytosis X in the lung. Hum Pathol 1983;14:847-856.
15. King TE Jr. Respiratory bronchiolitis-associated interstitial lung disease. Clin Chest Med 1993;4:693-698.
16. Claypool WD, Rogers RM, Matuschak GM. Update on the clinical diagnosis, management, and pathogenesis of pulmonary alveolar proteinosis (phospholipidosis). Chest 1984;85:550-558.
17. Copper JA Jr. Drug-induced lung disease. Adv Intern Med 1997;42:231.
18. Schwarz MI. The acute (noninfectious) interstitial lung diseases. Compr Ther 1996;22:622-637.

CHAPTER 49

Pulmonary Vascular Disease

Scott M. Palmer
Victor F. Tapson

CHAPTER OUTLINE

OBJECTIVES

1. Describe the physiology of the right ventricle and pulmonary circulation in normal and disease states.
2. Describe the signs and symptoms of pulmonary vascular diseases, including those present in pulmonary embolism (PE), cor pulmonale, and primary pulmonary hypertension (PPH).
3. Define the role of ventilation perfusion ($\dot{V}/\dot{Q}$) scanning, pulmonary angiography, and computed tomography (CT) in the diagnosis of PE.
4. Discuss the role of anticoagulation and thrombolytic therapy in the management of acute PE.
5. Describe the pathogenesis and treatment of cor pulmonale.
6. Discuss the role of pulmonary vasodilators and lung transplantation in the management of PPH.

KEY TERMS

Anticoagulation	Hypoxic Pulmonary Vasoconstriction	Pulmonary Embolism (PE)
Calcium Channel Blockers	Inferior Vena Cava (IVC) Filter	Pulmonary Vascular Resistance
Cor Pulmonale	Primary Pulmonary Hypertension (PPH)	Spiral Computed Tomography (CT)
Deep Vein Thrombosis (DVT)	Prostacyclin	Thrombolytic Therapy
Heparin-Induced Thrombocytopenia (HIT)	Pulmonary Angiogram	

Disorders of the pulmonary circulation include a large and heterogeneous group of conditions. Some pulmonary vascular diseases, such as pulmonary thromboembolism, occur quite commonly, whereas others, such as primary pulmonary hypertension (PPH), are extremely rare. Diseases of the pulmonary circulation occur as a result of intrinsic abnormalities of the pulmonary vessels, embolic complications from elsewhere in the vascular system, or secondary to underlying cardiac or pulmonary disease. Because the right ventricle (RV) is poorly suited to respond to elevations in pulmonary vascular pressure, similar pathologic consequences occur once pulmonary hypertension develops, regardless of the etiology. In this chapter the pathophysiology of pulmonary vascular disease is reviewed in light of the normal physiology and function of the RV and pulmonary circulation. Features common to many pulmonary vascular diseases are described in addition to issues related to the specific diagnosis and management of several common disorders of the pulmonary circulation.

Pathophysiology

Normal Pulmonary Vascular Physiology

The principal function of the pulmonary circulation is gas exchange. Venous blood low in oxygen and rich in carbon dioxide passes through the pulmonary capillaries, where oxygen is absorbed and carbon dioxide is eliminated, thus allowing the left ventricle to return oxygenated blood to the rest of the body. Under normal circumstances, the pulmonary circulation is a low-pressure, high-flow system, providing little resistance to the right ventricular outflow.[1] Mean pulmonary artery pressure and **pulmonary vascular resistance** at rest is approximately one sixth of that of the systemic circulation.[1] The RV serves primarily as a capacitance chamber for blood returning from the systemic veins. As long as pulmonary vascular resistance is normal, blood flows from the right side of the heart through the lungs to the left side of the heart as a result of left heart action. The contraction of the left ventricle and interventricular septum pulls the free wall of the RV against the septum and augments the flow of blood through the pulmonary circulation.[2] In addition, the phasic changes in intrathoracic pressure that accompany respiration also direct the forward flow of blood from the RV through the pulmonary circulation.[2]

Normally, the pulmonary vascular bed is able to accommodate large increases in blood flow without much change in pressure preventing RV overload. For example, cardiac output can increase substantially during exercise in normal individuals with increases of up to fivefold in pulmonary blood flow.[2,3] The thin-walled RV is highly compliant and able to accommodate large volumes and filling pressures. Recruitment of vessels in the poorly perfused upper lung and distention of the compliant vessels in the dependent areas allow the pulmonary circulation to accommodate these increases in cardiac output and pulmonary blood flow.[4,5]

Pulmonary Vascular Pathophysiology

The pulmonary vascular tree is a low resistance circulation that can absorb large changes in cardiac output without significant increases in pulmonary pressures. However, many pathologic conditions can give rise to pulmonary hypertension as summarized in Box 49-1. Depending on the specific disorder, different mechanisms are likely to contribute to the initial pathogenesis of pulmonary hypertension.

Destruction or obliteration of the pulmonary vascular bed is likely to play a key role in patients with pulmonary parenchymal diseases, such as chronic obstructive pulmonary disease (COPD).[6] In contrast, in patients with PPH, an intrinsic vascular abnormality appears to alter pulmonary vasoreactivity. Patients with PPH are thought to have decreased production of pulmonary vasodilators such as prostacyclin and overproduction of pulmonary vasoconstrictors such as thromboxane.[7] In addition, in many individuals with pulmonary vascular diseases, chronic alveolar hypoxia and associated hypoxic pulmonary vasoconstriction contribute to the development of pulmonary hypertension.[6]

Once pulmonary hypertension develops, independent of the inciting event, pulmonary vascular remodeling occurs, leading to medial hypertrophy and intimal fibrosis, which further reduces pulmonary vascular cross-sectional area and exacerbates pulmonary hypertension. Figure 49-1 illustrates vascular changes observed in a patient with pulmonary hypertension. As right ventricular afterload increases with worsening pulmonary hypertension, RV hypertrophy, dilation, or failure can occur. **Cor pulmonale** is right ventricular dysfunction resulting from pulmonary hypertension, which in turn results from an underlying pulmonary parenchymal disease.[6] COPD and idiopathic pulmonary fibrosis (IPF) are two diseases commonly associated with the development of cor pulmonale.

Box 49-1

Selected Causes of Pulmonary Hypertension

Obstruction of the Pulmonary Vasculature
Venous thromboembolism
Schistosomiasis
Malignancies
Foreign bodies (for example, talc)
Sickle cell disease

Pulmonary Parenchymal Disease
Chronic obstructive pulmonary disease (COPD)
Interstitial lung disease

Cardiac Disease
Congenital heart disease (Eisenmenger's syndrome)
Left-sided heart failure
Left-sided valvular disease

Intrinsic Disorders of the Pulmonary Vasculature
Primary pulmonary hypertension
Pulmonary veno-occlusive disease
Drugs
Anorexic agents
Crack cocaine

Pulmonary Hypertension Associated with Systemic Illness
Collagen vascular disease (for example, scleroderma)
Portal hypertension
Human immunodeficiency virus (HIV)
Hypoventilation/sleep apnea

Pathophysiology of Acute Pulmonary Emboli

The luminal area of the pulmonary circulation may be obstructed, leading to acute or chronic pulmonary hypertension. Venous thromboemboli that cause PE usually arise from **deep vein thrombosis (DVT)** in the lower extremities. When emboli acutely obstruct a significant portion of the pulmonary arterial bed, profound hemodynamic alterations occur. Hypoxemia occurs as a result of regions with low ventilation-perfusion ($\dot{V}/\dot{Q}$) ratios and shunting secondary to perfusion of atelectatic areas. The impact of the embolic event depends on the extent of reduction of the cross-sectional area of the pulmonary vasculature and on the presence or absence of underlying cardiovascular disease.[8] With massive emboli, cardiac output is diminished but may be sustained to a certain point. Increased pulmonary vascular resistance impedes right ventricular outflow and reduces left ventricular preload. More than 50% obstruction of the pulmonary arterial bed is usually present before substantial elevation of mean pulmonary artery pressure develops. When the extent of obstruction of the pulmonary circulation approaches 75%, a normal individual

cannot generate the right ventricle systolic pressures in excess of 50 mm Hg required to preserve pulmonary perfusion, and cardiac failure and death will occur.[9] Thus although supportive measures may sustain a patient with massive PE, any additional increment in embolic burden may be fatal.

Epidemiology

Disorders of the pulmonary circulation include a diverse group of clinical conditions that result in substantial morbidity and mortality. Pulmonary thromboembolism, for example, is recognized as the third most common cause of cardiovascular disease in the United States after ischemic heart disease and stroke.[10] Autopsy studies suggest that more than 600,000 patients in the United States develop DVT and/or PE each year, with over half of these cases not recognized before death. PE probably causes or contributes to the death of at least 100,000 of these patients each year.[11]

In addition, cor pulmonale appears to contribute substantially to mortality in patients with a variety of pulmonary parenchymal diseases, especially COPD. The exact incidence and prevalence of cor pulmonale in COPD is not known but recent estimates suggest that 10% to 40% of patients with COPD have evidence of right ventricular hypertrophy.[6] Cor pulmonale increases in prevalence with increased severity of lung disease and may occur in over 70% of COPD patients with an FEV_1 less than 0.6 L.[12] The development of cor pulmonale in these patients portends a significantly worse prognosis than in patients with normal right ventricular pressures. In patients with COPD, which causes an estimated 70,000 deaths each year in the United States, overt right heart failure is associated with a 5-year survival of only 30%.[6,13] In fibrotic lung disease, such as IPF, pulmonary artery pressures are also important predictors of survival.[14]

Primary pulmonary hypertension (PPH) is an uncommon disorder of the pulmonary vessels associated with severe elevation in pulmonary vascular resistance. The incidence of PPH is estimated at one to two cases per million people in the population.[15] PPH is most common among younger patients (ages 20 to 40 years) and occurs at least twice as frequently in women. PPH is associated with poor prognosis. In the PPH registry data, the median survival from the time of diagnosis was 2.8 years, with a 5-year survival of only 34%.[16] A mean pulmonary artery pressure of more than 85 mm Hg or a car-

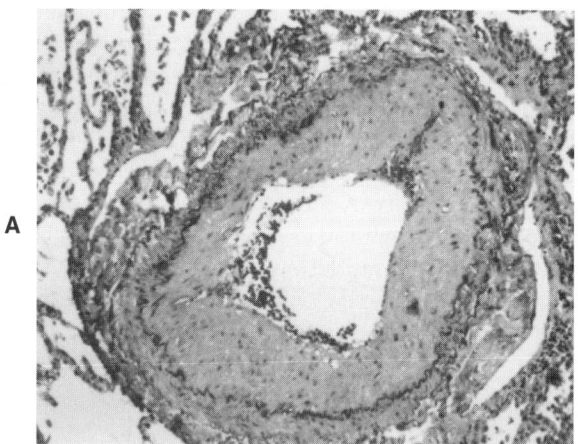

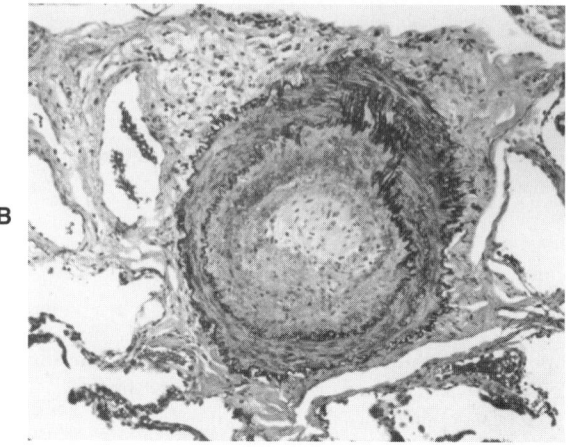

Figure 49-1 Pathologic changes of pulmonary hypertension. **A,** Lung specimen from a patient with primary pulmonary hypertension demonstrates medial hypertrophy and intimal proliferation in one pulmonary artery. **B,** Complete obliteration of another pulmonary artery (elastic stain).

Age-Specific Angle

PPH is most common among patients ages 20 to 40 years.

diac index less than 2.0 L/minute are associated with low survival. A lack of effective therapeutic options, until recently, contributed to the high mortality rate associated with PPH.

Pulmonary vascular disease clinically and pathologically indistinguishable from PPH can occur in association with a number of systemic illnesses, such as scleroderma and human immunodeficiency virus (HIV) infection, or in association with certain drugs, including appetite suppressants.[17-19] Recently, the use of the appetite suppressants fenfluramine and dexfenfluramine have been found to significantly increase the risk of pulmonary hypertension (odds ratio of greater than 20 with more than 3 months of use).[19] In general, the prognosis for patients with these secondary forms of pulmonary hypertension is similar to that in PPH and remains poor.

Diagnosis of Pulmonary Vascular Disease

Pulmonary Embolism

The history, physical exam, arterial blood gas, electrocardiogram, and chest radiograph are often useful in suggesting the presence or absence of **pulmonary embolism (PE).** The clinical evaluation alone, however, is not a reliable guide to the diagnosis of PE, as is underscored by the high incidence of unsuspected PE in autopsy series.[20] PE should be considered whenever unexplained dyspnea occurs. Common risk factors for PE are listed in Box 49-2. The presence of one or more risk factors should increase the clinical suspicion. Unexplained dyspnea in association with pleuritic chest pain or hemoptysis is suggestive of PE. PE also must be considered in the setting of unexplained syncope or sudden hypotension.

The physical examination may be unrevealing in patients with acute PE. Because patients with lower extremity DVT often do not exhibit erythema, warmth, pain, or swelling, physical exam may not provide clues to the presence of an underlying DVT. An increased pulmonic component of the second heart sound has been reported in massive PE, but the nonspecific findings of tachypnea and

$\mathcal{B}$OX 49-2
_____

Important Risk Factors for Pulmonary Embolism

Recent surgery
Malignancy
Pregnancy/postpartum
Immobilization/paralysis
Prior history DVT/PE
Hypercoagulable state
    Antithrombin III deficiency
    Protein C or S deficiency
    Factor V Leiden mutation
    Antiphospholipid antibody syndrome

tachycardia are the most common physical examination abnormalities described in PE.

Hypoxemia is common in acute PE but is not universally present. Young patients without underlying lung disease may have a normal PaO_2. In a retrospective analysis of hospitalized patients with proven PE, the PaO_2 was more than 80 mm Hg in 29% of patients less than 40 years old, compared with 3% in the older group.[21] The alveolar-arterial difference was abnormal in all patients, however. Thus the diagnosis of acute PE cannot be excluded based on a normal PaO_2.

Age-Specific Angle

Young patients with PE, but without underlying lung disease, may have a normal PaO_2.

Electrocardiographic findings in acute PE are generally nonspecific and include T-wave changes, ST segment abnormalities, and left or right axis deviation. Manifestations of acute right heart failure including the S1 Q3 T3 pattern, right bundle branch block, P-wave pulmonale or right axis deviation were present in only 32% patients with massive PE in the Urokinase Pulmonary Embolism Trial (UPET).[22]

The majority of patients with PE have nonspecific abnormalities on chest radiograph. Common radiographic findings include atelectasis, pleural effusion, pulmonary infiltrates, and elevation of a hemidiaphragm.[23] Classic radiographic findings of pulmonary infarction such as wedge-shaped pleural density (Hampton's hump) or decreased vascularity (Westermark's sign) are suggestive but infrequent. A normal chest radiograph in the setting of severe dyspnea and hypoxemia without evidence of bronchospasm or cardiac shunt is strongly suggestive of PE. In general, however, the chest radiograph cannot be used to conclusively prove or exclude PE.

Ventilation-perfusion ($\dot{V}/\dot{Q}$) scanning should be performed when PE is suspected. Normal and high probability scans are considered diagnostic. Figure 49-2 illustrates a high-probability $\dot{V}/\dot{Q}$ scan in a patient with PE. Unfortunately, the $\dot{V}/\dot{Q}$ scan is rarely diagnostic (that is, it is rarely interpreted as normal or high probability). A normal perfusion scan rules out the diagnosis of PE with a high enough degree of certainty that further diagnostic evaluation is unnecessary.

In the Prospective Investigation of Pulmonary Embolism Diagnosis (PIOPED) study, the utility of $\dot{V}/\dot{Q}$ scanning combined with clinical assessment of patients with suspected PE was prospectively evaluated in more than 700 patients.[24] Patients with PE had scans that were high, intermediate, or low probability, but so did most patients without PE. Although the specificity of high probability scans was 97%, the sensitivity was only 41%. Of interest, 33% of patients

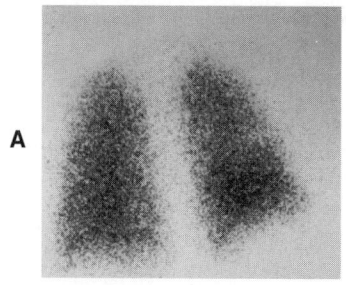
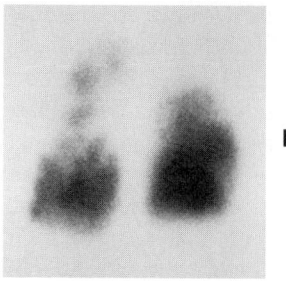

Figure 49-2 High-probability lung scan. This patient with metastatic cancer developed sudden dyspnea and unexplained hypoxemia after prolonged bed rest. The ventilation scan **(A)** is normal but the perfusion scan **(B)** demonstrates multiple bilateral perfusion defects, virtually diagnostic of pulmonary embolism.

with intermediate probability scans and 12% of patients with low probability scans were diagnosed definitively with PE by pulmonary arteriography. When the clinical suspicion of PE was considered high, PE was found to be present in 96% of patients with high probability scans, 66% of patients with intermediate scans, and 40% of patients with low probability scans. Thus additional diagnostic tests must be pursued when the $\dot{V}/\dot{Q}$ scan is of low or intermediate probability if the clinical scenario is suggestive of PE.

$\mathcal{R}$espiratory Recap

Diagnosis of Pulmonary Embolism
The physical exam may be unremarkable. Hypoxemia is common but not universally present. ECG findings are often nonspecific. The chest radiograph is often unremarkable; a normal chest radiograph with dyspnea and hypoxemia (and without bronchospasm) is suggestive of PE. High probability $\dot{V}/\dot{Q}$ scans are diagnostic of PE. Pulmonary angiography is the most diagnostic test for PE, but it is invasive and associated with significant risks. Spiral CT may be useful to diagnose proximal pulmonary emboli. The role of MRI remains investigational.

In patients requiring additional diagnostic testing, a **pulmonary angiogram** is usually performed. Figure 49-3 illustrates a pulmonary angiogram diagnostic of PE. However, in selected stable patients with suspected acute PE and nondiagnostic lung scans, serial noninvasive lower extremity testing to rule out DVT has been shown to be a reasonable alternative approach because a positive lower extremity study requires treatment without further testing.[25] However, in many cases, the lower extremity test is negative and pulmonary angiography is still required to provide a definite diagnosis. Serious complications of pulmonary angiography occur infrequently (less than 0.5% incidence in most series) but respiratory failure, renal failure, significant bleeding, and death have been reported.[26]

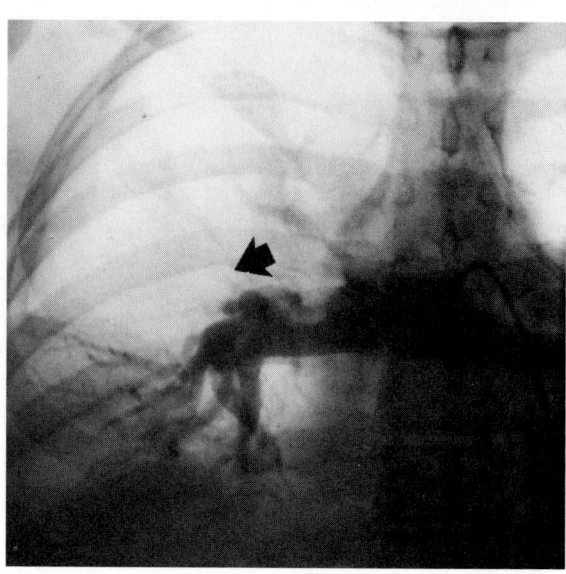

Figure 49-3 Pulmonary angiogram demonstrating acute pulmonary embolism. There is a large filling defect in the right pulmonary artery (*arrow*) and marked hypoperfusion to the right upper and middle lobes.

Thus although angiography is considered the most accurate diagnostic procedure for PE, it is invasive and carries small but significant risks. Angiography also requires the presence of experienced physicians to perform the test and interpret the results. Consequently, several less invasive imaging modalities such as **spiral computed tomography (CT)** have been investigated for the diagnosis of PE. Spiral (helical) CT involves continuous movement of a patient through the CT scanner with concurrent scanning by a constantly rotating gantry and detector system, allowing large volumes of data to be obtained quickly. Continuous scanning after contrast injection allows excellent visualization of the pulmonary arteries and direct visualization of arterial clot. Figure 49-4 illustrates spiral CT identification of a proximal pulmonary artery clot in a patient with PE. Although more data is needed to define the true utility of spiral CT for the diagnosis of PE, initial results suggest this modality allows detection of proximal pulmonary emboli with high degree of sensitivity and specificity.[27] Box 49-3 summarizes advantages and disadvantages of spiral CT in the diagnosis of PE. Recent studies have also investigated the use of magnetic resonance imaging (MRI) in the diagnosis of PE, but this work also remains quite preliminary.[28] In summary, although $\dot{V}/\dot{Q}$ scanning remains the most widely accepted initial diagnostic study in patients with suspected PE, increasing experience suggests spiral CT may eventually become the preferred study.

Pulmonary Hypertension (Primary or Secondary)

The clinical history and physical examination can provide important clues to the presence of primary or secondary pulmonary hypertension. Dyspnea is a common feature in most patients with pulmonary vascular disease but is non-

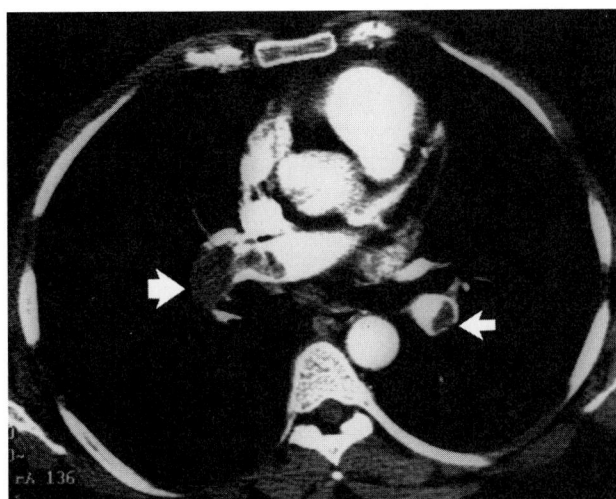

Figure 49-4 Spiral CT scan demonstrating acute pulmonary emboli. The large low density embolus is easily visualized in the right pulmonary arteries (*larger arrow*) surrounded by the dense white contrast. In addition, a smaller embolus is also evident in the left pulmonary artery (*smaller arrow*).

specific. Chest pain does occur in some patients with primary and secondary pulmonary hypertension but is often attributed to other etiologies such as panic attacks or gastroesophageal reflux. In the PPH registry, a period of 2 to 5 symptomatic years prior to diagnosis was documented.[29] In patients with PPH, Raynaud's phenomenon is common and may be associated with a poorer outcome. Presyncope and syncope are usually exertional in patients with severe pulmonary hypertension because of the inability to increase cardiac output in response to the increased demand.

Orthopnea is relatively common in patients with severe COPD, although it is not necessarily accompanied by worsening cardiac function. Orthopnea in these patients is believed to be related to hyperinflation of the lungs, and the subsequent effects on ventricular function and/or reduction in venous return. In patients with cor pulmonale and other forms of pulmonary hypertension, increased venous and hepatic congestion can occur in advanced disease and lead to the development of early satiety, increasing lower extremity edema and fluid overload. In all patients a careful history of current and prior medication use and concomitant medical conditions is essential.

The presence of a loud pulmonic valve closure sound is a common finding in patients with pulmonary hypertension, independent of the cause. It may be accompanied by a parasternal or epigastric lift resulting from a hypertrophied RV. Tricuspid valvular regurgitation also develops because of dilation of the RV, which causes a prominent jugular V wave. Progressive signs of chronic right ventricular dilation and failure include pulmonic valve insufficiency, a right ventricular third heart sound, jugular venous distention, hepatojugular reflux, hepatomegaly, lower extremity edema, ascites, and eventually anasarca.

Patients with cor pulmonale and pulmonary hypertension resulting from COPD also invariably have findings associated with their obstructive lung disease, including decreased breath sounds and hyperinflation. Individuals with cor pulmonale secondary to interstitial lung disease often have dry crackles at the lung bases. Auscultation of the lungs in PPH is generally unremarkable. Clubbing is also a common finding in patients with pulmonary fibrosis.

Hypoxemia is frequently observed in patients with significant pulmonary hypertension and cor pulmonale. Patients with PPH may have a normal arterial oxygen content until late in the disease. Pulmonary function tests may sometimes help identify the etiology of pulmonary vascular disease. The presence of significant pulmonary hypertension and cor pulmonale with mild abnormalities in pulmonary function tests should suggest a diagnosis of primary pulmonary vascular disease.

$\mathcal{R}$*espiratory Recap*

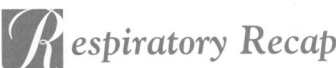

Diagnosis of Primary or Secondary Pulmonary Hypertension
Dyspnea is common but not specific.
Chest pain occurs in some patients.
Raynaud's phenomenon is common.
Exertional syncope may occur.
A loud pulmonic valve closure sound is common.
Hypoxemia is frequently present in patients with cor pulmonale.
ECG findings consistent with right heart strain are commonly observed.
Enlarged pulmonary arteries may be seen on the chest radiograph.
Echocardiography is often useful.
The gold standard for diagnosis of pulmonary hypertension is right heart catheterization.

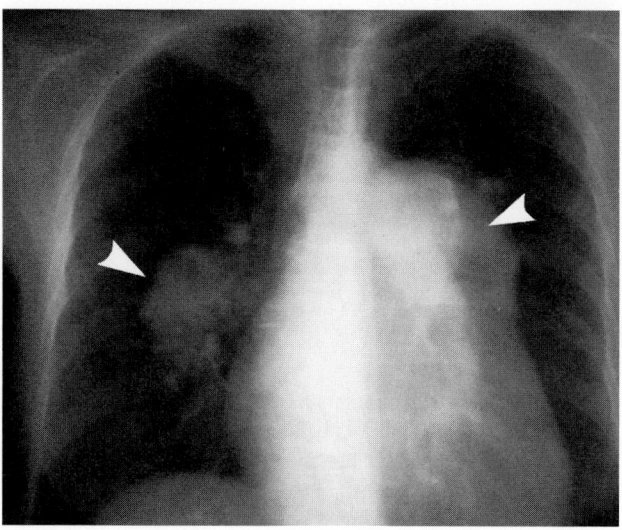

Figure 49-5 Chest radiograph in a patient with primary pulmonary hypertension. Enlarged right and left pulmonary arteries are evident (*arrows*).

In contrast to PE, in which nonspecific ECG changes are commonly observed, right heart strain, including P-pulmonale, right axis deviation, and right ventricular hypertrophy are typically present in patients with pulmonary hypertension or cor pulmonale. For example, in patients with PPH evidence of right heart strain occurs in approximately 80% of patients.[29]

Patients with longstanding pulmonary hypertension or cor pulmonale have markedly abnormal radiographs that suggest the presence of their disease. Enlarged pulmonary arteries with or without an enlarged RV are often evident. Figure 49-5 illustrates severe bilateral pulmonary artery and RV enlargement in a patient with PPH.

Echocardiography is quite useful in the diagnosis of pulmonary hypertension.[30] The echocardiogram also helps establish secondary causes for pulmonary hypertension, such as left ventricular dysfunction, mitral valve abnormalities, or congenital heart disease. Although echocardiography is not foolproof in the detection of mild to moderate pulmonary hypertension, it is sensitive in the detection of severe elevations in pulmonary artery pressure. The majority of such patients have tricuspid regurgitation, thereby allowing a reasonably accurate estimate of pulmonary artery systolic pressure. Because echocardiography is noninvasive, it is generally used early to determine the presence and severity of pulmonary hypertension and the presence or absence of cor pulmonale. It is also extremely useful in the following of patients with established pulmonary hypertension after therapeutic interventions. For evaluation of a patient with pulmonary hypertension, $\dot{V}/\dot{Q}$ scanning may be useful in the exclusion of chronic thromboembolic disease as a secondary cause of pulmonary hypertension.[31]

The gold standard for the diagnosis of pulmonary hypertension remains the right-heart catheterization. This technique utilizes a thermodilution balloon catheter to measure right ventricular, pulmonary artery, and pulmonary capillary wedge pressures.[32] Patients with PPH have normal wedge pressures. The presence of an abnormal capillary wedge pressure usually requires left heart catheterization for further evaluation. In addition, right heart catheterization allows for comparisons between the oxygen saturation in the central veins, right atrium, right ventricle, and pulmonary artery. This determines whether left-to-right or right-to-left shunting is present. The right heart catheterization may supplement the echocardiographic data in the diagnosis and evaluation of congenital heart disease.

In summary, in patients in whom pulmonary hypertension is suspected based on the clinical history or physical exam, a reasonable diagnostic approach may begin with a chest radiograph and electrocardiogram. Echocardiography serves as useful, noninvasive alternative to right heart catheterization and is often diagnostic in patients with more advanced pulmonary hypertension. A $\dot{V}/\dot{Q}$ scan is often performed to exclude PE in patients with evidence of pulmonary hypertension and right-heart catheterization. It is usually reserved for those patients in whom the diagnosis remains unclear after echocardiography.

Management of Selected Pulmonary Vascular Diseases

Pulmonary Thromboembolism

Once the diagnosis of PE is suspected, anticoagulation with intravenous heparin should be initiated (unless a contraindication to anticoagulation exists, such as recent surgery or internal bleeding). Heparin exerts a prompt antithrombotic effect, preventing thrombus growth and allows the fibrinolytic system to act unopposed to more readily reduce the size of the thromboembolic burden.[33] With the institution of continuous intravenous heparin, the activated partial thromboplastin time (aPTT) should be followed at 6 hour intervals until it is consistently in the therapeutic range of 1.5 to 2.0 times control values.[34] A heparin regimen consisting of a bolus of 80 u/kg followed by 18 u/kg/hr has been recommended.[34] This aggressive approach decreases the risk of subtherapeutic anticoagulation and although supratherapeutic levels are sometimes achieved initially, bleeding complications do not appear to be increased. More recent data continues to support aggressive heparin dosing, because several analyses suggest failure to achieve a therapeutic aPTT within 24 hours of initial therapy is associated with a substantially increased risk of recurrent thromboembolic events.[35] Low molecular weight heparins (LMWH) have been utilized for the treatment of DVT and may also prove effective for the treatment of PE. Advantages of LMWH include convenient subcutaneous dosing and the fact that aPTT monitoring is unnecessary.

Warfarin therapy may be initiated as soon as the aPTT is therapeutic and heparin should be maintained until a therapeutic international normalized ratio (INR) of 2.0 to 3.0 has been overlapped with a therapeutic aPTT for 3 consecutive days.[36] The duration of anticoagulation depends on the presence and/or persistence of risk factors, but in all cases, documented PE should be treated with anticoagulation for at least 3 months. In some cases, however, with underlying hypercoagulable states (see Box 49-2), lifetime anticoagulation may be indicated. Because diet and many drugs interact with warfarin, careful monitoring is necessary to keep the INR within the recommended therapeutic range of 2.0 to 3.0.

Complications of heparin include bleeding and **heparin-induced thrombocytopenia (HIT).** The rates of major bleeding in recent trials using heparin by continuous infusion are less than 5%.[37] Heparin-induced thrombocytopenia (defined as a platelet count less than 150,000 mm³) typically develops 5 to 10 days after the initiation of heparin therapy, occurring in 3% to 5% of patients. The syndrome is caused by heparin-dependent, IgG anti-platelet antibodies and can result in either paradoxical thrombus or bleeding.[38] If a patient is placed on heparin for venous thromboembolism and the platelet count progressively decreases to 100,000/mm³ or less, heparin therapy should be discontinued. A heparinoid (danaparoid) has been approved for use in the setting of HIT.

If heparin therapy cannot be continued, **inferior vena cava (IVC) filter** placement can be undertaken to prevent lower extremity thrombus from embolizing to the lungs. These devices have been widely used for nearly two decades. The primary indications for filter placement include contraindications to anticoagulation, recurrent embolism while on adequate therapy, and significant bleeding complications during anticoagulation.[39] Filters are sometimes placed in the setting of massive PE when it is believed that any further emboli might be lethal. A recent randomized study suggested that filter placement in patients with new DVT reduces the risk of acute PE at day 12 but increases the risk of recurrent DVT at 2 years.[40] A number of filter designs exist, but the Greenfield filter has been most widely used. Filters can be inserted via the jugular or femoral vein. These devices are effective and complications are unusual. Rare complications include clinically significant perforation of the IVC, cephalad migration, and displacement of the filter during insertion. Occasionally, IVC obstruction because of thrombosis at the filter site may occur. Deaths resulting from filter placement are exceedingly uncommon. In general, anticoagulation is continued when a filter is placed unless it is contraindicated.

The National Institutes of Health consensus guidelines for PE thrombolysis issued in 1980 suggested that **thrombolytic therapy** was appropriate for patients with obstruction of blood flow to a lobe or multiple pulmonary segments and for patients with hemodynamic compromise, regardless of the size of the PE.[41] Current guidelines also favor the use of thrombolytic therapy in patients with hemodynamic instability (hypotension) or severely compromised oxygenation. Stable patients with a significant embolic load are individualized, often receiving thrombolytic treatment in the absence of absolute or relative contraindications. Acceleration of clot lysis in PE with thrombolytic therapy was documented in several trials.[22,42] One trial demonstrated thrombolysis was accelerated in patients receiving urokinase compared with those on heparin when pulmonary arteriograms and lung perfusion scans were examined 24 hours after treatment.[22] At present, tPA (100 mg intravenous infusion delivered over 2 hours) may be the most commonly employed protocol when thrombolysis is used in PE.[43] Heparin should be withheld until the thrombolytic infusion is completed.

Cor Pulmonale

Cor pulmonale describes RV dysfunction in response to underlying pulmonary parenchymal disease. Therefore one goal of the treatment of cor pulmonale is to optimize medical management of the underlying lung disease. For example, several classes of drugs are used in patients with obstructive lung disease for their bronchodilator properties. β-receptor agonists, such as albuterol, produce bronchodilation and are used in acute exacerbations of COPD and for chronic maintenance therapy. Ipratropium bromide is another inhaled bronchodilator agent used in patients with airflow obstruction. Theophylline has some bronchodilator properties and is frequently used in patients with COPD. Finally, inhaled and/or systemic corticosteroids appear to benefit a subset of patients with COPD.

In addition, because **hypoxic pulmonary vasoconstriction** is thought to contribute to the pathogenesis of pulmonary hypertension in patients with cor pulmonale, supplemental oxygen therapy is often employed. Supplemental oxygen reduces hypoxic pulmonary vasoconstriction, thereby reducing pulmonary artery pressures. The reduction in such hemodynamic parameters might then allow right ventricular function to improve. Two large trials have demonstrated a survival benefit of supplemental oxygen therapy in COPD patients with hypoxemia and cor pulmonale.[44,45] Based on the results of these and other studies, long-term oxygen therapy is recommended in patients with an arterial oxygen tension (PaO_2) of 55 mm Hg or less, or in patients with a PaO_2 of 60 mm Hg or less and evidence of cor pulmonale or secondary polycythemia.

The use of inotropic agents or pulmonary vasodilators in cor pulmonale is controversial. Digoxin has been studied as an agent to improve RV cardiac contractility in patients with cor pulmonale. A randomized placebo-controlled trial demonstrated improvement in right ventricular ejection fraction (RVEF) after 8 weeks in patients treated with digoxin.[46] However, this benefit was seen in those patients with concomitant left ventricular dysfunction, but not in those individuals with isolated right ventricular dysfunction. Because patients with chronic lung disease tend to develop digoxin toxicity at lower serum levels than most patients, digoxin is generally avoided in these patients. Studies have also examined the utility of several pulmonary vasodilators in patients with secondary pulmonary hypertension and cor pulmonale.[6] Unfortunately, these studies failed to show any benefit and, in some cases, were associated with deleterious effects resulting from systemic vasodilation.

Primary Pulmonary Hypertension

Because pulmonary arterial muscularization and vasoconstriction are believed to be major pathophysiologic mechanisms for the development of PPH, a number of vasodilator agents have been studied in this disease. Initial studies focused on the use of **calcium channel blockers.** These agents appear to result in a sustained improvement in pulmonary hemodynamics in 25% to 30% of patients.[47] Nifedipine and diltiazem are the most commonly used, because verapamil has been shown to have negative inotropic effects. Typically, the patients that experience the most sustained improvement in hemodynamics during an acute vasodilator challenge are those that experience improvement in symptoms and prolonged survival.[47] Unfortunately, these agents may also result in significant adverse effects such as hypotension, which can be life-threatening in patients with severely compromised right ventricular function. Therefore indiscriminate use of these agents should be avoided.

Prostacyclin (epoprostenol, PGI_2) is a pulmonary vasodilator that has proven to be the most effective therapy available in the treatment of patients with PPH. Because prostacyclin has a short half-life and is rapidly inactivated by the low gastric pH, it is given as a continuous intravenous infusion via a permanent indwelling catheter with a portable infusion pump. A large, prospective, randomized, multicenter trial compared prostacyclin plus conventional therapy with conventional therapy alone in patients with Class III and IV PPH.[48] The patients treated with prostacyclin had significant improvements in exercise capacity, hemodynamics, and survival. Long-term benefits also have been reported, even in patients who have not demonstrated hemodynamic improvement during the acute infusion. The dose of the drug is increased, generally once or twice per week, because tolerance develops over time. The long-term effects have been suggested to be due to the vasodilator properties, and to antiplatelet or anti-smooth muscle proliferation properties. Dose-related side effects include diarrhea, jaw pain, flushing, and arthralgias. Because of the life-threatening nature of PPH, the management of prostacyclin should be restricted to physicians with considerable experience in this area.

Other options in the management of PPH include oxygen therapy in patients with a reduced arterial oxygen content. As in patients with cor pulmonale, supplemental oxygen can relieve hypoxic pulmonary vasoconstriction that can contribute to pulmonary hypertension. Diuretics may be useful in patients with PPH and severe right heart failure, but extreme caution is required because the RV is sensitive to preload. **Anticoagulation** is another option recommended in the treatment of patients with pulmonary hypertension. In a subgroup of these patients, microscopic thrombi may play a role in the pathogenesis of the disease. In addition, PPH patients appear to be at risk of thromboembolism due to right ventricular dilation and dysfunction as well as relative immobility. A retrospective clinical trial and a nonrandomized prospective study suggest improved survival with anticoagulation therapy.[47,49] When warfarin is used, an international normalized ratio of 1.5 to 2.5 is considered therapeutic. The risk-benefit ratio has to be considered on an individual basis when anticoagulant therapy is used in patients with PPH.

Lung transplantation represents a viable therapeutic option in patients with PPH. Because the waiting time at most transplant centers averages 14 to 18 months, patients should be referred for transplantation early in the course of disease. Most patients should undergo a trial of prostacyclin therapy by continuous infusion before actually proceeding to lung transplantation, because a response to prostacyclin may delay the need for surgery. In patients who fail to respond to medical therapy, single or bilateral lung transplantation, are options. Because the markedly depressed right ventricular function often improves considerably after lung transplantation heart-lung transplantation not necessary in most patients but is reserved for those with both severe left and right ventricular dysfunction.[50] One-year survival rates for lung transplantation are approximately 80%. Obliterative bronchiolitis is the major long-term complication of transplantation and is thought to represent a form of chronic allograft rejection. Patients with PPH appear to have higher mortality rates and increased frequency of obliterative bronchiolitis.

Secondary Pulmonary Hypertension

Many of the principles outlined in the management of patients with cor pulmonale and PPH apply to the management of patients with pulmonary hypertension resulting from other causes. In general, treatment of any underlying disease that may be contributing to the development of pulmonary hypertension and the use of supplemental oxygen to alleviate hypoxic pulmonary vasoconstriction remain important goals of therapy. Treatment of nonthrombotic obstruction of the pulmonary circulation is aimed at the treatment of the underlying etiology of the obstruction. The treatment of pulmonary hypertension resulting from cardiac disease is aimed at the treatment of the underlying cardiac defect. A detailed discussion of the treatment of pulmonary hypertension associated with cardiac disease is beyond the scope of this chapter. However, in some of these cases pulmonary hypertension may improve after treatment of the underlying cardiac defect, such as after valve replacement in pulmonary hypertension resulting from mitral stenosis. In other cases, such as complex congenital heart disease with a right to left shunt (Eisenmenger's syndrome), heart-lung transplantation is necessary.[50]

Patients with pulmonary hypertension associated with systemic disease or secondary to anorexic drugs often are managed similarly to patients with PPH, although in many cases, enough evidence does not yet exist to determine if these therapies are beneficial. An ongoing randomized trial is currently evaluating the use of continuous intravenous prostacyclin infusion in patients with secondary pulmonary hypertension due to scleroderma. Such ongoing prospective studies are needed to determine if vasodilator therapy offers as much benefit to patients with secondary pulmonary hypertension as in those with PPH.

CASE STUDIES

Case One
Acute Right Ventricular Failure

A 50-year-old man with a history of arthritis 5 days after left hip replacement suddenly developed shortness of breath and hypotension. The patient previously had been healthy and well. His postoperative course was uncomplicated, and Coumadin had been started for thromboembolism prophylaxis. The patient had just gotten out of bed to go to the bathroom when he suddenly felt short of breath and dizzy. On examination he looked pale and in moderate respiratory distress. Blood pressure was 85/palp, heart rate 120/min, respiratory rate 30/min, and oxygen saturation 90% on 15 L/min oxygen via nonrebreather mask. Physical exam was notable for clear lungs, an elevated jugular venous pressure with a prominent V wave, tachycardia with a prominent S_2, a systolic murmur at the left sternal border, and an S_3 that augmented with inspiration. The left leg was edematous. An arterial blood gas revealed a pH of 7.45, a $PaCO_2$ of 28 mm Hg, and a PaO_2 of 59 mm Hg. An ECG revealed tachycardia with a new right bundle branch pattern, and a chest radiograph disclosed bilateral lower lobe atelectasis.

The patient has had an acute event resulting in hypoxemia, hypotension, and signs of right heart failure. Given his recent hip surgery, the most likely etiology is acute PE. Hypotension is likely from acute right-sided heart failure. This results from an acute rise in the PVR leading to a decrement in RV stroke volume and an increase in the RVEDV. The increased RVEDV has multiple detrimental effects, including increased oxygen demands resulting in ischemia and decreased LV compliance via ventricular interdependence. The result is decreased cardiac performance and shock.

The approach to this patient will involve prompt, accurate diagnosis and treatment. Diagnostically, the patient could have a ventilation and perfusion radioisotope scan or a pulmonary angiogram. Given the instability of the patient an angiogram is preferred. The options for treatment include anticoagulation with heparin alone, anticoagulation with inferior vena cava filter placement, or fibrinolytic therapy. In the meantime the patient will require transfer to an intensive care unit for hemodynamic and respiratory support. In this case, the patient is defending his $PaCO_2$ and can be observed on high flow oxygen. Blood pressure should be supported with vasopressors. This patient would meet the indications for fibrinolytic therapy, but recent surgery increases the risk for bleeding complications. A careful assessment of the risks and benefits of fibrinolytic therapy is necessary in this case.

Case Two
Primary Pulmonary Hypertension

A 30-year-old woman developed progressive dyspnea over a 6-month period. The patient had been previously healthy and active until approximately 6 months before presentation when she noted dyspnea when walking to her third floor apartment. This was associated with occasional sharp chest pains but no wheezing or fevers. The dyspnea had progressed over the next few months such that the patient was getting short of breath with only a few stairs or walking on a hill. An evaluation had disclosed a normal chest radiograph, normal spirometry, a decreased diffusion capacity at 55% of predicted, and an ECG consistent with strain on the right ventricle. An echocardiogram disclosed a dilated, hypokinetic RV with an estimated RV systolic pressure of 76 mm Hg. The LV had normal size and function. No shunts were evident when contrast bubbles were injected.

On presentation, the patient was dyspneic with short walks on a flat surface. She had had a syncopal episode about 1 week before presentation. Further review of the history disclosed no history of prior lung disease, diet pill use, toxic oil ingestion, exotic travel, or previous thromboembolic disease. She denied symptoms of collagen vascular disease, had no history of smoking, and a noncontributory family history. Her oxygen saturation was 89% on room air. She had clear lungs on auscultation. Her cardiac exam was notable for elevated neck veins, a prominent RV heave, and PA tap. On auscultation she had a loud P_2 with a right-sided S_3. A prominent systolic murmur was detectable at the left lower sternal border that increased in intensity with inspiration. The patient also had 2+ edema of her lower extremities. A full laboratory evaluation was notable for normal serologies, a negative HIV test, normal coagulation profile, and normal liver function. A chest CT scan was normal. A $\dot{V}/\dot{Q}$ scan disclosed only small peripheral defects and was considered low probability for PE.

The patient was diagnosed with PPH and referred to a pulmonologist for additional diagnostic work-up and consideration for prostacyclin therapy.

𝒦ey 𝒫oints

- The low pressure pulmonary circulation normally offers little resistance to the flow of blood out of the right ventricle.
- Pulmonary vascular disease leads to increased pulmonary vascular resistance. When sustained over time, elevations in pulmonary vascular resistance lead to right ventricular hypertrophy, dilation, and failure.
- The diagnosis of pulmonary vascular disease based on clinical examination is often difficult because many signs and symptoms are nonspecific. Therefore when PE or pulmonary hypertension is suspected, additional diagnostic testing is indicated.
- Although ventilation perfusion scanning is the first diagnostic study often employed in patients with suspected PE, study results are frequently nondiagnostic. Pulmonary angiography should be pursued if a high clinical suspicion for PE exists.
- Anticoagulation with heparin is the primary therapy in acute PE, except in cases with hemodynamic instability or severe hypoxemia where thrombolytic therapy may be indicated.
- Treatment of cor pulmonale is directed at the reduction of hypoxic pulmonary vasoconstriction and the treatment of any underlying pulmonary disease that may be contributing to the pulmonary hypertension.
- Prostacyclin, a pulmonary vasodilator, decreases pulmonary vascular resistance and improves survival in patients with PPH. If medical therapy for PPH fails, lung transplantation is the best therapeutic option.

References

1. Schulman DS, Matthay RA. The right ventricle in pulmonary disease. Cardiol Clin 1992;10:111-138.
2. Weber K, Janicki J, Shroff S, et al. The right ventricle: physiologic and pathophysiologic considerations. Crit Care Med 1983;11:323-328.
3. D'Amato AN, Galante JF, Smith WM. Hemodynamic response to treadmill exercise in normal subjects. J Appl Physiol 1966;23:631-640.
4. Epstein SE, Reiser GD, Stampfer M, et al. Characterization of the circulatory response to maximal upright exercise in normal subjects and patients with heart disease. Circulation 1967;35:1049-1062.
5. Fishman AP. Chronic cor pulmonale. Am Rev Respir Dis 1976;114:775-794.
6. Klinger JR, Hill NS. Right ventricular dysfunction in chronic obstructive pulmonary disease: evaluation and management. Chest 1991;99:715-723.
7. Christman BW, McPherson CD, Newman JH, et al. An imbalance between the excretion of thromboxane and prostacyclin metabolites in pulmonary hypertension. N Engl J Med 1992;327:70-75.
8. McIntyre KM, Sasahara AA. The ratio of pulmonary artery pressure to pulmonary vascular obstruction. Chest 1977;71:692.
9. Benotti JR, Dalen JE. The natural history of pulmonary embolism. Clin Chest Med 1984;5:403.
10. Giuntini C, DiRocco G, Marini C, et al. Epidemiology. Chest 1995;107(Suppl):3-9.
11. Dalen JE, Alpert JS. Natural history of pulmonary embolism. Prog Cardiovasc Dis 1975;17:259-270.
12. Renzetti AD, McClement JH, Litt BD. The veterans administration cooperative study of pulmonary function. Am J Med 1966;41:115-129.
13. McFadden E, Braunwald E. Cor pulmonale. In: Braunwald E, editor. Heart disease: a textbook of cardiovascular medicine. 3rd ed. Philadelphia; Saunders; 1988. pp. 1597-1616.
14. Bishop J, Cross K. Physiologic variables and mortality in patients with various categories of chronic respiratory disease. Bull Eur Physiopathol Respir 1984;20;495-500.
15. Rubin LJ. Primary pulmonary hypertension. N Engl J Med 1998;336:111-117.
16. D'Alonzo GE, Barst RJ, Ayres SM, et al. Survival in patients with primary pulmonary hypertension. Results from a national prospective registry. Ann Intern Med 1991;115:343-349.
17. Petitpretz P, Brenot F, Azarian R, et al. Pulmonary hypertension in patients with human immunodeficiency virus infection: comparison with primary pulmonary hypertension. Circulation 1994;89:2722-2727.
18. Brenot F, Herve P, Petitpretz P, et al. Primary pulmonary hypertension and fenfluramine use. Br Heart J 1993;70:537-541.
19. Abenhaim L, Moride Y, Brenot F, et al. Appetite-suppressant drugs and the risk of primary pulmonary hypertension. N Engl J Med 1996;335:609-616.
20. Goldhaber SZ, Hennekens CH, Evans DA, et al. Factors associated with correct antemotem diagnosis of major pulmonary embolism. Am J Med 1982;73:822-826.
21. Green RM, Meyer TJ, Dunn M, Glassroth J. Pulmonary embolism in younger adults. Chest 1992;101:1507-1511.
22. The Urokinase Pulmonary Embolism Trial. A national cooperative study. Circulation 1973;47(Suppl II):1-108.
23. Stein PD, Terrin ML, Hales CA, et al. Clinical, laboratory, roentgenographic, and electrocardiographic findings in patients with acute pulmonary embolism and no preexisting cardiac or pulmonary disease. Chest 1991;100:598-603.
24. A Collaborative Study by the PIOPED Investigators. Value of the ventilation-perfusion scan in acute pulmonary embolism: results of the Prospective Investigation of Pulmonary Embolism Diagnosis (PIOPED). JAMA 1990;263:2753-2759.
25. Stein PD, Hull RD, Pineo G. Strategy that includes serial noninvasive leg tests for diagnosis of thromboembolic disease in patients with suspected acute pulmonary embolism based on data from PIOPED. Arch Intern Med 1995;155:2101-2104.
26. Stein PD, Athanasoulis C, Alavi A, et al. Complications and validity of pulmonary angiography in acute pulmonary embolism. Circulation 1992;85:462-469.
27. Remy-Jardin M, Remy J, Wattinne L, et al. Central PE: diagnosis with spiral volumetric CT with single-breath-hold technique: comparison with pulmonary angiography. Radiology 1992;185:381-387.
28. Grist TM, Sostman HD, MacFall JR, et al. Pulmonary angiography with MRI: preliminary clinical experience. Radiology 1993;189:523-530.
29. Rich S, Dantzker DR, Ayers SM. Primary pulmonary hypertension: a national prospective study. Ann Intern Med 1987;107:216-223.

30. Jaffe CC, Weltin G. Echocardiography of the right side of the heart. Cardiol Clin 1992;10:41-57.

31. D'Alonzo GE, Bower JS, Dantzker DR. Differentiation of patients with primary and thromboembolic pulmonary hypertension. Chest 1984;85:457-461.

32. Swan HJC, Ganz W, Forrester J, et al. Catheterization of the heart in man with the use of a flow-directed balloon-tipped catheter. N Engl J Med 1970;283:447-451.

33. Hirsh J, Dalen JE, Deykin D, et al. Heparin: mechanism of action, pharmacokinetics, dosing considerations, monitoring, efficacy and safety. Chest (Suppl) 1992;102:337-351.

34. Hull RD, Raskob GE, Rosenbloom D, et al. Optimal therapeutic level of heparin therapy in patients with venous thrombosis. Arch Intern Med 1992;152:1589-1595.

35. Hull RD, Raskob GE, Brant RF, et al. The importance of the initial heparin treatment on long term clinical outcomes of antithrombotic therapy. The emerging theme of delayed recurrence. Arch Intern Med 1997;157:2317-2321.

36. Dalen JE, Hirsh J. Fourth American College of Chest Physicians Consensus Conference on antithrombotic therapy. Chest 1995;108:225S-522S.

37. Clagett GP, Anderson FA Jr, Heit J, et al. Prevention of venous thromboembolism. Chest 1995;108(Suppl):312S.

38. Kelton JG, Sheridan D, Santos A, et al. Heparin-associated thrombocytopenia: laboratory studies. Blood 1988;79:925-930.

39. Greenfield LJ. Vena caval interruption and pulmonary embolectomy. Clin Chest Med 1984;5:495-505.

40. Decousus H, Leizorovicz A, Parent F, et al. A clinical trial of vena caval filters in the prevention of pulmonary embolism in patients with proximal deep vein thrombosis. N Engl J Med 1998;338:409-415.

41. Symposium: Thrombolytic therapy in thrombosis: a National Institutes of Health Consensus Development Conference. Ann Intern Med 1980;93:141-143.

42. Miller GAH, Gibson RV, Sutton GC. Treatment of pulmonary embolism with streptokinase. Br Med J 1969;1:812-815.

43. Goldhaber SZ, Kessler CM, Heit J, et al. A randomized controlled trial of recombinant tissue plasminogen activator versus urokinase in the treatment of acute pulmonary embolism. Lancet 1988;2:293-298.

44. Nocturnal Oxygen Therapy Trial Group. Continuous or nocturnal oxygen therapy in hypoxemic chronic obstructive lung disease. A clinical trial. Ann Intern Med 1980;93:391-398.

45. Medical Research Council Working Party. Long term domiciliary oxygen therapy in chronic hypoxic cor pulmonale complicating chronic bronchitis and emphysema: a clinical trial. Lancet 1981;1:681-685.

46. Mathur P, Powles P, Pugsley S, et al. Effect of digoxin on right ventricular function in severe chronic airflow obstruction. Ann Intern Med 1981;95:283-287.

47. Rich S, Brundage BH. High-dose calcium channel-blocking therapy for primary pulmonary hypertension: evidence for long-term reduction in pulmonary arterial pressure and regression of right ventricular hypertrophy. Circulation 1987;76:135-141.

48. Barst RJ, Rubin LJ, Long WA, et al. A comparison of continuous intravenous epoprostenol (prostacyclin) with conventional therapy for primary pulmonary hypertension. N Eng J Med 1996;334:296-301.

49. Fuster V, Steele PM, Edwards WD, et al. Primary pulmonary hypertension: natural history and the importance of thrombosis. Circulation 1984;70:580-587.

50. Katayama Y, Cremona G, Wallwork J, et al. Transplantation for primary pulmonary hypertension. In: Rubin LJ, Rich S, editors. Primary pulmonary hypertension. New York; Marcel Dekker; 1997. pp. 287-317.

CHAPTER 50

Pneumonia

Bekele Afessa
Bethany Weaver

CHAPTER **OUTLINE**

OBJECTIVES

1. Define pneumonia.
2. Compare community-acquired and hospital-acquired pneumonia.
3. Describe noninvasive and invasive diagnostic methods for pneumonia.
4. List causes of gram-positive bacterial pneumonia, gram-negative bacterial pneumonia, atypical organisms causing pneumonia, anaerobic bacterial pneumonia, viral pneumonia, mycobacterial pneumonia, fungal pneumonia, actinomycosis, and nocardiosis.
5. Discuss the etiology, diagnosis, and treatment of gram-positive bacterial pneumonia, gram-negative bacterial pneumonia, atypical organisms causing pneumonia, anaerobic bacterial pneumonia, viral pneumonia, mycobacterial pneumonia, fungal pneumonia, actinomycosis, and nocardiosis.
6. Discuss the etiology, initial management, and prognosis of community-acquired pneumonia.
7. Discuss the epidemiology, etiology, initial management, mortality, prognosis, and prevention of hospital-acquired pneumonia.

Continued

OBJECTIVES—cont'd

8. Describe the clinical and radiographic findings, diagnostic procedures, causes, and therapeutic considerations for pneumonia in the immunocompromised host.
9. Describe the management of pneumonia in patients with HIV.
10. Discuss the management of pneumonia in children.

KEY TERMS

Anaerobic Bacterial Pneumonia	Fungal Respiratory Infections	Protected Specimen Brush (PSB)
Antigen Detection and Polymerase Chain Reaction (PCR)	Gram's Stain	Transbronchial Lung Biopsy
	Gram-Negative Bacteria	Transthoracic Needle Aspiration (TTNA)
Atypical Organisms	Gram-Positive Bacteria	Transtracheal Aspiration (TTA)
Atypical Pneumonia	Hospital-Acquired Pneumonia	Tuberculosis
Bronchoalveolar Lavage (BAL)	Human Immunodeficiency Virus (HIV)	Typical Pneumonia
Community-Acquired Pneumonia (CAP)	Mycobacterial Pneumonia	Ventilator-Associated Pneumonia (VAP)
	Pneumonia	Viral Pneumonia

Respiratory infections are among the most common clinical problems respiratory therapists encounter in their practice. Pneumonia affects millions of people annually and is the sixth leading cause of death in the United States. Pneumonia and influenza have been responsible for most of the infectious disease deaths throughout this century.[1]

Pneumonia is the inflammation and consolidation of lung tissue caused by infectious agents. Aspiration, inhalation, and hematogenous dissemination are the mechanisms by which organisms gain access to the lower respiratory tract and cause pneumonia. Most authors have based the diagnosis of pneumonia on clinical criteria, which include radiographic appearance of new or progressive pulmonary infiltrates, fever, leukocytosis or increased immature neutrophils and purulent tracheal secretions. Unfortunately, the clinical criteria can lead to underdiagnosis or overdiagnosis of pneumonia, particularly in patients requiring endotracheal tubes and those with acute respiratory distress syndrome (ARDS).

Respiratory Recap

Pneumonia
Vaccinate if possible.
Identify the infecting organism.
Perform appropriate antimicrobial therapy.
Provide supportive care.

Community-acquired pneumonias (CAPs) are acquired outside the hospital. Classifications based on severity are important because the management strategies differ according to severity. The American Thoracic Society classifies patients with CAP into four subcategories based on the need for hospitalization, the severity of illness, the presence of coexisting disease, and the patient's age (Box 50-1).[2] The Pneumonia Patient Outcomes Research Team

Box 50-1

Categories of Community-Acquired Pneumonia According to Severity

1. Patients 60 years of age or less, with no comorbidity, who can be treated as outpatients
2. Patients older than 60 years of age, with comorbidity, who can be treated as outpatients
3. Patients requiring hospitalization but not in an intensive care unit
4. Severely ill patients requiring admission to an intensive care unit

From Niederman MS, Bass JB, Fein AM, et al. American Thoracic Society guidelines for the initial management of adults with community-acquired pneumonia: diagnosis, assessment of severity, and initial antimicrobial therapy. Am Rev Respir Dis 1993;148:1418-1426.

also has developed five severity classes of patients with CAP based on 19 variables, which include the patient's age, comorbid conditions, abnormal vital signs, mental status changes, and abnormal laboratory findings.[3]

Hospital-acquired pneumonia develops 48 hours or more after hospital admission, excluding any infection that is incubating at the time of admission. **Ventilator-associated pneumonia (VAP)** develops after at least 48 hours of mechanical ventilation. To minimize the inaccuracies associated with the clinical diagnosis of VAP, an International Consensus Conference has recommended several criteria and categories, as listed in Box 50-2.[4] Regardless of the criteria, antibiotic therapy given before obtaining respiratory samples modifies results. Even in the absence of prior antibiotic treatment, the bacterial burden of mechanically ventilated patients may be independent of the presence or absence of pneumonia.

Hospital-acquired pneumonia and VAP are further divided into the following two categories: early onset, occurring within less than 5 days of admission, and late onset, occurring

Box 50-2

Criteria Used in the Diagnosis of Ventilator-Associated Pneumonia

A. *Definite pneumonia:* New or persistent pulmonary infiltrates and purulent secretions in addition to one of the following:
1. Radiographic evidence of abscess and positive needle aspirate culture
2. Pathogenic evidence of pneumonia on histologic examination of lung tissue obtained by open lung biopsy or postmortem plus a positive quantitative culture of lung parenchyma ($>10^4$ CFU/g of lung tissue)

B. *Probable pneumonia:* New or persistent pulmonary infiltrate (in the absence of the above) and one of the following:
1. The presence of positive quantitative culture by protected specimen brush (PSB) or bronchoalveolar lavage (BAL)
2. Blood culture positive for the same organisms as respiratory sample

3. Positive pleural fluid culture as respiratory secretions
4. Pathologic evidence of pneumonia by open lung biopsy or autopsy

C. *Definitive absence of pneumonia:* One of the following:
1. No histologic evidence of pneumonia postmortem
2. Definitive alternate etiology
3. Cytologic identification of nonpneumonia diagnosis

D. *Probable absence of pneumonia:* Lack of significant growth from reliable specimen in addition to one of the following:
1. Resolution of fever, infiltrate or radiographic infiltrate without antibiotic, and a definite alternative diagnosis
2. Persistent fever and infiltrate with alternative diagnosis

From Pingleton SK, Fagon JY, Leper KV. Patient selection for clinical investigation of ventilator associated pneumonia. Chest 1992;102:553S-556S.

5 days or more after admission. Some have classified hospital-acquired pneumonia into three groups: primary endogenous, secondary endogenous, and exogenous. Primary endogenous pneumonias are community-acquired and caused by *Streptococcus pneumoniae* and *Haemophilus influenzae*. Secondary endogenous pneumonias are caused by *Pseudomonas aeruginosa* and *Enterobacter* species, organisms that have replaced the normal pharyngeal population and usually are of intrahospital origin. Exogenous pneumonias are caused by organisms acquired from colonized respiratory equipment.

Diagnostic Work-Up

Despite aggressive diagnostic work-up, the etiology of CAPs cannot be determined in more than 30% of cases. Etiologic diagnoses can simplify and optimize antibiotic treatment. However, treatment should not be delayed in critically ill patients because of diagnostic considerations. Controversy remains regarding aggressive microbiologic work-up in the setting of CAP. In areas where the prevalence of tuberculosis, **human immunodeficiency virus (HIV)** infection, and *S. pneumoniae* resistance to penicillin are high, the usual antibiotic regimens that are used empirically may not be good choices. It is also important to evaluate the local prevalence of respiratory pathogens and the state of resistance and to document the precise microbiologic etiology of each case when new antibiotics are assessed.

Noninvasive Diagnostic Methods

Sputum

Sputum is a mixture of lower respiratory secretions with oropharyngeal contamination. Despite criticism about its sensitivity, specificity, and reliability, sputum **Gram's stain**

and culture have been the cornerstones in the diagnosis of pneumonia. Inadequate sputum collection methods and oropharyngeal contamination are the main problems affecting the reliability of sputum. The sensitivity and specificity of sputum improve as the collection, quality, and manipulation of the samples improve. Many inpatients are unable to produce adequate sputum. Inducing sputum partly overcomes this problem. Specimens of lower respiratory secretions should contain 25 or more neutrophils and up to 10 epithelial cells per microscopic field (magnified $\times$ 100) before being subjected to Gram's stain. Culture of sputum is performed only after macromicroscopic evaluation. A predominant pathogen identified on a screened sputum, yielding 10^6 or more colony-forming units (CFU)/mL is considered positive. Both false-positive and false-negative results complicate the diagnosis of pneumococcal pneumonia. *S. pneumoniae* is commonly found in the pharynx of healthy subjects and can give false-positive results. Its growth can be hindered by stronger bacteria such as gram-negative bacilli and in patients pretreated with antibiotics. The presence of antibody-coated bacteria may help in the discrimination between true pathogens and colonizers. New techniques such as **antigen detection and polymerase chain reaction (PCR)** applied to sputum samples can help in the rapid identification of pathogens that may be difficult to culture or of pathogens barely growing because of prior antibiotic treatment.

Although the role of Gram's stain is controversial, it is a simple, rapid, and inexpensive first step in the diagnosis of patients not previously treated with antibiotics and who are able to produce an adequate sputum sample. Identifying the presence of a predominant bacterial morphology is helpful. The absence of organisms in a sample with neutrophils favors *Legionella* species, or an atypical agent. Cultures are accepted if they agree with the Gram's stain. Cultures are useful in the identification of *Legionella pneumophila* and *Mycobacterium tuberculosis*.

Induced sputum has been very helpful in the diagnosis of *Pneumocystis carinii* pneumonia (PCP). Before sputum induction, patients brush their teeth and gums and gargle with water to remove any debris. They then inhale 3% saline for 20 minutes from an ultrasonic nebulizer and are encouraged to cough every 5 minutes. β_2-Agonist inhalers are administered to patients prone to develop bronchospasm during sputum induction. Cytochemical stains (toluidine blue O, Papanicolaou, Giemsa, Methenamine silver nitrate), monoclonal antibody, and PCR are applied to the induced sputum to diagnose PCP.

Antigen detection can be applied to sputum, serum, urine, and body fluids. Pneumococcal antigen detection in sputum has not been proven to be cost effective. Antigen detection for *H. influenzae* is possible for strains capable of being typed. Antigen detection has been most valuable in the diagnosis of difficult to culture organisms, such as *M. pneumoniae*, *L. pneumophila*, *Chlamydia pneumoniae*, and viral pneumonias. Direct fluorescent antigen (DFA) detection for *L. pneumophila* has high specificity but low sensitivity.

Serology

Serologic testing for atypical bacteria is of minor help in the acute phase. Paired acute and convalescent serologic testing provide a reliable retrospective diagnosis, useful only for epidemiologic studies. Serology is used in *L. pneumophila*, *M. pneumoniae*, *C. pneumoniae*, and viral infections.

Blood Culture

The overall positivity of blood culture in CAP is 5%. However, the rate of bacteremia reaches 20% to 30% in pneumococcal pneumonia. Bacteremia complicates around 8% of hospital-acquired pneumonia. The overall cost-effectiveness of routine blood culture is questionable. Two blood cultures are routinely obtained before antibiotics are initiated in hospitalized patients with pneumonia. Blood culture has low sensitivity but high specificity in the diagnosis of pneumonia. The presence of bacteremia is associated with high morbidity and mortality.

Pleural Fluid

In patients with a significant amount of pleural effusion, diagnostic thoracentesis is needed to exclude empyema or complicated parapneumonic effusion. The pleural fluid should be analyzed for pH, protein, lactate dehydrogenase, and Gram's stain and culture.

Urine

Pneumococcal antigen detection has an acceptable sensitivity but is cumbersome. *L. pneumophila* antigen detection has a good diagnostic accuracy.

Invasive Diagnostic Methods

In CAP and nosocomial pneumonia in nonintubated patients, the diagnosis of pneumonia relies on clinical and radiologic signs with low risk of misdiagnosis. However, in mechanically ventilated patients, clinical and radiologic signs are poorly specific, and it is not easy to determine whether a patient has pneumonia and what the causative organisms are. Fever and new radiologic infiltrates are seen in many noninfectious conditions.[5] Culture of endotracheal aspirates has high sensitivity but low specificity in endotracheally intubated patients. Invasive diagnostic techniques are used in such conditions.

Bronchoscopy

Quantitative culture of bronchoscopic specimen has higher specificity than that of endotracheal aspirates. However, the sensitivity of **bronchoalveolar lavage (BAL)** and **protected specimen brush (PSB)** in the diagnosis of VAP is 36% to 58%. Because of the lack of data showing that the use of invasive methods in the diagnosis of VAP improves outcome, including survival, length of hospital stay, antibiotic resistance, complications, or costs, the use of bronchoscopy in the diagnosis of pneumonia has become controversial. Bronchoscopy is rarely performed in nonintubated patients for the diagnosis of bacterial pneumonia.

The double lumen brush catheter has been shown to bypass the nasopharyngeal and oropharyngeal flora, which contaminates the working channel of the fiberoptic bronchoscope. PSB samples need to be processed both qualitatively and quantitatively, and culture showing 10^3 CFU/mL is used as a cutoff point for positivity. False-positive and false-negative results can be seen with PSB. To eliminate false-positive results, the following actions are taken: suctioning through the working channel of the bronchoscope before the double lumen brush catheter is passed down to the subglottic airways is avoided, injection of lidocaine through the working channel below the vocal cords is avoided, the patient is premedicated with atropine, and the patient is placed in the supine Trendelenburg or lateral decubitus position with the lung to be sampled upright. In patients with chronic obstructive pulmonary disease (COPD), endobronchial disease, or acute bronchitis, the PSB can recover high counts of pathogens in the absence of pneumonia. To avoid false-negative results, bacterial processing is done within 2 hours of sampling, and antibiotics are not given before sampling.

BAL specimens are contaminated by oropharyngeal flora when used in nonintubated patients. However, quantitative cultures and direct examination for intracellular bacteria make it a useful diagnostic tool. BAL explores large areas of the lung and is more helpful than PSB in the diagnosis of opportunistic infections. In patients with focal disease, BAL is performed by wedging of the bronchoscope in the area of greatest involvement. In patients with diffuse disease, BAL is performed from two lobes, usually the upper lobe and the middle lobe or lingula. Dependent segments such as the anterior or apical segment of the upper lobe are preferred to increase the volume of lavage return. About 100 to 200 mL of sterile normal saline in 20 to 60 mL aliquots are instilled, and return of 40% to 50% of instilled volume, with a minimum of 50 mL, is considered acceptable. The BAL sample can be processed for Gram's stain, bacterial culture, *Pneumocystis* stain, mycobacterial and fungal stains and culture, and cytology. A threshold of 10^4 CFU/mL is used in the diagnosis of bacterial pneumonia.

Transbronchial lung biopsy is taken from the most involved lung segment. In diffuse diseases, the biopsy is taken from the lateral segment of the right lower lobe. Although the optimal number of biopsy specimens is not known, a minimum of five biopsy specimens should be taken. The biopsy sample can be processed for histology, Gram's stain and bacterial cultures, *Pneumocystis* stains, and mycobacterial and fungal stains and cultures. Because of its potential complications, transbronchial lung biopsies are rarely performed in patients receiving positive pressure ventilation.

Transthoracic Needle Aspiration and Transtracheal Aspiration

Transthoracic needle aspiration (TTNA) has good sensitivity and excellent specificity. **Transtracheal aspiration (TTA)** was used in the past to diagnosis pneumonia, especially anaerobic pneumonia. However, TTNA and TTA are rarely performed in clinical practice today.

Choosing Diagnostic Methods

The choice of the diagnostic method to be used depends on cost effectiveness, availability, expertise, severity, and likelihood of changing empirical treatment. An attempt should be made to establish the etiologic diagnosis of pneumonia to permit optimal antibiotic selection and identify pathogens of potential epidemiologic signficance.[6] In a patient with mild pneumonia who is treated as an outpatient, sputum Gram's stain should be performed if possible. In severe and presumed pneumococcal pneumonia, sputum Gram's stain, culture, and antibiotic sensitivity; two blood cultures; and pleural fluid (if significantly present) Gram's stain and culture should be obtained. In severe pneumonia of unknown etiology, sputum Gram's stain and cultures (including *Legionella* species), two blood cultures, acute phase serology for *Legionella* species and atypical agents, urine *Legionella* antigen, and pleural fluid stains and cultures should be performed. In the appropriate clinical setting, a respiratory specimen should be examined for acid-fast bacilli (AFB), *Pneumocystis* stains, and mycobacterial cultures. Bronchoscopy, TTA, and TTNA can be used to obtain specimens for the diagnostic work-up. Many clinicians consider these invasive procedures to be the last step in nonresponding cases, whereas others consider them earlier in the course of treatment

when the patient is not yet in critical condition in order to have a higher impact on outcome.

Bacterial Causes of Pneumonia

Gram-Positive Bacteria

Streptococcus pneumoniae *Streptococcus pneumoniae* is the most common cause of pneumonia. *S. pneumoniae* is a lancet-shaped diplococcus, described as a **gram-positive bacteria** because it retains the stain, or resists decolorization, by Gram's staining method. It is found worldwide and causes 40% to 50% of all CAP. Risk factors for pneumococcal disease include anatomic or functional asplenia, HIV infection, alcoholism, cirrhosis of the liver, hypogammaglobulinemia, and COPD.

The typical presentation of pneumococcal pneumonia includes fever, rigor, cough productive of rusty sputum, and chest pain. The chest radiograph reveals a unilobar or multilobar infiltrate (Figure 50-1). Complications of pneumococcal infection include lung abscesses, empyema, septic shock, pericarditis, endocarditis, meningitis, and brain abscesses.

Penicillin has been the drug of choice for treatment of *S. pneumoniae*. Third-generation cephalosporins, imipenem, and vancomycin are used to treat penicillin-resistant *S. pneumoniae*. The Centers for Disease Control and Prevention recommends the 23-valent pneumococcal vaccine for individuals at increased risk of pneumococcal disease. The current 23-valent pneumococcal vaccine covers 88% of the pneumococcal serotypes causing bacteremic infection in the United States, and its side effects are mild and self-limited. Revaccination is recommended in 6 years.

Staphylococcus aureus *Staphylococcus aureus* appears as clusters on Gram's stain. The incidence of *S. aureus* has been increasing recently. The risk factors for *S. aureus* pneumonia include endotracheal intubation, injection drug use, long-term intravenous catheters, arteriovenous shunts for hemodialysis, burns, infections of the skin, head trauma, chronic pulmonary diseases, quantitative or qualitative neutrophil dysfunction, HIV infection, and viral infections (especially influenza).

The clinical presentation of *S. aureus* pneumonia includes fever, cough productive of purulent sputum, and hemoptysis. *S. aureus* pneumonia can be complicated with abscess, empyema, hematogenous spread, rash, and septic shock. Neutrophilic leukocytosis is common. The chest radiograph reveals diffuse parenchymal infiltrates, occasionally with focal distribution and cavitation.

The incidence of *S. aureus* pneumonia is increased in neurosurgical patients receiving mechanical ventilation. *S. aureus* is the organism that most commonly causes pneumonia in critically ill comatose patients. More recently, the development of methicillin-resistant *S. aureus* (MRSA) has become a growing problem, especially in tertiary and teaching hospitals. Patients with MRSA infection are

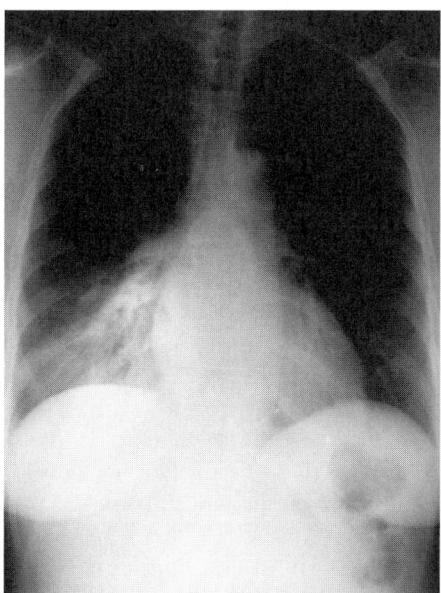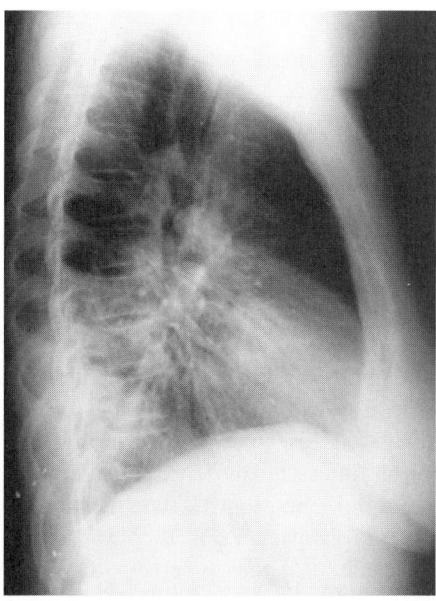

Figure 50-1   From left, posteroanterior (PA) and lateral chest radiograph of a patient with pneumococcal pneumonia showing right lower lobe infiltrate.

more likely to have received steroids, to have received antibiotics for more than 48 hours, to have been ventilated for more than 6 days, to be more than 25 years of age, and to have COPD. Compared to methicillin-sensitive *S. aureus* (MSSA), MRSA is associated with more frequent bacteremia, septic shock, and *Pseudomonas* species coinfection, and higher mortality.

The mortality of patients with staphylococcal pneumonia ranges from 30% to 40%. Nafcillin, clindamycin, and the first-generation cephalosporins are the drugs of choice for MSSA pneumonia. Vancomycin is used to treat MRSA. In treatment failure and severe cases, rifampin and aminoglycosides are added. Contact isolation and early hospital discharge of patients with MRSA, culture surveillance of staff and patients, and elimination of nasal carriage are necessary to prevent outbreaks of MRSA.

Enterococcus *Species*   Most cases of enterococcal pneumonia occur as superinfections in patients receiving broad-spectrum antibiotics or topical antimicrobial prophylaxis. Vancomycin is used for treatment if the organism is resistant to ampicillin.

Gram-Negative Bacteria

Haemophilus influenzae
Haemophilus influenzae is a common inhabitant of human pharyngeal flora. It appears as coccobacilli on Gram's stain. This **gram-negative bacteria**, so called because it "loses" the stain, or becomes decolorized by alcohol in Gram's method of staining, is the most common cause of bacteremia in children. *H. influenzae* serotype b is the most significant cause of serious disease. In addition to pneumonia, *H. influenzae* can cause meningitis, epiglottitis, arthritis, and bacteremia. Both type b and non-

typable strains of *H. influenzae* have been implicated in nosocomial pneumonia. Risk factors for *H. influenzae* infection include COPD, defects in B cell function, functional and anatomic asplenia, and HIV infection.

Encapsulated strains of *H. influenzae* cause severe pneumonia with acute onset of fever, pleuritic chest pain, productive cough, and hemoptysis. The nonencapsulated strains cause insidious, bronchitis-like disease. The typical chest radiograph finding is bronchopneumonia with small patchy infiltrates. Adults and most children without meningitis recover fully. In patients with severe underlying disease, respiratory and multiple organ failure may develop.

In cases in which the frequency of β-lactamase–producing *H. influenzae* is low, ampicillin and amoxicillin are used for treatment. In cases in which the frequency of β-lactamase–producing *H. influenzae* is high, amoxicillin-clavulanate potassium, fluoroquinolones, and second- and third-generation cephalosporins are the preferred treatment. Influenza vaccination protects against *H. influenzae* type b.

Moraxella catarrhalis
Moraxella catarrhalis is a natural inhabitant of the human pharynx. *M. catarrhalis* is the third most prevalent cause, following *S. pneumoniae* and *H. influenzae*, of acute exacerbation of chronic bronchitis in patients with COPD. In addition to pneumonia and acute bronchitis, it also causes bacteremia, endocarditis, pericarditis, and urinary tract infection.

Because most patients with *M. catarrhalis* pneumonia have underlying lung disease, their clinical presentation is similar to an acute exacerbation of chronic bronchitis. The chest radiograph usually reveals patchy infiltrates. Because most strains of *M. catarrhalis* are β-lactamase–producing, amoxicillin-clavulanate potassium, ampicillin-sulbactam, fluoroquinolones, macrolides, trimethoprim-sulfamethoxazole, and second- and third-generation cephalosporins are used to treat *M. catarrhalis* pneumonia.

Pseudomonas aeruginosa

Pseudomonas aeruginosa is ubiquitous in a moist environment, and it colonizes the gut, wounds, burns, and catheterized urinary tract. Factors that predispose one to *P. aeruginosa* infection include neutropenia, HIV infection, preexisting lung disease, endotracheal intubation, and prior antibiotic use.

P. aeruginosa is the gram-negative bacillus isolated most often in VAP and the leading cause of death among intubated patients with pneumonia. Less than 10% of cases of *P. aeruginosa* pneumonia are bacteremic. Risk factors for *P. aeruginosa* VAP include COPD, mechanical ventilation for more than 8 days, antibiotic use for more than 48 hours, poor nutritional status, and tracheostomy. Crude mortality rate among patients with *P. aeruginosa* VAP is 55.5%.

The clinical presentation of *P. aeruginosa* pneumonia includes fever, chill, and cough productive of yellow or green sputum. The chest radiograph usually shows diffuse infiltrates. Bacteremic *P. aeruginosa* pneumonia is more common in neutropenic patients and has a poor prognosis. Chronic *Pseudomonas* infection, seen in cystic fibrosis and chronic pulmonary disease, has a less severe clinical course.

The treatment of *P. aeruginosa* pneumonia includes antipseudomonal penicillin such as piperacillin or a cephalosporin such as ceftazidime combined with aminoglycoside, ciprofloxacin, meropenem, imipenem, or aztreonam. Although instillation of aminoglycosides via endotracheal tube does not improve clinical outcome, it has a higher bacterial eradication rate.

Klebsiella Species

Klebsiella pneumoniae is the most common *Klebsiella* species associated with pneumonia. In addition to nosocomial pneumonia, *Klebsiella* species can cause CAP in alcoholics. Presenting features include fever, productive cough, hemoptysis, and chest pain. Transmission from patient to patient occurs through water or via hands of personnel leading to hospital-acquired pneumonia. Chest radiograph shows lobar consolidation with bulging interlobular fissures.

The antibiotics of choice in the treatment of *Klebsiella* pneumonia include third-generation cephalosporins, the ureidopenicillins, such as piperacillin and aminoglycosides. Recent emergence of resistance to β-lactams such as ceftazidime and aztreonam, resulting from extended-spectrum β-lactamase production, has caused concern.

Escherichia coli

Escherichia coli normally is present in the intestinal tract. It is more commonly the cause of nosocomial pneumonia rather than CAP. Third-generation cephalosporins and fluoroquinolones are used for treatment.

Enterobacter Species

Enterobacter cloacae and *Enterobacter aerogenes* are the species most commonly implicated in pneumonia. Pneumonia caused by *Enterobacter* species is treated with a combination of third-generation cephalosporins and aminoglycosides.

Serratia Species

Serratia species are responsible for about 7% of cases of nosocomial pneumonia. It usually responds to treatment with imipenem, aztreonam, trimethoprim-sulfamethoxazole, or a combination of an extended penicillin and amikacin.

Acinetobacter Species

Acinetobacter species cause pneumonia in intensive care unit (ICU) patients receiving long-term mechanical ventilation. The clinical features and treatment are similar to *P. aeruginosa*. *Acinetobacter* species are transmitted on the hands of personnel. Most cases occur after the second week of hospitalization and after the patient has received a long course of broad-spectrum antibiotic therapy. It is associated with high mortality. Risk factors for its development include the severity of the patient's illness and previous infection.

Proteus mirabilis

Proteus mirabilis causes nosocomial pneumonia. It responds to third-generation cephalosporins and aminoglycosides.

Atypical Organisms

Legionellosis

Legionnaires' disease was first recognized among legionnaires attending a convention in a Philadelphia hotel. Although more than 30 species of *Legionella* have been identified, most infections are caused by *L. pneumophila*. This **atypical organism** colonizes domestic water and wet cooling systems, which have been implicated as sources in outbreaks of legionellosis. Infections by the *Legionella* species present as Pontiac fever or pneumonia. Pontiac fever is a transient, self-limiting, influenza-like illness. *Legionella* species can cause both community- and hospital-acquired pneumonia. Clinical symptoms include cough, fever, dyspnea, confusion, abdominal pain, and diarrhea. Nonpulmonary complications include pericarditis/myocarditis, encephalomyelitis, Guillain-Barré syndrome, rhabdomyolysis, acute renal failure, paralytic ileus, and pancreatitis. Quinolones and macrolides are used to treat legionellosis. Rifampin is added to erythromycin to treat severe legionellosis.

Mycoplasma pneumoniae

Mycoplasma pneumoniae is acquired by inhalation of respiratory droplets. It causes infection in closed populations such as those in military recruit camps and boarding schools. Epidemics of *Mycoplasma* pneumonia occur in 4-year cycles. Symptoms include fever, malaise, headache, and cough. Extrapulmonary manifestations can involve any organ. Myringitis is associated with *Mycoplasma* infection. Elevated cold hemagglutinins are seen in *Mycoplasma* infection but are nonspecific. The treatment includes fluoroquinolones, doxycyclines, and macrolides.

Chlamydia psittaci

Psittacosis (caused by *Chlamydia psittaci*) occurs in people who have contact with birds and bird products. Symptoms include fever, cough, dyspnea, headache, and myalgia. Extrapulmonary manifestations are common and involve the skin, blood, kidney, liver, central nervous system, and heart. The treatment of choice is doxycycline.

Chlamydia pneumoniae Outbreaks of *Chlamydia pneumoniae* infection have occurred in schools, military institutions, and within families. The clinical manifestations include fever, cough, and pharyngitis. Extrapulmonary manifestations of *C. pneumoniae* include arthritis, meningoencephalitis, myocarditis, endocarditis, coronary artery disease, and Guillain-Barré syndrome. Treatment includes fluoroquinolones, doxycycline, and macrolides.

Coxiella burnetii Cattle are the reservoir for *Coxiella burnetii*, which causes Q fever. The clinical manifestations include fever, chills, cough, fatigue, myalgia, and diarrhea. The nonpulmonary manifestations include endocarditis, hepatitis, meningoencephalitis, and osteomyelitis. Tetracyclines and fluoroquinolones are used for treatment.

Anaerobic Bacterial Infection

The major anaerobic pathogens implicated in pneumonia are *Peptostreptococcus* species, *Bacteroides melaninogenicus*, *Fusobacterium necrophorum*, *Bacteroides asaccharolyticus*, *Porphyromonas endodontalis*, and *Porphyromonas gingivalis*.[7] Aspiration of oropharyngeal secretions, which contain large numbers of anaerobic bacteria, is the major mechanism of anaerobic lung infection. Anaerobic pneumonia caused by hematogenous spread from septic phlebitis and contiguous spread from subdiaphragmatic abscess are less common. Predisposing factors for anaerobic lung infections include decreased level of consciousness, impaired swallowing, and gastrointestinal dysfunction. Anaerobic pneumonia is usually multimicrobial.

Patients with anaerobic pneumonia may have poor dental hygiene and longer duration of symptoms compared to those with pneumococcal pneumonia. Radiographically, the posterior segment of the right upper lobe and the superior segment of the right lower lobe are commonly involved. The diagnosis of anaerobic lung infection is made by positive culture of a transtracheal aspirate or empyema. Unless promptly treated, anaerobic pneumonia can lead to necrotizing pneumonia, lung abscess, and empyema.

Clindamycin is the drug of choice to treat anaerobic pneumonia. Amoxicillin-clavulanate, ticarcillin-clavulanate, ampicillin-sulbactam, imipenem, meropenem, and a metronidazole–penicillin combination are other alternatives.

Viral Causes of Pneumonia

Viruses usually cause trivial disease limited to the upper respiratory tract. **Viral pneumonias** are uncommon but often severe. The major viruses causing pneumonia include influenza, parainfluenza, respiratory syncytial virus (RSV), cytomegalovirus (CMV), adenovirus, measles, varicella zoster, herpes simplex, Epstein-Barr, and *Hantavirus* species.

Influenza Virus

Influenza infection is characterized by yearly outbreaks, usually in the winter, and less frequent irregular cycles of pandemics. Attack rates for influenza are highest in young children. Hospital admission and mortality rates are highest in the elderly, especially in those with underlying chronic medical conditions. Secondary bacterial pneumonia, usually caused by *S. aureus* and *S. pneumoniae*, is a severe complication of influenza infection. Treatment of influenza infection is usually symptomatic, with rest and adequate fluid intake being prescribed. The antiviral drugs amantadine and rimantadine are used in selected cases. Annual influenza vaccination is used as prophylaxis against influenza infection. The influenza vaccines are made annually based on surveillance of strains that are prevalent in the community. The current inactivated influenza vaccines are highly purified and associated with few side effects. The vaccine is contraindicated in people who have an allergy to hen's eggs.

Age-Specific Angle

> Influenza rates are highest in young children. Hospital admission and mortality rates are highest among the elderly.

Other Viruses

Parainfluenza viruses rarely cause pneumonia in adults. Treatment is similar to that for influenza. No vaccination is available against parainfluenza infection.

RSV is more frequent in children. Outbreaks of RSV peak in the winter months. Clinical features are similar to influenza. Aerosolized ribavirin is the treatment of choice.

Age-Specific Angle

> RSV infection is frequent in children—particularly in the winter months.

CMV rarely causes a problem in an immunocompromised patient. However, it causes severe disease with high mortality in immunocompromised patients. The risk of primary CMV infection is high when a seronegative, immunocompromised patient with CMV receives blood products or tissue from a seropositive donor. The clinical presentations include fever, dry cough, and tachypnea with hypoxemia. Radiographic abnormalities include diffuse interstitial infiltrates. Most of the patients who have positive CMV culture in respiratory secretions do not have histologic evidence of CMV pneumonia. Ganciclovir is used to treat CMV pneumonitis. Acyclovir and ganciclovir are used as prophylaxis against CMV.

Adenoviruses can cause severe illness, especially in children. There is no effective antiviral agent that can be used against adenoviruses.

Patients with measles pneumonia usually have the classic measles rash. Measles pneumonia is characterized by prolonged fever, increased cough, and progressive respiratory failure requiring mechanical ventilation. Measles in pregnant women is associated with premature labor and spontaneous abortion. Intravenous ribavirin has been used to treat measles.

Varicella zoster pneumonia is more common in immunocompromised patients. Patients present with typical chicken pox rash followed by dry cough, dyspnea, and pleuritic chest pain. The chest radiograph usually shows diffuse nodular or reticular densities. Acyclovir is used to treat varicella zoster pneumonia. Vidarabine and foscarnet are alternatives.

Most cases of herpes simplex pneumonia occur in patients with severe immunosuppression, burns, or ARDS. Stomatitis, genital infection, ocular infection, and encephalitis are the main manifestations of herpes simplex infection. The presence of herpes simplex virus in respiratory secretions does not confirm the diagnosis of pneumonia. Histologic proof of parenchymal involvement on lung biopsy is required to confirm the diagnosis of herpes simplex pneumonia. Herpes simplex bronchitis has been associated with fever, wheezing, cough, and bronchospasm. Acyclovir, foscarnet, and vidarabine are used for treatment of herpes simplex pneumonia.

Epstein-Barr virus has been implicated in the etiology of lymphocytic interstitial pneumonitis, a disorder associated with hypergammaglobulinemia, autoimmune disorders, pediatric HIV infection, and malignancy. There is no effective antiviral therapy for Epstein-Barr infection. Corticosteroids are used in lymphocytic interstitial pneumonitis.

Hantavirus causes influenza-like illness with fever and myalgia, followed by dyspnea, hypoxemia, pulmonary edema, shock, and death. The major reservoir for the virus is the deer mouse. It was initially reported in the four corners region of Arizona, Colorado, New Mexico, and Utah.[8] There is no effective therapy to treat this virus.

Mycobacterial Causes of Pneumonia

In addition to *Mycobacterium tuberculosis*, about 19 other nontuberculous mycobacteria (NTM) can cause human disease. AFB smears and mycobacterial cultures are used in the diagnosis of **mycobacterial pneumonia** infections. Once mycobacteria are isolated, M. *tuberculosis*, M. *avium-intracelluare* complex, M. *gordonae*, and M. *kansasii* can be identified with nucleic acid probes.

Tuberculosis

The World Health Organization (WHO) has estimated that nearly one billion people worldwide will be newly in-fected, 200 million will become ill, and 35 million will die from **tuberculosis** between the years 2000 and 2020. In the United States, the number of cases of tuberculosis has increased each year since 1985; in the preceding 30 years, a 6% annual fall in the number of cases was reported. HIV infection, homelessness, drug abuse, overcrowding, and emigration are responsible for the current rise.

Tuberculous infections are transmitted by inhalation of organisms from infected, coughing individuals. In countries with a high prevalence of tuberculosis, primary tuberculosis occurs in childhood. When infection develops, the affected persons may have malaise and fever or exhibit no symptoms at all. In most children with primary tuberculosis, the primary complex heals, and calcification of the affected lymph node and the associated primary lesion occurs. In some patients, the primary infection can progress and cause cough productive of tubercle bacilli in sputum and, in some cases, pleural effusion. Lymphatic and hematogenous spread to other organs also can be seen. Postprimary pulmonary tuberculosis usually arises from reactivation of a previously dormant primary infection or sometimes as a result of a new exogenous infection. Symptoms include malaise, anorexia, fever, night sweats, weight loss, productive cough, and hemoptysis.

AFB smears and mycobacterial cultures are performed on expectorated and induced sputum, BAL, and lung tissues to diagnose pulmonary tuberculosis. Tuberculin skin test, with purified protein derivative (PPD), is used to determine an individual's exposure to mycobacterial infection, including past bacille Calmette-Guérin (BCG) vaccination. A positive test is defined as induration of 10 mm or more in diameter in high-risk individuals without HIV infection, and 5 mm in those with HIV infection. However, the test can be false-negative in overwhelming infections, sarcoidosis, lymphoma, malignancy, and treatment with immunosuppressive drugs and corticosteroids.

Primary pulmonary tuberculosis can involve any lobe and has no typical radiologic features. More advanced tuberculosis usually involves the upper lobes and the superior segments of the lower lobes with cavitation. Longstanding disease may cause fibrosis.

Treatment of tuberculosis should include at least 6 months of isoniazid and rifampin and 2 months of pyrazinamide. In areas where the incidence of isoniazid resistance is 4% or greater, ethambutol should be added. Directly observed therapy is recommended.

BCG vaccination and isoniazid are used to prevent tuberculosis. BCG may be beneficial in health care workers at risk and tuberculin-negative adults and infants from countries where tuberculosis is common.

Nontuberculous Mycobacteria

The most commonly isolated nontuberculous mycobacteria (NTM) are M. *avium-intracelluare* complex, M. *gordonae*, and M. *kansasii*. The NTM are widespread

$\mathcal{B}$ox 50-3

American Thoracic Society Diagnostic Criteria for Pulmonary Disease Caused
by Nontuberculous Mycobacteria

A. If three sputum/bronchial samples are available from the previous 12 months:
  1. Three positive cultures with negative AFB smear or
  2. Two positive cultures and one positive AFB smear
B. If only one bronchial wash is available:
  1. Positive culture with a 2+, 3+, or 4+ AFB smear or
  2. Positive culture with a 2+, 3+, or 4+ growth on solid media

C. If sputum/bronchial wash evaluations are nondiagnostic or another disease cannot be excluded:
  1. Transbronchial or open lung biopsy yielding a NTM or
  2. Biopsy showing mycobacterial histopathologic features (granulomatous inflammation and/or AFB) and one or more sputums or bronchial washings are positive for a NTM even in low numbers

From American Thoracic Society. Diagnosis and treatment of disease cause by nontuberculous mycobacteria. Am J Respir Crit Care Med 1997;156:S1-S25.
NTM, Nontuberculous mycobacteria; AFB, acid-fast bacilli.

worldwide and are found in soil and water. NTM are often isolated in the absence of clinical disease. The mode of transmission of NTM is not clear. Many cases of pulmonary disease caused by NTM occur in smokers with COPD, silicosis, malignancy, cystic fibrosis, HIV infection, and other immunocompromised conditions. The isolation of NTM without evidence of tissue involvement by biopsy does not differentiate between colonization and disease. The diagnosis of NTM pneumonia is even more difficult in immunocompromised patients because the classic histologic response may not occur. To overcome these diagnostic difficulties, the American Thoracic Society has published diagnostic criteria of NTM lung disease for patients with clinical and radiologic features compatible with mycobacterial disease (Box 50-3).[9]

Chronic pulmonary disease is the most common localized manifestation of NTM. M. *avium-intracellulare* complex, followed by M. *kansasii*, is the most frequent NTM causing lung disease in the United States. Symptoms at presentation include chronic cough, sputum production, fatigue, malaise, dyspnea, fever, hemoptysis, and weight loss. Radiographic features of NTM pneumonia are highly variable and range from upper lobe apical opacities with cavitation to nonspecific lower lobe infiltrates and nodules. High-resolution computerized tomography of the chest may show bronchiectasis in patients with M. *avium-intracellulare* complex. Skin testing is of limited use in the diagnosis of NTM.

When the AFB smear of a specimen from the respiratory tract is positive, the initial therapy should be directed against tuberculosis. When the culture reveals NTM in the appropriate clinical setting, specific therapy against NTM should be started. Treatment with isoniazid, rifampin, and ethambutol for 18 months is recommended for pulmonary disease caused by M. *kansasii*. Clarithromycin, ethambutol, and rifabutin for 18 to 20 months is recommended for the treatment of M. *avium-intracellulare* lung disease. Rifabutin combined with azithromycin is used for prophylaxis against M. *avium-intracellulare* complex.

Fungal Respiratory Infections

Histoplasmosis

The major endemic areas of histoplasmosis are in North and South America, especially in the Ohio and Mississippi River valleys of the United States. Cutting through logs contaminated with avian excrement, doing construction work, being exposed to a chicken coop or other bird roosts predisposes people to contracting histoplasmosis. The majority of **fungal respiratory infections** resulting from exposure to *Histoplasma capsulatum* are asymptomatic. Symptoms develop in individuals exposed to a large inoculum of the organism or in immunocompromised persons. The manifestations of acute pulmonary histoplasmosis include fever, headache, malaise, and nonproductive cough. An intense inflammatory response during an acute pulmonary histoplasmosis infection can cause mediastinal granulomatosis and fibrosis leading to life-threatening complications such as superior vena cava syndrome, esophageal compression, constrictive pericarditis, and lung collapse. Healed pulmonary foci of histoplasmosis can leave calcified coin lesions. Individuals with COPD are at risk for chronic pulmonary histoplasmosis, which is associated with extensive pulmonary infiltrates, cavitation, and volume loss. Disseminated histoplasmosis is life-threatening and is seen in immunocompromised patients.

H. capsulatum can be seen in blood smears, sputum, cerebrospinal fluid, bone marrow, and lung tissue. Fungal cultures of sputum, bronchial washing, and lung tissues are also used for the diagnosis of histoplasmosis. In disseminated histoplasmosis, urine and sputum *Histoplasma* polysaccharide antigen may be positive.

No specific treatment is needed for asymptomatic or mildly symptomatic acute pulmonary histoplasmosis. In patients with persistent or progressive acute pulmonary histoplasmosis, itraconazole can be used. In severe cases, amphotericin B is needed. Amphotericin B is also recommended for chronic pulmonary and disseminated histoplasmosis.

Blastomycosis

Blastomycosis is endemic in the southern and upper midwestern United States. The presence of both decaying organic debris and high humidity favors the growth of *Blastomyces dermatitidis*. Blastomycosis is acquired sexually or through inhalation.

Acute blastomycosis manifests as pneumonia with fever, chills, myalgia, and productive cough. Chronic blastomycosis manifests with fever, weight loss, cough productive of purulent sputum, and hemoptysis. Chronic blastomycosis can involve the skin, bones, joints, and central nervous system. The diagnosis is made by observation of the organism or by the obtaining of a positive culture from sputum, bronchial lavage, pleural fluid, skin lesion, cerebrospinal fluid, or urine. Blastomycosis is treated with itraconazole or amphotericin B.

Coccidioidomycosis

Coccidioides immitus lives in soil with arid and semiarid climates. It is endemic in southwestern Unites States and some countries of South America. Coccidioidomycosis peaks in the summer and late autumn. In 1994, there was an epidemic of coccidioidomycosis in the Los Angeles area among persons who were exposed to dust clouds after the earthquake.

Infection is generally initiated by inhalation of the organisms. Primary coccidioidomycosis is asymptomatic in the majority of cases. Clinical features include fever, malaise, anorexia, myalgia, cough, hemoptysis, and chest pain. An erythematous, macular rash is seen initially. The usual radiologic manifestations of primary coccidioidomycosis are patchy pulmonary infiltrates. Resolution of the infiltrates is followed by the development of a pulmonary nodule, which may cavitate. Miliary pulmonary infiltrates are seen in disseminated coccidioidomycosis. A minority of the patients with primary coccidioidomycosis may develop chronic, progressive coccidioidomycosis, characterized by apical fibronodular infiltrates. Hematogenous dissemination of coccidioidomycosis is more common in African-Americans and Filipinos than in whites and may involve the skin, bones, and meninges. Smear and fungal culture of sputum, bronchial washings, and lung tissues and complement fixation and immunodiffusion serology are used to diagnose coccidioidomycosis.

Primary pulmonary coccidioidomycosis is usually self-limited and does not require antifungal therapy. However, in cases of persistent and progressive symptoms and disseminated disease and in individuals at high risk for dissemination, such as African-Americans, Filipinos, immunosuppressed patients, and women in late pregnancy, antifungal therapy is indicated. Amphotericin B is the treatment of choice. Amphotericin B is also effective in chronic and disseminated coccidioidomycosis, although the disease relapses when treatment is stopped. Cavitary pulmonary lesions do not respond to antifungal therapy and may require surgical intervention.

Cryptococcosis

Cryptococcus neoformans has worldwide distribution. The organism is often found in areas contaminated with avian droppings. Infection occurs when aerosolized *Cryptococcus* organisms are inhaled. Most infections are asymptomatic. Cryptococcal disease can occur in normal or immunocompromised persons. Normal persons usually develop self-limited pneumonia without extrapulmonary manifestation, although cryptococcal meningitis can occur in some. Disseminated cryptococcosis occurs more often in patients with impaired cellular immunity, such as those with HIV infection; systemic, prolonged corticosteroid use; certain hematologic malignancies; and organ transplantation. The clinical manifestations of pulmonary cryptococcosis include dry cough, dyspnea, and chest pain. Although meningitis is the most common form of extrapulmonary cryptococcosis, skin, bones, and any other organ also can be involved. The diagnosis is made by direct visualization or culturing of the organism from sputum, bronchial washing, and lung tissue. The cryptococcal antigen test is good for the diagnosis of cryptococcal meningitis but not respiratory tract infection. Patients with severe cryptococcal pneumonia, extrapulmonary disease, and immunosuppression need treatment with amphotericin B, with or without flucytosine.

Aspergillosis

Aspergillus molds are ubiquitous, being found in soil, dust, and water. The most common *Aspergillus* species causing human disease is *Aspergillus fumigatus*. The organism is transmitted by inhalation from the environment, especially during hospital construction alterations. Qualitative and quantitative neutrophil defects predispose a person to invasive aspergillosis.

The pulmonary manifestations of *Aspergillus* infection include hypersensitivity type reaction, noninvasive infection, and invasive infection.[10] The hypersensitivity type reactions include asthma, extrinsic allergic alveolitis, and allergic bronchopulmonary aspergillosis. Noninvasive infection can present as aspergilloma and invasive infection as chronic necrotizing aspergillosis, acute invasive aspergillosis, and acute tracheobronchitis. The hypersensitivity type manifestations are treated with systemic corticosteroids. Aspergilloma usually develops in a preexisting cavity, and the infected person may be asymptomatic or present with cough and hemoptysis. Aspergillomas are usually managed conservatively but may require surgery if recurrent or life-threatening symptoms occur. Amphotericin B is used to treat invasive *Aspergillus* pulmonary infection.

Candidiasis

Candida species are found in soil and food and colonize the gastrointestinal tract, skin, and hospital environment. Candidal infections play a major role in nosocomial infections, particularly in the ICU and in patients with granulocytopenia. *Candida albicans* is the most common species causing human disease. The manifestations of *Candida* respiratory infections include bronchitis, laryngitis, epiglottitis, mycetoma, lung abscess, and pneumonia. *C. albicans* is a common cause of pharyngeal infection in persons using inhaled corticosteroids. Because *Candida* organisms colonize the respiratory tract, the diagnosis of *Candida* pneumonia requires lung biopsy demonstrating tissue invasion. Amphotericin B is the treatment of choice.

Actinomycosis and Nocardiosis

Actinomycosis

Actinomyces species are normally present in the mouth and have a tendency to form filaments as a result of failure to separate with growth. Actinomycosis affects men more often than women. *Actinomyces israelii* is the most commonly implicated species. After dental surgery, aspiration, or penetrating trauma, actinomycosis can involve the thoracic cage, bronchi, mediastinum, lungs, or pleura. Initial clinical features include cough, fever, hemoptysis, chest pain, weight loss, or malaise. Chest radiograph may reveal infiltrates, cavitation, lung abscess, mass lesions, or chest wall involvement. Penicillin is the drug of choice in the treatment of actinomycosis. Alternative antimicrobials include first generation cephalosporins, imipenem, clindamycin, erythromycin, chloramphenicol, tetracycline, trimethoprim-sulfamethoxazole, or ciprofloxacin. Surgical intervention is required in patients who fail to respond to medical therapy. Hyperbaric oxygen has been used as an adjunctive therapy.

Nocardiosis

Nocardia species are ubiquitous in soil. *Nocardia asteroides* is the most common *Nocardia* species causing human disease. Nocardial infection is acquired through inhalation. Pulmonary nocardiosis occurs in patients with immunosuppression, chronic pulmonary disease, steroid use, alcoholism, alveolar proteinosis, and autoimmune diseases. Patients with pulmonary nocardiosis present with productive cough of weeks' duration associated with fatigue, weight loss, fever, dyspnea, and chest pain. Extrapulmonary involvement can include the skin and central nervous system. The radiologic abnormalities include infiltrates, necrotizing pneumonia, cavitation, pulmonary nodules, abscesses, pleural effusion, and hilar and mediastinal lymphadenopathy. The diagnosis of pulmonary nocardiosis can be made from sputum, BAL, and transbronchial and open lung biopsies. Trimethoprim-sulfamethoxazole is the drug of choice used to treat nocardiosis. In addition to antimicrobials, surgical resection and drainage may be necessary for abscess and empyema.

Community-Acquired Pneumonia

Community-acquired pneumonia (CAP) is not a reportable condition, and its exact incidence cannot be determined from hospital discharge records because only 20% to 25% of patients require hospitalization. In the United States, two to three million cases of CAP occur annually, resulting in 10 million physician visits, 500,000 hospitalizations, and 45,000 deaths. Estimates of the incidence of CAP have ranged from 2 to 15 cases per 1000 persons per year. The incidence is highest in the winter months, especially in the very young and the very old.

> ## Age-Specific Angle
>
> In the very young and very old the incidence of CAP is highest in the winter months.

Risk factors for acquisition of CAP include age, cigarette smoking, COPD, congestive heart failure, alcoholism, injection drug use, impaired consciousness, neurologic disease, diabetes mellitus, steroid therapy, HIV infection, and prior history of pneumonia.

Etiology

Of those who contract CAP, 80% can be treated as outpatients. The most significant pathogens in this setting are *S. pneumoniae*, *H. influenzae*, and influenza A virus. The incidence of *M. pneumoniae* may vary according to the rapidity of its reproductive cycle and the age of the exposed population.

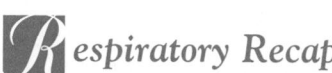

espiratory Recap

> **Community-Acquired Pneumonia**
>
> Most individuals can be treated as outpatients.
> CAP can be classified as typical and atypical.
> Antibiotic therapy aimed against likely pathogens should be started promptly.
> The decision to hospitalize is based on the presence of risk factors.
> Mortality is less than 15%.

Approximately 20% to 50% of patients with CAP require hospitalization. *S. pneumoniae* is the most common pathogen; it is responsible for 30% to 40% of these pneumonias and is associated with bacteremia in 20% to 30% of cases. *H. influenzae* and *M. pneumoniae* are the second most common pathogens, causing 10% to 20% of the episodes. The most important difference between out-patient and hospital-treated CAP is the higher incidence of *L. pneumophila* in the hospital-treated group. However, there are regional and annual variations in the incidence of *L. pneumophila*. Epidemic and endemic cases of *L. pneumophila* highlight the need to investigate the source of the infection. Mixed infections account for 10% to 20% of cases of CAP.

Admission to an ICU is required for 10% of patients hospitalized for CAP. In these critically ill patients, *S. pneumoniae* is the most common pathogen, followed by *L. pneumophila*.

The etiology of CAP is modified by age, coexisting illnesses, and geographic, seasonal, and individual factors. Elderly patients appear to suffer from a more severe course of infection. Patients with COPD are often colonized with *S. pneumoniae* and *H. influenzae*. Patients with alcohol abuse suffer more often from *S. pneumoniae* and *K. pneumoniae* infections and aspiration pneumonia. Patients with cystic fibrosis and bronchiectasis develop pneumonia caused by *P. aeruginosa*, *S. aureus*, and *H. influenzae*. Severe neurologic impairment predisposes a person to aspiration pneumonia. In the developing countries, *M. tuberculosis* is very common. Travel to certain endemic regions can lead to pneumonia caused by *Histoplasma capsulatum*, *Coccidioides immitis*, and *Blastomyces dermatitidis*. The incidence of pneumonia rises in the winter, coinciding with peaks of pneumococcal and influenza virus pneumonia. *Legionella* pneumonia is more common in the summer and autumn. *M. pneumoniae* has cyclic epidemics every 3 to 4 years. Contact with avian species is associated with *C. psittaci*. Domestic animals are the main source of *C. burnetii*. Injection drug users are at increased risk for pneumococcal and staphylococcal pneumonia.

Age-Specific Angle

Elderly patients suffer a more severe course of CAP.

Additional pathogens causing CAP include *C. pneumoniae* and *M. catarrhalis*. Even after an extensive microbiologic investigation, prospective studies of CAP fail to detect pathogens in up to 50% of the cases.

It is commonly accepted that persons living in nursing homes are at risk of suffering pneumonia caused by uncommon pathogens. In patients who are living in nursing homes but are self-sufficient, the etiologies are probably the same as in the community. In those who are severely limited and handicapped, pathogens causing hospital-acquired pneumonia should be considered.

Classically, the epidemiologic, clinical, and radiographic characteristics of each case have been considered to give a clue for the initial etiologic assessment. Based on these characteristics, pneumonias have been classified into "typical" and "atypical." However, the usefulness of a classification of CAP into "typical" and "atypical" has been questioned because no convincing association has been found between individual symptoms, physical findings or laboratory values, and specific etiologies.

Typical pneumonias are characterized by abrupt onset of chills, high fever, pleuritic chest pain, and cough productive of rusty or purulent sputum. Physical signs of consolidation such as bronchial breath sounds and inspiratory crackles are present. Lobar or segmental consolidation is seen on the chest radiograph. Leukocytosis is present. Pneumococcus (*Streptococcus pneumoniae*) is the most common cause of typical pneumonia, followed by *H. influenzae*, *Enterobacteriaceae* species, and *S. aureus*. Chronic debilitating diseases such as diabetes mellitus, COPD, hepatic cirrhosis, and alcoholism increase the risk of having the nonpneumococcal etiologies.

Age-Specific Angle

Atypical pneumonia is more common in younger patients.

Atypical pneumonia is more common in the young. It is characterized by a flulike disease with prodromal symptoms, dry cough, myalgia, malaise, rhinorrhea, and moderate fever. Chills are rare. The white blood cell count is usually normal. Chest radiograph shows diffuse infiltrate or a focal peribronchial pattern. Usual pathogens include *M. pneumoniae*, *C. psittaci*, *C. burnetii*, *C. pneumoniae*, and respiratory viruses.

Initial Management

When choosing empirical therapy for CAP, one should consider the geographic distribution of the causative organisms, the cyclic appearance of organisms such as *M. pneumoniae*, and the variable incidence of organisms such as *L. pneumophila*. Before initiating therapy, one should consider the most likely pathogen causing the pneumonia and the severity of the pneumonia.

Auscultation of the chest may reveal abnormal signs in the absence of pneumonia, particularly in febrile patients with COPD. Chest radiograph may show the characteristic distribution of consolidation, pleural effusion, and cavitation, which are useful to determine the implicated pathogen. The epidemiologic and the individual patient characteristics may give clues to the likely pathogen. Various medical societies have published guidelines for the management of CAP.[2,6,11,12] Sputum Gram's stain and culture is obtained in patients with CAP, and blood cultures are obtained from those requiring hospitalization.

Because a delay in antibiotic therapy has been associated with increased mortality, antibiotic therapy aimed against the likely pathogens should be started promptly. Empiric antibiotic therapy for patients who do not require hospitalization should include macrolide, fluoroquinolone, tetracycline, or doxycycline.[13] For patients requiring hospitalization, second- or third-generation cephalosporin or β-lactam/β-lactamase inhibitor should be used, with the addition of a macrolide or fluoroquinolone in cases with severe presentation or suspected atypical pathogens. In patients with structural lung disease, such as bronchiectasis, antipseudomonal antibiotics such as piperacillin, carbepenem, cefepime, or ciprofloxacin, should be added. In patients suspected of having anaerobic aspiration pneumonia, clindamycin or β-lactam/β-lactamase inhibitor should be used.

The decision to hospitalize should be based on the presence of risk factors that are associated with increased mortality and morbidity of patients with CAP.[3] These risk factors include age more than 50 years, coexistent chronic disease, alcoholism, illicit drug use, HIV infection, pulse rate 125 or more per minute, respiratory rate 30 or more per minute, systolic blood pressure less than 90 mm Hg, temperature lower than 35° C or 40° C or higher, altered mental status, lack of response after 3 days of antibiotics, metastatic infection, multilobar involvement, significant pleural effusion, cavitation, leukocyte count less than 4000/mL or more than 20,000/mL, hemoglobin less than 9g/dL, and acute renal failure.[2,3] Social problems, such as degree of compliance and quality of home support, should also be considered in the decision making process regarding hospitalization. Patients with severe respiratory failure, hemodynamic instability, acute renal failure, severe disseminated intravascular coagulation, meningitis, and coma should be considered for admission to an ICU.

Nonresponding CAP is characterized by persistent fever, tachypnea, leukocytosis, hypoxemia, progression of pulmonary infiltrates, and appearance of pleural effusion. Noninfectious pneumonitis, inadequate antibiotic coverage, bronchial obstruction, empyema, defects of the host defense, antibiotic resistance, distant infection, and drug toxicity should be included in the differential diagnosis of nonresponding cases. Bronchoscopy should be considered in the management of nonresponding pneumonia to detect localized bronchial obstruction and obtain a sputum sample.

Prognosis

The overall mortality rate of CAP is 13.7%, ranging from 5.1% for hospitalized and ambulatory patients to 36.5% for ICU patients.[13] There are many factors that influence the prognosis of CAP. Old age, coexisting illnesses, alcoholism, delay in antimicrobial therapy, and inappropriate initial antimicrobial therapy increase mortality. Tachypnea, hypotension, tachycardia, lack of fever, confusion, low arterial oxygen tension, leukopenia, low serum albumin, increased blood urea nitrogen, increased serum lactate dehydrogenase, multiple lobe infection, bacteremia, certain pathogens, and overall disease severity measured by the Acute Physiology and Chronic Health Evaluation (APACHE) prognostic system are indicators of poor outcome. The disease progression leading to requirement of mechanical ventilation, the development of septic shock, ARDS, renal failure, secondary gram-negative colonization, and radiographic spread of the pneumonia are also associated with poor outcome.

Hospital-Acquired Pneumonia

Although the secretions aspirated from the lungs may contain multiple organisms, hospital-acquired pneumonia is usually monomicrobial. The etiology in hospital-acquired pneumonia results from the selection of certain pathogens by local or systemic host factors, the virulence of the organism, underlying disease of the patient, and previous exposure to antimicrobials.

Epidemiology

Hospital-acquired pneumonia accounts for 13% to 18% of all nosocomial infections and occurs at a rate of 4 to 7 episodes per 1000 hospitalizations. Rates of VAP are approximately 15 per 1000 ventilator days in ICU patients. Hospital-acquired pneumonia is the second most common nosocomial infection in the United States and is associated with high expenditure, morbidity, and mortality. The highest incidence of hospital-acquired pneumonia is found in the intensive care units, and the incidence depends on the percentage of endotracheally intubated patients. VAP is the leading cause of nosocomial infection among intubated patients. The incidence of hospital-acquired pneumonia is higher in older patients and in large teaching hospitals. Independent risk factors for hospital-acquired pneumonia include age older than 60 years, APACHE II older than 16, trauma, head injury, impaired airway reflexes, coma, bronchoscopy, nasogastric tube, endotracheal tube, upper abdominal surgery, thoracic surgery, low serum albumin, and neuromuscular disease.[14,15] The risk factors for VAP include the presence of COPD, use of positive end-expiratory pressure (PEEP), the presence of intracranial pressure monitor, organ failure, large volume gastric aspirate, prior antibiotics, H_2-blockers and antacids, gastric colonization and high pH, reintubation, mechanical ventilation more than 2 days, tracheostomy, supine head position, failure of subglottic aspiration, and low intracuff pressure.[14,15]

Age-Specific Angle

The incidence of hospital-acquired pneumonia is higher in older patients.

Etiology

The incidence of the organisms causing hospital-acquired pneumonia varies from hospital to hospital and at times varies within different units of the same hospital. The time of onset of the pneumonia may give a clue to the most likely pathogen (Box 50-4). Most cases are caused by more than one species of bacteria. Certain risk factors are associated with specific pathogens: recent abdominal surgery and witnessed aspiration with anaerobes; coma, head trauma, diabetes mellitus, and renal failure with *S. aureus*; high-dose corticosteroid therapy with *Legionella*; prolonged ICU stay, steroid therapy, antibiotics, and structural lung disease with *P. aeruginosa*.

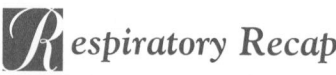

Respiratory Recap

Hospital-Acquired Pneumonia
Pneumonia accounts for 13% to 18% of nosocomial infections and is the second most common nosocomial infection. Nosocomial pneumonia has a high mortality rate (20% to 50%). The initial choice of antibiotic depends on severity of the infection, risk factors, and time of onset. Surveillance and infection control programs are important to lower nosocomial pneumonia rates.

Uncommon pathogens should be included as a possible etiology of hospital-acquired pneumonia under certain conditions. Clusters of legionellosis have been related to contamination of water and cooling towers as well as to soil movement in an area adjacent to the hospital. *P. carinii* and

Box 50-4

Common Pathogens Associated with Hospital-Acquired Pneumonia

Early Onset
    Streptococcus pneumoniae
    Nonpseudomonal *Enterobacter* species
    Escherichia coli
    Haemophilus influenzae
    Klebsiella species
    Proteus species
    Serratia marcescens
    MSSA
 	
Late Onset
    Pseudomonas aeruginosa
    MRSA
    Acinetobacter species
    Organisms listed under early onset

MRSA, *Methicillin-resistant* Staphylococcus aureus; MSSA, *methicillin-sensitive* Staphylococcus aureus.

viruses should be considered in immunocompromised patients. *Candida* species may cause pneumonia in patients on cancer chemotherapy or broad-spectrum antibiotics and in patients with neutropenia. *Aspergillus fumigatus* should be considered in patients with severe neutropenia, in those on steroid therapy, and in the presence of construction activity or a faulty ventilator system around a hospital.

Initial Management

In contrast to infections of more frequently involved organs such as the urinary tract and skin, mortality associated with hospital-acquired pneumonia in the lungs is very high. Therefore, more rapid identification of infected patients and accurate selection of antimicrobial agents for initial treatment are important. Successful treatment of hospital-acquired pneumonia is a difficult and complex undertaking. Conventional criteria such as fever, leukocytosis, purulent tracheal secretions, and presence of a new pulmonary infiltrate on chest radiographs are not very sensitive nor specific for the diagnosis of bacterial pneumonia in ICU patients. This makes the diagnosis of pneumonia problematic when the etiology of infection is not always identified.

Patient survival improves if pneumonia is correctly diagnosed and appropriately treated. The appropriate antibiotics are more likely to be prescribed if specific etiologic agents are identified. In one study evaluating the reliability of clinical judgment in the treatment of hospital-acquired pneumonia of patients receiving mechanical ventilation, only 33% of 131 therapeutic plans were subsequently found to be effective.[16]

Hospital-acquired pneumonia is likely to result from resistant organisms, especially in patients who have been treated with antibiotics. Multiple organisms are usually cultured from pulmonary secretions in patients with suspected pneumonia. These factors make it impossible to find an empirical regimen of antibiotics that will cover all organisms. Although appropriate antibiotics may improve survival of patients with hospital-acquired pneumonia, use of broad-spectrum antibiotics in patients without infection facilitates colonization and superinfection with multiresistant microorganisms.

The initial choice of antibiotic used for the management of hospital-acquired pneumonia depends on the severity, the presence of risk factors predisposing to certain organisms, and time of onset. The criteria for severe hospital-acquired pneumonia are admission to an ICU, respiratory failure requiring mechanical ventilator support or FiO_2 more than 35% to keep oxygen saturation greater than 90%, rapid radiographic progression, multilobar pneumonia, cavitation of infiltrate, acute renal failure requiring dialysis, and severe sepsis with hypotension or organ dysfunction. The antibiotics recommended for the initial, empirical therapy of hospital-acquired pneumonia based on severity and time of onset are listed in Table 50-1.[17] Regardless of the severity and time of onset, other specific antibiotics should be added for patients at risk for pneumonia due to anaerobic bacteria (**anaerobic bacterial pneumonia**), *P. aeruginosa, S. aureus,* and *Legionella* species.[17] In patients who have not received antibiotics, the morphology and Gram's stain of pulmonary secretions obtained by bronchoscopy enables early initiation of specific antimicrobial therapy before culture results are available. Because the microbial trends in hospital-acquired pneumonia are showing more resistant and more difficult to treat pathogens, including multiresistant gram-negative bacilli and MRSA, the medical community needs to be aware of each hospital's specific characteristics.

Antibiotic treatment of bacterial pneumonia depends on adequate delivery of the agents to the site of infection. Antibiotic levels in infected tissues are considered to be therapeutic if the free drug concentration level at least equals the minimum inhibitory concentration for the pathogen. The ratio of the concentration of drug in bronchial secretions to that in serum is 0.05 to 0.25 for penicillins and cephalosporins, 0.80 to 2.0 for fluoroquinolones, and 0.2 to 0.6 for aminoglycosides and tetracyclines. The tissue penetration may increase for the β-lactams in the presence of inflammation.

Mortality and Prognostic Factors

The crude mortality rates for hospital-acquired pneumonia range from 20% to 50%. High-risk organisms such as *Enterobacteriaceae* and *Pseudomonas* species and MRSA; bilateral infiltrates and respiratory failure are independent risk factors for mortality from hospital-acquired pneumonia.

Previous antibiotic therapy, transfer from another hospital or ward, duration of mechanical ventilation, severe underlying disease, and inappropriate antibiotic therapy also increase the mortality associated with hospital-acquired pneumonia.

Prevention

Prevention strategies result from an understanding of the epidemiology and pathogenesis of hospital-acquired pneumonia. Bacteria gain entry into the lower respiratory tract by aspiration, direct inoculation, or inhalation of airborne droplets or aerosols. The virulence of different pathogens is poorly understood in relation to pathogenesis and transmission. Age, underlying disease, medical treatments, and surgical procedures alter host resistance and lead to colonization and pneumonia.

Hospital-acquired pneumonia has changed with evolving differences in patient populations, the use of new invasive devices and respiratory equipment, and implementation of prevention strategies. Hospitals with effective surveillance and infection control programs have lower rates of pneumonia than hospitals without such programs. Surveillance targeted at high-risk patients coupled with staff education, use of proper isolation techniques, and infection control practices are important prevention strategies. Rates of nosocomial pneumonia should be based on the organism and adjusted for the duration of hospital stay and mechanical ventilation. Attention should be paid to hospital-acquired pneumonia caused by special pathogens or clusters of cases caused by multidrug resistant organisms.

Preventing hospital-acquired pneumonia is cost effective because it will decrease the duration of hospitalization. Organisms causing hospital-acquired pneumonia originate from the environment, devices, hospital staff, and other patients.[18] Although VAP may result from bacteremia or translocation from the gastrointestinal tract, direct inoculation or aspiration of bacteria, primarily from the oropharynx and less commonly from the stomach, are the most important routes of infection. In the patient with endotracheal tube, leakage of bacteria along the endotracheal cuff, with local trauma and tracheal inflammation from the endotracheal tube, increases colonization and reduces the clearance of organisms and secretions from the

TABLE 50-1

Empiric Antibiotic Therapy for Hospital-Acquired Pneumonia Based on Severity and Time of Onset

Antibiotics	Severity	Time of Onset
Second-generation cephalosporin	Mild or moderate	Any time
Non-antipseudomonas third-generation cephalosporin	Severe	Early
β-Lactam/β-lactamase inhibitor		
Fluoroquinolone		
Clindamycin+aztreonam		
Aminoglycoside or ciprofloxacin (and vancomycin, depending on the incidence of MRSA in the hospital) plus one of the following:	Severe	Late
Antipseudomonal penicillin		
β-Lactam/β-lactamase inhibitor		
Ceftazidime or cefepime		
Imipenem or meropenem		
Aztreonam		

MRSA, *Methicillin-resistant* Staphylococcus aureus.

lower respiratory tract. Tracheal colonization with bacteria and tracheobronchitis are common precursors of VAP. Stomach colonization increases in the presence of achlorhydria, gastrointestinal disease, malnutrition, and administration of antacids and H_2 blockers. Supine position, gastric tube, and enteral feeding may encourage colonization of the oropharynx and lower respiratory tract.

Risk factors for hospital-acquired pneumonia can be the result of host factors, conditions that favor colonization and aspiration, cross-infection, and complications from medications and devices. Measures recommended to prevent hospital-acquired pneumonia include tapering of steroids and cytotoxic agents, proper and judicious use of antibiotic prophylaxis, proper positioning of the patient, vaccines, surveillance for *L. pneumophila* infection, education of hospital personnel in proper aseptic and isolation techniques, respiratory isolation of patients with certain respiratory infections, proper hand washing, appropriate use of gown and gloves, feedback nosocomial infection surveillance data, appropriate cleaning and sterilization of equipment, avoidance of self-extubation/reintubation, infrequent change of ventilator circuits with humidifiers, continuous aspiration of subglottic secretions, use of aseptic technique during tracheal suctioning and sterilizing, and cleaning and disinfection of spirometers, O_2 sensors, and hand-powered resuscitation bags used among patients.[19]

Pneumonia in Immunocompromised Patients without HIV

Infectious pulmonary complications are common in immunocompromised patients.[20,21] The progress in the treatment of malignancies, connective tissue diseases, and organ transplantation have led to an increased number of patients with immunologic defect. The type of immunologic defect determines the kind of pneumonia that develops in these patients. Neutropenia and impaired granulocyte function compromise resistance to bacterial and fungal infections. Qualitative and quantitative defects of T-lymphocyte function facilitate the development of viral, fungal (including *P. carinii*), mycobacterial, and other intracellular microorganisms. B-lymphocyte dysfunction with impaired antibody formation increases patients' vulnerability to pneumonia by encapsulated bacteria.

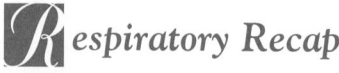

Respiratory Recap

Pneumonia in Immunocompromised Patients
Pulmonary infections are common in these patients. Bronchoalveolar lavage (BAL) is often diagnostic. Infections are caused by bacteria, mycobacteria, fungi, and viruses. Noninfectious causes account for about 25% of infiltrates.

Clinical and Radiographic Findings

The patient's history, including previous radiation therapy, medications, CMV status of recipient or donor, previous antibiotics, and prophylactic treatment may suggest the type of pulmonary complications that develop in the immunocompromised patient. The time and acuteness of onset also help in the differential diagnosis. In bone marrow transplant patients, bacterial and candidal pneumonia are often observed within 30 days of transplant, whereas CMV and *Aspergillus* species occur within 30 to 100 days. Acute onset is seen in bacterial or viral (influenza, adenovirus, RSV) infections, whereas subacute pneumonia occurring within 1 or 2 weeks is seen in CMV, aspergillosis, and mucormycosis. Nocardiosis and tuberculosis have chronic or insidious onset. PCP in non-HIV, immunocompromised patients has an acute onset.

Patients usually present with dyspnea, cough, and fever. Skin lesions are seen in mucormycosis, meningitis in cryptococcal and CMV infection, chorioretinitis in CMV, and choroidal lesions in *Candida* infections.

CMV and PCP produce diffuse reticulonodular patterns on chest radiograph, whereas extensive air space consolidation is seen in bacterial pneumonia, pulmonary edema, and hemorrhage. Focal infiltrates suggest bacterial or fungal pneumonia. Nodular or cavitating lesions are observed in nocardiosis, mycobacteriosis, or bacterial abscess. Infiltrates secondary to radiation pneumonitis are limited to the field of radiation. Air crescent sign is suggestive of invasive aspergillosis. Pleural effusions are rare in CMV and PCP. Mediastinal adenopathy is infrequent in PCP and more common in mycobacteriosis and nocardiosis.

Diagnostic Procedures

Diagnostic procedures should be able to give rapid and specific diagnoses. Blood culture helps identify dissemination of infection. Antibody detection for *Legionella* and *Aspergillus* species have low sensitivity and delayed results. CMV viremia, viruria, and antibody titers are useful markers of active infection but nonspecific for pneumonia. Detection of cryptococcal and *Aspergillus* antigens are highly specific but not sensitive.

Expectorated and induced sputum have low yield for PCP, mycobacteria, and *Legionella* species in non-HIV immunocompromised patients. *Aspergillus, Cryptococcus,* and *Nocardia* species are usually considered to be colonizing agents, except in severely immunocompromised patients. Transthoracic percutaneous needle aspiration is not routinely performed because of its potential complications.

BAL is diagnostic of *P. carinii, Toxoplasma gondii, Legionella* species, *M. tuberculosis,* influenza, *Mycoplasma* species, and RSV infections. Detection of herpes simplex and CMV in BAL fluid is not an accurate indicator of pneumonia unless there is cytologic or histologic evidence of infection. The presence of fungi, bacteria, and NTM need to be correlated with the clinical and radiographic findings. BAL can establish definite diagnosis in 33% to

66% of immunocompromised patients. Application of PCR to BAL fluid increases the sensitivity and is rapid in the detection of CMV, PCP, and mycobacterial pulmonary infection. Transbronchial lung biopsy is used in the diagnosis of CMV, *Aspergillus* species, rejection, and noninfectious etiologies. At times, open lung or thoracoscopic lung biopsies may be needed.

Causes of Pneumonia

Immunocompromised patients are vulnerable to infections caused by bacteria, mycobacteria, fungi, and viruses. Encapsulated organisms such as *S. pneumoniae* are common causes of pneumonia in patients with B-lymphocyte deficit such as multiple myeloma. Gram-negative organisms such as *P. aeruginosa* are common causes of pneumonia in neutropenic patients.

Fungal infections are common, especially in hematologic malignancies. Prolonged neutropenia, long duration of steroid therapy, broad spectrum antibiotic therapy, and central venous catheters are risk factors for the development of fungal infections. *Candida* pneumonia is the most common fungal pneumonia in the immunocompromised host. *Aspergillus* species cause extensive pneumonia with diffuse pulmonary hemorrhage. Pneumonias caused by *Mucor* and *Cryptococcus* species are reported occasionally. *Histoplasma*, coccidioidomycosis, and blastomycosis pneumonia should be considered in endemic areas.

CMV infection is the most common opportunistic infection after organ transplantation and is associated with poor prognosis. In the preprophylaxis era, CMV reactivation in seropositive patients was 80% in bone marrow transplant patients, and CMV pneumonitis was diagnosed in 10% to 35% of cases, with a mortality rate of 50%. In lung transplant patients, CMV pneumonitis is reported in 16% to 58% and is the most significant risk factor for early death and rejection. Herpes simplex viral pneumonitis occurs less often, and it is often associated with intraoral mucosal lesions.

Mycobacterial infections are rare in immunocompromised patients without HIV infection. PCP is a common opportunistic infection in immunocompromised patients. It also occurs in patients receiving methotrexate and systemic corticosteroids. However, its incidence has been decreasing since prophylaxis was started.

Noninfectious causes are responsible for about 25% of infiltrates in the immunocompromised patient. These causes include cytotoxic drugs, radiation, pulmonary edema, progression of underlying disease such as carcinomatous lymphangitis or tumor, alveolar hemorrhage, lung involvement resulting from connective tissue disease, graft-versus-host disease, or bronchiolitis obliterans organizing pneumonia (BOOP).

Therapeutic Considerations

Antimicrobial therapy is usually needed during the wait for results of diagnostic procedures. For bacterial pneumonia, a combination of antibiotics effective in the treatment of *P. aeruginosa* and *S. aureus* infections is usually necessary. Trimethoprim-sulfamethoxazole is used for PCP. When CMV pneumonitis is present, ganciclovir or foscarnet is used. Amphotericin B is used for invasive aspergillosis. In patients able to tolerate invasive procedures, bronchoscopy is needed when pulmonary infiltrates progress despite empirical treatment or when the diagnosis is uncertain.

Prophylaxis

Oral fluoroquinolones have been used to reduce the frequency of bacterial infection with gram-negative organisms in neutropenic patients. Acyclovir and ganciclovir have been used for CMV and trimethoprim-sulfamethoxazole for PCP.

Pneumonia in Patients with HIV

The WHO estimated more than 29 million adults to be living with HIV/AIDS worldwide at the end of 1997. In some sub-Saharan African countries, the prevalence of HIV infection in adults is higher than 25%. The cumulative incidence of AIDS in the United States was estimated to be 641,086 by the end of 1997. Infectious lung diseases are seen in 60% to 80% of patients with HIV infection. Coinfection with multiple pathogens is common. The common infectious agents causing pneumonia in patients with HIV infection are listed in Box 50-5. The type of pneumonia that develops in these patients depends on the CD_4 count, history of prior infection, HIV exposure category, and the virulence of the infecting organism. Pneumonias caused by bacteria, tuberculosis, influenza, and endemic mycoses are seen even with normal CD_4 count. PCP occurs more often when the CD_4 count drops below 200/μL.

Expectorated or induced sputum, nonbronchoscopic catheter lavage, specimen obtained by bronchoscopy and open lung biopsy are used in the diagnosis of pulmonary complications. BAL has an overall sensitivity of greater than 85% in the diagnosis of pulmonary disorders in patients with HIV infection. Transbronchial lung biopsy has an additive yield to BAL, especially in patients with non-

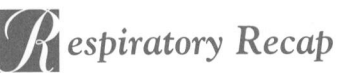

*R*espiratory Recap

Pneumonia in Patients with HIV
Pneumocystis carinii pneumonia (PCP) occurs more frequently when the CD_4 count is less than 200. Bronchoalveolar lavage (BAL) is often diagnostic. PCP is a common cause of mortality. Human immunodeficiency virus (HIV) has a major impact on the epidemiology of tuberculosis.

Box 50-5

Major Causes of Pneumonia in Patients with HIV

Bacterial
Streptococcus pneumoniae
Haemophilus influenzae
Staphylococcus aureus
Pseudomonas aeruginosa

Mycobacterial
Mycobacterium tuberculosis
Mycobacterium avium-intracellulare complex

Fungal
Pneumocystis carinii
Candida species
Aspergillus species

Viral
Cytomegalovirus
Herpes simplex virus

PCP pulmonary complications. Bronchoscopic brush biopsy is not used in patients with HIV infection because of its low additive yield. Open lung biopsy is rarely performed in patients with HIV infection because of the high diagnostic yield of BAL and transbronchial lung biopsy for treatable pulmonary complications. However, open lung biopsy is indicated when bronchoscopy is nondiagnostic or transbronchial biopsy cannot be performed because of a bleeding disorder or positive-pressure ventilation.

The differential diagnoses of pulmonary infiltrates in patients with HIV infection should include noninfectious causes such as nonspecific interstitial pneumonitis, lymphoid interstitial pneumonitis, Kaposi's sarcoma, and non-Hodgkin lymphoma. The application of primary prophylaxis has modified the approach to patients with HIV.

Causes of Pneumonia

Bacterial pneumonia is more common and is more likely to be bacteremic in patients with HIV compared to those without HIV infection. The most common organisms causing bacterial pneumonia are *S. pneumoniae* and *H. influenzae*. *P. aeruginosa* is being reported more often, especially in patients with low CD_4 and leukocyte count. Some patients develop recurrent bronchitis and sinusitis. Legionnaires' disease is rare in patients with HIV infection. *Nocardia asteroides* and *Rhodococcus equi* can cause pneumonia in these patients. Pneumococcal vaccination is recommended for patients with HIV infection.

PCP is the leading single cause of morbidity in patients with AIDS in developed countries. In Europe and North America, 30% to 60% of untreated patients with AIDS will have PCP at the time of AIDS diagnosis and an additional 20% to 35% will develop PCP thereafter. These rates are lower in patients who receive prophylactic therapy against PCP. The occurrence of PCP varies according to region, CD_4 count, nutritional status, and risk factors for HIV infection. Patients with HIV infection and PCP usually present with fever, dyspnea, and nonproductive cough of several weeks' duration. The chest radiograph often reveals diffuse, bilateral interstitial infiltrates. Atypical presentations are seen in patients receiving antiretroviral therapy and PCP prophylaxis. Extrapulmonary manifestations can be seen, especially in patients on aerosolized pentamidine for PCP prophylaxis. Arterial blood gas measurements are used to determine the severity of infection and guide management. Hypoxemia with wide alveolar-arterial oxygen tension gradient and elevated serum lactate dehydrogenase are seen in patients with PCP. Induced sputum has 80% yield in the diagnosis of PCP in some centers. BAL has high sensitivity in the diagnosis of PCP. In patients with endotracheal tubes, PCP can be diagnosed by the instilling of 60 mL of saline in 10 mL of aliquots and the collection of the specimen 30 seconds after each aliquot. Trimethoprim-sulfamethoxazole and intravenous pentamidine are the primary medications used for treatment of PCP. Other alternatives include clindamycin-primaquine, trimetrexate, and atovaquone. Corticosteroids are used as adjunctive therapy for AIDS patients with PCP. PCP prophylaxis should be given to all patients with HIV infection who have history of PCP, CD_4 count less than $200/\mu L$, oral thrush, or unexplained fever. Trimethoprim-sulfamethoxazole and inhaled pentamidine have been widely used for prophylaxis against PCP. However, inhaled pentamidine is more expensive and has been associated with breakthrough episodes and extrapulmonary *P. carinii* infection.

HIV infection has a major impact on the epidemiology of tuberculosis. In the United States, 52,100 excess cases of tuberculosis were reported during 1985 to 1992. At least 50% of these excess cases could be attributed to HIV infection. Among patients exposed to *M. tuberculosis*, those with HIV infection have a higher probability of progressing to clinical tuberculosis than those without HIV infection. Pulmonary tuberculosis can occur at any stage during HIV infection. However, extrapulmonary and disseminated tuberculosis are more common in patients with low CD_4 count. Chest radiographic manifestations of tuberculous pneumonia in patients with HIV infection are very variable. Even a normal chest radiograph does not exclude tuberculosis. In patients with advanced HIV disease, hilar and mediastinal lymphadenopathy, and lower lung field infiltrates are common and cavitation is less common. Because of their anergy, these patients are considered to have a positive tuberculosis skin test when induration is 5 mm.

Expectorated and induced sputum are used for the diagnosis of pulmonary tuberculosis. BAL, transbronchial lung biopsy, and postbronchoscopy sputum analysis are used to make the diagnosis when sputum smears are negative or when patients are unable to produce sputum. The isolation of M. *avium-intracellulare* complex does not correlate with pulmonary disease because it may represent colonization. Histologic evidence of tissue invasion is needed for the diagnosis of M. *avium-intracellulare* complex pneumonia. Both tuberculosis and M. *avium-intracellulare* complex can present as endobronchial lesions. Stool, urine, and blood specimens should be sent for mycobacterial culture because the incidence of extrapulmonary involvement is high, especially in advanced HIV infection. Because tuberculosis is more commonly smear-positive, communicable, and treatable, antituberculosis medications should be initiated when microscopy reveals AFB or caseating granulomas.

Patients with HIV infection have good response to standard antituberculosis treatment. Standard antituberculosis therapy includes 9 months of isoniazid and rifampin and 2 months of pyrazinamide. In areas where the incidence of isoniazid resistance is 4% or more, ethambutol or streptomycin is added to this regimen. Because of uncertainty about patients' adherence to therapy, direct observed therapy is preferred. One year of isoniazid is used as prophylaxis against tuberculosis in patients with positive skin test and in those exposed to potentially infectious cases of tuberculosis. Although the WHO recommends BCG vaccination for children with HIV infection, it is not used in the United States for fear of disseminating BCG infection.

Candida and *Aspergillus* pneumonia are uncommon in patients with HIV. Because the respiratory tract may be colonized with these organisms, a positive culture from a respiratory tract specimen is not sufficient. Histologic evidence from lung tissue is needed for the diagnosis of *Candida* and *Aspergillus* pneumonia. *Aspergillus* pneumonia is usually part of disseminated infection, and occurs in patients with advanced HIV infection and additional risk factors, such as neutropenia and steroid use.

In patients with HIV infection, pulmonary cryptococcosis is almost always part of a disseminated cryptococcal infection. A recent autopsy study has shown cryptococcal pneumonia to be the most common fungal pulmonary infection, affecting 10% of the cases.[22] Pulmonary histoplasmosis, coccidioidomycosis, and blastomycosis are seen in patients with HIV infection who have lived in or traveled to endemic areas. Although these endemic mycoses can develop during any stage of HIV infection, dissemination becomes more common when the CD_4 count becomes low. Amphotericin B remains the antifungal therapy of choice.

Although CMV can be cultured from the BAL of many patients with HIV infection, it has not been found to be an important pathogen causing pneumonia in these patients. The clinical manifestations of CMV pneumonia are similar to those of PCP. Histologic evidence from lung tissue is needed for the diagnosis of CMV pneumonia. However, the detection of CMV in BAL may predict an increased risk of developing CMV-associated disease in other organs. Ganciclovir is used to treat CMV pneumonia. Although rare, herpes simplex virus can cause pneumonia in patients with HIV infection. Acyclovir is used to treat herpes simplex virus pneumonia.

Pneumonia in Children

Most respiratory infections in children affect only the upper respiratory tract and are self-limiting. However, some children develop pneumonia leading to a more serious illness. Although mortality from respiratory infections has declined in developed countries, millions of children still die of acute respiratory infections in the developing world. The patterns of respiratory infection in children and the causative pathogens are different from those in adults. Compared to adults, children have smaller airways, more compliant thoracic cages, less efficient respiratory muscles, and underdeveloped immunologic systems that affect their response to respiratory infection. Several factors place children at increased risk for respiratory infection. These factors include male sex, passive smoking, low socioeconomic status, malnutrition, exposure to other children or adults with infections, premature birth, congenital respiratory diseases such as tracheoesophageal fistula and lobar sequestration, cystic fibrosis, bronchopulmonary dysplasia, congenital heart disease, neurologic impairment, and compromised immune system. Breast feeding has a protective effect against infection.

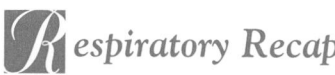
espiratory Recap ———————————

Pneumonia in Children
Respiratory infections in children often affect the upper respiratory tract and are self limiting.
No pathogen is identified in about 50% of cases of pneumonia in children.
Differential diagnosis includes asthma, bronchiolitis, bronchitis, bronchiectasis, foreign body aspiration, pulmonary sequestration, and atelectasis.
Most children recover fully.

The age of a child influences the type, frequency, and severity of the respiratory infection. Viral bronchiolitis is seen in infants aged between 4 weeks and 8 months; epiglottitis is uncommon in the first year of life and peaks in incidence in the third year. Most deaths caused by respiratory infections occur in infancy.

The incidence, etiology, and optimal management of pneumonia in children has not been well defined because of

$\mathcal{B}$OX 50-6

Pathogens Causing Pneumonia in Children
According to Age

Neonate
 Group B streptococci
 Escherichia coli
 Staphylococcus aureus
 Chlamydia trachomatis

1 Month to 2 Years
 Respiratory syncytial virus
 Parainfluenza viruses
 Influenza viruses
 Streptococcus pneumoniae
 Haemophilus influenzae

2 to 12 Years
 Streptococcus pneumoniae
 Mycoplasma pneumoniae
 Chlamydia pneumoniae

the lack of a practical definition of pneumonia, the wide spectrum of microorganisms causing pneumonia in the different age groups, and the difficulties in the identification of the causative pathogens. Many cases of CAP may not be diagnosed if the child is not seriously ill and chest-radiographs are not performed. The incidence of pneumonia peaks at 40 episodes/1000 children/year in children between 6 months and 5 years of age, and falls to 11 episodes/1000 children/year in children over the age of 9 years. Pneumonia is more common in the winter months.[23]

The age of a child influences the pathogen causing pneumonia. The common pathogens causing pneumonia in children are listed in Box 50-6. *S. aureus* pneumonia is seen in children with underlying congenital abnormality of the lung, prematurity, and recent measles.

Diagnosing pneumonia in a child is more difficult than in an adult. The typical features of pneumonia, such as bronchial breathing, dull percussion note and pleuritic pain, are uncommon in children. Fever, tachypnea, chest wall recession, and scattered crackles may be the only signs of pneumonia. The younger the child the less specific the clinical signs. The common presenting features of pneumonia in the newborn are recurrent apnea, hypotension, tachypnea, and lethargy. The absence of the symptom cluster of respiratory distress, tachypnea, crackles, and decreased breath sounds excludes pneumonia.[24] *C. trachomatis* causes afebrile pneumonia with dry cough in the first 2 months of life. Wheezing is more common in viral and *Mycoplasma* infection. However, it is difficult to determine the causative pathogen based on clinical findings. Respiratory rate greater than 50/minute in an infant less than 12 months old or greater than 40/minute in a child between 12 and 25 months old, recession of the lower chest wall, and cyanosis indicate severe pneumonia. Be-

cause cyanosis may not be detected in children with dark skin and anemia, and it is often a late sign of severe disease, oximetry should be used to assess the severity of pneumonia in children. Oximetry correlates with clinical outcome and length of hospital stay. The clinical presentation of pneumonia in older children and teenagers is similar to that in adults.

Despite extensive investigation, no pathogen is identified in 40% to 50% of pneumonia in children. Bacterial cultures of nasal and pharyngeal swabs cannot distinguish between infection and asymptomatic carriage. Most children cannot expectorate sputum, and even if they do, the sputum is contaminated with upper airway commensals. In the newborn with pneumonia, cultures of gastric and tracheal aspirates or maternal cervical swabs are performed but are often unhelpful. Blood cultures are positive in 40% of neonates and 10% to 20% of older children with bacterial pneumonia. The detection of pneumococcal and *H. influenzae* B antigen in serum or urine is more sensitive than blood culture in childhood pneumonia. However, it is associated with high false-positive and false-negative rates. Culture of pleural fluid, if present, may be diagnostic. In most cases of bacterial pneumonia, the white blood cell count is elevated with predominance of polymorphonuclear cells. Leukopenia can be seen in viral and severe bacterial infections.

A child with pneumonia who responds to treatment as an outpatient does not need further investigation. However, a child admitted to the hospital for pneumonia should have chest radiograph and blood culture. The chest radiographic finding of consolidation does not distinguish between viral and bacterial pneumonia. However, pleural effusion and abscess formation suggest bacterial infection.

The differential diagnosis of pneumonia in children should include asthma, bronchiolitis, acute bronchitis, acute exacerbation of bronchiectasis, aspiration of a foreign body, pulmonary sequestration, and atelectasis. Children with recurrent or persistent cough productive of purulent sputum should be evaluated for the presence of cystic fibrosis, bronchial obstruction, ciliary abnormalities, congenital abnormalities of the lung (lobar sequestration, lung cysts, bronchial stenosis, cystadenomatoid malformation), esophageal atresia, tracheoesophageal fistula, and immunodeficiency disorders.

There is a paucity of well-conducted, randomized, controlled trials comparing the efficacy of different antibiotics and their impact on outcome of pneumonia in children. The choice of antibiotic depends on the child's age and knowledge of the likely pathogen in that age group. Oral antibiotics are adequate for most mild to moderately severe pneumonias. Parenteral antibiotics are needed for neonates and other children with severe pneumonia. In neonates, the antibiotic regimen should cover group B streptococcus and gram-negative organisms. A macrolide should be added to cover *C. trachomatis* in certain areas. There is no specific treatment for viral pneumonia. Antibiotic usage for nonbacterial infections should be discouraged because it may lead to the development of resistance. Some children with RSV pneumonia respond to aerosolized ribavirin therapy. Children requiring hospitalization should receive a second- or third-generation cephalosporin, with or without a macrolide depending on the child's age. For children with pneumonia after viral infection, antistaphylococcal coverage should be included. In places where the incidence of penicillin-resistant *S. pneumoniae* is high, vancomycin should be considered. Supplemental oxygen, intravenous or nasogastric fluids, postural drainage, and percussion may be needed.

Most children with pneumonia recover fully. It takes longer for radiologic recovery than clinical recovery. Severe *Mycoplasma* infection and adenoviral pneumonia can lead to permanent lung damage such as persistent collapse, bronchiolitis obliterans, bronchiectasis, and Swyer-James syndrome, which is characterized by a small hyperlucent lobe with impaired perfusion and ventilation.

Children with HIV infection present most often with respiratory illnesses. PCP is the most common infection in these children. Other causes of pneumonia include CMV, RSV, adenovirus, influenza, parainfluenza, herpes simplex, varicella zoster, encapsulated bacteria, gram-negative bacteria, mycobacteria, and fungi.

CASE STUDIES

Case One
Community-Acquired Pneumonia

A 44-year-old African-American man was admitted to the hospital because of productive cough. The patient has a history of alcohol abuse and 20 pack-a-day years of smoking. He had been in good health until 3 days before admission, when he developed a cough productive of yellow sputum. The cough was associated with fever and chills. He also had dyspnea with minimal exertion. He denied weight loss, night sweats, and previous exposure to tuberculosis. He had no visit to a physician in the previous 30 years.

On presentation to the hospital, he was in mild respiratory distress with a temperature of 102.1° F, a respiratory rate of 34/min, a blood pressure of 125/79 mm Hg, and a pulse rate of 125/min. On physical examination, crackles were heard on auscultation, and dullness was present on percussion of the right lower chest. Pulse oximetry showed an oxygen saturation of 93% on room air. The serum electrolyte values, hematocrit, and platelet count were normal. His white blood cell count was 16,000/mm³, with 20% bands, 70% neutrophils, and 10% lymphocytes. Serum protein was 7 g/dL and lactate dehydrogenase (LDH) was 210 U/L. A radiograph of the chest showed right pleural effusion and alveolar infiltrate involving the right middle and lower lobes.

After blood and expectorated sputum were obtained for Gram-stain and culture, antibiotic therapy with intra-venous erythromycin and vancomycin was initiated. Diagnostic thoracentesis was performed. Pleural fluid analysis showed white cells 1000/mm³ with 95% neutrophils and 5% monocytes; protein 5 g/dL, LDH 198 U/L, and pH 7.37. The Gram's stain and culture of the pleural fluid showed no organisms. The sputum and blood culture grew *Streptococcus pneumoniae*, sensitive to penicillin.

On the second hospital day, the patient's symptoms improved and he became afebrile. On the third hospital day, the vancomycin and erythromycin were discontinued, and intravenous penicillin was initiated. The patient's condition continued to improve, and the intravenous penicillin was changed to oral penicillin on the fourth hospital day. He was discharged home on the fifth hospital day, on oral penicillin with follow-up appointment to outpatient clinic in one week.

Case Two
Pneumonia in an Immunocompromised Patient

A 26-year-old white woman was admitted to the hospital for dyspnea. The patient had a remote history of unprotected sex and injection drug use. She had weight loss of 25 pounds over a 3-month period, cough for 5 weeks, and night sweats and fever for 1 week. Her cough had been dry for the first 4 weeks, but productive of brown sputum for the last 7 days. She had dyspnea for 7 days that worsened on the day of admission. She denied exposure to tuberculosis.

On presentation to the hospital, the patient was in moderate respiratory distress with a temperature of 101.2° F, a respiratory rate of 39/min, a blood pressure of 90/55 mm Hg, and a pulse rate of 145/min. Diffuse crackles were heard on auscultation of the chest. Pulse oximetry showed an oxygen saturation of 82% on room air. The serum electrolyte values were normal. The hematocrit was 23%, platelet count 85,000 per mm³, white blood cell count was 5000 per mm³ with 10% bands, 80% neutrophils, and 10% lymphocytes. Serum protein was 6 g/dL and lactate dehydrogenase was 900 U/L. A radiograph of the chest showed diffuse interstitial infiltrate, with denser consolidation of the right upper lobe. Blood culture was obtained. Sputum was induced with 3% NaCl by use of an ultrasonic nebulizer for Gram's stain, routine culture, and sensitivity; acid fast bacilli (AFB) stain and mycobacterial culture; and *Pneumocystis carinii* stains.

Intravenous trimethoprim-sulfamethoxazole and oral prednisone were administered for treatment of suspected *P. carinii* pneumonia. On the second hospital day, her condition deteriorated, and she was transferred to the medical ICU. Her PaO₂ was 65 mm Hg breathing 100% O₂. She underwent endotracheal intubation and mechanical ventilation for hypoxemic respiratory failure. The induced sputum monoclonal antibody stain was positive for *P. carinii*. Both the ELISA and Western blot were positive for HIV. Her CD₄ count was 10/μL.

Because of failure to improve, bronchoscopy was performed on her fifth hospital day. The AFB stain of the bronchoalveolar lavage (BAL) was positive, and the polymerase chain reaction (PCR) was consistent with *Mycobacterium tuberculosis*, later confirmed with the culture result. Treatment with four antituberculosis drugs was initiated. The patient's condition gradually improved over the next 3 weeks. However, her condition deteriorated during the fourth week of her hospital stay. Repeat bronchoscopy was performed. The quantitative culture of the BAL showed 2.3×10^6/mL of methicillin resistant *Staphylococcus aureus*. Her blood culture also grew methicillin resistant *S. aureus*. She died of multiple organ failure secondary to septic shock on her thirty-fifth day of hospital stay.

$\mathcal{K}$EY $\mathcal{P}$OINTS

- Pneumonia is the inflammation and consolidation of lung tissue caused by infectious agents.
- Community-acquired pneumonia (CAP) occurs outside the hospital.
- Hospital-acquired pneumonia and ventilator-associated pneumonia (VAP) are acquired in the hospital.
- Noninvasive and invasive procedures are used to diagnose pneumonia.
- Organisms causing pneumonia include gram-positive bacteria, gram-negative bacteria, atypical organisms, anaerobic bacteria, viruses, mycobacteria, fungi, actinomycosis, and norcardiosis.
- Most CAP can be treated as an outpatient.
- Pneumonia is the second most common nosocomial infection and has a high mortality rate.
- Pulmonary infections are common in immunocompromised patients and BAL is often diagnostic.
- PCP is a common cause of mortality in patients with HIV; TB is also common in these patients.
- Children usually recover fully from pneumonia and no pathogen is identified in about half of all cases.

References

1. Armstrong GL, Conn LA, Pinner RW. Trends in infectious diseases mortality in the United States during the 20th century. JAMA 1999;281:61-66.
2. Niederman MS, Bass JB, Fein AM, et al. American Thoracic Society guidelines for the initial management of adults with community-acquired pneumonia: diagnosis, assessment of severity, and initial antimicrobial therapy. Am Rev Respir Dis 1993;148:1418-1426.
3. Fine MJ, Auble TE, Yealy DM, et al. A prediction rule to identify low-risk patients with community-acquired pneumonia. N Engl J Med 1997;336:243-250.
4. Pingleton SK, Fagon JY, Leeper KV. Patient selection for clinical investigation of ventilator associated pneumonia. Chest 1992;102:553S-556S.
5. Meduri GU, Mauldin GL, Wunderink RG, et al. Causes of fever and pulmonary densities in patients with clinical manifestations of ventilator-associated pneumonia. Chest 1994;106:221-235.
6. Bartlett JG, Breiman RF, Mandell LA, et al. Guidelines from the Infectious Diseases Society of America. Community-acquired pneumonia in adults: guidelines for management. Clin Infect Dis 1998;26:811-838.
7. Bartlett JG. Anaerobic bacterial infection of the lung. Chest 1987;91:901-909.
8. Duchin JS, Koster F, Peters CJ, et al. *Hantavirus* pulmonary syndrome: a clinical description of 17 patients with a newly recognized disease. N Engl J Med 1994;330:949-955.
9. American Thoracic Society. Diagnosis and treatment of disease caused by nontuberculous mycobacteria. Am J Respir Crit Care Med 1997;156:S1-S25.
10. Sharma OP, Chwogule R. Many faces of pulmonary aspergillosis. Eur Respir J 1998;12:705-715.
11. The British Thoracic Society. Guidelines for the management of community-acquired pneumonia in adults admitted to hospital. Br J Hosp Med 1993;49:346-350.
12. Mandell LA, Niederman M. The Canadian Community-Acquired Pneumonia Consensus Conference Group. Antimicrobial treatment of community-acquired pneumonia in adults: a conference report. Can J Infect Dis 1993;4:25.
13. Fine MJ, Smith MA, Carson CA, et al. Prognosis and outcome of patients with community-acquired pneumonia: a meta-analysis. JAMA 1995;274:134-141.
14. Craven DE, Steger KA. Epidemiology of nosocomial pneumonia: new perspective on an old disease. Chest 1995;108:1S-16S.
15. Torres A, Aznar R, Gatell JM, et al. Incidence, risk, and prognostic factors of nosocomial pneumonia in mechanically ventilated patients. Am Rev Respir Dis 1990;142:523-528.
16. Fagon JY, Chastre J, Hanes AJ, et al. Evaluation of clinical judgment in the identification and treatment of nosocomial pneumonia in ventilated patients. Chest 1993;103:547-553.
17. Campbell GD, Niederman MS, Broughton WA, et al. Hospital-acquired pneumonia in adults: diagnosis, assessment of severity, initial antimicrobial therapy, and preventive strategies: a consensus statement. Am J Respir Crit Care Med 1996;153:1711-1725.
18. Craven DE, Steger KA. Hospital-acquired pneumonia: perspective for the epidemiologist. Infect Control Hosp Epidemiol 1997;18:783-795.
19. Tablan OC, Anderson LJ, Arden NH, et al. Guidelines for prevention of nosocomial pneumonia. Part I. Issues on prevention of nosocomial pneumonia, 1994. Infect Control Hosp Epidemiol 1994;15:588-625.
20. Rosenow EC, Wilson WR, Cockerill FR. Pulmonary disease in the immunocompromised host. Mayo Clin Proc 1985;60:473-487.
21. Wilson WR, Cockerill FR, Rosenow EC. Pulmonary disease in the immunocompromised host. Mayo Clin Proc 1985;60:610-631.
22. Afessa B, Green W, Chiao J, et al. Pulmonary complications of HIV infection: autopsy findings. Chest 1998;113:1225-1229.
23. Murphy TH, Henderson FW, Clyde WA, et al. Pneumonia: an eleven-year study in a pediatric practice. Am J Epidemiol 1981;113:12-21.
24. Jadavi T, Law B, Lebel MH, et al. A practical guide for the diagnosis and treatment of pediatric pneumonia. Can Med Assoc J 1997;156(5):S703-S711.

CHAPTER 51

Cystic Fibrosis

Scott H. Donaldson
James R. Yankaskas

CHAPTER OUTLINE

OBJECTIVES

1. Describe the inheritance pattern of cystic fibrosis.
2. Describe the pathogenesis of cystic fibrosis.
3. List the diagnostic criteria for cystic fibrosis.
4. Describe the numerous extrapulmonary manifestations of cystic fibrosis.
5. Describe typical respiratory manifestations of cystic fibrosis.
6. Discuss the approach to common life-threatening respiratory complications of cystic fibrosis.
7. Describe the principles of preventive care for cystic fibrosis.
8. Outline an approach to the management of an acute exacerbation of cystic fibrosis lung disease.
9. Describe the role that lung transplantation plays in the management of cystic fibrosis.

KEY TERMS

Bronchial Artery Embolization (BAE)
Cepacia Syndrome
Cystic Fibrosis (CF)
Cystic Fibrosis-Related Diabetes (CFRD)

Cystic Fibrosis Transmembrane
   Conductance Regulator (CFTR)
Lung Transplantation
Meconium Ileus

Steatorrhea
Sweat testing

Andersen and colleagues[1] first described "cystic fibrosis of the pancreas" as a distinct disease entity in 1938. Affected infants presented with intestinal obstruction or malnutrition as a consequence of poor gastrointestinal absorption. Overwhelming respiratory infection commonly led to death. Patients with **cystic fibrosis (CF)** usually died within the first year of life. Postmortem studies revealed obstruction of pancreatic ducts, airways, and the gut with abnormally viscous mucus, prompting the term "mucoviscidosis."[2] In the 1950s, di Sant'Agnese and colleagues[3] investigated cases of severe dehydration in children with CF during a summer heat wave, and recognized for the first time that excessive salt loss occurred via the sweat. This observation led to the development of the pilocarpine iontophoresis sweat test as a standard diagnostic test for CF. In 1989 the gene responsible for CF was cloned and its protein product named the **cystic fibrosis transmembrane conductance regulator (CFTR).**[4]

Today CF is recognized as the most common lethal genetic disease in the Caucasian population. Within this population, one in 29 persons carries a mutant CFTR allele and one in 3300 live births has CF. Other ethnic populations have lower mutation carrier rates, and thus lower incidences of CF disease. The Hispanic birth incidence is 1 in 9500; Native American 1 in 11,200; African American 1 in 15,300; and Asian 1 in 32,100 live births. Although CF was previously a disease of infancy, survival now commonly extends into adulthood, with a median survival of more than 31 years (Figure 51-1).[5] More than 21,000 patients with CF have been identified in the United States, with more than a third being older than 18 years of age.

This chapter describes the pathogenesis, diagnosis, and clinical manifestations of CF. Although CF is a multisystem disease, the management of acute and chronic respiratory complications is emphasized.

Pathogenesis

Genetics of Cystic Fibrosis

CF is a monogenetic disorder that is inherited in an autosomal recessive pattern. Persons who carry a single mutated CFTR gene along with a normal CFTR allele are termed *carriers* and have no symptoms attributable to CF. Each offspring conceived from two CF carriers therefore has a one in four chance of being affected with CF, and a two in four chance of being a CF carrier.

The CFTR gene belongs to a family of membrane proteins that serve as molecular pumps, and itself functions as a cAMP-regulated chloride channel in epithelial tissues such as the lung, pancreas, gastrointestinal tract, sweat duct, and reproductive tract. Since the discovery of the CFTR gene in 1989, more than 920 individual mutations have been identified,[6] although the most common mutation (F508) accounts for 66% of CF alleles reported worldwide.[7] The exact prevalence of individual mutations also varies according to the ethnic group being studied, with the F508 mutation being less common among nonwhite populations.

Mutations in the CFTR gene may be divided into five groups, which reflect the mechanism by which loss of CFTR function occurs (Table 51-1). Class I mutations result in the loss of protein production and thus complete absence of full length CFTR. Class II mutations result in abnormal protein processing between the cell nucleus and plasma membrane. This class of mutations includes the common F508 mutation, in which improper protein glycosylation and folding prevents normal transport to

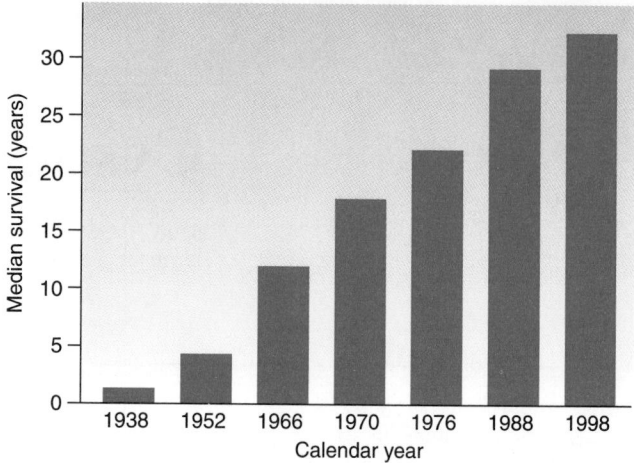

Figure 51-1 The overall median survival with CF expressed as a function of time.

the apical cell membrane. Class III mutations in the CFTR gene affect the regulation/activation of the CFTR chloride channel, although the channel itself successfully reaches the plasma membrane. Class IV mutations also reach the plasma membrane but affect the conductance of chloride through the channel pore. Class V CFTR mutations decrease the abundance of mature CFTR mRNA and protein levels and may include mutations in gene promoters or regions that influence mRNA splicing. These mutations may, however, permit the production of adequate CFTR levels to confer a less severe disease phenotype.[8]

Respiratory Recap ————————

Genetics of CF
CF is inherited in an autosomal recessive pattern.
CFTR is the gene responsible for CF.
It is difficult to predict phenotype from CFTR mutation.

Somewhat surprisingly, predicting an individual patient's clinical phenotype has been difficult based on the specific CFTR mutations present. Some genotype-phenotype correlation has been noted, principally among a group of mutations associated with pancreatic exocrine sufficiency, milder lung disease, and borderline or even normal sweat chloride values.[8,9] In addition, certain mutations have been found in men who present solely with infertility resulting from the congenital bilateral absence of the vas deferens (CBAVD), without other stigmata of typical CF disease.[10,11] The manifestations of CF in an individual depend upon other genetic factors (that is, modifier genes) and environmental factors.

CFTR Functions and Host Defense

CFTR is a chloride channel expressed in the apical membrane of epithelial cells lining the lung, pancreas, gut, sweat duct, and reproductive tract. As its name implies, however, CFTR regulates several other ion conductance pathways,[12] including sodium channels,[13-16] chloride channels other than CFTR,[17-19] and potassium channels.[20] The loss of a normally functioning CFTR therefore can have a profound impact on epithelial ion transport. In the lung, the absence of CFTR results in sodium hyperabsorption from the airway lumen[21,22] and a diminished capacity to secrete chloride ions via CFTR. This combination alters the local milieu and adequate defense against invading microbes is lost.

One hypothesis for the mechanism underlying this defect rests on data showing that increased isotonic volume absorption from the airway lumen (driven by sodium hyperabsorption) depletes the periciliary liquid layer and concentrates mucins in the mucus layer. Periciliary liquid depletion results in disruption of rotational mucus transport in vitro and is predicted to impair both ciliary and cough clearance of airway secretions in vivo.[23] Reduced airway clearance and retention of mucus plaques will in turn cause airway obstruction and allow the establishment of bacterial infection.

A second hypothesis proposes that NaCl concentrations in airway surface liquid (ASL) are normally low (<50 mM NaCl) but are high in CF (>100 mM) because of the inability to absorb chloride through CFTR. Elevated NaCl concentrations in ASL may inhibit the antimicrobial effects of defensins, which are small, salt-sensitive peptides produced by airway epithelia.[24] Challenges to this hypothesis are the scarcity of defensins in ASL relative to other salt-insensitive antimicrobial molecules (for example, lactoferrin, lysozyme)[25] and the absence of a physiologic mechanism for the generation of hypotonic fluids across the water-permeable airway epithelium.

Because CFTR expression in the lung is greatest within submucosal glands lining proximal conducting airways,[26] perhaps an alteration in glandular secretion resulting from absent CFTR is a cause of altered airway defense in CF. Indeed, CFTR is involved in generating airway surface liquid via submucosal glands in proximal airways.[27] A third hypothesis relating CFTR function and host defenses therefore emphasizes that deficient secretion of fluid containing sodium chloride or sodium bicarbonate from submucosal glands or serous cells lining small airways may lead to a volume-depleted ASL layer and/or an ASL layer with an altered composition.

Other hypotheses relating to the pathogenesis of CF lung disease describe differences in airway mucins[28-30] or the CF immune response.[31-35] These do not tightly link CFTR function with the resulting disease process and in most cases rest on observations that may be secondary to infection rather than the primary cause of it (for example, altered mucin properties, enhanced/prolonged airway inflammatory response). The greatest weight of evidence therefore rests on reduced clearance of airway secretions as the key pathophysiologic link between CFTR dysfunction and airway infection and inflammation in CF. Most therapies focus on airway clearance and fighting chronic bacterial infection.

Diagnosis

The diagnosis of CF is based on the combination of one or more typical phenotypic features and evidence for CFTR malfunction (Box 51-1).[36,37] Knowledge of the broad range of clinical features that may be present in CF and appro-

TABLE 51-1

Consequences of CFTR Mutations by Class

Class	Problem	Examples	Features
I	No synthesis of mature protein	G542X; 394delTT	Mutations cause premature stop codons (for example, frameshift, nonsense) or unstable mRNA.
II	Block in processing	ΔF508; N1303K	Mutations cause improper intracellular processing (folding, glycosylation), so protein may not reach plasma.
III	Abnormal regulation	G551D; G551S	Protein reaches plasma membrane but is not activated properly; mutation may be mild or severe.
IV	Altered conductance	R117H; R347P	Ionic conductance of the channel is altered. Partial functioning channel is associated with pancreatic sufficiency.
V	Reduced synthesis	3489+10kbC>7	Altered mRNA splicing sites results in reduced synthesis of normal protein; low levels of preserved synthesis may allow mild phenotype.

CFTR, *Cystic fibrosis transmembrane conductance regulator.*

Box 51-1

*Diagnostic Criteria for Cystic Fibrosis**

Phenotypic Feature
Chronic sinopulmonary disease
Persistent infection with typical CF pathogen (for example,
  S. aureus, P. aeruginosa)
Chronic cough/sputum
Persistent chest radiographic abnormality (for example,
  bronchiectasis, hyperinflation, atelectasis)
Airway obstruction (wheezing, PFTs)
Nasal polyps or radiographic sinus involvement
Digital clubbing
Gastrointestinal/nutritional abnormality
Intestinal: meconium ileus, rectal prolapse, distal intestinal
  obstruction syndrome
Pancreatic: pancreatic insufficiency, recurrent pancreatitis
Hepatic: focal biliary cirrhosis
Nutritional: malnutrition, hypoproteinemia, fat-soluble
  vitamin deficiency
Salt loss syndrome
Acute salt depletion
Chronic metabolic alkalosis
Male urogenital abnormality
Obstructive azoospermia resulting from congenital bilateral
  absence of the vas deferens (CBAVD)

CFTR Abnormality
Sweat chloride test
Result >60 mmol/L on two occasions (minimum 75 mg of
  sweat collected during 30 minutes)
CFTR mutational analysis
Two mutant CFTR alleles required
Nasal potential difference (PD) testing
Higher basal PD
Greater amiloride sensitive PD
Absent/minimal change in PD after isoproterenol in chloride
  free perfusion solution

CFTR, *Cystic fibrosis transmembrane conductance regulator.*
*The combination of one or more phenotypic abnormalities (or CF in a
sibling, or positive newborn screening test) with evidence for a CFTR
abnormality constitutes a CF diagnosis.*

priate access to specialized diagnostic testing are essential for an accurate diagnosis. Among the clinical features assessed are the presence of obstructive lung disease and infection with typical pathogens, chronic sinus disease or nasal polyposis, exocrine pancreatic insufficiency or recurrent pancreatitis, intestinal obstruction either at birth **(meconium ileus)** or later in life (distal intestinal obstruction syndrome), rectal prolapse, chronic liver disease, nutritional deficiencies including protein/caloric malnutrition and complications of fat-soluble vitamin deficiency, electrolyte abnormalities such as acute salt depletion or chronic metabolic alkalosis, absence of the vas deferens resulting in obstructive azoospermia in males, and digital clubbing. A family history of CF should also be sought in support of a clinical CF diagnosis.

Evidence for CFTR dysfunction is provided typically by **sweat testing,** which should reveal a chloride concentration of more than 60 mmol/L on two or more occasions. Values greater than 40 mmol/L are considered borderline and are more suggestive of CF in infants. Values between 60 and 80 mmol/L can be seen also in individuals with diseases other than CF. Laboratory errors are also common with this technique, which highlights the need to repeat all positive and borderline tests and negative tests when the clinical suspicion remains high.

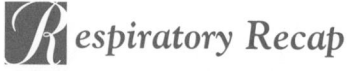
Respiratory Recap

Diagnosis of Cystic Fibrosis

Clinical features consistent with the disease Family history Sweat testing Mutational analyses to identify CF alleles	Nasal epithelial potential difference (PD) measurements in response to various pharmacologic agents

---

A complimentary approach to sweat testing is the use of CFTR mutational analyses to identify CF alleles. The identification of two CFTR mutations is highly specific for the diagnosis of CF, but this approach lacks sensitivity. Currently available CFTR mutational analyses screen for between 6 and 70 common mutations and detect up to 80% to 95% of CF alleles. The use of mutation panels customized for a given ethnic group or clinical situation (for example, African American, pancreatic sufficient) may increase the likelihood of the identification of CF alleles. No commercially available screening panel can rule out the diagnosis of CF, however, because none test for all the known mutations capable of causing CF.

When sweat testing and CFTR mutational analysis are inconclusive, the use of nasal epithelial potential difference (PD) measurements in response to various pharmacologic agents can be useful.[38,39] Using a small catheter to measure electrical potentials across the nasal epithelium, an increased basal PD, an increased amiloride-sensitive sodium conductance, and an absent cAMP-mediated chloride conductance suggest the diagnosis of CF. As with sweat testing, this procedure should be performed more than once by an experience laboratory to obtain reliable information.

Extrapulmonary Manifestations

Upper Respiratory Tract

Virtually all patients with CF have roentgenographic opacification of the paranasal sinuses,[40] and a large fraction report symptoms attributable to either nasal obstruction or chronic sinusitis.[41] Symptomatic nasal polyps occur in approximately 20% of patients[42] and are particularly common toward the end of the first decade and during the second decade of life. Manifestations include severe or complete airflow obstruction, rhinorrhea, and occasionally widening of the bridge of the nose. Despite the presence of roentgenographic abnormalities, acute or chronic symptoms attributable to sinusitis occur in less than 10% of children[43] and approximately 24% of adults.[44,45] Unfortunately, recurrence of polyps and sinus symptoms are extremely common after surgical interventions. Patients must be carefully selected therefore when a surgical intervention for nasal or sinus disease is considered.

Exocrine and Endocrine Pancreas

Exocrine pancreatic insufficiency is present from birth in a large majority of patients with CF.[46] Enzyme deficiency results in fat and protein maldigestion, producing **steatorrhea.** Uncorrected malabsorption results in failure to gain weight and ultimately a failure of linear growth. Exocrine pancreatic insufficiency and malnutrition are managed with oral pancreatic enzyme supplementation and dietary supplements. Impaired absorption of fat-soluble vitamins (A, D, E, and K) occasionally produces symptoms of vitamin deficiency, which can be prevented with adequate supplementation. Symptoms of pancreatitis are encountered in less than 1% of identified adolescent and adult CF patients and are limited to those who have retained some exocrine pancreatic function.[47] However, recurrent pancreatitis has been associated with mutations in CFTR and may be the presenting symptom in adults with CF.[48,49]

Age-Specific Angle

Exocrine pancreatic insufficiency is present from birth in most patients with CF.

Although the exocrine pancreas is frequently affected from birth, the gradual loss of insulin production from the endocrine pancreas occurs slowly over time in patients with CF. In the United States, the overall incidence of **cystic fibrosis-related diabetes (CFRD)** or glucose intolerance is reported to be 8.2%, with 14.2% of adult patients requiring chronic insulin therapy.[5] Because of the insidious onset of CFRD and the lack of routine screening, these figures likely underestimate the magnitude of this problem. In fact, when rigorous screening with oral glucose tolerance tests was undertaken in a CF population, 14% of patients were found to have CFRD and an additional 15% had glucose intolerance.[50] Manifestations of CFRD may include failure to gain or maintain weight despite nutritional intervention, poor growth, or an unexplained chronic decline in pulmonary function.[51] Insulin is the preferred hypoglycemic agent in CFRD, because limited islet cell reserve exists in most cases. Other facets of CFRD management, however, differ substantially from

that of either type 1 or 2 diabetes mellitus. Because all CF patients require a high-energy intake and generally malabsorb fat even with appropriate pancreatic enzyme supplementation, a high-calorie diet consisting of 40% fat is recommended. Caloric restriction never should be used to aid management of blood glucose. Insulin dosage is instead matched to the calorie and carbohydrate intake, whereas exercise regimes and the presence of intercurrent infections are factored in as needed.[52] Because patients are at risk for the usual microvascular complications of diabetes,[50] similar glucose targets are used as with type 1 and type 2 diabetes mellitus. Equally important, however, is the maintenance of optimal nutrition and growth, the avoidance of severe hypoglycemia, and the need to fit this additional treatment burden within the patient's already complicated CF regimen.

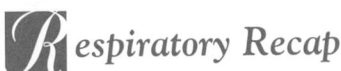

espiratory Recap

Extrapulmonary Manifestations of Cystic Fibrosis	
Upper airway	Hepatobiliary system
Exocrine and endocrine pancreas	Reproductive tract
	Sweat glands
Gastrointestinal tract	

Gastrointestinal Tract

Meconium ileus occurs in about 17% of newborns with CF and is nearly diagnostic for CF.[53] A barium enema usually demonstrates a small colon and a site of ileal obstruction may be identified. Occasionally, obstruction occurs in the colon and causes delayed stooling (the meconium plug syndrome), which is less specific for CF.[54] Later in life, intestinal obstruction may be caused by the distal intestinal obstruction syndrome (DIOS), which occurs in approximately 20% of patients and usually presents with constipation, right lower quadrant abdominal pain, and sometimes fever.[53,55,56] As with meconium ileus, obstruction usually occurs in the terminal ileum and is associated with copious, incompletely digested intestinal contents. Other causes of abdominal pain include intussusception, intestinal adhesions from previous abdominal surgery, or chronic appendicitis that has been partially suppressed by antibiotic therapy. Rectal prolapse occurs in nearly 20% of children but is an infrequent event for adults with CF.[57] Excessive pancreatic enzyme dosages have been associated with the occurrence of fibrosing colonopathy, especially in those pa-

Age-Specific Angle

Meconium ileus occurs in about 17% of newborns with CF and is diagnostic for CF.

tients taking at least 6000 units of lipase/kg/meal.[58-60] Pancreatic enzyme dosages 2500 units or less of lipase/kg/meal are recommended to avoid this complication. Gastroesophageal reflux disease is common and should be recognized and treated because this process may exacerbate lung disease.[61-63]

Hepatobiliary System

Focal biliary cirrhosis is characteristic of CF but produces symptoms in less than 5% of CF patients and is the cause of death in about 2%.[64,65] Unlike many complications of CF, hepatic disease has a peak incidence during adolescence and a decreased prevalence in patients over age 20.[66] Hepatic abnormalities can present as hepatosplenomegaly or as a persistent elevation of hepatic enzymes (particularly alkaline phosphatase). Rarely, patients may present with esophageal varices and hemorrhage resulting from portal hypertension. Fatty liver is also common and may improve with adequate nutrition. Dysfunctional gallbladders[67] or gallstones[68] are present in 10% to 30% of patients.

Reproductive Tract

More than 98% of male patients with CF have azoospermia resulting from obstruction of the vas deferens.[69] In fact, absence of a palpable vas deferens is a useful clue to the diagnosis of CF during the evaluation of a male patient with otherwise unexplained bronchiectatic lung disease or some other possible manifestation of CF. Semen analysis may be required to identify the 1% to 2% of male CF patients who are fertile. The volume of ejaculate is usually one third to one half of normal, completely void of spermatozoa, and possesses a number of semen chemical abnormalities that reflect the absence of secretions from the seminal vesicles.[70] Because spermatozoa do develop in the testis, despite being absent in the ejaculate, epididymal sperm microaspiration coupled with intracytoplasmic oocyte injection may allow successful conception.[71]

Although male infertility is nearly universal, female infertility is only about 20%.[70] Some women with CF are anovulatory because of chronic lung disease and malnutrition. In addition, mucus in the cervical os is dehydrated, has abnormal electrolyte concentrations, and can present an obstacle to conception by impeding normal sperm migration.[72] Nevertheless, more than 600 pregnancies in CF females have been reported. A longitudinal study of 325 pregnant women with CF demonstrated 258 live births (79%) and 67 therapeutic abortions. Pregnancy in women with CF did not have an independent negative effect on pulmonary status or mortality over 2 years.[73] However, females with CF must consider their own health and expected life span in the context of family planning.

Sweat Glands

Sweat chloride is elevated in most CF patients because of reduced NaCl reabsorption in the sweat duct.[37] This abnormality forms the basis for the diagnostic sweat chloride test and may predispose patients to salt depletion. Young children are most at risk for episodes of salt loss, especially in warm arid climates and in the setting of concomitant salt/volume loss resulting from vomiting or diarrhea. These children present with lethargy, anorexia, and hypochloremic alkalosis. Presentation with hypochloremic alkalosis is rare in older children and adults.[74] Salt restriction therefore is never indicated in CF, and increased salt intake should be encouraged when environmental or clinical circumstances place a patient at increased risk for salt depletion.

> *Age-Specific Angle*
>
> Young children with CF are most at risk for episodes of salt loss, especially in warm arid climates and in the setting of concomitant salt/volume loss resulting from vomiting or diarrhea.

Respiratory Manifestations

Symptoms

Newborns with CF appear to have normal lung function, implying normal intrauterine lung development. Clinical symptoms or evidence of increased airways resistance and gas trapping often develop very early in life, although they may not be apparent until adulthood in a minority of patients. Respiratory symptoms typically include a cough that becomes persistent and productive of thick, purulent sputum over time. Periods of clinical stability are inevitably interrupted by typical exacerbations, characterized by increased cough, sputum, fatigue, anorexia, weight loss, and loss of lung function. These exacerbations require more intensive therapy, with the goal to alleviate symptoms and restore lost lung function through the use of antibiotics and aggressive airway clearance maneuvers. Over time, these exacerbations become more frequent, respond less well to interventions, and result in the gradual onset of respiratory failure.

Chest Radiography

Chest radiographs in CF are often normal early in the course of disease. Hyperinflation may be the first radiographic finding in children, followed by increased interstitial markings. These increased interstitial markings progress to the typical findings of cystic bronchiectasis, which are usually most pronounced in the upper lobes. The right upper lobe is more frequently and severely affected than the left for unclear reasons. Despite high densities of bacteria in airways, findings of an alveolar filling process typical of bacterial pneumonia are not generally seen even during periods of acute illness. Segmental or subsegmental atelectasis and lobar collapse are common radiographic findings related to airway obstruction and retained secretions. Although the chest radiograph demonstrates the chronic progression of lung destruction and is useful for the detection of important complications such as lobar collapse and pneumothorax, little correlation between the radiograph and acute clinical changes might exist later in the course of disease. The use of chest CT scans may be useful to detect bronchiectasis and other early pathologic changes that are not visible on routine chest radiographs, especially during the evaluation of a patient with chronic cough and sputum production who is not otherwise known to have CF or other forms of bronchiectasis.[75] Chest CT also may be useful in the CF patient with a persistent, heavy burden of nontuberculous mycobacteria (NTM), because the presence of multiple, small parenchymal nodules predominating in the middle and lower lobes and patchy airspace disease are evidence of true NTM infection rather than airway colonization.[76,77]

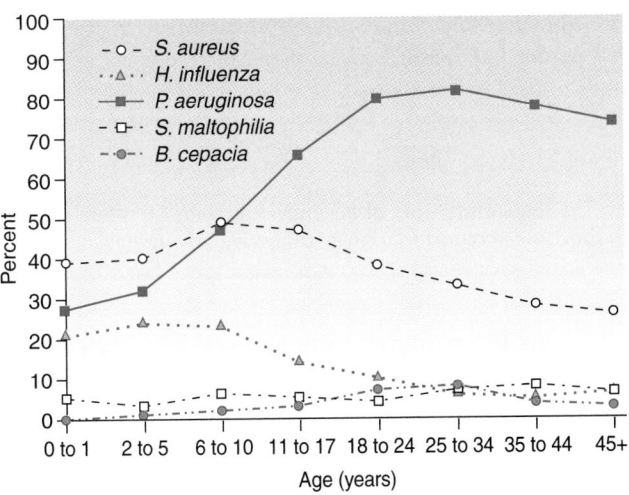

Figure 51-2 The prevalence of common bacterial organisms in different age groups. (Data from Cystic Fibrosis Foundation. Patient Registry. 1998 Annual Data Report. Bethesda, Md: The Foundation; 1999.)

 espiratory Recap ─────────

Respiratory Manifestations of CF

Clinical symptoms: cough, sputum, fatigue, anorexia, weight loss
Chest radiograph: hyperinflation
Pulmonary function: airflow obstruction

Respiratory microbiology: airways become persistently infected with gram-negative pathogens such as *Pseudomonas aeruginosa*

Pulmonary Function

Pulmonary function testing is a sensitive and reliable method used to evaluate the severity of CF lung disease and is an objective means to determine when a patient's clinical status has deteriorated and requires more intensive therapy. The first abnormality detected is obstruction of small airways, as indicated by reduced flow rates at low lung volumes (for example, $FEF_{25\%-75\%}$) and elevation of the residual volume to total lung capacity ratio (RV/TLC).[78,79] Later in the course of disease, pulmonary function tests demonstrate progressive reductions in FEV_1, followed by reductions in FVC. Importantly, the FEV_1 is the best indicator of exercise capacity and disability and is somewhat predictive of length of survival.[80-82] An FEV_1 of about 30% of predicted is therefore often used as an indication to initiate lung transplant evaluation, although other factors also should be considered.[83,84]

As airway obstruction worsens, hypoxemia develops as the result of ventilation/perfusion mismatching. Even when oxygenation is adequate at rest, the clinician should be cognizant that significant hypoxemia may occur during sleep and/or exercise in the setting of moderate to severe lung disease and should be screened for with exercise and sleep oximetry recordings.[85,86] Although significant hypoxemia tends to occur in patients with more advanced lung disease, spirometric parameters are poor predictors of the need for oxygen therapy.[86] Supplemental oxygen may improve exercise performance in patients found to desaturate during exercise[87,88] and is generally effective for the prevention of pulmonary hypertension and cor pulmonale.[89]

Severe airway disease causes retention of carbon dioxide due to an increased dead space to tidal volume ratio (V_D/V_T), which in turn may worsen hypoxemia. Carbon dioxide retention usually does not occur until severe airway obstruction is present. Along with resting hypoxemia it is a negative predictor of survival.[81]

Respiratory Microbiology

The respiratory tract of newborns is likely sterile and without inflammation but often becomes colonized with pathogens early in life.[90] Once infection is established, it is rarely, if ever, eradicated and consists of characteristic age-related bacteria (Figure 51-2). *Staphylococcus aureus* and *Haemophilus influenzae* are often the first organisms detected, though *H. influenzae* rarely persists beyond childhood.[91] *S. aureus* may not persist after its initial isolation during childhood or may be isolated for the first time during the adult years. The prevalence of *S. aureus* is 40% in newly diagnosed children, peaks at 46% in children 6 to 10 years of age, then gradually decreases to 25% in patients more than 35 years of age. Oxacillin resistant strains of *S. aureus*, likely acquired through nosocomial transmission, are also becoming increasingly prevalent, with the mean CF center rate being 3.2% of patients.[5]

For unclear reasons, the airways of CF patients have a peculiar propensity to become persistently infected with a small cadre of otherwise unusual gram-negative pathogens. Among these, *Pseudomonas aeruginosa* is the most common, with the prevalence ranging from approximately 25% during the first year of life to more than 80% by adulthood.[5] With the progression of lung disease, *P. aeruginosa* is often the only organism recovered from sputum and may be present in several types of colonies, usually with different antibiotic sensitivity patterns. The recovery of *P. aeruginosa*, particularly the mucoid form, from the lower respiratory tract of a child or young adult with chronic lung symptoms is highly suggestive of CF. Infection with *P. aeruginosa* is a negative predictor of lung function and survival,[92] making avoidance of initial colonization desirable. As a result, many clinics segregate infected patients from those who have never grown *P. aeruginosa* in sputum cultures.[93] Along similar lines of reasoning, the feasibility and efficacy of the eradication of pseudomonas on its initial isolation is being investigated.[93-95]

Other gram-negative rods that may infect CF airways include *Burkholderia cepacia*, *Alcaligenes xylosoxidans*, and *Stenotrophomonas maltophilia*.[91] These bacterial species may persist and lead to progressive lung destruction. *B. cepacia*, in particular, has been isolated in increasing frequency and is difficult to treat because it is often resistant to most antimicrobial drugs. A subset of patients with *B. cepacia* will manifest the **cepacia syndrome**,[96] a rapid clinical decline with fever and frank sepsis at some point after initial infection, although the precise pathogen/host factor(s) that trigger this dramatic decompensation are unknown. Because strong evidence exists that person-to-person spread of *B. cepacia* occurs, particularly with highly transmissible strains expressing the cable pilus,[97,98] stringent infection control measures are now advocated wherever CF care is provided.[99,100]

Fungi and molds are frequently cultured from the respiratory secretions of CF patients. In fact, *Aspergillus* species were reported in sputum cultures from 6% of children and 13% of adults in the 1997 CF Foundation Patient Registry,[101] although the prevalence is probably higher. Invasive aspergillosis has only rarely been reported in CF, but allergic bronchopulmonary aspergillosis (ABPA) develops in 2% to 11% of CF patients at some point in their lives.[102,103] Other fungi may colonize the airways and evoke similar allergic responses. The diagnosis of ABPA is based upon the presence of clinical features such as new infiltrates, wheezing, worsened cough, or an unexplained deterioration in lung function. The combination of these clinical findings plus evidence for immunologic sensitivity to aspergillus or other fungi, including elevated titers of aspergillus precipitating antibodies and high total IgE levels, should prompt consideration of this diagnosis.

Isolation of nontuberculous mycobacteria (NTM) from appropriately processed[104] CF sputum is relatively common and may occur in as many as 20% of CF adults.[105] Preliminary data from a multi-center study suggest an overall prevalence of about 13%, with *Mycobacterium avium* complex being most common and a significant prevalence of both *Mycobacterium abscessus* and *Mycobacterium fortuitum*. The role that these organisms play in the progression of CF lung disease are not clear, although some patients with high mycobacterial burdens and symptoms refractory to treatment of typical bacteria may benefit from antimycobacterial therapy.

Major Respiratory Complications

Hemoptysis, pneumothorax, and respiratory failure are major pulmonary complications that tend to occur in association with more severe lung disease. In the adult CF population, major hemoptysis and pneumothorax each occur in about 1% of patients per year. With proper management, most patients who suffer massive hemoptysis or pneumothorax can be treated successfully. Respiratory failure, as the result of progressive airway obstruction and destruction, is nearly universal and the cause of death in 94% of CF patients. Although improved therapies have delayed the development of respiratory failure, this eventual outcome can be prevented only by lung transplantation at this time.

Hemoptysis

Hemoptysis in CF may range from minor streaking of the sputum, requiring little intervention at all, to massive bleeding (more than 240 mL in 24 hours). Minor hemoptysis is common and usually self-limited. Massive hemoptysis in CF almost invariably stems from the bronchial artery circulation, which unlike the pulmonary vascular bed is under systemic arterial pressure. The new occurrence of any amount of bleeding may signal the presence of an increased infectious/inflammatory burden and the need for intensified treatment. The approach to a minor amount of hemoptysis therefore is aimed to determine whether the patient requires treatment with antibiotics and whether medication usage (NSAID, aspirin, penicillin) or vitamin K deficiency may be contributing to the new onset of bleeding.

Massive hemoptysis (more than 240 mL in 24 hours) from bronchiectatic airways occurs in approximately 5% of patients,[106] and may lead to airway obstruction and asphyxiation if left untreated. Hypotension, anemia, and chemical pneumonitis also may result from massive hemoptysis. Less voluminous hemoptysis that persists for several days (for example, 100 mL/day for 3 days) also should be considered a major bleeding event, because it may herald massive bleeding and often interferes with adequate chest physiotherapy. In addition to the correction of any hemostatic defects that may be present, these patients should be hospitalized and treated with appropriate antibiotics based on recent sputum culture results. Cough suppression and bed rest may be used during the acute presentation to lessen the likelihood of further bleeding but should not be continued for prolonged periods of time without more definitive therapy in patients with advanced lung disease who are likely to suffer from inadequate airway clearance.

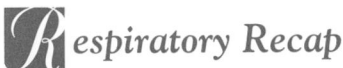

*R*espiratory Recap

Major Respiratory Complications of CF
Hemoptysis
Pneumothorax
Respiratory failure

When bleeding is rapid, positioning the patient with the bleeding lung in a dependent position may help prevent soiling of the nonbleeding lung. Endotracheal intubation may be required, however, if the patient is unable to maintain a patent airway. A large orotracheal tube, which can be advanced into the main bronchus serving the nonbleeding lung, is preferable to double-lumen tubes in this circumstance because the small lumens of these later devices limit airway suctioning. Attempts to localize the site of bleeding with chest radiography, CT scanning, and bronchoscopy may help direct invasive therapies aimed at the control of bleeding but often are not diagnostic and may delay definitive therapy.

When bleeding is from bronchiectatic airways, **bronchial artery embolization (BAE)** is the therapy of choice and is usually directed at any tortuous and hypertrophied bronchial artery when the precise location of bleeding is not known.[107] Nonbronchial systemic collateral vessels are also frequently involved, especially in cases of recurrent hemoptysis after BAE.[108] The use of nonionic contrast material, embolizing particles greater than 250 m in diameter (to prevent distal tissue ischemia), and avoidance of sclerosant agents have made BAE relatively safe and successful in experienced hands. Rebleeding after BAE is not uncommon and may require further attempts at BAE to achieve a successful outcome.[108] Surgical resection rarely is required for bleeding refractory to repeated attempts at BAE in patients with adequate pulmonary reserve.

Pneumothorax

The presence of subpleural air cysts is likely responsible for the increased incidence of spontaneous pneumothorax in CF. The incidence of this complication is approximately 1% per year overall, but it increases with age. Pneumothorax occurs in 5% to 8% of all CF patients at some time in their life, whereas 16% to 20% of adult patients will suffer this complication.[109,110] Most patients complain of a sudden increase in dyspnea or chest discomfort, although some patients are completely asymptomatic. The presence of a newly detected pneumothorax in a CF patient mandates hospitalization, whether or not chest tube insertion is planned at the outset. Asymptomatic pneumothoraces that occupy less than 20% of the hemithorax may be observed in the hospital, with follow-up radiographs and clinical monitoring to assess its progression. The small, asymptomatic pneumothorax that remains stable over a 24-hour period may be followed on an outpatient basis.

Larger pneumothoraces and those leading to symptoms should be treated with tube thoracostomy. Chest tubes may be removed once the pneumothorax has resolved and the air leak stopped. Additional tubes are occasionally required when significant air collections persist after the initial tube placement, in an effort to facilitate healing of the ruptured bleb through apposition of the parietal and visceral pleurae. When a pneumothorax has resolved but the air leak persists beyond 5 days, chest tube suction may be stopped, placed to water-seal for 24 hours, and removed if no recurrence of pneumothorax is detected radiographically. Further interventions may be necessary when a persistent air leak results in recurrent or persistent pneumothorax. Chemical or physical sclerosing agents (quinacrine, tetracycline, bleomycin, or talc) have been used to cause an inflammatory reaction that leads to obliteration of the pleural space. These approaches may hamper lung transplantation, however, because of the severity of adhesions between the lung and chest wall. A surgical approach, with either a small transaxillary thoracotomy or a thoracoscopic procedure, is preferred in the patient who may eventually require lung transplantation. Stapling across ruptured pleural blebs and pleural abrasion can be performed with a relatively low rate of recurrence, while the option of lung transplantation is preserved. Unfortunately, CF patients who are waiting for lung transplantation are often poor candidates for other major surgical procedures, and all options must be weighed carefully.[109,111]

Respiratory Failure

Hypoxemic and hypercapnic respiratory failure occurs in the late stages of CF and account for the majority of deaths. Evidence suggests that treatment of hypoxemia may improve both the quality and duration of life while preventing the development of cor pulmonale.[89,112,113] In addition, the era of lung transplantation and the development of improved methods of noninvasive ventilatory support have increased the rationale and feasibility of assisted ventilation for hypercapnic respiratory failure in certain defined clinical scenarios.

As infection and inflammation cause progressive airway obstruction and parenchymal destruction progress, ventilation/perfusion mismatch worsens and leads to hypoxemia. Other physiologic mechanisms also may contribute to hypoxemia, including an increased partial pressure of carbon dioxide, intrapulmonary shunt, and reduced mixed venous saturation resulting from increased oxygen consumption. Treatment of hypoxemic respiratory failure is first aimed at addressing all reversible processes. This includes optimization of the treatment of airway infection and clearance of retained secretions, as well as the addressing of other contributors that may be present, such as bronchospastic airways or allergic bronchopulmonary aspergillosis (ABPA). Supplemental oxygen via nasal cannula should be prescribed with the goal of continuous maintenance of an arterial hemoglobin oxygen saturation of at least 90%. Even when daytime oxygen saturation levels are adequate, hypoxemia during sleep and/or exercise may occur and should be assessed, especially in the setting of severe lung disease ($FEV_1 \leq 30\%$ of predicted), borderline resting oxygen saturation ($\leq 92\%$), or when signs of cor pulmonale are present. Because spirometric values poorly predict the occurrence of exercise or sleep induced hypoxemia, a low threshold for screening should exist.[86] This approach to the treatment of hypoxemic respiratory failure in CF is expected to improve exercise capacity[87,88] and prevent the development of cor pulmonale and significantly improve survival.[89,112]

Hypercapnic respiratory failure is the result of alveolar hypoventilation, primarily from airway obstruction and increased dead space ventilation. In addition, respiratory muscle weakness in association with muscle fatigue and malnutrition may be important contributors to this process. Acidosis that develops gradually from hypercapnia usually is well compensated by renal mechanisms, such that an adequate acid-base balance is maintained. Acute elevations in the P_{CO_2}, however, will lead to acidosis and an impaired sensorium. Although often the result of slowly progressive lung disease, a search for treatable causes of respiratory failure should be performed, and all reversible processes addressed. The decision to initiate assisted ventilation, whether via a noninvasive device or with endotracheal intubation, should then be based on whether a reversible precipitating process exists, the baseline severity of lung disease, and whether the patient has been accepted for lung transplantation.[114-116]

Although patients with irreversible respiratory insufficiency are unlikely to benefit from mechanical ventilation without the option of imminent lung transplantation, other patients may in fact benefit from this form of therapy. In the setting of an acute, reversible process such as pneumothorax, massive hemoptysis, bronchospasm, or prior suboptimal treatment of the underlying CF lung disease, assisted ventilation may provide the time needed to treat the acute, superimposed process. Once the decision

to intubate a patient has been made, an aggressive regimen of airway clearance with chest physiotherapy, suctioning, and bronchodilators should be implemented. In addition, prevention of muscle weakness through provision of adequate nutrition and exercise (including ambulation with assisted ventilation) should be instituted whenever possible. Successful weaning from mechanical ventilation depends primarily on the extent of the underlying lung disease in these scenarios, rather than the severity of the acute respiratory event. In the patient awaiting lung transplantation who has accrued enough seniority to make organ availability a possibility within several days or weeks, a trial of mechanical ventilation and intensive therapy may be reasonable, with the understanding that prolonged support of this kind will not be possible. This period of support may provide a bridge to successful transplantation and may allow the patient and family to address end-of-life issues in a more suitable fashion.

In the setting of chronic hypercapnic respiratory failure, it is unclear whether patients may benefit from nocturnal, noninvasive positive pressure ventilation (NPPV). In selected patients, NPPV may decrease the work of breathing, thus decreasing daytime respiratory muscle fatigue, while reducing hypercapnia and hypoxemia during sleep.[117] Results of studies examining the utility of NPPV in CF and other chronic obstructive lung diseases have yielded mixed results in terms of its ability to improve quality of life, daytime gas exchange, respiratory muscle function, and quality of sleep. As with conventional mechanical ventilation, NPPV may be able to help sustain patients with decompensated respiratory failure who are waiting for lung transplantation.[118] Because of these mixed results, NPPV use should be individualized and closely monitored. The use of a formal sleep study should be considered to document the degree of gas exchange deterioration during sleep and the frequency of respiratory disturbances, and to titrate airway pressures being delivered.

Standard Therapy of Lung Disease

Treatment of CF lung disease can be broken down into those therapies that are used to prevent deterioration of lung function and those used to treat acute exacerbations. Although a variety of therapies are being developed that are aimed at the correction of either the gene defect itself (that is, gene therapy) or the ion transport abnormalities that characterize CF epithelia, currently available therapies either promote the physical removal of airway secretions or reduce airway infection and inflammation. Several lines of therapy are often combined in an attempt to provide optimal care for patients. When multiple expensive and labor-intensive treatment modalities are prescribed, careful attention should be paid to correctness of technique and the order in which medications are given to realize maximal benefits (Table 51-2). Although not addressed in detail here, appropriate nutritional support

TABLE 51-2

*Optimal Sequencing of Inhaled Medications
and Airway Clearance Maneuvers*

Agent	Rationale
rhDNase	Decreases secretion viscosity by degrading free DNA; once daily appears equivalent to twice daily
Bronchodilator (β-adrenergic agonist; ipratropium bromide)	May aid subsequent secretion clearance by dilating airways; protects against bronchospasm induced by mucolytics and/or antibiotics later in treatment series
Hypertonic saline/mucolytic	May make secretions more mobile through improved hydration (hypertonic saline) or by disrupting disulfide bonds within mucin molecules (N-acetylcysteine)
Airway clearance maneuvers	Numerous available methods available and should be individualized to the patient; should be repeated two to four times daily depending on the clinical scenario
Antibiotic (TOBI, Colistin); corticosteroid	Maximal deposition of these agents achieved after bronchodilation and secretion clearance

BOX 51-2

*Respiratory Therapist Roles in Cystic Fibrosis
Management*

Monitoring of oxygen therapy (rest, nocturnal, exercise)
Administration of nebulized therapies
    Bronchodilators
    rhDNase
    Antibiotics
    Hypertonic saline
Assisted ventilation (via mask or endotracheal tube)
Performance of airway clearance maneuvers
Patient education
    Proper use of inhaled medications
    Instruction on airway clearance techniques
    Respiratory equipment care and maintenance

(aiming to achieve and maintain ideal body weight more than 90% of predicted) and treatment of complications such as CF-related diabetes are integral parts of the multidisciplinary care of patients and may directly impact the severity of lung disease and survival. The development of specialized CF care centers where expertise from multiple disciplines can be applied in an integrated fashion has greatly improved survival. Typical respiratory therapist roles in the management of patients with CF are listed in Box 51-2.

Maintenance Therapy

Airway Clearance Techniques

CF airway secretions are difficult to clear as the result of reduced water content (resulting from excessive sodium and water absorption) and the presence of high concentrations of DNA from degrading inflammatory cells. If left untreated, retained secretions lead to progressive airway obstruction and serve as a nidus for ongoing infection and inflammation. In an attempt to circumvent the relentless progression of infection, inflammation, and lung destruction, a variety of physical maneuvers have been developed to promote the movement of airway secretions from small airways toward central airways where they may be removed by cough. Even with the advent of medications developed specifically to treat CF lung disease, these techniques continue to be a cornerstone of therapy (Table 51-3).

Several means of airway clearance are available to patients with CF, with little other than systematic, individual trials to guide the clinician to the best choice for a given patient. Chest percussion and postural drainage (PD), the traditional means used to clear secretions, is usually effective although many patients consider this time and labor intensive. PD uses multiple body positions to facilitate drainage of individual lung segments via gravity in conjunction with chest percussion and vibration and has been shown to improve mucus clearance and pulmonary function in otherwise stable patients.[119,120] Because this method requires a second person and a significant amount of time to be performed correctly, many patients have turned to alternative means of airway clearance with good apparent efficacy and improved autonomy.

In addition to a variety of mechanical percussors that are available, a number of breathing techniques and respiratory devices are available to assist patients with airway clearance.[121] Several studies suggest that these alternatives to PD may be effective, including the use of forced expiratory maneuvers,[121] positive expiratory pressure (PEP) devices,[122] the Flutter valve,[123,124] and exercise.[125] Other devices and techniques include a high-frequency chest compression vest (ThAIRapy vest [American Biosystems, St. Paul, Minn.]),[126-128] autogenic drainage, and the active cycle of breathing technique. Because no single method has been shown to be consistently superior and great variability exists between patients, several of these methods should be tried until an optimal set of methods is identified. Clearly, patient acceptance of a technique is crucial if a sufficient degree of compliance can be expected.

TABLE 51-3

Airway Clearance Techniques

Technique	Description	Performed Independently?
Percussion, vibration, postural drainage	Hand percussion, shaking, and/or vibration is applied over individual lung segments in conjunction with postural drainage positions. Mechanical percussors provide limited patient autonomy and may decrease fatigue in the caregiver.	No
Active cycle of breathing (ACB)	Technique alternates (1) gentle breathing with the lower chest, (2) deep breathing with emphasis on inspiration, and (3) forced exhalation technique (FET) using the abdominal muscles and an open mouth/glottis (huff). ACB may be combined with postural positions.	Yes
Autogenic drainage	Technique alternates (1) breathing at low lung volumes to loosen peripheral secretions, (2) breathing at low-mid lung volumes to collect mucus from central airways, and (3) mucus evacuation by breathing at mid-high lung volumes. It is performed in the sitting position and requires significant teaching.	Yes
Positive expiratory pressure (PEP)	Pressure (10-20 cm H_2O) is applied via an expiratory resistor contained within a mask or mouthpiece. Tidal breathing with slightly active exhalation is used. Forced expirations and cough follow PEP to evacuate mucus. Nebulized medications may be delivered in conjunction with PEP device. PEP is a simple technique to learn and perform.	Yes
Flutter	This device delivers oscillating positive expiratory pressure with a hand-held device. Sufficient airflow may not be achieved in patients with very severe lung disease.	Yes
High-frequency chest compression (ThAIRapy vest)	An inflatable vest is linked to an air delivery system capable of providing air pulses at various frequencies. Several frequencies (6-25 Hz) are employed over 20-30 minutes in an upright position, followed by FET/cough. Nebulized medications may be administered simultaneously to assist secretion removal.	Yes
Exercise	Exercise has been shown to assist secretion removal, in addition to other beneficial effects on health and well-being. The need for supplemental oxygen during exercise should be assessed periodically.	Yes

Respiratory Recap

Maintenance Therapy for CF	
Airway clearance tecniques	Antibiotics
Aerosolized rhDNase	Antiinflammatory
Other mucus modifying agents	medications

Aerosolized rhDNase A second strategy used to facilitate secretion removal is to modify the transportability of the secretions themselves. Because DNA is a major component of CF secretions, which is extremely viscous and therefore poorly transportable within the airway, recombinant human DNase I (rhDNase; Pulmozyme) was developed and approved for use in CF in 1994.[129] Once daily use of this agent improved the FEV_1 by 6% above baseline and lessened the frequency of respiratory exacerbations by 28% in a well-controlled study lasting 6 months. The response to rhDNase is apparently variable, however, with some patients showing clear benefit, and others showing no change or actually worsening. Therefore individualized use and careful monitoring of the response are warranted. Because most patients who benefit show a response within 1 to 3 months of the initiation of the drug, a therapeutic trial should be considered in patients for this duration of time while the individual is monitored for improvement in lung function and clinical symptoms. The efficacy of rhDNase over longer time periods and its impact on mortality remain unknown.

Other Mucus Modifying Agents A variety of mucolytics have been used in CF through the years, although none have been shown to improve lung function or other clinical outcomes. Among these agents, N-acetylcysteine (Mucomyst) is perhaps the most commonly used. This agent reduces disulfide bonds in mucins, thus making them less viscous. Unfortunately, this agent may increase epithelial injury or inflammation and should be used only in selected patients for brief periods of time. Other mucolytic agents and expectorants also have been used but have not been well studied in CF. More recently, hypertonic saline solutions have been used to promote hydration of inspissated mucous secretions, although data supporting this approach are fairly limited. Studies examining the acute effect of hypertonic NaCl (3% to 12%) on mucociliary clearance[130-132] and short-term studies of lung function[133,134] do suggest, however, that this approach may be useful. A small fraction of CF patients with coexistent reactive airways may not tolerate hypertonic solutions because of bronchospasm,[135] although most do well with 3% NaCl after albuterol pretreatment. Because the beneficial effect of the addition of salt to airway surface liquid is predicted to be brief, administration immediately before some means of airway clearance may be the optimal method of use.

Antibiotics   Because airway infection is a critical step in the development and progression of CF lung disease, oral and inhaled antibiotics are an important part of a standard CF care regimen. In general, oral antibiotics are used episodically, when new respiratory symptoms develop, or a minor decline in lung function is detected. Scheduled cycles of oral antibiotics also may be used prophylactically in the patient having frequent exacerbations. Continuous use of an oral antibiotic designed to suppress infection with *Staphylococcus aureus* has been a common practice in the past but cannot be recommended as good practice except in individual cases. Studies examining the chronic use of anti-staphylococcal antibiotics have not demonstrated significant clinical benefit, suggest an association between their use and an increased density of *Pseudomonas aeruginosa*,[136] and could contribute to the already growing problem of resistant *S. aureus* infection in CF.[137] Similarly, long-term use of ciprofloxacin, the primary oral agent with good activity versus *P. aeruginosa*, should be avoided because of the rapid emergence of resistance after 3 to 4 weeks of use.

Because of the limited number of oral agents available to treatment of *P. aeruginosa*, inhaled aminoglycosides and other parenteral antibiotics have been employed. This route of administration has the additional benefit of achieving high drug levels in airway secretions, with minimal systemic levels or toxicity. High drug concentrations in secretions may be particularly helpful in the treatment of organisms that are resistant to antibiotic concentrations that may be achieved via the intravenous route. The best data for inhaled antibiotic efficacy is with high-dose tobramycin. A preservative-free, concentrated preparation of tobramycin (TOBI 300 mg, twice a day), taken during alternate months for three cycles clearly improved lung function, decreased bacterial burden, and lessened the relative risk of hospitalization or treatment with intravenous anti-pseudomonal antibiotics. The rate of acquired tobramycin resistance was 7% over the duration of the study.[138] Whether these beneficial effects will be sustained over longer time periods, without the development of significant resistance to this agent, is unknown. An alternative to inhaled tobramycin is colistin (75 to 150 mg, twice a day), which has good *in vitro* activity against *P. aeruginosa* but has been less well studied in clinical trials.[139] In addition, bronchospasm is more frequently encountered with this agent.

In general, inhaled antibiotics may be used in a variety of clinical scenarios. As described above, the prophylactic use of high-dose tobramycin improved lung function and lessened the need for hospitalization. Alternatively, inhaled antibiotics may be reserved for "minor exacerbations" of respiratory disease, with or without oral ciprofloxacin, in attempt to avoid the need for hospitalization and intravenous antibiotics. This approach may be especially beneficial in patients being followed closely, where signs of deterioration may be detected very early.

An alternative approach embraced by the Danish CF community stresses measures aimed at delaying the acquisition of *P. aeruginosa* and aggressive antibiotic treatment once encountered. These measures include the segregation of patients by microbiologic status and attempts to eradicate pseudomonas when initially cultured in a patient.[94] Scheduled courses of intravenous antibiotics are also employed every 3 months for patients who are chronically colonized with pseudomonas. This center claims that improved survival has resulted from this approach,[140] based on historical controls at their center, although this approach has not been widely adopted by other centers. Significant concerns include the earlier development of bacterial antibiotic resistance, the lack of proven efficacy by controlled trials, and the enormous health-care resources involved and personal impact this approach has on patients.

Bronchodilators   Bronchodilators, especially those delivered via the inhaled route, are commonly prescribed in CF. Approximately one quarter of patients have bronchial reactivity and will improve after bronchodilator administration.[141-144] In these patients, bronchodilators may improve respiratory symptoms and airway secretion clearance. Whether or not these agents provide long-term benefit in CF is unknown. In general, inhaled β-adrenergic agents are used in patients with documented reversibility on spirometric values, or who symptomatically benefit. Inhaled anticholinergic agents, especially ipratropium bromide, may also have a role in CF.[145] Oral preparations, including theophylline, are not routinely used, have not been shown to be efficacious, and must be monitored carefully because marked pharmacokinetic variability occurs with this agent.

Antiinflammatory Medications   A clear rationale exists for the use of antiinflammatory agents to lessen neutrophilic inflammation and the harmful effects of neutrophil products. Initial studies designed to test this approach used high doses of corticosteroids and yielded mixed results. Although patients receiving 1 to 2 mg/kg of prednisolone on alternate days had a slowed decline in lung function (ΔFEV_1 −2% versus −6% in placebo group, at 48 months), unacceptable side effects were encountered.[146-148] Glucose metabolism abnormalities, cataracts, and delayed linear growth limit chronic therapy with oral corticosteroids, although the risk-benefit ratio may favor their use in patients with ABPA, reactive airways, and with shorter courses of treatment. Inhaled steroids also have been studied in CF and are certain to have a much better safety profile. Efficacy, however, has not been proven by these studies, although individual patients with co-existent asthma or bronchial reactivity may benefit.[149]

An alternative means to lessen neutrophilic inflammation is high-dose ibuprofen. In a well-designed trial over the course of 4 years, young patients (5 to 13 years) with mild lung disease (FEV_1 ≥60% of predicted) benefited from twice daily ibuprofen at doses sufficient to achieve peak blood levels of 50 to 100 mg/L. In those who complied with therapy, the annual rate of change in FEV_1 was −1.5%, versus −3.5% in the placebo group. Nutritional status and radiographic indices of disease activity also were improved in the treated group, and few side effects were encountered.[150] Further studies are needed to determine whether even younger patients may benefit from ibuprofen therapy.

Acute Exacerbations

The course of CF lung disease is punctuated by periodic episodes of worsened airway infection, inflammation, and worsened lung function. These episodes occur more frequently and become more difficult to treat as lung disease progresses and bacterial resistance develops. This fact makes an effective preventive regimen for CF lung disease of paramount importance. When exacerbations inevitably occur, a similarly aggressive approach should be taken to reclaim lost lung function and to prevent early relapse with its associated risks.

Typical features of an infectious exacerbation of CF lung disease include an increase in the frequency of cough and amount of sputum, diminished appetite, weight loss, fatigue, and a decrease in the FEV_1. Fever is not uncommon, but high fever should prompt the search for other etiologies, including infection with *Burkholderia cepacia*, atypical organisms (for example, respiratory viruses, mycobacteria), or indwelling catheter infection. Leukocytosis is typically mild to moderate, and chest radiographs may show little or no acute change.

During the initiation of therapy for a CF exacerbation, consideration of potential precipitating causes should include the presence of environmental allergens or irritants, inadequate airway clearance measures, allergic bronchopulmonary aspergillosis, and medicine noncompliance. The adequacy of airway clearance at home, the severity of the exacerbation, the baseline severity of lung disease, and the complexity of the treatment regimen being instituted should be weighed during consideration of whether home therapy with intravenous antibiotics may be an option. In either environment, airway clearance maneuvers should be intensified, preferably to include at least thrice daily efforts to clear the airways. Antibiotics should be selected based on recent, pretreatment culture and sensitivity testing whenever possible.

Every isolated organism is often targeted when feasible, although patients often improve even when only selected organisms are targeted. *Pseudomonas aeruginosa*, *Burkholderia cepacia*, and other typical gram-negative organisms (*Stenotrophomonas maltophilia*, *Alcaligenes xylosoxidans*) should be treated with two antibiotics from different drug classes. When both a gram-negative organism and *Staphylococcus aureus* are cultured, the decision to add specific anti-staphylococcal therapy (for example, oxacillin, vancomycin) is not always easy and may be based on the past history of response to certain antibiotic regimens in that patient. The duration of therapy is typically around 2 weeks but may be longer when the clinical response is slow. Pulmonary function testing near the end of a planned antibiotic course may be useful as an objective measure of the adequacy of therapy. Although some further improvement in lung function may occur even after completion of the antibiotic course, the return of lung function parameters to preexacerbation levels is reassuring.

Lung Transplantation

Lung transplantation has become an accepted therapy for end-stage CF lung disease. The relative paucity of donor organs and subsequent long waiting times before organ availability mandate that patients be referred to transplant centers on a timely basis. With waiting times exceeding 2 years at some centers, close attention should be paid to clinical clues that suggest an expected duration of survival that approximates this time frame. These predictors include an FEV_1 of ~30% of predicted, the rate of decline in lung function, hypoxemia (at rest or induced by exercise/sleep), and hypercapnia (PCO_2 ≥45 mm Hg). The presence of an accelerated clinical decline, characterized by more frequent exacerbations that respond incompletely to aggressive therapy, recurrent pneumothoraces, recurrent massive hemoptysis, or pan-resistant organisms should prompt consideration for earlier referral.[80-83] Optimal transplant candidates should not have significant associated organ dysfunction (kidney, liver), should be motivated and compliant with therapy, and should have adequate psychosocial supports.

The surgical approach now preferred is sequential, bilateral transplantation rather than heart-lung transplantation. Alternatively, when a patient is not likely to survive until a cadaveric transplant can be performed, living donor lobar transplantation can be performed when healthy donors of sufficient size and correct blood type are available.[151] In either case, survival after transplant appears no different in CF than in transplantation for other indications. The 5-year survival rate is approximately 48% and is limited primarily by opportunistic infections and chronic graft rejection, manifesting as bronchiolitis obliterans.[152]

KEY POINTS

- Cystic fibrosis is a prevalent inherited disorder that causes significant morbidity and premature mortality in those who suffer from it.
- Cystic fibrosis is the most common lethal genetic disease affecting the Caucasian population; it is autosomal recessive.
- Mutations in the CFTR gene result in several ion transport abnormalities, which in turn impair mucociliary clearance and lung defense.
- Chronic infection and inflammation lead to progressive lung damage and respiratory failure in a majority of patients.
- Improvements in care, including better antibiotics and nutritional support, have greatly extended survival.
- Cystic fibrosis is a multi-organ disease, with a broad spectrum of clinical manifestations.
- The combination of a typical CF clinical manifestation with evidence for abnormal CFTR is required for the diagnosis of cystic fibrosis.
- Preventive care is the cornerstone of effective CF management.
- Close monitoring of lung function, aggressive therapies aimed at airway clearance and minimization of infection, and nutritional support are necessary elements in CF care.
- Lung transplantation is an appropriate therapy for patients with severe CF lung disease. Evaluation for transplant, in appropriate candidates, should occur before the local waiting time for donor availability exceeds the anticipated survival time.

References

1. Andersen DH. Cystic fibrosis of the pancreas and its relation to celiac disease: a clinical and pathologic study. Am J Dis Child 1938;56:344-399.
2. Farber S. Some organic digestive disturbances in early life. J Mich Med Sci 1945;44:587-594.
3. di Sant'Agnese PA, Darling RC, Perera GA, et al. Abnormal electrolyte composition of sweat in cystic fibrosis of the pancreas. Pediatrics 1953;12:549-563.
4. Riordan JR, Rommens JM, Kerem B-T, et al. Identification of the cystic fibrosis gene: cloning and characterization of complementary DNA. Science 1989;245:1066-1073.
5. Cystic Fibrosis Foundation, Patient Registry 1998 Annual Data Report. Bethesda, Maryland; 1999.
6. Tsui LC. Cystic fibrosis mutation database. http://www.genet.sickkids.on.ca/cftr/. 2000.
7. Population variation of common cystic fibrosis mutations. The cystic fibrosis genetic analysis consortium. Hum Mutat 1994;4:167-177.
8. Zielenski J, Tsui LC. Cystic fibrosis: genotypic and phenotypic variations. Annu Rev Genet 1995;29:777-807.
9. Correlation between genotype and phenotype in patients with cystic fibrosis. The cystic fibrosis genotype-phenotype consortium. N Engl J Med 1993;329:1308-1313.
10. Chillon M, Casals T, Mercier B, et al. Mutations in the cystic fibrosis gene in patients with congenital absence of the vas deferens. N Eng J Med 1995;332:1475-1480.
11. Dork T, Dworniczak B, Aulehla-Scholz C, et al. Distinct spectrum of CFTR gene mutations in congenital absence of vas deferens. Hum Genet 1997;100:365-377.
12. Greger R, Mall M, Bleich M, et al. Regulation of epithelial ion channels by the cystic fibrosis transmembrane conductance regulator. J Mol Med 1996;74:527-534.
13. Stutts MJ, Rossier BC, Boucher RC. Cystic fibrosis transmembrane conductance regulator inverts protein kinase A-mediated regulation of epithelial sodium channel single channel kinetics. J Biol Chem 1997;272:14037-14040.
14. Stutts MJ, Canessa CM, Olsen JC, et al. CFTR as a camp-dependent regulator of sodium channels. Science 1995;269:847-850.
15. Mall M, Bleich M, Greger R, et al. The amiloride-inhibitable Na^+ conductance is reduced by the cystic fibrosis transmembrane conductance regulator in normal but not in cystic fibrosis airways. J Clin Invest 1998;102:15-21.
16. Mall M, Bleich M, Kuehr J, et al. CFTR-mediated inhibition of epithelial Na^+ conductance in human colon is defective in cystic fibrosis. Am J Physiol 1999;277:G709-G716.
17. Gabriel SE, Clarke LL, Boucher RC, et al. CFTR and outward rectifying chloride channels are distinct proteins with a regulatory relationship. Nature 1993;363:263-268.
18. Egan M, Flotte T, Afione S, et al. Defective regulation of outwardly rectifying Cl^- channels by Protein Kinase A corrected by insertion of CFTR. Nature 1992;358:581-584.
19. Kunzelmann K, Mall M, Briel M, et al. The cystic fibrosis transmembrane conductance regulator attenuates the endogenous Ca^{2+} activated Cl^- conductance of Xenopus oocytes. Pflugers Arch 1997;435:178-181.
20. McNicholas CM, Guggino WB, Schwiebert EM, et al. Sensitivity of a renal K^+ channel (ROMK2) to the inhibitory sulfonylurea compound glibenclamide is enhanced by coexpression with the ATP-binding cassette transporter cystic fibrosis transmembrane regulator. Proc Natl Acad Sci USA 1996;93:8083-8088.
21. Boucher RC, Stutts MJ, Knowles MR, et al. Na^+ transport in cystic fibrosis respiratory epithelia. abnormal basal rate and response to adenylate cyclase activation. J Clin Invest 1986;78:1245-1252.
22. Cotton CU, Stutts MJ, Knowles MR, et al Abnormal apical cell membrane in cystic fibrosis respiratory epithelium. An *in vitro* electrophysiologic analysis. J Clin Invest 1987;79:80-85.
23. Matsui H, Grubb BR, Tarran R, et al. Evidence for periciliary liquid layer depletion, not abnormal ion composition, in the pathogenesis of cystic fibrosis airways disease. Cell 1998;95:1005-1015.
24. Smith JJ, Travis SM, Greenberg EP, et al. Cystic fibrosis airway epithelia fail to kill bacteria because of abnormal airway surface fluid. Cell 1996; 85:229-236.
25. Travis SM, Conway BA, Zabner J, et al. Activity of abundant antimicrobials of the human airway. Am J Respir Cell Mol Biol 1999;20:872-879.
26. Engelhardt JF, Yankaskas JR, Ernst SA, et al. Submucosal glands are the predominant site of CFTR expression in the human bronchus. Nat Genet 1992;2:240-248.

27. Ballard ST, Trout L, Bebok Z, et al. CFTR involvement in chloride, bicarbonate, and liquid secretion by airway submucosal glands. Am J Physiol 1999;277:L694-L699.

28. Davril M, Degroote S, Humbert P, et al. The sialylation of bronchial mucins secreted by patients suffering from cystic fibrosis or from chronic bronchitis is related to the severity of airway infection. Glycobiology 1999;9:311-321.

29. Wesley A, Forstner J, Qureshi R, et al. Human intestinal mucin in cystic fibrosis. Pediatr Res 1983;17:65-69.

30. Cheng PW, Boat TF, Cranfill K, et al. Increased sulfation of glycoconjugates by cultured nasal epithelial cells from patients with cystic fibrosis. J Clin Invest 1989;84:68-72.

31. Bonfield TL, Konstan MW, Berger M. Altered respiratory epithelial cell cytokine production in cystic fibrosis. J Allergy Clin Immunol 1999;104:72-78.

32. Bonfield TL, Konstan MW, Burfeind P, et al. Normal bronchial epithelial cells constitutively produce the anti-inflammatory cytokine interleukin-10, which is downregulated in cystic fibrosis. Am J Respir Cell Mol Biol 1995;13:257-261.

33. Bonfield TL, Panuska JR, Konstan MW, et al. Inflammatory cytokines in cystic fibrosis lungs. Am J Respir Crit Care Med 1995;152:2111-2118.

34. Muhlebach MS, Stewart PW, Leigh MW, et al. Quantitation of inflammatory responses to bacteria in young cystic fibrosis and control patients. Am J Respir Crit Care Med 1999; 160:186-191.

35. Noah TL, Black HR, Cheng PW, et al. Nasal and bronchoalveolar lavage fluid cytokines in early cystic fibrosis. J Infect Dis 1997;175:638-647.

36. Stern RC. The diagnosis of cystic fibrosis. N Engl J Med 1997;336:487-491.

37. Rosenstein BJ, Cutting GR. The diagnosis of cystic fibrosis: a consensus statement. Cystic Fibrosis Foundation Consensus Panel. J Pediatr 1998;132:589-595.

38. Knowles M, Gatzy J, Boucher R. Increased bioelectric potential difference across respiratory epithelia in cystic fibrosis. N Engl J Med 1981;305:1489-1495.

39. Knowles MR, Paradiso AM, Boucher RC. In vivo nasal potential difference: techniques and protocols for assessing efficacy of gene transfer in cystic fibrosis. Hum Gene Ther 1995;6:445-455.

40. Gharib R, Allen RP, Joos HA, et al. Paranasal sinuses in cystic fibrosis: incidence of roentgen abnormalities. Am J Dis Child 1964;108:499-502.

41. Stern RC, Jones K. Nasal and sinus disease. In Yankaskas JR, Knowles MR, editors. Cystic fibrosis in adults, Philadelphia: Lippincott-Raven; 1999. pp. 221-231.

42. Stern RC, Boat TF, Wood RE, et al. Treatment and prognosis of nasal polyps in cystic fibrosis. Am J Dis Child 1982;136: 1067-1070.

43. Cepero R, Smith RJ, Catlin FI, et al. Cystic fibrosis—an otolaryngologic perspective. Otolaryngol Head Neck Surg 1987; 97:356-360.

44. Jaffe BF, Strome M, Khaw KT, et al. Nasal polypectomy and sinus surgery for cystic fibrosis—a 10 year review. Otolaryngol Clin North Am 1977;10:81-90.

45. Shwachman H, Kowalski M, Khaw KT. Cystic fibrosis: a new outlook. 70 patients above 25 years of age. Medicine (Baltimore) 1977;56:129-149.

46. Durie PR, Forstner GG. The exocrine pancreas. In Yankaskas JR, Knowles MR, editors. Cystic fibrosis in adults. Philadelphia: Lippincott-Raven; 1999. pp. 261-287.

47. Shwachman H, Lebenthal E, Khaw KT. Recurrent acute pancreatitis in patients with cystic fibrosis with normal pancreatic enzymes. Pediatrics 1975;55:86-95.

48. Cohn JA, Friedman KJ, Noone PG, et al. Relation between mutations of the cystic fibrosis gene and idiopathic pancreatitis. N Engl J Med 1998;339:653-658.

49. Sharer N, Schwarz M, Malone G, et al. Mutations of the cystic fibrosis gene in patients with chronic pancreatitis. N Engl J Med 1998;339:645-652.

50. Lanng S, Thorsteinsson B, Lund-Andersen C, et al. Diabetes mellitus in Danish cystic fibrosis patients: prevalence and late diabetic complications. Acta Paediatr 1994;83:72-77.

51. Lanng S, Thorsteinsson B, Nerup J, et al. Diabetes mellitus in cystic fibrosis: effect of insulin therapy on lung function and infections. Acta Paediatr 1994;83:849-853.

52. Moran A, Hardin D, Rodman D, et al. Diagnosis, screening and management of cystic fibrosis related diabetes mellitus: a consensus conference report. Diabetes Res Clin Pract 1999;45:61-73.

53. di Sant'Agnese PA; Hubbard VS. The gastrointestinal tract. In Taussig LM, editor. Cystic fibrosis. New York: Thieme-Stratton; 1984. pp. 212-229.

54. Rosenstein BJ, Langbaum TS. Incidence of meconium abnormalities in newborn infants with cystic fibrosis. Am J Dis Child 1980;134:72-73.

55. di Sant'Agnese PA, Davis PB. Cystic fibrosis in adults. 75 cases and a review of 232 cases in the literature. Am J Med 1979;66:121-132.

56. Gaskin KJ: Intestines. In Yankaskas JR, Knowles MR, editors. Cystic fibrosis in adults. Philadelphia: Lippincott-Raven; 1999. pp. 325-342.

57. Stern RC, Izant RJ Jr, Boat TF, et al. Treatment and prognosis of rectal prolapse in cystic fibrosis. Gastroenterology 1982; 82:707-710.

58. Borowitz DS, Grand RJ, Durie PR. Use of pancreatic enzyme supplements for patients with cystic fibrosis in the context of fibrosing colonopathy. Consensus Committee. J Pediatr 1995; 127:681-684.

59. Fitzsimmons SC, Burkhart GA, Borowitz D, et al. High-dose pancreatic-enzyme supplements and fibrosing colonopathy in children with cystic fibrosis. N Engl J Med 1997;336:1283-1289.

60. Stevens JC, Maguiness KM, Hollingsworth J, et al. Pancreatic enzyme supplementation in cystic fibrosis patients before and after fibrosing colonopathy. J Pediatr Gastroenterol Nutr 1998;26:80-84.

61. Ledson MJ, Tran J, Walshaw MJ. Prevalence and mechanisms of gastro-oesophageal reflux in adult cystic fibrosis patients. J R Soc Med 1998;91:7-9.

62. Malfroot A, Dab I. New insights on gastro-oesophageal reflux in cystic fibrosis by longitudinal follow up. Arch Dis Child 1991;66:1339-1345.

63. Stringer DA, Sprigg A, Juodis E, et al. The association of cystic fibrosis, gastroesophageal reflux, and reduced pulmonary function. Can Assoc Radiol J 1988;39:100-102.

64. Colombo C, Crosignani A, Battezzati PM. Liver involvement in cystic fibrosis. J Hepatol 1999;31:946-954.

65. Colombo C, Crosignani A, Melzi ML, et al. Hepatobiliary system. In Yankaskas JR, Knowles MR, editors. Cystic fibrosis in adults. Philadelphia: Lippincott-Raven; 1999. pp. 309-324.

66. Scott-Jupp R, Lama M, Tanner MS. Prevalence of liver disease in cystic fibrosis. Arch Dis Child 1991;66:698-701.

67. Jebbink MC, Heijerman HG, Masclee AA, et al. Gallbladder disease in cystic fibrosis. Neth J Med 1992;41:123-126.

68. Nagel RA, Westaby D, Javaid A, et al. Liver disease and bile duct abnormalities in adults with cystic fibrosis. Lancet 1989;2:1422-1425.

69. Wilschanski M, Corey M, Durie P, et al. Diversity of reproductive tract abnormalities in men with cystic fibrosis. JAMA 1996;276:607-608.

70. Flume PA, Yankaskas JR. Reproductive issues. In Yankaskas JR, Knowles MR, editors. Cystic fibrosis in adults. Philadelphia: Lippincott-Raven; 1999. pp. 449-464.

71. Silber SJ. The use of epididymal sperm for the treatment of male infertility. Baillieres Clin Obstet Gynaecol 1997;11:739-752.

72. Kopito LE, Kosasky HJ, Shwachman H. Water and electrolytes in cervical mucus from patients with cystic fibrosis. Fertil Steril 1973;24:512-516.

73. Fiel SB, Fitzsimmons S. Pregnancy in patients with cystic fibrosis. Pediatr Pulmonol Suppl 1997;16:111-112.

74. Nussbaum E, Boat TF, Wood RE, et al. Cystic fibrosis with acute hypoelectrolytemia and metabolic alkalosis in infancy. Am J Dis Child 1979;133:965-966.

75. Santamaria F, Grillo G, Guidi G, et al. Cystic fibrosis: when should high-resolution computed tomography of the chest be obtained? Pediatrics 1998;101:908-913.

76. Moore EH. Atypical Mycobacterial infection in the lung: CT appearance. Radiology 1993;187:777-782.

77. Hartman TE, Swensen SJ, Williams DE. Mycobacterium avium-intracellulare complex: evaluation with CT. Radiology 1993;187:23-26.

78. Levison H, Godfrey, S. Pulmonary aspects of cystic fibrosis. In: Mangos JA, Talamo RE, editors. Cystic fibrosis: projections into the future. New York: Stratton Intercontinental Book Corporation; 1976. pp. 3-24.

79. Feher A, Castile R, Kisling J, et al. Flow limitation in normal infants: a new method for forced expiratory maneuvers from raised lung volumes. J Appl Physiol 1996;80:2019-2025.

80. Hayllar KM, Williams SG, Wise AE, et al. A prognostic model for the prediction of survival in cystic fibrosis. Thorax 1997;52:313-317.

81. Kerem E, Reisman J, Corey M, et al. Prediction of mortality in patients with cystic fibrosis. N Engl J Med 1992;326:1187-1191.

82. Milla CE, Warwick WJ. Risk of death in cystic fibrosis patients with severely compromised lung function. Chest 1998;113:1230-1234.

83. Doershuk CF, Stern RC. Timing of referral for lung transplantation for cystic fibrosis: overemphasis on FEV$_1$ may adversely affect overall survival. Chest 1999;115:782-787.

84. Nixon PA, Orenstein DM, Kelsey SF, et al. The prognostic value of exercise testing in patients with cystic fibrosis. N Engl J Med 1992;327:1785-1788.

85. Ballard RD, Sutarik JM, Clover CW, et al. Effects of non-REM sleep on ventilation and respiratory mechanics in adults with cystic fibrosis. Am J Respir Crit Care Med 1996;153:266-271.

86. Bradley S, Solin P, Wilson J, et al. Hypoxemia and hypercapnia during exercise and sleep in patients with cystic fibrosis. Chest 1999;116:647-654.

87. Marcus CL, Bader D, Stabile MW, et al. Supplemental oxygen and exercise performance in patients with cystic fibrosis with severe pulmonary disease. Chest 1992;101:52-57.

88. Nixon PA, Orenstein DM, Curtis SE, et al. Oxygen supplementation during exercise in cystic fibrosis. Am Rev Respir Dis 1990;142:807-811.

89. Fraser KL, Tullis DE, Sasson, Z, et al. Pulmonary hypertension and cardiac function in adult cystic fibrosis: role of hypoxemia. Chest 1999;115:1321-1328.

90. Khan TZ, Wagener JS, Bost T, et al. Early pulmonary inflammation in infants with cystic fibrosis. Am J Respir Crit Care Med 1995;151:1075-1082.

91. Gilligan PH. Microbiology of cystic fibrosis lung disease. In: Yankaskas JR, Knowles MR, editors. Cystic fibrosis in adults. Philadelphia: Lippincott-Raven; 1999. pp. 93-114.

92. Wilmott RW, Tyson SL, Matthew DJ. Cystic fibrosis survival rates: the influences of allergy and *Pseudomonas aeruginosa*. Am J Dis Child 1985;139:669-671.

93. Frederiksen B, Koch C, Hoiby N. Changing epidemiology of pseudomonas aeruginosa infection in Danish cystic fibrosis patients (1974-1995). Pediatr Pulmonol 1999;28:159-166.

94. Frederiksen B, Koch C, Hoiby N. Antibiotic treatment of initial colonization with *Pseudomonas aeruginosa* postpones chronic infection and prevents deterioration of pulmonary function in cystic fibrosis. Pediatr Pulmonol 1997;23:330-335.

95. Valerius NH, Koch C, Hoiby N. Prevention of chronic *Pseudomonas aeruginosa* colonisation in cystic fibrosis by early treatment. Lancet 1991;338:725-726.

96. Lewin LO, Byard PJ, Davis PB. Effect of *Pseudomonas cepacia* colonization on survival and pulmonary function of cystic fibrosis patients. J Clin Epidemiol 1990;43:125-131.

97. Holmes A, Nolan R, Taylor R, et al. An epidemic of *Burkholderia cepacia* transmitted between patients with and without cystic fibrosis. J Infect Dis 1999;179:1197-1205.

98. Sun L, Jiang RZ, Steinbach S, et al. The emergence of a highly transmissible lineage of cbl+ *Pseudomonas (Burkholderia) cepacia* causing CF centre epidemics in North America and Britain. Nat Med 1995;1:661-666.

99. Goldstein R, Sun L, Jiang RZ, et al. Structurally variant classes of pilus appendage fibers coexpressed from *Burkholderia (Pseudomonas) cepacia*. J Bacteriol 1995;177:1039-1052.

100. LiPuma JJ, Dasen SE, Nielson DW, et al. Person-to-person transmission of *Pseudomonas cepacia* between patients with cystic fibrosis. Lancet 1990;336:1094-1096.

101. Cystic Fibrosis Foundation, Patient Registry 1997 Annual Data Report. Bethesda, Md; 1998.

102. Geller DE, Kaplowitz H, Light MJ, et al. Allergic bronchopulmonary aspergillosis in cystic fibrosis: reported prevalence, regional distribution, and patient characteristics. Scientific advisory group, investigators, and coordinators of the epidemiologic study of cystic fibrosis. Chest 1999;116:639-646.

103. Knutsen A, Slavin RG. Allergic bronchopulmonary mycosis complicating cystic fibrosis. Semin Respir Infect 1992;7:179-192.

104. Whittier S, Hopfer RL, Knowles MR, et al. Improved recovery of mycobacteria from respiratory secretions of patients with cystic fibrosis. J Clin Microbiol 1993;31:861-864.

105. Kilby JM, Gilligan PH, Yankaskas JR, et al. Nontuberculous mycobacteria in adult patients with cystic fibrosis. Chest 1992;102:70-75.

106. Stern RC, Wood RE, Boat TF, et al. Treatment and prognosis of massive hemoptysis in cystic fibrosis. Am Rev. Respir Dis 1978;117:825-828.

107. Fellows KE, Khaw KT, Schuster S, et al. Bronchial artery embolization in cystic fibrosis; technique and long-term results. J Pediatr 1979;95:959-963.

108. Brinson GM, Noone PG, Mauro MA, et al. Bronchial artery embolization for the treatment of hemoptysis in patients with cystic fibrosis. Am J Respir Crit Care Med 1998;157:1951-1958.

109. Schidlow DV, Taussig LM, Knowles MR. Cystic fibrosis foundation consensus conference report on pulmonary complications of cystic fibrosis. Pediatr Pulmonol 1993;15:187-198.

110. Spector ML, Stern, RC. Pneumothorax in cystic fibrosis: a 26-year experience. Ann Thorac Surg 1989;47:204-207.

111. Yankaskas JR, Egan TM, Mauro MA. Major complications. In: Yankaskas JR, Knowles MR, editors. Cystic fibrosis in adults. Philadelphia: Lippincott-Raven; 1999. pp. 175-193.

112. Nocturnal oxygen therapy trial group. Continuous or nocturnal oxygen therapy in hypoxemic chronic obstructive lung disease: a clinical trial. Ann Intern Med 1980;93:391-398.

113. Spier S, Rivlin J, Hughes D, et al. The effect of oxygen on sleep, blood gases, and ventilation in cystic fibrosis. Am Rev Respir Dis 1984;129:712-718.

114. Davis PB, di Sant'Agnese PA. Assisted ventilation for patients with cystic fibrosis. JAMA 1978;239:1851-1854.

115. Garland JS, Chan YM, Kelly KJ, et al. Outcome of infants with cystic fibrosis requiring mechanical ventilation for respiratory failure. Chest 1989;96:136-138.

116. Sood S, Paradowski LJ, Yankaskas JR. Outcomes of ICU care in adults with cystic fibrosis. Am J Respir Crit Care Med 2000 (in press).

117. Piper AJ, Parker S, Torzillo PJ, et al. Nocturnal nasal IPPV stabilizes patients with cystic fibrosis and hypercapnic respiratory failure. Chest 1992;102:846-850.

118. Hodson ME, Madden BP, Steven MH, et al. Non-invasive mechanical ventilation for cystic fibrosis patients: a potential bridge to transplantation. Eur Respir J 1991;4:524-527.

119. Desmond KJ, Schwenk WF, Thomas E, et al. Immediate and long-term effects of chest physiotherapy in patients with cystic fibrosis. J Pediatr 1983;103:538-542.

120. Thomas J, Cook DJ, Brooks D. Chest physical therapy management of patients with cystic fibrosis: a meta-analysis. Am J Respir Crit Care Med 1995;151:846-850.

121. Mortensen J, Falk M, Groth S, et al. The effects of postural drainage and positive expiratory pressure physiotherapy on tracheobronchial clearance in cystic fibrosis. Chest 1991;100:1350-1357.

122. Oberwaldner B, Evans JC, Zach MS. Forced expirations against a variable resistance: a new chest physiotherapy method in cystic fibrosis. Pediatr Pulmonol 1986;2:358-367.

123. Gondor M, Nixon PA, Mutich R, et al. Comparison of flutter device and chest physical therapy in the treatment of cystic fibrosis pulmonary exacerbation. Pediatr Pulmonol 1999;28:255-260.

124. Konstan MW, Stern RC, Doershuk CF. Efficacy of the flutter device for airway mucus clearance in patients with cystic fibrosis. J Pediatr 1994;124:689-693.

125. Baldwin DR, Hill AL, Peckham DG, et al. Effect of addition of exercise to chest physiotherapy on sputum expectoration and lung function in adults with cystic fibrosis. Respir Med 1994;88:49-53.

126. Hansen LG, Warwick WJ. High-frequency chest compression system to aid in clearance of mucus from the lung. Biomed Instrum Technol 1990;24:289-294.

127. Warwick WJ, Hansen LG. The long-term effect of high-frequency chest compression therapy on pulmonary complications of cystic fibrosis. Pediatr Pulmonol 1991;11:265-271.

128. Arens R, Gozal D, Omlin KJ, et al. Comparison of high frequency chest compression and conventional chest physiotherapy in hospitalized patients with cystic fibrosis. Am J Respir Crit Care Med 1994;150:1154-1157.

129. Fuchs HJ, Borowitz DS, Christiansen DH, et al. Effect of aerosolized recombinant human DNase on exacerbations of respiratory symptoms and on pulmonary function in patients with cystic fibrosis. The Pulmozyme Study Group. N Engl J Med 1994;331:637-642.

130. Robinson M, Hemming AL, Regnis JA, et al. Effect of increasing doses of hypertonic saline on mucociliary clearance in patients with cystic fibrosis. Thorax 1997;52:900-903.

131. Robinson M, Regnis JA, Bailey DL, et al. Effect of hypertonic saline, amiloride, and cough on mucociliary clearance in patients with cystic fibrosis. Am J Respir Crit Care Med 1996;153:1503-1509.

132. Daviskas E, Anderson SD, Gonda I, et al. Inhalation of hypertonic saline aerosol enhances mucociliary clearance in asthmatic and healthy subjects. Eur Respir J 1996;9:725-732.

133. Ballmann M, Hardt H vd. Hypertonic saline and recombinant human DNase: a randomised cross-over pilot study in patients with cystic fibrosis. Pediatr Pulmonol Suppl 1998:A488.

134. Eng PA, Morton J, Douglass JA, et al. Short-term efficacy of ultrasonically nebulized hypertonic saline in cystic fibrosis. Pediatr Pulmonol 1996;21:77-83.

135. Rodwell LT, Anderson SD. Airway responsiveness to hyperosmolar saline challenge in cystic fibrosis: a pilot study. Pediatr Pulmonol 1996;21:282-289.

136. Loening-Baucke VA, Mischler E, Myers MG. A placebo-controlled trial of cephalexin therapy in the ambulatory management of patients with cystic fibrosis. J Pediatr 1979;95:630-637.

137. Branger C, Fournier JM, Loulergue J, et al. Epidemiology of *Staphylococcus aureus* in patients with cystic fibrosis. Epidemiol Infect 1994;112:489-500.

138. Ramsey BW, Pepe MS, Quan JM, et al. Intermittent administration of inhaled tobramycin in patients with cystic fibrosis. Cystic fibrosis inhaled tobramycin study group. N Engl J Med 1999;340:23-30.

139. Jensen T, Pedersen SS, Garne S, et al. Colistin inhalation therapy in cystic fibrosis patients with chronic pseudomonas aeruginosa lung infection. J Antimicrob Chemother 1987;19:831-838.

140. Frederiksen B, Lanng S, Koch C, et al. Improved survival in the Danish center-treated cystic fibrosis patients: results of aggressive treatment. Pediatr Pulmonol 1996;21:153-158.

141. Hordvik NL, Konig P, Morris D, et al. A longitudinal study of bronchodilator responsiveness in cystic fibrosis. Am Rev Respir Dis 1985;131:889-893.

142. Hordvik NL, Sammut PH, Judy CG, et al. Effects of standard and high doses of salmeterol on lung function of hospitalized patients with cystic fibrosis. Pediatr Pulmonol 1999;27:43-53.

143. Hordvik NL, Sammut PH, Judy CG, et al. The effects of albuterol on the lung function of hospitalized patients with cystic fibrosis. Am J Respir Crit Care Med 1996;154:156-160.

144. Konig P, Poehler J, Barbero GJ. A placebo-controlled, double-blind trial of the long-term effects of albuterol administration in patients with cystic fibrosis. Pediatr Pulmonol 1998;25:32-36.

145. Sanchez I, De Koster J, Holbrow J, et al. The effect of high doses of inhaled salbutamol and ipratropium bromide in patients with stable cystic fibrosis. Chest 1993;104:842-846.

146. Auerbach HS, Williams M, Kirkpatrick JA, et al. Alternate-day prednisone reduces morbidity and improves pulmonary function in cystic fibrosis. Lancet 1985;2:686-688.

147. Eigen H, Rosenstein BJ, Fitzsimmons S, et al. A multicenter study of alternate-day prednisone therapy in patients with cystic fibrosis. Cystic fibrosis foundation prednisone trial group. J Pediatr 1995;126:515-523.

148. Rosenstein BJ, Eigen H. Risks of alternate-day prednisone in patients with cystic fibrosis. Pediatrics 1991;87:245-246.

149. Bisgaard H, Pedersen SS, Nielsen KG, et al. Controlled trial of inhaled budesonide in patients with cystic fibrosis and chronic bronchopulmonary psuedomonas aeruginosa infection. Am J Respir Crit Care Med 1997;156:1190-1196.

150. Konstan MW, Byard PJ, Hoppel CL, et al. Effect of high-dose ibuprofen in patients with cystic fibrosis. N Engl J Med 1995; 332(13):848-854.

151. Cohen RG, Barr ML, Schenkel FA, et al. Living-related donor lobectomy for bilateral lobar transplantation in patients with cystic fibrosis. Ann Thorac Surg 1994;57:1423-1427.

152. Yankaskas JR, Mallory GB Jr. Lung transplantation in cystic fibrosis: consensus conference statement. Chest 1998;113: 217-226.

CHAPTER 52

Acute Respiratory Distress Syndrome

Margaret J. Neff
Kenneth P. Steinberg

CHAPTER OUTLINE

OBJECTIVES

1. Define the acute respiratory distress syndrome (ARDS).
2. List common risk factors for ARDS.
3. Discuss the difficulties in estimation of the incidence of ARDS.
4. Recognize the clinical, radiographic, and pathophysiologic features of ARDS.
5. Describe the pathogenesis of ARDS.
6. Discuss the experimental and proven therapeutic interventions for ARDS, including pharmacologic and mechanical therapies.
7. Describe how ARDS affects patients' long-term physical functioning and quality of life.

KEY TERMS

Acute Lung Injury (ALI)
Acute Respiratory Distress Syndrome (ARDS)

Diffuse Alveolar Damage
Fibroproliferative
Hydrostatic Pulmonary Edema

Hypoxic Pulmonary Vasoconstriction
Permeability Pulmonary Edema

Acute respiratory distress syndrome (ARDS)—the words roll off your tongue as you describe this disease to a family for whom ARDS is an entirely new concept. How can their 25-year-old son who survived a motorcycle collision, ruptured spleen, and fractured femur now be facing a life-threatening respiratory illness when his lungs were not injured? Although this may be an alien concept to the families involved, this scenario is familiar territory for most critical care practitioners. Having a solid understanding of the epidemiology, diagnosis, and management of ARDS will help practitioners communicate with patients and families during such conversations and will further their own understanding of this disease process.

Definition and Incidence

Critical to a description of the incidence of any process is the ability to accurately define the disease, in this case ARDS. Since the first clinical description of ARDS was established in 1967, efforts have been ongoing to better understand the pathophysiology leading to lung injury and to better define this process.[1] Inexact definitions can lead to the study of a heterogeneous population of patients with different clinical characteristics, outcomes, and responses to interventions. In an attempt to address this problem, an international conference was convened in 1992 to standardize the definition of **acute lung injury (ALI)** and ARDS. This meeting, the American-European

TABLE 52-1

American-European Consensus Conference Definition of ALI and ARDS

Condition	Pao_2/Fio_2*	CXR	PAWP
ALI	≤300 mm Hg	Bilateral infiltrates seen on frontal chest radiograph	≤18 mm Hg when measured or no clinical evidence of left atrial hypertension
ARDS	≤200 mm Hg	Bilateral infiltrates seen on frontal chest radiograph	≤18 mm Hg when measured or no clinical evidence of left atrial hypertension

From Bernard GR, Artigas A, Brigham KL, et al. The American-European Consensus Conference on ARDS: definitions, mechanisms, relevant outcomes, and clinical trial coordination. Am J Respir Crit Care Med 1994;149:818-824.
ALI, Acute lung injury; ARDS, acute respiratory distress syndrome; CXR, chest radiograph; PAWP, pulmonary artery wedge pressure.
*Regardless of level of PEEP.

Consensus Conference (AECC), resulted in criteria recommended for use in the identification of patients with ALI and ARDS.[2] ALI is characterized by the abrupt onset of respiratory distress and is associated with severe hypoxemia and diffuse pulmonary opacities on chest radiograph (CXR) that are not caused by congestive heart failure or volume overload. ARDS is a more severe form of this lung injury (Table 52-1). Pathologically, ALI/ARDS is characterized by acute alveolar inflammation, surfactant deficiencies, damage to the alveolar epithelium and capillary endothelium, and development of proteinaceous pulmonary edema and alveolar collapse. These definitions for ALI and ARDS refer to an acute process and, as such, exclude chronic lung disorders such as interstitial lung disease or sarcoidosis that might also meet the oxygenation and radiographic criteria for this process. Mechanical ventilation, although very common in patients with this degree of lung dysfunction, is not a requirement for the definition. Additionally, even though several risk factors are known to be associated with ALI/ARDS, a predisposing risk factor is not required for the diagnosis of ALI/ARDS.

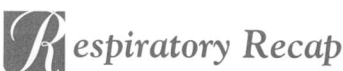

Respiratory Recap

Definitions of ALI and ARDS
Abrupt onset of respiratory distress
Severe hypoxemia
Diffuse pulmonary infiltrates
ARDS = more severe form of ALI

This effort to standardize the definition of ALI/ARDS was an important step toward the identification of a more homogeneous population of patients. However, several unresolved issues arose during these discussions that need further investigation. For example, neither the level of positive end-expiratory pressure (PEEP) nor lung compliance is incorporated into this definition despite these measures of function often being abnormal in these patients. In effect, other than the Pao_2/Fio_2 (P/F) ratio, the definition does not allow quantification of severity.

One potential solution to characterize the severity of lung injury is the use of the Lung Injury Score developed by Murray, et al.[3] It incorporates the level of PEEP, P/F ratio, a CXR score, and lung compliance into a summary score that can be used to describe the severity of lung injury and to follow the course of the disease.[3] Although not a part of the AECC ALI/ARDS definition, it could be useful when used in conjunction with this definition.

Another unresolved issue is the evaluation of the chest radiograph, which can be complicated by the presence of pleural effusions or atelectasis and the radiographic technique (Figure 52-1). A survey of experts reading a series of CXRs revealed a range of 36% to 71% of the CXRs being read as consistent with the AECC definition of ALI/ARDS.[4] The reading of CXRs has yet to be standardized.

Similarly, the requirement for a pulmonary artery wedge pressure (PAWP) of less than or equal to 18 mm Hg or no clinical evidence of left atrial hypertension (LAH) remains an inexact way to exclude those patients whose respiratory failure is due solely to heart failure. Although it can be a useful tool, the PAWP also can be fraught with inaccuracy. Variability in readings can occur as a result of catheter placement in the different branches of the pulmonary artery, interobserver variability,[5] and elevations in the pressure reading caused by increased intrathoracic pressure as occurs in the application of PEEP. As a result, under a variety of conditions PAWP may not provide a reliable estimate of intravascular volume.[6-8] The AECC stated that ALI/ARDS "cannot be explained by, but may coexist with, left atrial or pulmonary capillary hypertension."[2] However, excluding all patients with PAWP greater than 18 mm Hg eliminates patients with a falsely elevated PAWP as well as those with a combination of heart failure and lung injury. In one study, this amounted to nearly one-third of all patients meeting CXR and P/F criteria for ARDS.[9] Further, in those cases where no PAWP is available, the definition requires clinical evidence of no LAH, yet there are no guidelines to direct the application of this rule. The number of patients meeting ALI/ARDS criteria can vary greatly depending on the criteria used to define clinical LAH,[10] an area for further evaluation.

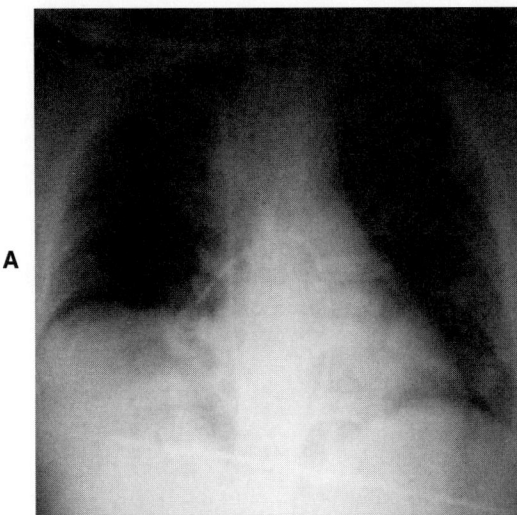

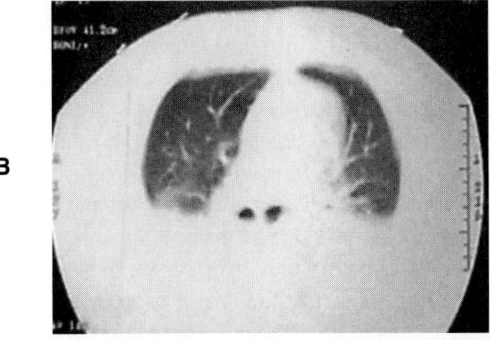

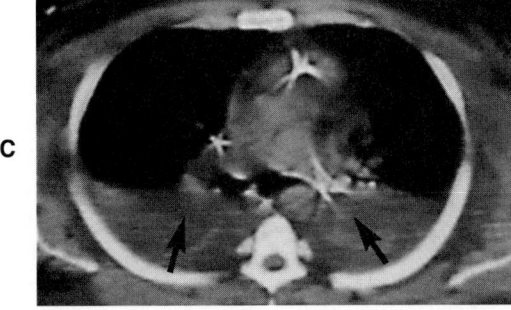

Figure 52-1 A, Chest x-ray film that meets the criteria for acute respiratory distress syndrome (ARDS), but when chest is viewed by computed tomography scan, **B** and **C,** abnormalities are shown to represent effusions without parenchymal involvement. (Arrows indicate pleural effusions.)

Although the current AECC definition of ALI/ARDS uses clinical criteria to identify patients, some investigators suggest that ALI/ARDS should be described as a syndrome characterized by alveolar inflammation and increased capillary permeability.[2,11-13] In addition to more closely reflecting the true pathophysiology of the disease, an approach focused on the underlying physiologic mechanisms may help identify a more homogeneous population of patients and may resolve issues related to PEEP, CXR interpretation, and volume status as described above. Ongoing efforts using analyses from edema fluid and bronchoalveolar lavage (BAL) fluid are attempting to address these issues.

Given these difficulties in the definition of ALI and ARDS, it is perhaps not surprising that studies attempting to describe the incidence of this disease have resulted in widely varying estimates. Many of the prior estimates of the incidence of ARDS preceded the AECC definition and as such used a variety of definitions, at times relying on investigator identification of cases and at other times using International Classification of Diseases (ICD9) coding. An initial report by the National Institutes of Health in 1972 estimated 75 cases of ARDS per 100,000 population (approximately 150,000 cases of ARDS per year) in the United States.[14] In contrast, more recent studies have found lower estimates of the incidence of ARDS, ranging from 3 to 13.5 cases per 100,000 population.[15-18]

Given the wide range of estimates for the incidence of ARDS, the need for better epidemiologic data is clear. Additional studies using AECC criteria and more exact definitions of the population at risk will help more accurately define the incidence of this disease. Ideally, it will also be possible to describe geographic and perhaps risk data that will help target research and clinical resources more effectively.

Clinical Risk Factors

Identification of patients at risk for the development of ALI/ARDS is important clinically for the purpose of research studies and for the application of potential therapeutic interventions. It is recognized that not all patients with ALI/ARDS have the same clinical course and outcome. In part, some of this variation is related to the initial insult. Risk factors can be described as those factors that cause direct injury to the lung, such as pneumonia, inhalation of toxic gases, or pulmonary contusion, and those that cause indirect injury to the lung, such as sepsis and multiple trauma. In the case of indirect injury, the insult is thought to be the result of systemic inflammation and is often associated with ARDS as well as other organ dysfunction. This distinction of pulmonary (direct injury) and extrapulmonary (indirect injury) is one that has been pursued by some investigators as a potential cause for different responses to interventions such as PEEP.[19] This distinction, although at times difficult to apply, was also adopted by the AECC.[2]

R̲espiratory Recap ———————————

Risk Factors for ARDS
Direct injury to the lungs such as pneumonia or aspiration Indirect injury to the lungs such as sepsis or nonthoracic trauma

Three studies, using patient populations from the early 1980s, attempted to identify the most common risk factors for ARDS.[20-22] Although each study was designed somewhat differently, taken as a whole they did identify

TABLE 52-2

*Frequency of ARDS Based on Risk Category**

Risk Factor	Number with ARDS/ Number at Risk (%)
Sepsis syndrome	56/136 (41.2)
Multiple transfusions (≥15 units of blood in 24 hr), trauma, and non-trauma–related	28/77 (36.4)
Trauma (pulmonary contusion, multiple fractures, and/or multiple transfusions)	45/188 (23.9)
Aspiration of gastric contents	13/59 (22.0)
Pulmonary contusion	12/55 (21.8)
Multiple fractures	7/63 (11.1)
Drug overdose	14/164 (8.0)
Near drowning	2/6 (33.0)

Hudson LD, Milberg JA, Anardi D, et al. Clinical risks for development of the acute respiratory distress syndrome. Am J Respir Crit Care Med 1995;151:293-301.
**Percentages are for each risk category.*
NOTE: *48 of 227 (21.1%) patients with ARDS did not have an identified risk factor.*

BOX 52-1

ARDS Risk Factors as Defined by the AECC

Direct Injury (Pulmonary Cause)	Indirect Injury (Extrapulmonary Cause)
Aspiration of gastric contents	Sepsis syndrome
Diffuse pulmonary infection	Severe, nonthoracic trauma
Near-drowning	Hypertransfusion for emergency resuscitation
Toxic inhalation	Cardiopulmonary bypass (rare cause)
Lung contusion	

From Bernard GR, Artigas A, Brigham KL, et al. The American-European Consensus Conference on ARDS: definitions, mechanisms, relevant outcomes, and clinical trial coordination. Am J Respir Crit Care Med 1994;149:818-824.
ARDS, Acute respiratory distress syndrome; AECC, American-European Consensus Conference.

the most common risk factors for ARDS: sepsis, aspiration of gastric contents, multiple transfusions, and severe trauma (Table 52-2).[22] Building on these data, the AECC developed a list of risk factors for ARDS (Box 52-1).[2]

In addition to their role in the identification of those patients at greatest risk of developing ALI/ARDS, the previously mentioned risk factors also help anticipate the onset of ALI/ARDS. One study revealed that among those patients with a risk factor of sepsis, trauma, or aspiration, approximately 50% of those patients who developed ARDS did so within 24 hours of meeting risk criteria.[22] Nearly 85% of those who ultimately developed ARDS did so within the first 72 hours. In contrast to sepsis, in which 20% of ARDS patients with a sepsis risk met ARDS criteria on day 1 of risk, trauma patients had a slower onset of ARDS. This is likely the result of the more acute event in trauma, whereas sepsis may be "smoldering" for a number of days before being detected.[22,23] Despite attempts to standardize these risks, difficulties in the application of these risk factors still exist. Approximately 20% of patients who ultimately develop ARDS were not identified by these risk factors,[22] and the exact definition of each risk factor is at times indistinct. This is particularly the case with sepsis and multiple trauma, which can be interpreted quite differently. Despite these limitations, having defined ARDS risk factors can help in the management of these patients and in the selection of certain subsets of patients for clinical studies in which a high incidence of patients with ARDS is desired.

Clinical Manifestations

At the most basic clinical level, ALI and ARDS are processes that result in acute hypoxemic respiratory failure and pulmonary opacities. Although we know that these abnormalities are the result of an intense inflammatory response and an increase in vascular permeability of the lungs, it is rare that pathology is available to confirm the diagnosis. As such, these processes are often diagnosed on a clinical level with the definitions and risk factors described previously to identify patients.

Most patients identified as having ALI/ARDS are symptomatic with progressive dyspnea. The profound hypoxemia, for example a PaO_2 of 60 mm Hg on 0.50 FIO_2 (P/F ratio of 120), is primarily the result, in the early stages of lung injury, of intrapulmonary shunt.[24] These areas of absent ventilation relative to perfusion (low $\dot{V}/\dot{Q}$ regions or shunt) appear to be caused by atelectasis and alveolar flooding caused by the intense inflammation and capillary permeability known to play a major role in this disease. In addition, some disturbance in the normally protective mechanism of **hypoxic pulmonary vasoconstriction** contributes to the shunt physiology and hypoxemia.

Patients in the first few days of ARDS also demonstrate a decrease in lung compliance, partly because of the alveo-

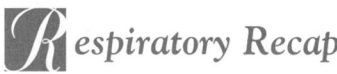

Respiratory Recap

Clinical Manifestations of ARDS	
Profound hypoxemia early in the disease course	Bilateral opacities on chest x-ray film
Decreased lung compliance	Heterogeneity of disease on chest computed tomography; dependent atelectasis
Rapid shallow breathing pattern	
Increased dead space	

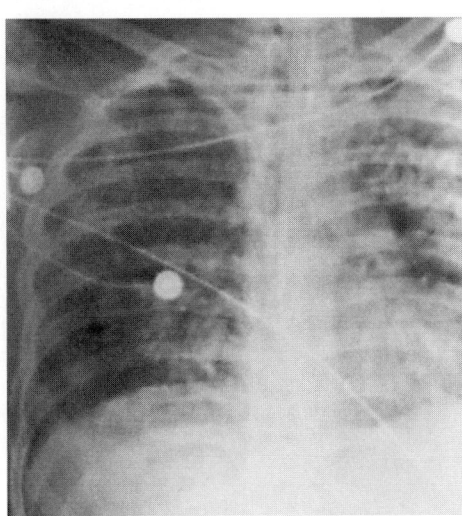

Figure 52-2   Chest radiograph taken 24 hours after severe trauma to the abdomen and lower extremity.

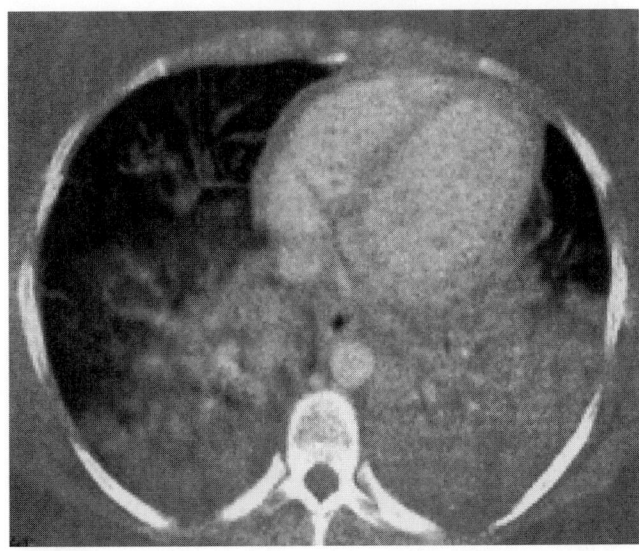

Figure 52-3   Computed tomography (CT) scan of chest demonstrating heterogeneity of acute respiratory distress syndrome (ARDS).

lar and interstitial edema, but also because of loss of surfactant function. Decreased compliance and hypoxemia together lead to rapid, shallow breaths in those still spontaneously breathing with increased minute ventilation and work of breathing. This combination of events usually culminates in the need for mechanical ventilatory support.

In patients for whom this process continues longer than 3 to 7 days, the clinical characteristics often change. Profound hypoxemia may subside, but poor compliance often continues, in part because of the initiation of fibrosis. Rather than intrapulmonary shunt, the problem at this phase, known as the **fibroproliferative** phase of ARDS, is increasing dead space (high $\dot{V}/\dot{Q}$ regions) resulting in increasing minute ventilatory requirements. It is not uncommon to see dead space calculations in excess of 70%. This increased dead space is in part the result of fibrosis, as well as obstruction and destruction of pulmonary capillaries from microthrombi and distortion from the fibrosis. These effects can lead to pulmonary hypertension and, in some cases, to right heart dysfunction.[25]

Unfortunately, no clearly identified systemic markers exist that are specific to ALI/ARDS. Although evidence of systemic inflammation and often dysfunction of other organ systems can be found, these are commonly caused by the underlying disease process and not solely a result of pulmonary dysfunction. Evaluation of lung fluids to more specifically investigate the presence of alveolar inflammation and edema has shown promise and is discussed below with regard to pathogenesis of the disease.

By definition, the CXR should show bilateral opacities consistent with pulmonary edema. The opacities may be confluent, patchy, or asymmetric but not fully explained by atelectasis or effusions—conditions that can complicate the interpretation of the CXR. Radiographic abnormalities may occur before profound hypoxemia or may lag behind clinical manifestations. Because ALI and ARDS represent a spectrum of disease, the CXR may also range from mild edema to profound white-out, both extremes meeting the CXR criterion for a diagnosis of ALI or ARDS. In the case of the 25-year-old trauma patient described at the beginning of this discussion, his initial CXR was clear but within 24 hours revealed diffuse alveolar infiltrates consistent with his hypoxemia and poor compliance (Figure 52-2). Subsequent chest x-ray films in patients with persistent ARDS may reveal evidence of barotrauma such as pneumothoraces, pneumomediastinum, or pneumatoceles.

Despite the diffuse appearance on CXR, ALI/ARDS is not a homogeneous process. Although not commonly obtained for the sole purpose of a diagnosis of ALI/ARDS, computed tomography (CT) of the chest has demonstrated the profound heterogeneity of this disease (Figure 52-3).[26,27] More dependent (posterior) portions of the lung often demonstrate greater atelectasis than the more anterior, better ventilated areas. This also may be reflected by the differential response to PEEP seen in these different regions of the lung.[28]

Pathogenesis

Despite more than 30 years of research attempting to identify the specific cause of the lung injury seen in ALI and ARDS, the exact molecular basis is still unclear. What is clear is the intense inflammation and increased permeability seen early in the course of the disease. Injury to the endothelium, epithelium, and interstitium is implicated. The preponderance of neutrophils in the pulmonary edema fluid and in BAL fluid has led to the suggestion that the neutrophil itself, the cytokines released, or other toxic products released from the neutrophil may be responsible for the direct injury to the lung. The exact mechanism, however, remains unknown.

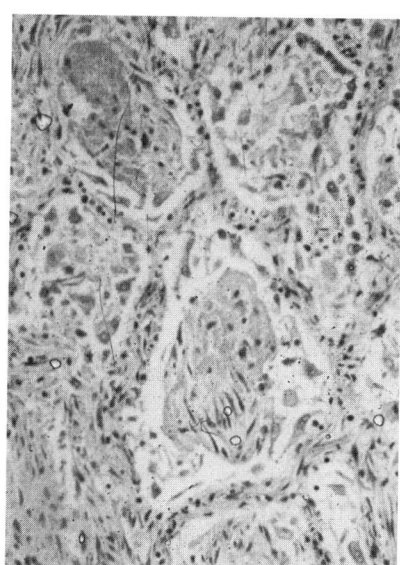

Figure 52-4   Diffuse alveolar damage noted on the biopsy of a patient with acute respiratory distress syndrome (ARDS).

Part of the initial injury is manifested by destruction of the type I alveolar epithelial cells, which are seen to become rapidly detached from the underlying basement membrane, contributing to the increased permeability and resultant influx of protein-rich edema fluid into the interstitium and alveolar space. Rapidly, this denuded basement membrane becomes covered with a layer of fibrin, known as the *hyaline membrane*. This constellation of findings is described pathologically as **diffuse alveolar damage** (Figure 52-4). In patients with persistent lung injury, this process progresses to a more fibrotic stage, generally 3 to 7 days after commencement of lung injury, which is characterized by proliferation of alveolar type II cells. This fibrosis, in addition to contributing to the poor compliance of the lung, can contribute to loss of the alveolar-vascular interface. Additional destruction of the pulmonary vasculature caused by fibrosis and in-situ thrombosis can lead to pulmonary hypertension.[13,25]

Although no clinically available systemic marker exists that correlates with lung injury, the study of pulmonary edema fluid and BAL fluid in patients with ALI and ARDS has been important in the acquisition of knowledge about the inflammatory response in the lungs of these patients. Comparison of the protein concentration in pulmonary edema fluid to the protein concentration in plasma soon after initiation of mechanical ventilation for respiratory failure has shown a consistently higher ratio in patients with **permeability pulmonary edema** (ALI and ARDS) than in patients with **hydrostatic pulmonary edema** (heart failure).[29] Bronchoscopy with BAL has been shown to be safe in this population[30] and has been used in an attempt to find cells or inflammatory mediators that may identify patients at risk for ALI/ARDS or may predict which patients have a worse prognosis.

No one marker has proven to be both sensitive and specific as a tool, but BAL results have provided a better understanding of the inflammation occurring in the alveolar space.[31-33] For instance, analysis of BAL fluid in patients with ARDS reveals a high percentage of neutrophils, usually present in only trace amounts in a normal lung lavage. As lung injury progresses, these neutrophils tend to be replaced with alveolar macrophages. However, patients noted to have a persistence of alveolar neutrophils have a higher mortality rate.[34,35]

Procollagen peptides, surfactant proteins, and other cellular mediators are also being explored in an attempt to better understand the inflammatory response and to identify more specific markers to reflect the actual injury to both the endothelial and epithelial surfaces.[36,37] As important as any one marker is, the balance of proinflammatory and antiinflammatory cytokines may be even more important.[38] These issues are targets for future study with edema fluid and BAL in patients who are both at risk for and have been diagnosed with ALI or ARDS.

Management

Even after years of clinical research and trials, there as yet remains no specific pharmacologic agent to cure ALI/ARDS. Encouraging are the recent results of a large, multicenter, randomized, controlled trial showing a 25% reduction in mortality based on how these patients were mechanically ventilated.[39] However, despite past or future clinical trial results, an important aspect of the care of patients with ALI/ARDS is paying close attention to detail while providing supportive care. Avoiding intensive care unit (ICU)–related complications such as stress gastritis, deep venous thrombosis, and ventilator-associated pneumonia can have a substantial impact on patients' outcomes.

An additional goal, as is true for all critically ill patients, is the maintenance of adequate end-organ perfusion. This is no different for patients with ALI/ARDS but can be complicated by the desire to keep the lungs dry.[40,41] Although the pulmonary edema seen on CXR in patients with lung injury is not solely the result of volume overload, the capillary permeability that is part of this syndrome can potentiate additional edema formation in the setting of elevated transalveolar pressures. On the other hand, aggressive restriction of fluids can lead to volume depletion, hypotension, and end-organ dysfunction with ultimately more serious consequences. There is no right answer about how much fluid to give or at what value to keep a patient's PAWP. The best approach is to maintain organ perfusion with the least volume necessary. In cases where this still results in an elevated PAWP, the secondary goal would be to facilitate diuresis as soon as the inflammatory response necessitating the volume resuscitation has resolved.

Pharmacologic Agents

Many potential medications have been proposed in the therapy of patients with ALI and ARDS. Common targets of these medications have included the inflammatory response, oxygen radical production, and physiologic abnormalities such as $\dot{V}/\dot{Q}$ mismatch. Although some of these agents have shown improvement in some surrogate endpoints, none have proven effective at reducing mortality in patients with ALI/ARDS.

Given the discussion of the intense inflammatory response used to describe the pathogenesis of this disease, the use of corticosteroids makes empiric sense given their function as potent inhibitors of inflammation. However, as is becoming more apparent through the study of inflammation, as important as any one inflammatory mediator is the balance of proinflammatory and antiinflammatory mediators.[38] This balance may, in part, help researchers understand the failure of trials to date. Corticosteroids used early in the course of ARDS have not proven beneficial,[42,43] and several recent, small studies have not convincingly proven the benefit of steroids in the late, fibroproliferative phase of ARDS. One of these trials demonstrated an improvement in lung injury score and mortality, but the small sample size and crossover design of the trial warrant further confirmation of the results.[44] In this regard, there is currently an ongoing randomized controlled trial sponsored by the National Institutes of Health of corticosteroids in late-stage ARDS that may provide more definitive evidence either for or against steroid use for this disease. Other antiinflammatory agents such as ibuprofen, ketoconazole, and lisophylline have been ineffective in large randomized trials.[45,46]

Some trials have pursued treatment with surfactant therapy.[47,48] Unlike in neonates where surfactant is depleted, in patients with ALI/ARDS not only is the surfactant decreased in amount but the remaining surfactant is also dysfunctional. Several different surfactant replacement products have been tried to date, including bovine or porcine preparations and synthetically derived preparations using recombinant DNA technology. In addition to different preparations, a variety of delivery devices have been used including aerosolization, direct segmental delivery by bronchoscopy, and instillation through the endotracheal tube. Trials to date have not had an impact on survival, but additional efforts are underway using different combinations of phospholipids and different surfactant proteins.

Given the necessary therapy with often high concentrations of oxygen, the development of oxygen-free radicals in the course of therapy for ALI/ARDS is likely unavoidable and makes antioxidant therapy an attractive option. Interventions with vitamin E or *N*-acetylcysteine have been pursued with varying results.[49-51] More recently reported were the results of a randomized trial comparing standard enteral feeding to a formula replete with antioxidants, fish oil, and borage oil.[52] The investigators saw less alveolar inflammation by BAL, shorter time on the ventilator and in the ICU, and fewer failures of other organs in those patients receiving the intervention. These results warrant further investigation to establish reproducibility and the ability to generalize these results to a broader patient population.

The agent that has engendered perhaps some of the most passionate discussion is the use of inhaled nitric oxide (NO). Physiologically this drug should be ideal in the setting of lung injury. It is a potent vasodilator that is delivered only to areas of adequate ventilation where it then crosses the capillary endothelium, causes site-specific vasodilation, and is then immediately inactivated. As a result of the rapid inactivation, this drug does not engender the systemic effects that can be seen by some other vasodilating agents, such as intravenous prostacyclin. As is seen in other uses of inhaled nitric oxide, for example, pulmonary hypertension of the newborn and right ventricular dysfunction after bypass surgery, inhaled nitric oxide can result in a decrease in pulmonary artery pressures, improved right ventricular function, and improved ventilation-perfusion matching leading to improved oxygenation.[53-55] Despite these advantages, when tested in two recent randomized trials of patients with ARDS, inhaled nitric oxide did not have an effect on mortality.[56,57]

Patient Position

Changes in body position could be expected to improve oxygenation and gas exchange, particularly in patients with very asymmetric disease where the lateral decubitus position may improve ventilation-perfusion matching. The use of prone positioning is based on its presumed ability to improve gas exchange by restoring ventilation to dorsal areas of the lung that were collapsed while in the supine position. This would only be of particular benefit if, when prone, the ventral areas of lung were not similarly compromised. Recent data suggest that this benefit is indeed achieved.[58] An alternate explanation is that prone positioning results in redirection of perfusion away from areas of shunt.[59] Several other studies also have shown improvement in oxygenation and ventilation.[60,61] In general, these and other studies have used varying regimens of the time spent prone. Clinical improvement appeared to be more predictable in those patients with pulmonary edema, that is, in those patients in the early, exudative phase of ARDS. In addition, although some studies have succeeded with this intervention in trauma patients, the potential for complications is higher.[62]

For all patients, this intervention should be done in a facility that is familiar with the procedure and that has the resources to safely perform the maneuver in order to lessen the chance of inadvertent removal of tubes and lines and the development of potentially debilitating pressure necroses, including ocular injury. As has been seen with other interventions, such as inhaled nitric oxide, prone position shows improvement in oxygenation without demonstrable effects on mortality. Further studies are required to determine if this intervention is likely to provide long-term benefits.

Ventilator Interventions

As ventilators have evolved, new modes and capabilities have been added to the management of patients with respiratory failure. By and large, there is no specific function so unique to one type of today's ventilators that would make it clearly the best ventilator or mode to use in all patients with ALI and ARDS. However, PEEP, available on all modern ventilators, is used so commonly in patients with ALI/ARDS as to warrant a review of its effects and goals.

In some of the initial descriptions of ARDS, PEEP was observed to provide marked improvements in arterial oxygenation.[1] It was then postulated, but subsequently proven incorrect, that early application of PEEP might help prevent the onset of ARDS.[63] What is known is that PEEP can increase functional residual capacity by recruiting alveoli that have collapsed either as the result of low lung volumes or of loss of surfactant. The potential beneficial effects of PEEP from this recruitment include improved oxygenation, decreased intrapulmonary shunt, and improved compliance. Additionally, it is proposed that the shear force that results when alveoli constantly open and close can be eliminated by application of adequate levels of PEEP.[28,64] However, PEEP has some potential negative effects as well. By increasing intrathoracic pressure, it can decrease venous return and subsequently decrease cardiac output. Additionally, especially in patients with more heterogeneous disease, PEEP can result in overdistention of more normal alveoli and can result in barotrauma.[65] Also, this overdistention can cause increased resistance to blood flow to these ventilated areas, resulting in an increase in dead space.

Respiratory Recap

Management of ARDS

Most pharmacologic interventions have not proven useful.
Steroids may be of value in the fibroproliferative phase of the disease.
The prone position improves oxygenation in many patients with ARDS.
Effective ventilatory strategies include PEEP to maintain alveolar recruitment and low tidal volumes to avoid alveolar overdistention.

In some studies, the appropriate level of PEEP has been established by means of pressure-volume curves. In other studies it has been chosen empirically. It is difficult to predict who will benefit from PEEP and how much PEEP is needed. Application of PEEP requires close attention to ensure either improved oxygen delivery or the same oxygen delivery at lower FIO_2 and ventilatory support. Attention to blood pressure, compliance, and cardiac output (di-

Box 52-2

Protocol for Positive End-Expiratory Pressure Wean

1. Perform clinical assessment:
   - Hemodynamically stable and no signs of sepsis
   - PaO_2 ≥80 mm Hg on FIO_2 ≤0.40
   - No change in PEEP during past 12 hours
2. Obtain baseline respiratory and hemodynamic data, including ABGs.
3. Reduce PEEP level by 5 cm H_2O (2.5 if borderline oxygenation).
4. After 3 minutes, obtain ABG and return PEEP to previous level while awaiting results.
5. Compare baseline and 3-minute PaO_2 values:
   - If PaO_2 falls more than 20%, reduction in PEEP is not recommended and patient should remain at baseline PEEP level at least 6-12 hours before PEEP wean tried again
   - If PaO_2 falls more than 20%, PEEP may be decreased by 5 cm H_2O with repeat assessment for further PEEP wean during the next several hours

From Steinberg KP, Pierson DJ. In: Pierson DJ, Kacmarek RM, editors. Foundations of respiratory care. New York: Churchill Livingstone; 1992. pp. 721-739; and Hudson LD, Weaver LJ, Haisch CE, et al. Positive end-expiratory pressure: reduction and withdrawal. Respir Care 1988;33:613-617.
PEEP, Positive end-expiratory pressure; ABGs, arterial blood gas values.

rectly or by assessment of end-organ perfusion) is critical to ensure that benefit is being achieved by increasing levels of PEEP.

As important as careful application of PEEP is the successful withdrawal of PEEP. When applied successfully in patients with ALI/ARDS, PEEP should subsequently be weaned and not abruptly discontinued. Studies at Harborview Medical Center in Seattle revealed that successful weaning was less likely to result in set-backs, which often would require more than 24 hours to re-recruit atelectatic alveoli that were not ready for a reduction in PEEP. The ultimate protocol included a clinical assessment of a patient's readiness followed by a 3-minute reduction in PEEP by 5 cm H_2O with the PEEP returned to the prior level while awaiting arterial blood gas results. This prevented extensive de-recruitment in those patients who would be found not ready for PEEP reduction. A drop in PaO_2 of less than 20% implied an acceptable response (Box 52-2).[65,66]

The use of a lung-protective ventilation strategy, on the other hand, has now been shown to reduce mortality and should be widely employed in patients with ALI and ARDS. Historically, there has been extensive evidence to suggest that lung overdistention, as can occur with large tidal volumes, can result in increased permeability and pulmonary edema, lung inflammation, and poor outcomes.[64,67] Four randomized controlled trials of tidal volume reduction in humans were reported over the last 2 years.[68-71] All four trials used slightly different tidal volumes and PEEP strategies. Only the Amato trial[70] showed evidence of mortality reduction. The Ranieri trial[71] was the only one to evaluate lung inflammation and to show a decrease in alveolar inflammation in the lung protective group.

The data on stretch as a mechanism for ventilator-induced lung injury are confirmed by the recently reported multicenter, randomized, controlled trial that showed a 25% reduction in mortality for patients with ALI managed with a lung-protective strategy;[39] 861 patients were enrolled in this study and were randomized to either a tidal volume of 6 mL/kg (lung-protective) or 12 mL/kg (traditional), with weight based on predicted body weight (PBW). Plateau pressures were limited to 30 cm H_2O in the lung-protective group and 50 cm H_2O in the traditional group. A significant mortality difference was noted: 31% mortality in the lung-protective group compared to 40% in the traditional group. In addition, plasma interleukin-6 levels were noted to show a greater decrease between day 0 and 3 and to be lower overall on day 3 in the lung-protective group as compared to the traditional group. This fact supports the data previously reported by many investigators that one main effect of lung stretch was a propagation of systemic inflammation that could subsequently lead to other organ dysfunction and death.

These results are very important in that they confirm previous work and are immediately applicable to patients. It should be noted, though, that this protocol applies to patients with documented ALI and that the use of low tidal volumes prophylactically is not supported by these results. In addition, there are aspects of the study that cannot be taken apart. For instance, the lung-protective group also had lower plateau pressures, making it difficult, from this one study, to separate the effect of tidal volume from pressure. In effect, to have the best chance to realize the mortality reduction, clinicians need to reproduce the study protocol as closely as possible (Box 52-3).[72]

Outcomes

A successful trial in this patient population effectively means a reduction in mortality. Although other endpoints, often referred to as *surrogate endpoints,* could be chosen, it is not always clear that these would adequately translate to ultimate improved survival. For instance, both inhaled nitric oxide and prone positioning have been shown to improve oxygenation and ventilation-perfusion matching, but without a discrete mortality benefit. Although this may be the result of a small sample size or the need for a composite of interventions, it is generally felt that improvement in intermediate markers without an overall improvement in mortality is essentially a negative trial. Put another way, it is not necessarily of benefit to shorten the duration of mechanical ven-

---

Box 52-3

Lung-Protective Ventilation for Patients with Acute Lung Injury

Patient population: patients with ALI, using AECC criteria
Tidal volume: 6 mL/kg; weight based on predicted body weight
 Men: 50 + [2.3 × (Height in inches − 60)]
 Women: 45.5 + [2.3 × (Height in inches − 60)]
Oxygenation goal: Pao_2 55-80 mm Hg (or Spo_2 88%-95%)
Plateau pressure: ≤30 cm H_2O
 Tidal volume decreased to minimum of 4 mL/kg if plateau pressures exceed 30 cm H_2O
 Tidal volume may increase in increments of 1 mL/kg if refractory acidemia (pH <7.15) regardless of plateau pressure

Data from Acute Respiratory Distress Syndrome Clinical Network (ARDSnet). http://www.ardsnet.org.
ALI, *Acute lung injury;* AECC, *American-European Consensus Conference.*

---

tilation or ICU stay but still end with the death of the patient.

Given this defined mortality endpoint, what would be the prognosis for the 25-year-old trauma patient? In answering his family's questions, it would be useful to keep the following facts in mind. Approximately one third of the patients who will ultimately die do so within the first 72 hours. The cause of death in these patients is usually related to their underlying risk, for example, sepsis or trauma. Only a minority (15%) die from insupportable respiratory failure. The vast majority of ARDS patients who die do so in the setting of sepsis or multisystem organ failure.[73,74] These trends were originally seen in the epidemiology study done at Harborview Medical Center in the early 1980s and were re-confirmed when the subsequent 10 years' worth of data were analyzed.

Also notable in this earlier study was a nearly three-fold higher mortality for any particular risk when ARDS was diagnosed compared to patients with similar risk who did not develop ARDS. Overall, though, mortality rates have declined from 60% to 70% in the early 1980s to 30% to 40% in the mid-1990s. This trend was seen in the more recently analyzed Harborview data, as well as in the incidence study conducted in Sweden, Denmark, and Iceland where the 90-day mortality for patients with ALI and ARDS was approximately 40%.[18,75] A subsequent analysis of ARDS survivors compared to a matched cohort of critically ill controls showed no difference in long-term survival between these groups.[76] Another study evaluating the effect of age on survival echoed previous results that showed advanced age as being an independent risk factor for increased mortality in patients with ARDS.[77]

Although not necessarily used for primary study outcomes, assessments of pulmonary function, neuropsychiatric testing, and quality of life are important markers of a survivor's overall outcome. Pulmonary function tests performed as part of a prospective study were completed within 2 weeks of extubation and showed substantial restrictive impairments.[78] Pulmonary function improved at 3 months, and further improvement was seen at 6 months. Little additional improvement was noted at that point, and no further gains were noted at 1 year. Most patients returned to normal range at 1 year or had mild-to-moderate restriction, with an abnormal diffusing capacity being seen most commonly. This abnormal diffusing capacity is consistent with the known vascular destruction that occurs as part of the acute process. Whereas many patients require oxygen at the time of hospital discharge, a persistent gas exchange abnormality at 1 year is uncommon, except for desaturation occasionally seen with exercise. Ultimate lung function is most consistently associated with the severity of the original lung injury and with length of mechanical ventilation.

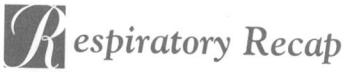espiratory Recap

---

ARDS Outcomes

Mortality is about 30% to 40%.

About one third of patients who die do so within the first 72 hours.

Mortality is usually not the result of inability to support lung function.

Most patients' lung function returns to near-normal within 1 year of discharge.

Many ARDS survivors have a lower than expected health-related quality of life and cognitive function.

The impact of ARDS on patients' quality of life also was assessed by comparison of these patients to non-ARDS patients with similar critical illness.[79] ARDS survivors were noted to have lower health-related quality of life scores, both generic and respiratory-specific, than the published data for normal subjects and lower scores than those for the critically ill control patients with severe sepsis and trauma. To assess less well–identified deficits, Hopkins, et al.[80] conducted neuropsychologic testing at discharge and then again 1 year later. When tested at the 1-year interval, one-third of the patients had generalized cognitive decline and three-fourths had at least one impairment in memory, attention, concentration, or mental processing speed. Although these outcomes of pulmonary function, quality of life, and cognitive functioning are not as clearly defined or as readily attainable as mortality, they do represent a significant impact on the lives of the sur-

vivors. Better understanding of these deficits will allow future research efforts to focus on these issues and will direct appropriate resources toward the care of these patients.

CASE STUDY

Case One
ARDS after Multiple Trauma

A 25-year-old man is admitted to the ICU after being in a motorcycle collision and sustaining a ruptured spleen and fractured femur. On admission his chest radiograph was clear but was noted to have bilateral infiltrates consistent with pulmonary edema by the next morning. With a PaO_2 of 50 mm Hg, a FIO_2 of 0.5 (P/F = 100), and a PAWP of 16 mm Hg, he was diagnosed with ARDS. This is not unexpected when more than one-third of patients with multiple transfusion (he received 20 units of blood within the first 24 hours as a result of his spleen and femur injuries) will develop ARDS. Initially his oxygenation was difficult to support but finally was responsive to PEEP. A PEEP trial revealed the best oxygenation at 15 cm H_2O. He was ventilated with a lung-protective strategy with a tidal volume of 410 mL. (He was 5'8" tall so his PBW = 50 + [2.3 × (68 − 60)] = 68.4 kg.) His plateau pressure was 28 cm H_2O, which was acceptable.

His mother appreciated all the information she was given and became interested in gaining a better understanding of this disease process. She was pleased that her son was benefiting from the results of past research, and she consented for her son to undergo serial bronchoscopy and lavage to help in ongoing research efforts. Consistent with his diagnosis of ARDS, his BAL fluid revealed a high percentage of neutrophils (80%) on day 3 of ARDS. On subsequent studies (days 7 and 14), this percentage steadily decreased and was replaced with alveolar macrophages. It was stressed to the mother that these results were not prognostic but that they were consistent with his overall improvement.

Despite problems with poor compliance (likely related to edema and fibrosis) and barotrauma, he did not develop sepsis. This single point likely led to his continued improvement and ultimate extubation at day 16. After learning about this disease process himself, he also wanted to take part in further studies and agreed to return to the hospital at regular intervals for evaluation of his pulmonary function and quality of life. It is hoped that ongoing, collaborative research will produce many more positive trials that will provide critical care practitioners with therapies and interventions that will improve mortality as well as subsequent function.

ℋℰ𝓨 𝒫ℴℐℕ𝒯𝒮

- Critical to any discussion or study of ALI/ARDS is an exact definition of the process. Current practice uses the AECC criteria for ALI and ARDS.
- Because of differences in definitions and study design, no clear national or worldwide incidence of ARDS can be estimated at this time.
- The most common risk factors for ARDS are sepsis, aspiration of gastric contents, multiple transfusions, and severe trauma.
- More than half of patients who develop ARDS will do so within 24 hours of the risk onset.
- ARDS is a heterogeneous disease and is characterized by an intense inflammation of the lung and increased permeability.
- There are no proven effective drug therapies for ARDS.
- The most important therapeutic advance for treatment of ARDS has been the identification of a lung-protective ventilatory strategy. This is based on the use of a tidal volume of 6 mL/kg PBW and plateau pressure less than 30 cm H_2O.
- Mortality for ARDS patients has decreased from nearly 70% in the 1980s to approximately 40% by the year 2000.
- Survivors are noted to have mild-to-moderate pulmonary restriction and decreased diffusing capacity on pulmonary function tests at 1 year. Additional decrements in quality of life and cognitive function also are noted.

References

1. Ashbaugh DG, Bigelow DB, Petty TL, et al. Acute respiratory distress in adults. Lancet 1967;12:319-323.
2. Bernard GR, Artigas A, Brigham KL, et al. The American-European consensus conference on ARDS: definitions, mechanisms, relevant outcomes, and clinical trial coordination. Am J Respir Crit Care Med 1994;149:818-824.
3. Murray JF, Matthay MA, Luce JM, et al. An expanded definition of the adult respiratory distress syndrome. Am Rev Resp Dis 1988;138:720.
4. Rubenfeld GD, Caldwell E, Granton J, et al. Interobserver variability in applying a radiographic definition for ARDS. Chest 1999;116:1347-1353.
5. Al-Kharrat T, Zarich S, Amoateng-Adjepong Y, et al. Analysis of observer variability in measurement of pulmonary artery occlusion pressures. Am J Respir Crit Care Med 1999;160:415-420.
6. Marinelli WA, Weinert CR, Gross CR, et al. Right heart catheterization in acute lung injury: an observational study. Am J Respir Crit Care Med 1999;160:69-76.
7. Dambrosio M, Fiore G, Brienza N, et al. Right ventricular myocardial function in ARF patients: PEEP as a challenge for the right heart. Intensive Care Med 1996;22:772-780.
8. Diebel LN, Myers T, Dulchavsky S. Effects of increasing airway pressure and PEEP on the assessment of cardiac preload. J Trauma 1997;42:585-591.
9. Neff MJ, Rubenfeld GD, Caldwell ES, et al. Exclusion of patients with elevated pulmonary capillary wedge pressure from acute respiratory distress syndrome. Am J Respir Crit Care Med 1999;159:A716.
10. Neff MJ, Caldwell ES, Hudson LD, et al. The effect of the definition of left atrial hypertension (LAH) on identification of patients with acute lung injury (ALI). American Thoracic Society International Conference 2001. Am J Respir Crit Care Med 2001;163:A449.
11. Abraham E, Matthay MA, Dinarello CA, et al. Consensus conference definitions for sepsis, septic shock, acute lung injury, and acute respiratory distress syndrome: time for a reevaluation. Crit Care Med 2000;28:232-235.
12. Abraham E. Toward new definitions of acute respiratory distress syndrome. Crit Care Med 1999;27:237-238.
13. Artigas A, Bernard GR, Carlet J, et al. The American-European Consensus Conference on ARDS. Part 2. Ventilatory, pharmacologic, supportive therapy, study design strategies, and issues related to recovery and remodeling. Am J Respir Crit Care Med 1998;157:1332-1347.
14. National Heart and Lung Institutes. Task force report on problems, research approaches, needs. Washington, DC: U.S. Government Printing Office; 1972. pp. 167-180.
15. Villar J, Slutsky AS. The incidence of the adult respiratory distress syndrome. Am Rev Respir Dis 1989;140:814-816.
16. Lewandowski K, Metz J, Deutschmann C, et al. Incidence, severity, and mortality of acute respiratory failure in Berlin, Germany. Am J Respir Crit Care Med 1995;151:1121-1125.
17. Thomsen GE, Morris AH. Incidence of the adult respiratory distress syndrome in the state of Utah. Am J Respir Crit Care Med 1995;152:965-971.
18. Luhr OR, Antonsen K, Karlsson M, et al. Incidence and mortality after acute respiratory failure and acute respiratory distress syndrome in Sweden, Denmark, and Iceland. The ARF Study Group. Am J Respir Crit Care Med 1999;159:1849-1861.
19. Gattinoni L, Pelosi P, Suter PM, et al. Acute respiratory distress syndrome caused by pulmonary and extrapulmonary disease: different syndromes? Am J Respir Crit Care Med 1998;158:3-11.
20. Pepe PE, Potkin RT, Reus DH, et al. Clinical predictors of the adult respiratory distress syndrome. Am J Surg 1982;144:124-130.
21. Fowler AA, Hamman RF, Good JT, et al. Adult respiratory distress syndrome: risk with common predispositions. Ann Intern Med 1983;98:593-597.
22. Hudson LD, Milberg JA, Anardi D, et al. Clinical risks for development of the acute respiratory distress syndrome. Am J Respir Crit Care Med 1995;151:293-301.
23. Hudson LD, Steinberg KP. Epidemiology of acute lung injury and ARDS. Chest 1999;116:74S-82S.
24. Steinberg KP. Diffuse pulmonary infiltrates and acute respiratory distress syndrome. In: Root RK, editor. Clinical infectious diseases: a practical approach. New York: Oxford University Press; 1999. pp. 557-564.
25. Maunder R, Pierson DJ. The acute respiratory distress syndrome. In: Pierson DJ, Kacmarek RM, editors. Foundations of respiratory care. New York: Churchill Livingstone; 1992. pp. 331-338.
26. Maunder RJ, Shuman WP, McHugh JW, et al. Preservation of normal lung regions in the adult respiratory distress syndrome: analysis by computed tomography. JAMA 1986;255:2463-2465.

27. Gattinoni L, Pesenti A. ARDS: the non-homogenous lung; facts and hypothesis. Crit Care Dig 1987;6:1-4.

28. Gattinoni L, Pelosi P, Crotti S, et al. Effects of positive end-expiratory pressure on regional distribution of tidal volume and recruitment in adult respiratory distress syndrome. Am J Respir Crit Care Med 1995;151:1807-1814.

29. Matthay MA, Wiener-Kronish JP. Intact epithelial barrier function is critical for the resolution of alveolar edema in humans. Am Rev Respir Dis 1990;142:1250-1257.

30. Steinberg KP, Mitchell DR, Maunder RJ, et al. Safety of bronchoalveolar lavage in patients with adult respiratory distress syndrome. Am Rev Respir Dis 1993;148:556-561.

31. Pugin J, Verghese G, Widmer M, et al. The alveolar space is the site of intense inflammatory and profibrotic reactions in the early phase of acute respiratory distress syndrome. Crit Care Med 1999;27:237-238.

32. Goodman RB, Strieter RM, Martin DP, et al. Inflammatory cytokines in patients with persistence of the acute respiratory distress syndrome. Am J Respir Crit Care Med 1996;154:601-611.

33. Martin TR. Lung cytokines and ARDS. Roger S. Mitchell lecture. Chest 1999;116:2S-8S.

34. Steinberg KP, Milberg JA, Martin TR, et al. Evolution of bronchoalveolar cell populations in the adult respiratory distress syndrome. Am J Respir Crit Care Med 1994;150:113-122.

35. Meduri GU, Headley S, Kohler G, et al. Persistent elevation of inflammatory cytokines predicts a poor outcome in ARDS. Plasma IL-1 and IL-6 levels are consistent and efficient predictors of outcome over time. Chest 1995;107:1062-1073.

36. Greene KE, Ye S, Mason RJ, et al. Serum surfactant protein-A levels predict development of ARDS in at-risk patients. Chest 1999;116:90S-91S.

37. Newman V, Gonzalez RF, Matthay MA, et al. A novel alveolar type I cell-specific biochemical marker of human acute lung injury. Am J Respir Crit Care Med 2000;161:990-995.

38. Martin TR. Cytokines and the acute respiratory distress syndrome (ARDS): a question of balance. Nature Med 1997;3:272-273.

39. The Acute Respiratory Distress Syndrome Network. Ventilation with lower tidal volumes as compared with traditional tidal volumes for acute lung injury and the acute respiratory distress syndrome. N Engl J Med 2000;342:1301-1308.

40. Simmons RS, Berdine GG, Seidenfeld JJ, et al. Fluid balance and the adult respiratory distress syndrome. Am Rev Respir Dis 1987;135:924-929.

41. Schrier RW, Abraham E. Aggressive volume expansion and pseudo-ARDS. Hosp Pract (Off Ed) 1995;30:19, 23.

42. Lefering R, Neugebauer EA. Steroid controversy in sepsis and septic shock: a meta-analysis. Crit Care Med 1995;23:1294-1303.

43. Cronin L, Cook DJ, Carlet J, et al. Corticosteroid treatment for sepsis: a critical appraisal and meta-analysis of the literature. Crit Care Med 1995;23:1430-1439.

44. Meduri GU, Headley AS, Golden E, et al. Effect of prolonged methylprednisolone therapy in unresolving acute respiratory distress syndrome: a randomized controlled trial. JAMA 1998;280:159-165.

45. The Acute Respiratory Distress Syndrome Network. Ketoconazole for early treatment of acute lung injury and acute respiratory distress syndrome: a randomized controlled trial. The ARDS Network. JAMA 2000;283:1995-2002.

46. Bernard GR, Wheeler AP, Russell JA, et al. The effects of ibuprofen on the physiology and survival of patients with sepsis. The Ibuprofen in Sepsis Study Group. N Engl J Med 1997;336:912-918.

47. Weg JG, Balk RA, Tharratt RS, et al. Safety and potential efficacy of an aerosolized surfactant in human sepsis-induced adult respiratory distress syndrome. JAMA 1994;272:1433-1438.

48. Gregory TJ, Steinberg KP, Spragg R, et al. Bovine surfactant therapy for patients with acute respiratory distress syndrome. Am J Respir Crit Care Med 1997;155:1309-1315.

49. Domenighetti G, Suter PM, Schaller MD, et al. Treatment with N-acetylcysteine during acute respiratory distress syndrome: a randomized, double-blind, placebo-controlled clinical study. J Crit Care 1997;12:177-182.

50. Jepsen S, Herlevsen P, Knudsen P, et al. Antioxidant treatment with N-acetylcysteine during adult respiratory distress syndrome: a prospective, randomized, placebo controlled study. Crit Care Med 1992;20:918-923.

51. Suter PM, Domenighetti G, Schaller MD, et al. N-acetylcysteine enhances recovery from acute lung injury in man. Chest 1994;105:190-194.

52. Gadek, JE, DeMichele SJ, Karlstad MD, et al. Effect of enteral feeding with eicosapentaenoic acid, gamma-linoleic acid, and antioxidants in patients with acute respiratory distress syndrome. Enteral Nutrition in ARDS Study Group. Crit Care Med 1999;27:1409-1420.

53. Rossaint R, Falke KJ, Lopez F, et al. Inhaled nitric oxide for the adult respiratory distress syndrome. N Engl J Med 1993;328:399-405.

54. Frostell CG, Blomqvist H, Hedenstierna G, et al. Inhaled nitric oxide selectively reverses human hypoxic pulmonary vasoconstriction without causing systemic vasodilation. Anesthesiology 1993;78:427-435.

55. Gerlach H, Rossaint R, Pappert D, et al. Time-course and dose-response of nitric oxide inhalation for systemic oxygenation and pulmonary hypertension in patients with adult respiratory distress syndrome. Eur J Clin Invest 1993;23:499-502.

56. Dellinger RP, Zimmerman JL, Taylor RW, et al. Effects of inhaled nitric oxide in patients with acute respiratory distress syndrome: results of a randomized phase II trial. Inhaled Nitric Oxide in ARDS Study Group. Crit Care Med 1998;26:15-23.

57. Michael JR, Barton RG, Saffle JR, et al. Inhaled nitric oxide versus conventional therapy: effect on oxygenation in ARDS. Am J Respir Crit Care Med 1998;157:1372-1380.

58. Albert RK, Hubmayr RD. The prone position eliminates compression of the lungs by the heart. Am J Respir Crit Care Med 2000;161:1660-1665.

59. Lamm WJE, Graham MM, Albert RK. Mechanism by which the prone position improves oxygenation in acute lung injury. Am J Respir Crit Care Med 1994;150:184-193.

60. Nakos G, Tsangaris I, Kostanti E, et al. Effect of the prone position on patients with hydrostatic pulmonary edema compared with patients with acute respiratory distress syndrome and pulmonary fibrosis. Am J Respir Crit Care Med 2000;161:360-368.

61. Jolliet P, Bulpa P, Chevrolet J. Effects of the prone position on gas exchange and hemodynamics in severe acute respiratory distress syndrome. Crit Care Med 1998;26:1977-1985.

62. Offner PJ, Haenel JB, Moore EE, et al. Complications of prone ventilation in patients with multisystem trauma with fulminant acute respiratory distress syndrome. J Trauma 2000;48:224-228.

63. Pepe PE, Hudson LD, Carrico CJ. Early application of positive end-expiratory pressure in patients at risk for the adult respiratory-distress syndrome. N Engl J Med 1984;311:281-286.

64. Webb HH, Tierney DF. Experimental pulmonary edema due to intermittent positive pressure ventilation with high inflation pressures: protection by positive end-expiratory pressure. Am Rev Respir Dis 1974;110:556-565.

65. Steinberg KP, Pierson DJ. Clinical approach to the patient with acute oxygenation failure. In: Pierson DJ, Kacmarek RM, editors. Foundations of respiratory care. New York: Churchill Livingstone; 1992. pp. 721-739.

66. Hudson LD, Weaver LJ, Haisch CE, et al. Positive end-expiratory pressure: reduction and withdrawal. Respir Care 1988; 33:613-617.

67. Dreyfuss D, Saumon G. Role of tidal volume, FRC, and end-inspiratory volume in the development of pulmonary edema following mechanical ventilation. Am Rev Respir Dis 1993; 148:1194-1203.

68. Brochard L, Roudot-Thoraval F, Roupie E, et al. Tidal volume reduction for prevention of ventilator-induced lung injury in acute respiratory distress syndrome. The Multicenter Trail Group on Tidal Volume reduction in ARDS. Am J Respir Crit Care Med 1998;158:1831-1838.

69. Stewart TE, Meade MO, Cook DJ, et al. Evaluation of a ventilation strategy to prevent barotrauma in patients at high risk for acute respiratory distress syndrome. N Engl J Med 1998; 338:355-361.

70. Amato MB, Barbas CS, Medeiros DM, et al. Effect of a protective-ventilation strategy on mortality in the acute respiratory distress syndrome. N Engl J Med 1998;338:347-354.

71. Ranieri VM, Suter PM, Tortorella C, et al. Effect of mechanical ventilation on inflammatory mediators in patients with acute respiratory distress syndrome: a randomized controlled trial. JAMA 1999;282:54-61.

72. Acute Respiratory Distress Syndrome Clinical Network (ARDSnet). http://www.ardsnet.org. 2001.

73. Hudson LD. Epidemiology of the adult respiratory distress syndrome. Semin Respir Crit Care Med 1994;15:254-259.

74. Montgomery AB, Stager MA, Carrico CJ, et al. Causes of mortality in patients with the adult respiratory distress syndrome. Am Rev Respir Dis 1985;132:485-489.

75. Milberg JA, Davis DR, Steinberg KP, et al. Improved survival of patients with acute respiratory distress syndrome (ARDS): 1983-1993. JAMA 1995;273:306-309.

76. Davidson TA, Rubenfeld GD, Caldwell ES, et al. The effect of acute respiratory distress syndrome on long-term survival. Am J Respir Crit Care Med 1999;160:1838-1842.

77. Sprenkle MD, Caldwell ES, Rubenfeld GD, et al. Mortality following acute respiratory distress syndrome (ARDS) among the elderly. Am J Respir Crit Care Med 1999;159:A717.

78. McHugh LG, Milberg JA, Whitcomb ME, et al. Recovery of function in survivors of the acute respiratory distress syndrome. Am J Respir Crit Care Med 1994;150:90-94.

79. Davidson TA, Caldwell ES, Curtis JR, et al. Reduced quality of life in survivors of acute respiratory distress syndrome compared with critically ill control patients. JAMA 1999;281:354-360.

80. Hopkins RO, Weaver LK, Pope D, et al. Neuropsychological sequelae and impaired health status in survivors of severe acute respiratory distress syndrome. Am J Respir Crit Care Med 1999;160:50-56.

CHAPTER 53

Postoperative Respiratory Care

Mark Simmons

OBJECTIVES

1. List the steps in preoperative assessment and management.
2. Identify factors that increase the risk of postoperative pulmonary complications.
3. List the studies commonly performed during preoperative testing.
4. Identify the intraoperative factors that contribute to postoperative pulmonary complications.
5. Describe the common assessment and management practices employed to combat postoperative respiratory failure.
6. Discuss the etiology, risk factors, clinical manifestations, diagnostic findings associated with atelectasis, and management of postoperative atelectasis.
7. Discuss the etiology, risk factors, clinical manifestations, diagnostic findings, and management of postoperative pulmonary embolism and thromboembolic disease.
8. Discuss the etiology, risk factors, clinical manifestations, diagnostic findings, and management of postoperative pneumonia.

KEY TERMS

Atelectasis	Myocardial Ischemia	Thrombolytic
Deep Vein Thrombosis (DVT)	Partial Thromboplastin Time (PTT)	Total Parenteral Nutrition (TPN)
Enteral Tube Feeding (ETF)	Patient-Controlled Analgesia (PCA)	Tissue Plasminogen Activator (TPA)
Heparin	Pulmonary Emboli (PE)	
Impedance Plethysmography	Pneumonia	

Over the past 25 years, great strides have been made in all aspects of care for the surgical patient including the preoperative, intraoperative, and postoperative phases. Despite these advances, however, pulmonary complications are the leading cause of postoperative morbidity and death.[1] Most patients having thoracic or upper abdominal surgery will have a decrease in pulmonary function after surgery. They experience decreased lung volumes, diaphragmatic dysfunction, and gas exchange abnormalities. However, many of these patients compensate for any decrease in pulmonary function with their pulmonary reserves. Postoperative pulmonary complications occur in approximately 6% to 8% of patients with normal preoperative lung function,[2] and respiratory failure is rare without preexisting cardiopulmonary or neuromuscular disorders. However, pulmonary complications with increased risk factors have been reported to be as high as 75%. This chapter addresses some of the preoperative, intraoperative, and postoperative factors that increase the risk of postoperative pulmonary complications and respiratory failure. Also included is management of the postoperative patient to prevent postoperative respiratory failure.

Preoperative Assessment and Management

The goal of preoperative evaluation is to identify patients who are at risk for intraoperative or postoperative complications. If a patient at risk is identified, the next step is to determine how complications can be prevented. In some cases it may mean a postponement in surgery or a change in the anesthesia or surgical plan. Other interventions include modification of risk factors such as smoking or obesity. The use of pulmonary medications and deep breathing exercises also may be appropriate for the prevention of postoperative complications.

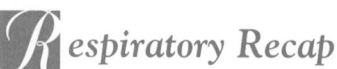
Respiratory Recap

Key Considerations in Preoperative Assessment and Management
A careful patient history
Detailed planning of surgery and postsurgical care and complications
Patient education

An important first step in preoperative management is a patient history. A careful history may identify conditions that could increase the risk of postoperative pulmonary complications and note indications for preoperative screening tests. Preoperative detailed planning of the surgery is necessary, including considerations for postoperative care and complications to avoid.

Preoperative patient education is important. The patient should be informed of the type of surgery planned, the pain intensity expected postoperatively, and the type of therapy after surgery. Preoperative instruction in planned postoperative respiratory care procedures is important for effective patient use after surgery.[3] When patients are educated about postoperative expectations, they require less analgesic in the postoperative period.[4]

Several factors have been identified as risk factors for postoperative complications (Box 53-1).

Age

Age is an independent morbidity and mortality risk for many diseases.[5] Increased postoperative complications occur in half of the patients more than 70 years old. In the elderly, evidence suggests a functional impact of Ca^{+2} blockers on mental function, so they should be avoided. Narcotics and sedatives can further compromise postoperative ventilatory function, leading to respiratory failure. Cardiopulmonary, hepatic, renal, and nervous system reserves are reduced in the elderly and this increases their susceptibility to decompensation.[6] Older people (more than 75 years) also have an augmented inflammatory response. These factors result in increased postoperative mortality rates.

Age-Specific Angle

The elderly are at increased risk for postoperative respiratory complications.

Box 53-2 lists pulmonary changes seen in the elderly patient. Because of these changes, the use of supplemental oxygen is suggested for any operative procedure in the elderly. The increased work of breathing that accompanies increased age compromises capacity to meet the additional workload demand following surgery and may contribute to postoperative respiratory failure.

Box 53-1

Patient Factors Increasing the Risk of Postoperative Pulmonary Complications

Increased age (>70 years)
Positive smoking history
Preexisting pulmonary disease (chronic bronchitis, emphysema, asthma)
Cardiac disease
Obesity
Poor nutritional status
Sputum production or chronic cough
History of shortness of breath
Low preoperative Pao_2

Box 53-2

Changes in Pulmonary and Thoracic Systems of Elderly Individuals

Increased rigidity of chest wall
Increased expenditure of energy to move chest wall
Decreased respiratory muscle strength (by 20% at age 70)
Decreased functional surface area for gas exchange (by 15% at age 70)
Increased $\dot{V}/\dot{Q}$ mismatch and decreased Pao_2 values
Diminished response to hypoxemia and hypercapnia
Decreased vital capacity
Increased closing volume

The elderly also have a decreased cardiac stress response and an increased association with coronary artery disease, placing them at high risk for cardiac complications. Factors influencing cardiovascular function (for example, hypotension, fluid volume, positive pressure ventilation) can have greater affects on the elderly than they do on the young.[6] Each of these factors increases the probability of pulmonary complications after surgery in the elderly.

Age-Specific Angle

Operative factors affecting cardiovascular function have a greater effect on the elderly.

Smoking

Smoking cessation has shown benefit in decreasing pulmonary complications of general anesthesia and surgery. People who stop smoking for 8 weeks yielded a significant decrease in pulmonary complications compared with those who continue to smoke.[7] Heavy smokers have a higher rate of pulmonary complications than light smokers do. Heavy smokers may benefit from refraining from smoking for even 1 day before surgery. This allows carboxyhemoglobin levels to decrease and improves oxygen-carrying capacity.

Preexisting Lung Disease

Patients with chronic bronchitis, airflow obstruction, asthma, and COPD are at increased risk for postoperative complications.[8,9] Chronic lung disease has been identified as the most significant factor for increased risk of postoperative pulmonary complications, including respiratory failure.[10] Patients with COPD have an increase in postoperative complications ranging from 26% to 78%.[8,11] People with symptomatic asthma also have an increased risk of morbidity from anesthesia.[12] Surgery on these patients

should occur when they are symptom free or when their symptoms are well controlled.

An increased residual volume, decreased forced expiratory volume in 1 second (FEV_1), decreased diffusing capacity for carbon monoxide ($DLCO$), and excessive sputum production are highly predictive for postop pulmonary complications.[13,14] Preoperative dyspnea also has been shown to correlate with increased postoperative complications. Each of these are common findings in patients with COPD. The use of antibiotics, bronchodilators, and steroids can reduce the risk of postoperative complications in high-risk patients. Antibiotics should be reserved for patients with evidence of infected sputum. A 10-day course of preoperative antibiotic therapy may reduce the risk of postoperative pneumonia. In one study, the use of preoperative bronchodilators and steroids decreased the risk of postoperative pneumonia with COPD.[15]

Patients with pulmonary disease and hypoxemia are at increased risk for **myocardial ischemia** and cardiac complications.[16] Pulmonary complications are also among the most common encountered in patients with cardiac compromise. Patients with cardiopulmonary disease who undergo elective surgery should have their lung function optimized, be free of pulmonary infections, and have their heart failure controlled.

Obesity

Surgical mortality has not been shown to be increased in obese patients.[17] Obese patients are, however, at increased risk for postoperative pulmonary complications such as atelectasis and persistent hypoxemia.[18] Complication rates are three times higher in obese patients than they are in patients who are of appropriate weight.[19] Weight loss has shown some benefit in decreasing pulmonary complications of general anesthesia and surgery. In morbidly obese patients, delaying surgery may be appropriate until some weight loss can be achieved.

Nutritional Status

Preoperative nutritional assessment for major operations is essential. Patients with serum albumin less than 2.5 g/dL and more than 10% weight loss should have nutritional repletion for 7 to 10 days before surgery.[20] If diet alone cannot correct the problem, nutritional support may be indicated. Preoperative **total parenteral nutrition (TPN)** for malnourished patients has had some good results but only in select patients. In general, postoperative administration of TPN has had dismal results. On the other hand, **enteral tube feeding (ETF)** via gastrointestinal administration is well tolerated as long as the patient has adequate gastric motility and emptying. ETF improves postoperative morbidity and mortality better than TPN when used for preoperative nutritional support.[21,22]

Poor nutritional status in critically ill patients undergoing major surgery is associated with reduced systemic immunity and an exaggerated stress response. Weight loss (more than 10% from baseline), low percentage of ideal body weight (less than 85%), hypoalbuminemia, and protein calorie malnutrition are all predictors of increased postoperative complications such as infection, organ system failure, delayed wound healing, and delayed functional recovery. Patients with at least one of the above abnormalities have a significant increase in incidence of overall surgical complications, major complications, and increased length of stay compared with patients who had all normal markers.[23,24] The severely malnourished carry the highest risk of postoperative complications.

Preoperative Testing

More than 40 million surgical operations and procedures are performed in the United States each year. An estimated $3 billion are spent in the United States each year on preoperative labs and diagnostic studies.[25] In general, these studies should be ordered for specific clinical indications and not as routine preoperative screens unless they will influence patient treatment and outcome. Little evidence exists that routine screening of patients with electrocardiography (ECG), chest radiographs, pulmonary function tests (PFT), echocardiograms, or blood chemistries significantly alter outcomes.

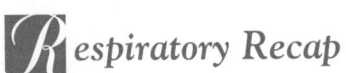
espiratory Recap

Typical Preoperative Laboratory and Diagnostic Studies	
ECG	Arterial blood gases
Chest radiograph	Pulmonary function testing

Electrocardiogram

The ECG is used to evaluate cardiac rhythm and conduction disturbances, ischemia, myocardial infarction, and metabolic disorders. ECGs are important for patients with clinical indications of circulatory and cardiac problems.[25] ECGs should not be performed as a routine preoperative screen or done based on patient age alone. Clinical indications for preoperative ECG are listed in Box 53-3.

Chest Radiograph

Chest radiographs are used to detect the presence of unknown conditions or clinically suspected processes in the chest. They also can be used to follow the progression of an active disease process. Chest radiographs are not recommended as part of a routine protocol. They should be individualized and based on clinical indications.[25] Chest radiographs are indicated in patients with acute, progressive, or chronic cardiopulmonary disease and in patients at high risk for developing postoperative pulmonary complications.[3] Chest radiographs should not be done based on age alone. Box 53-4 lists indications for preoperative chest radiographs.

Arterial Blood Gases

Arterial blood gases (ABGs) are used to evaluate the ventilatory, oxygenation, and acid-base status of a patient. They are not recommended as a general preoperative screening test. Arterial blood gases and oxygen saturation should be obtained before general anesthesia is initiated if the patient's respiratory symptoms have changed. ABGs are indicated in patients with new or changing lung disease and in patients at high risk for lung disease. Patients with increased $PaCO_2$ have an increased incidence of postoperative pulmonary complications. A chronically elevated $PaCO_2$ greater than 45 mm Hg predicts a high risk for pulmonary complications or death.[26,27] A PaO_2 of less than 50 mm Hg may be a relative contraindication to surgery.[3]

Pulmonary Function Tests

Pulmonary function tests (PFTs) assess the presence and severity of lung disease. However, the use of PFTs as a general preoperative screen for the presence of pulmonary disease in patients without a suggestive clinical history is not indicated. Spirometry should be obtained before the initiation of general anesthesia if the patient's respiratory

Box 53-3

Clinical Indications for Preoperative Electrocardiogram

Hypertension	Cerebral and peripheral
Congestive heart failure	vascular disease
Diabetes	Shortness of breath
Chest pain	Palpitations
Dizziness	Ankle edema
Syncope	Abnormal valvular murmurs

Box 53-4

Indications for Preoperative Chest Radiographs

Pneumonia	Cardiomegaly
Pulmonary edema	Pulmonary hypertension
Atelectasis	Chronic obstructive
Aortic aneurysm	pulmonary disease
Mediastinal or pulmonary	Pulmonary embolism
masses	Dextrocardia
Tracheal deviation	

symptoms have changed. In abdominal and cardiac surgery, the predictive value of spirometry and lung volumes determination is unproved as a general screening test. However, spirometry is indicated in patients in whom severe pulmonary dysfunction is evident to assess whether pulmonary rehabilitation is indicated to improve the pulmonary condition prior to surgery.[28] PFTs also are recommended on patients with neuromuscular disease, chest wall and spinal deformities, and in morbidly obese patients. With COPD, PFTs may help to assess the probability of early extubation.[3]

Intraoperative Risk Factors

Several intraoperative factors contribute to postoperative pulmonary complications. These include surgical incision site, duration of anesthesia, monitoring during anesthesia, intraoperative fluid management, and cardiac surgery.

Surgical Incision Site

Thoracic and upper abdominal incisions have been shown to have the most negative effects on pulmonary function and carry the highest rate of postoperative pulmonary complications. In general, the closer the incision to the diaphragm, the greater the risk of pulmonary complications. Upper abdominal procedures carry a 150% greater risk than lower abdominal surgeries.[29] Upper abdominal and thoracic surgeries carry a 20% to 70% pulmonary complication rate compared with a 4% pulmonary complication rate after urologic and orthopedic surgery.[8,11,30-32] The use of muscle sparing thoracotomy may improve postoperative muscle strength and lung function.[28]

Duration of Anesthesia

Supine positioning decreases the functional residual capacity (FRC) by 10% to 15%. General anesthesia decreases the FRC another 5% to 10%.[33] Postoperative complications reportedly double if surgery lasts longer than 3 hours.[2] Regardless of the site of surgery, anesthesia for at least 4 hours increases the risk of postoperative cardiac and pulmonary complications. The choice of anesthetic agent or technique used has little correlation to postoperative morbidity or mortality.

Cardiac Surgery

Coronary artery disease is common in the surgical population, with up to 50% of postoperative deaths resulting from cardiac events. Most of these events are ischemic. Catecholamine release during surgery can predispose the patient to arrhythmias and possible coronary plaque rupture. Recent data indicate that acute-adrenergic blockade during the perioperative period can decrease ischemia and the incidence of myocardial infarction.[34] Unique factors

contribute to the development of pulmonary complication after cardiac surgery. The use of a topical cooling slush to protect the myocardium results in phrenic nerve paralysis in more than 30% of patients (less than 5% without slush) and left lower collapse in more than 80% of patients (32% without slush).[35] These factors may lead to pulmonary compromise after surgery.

Monitoring

Intraoperative monitoring may decrease anesthetic risks of cardiopulmonary compromise, thus reducing postoperative complications. Although the evidence is scant, most clinicians would agree that the addition of physiologic monitoring intraoperatively, especially pulse oximetry and capnography, has improved postoperative outcomes.[36]

Fluid Management

Intraoperative fluid management is important in overall patient management. Proper fluid volume control is important for maintenance of renal function, ensuring gastrointestinal integrity, and maintaining oxygen delivery. Excessive fluids may lead to water accumulation (edema), CHF, and hypertension.[37] Blood loss and lack of fluids can lead to hypotension, poor organ perfusion, and insufficient oxygen delivery. Intraoperative blood loss greater than 1200 mL also has been associated with increased pulmonary complications.

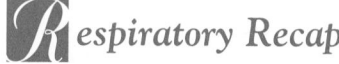
Respiratory Recap

Intraoperative Factors Contributing to Postoperative Pulmonary Complications	
Surgical incision site	Monitoring during anesthesia
Duration of anesthesia	Inoperative fluid
Cardiac surgery	management

Postoperative Respiratory Failure: Assessment and Management

Postoperative respiratory management includes pain control, early mobilization, deep breathing, chest physiotherapy, early ventilator weaning, early feeding, and use of oxygen.[38]

Hypoxemia

Mild hypoxemia is treated with low concentrations of oxygen. Nasal cannula is most commonly used for low-flow oxygen. Alternatively, air entrainment masks can be used if the delivery of a more constant and accurate oxygen concentration by a high-flow system is desired. The hazards of low-level oxygen therapy use are minimal. Severe cases of hypoxemia require more aggressive therapy with the use of continuous positive airway pressure (CPAP) or mechanical ventilation with PEEP and high oxygen levels. Postoperative patients with hypoxemia also may require treatment targeted at the underlying cause of the hypoxemia. Atelectasis is a major contributor to postoperative hypoxemia and lung volume expansion therapies may be required such as incentive spirometry (IS), IPPB (intermittent positive pressure breathing), and positive expiratory pressure (PEP) therapy.

$\mathcal{R}$espiratory Recap

Components of Postoperative Management	
Pain control	Early weaning from
Early mobilization	mechanical ventilation
Deep breathing exercises	Early feeding
Chest physiotherapy	Appropriate use of oxygen

Hypercapnia

Hypercapnic respiratory failure may be present in the postoperative patient. The central respiratory drive is blunted, an increased $PaCO_2$ will occur. The use of anesthetics and analgesics, during and after surgery, is the major reason for short-term acute respiratory failure after surgery. Once sedation has been terminated and the drug is metabolized or excreted, most postoperative patients can ventilate appropriately if pain control measures are utilized. Treatment is aimed at the underlying etiology. Supportive care (mechanical ventilation) can be maintained until the cause of respiratory failure is reversed.

Motor neuron disorders, respiratory muscle weakness, chest wall abnormalities, and diaphragmatic or abdominal conditions also can result in hypercapnia. Postoperative respiratory failure resulting from ventilatory pump or bellows dysfunction is uncommon except with preexisting preoperative factors. Diaphragmatic paralysis can occur after some surgeries (for example, cardiac) and may contribute to pump failure. Muscle weakness may result from drugs used intraoperatively or during the postoperative period. Pain can also be a factor preventing the normal use of the ventilatory bellows. Treatment is directed toward the underlying disorder and mechanical ventilation can be used for supportive care.

Nutrition

The integrity of the gut affects immune defenses, organ function, and whether the stress response is provoked or attenuated.[39] If a patient is unable to eat, initiation of ETFs may be desirable. Generally ETFs are well tolerated and improve postoperative morbidity and mortality better

$\mathcal{B}$OX 53-5

Positive Aspects of Enteral Tube Feedings Compared with Total Parenteral Nutrition

Increased integrity of gastrointestinal system	Improved return of cognitive function
Improved immune defenses	Decreased mortality
Improved organ function	Less expense
Attenuated immune response	Decreased septic complications
Decreased nosocomial infections	

than parenteral nutrition.[21] Box 53-5 lists the positive aspects of ETF. When compared with control subjects who received no feedings, nutritional intervention in the perioperative period has shown a benefit of reduced postoperative morbidity. A group of trauma patients receiving ETF for 5 to 7 days had a lower rate of sepsis compared with a group receiving intravenous fluid administration.[40] Patients with liver transplantation had a lower viral infection rate with administration of ETF.[41]

Pain Management

Pain management is essential after surgery, particularly for thoracic and abdominal surgery. Ineffective pain management may lead to serious pulmonary complications. Analgesia can be delivered orally, parenterally, or via epidural catheters. **Patient-controlled analgesia (PCA)** is a popular method of pain control.

Patient Temperature

Postoperative hypothermia causes vasoconstriction and may decrease tissue perfusion resulting in metabolic acidosis. If shivering is present, it will increase oxygen consumption and carbon dioxide production. This may increase the risk of myocardial ischemia and hypercapnic ventilatory failure.[42]

Muscle Strength

Postoperative sedation may lead to respiratory depression as a result of muscle weakness. The diaphragm is the last muscle to become paralyzed and the first to recover from neuromuscular blockade. A 5-second head-lift or leg-lift evaluation may be a good indicator of a patient's ability to maintain an adequate airway. If previously sedated patients who are alert and following commands can lift their extremities for 5 seconds, the diaphragm should be functional and they should be able to protect their airway. The 5-second lift test has correlated well with the maximal inspiratory pressure, which checks respiratory muscle strength.[43,44]

Deep Breathing

Pulmonary complications are the most common form of postoperative morbidity experienced by patients who undergo general surgical abdominal and thoracic procedures. The high incidence of pulmonary complications in the postoperative period is likely due to pain and the inability to take deep breaths because of decreased diaphragmatic function, chest wall dysfunction, and alterations in mechanics. Some studies have shown that forced vital capacity and peak flow can be decreased by as much as 50%. Functional residual capacity may be decreased by as much as 10% to 15% in lower abdominal surgery, 30% in upper abdominal surgery, and 35% in thoracic surgery in the postoperative period and may not return to normal for 3 to 6 days.[45-50] Transdiaphragmatic pressure has been shown to decrease by as much as 70% in abdominal surgery and normal function may not return for 1 week. In some cases, adequate pain management does not reduce this impairment, which seems to occur from diaphragm dysfunction itself.[51]

Another important element in the etiology of postoperative respiratory complications is the lung volume at which airway closure occurs. Factors that increase closing volumes include increased age, tobacco use, fluid overload, bronchospasm, and airway secretions.[28] With a decreased FRC or increased closing volume, the lungs are predisposed to airway closure and atelectasis, leading to $\dot{V}/\dot{Q}$ mismatch, hypoxemia, retained secretions, and respiratory failure. Deep breathing exercises and pulmonary hygiene are important postoperative considerations for impending pulmonary complications. Pulmonary complications, specifically atelectasis, pneumonia, and pulmonary embolism, represent the leading causes of postoperative morbidity and mortality.[31,52]

Atelectasis

Etiology and Risk Factors

Atelectasis is the incomplete expansion of the lung or the collapse of previously expanded lung tissue. Collapse may be minimal and diffuse, unseen on chest x-ray (microatelectasis) or involving whole segments, lobes, or a lung and easily seen on chest radiographs. Atelectasis is one of the most common noninfectious pulmonary complications after surgery. Studies have reported that 20% to 25% of lung tissue in the basal lung areas collapses after induction with general anesthesia. Furthermore, the use of high concentrations of oxygen (more than 40%) also contributes to the collapse.[53] Atelectasis is reported in a wide range of patients (6% to 75%) having abdominal or thoracic surgery.[54] The incidence of clinically significant atelectasis after abdominal surgery is 15% to 20%,[53] with the left lower lobe being the most common area for atelectasis.[55]

Atelectasis may be due to many factors, including small, monotonous tidal volumes and inadequate lung distending forces, airway obstruction with gas absorption,

and reduction in surfactant levels. These conditions are likely in postoperative patients who are sedated, have significant pain, and often have poor clearance of airway secretions. Any condition that interferes with the generation of negative pleural pressure predisposes to atelectasis. Examples include weak inspiratory muscles because of sedation, advanced age, obesity, chest wall deformities, pulmonary fibrosis, abdominal and thoracic surgery, and pain.

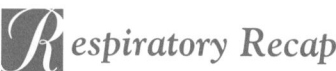

espiratory Recap

> **Atelectasis**
>
> Atelectasis is the incomplete expansion of the lung or the collapse of previously expanded lung tissue.

Age-Specific Angle

> Elderly patients are at greater risk for atelectasis.

Retained secretions may be the common factor in the development of postoperative atelectasis when the patient has an inadequate cough. Furthermore, anesthetics and a lack of humidity can diminish airway mucus transport during the intraoperative period. Surfactant levels may also be decreased in the lungs of postoperative patients as a result of the use of anesthetics, administration of high concentrations of oxygen, and the absence of deep breathing. Intraoperative aspiration may contribute to airway compromise as well.

Clinical Manifestations and Diagnostic Findings

Some of the signs and symptoms of atelectasis include fine late inspiratory crackles, bronchial type breath sounds, diminished breath sounds, increased breathing frequency and dyspnea, increased heart rate, and hypoxemia. The significance of each of these findings depends on the degree of atelectasis present. Atelectasis also can lead to respiratory failure and pneumonia. The presence of a fever in a patient with atelectasis is most often associated with infection resulting from retained secretions. Although contrary to common teaching, atelectasis without infection does not result in fever.[53,56]

Atelectasis is one of the most commonly encountered abnormalities on chest radiographs. At times it may be overlooked and at other times confused with other intrathoracic pathology such as **pneumonia.** Some of the radiographic signs of atelectasis include localized increase in density or opacity, air bronchograms, displacement of lobar fissures, elevation of the diaphragm, mediastinal shift, hilar displacement, regional change in rib spacing, hyperinflation of surrounding lung, and generalized volume reduction.

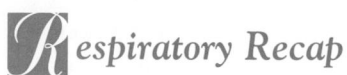

Pulmonary function tests reveal a decreased FRC, a decreased VC, and decreased compliance. An arterial blood sample often shows an uncompensated respiratory alkalosis with hypoxemia. The hypoxemia is a result of $\dot{V}/\dot{Q}$ mismatch and areas of right to left shunt. General anesthesia inhibits hypoxic pulmonary vasoconstriction, which further contributes to $\dot{V}/\dot{Q}$ mismatch and increased work of breathing.

Medical Management

Treatment for atelectasis varies, depending on the severity and etiology of the problem. Clearly, preventive treatment is best. Preoperative patient education and training, when the patient is alert, responsive to instruction, and without pain, may play a significant role in preventing postoperative complications. Smoking cessation at least 8 weeks before surgery has also been shown to improve postoperative outcomes.[54]

With minimal postoperative atelectasis, no special intervention is needed. Spontaneous coughing, deep breathing, and mobilization (walking) should be sufficient to reverse any pulmonary impairment. In moderate cases, incentive spirometry (IS), intermittent positive pressure breathing (IPPB), and PEP therapy can be used to help prevent or reverse atelectasis. Chest physiotherapy (CPT) and the use of bronchodilators may improve bronchial hygiene and aid in removal of secretions if present. Some studies have shown that deep breathing and coughing are as effective as other modes of therapy for the treatment of atelectasis and that no one form of lung inflation therapy is significantly superior to another. Other studies have pointed out that although treatments are

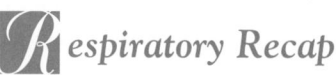

similar in their ability to prevent pulmonary complications, each has been shown to be better than no treatment at all. Some studies have demonstrated PEP and CPAP therapy to be more effective than the deep breathing of incentive spirometry.[3,54,56]

Low-risk surgical patients probably do not need therapy, but even with proper therapy, an estimated 25% of high-risk patients will suffer from postoperative pulmonary complications. Oxygen therapy is often indicated for at least short periods of time. In severe cases, mechanical ventilation with PEEP and high oxygen levels may be indicated to reinflate collapsed areas and support oxygenation until the patient has improved. Therapeutic fiberoptic bronchoscopy may be indicated to remove mucus plugs if they are the cause of airway obstruction and atelectasis.

Pulmonary Emboli—Pulmonary Thromboembolic Disease

Etiology and Risk Factors

The most common cause of **pulmonary emboli (PE)** is venous thromboembolism. Blood clots formed in the leg veins travel to the lungs where they obstruct pulmonary vessels. Blood clotting in the legs and pelvis, **deep vein thrombosis (DVT),** usually occurs as a result of venostasis common in surgical patients and other causes of immobility, damage to the endothelial wall of the blood vessels, and hypercoagulability states. Risk factors associated for DVT include age greater than 70 years, obesity, CHF, presence of malignancies, burns, use of estrogen-containing drugs, and postoperative states.[57]

Clinical Manifestations and Diagnostic Findings

Signs and symptoms of acute PE include abrupt onset of cough, pleuritic chest pain, anxiety, and tachycardia. Tachypnea and dyspnea are the most common findings present, even in patients without hypoxemia. Lung auscultation may reveal wheezing or crackles. Hemoptysis may occasionally occur. The lower extremities may reveal some tenderness or swelling associated with DVT, but PE often occurs as the first sign of DVT.

The severity of symptoms and degree of compromise depends on the magnitude of occlusion of the pulmonary vessels and the amount of preexisting cardiopulmonary disease. As a result of venous occlusion, hypoxemia usually occurs. This is due to $\dot{V}/\dot{Q}$ mismatch, bronchoconstriction, decreased surfactant production, atelectasis, and shunting. In healthy patients, right-sided heart dysfunction does not usually occur unless occlusion of 50% or more (massive occlusion) of the pulmonary vasculature occurs. In patients with cardiopulmonary disease, hemodynamic collapse can occur with less than massive occlusion. Although pulmonary occlusion can be extensive, pulmonary infarction is uncommon because the lung receives oxygen from three sources: pulmonary circulation, bronchial circulation, and the alveolar gas.

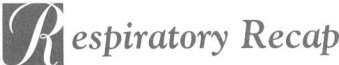

Signs and Symptoms of PE	
Abrupt onset of cough	Tachycardia
Pleuritic chest pain	Hypoxemia
Anxiety	

PE can occur with few symptoms or it may be mistaken for other diseases or coexist with them. PE is commonly mistaken for pneumonia.[58] The diagnosis of PE includes clinical suspicion, physical exam, chest radiograph, ECG, and arterial blood gases. Chest radiographs may be normal or an infiltrate may be present. X-rays are often not specific enough to be of great help. In some cases a wedge-shaped density called Westermark's sign may be present. The ECG may have nonspecific alterations. Arterial blood gases often show a respiratory alkalosis and hypoxemia.

Noninvasive studies used to diagnose DVT include **impedance plethysmography** and Doppler ultrasound. Contrast venography is gold standard in the diagnosis of DVT. The hazard associated with venography is mobilization of the clot. To diagnosis PE, the $\dot{V}/\dot{Q}$ scan is used to evaluate perfusion defects combined with areas of normal ventilation. The pulmonary angiogram, although considered the gold standard to determine the presence of PE, is invasive and carries with it a higher risk of complications than the $\dot{V}/\dot{Q}$ scan. Because of the increased risk of complications, pulmonary angiography is often used as a last resort.

Medical Management

Prophylaxis of PE involves prevention of DVT including compression wraps (stockings) or pneumatic boots with intermittent inflation and early ambulation and leg exercises. Anticoagulation therapy is also indicated. Anticoagulation therapy is considered therapeutic if the clotting time or **partial thromboplastin time (PTT)** is 2 to 2.5 times the control. If venous thrombosis is present, **heparin** will prevent further clot formation but it will not dissolve clots already present.

Thrombolytic therapy will help dissolve clots. Common thrombolytics include streptokinase, urokinase, and **tissue plasminogen activator (TPA).** The insertion of an inferior vena caval (IVC) filter (Greenfield or birds-nest filter) can be used to prevent clots originating in the lower extremities from reaching the lungs. These implanted filters intercept clots, thus preventing PE. Surgical removal of the embolus may rarely be attempted. Supportive ther-

apy includes supplemental oxygen and, in severe cases of acute respiratory failure, mechanical ventilation with PEEP and high oxygen levels.

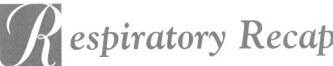

Management of PE	
Prophylaxis/prevention of DVT	Thrombolytic therapy
	Insertion of IVC filters
Anticoagulation therapy	Surgery

Pneumonia

Etiology and Risk Factors

Nosocomial pneumonia accounts for 15% of all hospital-acquired infections, with half occurring in surgical patients.[59] Postoperative pneumonia has been reported to occur in 18% of patients undergoing elective upper or lower abdominal and thoracic surgery.[60] Pneumonia carries the highest mortality rate from hospital-acquired infections.[56] It is the most common cause of death among surgical patients, with a reported mortality rate of 20% to 50% and up to 90% mortality in patients with ARDS.[58]

Risk factors for development of pneumonia include immunosuppression, malnutrition, COPD, and age greater than 65 years. Additional risk factors for development of nosocomial pneumonia include major thoracic and upper abdominal surgery, greater than 1200 mL blood loss during surgery, altered protective effects of the glottic area, ineffective cough, inhibition of ciliary motion, and impaired consciousness leading to increased chance of aspiration. Postoperative patients are at high risk especially when they are intubated, have a nasogastric tube in place, have had general anesthesia, have swallowing difficulties, or have regurgitation of gastric contents.

Clinical Manifestations and Diagnostic Findings

Signs and symptoms of pneumonia include fever, shaking chills, cough, hemoptysis, tachypnea, dullness to percussion, crackles, purulent sputum production, and pleuritic chest pain. However, some of the usual clinical manifestations are often less clear and may be overshadowed by an underlying illness when pneumonia develops while a patient is in the hospital. When a bacterial pneumonia is present, laboratory data includes increased white blood cell count (leukocytes), increased granulocytes (neutrophilia), and an increased percent of immature forms (shift to the left). Arterial blood gases show hypoxemia with respiratory alkalosis. Chest radiographs vary according to the type of pneumonia present. Lobar pneumonia presents as a homogenous infiltrate with air bronchograms. Nonhomogeneous, patchy, nonlobar densities occur with bronchopneumonia. A diffuse bilateral reticular density often indicates a viral infection.

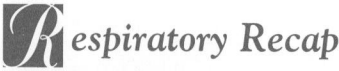espiratory Recap

Signs and Symptoms of Pneumonia	
Fever	Dullness to percussion
Shaking chills	Crackles
Cough	Purulent sputum
Hemoptysis	Pleuritic chest pain
Tachypnea	

Medical Management

The use of antibiotics is the most important therapy. If isolation of the causative agent is possible, culture and sensitivity tests should direct proper antimicrobial use. If the agent cannot be isolated, general antimicrobial therapy includes extended-spectrum penicillin, aminoglycosides, and the cephalosporins. Bronchopulmonary hygiene is used to help in the removal of secretions. This may include delivery of bronchodilators, chest physiotherapy, and deep breathing exercises. Therapeutic bronchoscopy may be used for secretion removal. Oxygen is often needed for hypoxemia. In severe cases, mechanical ventilation with PEEP may be indicated. Prevention is the best course of action. Proper hand washing is essential. Deep breathing maneuvers and coughing are indicated for secretion removal. The use of CPT and bronchodilator therapy may also be indicated.

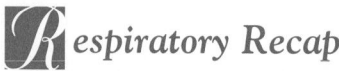espiratory Recap

Management of Pneumonia	
Antibiotics	Therapeutic bronchoscopy
Bronchodilators	Oxygen
Chest physiotherapy	Mechanical ventilation with
Deep breathing exercises	PEEP

Mechanical Ventilation

Postoperative mechanical ventilation occasionally is required. Most commonly, this is due to the residual respiratory depressant effects of anesthesia. This often involves several hours of ventilatory support in the postanesthesia care unit, after which the patient is extubated. After cardiac surgery, the patient is mechanically ventilated in the intensive care unit for several hours, after which fast-track weaning protocols are used to rapidly liberate the patient from the ventilator. After neurosurgery, mechanical ventilation may be needed because of respiratory depression and to assist with the control of intracranial pressure. After

thoracic surgery, mechanical ventilation is often required because of the extent of surgical trauma to the thorax.

The principles of mechanical ventilation are similar for the postoperative patient as for other patients requiring this therapy. Appropriate ventilatory support is provided, with attention to the prevention of iatrogenic injuries such as overdistention, auto-PEEP, and hemodynamic compromise. Some postoperative patients (for example, neurosurgery) may have relatively normal lungs and chest wall. Others may have relatively normal lung function, but surgical chest wall trauma (for example, cardiac surgery). Thoracic surgery patients may be difficult to manage because they have surgical chest wall trauma, lung resection with risk of pneumothorax, and underlying lung disease such as COPD.

𝒦ey 𝒫oints

- An important first step in preoperative management is a patient history.
- Age, smoking history, preexisting lung disease, obesity, and poor nutritional status are risk factors for postoperative respiratory complications.
- Little evidence exists that routine screening of patients with ECG, chest radiographs, PFTs, echocardiograms, or blood chemistries significantly alter outcomes.
- Intraoperative factors that affect postoperative pulmonary complications include surgical incision site, duration of anesthesia, monitoring during anesthesia, intraoperative fluid management, and cardiac surgery.
- Postoperative respiratory management includes pain control, early mobilization, deep breathing, CPT, early ventilator weaning, early feeding, and use of oxygen.
- Atelectasis, pulmonary embolism, and pneumonia are common postoperative problems.

References

1. Brooks-Brunn JA. Postoperative atelectasis and pneumonia. Heart Lung 1995;24:94-115.
2. Van Hoozer B, Albertson TE. Acute respiratory failure. In: Burton GG, Hodgkin JE, Ward JJ, editors. Respiratory care: a guide to clinical practice. 4th ed. Philadelphia: JB Lippincott; 1997.
3. Doyle RL. Assessing and modifying the risk of postoperative pulmonary complications. Chest 1999;115:77S-81S.
4. Eghert LD, Battit GE. Reduction of postoperative pain by encouragement and instruction of patients. N Engl J Med 1964;270:825-827.
5. Classen DC, Pestotnik SL, Evans RS, et al. Adverse drug events in hospitalized patients: excess length of stay, extra costs, and attributable mortality. JAMA 1997;277:301-306.
6. Oskuig RM. Special problems in the elderly. Chest 1999;115:158S-164S.

7. Warner MA, Divertie MB, Tinker JH. Preoperative cessation of smoking and pulmonary complications in coronary artery bypass patients. Anesthesiology 1984;60:380-383.

8. Gracey DR, Divertie MB, Didier EP. Preoperative pulmonary preparation of patients with chronic obstructive pulmonary disease. Chest 1979;76:123-129.

9. Tarhan S, Mottitt E, Sessler AD, et al. The risk of anesthesia and surgery in patients with chronic bronchitis and chronic obstructive pulmonary disease. Surgery 1973;74:720-726.

10. Wilkins RL, Dexter JR. Introduction to respiratory failure. In: Wilkins RL, Dexter JR, editors. Respiratory care, a case study approach to patient care. 2nd ed. Philadelphia: FA Davis; 1998.

11. Stein M, Cassara EL. Preoperative pulmonary evaluation and therapy for surgery patients. JAMA 1970;211:787-790.

12. Warner DO, Warner MA, Barnes RD, et al. Perioperative respiratory complications in patients with asthma. Anesthesiology 1996;82:460-467.

13. Barisione G, Rovida S, Gazzaniga GM, et al. Upper abdominal surgery: does a lung function test exist to predict early severe postoperative respiratory complications? Eur Respir J 1997;10:1301-1308.

14. Mitchell CK, Smoger SH, Pfeifer MP, et al. Multivariate analysis of factors associated with pulmonary complications following general elective surgery. Arch Surg 1998;133:194-198.

15. Garibaldi RA, Britt MR, Coleman ML, et al. Risk factors for postoperative pneumonia. Am J Med 1981;70:677-680.

16. Belzberg H, Rivkind AI. Preoperative cardiac preparation. Chest 1999;115:82S-95S.

17. Mohr DN, Jett JR. Preoperative evaluation of pulmonary risk factors. J Gen Intern Med 1988;3:277-287.

18. Latimer RG, Dickman M, Day WC, et al. Ventilatory patterns and pulmonary complications after upper abdominal surgery determined by preoperative and postoperative computerized spirometry and blood gas analysis. Am J Surg 1971;122:622-632.

19. Mircea N, Constantinescu C, Jianu E, et al. Risk of pulmonary complications in surgical patients. Resuscitation 1982;10:33-41.

20. Stack JA, Babineau TJ, Bristrian BR. Assessment of nutritional status in clinical practice. Gastroenterologist 1996;4:8S-15S.

21. McClave SA, Snider HL, Spain DA. Preoperative issues in clinical nutrition. Chest 1999;115:64S-70S.

22. Chan S, McCowen KC, Blackburn GL. Nutrition management in the ICU. Chest 1999;115:145S-148S.

23. Warnold I, Lundholm K. Clinical significance of preoperative nutritional status in 215 noncancer patients. Ann Surg 1984;199:299-305.

24. Windsor JA, Hill GL. Weight loss with physiologic impairment—a basic indicator of surgical risk. Ann Surg 1988;207:290-296.

25. Fischer SP: Cost-effectiveness preoperative evaluation and testing. Chest 1999;115:96S-110S.

26. Zibrak JD, O'Donnel CR. Indications for preoperative pulmonary function testing. Clin Chest Med 1993;14:227-236.

27. Tisi GM. Preoperative evaluation of pulmonary function: validity, indications and benefits. Am Rev Respir Dis 1979;119:293-310.

28. Ferguson MK. Preoperative assessment of pulmonary risk. Chest 1999;115:58S-63S.

29. Mitchell C, Garrahy P, Peake P. Postoperative respiratory morbidity: identification and risk factors. Aust N Z J Surg 1982;52:203-209.

30. Kroenke K, Lawrence VA, Theroux JF, et al. Operative risk in patients with severe obstructive pulmonary disease. Arch Intern Med 1992;152:967-971.

31. Wightman JA. A prospective survey of the incidence of postoperative pulmonary complications. Br J Surg 1968;55:85-91.

32. Pedersen T, Viby-Mogensen J, Ringsted C. Anaesthetic practice and postoperative pulmonary complications. Acta Anaesthesiol Scand 1992;36:812-818.

33. Price JA, Rizk NW. Postoperative ventilatory management. Chest 1999;115:130S-137S.

34. Hollenberg SM. Preoperative cardiac risk assessment. Chest 1999;115:51S-57S.

35. Efthimiou J, Butler J, Woodham C, et al. Diaphragm paralysis following cardiac surgery: role of phrenic nerve cold injury. Ann Thorac Surg 1994;52:1005-1008.

36. Pierce EC Jr. Monitoring instruments have significantly reduced anesthetic mishaps. J Clin Monit 1988;4:111-114.

37. Rosenthal MH. Intraoperative fluid management—what and how much? Chest 1999;115:130S-137S.

38. Peeters-Asdourian C, Gupta S. Choices in pain management following thoracotomy. Chest 1999;115:122S-124S.

39. Carrico CK. The elusive pathophysiology of the multiple organ failure syndrome [editorial]. Ann Surg 1993;218:109.

40. Moore EE, Jones TN. Benefits of immediate jejunostomy feeding after major abdominal trauma—a prospective, randomized study. J Trauma 1986;26:874-881.

41. Hasse JM, Blue LS, Liepa GU, et al. Early enteral nutrition support in patients undergoing liver transplantation. J Parenter Enteral Nutr 1995;19:437-443.

42. Mecca RS. Postoperative recovery. In: Barash PG, editor. Clinical anesthesia. Philadelphia: JB Lippincott; 1997. pp. 1279-1301.

43. Pavlin EG, Holle RH, Schoene RB. Recovery of airway protection compared with ventilation in humans after paralysis with curare. Anesthesiology 1996;70:381-385.

44. Stone DJ, Gal TJ. Airway management. In: Miller RD, editor. Anesthesia. New York: Churchill Livingstone; 1994.

45. Ali J, Weisel RD, Layug AB, et al. Consequences of postoperative alterations in respiratory mechanics. Am J Surg 1974;128:376-382.

46. Meyers JR, Lembeck L, O'Kane H, et al. Changes in functional residual capacity of the lung after operation. Arch Surg 1975;110:576-583.

47. Alexander JI, Spence AA, Parikh RK, et al. The role of airway closure in postoperative hypoxaemia. Br J Anaesth 1973;45:34-40.

48. Vaughan RW, Wise L. Choice of abdominal operative incision in the obese patient: a study using blood gas measurements. Ann Surg 1975;181:829-835.

49. Craig DB. Postoperative recovery of pulmonary function. Anesth Analg 1981;60:46-52.

50. Bastin R, Moraine JJ, Bardocsky G, et al. Incentive spirometry performance. Chest 1997;111:559-563.

51. Simonneau G, Vivien A, Saartene R, et al. Diaphragm dysfunction induced by upper abdominal surgery. Am Rev Respir Dis 1983;128:899-903.

52. Cina G, Marra R, Di Stasi C, et al. Epidemiology, pathophysiology and natural history of venous thromboembolism. Rays 1996;21:315-327.

53. Platell C, Hall JC. Atelectasis after abdominal surgery. J Am Coll Surg 1997;185:584-592.

54. Bakow ED. Atelectasis, pathophysiology and treatment. In: Dantzker DR, MacIntyre NR, Bakow ED, editor. Comprehensive respiratory care. Philadelphia: WB Saunders; 1995.

55. Lode HM, Schaberg T, Raffenberg M, et al. Nosocomial pneumonia in the critical care unit. Crit Care Clin 1998;14: 119-133.

56. Mayhill CG. Nosocomial pneumonia: diagnosis and prevention. Infect Dis Clin N Am 1997;11:427-457.

57. Tukstra F, Koopman MM, Buller HR. The treatment of deep vein thrombosis and pulmonary embolism. Thromb Haemostasis 1997;78:489-496.

58. Polk HC Jr, Heinzelmann M, Mercer-Jones MA, et al. Pneumonia in the surgical patient. Current Probl Surg 1997;34: 117-200.

59. Tapson VF, Kussin PS. Respiratory tract infections. In: Dantzker DR, MacIntyre NR, Bakow ED, editors. Comprehensive respiratory care. Philadelphia: WB Saunders; 1995.

60. Trofe J, Peterson AM. The role of H_2-receptor antagonists in the pathogenesis of nosocomial pneumonia in mechanically ventilated patients. Pharmacotherapy 1998;18:808-815.

CHAPTER 54

Cardiac Failure

Benjamin D. Medoff
Thomas G. DiSalvo

CHAPTER OUTLINE

OBJECTIVES

1. Discuss the epidemiology and etiology of cardiac failure.
2. Describe the physiology of normal cardiac function, the pathophysiology of abnormal cardiac function, and the pathophysiology of pulmonary edema.
3. List the symptoms and signs of cardiac failure.
4. Discuss the basic ways in which the heart and lungs interact.
5. Discuss the common causes of heart failure and their treatment, with an emphasis on respiratory failure.

KEY TERMS

Afterload	Echocardiography	Pulmonary Edema
Backward Heart Failure	Forward Heart Failure	Pulsus Paradoxus
Cardiac Output (Q̇c)	Heart Failure	Starling's Law of Cardiac Function
Cardiomyocytes	Hepatojugular Reflux	Stroke Volume
Cardiomyopathy	Intraaortic Balloon Pump (IABP)	Systole
Cardiomyoplasty	Isovolumic Contraction	Vascular Resistance
Contractility	Isovolumic Relaxation	Venous Return
Coronary Angiography	Oncotic Pressure	Ventricular Assist Device (VAD)
Coronary Artery Bypass Surgery	Orthopnea	Ventricular Interdependence
Diastole	Preload	

Cardiac failure is the final common pathway of almost all forms of heart disease. The high prevalence of heart disease has made cardiac failure one of the most common problems encountered in hospitalized patients. **Heart failure** results in a broad range of symptoms and presentations, and in extreme cases, respiratory failure requiring mechanical ventilation may occur. Mechanical ventilation of these patients can be challenging because of the complexity of the cardiopulmonary interactions and concomitant cardiac problems such as myocardial ischemia. Proper care of the ventilated patient with heart failure requires knowledge of the clinical manifestations and the pathophysiology of heart failure. This chapter reviews the clinical aspects of cardiac failure, the pathophysiology of impaired cardiac function, and the pathophysiology of pulmonary edema. Special attention is paid to general treatment measures and aspects of cardiopulmonary interactions. The final section gives examples of common causes of cardiac failure and specific therapeutic interventions.

Definition

Cardiac failure was defined by a National Heart, Lung, and Blood Institute task force as follows:[1]

> Heart failure occurs when an abnormality of cardiac function causes the heart to fail to pump blood at a rate required by the metabolizing tissues or when the heart can do so only with an elevated filling pressure. The heart's inability to pump a sufficient amount of blood to meet the needs of the body tissues may be due to insufficient or defective cardiac filling and/or impaired contraction and emptying. . . .

Others have defined cardiac failure in terms of symptoms such as effort intolerance, fluid retention, dyspnea, and fatigue that result from inadequate tissue perfusion and from an inability of the heart to fill or empty properly.[2,3]

Epidemiology

Cardiac failure is one of the most common causes of hospital admission in the United States and Europe and is as-

sociated with substantial costs to the health care system.[4,5] Despite overall declining mortality resulting from coronary disease, cardiac failure continues to be a major public health problem.[6]

Incidence and Prevalence

The incidence of heart failure is estimated to be 1 to 5 persons per 1000 population each year, but the incidence is more than 30 cases per 1000 population each year in people over age 75.[7,8] Prevalence is estimated at 3 to 20 individuals per 1000 and up to 160 individuals per 1000 among those over age 75.[7,8] Thus heart failure is predominantly a disease of the elderly.

Mortality

The mortality of established, symptomatic heart failure is similar to that of cancer and end stage AIDS. In the Framingham study a 25% 5-year survival was found in men, and a 38% 5-year survival was found in women with symptomatic heart failure.[9] Annual mortality for chronic heart failure is approximately 10% but increases to 30% to 50% in hospitalized patients.[7,10-13]

Etiology

Cardiac failure results from a large number of primary cardiac diseases as well as systemic diseases. The most common etiologies include coronary artery disease (CAD), hypertension, alcohol, and idiopathic dilated cardiomyopathy.[9] Box 54-1 lists many of the possible etiologies of cardiac failure.

Cardiac Physiology

The heart is often compared to a specialized mechanical pump that circulates blood through the pulmonary and systemic circulation. The intact performance of the heart requires a complex series of events that coordinates excitation at the individual myocyte to contraction of the heart muscle itself. To generate an adequate cardiac output, the heart must contract and pump blood out (systolic

$\mathcal{B}$OX 54-1

Diagnoses Associated with Cardiac Failure

Acute ischemia	Arrhythmia
Dilated cardiomyopathy	Tachycardia
Chronic ischemic disease	Bradycardia
Idiopathic	Pericardial disease
Tachycardia induced	Constrictive pericarditis
Myocarditis (viral, giant cell, etc.)	Constrictive/effusive pericarditis
Chagas	Pericardial tamponade
Toxin/drug-mediated (for example, Adriamycin, Cobalt)	Right heart failure
Sarcoidosis	Valvular (pulmonary stenosis/insufficiency, tricuspid regurgitation)
Hemochromatosis	Eisenmenger's syndrome (for example, atrial septal defect)
Thyroid disease	Pulmonary hypertension (pulmonary embolism, primary, etc.)
Heredity	High-output failure
Restrictive cardiomyopathy	Arterial-venous shunting
Hypertrophic cardiomyopathy	Paget's disease
Infiltrative disorders (amyloid, malignancy)	Thyroid disease
Idiopathic	Beri-Beri
Valvular/mechanical disease	Miscellaneous
Aortic stenosis	Vasculitis (Churg-Strauss, Wegener's, etc.)
Aortic insufficiency (acute and chronic)	Carcinoid
Mitral stenosis	Scleroderma
Mitral regurgitation (acute and chronic)	Eosinophilic cardiomyopathy (Löffler's endocarditis)
Ventricular septal defect (acute and chronic)	
Free wall rupture	

function) and also relax and refill the chambers with blood (diastolic function). Overall cardiac function is regulated by numerous neurohumoral and mechanical factors that can be manipulated with various pharmacologic agents.

Cellular Biology and Biochemistry of Cardiac Function

The heart comprises cardiac muscle cells (**cardiomyocytes**) organized into linear series called *myofibers*. The myocytes contain primarily the basic contractile apparatus of the heart (sarcomere), as well as numerous mitochondria for energy production. In addition the heart has specialized myocytes that initiate and propagate the action potential that causes contraction of the muscle cells. Each myocyte is bound by a cell membrane called the *sarcolemma* that invaginates into the cell at numerous sites, forming the T-tubules (Figure 54-1). Lying next to the sarcolemma and its T-tubules is another intracellular membrane structure called the *sarcoplasmic reticulum (SR)*.

The smallest unit of muscle that contracts is the sarcomere. Multiple sarcomeres make up a myofibril, and each muscle cell contains numerous myofibrils. The sarcomere itself contains the contractile proteins that interact to cause muscle shortening and/or force generation. The sarcomere is defined by two Z *lines* that act to anchor the contractile proteins. Long, thin protein complexes extend from the Z lines and interact with thick filaments that are oriented in the center of the sarcomere. The thin filament is composed of a complex of the proteins actin, troponin C, troponin I,

and troponin T, and tropomyosin (Figure 54-2, A). The thick filament is made up of myosin and is bound to the protein titin, which anchors the thick filament to the Z line. The orientation of these proteins allows myosin and actin to form cross bridges (Figure 54-2, B). However the configuration of tropomyosin on the actin molecules inhibits this interaction.

Contraction of the myocyte is initiated by cell membrane depolarization. The conducting cells of the heart initiate the action potential that propagates to the muscle cells. The action potential depolarizes the sarcolemma, which, in turn, depolarizes the SR. The SR initiates contraction by releasing calcium into the cytoplasm through extensive membrane channels (ryanodine receptor). The SR also controls cardiac relaxation by actively taking up calcium after contraction via an energy-dependent calcium pump. The calcium is then stored until the next contraction. The calcium released from the SR interacts with the contractile proteins, and in the presence of ATP the muscle cell will generate a force and/or shorten. The calcium is then pumped back into the SR and the muscle cell relaxes. Both the contraction and the relaxation of the myocyte are energy dependent functions.[14,15]

When calcium is released into the cytosol from the SR, it interacts with troponin C, which binds to troponin I and troponin T. This process repositions tropomyosin on the actin filament and removes its inhibitory effect from myosin binding to actin. Myosin and actin then interact and form a cross bridge. By dephosphorylating the high energy phosphate adenosine triphosphate (ATP), the myosin

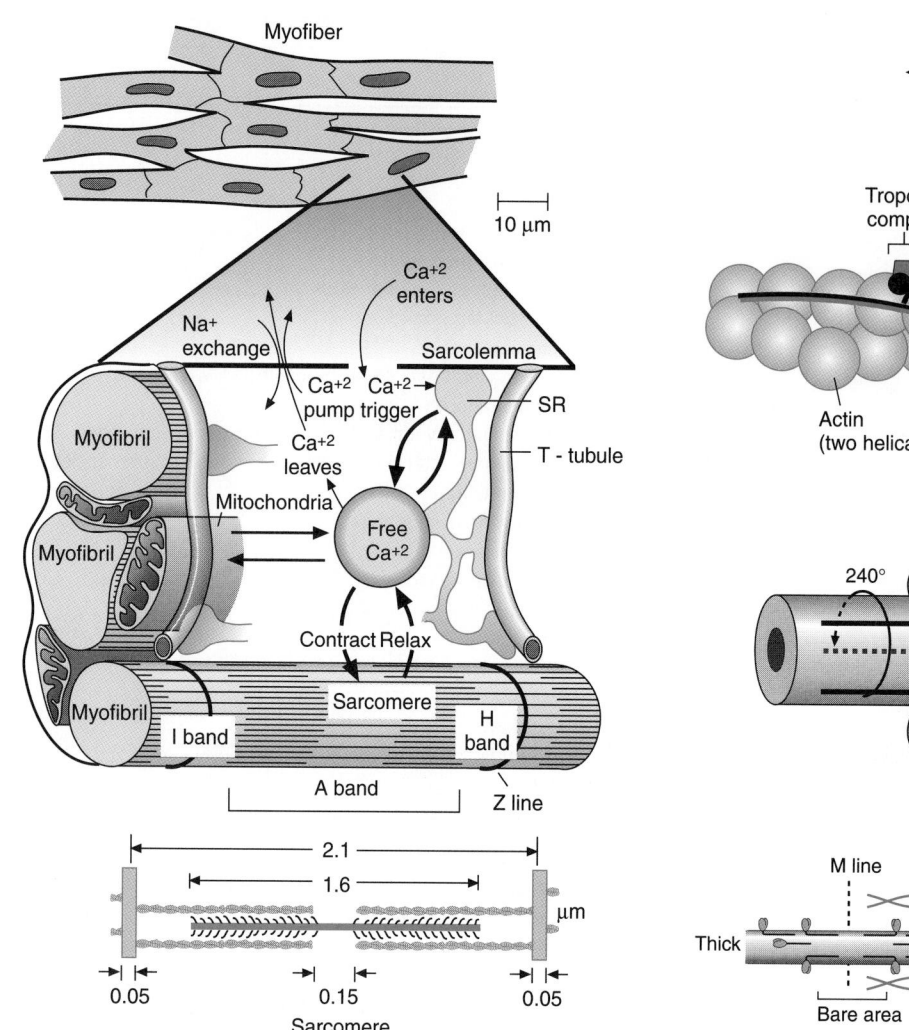

Figure 54-1   Microanatomy of the heart. The myofiber is made up of multiple sarcomeres. The sarcomere is the major contractile unit of the heart and is stimulated to shorten by the release of calcium. *SR,* Sarcoplasmic reticulum.

Figure 54-2   **A,** Thin filament structure. Actin forms a ropelike filament that has a troponin complex attached to it. **B,** Thick filament structure with multiple heads oriented around the core.

head changes configuration, and the two filaments slide over one another, thus pulling on the two Z lines. This action either shortens the sarcomere or generates an isometric force if there is tension on the muscle. A more detailed demonstration of this process is shown in Figure 54-3.

In the presence of calcium and adequate ATP, multiple cycles of cross bridge formation and sliding can occur, leading to marked sarcomere shortening. By coordinating the contraction of multiple sarcomeres, the muscle cells and thus the myofibers are able to shorten and generate force. When calcium is removed from the cytoplasm, the cross bridges are inhibited and the sarcomeres relax. Calcium is removed via an ATP-dependent calcium pump as well as a sodium-calcium exchanger on the sarcolemma. Sodium concentrations are kept low in the cytoplasm by various sodium pumps, including a sodium-potassium ATP-dependent exchanger.[15,16]

Cardiac Pump Function

By coordinating the complex events detailed previously, the heart rhythmically contracts and continually empties and fills with blood, thus propelling blood through the circulation. The cardiac cycle consists of a period of contraction (**systole**) during which the heart pumps blood into the pulmonary and systemic circulation followed by a relaxation period (**diastole**) during which venous blood returns to the heart. With each cardiac cycle, a volume of blood is ejected; this is termed the **stroke volume** of the heart (normal is 60 to 70 mL). The ejection fraction of the heart is the ratio of stroke volume to left ventricular end-diastolic volume (LVEDV) and is usually expressed as a percentage (normal values are 55% to 75%). The product of the stroke volume and heart rate (in beats per minute) gives the **cardiac output ($\dot{Q}c$),** expressed as L/min.

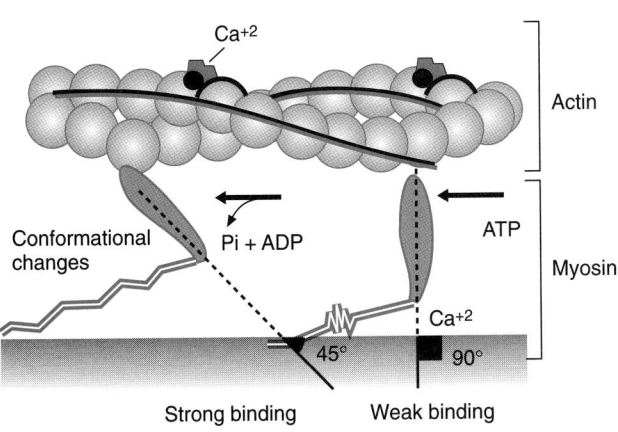

Figure 54-3 Proposed mechanism for sliding of the thick and thin filaments. The thick filament head undergoes a conformational change from the 90-degree configuration to the 45-degree configuration, a process that requires adenosine triphosphate (ATP). *ADP,* Adenosine diphosphate.

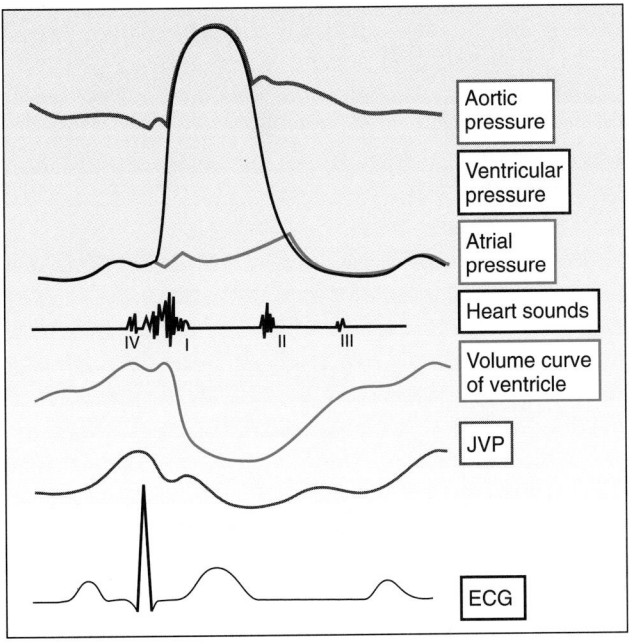

Figure 54-4 The Wiggers' diagram that explains the relationship between the pressure in the ventricle, aorta, and atria, the electrical activity in the heart, and the ventricular shape changes during a cardiac contraction. *JVP,* Jugular venous pressure; *ECG,* electrocardiogram.

After the blood is ejected, the heart quickly fills with blood from the venous circulation, termed **venous return.** In the steady state the venous return must equal the $\dot{Q}c$. The concept of matched venous return and $\dot{Q}c$ is important in the determination of overall function, because processes that effect the venous return must then effect $\dot{Q}c$ and vice versa. The importance of the venous return cannot be overemphasized. Significant changes in $\dot{Q}c$ must be reflected by changes in the venous return, right ventricular filling, and right atrial pressure.[17]

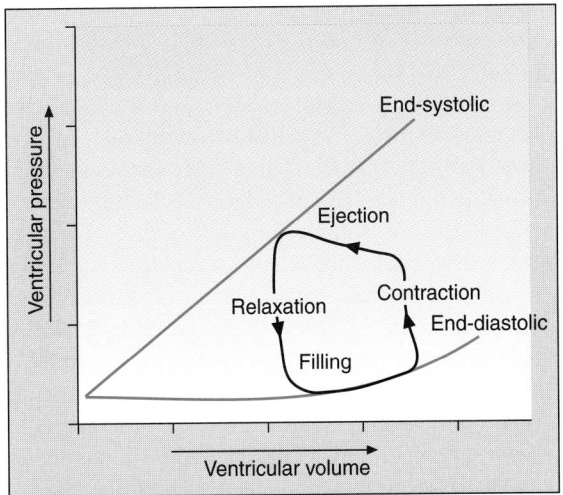

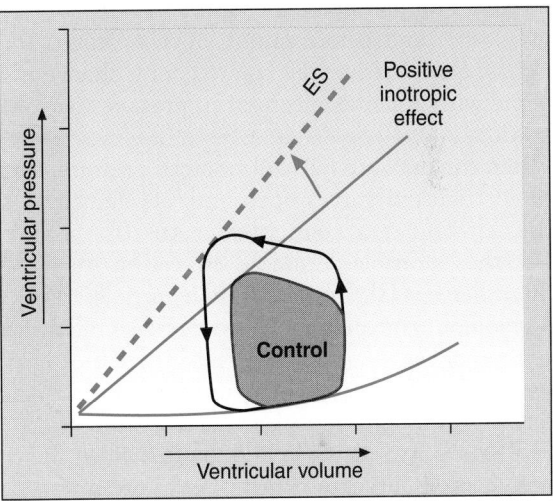

Figure 54-5 Normal left ventricular (LV) pressure-volume relationship during a cardiac cycle. *ES,* End-systolic.

The left ventricle (LV) and the right ventricle (RV) interact both in systole and diastole. The interaction between the LV and RV occurs through alterations in systemic and pulmonary venous return, LV and RV dimensional changes, and functional changes. This complex interplay is termed **ventricular interdependence** (see section on heart and lung interactions). Thus a complete understanding of the $\dot{Q}c$ must not only consider the performance of the LV but also take into account changes in RV dimensions and function.

Cardiac Cycle

The cardiac events can be illustrated by an examination of the pressure and volume changes of the ventricle versus time (Figure 54-4) and the changes in pressure as a function of changes in ventricular volume (P-V loop; Figure 54-5). At the onset of systole, the ventricular pressure rises, but the volume of the ventricle does not change until a pressure gradient is established (**isovolumic contraction**). When the pressure is greater than aortic pressure, the aortic valve opens and blood is ejected into the aorta. The mitral valve remains closed during systole since ventricular pressure is greater than atrial pressure. After the aortic valve opens, the ventricular pressure continues to rise at a decreased rate, then peaks and falls as the LV volume rapidly decreases. When the pressure falls below aortic pressure, the aortic valve closes and systole ends. This is seen on pressure tracings as a small increase in pressure called the *dicrotic notch* (see Figure 54-4).

Diastolic filling is crucial to the production of the circulation. The process of cardiac relaxation consists of an active energy-dependent component and a passive component that is dependent on the elastic properties of the ventricles. The first phase of diastole occurs after aortic valve closure and before mitral valve opening. During this phase the ventricle relaxes without a change in volume and with a marked decrease in pressure (**isovolumic relaxation**).

When the pressure falls below atrial pressure, the mitral and tricuspid valves open and the ventricles start to fill. This phase accounts for up to 70% of the filling of the ventricles[16] and is driven by the pressure gradient between the atria and the ventricles. The pressure gradient is augmented by energy-dependent active relaxation of the myocardium. This lowers the ventricular pressures and creates a suction-like effect that aids filling.

The next phase occurs in mid-diastole when the rising ventricular pressure approximates atrial pressure and filling slows markedly or may even cease for a brief moment (diastasis). This is followed by atrial contraction, which ejects the final portion of blood into the ventricles to complete filling.

The relative changes in atrial and ventricular diastolic pressure that occur as the ventricle fills determine the degree of filling, and the rate of rise of ventricular pressure depends on the elastic properties of the ventricle. This is represented by ventricular compliance (the ratio of change in volume with change in pressure). Processes that raise atrial pressure or improve relaxation will improve filling, whereas processes that impede relaxation or decrease the pressure gradient will decrease filling. In addition, a stiff noncompliant ventricle will require higher atrial pressures to achieve the same degree of diastolic filling. The importance of atrial contraction depends on the effectiveness of the previous filling phases. With impaired early diastole, more blood is in the atria, and the relative contribution of atrial systole is greater. In normal hearts the contribution of atrial contraction to LV filling is small. However, in most forms of cardiac failure, the atrial contraction plays an important role in the improvement of ventricular filling and thus the improvement of $\dot{Q}c$ and reduction of atrial pressures.

Determinants of Ventricular Function

Preload

Mechanical factors effect myocyte and myocardial contraction. **Starling's law of cardiac function** states that the longer the initial sarcomere length, the greater the force generated with contraction. The degree of precontraction stretch of the sarcomere is termed the **preload.** In general, as preload increases, $\dot{Q}c$ increases (Frank-Starling relationship). However, as preload continues to increase, the $\dot{Q}c$ eventually reaches a plateau. Increased sarcomere length likely leads to greater force of contraction by enhancing calcium availability and the sensitivity of the contractile proteins to the calcium.[15,16] The preload of the ventricle may be approximated by the ventricular end-diastolic volume (EDV; Figure 54-6). Unfortunately this is a difficult variable to measure clinically, and the end-diastolic pressure (EDP) is often used as a surrogate. The relationship between ven-

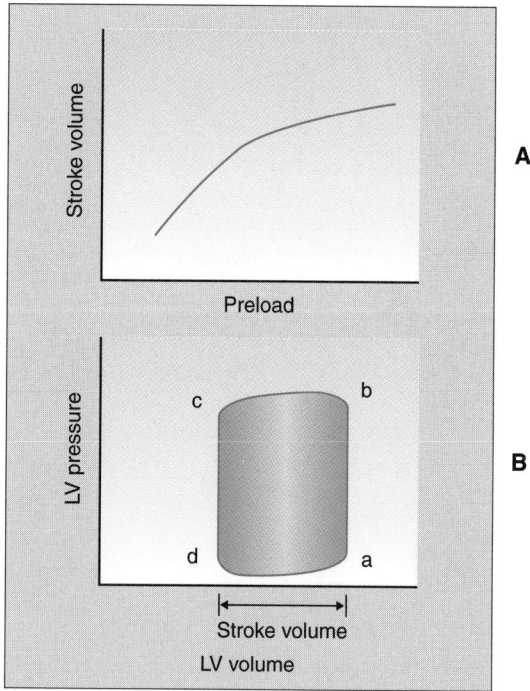

Figure 54-6 **A,** Relationship between preload and stroke volume. **B,** The pressure-volume loop. For a single cardiac cycle, left ventricular (LV) pressure is plotted against LV volume. Point *a* represents end-diastole and the start of isovolemic contraction. Ventricular pressure increases without a change in volume until ejection starts at point *b*, which represents the opening of the aortic valve. During ejection, ventricular volume decreases. Point *c* represents end-systole and the start of isovolemic relaxation. The aortic valve closes near end-systole. Ventricular pressure continues to fall until ventricular filling starts with the opening of the mitral valve at point *d.* Ventricular pressure increases very slightly during diastolic filling. (**A,** Modified from Nwasokwa ON. Cardiac function. In: Dantzker DR, Scharf SM, editors. Cardiopulmonary critical care. 3rd ed. Philadelphia: WB Saunders; 1998. **B,** Modified from Wannenburg T, Little WC. Regulation of cardiac output. In: Brown DL, editor. Cardiac intensive care. Philadelphia: WB Saunders; 1998.)

tricular EDV and EDP is affected by myocardial compliance (C) and the pressure surrounding the heart (P_{cs}) as related by the equation EDV = (EDP − P_{cs}) × C. Thus interpretations of filling pressures as a measure of preload must take into account the transmyocardial pressure (EDP − P_{cs}), as well as the ventricular compliance. The ventricular diastolic filling pressure also represents a back-pressure limiting venous return (Figure 54-7). The relationship between preload and $\dot{Q}c$ requires consideration of both intrinsic ventricular function and venous return (Figure 54-8).

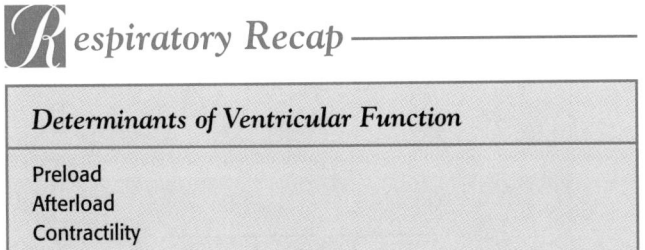

Respiratory Recap

Determinants of Ventricular Function
Preload
Afterload
Contractility

Afterload

The load that opposes myocardial shortening is called the **afterload.** There is a tight inverse relationship between the force generated by the cardiac muscle against a load and the degree and velocity of muscle shortening. As the afterload is increased at any fixed degree of contractility, there is less myocardial shortening and decreased cardiac output, a concept demonstrated graphically in Figure 54-9. Afterload is not easily quantified. The aortic input impedance has been suggested as the most accurate estimate of afterload, but this variable is difficult to measure.[16] The systolic wall stress of the ventricle can be used as a measure of afterload, but since wall stress depends on chamber radius, thickness, and pressure, it is also difficult to meas-

ure. For clinical purposes, the mean arterial blood pressure (MAP) may be a reasonable estimate of afterload. The calculated **vascular resistance** (SVR = [(MAP − CVP) ÷ $\dot{Q}c$] × 80) also may be used to follow relative changes in afterload after interventions but should not be used as a direct measurement of afterload.

Contractility

Contractility defines the intrinsic strength of contraction independent of preload and afterload. The myocardium can alter contractility in many ways. In general, measures that increase the concentration or availability of cytoplasmic calcium ions increase the contractility. The effect of changes in contractility can be demonstrated graphically as a change in the relationship between stroke volume and preload or afterload (Figure 54-10). An increase in contractility improves the relative cardiac performance for a given preload and afterload. Similarly, decrements in contractility will alter this relationship in a negative fashion.

Control of Preload, Afterload, and Contractility

The β-adrenergic nervous system is one of the most important regulators of contractility. β-Adrenergic receptors (types 1 and 2) in the heart are stimulated by catecholamines that circulate (for example, epinephrine) or are released from autonomic nerves. These receptors, when occupied, stimulate adenylate cyclase and increase the intracellular amount of the secondary messenger cyclic adenosine monophosphate (cAMP). This stimulates a cascade of events that result in the addition of phosphate (phosphorylation) to several key enzymes. These enzymes lead to greater calcium release from the SR as well as better re-uptake of cytosolic

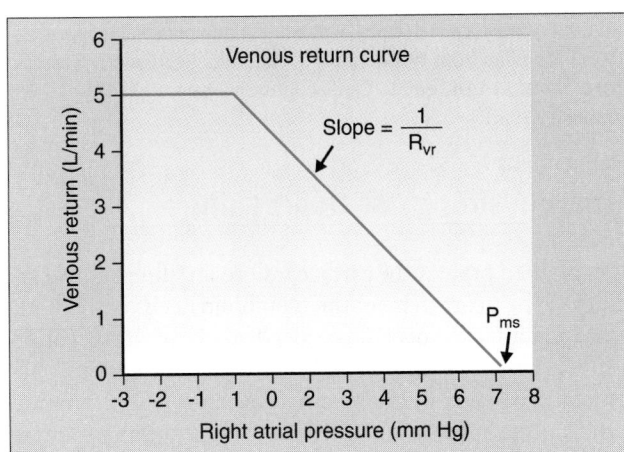

Figure 54-7 Relationship between right atrial pressure and the venous return. R_{vr}, Resistance to venous return; P_{ms}, mean systolic pressure. (Modified from Brienza N, Ayuse T, Revelly JP, et al. Peripheral control of venous return in critical illness: role of the splanchnic vascular compartment. In: Dantzker DR, Scharf SM, editors. Cardiopulmonary critical care. 3rd ed. Philadelphia: Saunders; 1998.)

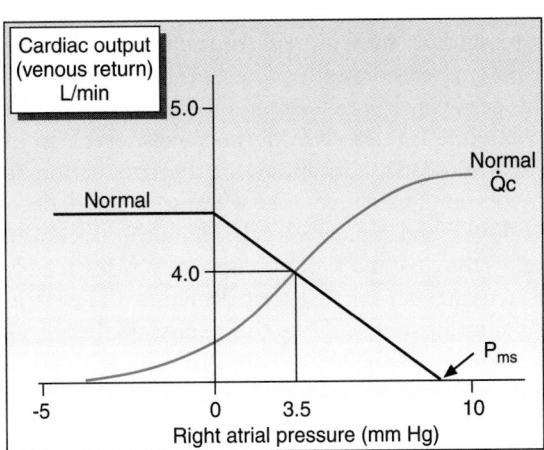

Figure 54-8 Venous return and cardiac output ($\dot{Q}c$) as a function of right atrial pressure. The intersection of the two curves represents the steady state $\dot{Q}c$ of the heart under the given loading conditions. (Modified from Jacobsohn E, Chorn R, O'Connor M. Can J Anesth 1997;44:849-867.)

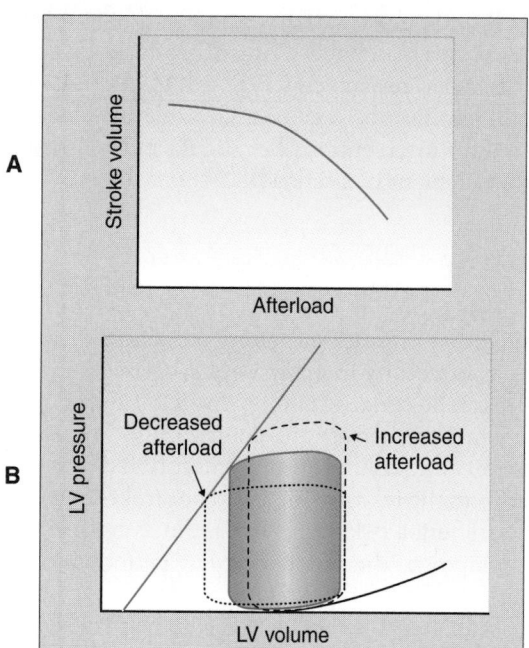

Figure 54-9 **A,** Effects of afterload on stroke volume. **B,** Effects of afterload on the pressure-volume curve of the left ventricle (LV). (**A,** Modified from Nwasokwa ON. Cardiac function. In: Dantzker DR, Scharf SM, editors. Cardiopulmonary critical care. 3rd ed. Philadelphia: WB Saunders; 1997. **B** Modified from Wannenburg T, Little WC. Regulation of cardiac output. In: Brown DL, editor. Cardiac intensive care. Philadelphia: WB Saunders, 1998. pp. 55-62.)

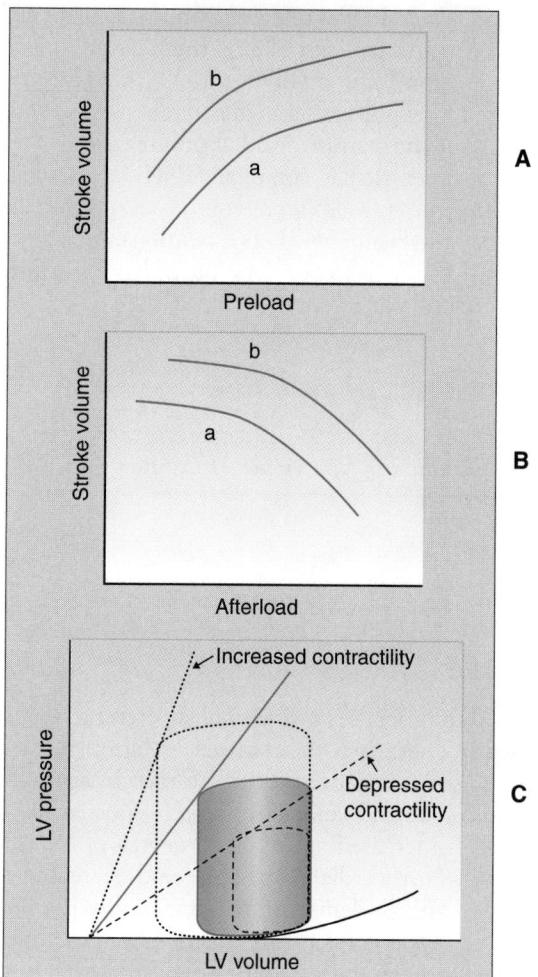

Figure 54-10 **A,** Effects of changes in contractility on stroke volume as shown as a function of preload. **B,** Effects of changes of contractility as a function of afterload. **C,** Effects of changes in contractility on the pressure-volume curve. *LV,* Left ventricle. (**A** and **B,** Modified from Nwasokwa ON. Cardiac function. In: Dantzker DR, Scharf SM, editors. Cardiopulmonary critical care. 3rd ed. Philadelphia: WB Saunders; 1997. **C,** Modified from Wannenburg T, Little WC. Regulation of cardiac output. In: Brown DL, editor. Cardiac intensive care. Philadelphia: WB Saunders; 1998.)

calcium. This results in enhanced contractility and relaxation. β-Receptors are also expressed on the conduction tissue of the heart and, when stimulated, increase heart rate. In the periphery, smooth muscle cells surrounding the vasculature can be stimulated by β-receptors to relax and dilate, thus reducing afterload and preload. Another sympathetic receptor, the β-receptor, leads to smooth muscle cell contraction and vasoconstriction (increased afterload and preload).[14]

The parasympathetic system also can effect the heart. Acetylcholine is released from the vagus nerve and interacts with muscarinic receptors on the conduction tissue and myocytes. These receptors, when stimulated, decrease cAMP levels and increase levels of another second messenger, cyclic guanine monophosphate (cGMP).[18] Cyclic GMP activates an enzyme that decreases the activity of the calcium channels. Thus the parasympathetic system leads to decreased heart rate and, to a lesser extent, decreased contractility.

The cardiomyocytes and the smooth muscle cells around the vasculature are influenced by nitric oxide (NO). NO can suppress myocardial function and leads to vasodilation in the periphery by upregulation of cGMP.[19] Other proteins such as angiotensin II and vasopressin are potent stimulators of vasoconstriction. They also have receptors on cardiomyocytes, but the exact nature of the effects of these proteins on cardiac performance is unclear.

Pathophysiology of Heart Failure

As explained previously, cardiac failure is defined as the inability of the heart to meet the metabolic needs of the body or the inability to meet those needs without an elevation in filling pressures. The complex interplay of various phenomena results in normal cardiac function. Coordination of the cardiac muscle function with venous filling, the rate and rhythm of contraction, and valvular competence is required. Abnormalities of any of these components can eventually lead to cardiac failure.

Mechanisms

Impairment of contractile function includes primary muscle disorders such as myocardial infarction and rhythm disorders.

TABLE 54-1

Pathophysiology of Heart Failure with Clinical Examples

Pathophysiology	Clinical Example
Restricted filling	Restrictive cardiomyopathy
	Constrictive pericarditis
	Tamponade
	Hypertrophic cardiomyopathy
	Mitral stenosis
	Tricuspid stenosis
Pressure overload	Hypertension
	Aortic stenosis
	Pulmonary embolism
	Pulmonary hypertension
	Pulmonary stenosis
Volume overload	Mitral regurgitation
	Aortic regurgitation
	Pulmonary regurgitation
	Tricuspid regurgitation
	Septal defects
Contractile impairment	Ischemia (chronic or acute)
	Dilated cardiomyopathy
	Myocarditis
Arrhythmia	Tachycardia
	Bradycardia

From Timmis AD, Nathan AW. Essentials of cardiology. Oxford: Blackwell Scientific; 1993.

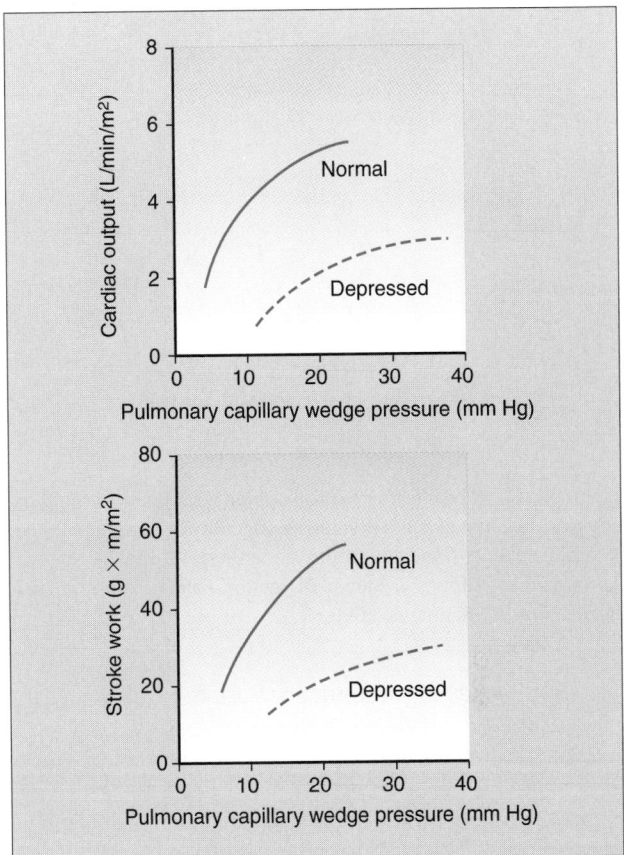

Figure 54-11 The effect of a decrease in contractility on the Starling relationship. (Modified from Little WC, Braunwald E. Assessment of cardiac function. In: Braunwald E, editor. Heart disease: a textbook of cardiovascular medicine. 5th ed. Philadelphia: WB Saunders; 1997)

A list of common cardiac disorders that can lead to heart failure via this pathway is shown in Table 54-1. In these disorders, the primary problem is the inability of the heart to pump because of either direct impairment in the force of contraction or in the frequency of contractions (as in arrhythmias). This form of heart failure is often called systolic dysfunction and can be represented graphically as a shift in the Starling curve downward (Figure 54-11). Cellular aspects of systolic dysfunction are discussed in a later section.

Respiratory Recap

Mechanisms of Heart Failure*
Primary impaired myocardial contractile function
Excessive ventricular load (pressure or volume)
Restricted ventricular filling

*These mechanisms of cardiac failure are not mutually exclusive and many forms of heart disease share components of all three pathways.

Many forms of heart disease impose an excessive load on the heart (see Table 54-1). This load can be either in the form of an excess pressure requirement or an excess volume requirement. In addition, the load may occur as an acute overload that rapidly causes deterioration in cardiac function or as a chronic load that slowly leads to cardiac failure.

An example of an acute volume overload is papillary muscle rupture and acute mitral regurgitation. In this situation, the heart suddenly ejects a large amount of blood through the mitral valve during systole, thus reducing the forward $\dot{Q}c$ and increasing left atrial pressure. As a result there is an acute rise in atrial pressure, LVEDP, and LVEDV. Compensation via increased contractility may not adequately augment forward stroke volume because of the low pressure of the left atrium relative to the systemic circulation. Thus these patients will often present in shock with pulmonary edema.

Chronic volume overload results from disorders such as progressive aortic or mitral valve regurgitation in which initially a small portion of the stroke volume is regurgitated back into the ventricle. The result is a decrease in the true forward $\dot{Q}c$ at a given LVEDV. Under such conditions the slow progression of the degree of regurgitation allows the heart to compensate with slow dilation and an increase in mass, which helps to normalize wall stress and preserve the forward stroke volume (Figure 54-12), al-

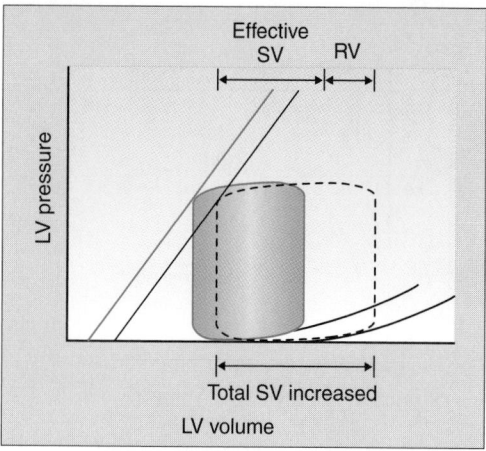

Figure 54-12   The effect of a chronic volume overload on the pressure volume curve of the left ventricle (LV). *RV,* Regurgitant volume; *SV,* stroke volume. (Modified from Wannenburg T, Little WC. Regulation of cardiac output. In: Brown DL, editor. Cardiac intensive care. Philadelphia: WB Saunders; 1998.)

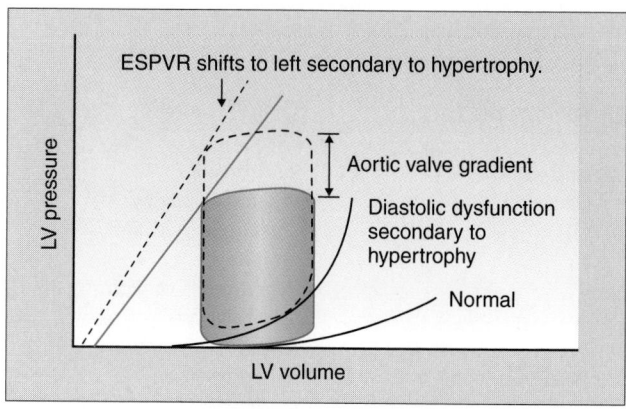

Figure 54-13   The effect of a chronic pressure overload (aortic stenosis) on the pressure volume curve of the left ventricle (LV). *ESPVR,* End-systolic pressure-volume relationship. (Modified from Wannenburg T, Little WC. Regulation of cardiac output. In: Brown DL, editor. Cardiac intensive care. Philadelphia: WB Saunders; 1998.)

though this leads to a chronic increase in LVEDV and LV wall thickness.

In acute pressure overload, the high afterload reduces the forward output of the heart. Because of the acute nature of the overload, the compensatory mechanisms of the heart (increased LVEDV and increased contractility) may be inadequate to augment forward flow, leading to elevated filling pressures with pulmonary edema.

Chronic pressure overload (for example, hypertension, aortic stenosis) results in a sustained increase in afterload and ventricular wall tension. This decreases the velocity of muscle shortening and eventually decreases intrinsic cardiac contraction. Graphically a pressure overload such as aortic stenosis can be demonstrated as shown in Figure 54-13. The subsequent decrease in stroke volume will be compensated by adaptive mechanisms.

As the increased load continues, the adaptive mechanisms will eventually fail to compensate and the signs of cardiac failure will become evident. The end result is systolic dysfunction. This differs from the previous mechanism described in that the original cause of the dysfunction is not a primary disorder of the contractile apparatus but, ultimately, is caused by exhausted compensation.

Alteration of ventricular filling may accompany a number of different cardiac disorders (see Table 54-1). The disorders range from myocardial valvular disease to pericardial disease. In these disorders, the abnormally high filling pressures are required to achieve the preload necessary to deliver an adequate stroke volume.

The failure of the cardiac muscle to relax normally often is called *diastolic dysfunction* and represents one of the most common and significant forms of cardiac failure. Diastolic dysfunction results in elevated filling pressures and symptoms of pulmonary and systemic congestion despite normal systolic function. Diastolic dysfunction is caused by processes that effect the active (energy-dependent) and

passive (compliance) relaxation of the ventricle. Many conditions cause diastolic dysfunction. As previously noted, early in diastole the ventricular relaxation is an energy-requiring process, so cardiac ischemia is a common cause of both diastolic and systolic dysfunction. Volume overload can cause relative diastolic dysfunction by increasing the LVEDV, thus increasing the LV filling pressures because of a shift of the diastolic pressure volume curve into a less compliant region (Figure 54-14). Diastolic dysfunction may also occur with an increase in afterload. Increased afterload has been shown to reduce the rate of both myocardial contraction and active relaxation.[20] With hypertrophy of the myocardium or in conditions of abnormal infiltration of the myocardium, the ventricles are less compliant, and the diastolic pressure volume curve will shift upward (see Figure 54-14). Extrinsic compression of the heart does not effect the intrinsic relaxation of the myocardium but reduces the distensibility of the heart and thus displaces the PV curve upwards.[21]

Classification

Heart failure can be further separated into a number of different forms. The clinical manifestations arise from either poor organ perfusion, so called **forward heart failure,** or

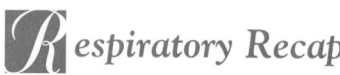

espiratory Recap ——————

Classification of Heart Failure
Forward versus backward heart failure
Acute versus chronic heart failure
Right versus left heart failure
High-output versus low-output failure

from accumulation of blood in the heart and increased filling pressures, so called **backward heart failure.** Although originally presented as opposing theories of heart failure pathophysiology, it is likely that both forms of heart failure occur in the majority of patients with chronic cardiac dysfunction.[22]

The acuity of heart failure is an important etiologic consideration. Myocardial infarction, myocarditis, and pulmonary emboli may cause acute cardiac failure. An acute, severe change in cardiac function can cause pulmonary edema and shock resulting from the inability of the heart to adapt rapidly to loss of myocardium or a dramatic increase in load. Chronic heart failure is seen in conditions such as CAD, hypertensive heart disease, and chronic valvular disease. Often long-standing compensation can lead to chronic heart failure in later years (for example, ischemic **cardiomyopathy**). As opposed to the severe symptoms of acute changes in cardiac function, chronic cardiac failure may manifest only relatively mild symptoms until late in the disease process because of the compensatory mechanisms.

The clinical effects of isolated left ventricular failure are largely attributed to venous congestion of the lungs. Similarly, RV failure leads to symptoms caused by congestion of the systemic veins. RV failure can occur in isolation (as with pulmonary embolism) or concurrent with LV failure (biventricular failure). RV failure most commonly results from LV failure. In cases of biventricular failure a patient may manifest symptoms of predominantly right or left ventricular failure, or both.

Most forms of heart failure are characterized by a reduction in the $\dot{Q}c$ either at rest or with exercise. In certain uncommon conditions, the tissue demand for oxygen cannot be met despite a high $\dot{Q}c$. This is called *high-output failure* and is seen in conditions of increased metabolic rate (for example, thyrotoxicosis), reduced oxygen-carrying capacity of blood (for example, anemia), and arteriovenous shunting, which reduces the effective $\dot{Q}c$ (for example, arteriovenous fistulas, beriberi, and Paget's disease).[4]

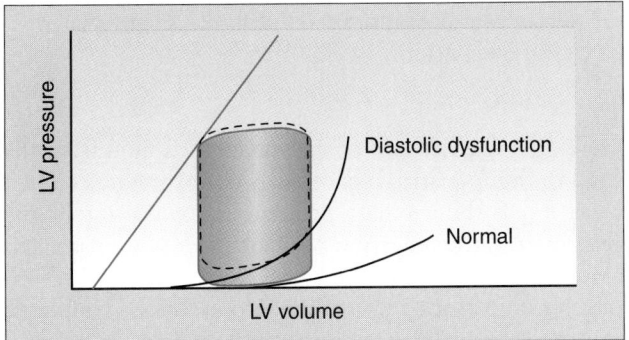

Figure 54-14 Diastolic dysfunction leads to an elevation in the diastolic pressure volume curve of the left ventricle (LV). (Modified from Wannenburg T, Little WC. Regulation of cardiac output. In: Brown DL, editor. Cardiac intensive care. Philadelphia: WB Saunders; 1998.)

Adaptive Mechanisms

Two general mechanisms are invoked to compensate for a reduction in cardiac contractility or abnormal filling dynamics: neurohumoral activation and ventricular remodeling. These compensatory mechanisms work to restore perfusion to the vital organs by augmenting $\dot{Q}c$ and supporting blood pressure. However, the compensatory mechanisms themselves are maladaptive over time.

Myocardial sympathetic stimulation via β-receptors can augment both the heart rate (chronotropy) and contractility (inotropy). In addition, sympathetic-induced contraction of peripheral arteries and veins increases blood pressure and venous return. By selectively vasoconstricting skin, muscle, and gut vessels, the $\dot{Q}c$ is redistributed to the brain and heart. Thus sympathetic augmentation of blood pressure and $\dot{Q}c$ may be an effective compensation for acute episodes of mild to moderate heart failure. In chronic heart failure, however, the number of myocardial β-receptors is down-regulated, as is their sensitivity to stimulation, thus decreasing the effectiveness of sympathetic stimulation.[23] A state of chronically increased sympathetic tone and decreased parasympathetic tone is usually found in chronic heart failure.[24] This is detrimental over time because of the induction of arrhythmias, apoptosis, and a chronic increase in afterload.[21]

A very important means to support the blood pressure is the renin-angiotensin system. If renal perfusion is decreased, the kidney releases an enzyme called *renin*. This enzyme acts to produce angiotensin I, which is cleaved by another enzyme, angiotensin-converting enzyme (ACE), into angiotensin II (AII), a potent arteriolar vasoconstrictor. In addition, AII stimulates the adrenals to release aldosterone, which acts on the distal part of the nephron to stimulate sodium reabsorption. Thus the renin-angiotensin system augments blood pressure via AII-mediated vasoconstriction and increases blood volume by sodium retention via aldosterone. Unfortunately, in chronic heart failure, this can lead to detrimental increases in afterload and preload that can adversely tax cardiac function. Although the increase in blood volume initially increases $\dot{Q}c$ by increasing preload, it also increases wall tension and imposes greater workload on the failing ventricle. The failing heart may be working on the flat portion of the Frank-Starling curve where $\dot{Q}c$ has reached a plateau; thus an increase in circulating volume will not necessarily augment $\dot{Q}c$ and may contribute to pulmonary and peripheral edema.

Two other systemic hormones, vasopressin and atrial natriuretic peptide (ANP), are up-regulated in cardiac failure. Vasopressin, just as is AII, is a potent vasoconstrictor and also increases circulating blood volume. ANP is a vasodilator and induces diuresis. Its role in cardiac failure is largely unknown.[25]

The ventricle remodels in response to the load placed on it. This remodeling can be in several different forms: (1) concentric hypertrophy, (2) eccentric hypertrophy, and (3) changes in chamber geometry (usually more spherelike). A prolonged pressure load on the myocardium leads to fundamental changes in cardiac muscle. In experimental models, increased systolic wall stress up-regulates growth factors that increase the number of mitochondria and increase myofibril mass. The new myofibrils are usually laid down in parallel leading to hypertrophied myocytes and, ultimately, to a concentrically thicker ventricle. Physiologically a thicker ventricle serves to normalize increased wall stress. Wall stress can be calculated by Laplace's law:

$$\text{Wall stress} = \frac{\text{Pressure} \times \text{Radius}}{2 \times \text{Wall thickness}}$$

Thus the pressure the ventricle contracts against is directly proportional to wall stress. As the ventricle increases its thickness, wall stress decreases, which in turn improves cardiac performance to a point.[15,21] However, this improved performance is at the price of increased oxygen demand and possible diastolic dysfunction.

The dilated ventricle has increased diastolic wall stress caused by increased diastolic volume (due to an increased radius). In an effort to accommodate the increased volume, myocytes increase the number of sarcomeres in series, thus increasing the radius and length of the ventricle. As the chamber radius increases, so does systolic wall stress, and the ventricle is therefore stimulated to increase in thickness. Thus volume overload induces ventricular dilation (eccentric) and hypertrophy to compensate for the increased diastolic wall stress. This initially allows compensation for increased diastolic load at normalized wall stress.[21]

The ventricle changes in shape in response to the specific, chronic load placed on it to optimize function. Chronic pressure loads induce thickened ventricles with small cavities, whereas chronic volume loads cause dilation of the ventricle. These ventricular shape changes have effects on both systolic and diastolic performance, as well as on oxygen use. These adaptive compensatory changes may become ineffective if the heart thickens or dilates excessively and heart failure may ensue.

Cellular Mechanisms

The cellular events associated with heart failure are complex and have been reviewed elsewhere.[15,21] These include abnormalities in excitation-contraction coupling, contractile protein interaction, and intrinsic alterations in protein expression. In some cases these are primary abnormalities that result from genetic defects or a direct insult to the myocardium (for example, myocardial ischemia). In other cases the abnormalities are likely secondary to the maladaptive responses and contribute to progression of cardiac failure.[26]

When an excessive load is presented to the ventricle, the compensatory mechanisms listed previously function to preserve $\dot{Q}c$. Often this compensation is inadequate and intrinsic problems with contractility persist.[27] Over time, cellular changes occur such as apoptosis of myocardiocytes, lysis of myofibrils, distortion of the SR, and capillary dropout.[21] This leads to a continued increase in wall stress and an exacerbated stimulus for hypertrophy and/or dilation. As the muscle thickens, portions become ischemic causing further progression of the cardiac failure.[21] A viscous positive feedback cycle may thus ensue.

Abnormalities in contraction, relaxation, and electrical properties of the failing myocardium are linked to abnormal calcium handling.[28] Calcium release and re-uptake by the SR are abnormal in the failing heart.[29,30] This may be caused by abnormalities in the calcium release channel,[29] the voltage-dependent calcium channel,[31] and the calcium ATPase enzyme.[32] These abnormalities have been demonstrated in many forms of heart failure and may represent a final common pathway of cardiac cellular dysfunction. Alterations in the contractile apparatus have also been demonstrated in cardiac failure. The overall myofibril protein content is reduced in heart failure.[33] In addition, there are abnormalities in the myosin ATPase activity and regulatory protein function.[34,35]

Pathophysiology of Pulmonary Edema

Pulmonary edema is the accumulation of excess fluid in the interstitial and alveolar spaces in the lung. The large capillary network of the pulmonary circulation has extensive interaction with the air-filled alveoli. The interstitium between the capillary endothelial cells and the alveolar epithelial cells is quite thin and made up of a basement membrane, connective tissue, and cellular elements (macrophages and fibroblasts). Normally a continuous flux of fluid and proteins is transported between the pulmonary circulation and the lung interstitium, with a net flow from the capillaries into the interstitial tissue.[36] Excess fluid is removed from the interstitium by the lymphatic system. Pulmonary edema develops when there is an increase in the flux of fluid going into the lung interstitium that overwhelms the lymphatic drainage.

The net rate of transudation of fluid can be related by the Starling equation:[37]

$$Q = K_f[(P_{cap} - P_{int}) - \sigma_f(\pi_{cap} - \pi_{int})]$$

where Q is the net rate of transudation of fluid from the blood to the interstitial space, K_f is the hydraulic conductance, P_{cap} is the capillary pressure, P_{int} is the interstitial pressure, σ_f is the reflection coefficient for proteins, π_{cap} is the **oncotic pressure** of the capillaries, and π_{int} is the oncotic pressure of the interstitium. Normally the lymphatic drainage actively takes up interstitial fluid and removes it from the interstitial space at about 20 mL/hour. With chronic pulmonary edema, the pulmonary lymphatics hypertrophy and increased amounts of fluid can be removed (up to 200 mL/hour).[21]

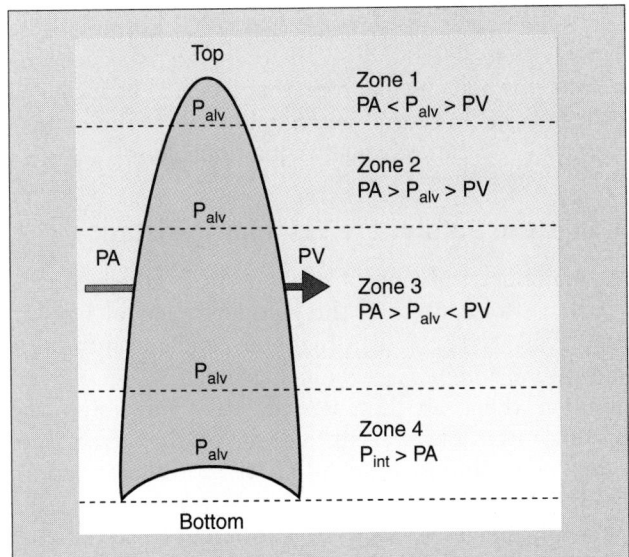

Figure 54-15   The four perfusion zones of the lung. The heights of the *thick black lines* represent pulmonary arterial (PA) and pulmonary venous (PV) pressures. P_{alv}, Alveolar pressure; P_{int}, interstitial pressure. (Modified from Gaine SP, Brower RG, Wiener CM. Pathophysiology of the pulmonary vascular bed. In: Dantzker DR, Scharf SM, editors. Cardiopulmonary critical care. 3rd ed. Philadelphia: WB Saunders; 1998.)

Given the previous equation, pulmonary edema can result from any of a number of causes that create an imbalance in the Starling equation. These include increased pulmonary capillary pressure as in heart failure, decreased blood oncotic pressure, and increased capillary permeability. Increased fluid flux into the interstitium eventually overwhelms the lymphatic drainage and fluid initially collects in the most compliant regions of the interstitium around vessels and airways. With increased accumulation, fluid begins to collect in the alveolar-capillary membrane and eventually floods the alveoli.[38]

Gravity directs the majority of lung blood flow toward the most dependent regions of the lung. Pulmonary perfusion pressure and pulmonary venous pressure increase from the apex to the base in the upright lung (Figure 54-15). Thus edema is most likely to form in the dependent regions (West zone III). As interstitial pressure increases, the lumen of the pulmonary vessels may be compressed in the dependent regions leading to a decrease in their perfusion (West zone IV) and redistribution of the blood flow into the nondependent regions. This is the cause of the increased apical vascular markings commonly seen on chest radiographs of patients with pulmonary edema.

In cardiac failure, pulmonary edema results from elevation in the pulmonary capillary pressure. This is a direct result of increased downstream pressure in the pulmonary veins, left atrium, and left ventricle that results from the various causes of heart failure. The development of pulmonary edema depends on the relationship between the capillary pressure, the oncotic pressures, and the lymphatic drainage. In acute heart failure, it has been esti-

mated that pulmonary capillary pressures in excess of 28 mm Hg are needed before edema forms.[39] In chronic conditions considerably higher pressures may be tolerated because of lymphatic hypertrophy (up to 40 mm Hg).

As the pulmonary capillary pressure rises, there is an increase in the caliber of vessels and engorgement of the lungs with blood. This increases the elasticity of the lung and commonly is associated with a sense of dyspnea. As edema forms in the interstitium, there is a further increase in lung elasticity. Ventilation-perfusion inequalities appear, leading to increased work of breathing and problems with oxygen uptake.[40] The edema also effects dyspnea receptors leading to the symptom of shortness of breath. As edema worsens and fluid begins to flood alveoli, early dependent airway closure and associated lung collapse occur. This leads to further abnormalities in gas exchange and a dramatic increase in elasticity and work of breathing. In addition, engorged blood vessels may reduce the caliber of small airways and increase airways' resistance. This can then cause a decreased vital capacity and air trapping. Often the airway edema predisposes patients to bronchospasm, and they may develop wheezing (cardiac asthma).[22,41] Gas exchange abnormalities may be quite severe, with hypoxia followed by hypercapnia as the patient begins to fatigue. In acute severe pulmonary edema, the patient may rapidly progress to respiratory failure. Rapid diagnosis and application of therapy can be life-saving and often can avoid the use of mechanical ventilation.

Heart-Lung Interactions

The heart and lungs are pressure-driven systems that share the primary responsibility for oxygen uptake and delivery to the body. They also share a common space (the thorax) and thus are linked anatomically. The heart and lung interactions based on these physiologic links often have profound consequences in critical illness. Extensive reviews of heart-lung interactions have been published elsewhere.[42-45]

With each breath the lungs and thorax change, both in volume and in intrathoracic pressure. These fluctuations can effect cardiac function by inducing changes in the heart rate, preload, afterload, venous return, and contractility of the heart. The heart-lung interactions in cardiac failure can be especially challenging because the heart is less likely to tolerate fluctuations in these physiologic variables. A basic understanding of these interactions is important in the guidance of therapy such as mechanical ventilation.

Changes in Intrathoracic Pressure

The changes in pleural pressure with ventilation also affect the pressures at the heart's surface. The cardiac surface pressure will affect cardiac filling pressures based on the compliance of the myocardium. In addition, cardiac filling volume is dependent on the transmural pressure or the distending stress across the wall of the cardiac chamber. Thus, the pleural pressure swings during respiration can affect preload and afterload of the heart. For example, a decrease in pleural pressure during inspiration will be transmitted to the surface of the heart. During inspiration, the right atrial pressure falls relative to the systemic extrathoracic venous circulation, and venous filling of the right atrium is enhanced. This leads to an increase in venous return and right atrial volume during inspiration. Similarly, assuming a constant arterial pressure, a decrease in the pleural pressure that also lowers cardiac surface pressure will increase afterload by increasing the LV transmural pressure. An increase in intrathoracic pressure can decrease afterload by a similar mechanism. Normally these are small changes, but if there are large swings in the pleural pressure (as with respiratory distress) or the cardiac function is reduced, the effects can be more significant. The cardiac surface pressure also depends on the pericardial compliance and pressure, which is sensitive to changes in the volume of the cardiac chambers. Thus the change in cardiac surface pressure with a change in pleural pressure can be quite variable.[45]

Changes in Lung Volume

Changes in lung volume can influence cardiovascular performance by a number of different mechanisms. These mechanisms include changes in autonomic tone, changes in pulmonary vascular resistance (PVR), direct mechanical compression of the cardiac fossa, increases in intraabdominal pressure, and ventricular interdependence.[42] Such effects are manifest with every breath and can become quite significant during periods of sustained inflation as with mechanical ventilation with high positive end-expiratory pressure (PEEP).

Autonomic Changes

With an increase in lung volume there is a reflex decrease in heart rate and vascular tone that seems to be mediated by alterations in central autonomic tone.[46] The clinical significance of these changes is questionable.[42]

Changes in Pulmonary Vascular Resistance

The major determinants of pulmonary blood flow are RV systolic performance and the pulmonary vascular resistance (PVR).[42] The PVR is highly dependent on the volume of the lungs. As alveoli expand, the vessels surrounding them are compressed, thus increasing the resistance to flow. Vessels outside of the alveoli are pulled open during lung inflation by radial traction, which decreases vascular resistance. The net effect of the opposing changes is that PVR is lowest at the functional residual capacity (FRC) of the lungs. Decreases or increases in lung volume cause increases in the PVR (Figure 54-16).[47] An increase in PVR increases RV afterload and thus may decrease cardiac performance. In cardiac failure, alveolar edema may cause lung collapse and an increase in PVR. The use of PEEP may restore resting lung volume to the normal FRC and decrease PVR. If applied in excess, PEEP can increase lung volume above FRC and increase the PVR.

Mechanical Effects of Lung Expansion

As the lungs expand, they can affect the heart by physically pushing against the cardiac fossa (Figure 54-17).[42,45] This will increase the pressure surrounding the heart and can effect filling of the ventricles. The effect is independent of the pleural pressure change and dependent on lung

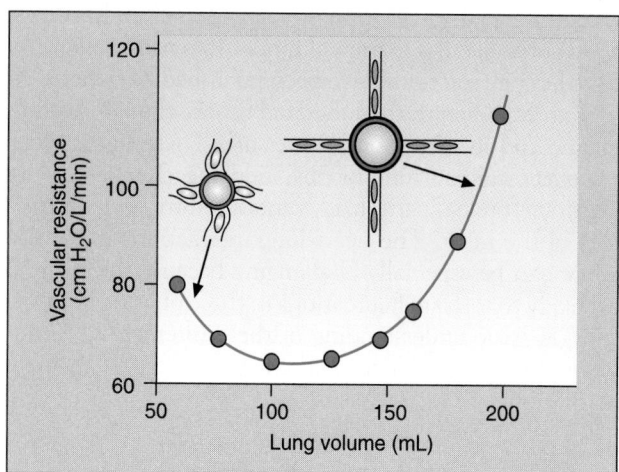

Figure 54-16   Effect of lung volume on the pulmonary vascular resistance. The effect of the lung volume on the caliber of extra-alveolar vessels is also shown. (Modified from West JB. Respiratory physiology. Baltimore: Williams & Wilkins; 1990.)

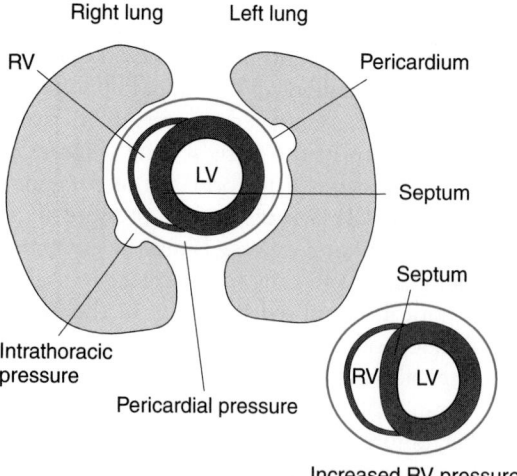

Figure 54-17   The anatomic relationship between the heart and lungs. *RV*, Right ventricle; *LV*, left ventricle. (Modified from Scharf SM. Mechanical cardiopulmonary interactions in critical care. In: Dantzker DR, Scharf SM, editors. Cardiopulmonary critical care. 3rd ed. Philadelphia: WB Saunders; 1998.)

volume. In patients with hyperinflation (as with chronic obstructive pulmonary disease [COPD]) the lungs can exert a fair amount of pressure around the heart and adversely effect ventricular filling.

Abdominal Pressure Changes

The descent of the diaphragm with respiration compresses the abdominal compartment and increases abdominal pressure. This increases the abdominal vascular pressures and increases the driving pressure for venous return.[48] If the patient is receiving positive pressure ventilation, the increase in abdominal pressure may partially compensate for the increase in right atrial pressure induced by the positive pressure.[42] Thus the application of PEEP can have complicated effects on the venous return depending on the change in abdominal pressure and previous filling pressure of the ventricle (Figure 54-18).[45]

Ventricular Interdependence

Although not a true heart-lung interaction, ventricular interdependence is often discussed in this setting. Changes in the volume and performance of one ventricle will affect the other ventricle through two general mechanisms. The filling of the LV depends on the output of the RV. Thus, a reduction in RV performance will reduce LV output by reducing LV preload. This is often called the *series interaction*.[45] In addition, the ventricles are both surrounded by the relatively nondistensible sac called the *pericardium*, and both ventricles share a common intraventricular septum. This anatomic coupling results in *parallel interactions* in which an increase in the volume of one ventricle reduces the compliance of the other.[45] For instance, the rise in the RVEDV that often accompanies an acute increase in the PVR will act to decrease LV compliance via effects on the septum. The net effect is a reduction in the LV preload and a decrease in LV output. This description is the general mechanism of the phenomenon of **pulsus paradoxus,** or an inspiratory decrease in systolic blood pressure.

Clinical Aspects of Cardiac Failure

The clinical manifestations of cardiac failure are related to inadequate organ perfusion and venous congestion from elevated ventricular filling pressures. The circulatory system has many compensatory mechanisms such that the signs and symptoms of heart failure may be manifest only during times of stress (that is, exercise).

Symptoms

The increased pulmonary capillary pressure and resulting interstitial edema seen in cardiac failure commonly leads to difficulty in breathing or an increased awareness of breathing. Most of the dyspnea can be attributed to an increased work of breathing resulting from decreased pulmonary function and increased ventilatory drive. Pulmonary edema decreases lung compliance and can increase airway resistance, thus increasing the pressure changes needed to move air in and out of the lungs. Ventilation and perfusion abnormalities lead to hypoxemia and hypercapnia, which increase the drive to breathe. With extreme decreases in $\dot{Q}c$, respiratory muscle fatigue can develop as a result of poor oxygen delivery and further exacerbate the patient's dyspnea.[22] Thus, dyspnea may be caused by either pulmonary congestion or a low-output state.

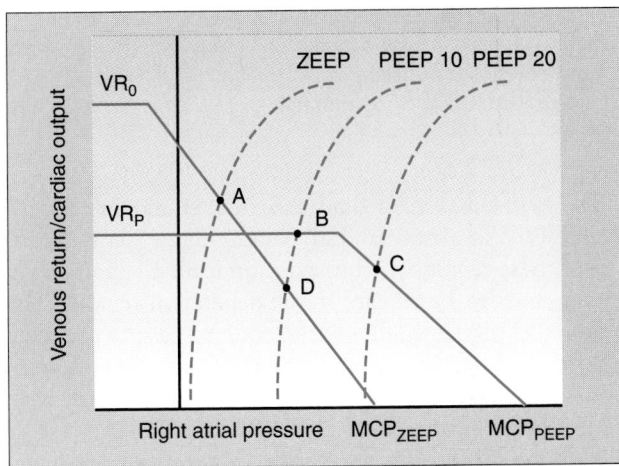

Figure 54-18 Effects of positive end-expiratory pressure (PEEP) on the determinants of venous return. *VR₀,* Venous return curve with zero PEEP (ZEEP); *VR_P,* venous return with PEEP; *MCP,* mean circulatory pressure. (Modified from Scharf SM. Mechanical cardiopulmonary interactions in critical care. In: Dantzker DR, Scharf SM, editors. Cardiopulmonary critical care. 3rd ed. Philadelphia: WB Saunders; 1998.).

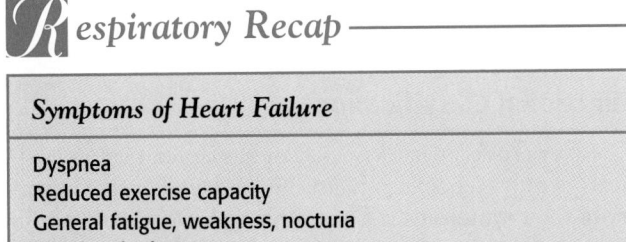

Respiratory Recap ————————

Symptoms of Heart Failure
Dyspnea Reduced exercise capacity General fatigue, weakness, nocturia Peripheral edema

The breathlessness of heart failure can manifest in many different ways. Most commonly the patient with heart failure has dyspnea on exertion. This can be a slowly progressive process, so it is important to ascertain the changes in the patient's exercise tolerance over time. Interestingly, the degree of limitation does not correlate with the degree of ventricular impairment and may have more to do with the degree of compensation for the cardiac dysfunction. As cardiac failure progresses, the patient may develop breathlessness when recumbent, a symptom called

orthopnea. This likely results from the decreased pooling of blood in the lower extremities in the supine position. This displaces blood into the central circulation, increases filling pressures, and increases interstitial edema. The patient may report a change in the number of pillows required to sleep or, in severe cases, the need to sleep in a chair. Breathlessness can occur suddenly during sleep, so called "paroxysmal nocturnal dyspnea" (PND). Patients will relate terrifying episodes of air hunger during the night that require them to sit upright and sometimes open a window for air. PND may result from sudden bronchospasm related to airway edema. Often the symptoms resolve once the patient is upright for a period of time. Finally, in its most severe forms, cardiac failure will lead to dyspnea at rest and, in acute situations, fulminate respiratory failure.[22]

Patients commonly complain of a reduction in their exercise capacity. The limitation can be primarily caused by shortness of breath or muscle fatigue. An insufficient augmentation of the stroke volume and heart rate leads to inadequate oxygen delivery to the working muscle.[49] The resulting oxygen debt leads to muscle fatigue. Patients may complain of leg pain or fatigue with exertion that resolves with rest.

A multitude of nonspecific symptoms are commonly seen in patients with heart failure. These include general fatigue, weakness, and nocturia. The occurrence of mental status changes or confusion are signs of a drastically reduced $\dot{Q}c$. Patients with right heart failure, either isolated or resulting from left heart failure, will commonly complain of peripheral edema. The legs are involved most commonly. Dyspnea is not a prominent feature of right heart failure and is usually seen only with severe RV dysfunction. The mechanisms are likely reduced $\dot{Q}c$ leading to acidosis and poor perfusion to respiratory muscles. Severe chronic right heart failure also can produce cardiac cirrhosis, which can lead to hepatic dysfunction and ascites.[22]

Functional Classification

The New York Heart Association has developed a classification of patients with heart disease based on the severity of their symptoms.[50] These criteria have proven useful for comparison studies of patients and following patients longitudinally:[22]

Class I—No limitation with ordinary activity
Class II—Slight limitation of physical activity; no symptoms at rest, but ordinary activity will result in fatigue, dyspnea, palpitation, or angina
Class III—Marked limitation of physical activity; less than ordinary activity resulting in symptoms but comfortable at rest
Class IV—Inability to carry on any physical activity without discomfort; symptoms present at rest

Physical Exam

The physical signs of cardiac failure are often nonspecific and can be absent in patients even with severe chronic heart failure.[51] In the correct clinical setting, signs of elevated cardiac filling pressures can be diagnostic of cardiac failure. The following physical signs are suggestive of cardiac failure.[52,53]

Fluid retention and elevated right filling pressures can lead to the extravasation of fluid into the extravascular space, which is usually seen in the legs or back. Commonly the edema is symmetrical and manifests over several days.

An enlarged and/or pulsatile liver can result from elevated filling pressures and tricuspid regurgitation. Ascites can be seen in severe cases.

In a recumbent patient with the head of bed at 45%, the upper excursion of the pulsations in the internal jugular vein are normally not more than 3 cm above the sternal angle. With elevated right ventricular filling pressures, the level will be elevated. In addition, large waves correlating to ventricular contraction (V waves) may be seen in the neck with tricuspid regurgitation. Some patients will have a normal jugular venous pressure (JVP) but will elevate the JVP inappropriately when the abdomen is compressed for 1 minute over the liver. This is called **hepatojugular reflux** and, if abnormal (sustained increase in JVP during and after compression), suggests altered RV compliance and/or RV failure.

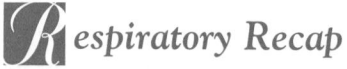

espiratory Recap

Physical Exam in Heart Failure
Peripheral edema
Congestive hepatomegaly
Elevated jugular venous pressure
Pulmonary auscultation: dependent lung crackles and wheezes
Cheyne-Stokes breathing pattern
Abnormal cardiac palpation
Cardiac auscultation: S_3, S_4, murmurs

The transudation of fluid into the pulmonary parenchyma leads to airway and alveolar collapse. The expansion of these regions with inspiration leads to characteristic wet crackles, best heard in the dependent regions. The presence of airway edema with bronchospasm will create high-pitched wheezes similar to those in patients with asthma. Crackles and wheezes together in a patient with sudden onset shortness of breath is highly suggestive of pulmonary edema. Cheyne-Stokes respirations are occasionally seen in cardiac failure. This characteristic pattern of alternating hyperpneas and apneas results from a slow circulation time between the lungs and brain. Patients are often unaware of the breathing pattern and it may manifest only during sleep.

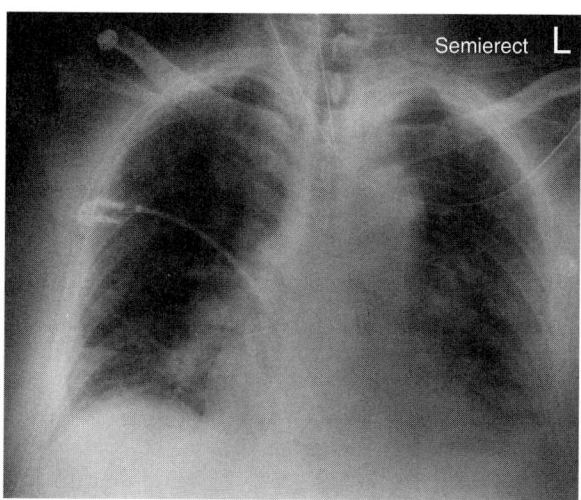

Figure 54-19 Anteroposterior chest radiograph of a patient with cardiac failure.

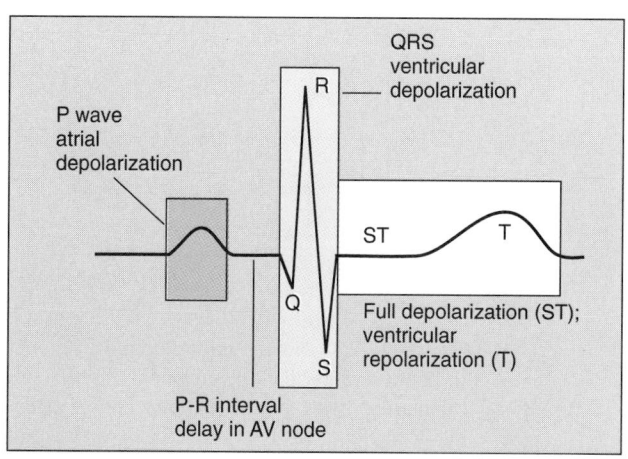

Figure 54-20   Normal ECG waveform. *AV,* Arteriovenous.

The contraction of the heart can normally be felt as a small impulse on the chest below the left nipple. With enlargement of the left ventricle, the point of maximal impulse will be displaced inferiorly and laterally on the chest. The impulse may become quite enlarged and diffuse with severe LV dilation. With hypertrophy of the left ventricle, the impulse may feel stronger and more sustained. Occasionally a smaller extra impulse may be felt preceding the major impulse, which corresponds to atrial contraction (so called *palpable* S_4). The right ventricular impulse is not usually felt, but with RV strain or dilation, a lift may be felt just to the left of the sternum. This parasternal lift is suggestive of RV enlargement or failure. With pulmonary hypertension, a tap may be felt over the left base of the heart, a so called *PA tap.* Finally, severe murmurs can occasionally be palpated as thrills over the precordium.

The presence of a third heart sound (S_3) after the closure of the aortic and pulmonary valves is suggestive of cardiac failure in patients older than 30 years of age. The sound likely represents the deceleration of blood in the right or left ventricle during early diastole. An S_3 can also be heard with mitral or tricuspid regurgitation, left to right shunts, pericarditis, and in normal hearts of young adults. A fourth heart sound (S_4) occurring in late diastole is found in patients with thick noncompliant ventricles and likely results from vibrations from atrial contraction. Other cardiac sounds such as murmurs, which result from turbulent flow, can result from stenosis or regurgitation of any of the four valves.

Radiography

The chest radiograph (Figure 54-19) provides a relatively inexpensive and easy way to assess the lung fields and the size of the heart. Pulmonary edema is often evident on a chest x-ray film as basilar infiltrates with pulmonary vascu-

lar redistribution. The infiltrates range from subtle interstitial markings to frank alveolar exudates. As blood flow is redistributed to the nondependent vessels, the upper lobe vasculature appears plump and indistinct. Bilateral pleural effusions and enlargement of the cardiac silhouette also are commonly seen. In chronic heart failure, the chest radiograph may be quite unremarkable apart from cardiomegaly. In addition, radiographic changes may lag behind clinical changes. Nevertheless, the chest radiograph remains a cornerstone for the diagnosis and follow-up of cardiac failure.

Measurement and Monitoring of Cardiac Function

Electrocardiography

The electrocardiogram (ECG) records the electrical impulses propagated in the heart (Figure 54-20). The impulses are recorded in two planes and at 12 different positions (leads). By examining the resulting complexes, one can determine the heart rate, the rhythm, and whether there are any abnormalities in conduction or repolarization. In addition, the patterns on the ECG may be diagnostic of certain cardiac disorders. Most notably, the syndrome of cardiac ischemia or infarction can be diagnosed by certain repolarization abnormalities on the electrocardiogram.[54]

Echocardiography

Echocardiography is a noninvasive form of cardiac imaging used extensively to diagnose a variety of valvular and myocardial diseases. An echo transducer converts electrical energy into an ultrasound beam that is then directed at the heart. The reflected beams or echoes are received by

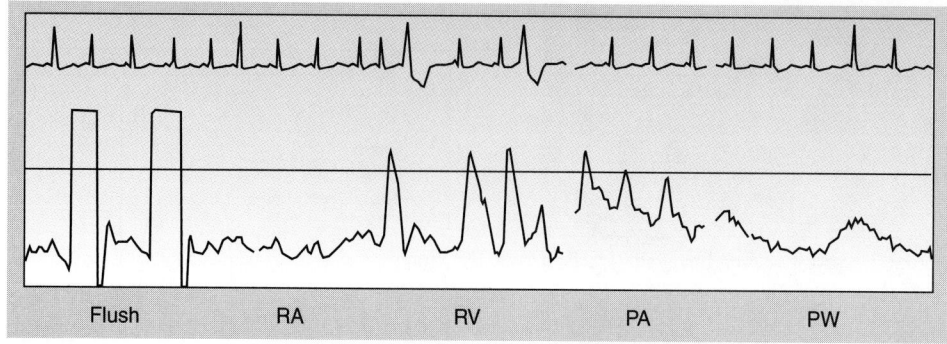

Figure 54-21 Normal tracing from a pulmonary artery catheter as it is advanced from the right atrium (RA), right ventricle (RV), pulmonary artery (PA), and into occlusion or "wedge" (PW). (Modified from Leatherman JW, Marini JJ. Pulmonary artery catheterization: interpretation of pressure recordings. In: Tobin MJ, editor. Principles and practice of intensive care monitoring. New York: McGraw-Hill; 1998.)

the transducer. The time delay and intensity of the returning echoes give information about distance and the density of the tissue. By radiating a fan of echoes, a two-dimensional image of the heart can be obtained in real time. The resulting images provide a wealth of information about cardiac pump function as well as valvular and pericardial morphology. Many forms of cardiac disease can be definitively diagnosed with echocardiography. Injection of small air bubbles into a vein provides contrast within the cardiac chambers. Crossover of bubbles into the left-sided chambers allows identification of intracardiac shunts. Recently, echocardiography during intravenous infusions of cardiac inotropes or vasodilators has been used as a screening test for CAD and to assess viability of dysfunctional myocardium.[55]

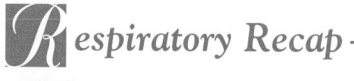

espiratory Recap ───────────

Measurement and Monitoring of Cardiac Function	
Electrocardiogram	Radionucleotide imaging
Echocardiogram	Coronary angiography
Exercise stress test	Hemodynamic monitoring

Exercise Stress Test

The exercise stress test is used to diagnose cardiac ischemia resulting from CAD as a cause of chest pain or cardiac dysfunction. The patient is exercised on a treadmill with electrocardiographic and blood pressure monitoring. ECG changes indicative of ischemia are a reasonably reliable method used to detect CAD.

Radionucleotide Imaging

The sensitivity and specificity of exercise ECG stress testing can be increased by imaging of myocardial perfusion with a radioisotope. The isotope (sestabmibi or thallium)

is injected during peak exercise, and the heart is imaged with a gamma camera. The heart is then re-imaged at rest. Alternatively, images can be taken during infusion of a chemical agent that can induce ischemia or changes in myocardial perfusion (that is, dobutamine or adenosine). Areas of myocardium that have altered perfusion caused by ischemia or infarction will not take up the isotope. At rest those areas that were ischemic during exercise (or chemical infusion) reperfuse and take up isotope, whereas infarcted areas remain devoid of isotope. Isotopes that remain intravascular (technetium) can be used to assess left ventricular function. The ratio of radioactive counts during systole to diastole allows an accurate estimation of ejection fraction and overall LV size.

Coronary Angiography

Direct imaging of the coronary arteries (**coronary angiography**) is possible by cardiac catheterization. This technique is used to assess the extent and severity of CAD as a cause for chest pain and/or cardiac dysfunction. Special catheters are inserted into the aorta and into the origins of the right and left coronary arteries. Contrast dye is injected as radiographic images are obtained. The information obtained can identify atherosclerotic lesions as well as coronary anomalies, areas of spasm, and acute thrombi. Contrast dye also can be injected into the left ventricle, and with subsequent imaging, the cardiac pump function (ejection fraction) can be assessed. In addition, valvular disease can be diagnosed and quantified by imaging and direct pressure measurements.

Hemodynamic Monitoring

Direct measurements of the intracardiac and pulmonary vascular pressures are possible through the use of the pulmonary artery catheter. This catheter is equipped with a balloon on the tip that allows it to float from a central vein (internal jugular, subclavian, or femoral) into the

TABLE 54-2

Classification of Different Hemodynamic Profiles Based on Three Primary Variables and One Derived Variable*

Hemodynamic Profile	CVP (mm Hg)	PAOP (mm Hg)	Cardiac Index (L/m²/min)	SVR Index (dynes/cm⁵/m²)
Normal	4 to 10	6 to 15	2.5 to 4.0	1900 to 2400
Hypovolemia	<4	<6	<2.5	>2400
Fluid overload	>10	>15	>2.5	<2400
Septic shock	<10	<15	>4.0	<1900
Left heart failure	Variable	>15	<2.5	>1900
Right heart failure	>10	Variable	<2.5	PVR elevated

Modified from Pinsky MR. Hemodynamic profile interpretation. In: Tobin MJ, editor. Principles and practice of intensive care monitoring. New York: McGraw-Hill; 1998.

CVP, Central venous pressure; PAOP, pulmonary artery occlusion pressure; SVR, stroke vascular resistance; PVR, pulmonary vascular resistance.

*Mixed disorders may not fit into the profiles listed in the table.

right atrium, right ventricle, pulmonary artery, and then into a pulmonary artery occlusion position (often called a *wedge*). A column of fluid within the catheter allows pressure fluctuations to be transmitted to a transducer and then displayed graphically for analysis. A normal set of tracings is shown in Figure 54-21.

The pulmonary artery occlusion ("wedge") technique creates a static column of blood in a section of the pulmonary vasculature. The measured pressure is a pulmonary venous pressure, which closely approximates left atrial pressure. The left atrial pressure can then be used to estimate the LVEDP, either by the taking of a mean value or the use of a pressure read shortly after the peak of the atrial contraction wave (the Z-point).[56] The mean left atrial pressure also estimates the pressure in the pulmonary capillary circulation. If elevated, fluid may move from the capillaries into the pulmonary interstitium. Most catheters are equipped with a temperature-sensitive probe that allows the calculation of $\dot{Q}c$ by the thermodilution method.[57,58] New generation catheters allow continuous monitoring of the $\dot{Q}c$ and mixed venous saturation.

Determination of the filling pressures and $\dot{Q}c$ can provide a wealth of information in the setting of pulmonary edema or hypotension. In the case of pulmonary edema, an elevated pulmonary artery occlusion pressure suggests a cardiac cause for the edema, whereas a low occlusion pressure suggests a capillary leak syndrome (as with ARDS or sepsis). In the setting of hypotension, a low $\dot{Q}c$ with high filling pressures is suggestive of cardiogenic failure or cardiogenic shock, whereas other syndromes will give different hemodynamic profiles (Table 54-2).[59]

General Treatment Guidelines

The initial approach to the patient with heart failure is to identify the underlying cause and, if possible, treat or remove it. Unfortunately, in the majority of cases of cardiac failure, the underlying cause cannot be easily reversed, so treatment of symptoms is a major goal of therapy. The management of heart failure is, however, no longer confined to symptom relief. Treatment to prevent or delay progression of disease and LV remodeling is now the primary focus of many interventions. In the last decade, there have been many studies on cardiac failure, and accumulating data suggests that we can not only improve quality of life but also reduce mortality. The vast majority of studies deal with cardiac failure from systolic dysfunction (dilated cardiomyopathies). Therapeutic options for pure diastolic dysfunction are limited at present to symptom relief and will be mentioned only briefly.

The goals of therapy are twofold. The first goal is symptom control and improvement in quality of life. Relieving circulatory congestion and increasing oxygen delivery are the major mechanisms employed to improve symptoms. The effectiveness of therapy is routinely assessed by physical exam and history. The second goal is to prevent or delay the progression of the cardiac dysfunction and to prevent the complications that increase mortality. Unfortunately no reliable clinical measure of the effectiveness of therapy for this goal is available.[3] The following discussion is a brief overview of general treatment measures.

Nonpharmacotherapy

Peripheral edema and pulmonary congestion often result from the fluid retention associated with cardiac failure. Restricting salt intake reduces volume overload and often improves symptoms. Efforts should be made to keep intake under 2 g of sodium per day and 2.5 L of fluid per day. Alcohol intake should be limited or avoided entirely. In cases of alcohol-induced cardiomyopathy, abstention may help reverse the process.[60]

Deconditioning is a common problem in cardiac failure. Regular exercise or cardiac rehabilitation programs can improve muscle conditioning and improve exercise capacity.[61] It is unknown if regular exercise effects the progression of the cardiac dysfunction.[3]

TABLE 54-3

Major Trials Favoring Use of ACE Inhibitors at Each Stage of Heart Failure

Stage of Heart Failure	Drugs	Trial (Patients Treated)	Outcome
NYHA I, II	Enalapril Diuretic 27% Digoxin 18%	SOLVD[a] (2111) prevention	Reduced overt CHF; death reduced 8% (NS)
NYHA I, II, III	Enalapril Diuretic 86% Digoxin 66%	SOLVD[b] (1285) treatment	Death reduced 16%; hospitalization reduced 22%
NYHA II, III	Enlapril Diuretic 100% Digoxin 100%	V-HEFT II[c] (403)	Death reduced 28% versus hydralazine-nitrate
NYHA IV	Enlapril Diuretic 77% Digoxin 72%	CONSENSUS[d] (127)	Death reduced 27%
Early postinfarct (3 to 16 days) LV dysfunction	Captopril Diuretic 35% Digoxin 25%	SAVE[e] (1115)	Death reduced 19%; 37% fewer cardiovascular deaths
Early postinfarct (3 to 10 days) clinical CHF	Ramipril Diuretic 58% Digoxin 12%	AIRE[f] (1986)	Death reduced 27%

Modified from Opie LH, Poole-Wilson PA, Sonnenblick E, et al. Angiotensin-converting enzyme inhibitors and conventional vasodilators. In: Opie LH, editor. Drugs for the heart. Philadelphia: WB Saunders; 1995.
NYHA, *New York Heart Association;* SOLVD, *Studies of Left Ventricular Dysfunction;* CHF, *congestive heart failure;* V-HeFT-11, *VA Cooperative Vasodilator Heart Failure Trial;* CONSENSUS, *Cooperative North Scandinavian Enalapril Survival Study;* LV dysfunction, *low ventricular ejection fraction;* SAVE, *survival and ventricular enlargement;* AIRE, *acute infarction ramipril efficacy.*
[a]*Investigators. Effect of enalapril on survival in patients with reduced left ventricular ejection fractions and congestive heart failure. N Engl J Med 1991;325:293-302.*
[b]*Investigators. Effect of enalapril on mortality and the development of heart failure in asymptomatic patients with reduced left ventricular ejection fractions. N Engl J Med 1992;327:685-691.*
[c]*Cohn JN, Johnson G, Ziesche S, et al. A comparison of enalapril with hydralazine-isosorbide dinitrate in the treatment of chronic congestive heart failure N Engl J Med 1991;325:303-310.*
[d]*Effects of enalapril on mortality in severe congestive heart failure. Results of the Cooperative North Scandinavian Enalapril Survival Study (CONSENSUS). The CONSENSUS Trial Study Group. N Engl J Med 1987;316:1429-1435.*
[e]*Pfeffer MA, Braunwald E, Moye LA, et al. Effect of captopril on mortality and morbidity in patients with left ventricular dysfunction after myocardial infarction: results of the survival and ventricular enlargement trial. The SAVE Investigators. N Engl J Med 1992;327:669-677.*
[f]*Effect of ramipril on mortality and morbidity of survivors of acute myocardial infarction with clinical evidence of heart failure. The Acute Infarction Ramipril Efficacy (AIRE) Study Investigators. Lancet 1993;342:821-828.*

Pharmacotherapy

The treatment of chronic cardiac failure has progressed greatly in the last decade. Treatment is directed not only at symptom control but also at long-term reductions in morbidity and mortality. Many treatments have been shown to delay or prevent progression of cardiac dysfunction and improve mortality. Thus even asymptomatic patients with LV dysfunction require thorough evaluation and aggressive treatment.

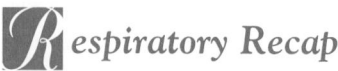 *espiratory Recap*

Pharmacotherapy for Cardiac Failure	
Vasodilators	β-Blockers
Diuretics	Antiarrhythmic agents
Digitalis	Anticoagulation
Inotropic agents	

Vasodilators Arterial vasodilation reduces afterload and increases Q̇c, whereas venodilation can decrease preload and improve symptoms of congestion. If mitral regurgitation is present, these effects may augment forward output considerably. Thus vasodilators may have many beneficial effects in improving the symptoms of cardiac failure caused by systolic or diastolic failure. In addition, certain vasodilators have been shown to slow or prevent progression of disease and improve mortality in patients with systolic dysfunction.

Hydralazine is an effective vasodilator that when combined with isosorbide dinitrate has been shown to modestly increase survival in patients with cardiac failure.[62] Hydralazine is primarily an arterial vasodilator whose mechanism of action is unclear. Nitrates such as isosorbide dinitrate work by releasing nitric oxide and work as venodilators at low doses, as well as arterial vasodilators at higher doses. Hydralazine is usually titrated to 300 mg or more a day (divided into 3 or 4 doses), and isosorbide

TABLE 54-4

ACE Inhibitors Used in Heart Failure

Drug	Target Dose*
Captopril	50 mg tid
Enalapril	10 mg bid
Lisinopril	—
Ramipril	5 mg bid
Quinapril	—
Zofenopril	30 mg bid
Trandolapril	4 mg qd

Modified from Cohn JN. The management of chronic heart failure. N Engl J Med 1996;335:490-498.
tid, Three times daily; bid, twice daily; qd, every day.
*Dose that was associated with increased survival in clinical trials.

dinitrate is titrated to 120 mg a day (divided into 3 doses).[63]

Angiotensin-converting enzyme (ACE) inhibitors prevent the formation of the potent vasoconstrictor angiotensin II and prevent the breakdown of the vasodilator bradykinin. Thus ACE inhibitors can reduce the deleterious effects of the chronic elevation of angiotensin II seen in heart failure. Several studies now document decreased morbidity and mortality with the use of ACE inhibition in heart failure (Table 54-3). Moreover, these drugs seem to be effective in all stages of heart failure.[64] When compared to other vasodilator regimens such as hydralazine and isosorbide dinitrate, ACE inhibitors confer a greater mortality reduction.[65] It is recommended that all patients with LV dysfunction be maintained on an ACE inhibitor regardless of symptoms. Angiotensin slows relaxation, so a reduction in its tissue levels can augment relaxation and improve diastolic filling. This suggests that ACE inhibitors may be beneficial in cases of heart failure resulting from diastolic dysfunction, but this has yet to be proven. Various ACE inhibitors and their target doses are shown in Table 54-4.

Other vasodilators include calcium channel blockers, α-antagonists (prazosin, doxazosin, terazosin), and the new angiotensin II receptor antagonists (losartan, irbesartan, candesartan, valsartan). Studies of the calcium channel blockers felodipine and amlodipine have shown no mortality benefit in patients with heart failure, but no adverse effects were found either.[66,67] The calcium channel blockers diltiazem and verapamil have negative inotropic actions and thus are not recommended in patients with systolic dysfunction. Their actions may also impede relaxation. However, clinically they seem to improve symptoms of diastolic failure (perhaps by slowing rate and contraction) and remain as first-line therapy for heart failure caused by diastolic dysfunction. No studies have been done that demonstrate benefit with the use of α-antagonists in heart failure.[64] The new angiotensin II receptor blockers have been shown to have favorable hemodynamic effects in cardiac failure.[68] They have the advantage

of inducing less cough than ACE inhibitors but also do not have some of the tissue effects and the increased bradykinin levels. A small randomized trial in the elderly compared captopril to losartan and demonstrated a mortality advantage with losartan.[69] These results need to be confirmed with further trials before firm conclusions can be drawn.

In the acute setting, patients can be treated with intravenous sodium nitroprusside or nitroglycerin. These drugs work to dilate arteries and veins via nitric oxide release. In patients with acute heart failure, these drugs allow rapid titration of blood pressure to achieve adequate perfusion with minimal afterload and preload. If the patient has pulmonary edema on the basis of cardiac ischemia, nitroglycerin may be particularly effective and is the drug of choice.[70] A pulmonary arterial catheter is occasionally inserted in these situations for optimal titration of the medications.

Diuretics Diuretics are a class of drugs that prevent sodium reabsorption in the kidney and promote sodium loss in the urine. This effect increases salt and water excretion and in heart failure helps reduce circulatory congestion. The physiologic effect of reduced circulating volume is a reduction in filling pressures and thus less transudation of fluid from the systemic and pulmonary circulation. No prospective controlled trials are currently in progress that would demonstrate the safety or efficacy of most diuretics in cardiac failure. Experience gained from the treatment of patients with hypertension suggests that diuretics are safe, but it is unclear whether they have any benefit other than symptom control.[63]

Diuretics are effective for symptoms in both diastolic and systolic heart failure. However, these drugs should be used only in patients with evidence of volume overload because use of diuretics in patients with euvolemia may lead to decreased organ perfusion and adverse reflex activation of the neurohormonal axis. For relatively compensated patients, occasional use of a diuretic may help them manage their symptoms of congestion. In patients with class III or IV failure, daily doses of a diuretic are usually necessary. Generally, loop diuretics (furosemide, bumetanide, torsemide) are used acutely and for daily maintenance doses. Thiazides or thiazide-like drugs (metolazone) may be added to a loop diuretic to enhance diuresis.

Spironolactone is an aldosterone antagonist with natriuretic properties. Aldosterone has several undesirable effects in cardiac failure including arrhythmogenicity, magnesium depletion, increased extracellular catecholamines, and induction of cardiac fibrosis. It has been suggested that spironolactone therapy would not only aid symptom control but also reduce mortality by reducing the deleterious effects of excess aldosterone found in heart failure.[71] Preliminary data clearly shows an improvement in heart failure symptoms,[72] and a recent randomized trial of spironolactone has shown a significant 27% reduction in mortality.[73]

In the patient with acute severe pulmonary edema and volume overload, intravenous dosing of a loop diuretic may be necessary. Bolus dosing is usually effective, however, continuous drips may be more effective and have been associated with fewer side effects.[74-76]

Digitalis Derived from the leaves of the digitalis plant, digoxin is one of the oldest medications in use. This cardiac glycoside is a potent inhibitor of sodium and potassium exchange across the cardiac cell membranes. The excess sodium available within the cell increases calcium flux into the cell. The increased availability of cytosolic calcium increases the velocity and force of muscle shortening. Digoxin thus has a positive inotropic effect. Digoxin also increases the sensitivity of the baroreceptors, leading to a decrease in the sympathetic activation seen in heart failure.[77]

The benefit of digoxin therapy is counterbalanced by the risk for toxicity. Increased serum levels of digoxin are associated with mental status changes, arrhythmias, and sinus arrest. Moreover, the drug has numerous interactions with other medications and has a reduced clearance in patients with renal failure. Studies of digoxin therapy in patients with systolic dysfunction have failed to show a mortality benefit, although digoxin did reduce symptoms and hospitalizations.[78-80] Based on available data, therapy with a daily dose of digoxin with serum levels of 0.5 to 1.2 are reasonable in patients with symptoms despite therapy with an ACE inhibitor.

Inotropic Agents The phosphodiesterase (PDE) inhibitors inhibit the enzymes that break down cAMP and cGMP and results in more forceful contraction and vasodilation. Agents such as milrinone and amrinone are used in acute systolic dysfunction for their inotropic and vasodilatory effects. These agents are used in acutely ill patients to bridge them to transplant or stabilize them until oral therapy can be started. In a long-term study, an oral preparation of milrinone increased mortality in patients with congestive heart failure (CHF).[81] A study of the oral agent vesnarinone in a low-dose and high-dose formulation showed decreased symptoms and mortality in the low-dose group and increased mortality in the high-dose group.[82] A more recent randomized trial of vesnarinone showed a dose-dependent decrease in symptoms but also an associated increase in mortality.[83] The PDE inhibitors are presently not standard therapy. Their main indication is for short-term intravenous use in patients with decompensated cardiac failure.[63]

Theophylline is a PDE inhibitor commonly used in pulmonary diseases such as asthma and emphysema. This drug has effects on the respiratory center that stimulate ventilation. In patients with heart failure and a periodic breathing pattern (Cheyne-Stokes) during sleep, theophylline was shown to reduce the number of apneic episodes and to decrease the degree of arterial oxygen desaturations.[84]

Intravenous agents such as dobutamine and dopamine stimulate β-receptors in the heart and vasculature. Dobutamine is a pure β-agonist and results in positive inotropy and vasodilation. These effects increase $\dot{Q}c$ by increasing contractility, increasing heart rate, and decreasing afterload. In patients with refractory cardiac failure, infusions of dobutamine are used to improve symptoms and reverse the chronic decompensated state. Long-term use of IV dobutamine has been reported, but no randomized controlled trials have been done that show sustained benefit.[63]

Dopamine has a wide range of effects depending on its dosing. At low doses (approximately 0 to 2 μg/kg/min), it exhibits relatively selective splanchnic and renal arterial vasodilation resulting from direct stimulation of dopaminergic receptors. This increases renal blood flow and has been shown to enhance natriuresis. Despite some claims to the contrary, no conclusive evidence shows that dopamine protects against renal failure.[85] At higher doses (approximately 2 to 10 μg/kg/min), dopamine enhances norepinephrine release leading to increased α-receptor activation. At the highest doses (approximately 5 to 20 μg/kg/min), dopamine directly stimulates α-receptors leading to vasoconstriction.[77] The individual response to dopamine infusions can be quite variable and often does not correlate to reported dosing ranges. Often patients will exhibit tachycardia and vasoconstriction at low doses leading to decreased cardiac function and decreased relaxation time.

The somewhat unpredictable effects of dopamine make it a less attractive agent in patients with cardiac failure. It may have a role in patients with volume overload unresponsive to conventional diuretics. A low-dose infusion in "renal range" can be attempted in such patients. If there is no increase in urine output or no tachyarrhythmias, the infusion should be discontinued.

β-Blockers β-Blockers have been used to treat heart failure caused by cardiac ischemia and diastolic dysfunction for many years. Although they slow relaxation, clinically they control symptoms of diastolic heart failure by slowing the heart rate and providing overall more time for filling during diastole. The use of β-blockers in systolic dysfunction seems counterintuitive but is clearly effective. Initial studies in the 1970s suggested that β-blockade improved symptoms and cardiac function in patients with systolic heart failure.[86,87] Smaller studies in the 1980s confirmed these results,[88,89] but β-blockade to treat heart failure caused by LV dysfunction had not become accepted therapy until recently. One reason for this is the lack of a mechanistic consensus on how β-blockers are beneficial in cardiac failure. β-Blockers alter the sympathetic axis and effect the β-receptor signaling cascade. Since excessive, sustained neurohumoral activation is common in cardiac failure and contributes to myocyte dysfunction and deleterious chamber remodeling, blockade of this pathway actually improves cardiac function, inhibits adverse remodeling, and improves survival.[90] β-Blockers also may improve ventricular arterial coupling by slowing contraction and heart rate.[77] Enthusiasm for β-blockers in severe heart failure (class IV) has been tempered by the negative results of the Xamoterol Study.[91] A more recent meta-analysis of trials involving over 3000 patients demonstrated that β-blocker therapy increased LV ejection fraction and reduced the risk of death by 32%.[92] The CIBIS-II trial involved 2647 patients with symptomatic class III and IV heart failure. The trial was stopped early because of an impressive mortality advantage (34% reduction) with β-blocker treatment.[93] Another trial (MERIT-HF) demonstrated a 35% reduction in mortality with metoprolol therapy.[90,94] Based on this data, investigators are recommending the use of β-blockers in all symptomatic patients with decreased ejection fractions except those with severely decompensated failure.[95]

Carvedilol is a β-adrenergic blocker with β-adrenergic blocking properties that was approved for use in symptomatic heart failure in the United States in 1997. This drug combines the usual benefits of a β-blocker with afterload reduction from α-receptor-mediated peripheral vasodilation. These properties would seem to make it an optimal drug for the management of heart failure.[96] Studies in patients with LV dysfunction have demonstrated decreased hospitalizations, decreased mortality, and improvement in the symptoms of heart failure.[96] Two small studies comparing the β-blocker metoprolol with carvedilol demonstrated greater improvement in symptoms in the carvedilol group.[97]

When the patient with cardiac failure is started on β-blocker therapy, the dose must be titrated slowly and carefully. Only compensated patients on stable doses of ACE inhibitors and diuretics should be considered for β-blockade. A low-dose β-blocker or carvedilol (that is, 3.125 mg twice daily) can be started and maintained for 2 weeks. If tolerated, the dose can be doubled at a minimum of every 2 weeks until the target dose is achieved (25 mg twice daily for carvedilol) or signs of toxicity are evident (bradycardia, hypotension, dizziness, or increased symptoms of heart failure).[96]

Antiarrhythmic Agents
Arrhythmias are a major cause of mortality in patients with cardiac dysfunction, especially in patients with the cardiomyopathy of CAD. Patients with prior episodes of cardiac arrest or ventricular arrhythmias are at especially high risk for sudden death (30% over the next 1 to 3 years).[63] Although many antiarrhythmic agents are available, most agents have a negative inotropic effect and are associated with worsening of cardiac failure[98] or increased mortality.[99] Amiodarone is an antiarrhythmic with predominantly class III activity. Unlike other agents, amiodarone is well tolerated even in severe LV dysfunction and may actually improve LV ejection fraction.[100] In patients with arrhythmias and CHF, one large study suggested a survival advantage with treatment.[101] In another study of patients with heart failure and without significant arrhythmias, amiodarone therapy was not associated with a change in mortality.[102]

Anticoagulants
Thromboembolism is a potential complication in patients with LV dysfunction. Although retrospective analysis have shown that the risk for embolic events is low,[3] many experts recommend anticoagulant therapy with warfarin for patients with severe LV systolic dysfunction (LVEF <30%).[103] Patients with a history of previous thromboembolism or atrial fibrillation should all receive anticoagulation.[3] Short of this, the decision to anticoagulate the patient with cardiac failure should be based on a case by case analysis.

Mechanical Treatments

Tailored Therapy
In patients with severely decompensated heart failure, aggressive intravenous therapy with diuretics and vasodilators can be administered with concurrent hemodynamic monitoring. A pulmonary arterial catheter can provide important information regarding serial determination of filling pressures and $\dot{Q}c$, allowing optimal titration of vasodilators and volume status. Occasionally, intravenous inotropes such as dobutamine or milrinone are needed to augment the $\dot{Q}c$ and help optimize hemodynamics. Such "tailored therapy" has been shown to reduce symptoms and hospitalizations in patients with heart failure refractory to oral therapy. Tailored therapy remains a useful intervention in patients with severe cardiac failure, especially in those awaiting cardiac transplantation.[63,104]

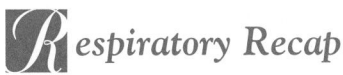

Respiratory Recap

Mechanical Treatments for Cardiac Failure	
Tailored therapy	Automated implantable cardioverter defibrillators
Intraaortic balloon pump	
Ventricular assist device	

Intraaortic Balloon Pump
The **intraaortic balloon pump (IABP)** uses the principle of counterpulsation to support the failing heart. The catheter-based balloon is inserted into the descending aorta just below the aortic arch. The balloon is then inflated during diastole causing increased coronary blood flow and deflated during systole causing decreased afterload. An IABP is especially effective in cardiogenic shock caused by myocardial ischemia as it decreases myocardial oxygen demand while increasing coronary perfusion. IABPs can be inserted safely in emergent situations and often can bridge a critically ill patient to corrective surgery.[105]

Ventricular Assist Device
Ventricular assist devices (VADs) are mechanical pumps that can completely assume the workload of the right or left ventricle and restore normal hemodynamics. A left ventricular assist de-

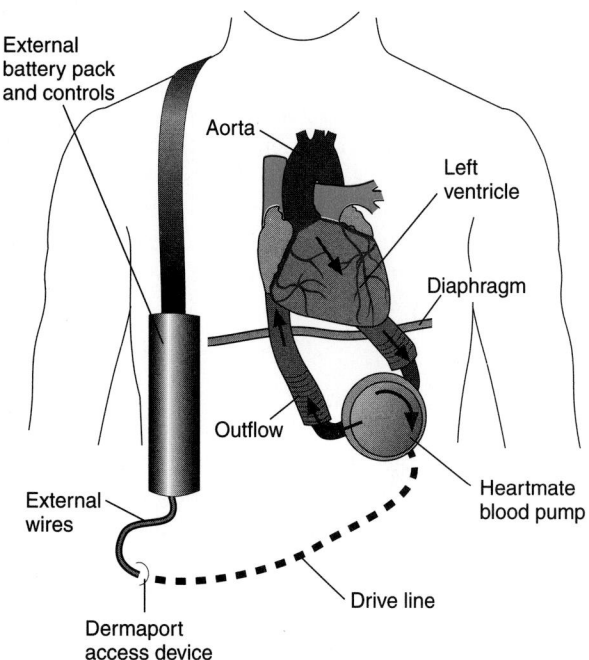

External battery pack and controls

Aorta

Left ventricle

Diaphragm

Outflow

External wires

Heartmate blood pump

Drive line

Dermaport access device

Figure 54-22 Example of a wearable left ventricular assist device and its components. The inflow cannula is inserted into the apex of the left ventricle, and the outflow cannula is anastomosed to the ascending aorta. A transcutaneous cable carries the electrical supply and air vent to the device. (Modified from Goldstein DJ, Oz MC, Rose EA. N Engl J Med 1998;339:1522-1533.)

vice (LVAD) is shown in Figure 54-22. Four systems are available for long-term circulatory support: the HeartMate (Thermo Cardiosystems Inc.), Novacor (Baxter Healthcare Corp.), Thoratec (Thoratec Laboratories Corp.), and the CardioWest Total Artificial Heart (TAH) (CardioWest Technologies, Inc.).[106] These devices allow long-term support of circulation in patients with refractory heart failure. Although primarily used as a bridge to transplantation, in the future portable implantable LVADs will be developed for long-term ambulatory hemodynamic support.[107]

Automatic Implantable Cardioverter Defibrillators

The use of automatic implantable cardioverter defibrillators (AICDs) has increased greatly in the last few years. Studies involving patients who have had myocardial infarction (MI) with LV dysfunction and arrhythmias have shown increased survival in patients treated with AICDs.[108] Recently a randomized trial that compared AICDs to amiodarone in patients with high-risk arrhythmias and LV dysfunction reported a mortality advantage with AICD placement.[109] Presently it is recommended that patients with cardiac failure and significant or symptomatic ventricular arrhythmias undergo evaluation for AICD placement. If the AICD is contraindicated, amiodarone therapy should be considered.

Surgical Treatments

Heart Transplantation   Advances in the techniques of heart transplantation and immunosuppression now allow an 85% to 90% survival at 1 year and 50% survival at 5 years.[110] Patients who undergo transplantation experience a near normal quality of life but remain at risk for rejection, increased rates of infection, and a unique coronary vasculopathy that leads to severe CAD.[110] The major limitation in cardiac transplantation is organ availability. It is estimated that 40,000 patients die every year that might have benefited from transplantation. Only 2500 hearts are available for transplant every year.[109]

*R*espiratory Recap

Surgical Treatments for Cardiac Failure	
Heart transplantation	Batista procedure
Cardiomyoplasty	Coronary revascularization

Cardiomyoplasty   The shortage of human organ donors has necessitated the search for alternative means to improve cardiac function. **Cardiomyoplasty** involves the surgical transposition of an electrically transformed piece of skeletal muscle to augment the failing myocardium (usually the latissimus dorsi is wrapped around the ventricles). Despite initial enthusiasm, a high mortality and an absence of hemodynamic improvement in most cases has limited the widespread use of this procedure.[110]

Batista Procedure   Recently a new surgical technique has been investigated for patients with dilated cardiomyopathies. The technique, pioneered by Dr. Randas Batista, involves removal of a large part of the myocardium to restore the heart to a normal volume. The theory is that the surgery will restore normal wall tension by reducing the radius of the ventricle and increasing wall thickness.[111] In observational studies this has resulted in some impressive improvement in some patients. Not all patients benefit, and the procedure appears equivalent in 1-year outcome to transplantation.[111,112] The mitral valve also is usually repaired in this procedure.

Coronary Revascularization   Coronary revascularization with **coronary artery bypass surgery** can improve myocardial function by reducing ischemia. In some cases so called "hibernating myocardium" (myocardium rendered hypocontractile because of chronic hypoperfusion) can return to normal contractile function after restoration of normal blood flow. Other surgical procedures considered for patients with cardiac failure include valvular repairs or replacements and limited septal myomectomies for patients with hypertrophic obstructive cardiomyopathy.

Ventilatory Support of the Patient with Cardiac Failure

Pulmonary edema is associated with decreased pulmonary compliance, increased airway resistance, and lung collapse. Thus pulmonary edema from any cause leads to increased work of breathing and hypoxemia. The large negative intrathoracic pressure swings may increase afterload for the strained left ventricle. Hypoxic pulmonary vasoconstriction will increase afterload of the right ventricle. In severe cases the patient may not be able to maintain adequate ventilation and oxygen delivery. This can then further exacerbate myocardial dysfunction because of cellular hypoxia and acidosis, especially when the heart failure is caused by cardiac ischemia. The increased work of the respiratory muscles also may "steal" oxygen from the working myocardium. Thus combined cardiac failure and respiratory distress begets more cardiac failure.

If the cycle of respiratory failure can be temporarily interrupted, therapy aimed at treating the cardiac abnormalities can be used and the process can be reversed. Positive pressure ventilation is an ideal mechanism used to stabilize the acutely decompensated patient. Positive pressure ventilation improves oxygenation by recruiting collapsed lung and decreases the work of breathing by unloading the respiratory muscles. In addition, positive intrathoracic pressure may improve forward $\dot{Q}c$.[45,113] Chronic therapy with noninvasive positive pressure ventilators may have a role in selected patients with sleep-disordered breathing and heart failure.

Noninvasive Ventilation

In the past, many patients with respiratory failure caused by heart failure were intubated for mechanical ventilation. However, recent experience with noninvasive positive pressure ventilation (NPPV) with a face mask has provided encouraging results. In some cases the patient can be stabilized and endotracheal intubation can be prevented by the use of mask continuous positive airway pressure (CPAP) at 5 to 10 cm H_2O.[114] Inspiratory pressure also can be applied to further unload the respiratory muscles. Although randomized studies demonstrating the added efficacy of inspiratory pressure support are currently lacking,[115] two recent case series have demonstrated the efficacy of the use of pressure support ventilation with face mask delivery in patients with pulmonary edema from multiple causes. In these series there was a low rate of intubation in the mask-ventilated patients, and the support reduced $PaCO_2$, increased pH, and increased oxygen saturation.[116,117]

In one of these studies, patients with acute myocardial ischemia had a high mortality compared to the other patients.[116] One study compared the effects of CPAP with NPPV in acute pulmonary edema.[118] In this study only NPPV reduced dyspnea score, acidosis, and $PaCO_2$, whereas

patients in the CPAP arm only had a reduced respiratory rate. The NPPV group had an increased incidence of infarction, but the significance of this finding is not clear.

Based on these studies, it is recommended that NPPV not be used in patients with cardiac failure caused by active myocardial ischemia.[119] In patients with active cardiac ischemia, heavy sedation and controlled mechanical ventilation through an endotracheal tube significantly reduces the work of breathing, reduces the work of the myocardium, and allows the most effective oxygen delivery to the ischemic myocardium. Patients with hemodynamic instability, arrhythmias, a depressed mental status, or some patients undergoing invasive procedures (such as cardiac catheterization) should also be managed with intubation and controlled mechanical ventilation.

Invasive Mechanical Ventilation

Intubation of the patient with cardiac failure may prove challenging because of underlying hemodynamic abnormalities. The necessary sedation for this procedure can potentially cause hypotension and arrhythmias. Thus monitoring of the rhythm and blood pressure is essential. Very few sedating medications do not have some cardiovascular depressive actions. One exception is etomidate. This drug is a hypnotic agent with minimal cardiovascular depressant actions.[120] Etomidate is the recommended induction agent for intubation of patients with cardiovascular instability. After intubation the patient will likely require continued sedation. Low doses of benzodiazepines and opiates are often sufficient. The general anesthetic propofol has a rapid onset and clearance allowing rapid sedation and emergence from sedation. However, this drug exhibits potent cardiovascular depressive effects and is often associated with hypotension.[121]

No controlled trials on various modes of ventilation in cardiac failure have been conducted. The practitioner should use the mode that provides the most effective and comfortable ventilation for the patient. Patients with mild or chronic heart failure and significant pulmonary edema may be managed with minimal ventilatory support and spontaneous ventilation with a mode such as inspiratory pressure support. Most patients with severe cardiac failure will benefit from complete ventilatory support. Pressure or volume ventilation can be used for cardiac failure as long as adequate ventilation and oxygenation are maintained without hyperinflation (peak alveolar pressures less than 35 cm H_2O) and significant lung collapse.

The pressure mode allows patients to set their own inspiratory flows and in many cases permits less sedation by providing a comfortable form of ventilation. In addition, pressure ventilation prevents a significant degree of hyperinflation by limiting the end-inspiratory pressure to a safe level. If pressure ventilation is used, the pressure level should be set to deliver 8 to 10 mL/kg tidal volumes with an inspiratory time of 0.8 to 1.2 seconds. An adequate rate should be provided if heavy sedation is used.

If volume ventilation is used, 8 to 10 mL/kg tidal volumes delivered with a decelerating waveform and moderate flow rates (40 to 80 L/min) are used. FiO_2 should be set at 1.0 and then weaned to the lowest level that maintains saturation greater than 90%. PEEP is initially set at 5 cm H_2O and titrated up as needed for oxygenation if tolerated hemodynamically.

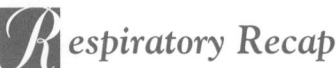
Respiratory Recap

Mechanical Ventilation for Cardiac Failure
A mode should be chosen that is most effective and comfortable for the patient.
Pressure or volume ventilation can be used, provided peak alveolar pressure is less than 35 cm H_2O.
An initial tidal volume of 8 to 10 mL/kg should be chosen.
An initial inspiratory time of 0.8 to 1.2 seconds should be chosen.
An initial FiO_2 of 1.0 should be chosen.
An initial PEEP of 5 cm H_2O should be chosen.

Cardiac Effects of Mechanical Ventilation

Positive pressure ventilation has many potential effects on the cardiovascular system. The filling of the ventricles is highly dependent on the pressures surrounding the heart. Cardiac surface pressure depends on the pericardial pressure, intrathoracic pressure, and lung volume around the heart. Changes in lung volume also will affect PVR and thus RV performance. In turn, the RV performance can effect LV performance via series and parallel interactions. Thus the overall effects of the application of positive pressure ventilation in the individual patient is highly unpredictable and can be beneficial (reduced work of breathing, reduced edema, increased $\dot{Q}c$) or potentially detrimental (hypotension, hyperinflation, ischemia). Therefore a careful titration of support during monitoring of all available aspects of cardiovascular performance (that is, blood pressure, heart rate, filling pressures, $\dot{Q}c$, arterial blood gases, electrocardiogram) may be the optimal method of ventilation in the patient with cardiac failure.

The most effective means to increase intrathoracic positive pressure is the application of PEEP. In addition to potentially reducing afterload and preload, PEEP prevents derecruitment of opened lung units. Collapsed lung units increase intrapulmonary shunt, increase PVR, and induce hyperinflation in open lung units by reducing the amount of available lung available to accommodate the delivered tidal volume. In addition, with each tidal breath collapsed, lung units are exposed to high pressures and some will open. If the pressure is decreased below the closing threshold of these units, they will again collapse. This cyclic opening and closing of lung units has been associated with lung injury in animal experiments.[122] Optimal ventilatory settings should thus attempt to open collapsed

lung units and then prevent derecruitment by ventilating above the closing pressures of the lung units.

This approach is most applicable to the patient with ARDS[123] but also may apply in a limited fashion to pulmonary edema from cardiac failure. The edema resulting from cardiac failure is different from that of the capillary leak from ARDS. Cardiogenic edema has lower protein levels and relatively normal surfactant function when compared to edema from patients with ARDS.[124] Thus the alveolar collapse associated with heart failure may be less refractory and require lower pressures to re-open. Modest levels of PEEP (5 to 10 cm H_2O) may be all that is required to prevent subsequent derecruitment of opened airways.

PEEP has been shown to improve $\dot{Q}c$ without increasing the oxygen requirements of the LV.[125] It is widely believed that this effect is from a reduced afterload on the LV induced by the positive intrathoracic pressure.[113] The afterload on the heart can be estimated by the transmural pressure across the LV, and since PEEP can increase cardiac surface pressure, it will reduce afterload assuming the arterial pressure does not increase. However, direct pressure measurements on the surface of the heart have failed to demonstrate an increase in cardiac surface pressure with increases in intrathoracic pressure when the LV is dilated.[126] It is hypothesized that the increase in $\dot{Q}c$ that occurs in patients with cardiac failure when placed on positive pressure ventilation may be caused by displacement of blood from the thorax.[127]

This increase in $\dot{Q}c$ is not seen in patients with normal cardiac function or normal volume status. Exactly how this leads to improved myocardial performance in patients with dilated cardiomyopathies is unclear, but a similar effect has been demonstrated previously with the analogous scenarios of phlebotomy or rotating tourniquets.[127] PEEP can also redistribute edema to the perivascular spaces and reduce PVR by reducing lung collapse.[128] However, PEEP can potentially lead to hypotension by decreasing preload and $\dot{Q}c$. In general hypotension does not occur in patients with elevated filling pressures.[129,130] Positive pressure ventilation has been shown to reduce coronary perfusion,[131] but this effect did not occur until pressures were greater than 40 cm H_2O. Based on these clinical effects of PEEP, a careful increase in PEEP is recommended, while simultaneously monitoring oxygenation, blood pressure, the electrocardiogram, and the $\dot{Q}c$ if possible. Arterial blood gases and mixed venous blood gases can also be helpful to determine oxygen delivery and pulmonary shunt. PEEP can be increased to 10 to 15 cm H_2O if necessary to reduce FiO_2 and lung collapse. The degree of pulmonary shunt can be used as an estimate of lung collapse.

Weaning from Mechanical Ventilation

Acute respiratory failure from pulmonary edema is often rapidly reversible and does not usually require prolonged mechanical ventilation. Weaning these patients from the ventilator tends to be fairly straightforward. Often the pa-

$\mathcal{B}$OX 54-2

Effects of Obstructive Sleep Apnea on Cardiovascular Function

Negative Intrathoracic Pressure
Increased left ventricular systolic transmural pressure (that is, afterload)
Reduced stroke volume and cardiac output

Hypoxemia and Hypercapnia
Increased respiratory drive and sympathetic nervous system activity
Pulmonary vasoconstriction and hypertension leading to increased right ventricular afterload

Systemic vasoconstriction and hypertension
Cardiac arrhythmias (bradycardia, heart block, ventricular and supraventricular tachycardias)

Arousal
Increased central sympathetic nervous system activity
Increased systemic blood pressure
Increased heart rate

From Naughton MT, Bradley TD. Sleep apnea in congestive heart failure. Clin Chest Med 1998;9:99-113.

tients can be extubated without a prolonged wean of support. However, the sudden loss of positive pressure in the thorax can lead to acute edema and rapid failure in fragile patients.[132] Ongoing cardiac ischemia is associated with failure to wean and should be corrected before ventilatory support is removed.[133]

Recent clinical trials of ventilator weaning have demonstrated that a spontaneous breathing trial early in the patient's course can rapidly identify those patients who can be extubated without weaning.[134] It is recommended that a spontaneous breathing trial be performed early on awake patients when the underlying cardiac problems are controlled. The patient can breath spontaneously through a T-tube or through the ventilator with 0 cm H_2O CPAP to ensure the patient will not develop pulmonary edema when removed from positive pressure ventilation. If the ventilator is used, then flow triggering is used to reduce the imposed load to breathing from the ventilator tubing. If the patient fails a spontaneous breathing trial, attempts to optimize cardiac function should be undertaken before additional changes in the ventilatory strategy are made. Daily spontaneous breathing trials are likely to be as effective as other methods to wean patients from the ventilator.[134] NPPV can be used to treat patients if they develop respiratory distress after extubation.

Chronic Noninvasive Ventilation in Sleep-Disordered Breathing

Many patients with chronic cardiac failure have sleep-disordered breathing including Cheyne-Stokes and sleep apnea. In a reported series of stable outpatients with heart failure, 40% to 50% of patients had obstructive sleep apnea (OSA) or Cheyne-Stokes respiration with central sleep apnea (CSR-CSA).[135-137] In patients with heart failure, the presence of sleep-disordered breathing is associated with a poor prognosis and a higher mortality.[138-140] The extensive cardiovascular effects of apneic episodes are shown in Box 54-2.

It is clear that these effects work in concert to increase afterload and overload the myocardium. It has been suggested that these pathophysiologic effects may contribute to the progression of cardiac failure.[137] There is increasing evidence that treatment of these disorders with nocturnal mask CPAP is associated with marked improvements in cardiac function and the symptoms of heart failure.[136,141,142]

The assessment of all patients with cardiac failure should include questions about sleep disorders and symptoms of sleep deprivation, snoring, and apneas. Any suggestion of sleep-disordered breathing should prompt a thorough evaluation with a sleep study and treatment if indicated.

CASE STUDIES

Case One
Ischemic Congestive Heart Failure

A 55-year-old man (100 kg) with a history of coronary artery disease (CAD) and prior infarction presented with chest pain and shortness of breath. The patient presented with an anterior myocardial infarction (MI) 6 months ago and underwent emergent coronary angioplasty with stent placement to his left anterior descending (LAD) coronary artery. His LV function after MI was moderately impaired at an LVEF of 40%. He was managed with aspirin, β-blockers, and an ACE inhibitor. Over the last 2 weeks he has noted return of his chest pain with exertion and on the day of presentation had two 20-minute episodes of pain at rest. The last one was associated with some mild dyspnea. Shortly before presenting he developed severe crushing chest pain and became quite dyspneic. An ambulance was called, and he was taken to the emergency department. On presentation he was in respiratory distress, sitting upright, and sweating with marked use of accessory muscles. His respiratory rate was 36/min, heart rate 110/min, and blood pressure 150/100 mm Hg, and oxygen saturation was 91% on 15 L/min oxygen via face mask. On exam the patient appeared to have distended neck veins. His chest had diffuse crackles and wheezes throughout. Cardiac exam was notable for tachycardia and a summation gallop. An ECG showed T-wave inversions and ST depression in leads V_2 to V_6, and a chest x-ray showed moderate pulmonary edema.

The patient clearly has CHF from myocardial ischemia. In this case the lack of oxygen delivery to the working myocardium led to depletion in ATP and dysfunction of both contraction and relaxation of cardiac muscle. This resulted in elevated LV filling pressures and pulmonary edema. He has evidence for marked increase in work of breathing that is likely contributing to the ischemia by increasing the oxygen demand on the circulation. If the patient begins to retain carbon dioxide, the resulting acidosis may lead to further myocardial dysfunction and increase the risk of arrhythmias. Efforts to restore oxygen supply to the heart might be more successful if the patient were intubated and heavily sedated.

The therapeutic strategy is to intubate the patient and provide full mechanical ventilatory support. Pressure or volume ventilation so that the volumes are 800 mL and inspiratory time is 0.8 to 1.2 seconds with a rate of 12 to 16 breaths/min is a good starting point. The FIO_2 should be 1.0 to start. PEEP of 5 cm H_2O should be applied, and if the blood pressure tolerates this, a slow increase to 10 cm H_2O could be attempted. In the meantime the patient should be treated with anticoagulation (aspirin, heparin, a II/IIIa inhibitor), intravenous nitroglycerin, and diuretics. Consultation with a cardiologist for possible cardiac catheterization also should be obtained.

Case Two
Acute Aortic Valve Insufficiency

A 28-year-old man complains of fevers, chills, and shortness of breath. The patient has a history of rheumatic fever as a child but has otherwise been in good health. Three days before presentation he injected intravenous heroin with a dirty needle. The day before presentation he noted chills and sweats. On the morning of presentation he had the rapid progression of dyspnea and nausea. He felt weak when standing and finally collapsed in his home. The patient was brought to the emergency room awake but in respiratory distress. His blood pressure was 110/40 mm Hg, heart rate 120/min, respiratory rate 30/min, temperature 102° F, and oxygen saturation was 88% on 10 L/min oxygen by face mask. Physical exam was notable for signs of increased work of breathing and crackles on chest auscultation. His cardiac exam disclosed an elevated jugular venous pressure (JVP), a hyperdynamic precordium on palpation, tachycardia, and a loud diastolic murmur at the left lower sternal border on auscultation. A summation gallop also was noted. The patient's extremities were cool and without edema. Laboratory evaluation disclosed an elevated white count; an ECG showed tachycardia with some nonspecific T-wave changes. The chest radiograph

showed pulmonary edema. An urgent echocardiogram showed 4+ aortic regurgitation with LV dilation. LV systolic function appeared intact. A large vegetation was seen on one of the aortic cusps, and the other cusps appeared thickened.

This patient has acute aortic valve endocarditis, likely from a staphylococcal infection. The infection was probably acquired from his IV drug use and involved his aortic valve, which may have been damaged previously from the episode of rheumatic fever. The infection has eroded his aortic valve and produced acute aortic insufficiency. In this case the LV acutely has a large regurgitant volume load. When the aortic valve eroded, there was an acute increase in diastolic volume caused by regurgitation of blood from the aorta. This led to LV dilation and increased diastolic wall stress and elevated filling pressures. The elevated filling pressures lead to pulmonary edema and dyspnea. The $\dot{Q}c$ is decreased because of the regurgitation of blood into the LV, but the heart has partially compensated by increasing its rate and augmenting its stroke volume. Unfortunately, the $\dot{Q}c$ is not adequate to meet the body's demands, and the patient is developing tissue hypoperfusion and cardiogenic shock.

Management in this case begins with stabilization of the respiratory system. Oxygen delivery and respiratory muscle unloading are required. Positive pressure ventilation also may help cardiac function by reducing the afterload and the amount of blood regurgitated into the LV. A trial of mask ventilation with pressure support and PEEP may be attempted in this case. If the patient does not tolerate this, he may require intubation, sedation, and ventilation with pressure support and PEEP. PEEP can be started at 5 cm H_2O and increased as tolerated to support oxygenation and reduce afterload. In the meantime, antibiotic therapy and intravenous afterload reducers (that is, sodium nitroprusside) can be administered. The patient should be considered for urgent surgical replacement of the aortic valve given the severity of heart failure.

Case Three
Diastolic Dysfunction from Hypertension

An 80-year-old woman with a long history of hypertension and chronic obstructive pulmonary disease (COPD) presented with a fractured hip after a fall. She underwent surgical fixation of the fracture that evening. Postoperatively she was observed to develop atrial fibrillation with a rapid ventricular response. Shortly after she complained of shortness of breath. The patient was sitting upright in bed, was diaphoretic, and was in moderate respiratory distress. Blood pressure was 180/100 mm Hg, heart rate was 140 to 160/min and irregular, and temperature was 101° F. Oxygen saturation was 90% on 8 L/min oxygen via nasal cannula. Physical exam disclosed slight wheezing and crackles on chest auscultation. A chest radiograph was consistent with pulmonary edema. An ECG revealed atrial fibrillation without ischemic changes. An echocardiogram disclosed a thickened and hyperkinetic LV with normal chamber dimensions and ejection fraction.

This patient has pulmonary edema from diastolic dysfunction. The cause of her pulmonary edema is multifactorial. First, the heart is thickened from long-standing hypertension and likely has baseline abnormalities in relaxation. With atrial fibrillation, the contribution to ventricular filling from the atrial contraction was lost. Normally, atrial contraction serves to increase LVEDP without a large concurrent rise in mean left atrial pressure (LAP). In patients with thickened ventricles, the LVEDP may be 8 mm Hg or more greater than the mean LAP.[143] Loss of atrial contraction causes a rise in the mean left atrial pressure and can contribute to pulmonary edema. The rapid ventricular rate that results from atrial fibrillation also may impede diastolic function by limiting the diastolic interval available for filling. Finally, any heart rate–related ischemia can impede relaxation by reducing the available ATP needed to relax the ventricle.

In this case, therapy should be directed at restoration of a normal sinus rhythm. The respiratory status is reasonably stable at present and can be managed with supplemental oxygen alone. The quickest and easiest method to restore a normal sinus rhythm is synchronized electric cardioversion. Usually an initial attempt with 100 joules of electricity is used, but often 360 joules are needed to convert to a sinus rhythm. If this is unsuccessful or the patient reverts to atrial fibrillation, an antiarrhythmic drug may help convert and stabilize the rhythm. The antiarrhythmics procainamide or amiodarone can be rapidly loaded intravenously before a second attempt at cardioversion. The antiarrhythmic propafenone recently has been shown to be effective in converting patients to sinus rhythm with a one-time oral dose of 600 mg.[144] This method was safe and over 70% effective in patients with hypertension and over 80% effective in those with structural heart disease. If attempts at cardioversion fail, the patient may be rate controlled with a variety of agents. Digoxin can slow conduction and reduce the ventricular response. The calcium channel blockers diltiazem or verapamil are effective at rate control. Both can be given by continuous intravenous infusion. β-Blockers also can be used and are ideal after myocardial infarction (MI). Further supportive therapy with nitroglycerin and diuretics also may be used in this situation. Effective pain control, treatment of bronchospasm (with a nonabsorbed anticholinergic, that is, ipratropium, that will not stimulate the heart), and reduction of fever are important methods to reduce the cardiac stimulation from catecholamine release.

Case Four
Chronic Congestive Heart Failure from Cardiomyopathy of Coronary Artery Disease

A 55-year-old man with a history of congestive heart failure (CHF) and multiple myocardial infarctions (MIs) presented with slowly progressive fatigue and shortness of breath over the last week. The patient had his first MI at age 45 years. He initially did well with medical management but at age 53 years had a large anterior MI. His course after this MI has been notable for multiple episodes of heart failure. After the MI he was found to have two-vessel coronary disease and a decreased ejection fraction at 20%. He has been managed with an ACE inhibitor, diuretics, and digoxin while he awaits cardiac transplantation. About 3 months ago he was started on carvedilol. The patient was traveling in Italy the last 3 weeks and admits to noncompliance with his low-salt diet. He also ran out of his lisinopril 10 days ago. About 1 week ago he noted some increased dyspnea with exertion and fatigue. The last 3 days he has been sleeping on 3 to 4 pillows instead of his usual 2, and last night he woke up twice very short of breath. He denies any chest pain but has had some pedal edema.

On exam he was in mild respiratory distress and had a periodic breathing pattern, especially when distracted or resting. Blood pressure was 110/70 mm Hg, heart rate 75/min, oxygen saturation 95% on 2 L/min nasal cannula. Auscultation of his chest was notable only for a few mild crackles at the bases. His neck veins were elevated to his jaw, there was a large displaced LV apical impulse, and on auscultation a loud S_3 was noted. His legs had 2+ to 3+ pitting edema. Laboratory evaluation was unremarkable and an ECG showed his usual left bundle branch pattern. A chest radiograph showed cardiomegaly and small bilateral effusions. No pulmonary edema was noted. He was transferred to the critical care unit and while sleeping was noted to desaturate during periods of apnea.

This patient has decompensated heart failure from medical and dietary noncompliance. Although conservative therapy with diuretics and restarting of his ACE inhibitor may work, an attempt at tailored therapy may provide better long-term results. In this patient a pulmonary artery catheter could be placed to guide therapy. Intravenous diuretics and vasodilators could be used to obtain the lowest filling pressures that provide an adequate $\dot{Q}c$. If needed, an inotrope such as dobutamine could be added. Once hemodynamics are optimized, oral therapy would begin. The presence of periodic breathing is the result of his heart failure. An attempt to treat this with noninvasive positive pressure ventilation (NPPV) may help his left ventricular function and overall well-being.

Case Five
Coronary Bypass Surgery

A 68-year-old man with a history of angina underwent coronary bypass surgery for three-vessel disease. When coming off the pump he experienced hypotension that required high doses of a norepinephrine infusion to stabilize his blood pressure. The patient remained intubated and sedated and was transported to the intensive care unit. He was ventilated with volume ventilation at 10 mL/kg, PEEP

5 cm H_2O, FIO_2 of 1.0, and a rate of 12/min. With this he was hypoxemic with a blood gas of pH 7.46, $PaCO_2$ 34 mm Hg, and PaO_2 50 mm Hg. The pulmonary artery catheter disclosed a right atrial pressure of 14 mm Hg, an RV pressure of 45/14 mm Hg, a pulmonary artery pressure (PAP) of 45/20 mm Hg, and a pulmonary artery occlusion pressure (PAOP) of 8 mm Hg. The $\dot{Q}c$ by thermodilution was 3.8 L/min. A chest radiograph and an ECG were within normal limits. An emergent echocardiogram was notable for a hypocontractile RV with preserved LV function. A patent foramen ovale with right-to-left shunting was noted when air contrast was injected.

This patient has shock from isolated RV dysfunction after cardiopulmonary bypass during cardiac surgery. RV dysfunction after bypass is a well described complication of cardiac surgery. Several possible etiologies for this dysfunction include air emboli, RV infraction, and stunned myocardium. Air embolism can be fatal and requires prompt treatment with removal of the air or hyperbaric oxygen therapy. The other forms of RV dysfunction after cardiac surgery can reverse if given enough time. The goal is to support the patient with vasoactive drugs until the RV function returns. Occasionally an RV assist device can be used to support the patient.

In this case the situation is complicated by an intra-cardiac shunt. The foramen ovale is a hole that exists in utero between the atria. It closes after birth and in most people is fused. A significant portion of the population has a nonfused foramen ovale that remains closed because the left-sided atrial pressure is greater than the right-sided atrial pressure. In this patient, when the pressure increased in the right atrium in association with the decreased compliance of the RV, the foramen ovale opened and shunted blood from the right atrium to the left atrium. This shunted blood is the cause of the refractory hypoxemia.

This patient was stabilized hemodynamically with norepinephrine. The challenge is to reduce the shunt. Increasing PEEP, which generally improves oxygenation in patients with lung disease, may actually be detrimental in this case because it can increase pulmonary vascular resistance (PVR) and thus increase the fraction of right-to-left shunted blood. Intravenous vasodilators such as nitroprusside and nitroglycerin can lower the PVR but also can lower systemic blood pressure. In addition, these agents will reduce hypoxic vasoconstriction and may potentially worsen hypoxemia. Inhaled nitric oxide (NO) is a potent vasodilator with a short half-life. When inhaled, it selectively dilates the pulmonary arteries and improves $\dot{V}/\dot{Q}$ matching by preferentially dilating the vasculature of ventilated lung units. Recent experience in patients with acute RV failure has shown that NO can improve oxygenation and $\dot{Q}c$.[145] In this case, a trial of NO reduced the shunt and improved RV function by reducing PVR.

KEY POINTS

- Heart failure is a common occurrence in hospitalized patients and it often causes respiratory failure.
- Although there are numerous causes for heart failure, it ultimately results from an abnormality of contraction, excessive load, and/or restricted filling.
- Symptoms vary from patient to patient but usually manifest with fatigue and dyspnea on exertion. Often the symptoms occur late in the disease process.
- Treatment for heart failure requires a knowledge of its complex pathophysiology.
- The majority of treatments for cardiac failure stabilize the disease and do not reverse the process.
- Vasodilators and diuretics remain the mainstay of therapy, but recent studies have demonstrated the efficacy of β-blockers in patients with heart failure.
- Mechanical ventilation for patients with respiratory failure can be very effective in reversing the abnormalities resulting from pulmonary edema.
- The interactions of the lungs and heart are complex in patients with heart failure, and the use of positive pressure ventilation can often lead to unpredictable results if not used carefully.

References

1. National Heart, Lung, and Blood Institute. Report of the task force on research in heart failure. Bethesda, Md: The Institute; 1994.
2. Packer M. Survival in patients with chronic heart failure and its potential modification by drug therapy. In: Cohn JN, editor. Drug treatment of heart failure. Secaucus: ATC International; 1988. p. 273.
3. Cohn JN. The management of chronic heart failure. N Engl J Med 1996;335:490-498.
4. Timmis AD, Nathan AW. Essentials of cardiology. Oxford: Blackwell Scientific Publications; 1993. p. 351.
5. McMurray J, Hart W, Rhodes G. An evaluation of the economic cost of heart failure to the national health service in the United Kingdom. Br Med Econ 1993;6:99-110.
6. Eriksson H. Heart failure: a growing public health problem. J Intern Med 1995;237:134-141.
7. Sharpe N, Doughty R. Epidemiology of heart failure and ventricular dysfunction. Lancet 1998;352:3-7.
8. Cowie MR, Mosterd A, Wood DA, et al. The epidemiology of heart failure. Eur Heart J 1997;18:208-225.
9. Ho KK, Anderson KM, Kannel WB, et al. Survival after the onset of congestive heart failure in Framingham Heart Study subjects. Circulation 1993;88:107-115.
10. Brophy JM, Deslauriers G, Rouleau JL. Long-term prognosis of patients presenting to the emergency room with decompensated congestive heart failure. Can J Cardiol 1994;10:543-547.
11. Doughty RN, Rodgers A, Sharpe N, et al. Effects of beta-blocker therapy on mortality in patients with heart failure: a systematic overview of randomized controlled trials. Eur Heart J 1997;18:560-565.

12. Franciosa JA, Wilen M, Ziesche S, et al. Survival in men with severe chronic left ventricular failure due to either coronary heart disease or idiopathic dilated cardiomyopathy. Am J Cardiol 1983;51:831-836.

13. Garg R, Yusuf S. Overview of randomized trials of angiotensin-converting enzyme inhibitors on mortality and morbidity in patients with heart failure. JAMA 1995;273:1450-1456.

14. Guyton AC. Textbook of medical physiology. Philadelphia: Saunders; 1991. p. 1014.

15. Opie LH. Mechanisms of cardiac contraction and relaxation. In: Braunwald E, editor. Heart disease: a textbook of cardiovascular medicine. Philadelphia: Saunders; 1997. pp. 360-393.

16. Nwasokwa ON. Cardiac function. In: Dantzker DR, Scharf SM, editors. Cardiopulmonary critical care. 3rd ed. Philadelphia: Saunders; 1998. pp. 145-171.

17. Magder S. More respect for the CVP. Intensive Care Med 1998;24:651-653.

18. Hartel S, Karczewski P, Krause EG. Protein phosphorylation and cardiac function: cholinergic adrenergic interaction. Cardiovasc Res 1993; 27:1948-1953.

19. Balligand JL, Kelly RA, Marsden PA, et al. Control of cardiac muscle cell function by an endogenous nitric oxide signaling system. Proc Natl Acad Sci USA 1993;90:347-351.

20. Spann JF, Buccino RA, Sonnenblick EH, et al. Contractile state of cardiac muscle obtained from cats with experimentally produced ventricular hypertrophy and heart failure. Circ Res 1967;21:341.

21. Colucci WS, Braunwald E. Pathophysiology of heart failure. In: Braunwald E, editor. Heart disease: a textbook of cardiovascular medicine. Philadelphia: Saunders; 1997. pp. 394-420.

22. Braunwald E, Colucci WS, Grossman W. Clinical aspects of heart failure: high-output heart failure; pulmonary edema. In: Braunwald E, editor. Heart disease: a textbook of cardiovascular medicine. Philadelphia: Saunders; 1997. pp. 445-470.

23. Chandler BM, Sonnenblick EH, Spann JR, et al. Association of depressed myofibrillar adenosine triphosphatase and reduced contractility in experimental heart failure. Circ Res 1967;21:717.

24. Floras JS. Clinical aspects of sympathetic activation and parasympathetic withdrawal in heart failure. J Am Coll Cardiol 1993;22:72A.

25. Opie LH. The heart: physiology and metabolism. New York: Raven; 1991. p. 513.

26. Mann DL, Urabe Y, Kent RL, et al. Cellular versus myocardial basis for the contractile dysfunction of hypertrophied myocardium. Circ Res 1991;68:402-415.

27. Aoyagi T, Fujii AM, Flanagan MF, et al. Transition from compensated hypertrophy to intrinsic myocardial dysfunction during development of left ventricular pressure-overload hypertrophy in conscious sheep: systolic dysfunction precedes diastolic dysfunction. Circulation 1993;88:2415-2425.

28. Gwathmey JK, Copelas L, MacKinnon R, et al. Abnormal intracellular calcium handling in myocardium from patients with end-stage heart failure. Circ Res 1987;61:70-76.

29. Arai M, Alpert NR, MacLennan DH, et al. Alterations in sarcoplasmic reticulum gene expression in human heart failure: a possible mechanism for alterations in systolic and diastolic properties of the failing myocardium. Circ Res 1993;72:463-469.

30. D'Agnolo A, Luciani GB, Mazzucco A, et al. Contractile properties and Ca^{++} release activity of the sarcoplasmic reticulum in dilated cardiomyopathy. Circulation 1992;85:518-525.

31. Takahashi T, Allen PD, Lacro RV, et al. Expression of dihydropyridine receptor (Ca^{++} channel) and calsequestrin genes in the myocardium of patients with end-stage heart failure. J Clin Invest 1992;90:927-935.

32. Mercadier JJ, Lompre AM, Duc P, et al. Altered sarcoplasmic reticulum Ca^{++}-ATPase gene expression in the human ventricle during end-stage heart failure. J Clin Invest 1990;85:305-309.

33. Hammond EH, Anderson JL, Menlove RL. Prognostic significance of myofilament loss in patients with idiopathic cardiomyopathy determined by electron microscopy. J Am Coll Cardiol 1986;7:204A.

34. Malhotra A, Sheuer J. Troponin-tropomyosin dysfunction in cardiomyopathy. Circulation 1988;78:179.

35. Solaro RJ, Powers FM, Gao L, et al. Control of myofilament activation in heart failure. Circulation 1993;87:38.

36. Guyton AC. Pulmonary circulation; pulmonary edema; pleural fluid: textbook of medical physiology. Philadelphia: Saunders; 1991. pp. 414-421.

37. Staub NC. Pulmonary edema due to increased microvascular permeability to fluid and protein. Circ Res 1978;43:143-151.

38. Staub NC, Nagano H, Pearce ML. Pulmonary edema in dogs especially the sequence of fluid accumulation in lungs. J App Physiol 1967;22:227-240.

39. Gaar KA, Jr, Taylor AE, Owens LJ, et al. Effect of capillary pressure and plasma protein on development of pulmonary edema. Am J Physiol 1967;213:79-82.

40. Stock MC, Davis DW, Manning JW, et al. Lung mechanics and oxygen consumption during spontaneous ventilation and severe heart failure. Chest 1992;102:279-283.

41. Meyer TE, Gaasch WH. Acute congestive heart failure and pulmonary edema. In: Brown DL, editor. Cardiac intensive care. Philadelphia: Saunders; 1998. pp. 375-390.

42. Miro AM, Pinsky MR. Heart-lung interactions. In: Tobin MJ, editor. Principles and practice of mechanical ventilation. New York: McGraw-Hill; 1994. pp. 647-671.

43. Pinsky MR. The hemodynamic consequences of mechanical ventilation: an evolving story. Intensive Care Med 1997;23:493-503.

44. Fessler HE. Heart-lung interactions: applications in the critically ill. Eur Respir J 1997;10:226-237.

45. Scharf SM. Mechanical cardiopulmonary interactions in critical care. In: Dantzker DR, Scharf SM, editors. Cardiopulmonary critical care. Philadelphia: Saunders; 1998. pp. 75-91.

46. Glick G, Wechsler A, Epstein S. Reflex cardiovascular depression produced by stimulation of pulmonary stretch receptors in the dog. J Clin Invest 1969;48:467-472.

47. Howell JBL, Permutt S, Proctor DF, et al. Effect of inflation of the lung on different parts of the pulmonary vascular bed. J App Physiol 1961;16:71-76.

48. Takata M, Robotham JL. Effects of inspiratory diaphragmatic descent on inferior vena caval venous return. J Appl Physiol 1992;72:597-607.

49. Weber K, Kinasewitz G, Janicki J, et al. Oxygen utilization and ventilation during exercise in patients with chronic cardiac failure. Circulation 1982;65:1213.

50. Criteria Committee NYHA. Disease of the heart and blood vessels: nomenclature and criteria for diagnosis. Boston: Little, Brown; 1964. p. 114.

51. Badgett RG, Lucey CR, Mulrow CD. Can the clinical examination diagnose left-sided heart failure in adults? JAMA 1997;277:1712-1719.

52. Levine SA, Harvey WP. Clinical auscultation of the heart. Philadelphia: Saunders; 1959.

53. Perloff JK. Physical examination of the heart and circulation. Philadelphia: Saunders; 1990. p. 292.

54. Marriott HJL. Practical electrocardiography. Baltimore: Williams & Wilkins; 1988.

55. Johns JP, Abraham SA, Eagle KA. Dipyridamole-thallium versus dobutamine echocardiographic stress testing: a clinician's viewpoint. Am Heart J 1995;130:373-385.

56. Leatherman JW, Marini JJ. Pulmonary artery catheterization: interpretation of recordings. In: Tobin MJ, editor. Principles and practice of intensive care monitoring. New York: McGraw-Hill; 1998. pp. 821-838.

57. Tulzo YL, Belghith M, Sequin P, et al. Reproducibility of thermodilution cardiac output determination in critically ill patients; comparison between bolus and continuous method. J Clin Monit 1996; 12:379-385.

58. Magder S. Cardiac output. In: Tobin MJ, editor. Principles and practice of intensive care monitoring. New York: McGraw-Hill; 1998. pp. 797-810.

59. Pinsky MR. Hemodynamic profile interpretation. In: Tobin MJ, editor. Principles and practice of intensive care monitoring. New York: McGraw-Hill; 1998. pp. 871-888.

60. Gould L, Zahir M, DeMartino A, et al. Cardiac effects of a cocktail. JAMA 1971;218:1799-1802.

61. Sullivan MJ, Higginbotham MB, Cobb FR. Exercise training in patients with severe left ventricular dysfunction: hemodynamic and metabolic effects. Circulation 1988;78:506-515.

62. Cohn JN, Archibald DG, Ziesche S, et al. Effect of vasodilator therapy on mortality in chronic congestive heart failure: results of a Veterans Administration Cooperative Study. N Engl J Med 1986;314:1547-1552.

63. Smith TW, Kelly RA, Stevenson LW, et al. Management of heart failure. In: Braunwald E, editor. Heart disease: a textbook of cardiovascular medicine. Philadelphia: Saunders; 1997. pp. 492-514.

64. Opie LH, Poole-Wilson PA, Sonnenblick E, et al. Angiotensin-converting enzyme inhibitors and conventional vasodilators. In: Opie LH, editor. Drugs for the heart. Philadelphia: Saunders; 1995. pp. 105-144.

65. Cohn JN, Johnson G, Ziesche S, et al. A comparison of enalapril with hydralazine-isosorbide dinitrate in the treatment of chronic congestive heart failure N Engl J Med 1991;325:303-310.

66. Cohn JN, Ziesche S, Smith R, et al. Effect of the calcium antagonist felodipine as supplementary vasodilator therapy in patients with chronic heart failure treated with enalapril: V-HeFT III. Vasodilator-Heart Failure Trial (V-HeFT) Study Group. Circulation 1997;96:856-863.

67. Packer M, O'Connor CM, Ghali JK, et al. Effect of amlodipine on morbidity and mortality in severe chronic heart failure. Prospective Randomized Amlodipine Survival Evaluation Study Group. N Engl J Med 1996;335:1107-1114.

68. Gottlieb SS, Dickstein K, Fleck E, et al. Hemodynamic and neurohormonal effects of the angiotensin II antagonist losartan in patients with congestive heart failure. Circulation 1993;88:1602-1609.

69. Pitt B, Segal R, Martinez FA, et al. Randomised trial of losartan versus captopril in patients over 65, with heart failure (ELITE). Lancet 1997;349:747-752.

70. Cotter G, Metzkor E, Kaluski E, et al. Randomised trial of high-dose isosorbide dinitrate plus low-dose furosemide versus high-dose furosemide plus low-dose isosorbide dinitrate in severe pulmonary edema. Lancet 1998;351:389-393.

71. Barr CS, Lang CC, Hanson J, et al. Effects of adding spironolactone to an angiotensin-converting enzyme inhibitor in chronic congestive heart failure secondary to coronary artery disease. Am J Cardiol 1995;76:1259-1265.

72. Struthers AD. Aldosterone escape during angiotensin-converting enzyme inhibitor therapy in chronic heart failure. J Card Fail 1996;2:47-54.

73. Pitt B. RALES. Clinical trial results, American Heart Association's 71st Scientific Sessions; 1998 Nov 8-11; Dallas.

74. Dormans TP, van Meyel JJ, Gerlag PG, et al. Diuretic efficacy of high dose furosemide in severe heart failure: bolus injection versus continuous infusion. J Am Coll Cardiol 1996;28:376-382.

75. Martin SJ, Danziger LH. Continuous infusion of loop diuretics in the critically ill: a review of the literature. Crit Care Med 1994;22:1323-1329.

76. Yelton SL, Gaylor MA, Murray KM. The role of continuous infusion loop diuretics. Ann Pharmacother 1995;29:1010-1014.

77. Kelly RA, Smith TW. Drugs used in the treatment of heart failure. In: Braunwald E, editor. Heart disease: a textbook of cardiovascular medicine. Philadelphia: Saunders; 1997. pp. 471-491.

78. Uretsky BF, Young JB, Shahidi FE, et al. Randomized study assessing the effect of digoxin withdrawal in patients with mild to moderate chronic congestive heart failure: results of the PROVED trial. PROVED Investigative Group. J Am Coll Cardiol 1993;22:955-962.

79. Packer M, Gheorghiade M, Young JB, et al. Withdrawal of digoxin from patients with chronic heart failure treated with angiotensin-converting-enzyme inhibitors. N Engl J Med 1993;329:1-7.

80. The effect of digoxin on mortality and morbidity in patients with heart failure. The Digitalis Investigation Group. N Engl J Med 1997;336:525-533.

81. Packer M, Carver JR, Rodeheffer RJ, et al. Effect of oral milrinone on mortality in severe chronic heart failure. N Engl J Med 1991;325:1468-1475.

82. Feldman AM, Bristow MR, Parmley WW, et al. Effects of vesnarinone on morbidity and mortality in patients with heart failure. N Engl J Med 1993;329:149.

83. Cohn JN, Goldstein SO, Greenberg BH, et al. A dose-dependent increase in mortality with vesnarinone among patients with severe heart failure. N Engl J Med 1998;339:1810-1816.

84. Javaheri S, Parker TJ, Wexler L, et al. Effect of theophylline on sleep-disordered breathing in heart failure. N Engl J Med 1996;335:562-567.

85. Denton MD, Chertow GM, Brady HR. "Renal-dose" dopamine for the treatment of acute renal failure: scientific rationale, experimental studies, and clinical trials. Kidney International 1996;49:4-14.

86. Waagstein F, Hjalmarson A, Varnauskas E, et al. Effect of chronic beta-adrenergic receptor blockade in congestive cardiomyopathy. Br Heart J 1975;137:1022-1036.

87. Swedberg K, Hjalmarson A, Waagstein F, et al. Beneficial effects of long-term beta-blockade in congestive cardiomyopathy. Br Heart J 1980;44:117-133.

88. Engelmeier RS, O'Connell JB, Walsh R, et al. Improvement in symptoms and exercise tolerance by metoprolol in patients with dilated cardiomyopathy: a double-blind, randomized, placebo-controlled trial. Circulation 1985;72:536-546.

89. Anderson JL, Lutz JR, Gilbert EM, et al. A randomized trial of low-dose beta-blockade therapy for idiopathic dilated cardiomyopathy. Am J Cardiol 1985;55:471-475.

90. Krumholz HM. Beta-blockers for mild to moderate heart failure. Lancet 1999;353:2.

91. Group. Xamoterol in severe heart failure. Lancet 1990;336:1.

92. Lechat P, Packer M, Chalon S, et al. Clinical effects of beta-adrenergic blockade in chronic heart failure: a meta-analysis of double-blind, placebo-controlled, randomized trials. Circulation 1998;98:1184-1191.

93. Investigators. The cardiac insufficiency bisoprolol study II (CIBIS-II): a randomised trial. Lancet 1999;353:9-13.

94. Group. Effect of metoprolol CR/XL in chronic heart failure: Metoprolol CR/XL Randomised Intervention Trial in Congestive Heart Failure (MERIT-HF). Lancet 1999;353:2001-2007.

95. Stevenson LW. Inotropic therapy for heart failure. N Engl J Med 1998;339:1848-1850.

96. Frishman WH. Carvedilol. N Engl J Med 1998; 339: 1759-1765.

97. Gilbert EM, Abraham WT, Olsen S, et al. Comparative hemodynamic, left ventricular functional, and antiadrenergic effects of chronic treatment with metoprolol versus carvedilol in the failing heart. Circulation 1996;94:2817-2825.

98. Ravid S, Podrid PJ, Lampert S, et al. Congestive heart failure induced by six of the newer antiarrhythmic drugs. J Am Coll Cardiol 1989;14:1326-1330.

99. Echt DS, Liebson PR, Mitchell LB, et al. Mortality and morbidity in patients receiving encainide, flecainide, or placebo. The Cardiac Arrhythmia Suppression Trial. N Engl J Med 1991;324:781-788.

100. Hamer AW, Arkles LB, Johns JA. Beneficial effects of low dose amiodarone in patients with congestive cardiac failure: a placebo-controlled trial. J Am Coll Cardiol 1989;14:1768-1774.

101. Doval HC, Nul DR, Grancelli HO. Randomised trial of low-dose amiodarone in severe congestive heart failure. Lancet 1994;344:493-498.

102. Singh SN, Fletcher RD, Fisher SG, et al. Amiodarone in patients with congestive heart failure and asymptomatic ventricular arrhythmia. Survival Trial of Antiarrhythmic Therapy in Congestive Heart Failure. N Engl J Med 1995;333:77-82.

103. Dec GW, Fuster V. Idiopathic dilated cardiomyopathy. N Engl J Med 1994;331:1564-1575.

104. Stevenson LW. Tailored therapy before transplantation for treatment of advanced heart failure: effective use of vasodilators and diuretics. J Heart Lung Transplant 1991;10:468-476.

105. Torchiana DF, Hirsch G, Buckley MJ, et al. Intraaortic balloon pumping for cardiac support: trends in practice and outcome, 1968 to 1995. J Thorac Cardiovasc Surg 1997;113:758-769.

106. Hunt SA, Frazier OH. Mechanical circulatory support and cardiac transplantation. Circulation 1998;97:2079-2090.

107. Goldstein DJ, Oz MC, Rose EA. Implantable left ventricular assist devices. N Engl J Med 1998;339:1522-1533.

108. Moss AJ, Hall J, Cannom DS, et al. Improved survival with an implanted defibrillator in patients with coronary disease at high risk for ventricular arrhythmia. N Engl J Med 1996;335:1933-1940.

109. Investigators. A comparison of antiarrhythmic-drug therapy with implantable defibrillators in patients resuscitated from near-fatal ventricular arrhythmias. N Engl J Med 1997;337:1576-1583.

110. Taggart DP, Westaby S. Surgical management of heart failure. Br Med J 1997;314:453-454.

111. Carpentier A. Does surgical reduction of heart size reduce heart failure? Lancet 1997;350:456.

112. Angelini GD, Pryn S, Mehta D, et al. Left-ventricular-volume reduction for end-stage heart failure. Lancet 1997;350:489.

113. Fessler HE, Brower RG, Wise RA, et al. Mechanism of reduced LV afterload by systolic and diastolic positive pleural pressure. J Appl Physiol 1988;65:1244-1250.

114. Bersten AD, Holt AW, Vedig AE, et al. Treatment of severe cardiogenic pulmonary edema with continuous positive airway pressure delivered by face mask. N Engl J Med 1991;325:1825-1830.

115. Pang D, Keenan SP, Cook DJ, et al. The effect of positive pressure airway support on mortality and the need for intubation in cardiogenic pulmonary edema. Chest 1998;114:1185-1192.

116. Rusterholz T, Kempf J, Berton C, et al. Noninvasive pressure support ventilation with face mask in patients with acute cardiogenic pulmonary oedema. Intensive Care Med 1999;25:21-28.

117. Hoffmann B, Welte T. The use of noninvasive pressure support ventilation for respiratory insufficiency due to pulmonary oedema. Intensive Care Med 1999;25:15-20.

118. Mehta S, Jay GD, Woolard RH, et al. Randomized, prospective trial of bilevel versus continuous positive airway pressure in acute pulmonary edema. Crit Care Med 1997;25:620-628.

119. Wysocki M. Noninvasive ventilation in acute cardiogenic pulmonary edema: better than continuous positive airway pressure? Intensive Care Med 1999;25:1-2.

120. Giese JL, Stanley TH. Etomidate: a new intravenous anesthetic induction agent. Pharmocotherapy 1983;3:251-258.

121. Mirenda J, Broyles G. Propofol as used for sedation in the ICU. Chest 1995;198:539-548.

122. Muscedere JG, Mullen JBM, Gan K, et al. Tidal ventilation at low airway pressures can augment lung injury. Am J Respir Crit Care Med 1994;149:1327-1334.

123. Lachman B. Open up the lung and keep the lung open. Intensive Care Med 1992;18:319-321.

124. Gunther A, Siebert C, Schmidt R, et al. Surfactant alterations in severe pneumonia, acute respiratory distress syndrome, and cardiogenic edema. Am J Respir Crit Care Med 1996;153:176-184.

125. Huberfeld SI, Genovese J, Patel U, et al. Myocardial mechanics and energetics during continuous positive airway pressure in sedated pigs. Crit Care Med 1996;24:2027-2034.

126. Huberfeld S, Genovese A, Tarasiuk A, et al. Effects of CPAP on pericardial pressure, transmural pressure and respiratory mechanics in hypervolemic unanesthetized pigs. Am J Respir Crit Care Med 1995;152:142-147.

127. Multz A, Scharf SM. Pharmacologic and ventilatory support of the circulation in critically ill patients. In: Dantzker DR, Scharf SM, editors. Cardiopulmonary critical care. Philadelphia: Saunders; 1998. pp. 329-353.

128. Villar J, Slutsky A. PEEP or no PEEP? Clin Pulmonary Med 1996;3:279-287.

129. Calvin JE, Driedger AA, Sibbald WJ. PEEP does not depress left ventricular function in patients with pulmonary edema. Am Rev of Respir Dis 1981;124:121-128.

130. Grace MP, Greenbaum DM. Cardiac performance in response to PEEP in patients with cardiac dysfunction. Crit Care Med 1982;10:358-360.

131. Fessler HE, Brower RG, Wise R, et al. Positive pleural pressure decreases coronary perfusion. Am J Physiol 1990;258:H814-H820.

132. Lemaire F, Teboul JL, Cinotti L, et al. Acute left ventricular dysfunction during unsuccessful weaning from mechanical ventilation. Anesthesiology 1988;69:171-179.

133. Hurford WE, Favorito F. Association of myocardial ischemia with failure to wean from mechanical ventilation. Crit Care Med 1995;23:1475-1480.

134. Manthous CA, Schmidt GA, Hall JB. Liberation from mechanical ventilation. Chest 1998;114:886-901.

135. Javaheri S, Parker TJ, Wexler L, et al. Occult sleep-disordered breathing in stable congestive heart failure. Ann Intern Med 1995;122:487-492.

136. Naughton MT, Liu PP, Bernard DC, et al. Treatment of congestive heart failure and Cheyne-Stokes respiration during sleep by continuous positive airway pressure. Am J Respir Crit Care Med 1995;151:92-97.

137. Naughton MT, Bradley TD. Sleep apnea in congestive heart failure. Clin Chest Med 1998;19:99-113.

138. Lanfranchi PA, Braghiroli A, Bosimini E, et al. Prognostic value of nocturnal Cheyne-stokes respiration in chronic heart failure. Circulation 1999;99:1435-1440.

139. Andreas S, Hagenah G, Moller C, et al. Cheyne-Stokes respiration and prognosis in congestive heart failure. Am J Cardiol 1996;78:1260-1264.

140. Hanly PJ, Zuberi-Khokhar NS. Increased mortality associated with Cheyne-Stokes respiration in patients with congestive heart failure. Am J Respir Crit Care Med 1996;153:272-276.

141. Malone S, Liu PP, Holloway R, et al. Obstructive sleep apnoea in patients with dilated cardiomyopathy: effects of continuous positive airway pressure. Lancet 1991;338:1480-1484.

142. Takasaki Y, Orr D, Popkin J, et al. Effect of nasal continuous positive airway pressure on sleep apnea in congestive heart failure. Am Rev Respir Dis 1989;140:1578-1584.

143. Braunwald E, Frahm CJ. Studies on Starling's law of the heart. Circulation 1961;24:633-642.

144. Boriani G, Biffi M, Capucci A, et al. Oral propafenone to convert recent-onset atrial fibrillation in patients with and without underlying heart disease. A randomized, controlled trial. Ann Intern Med 1997; 126:621-625.

145. Bhorade S, Christenson J, O'Connor M, et al. Response to inhaled nitric oxide in patients with acute right heart syndrome. Am J Respir Crit Care Med 1999;159:571-579.

CHAPTER 55

Chest Trauma

Richard D. Branson
Robert S. Campbell
James M. Hurst

CHAPTER OUTLINE

OBJECTIVES

1. Compare blunt and penetrating chest trauma.
2. Discuss the etiology of blunt chest trauma.
3. Describe the management of flail chest, pulmonary contusion, hemothorax, and pneumothorax.
4. Discuss the role of tube thoracostomy in the treatment of hemothorax and pneumothorax.
5. Discuss the role of pain control in the management of blunt chest trauma.
6. Discuss the role of oxygen therapy, coughing, and deep breathing, and mask continuous positive airway pressure (CPAP) in the treatment of blunt chest trauma.
7. Describe the use of mechanical ventilation in patients with blunt chest trauma.
8. Discuss the use of independent lung ventilation in patients with unilateral lung injury.
9. Discuss the etiology, pathology, and treatment of penetrating chest trauma.

KEY TERMS

Blunt Chest Trauma	Mask CPAP	Pneumothorax
Cardiac Tamponade	Patient-Controlled Analgesia (PCA)	Pulmonary Contusion
Flail Chest	Penetrating Chest Trauma	Tube Thoracostomy
Hemothorax	Pericardiocentesis	

Trauma to the chest and damage to the contents of the thoracic cavity occur often with both blunt and penetrating injuries. Chest injuries account for about 16,000 deaths a year, or 20% to 25% of all trauma deaths, which makes them the second leading cause of death from trauma injury.[1-3] Traumatic chest injuries are also associated with prolonged disability and morbidity,[4-8] and because these injuries often occur in young, previously healthy patients, the economic impact on society is significant. For these reasons, early recognition and rapid treatment of chest injuries are crucial.[9,10]

Age-Specific Angle

Chest injuries often occur in young, previously healthy individuals.

Motor vehicle crashes (MVCs) are the most common cause of **blunt chest trauma,** accounting for 70% to 80% of all injuries. The mechanism of injury in blunt trauma is direct bruising of the lung, which results in alveolar hemorrhage and edema.[11] Because **penetrating chest trauma** is caused primarily by knife or gunshot wounds, the mechanism of injury depends on the velocity and size of the penetrating object. In low-velocity injuries, the affected area is predominantly confined to the tract of the wound. In high-velocity injuries, the affected area may be more extensive because of a blast effect, tumbling of the missile, deformation of the missile on impact, or secondary injury caused by fragmentation of the missile or creation of secondary missiles, such as pieces of the ribs. Penetrating trauma commonly occurs in urban areas, whereas blunt trauma most often is associated with highway travel and may occur in both urban and rural areas.[12] The spectrum of damage caused by chest trauma includes injury to the chest wall, lungs, heart, great vessels, and airways (Box 55-1). Isolated chest wall injury is relatively uncommon, occurring in only 16% of cases.[3]

Initial treatment of penetrating and blunt trauma includes the basics of the securing of an airway, provision of ventilation, and ensuring of adequate circulation. However, subsequent treatment differs significantly with the type and extent of injury.

Blunt Chest Trauma

Etiology

Blunt trauma to the chest results from motor vehicle and motorcycle crashes, falls, crush injuries, and assaults. The severity of injury may run the gamut from simple rib fracture to traumatic disruption of the heart or great vessels, resulting in immediate death. By far the most common injury with thoracic trauma is rib fracture. However, isolated chest injuries are the exception rather than the rule. Richardson and colleagues[13] found that in a group of 421 patients admitted for thoracic trauma, several concomitant injuries were common, including closed head injury (38%), shock (18%), long bone fracture (16%), rupture of the spleen (9%), liver laceration (7%), pelvic fracture (30%), and cervical spine fracture (3%). In this series, the most frequent causes of thoracic trauma (and their approximate incidence) were MVCs (268), falls (49), assaults (40), pedestrians hit by motor vehicles (28), motorcycle crashes (22), and crush injuries (14).[13]

Flail chest, which can be a life-threatening injury, usually results from multiple rib fractures on one side. Flail chest may also result from two or more rib fractures in two or more places, sternal fracture, or costochondral separation. The fourth to ninth ribs are most often fractured because of their protruding position. The term *flail* refers to the paradoxical motion of the chest caused by loss of chest wall stability. During inspiration the flail segment is drawn

Box 55-1

Spectrum of Injuries Seen with Blunt and Penetrating Chest Trauma

Penetrating Injuries
Cardiac
  Conducting system: Dysrhythmias, atrioventricular block
  Parenchyma: Hemopericardium, hemothorax, exsanguination, traumatic septal defects
  Vessels: Laceration of the coronary arteries
  Valves: Regurgitation, disruption
Pulmonary
  Nervous system: Laceration of the phrenic nerve
  Chest wall: Sucking chest wound
  Parenchyma: Laceration, contusion, pneumothorax, hemothorax
  Airways: Laceration of the trachea, bronchus, or larynx
Other
  Diaphragm: Laceration, perforation
  Great vessels: Laceration of the aorta or vena cava

Blunt Injuries
Cardiac
  Conducting system: Dysrhythmias, atrioventricular block
  Parenchyma: Contusion, hemopericardium, hemothorax, rupture
  Valves: Regurgitation, disruption
  Septum: Rupture
Pulmonary
  Chest wall: Rib fractures, contusion, flail chest, sternal fracture
  Parenchyma: Laceration, contusion, pneumothorax, hemothorax
  Airways: Tracheal, bronchial, or laryngeal disruption
Other
  Diaphragm: Rupture, diaphragmatic hernia
  Great vessels: Rupture or aneurysm of the aorta or vena cava
  Spinal cord: Compression fractures, subluxation, paralysis

inward by the negative intrapleural pressure, exactly the opposite of normal chest motion. During exhalation the flail segment is pushed outward. This seesaw motion is a characteristic physical finding in flail chest. Flail chest can be caused by trauma to the anterior chest, such as from a steering wheel during a motor vehicle crash, or as a complication of overzealous chest compressions during cardiopulmonary resuscitation. Figure 55-1 shows the site of flail injury based on the site of impact (that is, lateral or frontal).

Pathology

Injury to the chest wall from blunt chest trauma can affect lung function through a variety of mechanisms. For the most part. the gas exchange abnormalities that follow blunt chest injury occur secondary to pulmonary contusion.[2,14] The integrity of the chest wall is important to the normal bellows operation of the diaphragm and the move-

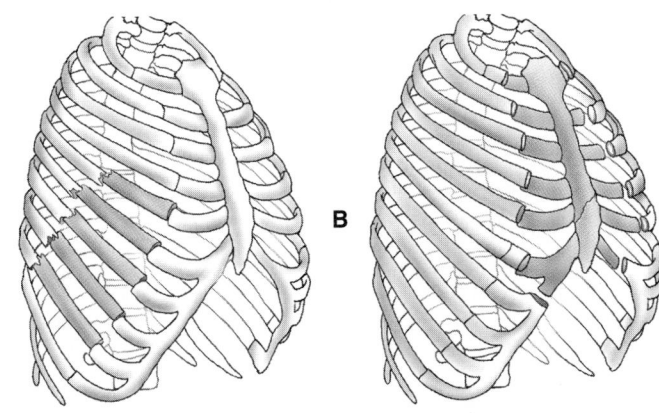

Figure 55-1 The anatomic location of the flail segment indicates the mechanism of injury. **A,** Lateral flail segments occur with broadside impacts and anteroposterior crush mechanisms. **B,** Anterior flail segments are caused by blows to the sternum.

ment of gases. However, patients with large flail segments but no underlying pulmonary injury rarely require ventilatory assistance.

Rib fractures and multiple rib fractures that create a flail segment are painful. Rapid, shallow breathing, splinting, and weak cough all lead to respiratory compromise. In these cases atelectasis and retention of secretions, particularly with hemoptysis, can cause hypoxemia. Flail segments may also compromise respiration by increasing the work of breathing. This happens when an unstable chest wall creates a paradoxical motion and results in inefficient air movement.[15-17]

Pulmonary contusion is the primary culprit in gas exchange abnormalities with chest trauma. A **pulmonary contusion** is a bruise of the lung, and it behaves much like other types of bruises. The initial trauma ruptures small blood vessels and disrupts the alveoli and terminal bronchioles, causing interstitial edema and intraalveolar hemorrhage.[18-20] This initial area of edema and hemorrhage is an isolated area of ventilation/perfusion mismatch. The size of the initial injury generally increases with time and administration of intravenous fluids. Pulmonary contusion often is said to "blossom" at 48 hours, with the height of gas exchange abnormalities occurring at this time.[21] Acute respiratory distress syndrome (ARDS) may develop after a pulmonary contusion, although no conclusive evidence suggests that pulmonary contusion causes ARDS. More likely, concomitant in-

ℜespiratory Recap

Blunt Chest Trauma
Flail chest
Pulmonary contusion
Hemothorax and pneumothorax

juries and the inflammatory response to injury precipitates ARDS.

In some cases of blunt chest injury, hemothorax or pneumothorax or both may result.[22-24] **Hemothorax** is the trapping of blood in the pleural space, which results in a space-occupying lesion. The blood typically comes from laceration of the lung or intercostal blood vessels by the fractured ribs. Hemothorax can cause hypotension and respiratory distress. **Pneumothorax,** or air in the pleural space, may occur with blunt chest injury because of direct puncture of the lung by a fractured rib, deceleration injuries that cause a tear in the lung tissue, or a crush injury that ruptures alveoli. Pneumothorax causes collapse of the lung and shortness of breath. *Tension pneumothorax* is a life-threatening condition in which air escapes the lung and is trapped in the pleural space with no means of escape. Tension pneumothorax most often is caused by application of positive pressure ventilation in a patient with a pneumothorax that occurred secondary to trauma. The lung on the side of the pneumothorax is collapsed, and the pressure in the pleural space forces the mediastinal structures toward the opposite lung. The result is hypotension and hypoxemia.

Management of the Unintubated Patient with Blunt Chest Trauma

Initial treatment of victims of blunt chest trauma should include the *ABCs* (that is, ensuring the airway, breathing, and circulation) and correction of life-threatening conditions, such as tension pneumothorax. Because chest trauma can produce a wide variety of injuries, treatment is dictated by the severity of injury. In general, chest trauma patients admitted to the intensive care unit (ICU) can be classified as intubated or unintubated patients. The treatment plans for both require judicious use of pain control, administration of oxygen, and aggressive respiratory care. Initial treatment of the unintubated patient includes pain control, proper positioning, oxygen therapy, secretion removal, and lung expansion techniques. Ideally, a respiratory care protocol to allow rapid delivery of these treatments should be in place.

Tube Thoracostomy

With pneumothorax or hemothorax, the first treatment is **tube thoracostomy,** or placement of a thoracostomy tube (chest tube) into the pleural space to evacuate the air or blood.[25] For pneumothorax, emergency decompression with a needle and syringe is accomplished by insertion of the needle in the midclavicular line into the third intercostal space. A chest tube (20 to 22 French [Fr]) should be placed into the third intercostal space along the midaxillary line. For hemothorax, a larger tube (38 to 40 Fr) is used, and the tube is placed in the midaxillary line into the fifth to sixth intercostal space. Drainage of blood requires

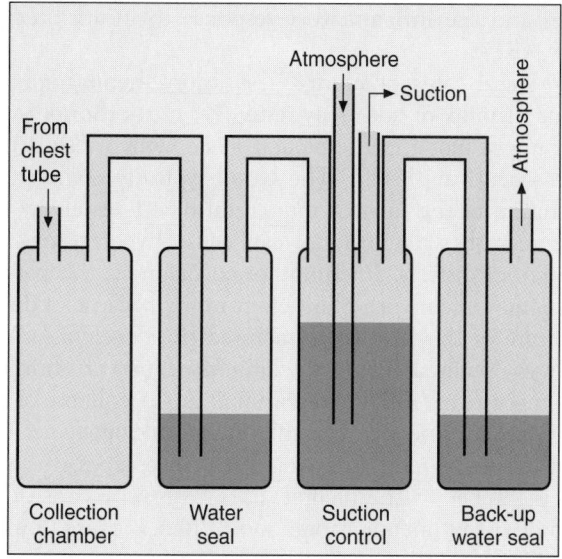

Figure 55-2   Schematic drawing of a chest drainage system. The collection chamber collects fluid drainage from the pleural space. The underwater seal serves as a one-way valve between the pleural space and the atmosphere. The suction control chamber controls the amount of pressure applied to the pleural space. The backup water seal is an added safety measure in case the suction control becomes obstructed.

placement of a larger tube in a gravity-dependent position. After insertion, the tube should be connected to a chest drainage system that uses an underwater seal and a continuous negative pressure of −20 cm H_2O (Figure 55-2).

Pain Control

Methods of pain control with chest trauma include parenteral techniques (intravenous and intramuscular injections), narcotics, epidural analgesia, intercostal nerve blocks, and administration of pain medication via an intrapleural or extrapleural catheter. These techniques can be controlled by the clinician or connected to **patient-controlled analgesia (PCA)** devices, which allow patients to dictate their pain relief by pushing a button.[26]

The goals of pain relief are to facilitate patient movement, enhance secretion clearance, and allow coughing and deep breathing.[13,19,27] Systemic narcotics given by intravenous or intramuscular injection are commonly used, but they present a predictable series of complications. Intermittent injections result in periods of pain (when the drug is requested) and periods of obtundation (Figure 55-3, A). Immediately before the drug is given, the patient has pain and anxiety and is unable to cough, breathe deeply, or change position. After administration of the narcotic, the patient may manifest confusion, depression of respiratory drive, and suppression of the cough reflex. This type of pain control regimen therefore leaves the patient unable to cooperate with respiratory care procedures at both ends of the dosing cycle. As an alternative, continuous low-level in-

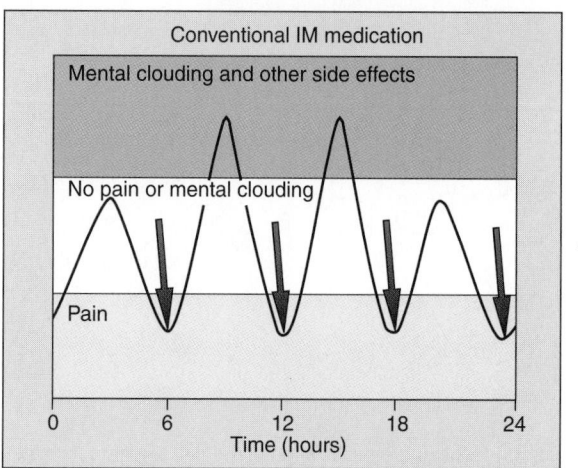

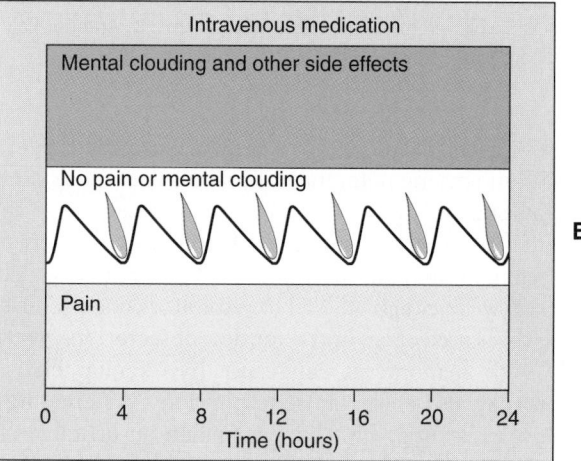

Figure 55-3   **A,** Delivery of narcotics for pain control by conventional intermittent dosing results in cycles of pain and mental clouding, making participation in respiratory care difficult. **B,** Continuous intravenous dosing of narcotics with a patient-controlled analgesia pump allows for more consistent pain control and fewer systemic side effects. (Modified from Haenel JB, Moore FA, Moore EE. Pulmonary consequences of severe chest trauma. Respir Care Clin N Am 1996;2:401-424.)

fusions of narcotics can be delivered and supplemented by additional dosing (Figure 55-3, B). This technique is preferred but still can result in respiratory depression.

$\mathcal{R}$ espiratory Recap

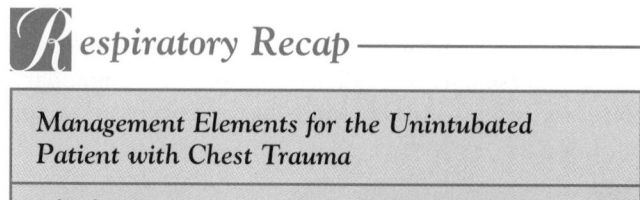

Management Elements for the Unintubated Patient with Chest Trauma	
Tube thoracostomy	Coughing and deep
Pain control	breathing
Oxygen therapy	Mask CPAP

Current state-of-the-art care of the patient with rib fractures and flail chest requires the use of regional anesthetics.[13,19,27-30] Continuous epidural infusions of narcotics

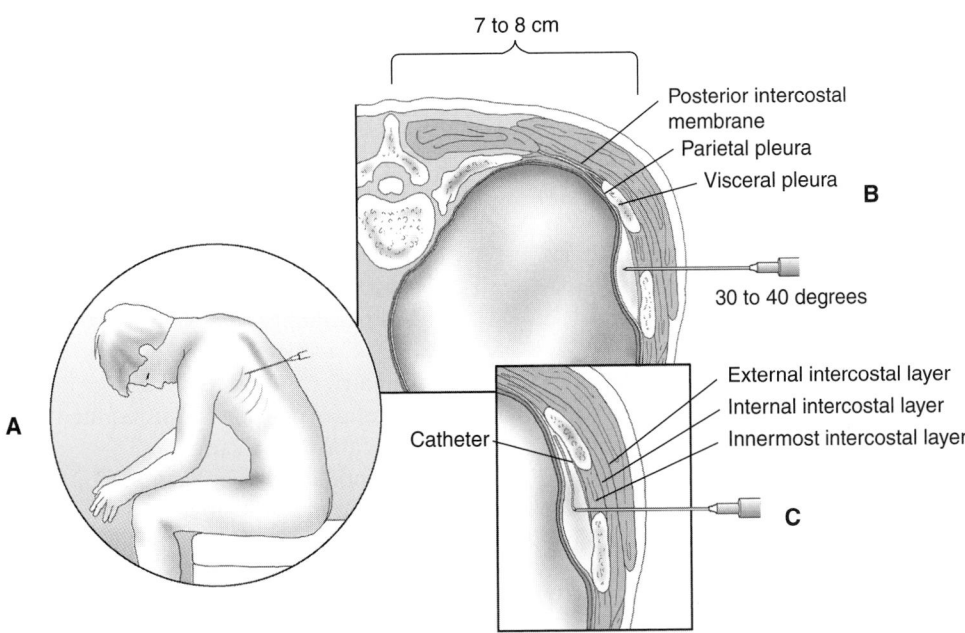

Figure 55-4   Proper placement of an intercostal catheter for pain control. **A,** With the patient in a sitting position, the needle is inserted above the most cephalad rib fracture. **B,** Saline (5 mL) is injected to disrupt the pleura from the chest wall. **C,** A catheter is inserted into the pleural space for injection of analgesics.

or local anesthetics have been used successfully to control pain and have resulted in improved respiratory function. Several authors who compared epidural analgesia to other pain control methods found that epidural analgesia provided longer pain relief in addition to improved respiratory function.[31-35] With epidural analgesia, the maximum inspiratory and expiratory pressures, vital capacity, and peak expiratory flow may improve as much as 40%. Compared to traditional intravenous narcotics, epidural analgesia has been shown to maintain normal arterial carbon dioxide ($PaCO_2$) and oxygen (PaO_2) pressures. The respiratory depression caused by intravenous administration of narcotics commonly causes a decrease in the PaO_2 and an increase in the $PaCO_2$.

Bolliger and Van Eeden[5] compared a group of patients treated with a combination of continuous positive airway pressure (CPAP) by face mask and epidural analgesia with a group treated with mechanical ventilation and traditional pain control. They found that the patients treated with **mask CPAP** and epidural analgesia had a shorter hospital stay, fewer days in the ICU, and a lower incidence of nosocomial pneumonia.

Haenel and coworkers[36] used an intercostal catheter to administer local anesthetic to 15 patients with multiple rib fractures from chest trauma. Figure 55-4 shows the proper placement of the intercostal catheter. A local anesthetic was placed into the pleural space to alleviate pain caused by the rib fractures. The researchers found that pain was significantly reduced within 15 minutes of administration of the anesthetic and that lung volumes achieved with incentive spirometry nearly doubled.

Respiratory Care

Despite conventional wisdom, bed rest is not a successful treatment for rib fractures, flail chest, and pulmonary contusion. Once pain control has been established, the patient should sit up, get into a chair, and ambulate if possible. Bed rest weakens muscles, contributes to reduced lung volumes, and causes venous stasis. Changes of position should be attempted early and often. Methods used to restrict the movement of the chest wall, including adhesive tape, sandbags, and rib belts, should be avoided. Restriction of chest wall movement worsens pulmonary dysfunction.

Oxygen therapy should be administered as required. Nasal cannulas may be used, but an air entrainment mask allows more precise control of the inspired oxygen concentration (FIO_2). There is no evidence that the addition of bland aerosol therapy improves secretion removal.

A regimen of coughing and deep breathing increases lung volume and removes secretions. Initially, if the patient is cooperative and pain has been controlled, only coughing and deep breathing are necessary. If the patient requires additional motivation, incentive spirometry may be helpful. Patients who cannot deep-breathe should be treated with other lung expansion techniques, including intermittent positive pressure breathing. Nasotracheal suctioning may be required for patients with retained secretions who are unable to generate a sufficient cough. Postural drainage can be helpful in the face of retained secretions, but chest percussion should not be performed. Clapping on the chest of a patient with rib fractures may lead to increased pain, further splinting, continued atelectasis, and hypoxemia.

Derangements in gas exchange with pulmonary contusion typically include hypoxemia and hypocarbia. The patient adopts a rapid, shallow breathing pattern in an attempt to provide sufficient gas exchange at the lowest metabolic cost of breathing.[35,36] When the patient's lungs are stiff, it takes less energy to breathe rapidly and at low tidal volumes than to attempt to expand the stiff lungs with a larger tidal volume. In an alert chest trauma patient who is able to protect the airway, mask CPAP is an excellent means of oxygenation support.[5,19,27-29,37,38]

CPAP increases the functional residual capacity (FRC), prevents alveoli from collapsing during expiration, and uses positive pressure to stabilize the chest wall in the presence of flail chest. This technique is useful for patients with hypoxemia but relies on the patient to perform ventilation. As such, mask CPAP is not useful in patients with hypercarbia or those with an unstable respiratory drive.

At least one study has reported the successful use of mask CPAP in the treatment of pulmonary contusion.[38] Of 33 patients with rib fractures and pulmonary contusion, 31 were treated successfully with mask CPAP and epidural analgesia. Success was defined as the prevention of intubation. All patients had an initial PaO_2/FiO_2 under 150. Other investigators have confirmed these findings. The criteria for use of mask CPAP and contraindications to this technique are shown in Table 55-1.

A clear, soft mask is attached to the patient's head by a four-tailed mask strap. The fit should be firm but not tight, because a too-tight fit makes the patient uncomfortable and less cooperative. A leak is permissible. CPAP can be provided via a homemade system, a commercially available CPAP system, or a mechanical ventilator. Regardless of the system used, the flow should be adequate to meet patient demand, and the CPAP valve should have a low flow resistance. Figure 55-5 depicts a system for mask CPAP. A humidifier that increases the gas temperature to 26° to 28° C reduces discomfort from the dry gas. Because the upper airway is intact, additional humidity is unnecessary. A nasogastric tube is not required unless there is another indication for its use.

CPAP should begin at 5 cm H_2O at an FiO_2 sufficient to maintain the oxygen saturation (SaO_2) more than 92%. CPAP can then be increased in increments of 2 to 3 cm H_2O while the respiratory frequency and the oxygen saturation as measured by pulse oximetry (SpO_2) are monitored. Observing the respiratory frequency and the patient's comfort level, along with the SpO_2, can predict which patients will be treated successfully.[39] When mask CPAP is successful, the SpO_2 increases and respiratory frequency decreases (Figure 55-6). If CPAP reaches 15 cm H_2O without relieving tachypnea, intubation should be considered. Blood gas measurements need not be taken during the titration of CPAP unless issues related to acid-base balance must be evaluated.

Table 55-1

Indications, Guide to Therapy, and Contraindications for Mask Continuous Positive Airway Pressure

Consideration	Rationale
Indications	
PaO_2/FiO_2 more than 100 but under 250	Patient must be treated before severe hypoxemia occurs.
Normal respiratory drive	Patient must provide all minute ventilation.
Patient able to protect upper airway	Patient should be able to clear secretions and prevent aspiration of gastric contents; a nasogastric tube is unnecessary at pressures below 15 cm H_2O.
Normocarbia	Mask continuous positive airway pressure (CPAP) will not aid ventilation.
Alert patient	Mask CPAP requires a cooperative patient.
Guide to Therapy	
Increase CPAP to maintain the SpO_2 above 92%.	As alveoli are stabilized, the SaO_2 increases.
Increase CPAP to maintain the respiratory frequency under 25 breaths/min.	As oxygenation and the lungs' position on the pressure-volume curve improve, the respiratory rate falls.
Contraindications	
Facial fractures or lacerations	Patient will be unable to wear the mask without discomfort.
Obtunded or uncooperative patient	These conditions may increase the risk of aspiration and prevent successful use of mask CPAP.
Uncontrolled vomiting	This condition increases the risk of aspiration.
Basilar skull fracture	Pneumocephalus has been reported with this injury.
Severe hypoxemia	This condition requires intubation and mechanical ventilation.

PaO_2, *Partial pressure of arterial oxygen*; FiO_2, *inspired oxygen concentration*; SpO_2, *oxygen saturation as measured by pulse oximetry*; SaO_2, *arterial oxygen saturation*; *CPAP, continuous positive airway pressure.*

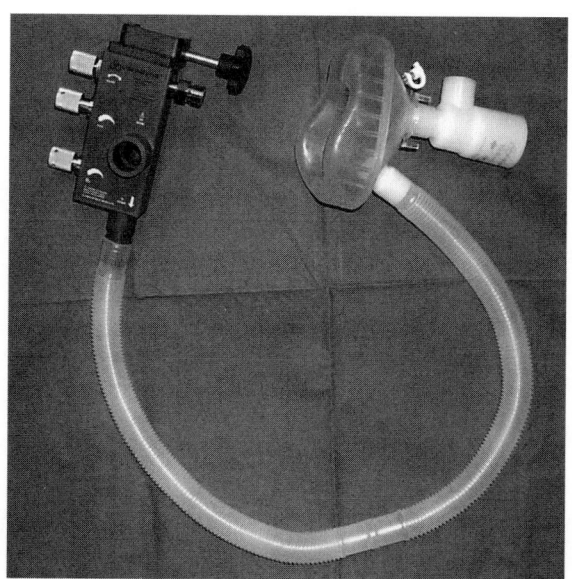

Figure 55-5 The Caradyne CPAP system. The flow generator is a large venturi that allows an F_{IO_2} of 0.3 to 1 at a flow up to 160 L/min. Standard aerosol tubing connects to a clear face mask, to which a CPAP valve is attached. (Courtesy Caradyne Limited, Galway Ireland.)

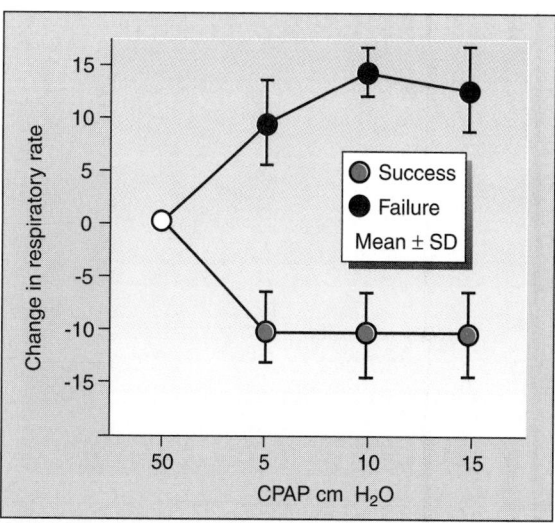

Figure 55-6 Changes in the respiratory rate seen in patients after application of mask CPAP. Failures demonstrate an increase in rate, whereas successful treatment demonstrates relief of tachypnea. (Modified from Branson RD. PEEP without endotracheal intubation. Respir Care 1988;33:598-610.)

Management of the Intubated Patient with Blunt Chest Trauma

Mechanical ventilation should be instituted when mask CPAP fails, hypercarbia ensues, or the patient meets the criteria for intubation. Many chest trauma patients with concomitant injuries, such as a pelvic fracture or a head injury, are intubated at the scene of the accident and arrive in the emergency department with an artificial airway. After intubation, pain control, secretion removal, and maintenance of the FRC with positive end-expiratory pressure (PEEP) remain important tenets.

Mechanical ventilation typically is provided in the pressure-controlled, synchronized intermittent mandatory ventilation (PC-SIMV) mode. PEEP is set to maintain an SpO_2 more than 92% with an F_{IO_2} below 0.6. Best compliance or inflection point determination also may be used in these patients to determine the best PEEP. PEEP chosen by inflection point determination is often within 2 to 3 cm H_2O of the PEEP chosen by best oxygenation. A pressure control level that provides a tidal volume of 10 mL/kg typically is used, with modifications made based on plateau pressure measurements. A plateau pressure above 35 cm H_2O should be avoided, because it may lead to volutrauma and progressive deterioration in lung function.[40-42] However, in a chest trauma patient with diminished chest wall compliance, higher plateau pressures are not only safe but required. Unfortunately, there is no simple method used to calculate the transpulmonary pressure (that is, the alveolar pressure minus the pleural pressure), which is the important pressure in the determination of the risk of overdistention lung injury.

Esophageal manometry can be used to measure the pleural pressure and calculate the transpulmonary pressure, but this is not practical for routine use. Clinical judgment, assessment of the chest wall, and the pressure-volume curve are used to choose the appropriate peak pressure in the most difficult cases. The respiratory rate is set to maintain a pH above 7.25 and a spontaneous respiratory frequency below 25 breaths/min. In patients who remain tachypneic, correction of acid-base disorders or sedation (or both) can be helpful. The inspiration to expiration (I:E) ratio is selected to prevent auto-PEEP. This is done by ensuring that the expiratory flow returns to baseline before delivery of the next mechanical breath. The inspiratory time is set to enhance synchrony or increase the mean airway pressure (or both) to improve oxygenation. An inspiratory time of 1 to 1½ seconds typically is used. Longer inspiratory times further increase the mean airway pressure but may contribute to reduced cardiac output and patient/ventilator dyssynchrony.

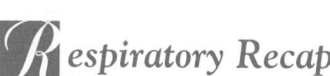espiratory Recap

Management Elements for the Intubated Patient with Chest Trauma	
Avoidance of overdistention lung injury	Prone positioning
	Inhaled nitric oxide
PEEP to maintain lung recruitment	Independent lung ventilation

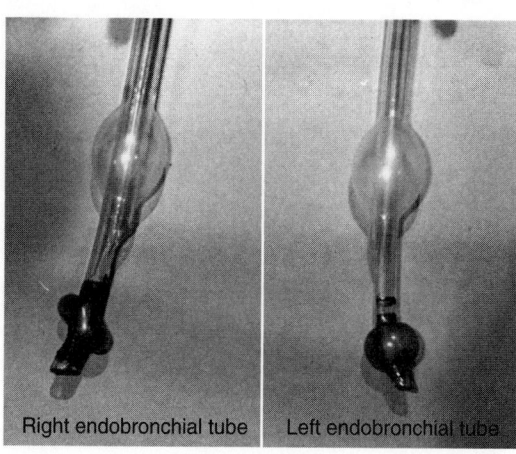

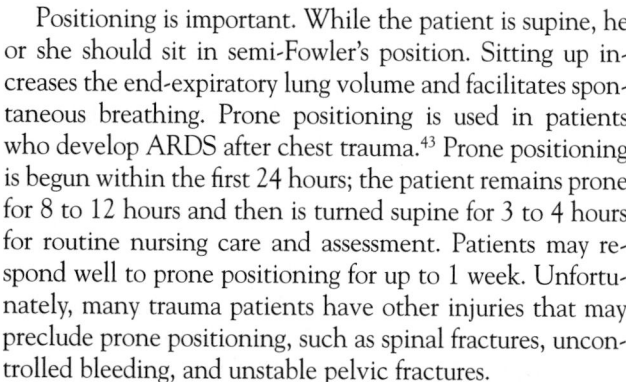

Right endobronchial tube   Left endobronchial tube

Figure 55-7   Right-sided and left-sided endobronchial tubes. The right-sided tube has a sigmoid-shaped cuff and Murphy eye to prevent accidental occlusion of the right upper lobe bronchus.

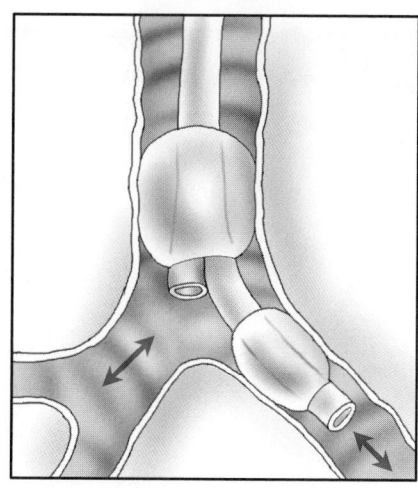

Figure 55-8   Position of the left-sided endobronchial tube, showing the inflated cuffs and direction of gas flow.

Positioning is important. While the patient is supine, he or she should sit in semi-Fowler's position. Sitting up increases the end-expiratory lung volume and facilitates spontaneous breathing. Prone positioning is used in patients who develop ARDS after chest trauma.[43] Prone positioning is begun within the first 24 hours; the patient remains prone for 8 to 12 hours and then is turned supine for 3 to 4 hours for routine nursing care and assessment. Patients may respond well to prone positioning for up to 1 week. Unfortunately, many trauma patients have other injuries that may preclude prone positioning, such as spinal fractures, uncontrolled bleeding, and unstable pelvic fractures.

With refractory hypoxemia, inhaled nitric oxide (iNO) may restore oxygenation in the patient with ARDS after chest trauma. The change in oxygenation with administration of 1 ppm iNO is assessed. A change in the PaO_2/FIO_2 of more than 20% is considered a positive response. There is no evidence that iNO affects mortality in ARDS, but it does improve oxygenation while resuscitative and operative care are rendered.[44,45]

Blunt thoracic trauma can also present unique problems when the pattern of injury is unilateral. In unilateral lung injury, the injured lung has reduced compliance, whereas the contra-lateral lung remains relatively unaffected. In this situation positive pressure ventilation over-inflates the uninjured lung, shifting the blood flow to the injured lung. Thus the unequal distribution of ventilation and perfusion is worsened by positive pressure ventilation.[46]

Independent lung ventilation (ILV) requires use of a double lumen endobronchial tube to separate ventilation of the lungs. The endobronchial tube has two lumens and two cuffs, one for the trachea and one for the bronchus. There are left-sided and right-sided endobronchial tubes (Figure 55-7). The right-sided tube uses a sigmoid-shaped cuff and Murphy eye on the bronchial tube to prevent accidental blockage of the right upper lobe bronchus.

Figure 55-8 shows the position of the endobronchial tube. Tube placement can be verified by measurement of inspired and expired volumes. If inspired volumes do not match expired volumes, incomplete separation of the lungs may be suspected. For example, if 400 mL is delivered to the right lung and 350 mL to the left lung, yet 600 mL is returned from the right lung and only 150 mL from the left lung, either the tube has not been placed properly or the cuffs are not fully inflated. Bronchoscopy can be used to assess proper tube placement. Because the double lumen tube has two smaller lumens (4 to 5 Fr each), suctioning usually is accomplished with a special suction catheter. This catheter is longer, has a smaller diameter, and is more rigid than a standard catheter. These small lumens are prone to obstruction; therefore adequate humidity and frequent suctioning are recommended.

ILV is not commonly used, but it can be lifesaving when necessary.[47-49] Indications for ILV include a mechanism of injury consistent with a unilateral injury, radiographic findings of unilateral involvement, and a paradoxical PEEP effect. The paradoxical PEEP effect is a continued deterioration in PaO_2 when PEEP is increased. This is caused by the worsening of ventilation/perfusion mismatching. A positioning test can help determine whether ILV should be used. The patient is placed in the lateral decubitus position with the good lung down.[50] If blood gas values improve in this position, a trial of ILV may be warranted.

Early studies suggested that ILV should be done with synchronized ventilators.[51,52] However, more recent work demonstrates that this is not necessary.[53] Once the double lumen tube has been placed and its position verified, two ventilators should be used. They should be set to the same FIO_2. Tidal volume and PEEP should be selected based on the compliance characteristics of each lung. This often results in a smaller tidal volume and higher PEEP in the injured lung. Many recommendations have been made to choose the settings for ILV, including matching of end-tidal carbon dioxide concentrations, matching of dead space to tidal volume ratios, and use of the best compliance for each lung. Treating each lung individually (individual PEEP trials) and monitoring lung compliance and oxygenation are the simplest methods used to choose appropriate ventilator settings. ILV commonly is necessary only for 48 to 72 hours. After this interval the patient either improves and can make the transition to a single lumen tube, or multisystem injury results in ARDS involving both lungs, which also requires transition to a single lumen tube.

Penetrating Chest Trauma

Etiology

Penetrating chest trauma usually is caused by stab and gunshot wounds. These types of injuries are further classified as low-velocity or high-velocity injuries. By nature, stab wounds and small-caliber gunshot wounds are low-velocity injuries. High-velocity injuries involve projectiles traveling more than 1500 feet/second. High-velocity gunshot wounds usually are seen in combat but increasingly are seen in inner cities. Defining injuries as low velocity or high velocity aids in determining the severity of tissue damage and the potential for collateral injury.[25]

Pathology

Low-velocity penetrating injuries cause injury along the path of the projectile. Local tissue injury, laceration of blood vessels, and violation of the pleural space commonly result in hemothorax or pneumothorax or both. Direct injury to the heart or great vessels can cause massive bleeding, pericardial tamponade, hypotension, and death.

High-velocity penetrating injuries also cause damage along the path of the projectile, but in addition, further damage results from a blast effect, which causes local tissue destruction and areas of contusion (in the lung, alveolar hemorrhage) stretching far beyond the tract of the projectile. The projectile may tumble and shatter in the thoracic cavity, causing several perforations and sites of bleeding, and secondary projectiles, such as rib fragments, may contribute to the injury. High-velocity injuries are more likely to require surgical intervention, including thoracotomy, pulmonary resection, and debridement of devitalized tissue.

Cardiac tamponade is a life-threatening complication of penetrating wounds to the heart. In **cardiac tamponade,** blood accumulates in the pericardial sac and prevents the heart from expanding to fill with blood; consequently, it cannot pump blood to the tissues. The result is a low cardiac output and hypotension. The symptoms of cardiac tamponade comprise *Beck's triad*: distention of the neck veins, muffled heart sounds, and hypotension. Elevated central venous pressure may also be noted with central venous access. Cardiac tamponade should be suspected in cases of penetrating chest wounds when hypotension persists without evidence of other blood loss.[25]

Treatment

Treatment of penetrating chest wounds includes tube thoracostomy, pain relief, lung expansion techniques, proper positioning, oxygen therapy, mask CPAP, and mechanical ventilation as required. These therapies should be used as described for blunt chest trauma. Because hemothorax is more common in penetrating injuries, a large-bore chest tube should be placed in the midaxillary line.

Treatment of cardiac tamponade requires removal of the collected blood in the pericardial sac. This can be accomplished by pericardiocentesis or by the creation of a subxiphoid pericardial window. The latter technique, which should be performed only by surgical specialists, requires a surgical opening in the chest wall and creation of an opening in the pericardial sac. **Pericardiocentesis** involves placement of a needle into the pericardium and withdrawal of the accumulated blood. Vital signs and the electrocardiogram (ECG) should be monitored before, during, and after the procedure. A 16- to 18-gauge over-the-needle catheter (15 cm or longer), a three-way stopcock, and a 35-mL syringe should be assembled for the procedure. The needle is directed at a 45-degree angle and inserted 1 to 2 cm below the xiphochondral junction. It is moved in a cephalad direction until the heart is encountered. If the needle is advanced too far, the ECG will demonstrate a rhythm known as the *current of injury,* which is characterized by extreme ST-T wave changes and an enlarged QRS complex. If this rhythm is seen, the needle should be withdrawn. After the procedure has been completed, a stopcock should be left on the catheter in case additional aspirations are needed.

CASE STUDIES

Case One
Pulmonary Contusion

A 30-year-old white man was admitted to the emergency department after a motor vehicle accident. He was an unrestrained passenger in a car broadsided by a

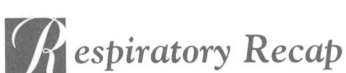

espiratory Recap

Penetrating Chest Trauma
Low velocity: Stab wounds and small-caliber gunshot wounds
High velocity: Gunshot wounds

vehicle running a red light. The impact occurred on the passenger side. Upon arrival in the emergency department, the patient was diaphoretic, tachypneic, and tachycardic. He complained of chest pain, and his SpO_2 on a partial rebreathing mask (10 L/min) was 90%. Breath sounds were diminished on the left, and a large area of ecchymosis could be seen over his left chest. Upon palpation, subcutaneous emphysema was noted, and further complaints of chest pain were elicited. The chest radiograph showed multiple rib fractures and a 15% pneumothorax on the left.

A 24-Fr chest tube was inserted into the fourth intercostal space along the midaxillary line. The patient was placed on an air entrainment mask (60%) and transferred to the surgical ICU. Upon arrival in the ICU, an epidural catheter was placed and a bolus of bupivacaine was given via the catheter, followed by continuous infusion. An intravenous infusion of morphine was connected to a PCA device, and the patient was instructed in its use. Pain relief from the epidural analgesia improved the patient's comfort, and he was placed in semi-Fowler's position for coughing and deep breathing. A brief period of hypotension was relieved by crystalloid infusion. The patient's SpO_2 remained at 90% to 91%. A chest radiograph to confirm the placement of the chest tube and epidural catheter showed a moderate pulmonary contusion of the left lower lobe.

Over several hours the patient became increasingly tachypneic, with a respiratory rate of 34 breaths/min, and his pain control continued to cause some hypotension, which was treated with fluid boluses. His arterial blood gas values after 6 hours in the ICU were as follows: pH, 7.34; $PaCO_2$, 38 mm Hg; PaO_2, 74 mm Hg; and bicarbonate (HCO_3^-), 18 mEq/L. With an FIO_2 of 0.6, this was a PaO_2/FIO_2 of 123. The patient was drowsy but aware of his surroundings, and a nasogastric tube was in place.

A decision was made for a trial of mask CPAP. The patient was instructed in the use of the mask, in how the CPAP would feel, and in ways to communicate if he became uncomfortable. The CPAP system was set to deliver an FIO_2 of 0.6, and CPAP was begun at 5 cm H_2O. The CPAP was increased every 10 to 15 minutes until the SpO_2 was more than 92% and the respiratory frequency was under 25 breaths/min. The results of this trial were as follows:

Time	CPAP	FIO_2	SpO_2	Respiratory Rate
1730	5 cm H_2O	0.6	92%	33 breaths/min
1745	8 cm H_2O	0.6	94%	29 breaths/min
1800	10 cm H_2O	0.6	95%	24 breaths/min

At 1830 the arterial blood gas values were as follows: pH, 7.37; $PaCO_2$, 38 mm Hg; PaO_2, 118 mm Hg; and HCO_3^-, 20 mEq/L. The PaO_2/FIO_2 was now 197. Pain control, coughing, deep breathing, and occasional nasotracheal suctioning were continued. After 48 hours the FIO_2 was reduced to 0.4, and CPAP was reduced to

5 cm H_2O. On day 3 the patient was returned to an air entrainment mask at an FIO_2 of 0.4. The chest tube was removed on day 4 and the epidural catheter on day 5. The patient was transferred to the floor and discharged home on day 7.

Case Two
Intubated Patient with Blunt Chest Trauma

A 19-year-old African-American woman was admitted to the hospital after falling approximately 20 feet from a second story platform to the pavement. She briefly lost consciousness after the fall but was oriented on admission. The physical examination revealed multiple lacerations and contusions on the right side. Radiographs detected fractures of the right wrist, humerus, femur, and pelvis. The initial chest radiograph was within normal limits. The patient was transferred to the ICU for observation and pain control.

On admission to the ICU the patient's respiratory rate was shallow at 18 breaths/min, and her breath sounds were clear but diminished on the right. She was receiving oxygen via an air-entrainment mask at an FIO_2 of 0.35. Her first arterial blood gas values were as follows: pH, 7.45; $PaCO_2$, 33 mm Hg; PaO_2, 89 mm Hg; and HCO_3^-, 20 mEq/L. Over the next 16 hours, her respiratory rate increased to 30 breaths/min because she required additional fluids and blood to treat blood loss caused by the pelvic fracture. A blood gas measurement at this time showed a PaO_2 of 59 mm Hg on an FIO_2 of 0.35 (PaO_2/FIO_2 of 169). She was placed on mask CPAP at 5 cm H_2O, and after 20 minutes the PaO_2 was 69 mm Hg (FIO_2 of 0.45). A second chest radiograph showed complete collapse of the right lung. Bronchoscopy was performed, and no evidence of mucus plugging was seen. The patient was intubated and placed on mechanical ventilation, and PEEP was increased over several hours to 15 cm H_2O. The PaO_2 remained 60 mm Hg on an FIO_2 of 0.45.

When the patient was placed in the right lateral decubitus position, the SpO_2 increased from 91% to 94%. A trial of ILV was decided upon, and a 39-Fr double lumen endobronchial tube was placed and its position confirmed. Compliance of the left lung was 58 mL/cm H_2O, and compliance of the right lung was 32 mL/cm H_2O. The left lung was ventilated with a tidal volume of 500 mL and 8 cm H_2O PEEP, and the right lung was ventilated with a tidal volume of 350 mL and 15 cm H_2O PEEP. After 1 hour the patient's arterial blood gas values were as follows: pH, 7.42; $PaCO_2$, 34 mm Hg; PaO_2, 124 mm Hg; and HCO_3^-, 21 mEq/L. A chest radiograph revealed reinflation of the right lung and normal expansion of the left lung. (Table 55-2 summarizes other blood gas values, respiratory mechanics, and ventilator settings.)

Over a 24-hour period, lung compliance improved on the right side, and PEEP in both lungs was set to 10 cm H_2O.

TABLE 55-2

Changes in Ventilation and Blood Gas Variables during Mechanical Ventilation with and without Independent Lung Ventilation

Value	8 Hours after Admission	Conventional Ventilation	Independent Lung Ventilation	Independent Lung Ventilation
FIO_2	1	0.6	0.6	0.4
PEEP (cm H_2O)	N/A	12	Left lung: 6 Right lung: 15	Left lung: 5 Right lung: 8
V_T (L)	N/A	0.8	Left lung: 0.5 Right lung: 0.35	Left lung: 0.4 Right lung: 0.4
pH	7.34	7.31	7.36	7.37
$PaCO_2$ (mm Hg)	33	39	40	43
PaO_2 (mm Hg)	61	57	127	92
SpO_2 (%)	91	89	97	94
Compliance (mL/cm H_2O)	N/A	32	Left lung: 59 Right lung: 26	Left lung: 61 Right lung: 56
Action taken	Patient intubated	ILV initiated	PEEP reduced	Switch made to conventional ventilation

FIO_2, *Fractional inspired oxygen concentration;* PEEP, *positive end-expiratory pressure;* V_T, *tidal volume;* $PaCO_2$, *partial pressure of arterial carbon dioxide;* PaO_2, *partial pressure of arterial oxygen;* SpO_2, *oxygen saturation as measured by pulse oximetry;* ILV, *independent lung ventilation;* N/A, *not available.*

At this point a single lumen tube was inserted, and the patient was ventilated conventionally until extubated without further problems.

KEY POINTS

- Chest trauma is a common injury that requires early correction of life-threatening conditions followed by intensive respiratory care.
- Pneumothorax or hemothorax requires placement of a thoracostomy tube.
- Early use of pain control, mask CPAP, and lung expansion techniques can improve the outcome and shorten the hospital stay.
- Pain control techniques with chest trauma include parenteral narcotics, epidural analgesia, intercostal nerve blocks, and pleural catheters.
- Mask CPAP can improve oxygenation in patients with lung contusion.
- In multiple trauma patients who develop ARDS and require mechanical ventilation, approaches that avoid alveolar overdistension and maintain lung recruitment should be used.
- Prone positioning, inhaled nitric oxide, and independent lung ventilation are useful in certain patients.
- Penetrating injuries can be classified as low velocity or high velocity.
- Treatment of cardiac tamponade requires pericardiocentesis or creation of a subxiphoid pericardial window.

References

1. LoCicero III J, Mattox KL. Epidemiology of chest surgery. Surg Clin North Am 1989;69:15-19.
2. Duff JH, Goldstein M, McLean AP, et al. Flail chest: a clinical review and physiological study. J Trauma 1986;8:63-74.
3. Relihan M, Litwin MS. Morbidity and mortality associated with flail chest injury. J Trauma 1973;13:663-671.
4. Johnson JA, Cogbill TH, Winga ER. Determinants of outcome after pulmonary contusion. J Trauma 1986;26:695-697.
5. Bolliger CT, Van Eeden SF. Treatment of multiple rib fractures: randomized controlled trial comparing ventilatory with non-ventilatory management. Chest 1990;97:943-948.
6. Gaillard M, Herve C, Mandin L, et al. Mortality prognosis factors in chest injury. J Trauma 1990;30:93-96.
7. Beal SL, Oreskovich MR. Long-term disability associated with flail chest injury. Am J Surg 1985;150:324-326.
8. Landercasper J, Cogbill TH, Lindesmith LA. Long-term disability after flail chest injury. J Trauma 1984;24:410-414.
9. Clark GC, Checter WP, Trunkey DD. Variables affecting outcome in blunt chest trauma: flail chest versus pulmonary contusion. J Trauma 1988;28:298-304.
10. Dougall AM, Paul ME, Finley RJ, et al. Chest trauma: current morbidity and mortality. J Trauma 1977;17:547-553.
11. Gerblich AA, Kleinerman J. Blunt chest trauma and the lung. Am Rev Respir Dis 1977;115:369-370.
12. Oparah SS, Mandal AK. Operative management of penetrating wounds of the chest in civilian practice: review of indications in 125 consecutive patients. J Thorac Cardiovasc Surg 1979; 77:162-168.
13. Richardson JD, Adam LA, Flint LM. Selective management of flail chest and pulmonary contusion. Ann Surg 1982;196:481-487.
14. Jonsson A, Clemedson CJ, Sunquist AB, et al. Dynamic factors influencing the production of lung injury in rabbits subjected to blunt chest wall impact. Aviat Space Environ Med 1979;50: 325-337.

15. Trinkle JK, Furman RW, Hinshaw MA, et al. Pulmonary contusion. Ann Thorac Surg 1973;16:568-573.

16. Shin B, McAslan TC, Hankins JR, et al. Management of lung contusion. Am Surg 179;45:168-175.

17. Shackford SR, Smith DE, Zarins CK, et al. The management of flail chest. Am J Surg 1976;132:759-762.

18. Fulton RL, Peters ET. Compositional and histologic effects of fluid therapy following pulmonary contusion. J Trauma 1974;14:783-790.

19. Freedland MA, Wilson RF, Bender J. The management of flail chest injury. J Trauma 1990;30:1460-1468.

20. Oppenheimer L, Craven KD, Fokert L, et al. Pathophysiology of pulmonary contusion in dogs. J Appl Physiol 1979;47:718-728.

21. Fulton RL, Peters ET. The progressive nature of pulmonary contusion. Surgery 1979;67:499-506.

22. Shorr RM, Crittenden M, Indeck M, et al. Blunt thoracic trauma: analysis of 515 patients. Ann Surg 1987;206:200-205.

23. Shackford SR. Blunt chest trauma in the intensivist's perspective. Intensive Care Med 1986;1:125.

24. Moghissi K. Laceration of the lung following blunt trauma. Thorax 1971;26:223-228.

25. Moore EE, Mattox KL, Feliciano DV. Trauma. 2nd ed. Norwalk, Conn: Appleton & Lange; 1991.

26. White PF. Use of patient-controlled analgesia for management of acute pain. JAMA 1988;259:243-247.

27. Linton DM, Polgieter PD. Conservative management of blunt chest trauma. S Afr Med J 1982;12:917-919.

28. Hankins JR, Shin B, McAslan TC, et al. Management of flail chest: an analysis of 99 cases. Am Surg 1979;45:176-181.

29. Mackersie RC, Shackford SR, Hoyt DB, et al. Continuous epidural fentanyl analgesia: ventilatory function improvement with routine use in treatment of blunt chest injury. J Trauma 1987;27:1207-1212.

30. Shackford SR, Virgillo RW, Peters RM. Selective use of ventilatory therapy in flail chest injury. J Thorac Cardiovasc Surg 1981;81:194-201.

31. Luchette FA, Radafshar SM, Kaiser R, et al. Prospective evaluation of epidural versus intrapleural catheters for analgesia in chest wall trauma. J Trauma 1994;36:865-870.

32. McIlvaine WB, Knox RF, Fennessey PV. Continuous infusion of bupivacaine via intrapleural catheter for analgesia after thoracotomy in children. Anesthesiology 1988;69:261-264.

33. Bachman-Mennega B, Biscoping J, Kuhn DFM, et al. Intercostal nerve block, intrapleural analgesia, thoracic epidural block, or systemic opioid application for pain relief after thoracotomy? Eur J Cardiothorac Surg 1993;7:12-18.

34. Crossley AWA. Intercostal catheterization: an alternative approach to the paravertebral space? Anesthesia 1988;43:163-164.

35. Middaugh RE, Menk EJ, Reynolds WJ, et al. Epidural block using large volumes of local anesthetic solution for intercostal nerve block. Anesthesiology 1984;63:214-216.

36. Haenel JB, Moore FA, Moore EE, et al. Extrapleural bupivacaine for amelioration of rib fracture pain. J Trauma 1995;38:22-27.

37. Trinkle JK, Richardson JD, Franz JL, et al. Management of flail chest without mechanical ventilation. Ann Thorac Surg 1975;19:355-363.

38. Hurst JM, Dehaven B, Branson RD. Use of CPAP mask as the sole mode of ventilatory support in trauma patients with mild to moderate respiratory insufficiency. J Trauma 1985;25:1065-1068.

39. Branson RD. PEEP without endotracheal intubation. Respir Care 1988;33:598-610.

40. Amato MBP, Barbas CSV, Medeiros DM, et al. Beneficial effects of the "open lung" approach with low distending pressures in acute respiratory distress syndrome. Am J Respir Crit Care Med 1995;152:1835-1846.

41. Amato MBP, Barbas CS, Medeiros DM, et al. Effect of a protective ventilation strategy on mortality in the acute respiratory distress syndrome. N Engl J Med 1998;338:347-354.

42. Stewart TE, Meade MO, Cook DJ, et al. Evaluation of a ventilation strategy to prevent barotrauma in patients at high risk for acute respiratory distress syndrome. N Engl J Med 1998;338:355-361.

43. Johannigman JA, Davis K Jr, Campbell RS, et al. Prone positioning for acute respiratory distress syndrome (ARDS) in the surgical intensive care unit: Who, when, and how long? Surgery 2000;128:708-716

44. McIntyre RC, Moore FA, Moore EE, et al. Inhaled nitric oxide variably improved oxygenation and pulmonary hypertension in patients with acute respiratory distress syndrome. J Trauma 1995;39:418-425.

45. Johannigman JA, Davis K Jr, Campbell RS, et al. Inhaled nitric oxide in ARDS. J Trauma 1997;43:904-909.

46. Hurst JM, Dehaven B, Branson RD. Comparison of conventional mechanical ventilation and synchronous independent lung ventilation (SILV) in the treatment of unilateral lung injury. J Trauma 1985;25:766-770.

47. Geiger K. Differential lung ventilation. In: Geiger K, editor. European advances in intensive care. Int Anesthesiol Clin 1983;21:83-96.

48. Carlon GC, Kahn R, Howland WS, et al. Acute life-threatening ventilation/perfusion inequality: an indication for independent lung ventilation. Crit Care Med 1978;6:380-383.

49. Rafferty TD, Palma J, Motoyanna EK, et al. Management of bronchopleural fistula with differential lung ventilation and positive end-expiratory pressure. Respir Care 1980;25:654-657.

50. Faysal HM, Beller TA, Sobonya RE, et al. Effect of body positive end-expiratory pressure and body position in unilateral lung injury. J Appl Physiol 1982;52:147-154.

51. Gallagher TJ, Banner MS, Smith RA. A simplified method of independent lung ventilation. Crit Care Med 1980;8:396-399.

52. Carlon GC, Ray C, Klein R, et al. Criteria for selective positive end-expiratory pressure and independent lung ventilation of each lung. Chest 1978;74:501-507.

53. Siegel JH, Stoklosa J, Borg U, et al. Quantification of asymmetric lung pathophysiology as a guide to the use of simultaneous independent lung ventilation in posttraumatic and septic adult respiratory distress syndrome. Ann Surg 1985;202:425-439.

CHAPTER 56

Burn and Inhalation Injuries

Robert L. Sheridan
Ray Ritz

CHAPTER **OUTLINE**

Burn Injury
    Phases of Burn Care
    Physiology of Burn Injury
Inhalation Injury
    Physiology of Inhalation Injury
    Diagnosis of Inhalation Injury
Management of Inhalation Injury
    Acute Upper Airway Obstruction
    Bronchospasm

    Small Airway Obstruction
    Pulmonary Infection
    Respiratory Failure
    Carbon Monoxide Exposure
Case Studies
    Case One: Minor Burn with Smoke Inhalation
    Case Two: Second- and Third-Degree Burns (70% BSA)
       with Severe Inhalation Injury

OBJECTIVES

1. Describe the four phases of burn management.
2. Use the Lund-Browder chart to evaluate the extent of a burn injury.
3. Compare first-, second-, third-, and fourth-degree burns.
4. Discuss issues related to fluid resuscitation of patients with a burn injury.
5. Describe the effect of circumferential burn wounds of the torso on ventilatory function.
6. Discuss issues related to cutaneous heat and water loss in patients with a burn injury.
7. Discuss the physiology of inhalation injury.
8. Describe the diagnosis of inhalation injury.
9. List five predictable events in patients with inhalation injury.
10. Describe the management of upper airway obstruction, bronchospasm, small airway obstruction, pulmonary infection, and respiratory failure in patients with an inhalation injury.
11. Describe the treatment of patients with carboxyhemoglobinemia.

KEY TERMS

Carboxyhemoglobin (COHb)	Escharotomy	Rule of Nines
CO Oximetry	Hyperbaric Oxygen (HBO)	Volumetric Diffusive Respiration
Eschar	Inhalation Injury	

The outcome for burn patients, both in survival and quality of life, has improved dramatically over the past 20 years.[1,2] This change began with a realization that the natural history of burns can be changed by prompt surgery; the early removal of **eschar** and immediate biologic closure of the resulting open wounds prevents the otherwise inevitable development of burn wound sepsis. However, to support a patient with a serious burn and associated respiratory failure through the physiologic trial of staged wound closure is not a simple undertaking.[3]

Burn Injury

Phases of Burn Care

Patients with large burns typically have a deep, painful wound at risk of sepsis and progressive multiorgan dysfunction. Immediate needs must be met, but an organized, overall plan of care must also be created. This organized plan of care has four phases (Table 56-1).[4] The first phase, the initial evaluation and resuscitation, extends from day

TABLE 56-1

Four Phases of Burn Care

Phase	Timing	Treatment Objectives
Initial evaluation and resuscitation	First 72 hours	To achieve accurate fluid resuscitation and perform a thorough evaluation
Initial wound excision and biologic closure	Days 1 through 7	To identify and remove all full-thickness wounds and obtain biologic closure
Definitive wound closure	Day 7 through week 6	To replace temporary covers with definitive ones and close small complex wounds
Rehabilitation, reconstruction, and reintegration	Entire hospitalization	Initially to maintain range of motion and reduce edema; subsequently to strengthen and prepare for return to community

1 through day 3. Accurate fluid resuscitation must be performed, and the patient must be thoroughly evaluated for other injuries and comorbid conditions. The second phase, initial wound excision and biologic closure, extends from day 1 through day 7. During this phase, the surgery is performed that changes so profoundly the natural history of the disease. Typically it involves a series of staged operations. The third phase, definitive wound closure, lasts from day 7 through week 6. It involves replacement of temporary wound covers with definitive cover, as well as closure and acute reconstruction of burns that have a small surface area but are highly complex, such as wounds on the face and hands. The final stage involves rehabilitation, reconstruction, and reintegration. Although this begins during the resuscitation period, it becomes very time-consuming and involved toward the end of the acute hospital stay.

Physiology of Burn Injury

An extensive cutaneous burn wound has a profound influence on pulmonary function, and accurate evaluation of the wound is important (Box 56-1). Wounds should be evaluated for extent, depth, and circumferential components. The extent is best estimated with a Lund-Browder chart,[5] which accounts for the variance in body proportions with growth (Figure 56-1). An alternative in adults is the **rule of nines.**[6] In addition to these methods, with an irregular pattern burn, the palmar surface of the hand (without fingers) can be used to represent approximately 0.5% of the body surface.[7]

Burns are classified as first, second, third, or fourth degree (Figure 56-2). It can be difficult even for an experienced examiner to accurately determine the depth of a burn early on.[8] As a general rule, depth usually is underestimated on the initial examination.

An understanding of the physiologic aberrations that occur with serious burns allows clinicians to provide respiratory care in the burn unit. Successfully resuscitated burn patients manifest a sequence of predictable physiologic changes (Table 56-2). These changes can be anticipated, which aids in patient management.

BOX 56-1

Evaluation of the Burn Wound

Extent
   Lund-Browder chart: An age-specific chart that accounts for changes in body proportions. This is the preferred method used to determine the extent of a burn injury.
   Rule of nines: A rough method of estimation that assumes adult body proportions. The head and neck are roughly 9%; the anterior and posterior chest are 9% each; the anterior and posterior abdomen (including buttocks) are 9% each; each upper extremity is 9%; each thigh is 9%; each leg and foot is 9%; and the genitals are 1%.
   Palmar surface of the hand: The palmar surface of a person's hand (without the fingers) is approximately 0.5% of the body surface over all age groups.

Depth
   First-degree: Red, dry, painful wounds that often are deeper than they appear; sloughing occurs the next day.
   Second-degree: Red, wet, very painful wounds. Their depth, ability to heal, and propensity to form hypertrophic scars vary immensely.
   Third-degree: Leathery, dry, insensate, waxy wounds that do not heal.
   Fourth-degree: Wounds that involve underlying subcutaneous tissue, tendon, or bone.

Individuals who suffer serious burns have massive diffuse capillary leakage, which occurs secondary to wound-released mediators. The result is extravasation of fluids, electrolytes, and moderate-size colloid molecules, which explains the enormous fluid resuscitation requirements of burn patients. A number of formulas have been developed that attempt to predict resuscitation volume requirements based on body weight or surface area and burn size.[9] However, a number of variables affect resuscitation requirements, including delay in initiation of resuscitation, inhalation injury, and the depth and vapor transmission characteristics of the wound itself. No two injuries are exactly alike, and no formula has yet been developed that can predict with acceptable accuracy the

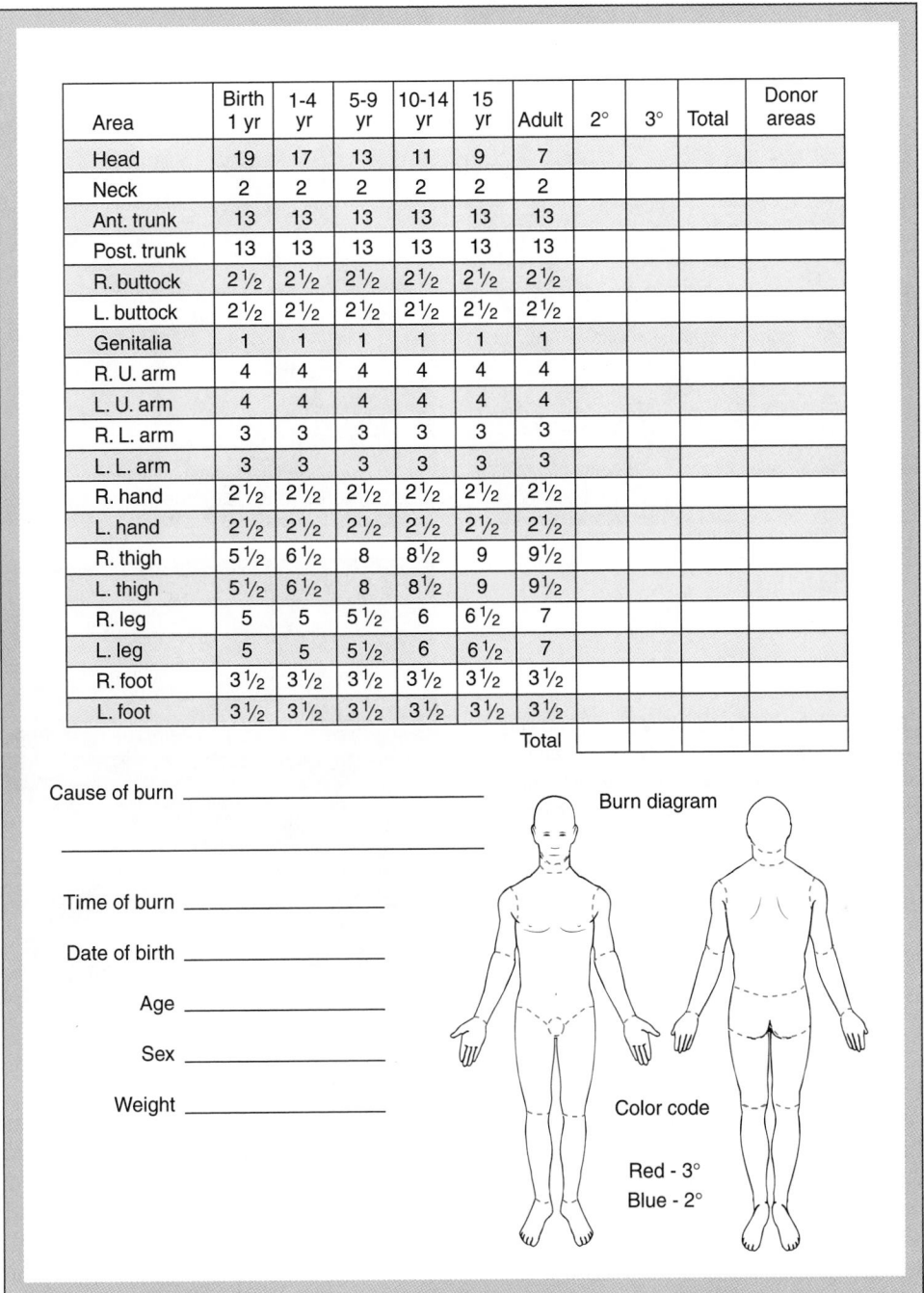

Area	Birth 1 yr	1-4 yr	5-9 yr	10-14 yr	15 yr	Adult	2°	3°	Total	Donor areas
Head	19	17	13	11	9	7				
Neck	2	2	2	2	2	2				
Ant. trunk	13	13	13	13	13	13				
Post. trunk	13	13	13	13	13	13				
R. buttock	2½	2½	2½	2½	2½	2½				
L. buttock	2½	2½	2½	2½	2½	2½				
Genitalia	1	1	1	1	1	1				
R. U. arm	4	4	4	4	4	4				
L. U. arm	4	4	4	4	4	4				
R. L. arm	3	3	3	3	3	3				
L. L. arm	3	3	3	3	3	3				
R. hand	2½	2½	2½	2½	2½	2½				
L. hand	2½	2½	2½	2½	2½	2½				
R. thigh	5½	6½	8	8½	9	9½				
L. thigh	5½	6½	8	8½	9	9½				
R. leg	5	5	5½	6	6½	7				
L. leg	5	5	5½	6	6½	7				
R. foot	3½	3½	3½	3½	3½	3½				
L. foot	3½	3½	3½	3½	3½	3½				
						Total				

Cause of burn _____

_____

Time of burn _____

Date of birth _____

Age _____

Sex _____

Weight _____

Burn diagram

Color code

Red - 3°
Blue - 2°

Figure 56-1   Burn size is best estimated with the Lund-Browder chart, which corrects for changes in body proportions that occur with aging.

Respiratory Recap

Diffuse Capillary Leakage

Burn patients require enormous fluid resuscitation.
An abrupt decline in fluid requirement occurs 18 to 24 hours after injury.
After 24 hours tissue edema begins to subside and urine output increases as excess fluid is reabsorbed and cleared.

volume requirements in all patients. For these reasons, a resuscitation formula can only help determine the initial volume infusion rate and roughly predict overall requirements. Because inaccurate volume administration is associated with substantial morbidity, it is essential that burn resuscitation be guided by hourly reevaluation of resuscitation end points.

Circumferential or near-circumferential burn wounds of the torso are areas that require special monitoring; such wounds can interfere with ventilation as soft tissues swell

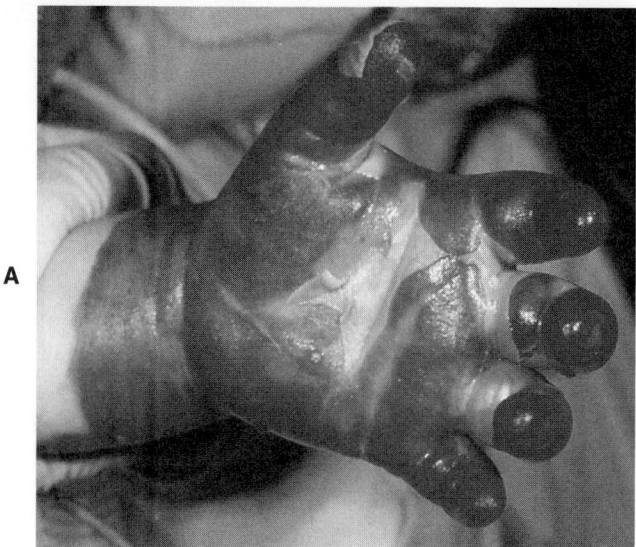

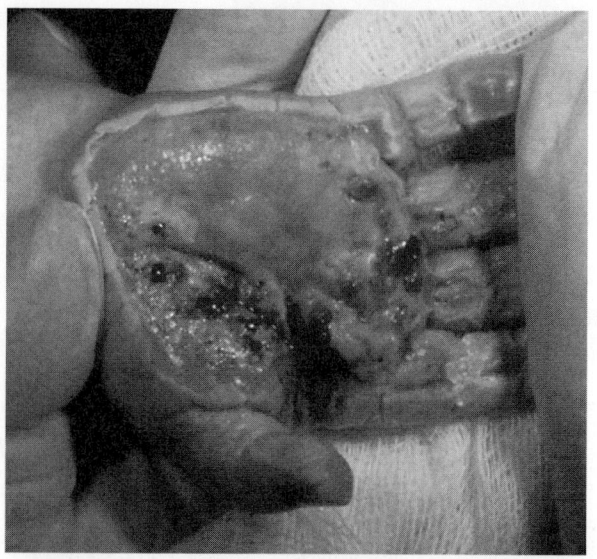

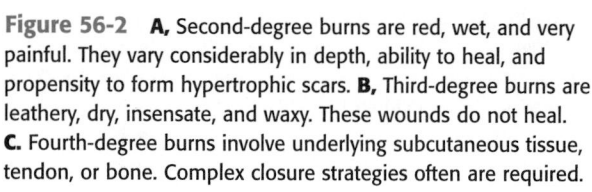

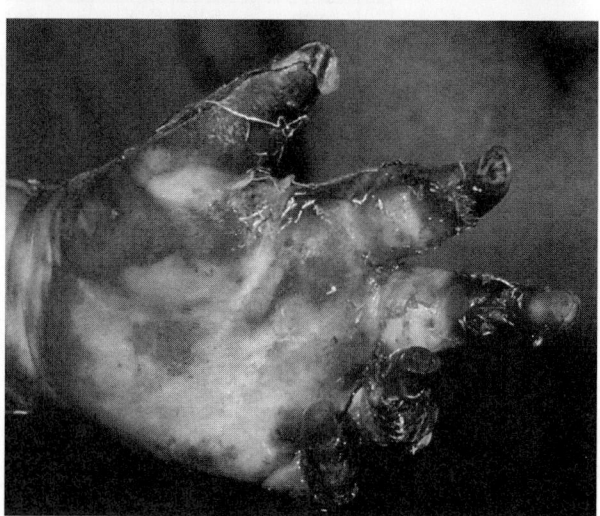

Figure 56-2 **A,** Second-degree burns are red, wet, and very painful. They vary considerably in depth, ability to heal, and propensity to form hypertrophic scars. **B,** Third-degree burns are leathery, dry, insensate, and waxy. These wounds do not heal. **C.** Fourth-degree burns involve underlying subcutaneous tissue, tendon, or bone. Complex closure strategies often are required.

beneath the inelastic eschar and may require **escharotomy** (Figure 56-3). The need for escharotomy must be recognized in a timely way to allow effective intervention. A dramatic improvement in ventilation is common after needed escharotomy of the chest and abdomen.

With successful resuscitation, volume requirements decline abruptly 18 to 24 hours after injury as the diffuse capillary leakage abates. A systemic inflammatory state then evolves, characterized clinically by a hyperdynamic circulation, fever, and massively increased protein catabolism. This physiologic state is thought to be caused by a combination of wound colonization, with release of bacteria and their byproducts; translocation of similar substances through a compromised gastrointestinal barrier; foci of infection; and augmented release of the counterregulatory hormones cortisol, catecholamines, and glucagon.

The metabolic stress associated with a large burn is enormous, and an important part of burn critical care is support of this physiologic condition. This therapy takes the form of accurate fluid repletion, nutritional support, control of environmental temperatures, prompt removal of nonviable tissue with physiologic wound closure, support of the gastrointestinal barrier, and proper management of pain and anxiety. An additional and critical component is support of body temperature. Burn patients have enormous and invisible evaporative water and energy losses if they are maintained in the typical cool, dry air of a general hospital. Burn units and operating rooms must be engineered to maintain a high ambient temperature and humidity level to avoid the difficult problem of hypothermia.

Inhalation Injury

Inhalation injury is defined as the sequela of aspiration of superheated gases, steam, or noxious products of incomplete combustion. It adversely affects both gas exchange and hemodynamics.[10] Approximately 20% of the patients

TABLE 56-2

Predictable Physiologic Changes in Burn Patients

Time Frame	Change	Treatment Steps
Resuscitation period (days 0 to 3)	Massive capillary leakage	Fluid resuscitation
Postresuscitation period (day 3 to 95% definitive wound closure)	Hyperdynamic and catabolic state with high risk of infection	Early wound closure to prevent sepsis (nutritional support is essential)
Recovery period (95% definitive wound closure to 1 year after injury)	Continuing catabolic state and risk of nonwound sepsis	Nutritional support essential; complications anticipated and treated

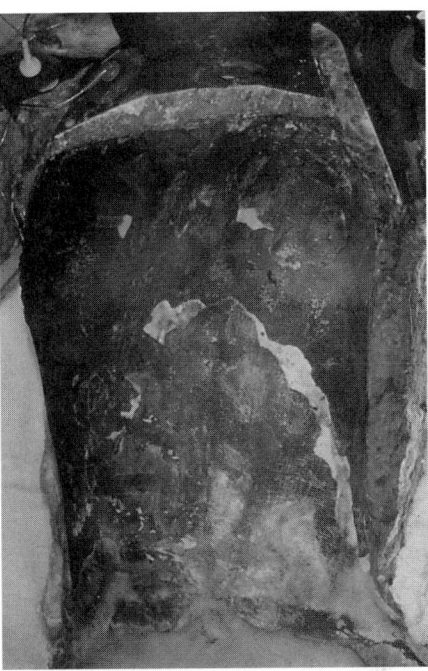

Figure 56-3 Circumferential wounds of the torso can interfere with ventilation and may require escharotomy.

admitted to regional burn centers have suffered inhalation injury. The severity of inhalation injury varies widely and cannot be predicted at the initial evaluation because of the poor correlation between diagnostic criteria and severity of injury. Several institutional reviews[2,11] have shown that inhalation injury has a profound effect on mortality, with the diagnosis as much as doubling mortality from that predicted based on age and burn size alone. There is no specific treatment for inhalation injury; management involves provision of the support required to compensate for decrements in gas exchange while the injured endobronchial and alveolar mucosae regenerate.

Physiology of Inhalation Injury

Inhalation injury involves the entire respiratory system, from the upper airway to the alveoli, to a variable and unpredictable degree. Superheated gas and liquid burn the upper airway, with resultant mucosal edema and airway obstruction. Irritating gases trigger bronchospasm. The major airways are denuded of their normal mucosal layer, which impairs the ciliary transport mechanism until resurfacing occurs. The smaller airways become obstructed with sloughed endobronchial debris and accumulated secretions. Pneumonia and tracheobronchitis frequently occur in partially obstructed lung units. The alveolar epithelium is disrupted by toxic products released by burning of synthetic products, resulting in alveolar flooding. The clinically important sequelae include loss of airway patency secondary to mucosal edema, bronchospasm, intrapulmonary shunting from small airway occlusion, diminished compliance secondary to alveolar flooding and collapse, pneumonia secondary to loss of ciliary clearance, and respiratory failure secondary to a combination of the previously stated factors.

Diagnosis of Inhalation Injury

A limited number of tests have been proposed to aid in the diagnosis inhalation injury. They include the history, physical examination, chest radiograph, bronchoscopy, the admission arterial oxygen pressure to inspired oxygen concentration (PaO_2/FIO_2) ratio, and radioisotope scanning. Because there are no specific preemptive therapies for inhalation injury and because current diagnostic measures only loosely predict the degree of subsequent pulmonary dysfunction, diagnostic tests are used only for general evaluation and prognosis. The underlying difficulty with diagnosis is that, unlike with a cutaneous burn, inhalation injuries evolve over time and involve the entire respiratory system to a variable degree. For these reasons, patients at risk of this diagnosis generally are classified as having or not having sustained inhalation injury, with no effort made to quantify the degree of injury.

Most authors have based the diagnosis of inhalation injury on the history, physical examination, and bronchoscopic findings. Burns sustained in a closed space or aspiration of hot steam or liquid have been the pertinent points of the history. Physical findings suggesting the diagnosis have included carbonaceous debris in the mouth or sputum, singed nasal hairs, and facial burns. The chest radiograph generally is normal initially, which is consistent with the evolution of these injuries over time.

In addition to bronchoscopy, invasive measures sometimes used include radioisotope scanning and determination of the serum carboxyhemoglobin level. Although logistically more complicated in young children, most

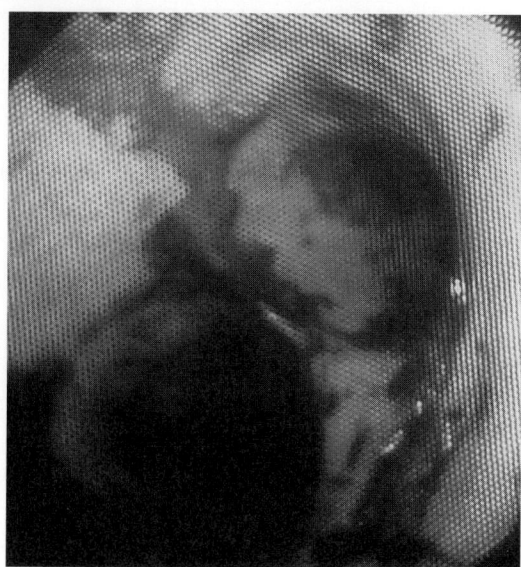

Figure 56-4   Bronchoscopic findings in inhalation injury include mucosal ulceration and carbonaceous debris.

clinicians use bronchoscopy as the gold standard for diagnosis of inhalation injury. Bronchoscopic findings consistent with this diagnosis include carbonaceous endobronchial debris and mucosal pallor and ulceration (Figure 56-4).[12-14] Two types of radioisotope imaging have been used to diagnose inhalation injury: intravenous administration of xenon-133 or inhalation administration of technetium-99. Both radioisotopes are rapidly cleared by normal lungs,[15] and asymmetric or delayed clearance is consistent with the diagnosis of inhalation injury.[16] Although physiologically sound, xenon and technetium scanning have not been widely used because of logistic difficulty and expense. In small clinical series tracheobronchial cytologic studies[17] and biopsy[18] have been reported to facilitate the diagnosis of inhalation injury, but because of logistic difficulties and potential complications, these techniques have not been widely used.

Management of Inhalation Injury

When a diagnosis of inhalation injury is suspected or confirmed, management is supportive only. As noted before, there are no prophylactic or preemptive therapies for inhalation injury. Prophylactic administration of antibiotics and steroids has no value. Although many patients demonstrate reactive bronchospasm[19] and benefit from early institution of nebulized β-agonists, steroids are infrequently required to treat bronchospasm. The only large clinical experience available suggests no benefit from the potentially risky administration of prophylactic steroids.[20] There also is no known benefit from prophylactic administration of antibiotics in these patients,[21] and cavalier use of these drugs may select for resistant species.

In patients with inhalation injury, five predictable events occur that have important clinical implications and require intervention: acute upper airway obstruction, bronchospasm, small airway obstruction, infection, and respiratory failure.

Acute Upper Airway Obstruction

Airway obstruction caused by mucosal edema evolves over time and ideally is anticipated and managed with intubation. In most cases intubation of these often difficult airways can be approached in a studied manner if the impending obstruction is anticipated. Failure to recognize impending airway obstruction can result in serious morbidity and even mortality in burn patients. Clinicians should be alert for the possibility of hot liquid aspiration that can lead to sudden loss of airway patency early[22,23] and to the late occurrence of the sequelae of upper airway burns.[24,25] The critical importance of initial airway evaluation and proper control cannot be over emphasized, and this need continues throughout the period of intubation.

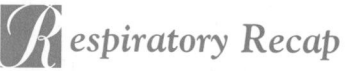

espiratory Recap

Management of Inhalation Injury	
Upper airway obstruction should be bypassed with endotracheal intubation or a tracheostomy; careful attention must be given to the endotracheal tube's position and patency. Bronchospasm should be treated with inhaled bronchodilators.	Aggressive pulmonary toilet is necessary to clear small airway obstruction. Pulmonary infection should be managed with a focus on organisms identified by sputum culture. Respiratory failure is managed with PEEP and efforts to avoid overdistention lung injury.

Oral endotracheal tubes are often used because they are easy to place. Tubes should be cut conservatively to allow for room for stabilization as facial edema changes. They must be stabilized in a fashion that allows easy adjustment as facial edema worsens and resolves. Because the lips are not reliable landmarks, the placement of the endotracheal tube must be monitored by notation of the centimeter mark at the incisor or gum. It is useful if this information is posted near the head of the bed for quick reference during routine and emergency airway care.

The security of the endotracheal tube should be verified regularly, because reintubation after accidental extubation can be incredibly difficult in burn patients, who commonly have massive facial and oropharyngeal edema (Figure 56-5). Clinicians who care for these patients should be equipped to deal with sudden airway emergencies.[23] Maintenance of endotracheal tubes in burn patients is compli-

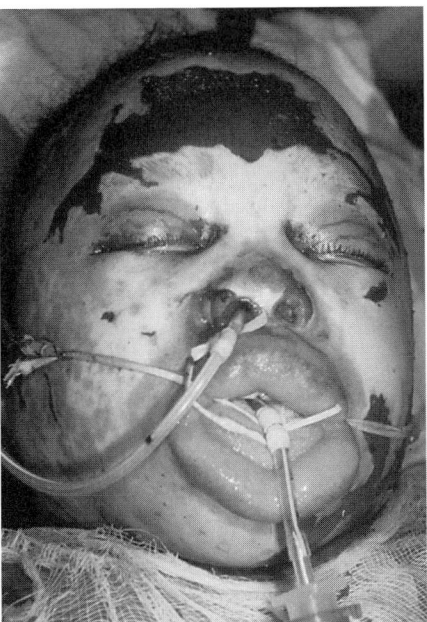

Figure 56-5   The security of the endotracheal tube should be verified regularly, because reintubation can be incredibly difficult in burn patients, who commonly have massive facial and oropharyngeal edema.

cated by shifts in extravascular volume. The method used to secure the tube should facilitate simple loosening and tightening as needed. When facial burns are present, adhesive tape is seldom useful. Cloth ties can be effectively used to secure tubes.

The proper indication and optimum timing for tracheostomy in the burn patient remain the subject of wide debate. However, the consensus is that adult burn patients in whom protracted intubation is expected are proper candidates, ideally after anterior neck burns have been addressed.

Bronchospasm

Intense bronchospasm from aerosolized irritants is common during the first 24 to 48 hours after injury, especially in young children. This condition is well managed with inhaled β-agonists in most patients, although some require intravenous bronchodilators, such as terbutaline or low-dose epinephrine infusions, or parenteral steroids. Another option is to provide continuous nebulization[26] or high-dose β-agonists.[27] Ventilatory strategies should be designed to minimize auto-PEEP in this setting, much as would be done to ventilate a patient with status asthmati-

---

Age-Specific Angle

Intense bronchospasm caused by aerosolized irritants is a particular problem in children.

Box 56-2

Evaluation and Initial Management of Deterioration of the Patient-Ventilator System

A sudden deterioration in the patient-ventilator unit requires immediate assessment for any of four problems: mechanical malfunction, obstruction of the artificial airway, displacement of the endotracheal tube from the trachea or into the mainstem bronchus, or pneumothorax, as follows:

1. Disconnect the patient from the ventilator and bag the individual with a self-inflating bag (remember the pop-off valve) and maximum inspired oxygen concentration (FIO_2). This eliminates or treats a mechanical problem.
2. Bag ventilate the patient. If the ventilations do not reach the airway, endotracheal tube obstruction is a possibility. If the patient's condition is stable, suction the tube. If it cannot be cleared quickly, extubate the patient, mask ventilate, and reintubate the airway.
3. If bilateral breath sounds are not heard, displacement of the airway or pneumothorax is possible. Auscultate in the axillae. If breath sounds are heard louder on the right than on the left, mainstem intubation is likely. Back the tube out cautiously and reassess. If gurgling is heard in the hypopharynx, the tube probably has been displaced from the airway. Extubate the patient, mask ventilate, and reintubate the airway.
4. If unilateral breath sounds are heard, pneumothorax may be present. This condition sometimes can be difficult to differentiate from mainstem intubation, but it often is accompanied by hemodynamic deterioration or hyperresonance (or a recent attempt to insert a subclavian line). If pneumothorax is suspected, insert a 14- or 16-gauge catheter into the second intercostal space in the midclavicular line and later place a chest tube.
5. The final common pathway is extubation, mask ventilation, and reintubation of the airway. The rule is: oxygen buys time.

If reintubation is impossible or mask ventilation is ineffective, the options are a laryngeal mask airway, needle cricothyroidotomy, surgical cricothyroidotomy or tracheostomy, or percutaneous cricothyroidotomy.

---

cus. Short inspiratory times and high inspiratory flow rates often may be necessary, but if air trapping is severe, some degree of carbon dioxide retention is acceptable.

Small Airway Obstruction

As necrotic endobronchial debris sloughs, pulmonary toilet often become increasingly difficult. An aggressive program of chest physiotherapy and pulmonary toilet is an important component of care. Toilet bronchoscopy can greatly facilitate clearance of the airways. Small endotracheal tubes can suddenly become occluded; staff members ideally are prepared to respond promptly (Box 56-2; Figure 56-6). Vigilant pulmonary toilet is an essential component of the management of patients with inhalation injury.

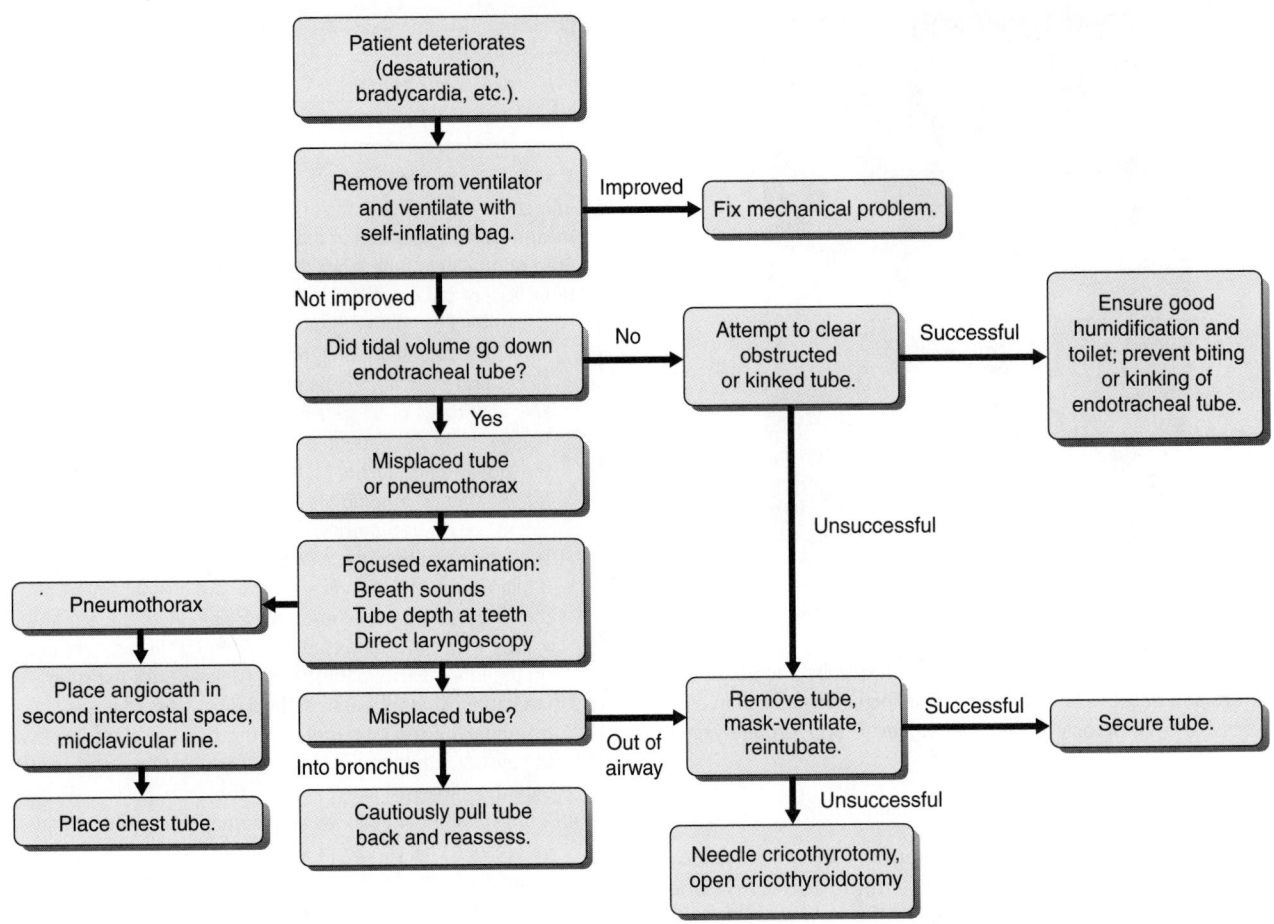

Figure 56-6 Algorithm for evaluation of a burn patient who suddenly deteriorates during mechanical ventilation.

Pulmonary Infection

Pulmonary infection develops in 30% to 50% of patients with inhalation injury. It frequently is difficult to distinguish between pneumonia and tracheobronchitis (purulent infection of the denuded tracheobronchial tree), but the difference often has little practical clinical importance. Infection typically occurs toward the end of the first postinjury week, patients with serious inhalation injuries often are seen to deteriorate at this time. A patient with newly purulent sputum, fever, and perhaps diminished gas exchange should be treated with antibiotics, which should be focused after sputum culture information has been obtained. To repeat an important point: the physiology of inhalation injury, which involves injury to endobronchial mucosa with hampered mucociliary clearance, makes good pulmonary toilet a particularly important component of management.

Respiratory Failure

Respiratory failure is not uncommon in individuals with inhalation injury, and its management is discussed elsewhere in this book. Respiratory failure among these pa-

tients is caused as often by sepsis as by inhalation injury. As in other forms of respiratory failure, recruitable lung volume is limited,[28] and overvigorous attempts to force high pressures into these lungs exacerbates the underlying injury.[29,30] These patients do well with a pressure-limited ventilation strategy based on permissive hypercapnia (Box 56-3; Figure 56-7).[31-34] If this approach fails, innovative methods of support should be considered, such as extracorporeal membrane oxygenation[35] or inhaled nitric oxide.[36] Prone positioning also has been shown to improve oxygenation.[37,38] In this position the posterior portions of the lungs, which are compressed by the diaphragm and heart, can be recruited through provision of a more uniform pleural pressure gradient. With adequate personnel, the patient can be quickly and safely repositioned while special attention is given to maintenance of the airway and central lines.

Enthusiasm has arisen for prophylactic use of **volumetric diffusive respiration** in burn patients.[39-43] This is essentially pressure-controlled ventilation with a superimposed subtidal oscillation that facilitates clearance of endobronchial debris. Although the initial data have been encouraging, burn patients with inhalation injury and res-

Box 56-3

Therapeutic Responses to Progressive Respiratory Failure

Address bronchospasm with nebulized β-agonist agents.

Address poor chest wall compliance that occurs secondary to overlying eschar with escharotomies.

Ensure ventilator synchrony with adequate opiate and benzodiazepine infusions. Neuromuscular blockade occasionally may be required.

Reset end point of ventilation to a physiologic pH (7.2 or higher). Allow gradual onset of hypercapnia as long as the patient does not have a head injury.

Reset end point of oxygenation to an arterial saturation of at least 90%, typically associated with an arterial oxygen content of 60 mm Hg or higher.

Optimize inflating pressures.

Choose optimum positive end-expiratory pressure (PEEP).

Choose optimum peak inflating pressure. This is best done with pressure-controlled ventilation and a total inflating pressure less than 40 cm H$_2$O. If this does not allow the reset end points of oxygenation and ventilation to be met, the pressure cap should be violated.

Choose optimum mean airway pressure. Lengthen expiratory time to a target mean airway pressure of 20 to 25 cm H$_2$O, as long as auto-PEEP is not detectable.

If these measures are inadequate, consider the use of innovative adjuncts, such as inhaled nitric oxide, or extracorporeal support.

Box 56-4

Important Considerations in the Weaning and Extubation of a Patient with a Burn Injury

Sensorium: The patient must be awake and alert enough to guard the airway.

Airway patency: Upper airway edema must be resolved to the extent that an air leak is audible around the endotracheal tube (with the cuff deflated if the tube is cuffed) at a moderate inflating pressure (20 to 30 cm H$_2$O).

Muscle strength: Strength must be adequate for ventilation. An indirect measure of this is a tidal volume of 6 to 10 mL/kg with continuous positive airway pressure of 5 cm H$_2$O and a negative inspiratory force less than −20 cm H$_2$O.

Compliance: Combined chest wall and lung compliance must be high enough that work of spontaneous breathing is not excessive. Indirect measures of this are a measured static compliance of at least 50 mL/cm H$_2$O and a tidal volume of at least 10 mL/kg with moderate inflating pressures (less than 25 cm H$_2$O).

Gas exchange: An intrapulmonary shunt less than 20% should be documented. This is indicated by a ratio of arterial oxygen pressure to inspired oxygen concentration (Pao$_2$ to Fio$_2$ ratio) more than 200.

piratory failure can be very well managed with a combination of careful pressure-limited ventilation and aggressive pulmonary toilet.[34]

Weaning and extubation of burn patients follow the general guidelines applicable to other patients. However, this patient group has some unique aspects that must be taken into consideration (Box 56-4). Of particular importance is the balance of the pain medication needs of patients with large wounds and donor sites with the need for an alert sensorium for extubation.

Carbon Monoxide Exposure

Many patients injured in structural fires inhale carbon monoxide (CO), and many are obtunded from a combination of CO, anoxia, and hypotension. CO binds avidly to heme-containing enzymes, particularly hemoglobin and the cytochromes, which it inactivates. The formation of **carboxyhemoglobin (COHb)** results in an acute physiologic anemia, much like an isovolemic hemodilution. A COHb concentration of 50% is physiologically similar to an isovolemic hemodilution to 50% of a baseline hemoglobin; therefore the routine occurrence of unconsciousness at this COHb level makes it clear that other mechanisms are involved in the pathophysiology of CO injury. It is likely that CO binding to the cytochrome system in the mitochondria, which interferes with oxygen utilization, is

more toxic than CO binding to hemoglobin. Many patients with severe CO exposure also have been exposed to cyanide, which is released from burning synthetics. However, the degree of exposure rarely is such that specific treatment is required.[44]

*R*espiratory Recap

Carboxyhemoglobinemia

Measure carboxyhemoglobin (COHb) with CO oximetry.

Administer 100% oxygen.

Consider hyperbaric oxygen therapy, particularly in patients with neurologic depression or delayed neurologic sequelae.

For unknown reasons 5% to 25% of patients with serious CO exposure have been reported to develop delayed major neurologic sequelae.[45,46] These patients can be managed with 100% isobaric oxygen or with **hyperbaric oxygen (HBO).** The half-life of COHb is about 5 hours breathing 21% oxygen at ambient pressure, about 74 minutes breathing 100% oxygen at ambient pressure (range is 26 to 148 min),[47] and less than 30 minutes breathing 100% oxygen at 3 atm. If serious exposure has occurred and is manifested by overt neurologic impairment or a high COHb level, HBO treatment probably is reasonable if it can be safely administered. With inhalation injury, 100% oxygen should be administered until a safe COHb level is reached.

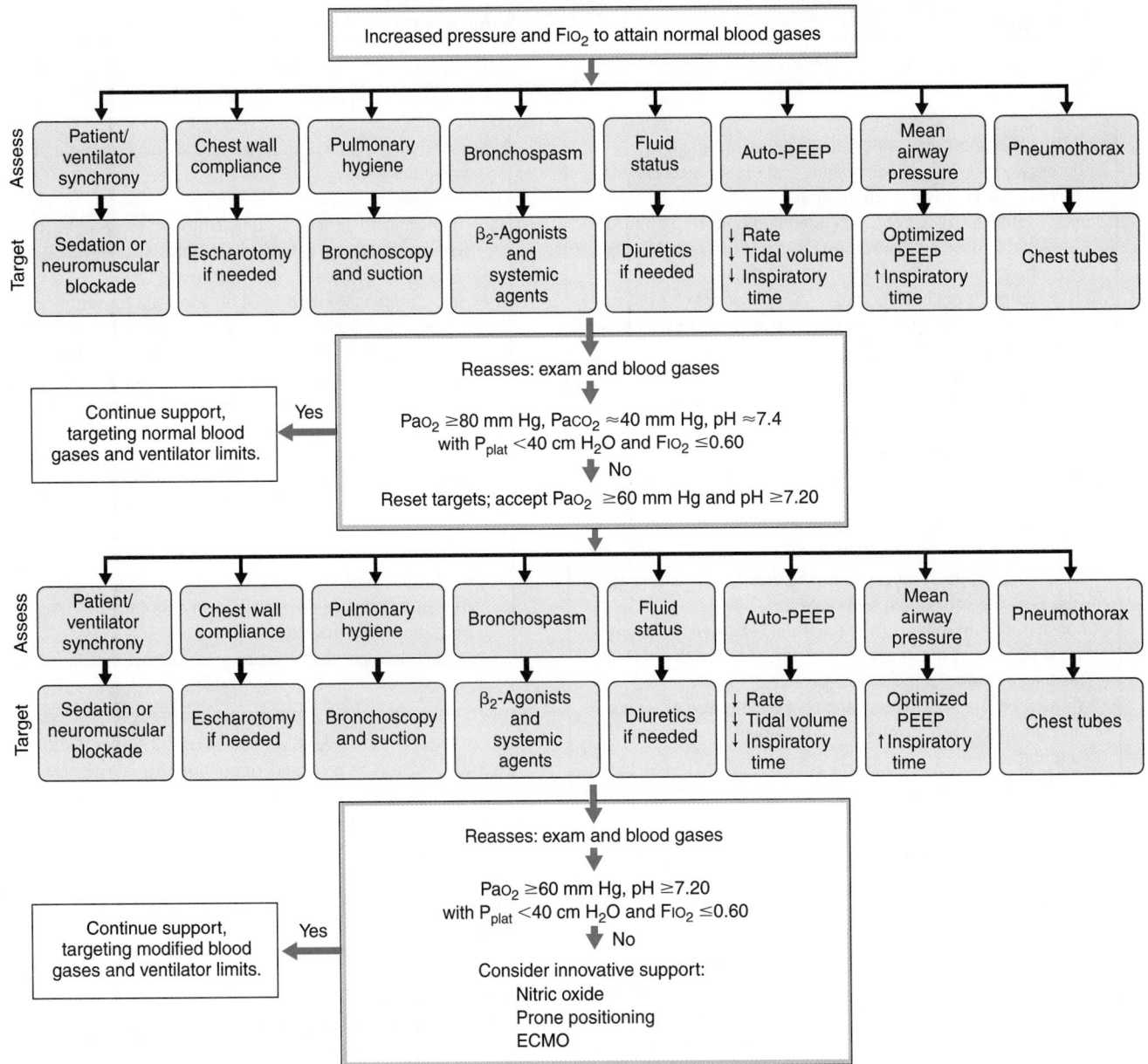

Figure 56-7 Algorithm for management of progressive respiratory failure in a burn patient with inhalation injury.

With inhalation injury the COHb level should be measured with **CO oximetry.** In the presence of COHb, pulse oximetry is unreliable and potentially misleading. Because pulse oximetry does not measure COHb, the pulse oximeter displays a high oxygen saturation (SpO_2) despite significant COHb, misleading the clinician to believe that COHb is not present. Because COHb does not affect gas exchange in the lungs, a patient with COHb who is breathing 100% oxygen may have a very high PaO_2 (more than 400 mm Hg) despite a low hemoglobin oxygen saturation as measured by CO-oximetry. The high PaO_2 competes with CO for hemoglobin binding sites, resulting in eventual displacement of CO from the hemoglobin.

HBO therapy has been proposed as a means to improve the prognosis of those who suffer serious CO exposure, but its use remains controversial. On a busy burn service the question of which patient to treat in the hyperbaric chamber commonly arises. Most patients who undergo hyperbaric oxygen therapy are treated in a monoplace hyperbaric chamber. Treatment regimens vary, but a typical one is 2 or 3 atm for 90 minutes, with three 10-minute air breaks to reduce the incidence of oxygen toxicity seizures. Because patient access is compromised in a monoplace chamber, patients in unstable condition are poor candidates. Other relative contraindications are wheezing or air trapping, which increases the risk of pneumothorax, and high fever, which increases the risk of seizures.

If a patient must be mechanically ventilated during HBO therapy, adequate preparation before the chamber door is closed can prevent most complications. Before the patient is placed in the chamber, the endotracheal tube cuff must be deflated and refilled with an appropriate volume of saline; this prevents collapse of the cuff during the compression phase of the treatment. The airway must be well positioned and adequately stabilized, because patients who inadvertently awaken during the therapy may attempt self-extubation. For the same reason, patients must be well restrained before HBO treatment regardless of their mental status. They must be well evaluated for bronchospasm and aggressively treated with bronchodilators just before treatment. Suctioning of both the lower respiratory tract and the oral pharynx is helpful, because this cannot be done while the patient is in the chamber. Prophylactic myringotomies are recommended for unconscious patients to prevent tympanic membrane rupture.

Ventilators used with monoplace HBO chambers are modified versions of a pressure-limited, time-cycled device. A base rate is maintained, but all spontaneous breathing efforts are unassisted. Patients who suddenly awaken during therapy and who cough or inspire vigorously can aspirate oral secretions, leading to an increase in airway pressure and a reduction in tidal volume (V_T). These same clinical signs occur with other clinical complications such as a kinked endotracheal tube, mainstem intubation, pneumothorax, or bronchospasm. Because the clinician is isolated from the patient, assessment can be very difficult. It may be best, if clinically appropriate, to adequately sedate the patient and avoid spontaneous breathing during the course of treatment.

CASE STUDIES

Case One
Minor Burn with Smoke Inhalation

A 47-year-old man was found unconscious on a smoldering mattress with minor burns to the right arm, chest, and thigh. Respirations were shallow and erratic; pulse was 110 beats/min; blood pressure was 140/90 mm Hg; and there was no apparent cyanosis. The patient could not be roused and was orally intubated at the scene. He was manually ventilated at an FIO_2 of 1 and transported to the emergency department.

On admission, the patient was mechanically ventilated in the synchronized intermittent mandatory ventilation (SIMV) mode at a tidal volume of 800 mL, a respiratory rate of 12 breaths/min, a positive end-expiratory pressure (PEEP) of 5 cm H_2O, and an FIO_2 of 1. Pressure support of 8 cm H_2O was available for any spontaneous breathing, but the patient made no inspiratory efforts above the set rate. A chest radiograph revealed the endotracheal tube to be 3.5 cm above the carina, with no evidence of pneumothorax or other chest trauma. The patient's pupils were sluggish but reactive. The heart rate and blood pressure remained 110 beats/min and 140/90 mm Hg, respectively. The SpO_2 was 100%. A toxicology screen was drawn. The arterial blood gas values were: pH, 7.45; arterial carbon

dioxide pressure ($PaCO_2$), 34 mm Hg; and PaO_2, 360 mm Hg. The COHb level as assessed by CO oximetry was 38%. Auscultation of the chest revealed mild diffuse bronchospasm, which resolved with administration of albuterol (six puffs via metered dose inhaler [MDI]). There was no evidence of air trapping or auto-PEEP. Because of the patient's depressed level of consciousness and elevated CO level, the decision was made to treat him with HBO.

At the HBO treatment center, the endotracheal cuff was deflated and refilled with saline. The airway was restabilized, and the patient was suctioned and given an additional four puffs of albuterol via MDI. Bilateral myringotomies were performed to avoid inadvertent rupture of the ear drums. All intravenous fluids and medications were transferred to specialized infusion pumps designed to operate with the HBO chamber. The patient was connected to a specialized HBO mechanical ventilator at the following settings: V_T, 700 mL; respiratory rate, 10 breaths/min; FIO_2, 1; and PEEP, 0. The patient was well restrained and placed in the HBO monochamber, and the chamber was pressurized to 3 atm. After approximately 15 minutes at this pressure, the V_T became erratic, and the peak inspiratory pressure increased by 15 cm H_2O. The patient became progressively more awake and attempted to remove the endotracheal tube. Initial attempts to sedate the patient failed, and anesthesia was induced with propofol. The patient was maintained with periodic boluses of propofol for the duration of the treatment, and there were no further complications.

After the HBO treatment, the patient was admitted to the burn intensive care unit (ICU), and all sedation was withdrawn. Assessment of ventilatory mechanics and level of consciousness demonstrated intact ventilatory function and responsiveness to commands. The patient was extubated and observed for 12 hours before being transferred to a non-ICU floor and subsequently discharged.

Case Two
Second- and Third-Degree Burns (70% BSA) with Severe Inhalation Injury

A 67-year-old unconscious woman was rescued from a kitchen fire with severe burns over much of her body. Assessment at the scene found significant facial burns and carbonaceous debris in the upper airway. The respiratory rate was 46 breaths/min and labored. The patient was orally intubated, manually ventilated with 100% oxygen, and transported to the emergency department. On admission the heart rate was 135 beats/min and the blood pressure was 150/100 mm Hg with profound wheezing throughout all lung fields. The patient was mechanically ventilated in the volume-controlled SIMV mode with a V_T of 800 mL; a respiratory rate of 18 breaths/min; a decelerating inspiratory flow of 60 L/min (which produced an inspiratory time of 1.46 seconds and an inspiration to expiration [I:E] ratio of 1.3); a PEEP of 5 cm H_2O; and an FIO_2 of 1. The arterial blood gas values with these settings were: pH, 7.35; $PaCO_2$, 66 mm Hg; and PaO_2, 82 mm Hg. The CO level was 27%. Ventilator graphics (flow and pressure) indicated significant flow present at end-exhalation. Total PEEP was measured and found to be 17 cm H_2O (12 cm H_2O of auto-PEEP). Albuterol was administered via nebulizer continuously over the next hour with little effect on the total PEEP.

The ventilator was adjusted to provide similar settings except for the flow pattern, which was changed from decelerating to square. This change reduced the inspiratory time to 0.8 second and increased the expiratory time from 1.9 to 2.5 seconds. On reassessment the total PEEP was 10 cm H_2O. Although air trapping was reduced, the diffuse bronchospasm remained refractory to aggressive β-agonist therapy. HBO therapy was rejected because of the significant risk of barotrauma. The applied PEEP was increased to match the total PEEP, and the FIO_2 was titrated to maintain an SpO_2 of 90% or higher. Over the next several days, the patient's arterial blood gas values deteriorated, requiring increases in applied PEEP up to 17 cm H_2O and an FIO_2 between 0.6 and 1. Air trapping continued to be a problem, and ventilator strategies were modified to include permissive hypercapnia. Bronchoscopy was performed several times to facilitate pulmonary toilet. The bronchoscopy also revealed significant airway injury and edema. By the fifth day of hospitalization, the patient showed signs of sepsis (increased fever and labile blood pressure) and purulent sputum. Appropriate antibiotic therapy was instituted, and the blood pressure was supported with vasopressor. Oxygenation worsened dramatically on day 6 despite various maneuvers to recruit lung volumes and increase the mean airway pressure. The blood pressure became progressively more unstable until the patient suffered cardiopulmonary arrest. Cardiopulmonary resuscitation was performed but was unsuccessful.

*K*EY *P*OINTS

- Respiratory failure is a leading cause of morbidity and mortality in the burn unit.
- An organized plan of care for patients with burn injury has four phases: initial evaluation and resuscitation, initial wound excision and biologic closure, definitive wound closure, and rehabilitation.
- Burn wounds should be evaluated for extent, depth, and circumferential components.
- Approximately 20% of burn injury patients suffer inhalation injury.
- Five predictable events occur in patients with inhalation injury: acute upper airway obstruction, bronchospasm, small airway obstruction, infection, and respiratory failure.
- All clinicians who care for burn patients should be prepared to deal with airway emergencies.
- Carboxyhemoglobin is treated with 100% oxygen and hyperbaric oxygen therapy.

References

1. Sheridan RL, Tompkins RG, Burke JF. Management of burn wounds with prompt excision and immediate closure. J Intensive Care Med 1994;9:6-19.
2. Ryan CM, Schoenfeld DA, Thorpe WP, et al. Objective estimates of the probability of death from burn injuries. N Engl J Med 1998;338:362-366.
3. Pruitt BA Jr, Erickson DR, Morris A. Progressive pulmonary insufficiency and other pulmonary complications of thermal injury. J Trauma 1975;15:369-379.
4. Sheridan RL. The seriously burned child: resuscitation through reintegration. I. Curr Probl Pediatr 1998;28:105-127.
5. Lund C, Browder N. The estimation of areas of burns. Surg Gynecol Obstet 1944;79:352-358.
6. Knaysi GA, Crikelair GF, Cosman B. The rule of nines: its history and accuracy. Plast Reconstr Surg 1968;41:560-563.
7. Sheridan RL, Petras L, Basha G, et al. Planimetry study of the percent of body surface represented by the hand and palm: sizing irregular burns is more accurately done with the palm. J Burn Care Rehabil 1995;16:605-606.
8. Heimbach D, Engrav L, Grube B, et al. Burn depth: a review. World J Surg 1992;16:10-15.
9. Scheulen JJ, Munster AM. The Parkland formula in patients with burns and inhalation injury. J Trauma 1982;22:869-871.
10. Pascuzzi TA, Storrow AB. Mass casualties from acute inhalation of chloramine gas. Mil Med 1998;163:102-104.
11. Wolf SE, Rose JK, Desai MH, et al. Mortality determinants in massive pediatric burns: an analysis of 103 children with ≥80% TBSA burns (≤70% full thickness). Ann Surg 1997;225:554-569.
12. Moylan JA, Adib K, Birnbaum M. Fiberoptic bronchoscopy following thermal injury. Surg Gynecol Obstet 1975;140:541-543.
13. Masanes MJ, Legendre C, Lioret N, et al. Fiberoptic bronchoscopy for the early diagnosis of subglottal inhalation injury: comparative value in the assessment of prognosis. J Trauma 1994;36:59-67.
14. Masanes MJ, Legendre C, Lioret N, et al. Using bronchoscopy and biopsy to diagnose early inhalation injury. Chest 1995;107:1365-1369.
15. Lull RJ, Anderson JH, Telepak RJ, et al. Radionuclide imaging in the assessment of lung injury. Semin Nucl Med 1980;10:302-310.
16. Lull RJ, Tatum JL, Sugerman HJ, et al. Radionuclide evaluation of lung trauma. Semin Nucl Med 1983;13:223-337.
17. Khoo AK, Lee ST, Poh WT. Tracheobronchial cytology in inhalation injury. J Trauma 1997;42:81-85.
18. Masanes MJ, Legendre C, Lioret N, et al. Using bronchoscopy and biopsy to diagnose early inhalation injury: macroscopic and histologic findings. Chest 1995;107:1365-1369.
19. Stenton SC, Kelly CA, Walters EH, et al. Induction of bronchial hyperresponsiveness following smoke inhalation injury. Br J Dis Chest 1988;82:436-438.
20. Robinson NB, Hudson LD, Riem M, et al. Steroid therapy following isolated smoke inhalation injury. J Trauma 1982;22:876-879.
21. Levine BA, Petroff PA, Slade CL, et al. Prospective trials of dexamethasone and aerosolized gentamicin in the treatment of inhalation injury in the burned patient. J Trauma 1978;18:188-193.
22. Hudson DA, Jones L, Rode H. Respiratory distress secondary to scalds in children. Burns 1994;20:434-437.
23. Sheridan RL. Recognition and management of hot liquid aspiration in children. Ann Emerg Med 1996;27:89-91.

24. Calhoun KH, Deskin RW, Garza C, et al. Long-term airway sequelae in a pediatric burn population. Laryngoscope 1988; 98:721-725.

25. Lund T, Goodwin CW, McManus WF, et al. Upper airway sequelae in burn patients requiring endotracheal intubation or tracheostomy. Ann Surg 1985;201:374-382.

26. Rudnitsky GS, Eberlein RS, Schoffstall JM, et al. Comparison of intermittent and continuously nebulized albuterol for treatment of asthma in an urban emergency room. Ann Emerg Med 1993;22:1842-1846.

27. Shrestha M, Bidali K, Gourlay S, et al. Continuous versus intermittent albuterol, at high and low doses, in the treatment of severe acute asthma in adults. Chest 1996;10:42-47.

28. Gattinoni L, Pesenti A, Bombino M, et al. Relationships between lung computed tomographic density, gas exchange, and PEEP in acute respiratory failure. Anesthesiology 1988;69: 824-832.

29. Parker JC, Hernandez LA, Peevy KJ. Mechanisms of ventilator-induced lung injury. Crit Care Med 1993;21:131-143.

30. Corbridge TC, Wood LD, Crawford GP, et al. Adverse effects of large tidal volume and low PEEP in canine acid aspiration. Am Rev Respir Dis 1990;142:311-315.

31. Kacmarek RM, Hickling KG. Permissive hypercapnia. Respir Care 1993;38:373-387.

32. Hickling KG, Walsh J, Henderson S, et al. Low mortality rate in adult respiratory distress syndrome using low-volume, pressure-limited ventilation with permissive hypercapnia: a prospective study. Crit Care Med 1994;22:1568-1578.

33. Bidani A, Tzouanakis AE, Cardenas VJ Jr, et al. Permissive hypercapnia in acute respiratory failure. JAMA 1994;272:957-962.

34. Sheridan RL, Kacmarek RM, McEttrick MM, et al. Permissive hypercapnia as a ventilatory strategy in burned children: effect on barotrauma, pneumonia, and mortality. J Trauma 1995;39: 854-859.

35. Goretsky MJ, Greenhalgh DG, Warden GD, et al. The use of extracorporeal life support in pediatric burn patients with respiratory failure. J Pediatr Surg 1995;30:620-623.

36. Sheridan RL, Hurford WE, Kacmarek RM, et al. Inhaled nitric oxide in burn patients with respiratory failure. J Trauma 1997; 42:641-646.

37. Chatte G, Sab JM, Dubois JM, et al. Prone position in mechanically ventilated patients with severe acute respiratory failure. Am J Respir Crit Care Med 1997;155:473-478.

38. Fridrich P, Krafft P, Hochleuthner H, et al. The effects of long-term prone positioning in patients with trauma-induced adult respiratory distress syndrome. Anesth Analg 1996;83:1206 1211.

39. Cioffi WG, Graves TA, McManus WF, et al. High-frequency percussive ventilation in patients with inhalation injury. J Trauma 1989;29:350-354.

40. Cioffi WG, Rue LW, Graves TA, et al. Prophylactic use of high-frequency percussive ventilation in patients with inhalation injury. Ann Surg 1991;213:575-580.

41. Mlcak R, Cortiella J, Desai M, et al. Lung compliance, airway resistance, and work of breathing in children after inhalation injury. J Burn Care Rehabil 1997;18:531-534.

42. Rodeberg DA, Maschinot NE, Housinger TA, et al. Decreased pulmonary barotrauma with the use of volumetric diffusive respiration in pediatric patients with burns. J Burn Care Rehabil 1992;13:506-511.

43. Rodeberg DA, Housinger TA, Greenhalgh DG, et al. Improved ventilatory function in burn patients using volumetric diffusive respiration. J Am Coll Surg 1994;179:518-522.

44. Barillo DJ, Goode R, Esch V. Cyanide poisoning in victims of fire: analysis of 364 cases and review of the literature. J Burn Care Rehabil 1994;15:46-57.

45. Thom SR, Taber RL, Mendiguren II, et al. Delayed neuropsychologic sequelae after carbon monoxide poisoning: prevention by treatment with hyperbaric oxygen. Ann Emerg Med 1995; 25:474-480.

46. Hardy KR, Thom SR. Pathophysiology and treatment of carbon monoxide poisoning. J Toxicol Clin Toxicol 1994;32:613-629.

47. Weaver LK, Howe S, Hopkins R, et al. Carboxyhemoglobin half-life in carbon monoxide–poisoned patients treated with 100% oxygen at atmospheric pressure. Chest 2000;117:801-808.

CHAPTER 57

Neuromuscular Dysfunction

Francis C. Cordova
Gerard J. Criner

CHAPTER OUTLINE

OBJECTIVES

1. Discuss the pathophysiology of neuromuscular disease on respiratory function.
2. Discuss the role of clinical history, physical examination, routine pulmonary function evaluation, and assessment of respiratory muscle function in the evaluation of respiratory function in patients with neuromuscular disease.
3. Describe neuromuscular disease associated with upper neuron lesions, lower motor neuron lesions, disorders of peripheral nerves, disorders of the neuromuscular junction, and inherited and acquired myopathies.
4. Discuss the treatment of respiratory dysfunction in patients with neuromuscular diseases.
5. Describe the role of the following in the management of neuromuscular disease: respiratory muscle training, assisted coughing, glossopharyngeal breathing, mechanical ventilation, positive pressure breathing, and diaphragmatic pacing.

KEY TERMS

Acid-Maltase Deficiency	Glossopharyngeal Breathing	Neuromuscular Disease
Amyotrophic Lateral Sclerosis (ALS)	Guillain-Barré Syndrome (GBS)	Parkinson's Disease
Botulism	Limb-Girdle Muscular Dystrophy	Poliomyelitis
Cheyne-Stokes Breathing	Maximum Expiratory Pressure (PE_{max})	Postpoliomyelitis Dystrophy
Chronic Steroid Myopathy	Maximum Inspiratory Pressure (PI_{max})	Sniff Test
Critical Care Polyneuropathy	Mitochondrial Myopathy	Stroke
Diaphragmatic Pacing	Mouth Occlusion Pressure	Systemic Lupus Erythematosus (SLE)
Duchenne Muscular Dystrophy (DMD)	Multiple Sclerosis (MS)	Tetraplegia
Eaton-Lambert Syndrome	Muscular Dystrophy	Transdiaphragmatic Pressure (P_{di})
Fascioscapulohumeral Dystrophy (FSHD)	Myasthenia Gravis (MG)	
	Myotonic Dystrophy	

The respiratory system can be divided into two functional parts: the lungs, where gas exchange occurs, and the respiratory muscles and rib cage, which act as a pump to enable normal gas exchange. **Neuromuscular diseases** are a diverse group of disorders that range from primary muscle diseases that impair all skeletal muscle functions to selected involvement of the diaphragm. The severity of respiratory muscle dysfunction depends on the type of neuromuscular disease, the pattern of respiratory muscle involvement (inspiratory or expiratory muscle), and whether or not effective medical therapies (for example, plasmapheresis in Guillain-Barré syndrome) are available. The respiratory pump may be impaired at the level of the central nervous system, spinal cord, peripheral nerve, neuromuscular junction, or respiratory muscles. Although the list of diseases usually classified under neuromuscular disorders includes a heterogenous and pathologically diverse composite of neurologic and muscular diseases (Table 57-1), they all commonly lead to a typical clinical course of ineffective cough, recurrent pulmonary infections, and ventilatory insufficiency in advanced disease. Chronic respiratory failure, in association with pulmonary sepsis, is the most common cause of death in these patients.

Some neuromuscular disorders are unrecognized by patients and physicians until an intercurrent illness leads to acute respiratory failure. In such cases, neuromuscular dysfunction is suspected only once the patient fails to wean from mechanical ventilation. In a recent report involving 293 chronic ventilator-dependent patients, 17% had an underlying neuromuscular disease as the major factor contributing to the development of respiratory failure.[1] The experience of the Temple University Hospital Ventilator Rehabilitation Unit also suggests that neuromuscular dysfunction frequently contributes to the need for prolonged mechanical ventilation.[2] Overall, the incidence of neuromuscular disease resulting in prolonged mechanical ventilation has been reported to range from 10% to 25% in various ventilator rehabilitation units across the United States.[1-3]

A thorough understanding of the neuroanatomic and pathologic changes brought on by the different neuromuscular disorders are important in the diagnosis and the treat-

TABLE 57-1

Levels of Pathologic Injury in Neuromuscular Diseases

Level	Disease
Upper Motor Neuron	
Cerebral spinal cord	Stroke trauma
Lower Motor Neuron	
Anterior horn cells	Poliomyelitis
	Amyotrophic lateral sclerosis
Peripheral nerves	Phrenic nerve injury
	Diabetes mellitus
	Guillain-Barré syndrome
	Critical illness polyneuropathy
Neuromuscular junction	Myasthenia gravis
	Eaton-Lambert syndrome
	Botulism
	Aminoglycosides

ment of these diseases. In this chapter, the etiology, pathophysiology, and treatment of ventilatory dysfunction in the setting of neuromuscular disease are discussed in detail.

Pathophysiology of Neuromuscular Disease and Respiratory Function

The changes that occur in ventilation with chronic neuromuscular disorders can best be understood through study of the impact of neuromuscular disease on the respiratory system's different functional components. Neuromuscular diseases can affect the integrity of the respiratory system by affecting its closely interrelated functional parts such as control of breathing, respiratory muscle function, lung and chest wall mechanics, and upper airway function. The commonly observed changes in respiratory function found in patients with moderately advanced chronic neuromuscular dysfunction are normal or high central respiratory drive except in certain diseases that affect the brain stem

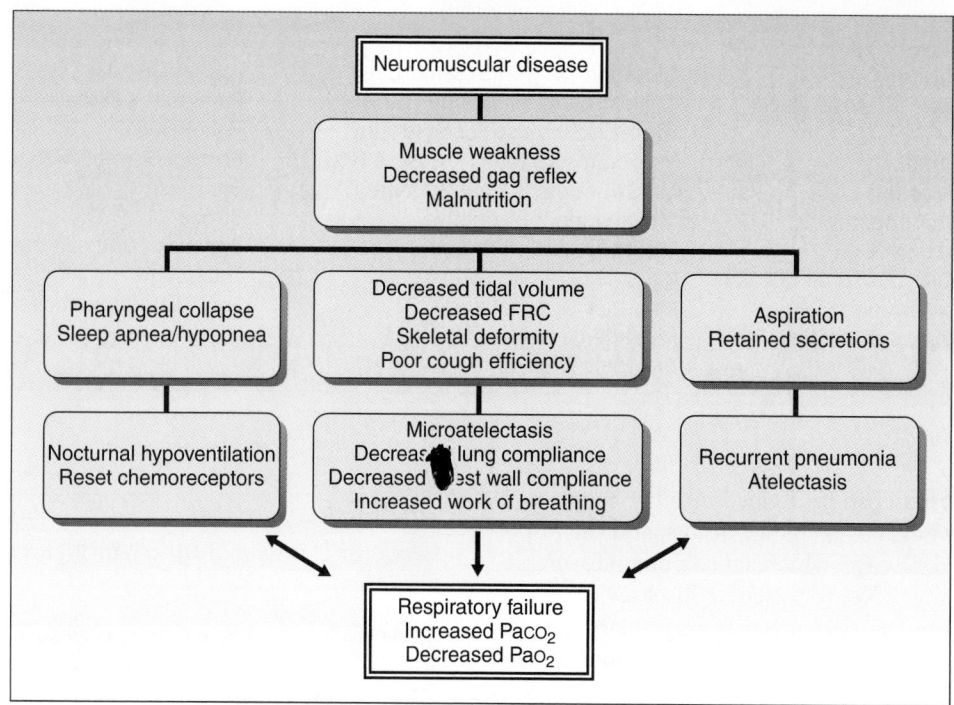

Figure 57-1   Pathophysiology of respiratory failure in patients with neuromuscular diseases. *FRC,* Functional residual capacity. (Modified from Hill NS, Braman S. Noninvasive ventilation in neuromuscular disease. In: Cherniack NS, Altose MD, Homma I, editors. Rehabilitation of the patient with respiratory disease. New York: McGraw-Hill; 1999.)

(that is, poliomyelitis), a restrictive ventilatory pattern manifested as a reduction in forced vital capacity (FVC) and an increase in residual volume (RV), and a reduction in respiratory muscle strength. Upper airway dysfunction may present as upper airway obstruction, recurrent aspiration pneumonia, and obstructive sleep apnea. All of these pathologic changes may present as subtle signs and symptoms during restful breathing but become more magnified during sleep and exercise (Figure 57-1).

Control of Breathing

The ventilatory responses to hypoxia and hypercapnia are used to assess the response of the peripheral and central chemoreceptors to chemical stimuli. In healthy individuals, the relationship between oxygen desaturation and ventilation is linear such that a fall in oxygen saturation by 1% will trigger an increase of approximately 1 L/min in minute ventilation. A much steeper linear increase in minute ventilation is seen during the hypercapnic breathing test. For every 1 mm Hg rise in PCO_2, ventilation increases by 2.5 to 3 L/min. The normally predictable increases in ventilation that occur in response to hypoxia and hypercapnia become disturbed in some neuromuscular disorders.

Several studies have shown that patients with neuromuscular disorders exhibit hypoventilation out of proportion to the severity of the respiratory muscle weakness.[4-6] However, definite conclusions cannot be drawn from these

studies because the ventilatory response to metabolic stress is not considered a good index of central respiratory drive in the presence of respiratory muscle weakness. The blunted ventilatory responses to hypoxic and hypercapnic challenges observed in patients with chronic neuromuscular disease may be related to inability of the respiratory pump to increase the work of breathing in response to increases in respiratory drive resulting from respiratory muscle weakness. Alternatively, abnormal chest wall and lung mechanics, defective afferent input from diseased respiratory muscles,[7] upper airway involvement,[8,9] and upper motor neuron disorders[10] may contribute to hypoventilation in selected neuromuscular disorders. A more accurate test of central respiratory drive that is independent of underlying respiratory mechanics is the **mouth occlusion pressure** or $(P_{0.1})$. $P_{0.1}$ refers to the maximum negative mouth pressure generated during the first 100 milliseconds of inspiration measured during complete airway occlusion.

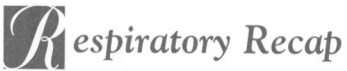 *espiratory Recap*

Control of Breathing
Patients with neuromuscular disease have hypoventilation out of proportion to the severity of respiratory muscle weakness. Respiratory drive is preserved in patients with neuromuscular disease.

TABLE 57-2

Innervation of the Respiratory Muscles

Muscle Group	Nerve
Upper Airway	
Palate, pharynx	Glossopharyngeal, vagus, spinal accessory
Genioglossus	Hypoglossal
Inspiratory	
Diaphragm	Phrenic
Scalenes	Cervical C4-C8
Parasternal intercostals	Intercostal T1-T12
Sternocleidomastoid	Spinal accessory
Lateral external	Intercostal T1-T12
Intercostal T1-T7	
Expiratory	
Abdominal	Lumbar T7-L1
Internal intercostals	Intercostal T1-T12

C, Cervical; T, thoracic; L, lumbar.

Because $P_{0.1}$ is obtained during early inspiration, a small fraction of total inspiratory time, it is not influenced by volitional effort. In addition, because $P_{0.1}$ requires only a fraction of maximum inspiratory muscle strength, it remains valid even in the presence of moderately severe inspiratory muscle weakness.

In contrast to studies that have used ventilation to assess central respiratory drive, $P_{0.1}$ has been found to be normal, or increased, in patients with neuromuscular diseases despite the presence of substantial muscle weakness.[11] Several studies have shown that despite significant reductions in respiratory muscle strength, $P_{0.1}$ values in patients with Duchenne muscular dystrophy, myotonic dystrophy, and a variety of other neuromuscular diseases are one to two fold higher than in normal controls.[12,13] Paton and Aaimia[14] also found that partial paralysis of the spontaneously breathing cat produced a marked increase in phrenic nerve discharge despite a significant decrease in minute ventilation. Similar increases in $P_{0.1}$ were observed in normal human volunteers after severe muscle weakness was induced by curare.[15] Thus it appears that central respiratory drive, as measured by $P_{0.1}$, usually is preserved in patients with underlying neuromuscular diseases.

Respiratory Muscle Function

The respiratory muscles include the muscles of the upper airway, the diaphragm, chest wall muscles, and abdomen muscles. The respiratory muscles can be further functionally divided into the inspiratory and expiratory muscles. The inspiratory muscles produce rib cage expansion and generate negative intrathoracic pressure, thereby facilitating inspiratory airflow. During rest, exhalation is passive and is driven

by the lung and chest wall elastic recoil pressures. However, active contraction of the expiratory muscles occurs under conditions when increased expiratory airflow is required such as coughing, exercise, and airway obstruction. The innervation of the different respiratory muscles and their major functions are shown in Table 57-2.

Patients with moderate to severe respiratory muscle weakness resulting from neuromuscular disease often complain of fatigue, poor sleep quality, and dyspnea on exertion. However, a significant percentage of these patients may be asymptomatic despite moderate to severe weakness of the inspiratory and expiratory muscles. Demedts and colleagues[16] reported that 27% of the patients with moderately advanced neuromuscular disease who had severe reduction in both the inspiratory and expiratory muscles had no respiratory complaints. Similarly, Vincken and colleagues[17] reported that as many as 50% of patients with severe respiratory muscle weakness resulting from chronic neuromuscular disease were asymptomatic. It is unclear why such poor correlation exists between the extent of respiratory muscle weakness and clinical symptoms exhibited by the patients. The presence of significant respiratory muscle weakness may be masked by the inability to achieve significant exercise because the generalized muscle weakness enforces a sedentary lifestyle. Whatever the case, a substantial number of patients may have significant neuromuscular impairment of the respiratory system that may go initially unnoticed.

The particular type of underlying neuromuscular disorder determines the pattern and severity of respiratory muscle weakness. Some diseases cause global respiratory muscle dysfunction, whereas others cause preferential weakness of the inspiratory or expiratory muscles. In addition, decreases in inspiratory and expiratory muscle strength may not correlate with general muscle strength assessment.[17] Primary muscle diseases (for example, polymyositis) may cause more significant impairment of the respiratory muscles compared with the neuropathies. The relationship between inspiratory muscle strength and the onset of ventilatory insufficiency is not linear. Hypercapnia ensues once maximum inspiratory mouth pressure decreases to less than 30% of predicted (Figure 57-2).[18] The clinical course of respiratory muscle dysfunction in different neuromuscular diseases also may vary. They can be relentlessly progressive (amyotrophic lateral sclerosis), reversible with therapy (Guillain-Barré syndrome, myasthenia gravis), or improve with time (critical care polyneuropathy).

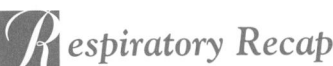

*R*espiratory Recap

Respiratory Muscle Weakness
Relentlessly progressive in some neuromuscular diseases
Reversible with therapy in some neuromuscular diseases
Improves with time in some neuromuscular diseases

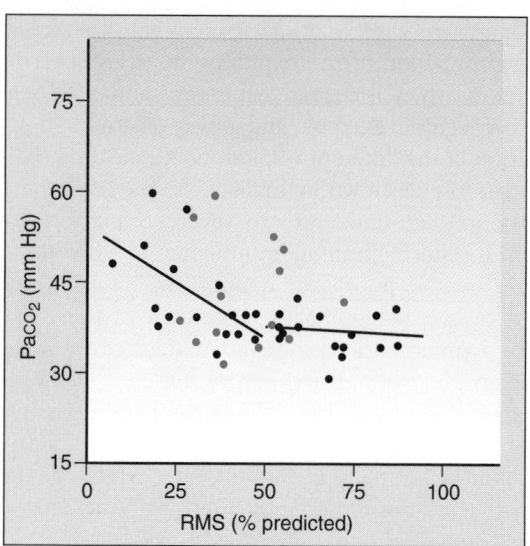

Figure 57-2 Relationship between respiratory muscle strength (RMS) and arterial $Paco_2$ in patients with myopathies. The data suggests that hypercapnia does not occur until the respiratory muscle strength is less than 30%. Red and black circles represent patients with and without concomitant lung disease, respectively. (Modified from Braun NMT, Arora NS, Rochester DF. Respiratory muscle and pulmonary function in polymyosities and other proximal myopathies. Thorax 1983;38:616-623.)

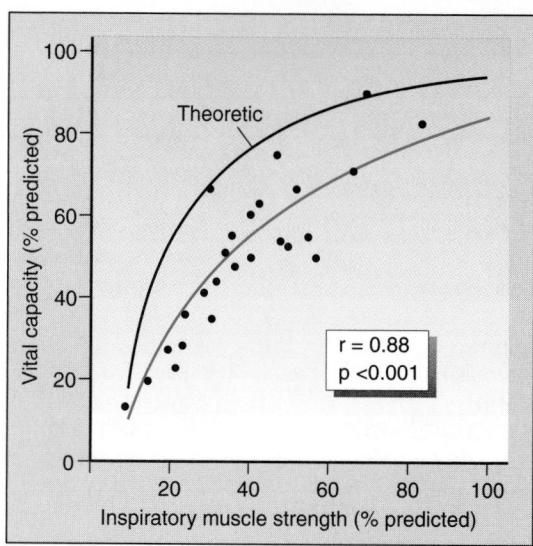

Figure 57-3 Relationship between inspiratory muscle strength and vital capacity. The red line represents the regression line calculated in 25 patients with neuromuscular diseases showing the disproportionate fall in vital capacity for the given degree of inspiratory muscle weakness. The black line represents the predicted relationship between vital capacity and inspiratory muscle strength. (Modified from De Troyer A, Borenstein S, Cordier R. Analysis of lung volume restriction in patients with respiratory muscle weakness. Thorax 1980;35:603-610.)

Lung and Chest Wall Mechanics

Lung volume studies in patients with chronic respiratory muscle weakness often show a restrictive ventilatory pattern with a reduction in total lung capacity (TLC) and FVC. Inspiratory and expiratory reserve volume both decrease moderately. The decrease in FVC is due primarily to respiratory muscle weakness and its decrease generally parallels the progression of the underlying neuromuscular disease. However, because of the sigmoidal shape of the pressure-volume curve of the respiratory system, vital capacity is relatively well preserved until respiratory muscle is well advanced (Figure 57-3).[18] Indeed, the fall in FVC has been shown to be out of proportion to the reduction in inspiratory muscle strength. De Troyer and colleagues[19] found an average reduction in lung compliance of 40% in 25 patients with moderate to severe neuromuscular disease. Additionally, respiratory muscle weakness may account for a lower vital capacity in these patients. The exact cause of reduced lung compliance in neuromuscular disease patients remains speculative. Several proposed explanations include the following:

1. Failed maturation of normal lung tissue in congenital neuromuscular diseases
2. Presence of micro- or macroatelectasis
3. Increased alveolar surface tension caused by breathing chronically at low tidal volumes
4. Alteration in lung tissue elasticity

Patients with neuromuscular disease have a rapid shallow breathing pattern similar to patients with interstitial lung disease. The exact mechanism(s) of this abnormal breathing pattern is unclear but is thought to be secondary to changes in lung and chest wall elastic recoil. Animal studies demonstrate that breathing at small tidal volumes is associated with reductions in lung compliance and may lead to increased alveolar surface tension.[20,21] In addition, the lower ventilatory demand induced by a sedentary lifestyle leads to lower lung mechanical stress and overtime may result in a reduction in lung tissue elasticity.

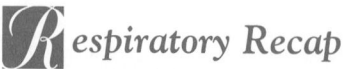

Respiratory System Mechanics

Lung volume shows a restrictive pattern.
The fall in FVC is out of proportion to the reduction in muscle strength.
Rapid shallow breathing pattern is present.
Chest wall compliance is reduced.

Similar to the changes seen in the lungs, a significant reduction in chest wall compliance also has been reported in patients with chronic neuromuscular disease.[22,23] The mechanisms of the reduction in chest wall compliance are unclear but may be due to increased rib cage stiffness resulting from decreased distensibility of chest wall structures (that is, tendons, ligaments, costovertebral and costosternal articulations).

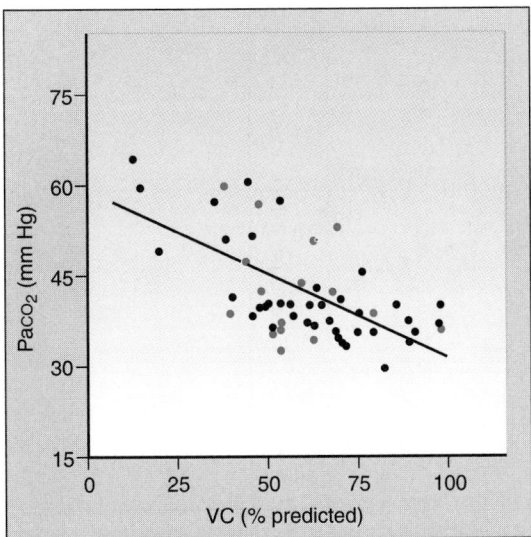

Figure 57-4 Relationship between vital capacity (VC) and arterial $PaCO_2$ showing that hypercapnia occurs when the vital capacity is less than 55% of predicted. Red and black circles represent patients with and without concomitant lung disease respectively. (Modified from Braun NMT, Arora NS, Rochester DF. Respiratory muscle and pulmonary function in polymyosities and other proximal myopathies. Thorax 1983;38:616-623.)

Although a low vital capacity is almost always seen in moderately advanced neuromuscular disease, the changes in functional residual capacity (FRC) and residual volume (RV) are variable and depend upon the type, severity, and stage of neuromuscular disease. Most studies report FRC to be unchanged or decreased.[19,24-27] Similar variable findings have been reported in RV.[19,24,25,28] In general, patients with neuromuscular diseases have moderate reductions in TLC and FRC, with a normal RV.

Gas Exchange Abnormalities

The presence of hypercapnia and hypoxemia is a late finding in patients with neuromuscular disease. Hypercapnia with a relatively normal FVC and static maximum respiratory pressures should raise the possibility of sleep-related breathing disorders (obstructive sleep apnea, obesity hypoventilation syndrome), the presence of parenchymal lung disease such as chronic obstructive airway disease, or problems with central respiratory drive such as chronic hypoventilation syndrome or hypothyroidism. Even with normal daytime gas exchange parameters, significant hypoxemia and alveolar hypoventilation may occur during sleep, especially during rapid eye movement (REM) sleep when the activity of the accessory muscles is diminished. In advanced neuromuscular diseases, evidence of alveolar hypoventilation on blood gas examination is likely when the FVC is less than 55% of predicted (Figure 57-4) and PI_{max} and PE_{max} are less than 30 cm H_2O.[18] However, the onset of hypercapnia in the setting of advanced neuro-

muscular disease may be abrupt.[29] Ventilation-perfusion inequality resulting from atelectasis is the most common cause of hypoxemia in these patients.

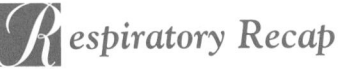

Gas Exchange Abnormalities

Hypercapnia and hypoxemia are late findings in neuromuscular disease.

Sleep Breathing Dysfunction

Sleep-related breathing disorders such as impaired sleep quality and REM-related hypopnea are common in patients with a variety of different neuromuscular diseases. Indeed, significant gas exchange abnormalities may be present and even unsuspected when daytime hypoxemia and hypercapnia are absent.

Several physiologic changes occur in the respiratory system during sleep, especially during REM sleep. Alveolar hypoventilation, causing a 2 to 3 mm Hg rise in $PaCO_2$, occurs during sleep in normal individuals. An inhibition of accessory inspiratory muscle activity during REM sleep may lead to a significant reduction in alveolar ventilation in patients with underlying diaphragm weakness.

Recent studies have shown that hypoventilation during sleep is the major cause of sleep-related oxygen desaturation. In a study of 26 patients with chronic respiratory failure and nocturnal oxygen desaturation (for example, patients with chronic airways obstruction, obesity hypoventilation, neuromuscular disease), minute ventilation decreased by 21% during non-REM eye sleep, and by 39% during REM sleep compared with wakefulness (Figure 57-5).[30] The decrease in minute ventilation was due primarily to a decrease in tidal volume and was found to be independent of the underlying lung disease. Phasic REM sleep-induced changes in breathing pattern superimposed on the rapid shallow breathing pattern commonly observed in patients with neuromuscular disease lead to further increases in dead space ventilation, resulting in more profound degrees of hypoxemia and hypercapnia. In addition to these sleep-induced breathing abnormalities, weakness of the pharyngeal muscles in certain neuromuscular diseases may predispose patients to obstructive sleep apnea and hypopnea because of loss of upper airway tone, especially during REM sleep.

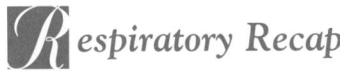

Sleep-Disordered Breathing

Sleep disorders are common in patients with neuromuscular disease.

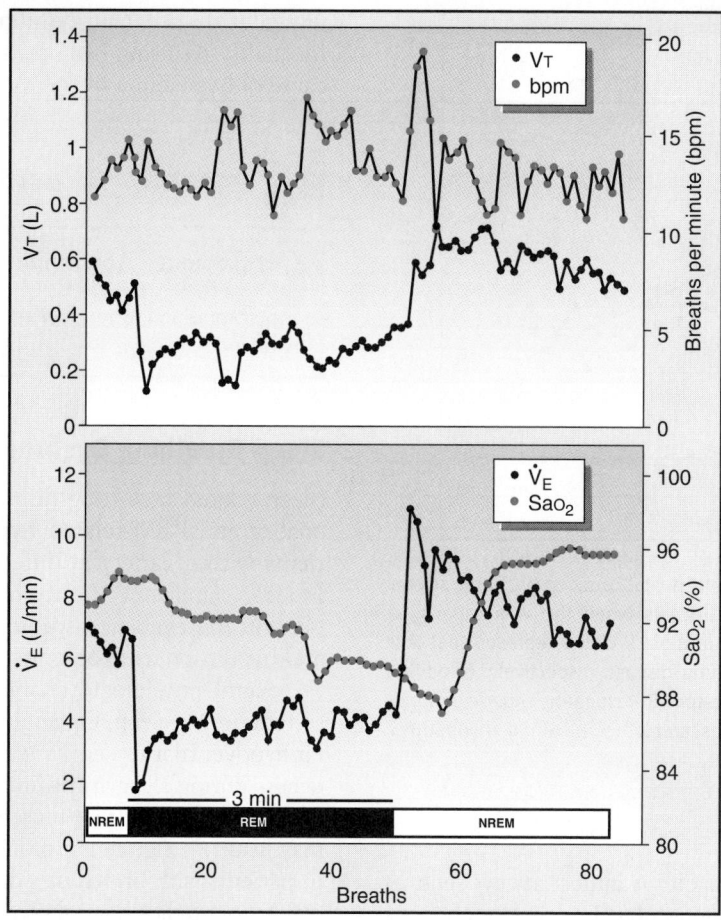

Figure 57-5 Both the upper and lower panel show the decrease in tidal volume (VT) and minute ventilation ($\dot{V}_E$) with no change in respiratory rate (bpm) during transition from non-rapid eye movement (NREM) sleep to rapid eye movement (REM) sleep. Hypoventilation due to decrease in VT during REM sleep appears to be the main reason leading to nocturnal oxygen desaturation in patients with limited pulmonary reserve. (Modified from Becker H, Piper A, Flynn W, et al. Breathing during sleep in patients with nocturnal desaturation. Am J Respir Crit Care Med 1999;159:112-118.)

If nocturnal hypoventilation is severe and remains clinically unrecognized, daytime hypercapnia and hypoxemia may ensue even in the absence of severe respiratory muscle dysfunction. Nocturnal gas exchange abnormalities usually precede abnormalities in daytime arterial blood gas results.[31,32] Indeed, most patients with normal nocturnal gas exchange are unlikely to have abnormal daytime values.

Abnormalities in daytime gas exchange and certain parameters of respiratory mechanics are useful in predicting the subset of patients with neuromuscular disease who are at risk for severe nocturnal oxygen desaturation. Bye and colleagues[31] studied 20 patients with a variety of moderately advanced neuromuscular diseases and showed that the degree of REM-related oxygen desaturation is directly related to the severity of daytime hypercapnia and hypoxemia. Absolute values for vital capacity and the decrement in vital capacity measured in the supine compared with the seated position also correlate with the nadir in oxygen saturation measured during REM sleep. The mean

decrease in VC measured in the supine compared with seated posture was 21%.

Upper Airway Dysfunction

Some neuromuscular diseases involve the bulbar muscles and therefore impair upper airway function. Upper airway dysfunction is manifested commonly by repeated pulmonary aspiration, stridor, obstructive sleep apnea, and hypopnea. In patients with chronic neuromuscular disorders, upper airway dysfunction is more common in pa-

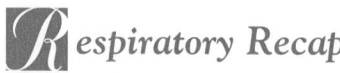*espiratory Recap*

Upper Airway Function

Upper airway function is impaired in patients with bulbar muscle dysfunction.

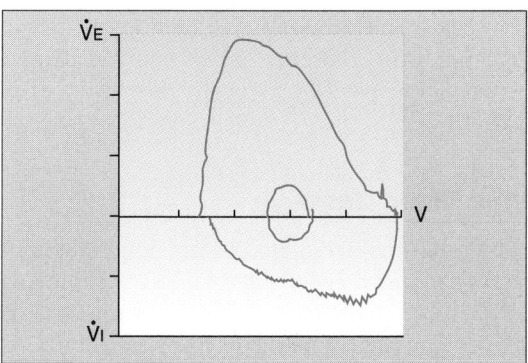

Figure 57-6 An example of flow-volume loop in a patient with motor neuron disease showing inspiratory flow limitation suggestive of partial upper airway obstruction. $\dot{V}_E$, Expiratory flow; $\dot{V}_I$, inspiratory flow; V, volume. (Modified from Vincken W, Ellecker G, Cosio M. Detection of upper airway muscle involvement in neuromuscular disorders using flow-volume loop. Chest 1986;90:52-57.)

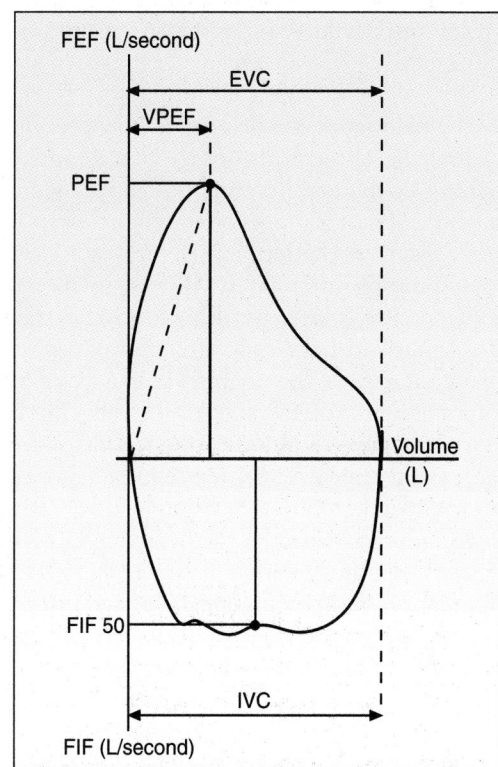

Figure 57-7 Analysis of the effort-dependent portion of the flow-volume loop to detect respiratory muscle weakness. These four parameters include (1) peak expiratory flow (PEF); (2) ratio of PEF to the exhaled volume at which PEF was achieved (VPEF); (3) rapid vertical drop of forced expiratory flow (FEF) at residual volume; and (4) forced midinspiratory flow. *EVC*, Expired vital capacity; *IVC*, inspired vital capacity; *FIF*, forced inspiratory flow. (Modified from Vincken WG, Elleker MG, Casio MG. Flow-volume loop changes reflecting respiratory muscle weakness in chronic neuromuscular disorders. Am J Med 1987;83:673-680.)

tients who exhibit respiratory muscle weakness compared with those without such weakness.

The flow-volume loop is a useful screening tool to detect significant upper airway dysfunction. Indeed an abnormal flow-volume loop has a high sensitivity[33] and specificity[34] in the prediction of bulbar and upper airway involvement in patients with neuromuscular dysfunction.[9] A typical flow-volume loop in a patient with motor neuron disease with bulbar involvement is shown in Figure 57-6. Vincken described a sawtoothing of the flow contour in patients with Parkinson's disease.[8,35] In addition, variable extrathoracic obstruction that reverses with drug therapy has been described in patients with myasthenia gravis.[36] Certain features of the flow-volume contour have been shown to correlate with reduced maximum static inspiratory and expiratory mouth pressures: a reduced peak expiratory flow, decreased slope of the ascending limb of the maximum expiratory curve, a drop off of the forced expiratory flow near residual volume, and a reduction in forced inspiratory flow at 50% of vital capacity (Figure 57-7).[9,37]

Evaluation of Respiratory Function in Patients with Neuromuscular Disease

Clinical History

The diagnosis of muscle weakness may not be made readily on initial clinical evaluation because of the overlapping syndromes among the different neuromuscular diseases. The predominant signs and symptoms of a particular neuromuscular disease depend on the acuity, severity, and the clinical course of the disease and the pattern of neuromuscular weakness. Diseases that predominantly affect the pump function of the respiratory system present as dyspnea, weak cough, and recurrent respiratory tract infections, whereas diseases that affect primarily the limb muscles present as impaired mobility

early in its disease evolution. Once respiratory muscles are affected in advanced neuromuscular disease, respiratory failure may occur abruptly because of an intercurrent illness or slowly over months and years culminating in chronic hypercapnic respiratory failure. However, in some neuromuscular diseases, a typical presentation leads to the correct diagnosis. For example, an acute ascending paralysis of the lower extremities suggests Guillain-Barré syndrome, waxing and waning of neurologic symptoms is commonly seen in multiple sclerosis, and skeletal muscle weakness with repetitive action of a particular muscle group is highly suspicious of myasthenia gravis.

In the majority of the neuromuscular diseases, respiratory muscle weakness usually occurs insidiously and is typically associated with weakness of other skeletal muscle groups. However, as many as 50% of patients with significant respiratory muscle weakness are asymptomatic until they develop respiratory failure.[17] In clinical practice, physicians and respiratory therapists are involved in the care of these patients when these patients develop either acute respiratory failure, chronic hypercapnic respiratory failure, or acute on chronic respiratory failure.

In patients who develop acute respiratory failure, the nature of the neuromuscular disease is often not clinically apparent and the clinical history is often dominated by the symptoms of the precipitating illness that led to respiratory failure. These patients often require early intubation, mechanical ventilation, and appropriate treatment of the precipitating intercurrent illness. In most cases, respiratory muscle weakness resulting from a neuromuscular disease comes to light only after the patients failed multiple weaning trials. In patients who have chronic stable neuromuscular diseases (ALS, congenital myopathies), progressive respiratory muscle weakness occurs over months and years eventually leading to chronic progressive hypercapnic respiratory failure. The challenge to both physicians and respiratory therapists is to detect early signs of respiratory muscle weakness before the onset of fulminant respiratory failure and to prevent complications (such as aspiration, recurrent respiratory tract infections, and cor pulmonale) and to preserve remaining lung function. The common symptoms of respiratory muscle weakness are dyspnea with activity, inability to clear secretions, weak cough, frequent respiratory tract infections, and choking episodes. These symptoms are often elicited several months before these patients seek medical attention. The presence of chronic headache, lethargy, somnolence suggest significant daytime and nocturnal hypercapnia. As previously discussed, nocturnal hypercapnia usually heralds the onset of chronic respiratory failure.

Physical Examination

A thorough physical examination and a detailed neurologic assessment may reveal a previously undiagnosed neuromuscular disorder. This is particularly true in patients who have mild respiratory muscle weakness but develop acute respiratory failure resulting from increased ventilatory demand from an acute illness such as an infection. In patients with early or mild neuromuscular weakness, respiratory muscle weakness may not be detected on routine physical examination. Limb muscle weakness is often recognized only after the patients fail multiple weaning attempts. Nevertheless, certain physical examination findings indicate significant respiratory muscle weakness. Tachypnea at rest is common with the onset of respiratory muscle weakness. As the respiratory muscle weakness progresses, the increase in respiratory rate is followed by signs of increased respiratory workload such as nasal flaring, recruitment of the accessory muscles, and intercostal and subcostal retractions. Further progression in respiratory muscle weakness will eventually lead to paradoxic inward motion of the rib cage and outward displacement of the abdomen during inspiration. Abnormal paradoxic motion of the rib cage, and abdomen may indicate either impending respiratory failure or diaphragm weakness. Indeed, paradoxic inward movement of the abdomen on inspiration that worsens with recumbent position typically is seen in diaphragm weakness.

Arterial Blood Gases

Abnormalities in arterial blood gases occur late in patients with severe respiratory muscle weakness and should not be relied upon before ventilatory support is initiated. Hypoxemia is commonly the result of microatelectasis resulting from ineffective cough and retained secretions causing ventilation-perfusion mismatch or intrapulmonary shunting. More important, alveolar hypoventilation resulting from respiratory muscle weakness, or decreased central respiratory drive may also contribute significantly to hypoxemia. Hypoxemia resulting from alveolar hypoventilation may be detected by a normal alveolar-arterial oxygen gradient. Pulse oximetry, which is a measure of arterial oxyhemoglobin saturation, helps detect hypoxemia but is an insensitive indicator of hypoventilation.

Hypercapnia is a late finding in severe respiratory muscle weakness. In fact, hypercapnia does not occur until the respiratory muscle strength is less than 50% of predicted. Careful analysis of the pH and bicarbonate level helps detect the presence of acute or chronic hypercapnic respiratory failure. Sleep-induced breathing disturbances also may lead to hypercapnia as previously discussed and should be carefully studied in susceptible patients.

Pulmonary Function Tests

Spirometry and lung volume studies are helpful in the initial evaluation and the follow-up of patients with neuromuscular disease during therapy. In general, spirometry produces a restrictive pattern characterized by a reduction in FVC and a normal FEV_1/FVC. Effort-dependent expiratory flow also decreases, such as the peak expiratory airflow measurement, whereas forced expiratory volume in 1 second (FEV_1) and measurement of mid expiratory flow rates (FEF_{25-75} or FEF_{50}) are often greater than normal predicted values because of decreased lung compliance, resulting in increased lung elastic recoil. Lung volume study shows low total lung capacity but high residual volume as a result of expiratory muscle weakness. Diffusion capacity is usually normal.

Serial measurement of FVC is helpful in following of the progression of respiratory muscle weakness in patients with chronic neuromuscular disease and in timing of the institution of noninvasive positive pressure ventilation. In patients with rapidly progressive respiratory muscle weakness such as seen in Guillain-Barré syndrome, daily measurement of FVC (10 mL/kg or 1 L) helps determine when to consider elective airway intubation and mechanical ventilation. Alternatively, FVC also can be used as one of the criteria for the initiation of weaning trials and liberation from mechanical ventilation.

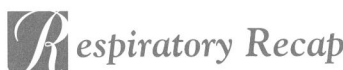espiratory Recap

Evaluation of Respiratory Function with Neuromuscular Disease

History: Respiratory weakness usually occurs insidiously.
Physical examination: Symptoms include tachypnea and paradoxic movement of the rib cage and abdomen, particularly with diaphragm weakness.
Arterial blood gases: Hypoxemia may occur secondary to retained secretions; hypercapnia is a late finding.
Pulmonary function tests: Serial measurement of vital capacity is helpful in following the progression of respiratory muscle weakness.
Chest radiograph: Lung volume is reduced and atelectasis may be present.

TABLE 57-3

Selected Normal Maximum Static Airway Pressures Values in Adults

Study	Sex	PI_{max} (cm H_2O)	PE_{max} (cm H_2O)
Black and Hyatt (1969)	Male	124 ± 22	233 ± 42
	Female	87 ± 16	152 ± 27
Rochester and Arora (1983)	Male	127 ± 28	216 ± 41
	Female	91 ± 25	138 ± 39
Vincken and colleagues (1987)	Male	105 ± 25	140 ± 38
	Female	71 ± 23	89 ± 24

Upper airway dysfunction commonly seen in chronic neuromuscular diseases may be detected easily through analysis of the flow-volume curve. For example, inspiratory plateau of the flow waveform is indicative of extrathoracic upper airway obstruction. In patients with Parkinson's disease, instability of the upper airway muscles is often reflected in a sawtoothing of the contour of the flow-volume loop. An abnormal flow-volume loop in patients with neuromuscular disease is both highly sensitive and specific in the prediction of bulbar dysfunction in these patients.[9]

Radiographic Assessment

In patients with inspiratory muscle weakness, lung volume often appears decreased on chest radiograph because of elevated bilateral hemidiaphragms. This radiographic picture can be easily dismissed as a poor inspiratory effort. The presence of bilateral basal platelike atelectasis is suggestive of chronic loss of lung volume resulting from weak respiratory muscles. Unilateral hemidiaphragm paralysis is recognized easily on routine chest radiograph as a unilateral elevated hemidiaphragm. The elevation of a hemidiaphragm resulting from paralysis can be confirmed by performance of a **sniff test** under fluoroscopy, which demonstrates paradoxic upward movement of the affected hemidiaphragm during a rapid sniff maneuver.

Assessment of Respiratory Muscle Function

Maximum Mouth Pressures

Maximum static respiratory pressures, measured at the airway opening during a voluntary contraction against an occluded airway, are the most sensitive tests to assess respiratory muscle dysfunction in patients with moderately advanced neuromuscular disease even in the absence of symptoms and normal ventilatory function.[16] The extent of respiratory muscle weakness can be quantified by measurement of the **maximum inspiratory pressure (PI_{max})** and **maximum expiratory pressure (PE_{max})** that can be generated by the respiratory muscles. Measurement of static mouth pressures are affected by lung volume. PI_{max} is greatest when measured near residual volume where the inspiratory muscles are at their optimum precontraction operating length. In contrast, PE_{max} is greatest when measured near total lung capacity, where the inward recoil of the respiratory system and the ability of the expiratory muscles to generate force is greatest. Table 57-3 shows normal values for maximum static inspiratory and expiratory muscle strength in adults. Reported values vary widely in different studies and may be due to differences in techniques utilized, or repeated measurements inducing a learning effect.

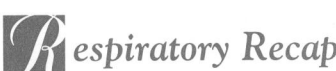espiratory Recap

Assessment of Respiratory Muscle Function

Maximum mouth pressures (inspiratory and expiratory)
Maximum voluntary ventilation
Transdiaphragmatic pressure measurement

In chronic neuromuscular disease, PI_{max} and PE_{max} are frequently decreased and range from 37% to 52% of normal.[12,28] In one study of 16 patients with a variety of chronic neuromuscular diseases, the mean static inspiratory pressure measured with an esophageal balloon was 43% of predicted.[22] Braun and colleagues[18] showed that in patients with proximal myopathies, hypercapnic respiratory failure was likely when the average PI_{max} and PE_{max} values were less than 30%, or vital capacity was less than

55% of predicted. A reduction in maximum static respiratory pressures also may be seen in patients with mild generalized nonrespiratory muscle weakness. Vincken and colleagues[17] evaluated 30 patients with stable chronic neuromuscular weakness and found that up to 30% of patients with relatively preserved general muscle strength had unsuspected severe respiratory muscle weakness (50% predicted). Based on Vincken's study, measurement of maximum static respiratory pressures should be routine in the assessment of respiratory status in neuromuscular disease patients regardless of the severity of the underlying neurologic disease or absence of respiratory symptoms.

Forced vital capacity (FVC) is also a useful index of global respiratory muscle function. It is also easy to measure and can be done serially at the bedside to predict impending respiratory failure and the need for ventilatory support. Ventilatory support is often required once FVC is less than 10 to 15 mL/kg or a PI_{max} less than 20 to 25 cm H_2O.[38] Mechanical ventilation may be required in select patients above these threshold values in the presence of additional respiratory loads such as occur with pneumonia, atelectasis, or inability to clear secretions. Although measurement of maximum static respiratory pressures or FVC is useful in quantification of global respiratory muscle strength, it does not distinguish selective weakness of certain respiratory muscle groups.

Maximum Voluntary Ventilation

Maximum voluntary ventilation (MVV) is a commonly performed maneuver, in which the subject is asked to breathe in and out as deep and as fast as possible for 12 to 15 seconds. It is a reflection of the global integrity of the respiratory system. MVV decreases with loss of coordination of the respiratory muscles, deformity of the thoracic bellows, neurologic diseases, and deconditioning. MVV is a useful test to assess respiratory muscle endurance. The MVV maneuver, however, is dangerous in patients with myasthenia gravis because it may precipitate acute respiratory failure.

Transdiaphragmatic Pressure Measurement

In contrast to maximum static pressures that measure global respiratory function, **transdiaphragmatic pressure (P_{di})** specifically measures diaphragm strength. Although transdiaphragmatic pressure measurement is more invasive and is not readily available in clinical practice, it may be useful in certain clinical conditions such as phrenic nerve paralysis after cardiac surgery or in cases of idiopathic diaphragm paralysis.

Measurement of P_{di} is made by measurement of esophageal (P_{es}) and gastric (P_{ga}) pressures via balloon-tipped catheters placed in the mid-esophagus and in the stomach, respectively. P_{di} is then calculated as the algebraic sum of P_{es} from P_{ga} [$P_{di} = P_{ga} - P_{es}$]. Several maneuvers with varying degrees of difficulty have been used during the measurement of P_{di} to obtain maximal voluntary activation of the diaphragm. P_{di} obtained during a maximal sniff maneuver is the easiest to perform, whereas maximal P_{di} obtained via a Mueller maneuver combined with active expulsive appears to be the most reproducible and maximal maneuver to measure transdiaphragmatic pressure.[8] Transdiaphragmatic pressure measurement is limited by the need for esophageal and gastric balloon placement and a variation in measured values as high as 40%.[39] The wide intrasubject variability of P_{di} is due to submaximal efforts or activation of the intercostal and accessory muscles, which results in falsely low P_{di} values.

Direct stimulation of the phrenic nerve, by consistent obtaining of maximal stimulation of the diaphragm, avoids variability in measured P_{di} when only volitional effort is used. The phrenic nerve is easily stimulated in the neck as it traverses the posterior border of the sternocleidomastoid-muscle at the level of the cricoid cartilage. Phrenic nerve stimulation may be performed with either a transcutaneous electrode or a magnetic coil.[40,41] Care should be taken to ensure supramaximal stimulation as indicated by the amplitude of the maximum diaphragm muscle action potential.

A single, unfused twitch contraction of the diaphragm following electrophrenic stimulation is known as $P_{diTWITCH}$. In a study involving 10 patients with diaphragm weakness and 20 normal subjects as controls, there was a large overlap in $P_{diTWITCH}$ between patients with diaphragm weakness (3 to 27 cm H_2O) and control subjects (9 to 33 cm H_2O).[42] The $P_{diTWITCH}$ was only consistently decreased when diaphragm weakness was severe. The appropriate role of electrophrenic stimulation in the assessment of respiratory muscle weakness is unclear and is considered a research tool.

Upper Motor Neuron Lesions

Stroke

Stroke, after an embolic or thrombotic vascular event, is one of the major causes of morbidity and mortality in developed countries. Because of the neuroanatomic and functional organization of the brain, different stroke syndromes have a predictable effect on the respiratory system that can be clinically recognized. For example, an acute hemispheric stroke may lead to loss of upper airway function and Cheyne-Stokes breathing, whereas a small stroke in the dorsolateral area of the medulla leads to sudden death because of respiratory arrest. The pulmonary consequences of the different stroke syndromes includes loss of upper airway function, abnormal breathing pattern, decreased diaphragmatic excursion, and loss of automatic or voluntary control of breathing.

Upper airway dysfunction resulting in swallowing incoordination is a common finding after stroke. This frequently leads to aspiration of oropharyngeal contents resulting in aspiration pneumonia. Different abnormal breathing patterns may be observed after an acute hemispheric stroke or in rostro-caudal loss of brain stem function, as in brain herniation, because of elevated intracerebral pressure. Hemispheric stroke often results in Cheyne-Stokes breathing, which is a breathing pattern characteristically described as cyclic hyperpnea and hypopnea often terminating in apnea. **Cheyne-Stokes breathing** is thought to be due to increased responsiveness to carbon dioxide as a result of interruption of normal cortical inhibition.[43] Brain stem stroke located in the midbrain may lead to central neurogenic hyperventilation, whereas apneustic and ataxic breathing may be seen after injury to the pontomedullary area of the brainstem. After an acute hemispheric stroke, voluntary contraction of the respiratory muscles is reduced on the side of hemiparesis as shown by EMG activity of the diaphragm and intercostal muscles.[11,44]

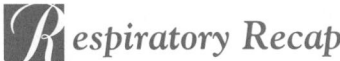 *espiratory Recap*

Stroke
Upper airway dysfunction results in swallowing incoordination. Cheyne-Stokes breathing may be present.

Respiration is under both voluntary and automatic control. The loss of automatic control of respiration (Ondine's curse) occurs after injury to the descending reticulospinal tract in the pons or the nucleus of the vagus, ambiguous, and para-ambiguous. The most common stroke syndrome associated with Ondine's curse is unilateral lateromedullary infarction.[45] A midpontine lesion, which results in the locked-in syndrome, may lead to a loss in the voluntary control of breathing.

Spinal Cord Injury

The degree of respiratory impairment and the need for chronic ventilator support depends on the level and extent of the spinal cord injury. After traumatic injury to the spinal cord, paresis or paralysis can be elicited easily at or below the level of spinal injury. High cervical cord injury above the origin of the phrenic nerve (C1-C3) leads to paralysis of all the major respiratory muscles except the accessory and bulbar muscles. All patients with high cervical injury invariably require chronic ventilator support. Injury at the level of the phrenic nerve roots (C3-C5) results in weakness or total paralysis of the diaphragm, requiring continuous ventilatory support. Lower cervical cord injury below the origin of the phrenic nerve (C5-C6) causes paralysis of the intercostal and abdominal muscles. However, because diaphragm function remains intact, the need for long-term ventilator support is obviated. However, these patients often require ventilatory support in the acute setting. Thus the requirement for chronic ventilatory support depends on the level of spinal injury, the ability of the accessory muscles to support ventilation, and the response to strengthening deconditioned muscles.

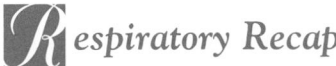 *espiratory Recap*

Spinal Cord Injury
All patients with high spinal cord injury require chronic respiratory support.
In patients with low cervical spinal cord injury, an ineffective cough leads to mucus retention, atelectasis, and pneumonia.

The effect of the level of spinal cord injury on the mechanical properties of the respiratory system is the same as in patients with chronic neuromuscular disease. Among the changes that may be seen on the respiratory system are (1) a reduction in inspiratory muscle strength to 60% of predicted; (2) a 20% to 30% reduction in both lung and chest wall compliance; and (3) a 50% to 80% reduction in predicted vital capacity with total lung capacity also moderately reduced.[46,47] The reduction in lung and chest wall compliance can be observed as early as the first week of injury and usually reaches its nadir by the first month after injury.[47] The reduction in lung compliance may be partly explained by the presence of small lung volumes resulting from airway closure and atelectasis. On the other hand, the reduction in chest wall compliance is thought to be due to stiffness and ankylosis of the rib cage resulting from a rapid-shallow breathing pattern and limited chest wall excursion.

In **tetraplegia** a paradoxic increase in FVC is measured in the supine compared with the seated position, without a significant increase in total lung capacity. The increase in FVC observed during the supine position is due to cephalad displacement in the end-expiratory position of the diaphragm as a result of gravitational effects of the abdominal visceral organs. The overall effect of these changes is to enable the diaphragm to operate on an optimal portion of its length-tension curve. Alternatively, the increase in FVC in the supine position may be due to a decrease in residual volume because total lung capacity is slightly decreased or unchanged. Estenne and De Troyer[49] reported that residual volume in both tetraplegia and paraplegia decreased by 30% to 38% of seated values, respectively. They showed that the decrease in RV was due to paralysis of the abdominal muscles and the effect of gravity on the abdominal contents. They further showed that the decrease in RV was not related to an abnormal increase in intrathoracic blood volume as a result of gravitational-induced fluid shifts.

In tetraplegic patients with relatively intact diaphragm function, paradoxic inward motion of the upper rib cage during inspiration occurs as a result of parasternal and

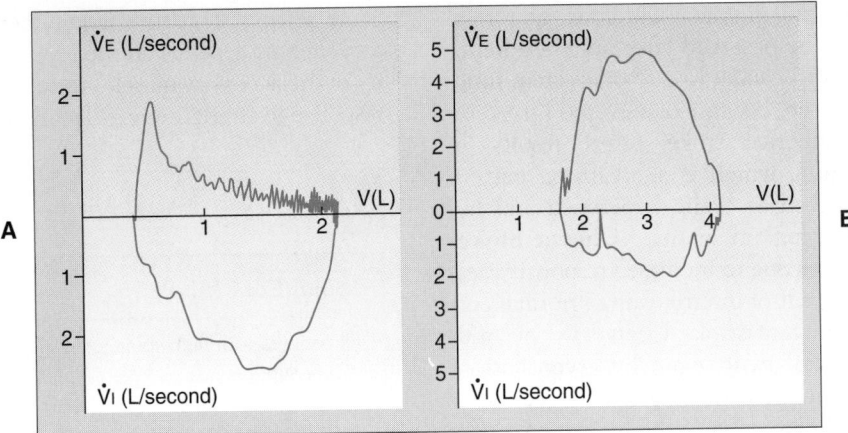

Figure 57-8   Two types of abnormal flow-volume loop in patients with extrapyramidal disorders. **A,** Type A flow-volume loop is characterized respiratory flutter, a regular consecutive flow deceleration and acceleration representing alternating abduction and adduction of the glottic opening. **B,** Type B flow-volume loop is characterized by grossly abnormal pattern with abrupt changes in flow indicating intermittent upper airway obstruction resulting from irregular jerky movements of the glottic structures $\dot{V}_E$, Expiratory flow; $\dot{V}_I$, inspiratory flow. (Modified from Vincken WG, Gauthier SG, Dollfuss RE, et al. Involvement of upper airway muscles in extrapyramidal disorders: a cause of airflow limitation. N Engl J Med 1984;311:438-442.)

scalene muscle weakness.[49,50] This abnormal pattern of breathing is even more marked in the supine position in contrast to when the subject is seated. In high tetraplegic patients (above C3-C5), short periods of spontaneous respiration are possible because of contraction of the sternocleidomastoid and trapezius muscles. Analysis of rib cage motion in these patients shows an increase in upper rib cage diameter because of the action of the neck accessory muscles in pulling the sternum cranially and expanding the upper rib cage.[46]

A common belief is that all of the expiratory muscles are paralyzed in low cervical cord injury. As a result, both cough and other expiratory maneuvers are passive and rely solely upon chest wall elastic recoil. An ineffective cough leads to mucus retention, atelectasis, and pneumonia.[51] Indeed pneumonia is still the leading cause of death in this subset of neurologically impaired patients.[52] Recently, De Troyer and colleagues[53] showed EMG activity of the clavicular portion of the pectoralis major during voluntary expiration and cough in patients with traumatic low cervical cord injury. Contraction of the clavicular portion of the pectoralis major decreases upper rib cage diameter during cough and can decrease expiratory reserve volume by 60% with the shoulders maintained in abduction. These findings suggest that an active cough can be generated by the clavicular portion of the pectoralis muscles in some tetraplegic patients. The authors concluded that abdominal binding with nonelastic straps to minimize dissipation of intrathoracic forces and training of the clavicular portion of the pectoralis muscle could further improve the effectiveness of cough in tetraplegic patients. Furthermore, 6 weeks of isometric training of the pectoralis muscle increases maximum pectoralis muscle isometric strength and thereby improves cough effectiveness.[54]

Parkinson's Disease

Parkinson's disease was first coined by James Parkinson in 1817 to describe a symptom complex of cogwheel rigidity, resting tremors, bradykinesia, shuffling gait, and postural instability. The disease affects about 1% of the population over 50 years of age and has a prevalence of 200 cases per 100,000 individuals.[55] Parkinsonism may be categorized as primary (for example, idiopathic) or secondary because of a variety of causes such as viral encephalitis and drugs. The pathologic findings in primary and secondary Parkinsonism are the same and are characterized by the degeneration of pigmented neurons in the substantia nigra resulting in disruptions of dopaminergic neural pathways.

Ventilatory failure, upper airway obstruction, and aspiration can complicate the clinical course of patients with Parkinson's disease. In fact, respiratory infection is the most common cause of death in these patients.[56] Both obstructive and restrictive ventilatory patterns have been noted on pulmonary function testing with about one third of patients with Parkinson's disease having an obstructive ventilatory defect. Both peak inspiratory and expiratory flows are reduced, which may be related to upper airway dysfunction. A concomitant restrictive ventilatory defect appear to be due to weakness and stiffness of the respiratory muscles.

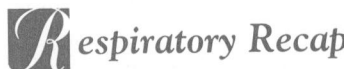

*R*espiratory Recap

Parkinson's Disease
Respiratory muscle dysfunction is common. Upper airway muscle dysfunction may occur. Aspiration is a common problem.

Respiratory muscle dysfunction is common in patients with Parkinson's disease. This is manifested usually as either a decrease in respiratory muscle strength or poor coordination, especially when repetitive ventilatory tasks are performed, similar to those observed in the limb muscles. Vincken and colleagues[8] showed that both maximum static inspiratory and expiratory pressures are reduced in Parkinson's disease. Poor muscle control as manifested by difficulty in the performance of repetitive inspiratory resistive efforts may be seen even in patients with normal pulmonary function and respiratory muscle strength. In addition, the performance of this maneuver was associated with a higher oxygen cost of breathing and a reduced efficiency of breathing.[57]

Vincken and colleagues[8] showed that upper airway muscles dysfunction is most likely the cause of the obstructive ventilatory pattern in patients with extrapyramidal disorders. In this study 24 out of 27 patients studied showed either regular (Type A, Figure 57-8, A) or irregular (Type B, Figure 57-8, B) flow oscillations on both the inspiratory and expiratory flow-volume loops. Oscillations on the flow-volume loop were due to upper airway muscle dyskinesia, which were confirmed by direct endoscopic evaluation. Some patients showed frank intermittent airway closure causing signs and symptoms of upper airway obstruction. A reduction in FEV_1 should alert the possibility of upper airway muscles dysfunction in patients with parkinsonism. The same group of authors reported improvement in upper airway obstruction after levodopa therapy in a patient with Parkinson's disease.[35] However, levodopa therapy may uncommonly induce respiratory dyskinesia that may be managed by a decrease in the dose of the medication or the use of dopamine antagonists.[58]

Patients with Parkinson's disease often complain of dyspnea and chronic tachypnea. The abnormal ventilatory pattern discussed above improves with levodopa treatment[59] and returns to baseline once therapy is stopped. Mehta and colleagues[60] reported modest improvement in FEV_1, FVC, and PEFR after 1 week of levodopa therapy in 9 out of 10 patients with Parkinson's disease. Four patients continued to have small sustained improvements in expiratory flow after 2 weeks of therapy. Patients who did not respond to levodopa therapy did not show improvement in ventilatory function.

Medications commonly used in the treatment of Parkinson's disease can cause pulmonary complications. Levodopa has been reported to cause dyspnea and respiratory distress, presumably because of respiratory muscle dyskinesia. Ergot derivatives such as bromocriptine can cause pleural effusion, pleural thickening, or pulmonary infiltrates.

Multiple Sclerosis

Multiple sclerosis (MS) is a demyelinating disease of the central nervous system clinically characterized by repeated remissions and exacerbations of symptoms. Multiple sclerosis is the most common neurologic disease affecting

Box 57-1

Patterns of Respiratory System Involvement in Multiple Sclerosis

> Paralysis of voluntary respiration
> Paralysis of automatic respiration
> Diaphragmatic paralysis
> Apneustic breathing
> Paroxysmal hyperventilation
> Obstructive sleep apnea
> Neurogenic pulmonary edema

young adults with an estimated prevalence of 250,000 to 300,000 cases in 1990.[61] The exact etiology of the disease remains elusive, although epidemiologic evidence points to both genetic and environmental factors. Classic clinical symptoms include paresthesias, motor weakness, diplopia, blurred vision, bladder incontinence, and ataxia. Symptoms are typically aggravated by an increase in temperature, which causes conduction block in partially demyelinated fibers. The disease may demonstrate remissions and relapses or follow a chronic progressive course. Pathologically, lesions or plaques have a predilection to involve the periventricular white matter of the cerebral hemisphere, the optic nerve, brain stem and the cervical spinal cord. Because multiple sclerosis can cause focal lesions anywhere in the central nervous system, different patterns of respiratory impairment can occur. Involvement of the respiratory centers in the medulla can affect either the voluntary or automatic breathing (Ondine's curse)[62,63] and produce apneustic breathing, paroxysmal hyperventilation, obstructive sleep apnea, or neurogenic pulmonary edema.[64] Box 57-1 lists the different patterns of respiratory involvement and their anatomic localization. The three most common patterns of respiratory involvement in multiple sclerosis includes respiratory muscle weakness, bulbar dysfunction, and abnormalities in respiratory control.[65]

Acute respiratory failure is rarely encountered in MS but can occur as a result of severe demyelination of the cervical cord.[66] Diaphragmatic paralysis resulting in respiratory insufficiency has also been reported.[67] More commonly, respiratory failure presents insidiously, affecting those only with

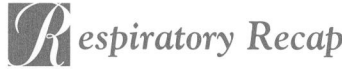

Respiratory Recap

Multiple Sclerosis
Expiratory muscles are more frequently involved than inspiratory muscles.
Advanced multiple sclerosis can be complicated by aspiration, atelectasis, and pneumonia.
Noninvasive ventilation may be useful in patients who do not have bulbar dysfunction.

advanced MS. Even with severe disability and impaired respiratory muscle function, patients with multiple sclerosis seldom complain of dyspnea. The paucity of respiratory complaints may be due to restricted motor activities and greater expiratory than inspiratory muscle weakness. Clinical signs that may help predict respiratory muscle involvement are a weak cough and the inability to clear secretions, a limited ability to count on a single exhalation, and the presence of upper extremity weakness.[68] Pulmonary dysfunction depends to a large extent on the severity of the disease and the functional capacity of the patient.

Expiratory muscles appear to be more frequently involved than the inspiratory muscles in patients with MS. Analysis of pulmonary function tests in 25 patients with varying severity of multiple sclerosis showed that FVC, MVV, and PE_{max} are normal in ambulatory MS patients but were severely reduced (39%, 32%, 36%, respectively) in bedridden patients.[68] Those patients who were wheelchair bound with upper extremity involvement also showed moderate reductions in FVC, MVV, and PE_{max}. In addition, patients who were quadriplegic and who exhibited prominent bulbar muscle involvement were at high risk for acute respiratory failure. Close respiratory monitoring is required in these patients. Arterial blood gas results are frequently normal even with abnormal respiratory muscle function results. Advanced multiple sclerosis is frequently complicated by aspiration, atelectasis, and pneumonia.

Treatment of multiple sclerosis includes adrenocorticotropic hormone (ACTH), high-dose corticosteroids, immunosuppressive agents such as cyclophosphamide and azathioprine, intravenous immunoglobulin therapy, and plasmapheresis. ACTH and prednisone have been shown to hasten the resolution of clinical symptoms in controlled studies.[69] Methylprednisolone 1 g daily for 5 days with or without prednisone taper may be helpful in MS patients with severe respiratory complications. Plasmapheresis has been shown to improve clinical symptoms in patients with severe acute exacerbation[33] and in the relapsing/remitting variety of MS with acute exacerbation.[70] A beneficial effect of intravenous immunoglobulin has been reported in patients with quadriplegia and respiratory failure after an attack of MS.

Both positive and negative noninvasive pressure ventilation have been successfully used in MS patients with intact bulbar function.[71,72] In the presence of bulbar dysfunction and respiratory failure, tracheostomy and positive pressure ventilation are usually required.

Lower Motor Neuron Lesions

Amyotrophic Lateral Sclerosis

Amyotrophic lateral sclerosis (ALS) is a progressive neurodegenerative disorder of both upper and lower motor neurons leading to a loss of skeletal muscle strength, including the respiratory muscles. The incidence of ALS is

one to two cases per 100,000 people. Males are more commonly affected than females with a ratio of 2:1 involvement. The majority of ALS cases are sporadic (classical ALS), but 5% to 10% of cases are due to an autosomal dominant inheritance (familial ALS). Death usually is due to progressive respiratory failure and repeated respiratory infections. Approximately 80% of ALS patients die within 5 years of initial diagnosis.

The exact etiology of ALS is unknown. A genetic mutation encoding copper-zinc superoxide dismutase, a free oxygen radical scavenger, has been identified in 10% to 15% of familial ALS patients, thus suggesting a susceptibility of the neurons to oxidative stress.[1] Recent evidence suggests that the motor neurons are susceptible to glutamate-induced neurotoxicity.[3] Glutamate is the principal excitatory brain neurotransmitter. A decreased uptake of glutamate may lead to overstimulation of the glutamate receptors leading to an increase in intracellular calcium, which then triggers proteolytic enzymes causing cell membrane injury.

The usual clinical presentation in two thirds of ALS patients is progressive weakness of the distal extremities, although early involvement of the bulbar muscles occurs in 25% of cases. Acute respiratory failure[29,73] and nocturnal hypoventilation[74] have been described as initial presentations of ALS. Early involvement of the phrenic nerve neurons within the cervical cord is implicated in this type of presentation.

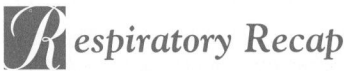
Respiratory Recap

ALS
Two thirds of patients with ALS present with progressive weakness of distal extremities; early involvement of bulbar muscles occurs in one fourth of patients.
Patients with ALS have progressive reductions of vital capacity and inspiratory and expiratory mouth pressures.
Despite optimal medical therapy, disease progression occurs and results in respiratory insufficiency.
The risk of death is decreased with the use of noninvasive ventilation.

Although respiratory muscle impairment is evident only in advanced stages of the disease, abnormalities in the pulmonary function tests are apparent even in patients with mild weakness of the extremities. Serial lung function studies in ALS patients who die show progressive reductions in FVC and MVV and progressive increases in RV compared with patients who survive.[10] Both PI_{max} and PE_{max} are reduced to 34% and 47% of predicted, respectively.[10,75] In ALS patients who are dyspneic but with relatively preserved pulmonary function tests, PI_{max} and PE_{max} are frequently abnormal.[75] A maximum static inspiratory pressure less negative than $^{-}60$ cm H_2O is 100% sensitive for the prediction of less than 18-month survival. However, FVC is the most specific test used to predict survival.[60]

Flow-volume curve shape may identify a subset of patients with greater expiratory muscle weakness. In patients with severe weakness of the expiratory muscles, the flow-volume loop will show a concavity of the maximal expiratory curve, with a sharp drop-off in flow at lower lung volumes. This group of ALS patients exhibit a lower PE_{max}, smaller VC, and higher RV compared with patients with more normal flow-volume loop contours.[76] Upper airway dysfunction may be detected by oscillations of the flow-volume loop or by direct laryngoscopy.[77,78] As the disease advances, FVC is reduced and RV is elevated, however, in contrast to other chronic neuromuscular diseases, TLC and FRC are relatively well preserved. These changes are due to earlier involvement of the abdominal muscles with preservation of intercostal and diaphragm function. Weakness of the abdominal muscles causes a reduction in MEP and an increase in RV. In addition, spasticity of the intercostal muscles may attenuate the stiffness of the chest wall, thus preserving lung volumes. More recent studies show that expiratory muscle weakness is often associated with inspiratory muscle weakness.[78] Adequate oxygenation is usually well maintained even with severe deterioration in spirometry. Arterial blood gas analysis is not useful in early disease. Spirometry, however, is still important in the initial evaluation of patients with ALS, because impairment in ventilatory function is frequently underestimated even by experienced examiners.[6]

The comprehensive management of ALS patients should include measures to alleviate symptoms and specific drug therapy to alter the progressive clinical course. Riluzole, an FDA-approved antiglutamate drug, is the only treatment that has shown to prolong survival in ALS.[79,80] It should be administered to patients once a diagnosis of ALS is made. Other antiglutamate drugs such as gabapentin or neurotrophic factors such as insulin-like growth factors, or glial-derived neurotrophic factor are currently under investigation.

Despite optimal medical therapy, disease progression invariably occurs, resulting in respiratory insufficiency that requires some form of ventilatory assistance. The onset of respiratory failure often signals a rapid decline in global and functional status. The need for mechanical ventilation should be discussed with the patient and family early to prevent rapid decline in lung function. In a survey of ALS patients, the majority of the patients considered mechanical ventilation during the early phase of their disease but eventually declined artificial ventilation as the disease progressed.[81] In ALS patients who develop respiratory symptoms or have a moderate or rapid reductions in lung function, noninvasive forms of ventilation should be considered. In patients who can tolerate nasal noninvasive positive pressure ventilation (NPPV), the risk of death is decreased a factor of 3:1.[82] More recently, Sherman and colleagues[83] studied 122 patients with ALS who were offered NPPV once they developed dyspnea, or

an FVC less than 50% or a fall of more than 15% in FVC in 3 months follow-up. Those patients who used NPPV more than 4 hours per day showed a slower decline in lung function and decreased mortality. Some patients with acute respiratory decompensation may have a partial improvement in respiratory muscle strength after a period of ventilatory assistance.[49]

Aminophylline has also been reported to improve respiratory muscle strength in ALS patients. Schiffman and Belsh[84] showed that theophylline significantly increased respiratory muscle strength after resistive breathing. The negative inspiratory pressure, FVC, and peak inspiratory flow increased by 28%, 10%, and 12%, respectively, in that study.

Poliomyelitis and Postpoliomyelitis Dystrophy

Poliomyelitis was the most common cause of respiratory failure in the early part of the twentieth century before the advent of the widespread use of the oral polio vaccine. Acute poliomyelitis is now rare in the United States and recent cases of poliomyelitis are due to exposure to oral polio vaccine and unimmunized individuals. Although most cases of acute polio infections are non-paralytic, as many as 25% of cases are the paralytic form of poliomyelitis, which leads to respiratory muscle weakness requiring assisted ventilation. In most cases, respiratory muscle function improves after the acute episode so that assisted ventilation is no longer required. However, progressive muscle weakness may occur years later.

Postpoliomyelitis dystrophy is recognized as a progressive muscle weakness occurring on average 29 years after recovery from an acute episode of acute poliomyelitis. Approximately 20% to 60% of poliomyelitis survivors will develop postpoliomyelitis syndrome with a mean age of onset of 51 years. These patients may complain of dyspnea, exercise intolerance, sleep-related symptoms such as daytime hypersomnolence, morning headaches, and muscle weakness. Muscles that were previously involved are primarily involved in this syndrome although other muscle groups may also be affected because of previous subclinical involvement.[85,86]

Several theories have been proposed to explain the pathogenesis of the postpolio syndrome, including susceptibility to aging of reinnervated motor units,[85-88] chronic

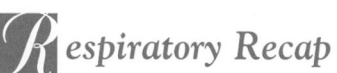

Respiratory Recap

Postpolio Syndrome
Approximately 20% to 60% of polio survivors develop this syndrome about 30 years after recovery from the acute episode.
It presents insidiously resulting from respiratory muscle weakness.
Sleep-disordered breathing is common with this syndrome.
Many of these patients benefit from NPPV.

compensatory overused of damage muscle fiber,[86,89] and immune-mediated attack on the abnormal motor units. The basic pathophysiology appears to be denervation and aberrant reinnervation of motor units.[86]

Postpoliomyelitis syndrome often presents insidiously as chronic respiratory failure secondary to respiratory muscle weakness. Serial monitoring of FEV_1, FVC and static respiratory pressures may help predict which subset of patients with a history of polio develop chronic respiratory failure.[70] The average yearly decline in FVC has been estimated at 18.6 mL/year or 1.9%. Once the VC is less than 1 L, assisted ventilation is often required.[34] Noninvasive ventilatory support is effective in reversing chronic hypoventilation and its associated symptoms.[34,90] Nocturnal noninvasive ventilation may also improve respiratory muscle strength and exercise capacity.[91]

Sleep-related breathing disorders are common in patients with postpolio syndrome,[85,92,93] even in patients who are already on nocturnal ventilatory support.[94] Hypersomnolence was the most common presenting symptom, present in 32 of 35 postpoliomyelitis patients.[95] The most frequently identified sleep-related breathing disorders were obstructive sleep apnea (19 of 35 patients), hypoventilation (7 of 35 patients), and mixed apnea and hypopnea (9 of 35 patients). Patients with bulbar dysfunction have a greater frequency of sleep apnea compared with those with intact bulbar muscle function.[93] Detailed questioning of sleep related symptoms during initial evaluation will select those patients with postpoliomyelitis syndrome who may benefit from a formal sleep study evaluation. Even patients who are already on nocturnal assisted ventilation may benefit from a sleep study, especially if they have daytime hypersomnolence, fatigue, and morning headache.

Postpoliomyelitis syndrome may also present as recurrent aspiration resulting from upper airway muscle weakness and vocal cord paralysis.[96] Asymmetric involvement of the thoracic muscles may lead to kyphoscoliosis and may further compromise respiratory muscle function. Central hypoventilation resulting from involvement of the brain stem respiratory center also has been reported.[97]

Disorders of the Peripheral Nerves

Phrenic Nerve Injury

Unilateral or bilateral diaphragm paralysis can occur after phrenic nerve injury. Phrenic nerve injury may be seen after cardiac surgery, trauma, mediastinal tumors, pleural space infection, or forceful neck manipulation.[98] Phrenic nerve injury during cardiac surgery is due to either cold exposure[97] or mechanical stretching of the nerve during surgery.[99] Diaphragm paralysis also may be seen with motor neuron disease, myelopathies, neuropathies, and myopathies. However, the majority of cases of diaphragm weakness are idiopathic.

Dyspnea is the main complaint of patients with bilateral diaphragm weakness, especially when they are lying down. Cranial displacement of the diaphragm by the abdominal visceral contents in the supine position can further impair the pump function of an already weakened diaphragm. Thus the presence of unexplained severe orthopnea and thoracoabdominal paradoxic breathing, especially in the supine position, are clinical clues to the presence of diaphragm dysfunction. Unilateral diaphragm weakness is usually well tolerated by patients even when the FVC and TLC are mildly reduced.

Bilateral diaphragm paralysis is identified as a restrictive ventilatory defect on pulmonary function testing. The VC is typically less than 50% of predicted in the erect posture. The chest radiograph typically shows either a unilateral or bilateral elevated hemidiaphragm(s), depending on the location of the phrenic nerve injury. However, both parenchymal and pleural diseases such as atelectasis, pulmonary fibrosis, or subpulmonic fluid collections may mimic the radiographic picture of diaphragm paralysis, making the diagnosis difficult and frequently even delayed.[100]

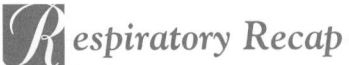

espiratory Recap

> **Phrenic Nerve Injury**
>
> Can be bilateral or unilateral
> Increased dyspnea in supine position
> Fluoroscopy (sniff test) useful for the diagnosis

Fluoroscopy can confirm diaphragmatic weakness or paralysis. The diaphragm is viewed under fluoroscopy while the patient performs a sniff (sniff test). The rapid decrease in intrapleural pressure during the sniff maneuver will cause a paradoxic cephalad movement of the weak hemidiaphragm. Fluoroscopy is not useful in bilateral diaphragm weakness because both hemidiaphragms may descend normally during a sniff maneuver despite profound weakness resulting from sudden relaxation of the abdominal muscles. The sniff test should be interpreted with caution because paradoxical diaphragmatic movement can be seen in up to 6% of normal individuals. The paradoxic movement should be at least 2 cm to increase the specificity of the test.

More recently ultrasound examination of the diaphragm has been reported as useful in the assessment of diaphragm contractile function.[101,102] This technique has the advantage of being rapid, easy to use, noninvasive, and avoids radiation exposure. The utility of this technique to assess diaphragm function in a variety of clinical scenarios is unclear at the present time and needs further study.

In patients with mild diaphragm weakness, both pulmonary function tests and radiographic examinations may be reported as normal. In this case, measurement of transdiaphragmatic pressure P_{di}, with all of its limitations (intersubject variability, invasive procedure, need for full patient cooperation), is useful in the diagnosis and quantitation of diaphragm weakness.[103] Total diaphragm paralysis is diagnosed when no pressure difference occurs across the two sides of the diaphragm (P_{di}=0) during forceful inspiratory maneuvers against an occluded airway.

Sleep may worsen ventilatory failure in patients with bilateral diaphragm paralysis because of a loss of respiratory accessory muscle activity during REM sleep. However, Laroche and colleagues[104] reported six patients with isolated bilateral diaphragm paralysis in whom significant nocturnal hypoventilation or daytime hypercapnia was not present. Recovery of diaphragm weakness depends on the etiology. In phrenic injury after cardiac surgery, 80% of patients will recover nerve function in 6 months and 90% in 1 year.[39]

Guillain-Barré Syndrome

Guillain-Barré syndrome (GBS) is an acute idiopathic polyneuritis usually presenting as an ascending symmetric paralysis of the lower extremities associated with absent tendon reflexes. The degree of motor weakness is variable, ranging from mild paresis to complete paralysis. Maximum weakness of the lower extremities occurs within 2 weeks in 50% of cases and 80% in 4 weeks. Facial (60%), ocular (15%), and oropharyngeal (50%) muscles may be involved. Pain over the extremities or flank is commonly reported as a "charlie horse." The objective findings of sensory loss are variable occurring in 40% to 70% of patients. Varying degrees of autonomic dysfunction such as cardiac arrhythmia, blood pressure lability, gastrointestinal dysfunction, pupillary dysfunction, sweating abnormalities, and urinary retention can occur in as many as 65% of patients as reported in one series.

Diagnostic criteria for GBS have been reported.[105] Other variants of GBS with asymmetric involvement of the extremities, presence of ataxia or the absence of paresthesia, also have been described. In more than 50% of cases, the syndrome is preceded by a history of a recent up-

per respiratory tract infection. The diagnosis of GBS is confirmed by abnormal CSF examination and nerve conduction studies. The cerebrospinal fluid examination characteristically shows an increased protein content with a paucity of cells commonly referred to as *albuminocytologic dissociation*. Nerve conduction study typically shows multifocal demyelination.

Although the exact etiology of GBS is unknown, several risk factors have been identified that may precipitate the disease. These risk factors include viral illnesses (cytomegalovirus, Epstein-Barr virus), *Mycoplasma pneumoniae* infection, influenza vaccination, recent surgery, and malignancy (lymphoma). A strong association between antecedent *Campylobacter jejuni* infection and GBS has also been found.

Respiratory failure requiring assisted ventilation occurs in 15% to 30% of cases.[106,107] However, once respiratory muscle dysfunction is evident and requires ICU care, up to 62% of patients will require ventilatory assistance. The average duration of mechanical ventilation in two large series was 50 to 55 days.[106,108,109] Most patients require tracheostomy because of the need for prolonged mechanical ventilation and to facilitate pulmonary hygiene. Ropper[108] suggested that tracheostomy be delayed up to 10 days to avoid the procedure in patients who rapidly improve.

A severe reduction in maximum P_{di} has been documented during acute ventilatory failure and during recovery from the illness.[110] Among the pulmonary function tests, serial VC measurement is the most useful test used to predict the need for mechanical ventilation. Several studies have shown that a VC of 12 to 15 mL/kg is a sign of imminent respiratory failure.[106,108,109,111] In patients who developed respiratory failure resulting from Guillain-Barré syndrome, the VC measured serially decreased from a mean of 2.5 L to 0.9 L within 2 weeks. Other indications for intubation and ventilatory support include respiratory distress, inability to handle oral secretions, hypoxemia (PaO_2 70 mm Hg breathing room air or alveolar-arterial O_2 difference of 300 mm Hg with FIO_2 of 100%) and hypercapnia. Early intubation and assisted ventilation is preferred as previously outlined to avoid complications that may arise from emergent intubation. Arterial blood gas analysis is used to ensure adequate oxygenation and ventilation. Hypercapnia is a late sign of ventilatory failure. The average PCO_2 at the time of intubation when VC is less than 12 mL/kg was 43 mm Hg in two large series of GBS patients.[109]

Upper airway dysfunction resulting from bulbar involvement may occur in GBS. This may lead to inability to swallow oral secretions, increasing the risks of aspiration. The presence of nasal voice, abnormal gag reflex, dysarthria, and poor mobility of pharyngeal muscles suggest significant bulbar muscle dysfunction. The swallowing mechanism can be assessed roughly at the bedside when the patient is asked to drink sips of water and then is observed for coughing. Once significant bulbar dys-

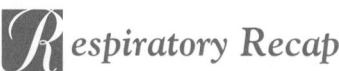

*R*espiratory Recap

Guillain-Barré Syndrome
It presents as an ascending symmetric paralysis.
15% to 30% of patients develop respiratory failure requiring assisted ventilation.
Upper airway dysfunction due to bulbar involvement may occur.
Measurements of vital capacity and maximum mouth pressure are useful to follow the course of disease.
Aggressive pulmonary toilet is an important part of the care of these patients.

function is observed, early intubation may be necessary to protect the airway even if respiratory muscle strength is adequate.

Aggressive pulmonary toilet is indicated to prevent and treat atelectasis. Atelectasis may require repeated bronchoscopy and may decrease the incidence of nosocomial pneumonia.[106] Subcutaneous heparin is preferred for deep venous thrombosis prophylaxis compared with pneumatic boots to avoid prolonged foot dropped because of compression of the peroneal nerve. Corticosteroids are not beneficial and may be harmful. Weaning may be started once VC exceeds 8 to 10 mL/kg, adequate oxygenation can be achieved with FIO_2 of 40% or less, and patients are able to double their minute ventilation. The PI_{max} at the time of successful weaning is more negative than 40 cm H_2O. In two multicenter trials, plasmapheresis (250 mL/kg every 2 days for a total of five treatments) with either albumin or fresh frozen plasma as replacement fluids showed short-term benefits in early motor recovery and ambulation, reduced the number of patients who required assisted ventilation and shortened the duration of mechanical ventilation.[112,113] Immunotherapy should be started within 2 weeks of onset of symptoms or as early as possible. However, in patients with rapidly deteriorating clinical symptoms, plasmapheresis may still offer some benefit even if the duration of the disease is more than 3 weeks.[108] Intravenous immunoglobulin (IVIG) given within 2 weeks of the onset of GBS may be as effective as plasma exchange therapy.[114] Further study is needed before IVIG will be the preferred treatment modality in GBS.

With the advent of modern ICU care, mortality from Guillain-Barré syndrome has dropped from 15% in the 1970s to 3% to 4% in the 1980s. Common complications are pneumonia, recurrent aspiration, and pulmonary thromboembolic disease. Prognosis for recovery is generally good, but 15% of patients have neurologic residuals. Factors associated with poor prognosis are older age, lower mean compound muscle action potential amplitudes during distal stimulation, and need for ventilatory support.

Critical Illness Polyneuropathy

Acute weakness syndrome acquired in the ICU is now increasingly recognized as a common sequelae of sepsis and multiorgan failure since its initial description 2 decades ago. Four categories of the syndrome are recognized and are shown in Table 57-4. The syndrome is often suspected initially because of failure to wean from mechanical ventilation as patients recover from their life-threatening illnesses or the development of flaccid and areflexic limbs.[115] Patients with this syndrome have no history of neuropathy or myopathy. They usually have prolonged ICU stay, documented evidence of sepsis, and clinical and laboratory findings of multisystem organ failure.[65] About one third of these patients have difficulty weaning from the ventilator, whereas 70% have evidence of peripheral neuropathy.[116]

TABLE 57-4

Acute Weakness Syndrome in the Intensive Care Unit

Mechanism	Manifestation
Myopathy	Acute necrotizing myopathy, disuse atrophy
Neuromuscular junction abnormalities	Myasthenia-like syndrome, prolonged neuromuscular blockade
Neuropathy	Critical illness polyneuropathy Acute motor neuropathy
Polyneuro-myopathy	Combination of neuropathy and myopathy

The diagnosis of **critical care polyneuropathy** is confirmed by EMG studies, which show primary axonal polyneuropathy rather than demyelination as suggested by the reduction in the amplitude of the compound action potential without significant prolongation of the conduction latency period.

For those patients who survive their critical illness, the clinical course of ICU acquired polyneuropathy or myopathy is usually benign, although clinical recovery of nerve function is usually prolonged but complete in 6 months to 1 year. Possible etiologies of critical care polyneuropathy include toxic metabolic causes such as hyperglycemia causing nerve ischemia by endovascular shunting[117] or nerve toxins generated from multiple organ failure. Possible causes of myopathy includes delayed clearance of the 3-desacetyl metabolite of vecuronium resulting from renal failure, steroid induced myopathy, and protracted use of neuromuscular blocking agents.[118]

Disorders of the Neuromuscular Junction

Myasthenia Gravis

Myasthenia gravis (MG) is an autoimmune disorder characterized by impaired transmission of neural impulses across the neuromuscular junction resulting from the destruction of the postsynaptic acetylcholine receptors. The typical presentation of the myasthenic patient is fluctuating weakness of the involved voluntary muscles, improvement with rest and/or with the administration of anticholinesterase agents (positive Tensilon test). The prevalence of the disease is estimated at 43 to 84 patients per million. The disease typically affects younger women and older men. Ocular, facial, and neck muscles are commonly involved. Generalized weakness is seen in advanced cases with involvement of the diaphragm and other respiratory muscles. Thymic tumors are seen in 10% of cases, mostly in older men. Antibodies to acetylcholine receptors are seen in 80% of patients with generalized myasthenia and 60% of ocular myasthenia. Electrodiagnostic study is nonspecific for MG but characteristically shows a 10% to 15% decrease in amplitude of the action potential during slow repetitive stimulation. The major cause of death in patients with MG is pulmonary infections.

Respiratory muscle weakness can occur in the absence of peripheral muscle weakness.[119,120] However, respiratory muscle weakness in MG typically occurs late in the disease process. In patients with moderately generalized MG, performance of pulmonary function tests before the administration of Mestinon reveal mild reduction in FVC and moderate reduction in both maximum static inspiratory (46% of predicted) and expiratory pressures (48% of predicted). No evidence exists of restrictive or obstructive lung disease. Like other chronic neuromuscular diseases, the breathing pattern of patients with MG is rapid and shallow. After Mestinon treatment, FVC, FEV$_1$, PI$_{max}$, and PE$_{max}$ show significant improvement, although respiratory muscle strength does not completely normalize.[5] Arterial blood gas examination is unreliable in predicting the severity of respiratory muscle weakness.

Acute respiratory failure usually occurs in the setting of either myasthenic, cholinergic, brittle crisis, or as the initial presentation of the disease.[121] Myasthenic crisis refers to the worsening of the basic underlying disease process. This is precipitated usually by discontinuation or decrease in the dosage of anticholinergic medications, surgery (thymectomy), administration of neuromuscular blocking medications (aminoglycosides, curare-like drugs), and emotional crisis. Myasthenic crisis can be confirmed with tensilon testing, which results in an improvement in muscle strength. Cholinergic crisis refers to the worsening of motor weakness as a result of an excess of anticholinesterase medications, which causes depolarizing blockade at the myoneural junction. This can be diagnosed and differentiated from myasthenic crisis by the presence of muscarinic symptoms such as hypersalivation, sweating, an increase in bronchial secretions, nausea and vomiting, and diarrhea. In addition, these symptoms may worsen with tensilon testing. Nicotinic symptoms such as fasciculations and cramps are rare. A brittle crisis occurs when the disease is difficult to treat, and the patient alternates between myasthenic and cholinergic crises.

The most common cause of respiratory failure is surgery (usually after thymectomy) followed by myasthenic and cholinergic crises. In a series of 22 patients reported by Gracey and colleagues,[122] the mean duration of mechanical ventilation was 8 days with six patients (32%) requiring tracheostomy for prolonged mechanical ventilation. Postoperative care of these patients is important because respiratory failure occurs usually within 24 hours of surgery in more than 50% of patients. Serial measurements of VC and PI$_{max}$ can help detect the onset of respiratory failure. It is important to remember that the dosing schedule of anticholinesterase medications will affect the measurement of respiratory parameters. The maximum improvement in respiratory muscle strength occurs about

2 hours after the drug is given and slowly declines before the next dose is given. Consequently, VC, PI$_{max}$, and PE$_{max}$ should be measured 30 minutes before the next dose of anticholinesterase agents. Once VC is less than 15 mL/kg, and PI$_{max}$ is less than 30 cm H$_2$O, assisted ventilation should be considered.

Upper airway obstruction resulting from vocal cord paralysis and recurrent aspiration resulting from bulbar involvement may occur in myasthenia gravis. Flow-volume loop analysis may show variable extrathoracic airway obstruction with the characteristic inspiratory plateau in cases of upper airway obstruction. Several clinical parameters were proposed as predictors of postoperative respiratory failure after thymectomy.[122] Severity of disease, especially with the presence of bulbar symptoms and low VC, appears to be the most important factor in the prediction of postoperative respiratory failure.

Respiratory Recap

Myasthenia Gravis

- Presentation is fluctuating weakness of the involved voluntary muscles, improvement with rest and/or administration of anticholinesterase agents.
- Respiratory muscle involvement is common and can be assessed with pulmonary function testing before and after administration of anticholinesterase agents.
- A myasthenic crisis is confirmed with a tensilon test.
- A cholinergic crisis occurs because of an excess of anticholinesterase medications.
- A brittle crisis occurs when the disease is difficult to treat.
- The most common cause of respiratory failure is surgery.
- Treatment involves anticholinesterase agents, high dose steroids, and plasmapheresis.

Sleep-related breathing disturbances may occur in patients with myasthenia gravis. Abnormal sleep study results in MG patients usually reveal mixed central apneas and hypopneas. Patients should be asked for sleep-related symptoms such as daytime hypersomnolence, nocturnal and early morning awakening, and morning headaches. Older patients with moderate obesity and daytime alveolar hypoventilation, and restrictive lung defect should undergo sleep study to screen for sleep apnea and nocturnal hypoventilation. A recent study suggests that the incidence of sleep apnea is higher in patients with a longer duration of MG.[123]

Treatment of MG includes anticholinesterase agents, high-dose corticosteroids, and plasmapheresis in patients who are refractory to steroids and immunosuppressive therapy. Anticholinesterase agents are the first line of treatment. Most patients will improve significantly with this treatment, but only a few patients will regain normal function. Remission can be induced in up to 80% of patients with corticosteroids. However, initiation of corticosteroid therapy may cause temporary worsening of muscle weakness, usually on the sixth to tenth day of therapy. Close observation for signs of respiratory insufficiency is advisable. Other immunosuppressive agents (azathioprine, cyclosporin) are also useful in MG either alone or in combination with steroids. Thymectomy also has been shown, in retrospective study, to improve survival and clinical symptoms even in the absence of thymoma in patients with myasthenia gravis compared with patients who were treated medically.[124] In patients who are less than 55 years old, thymectomy is recommended to prevent malignant transformation of the thymoma. Up to 80% of patients with no thymoma improve clinically following thymectomy, but the response may be delayed. Plasmapheresis may be beneficial in patients with fulminant MG who are not responding to conventional treatment.[125]

Eaton-Lambert Syndrome

Eaton-Lambert syndrome is a rare, myasthenic-like disorder resulting from a reduction of transmitter release from presynaptic terminals. The disease is commonly associated with small cell carcinoma of the lung. Unlike MG, limb and girdle muscles predominantly are involved instead of ocular and bulbar muscles. Although respiratory failure is infrequent, respiratory muscle weakness is often detected on pulmonary function tests.

Botulism

Botulism is a rare disorder caused by toxin produced by *Clostridium botulinum*. The toxin may be ingested by improperly cooked food, wound contamination by the organisms, or absorption of the toxin from the gastrointestinal tract, particularly in infants. There are eight types of toxins, although human disease is caused by types A, B, or E. Botulinum toxin binds with calcium channel in the presynaptic terminals, impairing neuromuscular transmission of acetylcholine. Gastrointestinal symptoms predominate early in the course of the disease, followed by neurologic impairment including descending paralysis of the neck, trunk, and limb muscles. Weakness of the respiratory muscles requiring ventilatory support is frequent especially with botulinum type A toxins. Spirometry usually reveals a restrictive ventilatory defect. Recovery from respiratory muscle weakness may take months, requiring prolonged ventilatory support. The average duration of ventilatory support for type A poisoning is 58 days, in contrast to 26 days in type B botulism.[48] Exertional dyspnea and poor exercise tolerance may persist even with normal lung function.

Inherited Myopathies

Muscular dystrophy refers to a heterogeneous group of progressive, hereditary degenerative skeletal muscle diseases. The respiratory muscles, like any skeletal muscle, be-

come progressively weak, eventually culminating in respiratory failure and death. In fact, respiratory complications are the most common cause of death in these diseases.

Duchenne Muscular Dystrophy

Duchenne muscular dystrophy (DMD) is the most well characterized of the hereditary familial muscle diseases. The disease is transmitted via an X-linked recessive gene, although about one third of cases may be due to spontaneous mutation. The disease is due to the mutation of the gene for skeletal protein dystrophin. The diagnosis can be confirmed by a mutation of the dystrophin gene in DNA from peripheral leukocytes or by the absence or abnormal dystrophin gene in muscle biopsy. Patients are usually symptomatic early in life. Early presenting symptoms are gait disturbances and delayed motor development. Cardiomyopathy is common but only rarely leads to significant cardiac dysfunction. Physical examination shows limb-girdle muscle weakness and pseudohypertrophy of the calf muscles. Most of the patients are wheelchair bound by the age of 15 years. Despite modern respiratory care and better understanding of the abnormal pulmonary mechanics of this disease, survival after the age of 25 is rare.

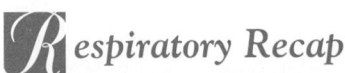
espiratory Recap

Duchenne Muscular Dystrophy
This sex-linked recessive disorder produces muscle weakness.
Progression of the disease is followed with measurements of vital capacity and maximum mouth pressures.
Kyphoscoliosis is common and can contribute to the respiratory failure.
Respiratory muscle weakness is progressive and ultimately requires ventilatory assistance.
NPPV is initially used, but many patients ultimately require tracheostomy.

Pulmonary symptoms are often minimal early in the course of disease despite significant weakness of the respiratory muscles. Serial pulmonary function tests and few select ancillary procedures such as chest radiograph and polysomnography can detect the severity of respiratory muscle weakness and the onset of secondary complications such as scoliosis, abnormal chest wall mechanics, atelectasis resulting from ineffective cough, and sleep-related breathing disorders. Forced vital capacity and maximum static respiratory pressures when done correctly and in serial fashion are simple and reproducible tests that are useful in the assessment of respiratory muscle strength. However, VC increases with growth during the first decade and may mask early respiratory muscle dysfunction before it plateaus and progressively decreases after 12 years of age, with VC decreasing by about 5% to 6% per year. PI_{max} is more useful during the formative years because it declines gradually despite body growth. Once the initial screening tests showed respiratory muscle dysfunction, a more complete battery of pulmonary tests may be needed to further define respiratory muscle endurance, the extent of expiratory muscle weakness, selective weakness of specific respiratory muscle groups, and abnormalities in lung and chest wall mechanics. Kyphoscoliosis is common and may contribute to restrictive ventilatory defect.

Maximum voluntary ventilation can help detect respiratory muscle fatigue but should be avoided in severely weakened patients. Measurement of PE_{max} is important because involvement of the expiratory muscles will lead to ineffective cough and inability to handle airway secretions. Because PI_{max} measures global inspiratory muscle strength, predominant involvement of the diaphragm may be missed unless P_{di} is measured. This procedure, however, is invasive and many patients may not be able to tolerate the procedure. Alternatively, weakness of the diaphragm could be in inferred noninvasively by greater than 25% decrement in VC from the seated to supine position and by fluoroscopic visualization of diaphragmatic excursion (sniff test). These noninvasive tests, however, are not sensitive in mild diaphragm weakness.

Although respiratory muscle weakness is progressive, hypercapnia is uncommon in the absence of complicating pulmonary infections. The maintenance of alveolar ventilation in early disease suggests that patients with DMD have intact diaphragm function until late in the course of the disease.[26,126] Once hypercapnia occurs, the course is rapidly progressive and prognosis is poor. Mean duration of survival after onset of hypercapnia is about 10 months.[127] Hypoxemia resulting from ventilation perfusion inequality is common in moderate to severe disease states.

Because ventilation is accomplished primarily by the diaphragm in patients with muscular dystrophy, nocturnal hypoventilation may occur during sleep, especially during REM sleep when activity of the chest wall and neck muscles are abolished. Indeed REM-induced hypoventilation has been documented in patients with normal daytime gas exchange.[91,128,129] Sleep-related hypoxemia may contribute to respiratory insufficiency and to the development of cor pulmonale. Hypoxemia is worse during REM sleep when the contribution of the accessory muscles are abolished. Supplemental oxygen may prolong the episode of hypopnea and apnea but does not appear to be clinically significant.[128] Noninvasive positive pressure ventilation (NPPV) has been used successfully in patients with sleep-disordered breathing and DMD.[129,130] In a study of 10 patients with DMD who had pronounced nocturnal oxygen desaturation but with normal daytime blood gases, nocturnal NPPV was successfully used to prevent nocturnal oxygen desaturation. The progressive decline in lung function appeared to be attenuated with NPPV up to 2 years in follow-up.[129]

Management of DMD is mainly supportive. Ambulation should be maintained and encouraged as long as pos-

sible to retard the development of scoliosis. Surgical correction of severe scoliosis may help partially correct the restrictive ventilatory defect, although recent studies show no significant improvement in respiratory function in patients who underwent spinal fusion surgery. Physiotherapy is important in the prevention of contractures. Patients with chronic neuromuscular disease are at risk for respiratory muscle fatigue, because weakened respiratory muscles are working against a high elastic load to maintain the same degree of alveolar ventilation. Inspiratory resistive breathing may be beneficial in this regard but awaits further study.[131] Certainly, vigorous respiratory training could be hazardous in patients with advanced disease, because it may increase the ventilatory burden on already weakened respiratory muscles.

Proper nutrition is important in the maintenance of respiratory muscle function; VC declines as nutritional status deteriorates. In addition, maximum static respiratory pressures correlate with body mass in both healthy and malnourished persons.[132] High-protein, low-calorie diets aiming to achieve ideal weight may be beneficial.[133,134]

Assisted ventilation is required once signs of respiratory insufficiency or symptoms of sleep-related breathing disorders are present. Once VC falls between 300 to 950 mL, assisted ventilation is often required. Chronic hypercapnic respiratory failure usually develops when VC is between 500 to 700 mL. Intermittent nasal positive pressure ventilation has been shown to prolong survival and attenuate the decline in VC and MVV in a small controlled study involving patients with advanced DMD.[127] Successful long-term assisted ventilation has been reported in DMD. Intermittent NPPV may be used initially for chronic alveolar ventilation, but all patients eventually require positive pressure ventilation via a tracheostomy as the disease advances. Tracheostomy is eventually needed to provide access to the airway secretions in patients who are too weak to cough. The use of prednisone has recently been shown to increase the number of years of effective ambulation and to prevent the decline in VC and PI_{max}.[135,136]

Myotonic Dystrophy

Myotonic dystrophy is the most common form of hereditary muscular dystrophy in adults with an estimated incidence of 1 in 8000 persons. The myotonic dystrophy gene, which is transmitted in autosomal dominant pattern, is located on the long arm of chromosome 19.[137] Symptoms usually present during adolescence and early adulthood, although the syndrome may be recognized in infancy.

Chronic respiratory failure is common in myotonic dystrophy even in the presence of mild limb muscle weakness.[138] This is due to the presence of several factors other than respiratory muscle weakness such as decreased respiratory system compliance, low central ventilatory drive, and sleep-related breathing disorders that act in concert to impair lung function. Myotonic respiratory muscles can contribute to an increased work of breathing by increasing the impedance to breathing. Weakness of the expiratory muscles are much more severe compared with the inspiratory muscles in these patients. However, weakness of the inspiratory muscles becomes severe once proximal muscle weakness becomes apparent, heralding the onset of alveolar hypoventilation.[138]

Early studies showed a high incidence of hypercapnia and blunted ventilatory response to CO_2 suggesting abnormal central respiratory drive.[139] However, subsequent studies have shown that these patients have either normal or high central ventilatory drive.[7,12] The abnormal ventilatory response to both hypoxia and hypercapnia has been attributed to respiratory muscle weakness and fatigue. In addition, these patients may have a chaotic breathing pattern resulting from impaired afferent input from the respiratory muscles. Daytime hypersomnolence, possibly resulting from a low central ventilatory drive or sleep apnea, may contribute to the high prevalence of chronic hypercapnia in these patients.[138]

Patients with myotonic dystrophy are particularly susceptible to general anesthesia and respiratory depressants. Avoidance of general anesthesia and muscle relaxants are recommended. If surgery is required, postoperative respiratory monitoring is required. The presence of pharyngeal and laryngeal dysfunction manifesting as nasal speech increases the risks of aspiration. Sleep-related breathing disorders are common in myotonic dystrophy. Central and obstructive sleep apnea may occur.[140] Nocturnal nasal positive pressure ventilation should be tried once hypercapnia (PCO_2 greater than 50 mm Hg) and hypoxemia occur (arterial O_2 saturation less than 85%).

Acid Maltase Deficiency

The muscle cell, similar to all metabolically active cells in the body, requires chemical energy stored in adenosine triphosphate (ATP). The regeneration of ATP high-energy phosphate bonds requires the availability of carbohydrate, fatty acids, and ketones. Enzymatic defects in the metabolism of carbohydrates (glycogen) leads to an abnormal accumulation of glycogen in the liver, kidney, and cardiac and skeletal muscles.

Acid maltase deficiency is a type II glycogen storage disease that arises because of a deficiency of the lysosomal enzyme responsible for the hydrolysis of both the α_{1-4} and α_{1-6} linkages of the glycogen. The disease presents in three clinical forms: infantile, childhood, and adult form. In adult onset disease, the age of onset is usually after 20 years of age. The syndrome typically presents with truncal and proximal limb weakness. Respiratory muscle weakness invariably leads to respiratory failure and REM-associated breathing disturbances. Severe weakness of the diaphragm, out of proportion to limb muscle weakness, may be the predominant clinical manifestation of the disease, which results in respiratory failure. These patients are often misdiagnosed because of the presence of non-specific symptoms of fatigue, hypersomnolence, morning

headaches, and orthopnea. The diagnosis of diaphragm weakness is suspected when paradoxic motion of the abdomen on inspiration is evident, leading to additional neurologic evaluation.[141] Autopsy studies have shown predominant involvement of the proximal respiratory muscles reflecting predominance of type 1 muscle fibers, which are less efficient in the synthesis and storage of glycogen than type 2 muscle fibers.

Diagnostic studies reveal elevated serum muscle enzymes, myopathic changes on EMG, and vacuoles with glycogen content on muscle biopsy. The diagnosis is confirmed by reduced acid maltase content in muscle and urine assays. Inspiratory muscle training and a high-protein diet may be beneficial.[142]

Fascioscapulohumeral Dystrophy

Fascioscapulohumeral dystrophy (FSHD) is an autosomal dominant dystrophy that affects primarily the face and the proximal portion of the upper extremities. The defective gene has been localized to chromosome 4q35. The disease is slowly progressive with long periods of disease inactivity. The disease usually affects children and young adults between the ages of 6 and 20. The initial manifestations of the disease usually are difficulty in raising of the arms above the head and winging of the scapula (angel-wing appearance). Facial weakness is manifested by the inability to close the eyes, purse the lips, and whistle. In 20% of the patients with FSHD, the disease also affects pelvic girdle and trunk muscles, which may impair respiratory function. Spirometry often shows decreased FVC but facial weakness makes the test unreliable because of poor lip seal.

Limb-Girdle Muscular Dystrophy

Limb-girdle muscular dystrophy is a heterogenous group of muscle dystrophies that is characterized mainly by weakness of the shoulder and pelvic girdles with sparing of the facial muscles. The mode of inheritance is variable, but the recessive forms are the most common. Similar to other congenital myopathies, symptoms usually become evident during childhood or early adult life. Late onset disease usually has a benign course. Hypercapnic respiratory failure is uncommon even with moderate respiratory muscle weakness. However, bilateral paresis of the diaphragm may lead to ventilatory failure. Cardiac involvement is rare.

Mitochondrial Myopathy

Mitochondrial myopathy, one of the manifestations of hereditary mitochondrial disorders, results from a point mutation in mitochondrial DNA (gene mutation at 3250). This group of mitochondrial disorders also can affect other organ systems, particularly the brain. The mitochondrial disorders that manifest polymyopathy as part of the syndrome include (1) myoneural-gastrointestinal encephalopathy; (2) myoclonic epilepsy, ragged red fibers; and (3) mitochondrial encephalomyopathy, lactic acidosis, and stroke. The disease may present initially in childhood or adulthood. The usual clinical manifestations are symmetric proximal muscle weakness that occurs in isolation or in association with central nervous system dysfunction or metabolic derangements as described in the syndromes listed above. Acute respiratory failure as the initial presentation of the disorder also has been reported.[143] Muscle biopsy is often required to confirm the diagnosis. Modified trichome stains show-marked enlargement of the mitochondria with a reddish tinge, the ragged red fibers. No specific treatment is available. The use of sedative drugs should be avoided.

Acquired Inflammatory Myopathies

Systemic Lupus Erythematosus

Systemic lupus erythematosus (SLE) is an autoimmune disease that can affect almost all of the organ systems. The pulmonary complications of SLE can be classified as (1) pleuritis and pleural effusions, (2) acute lupus pneumonitis, (3) interstitial lung disease, and (4) respiratory muscle weakness. Respiratory muscle weakness and diaphragm muscle dysfunction may occur without significant limb weakness. Up to 25% of patients with SLE may have significant diaphragm weakness even in the absence of generalized myopathy.[144] The diaphragm weakness can be apparent on the chest radiograph, which shows bilateral diaphragm elevation, coined by Hoffbrand as the shrinking lung syndrome.[145]

Acute ICU Myopathy

Acquired ICU myopathy is increasingly recognized as an important cause of weakness in the ICU, contributing to weaning failure from mechanical ventilation. In a recent study evaluating the causes of neuromuscular weakness in the intensive care unit, Lacomis and colleagues[146] retrospectively reviewed the clinical data of 92 patients who had EMG studies for the evaluation of muscle weakness; 89 had evidence of a neuromuscular abnormality. The most common causes of weakness in these patients by EMG criteria was myopathy (46%) and peripheral neuropathy (28%). Only four of the patients in this group had a preexisting myopathy that contributed to their admission to the ICU. Various neuromuscular diseases such as Guillain-Barré syndrome, myasthenia gravis, amyotrophic lateral sclerosis, and myopathy (acquired before ICU admission) accounted for only 28% of all patients. Thus 75% of the patients studied in this series had an acquired ICU weakness syndrome. Similar to previous studies, sepsis and multiple organ dysfunction are risk factors for the development of critical care myopathy and polyneuropathy. In addition, organ transplant recipients who suffer organ re-

jection also appear to be at increased risk for an ICU acquired myopathic syndrome. High-dose intravenous corticosteroids and prolonged used of neuromuscular blockade have been implicated in ICU acquired myopathy, especially in the presence of renal failure.[147,148] The use of corticosteroids and neuromuscular blocking agents is associated with a higher incidence of muscle weakness (129%) compared with the use of corticosteroids alone (0%).[149] In addition, the risk of muscle weakness increases with the duration of paralysis. Biopsy of the involved muscle usually reveals muscle fiber atrophy, vacuolar muscle necrosis, and loss of myosin thick filaments.

Chronic Steroid Myopathy

Unlike the acute myopathy recently described in the ICU setting, **chronic steroid myopathy** results from the prolonged use of corticosteroids. It usually manifests itself as proximal limb and girdle muscle weakness. Affected patients have difficulty combing their hair, reaching overhead for an object, and climbing stairs. Muscle enzymes are usually normal. EMG is either normal or reveals only slight myopathic changes. Muscle biopsy usually shows loss of type IIa muscle fibers with no evidence of inflammation or fiber necrosis. A poor correlation exists between the total dose of steroids given and the severity of muscle weakness. A gradual improvement in muscle strength is usually observed with the discontinuation or significant reduction in corticosteroid dosage.

Treatment of Neuromuscular Dysfunction

The proper care of these complicated patients often requires a multidisciplinary team of health care workers consisting of pulmonary specialists, respiratory therapists, pulmonary trained nurses, physiatrists, physical therapists, nutritionists, social workers, and clinical psychologists. Depending on the acuity, patients can be initially treated in an ICU setting until the resolution of their acute illness and then transferred in a respiratory rehabilitation unit specializing in the care of these patients. Frequent family interaction with the health care team is beneficial to facilitate the transition of care from the hospital to home. In

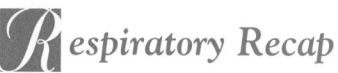

R̸espiratory Recap

Treatment of Neuromuscular Dysfunction
Respiratory muscle training: benefit controversial
Assisted coughing: use of maximum insufflation capacity
Glossopharyngeal breathing (frog breathing)
Noninvasive ventilation: positive pressure devices, negative pressure devices, rocking beds, pneumobelts
Diaphragmatic pacing

patients with stable chronic respiratory failure, the authors prefer to admit them into the noninvasive respiratory rehabilitation unit for a few days to familiarize them with the different types of ventilator support available (that is, noninvasive forms) in a relaxed and supportive environment.

The goals of therapy in the treatment of patients with chronic neuromuscular diseases are similar to other groups of patients with chronic lung disease (that is, to maintain lung function and to restore independent and functional lifestyle as long as possible). Clearly some patients with advanced disease will not be able to achieve these goals. Nevertheless, a rapid decline in lung function may be avoided by following of judicious pulmonary rehabilitation techniques such as the use of respiratory aid devices to facilitate clearance of airway secretions, early use of NPPV to augment alveolar ventilation during periods of acute decline, and the timely treatment of respiratory infections with appropriate antibiotics. Maintenance of proper nutrition is of utmost importance. Both obesity and undernutrition can contribute further to respiratory muscle dysfunction. The decreased chest wall compliance observed in obese patients leads to an increased work of breathing and may induce respiratory muscle fatigue in already weakened respiratory muscles. Undernutrition has also been shown to decrease respiratory muscle strength in a variety of chronic lung diseases.[132]

Respiratory Muscle Training

Respiratory muscle training improves strength and ventilatory endurance in normal subjects and in patients with pulmonary diseases. The clinical benefits of regular exercise training aim specifically to improve ventilatory capacity and to facilitate the clearance of airway secretions in patients with chronic neuromuscular diseases. Several uncontrolled studies performed in patients with muscular dystrophy have shown that inspiratory muscle training may improve respiratory muscle endurance and strength.[131,142,150] In a prospective, controlled trial of 19 patients with DMD, nine patients who received respiratory muscle training 30 minutes a day, 5 days/week for 2 months showed no significant improvements in VC or in PI_{max}, and PE_{max} pressures at the end of a 2-month training period compared with baseline. However, both increased inspiratory and expiratory times during loaded breathing suggest an improvement in respiratory muscle endurance.[151] In contrast, studies evaluating the effect of inspiratory resistive training in tetraplegic patients showed an improvement in inspiratory muscle strength and endurance after 6 to 16 weeks of exercise.[152,153] Furthermore, Estenne and colleagues[54] showed that 6 weeks of pectoralis muscle isometric training significantly increased ERV in patients with C6-C8 injury. The increase in ERV in these patients may have improved effective cough and diminished the incidence of lower respiratory tract infections.

Concerns have been raised about the potential detrimental effects of respiratory muscle training in patients with advanced neuromuscular weakness. Breathing through resistive loads during respiratory muscle training may potentially lead to muscle fiber damage and fatigue already weakened respiratory muscles. In addition, no study has correlated any improvement in respiratory mechanics to an improvement in clinical outcome. Thus the beneficial effect of respiratory muscle training remains unresolved.

Assisted Coughing

Ineffective cough is commonly seen in patients with moderate to advanced chronic neuromuscular disease. Diminished cough flows occur when (1) FVC is less than 1.5 L, (2) the upper airway is unstable, and (3) the patient is unable to generate high thoracoabdominal pressures because of respiratory muscle weakness. Effective clearance of airway secretions requires at least 5 to 6 L/second of peak cough expiratory flow (PCEF). Peak cough expiratory flow can be augmented by performance of manually assisted coughing techniques such as anterior chest compression and abdominal thrusts. The maximum insufflation capacity (MIC) is the maximum volume of air that the patient can hold before performing the cough maneuver. The MIC may be achieved either by air stacking ventilator delivered breaths or by glossopharyngeal breathing. Further improvement in PCEF can be obtained by combination of insufflation maneuvers and manually assisted coughing techniques.[154] In patients who have significant upper airway dysfunction, tracheostomy should be considered to facilitate pulmonary toilet.

Glossopharygeal Breathing

Glossopharyngeal breathing, also known as *frog breathing*, is a technique involving the use of oropharyngeal muscles to inject air into the trachea and thus augment ventilation to provide short periods of spontaneous ventilation, to improve effective cough, and to increase the volume of the voice.[55,56] With this technique, the patient gulps air by lowering and raising the tongue against the palate in a piston-like fashion, thereby injecting air into the trachea. With practice, patients may be able to gulp in 50 to 150 mL of air every half second. With six to eight successive gulps, a tidal volume of approximately 500 to 600 mL may be achieved and sustained for several hours, thus liberating the patients from ventilatory support. Although some patients have difficulty learning and mastering the technique, patients with spinal cord injuries, postpolio syndrome and other neuromuscular diseases have successfully utilized it.[55,155]

Mechanical Ventilation

Although ventilatory insufficiency leading to chronic respiratory failure is a common sequelae of progressive neuromuscular diseases, acute respiratory failure also is com-

TABLE 57-5

Indications for Mechanical Ventilation in Patients with Neuromuscular Disorders

Indication	Symptoms
Acute respiratory failure	Severe dyspnea
	Marked accessory muscle use
	Inability to handle secretions
	Unstable hemodynamic status
	Hypoxemia refractory to supplemental oxygen
	Acute respiratory acidosis
Chronic respiratory failure	
Nocturnal hypoventilation	Morning headache
	Lethargy
	Nightmares
	Enuresis
Nocturnal oxygen desaturation	Sao_2 <88% despite supplemental O_2
Cor pulmonale	Hypoventilation with $Paco_2$ >45 mm Hg, pH <7.32

BOX 57-2

Comparison of Clinical Factors Favoring Invasive Versus Noninvasive Mechanical Ventilation in Patients with Neuromuscular Disease

Invasive Ventilation (Endotracheal Intubation)
Copious secretions
Poor airway control
Inability to tolerate or failure of noninvasive ventilation
Impaired cognition
Unstable hemodynamics

Noninvasive Ventilation
Awake, cooperative patient
Good airway control
Minimal secretions
Hemodynamic stability

---

monly seen after recurrent aspiration, lower respiratory tract infection, or other acute illnesses place an additional burden on already compromised ventilatory reserve. Pneumonia is the most common cause of increased morbidity and mortality in patients with advanced chronic neuromuscular disease. Once impeding respiratory failure is recognized, mechanical ventilation should be used early to support spontaneous breathing until the acute precipitating event is identified and treated. The indications for mechanical ventilation are shown in Table 57-5. In patients who present with severe dyspnea, acute hypercapnia with respiratory acidosis, moderate to severe hypoxemia, and hemodynamic instability, translaryngeal intubation and mechanical ventilation are often necessary and are preferred over noninvasive mechanical ventilation. In certain clinical situations, NPPV may be used to augment minute ventilation in patients who present with acute hypercapnic respiratory failure who remain alert, cooperative, with intact upper airway function and minimal airway secretions. Comparisons of clinical scenarios in which invasive and noninvasive mechanical ventilation can be successfully used are shown in Box 57-2.

In patients who present with chronic respiratory failure or acute on chronic respiratory failure resulting from progression of their underlying neuromuscular disorder, NPPV has been effective in reversing hypercapnia and hypoxemia and is the treatment of choice because of patient comfort, effectiveness, and portability.[156] In addition, NPPV has been shown to decrease the incidence of pneumonia and reduce hospitalization rates in a survey of 654 patients with neuromuscular diseases with up to 20 years of follow-up.[156] In this group of patients, the manifestation of chronic respiratory insufficiency may be subtle with the onset of dyspnea occurring gradually over days to weeks. Common com-

plaints include lethargy, fatigue, daytime sleepiness, morning headache, and occasionally nightmares and enuresis. Nocturnal oximetry or polysomnogram may be indicated to detect the presence of nocturnal oxygen desaturation and hypercapnia, which may contribute to daytime symptoms.

Several forms of noninvasive ventilation are now available but in general, noninvasive mechanical ventilation can be divided into noninvasive positive pressure ventilation and noninvasive negative pressure ventilation. The benefits and limitations of both forms of noninvasive mechanical ventilation are listed in Table 57-6.

NPPV is preferred first over negative pressure ventilators because of the ease of use, portability, and maintenance of upper airway patency during sleep. In addition, NPPV provides better maintenance of alveolar ventilation and airway stability during sleep. Different types of masks may be used (nasal, oronasal, full face mask) depending on the patient's comfort and preference, as well as to minimize air leaks. In patients with significant mouth air leaks, the use of a chin strap or changing to an oronasal or full face mask often will solve the problem.[157] In chronic NPPV use, facial ulcers may rarely develop because of contact pressure from a particular mask interface. In this situation, using two different mask interfaces and rotating their use may promote healing of the facial ulcers and prevent recurrence. Alternatively, mouthpiece interfaces, either a generic mouthpiece with plastic lipseals or one custom fitted by an orthodontist, may be used to administer continuous ventilatory support in some patients.[155]

Once a proper mask interface has been chosen, a wide variety of positive pressure ventilators may be used to deliver NPPV. In the intensive care setting, the use of standard ICU ventilators is preferred because of the option of either assist/control or pressure-support mode or the combination of the two depending on the clinical situation and the patient's preference. For example, synchro-

TABLE 57-6

Advantages and Disadvantages of Positive and Negative Pressure Ventilation Used in Patients with Neuromuscular Disease

Type	Advantages	Disadvantages
Negative pressure ventilators (tank, pulmowrap, cuirass)	Dependability	Cumbersome
	Airway cannulation not required	Predisposition to obstructive apnea
	Minimal hemodynamic effect	Limit to nursing care
	Maintenance of speech	Controlled ventilation
Positive pressure by mask or mouthpiece	Avoidance of upper airway obstruction	Aerophagia
	Pressure preset, compensates leak	Pressure sores
	Patient initiated machine breaths	Leaks
		Problems with interface

nous intermittent mandatory ventilation (SIMV) combined with pressure support is useful in patients with nocturnal hypoventilation with decreased spontaneous respiratory rate during sleep. Some useful features available in standard ventilators and useful in the acute care setting are the ability to monitor respiratory pattern and to supply different amounts of supplemental oxygen. In patients with stable chronic respiratory failure, portable pressure ventilators are widely used. These devices are particularly useful in home use because of their low cost, simplicity in operation, portability, and ability to compensate for air leaks.

The initial ventilator setting (that is, preset tidal volume or inspiratory pressure) should be started low and slowly increased to achieve a tidal volume of 30% to 50% above baseline and/or a decrease in 5 to 10 mm Hg in $PaCO_2$. The expiratory airway pressure during is usually set at 4 cm to ensure continuous flow of gas during expiration, thus flushing out the expired gas from the breathing circuit. If supplemental oxygen is required, oxygen is connected to the ventilator tubing using a T-connector. Expiratory airway pressure also may be titrated to increase functional residual capacity and improve oxygenation. The initial duration of ventilatory assistance depends on the severity of respiratory failure and patient tolerance. In the acute setting, ventilatory assistance for more than 20 hours the first day may be needed. In the chronic setting, the patient uses NPPV during daytime for few hours followed by nocturnal use of 6 to 8 hours once the patient becomes accustomed to the NPPV settings.

Negative pressure ventilators intermittently apply subatmospheric pressure to the thorax and abdomen, thus increasing transpulmonary pressure and inflating the lung. The efficacy of negative pressure ventilation is determined by thoracic and abdominal compliance and the surface area over which the negative pressure is applied. Thus tank ventilators are the most efficient form of negative pressure ventilators because of the amount of body surface area it covers compared with cuirass ventilators, which cover only the upper torso. Although tank ventilators are

reliable, they are seldom used today because they are large, cumbersome, and some patients may complain of claustrophobia. In addition, they interfere with nursing care. Chest cuirass and poncho-wrap ventilators are more portable than tank ventilators, but they have to be used in the recumbent position to be effective. The slow but constant motion induced by these ventilators may cause low back pain and pressure sores at areas of skin contact. A common limitation to all forms of negative pressure ventilators is that they may induce obstructive sleep apnea because of upper airway collapse during a mechanically delivered breath.

In patients with mild to moderate ventilatory failure, several ventilatory assist devices such as rocking beds and pneumobelts may be used depending on patient preference, comfort, and the amount of ventilatory support required. Both devices act as abdominal displacement devices that augment diaphragmatic motion by displacing abdominal viscera against gravity. The rocking bed consists of a mattress on a motorized platform that rocks in an arc of 40 degrees with the patient laying recumbent. As the bed moves with the head dependent, gravity induces the abdominal contents and diaphragm to move cranially, assisting exhalation. In the next cycle, as the bed tilts upward, gravity moves the diaphragm and abdominal contents in a caudad direction assisting inspiration. The bed rocks between 12 to 24 times per minute and may be adjusted to optimize patient comfort to achieve the desired minute ventilation.

The pneumobelt is an inflatable bladder worn over the anterior abdomen and connected to a positive pressure ventilator that intermittently inflates it. With the patient seated upright, bladder inflation increases intraabdominal pressure, forcing the diaphragm cephalad and thereby inducing active exhalation. When the bladder deflates, gravity moves the abdominal contents and diaphragm caudally, thereby facilitating passive inspiration. Tidal volume can be augmented by increasing bladder inflation pressures to target goals.

Rocking beds and pneumobelts are limited by their constraint on patient and posture and thus the amount of ventilatory assistance provided. The rocking bed is bulky and stationary. Similarly, the pneumobelt requires that the patient use it in the upright position. Some patients complain of pain and discomfort when high bladder inflation pressures are required to sufficiently augment ventilation.

With the increasing popularity of noninvasive ventilation, several studies have showed impressive improvements in daytime gas exchange even though noninvasive ventilation was given only at night, or intermittently throughout the 24-hour period. At the end of 3 months of NPPV, the PaO_2 increased by approximately 15 mm Hg, whereas $PaCO_2$ decreased by approximately 14 mm Hg.[34,158-160] These patients have a significant improvement in their symptoms and functional capacity. The exact mechanism(s) responsible for the improvement with chronic intermittent noninvasive ventilation on daytime gas exchange in patients with neuromuscular diseases are unknown. Some of the proposed mechanisms are (1) intermittent ventilatory assistance rests already fatigued respiratory muscles, (2) resetting of the $PaCO_2$ central threshold by preventing nocturnal alveolar hypoventilation, (3) improved ventilation-perfusion matching, and (4) the higher lung volume achieved during assisted ventilation improves lung and chest wall compliance, which decreases the work of breathing.

Diaphragmatic Pacing

Phrenic nerve pacing via an external stimulator was introduced in the late 1940s. Its long-term use did not become a reality until the development of a small implantable electrode and receiver by Judson and Glenn[71] and in the late 1960s. **Diaphragmatic pacing** consists of a radio frequency transmitter and an antenna that discharges signals to a receiver to transmit electrical impulses to an electrode placed over the phrenic nerve. Both the electrodes and receiver are surgically implanted. Electrode implantation around the phrenic nerves can be divided via a cervical and thoracic approach. However, the thoracic approach is preferred to ensure stimulation of all phrenic nerve roots while the brachial plexus is avoided. The subcutaneous receiver usually is placed in the lower anterolateral rib cage to allow it to be superficial but placed in an area where soft tissue movement is limited.

The widespread use of diaphragmatic pacing is limited by its high cost, the potential for sudden failure, the development of upper airway obstruction, and the induction of diaphragm fatigue. The group of patients who appear to benefit most from this technology are ventilator-dependent patients with high cervical cord injury. Approximately one third of patients with this type of injury may be suitable for this type of treatment. Successful implantation and conditioning of the diaphragm allows the patients to be independent from ventilator support for prolonged periods of time and enables them to regain speech.[72]

CASE STUDIES

Case One
Amyotrophic Lateral Sclerosis

A 52-year-old male recently diagnosed with amyotrophic lateral sclerosis was referred to the Temple Lung Center for evaluation of his respiratory function. On initial consultation, the patient denied any respiratory complaints except for occasional cough productive of white phlegm. He did not smoke and had no history of lung disease. The patient remained ambulatory but he experienced progressive weakness of both upper extremities. He complained of fatigue and frequent headaches as well as nonrestful sleep. He denied any swallowing difficulty.

On physical examination, his respiratory rate was 22/min with no obvious signs of respiratory distress. Examination of his mouth revealed normal pharyngeal mobility. On auscultation of the chest, he had bilateral breath sounds with fine end-inspiratory crackles over both lung bases that diminished after coughing. Cardiac examination was within normal limits. No paradoxic abdominal rib cage motion was detected. No clubbing or cyanosis was detected. Motor strength of the right upper extremity was 3/5, whereas the left upper extremity was 2-3/5. Marked atrophy of the interosseus muscles was noted and loss of muscle bulk of the thenar and hypothenar eminences of both hands. Brisk reflexes were elicited in both upper and lower extremities. No sensory deficits were noted.

Initial hemogram showed a hemoglobin of 15 g/dL and white blood cell count of 7000/mm³ with normal differential. Chest x-ray showed small lung volumes and bibasilar plate-like atelectasis. Arterial blood gas analysis showed a pH 7.38, $PaCO_2$ of 42 mm Hg, and PaO_2 of 85 mm Hg. Pulmonary function tests revealed a FVC 75% of predicted and FEV_1 80% of predicted. Lung volumes revealed a TLC 70% of predicted and RV 110% of predicted. PI_{max} and PE_{max} were 75 and 88 cm H_2O. Polysomnogram revealed frequent episodes of hypopnea associated with oxygen desaturation as low as 80%, frequent arousals and poor overall sleep architecture. The respiratory disturbance index was 21/min. A repeat polysomnogram with CPAP titration was performed.

After the initial work-up, the patient was started on oral theophylline and was placed on nocturnal noninvasive ventilation with BiPAP using the spontaneous mode with an inspiratory pressure of 14 cm H_2O and expiratory pressure of 5 cm H_2O for 6 to 8 hours nightly. He received pneumococcal vaccine and the yearly influenza vaccine.

Case Two
Guillain-Barré Syndrome

A 24-year-old man was admitted to the hospital with the chief complaint of weakness of both lower extremities. Two months before admission, the patient recalled having cold symptoms that he described as dry cough, malaise, and myalgia. This was followed a few days later by watery diarrhea that resolved spontaneously. A few days before admission, he also experienced numbness and a tingling sensation in both lower extremities. A day prior to admission, he began to experience weakness on the right leg that eventually also affected the left leg. He denied any dyspnea, cough, or chest pain.

On physical examination, he was alert and oriented to person, place, and time. Respiratory rate was 15/min. Cardiopulmonary examination was within normal limits. Neurologic examination revealed diminished motor strength on both lower extremities (3/5) with absent tendon reflexes. No spinal tenderness was elicited over the back.

Magnetic resonance imaging of the spine showed no evidence of mass lesion or abscess. Lumbar puncture and analysis of the cerebrospinal fluid showed a protein level of 89 g/dL, glucose of 70 mg/dL and two white blood cells, 100% lymphocytes. A nerve conduction study showed prolonged latency with a normal amplitude suggestive demyelination. A diagnosis of Guillain-Barré syndrome was made and the patient was transferred to the intensive care unit for closer monitoring.

While in the intensive care unit, the patient received plasmapheresis. Arterial blood gas analysis revealed a pH of 7.45, $PaCO_2$ of 36 mm Hg, and PaO_2 of 90 mm Hg. The initial chest radiograph was unremarkable. Serial measurement of forced vital capacity (FVC) was performed every 8 hours. The initial FVC was 2.5 L. On the third ICU day, his FVC fell to 1.8 L. He had multiple episodes of coughing after drinking a glass of juice and had increased difficulty swallowing his secretions. He also developed a nasal voice and was noted to have a poor gag reflex. His oxygen saturation remained adequate on 3 L/min of oxygen supplementation but was electively intubated because of an increased risk of aspiration resulting from impaired bulbar function. He received a total of five sessions of plasmaphoresis. On the twelfth hospital day, he was extubated after a short spontaneous breathing trial.

Case Three
Duchenne Muscular Dystrophy

A 15-year-old boy diagnosed with Duchenne muscular dystrophy at age 5 years was referred to the Ventilator Rehabilitation Unit for initiation of NPPV. The patient has been wheelchair bound for about 1 year and was doing relatively well until 1 month ago when his mother noted him to be drowsy during the day despite an apparent full night of sleep.

An arterial blood gas revealed a pH of 7.34, $PaCO_2$ of 57 mm Hg, and PaO_2 of 56 mm Hg. On physical examination, the patient was afebrile and mildly tachypneic with a respiratory rate of 22/min. Examination of the rib cage revealed mild kyphoscoliosis and decreased breath sounds at the left base with dullness on percussion. Cardiac examination was within normal limits. His nail beds were slightly dusky but without clubbing. Atrophic changes were noted in both upper and lower extremities.

A repeat arterial blood gas on admission showed a pH of 7.32, $PaCO_2$ of 60 mm Hg, and PaO_2 of 63 mm Hg while breathing oxygen at 2 L/min via nasal cannula. A chest radiograph showed kyphoscoliosis of the thoracolumbar spine and a retrocardiac opacity. The patient was unable to perform spirometry and mouth pressures because of significant mouth leak. He was started on BiPAP with spontaneous/timed mode, rate 8/min, inspiratory pressure 18 cm H_2O, expiratory pressure 4 cm H_2O, and 2 L/min oxygen. A repeat arterial blood gas on these settings was a pH 7.44, $PaCO_2$ 48 mm Hg, PaO_2 88 mm Hg. The patient tolerated these settings. He was initially encouraged to use the BiPAP 2 to 3 hours during the day while awake to acclimate him to the mask and pressure, and 6 to 8 hours while sleeping. Repeat arterial blood gases two months later while off BiPAP showed a sustained improvement in gas exchange.

KEY POINTS

- Neuromuscular diseases impair the pump function of the respiratory muscles, leading to chronic respiratory failure or failure to wean from mechanical ventilation.
- Severe respiratory muscle weakness may occur in the absence of clinical symptoms.
- Measurements of static respiratory muscle strength and vital capacity help predict impending respiratory failure.
- Sleep-related breathing disorders and nocturnal oxygen desaturation may occur and often precede changes in daytime gas exchange abnormalities.
- A strong clinical suspicion is often required for the proper diagnosis and treatment of neuromuscular diseases.
- Upper motor neuron lesions include stroke, spinal cord injury, Parkinson's disease, and multiple sclerosis.
- Lower motor neuron lesions include amyotrophic lateral sclerosis, poliomyelitis and postpoliomyelitis muscular dystrophy.
- Disorders of peripheral nerves include phrenic nerve injury, Guillain-Barré syndrome, and critical care polyneuropathy.
- Disorders of the neuromuscular junction include myasthenia gravis, Eaton-Lambert disorder, and botulism.
- Inherited myopathies include Duchenne muscular dystrophy, myotonic dystrophy, acid maltase deficiency, fascioscapulohumeral muscular dystrophy, limb-girdle muscular dystrophy, and mitochondrial myopathy.
- Acquired inflammatory myopathies include systemic lupus erythematosus, acute ICU steroid myopathy, and chronic steroid myopathy.
- Noninvasive mechanical ventilation is the preferred mode of ventilatory assistance in patients with respiratory insufficiency who have intact bulbar function.

References

1. Votto J, Brancifort J, Scalise P, et al. COPD and other diseases in chronically ventilated patients in a prolonged respiratory care units. Chest 1998;113:86-90.
2. Criner G, Kreimer D. Patient outcome following prolonged mechanical ventilation via tracheostomy (abstract). Am Rev Respir Dis 1993;147:A874.
3. Scheinhorn D, Artinian B, Chan CK. Weaning from prolonged mechanical ventilation. Chest 1994;105:534-539.
4. Johnson DC, Kazemi H. Central control of ventilation in neuromuscular disease. Clin Chest Med 1994;15:607-617.
5. Spinelli A, Marconi G, Gorini M, et al. Control of breathing in patients with myasthenia gravis. Am Rev Respir Dis 1992; 145:1359-1366.
6. Riley D, Santiago T, Daniele R, et al. Blunted respiratory drive in congenital myopathy. Am J Med 1977;63:459-466.
7. Begin R, Bureau MA, Lupien L, et al. Control and modulation of respiration in Steinert's yotonic dystrophy. Am Rev Respir Dis 1980;121:281-289.
8. Vincken WG, Gauthier SG, Dollfuss RE, et al. Involvement of upper airway muscles in extrapyramidal disorders: a cause of airflow limitation. N Engl J Med 1984;311:438-442.
9. Vincken W, Ellecker G, Cosio M. Detection of upper airway muscle involvement in neuromuscular disorders using flow-volume loop. Chest 1986;90:52-57.
10. Mier-Jedrzejowicz A, Green M. Respiratory muscle weakness associated with cerebellar atrophy. Am Rev Respir Dis 1988; 137:673-677.
11. De Troyer A, Beyl DD. Function of the respiratory muscles in acute hemiplegia. Am Rev Respir Dis 1981;123:631-632.
12. Baydur A. Respiratory muscle strength and control of ventilation in patients with neuromuscular disease. Chest 1991;99:330-338.
13. Begin R, Bureau MA, Lupien L, et al. Control of breathing in Duchenne muscular dystrophy. Am J Med 1980;69:227-234.
14. Paton W, Aaimia E. The action of tubocurarine and of decamethonium on respiratory and other muscles in the cat. J Physiology 1951;112:311-331.
15. Holle R, Shoene R, Pavlin E. Effect of respiratory muscle weakness in P 0.01 induced by partial curarization. J Appl Physiol 1984;57:1150-1157.
16. Demedts M, Beckers J, Rochette F, et al. Pulmonary function in moderate neuromuclar disease without respiratory complaints. Eur J Respir Dis 1982;63:62-67.
17. Vincken W, Elleker MG, Cosio M. Determinants of respiratory muscle weakness in stable neuromuscular disorders. Am J Med 1987;82:53-58.
18. Braun NMT, Arora NS, Rochester DF. Respiratory muscle and pulmonary function in polymyosities and other proximal myopathies. Thorax 1983;38:616-623.
19. De Troyer A, Borenstein S, Cordier R. Analysis of lung volume restriction in patients with respiratory muscle weakness. Thorax 1980;35:603-610.
20. Young S, Tierney D, Clements J. Mechanism of compliance change in excised rat lungs at low transpulmonary pressure. J Appl Physiol 1970;29:780-785.
21. Mead J, Collier C. Relation of volume history of lungs to respiratory mechanics in anesthetized dogs. J Appl Physiol 1959;14:669-678.
22. Estenne M, Heilporn A, Delhez L, et al. Chest wall stiffness in patients with chronic respiratory muscle weakness. Am Rev Respir Dis 1983;128:1002-1007.
23. McCool R, Mayweski R, Shayne D, et al. Intermittent positive pressure breathing in patients with respiratory muscle weakness. Chest 1986;90:546-551.
24. Affeldt J, Whittenberger J, Mead J, et al. Pulmonary function in convalescent poliomyelitic patients. The pressure-volume relations of the thorax and lungs of chronic respiratory patients. N Engl J Med 1952;247:43-47.
25. Kilburn K, Eagan J, Sieker H, et al. Cardiopulmonary insufficiency in myotonic and progressive muscular dystrophy. N Engl J Med 1959;261:1089-1096.
26. Hapke EJ, Meek JC, Jacobs J. Pulmonary function in pregressive muscular dystrophy. Chest 1972;61:41-47.
27. De Troyer A, Deisser P. The effects of intermittent positive pressure breathing on patients with respiratory muscle weakness. Am Rev Respir Dis 1981;124:132-137.
28. Gibson GJ, Pride NB, Newsom D, et al. Pulmonary mechanics in patients with respiratory muscle weakness. Am Rev Respir Dis 1977;115:389-395.
29. Hill R, Martin J, Hakim A. Acute respiratory failure in motor neuron disease. Arch Neurol 1983;40:30-32.
30. Becker H, Piper A, Flynn W, et al. Breathing during sleep in patients with nocturnal desaturation. Am J Respir Crit Care Med 1999;159:112-118.
31. Bye PTP, Ellis ER, Issa FG, et al. Respiratory failure and sleep in neuromuscular disease. Thorax 1990;45:241-247.
32. Goldstein R, Molotiu N, Skrastins R, et al. Reversal of sleep-induced hypoventilation and chronic respiratory failure by nocturnal negative pressure ventilation in patients with restrictive ventilatory impairment. Am Rev Respir Dis 1987; 135:1049-1055.
33. Rodriquez M, Karnes W, Bartleson JD, et al. Plasmapheresis in acute episodes of fulminant CNS inflammatory demyelination. Neurology 1993;43:1100-1104.
34. Bach JR, Alba AS, Bohatiuk G, et al. Mouth intermittent positive pressure ventilation in the management of postpolio respiratory insufficiency. Chest 1987;91:859-864.
35. Vincken WG, Darauay CM, Cosio MG. Reversibility of upper airway obstruction after levodopa therapy in Parkinson's disease. Chest 1989;96:210-212.
36. Schmidt-Nowara W, Marder E, Feil P. Respiratory failure in myasthenia gravis due to vocal cord paralysis. Arch Neurol 1984;41:567-568.
37. Vincken W, Elleker MG, Cosio MG. Flow-volume loop changes reflecting respiratory muscle weakness in chronic neuromuscular changes. Am J Med 1987;83:673-680.
38. Ponte J. Indications for mechanical ventilation. Thorax 1990; 45:885-890.
39. De Troyer A, Estenne M. Limitations of measurement of transdiaphragmatic pressure in detecting diaphragmatic weakness. Thorax 1981;36:169-174.
40. Hubmayr R, Litchy W, Gay P, Nelson S. Transdiaphragmatic twitch pressure: effects of lung volume and chest wall shape. Am Rev Respir Dis 1989;139:647-652.
41. Laporta D, Grassino A. Assessment of transdiaphragmatic pressure in humans. J Appl Physiol 1996;58:1469-1476.
42. Mier A, Brophy C, Moxham J, Green M. Twitch pressures in the assessment of diaphragm weakness. Thorax 1989;44:990-996.
43. Klassen AC, Heaney LM, Lee MC, Kronenberg RS. Altered cerebral inhibition of respiratory and cardiac responses to hypercapnea in acute stroke. Neurology 1980;30:951-955.
44. Maskill D, Murphy K, Mier A. Motor cortical representation of diaphragm on man. J Physiol 1991;443:105-121.

45. Vingerhoets F, Bogousslavsky J. Respiratory dysfunction in stroke. Clin Chest Med 1994;15:729-737.

46. De Troyer A, Estenne M, Vincken W. Rib cage motion and muscle use in high tetraplegics. Am Rev Respir Dis 1986;133:1115-1119.

47. Scanlon PD, Loring SH, Pichurko BM, et al. Respiratory mechanics in acute quadriplegia. Am Rev Respir Dis 1989;139:615-620.

48. Hughes JM, Blumenthal JR, Merson MH, et al. Clinical features of type A and type B food-borne botulism. Ann Intern Med 1981;95:442-445.

49. Estenne M, De Troyer A. Relationship between respiratory muscle electromyogram and rib cage motion in tetraplegia. Am Rev Respir Dis 1985;1985:53-59.

50. Urmey W, Mead LJ, Slutsky AS, et al. Upper and lower rib cage deformation during breathing in quadriplegics. J Appl Physiol 1986;60:618-622.

51. Fishburn MJ, Marino RJ, Ditunno JF. Atelectasis and pneumonia in acute spinal cord injury. Arch Phys Med Rehabil 1990;71:197-200.

52. De Vivo MJ, Kartus PL, Stover SL, et al. Cause of death for patients with spinal cord injuries. Arch Intern Med 1989;149:1761-1766.

53. De Troyer A, Estenne M, Heilporn A. Mechanism of active expiration in tetraplegic subjects. N Engl J Med 1986;314:740-744.

54. Estenne M, Knoop C, Vanvaerenbergh J, et al. The effect of pectoralis muscle training in tetraplegic subjects. Am Rev Respir Dis 1989;139:1218-1222.

55. Dail CW, Affeldts JE, Collier CR. Clinical aspects of glossopharyngeal breathing. JAMA 1953;158:445-449.

56. Bach J, Alba A, Bodosky E, et al. Glossopharyngeal breathing and noninvasive aids in the management of post-polio respiratory insufficiency. Birth Defects 1987;23:99-103.

57. Estenne M, De Troyer A. Mechanism of the postural dependence of vital capacity in tetraplegic subjects. Am Rev Respir Dis 1987;135:367-371.

58. Jankovic J, Nour F. Respiratory dyskinesia in Parkinson's disease. Neurology 1986;36:303-304.

59. Paulson G, Tatrate R. Some "minor" aspects of parkinsonism, especially pulmonary function. Neurology 1970;20:14-17.

60. Mehta AD, Wright WB, Kirby BJ. Ventilatory function in Parkinson's disease. BMJ 1978;1;1456-1457.

61. Anderson D, Ellenberg J, Leventhal C, et al. Revised estimate of the prevalence of multiple sclerosis in the United States. Ann Neurol 1992;31:333-336.

62. Boor J, Johnson R, Canales L, et al. Reversible paralysis of automatic respiration in multiple sclerosis Arch Neurol 1977;34:686-689.

63. Rizvi S, Ishikawa S, Faling L, et al. Defect in automatic respiration in a case of multiple sclerosis. Am J Med 1974;56:433-436.

64. Carter JL, Noseworthy JH. Ventilatory dysfunction in multiple sclerosis. Clin Chest Med 1994;15:693-703.

65. Bolton C, Gilbert J, Hahn A, et al. Polyneuropathy in critically ill patients. J Neurol Neurosurg Psychiatry 1984;47:1223-1231.

66. Kuwahira I, Kondo T, Ohta Y, et al. Acute respiratory failure in multiple sclerosis. Chest 1990;97:246.

67. Balbierz J, Ellenberg M, Honet J. Complete hemidiaphragmatic paralysis in a patient with multiple sclerosis. Am J Phys Med Rehabil 1988;67:161-165.

68. Smeltzer S, Utell M, Rudick R, et al. Respiratory function in multiple sclerosis. Arch Neurol 1988;45:1245.

69. Carter JL, Rodriquez M. Immunosuppressive treatment of multiple sclerosis. Mayo Clin Proc 1984;64:664-669.

70. Deans E, Ross J, Road JD, et al. Pulmonary function in individuals with a history of poliomyelitis. Chest 1991;100:118-123.

71. Judson J, Glenn W. Radiofrequency electrophenic respiration: long term application to a patient with primary hypoventilation. JAMA 1968;203:1033-1037.

72. Glenn W, Hogan J, Phelps M. Ventilatory support of the quadriplegic patient with respiratory paralysis by diaphragm pacing. Surg Clin North Am 1980;60:1055-1078.

73. Fromm GB, Wisdom PJ, Block AJ. Amyotrophic lateral sclerosis presenting with respiratory failure. Chest 1977;71:612-614.

74. Carre PC, Didier AP, Tiberge YM, et al. Amyotrophic lateral sclerosis presenting with sleep hypopnea syndrome. Chest 1988;93:1309-1312.

75. Black LF, Hyatt RE. Maximal static respiratory pressures in generalized neuromuscular disease. Am Rev Respir Dis 1971;103:641-649.

76. Kreitzer SM, Saunders NA, Tyler HR, et al. Respiratory muscle function in amytrophic lateral sclerosis. Am Rev Respir Dis 1978;117:437-447.

77. Garcia-Pachon E, Marti J, Mayos M, et al. Clinical significance of upper airway dysfunction in motor neuron disease. Thorax 1994;49:896-900.

78. Polkey M, Lyall R, Green M, et al. Expiratory muscle function in amyotrophic lateral sclerosis. Am J Respir Crit Care Med 1998;158:734-741.

79. Bensimon G, Lacomblez L, Meininger V, and the ALS/riluzole study group. A controlled trial of riluzole in amyotrophic lateral sclerosis. N Engl J Med 1994;330:585-591.

80. Lacomblez L, Bensimon G, Leigh PN, et al, for the Amyotrophic Lateral Sclerosis/Riluzole Study Group II. Dose-ranging study of riluzole in amyotrophic lateral sclerosis. Lancet 1996;347:1425-1431.

81. Silverstein M, Stocking C, Antel J. Amyotrophic lateral sclerosis and life-sustaining therapy: Patient's desires for information, participation in decision making, and life-sustaining therapy. Mayo Clin Proc 1991;66:906-913.

82. Aboussouan L, Khan S, Meeker D, et al. Effect of noninvasive positive pressure ventilation on survival in amyotrophic lateral sclerosis. Ann Intern Med 1997;6:450-453.

83. Sherman M, Kleopa K, Neal B, et al. Noninvasive ventilation improves survival and slows decline of pulmonary function in patients with amyotrophic lateral sclerosis (abstract). Am J Respir Crit Care Med 1999;159:A295.

84. Schiffman PL, Belsh JM. Effect of inspiratory resistance and theophylline on respiratory muscle strength in patients with amyotrophic lateral sclerosis. Am Rev Respir Dis 1989;139:1418-1423.

85. Cosgrove JL, Alexander MA, Kitts EL, et al. Late effects of poliomyelitis. Arch Phys Med Rehabil 1987;68:4-7.

86. Dalakas MC, Elder G, Hallett M, et al. A long term follow-up study of patients with post-poliomyelitis neuromuscular symptoms. N Engl J Med 1986;314:959-963.

87. Cashman N, Maselli R, Wollman R, et al. Late denervation in patients with antecedent paralytic poliomyelitis. N Engl J Med 1981;317:7-12.

88. Klingman J, Chui H, Corgiat M, Perry J. Functional recovery: a major risk factor for the development of poliomyelitis muscular atrophy. Arch Neurol 1988;45:645-647.

89. Perry J, Barnes G, Gronley J. The postpolio syndrome: an overuse phenomenon. Clin Orthop 1988;223:145-162.
90. Curran FJ, Colbert AP. Ventilator management in Duchenne muscular dystrophy and post-myelitis syndrome: a twelve years' experience. Arch Phys Med Rehabil 1989;70:180-185.
91. Smith PEM, Calverley PMA, Edwards RHT. Hypoxemia during sleep in Duchenne muscular dystrophy. Am Rev Respir Dis 1988;137:884-888.
92. Hill R, Robbins AW, Messing R, et al. Sleep apnea syndrome after poliomyelitis. Am Rev Respir Dis 1983;127:129-131.
93. Dean A, Graham B, Dalakas M, et al. Sleep apnea in patients with postpolio syndrome. Ann Neurol 1998;43:661-664.
94. Steljes DG, Kryger MH, Kirk BW, et al. Sleep in postpolio syndrome. Chest 1990;98:133-140.
95. Hsu A, Staats B. "Postpolio" sequelae and sleep-related disordered breathing. Mayo Clin Proc 1998;73:216-224.
96. Canon S, Ritter FN. Vocal cord paralysis after post-myelitis syndrome. Laryngoscope 1987;97:981-983.
97. Solliday N, Gaensler E, Schwaber J, et al. Impaired central chemoreceptor function and chronic hypoventilation many years following poliomyelitis. Respiration 1974;31:177-192.
98. Pandit A, Kalra S, Woolcock A. An unsual cause of bilateral diaphragm paralysis. Thorax 1992;47:201.
99. Markand ON, Moorthy SS, Mahomed Y, et al. Postoperative phrenic nerve palsy in patients with open-heart surgery. Thorax 1985;35:603-610.
100. Chan CK, Loke J, Virgulto JA, et al. Bilateral diaphragmatic paralysis: clinical spectrum, prognosis, and diagnostic approach. Arch Phys Med Rehabil 1988;69:976-979.
101. Gottesman E, McCool FD. Ultrasound evaluation of the paralyzed diaphragm. Am J Respir Crit Care Med 1997;155:1570-1574.
102. McCool FD, Benditt JO, Conomos P, et al. Variability of diaphragm structure among healthy individuals. Am J Respir Crit Care Med 1997;155:1323-1328.
103. Mier-Jedrzejowicz A, Brophy C, Moxham J, et al. Assessment of diaphragm weakness. Am Rev Respir Dis 1988;137:877-883.
104. Laroche CM, Carroll N, Moxham J, et al. Clinical significance of severe isolated diaphragm weakness. Am Rev Respir Dis 1988;138:862-866.
105. Asbury A, Cornblath D. Assessment of current diagnostic criteria for Guillain-Barré syndrome. Ann Neurol 1990;27(suppl):S21-S24.
106. Gracey DR, McMihan JC, Divertie MB, et al. Respiratory failure in Guillain-Barré syndrome. Mayo Clin Proc 1982;57:742-746.
107. Moore P, James O. Guillain-Barré syndrome: incidence, management, and outcome of major complications. Crit Care Med 1981;9:549-555.
108. Ropper AH. The Guillain-Barré syndrome. N Engl J Med 1992;326:1130-1136.
109. Ropper AH, Kehne SM. Guillain-Barré syndrome: management of respiratory failure. Neurology 1985;35:1662-1665.
110. Borel CO, Tilford C, Nichols DG, et al. Diaphragmatic performance during recovery from acute ventilatory failure in Guillain-Barré syndrome and myasthenia gravis. Chest 1991;99:444-451.
111. Chevrolet J, Deleamont P. Repeated vital capacity measurements as predictive parameters for mechanical ventilation need and weaning success in the Guillain-Barré syndrome. Am Rev Respir Dis 1991;144:814-818.
112. Guillain-Barré Syndrome Study Group. Plasmapheresis and acute Guillain-Barré syndrome. Neurology 1985;35:1096-1104.
113. French Cooperative Group on Plasma Exchange in Guillain-Barré Syndrome. Efficiency of plasma exchange in Guillain-Barré Syndrome: role of replacement fluids. Ann Neurol 1987;22:753-761.
114. van der Meche FGA, Schmitz PIM, The Dutch Guillain-Barré Study Group. A randomized trial comparing intravenous immune globulin and plasma exchange in Guillain-Barré syndrome. N Engl J Med 1992;326:1123-1129.
115. Leijten F, De Weerd A, Poortvliet D, et al. Critical illness polyneuropathy in multiple organ dysfunction syndrome and weaning from the ventilator (abstract). Intensive Care Med 1996;22:856-861.
116. Witt N, Zochodne D, Bolton C. Peripheral nerve function in sepsis and multiple organ failure. Chest 1991;199:176-184.
117. Low P. Endoneural fluid pressure and microenvironment of nerve. In: Dyck P, Thomas P, Lambert E, Bunge R, editors. Peripheral neuropathy. 2nd ed. vol. 1. Philadelphia: WB Saunders 1984. pp. 599-617.
118. Zochodne D, Bolton C, Wells G, et al. Critical illness polyneuropathy: a complication of sepsis and multiple organ failure. Brain 1987;110:819-842.
119. Dushay KM, Zibrak JD, Jensen WA. Myasthenia gravis presenting as isolated respiratory failure. Chest 1990;97:232-234.
120. Mier-Jedrzejowicz A, Brophy C, Green M. Respiratory muscle function in myasthenia gravis. Am Rev Respir Dis 1988;138:867-873.
121. Mier A, Laroche C, Green M. Unsuspected myasthenia gravis presenting as respiratory failure. Thorax 1990;45:422-423.
122. Gracey DR, Divertie MB, Howard FM Jr. Mechanical ventilation for respiratory failure in myasthenia gravis. Mayo Clin Proc 983;58:597-602.
123. Amino A, Shiozawa Z, Nagasaka T, et al. Sleep apnea in well-controlled myasthenia gravis and the effect of thymectomy. J Neurol 1998;245:77-80.
124. Buckingham JM, Howard FM Jr, Bernatz PE, et al. The value of thymectomy in myasthenia gravis. Ann Surg 1976;184:453-458.
125. Gracey DR, Howard FM Jr, Divertie MB. Plasmapheresis in the treatment of ventilator-dependent myasthenia gravis patients. Chest 1984;6:739-743.
126. Inkley SR, Oldenburg FC, Vignos PJ. Pulmonary function in Duchenne muscular dystrophy related to stage of disease. Am J Med 1974;56:297-306.
127. Vianello A, Bevilacqua M, Salvador V, et al. Long-term nasal intermittent positive pressure ventilation in advanced Duchenne muscular dystrophy. Chest 1994;105:445-449.
128. Smith PEM, Edwards RHT, Calverley PMA. Ventilation and breathing pattern during sleep in Duchenne muscular dystrophy. Chest 1989;96:1346-1351.
129. Fanfulla F, Berardinelli A, Gaultieri G, et al. The efficacy of noninvasive mechanical ventilation on nocturnal hypoxemia in Duchenne muscular dystrophy. Monaldi Arch Chest 1998;53:9-13.
130. Guilleminault C, Philip P, Robinson A. Sleep and neuromuscular disease: bilevel positive airway pressure by nasal mask as a treatment for sleep disordered breathing in patients with neuromuscular disease. J Neurol Neurosurg Psychiatry 1998;65:225-232.
131. DiMarco A, Kelling J, DiMarco M, et al. The effects of inspiratory resistive training on respiratory muscle function in patients with muscular dystrophy. Muscle Nerve 1985;8:284-290.

132. Arora NS, Rochester DF. Respiratory muscle strength and maximal voluntary ventilation in undernourished patients. Am Rev Respir Dis 1982;126:5-8.

133. Margolis ML, Hill AR. Acid maltase deficiency in an adult: evidence for improvement in respiratory function with high-protein dietary therapy. Am Rev Respir Dis 1986;134:328-331.

134. Smith PEM, Calverley PMA, Edwards RHT, et al. Practical problems in the respiratory care of patients with muscular dystrophy. N Engl J Med 1987;316:1197-1205.

135. Fenichel G, Mendell J, Moxely R. A comparison of daily and alternate-day prednisone therapy in the treatment of Duchenne muscular dystrophy. Arch Neurol 1991;48:575-579.

136. Mendell J, Moxley R, Griggs R, et al. Randomized, double blind six month trial of prednisone in Duchenne muscular dystrophy. N Engl J Med 1989;320:1592-1597.

137. Harley H, Brook J, Rundle S, et al. Expansion of the unstable DNA region and phenotypic variation in myotonic dystrophy. Nature 1992;355:547-548.

138. Begin P, Mathieu J, Almirall J, Grassino A. Relationship between chronic hypercapnia and inspiratory-muscle weakness in myotonic dystrophy. Am J Respir Crit Care Med 1997;156:133-139.

139. Begin R, Bureau MA, Lupien L, et al. Pathogenesis of respiratory insufficiency in myotonic dystrophy. Am Rev Respir Dis 1982;125:312-318.

140. Guilleminault C, Cummisky J, Motta J, et al. Respiratory and hemodynamic studies during wakefulness and sleep in myotonic dystrophy. Sleep 1978;1:19-31.

141. Sivak E, Ahmad M, Hanson M, et al. Respiratory insufficiency in adult-onset acid maltase deficiency. South Med J 1987;80:205-208.

142. Martin R, Sufit R, Ringel S, et al. Respiratory muscle improvement by muscle training in adult-onset acid maltase deficiency. Muscle Nerve 1983;6:201-203.

143. Rosenow E III, Engel A. Acid maltase deficiency in an adults presenting as respiratory failure. Am J Med 1978;64:458-491.

144. Lynn DJ, Woda RP, Mendell JR. Respiratory dysfunction in muscular dystrophy and other myopathies. Clin Chest Med 1994;15:661-674.

145. Hoffbrand B, Beck E. "Unexplained" dypnea and shrinking lungs in systemic lupus erythematosus. Br Med J 1965;1:1273-1277.

146. Lacomis D, Petrella J, Giuliani M. Causes of neuromuscular weakness in the intensive care unit: a study of ninety-two patients. Muscle Nerve 1998;21:610-617.

147. Hansen-Flaschen J, Cowen J, Raps E. Neuromuscular blockade in the intensive care unit. Am Rev Respir Dis 1993;147:234-236.

148. Hirano M, Ott BP, Raps EC, et al. Acute quadriplegic myopathy: a complication of treatment with steroids, nondepolarizing blocking agents, or both. Neurology 1992;42:2082-2087.

149. Leatherman J, Fluegel W, David W, et al. Muscle weakness in mechanically ventilated patients with severe asthma. Am J Respir Crit Care Med 1996;153:1686-1690.

150. Adams M, Chandler L. Effects of physical therapy program on vital capacity of patients with muscular dystrophy. Physical Therapy 1974;54:160-162.

151. Martin A, Stern L, Yeates J, et al. Respiratory muscle training in Duchenne dystrophy. Med Child Neurol 1986;8:284-290.

152. Gross D, Ladd H, Riley E, et al. The effect of training on strength and endurance of the diaphragm in quadriplegia. Am J Med 1980;68:27-35.

153. Huldtgren A, Fugl-Myers A, Jonasson E, et al. Ventilatory dysfunction and respiratory rehabilitation in post-traumatic quadriplegia. Eur J Respir Dis 1980;61:347-356.

154. Massery M, Frownfelter D. Assisted coughing techniques: there's more than one way to cough. Phys Ther Forum 1990;9:1-4.

155. Bach J, Alba A, Saporito L. Intermittent positive pressure ventilation via the mouth as an alternative to tracheostomy for 257 ventilator users. Chest 1993;103:174-182.

156. Bach JR, Rajaraman R, Ballanger F, et al. Neuromuscular ventilatory insufficiency: effect of home mechanical ventilator use vs oxygen therapy on pneumonia and hospitalization rates. Am J Phys Med Rehabil 1998;77:8-19.

157. Criner G, Travaline J, Brennan K, Kreimer D. Efficacy of a new full face mask for noninvasive positive pressure ventilation. Chest 1994;106:1109-1115.

158. Bach J, Alba A. Management of chronic alveolar ventilation by nasal ventilation. Chest 1990;97:52-57.

159. Gay P, Patel A, Viggiano R, et al. Nocturnal nasal ventilation for treatment of patients with hypercapneic respiratory failure. Mayo Clin Proc 1991;144:1234-1239.

160. Heckmatt J, Loh L, Dubowitz V. Nighttime nasal ventilation in neuromuscular disease. Lancet 1990;335:579-581.

CHAPTER 58

Management of Obstructive Sleep Apnea Syndrome

Dennis H. Auckley
David W. Hudgel

CHAPTER OUTLINE

Weight Loss
Pharmacotherapy
Nasal Continuous Positive Airway Pressure

Oral Appliances
Oropharyngeal Surgery

OBJECTIVES

1. Define obstructive sleep apnea.
2. Describe the role of weight loss in the treatment of obstructive sleep apnea.
3. Discuss the role of pharmacology in the treatment of obstructive sleep apnea.
4. Describe the use of nasal continuous positive airway pressure for the treatment of obstructive sleep apnea.
5. Discuss the role of oral appliances and surgical approaches to the treatment of obstructive sleep apnea.
6. Compare the advantages and disadvantages of various treatment strategies for obstructive sleep apnea.

KEY TERMS

Mandibular Advancing Device (MAD)	Nasal Continuous Positive Airway	Sleep Apnea
Laser-Assisted Uvulopalatoplasty	Pressure (nCPAP)	Tongue Retaining Device (TRD)
(LAUP)	Oral Appliance (OA)	Uvulopalatopharyngoplasty (UPPP)

Sleep apnea is a disease process that is relatively common in Western society[1] and is associated with significant morbidity and mortality. The most important factor for treatment of this disorder is recognition. Physicians and the public are becoming increasingly aware of the clinical significance of a history of heavy snoring, excessive daytime sleepiness, and pulmonary hypertension in obese individuals. In this chapter, various treatment modalities available for obstructive sleep apnea (OSA) are discussed in an evidence-based format. The indications, efficacy, and drawbacks for each treatment will be discussed. Attention will be focused on weight loss, medications, **nasal continuous positive pressure (nCPAP), oral appliances (OAs),** and upper airway surgery.

Basic to successful treatment of OSA is good patient-clinician interaction. The patient must work with a sleep disorders specialist on designing an appropriate therapeutic program. Patients should be allowed to choose the therapeutic modality that best suits their interest and lifestyle. Patients need to commit to therapy, because treatment success is highly dependent upon their efforts. The patient must be followed closely after the initiation of treatment, because modifications to the program or a complete change in the chosen therapy are sometimes needed. Long-term follow-up determines the patient's compliance to the chosen treatment and whether modifications to the program are indicated, as dictated by such factors as changes in the patient's weight, medication, or living situation.

Weight Loss

Most often adults with OSA are obese.[2,3] Weight gain is the most important etiologic factor in the development of OSA.[4] In this community-based 4-year follow-up

TABLE 58-1

Pharmacologic Agents Used in OSA Treatment

Indication	Agent	Study Grade	Subjects Studied
Hypercapnia in obesity-hypoventilation	Medroxyprogesterone	A, B	31
Myxedema	Thyroid hormone replacement (may not be totally effective in obesity)	B	26
Central apnea	Acetazolamide	A, B	53
Periodic breathing in heart failure	Theophylline	A	15
REM-specific OSA	Tricyclic antidepressant	A, B	62
	Serotonin reuptake inhibitor	A, B	62
	Clonidine	A	8

OSA, Obstructive sleep apnea; A, randomized, controlled study; B, case-controlled study.

evaluation of 690 Wisconsin state employee volunteers, Peppard and colleagues[4] found that a 10% increase in weight was associated with a sixfold increase in the risk of developing significant sleep disorders breathing, defined by an apnea/hypopnea index (AHI) of at least 15/hours of sleep. For every 1 kg/m² increase in BMI, a 1% increase in the AHI occurred. In contrast, an average 26% decrease in the AHI was found in those subjects who lost 10% of their baseline BMI. In controlled and observational studies, a 10% decrease in body weight has been associated with an approximately 50% decrease in the AHI.[5-8] Pharyngeal function also improves with weight loss.[6,9] Extensive weight loss attained with gastric reduction or bowel bypass surgery resulted in dramatic improvement in the OSA, but operative mortality must be considered.[10-13] Thus body weight fluctuations are vitally important in the pathophysiology of OSA. These findings necessitate that dietary counseling and regular follow-up by a nutritionist are extremely important in the management of OSA patients. Institution of an exercise program also may be helpful in weight loss for OSA, although this has not been studied. For morbidly obese individuals, water aerobics may be a feasible form of exercise.

Weight loss should be combined with other therapies for OSA. Patients should not be placed on a weight loss regimen without simultaneous therapy with another modality. The fatigue and depression often present with OSA impair the potential success of weight loss, which is difficult in the best of circumstances. With improved mood induced by nCPAP, or other forms of therapy, the patient is more likely to lose weight, especially with the support and encouragement of caregivers. If successful with weight loss, patients may be able to eliminate other modes of therapy, such as nCPAP, from their regimen.

Based on the available literature, weight loss counseling must be an integral part of an OSA therapy program design. A nutritionist with knowledge of OSA and various weight loss treatment modalities should administer this therapy. Emphasis on this topic should extend over a long

duration of follow-up, because otherwise these patients tend to regain weight.

Pharmacotherapy

Ideally, the treatment of OSA would be improved if pharmacotherapy can be substituted for weight loss, nCPAP, or surgery. If a truly effective medication were available, then it may improve the rather poor success of weight loss in an obese population, the approximate 50% success rate of surgery, and the low compliance with nCPAP. Unfortunately, no such pharmacologic agent exists to improve the treatment of OSA.

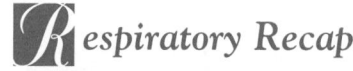
Respiratory Recap

> **Weight Loss and Pharmacotherapy**
>
> Weight gain is the most important etiologic factor in development of OSA.
> Weight reduction should be an integral part of OSA therapy program.
> Role of pharmacologic approaches to treatment of OSA is unclear.

The pharmacotherapy of OSA was recently reviewed in an evidenced-based format.[14] This review indicated that the quality of studies examining the effect of these agents on OSA is, in general, suboptimal: few randomized controlled trials exist of the pharmacologic treatment of OSA. Therefore making therapeutic recommendations is difficult based on many randomized, double blind clinical trials of pharmacologic agents. Table 58-1 summarizes the quality of studies on various pharmacologic agents used in the treatment of OSA. High-dose progesterone may be helpful in those patients with a strong component of central apnea or obesity hypoventilation. One trial of theophylline demonstrated its usefulness in periodic breathing during sleep present in patients with congestive heart failure. It also may be beneficial to OSA, but it significantly disturbs sleep, which renders it not useful in OSA patients. Surprisingly, treatment of hypothyroidism has not been uniformly shown to be efficacious in resolving the OSA of hypothyroid patients when larger numbers of patients have been studied. Acetazolamide, a known ventilatory stimulant resulting from the production of metabolic acidosis, may be helpful in patients with central sleep apnea and periodic breathing. However, acetazolamide may induce obstructive apneas in some patients, although this has not been universally found. Uncontrolled trials of β-adrenergic blocking agents, ACE inhibitors, and serotonin active agents show some early promise but are not universally effective. Further research is needed to determine which patient characteristics may predict a potential favorable response to particular pharmacologic agents. Combination of agents with different effects also may be beneficial, but have not been studied.

Nasal Continuous Positive Airway Pressure

Nasal CPAP can be an effective treatment for sleep-disordered breathing and is generally recommended as first-line therapy.[15] By creating a pneumatic splint to maintain airway patency throughout the respiratory cycle, nCPAP normalizes breathing during sleep for the majority of patients with OSA. Unfortunately, the practical use of nCPAP is limited by poor patient compliance, often resulting in a search for alternative therapies. The inability to wear and tolerate nCPAP appears related to many factors, including side effects, patient education, and the perceived benefits from treatment.[16]

The primary mechanism by which nCPAP relieves airway obstruction is by the production of a pressurized upper airway,[17] which prevents airway collapse during sleep. Sustaining airway patency during both the inspiratory and expiratory phases of respiration appears necessary to adequately control OSA,[18] and nCPAP accomplishes this. Other potential mechanisms by which nCPAP improves OSA have been proposed, although conclusive data are lacking.[17] The optimal nCPAP pressure for each individual

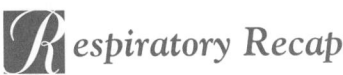

Respiratory Recap

Nasal Continuous Positive Airway Pressure
Recommended as first line therapy
Creates a pneumatic splint of the upper airway
Patient compliance problematic
Side effects common and varied

is typically determined by an attended polysomnogram, during which the pressure level is titrated to abolish respiratory disturbances. Positive airway pressure can be delivered via a nasal mask, nasal pillows (tubing that seals at the nostrils), or an oronasal mask.[19] Patient comfort and the ability to achieve an adequate mask seal are the main determinants as to which arrangement will work best for each individual.

The knowledge that nCPAP decreases daytime symptoms[19-21] and improves sleep-disordered breathing[22-24] resulting from OSA is not new. However, only recently have randomized placebo-controlled trials confirmed these findings (Table 58-2).[25-27] The studies consistently find that nCPAP enhances daytime alertness, vigilance, and sense of well being. This appears to be the case even in patients with mild disease.[25] Therefore one can reasonably conclude that nCPAP improves sleep and daytime functioning in patients with a wide spectrum of sleep-disordered breathing. Additional data from uncontrolled studies suggest that nCPAP also may improve several functional and physiologic parameters, including neuropsychiatric functioning,[22] daytime oxygenation,[28] exercise performance,[21] and hematocrit.[29] As might be expected, nCPAP therapy potentially can reduce the rate of traffic accidents[30] and hospitalizations[31] in patients with OSA. Even more intriguing are recent observations that treatment of OSA with nCPAP enhances plasma levels of nitric oxide derivatives[32] and attenuates neutrophil superoxide generation.[33] These findings, if confirmed, offer possible molecular mechanisms by which nCPAP may reduce the cardiovascular complications of OSA, a long suspected but not yet proven benefit of nCPAP therapy. Perhaps most significant, two retrospective studies have suggested that nCPAP improves survival in patients with OSA relative to the results of conservative therapy.[34,35] Prospective studies are needed to verify this important finding.

Compliance with nCPAP remains the limiting factor for successful implementation. It is not difficult to understand why sleeping with an obtrusive mask on one's face would be considered cumbersome and undesirable. However, because nearly all patients can tolerate nCPAP beyond the sleep laboratory (85% to 92% of patients[36]), and because most appreciate a beneficial effect after a night on nCPAP, the reasons for noncompliance become less obvious. Early reports, based on subjective data, suggested patients were reasonably adherent to their prescribed regimens.[36-38] With advances in technology, built-in timers have become standard and allow for more objective quantification of nCPAP usage. Studies reporting on this measure have yielded less than encouraging results.[39-42] Time on nCPAP generally ranges from 4 to 6 hours per night in most studies, with individuals rarely using nCPAP for 7 or more hours per night.[40] However, available data suggests that even 4 hours or less of nCPAP therapy per night may be enough to relieve daytime symptoms.[43] In addition, if nCPAP is discontinued

*T*ABLE 58-2

Placebo-Controlled Trials with Nasal CPAP

Study	Placebo	n Per Trial/Methods	Outcomes*		
			ESS	MWT	Psych
Engleman and colleagues[a]	Inactive ranitidine analogue	n = 34 4 weeks random- ized, crossover	p <0.001	p >0.2	p <0.02[d] p <0.03[e]
Jenkinson and colleagues[b]	Subtherapeutic nCPAP	Placebo = 49 nCPAP = 52 4 weeks randomized	p <0.0001	p = 0.005	p = 0.002[f] p = 0.08[g]
Hack and colleagues[c]	Subtherapeutic nCPAP	Placebo = 33 nCPAP = 22 4 weeks randomized	p = 0.0006	p = 0.003	p <0.04[h] p <0.05[i]

ESS, *Epworth Sleepiness Score;* MWT, *Maintenance of Wakefulness Test;* Psych, *neuropsychiatric measures (see each article for specific tests);* n, *number of subjects in trial;* p, *probability of findings due to chance;* nCPAP, *nasal continuous positive airway pressure.*
*All p values are for differences between nCPAP and placebo.
[a]*Engleman HM, Kingshall RM, Wraith PK, et al. Randomized placebo-controlled crossover trail of continuous positive airway pressure for mild sleep apnea/hypopnea syndrome. Am J Respir Crit Care Med 1999;159:461-467.*
[b]*Jenkinson C, Davies RJO, Mullins R, et al. Comparison of therapeutic and subtherapeutic nasal continuous positive airway pressure for obstructive sleep apnea: a randomized prospective parallel trial. Lancet 1999;353:2100-2105.*
[c]*Hack M, Davies RJO, Mullins R, et al. Randomized prospective parallel trial of therapeutic versus subtherapeutic nasal continuous positive airway pressure on steering snoring performance in patients with obstructive sleep apnea. Thorax 2000;55:224-231.*
[d]*For 2 of 7 cognitive tests.*
[e]*For 5 of 9 mood measures.*
[f]*For SF-36 mental summary.*
[g]*For SF-36 physical summary.*
[h]*For steering simulation-road positioning.*

after 4 hours, nocturnal oxygenation and sleep continuity appear to be improved during the remaining sleep time.[44] Whether this limited use of nCPAP is sufficient to prevent the long-term sequelae of OSA remains to be determined.

The factors affecting compliance appear to be numerous and varied. Acceptance of nCPAP by the patient is often the major initial obstacle to successful long-term treatment. In a placebo-controlled trial examining the efficacy of nCPAP as compared with a pill placebo, more than a third of the subjects preferred the placebo despite both objective and subjective improvement after nCPAP.[43] The success of nCPAP may therefore be directly linked to an individual's willingness to wear it. Rosenthal and colleagues[45] suggest that a 1-week trial of therapy at home may be sufficient to determine long-term compliance with nCPAP. In another study of 575 patients, those who initially accepted nCPAP therapy were found to have compliance above 85% at both 3 and 7 years follow-up.[41] Additional factors influencing acceptance and compliance include the perceived benefit of nCPAP and the level of patient education.[40,46] Group sessions geared toward the improvement of patient understanding of OSA and nCPAP also positively affect compliance.[47] The severity of OSA has been suggested to affect nCPAP usage,[41,48] although not all studies are in

agreement.[49] Side effects and complications resulting from nCPAP also may play a role in undermining long-term adherence to treatment.

Side effects related to nCPAP are common and varied. More than 50% of patients may experience nasal symptoms in the form of nasal dryness, congestion, or drip.[50-52] An assortment of nasal sprays or inhalers are available to address these problems. Recently, attention has focused on the use of heated humidifiers to reduce symptoms and improve compliance.[50,53,54] A randomized, crossover study comparing nCPAP systems with heated humidification, cold humidification, and no humidification found improvements in compliance (0.6 hours/night) and patient satisfaction accompanied by decreased nasal symptoms only in those using heated humidifiers.[53] These results were confirmed in a prospective cohort study in which heated humidifiers significantly improved compliance with nCPAP in those with persistent nasal symptoms despite the use of a cold humidifier.[54] Currently controversy exists over whether changes in temperature, humidity, or both result in the noted benefits.[55] External nasal irritation and skin breakdown also can occur, although with the availability of delivery devices, these problems are being encountered less frequently and, should they arise, are relatively easy to overcome. Less common side effects, such as claustrophobia, aerophagia, and recurrent sinusitis[51,52] may be particularly problematic and trigger a search for alternative therapies.

Relatively newer modes of positive pressure delivery have generated interest in the possible reduction of side effects and the improvement in compliance. Investigators have focused primarily on self-adjusting nCPAP and devices capable of delivering separate inspiratory and expiratory pressures (bilevel positive airway pressure). Changing body position, sleep stage, or other factors (that is, sedative or alcohol use) may influence upper airway dynamics such that variable pressures are required to maintain airway patency at different times during sleep.[17] Autotitration or self-adjustment of nCPAP allows for minute to minute fluctuations in the nCPAP level in response to changes in airway conditions. This continuous titration has been shown to be equivalent to manual titration of nCPAP while achieving a lower mean nCPAP level.[56-58] In a 3-month randomized, crossover trial comparing standard nCPAP to auto-titrating nCPAP, compliance (0.5 hours/night) and adherence to therapy (fewer dropouts) were found to be significantly improved while on auto-titrating nCPAP.[56] Whether these modest improvements justify the added expense of self-adjusting nCPAP as a long-term treatment option has not been determined. One potential use of this modality appears to be the ability to perform unattended nCPAP titration studies.[59,60] However, this approach needs further examination before widespread implementation, because up to 35% of patients titrated by self-adjusting devices may receive inadequate levels of support and thus suboptimal therapy.[58]

Bilevel pressure support supplies independent pressure levels to the patient during inspiration and expiration. This enables titration of the expiratory pressure to the minimum setting necessary to prevent airway collapse during expiration, found to be important in the management of OSA.[18] This pressure is often lower than that needed during inspiration[61] and thus bilevel pressure support was hoped to enhance compliance and potentially reduce side effects. Although improved acceptance is often noted in the laboratory setting, better long-term compliance has not been shown with bilevel pressure support versus nCPAP,[62] and a reduction in side effects remains to be proven. These disappointing findings, coupled with the increased cost of bilevel pressure support devices, have limited its utility in OSA.

Oral Appliances

The use of OAs for the treatment of OSA has gained popularity in recent years and is now considered as a viable alternative to nCPAP for mild to moderate sleep apnea.[63] A large variety of dental devices exists for clinical use, although they all can be characterized as primarily either **tongue retaining devices (TRDs)** or **mandibular advancing devices (MADs)**. Although at least one brand can be made in a physician's office,[64] the majority of OAs are

fashioned by dentists, stressing the need for close cooperation between sleep physicians and their dental colleagues. For the sake of efficacy and comfort, most devices are adjustable.

Oral appliances enlarge the pharyngeal cross-sectional area in most individuals[65] and thereby decrease the propensity for airway collapse. It may seem that the forward traction on the tongue (TRD), downward rotation on the mandible (TRD, MAD), and anterior protrusion of the mandible (MAD)[63] would serve primarily to increase the retrolingual[66,67] and hypopharyngeal[66] air spaces. However, some have found that OA can induce changes in the velopharynx[66,68,69] and the shape of the tongue and the soft palate.[63,66] Therefore the precise mechanism of action from an anatomic standpoint remains controversial. Furthermore, none of these studies evaluated patients during sleep. One report examined the site of airway collapse during sleep and correlated this with response to OA in a small number of subjects (n = 12).[70] Although all subjects with lower pharyngeal collapse (that is retrolingual or hypopharyngeal) responded to OA, the majority of subjects with velopharyngeal collapse also clearly benefited.[70] The authors concluded that the site of airway compromise should not deter the use of an OA in a given patient.

The American Academy of Sleep Medicine (AASM, formerly the American Sleep Disorders Association) reviewed the clinical efficacy of OA in 1995.[63] At that time, the only available data were in the form of case series. Through collective analysis of the data, OA were found to effectively control OSA, as defined by an AHI less than 10, in 51% of individuals. This was accompanied by both subjective and, in two studies, objective improvement in daytime symptoms. Patients with mild to moderate OSA, as defined by an AHI less than 50, appeared most likely to benefit.[63] The type of device (TRD vs. MAD) did not affect results. However, in 13% of patients, sleep-disordered breathing worsened, highlighting the need for objective documentation of treatment efficacy.

*R*espiratory Recap

Oral Appliances

Tongue retaining devices or mandibular advancing devices are available.

Propensity for airway collapse is decreased.

Sleep-disordered breathing may worsen in some persons using these devices.

Common side effect is TMJ pain.

Since the AASM review, several uncontrolled trials have been published with similar results.[69,71-78] Two of these studies warrant further comment. Marklund and colleagues[73] examined response to OA therapy as categorized by the severity of pretreatment OSA. They found an in-

*T*ABLE 58-3

Oral Appliances in the Treatment of OSA

Trial	Number of Subjects	Design	AHI (before/after)	Responders (%)*	Symptoms (before/after)	Satisfaction
Clark and colleagues[a]	21	Randomized, cross-over OA vs. nCPAP	OA: 39% decrease nCPAP: 52% decrease	OA: 43% nCPAP: 57%	Subjective improvement for both treatments	94% chose OA over nCPAP
Ferguson and colleagues[b]	25	Randomized, cross-over OA vs. nCPAP	OA: 20/10 nCPAP: 18/4	OA: 48% nCPAP: 62%	Subjective improvement for both treatments	OA: 68% nCPAP: 62%
Ferguson and colleagues[c]	20	Randomized, crossover OA vs. nCPAP	OA: 25/14 nCPAP: 24/4	OA: 55% nCPAP: 70%	ESS: 10/15 ESS: 11/5	OA: 80% nCPAP: 70%
Hans and colleagues[d]	18	Randomized, placebo-controlled	OA: 36/21 Placebo: 37/47	OA: 40% Placebo: 0%	ESS: 12/8 ESS: 13/12	NA NA NA
Wilhelmsson and colleagues[e]	80	Randomized OA vs. UPPP	OA: 18/6 UPPP: 20/10	OA: 81% UPPP: 60%	Subjective improvement for both treatments	NA

OSA, *Obstructive sleep apnea;* AHI, *apnea/hypopnea index before and after treatment;* OA, *oral appliance;* nCPAP, *nasal continuous positive airway pressure;* ESS, *Epworth Sleepiness Scale before and after treatment;* NA, *data not available;* UPPP, *uvulopalatopharyngoplasty.*
Responders defined differently for each study.
[a]*Clark GT, Blumenfeld I, Yoffe N, et al. A crossover study comparing the efficacy of CPAP with anterior mandibular positioning devices on patients with obstructive sleep apnea. Chest 1996;109:1477-1483.*
[b]*Ferguson KA, Ono T, Lowe AA, et al. A randomized crossover study of an oral appliance versus nasal-CPAP in the treatment of mild-moderate obstructive sleep apnea. Chest 1996;109:1269-1275.*
[c]*Ferguson KA, Ono T, Lowe AA, et al. A short-term controlled trial of an adjustable oral appliance for treatment of mild to moderate obstructive sleep apnea. Thorax 1997;52:362-368.*
[d]*Hans MG, Nelson S, Luks VG, et al. Comparison of two dental devices for treatment of obstructive sleep apnea syndrome. Am J Orthod Dentofacial Orthop 1997;111:562-570.*
[e]*Wilhelmsson B, Tegelberg A, Walker-Engstrom MC, et al. A prospective randomized study of a dental appliance compared with uvulopalatopharyngoplasty in the treatment of obstructive sleep apnea. Acta Otolaryngol 1999;119(4):503-509.*

verse correlation between the severity of OSA and the likelihood of a treatment response. Of those with a pretreatment AHI greater than 20, 81% were successes as defined by an AHI of less than 10 or at least a 50% reduction in the original index. However, only 25% of subjects with an AHI greater than 40 before therapy were successfully controlled by an OA. In contrast, Raphaelson and colleagues[78] demonstrated that, by slowly advancing the mandible over the course of a sleep study, they were able to successfully treat six of six patients, including an individual whose AHI decreased from 89 to 15. The mean AHI for the group improved from 37 to 4 with this approach, suggesting that optimal advancement may best be accomplished under controlled conditions. In concert with the AASM review, most studies continue to report a subset of patients who experience worsening of their sleep apnea with the use of an oral appliance. No mechanism to explain why this occurs in some patients has been clearly established.

Five controlled trials examining the utility of OA in OSA have now been published, although only one of these is a placebo-controlled trial. Three of the remaining four studies compare the efficacy of OA with that of nCPAP, long considered first line therapy for this condition (Table 58-3).[15] Hans and colleagues[79] used a dental device that did not advance the mandible as a placebo and compared this with a MAD. They found that the MAD was more effective at controlling OSA than the placebo device as assessed by both subjective and objective measurements. The small sample size limits the strength of these findings, however, and a larger trial of this nature should be considered. Closer inspection of the individual data from this study finds a marked variability in treatment response for those with more severe OSA. An explanation for these differences is not provided, though perhaps radiographic examination of upper airway changes after placement of the OA may have offered some clues.

The three crossover design studies comparing OA with nCPAP are remarkably consistent in their conclusions that nCPAP appears more effective than OA in normalizing the AHI, subjective improvement in daytime sleepiness is equally improved by OA and nCPAP, and patient satisfaction is greater with OA therapy.[80-82] The above findings raise the question of whether true normalization of breathing during sleep is the optimal endpoint by which to measure treatment success. If the treatment offered is unpalatable to most individuals, then compliance will be poor and little is gained. On the other hand, if a suboptimal treatment response results (as measured objectively) but the patient's quality of life is improved, will the long-term sequelae of untreated OSA be averted? Only prospective, longitudinal studies, analyzing objective measures, compliance and quality of life can provide these answers. One group has developed a hybrid OA/CPAP device in hopes of achieving the success of nCPAP with the satisfaction of OA.[84] This device, termed *oral positive airway pressure* or OPAP, delivers positive pressure via an MAD. Preliminary data indicates this device can be as effective as nCPAP at lowering the AHI while achieving this at a lower pressure than nCPAP.[84]

The response to OA is highly variable and a subset of individuals will worsen with this treatment modality.[63,74] Thus it would be desirable to predict which individuals are likely to benefit from OA before time and resources are invested in empiric trials. Studies investigating this question have analyzed primarily cephalographs, or lateral skull films, to identify anatomic variants that might be amenable to alteration. Unfortunately, conflicting results preclude firm conclusions and guidelines from being established. Some authors have found no correlation between anatomic measures and treatment response,[75,82] whereas others have found a variety of specific measures indicative of success.[68,74,85] In this latter group, agreement as to which variable or set of variables is most predictive is lacking. Furthermore, Henke and colleagues[70] noted that the site of airway collapse during sleep does not exclude a successful treatment response and therefore other factors may play a role in determining results with this therapy.

Patients who are being considered for an OA need an adequate dental examination. They should have reasonable dentition with at least six teeth in each arch to anchor the device.[86] Temporomandibular joint (TMJ) function should be assessed and individuals should be able to protrude their mandibles at least 5 mm without discomfort.[86] Collaboration with dental colleagues will help to ensure patients are appropriately selected.

Side effects related to OA can be categorized into early and late complications. Early side effects are usually transient and resolve with continued use of the devices. These effects include jaw and teeth discomfort, excessive salivation, dry mouth, and difficulty chewing in the morning.[63,81,82] Problems that arise after longer use of OA include TMJ pain and occlusive alignment alterations.[63] Ferguson and colleagues[81,82] found that 20% to 24% of patients had moderate to severe side effects after 4 months of treatment, although none of these included TMJ syndrome. In the longest reported follow-up to date (average 3.4 years), Menn and colleagues[75] found 30% of patients prescribed OA for OSA had discontinued use. Four of the seven experienced TMJ discomfort while the remaining three chose alternative treatments. Of particular interest was a study by Bondemark that found that in 30 patients using an MAD for 2 years, mandibular position changed by an average of 0.4 mm.[87]

However, 43% of the group had no change in mandibular position and none of the patients in the study complained of an altered sense of occlusion. Longer-term studies are necessary to better define the risks and complications of this therapy.

Compliance data are somewhat limited. Most data have come from self-reported compliance, previously shown to overestimate actual compliance with OSA therapies.[49] In these studies, compliance data ranged from 50% to 100% and, in some studies, appear inversely correlated with length of follow-up.[63,78,80] Recently, a heat-sensitive sensor embedded in an OA was used to objectively measure compliance in eight OSA patients treated with a MAD.[69] Over 2 weeks, mean OA usage was 6.8 hours, an improvement over what is typically seen with nCPAP. Larger longitudinal studies using this covert monitoring device are needed.

Oropharyngeal Surgery

Oropharyngeal surgery has been used in the treatment of OSA since the early 1980s. Numerous approaches have been developed, although success rates have been highly variable. In addition, modifications of traditional procedures are continually being introduced and, despite a lack of supporting data, enjoy widespread practice. The oldest and most commonly performed surgery, the **uvulopalatopharyngoplasty (UPPP),** is successful in only approximately 50% of patients as documented in numerous studies.[16] In addition, this procedure may worsen OSA in some patients[88] and a significant number of individuals may relapse within 18 months after surgery.[89] Some, but not all, of these cases can be explained by postoperative weight gain. More extensive surgery may include genioglossus advancement with hyoid repositioning, maxillomandibular advancement (MMA), laser midline glossectomy, and radiofrequency tongue ablation. These surgeries, when performed simultaneously or staged, address additional sites of airway collapse and may significantly improve outcomes.[90-92]

The surgical literature was reviewed in a meta-analysis format performed by the AASM.[93] On whole, small subject groups, limited follow-up, and biased patient selection prevented firm guidelines from being issued. The researchers determined that the site of pharyngeal collapse was important in helping to predict the success of UPPP.[94] They also recommended preoperative and postoperative polysomnograms to assess response to any surgical intervention. Patients must be told that only one procedure may not be curative and that a stepwise approach may be necessary to resolve the sleep apnea.

Despite the rather poor success rate of UPPP for treatment of OSA, office-based **laser-assisted uvulopalatoplasty (LAUP)** was developed as an alternative surgical approach. The advantages of LAUP over UPPP are that general anesthesia is not required, it may have a lower complication rate, and it is less costly.[95] Most studies have demonstrated that, compared with UPPP, LAUP has a similar success rate (approximately 40% to 50%) in decreasing the AHI by 50%.[95-100] However, several of these same studies also have found that up to 10% to 30% of patients undergoing LAUP will develop worsening of their disease.[95,98,100] Circumferential scarring may narrow the velopharyngeal airway in these patients.[101] Finkelstein and colleagues have shown that LAUP often decreased the cross-sectional area and the distensibility of the velopharynx.[101] These observations validate the need for postoperative polysomnogram on all patients. More importantly, the findings emphasize the necessity for further research to determine reliable, easy-to-use predictors of treatment outcomes before individuals are subjected to invasive therapies. Work to date has yielded conflicting results,[98,102] although specific cephalometric measurements (that is, mandibular hyoid distance) may hold promise.[102]

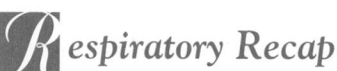

Respiratory Recap

Oropharyngeal Surgery
UPPP is most common.
Lack of controlled trials exists to support its effectiveness.

Surgical management of OSA with UPPP has recently been compared with OA in a randomized, controlled fashion.[83] Eighty individuals with mild OSA were randomized to treatment with an OA or UPPP and tonsillectomy and then followed for 1 year. Despite the uncommonly high 60% rate of improvement (defined as a 50% reduction in the AHI) for UPPP, the use of an OA was more likely to improve (81%) and resolve (78% versus 51%) OSA.[83] Measures of contentment and vitality were higher in those who had a UPPP, although all quality of life measures improved in both groups after treatment.[103] Randomized, controlled trials of UPPP compared with nCPAP have not been performed. Limited data suggests nCPAP is more effective than UPPP in controlling OSA, although compliance with nCPAP remains a problem.[104,105]

Frequently, additional surgical interventions such as septoplasty, tonsillectomy, and mandibular osteotomy are combined with UPPP.[88,102,104,105] The inclusion of these patients in data sets unfortunately limits the interpretation of results and may well overestimate the effectiveness of a UPPP. In support of this notion, a small case series of 9 adults with OSA and substantial tonsillar hypertrophy found a greater than 80% success rate after bilateral tonsillectomy alone.[106] Thus these adjunctive procedures, alone or in combination with UPPP, and not the UPPP itself may be responsible for the improvements in sleep disordered breathing seen in some patients.

Additional approaches and techniques to enlarge the airway have been investigated and reported. Those receiving the most attention are radiofrequency volumetric tissue reduction of the palate and transpalatal advancement pharyngoplasty. Radiofrequency ablation of palatal tissue has been demonstrated to improve snoring and possibly decrease symptoms related to upper airway resistance syndrome.[107] Its effects on OSA have not been fully evaluated, but presumably the results would be no better than that obtained with LAUP or UPPP. On the other hand, transpalatal advancement pharyngoplasty has shown some promise as an alternative surgical approach for OSA. In this procedure, a portion of the posterior hard palate is resected and the soft palate is advanced anteriorly. Woodson endoscopically examined six patients after this procedure and found the average cross-section area of the retropalatal airspace increased by 321% and the AHI decreased significantly.[108] All patients had previously undergone UPPP. The additional improvement seen with this procedure over UPPP may be the direct result of an increase in lateral airway dimensions and not just anteroposterior air space.[109]

Utley and colleagues[110] recommended a step-wise surgical approach with LAUP for snorers without OSA, upper airway resistance, and mild OSA. For patients with more severe OSA or multiple sites of airway collapse, UPPP and genioglossus advancement with hyoid myotomy were used. Although this protocol appeared effective in the elimination of snoring, only 50% of the patients with OSA had a 50% or greater decrease in the AHI. This is a much lower response rate than when MMA was used.[111,112] Li and colleagues[90,91] have advocated MMA for those who fail UPPP with genioglossus advancement and hyoid myotomy. They found a success rate of greater than 90% with this approach, even in those without evidence of maxillomandibular deficiency.[91] In addition, patient satisfaction appears high and complications seem uncommon. Impressive results after MMA with or without adjunctive procedures have been duplicated in a private practice setting,[92] suggesting that the procedure may be able to be generalized. Unfortunately, follow-up in all studies was limited to 6 months. This highlights the problem of limited long-term data prevalent in the surgery literature. Conradt and colleagues[113] objectively documented the relapse of OSA in 2 of 15 (13%) patients 2 years after MMA. Larger, longitudinal studies are necessary to assess efficacy.

The surgical literature continues to suffer from lack of controlled studies. Adequate comparison studies with nCPAP have not been performed and more longitudinal data is needed. Two conclusions appear apparent from the literature to date: (1) the site of pharyngeal collapse should be determined preoperatively and the specific surgical procedures(s) to be used should be determined based on this evaluation and (2) immediate and long-term objective assessments are necessary to evaluate the success of the surgery.

KEY POINTS

- Weight loss offers the potential to cure OSA in many individuals, but attempts at this conservative therapy are successful in only a minority.
- The role of medications in the treatment of OSA is unclear.
- Although it is an extremely effective treatment, nCPAP is cumbersome and subject to poor compliance.
- Oral devices are more convenient than nCPAP but may be limited to those with milder forms of OSA.
- Surgery has not been shown to be universally beneficial, although the maxillomandibular advancement procedure offers some promise.
- Treatment options should be discussed with each patient and it is best if the patient has a choice in deciding his or her treatment.
- Involvement of the patient in the decision-making process should help improve compliance.

References

1. Young T, Palta M, Dempsey J, et al. The occurrence of sleep-disordered breathing among middle-aged adults. N Engl J Med 1993;328:1230-1235.
2. Browman CP, Sampson MG, Yolles SF, et al. Obstructive sleep apnea and body weight. Chest 1984;85:435-436.
3. Shelton KE, Woodson H, Gay S, et al. Pharyngeal fat in obstructive sleep apnea. Am Rev Respir Dis 1993;148:462-466.
4. Peppard PE, Young T, Palta M, et al. Longitudinal study of moderate weight change and sleep-disordered breathing. JAMA 2000;284:3015-3021.
5. Loube MI, Loube AAS, Mitler MM. Weight loss for obstructive sleep apnea: the optimal therapy for obese patients. J Am Diet Assoc 1994;94:1291-1295.
6. Rubinstein I, Colapinto N, Rotstein LE, et al. Improvement in upper airway function after weight loss in patients with obstructive sleep apnea. Am Rev Respir Dis 1968;138:1192-1195.
7. Smith PL, Gold AR, Meyers DA, et al. Weight loss in mildly to moderately obese patients with obstructive sleep apnea. Ann Intern Med 1985;103:850-855.
8. Suratt PM, McTier RF, Findley LJ, et al. Changes in breathing and the pharynx after weight loss in obstructive sleep apnea. Chest 1987;92:631-638.
9. Schwartz DA, Gold AR, Schubert N, et al. Effect of weight loss on upper airway collapsibility in obstructive sleep apnea. Am Rev Respir Dis 1991;144:494-498.
10. Charuzi I, Ovnat A, Peiser J, et al. The effect of surgical weight reduction on sleep quality in obesity-related sleep apnea syndrome. Surgery 1985;97(5):535-538.
11. Harman EM, Wynne JW, Block AJ. The effect of weight loss on sleep-disordered breathing and oxygen desaturation in morbidly obese men. Chest 1982;82:291-294.
12. Peiser J, Lauie P, Ovnat A, et al. Sleep apnea syndrome in the morbidly obese as an indication for weight reduction surgery. Ann Surg 1984;199:112-115.
13. Sugerman HJ, Fairman RP, Sood RK, et al. Long-term effects of gastric surgery for treating respiratory insufficiency of obesity. Am J Clin Nutr 1992;55(Suppl):597S-601S.
14. Hudgel DW, Thanakitcharu S. Clinical controversy. Pharmacologic treatment of sleep-disordered breathing. Am J Respir Crit Care Med 1998;158:691-699.
15. McNicholas WT. Obstructive sleep apnea syndrome: who should be treated? Sleep 2000;23:S187-S190.
16. Hudgel DW. Treatment of obstructive sleep apnea: a review. Chest 1996;109:1346-1358.
17. Strollo PJ, Sanders MH, Atwood CW. Positive pressure therapy. Clin Chest Med 1998;19:55-68.
18. Reith O, Guido P, Picca V, et al. The role of the expiratory phase in obstructive sleep apnea. Respir Med 1999;93:190-195.
19. Sullivan CE, Grunstein RR. Continuous positive airway pressure in sleep-disordered breathing. In: Kryger M, Roth T, Dement W, editors. Principles and practice of sleep medicine. 2nd edition. Philadelphia: W.B. Saunders; 1994. pp. 694-705.
20. Hardinge FM, Pitson DJ, Stradling JR. Use of the Epworth Sleepiness Scale to demonstrate response to treatment with nasal continuous positive airway pressure in patients with obstructive sleep apnea. Resp Med 1995;89:617-620.
21. Taguchi O, Hida W, Okabe S, et al. Improvement in exercise performance with short-term nasal continuous positive airway pressure in patients with obstructive sleep apnea. Tohoku J Exp Med 1997;183:45-53.
22. Dederian SS, Bridenbaugh RH, Rajagopal KR. Neuropsychological symptoms in obstructive sleep apnea improve after treatment with continuous positive airway pressure. Chest 1988;94:1023-1027.
23. Sanders MH. Nasal CPAP effect on patterns of sleep apnea. Chest 1988;86:839-844.
24. Sullivan CE, Issa FG, Berthan-Jones M, et al. Reversal of obstructive sleep apnea by CPAP applied through the nares. Lancet 1981;1:862-865.
25. Engleman HM, Kingshall RM, Wraith PK, et al. Randomized placebo-controlled crossover trail of continuous positive airway pressure for mild sleep apnea/hypopnea syndrome. Am J Respir Crit Care Med 1999;159:461-467.
26. Hack M, Davies RJO, Mullins R, et al. Randomized prospective parallel trial of therapeutic versus subtherapeutic nasal continuous positive airway pressure on steering snoring performance in patients with obstructive sleep apnea. Thorax 2000;55:224-231.
27. Jenkinson C, Davies RJO, Mullins R, et al. Comparison of therapeutic and subtherapeutic nasal continuous positive airway pressure for obstructive sleep apnea: a randomized prospective parallel trial. Lancet 1999;353:2100-2105.
28. Leech JA, Onal E, Lopata M. Nasal CPAP continues to improve sleep-disordered breathing and daytime oxygenation over long-term follow-up of occlusive sleep apnea syndrome. Chest 1992;102:1651-1655.
29. Krieger J, Sforza E, Delanoe C, et al. Decrease in haematocrit with continuous positive airway pressure treatment in obstructive sleep apnea patients. Eur Respir J 1992;5:228-233.
30. Krieger J, Meslier N, Lebrun T, et al. Accidents in obstructive sleep apnea patients treated with nasal continuous positive airway pressure: a prospective study. Chest 1997;112:1561-1566.
31. Peker Y, Hedner J, Johansson A, et al. Reduced hospitalization with cardiovascular and pulmonary disease in obstructive sleep apnea patients on nasal CPA treatment. Sleep 1997;20:645-653.

32. Schulz R, Schmit D, Blum D, et al. Decreased plasma levels of nitric oxide derivatives in obstructive sleep apnea: response to CPAP therapy. Thorax 2000;55:1046-1051.

33. Schulz R, Mahmardi S, Hattar K, et al: Enhanced release of superoxide from polymorphonuclear neutrophils in obstructive sleep apnea. Impact of continuous positive airway pressure therapy. Am J Respir Crit Care Med 2000;162:566-570.

34. He J, Kryger MH, Zorick FJ, et al. Mortality and apnea index in obstructive sleep apnea: experience with 385 male patients. Chest 1988;94:9-14.

35. Keenan SP, Burt H, Ryan F, et al. Long-term survival of patients with obstructive sleep apnea treated by uvulopalato-pharyngoplasty or nasal CPAP. Chest 1994;105:55-59.

36. Waldhorn RE, Herrick W, Nguyen MC, et al. Long-term compliance with nasal continuous positive airway pressure therapy of obstructive sleep apnea. Chest 1990;97:33-38.

37. Rolfe I, Olson LG, Saunders NA. Long-term acceptance of continuous positive airway pressure in obstructive sleep apnea. Am Rev Resp Dis 1991;141:130-133.

38. Sanders MH, Gruendel CA, Rogers RM. Patient compliance with nasal CPAP therapy for sleep apnea. Chest 1986;90:330-338.

39. Engleman HM, Martin SE, Douglas NJ. Compliance with CPAP therapy in patients with the sleep apnea/hypopnea syndrome. Thorax 1994;49:263-266.

40. Kribbs NB, Pack AI, Kline LR, et al. Objective measurement of patterns of nasal CPAP use by patients with obstructive sleep apnea. Am Rev Resp Dis 1993;147:887-895.

41. Krieger J, Kurtz D, Petiau C, et al. Long-term compliance with CPAP therapy in obstructive sleep apnea patients and in snorers. Sleep 1996;19(Suppl 9):S136-143.

42. Pepin JL, Krieger J, Rodenstein D, et al. Effective compliance during the first three months of continuous positive airway pressure. Am J Respir Crit Care Med 1999;160:1124-1129.

43. Engleman HM, Martin SE, Deary IJ, et al. Effect of continuous positive airway pressure treatment on daytime function in sleep apnea/hypopnea syndrome. Lancet 1994;343:572-575.

44. Hers V, Liisto G, Dury M, et al. Residual effect of CPAP applied for part of the night in patients with obstructive sleep apnea. Eur Respir J 1997;10:973-976.

45. Rosenthal L, Gehardstein R, Lumley A, et al. CPAP therapy in patients with mild OSA: implementation and treatment outcome. Sleep Med 2000;1:215-220.

46. Meurice J-C, Dore P, Paquereau J. Predictive factors of long-term compliance with nasal continuous positive airway pressure treatment in sleep apnea syndrome. Chest 1994;105:429-433.

47. Likar LL, Panciera TM, Erikson AD, et al. Group education sessions and compliance with nasal CPAP therapy. Chest 1997;111:1273-1277.

48. McArdle N, Devereux G, Heidarnejad H. Long-term use of CPAP therapy for sleep apnea/hypopnea syndrome. Am J Respir Crit Care Med 1999;159:1108-1114.

49. Reeves-Hoche MK, Meck R, Zwillich CW. Nasal CPAP: an objective evaluation of patient compliance. Am J Respir Crit Care Med 1994;149:149-154.

50. Brown L. Back to basics: if it's dry, wet it. Chest 2000;117:617-619.

51. Hoffstein V, Vimer S, Mateika S, et al. Treatment of obstructive sleep apnea with nasal continuous positive airway pressure: patient compliance, perception of benefits, and side effects. Am Rev Respir Dis 1992;145:841-845.

52. Pepin JL, Leger P, Veale D, et al. Side effects of nasal continuous positive airway pressure in sleep apnea syndrome: study of 193 patients in two French Sleep Centers. Chest 1995;107:375-381.

53. Massie CA, Hart RW, Perolez K. Effects of humidification on nasal symptoms and compliance in sleep apnea patients using continuous positive airway pressure (CPAP). Chest 1999;116:403-408.

54. Rakotonanahary D, Pelletier-Fleury N, Gagnadoux F, et al. Predictive factors for the need for additional humidification during nasal continuous positive airway pressure therapy. Chest 2001;119:460-465.

55. Winck JC, Delgado JC, Almeida J, et al. Communication to the editor. Chest 2001;119:310-312.

56. Hudgel DW, Fung C. A long-term randomized crossover comparison of autotitrating and standard nasal continuous airway pressure. Sleep 2000;23(5):645-648.

57. Scharf MB, Brannen DE, McDannold MD, et al. Computerized adjustable versus fixed NCPAP treatment of obstructive sleep apnea. Sleep 1996;19:491-496.

58. Sharma S, Wali S, Pouliot Z, et al. Treatment of obstructive sleep apnea with a self-titrating continuous positive airway pressure (CPAP) system. Sleep 1996;19:497-501.

59. Lloberes P, Ballester E, Montserrat JM, et al. Comparison of manual and automatic CPAP titration in patients with sleep apnea/hypopnea syndrome. Am J Respir Crit Care Med 1996;154:1755-1758.

60. Series F, Marc I: Efficacy of automatic continuous positive airway pressure therapy that uses an estimated required pressure in the treatment of the obstructive sleep apnea syndrome. Ann Intern Med 1997;127:588-595.

61. Sanders MH, Kern N. Obstructive sleep apnea treated by independently adjusted inspiratory and expiratory positive airway pressure via nasal mask. Chest 1990;98:317-324.

62. Reeves-Hoche MK, Hudgel DW, Meck R, et al. Continuous versus bilevel positive airway pressure for obstructive sleep apnea. Am J Respir Crit Care Med 1995;151:443-449.

63. Schmidt-Nowara W, Lowe A, Wiegard C, et al. Oral appliances for treatment of snoring and obstructive sleep apnea: review. Sleep 1995;18(6):501-511.

64. Schmidt-Nowara W, Meade T, Hays M. Treatment of snoring and obstructive sleep apnea with a dental orthosis. Chest 1991;99:1378-1385.

65. Gale DJ, Sawyer RH, Woodcock A, et al. Do oral appliances enlarge the airway in patients with obstructive sleep apnea? A prospective computerized tomographic study. Eur J Orthod 2000;22:159-168.

66. Ferguson K, Love L, Ryan CF. Effect of mandibular and tongue protrusion on upper airway size during wakefulness. Am J Respir Crit Care Med 1997;155:1748-1754.

67. Johnson L, Arnett W, Tamborello J, et al. Airway changes in relationship to mandibular posturing. Otolaryngol Head Neck Surg 1992;106:143-148.

68. Bonham PE, Currier GF, Orr WC, et al. The effect of a modified functional appliance on obstructive sleep apnea. Am J Orthodon Dentofacial Orthop 1988;94:384-392.

69. Lowe AA, Sjoholm TT, Ryan CF, et al. Treatment, airway and compliance effects of a titratable oral appliance. Sleep 2000;23:S172-178.

70. Henke KG, Frantz DE, Kuna ST. An oral mandibular advancement device for obstructive sleep apnea. Am J Respir Crit Care Med 2000;161:420-425.

71. Castro-Barbosa R, Aloe F, Tavares S, et al. Mandibular-lingual repositioning device—MRLD: preliminary results in 8 patients with obstructive sleep apnea. Revista Paulista de Medicina 1995;113(3):88-94.

72. Lamont J, Beldwin DR, Hay KD, et al. Effects of 2 types of mandibular advancement splints on snoring and obstructive sleep apnea. Eur J Orthod 1998;20:2923-2997.

73. Marklund M, Franklin KA, Sahlin C, et al. The effect of a mandibular advancing device on apneas and sleep in patients with obstructive sleep apnea. Chest 1988;113:707-713.

74. Mayer G, Meier-Ewert K. Cephalometric predictors for orthopaedic mandibular advancement in obstructive sleep apnea. Eur J Orthodon 1995;17:35-43.

75. Menn SJ, Loube DI, Morgan TD, et al. The mandibular repositioning device: role in the treatment of obstructive sleep apnea. Sleep 1996;19:794-800.

76. Millman RP, Rosenberg CL, Carlisle CC, et al. The efficacy of oral appliances in the treatment of persistent sleep apnea after uvulopalatopharyngoplasty. Chest 1998;113:992-996.

77. Pancer J, Al-Faifi S, Al-Faifi M, et al. Evaluation of variable mandibular advancement appliance for treatment of snoring and sleep apnea. Chest 1999;116:1511-1518.

78. Raphaelson MA, Alpher EJ, Bakker KW, et al. Oral appliance therapy of obstructive sleep apnea syndrome: progressive mandibular advancement during polysomnogram. J Craniomand Practice 1998;16:44-50.

79. Hans MG, Nelson S, Luks VG, et al. Comparison of two dental devices for treatment of obstructive sleep apnea syndrome. Am J Orthodon Dentofacial Orthop 1997;111:562-570.

80. Clark GT, Blumenfeld I, Yoffe N, et al. A crossover study comparing the efficacy of CPAP with anterior mandibular positioning devices on patients with obstructive sleep apnea. Chest 1996;109:1477-1483.

81. Ferguson KA, Ono T, Lowe AA, et al. A randomized crossover study of an oral appliance versus nasal-CPAP in the treatment of mild-moderate obstructive sleep apnea. Chest 1996;109:1269-1275.

82. Ferguson KA, Ono T, Lowe AA, et al. A short-term controlled trial of an adjustable oral appliance for treatment of mild to moderate obstructive sleep apnea. Thorax 1997;52:362-368.

83. Wilhelmsson B, Tegelberg A, Walker-Engstrom MC, et al. A prospective randomized study of a dental appliance compared with uvulopalatopharyngoplasty in the treatment of obstructive sleep apnea. Acta Otolaryngol 1999;119(4):503-509.

84. Hart WT, Duhamel J, Guilleminault C. Oral positive airway pressure by the OPAP® dental appliance reduces mild to severe obstructive sleep apnea. Sleep Research 1997;26:371.

85. Eveloff SE, Rosenberg CL, Carlisle CC, et al. Efficacy of a Herbst mandibular advancement device in obstructive sleep apnea. Am J Respir Crit Care Med 1994;149:905-909.

86. Millman RP, Rosenberg CL, Kramer NM. Oral appliances in the treatment of snoring and sleep apnea. Clinics in Chest Medicine 1998;19:69-75.

87. Bondemark L. Does two years' nocturnal treatment with a mandibular advancement splint in adult patients with snoring and obstructive sleep apnea cause a change in the posture of the mandible? Am J Orthod Dentofacial Orthop 1999;116:621-628.

88. Senior B, Rosenthal L, Lumely A, et al. Efficacy of uvulopalatopharyngoplasty in unselected patients with mild obstructive sleep apnea. Otolaryngol Head Neck Surg 2000;123:179-182.

89. Launois SH, Feroah TR, Campbell WN, et al. Site of pharyngeal narrowing predicts outcome of surgery for obstructive sleep apnea. Am Rev Respir Dis 1993;147:182-189.

90. Li KK, Riley RW, Powell NB, et al. Obstructive sleep apnea surgery: patient perspective and polysomnographic results. Otolaryngol Head Neck Surg 2000;123:572-575.

91. Li KK, Riley RW, Powell NB, et al. Maxillomandibular advancement for persistent obstructive sleep apnea after phase I surgery for patients without maxillomandibular deficiency. Laryngoscope 2000;110:1684-1688.

92. Prinsell J. Maxillomandibular advancement surgery in a site-specific treatment approach for obstructive sleep apnea in 50 consecutive patients. Chest 1999;116:1519-1529.

93. Standards of Practice Committee of the American Sleep Disorders Association. Practice parameters for the treatment of obstructive sleep apnea in adults: the efficacy of surgical modifications of the upper airway. Sleep 1996;19:152-156.

94. Sher AE, Shechtman KB, Piccirillo JF. The efficacy of surgical modification of the upper airway in adults with obstructive sleep apnea syndrome. Sleep 1996;19:156-177.

95. Walker RP, Grigg-Damberger MM, Gopalsami C. Laser-assisted uvulopalatoplasty for the treatment of mild, moderate, and severe obstructive sleep apnea. Laryngoscope 1999;109:79-85.

96. Handada T, Shireru S, Tateyama T, et al. Laser-assisted uvulopalatoplasty with Nd:YAG laser for sleep disorders. Laryngoscope 1996;106:1531-1533.

97. Mickelson SA. Laser-assisted uvulopalatoplasty for obstructive sleep apnea. Laryngoscope 1996;106:10-13.

98. Ryan CF, Love LL. Unpredictable results of laser assisted uvulopalatoplasty in the treatment of obstructive sleep apnea. Thorax 2000;55:399-404.

99. Walker RP, Grigg-Damberger MM, Gopalsami C. Laser-assisted uvulopalatoplasty for snoring and obstructive sleep apnea: results in 170 patients. Laryngoscope 1995;105:938-943.

100. Walker RP, Grigg-Damberger MM, Gopalsami C. Uvulopalatopharyngoplasty versus laser-assisted uvulopalatoplasty for the treatment of obstructive sleep apnea. Laryngoscope 1997;107:76-82.

101. Finkelstein Y, Shapiro-Feinberg S, Stein G, et al. Uvulopalatopharyngoplasty vs. laser-assisted uvulopalatoplasty: anatomical considerations. Arch Otolaryngol Head Neck Surg 1997;123:265-276.

102. Millman RP, Carlisle CC, Rosenberg C, et al. Simple predictors of uvulopalatopharyngoplasty outcome in the treatment of obstructive sleep apnea. Chest 2000;118:1025-1030.

103. Walker-Engstrom M, Wilhelmsson B, Tegelberg A, et al. Quality of life assessment of treatment with dental appliance or UPPP in patients with mild to moderate obstructive sleep apnea. A prospective randomized 1-year follow-up study. J Sleep Res 2000;9:303-308.

104. Anand VK, Ferguson PW, Schoen LS. Obstructive sleep apnea: a comparison of continuous positive airway pressure and surgical treatment. Otolaryngol Head Neck Surg 1991;105:382-387.

105. Lojander J, Maasilta P, Partinea M, et al. Nasal CPAP surgery and conservative management for treatment of obstructive sleep apnea syndrome. Chest 1996;110:114-119.

106. Verse T, Kroker BA, Dirsig W, et al. Tonsillectomy as a treatment of obstructive sleep apnea in adults with tonsillar hypertrophy. Laryngoscope 2000;110:1556-1559.

107. Powell NB, Riley RW, Troell RJ, et al. Radiofrequency volumetric tissue reduction of the palate in subjects with sleep-disordered breathing. Chest 1998;113:1163-1174.

108. Woodson BT. Retropalatal airway characteristics in uvulopalatopharyngoplasty compared with transpalatal advancement pharyngoplasty. Laryngoscope 1997;107:735-740.

109. Woodson BT. Acute effects of palatopharyngoplasty on airway collapsibility. Otolaryngol Head Neck Surg 1999;121:82-86.

110. Utley DS, Shin EJ, Clerk AA, et al. A cost-effective and rational surgical approach to patients with snoring, upper airway resistance syndrome, or obstructive sleep apnea syndrome. Laryngoscope 1997;107:726-734.

111. Hochbas W, Conradt R, Brandenburg U, et al. Surgical maxillofacial treatment of obstructive sleep apnea. Plast Reconst Surg 1997;99:619-626.

112. Riley RW, Powell NB, Guilleminault C. Maxillary, mandibular and hyoid advancement for the treatment of obstructive sleep apnea: a review of 40 patients. J Oral Maxillofac Surg 1990;48:20.

113. Conradt R, Hochban W, Branderburg U, et al. Long-term follow-up after surgical treatment of obstructive sleep apnea by maxillomandibular advancement. Eur Respir J 1997;10:123-128.

CHAPTER 59

Lung Cancer

Atul Malhotra
David R. Schwartz

CHAPTER OUTLINE

Classification
Epidemiology
Risk Factors and Etiology
Presentation
Solitary Pulmonary Nodule
Diagnosis
Work-Up and Staging
Treatment
    Small Cell Lung Cancer
    Non–Small Cell Lung Cancer
    Complications of Therapy

Prognosis
Prevention
Future Directions
Case Studies
    Case One: Lung Cancer Screening
    Case Two: Early Stage Lung Cancer
    Case Three: Metastatic Lung Cancer

OBJECTIVES

1. Discuss the magnitude of the worldwide problem of bronchogenic cancer.
2. Classify the different types of lung cancer.
3. Explain the importance of cigarette smoking as a risk factor for lung cancer.
4. Describe the approach to staging of small cell and non–small cell lung cancer.
5. List the different treatment options for lung cancer and the associated prognoses.
6. Discuss possible future advances in screening, diagnosis, and treatment of lung cancer.

KEY TERMS

Adenocarcinoma	Mediastinoscopy	Solitary Pulmonary Nodule (SPN)
Adjuvant Therapy	Metastasis	Squamous Cell Carcinoma
Benign	Neoadjuvant Therapy	Transbronchial Needle Aspiration
Bronchogenic Cancer	Non–Small Cell Lung Cancer (NSCLC)	(TBNA)
Chemotherapy	Radiotherapy	Tumor Suppressor Gene
Malignant	Small Cell Lung Cancer (SCLC)	

Bronchogenic cancer is a common disease with major health implications. Approximately 170,000 cases are diagnosed each year in the United States, and the 5-year survival rate is only 14%. Lung cancer causes as many as 1 million deaths annually worldwide, and it currently is the leading cause of death from cancer in adults. Although it is largely preventable, lung cancer kills more people than breast cancer, colon cancer, and prostate cancer combined. Despite extensive research, the mortality rate for lung cancer has not improved substantially over the past several decades. The cost of treatment is estimated to be 1% of the gross domestic product of the United States. New chemotherapeutic agents, recent advances in diagnostic technology, and novel treatment strategies offer some basis for optimism. However, the progressively rising lung cancer mortality rate among women in developed countries and among both women and men in developing countries shows that the disease has reached epidemic proportions, a substantial cause for concern.[1-3]

Classification

Lung tumors can be classified as primary or secondary, **benign** or **malignant,** endobronchial or parenchymal. Box 59-1 presents the World Health Organization's histologic classification of lung and pleural tumors.

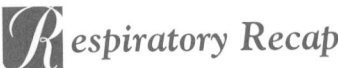 *espiratory Recap*

Lung Cancer Classification
Primary or secondary
Benign or malignant
Endobronchial or parenchymal

Bronchogenic carcinomas are classified as **small cell lung cancer (SCLC)** or **non–small cell lung cancer (NSCLC).** Although originally classified as histologically benign, bronchial adenomas include mucoepidermoid carcinomas, adenoid cystic carcinomas (cylindromas), and carcinoid tumors. NSCLC includes **squamous cell carcinoma** marked by histologic evidence of keratinization; **adenocarcinoma** marked by glandular organization and mucus secretion; and large cell undifferentiated cancer, a diagnosis of exclusion when there is no evidence of either squamous or glandular differentiation with light microscopy. Recent advances in electron microscopy and immunohistochemistry have led to an expansion of the original classification, providing subtypes of NSCLC. These subtypes do not have a major influence on management of the disease, although some differences in presentation and pattern of spread have been noted.

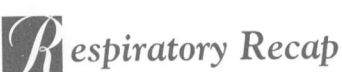 *espiratory Recap*

Types of Bronchogenic Carcinoma
Small cell lung cancer
Non–small cell lung cancer

Over the past 30 to 40 years, the percentage of adenocarcinomas has increased. These tumors most often are peripheral and include bronchoalveolar carcinoma, a subtype with unique behavior. The reason for the increased risk of adenocarcinoma is unclear but may be related to changes in smoking behavior (depth of inspiration, type of filter, nitrosamine content). Adenocarcinomas are the most common subtype in women and nonsmokers. They have a slightly greater propensity for early distant spread, especially to the brain, compared to squamous cell tumors. Large cell tumors also are most often peripheral and may be necrotic, leading to cavitation. Squamous cell tumors remain the most common histologic subtype in men. They

arise from the proximal respiratory epithelium and form large central masses, often with associated necrosis.

SCLC differs from NSCLC in its cell of origin and its aggressiveness. Although tumors with mixed histology have led to the idea of a pluripotent stem cell origin for all bronchogenic cancers, small cell cancers appear to be derived from the neuroendocrine cells of the airway, the so-called enterochromaffin or amine precursor uptake and decarboxylation (APUD) cells. SCLC is highly associated with tobacco smoking and accounts for 15% to 25% of all bronchogenic carcinomas. The name derives from the histologic appearance of the tumors, which are seen as small, round, blue cells with hematoxylin-eosin staining. These tumor cells are about twice as big as lymphocytes and have a high mitotic rate and metastatic potential. Small cell tumors have a rapid doubling time, and early distant spread is the rule. Although small cell cancers are sensitive to **chemotherapy** and **radiotherapy,** the survival rate remains dismal.

Epidemiology

As mentioned previously, the incidence of lung cancer in the United States is 170,000 new cases each year, and it is rising. The disease has reached epidemic proportions. As cigarette smoking increases in underdeveloped countries, the worldwide incidence of lung cancer may reach a staggering level.

Although traditionally considered a disease of men, lung cancer increasingly is seen in women, who account for 45% of new cases. These gender-specific trends are largely explained by smoking behaviors. The increase in tobacco use among girls and young women make these data a matter of particular concern.[1-4]

Risk Factors and Etiology

The major risk factor for lung cancer is cigarette smoking (Table 59-1). Given the dismal epidemiologic statistics, lung cancer differs from most other cancers because it is largely preventable. The relative risk of developing lung cancer is 10 to 30 times higher for smokers than for lifelong nonsmokers. For a heavy smoker the lifetime risk of developing lung cancer may be as high as 30% and is proportional to the total quantity and duration of cigarette use. Until recently the link between lung cancer and cigarette smoke was largely based on correlations and associations. However, a direct link recently was demonstrated by the induction of damage to specific loci of a **tumor suppressor gene** (p53, seen in roughly 60% of lung cancers) by benzopyrene (a chemical in tobacco smoke).[5] Moreover, proto-oncogenes can produce proteins that regulate cell growth and differentiation. For example, mutations of the ras proto-oncogenes have been identified in as many as one third of patients with NSCLC, with K-ras mutations commonly identified in adenocarcinomas in smokers.

Box 59-1

World Health Organization's Histologic Classification of Lung and Pleural Tumors

Epithelial Tumors
Benign
Papillomas
Squamous cell papilloma
    Exophytic
    Inverted
Glandular papilloma
Mixed squamous cell and glandular papilloma
Adenomas
Alveolar adenoma
Papillary adenoma
Adenomas of salivary gland type
    Mucous gland adenoma
    Pleomorphic adenoma
    Others
Mucinous cystadenoma
Others
Preinvasive lesions
Squamous dysplasia/carcinoma in situ
Atypical adenomatous hyperplasia
Diffuse idiopathic pulmonary neuroendocrine cell hyperplasia
Malignant
Squamous cell carcinoma
Variants
    Papillary
    Clear cell
    Small cell
    Basaloid
Small cell carcinoma
Variant
    Combined small cell carcinoma
Adenocarcinoma
Acinar
Papillary
Bronchoalveolar carcinoma
    Nonmucinous
    Mucinous
    Mixed mucinous and nonmucinous or indeterminate
Solid adenocarcinoma with mucin
Adenocarcinoma with mixed subtypes
Variants
    Well-differentiated fetal adenocarcinoma
    Mucinous ("colloid") adenocarcinoma
    Mucinous crystadenocarcinoma
    Signet ring adenocarcinoma
    Clear cell adenocarcinoma
Large cell carcinoma
Variants
    Large cell neuroendocrine carcinoma
      Combined large cell neuroendocrine carcinoma
    Basaloid carcinoma
    Lymphoepithelioma-like carcinoma
    Clear cell carcinoma
    Large cell carcinoma with rhabdoid phenotype
Adenosquamous carcinoma
Carcinomas with pleomorphic, sarcomatoid, or sarcomatous elements
Carcinomas with spindle and/or giant cells
    Pleomorphic carcinoma
    Spindle cell carcinoma
    Giant cell carcinoma
Carcinosarcoma

Pulmonary blastoma
Other
Carcinoid tumor
Typical carcinoid
Atypical carcinoid
Carcinomas of salivary gland type
Mucoepidermoid carcinoma
Adenoid cystic carcinoma
Others
Unclassified carcinoma

Soft Tissue Tumors
Localized fibrous tumor
Epithelioid hemangioendothelioma
Pleuropulmonary blastoma
Chondroma
Calcifying fibrous pseudotumor of the pleura
Congenital peribronchial myofibroblastic tumor
Diffuse pulmonary lymphangiomatosis
Desmoplastic round cell tumor
Others

Mesothelial Tumors
Benign
    Adenomatoid tumor
Malignant mesothelioma
    Epithelioid mesothelioma
    Sarcomatoid mesothelioma
      Desmoplastic mesothelioma
    Biphasic mesothelioma
    Other

Miscellaneous Tumors
Hamartoma
Sclerosing hemangioma
Clear cell tumor
Germ cell tumors
    Teratoma, mature or immature
    Other germ cell tumors
Thymoma
Malignant melanoma
Others

Lymphoproliferative Diseases
Lymphoid interstitial pneumonia
Nodular lymphoid hyperplasia
Low-grade marginal zone B-cell lymphoma of the mucosa-associated lymphoid tissue (MALT)
Lymphomatoid granulomatosis

Secondary Tumors
Unclassified Tumors
Tumorlike Lesions
Tumorlet
Minute meningothelioid nodule
Langerhans' cell histiocytosis
Inflammatory pseudotumor (inflammatory myofibroblastic tumor)
Localized organizing pneumonia
Amyloid tumor
Hyalinizing granuloma
Lymphangioleiomyomatosis
Micronodular pneumocyte hyperplasia
Endometriosis
Bronchial inflammatory polyp
Others

Modified from Travis WD, Colby TV, Corrin B, et al. World Health Organization Pathology Panel: World Health Organization histological typing of lung and pleural tumors: international histological classification of tumors. 3rd ed. Berlin, Springer-Verlag (in press).

TABLE 59-1

Relative Risk of Lung Cancer

Patient History	Risk Ratio*
Never smoked; no significant industrial contact	1
Cigarette smoker	
½ pack/day	15
½ to 1 pack/day	17
1 to 2 packs/day	42
More than 2 packs/day	64
Cigar smoker	3
Pipe smoker	8
Former smoker	2 to 10
Nonsmoking woman exposed to second-hand smoke	1.4 to 1.9
Asbestos worker	
Nonsmoker	5
Cigarette smoker	92
Uranium miner	
Nonsmoker	7
Cigarette smoker	38
Relatives of lung cancer patients	
Nonsmoker	4
Cigarette smoker	14

From Murray JF, Nadel JA: Textbook of respiratory medicine. 2nd ed. Philadelphia: WB Saunders; 1994.
*The risk ratio is the relative risk of an individual developing lung cancer compared with the risk faced by a comparable individual without the listed exposure.

Clearly evidence is emerging to explain the mechanisms underlying smoking-induced carcinogenesis.[6-10]

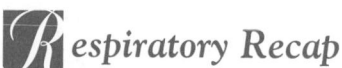

Respiratory Recap

> **Primary Risk Factor for Lung Cancer**
>
> The major risk factor for lung cancer is cigarette smoking

Second-hand smoke (environmental tobacco smoke [ETS]) may have important health effects. Although the amount of exposure is clearly less than in smokers, the onset of exposure generally occurs at a younger age. Although it varies across studies, the relative risk of lung cancer increases above that of lifelong nonsmokers in a dose-dependent fashion. Because most lung cancer victims are smokers, the number of cases of lung cancer attributable to ETS alone is small. Some have estimated that 1250 people would have to stop smoking to prevent one case of ETS-induced bronchogenic cancer. However, this issue requires further research.[11-13]

Risk factors unrelated to tobacco use have been reported, including exposure to chromium, asbestos, bischloromethyl ether, ionizing radiation, nickel, mustard gas, arsenic, radon,

BOX 59-2

Occupational Carcinogens for Lung Cancer

Proven Carcinogens
Arsenic
Asbestos
Bischloromethyl ether
Chromium
Mustard gas
Nickel
Polycyclic aromatic hydrocarbons
Ionizing radiation

Suspected Carcinogens
Acrylonitrile
Beryllium
Vinyl chloride
Silica
Iron ore
Wood dust

From Murray JF, Nadel JA: Textbook of respiratory medicine. 2nd ed. Philadelphia: WB Saunders; 1994.

and polycyclic aromatic hydrocarbons (Box 59-2).[14-20] Risk factors may act in concert to increase the risk of lung cancer substantially. For example, smoking and asbestosis increase the relative risk of lung cancer by 60- to 80-fold.[21,22] Low-level exposure to asbestos (for example, nonoccupational exposure) does not significantly change the risk of lung cancer.[23]

Genetic and dietary factors may also increase the risk of lung cancer.[24] First degree relatives of patients with lung cancer have a twofold to threefold higher risk. Females also appear to be at increased risk of lung cancer at all levels of tobacco use. In addition, numerous recent studies suggest that certain benign diffuse parenchymal lung diseases (for example, scleroderma, sarcoidosis, idiopathic pulmonary fibrosis, and emphysema) may increase the relative risk of developing lung cancer.[25-32]

Some have suggested that infection with the human immunodeficiency virus (HIV) may influence the development and progression of lung cancer. This theory is based primarily on small case series that have documented the development of particularly aggressive lung cancers in patients under 40 years of age.[33,34]

Presentation

Bronchogenic cancers may be found incidentally, through active screening, or because of local or systemic symptoms.[35] Because the outcome for individuals with symptomatic lung cancer is dismal, prevention and early diagnosis have been emphasized. Unfortunately, roughly 90% of patients found to have lung cancer are symptomatic at presentation.

Symptoms related to the primary lesion, such as cough, are common at presentation (Table 59-2). Along with dyspnea and hemoptysis, cough often is thought to indicate a

TABLE 59-2

Initial Symptoms of Bronchogenic Carcinoma in 100 Patients*

Symptom	Occurrence (%)
Cough	21
Hemoptysis	21
Chest pain	16
Dyspnea	12
Extrathoracic pain	6
Anorexia and weight loss	5
Cervical mass	5
Fatigue	3
Superior vena caval obstruction	3
Hoarseness	3
Central nervous system symptoms	3
Shoulder pain	2
Clubbing of the fingers	1

From Murray JF, Nadel JA: Textbook of respiratory medicine. 2nd ed. Philadelphia: WB Saunders; 1994.
*Patients were seen at M.D. Anderson Cancer Center, Houston, Texas.

central tumor. One confounder is the frequent concurrence of smoking-induced chronic obstructive pulmonary disease (COPD). A change in the quality or frequency of chronic cough in a patient with COPD should prompt consideration of the diagnosis of malignancy. Persistent pneumonic infiltrates or recurrent same-segment pneumonias should suggest an obstructing airway lesion. Similarly, a unifocal wheeze on physical examination may be a diagnostic clue to an obstructing airway lesion.

Respiratory Recap

Presentation of Lung Cancer

Dyspnea	Clubbing of the fingers
Hemoptysis	Endocrine syndromes
Chest pain	Neurologic syndromes
Dysphagia	Signs of metastases

Dyspnea that occurs as a direct result of lung cancer may be caused by airway obstruction with atelectasis, postobstructive pneumonitis, lymphangitic spread of the tumor, or a compressive malignant pericardial or pleural effusion. Local invasion of the phrenic nerve or the diaphragm may contribute to dyspnea related to diaphragmatic dysfunction.

Hemoptysis is a common symptom in patients with lung cancer, to some extent reflecting concurrent chronic bronchitis. Although lung cancer is in the differential diagnosis of massive hemoptysis because in rare cases tumors may erode into hilar vessels, low-volume but recurrent hemoptysis is most characteristic of bleeding tumors. High-resolution computed tomography (HRCT) scanning has facilitated the

work-up of submassive hemoptysis when routine radiography is not helpful. In patients at lower risk for malignancy (those under 35 years of age) who have a normal or nonlocalizing radiograph, HRCT can help identify suspicious lesions, direct bronchoscopy, and define common benign etiologies such as bronchiectasis. The prevalence of mild hemoptysis in hospitalized patients is increasing, probably secondary to bleeding diatheses related to anticoagulation, antiplatelet therapies, thrombolytics, or severe thrombocytopenia; prospective studies are required to determine the proper work-up. High-risk patients with hemoptysis for whom there is no clear cause should undergo a thorough bronchoscopy before or soon after hospital discharge.[36-39]

Substantial chest pain in lung cancer patients usually represents extension of a peripheral mass to the pleura or the chest wall. Pancoast's syndrome is chest wall and spinal nerve root/sympathetic chain invasion by an apical bronchogenic tumor, the so-called superior sulcus tumor.[40] The syndrome consists of pain in the shoulder and medial scapula, an ulnar distribution of radicular pain or muscle atrophy (or both), and Horner's syndrome (unilateral ptosis, miosis, anhydrosis, and enopthalmos). Superior sulcus tumors are most commonly squamous cell carcinomas.

Local spread of proximal tumors or lymph node masses may cause dysphagia related to esophageal compression, hoarseness related to recurrent laryngeal nerve involvement, chylothorax secondary to thoracic duct compromise, or superior vena caval (SVC) syndrome related to central venous obstruction. Although the differential diagnosis is wide, the most common cause of the SVC syndrome is intraluminal thrombosis related to extrinsic compression by bronchogenic cancer, usually SCLC. Patients with SVC syndrome have symptoms and signs of upper body venous congestion, such as headache or flushing, plethora, and a prominent upper body pattern of venous collaterals. Although controversy exists as to whether SVC syndrome is a true emergency, chemoradiotherapy in SCLC promptly resolves the syndrome.[41]

Extrathoracic symptoms may be related to hematogenous spread of the cancer itself. Common sites include the central nervous system (CNS), bone (axial more often than appendicular skeleton), liver, and adrenal glands. CNS and bone lesions are exceedingly important, because they may lead to substantial pain and disability and often are amenable to palliation, usually through radiotherapy. Liver and adrenal metastases, however, are often asymptomatic and may be suspected because of an infiltrative picture of elevated liver enzymes or on a CT scan of the chest or abdomen.

Lesions in the lung that represent the spread of a primary lung cancer consist of secondary nodules, lymphangitic spread, and tumor emboli. Tumor emboli increasingly recognized as a syndrome, may result in subacute or acute dyspnea, disseminated intravascular coagulation, and obstructive shock. The diagnosis may be made by cytologic analysis of a wedged sample obtained by pulmonary artery catheter. Lymphangitic spread, which causes dry cough, weight loss, and progressive dyspnea, may manifest as

TABLE 59-3

Endocrine and Hematologic Syndromes Associated with Lung Tumors

Syndrome	Tumor	Proteins/Cytokines Involved
Hypercalcemia of malignancy	Non–small cell	Parathyroid hormone–related peptide, parathormone
Hyponatremia of malignancy	Small cell	Arginine vasopressin
	Non–small cell	Atrial natriuretic peptide
Ectopic ACTH syndrome	Small cell	Adrenocorticotropic hormone
	Carcinoid	Corticotropin-releasing hormone
Acromegaly	Carcinoid, small cell	Growth hormone–releasing hormone
Granulocytosis	Non–small cell	C-CSF, GM-CSF, IL-6
Thrombocytosis	Non–small cell, small cell	IL-6
Thromboembolism	Non–small cell, small cell	Unknown

ACTH, *Adrenocorticotropic hormone;* C-CSF, *granulocyte colony-stimulating factor;* GM-CSF, *granulocyte-macrophage colony-stimulating factor;* IL-6, *interleukin 6.*

asymmetric pulmonary edema on the chest radiograph. In the appropriate clinical context, the presence of Kerley's B lines on the chest radiograph is suspicious for this diagnosis (especially if unilateral) and are highly characteristic on HRCT if seen as thickened, beaded, intralobular septae. The diagnosis also is made with high sensitivity and specificity by transbronchial biopsy. As can be seen, spread of the tumor itself can result in a variety of manifestations, depending on the mechanism.[42]

The paraneoplastic manifestations of bronchogenic carcinoma are those that are unrelated to the mechanical effects of primary or metastatic tumor. These paraneoplastic syndromes may occur in at least 10% of lung cancer patients (Table 59-3). Several specific syndromes deserve mention. Weight loss is a common feature of lung cancer. Thought to be a paraneoplastic syndrome associated with enhanced inflammatory cytokine production, which results in anorexia and hypermetabolism, the debility associated with weight loss is an important negative prognostic factor.[43-46]

Clubbing of the fingers, which is caused by an increase in subungual soft tissue with associated straightening of the nail bed (Lovibond's angle), is an important albeit nonspecific finding in lung cancer. Other causes of clubbing include chronic pulmonary infections (bronchiectasis, lung abscess, or empyema), restrictive lung diseases (idiopathic pulmonary fibrosis, pulmonary alveolar phospholipoproteinosis), cyanotic congenital heart disease, infective endocarditis, inflammatory bowel disease, and alcoholic cirrhosis.[47] Both clubbing and the related hypertrophic pulmonary osteoarthropathy (HPO), a symmetric, painful syndrome involving the long bones, are less commonly seen in SCLC than NSCLC. Both signs may disappear with successful tumor therapy. One interesting association has been made between unilateral facial pain and HPO in a small number of patients with lung cancer. Both syndromes have been postulated to result from afferent vagal nerve compression from an intrathoracic tumor.[48]

Endocrine syndromes are another relatively common feature of lung cancer, especially SCLC. The syndrome of inappropriate antidiuretic hormone secretion (SIADH, manifesting with hyponatremia) and ectopic Cushing's syndrome (manifesting with weakness, glucose intolerance, and hypokalemia related to an excess of adrenocorticotropin hormone) may be found in patients with established malignancy or may be the first clue to a previously occult tumor. Hypercalcemia, seen most often with squamous cell carcinoma, manifests with malaise, dehydration, and gastrointestinal and neurologic abnormalities. Differentiating paraneoplastic hypercalcemia from metastatic bone hypercalcemia that occurs secondary to osseous metastases (through identification of excess parathyroid hormone–related peptide) may be important in the determination of therapy. Hypercalcemia is a very poor prognostic factor in patients with bronchogenic carcinoma.[49]

Neurologic syndromes are increasingly recognized and devastating paraneoplastic manifestations of lung cancer. The antibody ANNA-1 (anti-Hu) is associated with SCLC and can have a variety of clinical manifestations. In addition to cerebellar ataxia and a sensory neuropathy, ANNA-1 can lead to alterations in gastric motility, manifesting with nausea, anorexia, and weight loss. Although SCLC often is localized to the chest at the time of diagnosis, the overall survival rate is still dismal. Although some authors report slower tumor growth in patients with ANNA-1, the prognosis remains poor because of the associated weight loss, malnutrition, and immobility from gait ataxia.[45,46,50]

Solitary Pulmonary Nodule

A **solitary pulmonary nodule (SPN),** a lesion seen on the chest radiograph, is completely surrounded by lung parenchyma, without other radiographic abnormalities such as pleural effusion or adenopathy. An arbitrary size cutoff of 3 cm distinguishes SPN from masses, which generally are malignant. SPNs, or *coin lesions,* usually are asymptomatic and generally are found on routine radiographs. In adults an SPN is considered malignant until proven otherwise, but a number of alternative etiologies are included in the differential diagnosis (Box 59-3 and Table 59-4).[51]

Diagnostic algorithms and recent advances in imaging have focused on differentiation of benign lesions from malignant ones. This distinction is important, because an SPN is the most curable presentation of bronchogenic carcinoma. The 5-year survival rate for these resected T1N0M0 lesions ranges from 60% to 90%. In addition, nonsurgical identification of a benign lesion may eliminate the need for thoracotomy or thoracoscopy. The U.S. Veterans Administration (VA) Cooperative Armed Forces Study reported in 1975 that only one third of resected SPNs were malignant.[52] However, a more recent VA study from Minnesota in 1996 reported that the percentage of resected SPNs found to be malignant had increased.[53] The percentage ranged from 55% to 60% from 1981 to 1983 to 90% to 100% from 1990 to 1994. This undoubtedly reflects the greater ability of computed tomography (CT) to identify benign lesions. In the community, the local frequency of malignant SPN depends to a large extent on the likelihood of obtaining chest radiographs in young people, the population's age distribution, the smoking prevalence, and the prevalence of infectious granulomatous disease, such as endemic fungi and tuberculosis. In the Minnesota VA study, 53% of benign lesions were granulomata, most of uncertain etiology. The differential diagnosis of an SPN also includes metastatic nodules, adenomas and other benign tumors, hamartomas, embolic phenomena, and nodules associated with rheumatologic lesions.

Historical risk factors for a malignant cause of an SPN include age over 35 years, exposure to tobacco or another known lung carcinogen, and previous malignancy (or metastatic disease). Radiographic signs of malignancy include larger size (more than 3 cm in diameter) and a spiculated border (Figures 59-1, 59-2, and 59-3). Most important, when comparison of current radiographs with previous ones shows growth of the nodule, with a volumetric doubling time of 20 to 400 days, malignancy is likely. Signs of benignity include stable lesions (that is, no growth over a 2-year period) and calcification. Although not 100% specific, an increased calcium content of nodules correlates with benign diagnoses, and certain patterns (popcorn, laminated, diffuse, and central calcification) are very suggestive of benignity. On the other hand, peripheral eccentric calcification is thought to be compatible with a diagnosis of malignancy.

Possible approaches to clinically indeterminate nodules include serial follow-up, transthoracic or bronchoscopic lung biopsy, phantom or contrast CT scanning, and positron emission tomography (PET) scanning. The choice of approach depends on the pretest probability of a diagnosis of malignancy, local practice patterns, and the patient's values (that is, the individual's comfort or discomfort in observing a lesion with a low likelihood of ma-

Box 59-3

Causes of Solitary Pulmonary Nodules

Malignant Nodules
Bronchogenic
  carcinoma
  Adenocarcinoma
  Squamous cell carcinoma
  Small cell
    carcinoma
Metastatic lesions
  Breast
  Head and neck
  Melanoma
  Colon
  Kidney
  Sarcoma
  Germ cell tumor
  Others
Pulmonary carcinoid

Benign Nodules
Infectious granuloma
  Histoplasmosis
  Coccidioidomycosis
  Tuberculosis
  Atypical mycobacteria
  Cryptococcosis
  Blastomycosis

Other infections
  Bacterial abscess
  Dirofilaria immitis
  Echinococcus cyst
  Ascariasis
  Pneumocystis carinii
  Aspergilloma
Benign neoplasms
  Hamartoma
  Lipoma
  Fibroma
Vascular
  Arteriovenous malformation
  Pulmonary varix
Developmental
  Bronchogenic cyst
Inflammatory
  Wegener's granulomatosis
  Rheumatoid nodule
Other
  Amyloidoma
  Rounded atelectasis
  Intrapulmonary lymph nodes
  Hematoma
  Pulmonary infarct
  Pseudotumor (loculated fluid)
  Mucoid impaction

lignancy). In general, serial follow-up is acceptable for low-risk nodules in patients who find diagnostic uncertainty acceptable. For high-risk lesions, definitive diagnosis is required. In many institutions the need for open thoracotomy has been largely replaced by video-assisted thoracoscopic surgery (VATS) techniques. The accuracy of bronchoscopic or transthoracic needle techniques used to diagnose SPN varies widely based on the size of the lesion, its position in the chest, local practice patterns, and the practitioner's skill.[54]

A diagnosis of malignancy made by transthoracic needle aspiration (TTNA) or transbronchial biopsy might eliminate the need for thoracoscopic or open biopsy or resection if surgical therapy is not otherwise required. In addition, in cases in which **neoadjuvant therapy** is given (that is, chemotherapy or radiotherapy or both are given before surgical resection), transbronchial needle aspiration (TBNA) or TTNA helps avoid serial thoracotomy. For patients or physicians who want to avoid thoracotomy for lesions that are not amenable to TBNA or TTNA, or after a negative biopsy result, certain imaging modalities may be used to better evaluate the likelihood of malignancy. Again, the potential for thoracoscopic biopsy or resection has changed the approach of many physicians in these cases.[55]

TABLE 59-4

Clinical and Radiologic Criteria in the Differentiation of Benign and Malignant Solitary Pulmonary Nodules

Criteria	Benign Nodule	Malignant Nodule
Clinical		
Age	Under 35 years of age; exception is hamartoma	Over 35 years of age
Symptoms	Absent	Present
Past history and functional enquiry	High incidence of granuloma in area; exposure to tuberculosis; nonsmoker	Diagnosis of primary lesion elsewhere; smoker; exposure to carcinogens
Radiographic		
Size	Small (<3 cm in diameter)	Large (>3 cm in diameter)
Location	No predilection except for tuberculosis (upper lobes)	Predominantly upper lobes except for lung metastases
Contour	Margins smooth	Margins spiculated
Calcification	Almost pathognomonic of a benign lesion if laminated, diffuse, or central	Rare, may be eccentric (engulfed granuloma)
Satellite lesions	More common	Less common
Serial studies showing no change over 2 years	Almost diagnostic of benign lesion	Most unlikely
Doubling time	<30 or >490 days	Between these extremes
Computed Tomography		
Calcification	Diffuse or central	Absent or eccentric
Fat	Virtually diagnostic or hamartoma	Absent
Bubble-like lucencies	Uncommon	Common in adenocarcinomas
Enhancement with intravenous contrast material	<15 Hounsfield units (HU)	>25 HU

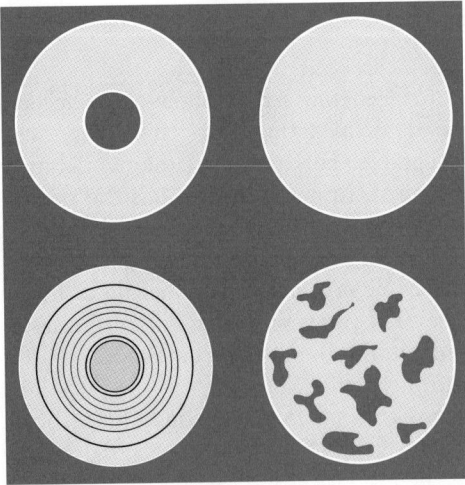

Figure 59-1 Patterns of benign calcification. Clockwise from top left: Target, diffuse, popcorn, and laminated concentric calcification. (Modified from Stark P. Computed and positron emission tomographic scanning of pulmonary nodules. In: Rose BD, editor. Up-to-date [CD-ROM]. Wellesley, Mass: Up-To-Date; 2000.)

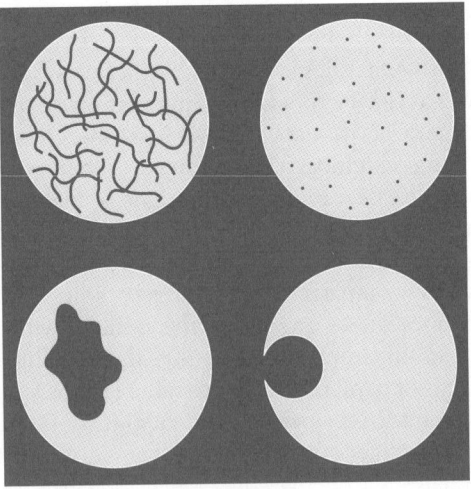

Figure 59-2 Patterns of malignant calcification. Clockwise from top left: Reticular, psammomatous (punctate), eccentric, and amorphous calcification. (Modified from Stark P. Computed and positron emission tomographic scanning of pulmonary nodules. In: Rose BD, editor. Up-to-date [CD-ROM]. Wellesley, Mass: Up-To-Date; 2000.)

With phantom CT scanning, a lung nodule can be compared to one of known density to risk stratify the likelihood of malignancy. Although phantom scanning was popular in some institutions, it has largely fallen out of favor. Contrast-enhanced CT scanning is based on the fact that malignant tissue is more metabolically active than nonmalignant tissue and therefore associated with greater blood flow. In a number of studies[56-60] the cutoff defined as substantial enhancement is +15 to 25 Hounsfield units. By use of intravenous contrast, the presence or absence of nodule enhancement yielded a sensitivity of 98% and a specificity of 58% to 73%. The authors concluded that the

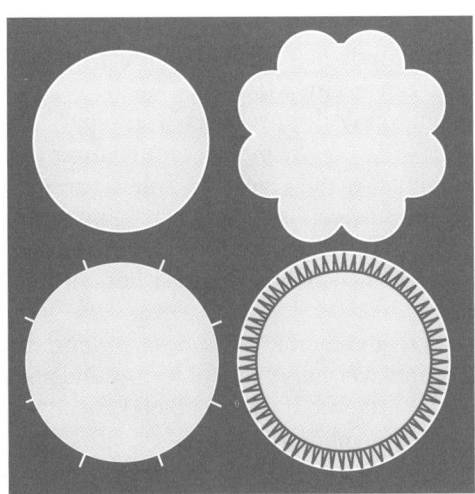

Figure 59-3   Margins of pulmonary nodules. Clockwise from top left: Smooth, scalloped, corona radiata, and spiculated margins. (Modified from Stark P. Computed and positron emission tomographic scanning of pulmonary nodules. In: Rose BD, editor. Up-to-date [CD-ROM]. Wellesley, Mass: Up-To-Date; 2000.)

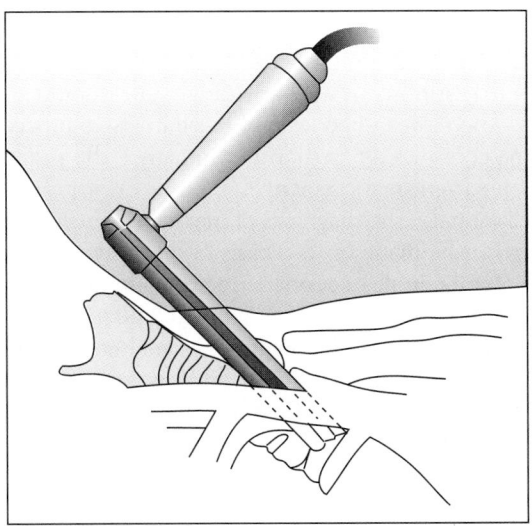

Figure 59-4   Mediastinoscope in place demonstrating the superior mediastinal plane.

degree of enhancement seen with spiral CT scanning was related to the likelihood of malignancy and the vascularity of the nodule. More experience with this technique at various institutions could make this a viable means to eliminate the need for tissue diagnosis in some cases.

PET scanning with fluorodeoxyglucose (FDG) has been advocated for risk stratification of SPNs. Highly metabolically active tissues, such as tumors, should have the greatest affinity for glucose and hence the greatest signal on PET scanning. Malignant nodules therefore would be expected to have substantially greater uptake than benign ones. Although the data on this subject are still emerging, several studies[61-64] estimate a sensitivity of up to 95% and a specificity in the range of 70% to 90%. The subgroup of patients that may benefit from this type of risk stratification has not yet been clearly identified.

A clinical prediction model recently was published that uses clinical and radiologic variables to achieve 98% sensitivity and 87% specificity for lung nodules. Independent predictors of malignancy were age, cigarette smoking, history of cancer, nodule diameter, spiculation of the nodule, and upper lobe location.[59] However, diagnostic certitude for an SPN still requires surgical resection or documented 2 years of stability. Advances in technology and improvements in statistical models may change this in the future.

Diagnosis

The diagnosis of bronchogenic cancer may be based on symptoms, the results of asymptomatic screening, or an incidental radiographic abnormality. Induced sputum is particularly useful to reach a diagnosis in patients with a central lung mass on the chest radiograph. Induced sputum

can be pooled over 24 hours, which increases the diagnostic yield of this study. Although the popularity of induced sputum has declined in recent years, it is recommended in hospitals with adequate experience if it does not lead to prolonged delays in the diagnostic work-up.

Bronchoscopy can be helpful in the work-up of central and mediastinal lesions. Different biopsy techniques are available, depending on the location of the abnormality. **Transbronchial needle aspiration (TBNA)** is useful for biopsy of lesions close to the tracheobronchial tree, with diagnostic yields of 80% to 90% reported in skilled hands. Endobronchial biopsies can be performed for amenable lesions, a technique also associated with excellent yields.[65]

Respiratory Recap

Diagnosis of Lung Cancer
Sputum tests
Bronchoscopy
Mediastinoscopy
Biopsy

A recent advance in the field of bronchoscopy is autofluorescence bronchoscopy for the detection of metaplasia and dysplasia in the tracheobronchial tree of individuals at risk. The laser-induced fluorescence emission (LIFE) system was developed to supplement standard bronchoscopy (white light) in the diagnosis of early malignant lesions in the central airways. Although recent reports suggest that LIFE can increase the diagnostic yield over standard white light bronchoscopy, the improvements are rather modest. Therefore LIFE remains an investigational technique.[66]

Mediastinoscopy can be used for individuals with mediastinal lymphadenopathy (Figure 59-4). This technique is useful for diagnostic purposes if transbronchial needle aspiration fails and for staging once the diagnosis of NSCLC has been established. The morbidity and mortality of mediastinoscopy are exceedingly low in most skilled hands. The risks and benefits of these invasive procedures must be considered based on the influence the result will have on patient management.[67,68]

Occasionally the diagnosis of metastatic bronchogenic cancer can be made on the basis of a biopsy of a remote lesion (for example, a cervical node or adrenal gland). In addition, pleural fluid may be sampled, and pleural biopsy can be performed for the diagnosis of malignant effusion. The advantage of pleural fluid sampling is that it can provide both diagnostic and staging information, because malignant effusion implies a lesion that is at least T_4 (stage IIIB).

Work-Up and Staging

Once the diagnosis has been established, the staging of lung cancer can begin. Knowledge of the staging system can help determine the necessary work-up.[69-74] Box 59-4 and Table 59-5 reflect the most recent changes in NSCLC staging. Table 59-6 and Figure 59-5 illustrate survival according to the stage of lung cancer. Staging for SCLC remains simple: limited or extensive. Limited disease is defined as a case in which all disease lies within a single radiation port.

The tests required after a diagnosis of lung cancer are somewhat controversial. A careful history and physical examination are followed by tests of blood chemistry (serum calcium, alkaline phosphatase [ALP], aspartate amino-

$\mathcal{B}$ox 59-4

TNM Descriptors

Primary Tumor (T)	
TX	Primary tumor cannot be assessed, or tumor proven by the presence of malignant cells in sputum or bronchial washings but not visualized by imaging or bronchoscopy
T0	No evidence of primary tumor
Tis	Carcinoma in situ
T1	Tumor ≤3 cm in greatest dimension, surrounded by lung or visceral pleura, without bronchoscopic evidence of invasion more proximal than the lobar bronchus* (that is, not in the main bronchus)
T2	Tumor with any of the following features of size or extent: >3 cm in greatest dimension Involves main bronchus, ≥2 cm distal to the carina Invades the visceral pleura Associated with atelectasis or obstructive pneumonitis that extends to the hilar region but does not involve the entire lung
T3	Tumor of any size that directly invades any of the following: chest wall (including superior sulcus tumors), diaphragm, mediastinal pleura, parietal pericardium; or tumor in the main bronchus <2 cm distal to the carina, but without involvement of the carina; or associated atelectasis or obstructive pneumonitis of the entire lung
T4	Tumor of any size that invades any of the following: mediastinum, heart, great vessels, trachea, esophagus, vertebral body, carina; or tumor with a malignant pleural or pericardial effusion,† or with satellite tumor nodule(s) within the ipsilateral primary-tumor lobe of the lung
Regional Lymph Nodes (N)	
NX	Regional lymph nodes cannot be assessed
N0	No regional lymph node metastasis
N1	Metastasis to ipsilateral peribronchial and/or ipsilateral hilar lymph nodes, and intrapulmonary nodes involved by direct extension of the primary tumor
N2	Metastasis to ipsilateral mediastinal and/or subcarinal lymph node(s)
N3	Metastasis to contralateral of mediastinal, contralateral hilar, ipsilateral or contralateral scalene, or supraclavicular lymph node(s)
Distant Metastasis (M)	
MX	Presence of distant metastasis cannot be assessed
M0	No distant metastasis
M1	Distant metastasis present‡

From Mountain CF. Revisions in the International System for Staging Lung Cancer. Chest 1997;111:1710-1717.

*The uncommon superficial tumor of any size with its invasive component limited to the bronchial wall, which may extend proximal to the main bronchus, is also classified T1.

†Most pleural effusions associated with lung cancer are due to tumor. However, there are a few patients in whom multiple cytopathologic examinations of pleural fluid show no tumor. In these cases, the fluid is nonbloody and is not an exudate. When these elements and clinical judgment dictate that the effusion is not related to the tumor, the effusion should be excluded as a staging element and the patient's disease should be staged T1, T2, or T3. Pericardial effusion is classified according to the same rules.

‡Separate metastatic tumor nodule(s) in the ipsilateral nonprimary-tumor lobe(s) of the lung also are classified MI.

transferase [AST], alanine aminotransferase [ALT], and a complete blood count [CBC]) and CT scanning of the entire chest, extending caudally to the level of the adrenal

TABLE 59-5

*Stage Grouping—TNM Subsets**

Stage	TNM Subset
0	Carcinoma in situ
IA	T1N0M0
IB	T2N0M0
IIA	T1N1M0
IIB	T2N1M0
	T3N0M0
IIIA	T3N1M0
	T1N2M0
	T2N2M0
	T3N2M0
IIIB	T4N0M0
	T4N1M0
	T4N2M0
	T1N3M0
	T2N3M0
	T3N3M0
	T4N3M0
IV	Any T Any N M1

From Mountain CF. Revisions in the International System for Staging Lung Cancer. Chest 1997;111:1710-1717.
**Staging is not relevant for occult carcinoma, designated TXN0M0.*

glands. Additional tests that may be useful are CT or magnetic resonance imaging (MRI) scans of the head and a bone scan. However, the yield on these tests for **metastasis** is somewhat low if the patient has no symptoms. Many of the lesions found in this setting are false positives, which makes the utility of these tests questionable. With SCLC some advocate complete staging, including a head MRI scan, bone scan, and unilateral or bilateral bone marrow biopsies; others perform a sequential, symptom-based work-up.

With NSCLC, mediastinoscopy is recommended to assess the extent of mediastinal node involvement because CT scanning can be misleading (false positives and false negatives) in the mediastinum. Evolving data suggest that PET scanning may be superior to CT scanning. However, the data are insufficient to determine in which patients it may obviate the need for mediastinoscopy. In patients who undergo neoadjuvant chemoradiotherapy, PET scanning is an attractive option for restaging, because mediastinoscopy is somewhat difficult in this setting (previous mediastinal radiation). Further data on the use of PET scanning are required before appropriate recommendations can be made.[62,75-78]

For patients who may be candidates for surgery, pulmonary function testing is useful to determine the patient's ability to undergo such a procedure. Ideally, a postoperative forced expiratory volume in 1 second (FEV_1) of 800 mL or 40% of predicted should be sought. However, this value is based largely on empiric data. In borderline cases a quantitative ventilation/perfusion scan can help estimate the

TABLE 59-6

Clinical (Top) and Surgical-Pathologic (Bottom) Stages

	Months after Treatment (Cumulative Percent Surviving)				
	12 (%)	24 (%)	36 (%)	48 (%)	60 (%)
cStage*					
cIA	91	79	71	67	61
cIB	72	54	46	41	38
cIIA	79	49	38	34	34
cIIB	59	41	33	26	24
cIIIA	50	25	18	14	13
cIIIB	34	13	7	6	5
cIV	19	6	2	2	1
pStage†					
pIA	94	86	80	73	67
pIB	87	76	67	62	57
pIIA	89	70	66	61	55
pIIB	73	56	46	42	39
pIIIA	64	40	32	26	23

From Mountain CF. Revisions in the International system for strike raw numbers Staging Lung Cancer. Chest 1997;111:1710-1717.
**Percentage distribution of cell types: adenocarcinoma, 47.2%; squamous cell carcinoma, 33.9%; large cell carcinoma, 3.1%; small cell carcinoma, 11.9%; NOS (carcinoma not specified), 3.9%.*
†Percentage distribution of cell types: adenocarcinoma, 53.0%; squamous cell carcinoma, 41.6%; large cell carcinoma, 3.6%; NOS (carcinoma not specified), 1.9%.

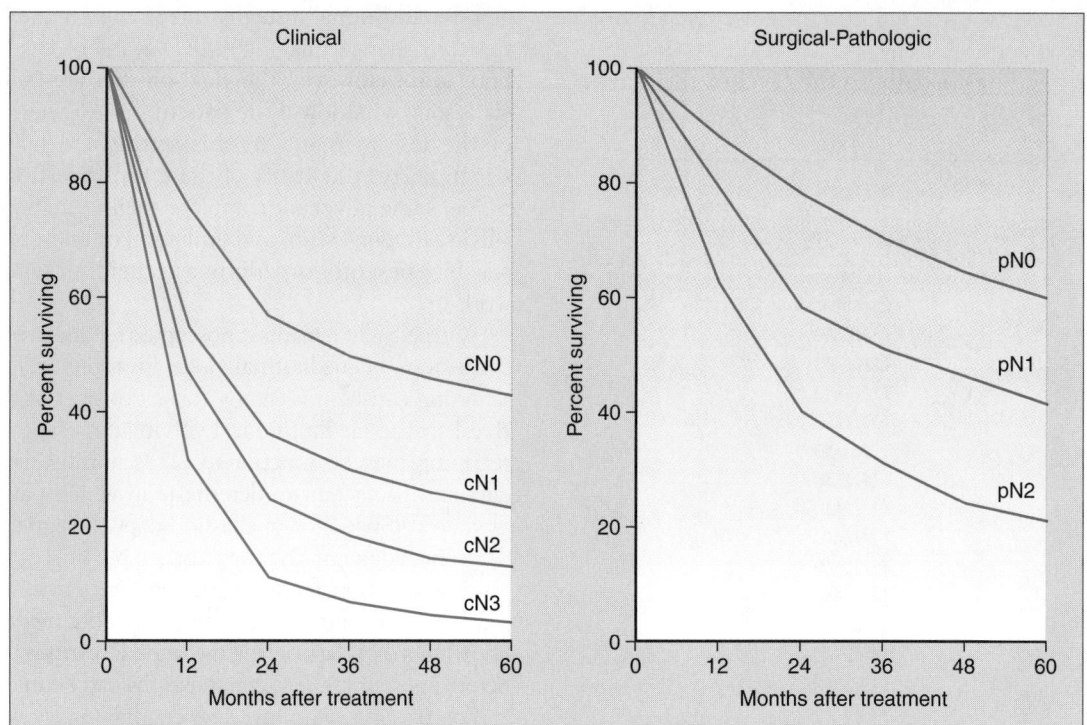

Figure 59-5 Cumulative percent of patients surviving 5 or more years after treatment to the status of lymph nodes. By clinical criteria: cT1-4 N0M0, no evidence of metastasis; cT1-4 N1M0, hilar and intrapulmonary metastasis; cT1 = 4 N2M0, ipsilateral mediastinal lymph node metastasis; cT1-4 N3M0, contralateral mediastinal, contralateral hilar, ipsilateral and contralateral supraclavicular/scalene lymph node metastasis. By surgical-pathologic criteria (small cell carcinoma excluded), pT1-4 N0M0, pT1-4 N1M0, pT1-4 N2M0. Collected database: M.D. Anderson Cancer Center, 1975 to 1988, Reference Center for Anatomic and Pathologic Classification of Lung Cancer (patients treated by the North American LCSG and submitted to the Reference Center for Anatomic and Pathologic Classification of Lung Cancer for confirmation of staging and histology, 1977 to 1982). (Modified from Mountain C, Dresler C. Regional lymph node classification for lung cancer staging. Chest 1997;111:1718-1723.)

amount of resection a patient could physiologically tolerate. Exercise testing may also help predict morbidity associated with thoracotomy; for example, patients with a maximum oxygen consumption under 10 mL/kg do poorly. Improvements in surgical and anesthetic techniques and the reemergence of lung volume reduction surgery (LVRS) have helped lower the threshold for surgical resection of NSCLC.[79-83] Many of the patients currently under study in the LVRS trials have FEV_1 values below the traditional thresholds for lung cancer resection. Some experts therefore have advocated a postoperative FEV_1 goal as low as 20% (with less than 5% mortality reported). However, further study clearly is required to establish this nadir threshold.

Treatment

Treatment options include surgery, radiation, and chemotherapy. Newer options, although not the mainstays of treatment, include immunotherapy, brachytherapy, gene therapy, bronchoscopic treatments, and photodynamic therapy (PDT).[84] Because the staging of NSCLC changed in 1997 to more accurately reflect prognostic data, some of the

stage-specific studies must be reinterpreted in this light. For example, stage II lung cancer now includes T3N0 lesions, which previously were considered stage IIIA. Because the individual chemotherapeutic agents and combinations of agents tend to change frequently, the underlying therapeutic principles in the treatment of lung cancer are emphasized.

$\mathcal{R}$espiratory Recap

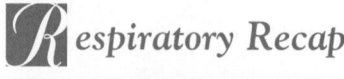

Treatment of Lung Cancer
Surgery
Radiotherapy
Chemotherapy

Small Cell Lung Cancer

Because of the aggressive nature of these tumors, most patients with SCLC who seek medical treatment have extensive disease at the time of diagnosis. Without treatment, patients with limited SCLC survive an average of 12 weeks; for extensive disease, survival is only 5 weeks. In addition to moderate improvements in survival, combination chemotherapy in some cases can lead to substantial improvements in the patient's quality of life.[85]

Chemotherapeutic agents have long been known to affect SCLC tumors in patients with both limited (90% of patients) and extensive (70% of patients) disease. However, despite the sensitivity of these tumors to chemotherapeutic agents, relapse is the rule. There has been no substantial improvement in survival in this disease over the past 20 to 30 years. Commonly used agents include etoposide, cisplatinum, carboplatin, ifosfamide, vincristine, and anthracyclines. Controversy exists regarding dose intensity, frequency, alternating therapies, sequential regimens, and bone marrow support, among other issues. Commonly used strategies include six cycles of one of the following combinations: cisplatinum plus etoposide, cyclophosphamide plus doxorubicin plus vincristine, or cyclophosphamide plus doxorubicin plus etoposide.[86] In general, multiple agents appear to be more effective than single agents, and higher dose regimens appear preferable to lower dose, but no one group of medications has emerged as the treatment of choice.[87-94]

Radiation therapy can be used for primary treatment of the intrathoracic tumor or for metastatic disease. Radiotherapy has been shown to improve mortality in the treatment of patients with limited stage SCLC. Generally these patients are given radiotherapy and chemotherapy, because trials indicate some benefit to the combination over chemotherapy alone in limited SCLC.[95] Although early radiotherapy appears to substantially improve long-term survival compared with delayed radiation treatment, considerable controversy exists regarding concurrent versus sequential radiotherapy, as well as the timing and dosages of therapy.[86,96-98]

Another possible role for radiation in SCLC is prophylactic cranial irradiation (PCI). The brain, which is poorly penetrated by chemotherapeutic agents, is a frequent site of tumor recurrence. A number of trials have shown that PCI probably postpones the development of intracranial metastases and may improve overall survival.[99] Substantial neurocognitive sequelae of the radiation treatment also have been reported. In limited stage SCLC patients, PCI should be considered for those who achieve a complete response to combination chemotherapy.[85,100-102] Patient preferences vary regarding this modest survival benefit and must be considered when this decision is made.

Surgery traditionally has not been considered useful for SCLC because of the disease's systemic nature at the time of diagnosis. With improvements in chemotherapeutic regimens, however, there has been some improvement in control of systemic disease, consequently local and regional recurrences have received increased attention. This has led to reconsideration of the role of surgery to facilitate control of local disease. Furthermore, the frequent occurrence of NSCLC elements in the histology of SCLC tumors has led to speculation that chemotherapy may treat the SCLC elements, whereas the NSCLC elements may persist. Therefore surgery for local regional control of the NSCLC elements has been suggested, an approach that has some support from uncontrolled series. Data in this area are evolving, but currently surgery cannot be recommended in SCLC outside the setting of a clinical trial. The one exception seems to be SCLC patients with a solitary pulmonary nodule who do well after complete resection (approximately 50% survival at 5 years).[103-106] In these cases postoperative chemotherapy often is recommended.

Non–Small Cell Lung Cancer

Several principles are important in the approach to treatment of patients with NSCLC. First, surgical resection is used much more commonly in NSCLC than in SCLC, particularly for early stage disease. Second, the probability of achieving cure in early stage NSCLC is quite good (60% to 80% for stage I disease). Third, in stage IIIA disease, there is an increasingly recognized role for multimodality therapy (that is, neoadjuvant chemotherapy and radiotherapy followed by surgical resection).[107-112] Fourth, stage-specific studies may be difficult to compare because of changes in staging systems and differences in local staging practices. For example, the routine performance of mediastinoscopy in some centers gives the subgroup of patients with no mediastinal adenopathy a much better prognosis than a patient with N0 disease based on CT scanning alone.

For early stage NSCLC, surgical resection is the treatment of choice, with excellent long-term survival reported in several series (weighted average is 74.25% for stage IA 5-year survival).[113-115] Most deaths that do occur are caused by recurrent disease. Although largely based on empirical evidence, radiation therapy alone appears to provide inferior cure rates (approximately 30% for stage I, 20% for stage II). After resection there is no clear role for **adjuvant therapy,** with several reports suggesting an increase in mortality with postoperative radiotherapy.[116] Recent data similarly do not support the use of adjuvant chemotherapy or chemoradiotherapy after surgical resection. Improvements in staging (for example, PET scanning) may help risk stratify patients at high risk of recurrent disease. Survival is clearly better for stage IA compared with stage IB and stage II. Therefore, future trials may need to study the highest risk patients to demonstrate the benefits of more aggressive therapy. The need for treatment advances is highlighted by the fact that patients with breast, colon, and prostate cancer (the next three most common causes of cancer deaths) have better 5-year survival rates than patients with stage I NSCLC.

The treatment of locally advanced NSCLC with multimodality therapies has become increasingly popular. The most controversial issue is the treatment of stage IIIA NSCLC, for which no clear consensus has yet emerged. One reason for this controversy is the potential variability in prognosis for N2 disease, depending on its nature (that is, incidental, bulky, or microscopic).[115] Most trials have had small sample sizes and have not subdivided these patients according to the nature of the adenopathy, which makes any general conclusions difficult. Surgical resection can be considered for those with nonbulky adenopathy, but the trend increasingly is toward treatment with platinum-based chemotherapy before attempted surgical resection. This allows control of micrometastatic disease and possibly improves the resectability of the tumor. Although improvements in surgical techniques have also allowed the resection of some disease previously deemed unresectable (for example, that involving the esophagus and vena cava, as well as T4 stage IIIB lesions), cure of stage IIIA disease by surgery alone is quite uncommon. Ongoing trials will help determine the relative roles of surgery, radiation therapy, and chemotherapy in the treatment of stage IIIA lung cancer. Currently, only phase II data are available for this trimodality approach. These patients are offered participation in randomized clinical trials, but neoadjuvant chemoradiotherapy followed by surgical resection is possible for those not involved in protocols.

Surgical resection is difficult for stage IIIB and bulky N2 stage IIIA tumors, making chemotherapy followed by radiation therapy the usual treatment.[117,118] Several trials have focused on concurrent administration of chemotherapy and radiotherapy. Although this strategy may help improve local control, the toxicities of treatment limit its utility. One investigational approach to these patients is the administration of chemotherapy or radiotherapy (or both) with the goal of making the tumor resectable. This neoadjuvant strategy for otherwise unresectable disease is the subject of research studies.

For metastatic NSCLC, a number of trials have examined the role of palliative chemotherapy compared with best supportive care. Because these patients are essentially incurable, the goal of treatment is to prolong life without increasing suffering or side effects.[119] Statistically significant improvements in survival have been reported with the use of chemotherapy in this patient group. However, the optimum therapy for an individual patient must be carefully considered and discussed. Some data also indicate preservation of the quality of life and cost-effectiveness for those who undergo palliative chemotherapy in this setting. However, most clinical trials have focused on younger patients with good performance status. Newer, relatively well-tolerated chemotherapeutic agents, such as vinorelbine, provide some basis for enthusiasm regarding this palliative therapy.

Complications of Therapy

The complications of the individual chemotherapeutic drugs are beyond the scope of this chapter.[120] Current estimates suggest a roughly 1% treatment-associated mortality from chemotherapy itself. Several important general points can be made, as follows:

1. In the week or two after chemotherapy, neutropenia can occur and greatly increases the risk of superimposed bacterial and opportunistic fungal pneumonias and sepsis. Growth factors can be used to prevent neutropenia in a susceptible or previously afflicted patient.
2. Mucositis, which represents acute toxicity of the highly active lining cells of the gastrointestinal tract, leads to substantial discomfort and can increase infectious sequelae as a result of an increased risk of aspiration and altered gastrointestinal permeability.
3. Various chemotherapeutic agents have acute or chronic pulmonary sequelae, which complicate the distinction between tumor spread or recurrence, infection, and drug toxicity; early invasive diagnostic attempts often are warranted in these cases. Fortunately the chemotherapeutic agents typically used for lung cancers do not, for the most part, have major pulmonary toxicities. Current trials are assessing the interaction of chemotherapeutic agents such as paclitaxel and radiotherapy.
4. Platinum-based chemotherapeutic drugs are commonly used in lung cancer and are frequently associated with neurologic toxicities, specifically peripheral neuropathy. This side effect can range from asymptomatic to nuisance to severe and disabling; therefore it must be considered and discussed with patients undergoing chemotherapy.

Radiation damage to the lung parenchyma remains the limiting factor in chest radiotherapy. The complications of radiation therapy may be characterized as acute or chronic. The incidence of acute radiation pneumonitis is higher for patients receiving larger daily or cumulative doses and to a larger amount of tissue. In addition, certain chemotherapeutic drugs used in lung cancer regimens, such as doxorubicin and vincristine, are radiosensitizers and can increase radiation-induced injury. Acute pneumonitis occurs within the first 6 months of therapy (mean is approximately 1 to 3 months) and is manifested by cough and dyspnea. It typically but not exclusively is confined to the radiation port, and the histopathology may be consistent with a lymphocytic alveolitis or diffuse alveolar damage. In addition, a nonspecific reaction, bronchiolitis obliterans with organizing pneumonia (BOOP), can occur in the lung in response to radiation injury. Corticosteroid therapy usually is given for acute pulmonary radiation toxicity, although human data are lacking. Chronic complications of radiotherapy include injury to lung and mediastinal structures. Lung fibrosis can be seen 6 months after discontinuation of radiotherapy and manifests with progressive dyspnea and restrictive pulmonary function tests. Mediastinal radiotherapy has been associated with a number of complications, including mediastinal fibrosis, constrictive pericarditis, restrictive cardiomyopathy, accelerated coronary artery disease, and valvular fibrosis.[121-123]

With thoracotomy, mortality rates as low as 1% are now reported, a considerable improvement compared with 20 to 30 years ago. Smoking cessation at least 2 months before surgery has been associated with an improved outcome in elective coronary artery bypass patients. These data are generally extrapolated to thoracotomy patients as well.[124] Other preoperative measures, such as exercise, good nutrition, pulmonary rehabilitation, and deep breathing regimens, may help smooth the perioperative

TABLE 59-7

Karnofsky Performance Scale

Definition	Percentage	Criteria
Able to carry on normal activity	100	Normal; no complaints; no evidence of disease
and to work; no special care	90	Able to carry on normal activity; minor signs or symptoms of disease
needed	80	Normal activity with effort; some signs or symptoms of disease
Unable to work; able to live at	70	Cares for self; unable to carry on normal activity or do active work
home and care for most per-	60	Requires occasional assistance but is able to care for most needs
sonal needs; varying amount	50	Requires considerable assistance and frequent medical care
of assistance needed		
Unable to care for self; requires	40	Disabled; requires special care and assistance
equivalent of institutional or	30	Severely disabled; hospitalization indicated, although death may not be imminent
hospital care; rapid progres-	20	Very sick; hospitalization necessary; active supportive treatment required
sion of disease possible	10	Moribund; fatal processes progressing rapidly

course. Meticulous attention must be paid to postsurgical pulmonary toilet to prevent and treat respiratory complications of atelectasis, lobar collapse, and pneumonia. Care after discharge from the hospital, through transitional care units and visiting nurses, also is crucial in many cases. Late complications, such as postthoracotomy pain syndromes, which occur in as many as 50% of patients, are somewhat underappreciated.

Prognosis

The prognosis for lung cancer is still quite poor; the 5-year survival rate is only 14%. The following are some prognostic or useful variables:

1. *Tumor stage, including size.* In addition to the tumor's stage, its size appears to linearly predict survival, with increasing mortality associated with larger size.
2. *Resectability (NSCLC).* Surgery clearly offers the best chance of cure for patients with NSCLC. In addition, patients who have undergone lobectomy appear to have a better prognosis than those with wedge resection or segmentectomy. Limited resection therefore should be reserved for patients unable to tolerate more extensive resections.
3. *Weight loss.* As with many diseases and other cancers, weight loss is an important prognostic indicator. The poor outcome associated with patients with lung cancer who lose weight has prompted some to aggressively place percutaneous gastrostomy feeding tubes. Thus even when oral intake is poor, caloric requirements can be met. Appetite stimulants such as megestrol acetate can help increase body weight. However, minimal outcome data support these approaches. Other systemic symptoms similarly predict a poor outcome.
4. *Performance status.* The Karnofsky Performance Scale (Table 59-7) provides a quantitative measure of patient performance as a percentage of normal activities. As with many tumors, a lung cancer patient with good performance status has a much better outcome.
5. *Histologic subtype.* In NSCLC, a few studies have suggested a superior outcome for squamous cell carcinoma compared with adenocarcinoma. However, several other studies have not shown important differences in survival or recurrence risk. Therefore the histologic subtype probably is not a major prognostic factor in NSCLC. However, subtyping of adenocarcinomas may be useful, because bronchoalveolar cell carcinoma appears to have an improved outcome compared with other adenocarcinomas.
6. *Tumor differentiation.* Variable results have been published in different papers regarding the importance of this factor. Although some data suggest a worse outcome for patients with undifferentiated cancers, others report no important differences in survival on this basis.
7. *Vascular or lymphatic invasion.* A resected tumor that demonstrates invasiveness may warrant more aggressive treatment than one that does not.
8. *Molecular markers.* Molecular markers, such as K-ras mutations, have not yet had a major impact on prognostication or prediction of relapse. However, combinations of molecular markers may make this type of strategy feasible in the near future for risk stratification and determination of the aggressiveness of therapy.[125]

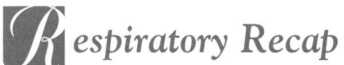

Respiratory Recap

Prognosis for Lung Cancer
The 5-year survival rate for lung cancer is only 14%.

9. *Male gender.* Disease in men is associated with a worse outcome than disease in women.
10. *African-American race.* This factor is also associated with worse outcome for all stages of lung cancer. This appears to be at least partly related to less aggressive therapy in this population.[126]

Prevention

The most important cause of cancer death in North America is preventable. Prevention of lung cancer requires smoking cessation, avoidance of exposures, and early detection. Evidence clearly suggests a decline in the risk of lung cancer among former smokers compared with current smokers. Although statistics vary, the lung cancer risk falls by 5 years after smoking cessation and continues to decline thereafter. However, these individuals probably do not completely return to the baseline risk seen in those who have never smoked.

Prevention generally is classified as primary, secondary, and tertiary in nature. *Primary prevention* refers to modification of potentially injurious behaviors. In the case of lung cancer, smoking cessation is the best defense. The onus is on the health care provider both to encourage and to facilitate the cessation of tobacco use. The modest success of tobacco control programs in North America should not distract health professionals from the huge problem of an estimated 1.1 billion smokers worldwide. For example, estimates suggest that 77% of all young men in China currently are smokers. Primary prevention must target the problem on both a global and an individual level. Emphasis is placed on the need for repeated discussions with smokers and planned follow-up. Despite this, most studies suggest that few health care providers address the issue of tobacco cessation. Furthermore, several attempts by patients and health care providers often are required to successfully overcome this addiction. Group or family therapy may be useful for some smokers. Recent data support the usefulness of nicotine replacement therapies to facilitate smoking cessation. Bupropion (150 mg given orally twice a day) has been shown to facilitate withdrawal from nicotine. However, only 23.1% of participants in one study were tobacco free at 1 year compared with 12.4% in the placebo group.[135] The combination of nicotine replacement and bupropion may have the highest probability of success.

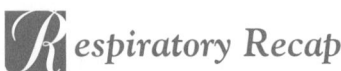

Lung Cancer Prevention
Smoking cessation
Screening
Interventions to prevent disease progression

Studies suggesting a possible genetic basis for nicotine addiction should help health care providers focus on patient education and support rather than blame or criticism.[127-135]

The Mayo Clinic recently published a cost-effectiveness analysis of its smoking cessation program. The authors estimated a cost of $6,828 per year of life gained, which is well below most other health care interventions.[135-139] One of the keys to cost containment was the use of personnel who were not physicians in their program.

Secondary prevention refers to early detection or the screening of asymptomatic disease. Because lung cancer screening trials have thus far failed, secondary prevention is not generally recommended. Improvements in technology, with spiral CT scanning and possibly PET scanning, may make secondary prevention of lung cancer feasible. Although spiral CT scanning allows complete evaluation of the chest during a single breath hold, the possible cost for detection of false positives must not be overlooked. For example, a small peripheral granulomatous lesion that otherwise would have gone undetected may lead the patient to open lung biopsy to exclude lung cancer. However, a number of reports have suggested that spiral CT scanning can detect early stage lung cancers in at-risk populations with yields comparable to those of mammography in breast cancer. Currently the precise role and ideal technique for lung cancer screening are unclear. A number of radiologic studies underway should help define the role of secondary prevention in lung cancer.[140]

Another example of secondary prevention is the use of molecular genetic analysis on bronchial biopsies or possibly sputum samples. By demonstrating genetic changes similar to those seen in lung cancer patients, individuals at high risk of developing lung cancer can be identified. These patients can then be followed closely or perhaps entered into clinical trials on chemoprevention. Technologic advances are being made in the early diagnosis and detection of lung cancer, but they must be evaluated for feasibility and cost-effectiveness before they can be widely recommended.

Tertiary prevention refers to interventions to prevent disease progression once a diagnosis has been made. Although limited data support the use of antioxidants (for example, vitamin E) to prevent secondary malignancies, these cannot be recommended until further data are available.[141-143]

Future Directions

As stated previously, worldwide smoking trends dictate that bronchogenic carcinoma will continue to be major health problem in the foreseeable future. Current epidemiologic statistics likely will be eclipsed. Although advances in imaging and chemotherapy and radiotherapy or even immunotherapy protocols may produce some incremental benefit, prevention is the only secure answer. Primary prevention, through political and financial pressure on tobacco companies, would help limit the supply of to-bacco and related products. Worldwide education programs through mass media could help limit the demand. Secondary prevention programs for early detection of lung cancer may benefit from advances in technology, such as spiral CT scanning and possibly PET scanning. Tertiary prevention through the use of antioxidants for previously diagnosed patients or high-risk groups may also become possible. Gene therapy to manipulate proto-oncogenes and tumor suppressor genes may also come to fruition.[125,144-151]

CASE STUDIES

Case One
Lung Cancer Screening

A 45-year-old man who smoked two packs a day for 20 years but who quit 2 years ago consults his physician. A friend of the patient recently was diagnosed with lung cancer, and the patient is concerned that he might develop the same condition. He otherwise is healthy and has no diagnosed lung disease. The review of systems is negative for weight loss, chest pain, and hemoptysis. The patient is taking no medications, and his family history also is negative for cancer. The patient works in an office and has never been exposed to any dusts, fumes, or toxic chemicals. His physical examination is normal.

This individual, although asymptomatic, is clearly at risk of developing lung cancer, given his 40 pack-year history of smoking. He has no additional risk factors from other exposures, from his family history, or from chronic obstructive pulmonary disease. He has no active symptoms or signs suggestive of lung cancer. However, this frequently is the case until the cancer becomes quite advanced. By the time a patient develops symptomatic lung cancer, the prognosis is quite poor because of the advanced disease. The emphasis thus has been placed on attempts at early diagnosis, before the onset of symptoms and signs.

Unfortunately, trials of screening for lung cancer in populations at risk have been largely unsuccessful. Sputum cytology and chest radiography have yielded some benefit in terms of increased detection of early stage tumors but have had no substantial impact on patient outcome. Therefore the general recommendation has been not to screen previous or current smokers.[152-155] Similarly, there is no proven role for antioxidants or other secondary prevention strategies.[156-159]

However, newer technologies may change this practice. A recent study using spiral computed tomography (CT) scan has provided some encouraging preliminary data in this field. These scans can be performed quickly, with minimal radiation exposure, and at relatively low cost.[140] However, false positive results (for example, identification of benign lesions that would not otherwise have been detected) could limit the utility of this technique. Further

data are required before spiral CT scans can be generally recommended for lung cancer screening.

Case Two
Early Stage Lung Cancer

A 63-year-old woman seeks medical attention after an abnormality is noted on a chest radiograph. She is a former smoker of 38 pack-years who quit smoking 5 years ago. She otherwise is quite healthy and has no active medical problems. Her exposure history, social history, and family history are unremarkable, as is her physical examination. The chest radiograph shows a 2-cm peripheral lesion in the right upper lobe. No other abnormalities are seen on the film, specifically no pleural effusion, no bony invasion, and no evidence of mediastinal adenopathy.

A transthoracic needle aspirate tests positive for squamous cell carcinoma. A CT scan of the chest to the level of the adrenal glands reveals no abnormalities apart from the 2-cm lesion. A complete blood count (CBC), as well as serum calcium and liver enzyme values, were all within normal limits. Mediastinoscopy revealed no evidence of adenopathy. Pulmonary function testing revealed a forced expiratory volume in 1 second (FEV_1) of 2.2 L (70% predicted). Because of the absence of symptoms, a bone scan and a CT scan of the head were not performed.

This patient has T1N0M0 disease, which represents stage 1A non–small cell lung cancer. The treatment of choice is surgical resection. The patient's pulmonary function tests are quite good and should easily allow resection of a single lobe. There is no proven role for (that is, postoperative chemotherapy or radiotherapy) in this setting.[160] The 5-year survival rate for this type of patient after resection is 70%. Enrollment in a trial for prevention of recurrence or a second primary lung cancer could be considered.

Case Three
Metastatic Lung Cancer

A 72-year-old Caucasian man sees his physician because of new onset of headaches. The patient currently smokes and has smoked two packs of cigarettes a day for the past 40 years. His past medical history is remarkable for two myocardial infarctions. His medications include daily aspirin, atenolol, and captopril (all for his heart). His family history and social history are unremarkable. His physical examination is remarkable for marked gait instability and asymmetric deep tendon reflexes, which are consistent with a pathologic condition in the central nervous system.

His chest radiograph reveals a 5-cm mass in the right midlung zone with enlargement of the mediastinum, which is consistent with substantial adenopathy in the paratracheal region and the aorticopulmonary window. A right-sided pleural effusion also is present. A CT scan of the head reveals three intracranial lesions, a finding consistent with metastatic disease. A diagnostic thoracentesis yields a positive result for adenocarcinoma of the lung.

This patient has metastatic non–small cell lung cancer. The staging would be T4N3M1. The T4 status is based on the malignant pleural effusion, whereas the N3 status is based on the radiographic evidence of contralateral mediastinal adenopathy. The metastatic lesion is evident from the head CT scan. For diagnostic certitude, a biopsy of the mediastinal nodes or the intracranial lesions could be performed, but it would be unlikely to alter the management of this patient.

The therapeutic goal in this situation should be palliation. The patient sought attention for his headaches, and cranial irradiation could be performed to control these symptoms. Because the patient has several intracranial metastases, surgical resection of these lesions is not recommended. Although somewhat controversial, most would advocate offering chemoradiotherapy for palliative purposes. This decision is based on discussion with the patient and his family regarding his wishes. Although treatment would not offer hope for a cure, some data suggest that survival is improved with chemoradiotherapy. However, the median survival still is likely to be less than 1 year.[161-164]

KEY POINTS

- Lung cancer is common but preventable.
- A tissue diagnosis generally is required. This can be obtained by analysis of sputum or pleural fluid or of bronchoscopic, surgical, or needle biopsy specimens.
- Lung cancer generally is classified as small cell or non–small cell cancer.
- Small cell lung cancer generally is treated with chemotherapy or radiotherapy or both but rarely with surgery.
- Surgical resection is the preferred treatment for non–small cell lung cancer.
- The role of chemotherapy and radiotherapy in non–small cell lung cancer is controversial, but these treatments probably have a role in stages 3 and 4. In stage 3A, neoadjuvant therapy (that is, that provided before surgical resection) probably will emerge as the preferred treatment. For stage 3B and stage 4, chemoradiotherapy can improve the duration and quality of life if the patients are carefully chosen.
- Prevention and early diagnosis are future areas of emphasis in lung cancer.

References

1. Andre F, Jacot W, Pujol JL, et al. Epidemiology, prognostic factors, staging, and treatment of non–small cell lung cancer. Bull Cancer (Paris) Suppl 1999;3:17-41.
2. Charloux A, Rossignol M, Purohit A, et al. International differences in epidemiology of lung adenocarcinoma. Lung Cancer 1997;16:133-143.
3. Christiani DC. Smoking and the molecular epidemiology of lung cancer. Clin Chest Med 2000;21:87-93.
4. Charloux A, Quoix E, Wolkove N, et al. The increasing incidence of lung adenocarcinoma: reality or artifact? A review of the epidemiology of lung adenocarcinoma. Int J Epidemiol 1997;26:14-23.
5. Denissenko M, Pao A, Tang M, et al. Preferential formation of benzo[a]pyrene adducts at lung cancer mutational hotspots in p53. Science 1996;274:430-432.
6. Bartsch H, Petruzzelli S, De Flora S, et al. Carcinogen metabolism in human lung tissues and the effect of tobacco smoking: results from a case-control multicenter study on lung cancer patients. Environ Health Perspect 1992;98:119-124.
7. Wang X, Christiani D, Wiencke JK, et al. Mutations in the p53 gene in lung cancer are associated with cigarette smoking and asbestos exposure. Cancer Epidemiol Biomarkers Prev 1995;4:543-548.
8. Komiya T, Hirashima T, Kawase I. Clinical significance of p53 in non–small cell lung cancer. Oncol Rep 1999;6:19-28.
9. Brambilla E, Brambilla C. p53 and lung cancer. Pathol Biol 1997;45:852-853.
10. Rosell R, Monzo M, Pifarre A, et al. Molecular staging of non–small cell lung cancer according to K-ras genotypes. Clin Cancer Res 1996;2:1083-1086.
11. Nyberg F, Agrenius V, Svartengren K, et al. Environmental tobacco smoke and lung cancer in nonsmokers: does time since exposure play a role? Epidemiology 1998;9:301-308.
12. Boffetta P, Agudo A, Ahrens W, et al. Multicenter case-control study of exposure to environmental tobacco smoke and lung cancer in Europe. J Natl Cancer Inst 1998;90:1440-1450.
13. Copas J, Shi J. Reanalysis of epidemiological evidence on lung cancer and passive smoking. Br Med J 2000;320:417-418.
14. Pershagen G, Akerblom G, Axelson O, et al. Residential radon exposure and lung cancer in Sweden. N Engl J Med 1994;330:159-164.
15. Churg A. Lung cancer cell type and asbestos exposure. JAMA 1985;253:2984-2985.
16. Svensson C, Pershagen G, Klominek J. Lung cancer in women and type of dwelling in relation to radon exposure. Cancer Res 1989;49:1861-1865.
17. Yngveson A, Williams C, Hjerpe A, et al. p53 Mutations in lung cancer associated with residential radon exposure. Cancer Epidemiol Biomarkers Prev 1999;8:433-438.
18. Lagarde F, Pershagen G. Indoor radon exposure and risk of lung cancer: a nested case-control study in Finland. J Natl Cancer Inst 1997;89:584-585.
19. Little JB. What are the risks of low-level exposure to α-radiation from radon? Proc Natl Acad Sci USA 1997;94:5996-5997.
20. Lubin J, Liang Z, Hrubec Z, et al. Radon exposure in residences and lung cancer among women: combined analysis of three studies. Cancer Causes Control 1994;5:114-128.
21. Saracci R. Asbestos and lung cancer: an analysis of the epidemiological evidence on the asbestos-smoking interaction. Int J Cancer 1977;20:323-331.
22. Saracci R. The interactions of tobacco smoking and other agents in cancer etiology. Epidemiol Rev 1987;9:175-193.
23. Demiroglu H. Nonoccupational exposure to chrysotile asbestos and the risk of lung cancer. N Engl J Med 1998;339:999-1000.

24. Du Y, Zhou BS, Wu JM. Lifestyle factors and human lung cancer: an overview of recent advances. Int J Oncol 1998;13:471-479.

25. Lynch H, Guirgis H, Harris RE. Familial susceptibility to lung cancer and chronic obstructive pulmonary disease. Lancet 1977;2:815.

26. Hubbard R, Venn A, Lewis S, et al. Lung cancer and cryptogenic fibrosing alveolitis: a population-based cohort study. Am J Respir Crit Care Med 2000;161:5-8.

27. Yamasawa H, Ishii Y, Kitamura S. Concurrence of sarcoidosis and lung cancer: a report of four cases. Respiration 2000;67:90-93.

28. Askling J, Grunewald J, Eklund A, et al. Increased risk for cancer following sarcoidosis. Am J Respir Crit Care Med 1999;160:1668-1672.

29. Yanagawa H, Goto H, Maniwa K, et al. A case of resectable lung adenocarcinoma associated with sarcoidosis. Med Oncol 1999;16:216-220.

30. Reich JM. Sarcoidosis and cancer revisited. Eur Respir J 1999;14:482-483.

31. Paksoy N, Elpek O, Ozbilim G, et al. Bronchoalveolar carcinoma in progressive systemic sclerosis: report of a case diagnosed by fine needle aspiration cytology. Acta Cytol 1995;39:1182-1186.

32. Rosenthal A, McLaughlin J, Gridley G, et al. Incidence of cancer among patients with systemic sclerosis. Cancer 1995;76:910-914.

33. Katariya K, Thurer R. Malignancies associated with the immunocompromised state. Chest Surg Clin North Am 1999;9:63-77.

34. Katariya K, Thurer R. Thoracic malignancies associated with AIDS. Semin Thorac Cardiovasc Surg 2000;12:148-153.

35. Patel A, Peters S. Clinical manifestations of lung cancer. Mayo Clin Proc 1993;68:273-277.

36. Colice GL. Detecting lung cancer as a cause of hemoptysis in patients with a normal chest radiograph: bronchoscopy versus CT. Chest 1997;111:877-884.

37. DiLeo M, Gianoli G. Diagnosis and management of hemoptysis. J La State Med Soc 1994;146:115-118.

38. Jackson C, Savage P, Quinn D. Role of fiberoptic bronchoscopy in patients with hemoptysis and a normal chest roentgenogram. Chest 1985;87:142-144.

39. Jenkinson S, Hubbard L, Burford J. Abnormal chest roentgenogram in a patient with hemoptysis. JAMA 1979;241:2429-2430.

40. Arcasoy SM, Jett J. Superior pulmonary sulcus tumors and Pancoast's syndrome. N Engl J Med 1997;337:1370-1376.

41. Yano S, Shimada K. Changes in superior vena cava pulsed Doppler flow patterns: possible indicator of improvement of superior vena cava syndrome due to lung cancer. J Ultrasound Med 1997;16:707-710.

42. Kashitani N, Eda R, Masayoshi T, et al. Lobar extent of pulmonary lymphangitic carcinomatosis: Tl-201 chloride and Tc-99m MIBI scintigraphic findings. Clin Nucl Med 1996;21:726-729.

43. Richardson G, Johnson B. Paraneoplastic syndromes in lung cancer. Curr Opin Oncol 1992;4:323-333.

44. Oh SJ. Paraneoplastic vasculitis of the peripheral nervous system. Neurol Clin 1997;15:849-863.

45. Patel A, Davila D, Peters S. Paraneoplastic syndromes associated with lung cancer. Mayo Clin Proc 1993;68:278-287.

46. Lennon V, Kryzer TJ, Griesmann G, et al. Calcium channel antibodies in the Lambert-Eaton syndrome and other paraneoplastic syndromes. N Engl J Med 1995;332:1467-1474.

47. Sridhar K, Lobo C, Altman RD. Digital clubbing and lung cancer. Chest 1998;114:1535-1537.

48. Schoenen J, Broux R, Moonen G. Unilateral facial pain as the first symptom of lung cancer: are there diagnostic clues? Cephalalgia 1992;12:178-179.

49. Strewler GJ. The physiology of parathyroid hormone–related protein. N Engl J Med 2000;342:177-185.

50. Hammack J, Kotanides H, Rosenblum MK, et al. Paraneoplastic cerebellar degeneration. II. Clinical and immunologic findings in 21 patients with Hodgkin's disease. Neurology 1992;42:1938-1943.

51. Kagan A, Steckel R, Braun R. Asymptomatic peripheral lung nodule. AJR Am J Roentgenol 1980;135:417-420.

52. Higgins GA, Shields TW, Kechn RJ. The solitary pulmonary nodule: 10-year follow-up of Veterans Administration Armed Forces Cooperative Study. Arch Surg 1975;110:570-575.

53. Rubins JB, Rubins HB. Temporal trends in the prevalence of malignancy in solitary pulmonary lesions. Chest 1996;109:100-103.

54. Sagel S, Ferguson T, Forrest JV, et al. Percutaneous transthoracic aspiration needle biopsy. Ann Thorac Surg 1978;26:399-405.

55. Swanson S, Jaklitsch M, Mentzer SJ, et al. Management of the solitary pulmonary nodule: role of thoracoscopy in diagnosis and therapy. Chest 1999;116:523-524.

56. Swensen S, Morin R, Schueler BA, et al. Solitary pulmonary nodule: CT evaluation of enhancement with iodinated contrast material: a preliminary report. Radiology 1992;182:343-347.

57. Swensen SJ. Thoracic neoplasms. Curr Opin Radiol 1990;2:355-359.

58. Swensen S, Brown L, Colby TV, et al. Lung nodule enhancement at CT: prospective findings. Radiology 1996;201:447-455.

59. Swensen S, Silverstein M, Edell ES, et al. Solitary pulmonary nodules: clinical prediction model versus physicians. Mayo Clin Proc 1999;74:319-329.

60. Swensen S, Viggiano R, Midthun DE, et al. Lung nodule enhancement at CT: multicenter study. Radiology 2000;214:73-80.

61. Lowe V, Fletcher J, Gobar L, et al. Prospective investigation of positron emission tomography in lung nodules. J Clin Oncol 1998;16:1075-1084.

62. Gupta N, Graeber G, Rogers JS, et al. Comparative efficacy of positron emission tomography with FDG and computed tomographic scanning in preoperative staging of non–small cell lung cancer. Ann Surg 1999;229:286-291.

63. Duhaylongsod F, Lowe V, Patz EF Jr, et al. Lung tumor growth correlates with glucose metabolism measured by fluoride-18 fluorodeoxyglucose positron emission tomography. Ann Thorac Surg 1995;60:1348-1352.

64. Duhaylongsod F, Lowe V, Patz EF Jr, et al. Detection of primary and recurrent lung cancer by means of F-18 fluorodeoxyglucose positron emission tomography (FDG PET). J Thorac Cardiovasc Surg 1995;110:130-139.

65. Prakash UB. Advances in bronchoscopic procedures. Chest 1999;116:1403-1408.

66. Khanavkar B, Gnudi F, Muti A, et al. Basic principles of LIFE autofluorescence bronchoscopy: results of 194 examinations in comparison with standard procedures for early detection of bronchial carcinoma: overview. Pneumologie 1998;52:71-76.

67. Preciado M, Duvall A, Koop SH. Mediastinoscopy: a review of 450 cases. Laryngoscope 1973;83:1300-1310.

68. Trastek V, Pichler J, Pairolero PC. Mediastinoscopy. Br Med Bull 1986;42:240-243.

69. Mountain C, Greenberg S, Fraire AE. Tumor stage in non–small cell carcinoma of the lung. Chest 1991;99:1258-1260.

70. Mountain C, Dresler C. Regional lymph node classification for lung cancer staging. Chest 1997;111:1718-1723.

71. Mountain CF. Lung cancer staging classification. Clin Chest Med 1993;14:43-53.

72. Mountain CF. Surgery for stage IIIA-N_2 non–small cell lung cancer. Cancer 1994;73:2589-2598.

73. Mountain CF. New prognostic factors in lung cancer: biologic prophets of cancer cell aggression. Chest 1995;108:246-254.

74. Mountain CF. Revisions in the International System for Staging Lung Cancer. Chest 1997;111:1710-1717.

75. Bone R, Balk R. Staging of bronchogenic carcinoma. Chest 1982;82:473-480.

76. Lau CL, Harpole D. Noninvasive clinical staging modalities for lung cancer. Semin Surg Oncol 2000;18:116-123.

77. Ferguson MK. Diagnosing and staging of non–small cell lung cancer. Hematol Oncol Clin North Am 1990;4:1053-1068.

78. Kaplan D, Goldstraw P. New techniques in the diagnosis and staging of lung cancer. Cancer Treat Res 1995;72:223-254.

79. Bae K, Slone R, Gierada DS, et al. Patients with emphysema: quantitative CT analysis before and after lung volume reduction surgery: work in progress. Radiology 1997;203:705-714.

80. Lefrak S, Yusen R, Trulock EP, et al. Recent advances in surgery for emphysema. Annu Rev Med 1997;48:387-398.

81. Cooper J, Patterson G, Sundaresan RS, et al. Results of 150 consecutive bilateral lung volume reduction procedures in patients with severe emphysema. J Thorac Cardiovasc Surg 1996;112:1319-1329.

82. Mentzer S, Swanson SJ. Treatment of patients with lung cancer and severe emphysema. Chest 1999;116:477S-479S.

83. Gierada D, Yusen R, Villanueva IA, et al. Patient selection for lung volume reduction surgery: an objective model based on prior clinical decisions and quantitative CT analysis. Chest 2000;117:991-998.

84. Sutedja G, Postmus P. Bronchoscopic treatment of lung tumors. Lung Cancer 1994;11:1-17.

85. Johnson B, Patronas N, Hayes W, et al. Neurologic, computed cranial tomographic, and magnetic resonance imaging abnormalities in patients with small cell lung cancer: further follow-up of 6- to 13-year survivors. J Clin Oncol 1990;8:48-56.

86. Hoffman P, Mauer AM, Vokes EE. Lung cancer. Lancet 2000;355:479-485.

87. Jett J, Everson L, Therneau TM, et al. Treatment of limited-stage small-cell lung cancer with cyclophosphamide, doxorubicin, and vincristine with or without etoposide: a randomized trial of the North Central Cancer Treatment Group. J Clin Oncol 1990;8:33-38.

88. Evans W, Feld R, Murray N, et al. The use of VP-16 plus cisplatin during induction chemotherapy for small cell lung cancer. Semin Oncol 1986;13:10-16.

89. Evans W, Feld R, Murray N, et al. Superiority of alternating non-cross-resistant chemotherapy in extensive small cell lung cancer: a multicenter, randomized clinical trial by the National Cancer Institute of Canada. Ann Intern Med 1987;107:451-458.

90. Murray N, Grafton C, Shah A, et al. Abbreviated treatment for elderly, infirm, or noncompliant patients with limited stage small cell lung cancer. J Clin Oncol 1998;16:3323-3328.

91. Murray N, Livingston R, Shepherd FA, et al. Randomized study of CODE versus alternating CAV/EP for extensive stage small cell lung cancer: an Intergroup Study of the National Cancer Institute of Canada Clinical Trials Group and the Southwest Oncology Group. J Clin Oncol 1999;17:2300-2308.

92. Jett J, Kirschling R, Jung SH, et al. A phase II study of paclitaxel and granulocyte colony-stimulating factor in previously untreated patients with extensive stage small cell lung cancer: a study of the North Central Cancer Treatment Group. Semin Oncol 1995;22:75-77.

93. Jensen P, Sehestad M, Langer SW, et al. Twenty-five years of chemotherapy in small cell lung cancer sends us back to the laboratory. Cancer Treat Rev 1999;25:377-386.

94. Arriagada R, Le Chevalier T, Pignon JP, et al. Initial chemotherapeutic doses and survival in patients with limited small cell lung cancer. N Engl J Med 1993;329:1848-1852.

95. Bunn P, Lichter AS, Makuch RW. Chemotherapy alone or chemotherapy with chest radiation therapy in limited stage small cell lung cancer: a prospective, randomized trial. Ann Intern Med 1987;106:655-662.

96. Murray N, Coy P, Pater JL, et al. Importance of timing for thoracic irradiation in the combined modality treatment of limited stage small cell lung cancer: the National Cancer Institute of Canada Clinical Trials Group. J Clin Oncol 1993;11:336-344.

97. Arriagada R. How should thoracic radiotherapy be given in limited small cell lung cancer? Chest 1989;96:78S-80S.

98. Arriagada R, Le Chevalier T, Baldeyrou P, et al. Alternating radiotherapy and chemotherapy schedules in small cell lung cancer, limited disease. Int J Radiat Oncol Biol Phys 1985;11:1461-1467.

99. Auperin A, Arriagada R, Pignon J. Prophylactic cranial irradiation for patients with small cell lung cancer in complete remission: Prophylactic Cranial Irradiation Overview Collaborative Group. N Engl J Med 1999;341:476-484.

100. Arriagada R, Pignon JP, Laplanche A, et al. Prophylactic cranial irradiation for small cell lung cancer. Lancet 1997;349:138.

101. Lee J, Umsawasdi T, Lee YY, et al. Neurotoxicity in long-term survivors of small cell lung cancer. Int J Radiat Oncol Biol Phys 1986;12:313-321.

102. Herskovic A, Orton C. Elective brain irradiation for small cell anaplastic lung cancer. Int J Radiat Oncol Biol Phys 1986;12:427-429.

103. Kreisman H, Wolkove N, Quoix E. Small cell lung cancer presenting as a solitary pulmonary nodule. Chest 1992;101:225-231.

104. Mountain CF. Operation for small cell carcinoma revisited. J Clin Oncol 1987;5:687-688.

105. Quoix E, Fraser R, Wolkove N, et al. Small cell lung cancer presenting as a solitary pulmonary nodule. Cancer 1990;66:577-582.

106. Lad T, Piantadosi S, Thomas P, et al. A prospective randomized trial to determine the benefit of surgical resection of residual disease following response of small cell lung cancer to combination chemotherapy. Chest 1994;106:320S-323S.

107. Roth J, Fossella F, Komaki R, et al. A randomized trial comparing perioperative chemotherapy and surgery with surgery alone in resectable stage IIIA non–small cell lung cancer. J Natl Cancer Inst 1994;86:673-680.

108. Rosell R, Gomez-Codina J, Camps C. Preresectional chemotherapy in stage IIIA non–small cell lung cancer: a 7-year assessment of a randomized controlled trial. Lung Cancer 1999;26:7-14.

109. Rosell R, Lopez-Cabrerizo M, Astudillo J. Preoperative chemotherapy for stage IIIA non–small cell lung cancer. Curr Opin Oncol 1997;9:149-155.

110. Rosell R. New approaches in the adjuvant and neoadjuvant therapy of non–small cell lung cancer, including docetaxel (Taxotere) combinations. Semin Oncol 1999;26:32-37.

111. Sugarbaker D, Strauss GM. Advances in surgical staging and therapy of non–small cell lung cancer. Semin Oncol 1993; 20:163-172.

112. Sugarbaker D, Herndon J, Kohman LJ, et al. Results of cancer and leukemia group B protocol 8935: a multiinstitutional phase II trimodality trial for stage IIIA (N_2) non–small cell lung cancer: Cancer and Leukemia Group B Thoracic Surgery Group. J Thorac Cardiovasc Surg 1995;109:473-483.

113. Martini N, Beattie EJ. Results of surgical treatment in stage I lung cancer. J Thorac Cardiovasc Surg 1977;74:499-505.

114. Little A, DeMeester TR, Ferguson MK, et al. Modified stage I (T_1-N_0-M_0, T_2-N_0-M_0), non–small cell lung cancer: treatment results, recurrence patterns, and adjuvant immunotherapy. Surgery 1986;100:621-628.

115. Reif M, Socinski M, Rivera MP. Evidence-based medicine in the treatment of non–small cell lung cancer. Clin Chest Med 2000;21:107-120.

116. PORT Meta-analysis Trialists Group. Postoperative radiotherapy in non–small cell lung cancer: systematic review and meta-analysis of individual patient data from nine randomised controlled trials. Lancet 1998;352:257-263.

117. Marino P, Preatoni A, Cantoni A. Randomized trials of radiotherapy alone versus combined chemotherapy and radiotherapy in stages IIIA and IIIB non–small cell lung cancer: a meta-analysis. Cancer 1995;76:593-601.

118. Pritchard R, Anthony S. Chemotherapy plus radiotherapy compared with radiotherapy alone in the treatment of locally advanced, unresectable, non–small cell lung cancer: a meta-analysis. Ann Intern Med 1996;125:723-729.

119. Bruera E, de Stoutz N, Velasco-Leiva A, et al. Effects of oxygen on dyspnoea in hypoxaemic terminal-cancer patients. Lancet 1993;342:13-14.

120. Byhardt R, Scott C, Sause WT, et al. Response, toxicity, failure patterns, and survival in five Radiation Therapy Oncology Group (RTOG) trials of sequential and/or concurrent chemotherapy and radiotherapy for locally advanced non–small cell carcinoma of the lung. Int J Radiat Oncol Biol Phys 1998; 42:469-478.

121. Kwa S, Theuws J, Wagenaar A, et al. Evaluation of two dose-volume histogram reduction models for the prediction of radiation pneumonitis. Radiother Oncol 1998;48:61-69.

122. Monson J, Stark P, Reilly JJ, et al. Clinical radiation pneumonitis and radiographic changes after thoracic radiation therapy for lung carcinoma. Cancer 1998;82:842-850.

123. Braun S, doPico A, Olson CE, et al. Low-dose radiation pneumonitis. Cancer 1975;35:1322-1324.

124. Warner MA, Offord K, Warner ME, et al. Role of preoperative cessation of smoking and other factors in postoperative pulmonary complications: a blinded prospective study of coronary artery bypass patients. Mayo Clin Proc 1989;64: 609-616.

125. Rom W, Hay JG, Lee TC, et al. Molecular and genetic aspects of lung cancer. Am J Respir Crit Care Med 2000;161:1355-1367.

126. Bach P, Cramer LD, Warren JL, et al. Racial differences in the treatment of early stage lung cancer. N Engl J Med 1999; 341:1198-1205.

127. Fiore MC. How to prevent the progression of chronic bronchitis: the role of smoking cessation in prevention. Monaldi Arch Chest Dis 1994;49:13-16.

128. Fiore MC. Treatment options for smoking in the '90s. J Clin Pharmacol 1994;34:195-199.

129. Fiore MC. AHCPR smoking cessation guideline: a fundamental review. Tob Control 1997;6(Suppl 1):S4-8.

130. Fiore M, Novotny T, Pierce JP, et al. Trends in cigarette smoking in the United States: the changing influence of gender and race. JAMA 1989;261:49-55.

131. Fiore M, Baker TB. Smoking cessation treatment and the good doctor club. Am J Public Health 1995;85:161-163.

132. Fiore M, Jorenby DE, Baker TB. Smoking cessation: principles and practice based upon the AHCPR guideline, 1996. Agency for Health Care Policy and Research. Ann Behav Med 1997;19:213-219.

133. Carmelli D, Swan G, Robinette D, et al. Genetic influence on smoking: a study of male twins. N Engl J Med 1992;327:829-833.

134. Henningfield JE. Nicotine medications for smoking cessation. N Engl J Med 1995;333:1196-1203.

135. Hurt R, Sachs D, Glover ED, et al. A comparison of sustained-release bupropion and placebo for smoking cessation. N Engl J Med 1997;337:1195-1202.

136. Hurt R, Dale L, Croghan GA, et al. Nicotine nasal spray for smoking cessation: pattern of use, side effects, relief of withdrawal symptoms, and cotinine levels. Mayo Clin Proc 1998;73:118-125.

137. Hurt R, Croghan G, Beede SD, et al. Nicotine patch therapy in 101 adolescent smokers: efficacy, withdrawal symptom relief, and carbon monoxide and plasma cotinine levels. Arch Pediatr Adolesc Med 2000;154:31-37.

138. Croghan I, Offord K, Evans RW, et al. Cost-effectiveness of treating nicotine dependence: the Mayo Clinic experience. Mayo Clin Proc 1997;72:917-924.

139. Croghan I, Offord K, Patten CA, et al. Cost-effectiveness of the AHCPR guidelines for smoking. JAMA 1998;279:836-837.

140. Henschke CI, McCauley D, Yankelevitz DF, et al. Early Lung Cancer Action Project: overall design and findings from baseline screening. Lancet 1999;354:99-105.

141. Omenn G, Goodman G, Thornquist MD, et al. Risk factors for lung cancer and for intervention effects in CARET, the β-Carotene and Retinol Efficacy Trial. J Natl Cancer Inst 1996;88:1550-1559.

142. Omenn G, Goodman G, Thornquist MD, et al. Effects of a combination of β-carotene and vitamin A on lung cancer and cardiovascular disease. N Engl J Med 1996;334:1150-1155.

143. Omenn G, Goodman G, Thornquist M, et al. Chemoprevention of lung cancer: the β-Carotene and Retinol Efficacy Trial (CARET) in high-risk smokers and asbestos-exposed workers. IARC Sci Publ 1996;136:67-85.

144. Swisher S, Roth J, Nemunaitis J, et al. Adenovirus-mediated p53 gene transfer in advanced non–small cell lung cancer. J Natl Cancer Inst 1999;91:763-771.

145. Elias AD. Future directions in lung cancer research and therapeutics. Hematol Oncol Clin North Am 1997;11:519-527.

146. Dubinett S, Kradin RL. Cytokine immunotherapy of non–small cell lung cancer. Reg Immunol 1993;5:232-243.

147. Dubinett S, Miller P, Sharma S, et al. Gene therapy for lung cancer. Hematol Oncol Clin North Am 1998;12: 569-594.

148. Jenks S. RAC conditionally approves lung cancer gene therapy. J Natl Cancer Inst 1994;86:964-965.

149. Jenks S. Gene therapy for lung cancer still on hold. J Natl Cancer Inst 1994;86:486.

150. Jenks S. Gene therapy trial for lung cancer: caught between the RAC and a hard place. J Natl Cancer Inst 1994;86:332-333.

151. Morton D, Goodnight JE. Clinical trials of immunotherapy: present status. Cancer 1978;42:2224-2233.

152. Eddy DM. Screening for lung cancer. Ann Intern Med 1990;112:73-74.

153. Strauss G, Gleason R, Sugarbaker DJ. Screening for lung cancer reexamined: a reinterpretation of the Mayo Lung Project randomized trial on lung cancer screening. Chest 1993;103:337S-341S.

154. Melamed M, Flehinger B, Zaman MB, et al. Screening for early lung cancer: results of the Memorial Sloan-Kettering study in New York. Chest 1984;86:44-53.

155. Fontana R, Sanderson D, Woolner LB, et al. Screening for lung cancer: a critique of the Mayo Lung Project. Cancer 1991;67:1155-1164.

156. Battey J, Brown P, Gritz ER, et al. Primary and secondary prevention of lung cancer: an International Association for the Study of Lung Cancer workshop. Lung Cancer 1995;12:91-103.

157. Hong WK. Chemoprevention of lung cancer. Oncology (Huntingt) 1999;13:135-141.

158. Huber M, Lee J, Hong WK. Chemoprevention of lung cancer. Semin Oncol 1993;20:128-141.

159. Omenn GS. Chemoprevention of lung cancer: the rise and demise of β-carotene. Ann Rev Public Health 1998;19:73-99.

160. Jett JR. Is there a role for adjuvant therapy for resected non–small cell lung cancer? Thorax 1999;54(Suppl 2):S37-41.

161. Jett JR. Current treatment of unresectable lung cancer. Mayo Clin Proc 1993;68:603-611.

162. Carrato A, Rosell R, Camps C, et al. Modified weekly regimen with vinorelbine as a single agent in unresectable non–small cell lung cancer. Lung Cancer 1997;17:261-269.

163. Le Chevalier T, Arriagada R, Quoix E, et al. Radiotherapy alone versus combined chemotherapy and radiotherapy in unresectable non–small cell lung carcinoma. Lung Cancer 1994;10(Suppl 1):S239-244.

164. Sause W, Scott C, Taylor S, et al. Radiation Therapy Oncology Group (RTOG) 88-08 and Eastern Cooperative Oncology Group (ECOG) 4588: preliminary results of a phase III trial in regionally advanced, unresectable non–small cell lung cancer. J Natl Cancer Inst 1995;87:198-205.

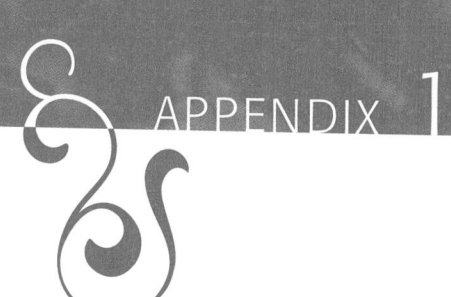

Formulary of Common Drugs Used in Respiratory Therapy

Christopher Carter
Christine Solberg

Albuterol (Proventil, Ventolin, Volmax)

Class:	Selective β_2-agonist
Indications:	Asthma/bronchospasm, COPD
Forms available:	MDI (90 µg/actuation)
	DPI (200 µg/actuation)
	Nebulized (0.083%, 0.5%)
	PO (2-, 4-, 8-mg tablets, 2-mg/5-mL syrup)
Onset/duration:	5 minutes (inhaled), 30 minutes (oral)/4 to 6 hours
Typical dose:	Outpatient MDI use: 2 puffs q4h prn
	Outpatient nebulizer use: 2.5 mg in 2-mL saline q4h prn
	Intubated patients: 4 to 8 puffs q1-4h
	Emergency treatment: 2 to 4 puffs q15min, or continuous nebulized
	Oral maintenance: 4 mg PO tid
Side effects and toxicity:	Tachycardia, palpitations, hypokalemia, lactic acidosis

Aminophylline (Phyllocontin, Truphylline)

Class:	Methylxanthine
Indications:	Asthma or other obstructive lung disease exacerbation, respiratory muscle weakness
Forms available:	PO (100-, 200-mg tablets; 225-mg sustained release, 105 mg/5-mL elixir)
	Rectal (250, 500 mg; 300-mg/5-mL liquid) IV
Onset/duration:	Minutes (IV)/approx. 6 hours
Typical dose:	Emergency treatment: Load 6 mg/kg, then 0.5-1.2 mg/kg/h infusion IV
	Maintenance, adult: 400 mg PO daily, divided tid-qid
	Maintenance, child: 16 mg/kg daily, divided tid-qid
Side effects and toxicity:	Tachycardia and palpitations, nausea, agitation and seizures

Amphotericin B (Liposomal Preparations Amphotec and AmBisome)

Class:	Antifungal antibiotic
Indications:	Prevention and treatment of invasive pulmonary aspergillosis in immunocompromised patients
Forms available:	Nebulized
	IV
Onset/duration:	N/A
Typical dose:	0.1 mg/kg/d, or 3 mL of 10-mg/mL solution or 10 mg by nebulizer bid
Actions:	Binds to ergosterol, disrupting fungal cell membrane
Side effects and toxicity:	Bronchospasm; potential for nephrotoxicity and ototoxicity

Aspirin (ASA)

Class:	Nonsteroidal antiinflammatory drug (NSAID)
Indications:	Diverse inflammatory processes, pain, fever, thrombotic syndromes
Forms available:	Oral (81-, 325-, 500-, 650-, 975-mg tablet)
	Rectal (120-, 200-, 300-, 600-mg suppository)
Duration:	6 hours
Typical dose:	MI and stroke prevention: 81 to 325 mg PO qd
	Antiinflammatory/analgesic: 650 PO q6h
Side effects and toxicity:	Peptic ulcer disease, increased bleeding, bronchospasm, nephropathy, tinnitus, nausea

Atropine

Class:	Anticholinergic
Indications:	Reduction of excessive secretions, especially before procedures such as bronchoscopy and intubation
Forms available:	Oral (0.4, 0.6 mg)
	IV, IM
Onset/duration:	5 minutes/1 to 2 hours
Typical dose:	0.4 to 0.6 mg PO/IV/IM q2h prn
Actions:	Reduces secretion of the liquid component of mucous
Side effects and toxicity:	Dry mouth, blurred vision, mydriasis, urinary retention, confusion

Beclomethasone Dipropionate (Beclovent, Vanceril, Beconase, Vancenase)

Class:	Inhaled corticosteroid
Indications:	Asthma and COPD maintenance therapy, rhinitis, sinusitis
Forms available:	MDI (42 μg/actuation)
	Nasal (42 μg/actuation)
Duration:	~8 hours
Typical dose:	2 to 3 puffs tid-qid (age >12)
	1 to 2 puffs tid-qid (children ages 6 to 12)
Side effects and toxicity:	Hoarseness, thrush, sore throat, possible growth retardation

Beractant (Survanta)

Class:	Surfactant replacement
Indications:	Treatment of neonatal respiratory distress syndrome (RDS), prophylaxis of RDS in neonates weighing less than 1250 g
Form available:	Intratracheal liquid instillation (25 mg phospholipid/mL)
Onset/duration:	Minutes/12 hours
Typical dose:	4 mL/kg; repeat doses q6h prn
Actions:	Reduces surface tension
Side effects and toxicity:	Mucous plugging, transient decrease in PaO_2 and hemodynamic instability

Bitolterol (Tornalate)

Class:	Selective β_2-agonist
Indications:	Bronchospasm/asthma, COPD
Forms available:	MDI (370 μg/actuation)
	Nebulized (0.2%)
Onset/duration:	5 minutes/5 hours
Typical dose:	MDI: 2 puffs q6h prn
	Nebulized: 1.25 mL in 1.25 mL saline q6h prn
Side effects and toxicity:	Tachycardia, palpitations, tremor

Budesonide (Pulmicort, Rhinocort)

Class:	Inhaled corticosteroid
Indications:	Asthma and COPD maintenance therapy, rhinitis, sinusitis
Forms available:	DPI (200 μg/actuation)
	Nasal (32 μg/actuation)
Duration:	~12 hours
Typical dose:	1 to 4 puffs bid
Side effects and toxicity:	Hoarseness, thrush, sore throat, possible growth retardation

Colfosceril Palmitate, Cetyl Alcohol, Tyloxapol (Exosurf)

Class:	Surfactant replacement
Indications:	Treatment of neonatal respiratory distress syndrome (RDS), prophylaxis of RDS in neonates weighing less than 1350 g
Form available:	Intratracheal liquid instillation (13.5 mg/mL when reconstituted)
Onset/duration:	Minutes/12 hours
Typical dose:	5 mL/kg q12h, three doses
Actions:	Reduces surface tension
Side effects and toxicity:	Pulmonary hemorrhage, mucous plugging, transient decrease in PaO_2

Colistimethate (Colistin, Coly-Mycin)

Class:	Polypeptide antibiotic
Indications:	Gram-negative pneumonia, especially *Pseudomonas* species
Forms available:	Nebulized (75 mg/mL)
	IV
Onset/duration:	N/A
Typical dose:	150 mg by nebulizer bid
Actions:	Binds phospholipids, disrupting bacterial cell membranes
Side effects and toxicity:	Nephrotoxicity, neurotoxicity including neuro-muscular blockade

Cromolyn Sodium (Intal, Nasalcrom)

Class:	Cromone
Indications:	Asthma, allergic rhinitis, conjunctivitis, mastocytosis
Forms available:	MDI (800 μg/actuation)
	DPI (20 mg/actuation)
	Nebulized (20 mg/2 mL)
	Nasal (5.2 mg/actuation)
	Oral (100 mg)
	Ophthalmic
Onset/duration:	10 minutes/2 to 6 hours
Typical dose:	MDI: 2 puffs qid
	DPI: 20 mg qid
	Nebulized: 20 mg qid
Actions:	Mast cell stabilization?
Side effects and toxicity:	Bronchospasm, arthralgia, angioedema, eosinophilic pneumonia, pulmonary infil-trates, mucosal irritation

Dexamethasone (Decadron, Dexacort)

Class:	Systemic (or inhaled) corticosteroid
Indications:	Multiple
Forms available:	MDI (dexamethasone sodium phosphate, 100 μg/actuation)
	Nasal (dexamethasone sodium phosphate, 100 μg/actuation)
	PO (0.25-, 0.5-, 0.75-, 1-, 1.5-, 2-, 4-, 6-mg tablets; 0.5 mg/5-mL elixir and solution; 0.5-mg/0.5-mL solution)

	IV
	Topical
	Ophthalmic
Duration:	More than 48 hours
Typical dose:	Systemic: varies
	Inhaled maintenance therapy: 3 puffs tid-qid
Side effects and toxicity:	Multiple

Dornase Alfa (DNAase, Pulmozyme)

Class:	Enzyme/secretion thinner
Indications:	CF and other conditions with thick purulent secretions
Form available:	Nebulized (1 mg/mL)
Onset/duration:	15 minutes/2 hours
Typical dose:	2.5 mg qd-bid
Action:	Digests DNA in purulent secretions
Side effects and toxicity:	Dyspnea, pharyngitis, cough, chest pain, hoarseness

Dyphylline (Lufyllin)

Class:	Methylxanthine
Indications:	Asthma or other obstructive lung disease ex-acerbation, respiratory muscle weakness
Form available:	PO (200, 400 mg)
Onset/duration:	30 minutes/6 hours
Typical dose:	Up to 15 mg/kg q6h
Side effects and toxicity:	Tachycardia and palpitations, nausea, agitation, and seizures

Ephedrine

Class:	Nonselective adrenergic agonist
Indications:	Asthma/bronchospasm
Forms available:	Nasal (0.25% spray, 0.5% drops, 1% jelly)
	PO (25, 50 mg)
	SC/IM/IV (25, 50 mg/mL)
Onset/duration:	15 minutes/4 hours
Typical dose:	Maintenance bronchodilator: 25 to 50 mg PO q4h prn
	Severe bronchospasm: 12.5 to 25 mg SC, IM, or IV
Side effects and toxicity:	Tachycardia, palpitations, cardiac ischemia, hypertension, tremor

Flunisolide (AeroBid, Nasalide)

Class:	Low-potency inhaled corticosteroid
Indications:	Asthma and COPD maintenance therapy, rhinitis, sinusitis
Forms available:	MDI (250 μg/actuation)
	Nasal (25 μg/actuation)
Duration:	~12 hours
Typical dose:	2 to 4 puffs bid
Side effects and toxicity:	Hoarseness, thrush, sore throat, possible growth retardation

Fluticasone (Flovent, Flonase)

Class:	High-potency inhaled corticosteroid
Indications:	Asthma and COPD maintenance therapy, rhinitis, sinusitis
Forms available:	MDI (44, 110, 220 μg/actuation)
	DPI (50, 100, 250 μg/actuation)
	Nasal (50 μg/actuation)
	Topical
Duration:	~12 hours
Typical dose:	MDI: 220-880 μg (1 to 4 puffs) bid
	DPI: 100-500 μg (1 to 2 doses) bid
	Nasal: 1 spray per nostril bid
Side effects and toxicity:	Hoarseness, thrush, sore throat, possible growth retardation

Glycopyrrolate (Robinul)

Class:	Anticholinergic
Indications:	Reduction of excessive secretions, especially before procedures such as bronchoscopy and intubation
Forms available:	Oral (1, 2 mg)
	IV, IM
Onset/duration:	5 minutes/1 to 2 hours
Typical dose:	Oral: 1 to 2 mg q4-6h
	IV/IM: 0.1 to 0.2 mg prn
Actions:	Reduces secretion of the liquid component of mucous
Side effects and toxicity:	Dry mouth, blurred vision, urinary retention, confusion

Heparin

Class:	Anticoagulant
Indications:	Prophylaxis and treatment of deep venous thrombosis and pulmonary embolism
Forms available:	IV
	SC
Onset/duration:	Minutes/~2 hours
Typical dose:	DVT prophylaxis: 5000 units SC q12h
DVT treatment:	IV infusion, dose variable
Actions:	Activates antithrombin III
Side effects and toxicity:	Excessive bleeding and bruising; contraindicated in active hemorrhage, recent intracranial hemorrhage, active pericarditis

Hydrocortisone (A-HydroCort, Cortef, Hydrocortone, Solu-Cortef, Cortisol)

Class:	Systemic corticosteroid
Indications:	Multiple
Forms available:	PO (5, 10, 20 mg; 10-mg/5-mL suspension)
	Rectal (10% foam = 90 mg/application; 100 mg/60 mL)
	IV
Duration:	~8 hours
Typical dose:	Adrenal insufficiency: 100 mg IV q6h
	Asthma/COPD exacerbation: 100 to 200 mg PO/IV q6h
	Pediatric: 1 mg/kg PO bid
Side effects and toxicity:	Multiple

Ibuprofen (Advil, Motrin, Nuprin, Rufen)

Class:	Nonsteroidal antiinflammatory drug (NSAID)
Indications:	Diverse inflammatory processes; pain; fever
Forms available:	Oral (200-, 800-mg tablet)
	Rectal (120-, 200-, 300-, 600-mg suppository)
Duration:	6 hours
Typical dose:	Antiinflammatory/analgesic: 600 PO q4-6h
Side effects and toxicity:	Peptic ulcer disease, increased bleeding, bronchospasm, nephropathy, nausea

Indomethacin (Indameth, Indocin)

Class:	Nonsteroidal antiinflammatory drug (NSAID)
Indications:	Diverse inflammatory processes; pain; fever
Forms available:	Oral (25-, 50-mg tablet, 25-mg/5-mL suspension)
	Rectal (50 mg suppository)
	IV
Duration:	6 hours
Typical dose:	Antiinflammatory/analgesic: 50 mg PO q6h
Side effects and toxicity:	Peptic ulcer disease, increased bleeding, bronchospasm, nephropathy, nausea

Infrasurf

Class:	Surfactant replacement
Indications:	Treatment of neonatal respiratory distress syndrome (RDS), prophylaxis of RDS in neonates weighing less than 1250 g
Form available:	Intratracheal liquid instillation
Onset/duration:	Minutes/12 hours
Typical dose:	3 mL/kg q12h
Actions:	Reduces surface tension
Side effects and toxicity:	Mucous plugging, transient decrease in PaO_2 and hemodynamic instability

Ipratropium (Atrovent)

Class:	Anticholinergic bronchodilator
Indications:	COPD, asthma and other obstructive lung diseases; rhinorrhea
Forms available:	MDI (18 μg/actuation)
	Nebulized (0.02%)
	Nasal spray (0.03%, 0.06%)
Onset/duration:	1 minute/6 hours
Typical dose:	MDI: 2 puffs q6h prn
	Nebulized: 2.5 mL (0.5 mg) q6h prn
	Nasal: 2 sprays per nostril q6h prn
Side effects and toxicity:	Palpitations, dry mouth, blurred vision, acute exacerbation of narrow-angle glaucoma, urinary retention

Isoproterenol (Isuprel)

Class:	β-Adrenergic agonist
Indications:	Asthma/bronchospasm
Forms available:	MDI (80, 120, 131 μg/actuation)
	Nebulized (0.25%, 0.5%, 1%)
	Sublingual (10, 15 mg)
	IV (200 μg/mL)
Onset/duration:	2 minutes/2 hours
Typical dose:	MDI: 1 to 2 puffs q4h prn
	Nebulized: 2 mL of 0.25% solution in 2-mL saline q4h prn
	Sublingual: 10 to 20 mg PO qd
	IV: 0.01 to 0.02 mg IV q2h prn
Side effects and toxicity:	Tachycardia, palpitations, tremor, hypo- or hypertension, flushing

Ketorolac (Toradol)

Class:	Nonsteroidal antiinflammatory drug (NSAID)
Indications:	Diverse inflammatory processes; pain; fever
Forms available:	Oral (10-mg tablet)
	IV, IM
Onset/duration:	30 minutes/6 hours
Typical dose:	Antiinflammatory/analgesic: 60 mg IM
	May repeat q6h × 1
Side effects and toxicity:	Peptic ulcer disease, increased bleeding, bronchospasm, nephropathy, nausea

Levalbuterol (Xopenex)

Class:	Selective β_2-agonist
Indications:	Asthma/bronchospasm, COPD, especially in patients bothered by side effects of racemic albuterol
Form available:	Nebulized (0.625- and 1.25-mg unit doses)
Onset/duration:	5 minutes/6 hours
Typical dose:	0.625 to 1.25 mg q4h prn
Side effects and toxicity:	Tachycardia, palpitations, tremor

Lidocaine

Class:	Topical anesthetic
Indications:	Cough, before bronchoscopy
Forms available:	Nebulized
	Intratracheal instillation
Onset/duration:	10 seconds/30 minutes
Typical dose:	Nebulized: 2 mL of 4% solution
	Intratracheal instillation: 2 mL of 1% solution
Actions:	Local anesthesia
Side effects and toxicity:	Cardiac arrhythmia, decreased level of consciousness, increased risk of aspiration

Low–Molecular-Weight Heparins

Class:	Anticoagulant
Indications:	Prophylaxis and treatment of deep venous thrombosis and pulmonary embolism
Form available:	SC
Onset/duration:	Hours
Typical dose:	Prophylaxis: 40 mg SC q12h
Treatment:	1.5 mg/kg SC q12h
Actions:	Activates antithrombin III
Side effects and toxicity:	Excessive bleeding and bruising; contraindicated in active hemorrhage, recent intracranial hemorrhage, active pericarditis

Metaproterenol (Alupent, Metaprel)

Class:	β-Adrenergic agonist (some β_2-selectivity)
Indications:	Asthma/bronchospasm, COPD
Forms available:	MDI (650 μg/actuation)
	Nebulized (0.4%, 0.6%, 5%)
	PO (10-, 20-mg tablets, 10-mg/5-mL syrup)
Onset/duration:	5 to 30 minutes/4 hours
Typical dose:	MDI: 2 to 3 puffs q3-4h prn
	Nebulized: 2.5 mL of 0.6% solution q4-6h prn
	Oral, adult: 20 mg q6h prn
	Oral, children >27 kg: 10 mL q6h prn
	Oral, children <27 kg: 5 mL q6h prn
Side effects and toxicity:	Tachycardia, palpitations, cardiac ischemia, tremor

Methylprednisolone (Medrol, Solu-Medrol)

Class:	Systemic corticosteroid
Indications:	Multiple
Forms available:	PO (2-, 4-, 8-, 16-, 24-, 32-mg)
	IV (injection and slowly absorbed suspension)
Duration:	12 to 24 hours
Typical dose:	Asthma or COPD exacerbation: 125 mg IV, then 60 mg q6h
	Pediatric: 1 to 2 mg/kg/day IV q6h
	Systemic: varies
Side effects and toxicity:	Multiple

Montelukast (Singulair)

Class:	Leukotriene synthesis inhibitor
Indications:	Asthma, allergic rhinitis
Form available:	PO (5-mg chewable, 10-mg tablet)
Onset/duration:	3 hours/24 hours
Typical dose:	10 mg qd (adults)
	5 mg qd (children)
Side effects and toxicity:	Churg-Strauss syndrome?

N-acetylcysteine (Mucomyst, Mucosil, NAC)

Class:	Secretion thinner
Indications:	Cystic fibrosis and other conditions with thick secretions; acetaminophen overdose
Form available:	Nebulized or oral solution (10%, 20%)
Onset/duration:	5 minutes/1 to 2 hours
Typical dose:	3 to 10 mL of 20% solution tid-qid
Actions:	Cleaves disulfide bonds in mucous
Side effects and toxicity:	Bronchospasm (usually administered with a bronchodilator), rhinitis, nausea, mild elevation in liver enzymes with oral administration

Nedocromil (Tilade)

Class:	Cromone
Indications:	Asthma, allergic rhinitis
Form available:	MDI (1.75 mg/actuation)
Onset/duration:	30 min/6 to 12 hours
Typical dose:	2 puffs qid, then reduce to bid as tolerated
Actions:	Mast cell stabilization?
Side effects and toxicity:	Bronchospasm, eosinophilic pneumonia

Pentamidine (NebuPent)

Class:	Antibiotic
Indications:	Prophylaxis against (nebulized) or treatment of (IV) PCP in sulfa-allergic patients
Forms available:	Nebulized
	IV
Onset/duration:	N/A
Typical dose:	PCP prophylaxis: 300 mg in 5 mL saline, nebulized monthly
	PCP treatment: 4 mg/kg IV qd
Actions:	Unknown
Side effects and toxicity:	Cough, bronchospasm

Pirbuterol (Maxair)

Class:	Selective β_2-agonist
Form available:	MDI (200 μg /actuation)
Onset/duration:	5 minutes/5 hours
Typical dose:	1 to 2 puffs q4h prn
Indications:	Bronchospasm/asthma, COPD
Side effects and toxicity:	Tachycardia, palpitations, tremor

Prednisolone (Delta-Cortef, Hydeltrasol, Prelone, Pediapred, Predicort)

Class:	Systemic corticosteroid
Indications:	Multiple
Forms available:	PO (5-mg tablet; 15-mg/5-mL, 5-mg/5-mL liquid)
	Ophthalmic
Duration:	12 to 24 hours
Typical dose:	Varies
Side effects and toxicity:	Multiple

Prednisone (Deltasone, Meticorten, Orasone, Sterapred)

Class:	Systemic corticosteroid
Indications:	Multiple
Forms available:	PO (1, 2.5, 5, 10, 20, 25, 50 mg; 5-mg/5-mL syrup and solution; 5-mg/1-mL solution)
	IV
Duration:	12 to 24 hours
Typical dose:	Varies
Side effects and toxicity:	Multiple

Racemic Epinephrine (Adrenalin, Asthma-Haler, AsthmaNefrin, Bronkaid, Epinal, Primatene Mist, Vaponephrine)

Class:	Nonselective adrenergic agonist
Indications:	Anaphylaxis; asthma/bronchospasm; upper airway edema and laryngospasm
Forms available:	MDI (160, 200, 250 μg/actuation)
	Nebulized (1%, 1.25%, 2.25% solution)
	SC (1:1000)
	IV (1:10,000 and 1:100,000)
Onset/duration:	1 minute/1 hour
Typical dose:	MDI: 1 puff q4h prn
	Nebulized: 0.5 mL of 2.25% solution in 2 mL saline, q6h prn
	Anaphylaxis: 0.4 mg SC
Actions:	Bronchodilation; blocks histamine release by mast cells; vasoconstriction
Side effects and toxicity:	Tachycardia, palpitations, cardiac ischemia, hypertension, tremor

Ribavirin (Virazole)

Class:	Antiviral
Indications:	RSV and severe influenza infection
Form available:	Nebulized
Onset/duration:	60 minutes/7 hours (children) to 24 hours (adults)
Typical dose:	6 g in 300 mL saline, continuous nebulization 18/24 hr for 3 to 7 days
Actions:	Unknown
Side effects and toxicity:	Bronchospasm, pulmonary edema, hypoxia, hypotension, cardiac arrhythmia (drug contraindicated in pregnancy; should be used with extreme caution with mechanical ventilators)

Salmeterol (Serevent)

Class:	Long-acting selective β_2-agonist
Indications:	Maintenance therapy of asthma, COPD and other obstructive diseases; especially useful in preventing overnight exacerbation
Forms available:	MDI (25 μg/actuation)
	DPI (50 μg/actuation)
Onset/duration:	10 minutes/12 hours
Typical dose:	MDI: 2 to 4 puffs bid
	DPI: 1 inhalation bid
Side effects and toxicity:	Tachycardia, palpitations (less than short-acting agents), paradoxic bronchospasm

Terbutaline (Brethine, Bricanyl, Brethaire)

Class:	Selective β_2-agonist
Indications:	Asthma/bronchospasm
Forms available:	MDI (200 μg/actuation)
	PO (2.5, 5 mg)
	IV (1 mg/mL)
Onset/duration:	5 to 30 minutes/4 hours
Typical dose:	Emergency nebulized treatment: 1 mg in 2 mL saline q4h prn
	Emergency parenteral treatment: 0.25 to 0.5 mg SC or IV q4h prn
	Inhaled maintenance therapy: 2 puffs q4-6h prn
	Oral maintenance therapy: 5 to 15 mg PO tid
Side effects and toxicity:	Tachycardia, palpitations, tremor, paradoxic bronchospasm

Theophylline (Accurbron, Aerolate, Aquaphyllin, Asmalix, Bronkodyl, Constant-T, Elixophyllin, Lanophyllin, Quibron-T, Respbid, Slo-Bid, Slo-Phyllin, Sustaire, Theobid, Theochron, Theoclear, Theo-Dur, Theolair, Theospan, Theostat, Theovent, Theox, T-Phyl, Uniphyl)

Class:	Methylxanthine
Indications:	Asthma, especially for nocturnal symptoms and in children; COPD and respiratory muscle weakness
Forms available:	PO (100-, 200-mg capsules; 100-, 125-, 200-, 250-, 300-mg tablet; 50-, 60-, 65-, 75-, 100-, 125-, 130-, 200-, 250-, 260-, 300-, 400-, 450-, 500-mg extended-release; 50-mg/5-mL, 80-mg/15-mL elixir; 50-mg/5-mL, 80-, 150-mg/15-mL syrup)
	IV
Onset/duration:	30 minutes/varies widely
Typical dose:	Maintenance therapy: 13 to 24 mg/kg/day, divided q6-8h
	Emergency treatment: Load 4.7 mg/kg, then 0.24 to 0.55 mg/kg/h infusion IV
Side effects and toxicity:	Tachycardia and palpitations, nausea, agitation and seizures

Thrombin

Class:	Coagulant
Indications:	Hemorrhage
Form available:	Topical
Onset/duration:	Seconds/hours
Typical dose:	1 mL reconstituted
Actions:	Converts fibrinogen to fibrin clot
Side effects and toxicity:	Large clot formation may cause airway obstruction

Tobramycin (TOBI)

Class:	Aminoglycoside antibiotic
Indications:	Patients with cystic fibrosis, and possibly other forms of bronchiectasis, colonized with *Pseudomonas* species
Forms available:	Nebulized (300 mg/5 mL unit dose)
	IV
	Ophthalmic
Onset/duration:	Hours/weeks
Typical dose:	300 mg bid × 28 days, then off × 28 days
Actions:	Interferes with bacterial protein translation; reduces pulmonary levels of *Pseudomonas* species and other gram-negative bacteria
Side effects and toxicity:	Ototoxicity, nephrotoxicity

Triamcinolone Acetonide (Azmacort)

Class:	Inhaled corticosteroid
Indications:	Asthma and COPD maintenance (and rarely, exacerbation) therapy; rhinitis, sinusitis
Forms available:	MDI (100 µg/actuation)
	Nasal (55 µg/actuation)
	Oral (1-, 2-, 4-, 8-mg tablets; 2-mg/mL, 4-mg/mL suspension)
	IV
Duration:	~8 hours
Typical dose:	MDI: 2 to 4 puffs tid-qid, tapered to bid as tolerated
	Pediatric MDI: 1 to 2 puffs tid-qid, tapered to bid as tolerated
	Systemic: varies
Side effects and toxicity:	Hoarseness, thrush, sore throat, possible growth retardation

Warfarin (Coumadin)

Class:	Anticoagulant
Indications:	Prophylaxis and treatment of deep venous thrombosis and pulmonary embolism
Form available:	PO
Onset/duration:	2 to 3 days/approx. 1 week
Typical dose:	2 to 8 mg PO qd
Actions:	Inhibits production of vitamin K-dependent factors V, VII, IX, X
Side effects and toxicity:	Excessive bleeding and bruising; contraindicated in active hemorrhage, recent intracranial hemorrhage, active pericarditis

Zafirlukast (Accolate)

Class:	Leukotriene receptor antagonist
Indications:	Asthma, allergic rhinitis
Form available:	PO (20-mg tablet)
Onset/duration:	3 hours/12 hours
Typical dose:	20 mg PO bid
Side effects and toxicity:	Churg-Strauss syndrome?

Zileuton (Zyflo)

Class:	5-Lipoxygenase inhibitor
Indications:	Asthma, allergic rhinitis
Form available:	PO (600 mg)
Onset/duration:	1½ hours/6 hours
Typical dose:	600 mg PO qid
Side effects and toxicity:	Hepatotoxicity

American Heart Association Algorithms for Cardiopulmonary Resuscitation

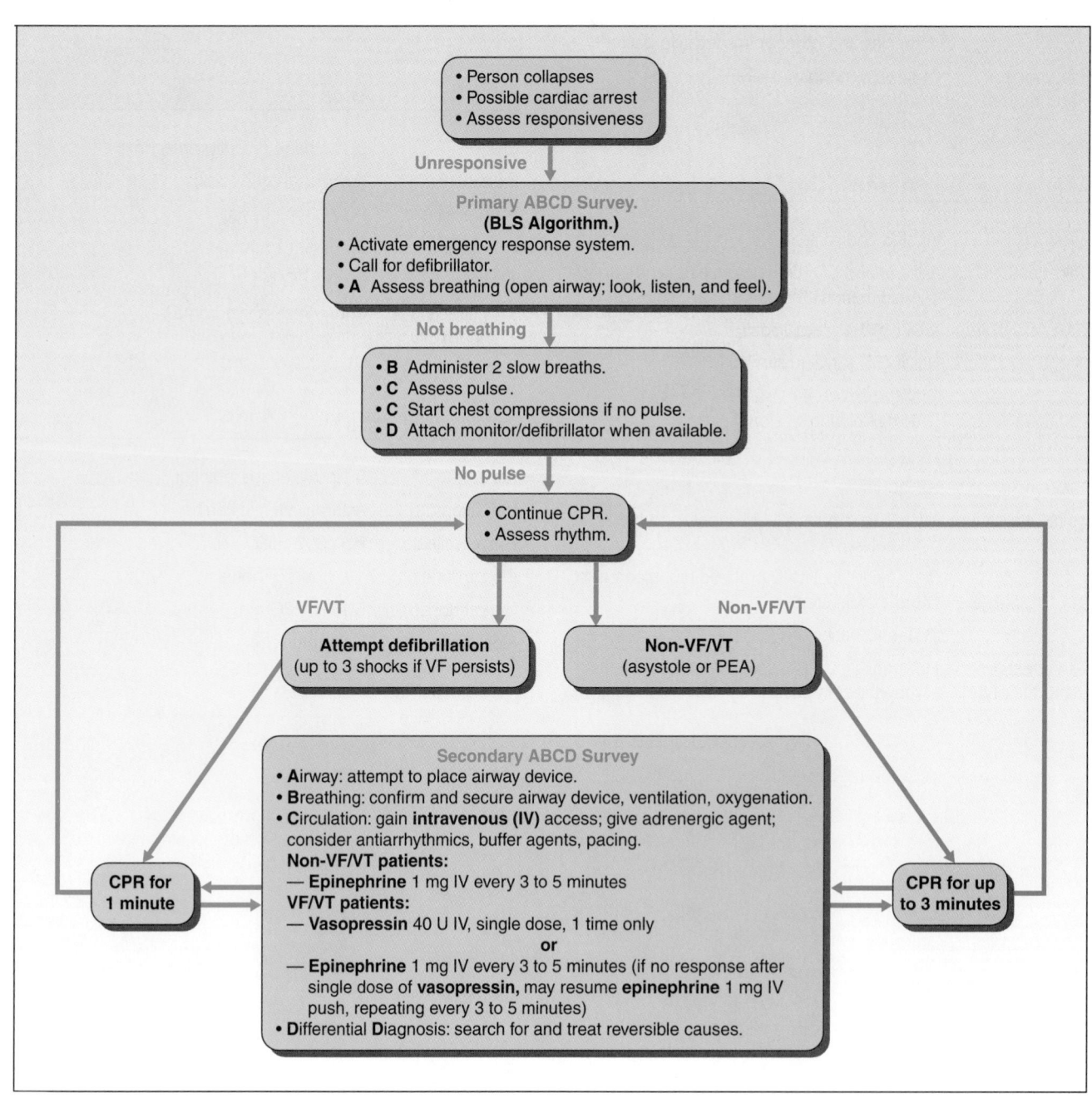

Comprehensive emergency cardiac care algorithm. *ABCD,* Airway, breathing, circulation, and defibrillation; *BLS,* basic life support; *VF/VT,* ventricular fibrillation/ventricular tachycardia; *CPR,* cardiopulmonary resuscitation; *PEA,* pulseless electrical activity. (Modified from Algorithm approach to ACLS emergencies. Part 7. Circulation 2000;102:I-136.)

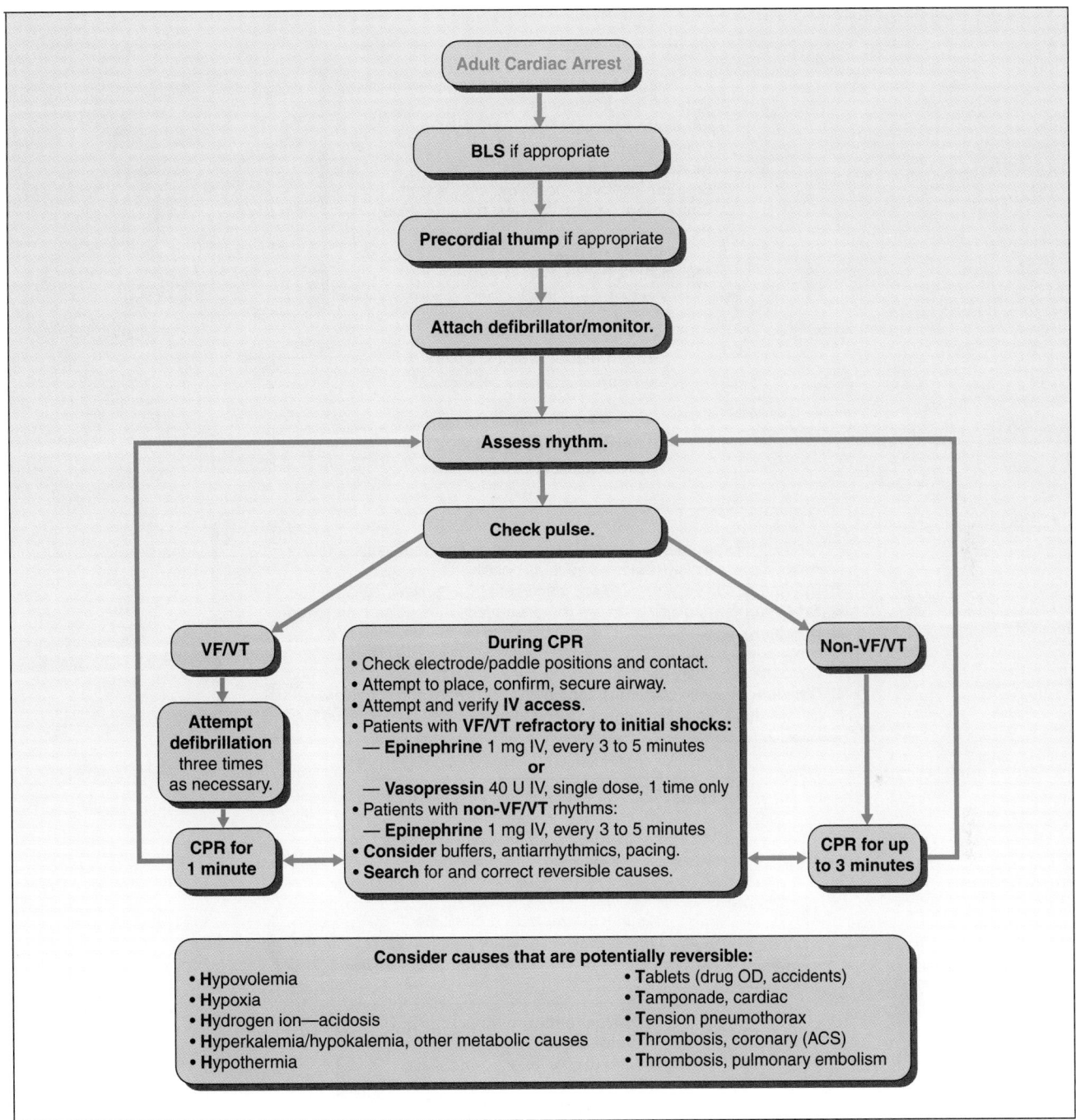

Universal advanced cardiac life support algorithm. *BLS,* Basic life support; *VF/VT,* ventricular fibrillation/ventricular tachycardia; *CPR,* cardiopulmonary resuscitation; *IV,* intravenous; *OD,* overdose; *ACS,* acute coronary syndromes. (Modified from Algorithm approach to ACLS emergencies. Part 7. Circulation 2000;102:I-136.)

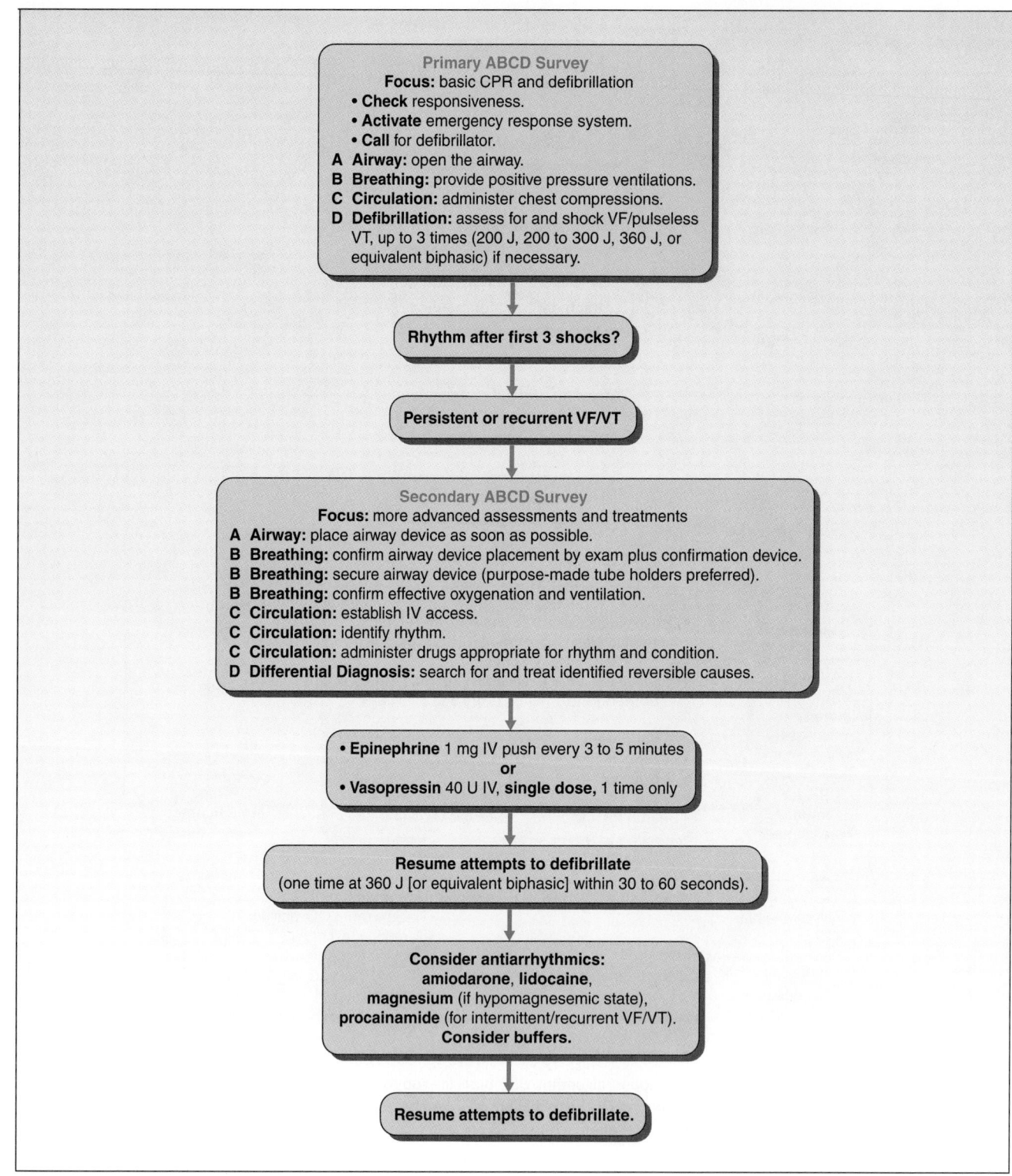

Ventricular fibrillation/pulseless ventricular tachycardia algorithm. *ABCD,* Airway, breathing, circulation, and defibrillation; *CPR,* cardiopulmonary resuscitation; *VF/VT,* ventricular fibrillation/ventricular tachycardia; *IV,* intravenous. (Modified from Algorithm approach to ACLS emergencies. Part 7. Circulation 2000;102:I-136.)

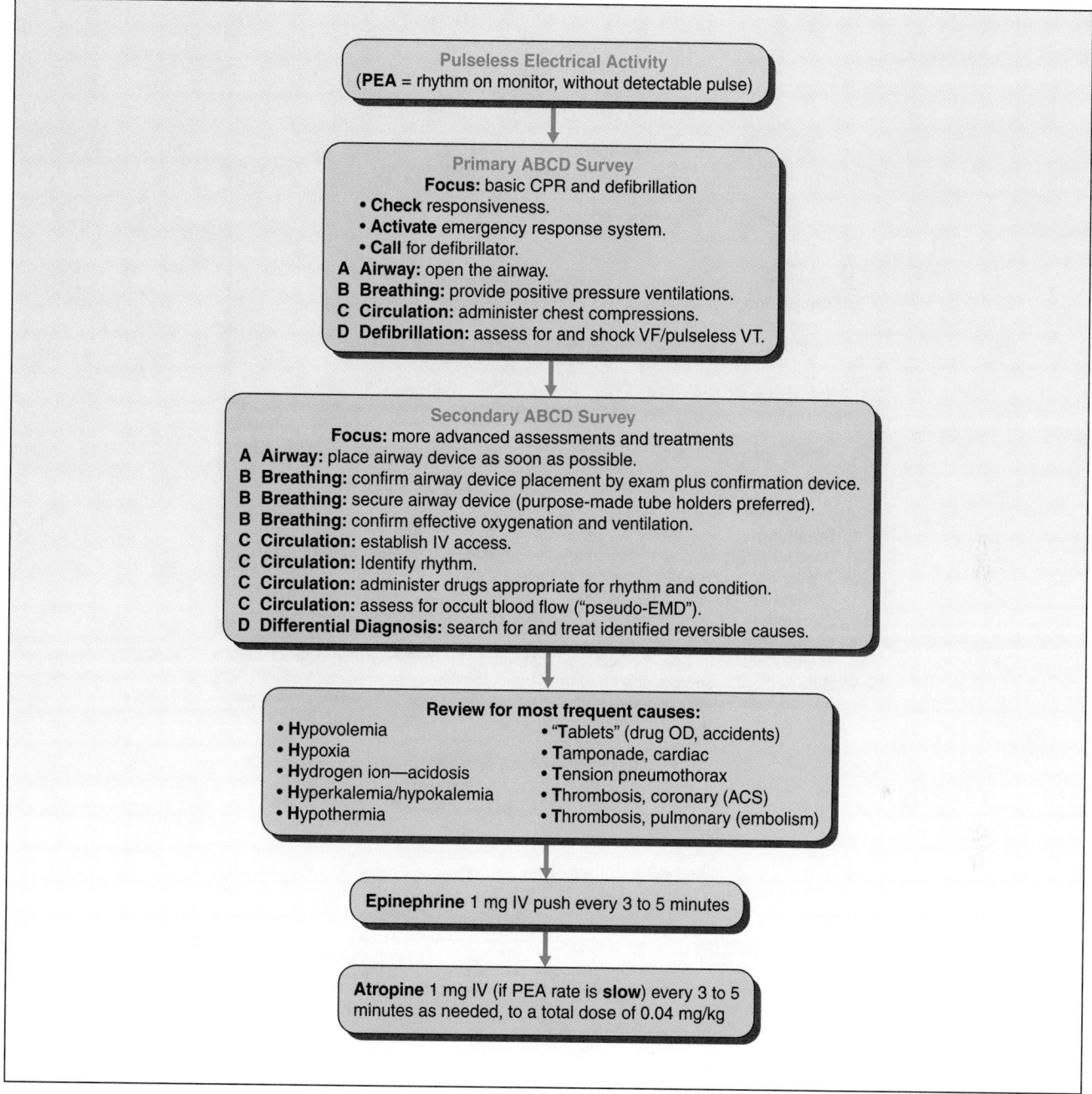

Pulseless electrical activity algorithm. *PEA,* Pulseless electrical activity; *ABCD,* airway, breathing, circulation, and defibrillation; *CPR,* cardiopulmonary resuscitation; *VF,* ventricular fibrillation; *VT,* ventricular tachycardia; *EMD,* electromechanical dissociation; *OD,* overdose; *ACS,* acute coronary syndromes; *IV,* intravenous. (Modified from Algorithm approach to ACLS emergencies. Part 7. Circulation 2000;102:I-136.)

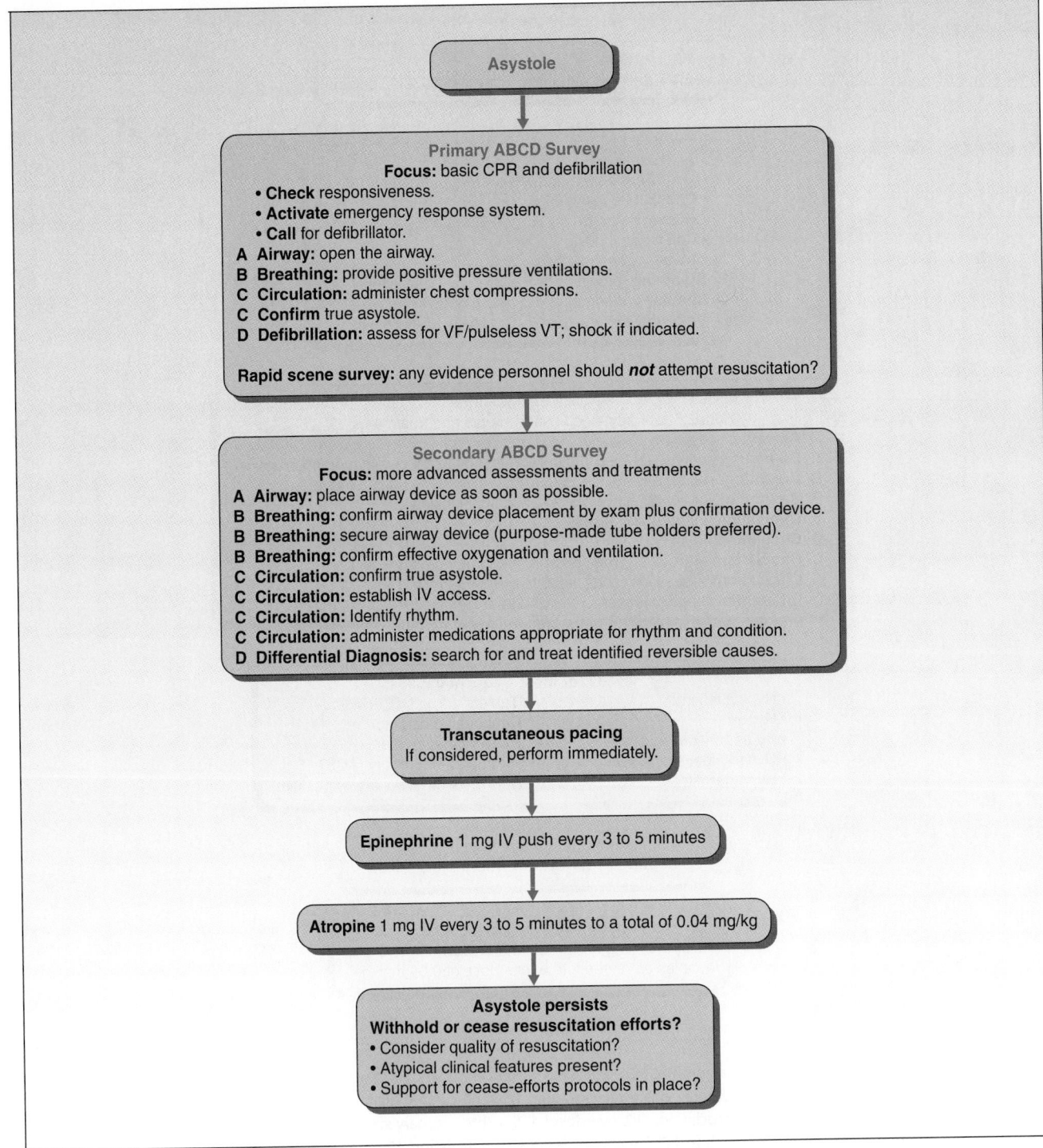

Asystole algorithm. *ABCD,* Airway, breathing, circulation, and defibrillation; *CPR,* cardiopulmonary resuscitation; *VF,* ventricular fibrillation; *VT,* ventricular tachycardia; *IV,* intravenous. (Modified from Algorithm approach to ACLS emergencies. Part 7. Circulation 2000;102:I-136.)

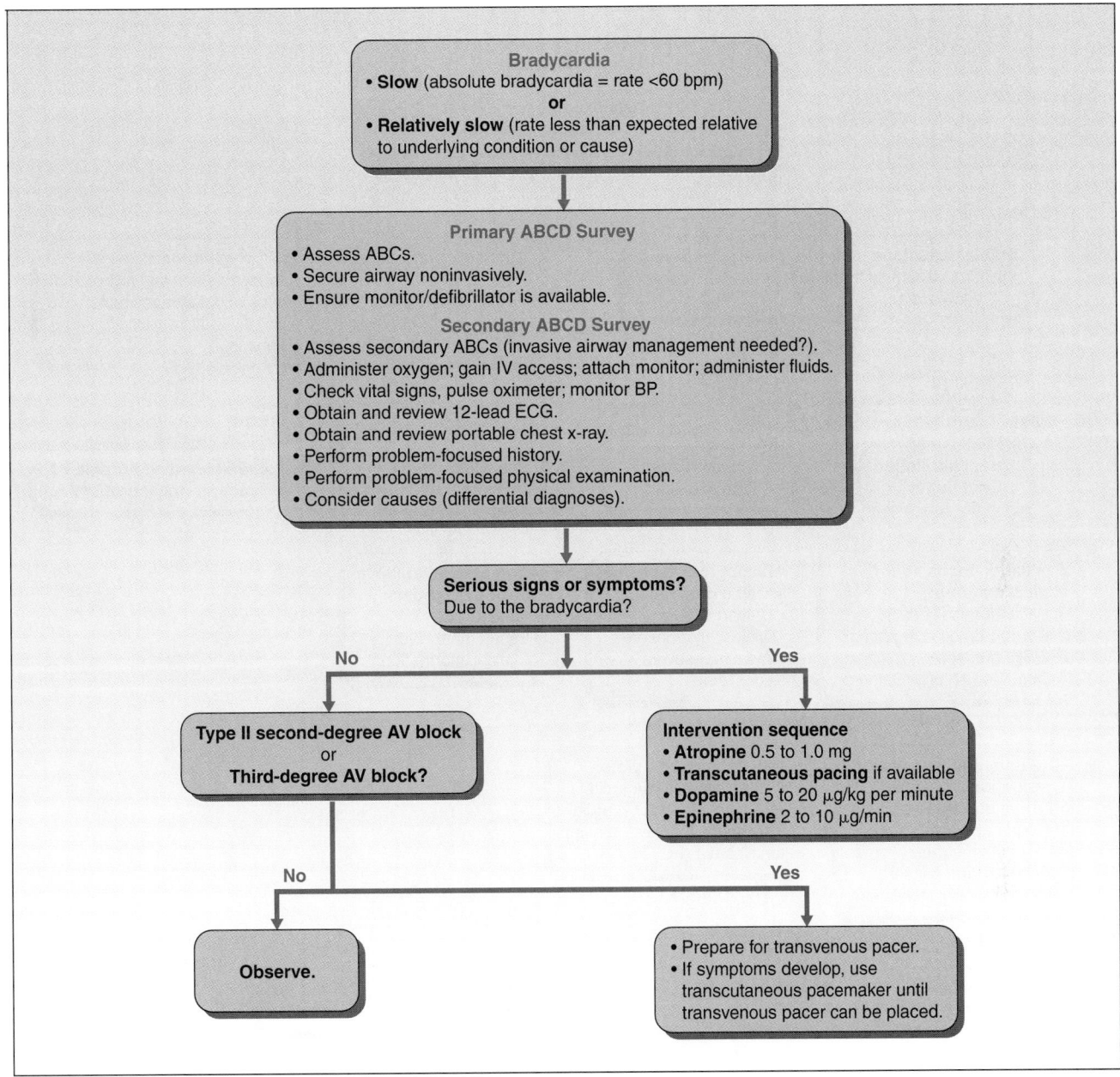

Bradycardia algorithm. *ABCD,* Airway, breathing, circulation, and defibrillation; *ECG,* electrocardiogram; *IV,* intravenous; *AV,* atrioventricular. (Modified from Algorithm approach to ACLS emergencies. Part 7. Circulation 2000;102:I-136.)

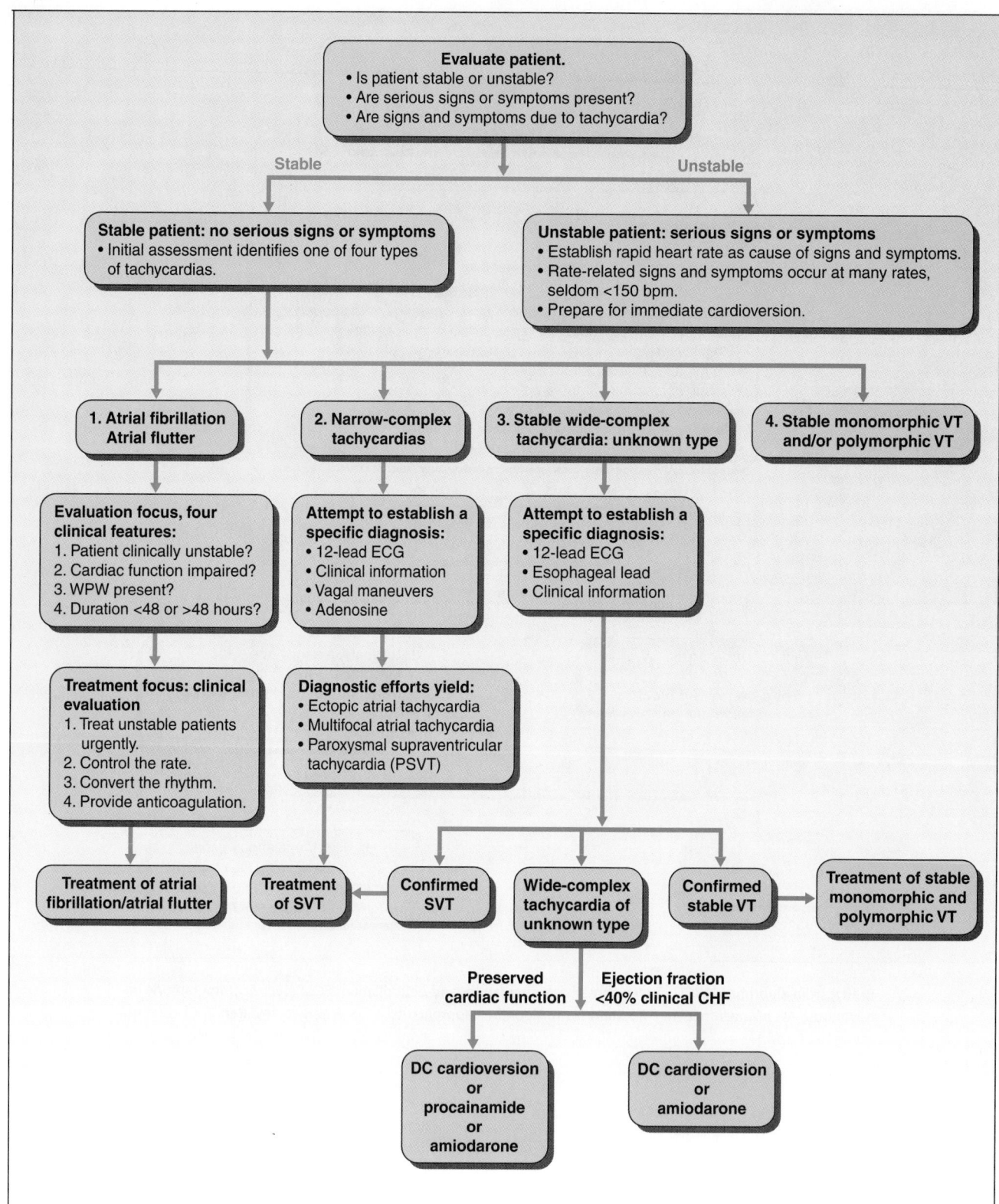

Tachycardia overview algorithm. *bpm,* Beats per minute; *VT,* ventricular tachycardia; *WPW,* Wolff-Parkinson-White (syndrome); *ECG,* electrocardiogram; *SVT,* supraventricular tachycardia; *DC,* direct current; *CHF,* congestive heart failure. (Modified from Algorithm approach to ACLS emergencies. Part 7. Circulation 2000;102:I-136.)

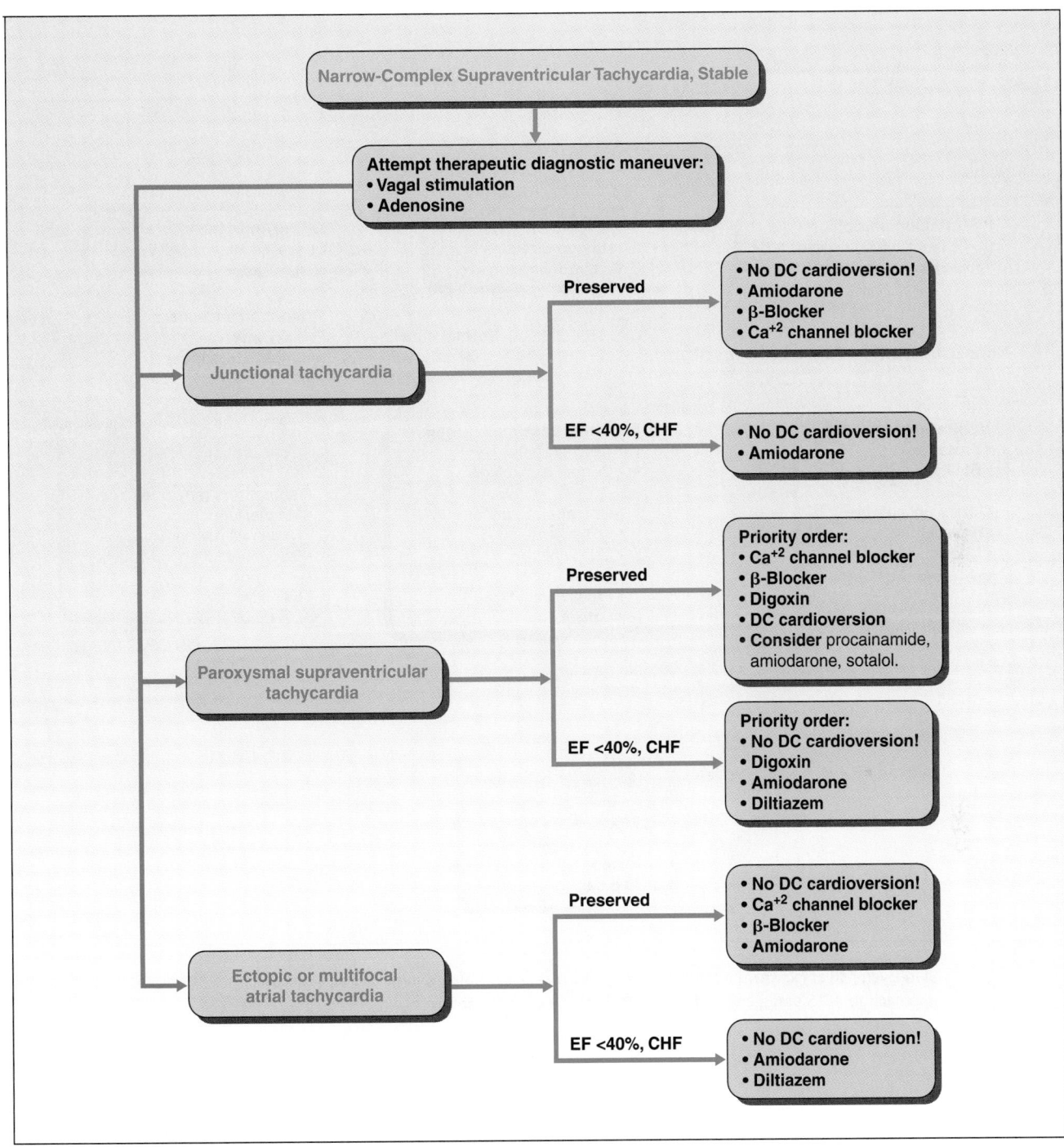

Narrow-complex supraventricular tachycardia algorithm. *EF,* Ejection fraction; *CHF,* congestive heart failure; *DC,* direct current. (Modified from Algorithm approach to ACLS emergencies. Part 7. Circulation 2000;102:I-136.)

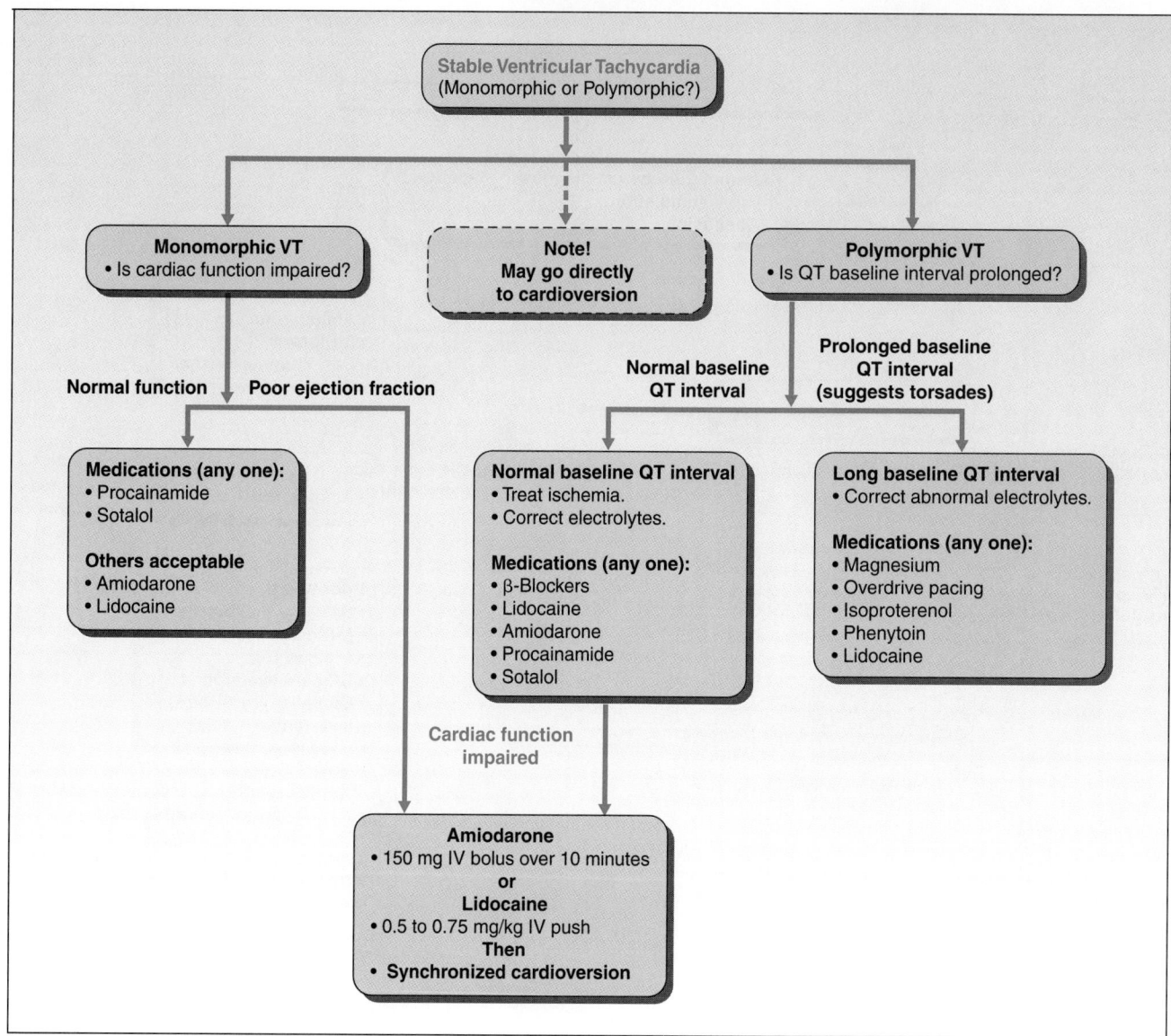

Stable ventricular tachycardia algorithm. *VT,* Ventricular tachycardia; *IV,* intravenous. (Modified from Algorithm approach to ACLS emergencies. Part 7. Circulation 2000;102:I-136.)

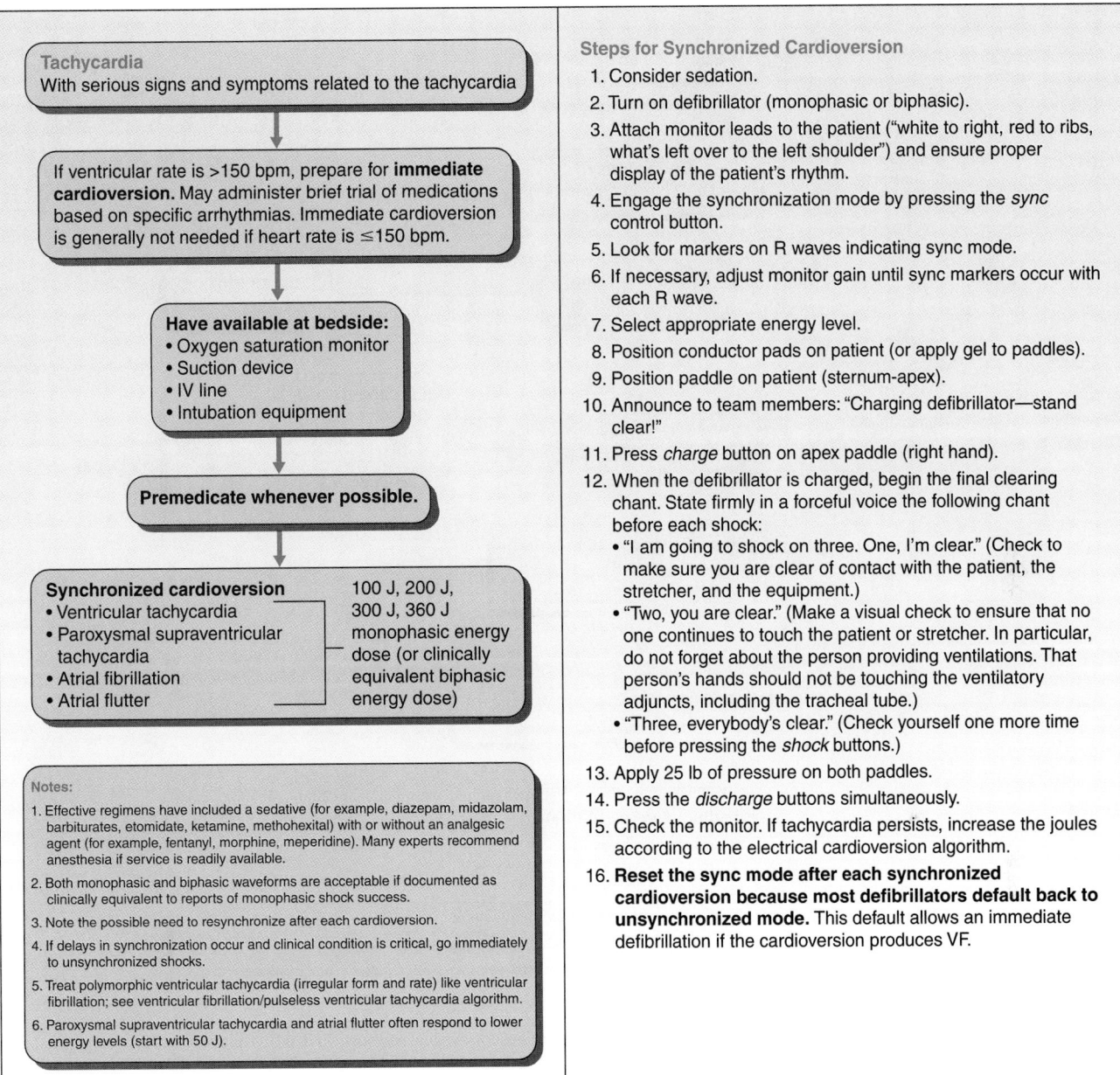

Tachycardia
With serious signs and symptoms related to the tachycardia

If ventricular rate is >150 bpm, prepare for **immediate cardioversion.** May administer brief trial of medications based on specific arrhythmias. Immediate cardioversion is generally not needed if heart rate is ≤150 bpm.

Have available at bedside:
- Oxygen saturation monitor
- Suction device
- IV line
- Intubation equipment

Premedicate whenever possible.

Synchronized cardioversion
- Ventricular tachycardia
- Paroxysmal supraventricular tachycardia
- Atrial fibrillation
- Atrial flutter

100 J, 200 J, 300 J, 360 J monophasic energy dose (or clinically equivalent biphasic energy dose)

Notes:
1. Effective regimens have included a sedative (for example, diazepam, midazolam, barbiturates, etomidate, ketamine, methohexital) with or without an analgesic agent (for example, fentanyl, morphine, meperidine). Many experts recommend anesthesia if service is readily available.
2. Both monophasic and biphasic waveforms are acceptable if documented as clinically equivalent to reports of monophasic shock success.
3. Note the possible need to resynchronize after each cardioversion.
4. If delays in synchronization occur and clinical condition is critical, go immediately to unsynchronized shocks.
5. Treat polymorphic ventricular tachycardia (irregular form and rate) like ventricular fibrillation; see ventricular fibrillation/pulseless ventricular tachycardia algorithm.
6. Paroxysmal supraventricular tachycardia and atrial flutter often respond to lower energy levels (start with 50 J).

Steps for Synchronized Cardioversion
1. Consider sedation.
2. Turn on defibrillator (monophasic or biphasic).
3. Attach monitor leads to the patient ("white to right, red to ribs, what's left over to the left shoulder") and ensure proper display of the patient's rhythm.
4. Engage the synchronization mode by pressing the *sync* control button.
5. Look for markers on R waves indicating sync mode.
6. If necessary, adjust monitor gain until sync markers occur with each R wave.
7. Select appropriate energy level.
8. Position conductor pads on patient (or apply gel to paddles).
9. Position paddle on patient (sternum-apex).
10. Announce to team members: "Charging defibrillator—stand clear!"
11. Press *charge* button on apex paddle (right hand).
12. When the defibrillator is charged, begin the final clearing chant. State firmly in a forceful voice the following chant before each shock:
    - "I am going to shock on three. One, I'm clear." (Check to make sure you are clear of contact with the patient, the stretcher, and the equipment.)
    - "Two, you are clear." (Make a visual check to ensure that no one continues to touch the patient or stretcher. In particular, do not forget about the person providing ventilations. That person's hands should not be touching the ventilatory adjuncts, including the tracheal tube.)
    - "Three, everybody's clear." (Check yourself one more time before pressing the *shock* buttons.)
13. Apply 25 lb of pressure on both paddles.
14. Press the *discharge* buttons simultaneously.
15. Check the monitor. If tachycardia persists, increase the joules according to the electrical cardioversion algorithm.
16. **Reset the sync mode after each synchronized cardioversion because most defibrillators default back to unsynchronized mode.** This default allows an immediate defibrillation if the cardioversion produces VF.

Synchronized cardioversion algorithm. *bpm,* Beats per minute; *IV,* intravenous; *VF,* ventricular fibrillation. (Modified from Algorithm approach to ACLS emergencies. Part 7. Circulation 2000;102:I-136.)

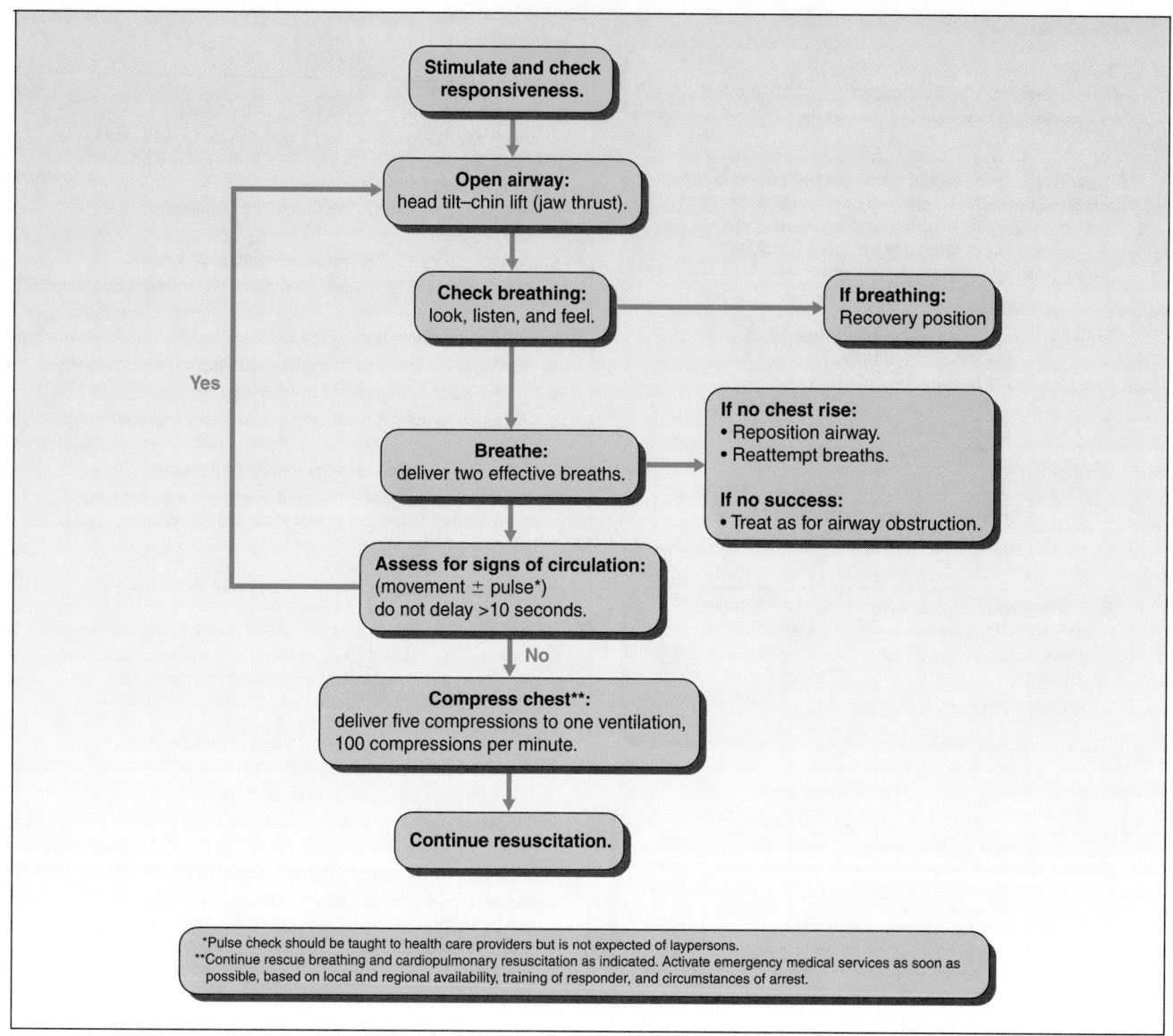

Pediatric basic life support algorithm. (Modified from Pediatric basic life support. Part 9. Circulation 2000; 102:I-136.)

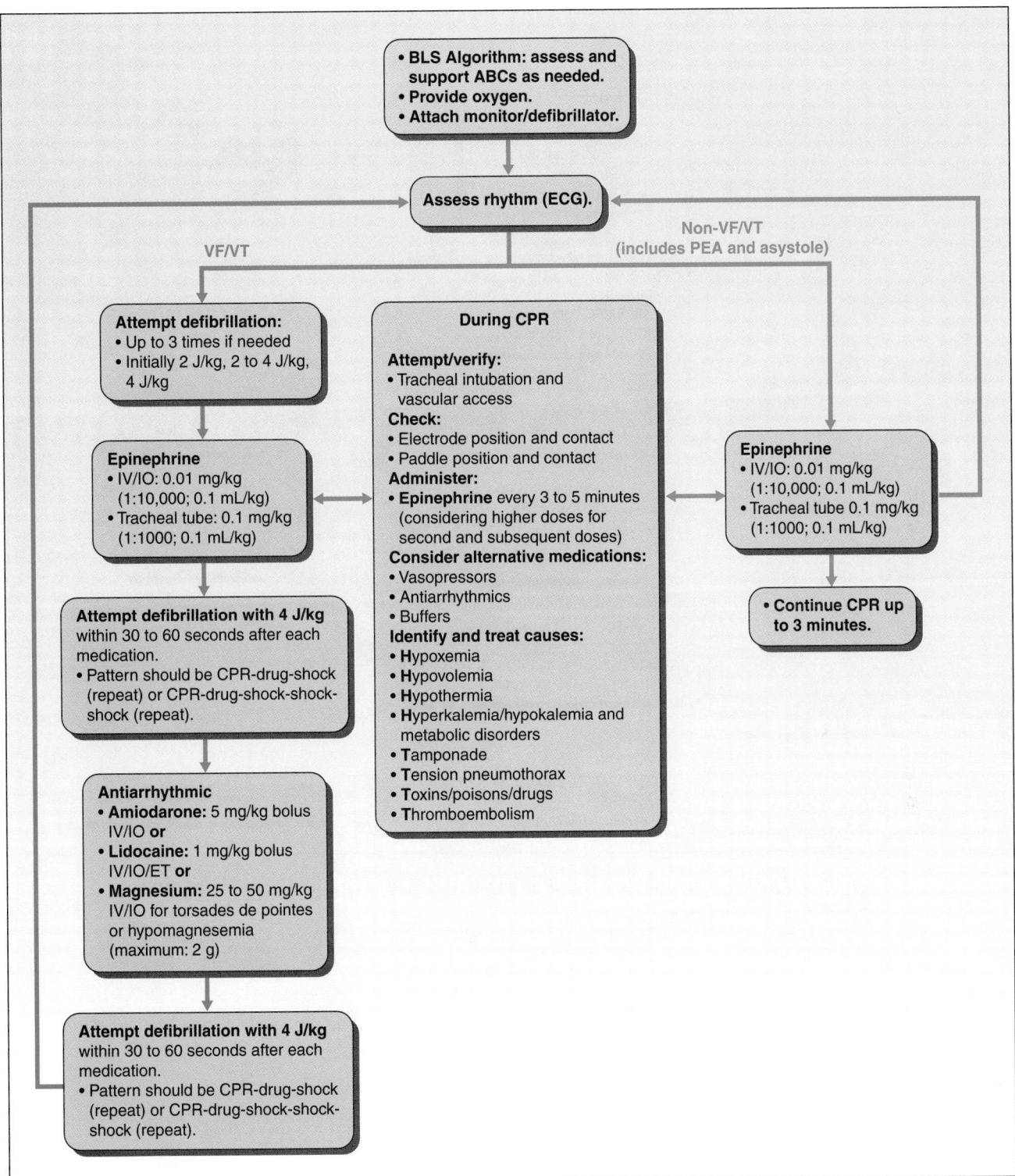

- BLS Algorithm: assess and support ABCs as needed.
- Provide oxygen.
- Attach monitor/defibrillator.

Assess rhythm (ECG).

VF/VT

Non-VF/VT
(includes PEA and asystole)

Attempt defibrillation:
- Up to 3 times if needed
- Initially 2 J/kg, 2 to 4 J/kg, 4 J/kg

During CPR

Attempt/verify:
- Tracheal intubation and vascular access

Check:
- Electrode position and contact
- Paddle position and contact

Administer:
- **Epinephrine** every 3 to 5 minutes (considering higher doses for second and subsequent doses)

Consider alternative medications:
- Vasopressors
- Antiarrhythmics
- Buffers

Identify and treat causes:
- **H**ypoxemia
- **H**ypovolemia
- **H**ypothermia
- **H**yperkalemia/hypokalemia and metabolic disorders
- **T**amponade
- **T**ension pneumothorax
- **T**oxins/poisons/drugs
- **T**hromboembolism

Epinephrine
- IV/IO: 0.01 mg/kg (1:10,000; 0.1 mL/kg)
- Tracheal tube: 0.1 mg/kg (1:1000; 0.1 mL/kg)

Epinephrine
- IV/IO: 0.01 mg/kg (1:10,000; 0.1 mL/kg)
- Tracheal tube 0.1 mg/kg (1:1000; 0.1 mL/kg)

- **Continue CPR up to 3 minutes.**

Attempt defibrillation with 4 J/kg within 30 to 60 seconds after each medication.
- Pattern should be CPR-drug-shock (repeat) or CPR-drug-shock-shock-shock (repeat).

Antiarrhythmic
- **Amiodarone:** 5 mg/kg bolus IV/IO **or**
- **Lidocaine:** 1 mg/kg bolus IV/IO/ET **or**
- **Magnesium:** 25 to 50 mg/kg IV/IO for torsades de pointes or hypomagnesemia (maximum: 2 g)

Attempt defibrillation with 4 J/kg within 30 to 60 seconds after each medication.
- Pattern should be CPR-drug-shock (repeat) or CPR-drug-shock-shock-shock (repeat).

Pediatric advanced life support (pulseless arrest) algorithm. *BLS,* Basic life support; *ABCs,* airway, breathing, circulation; *ECG,* electrocardiogram; *VF/VT,* ventricular fibrillation/ventricular tachycardia; *CPR,* cardiopulmonary resuscitation; *IV/IO/ET,* intravenous/intraosseous/endotracheal. (Modified from Pediatric basic life support. Part 9. Circulation 2000;102:I-291.)

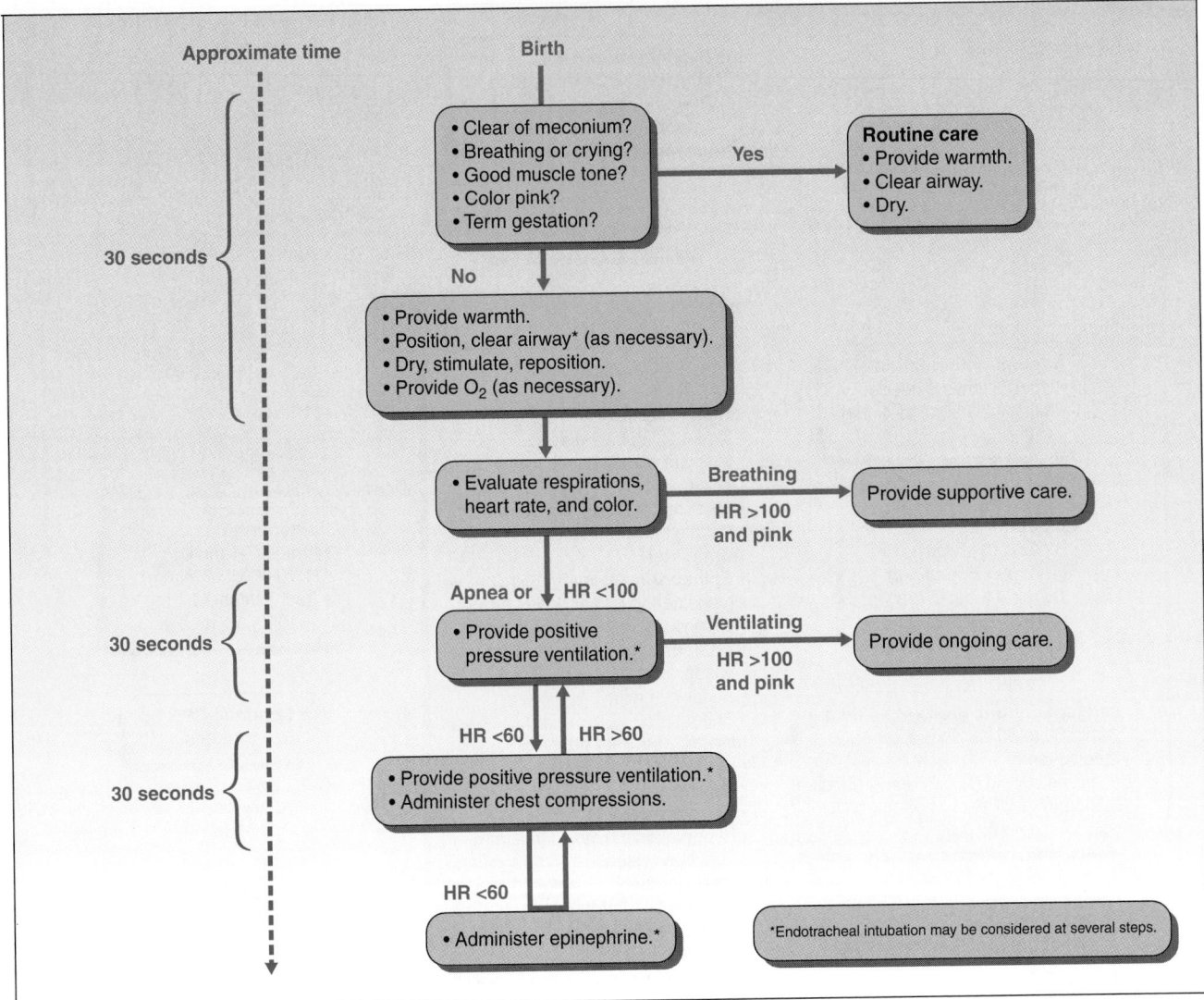

Resuscitation of the newborn infant algorithm. *HR,* Heart rate. (Modified from Neonatal resuscitation. Part 11. Circulation 2000;102:I-343.)

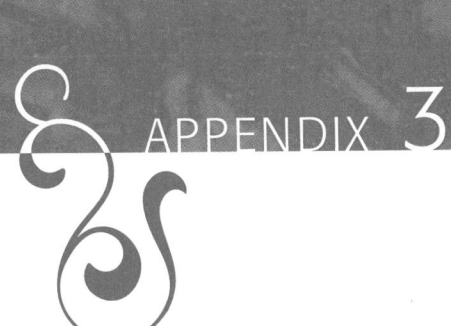

ECG Monitoring and Dysrhythmia Recognition*

Locations for Chest Electrodes

Lead I

- Positive electrode placed just below the left clavicle
- Negative electrode placed just below the right clavicle
- Provides information about the left lateral wall of the heart

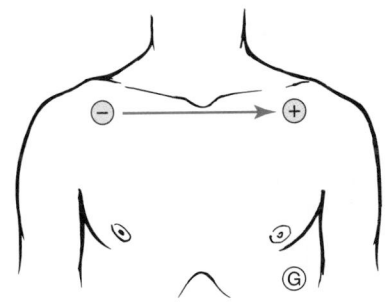

Lead I. *G,* Ground. (From Aehlert B. ACLS quick review study guide. St Louis: Mosby; 1994.)

Lead II

- Positive electrode just below the left pectoral muscle
- Negative electrode just below the right clavicle
- Provides information about the inferior wall of the heart

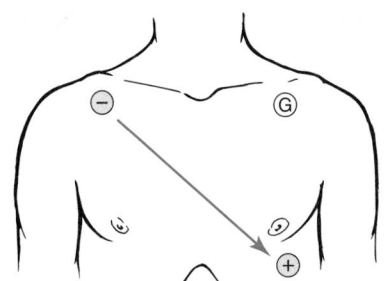

Lead II. *G,* Ground. (From Aehlert B. ACLS quick review study guide. St Louis: Mosby; 1994.)

Lead III

- Positive electrode placed just below the left pectoral muscle
- Negative electrode placed just below the left clavicle
- Provides information about the inferior wall of the heart

- P waves seen in this lead usually of lower amplitude than in leads I and II and are more likely to be biphasic (partly positive and partly negative)

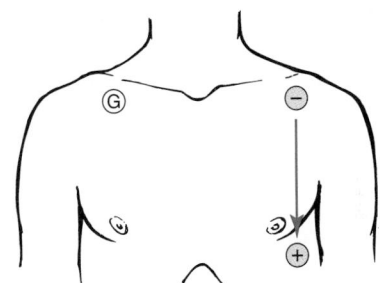

Lead III. *G,* Ground. (From Aehlert B. ACLS quick review study guide. St Louis: Mosby; 1994.)

Lead MCL₁ (Modified Chest Lead)

- Negative electrode placed just below the left clavicle
- Positive electrode placed to the right of the sternum at the fourth intercostal space
- Provides information about the anterior wall of the heart
- May prove useful in assessment of the width of the QRS complex to differentiate supraventricular tachycardia (SVT) from ventricular tachycardia (VT)

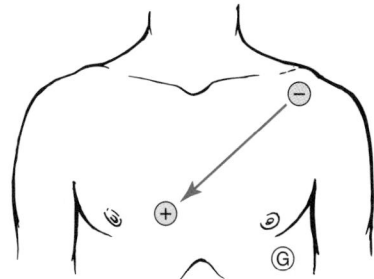

Lead MCL₁. *G,* Ground. (From Aehlert B. ACLS quick review study guide. St Louis: Mosby; 1994.)

Because the speed of ECG paper is 25 mm/second, the distance between two vertical lines is 1 mm and represents 0.04 seconds. Thus the time between two bold vertical lines (five small lines or 5 mm) represents 0.2 seconds. The distance between two horizontal lines is also 1 mm. An upward deflection of 10 small lines (or two bold lines) represents 1 mV.

*Modified from Aehlert B. ACLS quick review study guide. St. Louis: Mosby; 1994.

Dysrhythmia Recognition

Normal Sinus Rhythm (NSR)

Rate: 60 to 100 beats/min

Rhythm: Regular

P waves: Uniform and upright in appearance
One preceding each QRS complex

PRI: 0.12 to 0.20 seconds

QRS: <0.10 seconds

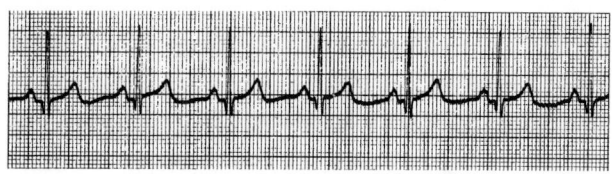

Normal sinus rhythm. (From Aehlert B. ACLS quick review study guide. St Louis: Mosby; 1994.)

Sinus Bradycardia

Rate: <60 beats/min

Rhythm: Regular

P waves: Uniform and upright in appearance
One preceding each QRS complex

PRI: 0.12 to 0.20 seconds

QRS: <0.10 seconds

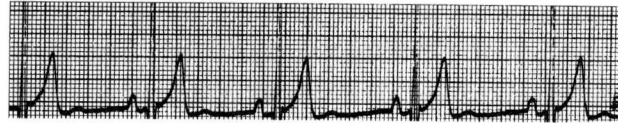

Sinus bradycardia. (From Aehlert B. ACLS quick review study guide. St Louis: Mosby; 1994.)

Sinus Tachycardia

Rate: 100 to 160 beats/min

Rhythm: Regular

P waves: Uniform and upright in appearance
One preceding each QRS complex

PRI: 0.12 to 0.20 seconds

QRS: <0.10 seconds

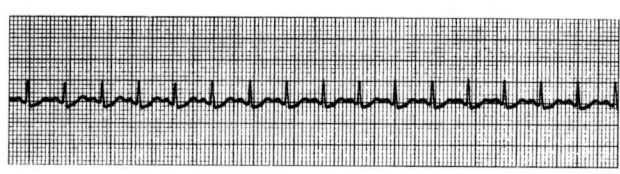

Sinus tachycardia. (From Aehlert B. ACLS quick review study guide. St Louis: Mosby; 1994.)

Sinus Arrhythmia

Rate: Usually 60 to 100 beats/min but may be faster or slower

Rhythm: Irregular

P waves: Uniform and upright in appearance
One preceding each QRS complex

PRI: 0.12 to 0.20 seconds

QRS: <0.10 seconds

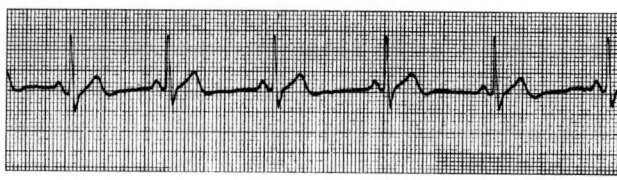

Sinus arrhythmia. (From Aehlert B. ACLS quick review study guide. St Louis: Mosby; 1994.)

Premature Atrial Complexes (PACs)

Rate: Usually normal, but depends on underlying rhythm

Rhythm: Irregular because of PACs

P waves: P wave of the early beat differs from sinus P waves
Is premature
May be flattened or notched
May be lost in the preceding T wave

PRI: Varies from 0.12 to 0.20 when the pacemaker site is near the SA node, to 0.12 seconds when the pacemaker site is nearer the AV node

QRS: Usually <0.10 seconds but may be prolonged

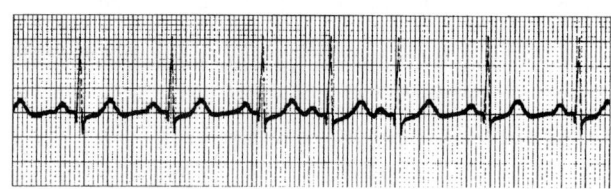

Premature atrial complexes (PACs). (From Aehlert B. ACLS quick review study guide. St Louis: Mosby; 1994.)

Supraventricular Tachycardia

Rate: 150 to 250/min

Rhythm: Regular

P waves: Atrial P waves different from sinus P waves
            P waves usually identifiable at the lower end of the rate range but seldom identifiable at rates >200
            May be lost in preceding T wave

PRI: Usually not measurable because the P wave is difficult to distinguish from the preceding T wave; if measurable, is 0.12 to 0.20 seconds

QRS: <0.10 seconds

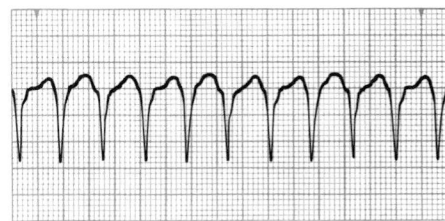

Supraventricular tachycardia (SVT). (From Huszar RJ. Basic dysrhythmias: interpretation and management. 2nd ed. St Louis: Mosby; 1994.)

Atrial Flutter

Rate: Atrial rate 250 to 350/min
            Ventricular rate variable

Rhythm: Atrial rhythm regular
            Ventricular rhythm usually regular but may be irregular

P waves: Saw-toothed flutter waves

PRI: Not measurable

QRS: Usually <0.10 but may be widened if flutter waves are buried in the QRS complex

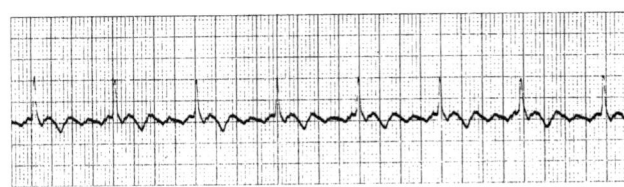

Atrial flutter. (From Aehlert B. ACLS quick review study guide. St Louis: Mosby; 1994.)

Atrial Fibrillation

Rate: Atrial rate usually >400
            Ventricular rate variable

Rhythm: Atrial and ventricular very irregular (regular, bradycardic ventricular rhythm may occur as a result of digitalis toxicity)

P waves: No identifiable P waves
            Erratic, wavy baseline

PRI: None

QRS: Usually <0.10 seconds

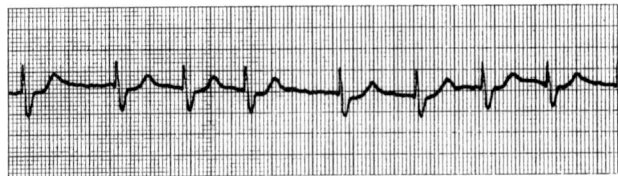

Atrial fibrillation. (From Aehlert B. ACLS quick review study guide. St Louis: Mosby; 1994.)

Premature Junctional Complexes (PJCs)

Rate: Atrial and ventricular rates dependent upon underlying rhythm

Rhythm: Irregular because of premature complex

P waves: May occur before, during, or after the QRS; if seen, will be inverted (retrograde)

PRI: If the P wave occurs before the QRS, the PRI will usually be ≤0.12 seconds

QRS: <0.10 seconds

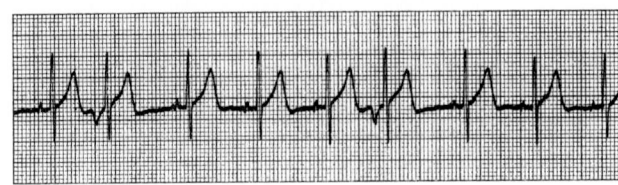

Premature junctional complexes (PJCs). (From Aehlert B. ACLS quick review study guide. St Louis: Mosby; 1994.)

Junctional Rhythm

Rate: 40 to 60 beats/min

Rhythm: Atrial and ventricular very regular

P waves: May occur before, during, or after the QRS; if seen, will be inverted (retrograde)

PRI: Not measurable unless the P wave precedes the QRS; when present, will usually be ≤0.12 seconds

QRS: <0.10 seconds

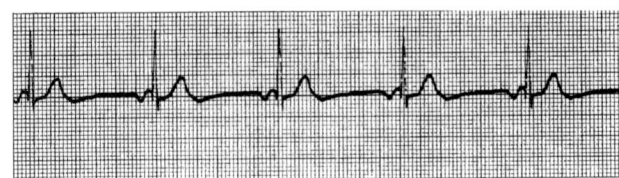

Junctional rhythm. (From Aehlert B. ACLS quick review study guide. St Louis: Mosby; 1994.)

Accelerated Junctional Rhythm

Rate: 60 to 100 beats/min

Rhythm: Atrial and ventricular very regular

P waves: May occur before, during, or after the QRS; if seen, will be inverted (retrograde)

PRI: Not measurable unless the P wave precedes the QRS; when present, will usually be ≤0.12 seconds

QRS: <0.10 seconds

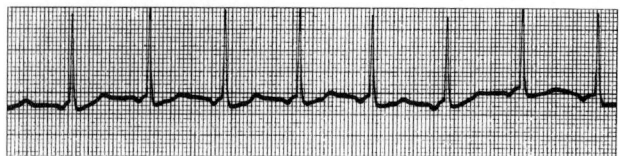

Accelerated junctional rhythm. (From Aehlert B. ACLS quick review study guide. St Louis: Mosby; 1994.)

Junctional Tachycardia

Rate: 100 to 180 beats/min

Rhythm: Atrial and ventricular very regular

P waves: May occur before, during, or after the QRS; if seen, will be inverted (retrograde)

PRI: Not measurable unless the P wave precedes the QRS; when present, will usually be ≤0.12 seconds

QRS: <0.10 seconds

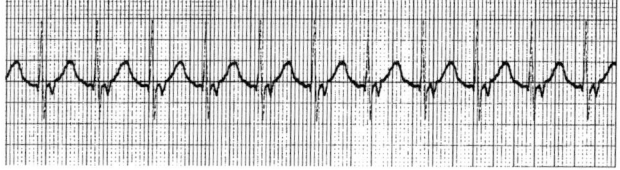

Junctional tachycardia. (From Aehlert B. ACLS quick review study guide. St Louis: Mosby; 1994.)

Premature Ventricular Complexes (PVCs)

Rate: Atrial and ventricular rate dependent upon the underlying rhythm

Rhythm: Irregular because of PVC
If the PVC is interpolated (sandwiched between two normal beats), the rhythm will be regular

P waves: No P wave is associated with the PVC

PRI: None with the PVC because the ectopic originates in the ventricles

QRS: >0.12 seconds
Wide and bizarre
T wave frequently in opposite direction of the QRS complex

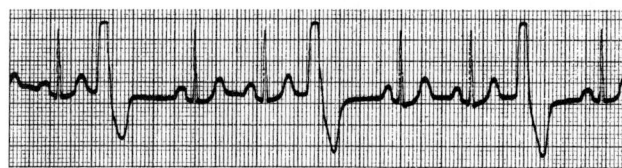

Premature ventricular complexes (PVCs). (From Aehlert B. ACLS quick review study guide. St Louis: Mosby; 1994.)

Ventricular Escape Rhythm (Idioventricular Rhythm [IVR])

Rate: Atrial not discernible; ventricular 20 to 40 beats/min

Rhythm: Atrial not discernible, ventricular essentially regular

P waves: Absent

PRI: None

QRS: >0.12 seconds

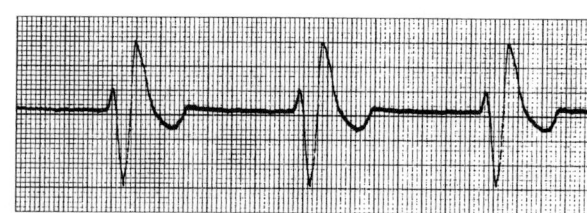

Ventricular escape (Idioventricular) rhythm. (From Aehlert B. ACLS quick review study guide. St Louis: Mosby; 1994.)

Accelerated Idioventricular Rhythm (AIVR)

Rate: Atrial not discernible; ventricular 40 to 100 beats/min

Rhythm: Atrial not discernible, ventricular essentially regular

P waves: Absent

PRI: None

QRS: >0.12 seconds

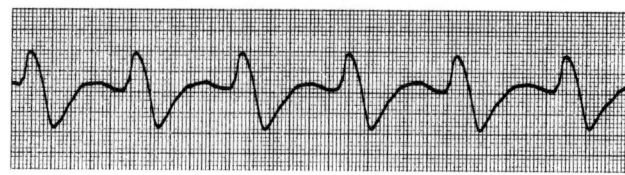

Accelerated idioventricular rhythm (AIVR). (From Aehlert B. ACLS quick review study guide. St Louis: Mosby; 1994.)

Ventricular Tachycardia (Monomorphic VT)

Rate: Atrial not discernible; ventricular 100 to
             250 beats/min

Rhythm: Atrial not discernible, ventricular essentially
             regular

P waves: May be present or absent; if present they have
             no set relationship to the QRS complexes—
             appearing between the QRSs at a rate different
             from that of the VT

PRI: None

QRS: >0.12 seconds
             Often difficult to differentiate between the QRS
             and the T wave

Note: Three or more PVCs occurring sequentially are
             referred to as a "run" of VT

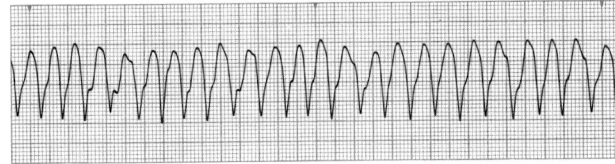

Ventricular tachycardia. (From Huszar RJ. Basic dysrhythmias: interpretation and management. 2nd ed. St Louis: Mosby; 1994.)

Torsades de Pointes (TdP) (a Type of Polymorphic VT)

Rate: Atrial not discernible; ventricular
             150 to 250 beats/min

Rhythm: Atrial not discernible, ventricular may be regular
             or irregular

PRI: None

QRS: >0.12 seconds
             Gradual alteration in the amplitude and direction
             of the QRS

Torsades de Pointes (French for *twisting of the points*; TdP) is a type of polymorphic VT associated with a prolonged QT interval. Symptoms associated with TdP are related to the decrease in cardiac output, which occurs as a result of the fast ventricular rate. Patients may complain of palpitation or lightheadedness or experience seizures or a syncopal episode. TdP is usually initiated by a PVC and may occasionally terminate spontaneously and recur after several seconds or minutes or it may deteriorate into VF.

The causes of long QT are many and include the following:

1. Drug-induced
   - Cyclic antidepressants (doxepin, imipramine, amitriptyline)
   - Phenothiazines (haloperidol, chlorpromazine, thioridazine)
   - Type I antidysrhythmics (quinidine, procainamide, disopyramide, tocainide, mexiletine)
   - Organophosphate insecticides
2. Eating disorders (bulimia, anorexia)
3. Electrolyte abnormalities (hypomagnesemia, hypokalemia, hypocalcemia)

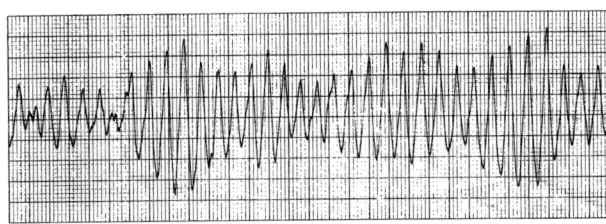

Torsades de Pointes. (From Aehlert B. ACLS quick review study guide. St Louis: Mosby; 1994.)

Ventricular Fibrillation

Rate: Cannot be determined because waves or
             complexes are discernible to measure

Rhythm: Rapid and chaotic with no pattern or regularity

P waves: Not discernible

PRI: Not discernible

QRS: Not discernible

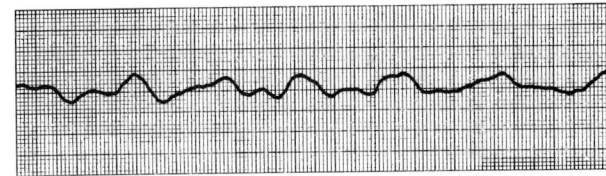

Ventricular fibrillation. (From Aehlert B. ACLS quick review study guide. St Louis: Mosby; 1994.)

Asystole (Ventricular Asystole, Ventricular Standstill)

Rate: Ventricular usually indiscernible but may see
             some atrial activity

Rhythm: Atrial may be discernible, ventricular indiscernible

P waves: Usually not discernible

PRI: Not measurable

QRS: Absent

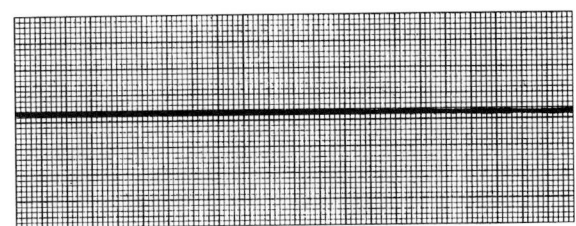

Asystole. (From Aehlert B. ACLS quick review study guide. St Louis: Mosby; 1994.)

First-Degree AV Block

Rate: Atrial and ventricular within normal limits and the same

Rhythm: Atrial and ventricular regular

P waves: Normal in size and configuration
           One P wave for each QRS

PRI: Prolonged (>0.20 seconds) but constant

QRS: <0.10 seconds

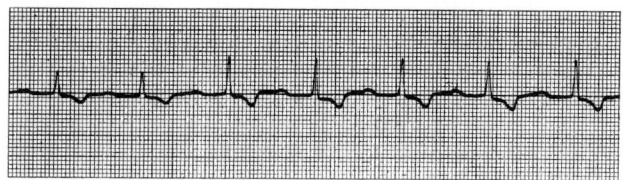

Sinus rhythm with first-degree AV block. (From Aehlert B. ACLS quick review study guide. St Louis: Mosby; 1994.)

Second-Degree AV Block, Type I (Wenckebach, Mobitz I)

Rate: Atrial rate > ventricular rate, both are usually within normal limits

Rhythm: Atrial regular (P waves plot through)
           Ventricular irregular

P waves: Normal in size and configuration
           Some P waves are not followed by a QRS (more P waves than QRS complexes)

PRI: Lengthens with each cycle (although lengthening may be slight) until a P wave appears without a QRS

QRS: <0.10 seconds but is dropped periodically

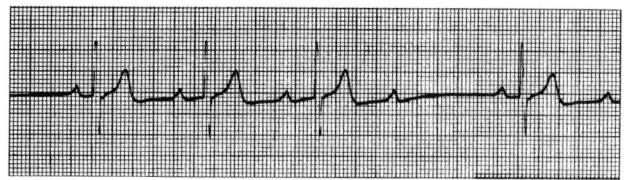

Second-degree AV block, type I. (From Aehlert B. ACLS quick review study guide. St Louis: Mosby; 1994.)

Second-Degree AV Block, Type II (Mobitz II)

Rate: Atrial rate > ventricular rate

Rhythm: Atrial regular (P waves plot through)
           Ventricular irregular

P waves: Normal in size and configuration
           Some P waves are not followed by a QRS (more P waves than QRS complexes)

PRI: May be within normal limits or prolonged but is constant for each conducted QRS

QRS: >0.10 seconds but is dropped periodically

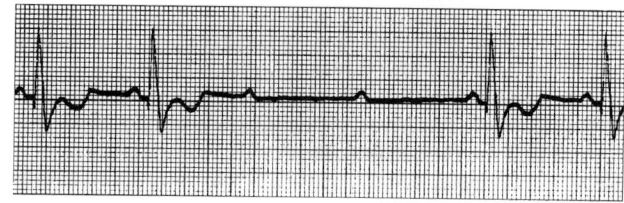

Second-degree AV block, type II. (From Aehlert B. ACLS quick review study guide. St Louis: Mosby; 1994.)

Second-Degree AV Block, 2:1 Conduction

Rate: Atrial rate > ventricular rate

Rhythm: Atrial regular (P waves plot through)
           Ventricular regular

P waves: Normal in size and configuration
           Every other P wave is followed by a QRS (more P waves than QRS complexes)

PRI: Constant

QRS: Within normal limits if the block occurs above the bundle of His (probably Type I)
           Wide if the block occurs at or below the bundle of His (probably Type II)
           Absent after every other P wave

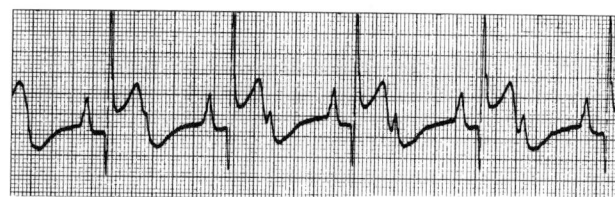

Second-degree AV block, 2:1 conduction; probably type I. (From Aehlert B. ACLS quick review study guide. St Louis: Mosby; 1994.)

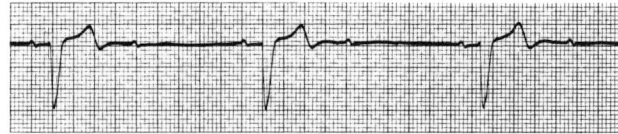

Second-degree AV block, 2:1 conduction; probably type II. (From Conover MB. Understanding electrocardiography: arrhythmias and the 12-lead ECG. 6th ed. St Louis: Mosby; 1992.)

Complete (Third-Degree) AV Block

Rate: Atrial rate > ventricular rate; ventricular rate determined by the origin of the escape rhythm

Rhythm: Atrial regular (P waves plot through)
Ventricular regular

P waves: Normal in size and configuration
Some P waves are not followed by a QRS (more P waves than QRS complexes)

PRI: None—the atria and ventricles beat independently of each other; no relationship between the P waves and QRS complexes

QRS: Narrow or wide depending on the location of the escape pacemaker and the condition of the interventricular conduction system

Narrow → junctional pacemaker
Wide → ventricular pacemaker

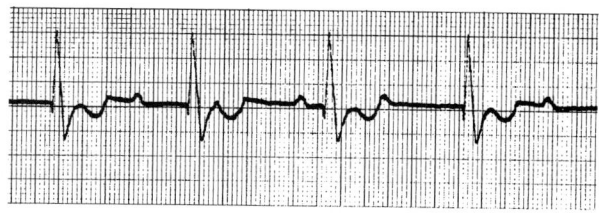

Complete (third-degree) AV block. (From Aehlert B. ACLS quick review study guide. St Louis: Mosby; 1994.)

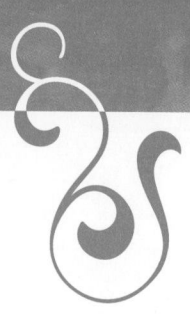

Glossary

AARC Code of Ethics   Professional policy document that describes the ethical behaviors for respiratory therapists to guide professional practice.

ABCD survey   Primary patient assessment/treatment steps to be taken in emergency or resuscitation situations, including Airway, Breathing, Circulation, and Defibrillation, focusing on basic CPR and defibrillation. Time drives all aspects of emergency cardiovascular care (ECC), and important preliminary first actions such as assessing unresponsiveness and calling for help are performed just before the "A" (airway) of the primary ABCD survey.

abdominal muscles   Muscles in addition to those directly involved in respiration that nevertheless aid in expiration, including the rectus abdominis, external and internal oblique muscles, and the transversus abdominis muscles, which depress the lower ribs, increase intraabdominal pressure, and flex the thoracic spine.

accessory muscles   Muscles outside the principal respiratory muscles that nevertheless affect inspiration, including the pectoralis minor and major (innervated by C5-C8 and T1), the serratus anterior (innervated by C5-C7), and the erector spinae, which all help raise ribs, push the sternum forward and upward, and straighten the concavity of the thoracic spine.

accreditation   Voluntary process intended to help establish and maintain the standards and expectations for all allied health education programs; although this is voluntary, the National Board for Respiratory Care requires graduation from an accredited educational program for eligibility for its credentialing examinations for individual professionals.

acid   Compound that donates or yields a hydrogen ion (H+) in an aqueous solution; a substance that donates a proton in a proton-transfer reaction.

acid-fast bacilli (AFB)   Bacteria in which the cell wall, because of the presence of waxes such as mycolic acid, retains red carbolfuschin stain despite rinsing with hydrochloric acid, making these bacteria acid-fast; acid-fast bacteria are considered neither gram-positive nor gram-negative.

acid-maltase deficiency   Type II glycogen storage disease that arises because of a deficiency of the lysosomal enzyme responsible for the hydrolysis of the glycogen.

activated partial thromboplastin time (APTT)   Direct way of evaluating overall coagulation status; used to assess the intrinsic clotting pathway, especially the early stages involving factors XII, XI, IX and VIII; often used for monitoring patients on heparin therapy.

active cycle of breathing   Breathing maneuver that combines breathing control, thoracic expansion control, and forced expiration technique.

active humidification   Humidification system in which energy (heat) is used to add water to the inspired gas.

acute exacerbation   Sudden worsening of respiratory symptoms accompanied by deteriorating lung function; most often, patients will present with increased dyspnea, cough, and changes in the quality or quantity of sputum.

acute lung injury (ALI)   Respiratory disorder characterized by the abrupt onset of respiratory distress; associated with severe hypoxemia and diffuse pulmonary opacities on chest radiograph (CXR) that are not caused by congestive heart failure or volume overload.

acute respiratory distress syndrome (ARDS)   Respiratory disorder characterized by fulminant pulmonary interstitial and alveolar edema, respiratory insufficiency, and hypoxemia.

adenocarcinoma   Any one of a large group of malignant, epithelial cell tumors.

adenosine triphosphate (ATP)   High-energy triphosphate that is the main molecule used to store energy; supplies energy directly to the energy-using reactions of all cells in all kinds of living organisms.

adjuvant   Substance, especially a drug, added to a prescription to assist in the action of the main ingredient; also, an additional treatment or therapy.

adrenergic receptor   Site in a sympathetic effector cell that reacts to adrenergic stimulation.

adsorption   Ability to hold substances to a surface.

advance directive   Document to be used on the patient's behalf, in the absence of competency, specifying what treatments a patient does or does not want in such a case and sometimes, in some states, specifying a surrogate to make decisions in the event that the patient cannot (see *medical power of attorney*).

advanced cardiac life support (ACLS)   Postarrest treatment after a cardiac arrest; includes (1) maintaining the airway with equipment and advanced techniques, (2) monitoring electrocardiogram (ECG) and recognizing dysrhythmias, (3) using conventional defibrillators, (4) administration of supplemental oxygen and drugs via parenteral or endotracheal routes.

aerobe   Free-living organism that requires oxygen for survival.

aerobic   Pertaining to the presence of air or oxygen.

aerosol   A suspension of solid or liquid particles in a gas.

affective characteristics   Common traits, attributes, qualities, and abilities found in those who share a condition or pattern of behavior or thinking.

afterload   Resistance in the circulation against which the ventricle must eject blood during contraction; the load that opposes myocardial shortening.

agonist Agent that stimulates a receptor.

air bronchogram Radiographic abnormality in the image of the bronchi occurring when the alveolar air spaces become filled with fluid, causing increased contrast between the air-filled bronchi and adjacent fluid-filled lung parenchyma, rendering the bronchi lucent and projecting them as branching tubular air-filled structures.

air liquefaction Process by which air is made into a liquid.

air trapping Condition in the lung in which air is not exhaled because of decreased lung elasticity and increased expiratory airway resistance; accompanied by hyperinflation.

air space disease Condition characterized by parenchymal opacification, the silhouette sign, and air bronchograms.

airway hyperresponsiveness Marker associated with asthma that is responsive to both specific and nonspecific factors (such as environment, exercise, allergens, and viral infections), whereby the airways constrict too easily and frequently.

airway inflammation Condition that exacerbates asthmatic reactions by the release of mediators including mast cells, eosinophils, macrophages, epithelial cells, and T lymphocytes, resulting in recurrent exacerbations that manifest as wheezing, progressive shortness of breath, chest tightness, and coughing; may be classified as acute, subacute, or chronic.

airways resistance (R_{aw}) Pressure difference developed per unit flow as gas flows into or out of the lungs; normally, 2.4 cm H_2O/L/s at 0.5 L/s. R_{aw} measurements can complement other tests evaluating airway responsiveness to bronchial provocation or bronchodilation.

algebraic Quality or property of a function that relies on its being constructed using the basic operations of algebra (addition, subtraction, multiplication, or division), either linear or quadratic.

algebraic relationship Association between measured values that use or reflect the basic operations of algebra; for example, additive, multiplicative, linear, parabolic, exponential, curvilinear, or sigmoidal relationships.

algorithm Specific protocol that provides explicit rules for solving a health care problem.

Allen's test Test performed before radial arterial puncture or cannulation to ascertain adequate ulnar artery perfusion to the hand.

allergen Common triggering mechanism for asthmatic reactions; can be indoor factors (that is, mold, animal dander, cleaning chemicals, cockroach antigen, dust mites) or outdoor factors (that is, noxious fumes, grass, and tree pollens).

allergy Specific type of hypersensitivity reaction; in adverse drug reactions, this is defined as an immune-mediated hypersensitivity reaction, which may be an immediate-type reaction or a delayed-type hypersensitivity reaction.

alpha₁-antitrypsin (AAT) Plasma protein produced in the liver that inhibits trypsin and other proteolytic enzymes; deficiency is associated with the development of emphysema.

α-adrenergic receptor Type of adrenergic receptor that acts in response to sympathomimetic stimuli.

alternate site mechanical ventilation (ASMV) Use of an artificial device to assist patient breathing at a location other than the hospital ICU—usually the home setting or a long-term care facility.

alveoli Small sacs or outpouchings through which gas exchange takes place between alveolar gas and capillary blood; composed of Type I and Type II cells.

American Association for Respiratory Care (AARC) Primary professional organization for respiratory care; the AARC and related organizations contribute to the scientific basis, governance, stature, and future growth of respiratory care; assists chartered affiliates in their efforts to pursue meaningful, nonrestrictive licensure and promotes the sequential functions of higher education: research, archiving, and dissemination of knowledge.

American Association of Inhalation Therapists (AAIT) Organization formerly called the *Inhalation Therapy Association (ITA)* and now known as *the American Association for Respiratory Care (AARC)*.

American Registry of Inhalation Therapists (ARIT) Organization established to oversee the processing, registration, and maintenance of the registry. In 1974 the ARIT, Inc., and the AART Technician Certification Board merged to form the National Board for Respiratory Therapy.

American Respiratory Care Foundation (ARCF) Trusteeship administering more than $20,000 annually in awards, education recognition, fellowships, and grants, as well as providing financial support of the AARC consensus and special proceedings conferences.

American Standard Safety System One of three indexed safety systems for medical gases. This system uses a combination of the following factors specific for each gas or gas combination: diameter of the outlet, number of threads per inch, whether outlet has right-handed or left-handed threads, whether the threads are external or internal, the shape of the mating nipple on the corresponding regulator.

amino acid Basic protein unit or building block of proteins; the basic structure of an amino acid consists of a carbon atom (called the *alpha carbon*) to which are bonded an amino group (NH₂), a carboxyl group (COOH), a hydrogen atom, and a side chain that constitutes the unique and identifying characteristic of the amino acid.

amyotrophic lateral sclerosis (ALS) Progressive neurodegenerative disorder of both upper and lower motor neurons leading to a loss of skeletal muscle strength, including the respiratory muscles.

anabolism Synthesis process that assembles precursor molecules, such as amino acids, sugars, fatty acids, and nitrogenous bases into cell macromolecules such as proteins, polysaccharides, lipids, and nucleic acids.

anaerobe Free-living organism that requires an absence of oxygen; thought to be a minor cause of community-acquired pneumonia but becomes increasingly important in nosocomial pneumonia and ventilator-associated pneumonia.

anaerobic bacterial pneumonia Pneumonia, usually multimicrobial, caused by anaerobic pathogens such as *Peptostreptococcus* spp., *Bacteroides melaninogenicus*, *Fusobacterium necrophorum*, *Bacteroides asaccharolyticus*, *Porphyromonas endodontalis*, and *Porphyromonas gingivalis*.

analgesic Pain reduction property, typically demonstrated in nonsteroidal antiinflammatory agents.

analog-to-digital converter Machine that samples an analog signal at short intervals and assigns a digit to the analog value at each time point; after transmission the digital information can be converted back to analog for display.

analysis method Ethics theory that combines key components from teleological and deontological theories, asserting that in the final analysis, most ethical decisions are made by a systematic analytic process devised by the individual.

analytic paradigm Traditional teaching method designed to convey scientific and medical knowledge, derived from research, through the accomplishment of specific, set learning objectives. Instructor retains control over the learning process from setting objectives to determining evaluation. Learners remain in largely passive roles for a highly structured educational experience that emphasizes the lecture method and competency- or performance-centered coursework based on research, expert opinion, and task analysis.

anesthetic Drug or agent capable of producing a complete or partial loss of feeling.

angina Choking, crushing, painful feeling most often associated with cardiac pain caused by hypoxia of the myocardium.

animal studies Use of animals for medical research to establish and study models or simulations of human disease.

anion Negatively charged ion that is attracted to the positive electrode (anode) in electrolysis; negatively charged atom, molecule, or radical.

anion gap Difference between the concentrations of serum cations and anions such that: anion gap = $([Na^+] + [K^+]) - ([HCO_3^-] + CL^-])$. If the anion gap exceeds 12 mmol/L, excessive unmeasured anions are likely present. Because its concentration is normally low, $[K^+]$ is often omitted from this calculation.

antagonist Drug that blocks a receptor.

anthropometry Study of human body measurements and components, including measurement of height, weight, body-mass index, mid-arm muscle circumference, skinfold thicknesses, and skeletal breadths.

antibiotic Chemical substance capable of inhibiting the growth of, or killing, certain microorganisms but generally nontoxic enough to be used chemotherapeutically in the treatment of infectious diseases.

anticholinergic Class of bronchodilators that decreases both bronchial and upper airway secretions; pertains to a blockade of acetylcholine receptors that results in the inhibition of the transmission of parasympathetic nerve impulses; the drug functions by competing with the neurotransmitter acetylcholine for its receptor sites at synaptic junctions.

anticholinergic agent Any agent that blocks the parasympathetic nerves; often used as bronchodilators, delivered by inhalation (for example, ipratropium bromide for chronic obstructive pulmonary disease, or COPD).

anticipating Key skill used in critical thinking; involves the ability to think ahead and envision possible problems; sometimes referred to as "future think."

anticoagulant Drug that blocks or delays blood coagulation, specifically the formation of a new blood clot (thrombus), allowing the existing thrombus to be slowly broken down by serum thrombolytic enzymes.

anticoagulation Use of an agent that prevents or delays coagulation of the blood.

antiderivative Indefinite integral, denoted by the fact that it produces a function rather than a number.

antiemetic Substance or procedure that prevents or alleviates nausea or vomiting.

antigen detection Newer technique that, along with PCR, is applied to sputum samples to help in the rapid identification of pathogens that may be difficult to culture or pathogens scarcely growing due to prior antibiotic treatment; can be applied to sputum, serum, urine, and body fluids; most valuable in the diagnosis of difficult-to-culture organisms, such as M. pneumoniae, L. pneumophila, C. pneumoniae, and viral pneumonias. (See also polymerase chain reaction [PCR].)

antihistamine Drug or substance capable of reducing the physiologic and pharmacologic effects of histamine, including a wide variety of drugs that block histamine receptors.

antimicrobial Drug or substance that kills microorganisms or inhibits their growth or replication.

antioxidant Agent that inhibits oxidation of a substance when added to it; those such as beta-carotene, alpha-tocopherol (vitamin E), and ascorbic acid (vitamin C) can help prevent lipid peroxidation triggered by free radicals and can assist in the repair of tissue damaged by oxidative stress.

antipyretic Fever-reducing agent.

antitussive Any drug that acts on the central and peripheral nervous systems to suppress the cough reflex.

anxiolytic Sedative or minor tranquilizing agent used primarily to treat episodes of anxiety.

apnea Absence of spontaneous respiration.

apnea of infancy Category or type of cessation of air flow in breathing in the full-term infant; resolution may be determined more by the maturation of the respiratory control center than an underlying disease process.

apnea of prematurity (AOP) Category or type of cessation of airflow in breathing in the premature infant; resolution may be determined more by the maturation of the respiratory control center than an underlying disease process; prevalence is higher at lower gestational ages and may be the result of an immature respiratory control system manifested by frequent periodic breathing, a decreased ventilatory response to CO_2, and a depression of respiration produced by hypoxemia.

apparent life-threatening event (ALTE) One of several most frequently diagnosed breathing disorders that call for home monitoring, including apnea of prematurity, sudden infant death syndrome, and GER.

arousal index Value derived from the data gathered during the polysomnogram: the number of arousals divided by the total sleep time, expressed in arousals/hour, which normally should be less than 15.

arterial blood gas Blood component whose primary measurements (P_{O_2}, P_{CO_2}, and pH) provide important information about oxygenation, ventilation, and acid-base status and also guide respiratory and metabolic interventions.

arterial blood pressure One of the four vital signs; monitoring techniques range from intermittent manual determinations using sphygmomanometry to automated noninvasive devices and indwelling arterial cannulae, providing continuous pressure measurements and waveform graphics.

arterial gas embolism   Disease that occurs from pulmonary over-pressurization; if the pressure in the lungs exceeds the integrity of the lung parenchyma, the lung will tear and the air escapes into either the pleura, resulting in a pneumothorax; into the mediastinum, resulting in pneumomediastinum or subcutaneous emphysema; or, in the worst scenario, into pulmonary vessels, carrying air into the heart.

artificial nose   Passive humidifier, also known as a *heat and moisture exchanger (HME)*, that captures exhaled heat and moisture and transfers part of that heat and humidity to the next inspired breath; can include condensers, hygroscopic condensers, and hygrophobic condensers.

assisted inspiration   Externally applied transrespiratory pressure change acting in synchrony with muscle pressure (if present) to increase tidal volume and flow.

assisted ventilation   A ventilator's function, occurring whenever airway pressure (that is, ventilator pressure) rises above baseline during inspiration; thus the breath is said to be assisted, independent of other breath characteristics (that is, whether the breath is classified as spontaneous or mandatory); not to be confused with the meaning of the word *assist* in specific names of modes of ventilation (for example, assist/control mode) sometimes used by ventilator manufacturers for modes without regard to consistency or theoretical relevance.

asthma   Chronic inflammatory disorder of the airways in which many cells and cellular elements play a role in particular, mast cells, eosinophils, T lymphocytes, macrophages, neutrophils, and epithelial cells; causes recurrent episodes of wheezing, breathlessness, chest tightness, and coughing, particular at night or in the early morning.

asthma education program   Plan implemented by clinicians to ensure patient and caregiver compliance, thereby minimizing exacerbations and health care costs by providing maximum understanding of current asthma treatment and management.

asthma trigger   Any mechanism that can cause asthmatic reactions, including allergens, pollution, food and drug additives, and viral agents.

asthmatic bronchitis   Type of chronic obstructive pulmonary disease (COPD), producing cough, dyspnea, and wheezing with expiratory airflow limitation.

atelectasis   Incomplete expansion of the lung or the collapse of previously expanded lung tissue, one of the most common noninfectious pulmonary complications after surgery; may be due to many factors, including small, monotonous tidal volumes and inadequate lung distending forces, airway obstruction with gas absorption, and reduction in surfactant levels.

atomic number   Number of protons contained inside the nucleus of an atom, determining the actual element.

atomic weight   Relative weight of an atom; often used interchangeably with the term *mass number*.

atria   Chambers of the heart; the left atrium in particular receives blood from the pulmonary veins and delivers it to the left ventricle.

atypical organisms   Strains of unusual type; for example, *Legionella* spp., *Mycoplasma pneumoniae*, *Chlamydia psittaci*, *Chlamydia pneumoniae*, and *Coxiella burnetti*.

atypical pneumonia   Pneumonia caused by any strain of unusual type (see *atypical organisms*) and characterized by a flulike disease with prodromal symptoms, dry cough, myalgia, malaise, rhinorrhea, and moderate fever; usual pathogens include *M. pneumoniae, C. psittaci, C. burnetti, C. pneumoniae,* and respiratory viruses.

audiovisual aids   Tools used to enhance the teaching of cognitive learning objectives; these aids create a synergistic effect when used to augment a discussion or lecture.

auscultation   Most commonly used physical assessment technique, involving listening to sounds produced by the body with the aid of a stethoscope placed on bare skin.

authentication   Process used to verify that an entry is complete, accurate, and final, including the date and the author identified.

autogenic drainage   Technique that aims to achieve the highest possible airflow in the different generations of bronchi to move secretions.

autonomy   Right and ability to govern one's self, particularly in regard to medical treatment and personal and financial care.

backward heart failure   Heart failure arising from accumulation of blood in the heart and increased filling pressures.

barotrauma   Injury to the lungs caused by alveolar overdistention, often due to a high intraalveolar pressure, such as may occur during positive pressure ventilation; results in pneumothorax, pneumomediastinum, and subcutaneous emphysema; in hyperbaric medicine, an all-inclusive term used to describe injury to the body and breakage of equipment due to pressure changes.

barrel chest   Chest configuration in which the individual's anterior-posterior chest is equal to the lateral diameter.

basal metabolic rate (BMR)   Amount of energy required to maintain the most basic bodily functions, expressed as kilocalories per day and having a fixed relationship with gender, weight, height, and age.

base   Solution that yields a hydroxide ion (OH^-) in an aqueous solution; species accepting the proton in a proton-transfer reaction.

basic life support (BLS)   Primary patient assessment/treatment procedure to be taken to stabilize the emergency patient, including preliminary first actions such as assessing unresponsiveness and conducting the primary ABCD survey.

Beer-Lambert law   Law defining the relationship between the concentration of a substance and the amount of light (I) transmitted through it: $I_{out} = I_{in} e^{-A}$ and $A = L \times C \times \epsilon$, where L is the optical path length, C is the concentration of the substance, and ϵ is the absorption of the particular wavelength used.

behavior contracting   Teaching technique creating a higher level of learner accountability and responsibility and calling on one's own integrity and autonomy.

benchmarking   Process of peer comparison that includes all efforts to determine not the average utilization of a particular diagnosis but the most medically appropriate utilization per diagnosis. This process is foundational to the standardization of health care delivery and the maximization of its benefits.

benign tumor   Noncancerous tumor.

Bernoulli principle   "First Law of Fluid Dynamics" used in 1738 by David Bernoulli to describe the relationship of fluid flow through a tube and to thus explain the pressure drop when fluid passes through a constriction in a rigid tube by showing how potential energy, kinetic energy, and pressure energy interact.

β-receptor Adrenergic component of receptor tissue that, when activated, causes various physiologic reactions such as relaxation of the bronchial muscles and an increase in the rate and force of cardiac contraction.

bicarbonate buffer system System influenced by the independent and direct effect of P_{CO_2} on $[HCO_3^-]$; made up of two components—hydration of CO_2 into carbonic acid (H_2CO_3) and the dissociation of carbonic acid into HCO_3^- and hydrogen ion: $H_2O + CO_2 \rightarrow H_2CO_3 \rightarrow H^+ + HCO_3^-$.

bilevel positive airway pressure A term used to describe noninvasive positive pressure ventilation in which the inspiratory positive airway pressure (IPAP) is set greater than the expiratory positive airway pressure (EPAP).

bilirubin Breakdown product of hemoglobin that is metabolized in the liver.

biopsy Removal of a small piece of living tissue from an organ or other part of the body for microscopic examination to confirm or establish a diagnosis, estimate prognosis, or follow the course of a disease.

Biot's respirations Pattern of breathing symptomatic of elevated intracranial pressure and meningitis; characterized by short burst of uniform, deep respirations followed by period of apnea lasting 10 to 30 seconds.

bite block Device that is placed between the teeth to prevent the patient from biting an orotracheal airway or from biting the tongue or lips, causing bleeding and trauma to the mouth; also used during bronchoscopy.

bland aerosol Inspired gas consisting of water, saline solution, or other substances without important pharmacologic action; used primarily to humidify, liquefy, or otherwise change the character of thick sections.

blinding Research technique for ensuring that the investigators and/or the participants are as aware as possible of the treatment being studied to avoid any tendency to prefer a specific outcome (bias).

blood urea nitrogen (BUN) Most common nonprotein nitrogenous compound in the blood; measurement used to assess renal function; in the adult, normal values for BUN are between 7 and 21 mg/dL.

blunt chest trauma Injury characterized by a direct bruise of the lung resulting in alveolar hemorrhage and edema; most often associated with automobile accidents.

Board of Directors (BOD) One of several governance and advisory entities of the AARC, composed of an executive committee consisting of the president, president-elect, immediate past president, vice president, treasurer, secretary, immediate past speaker of the House of Delegates, and chairperson of the Board of Medical Advisors.

Board of Medical Advisors One of several governance and advisory entities of the AARC; consists of four AARC sponsoring professional medical societies (the American Society for Anesthesia [ASA], the American College of Chest Physicians [ACCP], the American Thoracic Society [ATS], and the Society of Critical Care Medicine [SCCM]) that provide significant input concerning the art and science of the profession of respiratory care;

provides medical guidance in the art and science of respiratory care through service to the AARC.

body plethysmography Diagnostic tool that is used to achieve measurements of airway resistance (R_{aw}), airway conductance (G_{aw}), and static lung volumes; based on Boyle's law. In practice, the patient is placed inside a fixed-volume, air-sealed body box where the effects of excursion of the chest wall can be measured by small pressure changes in the box and airway.

Bohr effect The relationship between hydrogen ion concentration and hemoglobin affinity for oxygen. An increase in hydrogen ion concentration decreases the affinity of hemoglobin for oxygen.

boiling point Temperature required to raise the vapor pressure of a solution to atmospheric pressure; a colligative property of a solution.

Borg Scale of Perceived Exertion Numeric scale for assessing dyspnea, from 0 representing no dyspnea to 10 as maximal dyspnea.

botulism Rare disorder caused by toxin produced by *Clostridium botulinum,* often ingested by improperly cooked food, wound contamination by the organisms, or absorption of the toxin from the gastrointestinal tract, particularly in infants; GI symptoms predominate initially, followed by neurologic impairment.

Bourdon gauge flowmeter Flow control device with a fixed outlet orifice that allows an adjustable inlet pressure.

Boyle's law Observation credited to Robert Boyle, early in the 18th century, that predicts the relation of a volume of a fixed mass of gas to a pressure change.

brachytherapy Radiotherapy treatment that involves applying an ionizing radiation source near the body area being treated; in respiratory treatment, this usually entails the endobronchial placement of encapsulated radionuclide in close proximity to an endobronchial malignancy.

bradypnea Breathing rate slower than 12 breaths per minute.

bronchi Larger air passages of the lungs.

bronchial artery embolization (BAE) Method used to occlude or restrict blood flow within the bronchial artery; the therapy of choice when bleeding is from the bronchiectatic airways.

bronchial breath sounds Auscultation sounds normally heard over the trachea, at the manubrium anteriorly and between the scapulae posteriorly; heard over the periphery of the lungs, this suggests consolidation of lung tissue.

bronchial challenge testing Use of either methacholine or histamine to measure responsiveness to general stimuli, usually administered in a pulmonary function lab and followed (usually within 15 minutes) with a short-acting, β-agonist that results in a 12% to 15% increase in a patient's forced expiratory volume in 1 second (FEV_1).

bronchial circulation Regular or circuitous movement of the blood through the lungs; provides nutritional support for the lungs.

bronchiolitis obliterans organizing pneumonia (BOOP) Acute interstitial lung disease that appears to be a response of the lung to a variety of injuries affecting the smaller airways and alveoli as a unit (including infections, exposures to toxic gases, radiation therapy, drug toxicity, eosinophilic pneumonia, Wegener's granulomatosis, and hypersensitivity pneumonitis).

bronchoalveolar lavage (BAL) Irrigation of broncho-alveolar specimen, used in the diagnosis of ventilator-associated pneumonia.

bronchodilation Relaxation of the smooth muscles of the airways.

bronchodilator Substance, especially a drug, that relaxes contractions of the smooth muscle of the bronchioles to improve ventilation to the lungs.

bronchogenic carcinoma A malignant lung tumor that originates in the bronchi.

bronchophony Auscultation sound typical in consolidation of lung tissue, meaning that the normally aerated tissue has been filled with fluid, mucus, pus, or cellular debris; in bronchophony, the patient's repetition of "99" becomes easily audible, as opposed to its normal muffling.

bronchopulmonary dysplasia Chronic iatrogenic lung disease caused by oxygen toxicity and barotrauma resulting from positive pressure ventilation; incidence is greater in premature infants, perhaps related to the increased requirement for oxygen therapy and mechanical ventilation in this patient population.

bronchoscopic washing Technique designed to sample the airway, rather than the alveolar space, particularly in cytologic sampling when a patient has an exophytic lesion obstructing a lobar or segmental orifice.

bronchoscopy Examination using a bronchoscope that enables inspection of the interior of the tracheobronchial tree and related diagnostic and therapeutic maneuvers, including taking specimens for culture, biopsy, and removal of foreign bodies.

bubble humidifier System in which dry gas is directed toward the bottom of a water-filled reservoir, where the stream of gas is broken into bubbles that gain humidity as they rise through the water.

buffer Substances that maintain a relatively constant pH level when strong acids or strong bases are added.

bullae Air space enlargements greater than 1 cm; can progressively enlarge and compress adjacent lung tissue, impairing respiratory function.

bullectomy Removal of giant bullae (airspace enlargements that occupy one-third of a hemithorax), a reversible cause of pulmonary decompensation, particularly in patients with emphysema.

calcium channel blocker Drug that inhibits the flow of calcium ions across smooth muscle cell membranes, thus relaxing smooth muscles and reducing muscle spasm risk, particularly in heart disease with coronary artery spasm; appears to result in sustained improvement in pulmonary hemodynamics in 25% to 30% of patients.

calorie Amount of heat required to change the temperature of 1 g of water 1 degree Celsius.

cancer Neoplasm with uncontrolled anaplastic cell growth, usually involving invasion into surrounding tissue and metastasis to distant body sites.

capitation Prepaid and fixed amount that is negotiated in advance by the payer or plan and the provider; involves payment for each person for a particular period of time regardless of the care or services provided.

capnogram Assessment of gas at the proximal airway that plots CO_2 on the vertical axis and time on the horizontal axis.

capnography Noninvasive technique that measures carbon dioxide levels in inspired and expired gas and displays a capnogram.

capnometry Numeric display of CO_2 measurements taken from the proximal airway.

carbogen Oxygen/carbon dioxide mixture, usually consisting of 90% O_2/10% CO_2 or 95% O_2/5% CO_2.

carbohydrate Organic compound containing the elements carbon, hydrogen, and oxygen.

carbon monoxide poisoning Exposure to excessive levels of carbon monoxide in the atmosphere; the most common type of poisoning in the United States.

carbonic acid (H_2CO_3) Product of the hydration of CO_2 that almost completely ionizes to H^+ and bicarbonate in the blood because the pK of carbonic acid (~3.8) is much lower than blood pH; carbonic acid then forms bicarbonate, which is essential for blood CO_2 transport.

carboxyhemoglobin (COHb) Compound produced by exposing hemoglobin to carbon monoxide, usually inhaled into the lungs and subsequently bound to hemoglobin in the blood, blocking the sites for oxygen transport.

cardiac catheterization Invasive means to quantify valvular stenosis and regurgitation and assess coronary artery blood flow.

cardiac compression The technique by which circulaton is provided during CPR through compression directly on the sternum.

cardiac enzymes Group of enzymes that are released from myocardial tissue and appear in the serum during myocardial injury (usually ischemia); the initial panel of cardiac enzymes included serum lactate dehydrogenase (LDH), glutamic-oxaloacetic transaminase (SGOT), and creatinine kinase (CK). The myocardial-specific (MB isoform) creatinine kinase (CKMB) has become the standard; many centers now are also measuring troponin I or T isoforms.

cardiac output ($\dot{Q}c$) Volume of blood expelled by the heart's ventricles, equal to the amount of blood ejected at each beat multiplied by the heart rate (in beats per minute).

cardiac pacing Use of either an internal or external electric apparatus (pacemaker) to increase the heart rate in symptomatic bradycardia by stimulating the heart muscle.

cardiac tamponade Life-threatening complication of penetrating wounds to the heart, most often characterized by Beck's triad (distention of neck veins, muffled heart sounds, and hypotension), and often elevated central venous pressure.

cardiomyocytes Muscle cells that make up the heart.

cardiomyopathy Any disease that affects the heart's structure and function.

cardiomyoplasty Surgical transposition of an electrically transformed piece of skeletal muscle to augment the failing myocardium (usually the latissimus dorsi is wrapped around the ventricles).

cardiopulmonary resuscitation (CPR) All care required to treat life-threatening events, including basic life support (BLS) and advanced cardiac life support (ACLS).

cardioversion Synchronized electrical discharge that has been timed to occur during the nonvulnerable period of the cardiac cycle, when the heart is most susceptible to developing ventricular fibrillation if excited by an electrical stimulus; initially applied at energy levels lower than what is used for defibrillation (as low as 50 joules).

care management   Umbrella term referring to the coordination of patient interventions, comprising many loosely related terms: component management, demand management, case management, and disease management.

case control   Studies that involve, initially, the accumulation of a number of cases that are then matched as much as possible with those that do not have that condition so that both the cases and non-cases (controls) can be studied for differences that may account for why the cases contracted the disease.

case management   Collaborative process that assesses, plans, implements, coordinates, monitors, and evaluates the options and services required to meet an individual's health needs, using communication and available resources to promote quality, cost, and effective outcomes.

case mix   Relatively new form of reimbursement that refers to the overall intensity of conditions requiring medical and nursing intervention. It involves extensive assessment of the patient's condition followed by a determination of specific services or procedures considered necessary or essential to manage the patient effectively.

case report   Detailed, observational report of an unusual, interesting case. Case reports are observational and can be reported easily. The disease described in the case may be rare, the treatment may be unusual, or there may be specific instructional points. When several cases are reported over time, it constitutes a case series. Reports of cases or case series may lead to studies that clarify the disease or its treatment.

case series   Several case reports presented over time.

catabolism   Process of releasing chemical energy from food molecules in a decomposition process involving the oxidation of nutrient molecules, releasing energy (exergonic metabolism) in two forms, as either heat or as chemical energy.

cation   Positively charged ion; one of the most common serum electrolytes.

cell-mediated immunity   Primary component of the immune system involving lymphocytes; adversely affected by protein-calorie malnutrition.

central apnea   Loss of diaphragmatic and other respiratory muscle function, resulting in the cessation of respiratory effort.

central venous pressure (CVP)   Pressure measured in the superior vena cava and used to estimate intravascular volume status; single or multilumen catheters are positioned in the superior vena cava via the subclavian, internal, or external jugular veins to permit CVP monitoring, and venous blood sampling; the femoral vein is also a commonly used access site, especially during emergencies.

cepacia syndrome   Rapid clinical decline characterized by fever and frank sepsis at some point after initial infection by *B. cepacia*. The precise pathogen/host factor(s) that trigger this dramatic decompensation are unknown.

certified pulmonary function technologist (CPFT)   Individual, qualified by education and/or experience, who has successfully passed the pulmonary function certification examination of the NBRC.

certified respiratory therapist (CRT)   Respiratory therapist who has passed the entry-level certification exam of the NBRC.

Charles' law   Principle that predicts the effect of temperature on a fixed amount of dry gas, such that, at constant pressure, gas expands proportionally to changes in temperature, thus describing, at least at a qualitative level, the effect of kinetic energy on volume.

chemotherapy   Treatment of cancer, infections, and other diseases with chemical agents.

chest physiotherapy (CPT)   Technique used to help remove mucus and fluid from the lungs. Conventional CPT consists of postural drainage, percussion, and vibration.

Cheyne-Stokes breathing   Breathing consisting of a repeating pattern in which the rate and depth of breathing increases to a peak, followed by a decrease in the rate and depth of breathing, followed by a period of apnea.

cholesterol   Steroid lipid that combines with phospholipids in the cell membrane to help stabilize its bilayer structure; also used by the body as a starting point in making steroid hormones such as estrogen, testosterone, and cortisol.

chronic bronchitis   Type of chronic obstructive pulmonary disease (COPD) defined by the presence of cough and sputum production for 3 or more months in 2 successive years in patients who do not have other causes of cough.

chronic obstructive pulmonary disease (COPD)   Progressive, irreversible condition characterized by dyspnea, difficulty exhaling, and sometimes including chronic cough.

chronic steroid myopathy   Myopathy that results from the prolonged use of corticosteroids; manifests as proximal limb and girdle muscle weakness.

chronotrope   Substance that affects the regularity of a periodic function, especially with the rate of heartbeat.

CINAHL   Cumulative Index to Nursing and Allied Health Literature; database available through Ovid, which contains a wide variety of direct full-text articles in leading medical journals.

citric acid cycle   Aerobic process in stage 3 catabolism that converts two pyruvic acid molecules into six carbon dioxide molecules and six water molecules, taking place within the mitochondria of the cell.

Clark electrode P_{O_2} electrode, consisting of a platinum cathode and a silver anode immersed in a dilute, buffered potassium chloride solution; measures P_{O_2} using the principle of polarography.

clearance   Expulsion of a substance from the blood via the kidneys.

CLIA   Clinical Laboratory Improvement Act (CLIA); federal law regulating general aspects of quality control.

clinical outcomes   Use of any acuity-adjusted system to compile both clinical and financial information in assessing a hospital's care delivery.

clinical practice guideline (CPG)   Statement to assist clinicians with appropriate health care for specific clinical circumstances. CPGs are developed by professional associations and related clinical groups to address the appropriateness of health care by specifying indications for tests, procedures, and treatments by systematically using best available evidence. Clinical practice guidelines describe the "how to" for specific disciplines to treat certain conditions, diseases, or modalities.

clinical repository   Computer data storage that combines data from multiple entry points and visits into a single storage location available online.

Clinical Simulation Examination (CSE) Registry exam that accompanies a written examination to evaluate a candidate's qualifications for certification in respiratory care.

clinical trials Most important study of medical interventions, investigating a change in treatment or a new treatment in the clinical setting by comparing current (or usual) therapy with the new therapy in specific phases that examine its safety, effectiveness, and applicability to the public.

closed-loop control Means of mechanical system control in which information about output is used to modify input, which in turn improves the output; also called "feedback control" or "servo control."

clubbing Enlargement of the distal phalanges, particularly the fingers.

coagulant Substance, particularly a drug, that causes coagulation, or blood clot formation.

coagulation Blood's conversion from a free-flowing liquid into a semisolid gel, usually in response to tissue damage; begins with platelet clumping at the site, with prothrombin converted to thrombin to act as a catalyst for converting fibrinogen into an insoluble fibrin mesh.

coarctation of the aorta Congenital cardiac anomaly characterized by a localized narrowing of the aorta; results in increased pressure proximal to the defect and decreased pressure distal to it.

Cochrane Library Data base of controlled trials, systematic reviews of the effects of care, and critical assessments of effectiveness.

codon Sequence of three base pairs in an mRNA molecule that acts as the genetic code for a particular amino acid.

cohort Study that attempts to definitively answer an important question about the cause, treatment, or prevention of disease by enrolling a large number of participants and following them over time so that the study participants are measured, tested, or treated and followed up after years.

coliforms Members of the colon-aerogenes group, or *Escherichia coli*, which make up most of the intestinal flora; also, anything having the characteristics of a sieve or cribriform structure, such as certain porous bones.

collagen vascular disease Any of a group of diseases that can present with interstitial lung disease, including progressive systemic sclerosis, systemic lupus erythematosus, polymyositis and dermatomyositis, Sjögren's syndrome, and mixed connective tissue disease; clinical presentation and histopathologic features comparable to that of idiopathic pulmonary fibrosis with additional features of lymphoid hyperplasia, cellular interstitial pneumonitis, lymphoid interstitial pneumonitis, diffuse alveolar damage, and bronchiolitis obliterans with organizing pneumonitis.

colligative property Property of a solution that depends on the number of solute particles dissolved and not on chemical properties.

colloid Liquid mixture that consists of tiny particles suspended in a liquid.

Committee on Accreditation for Respiratory Care (CoARC) Constituency group sponsored by AARC as the successor to the Joint Review Committee for Respiratory Therapy Education (JRCRTE) and the Respiratory Care Accreditation Board (RCAB); CoARC receives validation from the Committee for Accreditation of Allied Health Education Programs (CAAHEP), reporting its accreditation findings for scrutiny by CAAHEP, which makes final accreditation decisions.

community-acquired pneumonia Pneumonia acquired outside the hospital.

competitive antagonism Interaction property of a drug in which increasing its concentration will force more of that drug onto the receptors, displacing the other agent.

competitive inhibitor Inhibitor of an enzyme reaction that competes with the substrate by binding at the active site.

compliance Lung characteristic that, with resistance, serves as a determinant in the mechanics of air flow in and out of the lungs; the ratio of volume change and pressure change.

component management Method of controlling health care costs that focuses on limiting the use of resources or services such as therapeutic procedures, diagnostic tests, medications, or hospital lengths of stay.

Compressed Gas Association (CGA) Industry technical trade organization that has developed numerous safety standards involving cylinders, fittings, and connections.

compressor A device whose internal volume can be changed to increase the pressure of the gas it contains.

computed tomography (CT) Radiographic technique that produces a film representing detailed cross sections of tissue using an array of detectors in a variety of angles and a collimated beam of x-rays that rotates in a continuous 360-degree motion around the patient to create cross-sectional images.

conchae Three curled bony plates or turbinates that project downward from the walls of the nasal cavity and greatly enlarge the surface area of the nose, move mucus towards the nasopharynx, and warm and humidify incoming air.

congenital diaphragmatic hernia Condition associated with a left posterolateral diaphragmatic defect and the failure of closure of the pleuroperitoneal canal early in gestation (fifth to tenth week of fetal life), resulting in compression of the developing lung by abdominal organs.

congenital heart disease Any functional or structural defect or abnormality of the heart or great vessels present at birth.

consequentialism See *teleological theory.*

constant Variable with an unchanging, fixed value.

continuous mandatory ventilation (CMV) System for delivering a set tidal volume (or pressure) and a minimum respiratory rate in which the patient can trigger additional breaths above the minimal rate, but the set volume or pressure is constant at the preset level.

continuous positive airway pressure (CPAP) A ventilation method by which a constant pressure greater than atmospheric pressure is applied to the airway through the respiratory cycle.

contractility Feature of muscle tissue, especially cardiac muscle, that allows it to contract by shortening the sarcomeres.

contrast venography Standard technique for the diagnosis of DVT, involving cannulation of a dorsal foot vein and injection of intravenous contrast to render the veins radiopaque.

control circuit Drive mechanism in a ventilator that transmits or transforms energy in a predetermined manner to assist or replace the patient's muscles in performing the work of breathing.

control variable   Factors that determine what controls breath delivery from a ventilator, such as pressure, volume, flow, and sometimes inspiratory and expiratory times.

controller medication   Any of a number of pharmacologic interventions whose goal is to maintain normal (or near normal) lung function and include inhaled corticosteroids, nonsteroidal antiinflammatory agents, long-acting β-agonists, methylxanthines, and leukotriene modifiers.

controls   Study participants who do not receive the new treatment but receive instead the usual treatment, a placebo, or sham treatment.

conventional ventilation   See *ventilation.*

CO-oximetry   Means for measuring COHb levels in inhalation injury. CO-oximetry is also the standard technique used to measure hemoglobin oxygen saturation and metHb.

copayment   Limited fee paid by enrollees of managed care organizations for each physician visit, prescription, or other service stipulated in the plan.

cor pulmonale   Hypertrophy and dilatation of the right ventricle.

coronary angiography   Direct imaging of the coronary arteries using cardiac catheterization and subsequent injection of contrast dye; can identify atherosclerotic lesions as well as coronary anomalies, areas of spasm, and acute thrombi.

coronary artery   Vessels that provide blood supply to the heart muscle.

coronary artery bypass surgery   Surgical procedure that can improve myocardial function by reducing ischemia after restoration of normal blood flow. An area of obstruction in a coronary artery is bypassed.

correlation   Statistical parameter used to measure the strength of the relationship between two variables.

corticosteroid   Major class of antiinflammatory drug that generally produces two types of effect: the *glucocorticoid effect,* which reduces inflammation, increases blood glucose and generally induces a catabolic state; and the *mineralocorticoid effect,* which is active primarily at the kidney, promoting sodium conservation.

cost outcomes   Categorization of outcomes of respiratory care that includes cost per respiratory modality, cost to recruit respiratory therapists, and cost of pulmonary rehabilitation program in relation to readmission rates.

covalent bond   Stable atomic configuration accomplished when each of the two bonding atoms shares one of its valance electrons.

crackles   Fine, high-pitched, discontinuous sounds heard during auscultation of the lungs.

creatinine   Substance formed from creatine metabolism and measured in blood and urine as an indicator of kidney function; creatinine levels are a function of skeletal muscle breakdown, and most creatinine is filtered in the glomeruli with little reabsorption.

credentialing   Formal identification of professionals who meet predetermined standards of professional skill or competence; can include both licensure and certification; the NBRC has established standards for the credentialing of practitioners who work under medical direction.

crenation   Process in which water leaves a cell, causing it to shrivel, as a result of greater osmotic pressure outside that cell.

criterion-referenced studies   Validation studies conducted by the NBRC on each health certification examination.

critical care polyneuropathy   Disease affecting several areas of the peripheral nervous system at once; diagnosis is confirmed by EMG studies, showing primary axonal polyneuropathy rather than demyelination as suggested by the reduction in the amplitude of the compound action potential without significant prolongation of the conduction latency period; may be caused by hyperglycemia causing nerve ischemia by endovascular shunting or nerve toxins generated from multiple organ failure.

critical pathway (CP)   Description of the probable sequence of events during a patient's course of health care; outlines all the tests, procedures, treatments, and teaching services that patients may use during a length of stay.

cromone   Class of antiinflammatory drug that appears to reduce the inflammatory response associated with asthma, principally through the inhibition of mast cell degranulation—the release of granules containing histamine and other proinflammatory factors.

crossover   Randomization, in research, of each patient to either a treatment or control group where, after measurements are made, the patient is then restudied in the other group (control or treatment).

cryogenic liquid   A gas that has been liquefied by a reduction in temperature and an increase in pressure. An example is liquid oxygen that is stored for medical use.

cryptography   Type of technical control process for information security that involves writing the information in a code.

cuirass   Type of body ventilator that consists of a lightweight rigid dome, which fits over the anterior chest wall and connects to a negative pressure generator; also called a *chest shell* or *turtle shell.*

cyanosis   Bluish hue to the skin that suggests hemoglobin is poorly saturated with oxygen.

cycle   In respiration, an inspiration followed by an expiration; period of time between the beginning of one breath and the beginning of the next.

cycle time   Ventilatory period; the reciprocal of ventilatory frequency (that is, 60 seconds per minute/number of breaths per minute).

cystic fibrosis   Disorder that is inherited in an autosomal recessive pattern and affects the exocrine glands, resulting in abnormally thick secretions of mucus, elevation of sweat electrolytes, increased organic and enzymatic constituents of saliva, and overactivity of the autonomic nervous system.

cystic fibrosis–related diabetes (CFRD)   Type of diabetes associated with cystic fibrosis and characterized by insidious onset, failure to gain or maintain weight despite nutritional intervention, poor growth, or an unexplained chronic decline in pulmonary function.

Dalton's law   Principle of partial pressures that describes the behavior of physical mixtures of gases and vapors such that each separate gas acts as predicted by the combined gas law, as if it were present alone; in such a mixture, the partial pressure of each particular gas is proportional to the fractional concentration of that gas and equal to the product of fraction concentration and total atmospheric pressure.

dative bond Atomic configuration accomplished when one of the atoms shares two of its valance electrons with another atom.

dead space volume Volume of the lungs that does not participate in gas exchange.

decannulation The removal of a tracheostomy tube.

decompression A decrease in the pressure of a gas; the opposite of compression.

decompression sickness (DCS) Painful, sometimes fatal syndrome caused by the formation of nitrogen bubbles in the tissues of divers, aviators, and others who move too rapidly from higher to lower atmospheric pressures; separated into categories, decompression sickness can be Type I, which involves pain only (usually in or around the joints), or Type II, which is neurological; also called *the bends*.

decompression table Schedule of depths at which anyone exposed to increased pressure must stop for a prescribed period of time to avoid decompression sickness.

deep sulcus sign Distinctive radiographic appearance of a pneumothorax in patients in the supine position, with free air in the pleural space rising to the highest portion of the thorax, usually the anterior costophrenic sulcus, and projecting over the upper abdomen and diaphragm.

deep venous thrombosis (DVT) Blood clotting in the legs and pelvis, which usually occurs as a result of venostasis; common in surgical patients and with other causes of immobility, damage to the endothelial wall of the blood vessels, and hypercoagulability states.

defibrillation Use of an electrical current passed through the heart in an attempt to eliminate the chaotic asynchronous activity of ventricular fibrillation by depolarizing cardiac cells and repolarizing them in a uniform manner with resumption of coordinated cardiac contraction; indicated for ventricular fibrillation, pulseless ventricular tachycardia, and asystole (with the possibility that the rhythm is actually fine ventricular fibrillation).

demand management Any organized effort or program designed to guide health care consumers into the most appropriate level of health care service by involving them in their own care.

dendritic cells Mobile, irregularly shaped cells derived from bone marrow stem cells that reside in small numbers within the airway epithelium and lung parenchyma as antigen-presenting cells, phagocytosing and processing antigens to present to T-lymphocytes, activating them; also produce adhesion molecules and cytokines and express class I and II major histocompatibility locus (HLA) molecules.

deontologic theory Ethical theory based on duty, asserting that an act is either right or wrong based on its intrinsic character rather than consequences.

deoxyribonucleic acid (DNA) Nucleic acid in which the sugar component is deoxyribose; largest molecule in the body, composed of two long polynucleotide chains running parallel to each other; carries the genetic information necessary for synthesis of proteins specific for a given species.

Department of Transportation (DOT) Government agency that regulates cylinder manufacture and testing and the transporting of hazardous materials, including compressed gases and cryogenic liquids.

dependent variable That variable in a function or relationship that is said to be *defined* in terms of the independent variable(s); the values of the independent variables and the function then assign the value for the dependent variable(s).

derivative Average rate of change of a function when the change of the independent variable is very small; the instantaneous rate of change of the function (in other words, a slope).

descriptive statistics Data or raw information obtained from conducting a study whose results are often presented more clearly and efficiently in tables, graphs, or figures.

determinant error Systematic or consistent error that occurs with each measurement.

dewar Container used to store liquid oxygen; each dewar has a capacity of several hundred liters of liquid oxygen; invented by Scottish chemist and physicist Sir James Dewar.

diagnostic-related groups (DRGs) Form of hospital reimbursement based on a patient classification system consisting of approximately 500 different groups, all entailing a predetermined amount of reimbursement. DRGs establish a rate based on bundled services for a particular diagnosis established at the time of admission. The provider receives this amount regardless of the medical care provided.

diagnostics A function that incorporates aspects of assessment and testing that include (1) blood gas analysis; (2) nutritional, cardiac, pulmonary, exercise, and sleep assessments; (3) chest radiology; (4) bronchoscopy; (5) pulmonary function testing; and (6) hemodynamics and gas exchange monitoring.

Diameter Index Safety System One of three indexed safety systems for medical gas distribution station outlets. In this system, a female nut and nipple is manually tightened onto the outlet until contact is made with the plunger, moving it forward until it seats on the stem, thus allowing gas to flow from the piping system.

diaphragm Membranous muscle separating the abdomen and thorax and serving as a major inspiratory muscle.

diaphragmatic pacing Use of a radio frequency transmitter and an antenna that discharges signals to a surgically implanted receiver to transmit electrical impulses to a surgically implanted electrode placed over the phrenic nerve to ensure stimulation of all phrenic nerve roots.

diastole Part of the cardiac cycle that consists of a period of relaxation during which venous blood returns to the heart.

diastolic dysfunction Impaired ventricular filling, recognized increasingly as a cause of congestive heart failure symptoms.

diffuse alveolar damage Constellation of findings including destruction of the Type I alveolar epithelial cells, which rapidly become detached from the underlying basement membrane, contributing to the increased permeability and resultant influx of protein-rich edema fluid into the interstitium and alveolar space.

diffusing capacity Number of milliliters of gas that transfer from the lungs across the alveolar-capillary membrane into the bloodstream each minute, for each 1 mm Hg difference in the pressure across the membrane. The average normal D_L value for oxygen is 20 ml/min/mm Hg.

dilute Relative concentration or strength of a solution indicating that it contains a small amount of solute.

disaccharide   Type of carbohydrate that is a double sugar.

disease management   Approach to patient care that emphasizes coordinated, comprehensive care along the continuum of disease and across health care delivery systems.

disease prevention   Individual's conscious choice to learn about and adopt healthy lifestyle practices, implementing behavior modification techniques as needed to reach a higher level of wellness and minimize certain health risks.

diuretic   Drug used to stimulate urine production.

documentation   Recording or charting individual patient education, including date and time of intervention, subject matter or content addressed, method of instruction, and response of learner or results of the learning.

documentation system   Rigorous recording of medical information into a patient's medical record, both paper and electronic records, and including such data as patient assessment, problem identification, care plans, treatments, and outcomes, as well as discharge summaries, progress notes, physician orders, laboratory results, flow sheets, and online reports, photographs, videotapes, films, and audio recordings.

documented event monitoring (DEM)   Digital recording of chest wall impedance, heart rate, and oxygen saturation.

Doppler   Echocardiography that uses ultrasound to detect the velocity of blood flow within the heart.

double blinding   Research technique in which both investigators and participants are unaware of the treatment being studied.

DRG   Diagnosis-related group system created by Medicare for establishing basis for payment for diagnostic testing.

dry powder inhaler (DPI)   Device that creates aerosols by drawing air through a dose of powdered medication. DPIs produce aerosols in which most of the drug particles are in the respirable range, with the distribution of particle sizes differing significantly among various DPIs.

dual control   Ventilatory mode that allows the ventilator to control pressure or volume (but not both at the same time) based on a feedback loop; can be classified as dual control within a breath or dual control breath-to-breath.

Duchenne's muscular dystrophy   Hereditary familial muscle disease transmitted via an X-linked recessive gene, although about one third of cases may be caused by spontaneous mutation; disease is due to the mutation of the gene for skeletal protein dystrophin; early presenting symptoms are gait disturbances and delayed motor development, as well as limb-girdle muscle weakness and pseudohypertrophy of the calf muscles.

ductus arteriosus   Vascular channel in the fetus that joins the pulmonary artery directly to the descending aorta; it normally closes after birth.

duplex ultrasound   Combination of real time B-mode and Doppler ultrasound, suitable for the ICU patient because the examination can be performed using a portable unit in the intensive care.

durable medical equipment (DME)   Umbrella term usually applied to medical equipment leased or borrowed for use outside the hospital by the patient.

durable power of attorney for health care   Document that names an individual or agent who can make decisions specifically related to health care for another individual.

dynamic airway compression   Condition occurring as a result of decreased lung elasticity and leading to increased expiratory airway resistance, which ultimately results in airtrapping and hyperinflation.

dyspnea   Shortness of breath or breathlessness; distressing feeling of inability to breathe or great effort required to breathe.

dyspnea index   Grading scale that measures the ratio of peak exercise ventilation to maximal voluntary ventilation.

Eaton-Lambert disorder   Rare myasthenic-like disorder resulting from a reduction of transmitter release from presynaptic terminals; commonly associated with small cell carcinoma of the lung; limb and girdle muscles predominantly are involved.

echocardiography   Diagnostic/assessment tool using ultrasound to examine the heart structures and function by transmission of high-frequency ultrasound waves through the chest and calibrating the velocity of sound waves in the medium under examination.

efficacy   Maximum achievable effect a drug is able to produce, regardless of concentration.

egophony   Auscultation sound typical in consolidation of lung tissue, meaning that the normally aerated tissue has been filled with fluid, mucus, pus, or cellular debris; in egophony, *e* sounds like *a*.

ejection fraction   Percentage of blood pumped from the ventricle during a single cardiac contraction; normal left ventricular ejection fraction is greater than 50%.

elastance   Ratio of pressure change to volume change (that is, the reciprocal of compliance).

elastic load   Pressure necessary to overcome the elastance (or compliance) of the respiratory system.

electrocardiography (ECG)   Insensitive and nonspecific test for the evaluation of ventricular function.

electron   Particle with a negative charge (-1) located outside the nucleus of an atom.

electron transport system   Movement of high-energy electrons (removed during glycolysis and TCA cycle in the form of reduced FAD and NAD) down a chain of carrier molecules imbedded in the inner membrane of the mitochondria, resulting in the production of some 90% of the ATP formed during carbohydrate catabolism.

electronic signature   Unique code or password that verifies the individual creating the entry and creates an individual "signature" on the record, then stores it on magnetic, optical, or some other computer storage media.

emotional filter   Nonverbal, internal interpretation of another's actions or communication as seen in light of a judgment, emotional reaction or opinion of the listener.

empathy   Characteristic essential to nurturing a relationship: envisioning oneself in the place of another and then verbally conveying that you understand what it must feel like to be in that person's situation.

emphysema   Type of COPD occurring in patients who experience damage to the lung parenchyma; results in histopathologic evidence of alveolar wall destruction without fibrosis and physiologic evidence of decreased lung elastic recoil, resulting in bullae that eventually enlarge and compress adjacent lung tissue, impairing respiratory function.

empowerment   Characteristic essential to nurturing a relationship providing the proper tools, resources and environment to build, develop, and increase the ability and effectiveness of others to set and reach goals for individual and social ends.

encoding Sender's act of assigning form to a message in either words, symbols, actions, pictures, numbers, or gestures.

endobronchial biopsy Method for sampling endoscopically visible exophytic central tumors or mucosal ulceration, irregularity, or infiltration.

endotracheal intubation Establishment of an artificial airway by placing a tube through the mouth or nose, through the glottis, and into the trachea.

endotracheal tube Large-bore catheter inserted through the mouth or nose and into the trachea.

end-tidal P_{CO_2} P_{CO_2} at end-exhalation (PET_{CO_2}).

enteral Oral route (PO) of drug administration, passing into the gastrointestinal system.

enteral nutrition Provision of nutrients through the GI tract when the patient is unable to chew or swallow.

enteral tube feeding (ETF) Nutrition administration via direct access to the gastrointestinal tract, bypassing the mouth and throat in a patient who cannot eat but who has adequate gastric motility and emptying.

enteric bacteria Intestinal bacteria.

entry and exclusion criteria Stipulations made before a study begins to determine how a subject or patient is to be entered into, excluded from, and withdrawn from a study.

eosinophilic granuloma Rare, predominantly pulmonary disorder that occurs almost exclusively in smokers or ex-smokers between 10 and 40 years old; likely an inflammatory response by Langerhans cells to a component of tobacco smoke.

epiglottis Cartilaginous structure overhanging the entrance to the larynx to prevent food from entering the larynx and trachea while swallowing.

equation Numeric representation of a chemical compound; in mathematics, the relationship among variables.

ergometer Bicycle-like apparatus used for measuring the respiratory, muscular, and metabolic effects of exercise.

eschar Scab or dry crust that develops after trauma, such as a thermal or chemical burn, infection, or excoriating skin disease.

escharotomy Surgical incision into necrotic tissue resulting from a severe burn to prevent edema from generating sufficient interstitial pressure to impair capillary filling, causing ischemia.

evidence-based medicine (EBM) Comprehensive approach to systematically document achievable health care outcomes across the disciplines; also called *evidence-based health care (EBH)*.

exclusive provider organization Managed care model in which choice is completely eliminated and enrollees must employ the physician and hospital stipulated in the plan; the most affordable but most restrictive of the managed care models.

exercise assessment This assessment performs two functions: (1) It quantitates the level of disability and provides information for setting initial exercise loads and program expectations. (2) It provides insight into the various cardiorespiratory factors that are involved in the functional disabilities.

exercise testing Testing method that measures physiologic reserve and functional capacity that cannot be determined from resting measurements; exercise testing delineates the reserve of each of the contributing subcomponents of respiration, and allows assessment of functional status through determination of maximal power output and oxygen consumption.

exercise-induced asthma Form of asthma characterized by transient airway obstruction, typically occurring 5 to 15 minutes after strenuous exertion; prevalent in 90% of individuals with asthma.

exhaled nitric oxide Marker of airway inflammation, particularly useful in both acute and chronic asthma in both children and adults.

expiratory flow time Interval from the start of expiratory flow to the end of expiratory flow.

expiratory pause time Interval from the end of expiratory flow to the start of inspiratory flow; often initiated to measure auto-PEEP.

expiratory phase Respiration period during which all mechanics from the start of expiratory flow to the end of expiratory flow occur, including those associated with expiratory hold or pause, until the start of inspiratory flow.

expiratory positive airway pressure (EPAP) Pressure applied to the airway during the expiratory phase with ventilators designed for noninvasive ventilation; synonomous with CPAP or PEEP.

expiratory time Time interval from the start of expiratory flow to the start of inspiratory flow; components include expiratory flow time and expiratory pause time.

exponent Useful means of abbreviating large or small (negative) numbers for convenience and ease of comparison, using superscripted numerals to indicate, for example, powers of 10, as seen in scientific notation; these superscripts, or exponents of 10, indicate where to move the decimal point to obtain the complete number.

external compressor Large, water-cooled, piston-type compressor that provides compressed gas from wall outlets.

extraalveolar air Distinctive radiographic indicator, in thoracic imaging, of pneumothorax, pneumomediastinum, or interstitial emphysema.

extracellular fluid (ECF) Body fluid comprising interstitial fluid and blood plasma.

extracorporeal life support (ECLS) Management technique for improving oxygenation and reducing ventilating pressures in selected full-term neonates through cannulation of the right heart; blood is drained from this cannula into a circuit containing a membrane oxygenator and a pump so that oxygen circulates through one side of the membrane and blood is pumped through the other side of the membrane, leading to oxygen diffusion into the blood and carbon dioxide elimination from the blood for its reinfusion into the infant.

extrinsic asthma Asthma associated with external allergens.

extubation Process of removal of an endotracheal tube.

face shield Apparatus used to provide emergency exhaled-gas ventilation; not as effective as masks, with or without nonrebreathing valves.

facilitation Technique in which words, postures, or actions encourage more detail if delivered with sincerity and genuineness.

fascioscapulohumeral (FSH) muscular dystrophy Autosomal dominant, slow-progressing dystrophy that affects primarily the face and the proximal portion of the upper extremities caused by a defective gene.

fetal hemoglobin   Hemoglobin F; has higher affinity to O_2 than adult hemoglobin (hemoglobin A), which can be attributed to the replacement of β chains in hemoglobin A by γ-chains.

FEV_1/FVC   Ratio that is a sensitive and reliable indicator of airway obstruction and a valuable tool for identifying the cause of a low FEV_1. FEV_1 is the volume of air exhaled in the first second of the FVC (forced expiratory vital capacity) maneuver and is the most reproducible measurement of airway obstruction.

fiberoptic plethysmography   Modification of inductance plethysmography, using optical fibers woven into elastic belts with light passing through the fibers into a photodetector; when rib cage or abdominal displacements stretch the elastic belt, large changes in light transmission through the fibers result, and the change in light transmission is electronically processed to provide data.

Fick equation   Equation that relates $\dot{V}O_2$ to cardiac output and arterial and mixed venous oxygen content, where $\dot{V}O_2$ is the product of the cardiac output and the arteriovenous oxygen content difference.

Fick's law   Description of the transfer by diffusion, demonstrating that the diffusion rate across a barrier is directly proportional to the cross-sectional area available for diffusion and the difference in concentration gradient per unit distance perpendicular to that cross section.

fidelity   See *role fidelity*.

flail chest   Potentially life-threatening injury, usually resulting from multiple rib fractures on one side or from two or more rib fractures in two or more places, from sternal fracture, or from costochondral separation; the term flail refers to the paradoxic motion of the chest resulting from loss of chest wall stability: a seesaw motion is a characteristic physical finding whereby the chest wall moves outward on expiration and inward on inspiration.

flexible fiberoptic bronchoscopy   Bronchoscopic procedure using a flexible instrument that transmits an image along flexible bundles of coated parallel glass or plastic fibers that make use of internal reflections to create more light to allow visualization of more distal airways.

flow restrictor   Specific size orifice that allows a specific flow of gas to pass through a flow control device, provided the inlet pressure is a constant 50 psig.

flow trigger   Alternative to pressure triggering, in which the ventilator responds to a change in flow rather than a pressure drop at the airway.

flow-inflating bag   Manual resuscitator that requires a continuous flow from an external gas source; pressure is determined by the flow and the pressure release valve with wide ranges of peak inspiratory pressure (PIP) and PEEP attainable.

flow-volume loop   System of testing pulmonary function in which a patient breathes into an electronic spirometer and performs forced inspiratory and expiratory vital capacity maneuvers while volume and flow are displayed.

Food and Drug Administration   Agency of the Department of Health and Human Services (HHS) that enforces regulations and standards concerning the purity of medical gases, their manufacture, packaging, and labeling.

foramen ovale   Opening in the septum between the right and left atria of the fetal heart; provides a bypass for blood that would otherwise flow to the fetal lungs.

forced expiratory technique   Breathing maneuver that consists of one or two forced expirations or huffs, combined with a period of controlled breathing.

forced vital capacity   Test of pulmonary function that measures the maximal volume gas which can be expelled forcibly after full inspiration.

foreign body obstruction   Presence of any object lodged in any part of the airway, interfering with the individual's ability to breathe and causing sudden choking.

forward heart failure   Heart failure causing poor organ perfusion.

fractional distillation of liquefied air   Process, first described in 1907 by Karl von Linde, by which the two major components of air (oxygen and nitrogen) are produced in bulk commercial quantities; the process relies on the Joule-Kelvin principle, which states that when gases under pressure are released into a vacuum, the gas molecules tend to lose their kinetic energy; in the vacuum, the reduction in kinetic energy causes a decrease in temperature and a reduction in the cohesive forces between the molecules, leading to liquefaction.

fractional oxygen saturation   Expression of oxyhemoglobin as a percentage of the *total* amount of hemoglobin.

freezing point   Temperature at which a liquid will enter the solid state and freeze; 0° C or 32° F at 1 atmosphere of pressure for water.

function   Rule associating two or more measurable quantities, which are called the variables for that function; in a mathematic function, the value of one variable is dependent on one or more other variables.

functional oxygen saturation   Expression of the amount of hemoglobin *bound* to oxygen expressed as a percentage of the amount of hemoglobin *available* for O_2 binding. Functional saturation provides an accurate measure of oxygen saturation if dysfunctional hemoglobins, notably COHb, are present only in negligible concentrations.

fundamental theorem of calculus   Specific connection in a function between the definite integral and the indefinite integral.

fungal respiratory infections   Respiratory infection caused by fungi and including the following: histoplasmosis, blastomycosis, coccidioidomycosis, cryptococcosis, aspergillosis, *Candida* respiratory infection.

gas gangrene   Tissue necrosis with gas bubbles in soft tissue after trauma or surgery, caused by anaerobic organisms and exhibiting a rapid rate of progression.

gastric tonometry   Technique that measures CO_2 in the gastric lumen using a catheter placed in the stomach.

Gay-Lussac's law   Proportional relationship of pressure and temperature at a constant volume and mass.

geometric standard deviation (GSD)   Measure of the magnitude of variation in particle size distribution—for example, a monodisperse aerosol in which all particles are basically the same size has a GSD < 1.2, whereas a heterodisperse aerosol, with a wider range of particle sizes, has a GSD > 1.2.

gestational age   Age of a fetus or a newborn, dating from the first day of the mother's last menstrual period; usually expressed in weeks.

glossopharyngeal breathing Also known as "frog breathing," a technique involving the use of oropharyngeal muscles to inject air into the trachea and thus augment ventilation to provide short periods of spontaneous ventilation, to improve effective cough, and to increase the volume of the voice.

glucose Six-carbon sugar with the formula of $C_6H_{12}O_6$; found in fruits and other foods; primary source of energy for cells.

glycolysis Anaerobic process necessary to glucose metabolism that begins with the breakdown of a six-carbon glucose chain ($C_6H_{12}O_6$) to two three-carbon pyruvate (pyruvic acid) molecules in the cytosol of the cell; prepares glucose for the second step in catabolism, the citric acid cycle.

Graham's law Principle predicting the rate of diffusion of a gas as inversely proportional to the square root of its density.

gram Metric standard of weight, equal to the weight of 1 ml of water at 4° C (its maximum density).

Gram's stain Test that stains microorganisms with crystal violet dye, followed by an iodine solution, decolorizing, and then counterstaining with safranin. The retention of either the violet color of the stain or the pink color of the counterstain serves as a primary means of identifying and classifying bacteria by revealing details of the cell wall structure.

gram-negative bacteria Bacteria that have a cell wall composed of a thin layer of peptidoglycan covered by an outer membrane of lipoprotein and lipopolysaccharide and which lose the stain or are decolorized by alcohol in Gram's stains; examples include the following: *Haemophilus influenzae*, *Moraxella catarrhalis*, *Pseudomonas aeruginosa*, *Klebsiella* species, *Escherichia coli*, *Enterobacter* species, *Serratia* species, *Acinetobacter* species, and *Proteus mirabilis*.

gram-positive bacteria Bacteria whose cell walls are composed of a thick layer of peptidoglycan with attached teichoic acids and which retain the stain or resist decolorization by alcohol in Gram's staining; examples include the following: *Streptococcus pneumoniae*, *Staphylococcus aureus*, and *Enterococcus* species.

Guillain-Barré syndrome (GBS) Acute idiopathic polyneuritis usually presenting as an ascending symmetrical paralysis of the lower extremities associated with absent tendon reflexes.

Hagen-Poiseuille equation Flow measure that calculates volume per unit time, not distance or flow velocity, relating volume flow to the fourth power of the radius, directly and inversely related to the viscosity of the fluid and the length of the tube through which the fluid passes, while directly related to the pressure gradient; if these variables are kept constant, the pressure gradient over the length of the tubular structure in question is directly proportional to flow.

Haldane effect Influence of O_2 on the CO_2 dissociation curve; ensures that the CO_2 content of deoxygenated blood is greater than oxygenated blood at any P_{CO_2}.

half-life Time required for a drug's concentration to be reduced by half.

health belief model Theory focusing on prevention of disease and asserting that taking action depends on one's perception of four issues: one's level of susceptibility to the condition, degree of severity of the consequences that might result from contracting the condition, potential benefits of the health action in preventing or reducing susceptibility, and the barriers or costs related to starting or continuing the proposed behavior.

Health Care Financing Administration (HCFA) Branch of the U.S. Department of Health and Human Services that administers the Medicare and Medicaid programs. HCFA is responsible for setting the coverage policy, payment, and other guidelines and directing the activities of government contractors.

health maintenance organization Type of group health care practice that provides basic and supplemental health maintenance and treatment services to voluntary enrollees who prepay a fixed periodic fee that is set without regard to the amount or kind of services received.

health promotion Individual's voluntary adoption of a wellness model and choice to gain an awareness and/or knowledge of healthy lifestyle practices, incorporating such practices into the daily routine, and ultimately reaching a higher level of well-being and wellness.

HEDIS Health Plan Employer Data and Information Set; set of standardized measures NCQA developed that allows purchasers to make comparisons among health plans.

helical diffusion Variant of spike theory that may also play a role in high-frequency ventilation (HFV).

heliox Gas mixture of helium and oxygen; used clinically because of its low density.

helium dilution One of the most commonly used methods for measuring functional residual capacity (FRC).

hematocrit Proportion of whole blood that is red blood cells (the hemoglobin-carrying cells).

hemoglobin Iron-containing globular protein consisting of two pairs of polypeptides; primary function is the transport of oxygen from the lungs to the tissues.

hemolysis Process in which water passes through a cell, possibly bursting it, as occurs when the water concentration is higher outside the cell, that is, osmotic pressure is lower outside the cell.

hemothorax Blood trapped in the pleural space, causing a space-occupying lesion; source of blood is typically from fractured ribs lacerating the intercostal blood vessels or lacerating the lung.

Henderson-Hasselbalch equation Assertion that the pH of a buffer is determined by the ratio of the concentration of base to the concentration of weak acid.

heparin Drug useful with venous thrombosis to prevent further clot formation.

heparin-induced thrombocytopenia (HIT) Complication of heparin use consisting of a platelet count less than 150,000 mm³ that typically develops 5 to 10 days after the initiation of heparin therapy.

hepatojugular reflux Inappropriate elevation of a usually normal jugular venous pressure (JVP) when the abdomen is compressed for 1 minute over the liver.

hertz Unit of measure for wave frequency; equal to 1 cycle per second.

high-frequency airway oscillation Technique used to enhance clearance of secretions through a variety of mechanisms, including alteration of mucus rheology, enhanced mucus-airflow interaction, and reflex mechanisms; oscillations can be mechanically generated and administered to the patient, or they can be self-generated by expiration through an oscillatory device.

high-frequency flow interrupter (HFFI) ventilation One of four general types of high-frequency ventilation; delivers inspiratory flow to the patient in short bursts via a rotating ball valve or microprocessor-controlled solenoid valve, producing breath rates of 2 to 22 Hz (1 Hz = 60 breaths/min); inspiration and exhalation are both active.

high-frequency jet ventilation (HFJV) One of four general types of high-frequency ventilation; delivers short pulses of gas directly into the trachea through a narrow-bore cannula or jet injector.

high-frequency oscillatory (HFO) ventilation One of four general types of high-frequency ventilation; essentially an airway vibrator, usually using piston pumps or a vibrating diaphragm that operates at frequencies ranging from 400 to 2400 breaths/min; both inspiration and expiration are active.

high-frequency positive-pressure ventilation (HFPPV) Conventional positive-pressure ventilation at high breath rates (>150/min) and small tidal volumes with short inspiratory time to facilitate the increased respiratory rate; exhalation is passive.

high-frequency ventilation (HFV) Widely accepted mode of mechanical ventilation in neonatal and pediatric critical care; positive pressure ventilation at rates greater than 150/minute and tidal volumes approximating anatomic dead space with an ability to deliver an adequate minute volume with a lower airway pressure—often when conventional mechanical ventilation has failed.

hilum Depression in the lung where the vessels and nerves enter.

home health Provision of services and equipment to the patient in the home for the purpose of restoring and maintaining his or her maximal level of comfort, function, and health; home health services fall into five different categories: home health agencies, hospice, home medical equipment, home infusion therapy, and homemaker services/private duty nursing.

hospital-acquired pneumonia Pneumonia that develops after hospital admission, excluding any infection that is incubating at the time of admission.

House of Delegates (HOD) One of several governance and advisory entities of the AARC, which exists as a representative body for the chartered affiliates to contribute to the growth, existence, governance and future of the respiratory care profession; the HOD exists to bring the wishes and concerns of the general membership to the national organization through local representation; serves as a communication bridge reporting activities, data, information, and needs back to the AARC chartered affiliates and members; serves an advisory role to the BOD and participates in governance of the AARC; and contributes to the governance of the AARC through approval of bylaws, budgets, nominations, and audits and through consideration of resolutions and motions that are forwarded to the BOD for consideration.

huff coughing Forced expiratory technique (FET) that is performed by sharply exhaling from high- to mid-lung volumes through an open glottis; used for patients unable to generate an effective cough.

hyaline membrane disease Acute lung disease affecting newborns (usually premature), characterized by airless alveoli, inelastic lungs, more than 60 respirations per minute, nasal flaring, intercostal and subcostal retractions, grunting on expiration, and peripheral edema.

hydrogen bond Connection holding adjacent water molecules together in a liquid state and requiring a significant amount of heat to be absorbed to change this water from a liquid to a gas.

hydrophilic Water-loving; describes molecules that tend to be attracted to, and mix well with, water molecules.

hydrophobic Water-hating.

hydrostatic pressure Static water pressure, generated by the water's weight and which varies on the basis of the density of fluid and height, reflecting the force of gravity; with other fluids, this pressure is called *manometric pressure*.

hydrostatic testing Process that measures the expansion characteristic of the cylinder when exposed to internal pressures two-thirds greater then normal; performed by totally suspending the cylinder in a tank of water and pumping water into the cylinder.

hyperbaric oxygen Treatment modality in which a patient breathes 100% oxygen intermittently while the pressure of the treatment chamber is increased to a point higher than sea-level pressure.

hyperbaric oxygenation Inhalation of oxygen at greater than normal atmospheric pressure in a specially designed chamber; considered a controversial means of improving the prognosis of those suffering serious CO exposures.

hypercalcemia Increased calcium serum levels characterized by anorexia, vomiting, polyuria, mental confusion, obtundation, and death.

hypercapnia Excess carbon dioxide in the blood; can be caused by hypoventilation, increased dead space, and increased CO_2 production.

hyperchloremia Excessive chloride in the blood.

hypercoagulability Tendency of the blood, to coagulate, or clot, more rapidly than is normal.

hyperinflation Condition in the lung in which air is not easily exhaled, resulting from decreased lung elasticity and subsequent increased expiratory airway resistance and air trapping as a result of dynamic airway compression.

hyperkalemia Serum potassium levels above normal; can produce hyporeflexia and muscle weakness; paralysis can occur in severe cases, but death because of cardiac arrhythmias usually takes place before this occurs.

hypermagnesemia High magnesium serum levels.

hypernatremia High sodium serum levels.

hyperoxygenation Mechanism of action, along with bubble reduction, in hyperbaric oxygen therapy, which is the primary therapy for decompression sickness and arterial gas embolism; a secondary effect of hyperbaric oxygen therapy.

hyperpnea Rapid, deep, labored breathing.

hyperresonance Sound, often produced in percussion technique, that is loud, low-pitched, and long; often heard over an emphysematous lung.

hypertonic Property existing in a solution with an osmotic pressure greater than that within the cell.

hyperventilation Rapid, deep, labored breathing resulting in a lowered P_{CO_2}.

hypocalcemia Low ionized serum calcium usually resulting from either decreased absorption or decreased mobilization of calcium from the bones.

hypochloremia Low levels of chloride in the extracellular space.

hypokalemia Low serum potassium level.

hypomagnesemia Low serum magnesium levels.

hyponatremia Low serum sodium levels, creating a significant shift in the relationship between intracellular and extracellular fluid compartments.

hypophosphatemia Low serum phosphorus levels primarily caused by decreased absorption, intracellular shifts, or increased excretion.

hypopneas Abnormally slow, shallow respiration.

hypotonic Property of any solution with an osmotic pressure less than that within the cell.

hypoxemia Deficiency in blood oxygenation; may be caused by inadequate ventilation relative to perfusion (that is, low $\dot{V}_A/\dot{Q}$ and shunt), which has a great effect on oxygen uptake by the lung; hypoxemia in adults is usually defined as PaO_2 of less than 80 mm Hg.

hypoxia Decreased tissue oxygenation below adequate levels, disabling adequate blood perfusion of the tissue.

hypoxic pulmonary vasoconstriction Narrowing of the lumen in a pulmonary blood vessel because of inadequate oxygen at the cellular level; a mechanism that is normally protective, but which, by some disturbance, can contribute to shunt physiology and hypoxemia.

ICU-acquired steroid myopathy Myopathy acquired in the ICU, becoming an important cause of weakness and contributing to weaning failure from mechanical ventilation.

ideal gas law Rule that $PV = nRT$, with the product of pressure (P) and volume (V) equal to the product of the number of molecules of gas (n), absolute temperature (T), and a gas constant (R).

idiopathic pulmonary fibrosis (IPF) Interstitial lung disease that affects predominantly males in the fifth to seventh decade of life; of unknown pathogenesis but likely to reflect an aberrant host response to injury of the alveolar epithelium and endothelium or a protracted response to the same; a history of a gradual onset of dyspnea with exercise is typical.

illness/wellness continuum Perspective of patient education in which health is viewed from a traditional perspective, and from a wellness perspective.

impedance plethysmography Noninvasive study for diagnosing deep venous thrombosis (DVT) by detecting volumetric changes in the limb through changes in the electric impedance.

impedance pneumography Method for measuring respiratory rate and excursion using two electrodes placed on the chest wall and then passing a high-frequency and low-ampere AC current between the electrodes on the chest surface.

incentive spirometry Technique designed to mimic natural sighing or yawning maneuvers; also referred to as *sustained maximal inspiration*; used to increase transpulmonary pressure and inspiratory volumes to near preoperative vital capacity, improve inspiratory muscle performance, and reestablish the normal pattern of periodic deep breathing.

incidence Factor that determines how often a disease or condition is contracted or diagnosed in a time period.

incident report Occurrence report filed for an untoward incident in a health care system, such as administration of an incorrect medication or a patient's falling, including specifics such as patient name, identification number, date, time, description of the incident, immediate action taken, and a signature of the reporting employee.

incubator Apparatus for keeping an infant in an environment of proper humidity and temperature.

indefinite integral Variable in a mathematical relationship that produces a function rather than a number; sometimes called the *antiderivative*.

indemnity insurance plan Type of commercial plan that provides a benefit only if and when a medical event occurs. Indemnity plans provide payment of a fixed sum for a covered benefit.

independent variable Variable in a specific function, or relationship, which, in the confines of that function, defines another, *dependent*, variable.

indeterminant error Inherent inaccuracy in a measurement.

Index Medicus Set of volumes that systematically organizes and allows access to articles from the major scientific journals, sorted and cited by author and topic; includes such journals as Chest, Critical Care Medicine, Respiratory Care, and American Journal of Respiratory and Critical Care Medicine.

indirect calorimetry Most commonly applied technique for measuring energy requirements in the clinical setting, based on the primary measurement of oxygen consumption ($\dot{V}O_2$); at the time of measurement, $\dot{V}O_2$ represents the actual rate of energy expenditure taking place for the measurement period.

inert gas narcosis Pressure reaction that is analogous to being intoxicated, caused by a pressure greater than 60 fsw, usually occurring in workers in multiplace chambers (which treat more than one individual at a time), particularly while treating divers for arterial gas embolism at depths of 165 fsw.

inertial impaction Deposition of large aerosol particles on the walls of an airway conduit; inertial impaction is the primary mechanism for deposition of aerosol particles of at least 5 μm and an important mechanism for particles as small as 2 μm.

infant apnea program (IAP) Treatment component whose recommendations form one of a list of clinical criteria used to consider discontinuation, based on the patient's clinical condition.

inferential statistics Data reported as averages (means) and variability (standard deviations) of the study measurements analyzed by statistical methods to allow inference to other settings or to explain "why this study means anything elsewhere."

inflammation Complex, protective immune response of body tissues to irritation or injury in the presence of an antigen or foreign substance.

information management System for developing, reviewing, and controlling all methods for capturing and recording patient information using both paper forms and computer forms.

information security Protection of the integrity, availability, and confidentiality of computer-based information and the resources used to enter, store, process, and communicate information.

informed consent Right of the patient to all information before undergoing or refusing treatments; includes the steps of disclosure, understanding, voluntary nature, competence, and permission giving.

inhalation injury Sequela of aspiration of superheated gases, steam, or noxious products of incomplete combustion, generating adverse effects on both gas exchange and on hemodynamics.

Inhalation Therapy Association (ITA) Association formed in 1946 as a precursor to the American Association of Inhalation Therapists (AAIT) to promote higher standards, professional advancement, to foster cooperation between the technician and physician, and to advance the knowledge of inhalation therapy.

inhaled nitric oxide (iNO) Gas shown to improve oxygenation in neonates with hypoxemia and pulmonary hypertension by lowering pulmonary vascular resistance by vasodilating pulmonary vasculature, resulting in decreased right-to-left shunting of blood; selective to pulmonary vasculature and not associated with a lowering of systemic blood pressure.

inoculum Substance introduced into the body to cause or to increase immunity to a specific disease or condition.

inotropic agent Substance that influences the force of muscular contractions.

inspiratory flow time Interval from the start of inspiratory flow to the end of inspiratory flow.

inspiratory pause time Interval from the end of inspiratory flow to the start of expiratory flow.

inspiratory phase Respiration phase during mechanical ventilation in which pressure, volume, and flow increase above their end-expiratory values; quantified by specifying the inspiratory time, defined as the time interval from the start of inspiratory flow to the start of expiratory flow, including the hold or pause time.

inspiratory positive airway pressure (IPAP) Level of pressure specified on ventilators designed to provide noninvasive positive-pressure ventilation. On such devices IPAP is usually the absolute inspiratory pressure and includes the expiratory pressure. The difference between IPAP and EPAP is the level of pressure support; if the EPAP level is changed, the IPAP level must be changed to maintain a constant pressure support level.

inspiratory time Time interval from the start of inspiratory flow to the start of expiratory flow, including the inspiratory hold (or pause) time.

Institutional Review Board (IRB) Facility group that officially approves proposed studies and ensures the safety of participants for a new treatment and that informed consent forms are signed by the patient, nearest relative, or guardian to approve the treatment or control.

integral Numeral or value that is part of a larger whole or set.

intermittent percussive ventilation (IPV) Therapeutic form of chest physical therapy using a pneumatic device called a *Percussionator*; the patient breathes through a mouthpiece, which delivers high-flow mini-bursts at rates of over 200 cycles/minute. IPV was designed to treat atelectasis, enhance the mobilization and clearance of retained secretions, and deliver nebulized medications to the distal airways.

intermittent positive pressure breathing (IPPB) Short-term or episodic mechanical ventilation for the primary purpose of assisting ventilation and providing short duration hyperinflation therapy; usually administered with pneumatically driven, pressure-triggered, and pressure-cycled ventilators.

internal compressor Small compressor linked to a motor within a ventilator and designed for use with a single ventilator.

Internet Grateful Med Free searching system provided by NLM for searching MEDLINE on Internet browsers.

interstitial lung disease (ILD) Term used to delineate approximately 200 distinct diseases in which the interstitium is altered by inflammation and/or fibrosis; may affect any of the following structures: the alveolar walls (and the lumens), pulmonary microvasculature, interstitial macrophages, fibroblasts, myofibroblasts, and matrix components of the lung.

intraaortic balloon pump (IABP) Catheter-based balloon inserted into the descending aorta just below the aortic arch and inflated during diastole, causing increased coronary blood flow, and deflated during systole, causing decreased afterload; uses the principle of counterpulsation to support the failing heart, especially in cardiogenic shock due to myocardial ischemia.

intracellular fluid (ICF) Fluid inside cell membranes that contains dissolved solutes essential to electrolytic balance and healthy metabolism.

intramuscular Administration (injection) of a bolus of drug into a muscle bed, where it is taken into the bloodstream by the local capillary bed.

intravenous Route of drug delivery to the inside of a vein; also pertaining to the inside of a vein.

intraventricular hemorrhage Bleeding within a ventricle; can develop in neonates who experience overventilation, hypocarbia, or hyperoxia.

intrinsic asthma Asthma associated with recent respiratory tract infection; inflammatory responses to viral infections (especially lower respiratory tract) may start the cascade of symptomatic wheezing from inflammatory debris or excessive mucus production in the airways.

ion Electrically charged atom or group of atoms.

ionic bond Stable atomic configurations accomplished by transferring electrons.

iron lung An airtight respirator that consists of a metal tank enclosing the whole body, except the head; the prototype negative pressure ventilator; also known as *tank ventilator* or *Drinker respirator*.

ischemia Decrease in oxygenated blood in a body part or organ; in heart disease, this is manifested as changes in the T wave, which reflects abnormalities of repolarization of the myocardium.

isothermic saturation boundary (ISB) The point at which inspired gas is fully saturated at body temperature (44 mg/L at 37° C), approximately 5 cm below the carina at the level of the third-generation airways. Above the ISB, temperature and humidity decrease during inspiration and increase during exhalation; there are no fluctuations in temperature or relative humidity below the ISB.

isotonic Property of a solution that occurs with an osmotic pressure that is equal to that found within cells, resulting in a solution with an osmotic pressure equal to that found within cells.

isotope Atom whose nuclei have the same number of protons (atomic number) but a different number of neutrons (mass number).

isovolumic contraction Early phase of systole in which the left ventricle generates enough tension to overcome the resistance of the aortic end-diastolic pressure.

isovolumic relaxation Marked decrease in pressure occurring during the first phase of diastole, after aortic valve closure and before mitral valve opening, when the ventricle relaxes without a change in volume.

IVC filter Filter placed in the inferior vena cava to prevent lower extremity thrombus from embolizing to the lungs; primary indications for filter placement include contraindications to anticoagulation, recurrent embolism while on adequate therapy, and significant bleeding complications during anticoagulation.

jaundice Yellowish skin color arising from an elevated serum bilirubin level.

jet nebulizer Device that uses a jet of compressed gas which passes through a restricted orifice, creating a low pressure area near the tip of a narrow tube, drawing fluid from a reservoir, which is then sheared or shattered into droplets by the airstream.

joule Unit of energy in the meter-kilogram-second system equivalent to the product pressure and volume, or equivalent to 10^7 ergs or 1 Watt/second.

kinesics Factor affecting communication on either a conscious or unconscious level through the use of body motion and gestures.

kinetic therapy Treatment that uses a special bed which rotates the patient continuously from one lateral position to another, reaching a 124-degree angle, every 4 minutes.

Kussmaul Hyperventilation as a compensatory mechanism for metabolic acidosis.

kyphosis Forward curvature of the spine.

lactate Anion of lactic acid most commonly formed in ischemic cells as a consequence of anaerobic glycolysis and the use of pyruvate for generation of ATP; frequently used as an indicator of the severity of shock and to give a rough idea of tissue perfusion, oxygen delivery, and oxygen utilization.

laminar flow A pattern of flow consisting of concentric layers of fluid flowing parallel to the tube wall at linear velocities that increase toward the center; considered smooth, uninterrupted flow.

large volume nebulizer An aerosol-producing device designed to deliver enough humidified inspired gases to provide adequate flow to meet patient inspiratory flow rates.

laryngeal mask airway (LMA) Device for both routine management of the airway during general anesthesia and as an emergency airway adjunct in the difficult airway.

larynx Musculocartilaginous structure behind the tongue and hyoid bone that acts as a sphincter to protect the entrance to the trachea; functions secondarily as the "voice box."

laser bronchoscopy Use of rigid bronchoscopy with laser technology to make use of a wider diameter of the working channel, which allows for simultaneous visualization, laser use, and suctioning; best applied to symptomatic centrally located, unresectable, endobronchial malignancies; appropriately located benign tumors without extrabronchial involvement (such as papillomas); luminal obstructions such as webs or tracheal granulomas; and noninflammatory tracheal stenoses.

leukocyte White blood cell.

leukocytosis Elevated white cell count; often a sign of significant infection but also can be associated with elevated glucocorticoids (for example, stress reaction, steroid administration) and in a number of hematologic malignancies.

leukopenia Decreased white cell count; often indicates overwhelming infection.

leukotriene Any one of several compounds that can act on smooth muscle cells through its own receptor to produce tonic bronchoconstriction.

limb-girdle muscular dystrophy Heterogenous group of muscle dystrophies characterized primarily by weakness of the shoulder and pelvic girdles with sparing of the facial muscles.

limit Rule or quality that establishes terms or confines in relating two quantities within a function or that affects the predictability of dependent variable(s) as the independent variable(s) approach a specific point; also, the behavior, or value, of the dependent variable as the independent variable approaches some point of interest.

limit variable Ventilation variable that rises no higher than a given preset value or increases to a preset value before inspiration ends.

lipid Organic biomolecule that is soluble in nonpolar organic solvents, such as ether, alcohol, or benzene but is not soluble in water; composed primarily, but not exclusively, of carbon, hydrogen, and oxygen.

liver enzymes Enzymes that are present in the liver and may indicate liver function, and dysfunction elsewhere (for example, alanine aminotransferase [ALT] is present in liver cells, and an increased serum level is an indicator of liver cell injury; aspartate aminotransferase [AST] is present in liver cells but is also present in cardiac, skeletal, kidney, and brain tissue; mildly elevated AST levels suggest alcoholic liver injury; elevation of liver ALP is indicative of intrahepatic or collecting system bile drainage abnormalities [cholestasis]; and elevated gamma-glutamyltransferase serum levels also indicate cholestasis).

lobes Upper, middle, and lower major divisions within each lung; further subdivided into bronchopulmonary segments that correspond to the distribution of a specific bronchus.

locus of control Attitude towards responsibility for one's behavior. Persons with an internal locus of control believe they can control their own destiny; those with an external locus of control tend to believe that their lives are controlled by forces outside themselves.

logarithm Extension of the use of scientific notation, originally invented to ease the difficulties of manual calculations of large or small numbers, in which logs (base 10) are the replacement of a whole number and an appropriate fraction for the real number (that is, log 10 = 1, log 15 = 1.176, log 150 = 2.176). The whole number position refers to the power of 10, and the decimals to the right refer to the actual numeric value.

long-term oxygen therapy (LTOT) Only pharmacologic intervention available for hypoxemic patients with COPD that has been shown to prolong survival.

lordosis Backward curvature of the spine.

Lund-Browder chart Tool used to evaluate the extent of cutaneous wounds and their potential influence on pulmonary function in patients with burn injuries.

lung protective ventilation strategy Ventilatory technique in which the plateau pressure is kept below 35 cm

H_2O, PEEP is applied to maintain alveolar recruitment, and F_{IO_2} is kept below 0.60.

lung transplantation   Transfer of a pulmonary organ system from a donor to a recipient; recognized as an accepted therapy for end-stage CF lung disease.

lung volume reduction surgery   Procedure that removes 20% to 30% of the lung tissue most severely affected by emphysema, encouraging the remaining lung to gain recoil elasticity and improve lung, chest wall, and diaphragmatic mechanics in addition to right ventricular performance.

macrophages   Cell type derived from blood monocytes or through local proliferation and that reside in many locations in the lung including the pleura, interstitium, and epithelial surface; associated with defending the lung against inhaled agents, and phagocytosing particulates and debris.

magnetic resonance imaging (MRI)   Useful imaging that takes advantage of nuclear magnetic resonance, in which nuclei with odd numbers of protons and a magnetic moment become aligned when they are placed in a strong magnetic field and are subsequently excited to a more energetic state with the addition of a radio frequency pulse; once allowed to relax, excited protons emit a resonance signal that is a reflection of the number of protons and their nuclear environment, and different relaxation signals are generated depending on the pulse sequence, the way in which the protons within the nuclei are excited.

malignant   Tending to become worse and to cause death; in the case of a cancer, it is anaplastic, invasive, and metastatic.

managed care   Health care system that seeks to eliminate redundant services and facilities, thereby reducing costs, through administrative control over primary health care services.

managed care organizations   Integrated network of doctors, hospitals and other health care providers that deliver health services to an insured population. The four different types of managed care organizations are the health maintenance organization (HMO), the preferred provider organization (PPO), the exclusive provider organization (EPO), and point-of-service plan (POS).

mandatory breath   Inspiration that is machine-triggered and/or machine-cycled.

manometric pressure   Static fluid pressure generated by the weight of the fluid and which varies on the basis of the density of fluid and height, reflecting the force of gravity.

Mantoux test   Placement of purified protein derivative (PPD) subcutaneously to detect the presence of an immune response to mycobacteria by eliciting a delayed-type hypersensitivity response.

manual resuscitator   Usually a ventilatory bag-valve device consisting of a self-inflating bag, an air-intake valve, a nonrebreathing valve, an oxygen inlet nipple, and oxygen reservoir to aid in resuscitation and breathing.

mask CPAP   Continuous positive airway pressure (CPAP) administered by face mask, relying on the patient to perform ventilation.

masking   Research technique for ensuring that the investigators and the participants are as aware as possible of the treatment being studied to avoid any tendency to prefer a specific outcome (bias).

mass medial aerodynamic diameter (MMAD)   Measurement that expresses the geometric size of the particles of an aerosol; for medical use, aerosol generators produce respirable particles with a mass median aerodynamic diameter (MMAD) between 1 to 5 µm.

mass number   Sum of the protons and neutrons inside the nucleus of an atom; often used interchangeably with the term "atomic weight."

mass spectrometer   Instrument capable of measuring all respiratory gases, including respiratory and anesthetic gases, breath by breath with greatest accuracy and with multichanneled units available to monitor several patients simultaneously; system aspirates sample gas into a vacuum chamber where it is ionized by an electron beam, accelerating the charged molecules through a magnetic field, where dispersion according to their mass and charge separates them before they reach a panel of detectors.

mast cells   Cells that produce histamine and leukotrienes which constrict airway smooth muscles; two types, classified according to neutral protease composition (chymase and/or tryptase).

matching   Research evaluation parameter of a study which asserts that the controls must be similar to the treatment group in as many respects as are feasible to avoid other factors from confounding (confusing) the results.

maximal expiratory pressure   After a full inhalation, the pressure generated by forced exhalation against an occluded airway.

maximal inspiratory pressure   After a full exhalation, the pressure generated by forced inhalation against an occluded airway.

MD Consult   Internet site designed to deliver authoritative medical information to physicians, available by subscription to its accesses; searches via MEDLINE, textbooks, practice guidelines, patient education handouts, and drug information.

mean airway pressure   Average pressure within the airway during one complete respiratory cycle; directly related to the inspiratory time, respiratory rate, peak inspiratory pressure, and positive end-expiratory pressure (PEEP).

mechanical insufflation-exsufflation   Technique in which a device inflates the lungs with positive pressure followed by a negative pressure to simulate a cough. Treatment consists of five cycles of MIE followed by 20 to 30 seconds of normal breathing, with repetitions until secretions are cleared.

meconium   Thick, dark green material that collects in the intestines of the full-term fetus and forms the first stools of a newborn; a mixture of intestinal gland secretions, some amniotic fluid, and intrauterine debris, such as bile pigments, fatty acids, epithelial cells, mucus, lanugo, and blood.

meconium aspiration syndrome   Condition that develops when the fetus or newborn inhales meconium; the most common cause of severe hypoxemic respiratory failure; can block the air passages and cause failure of the lungs to expand or other pulmonary dysfunction such as pneumonia or emphysema.

meconium ileus   Obstruction of the small intestine in the newborn resulting from an impaction of thick, dry, cohesive meconium, usually occurring at or near the ileocecal valve.

mediastinoscopy Examination of the mediastinum, using an endoscope with light and lenses inserted through an incision in the suprasternum.

mediastinum Area between the two pleural sacs that contains the heart, great vessels, esophagus, and thymus.

Medicaid Payment program funded jointly by federal and state governments to pay for medical services for the elderly, disabled, poor, and dependent children.

medical gas cylinders Containers used to store medical gas. They range from small, lightweight units containing a few cubic feet of gas to large cylinders of several hundred cubic feet. DOT regulations specify that high-pressure medical gas cylinders be made of seamless construction from high-quality steel, chromium-molybdenum alloy, or aluminum.

medical gases Gases used for medical purposes.

medical record Collection of documentation of patient assessments, problem identification, care plans, treatments, and outcomes, typically including discharge summaries, progress notes, physician orders, laboratory results, and flow sheets, as well as additional media, which may include online reports, photographs, videotapes, films, and audio recordings.

Medicare Federal government's health insurance program for the elderly, the disabled, and persons with certain diseases, such as end-stage renal disease.

MEDLINE Premier database of the National Library of Medicine (NLM), covering the fields of medicine, nursing, dentistry, veterinary medicine, the health care system, and preclinical sciences.

metabolic acidosis A decrease in pH associated with a loss of buffer (HCO_3^-).

metabolic alkalosis An increase in pH associated with an increase in buffer (HCO_3^-).

metastasis Process by which tumor cells spread to distant parts of the body.

methemoglobin Form of hemoglobin that is produced when the iron in heme is oxidized from Fe^{+2} to Fe^{+3}.

methylxanthine Traditional agent in the care of patients with COPD; declining in popularity for long-term care. Methylxanthines, however, provide significant bronchodilator effects in patients with COPD, although less than that observed with anticholinergic and beta$_2$-agonist agents.

MIGET Multiple inert gas elimination technique; based on the straightforward principles governing inert gas elimination by the lung, such that when an inert gas in solution is infused into systemic veins, the proportion of gas eliminated by ventilation from a lung unit depends only on the solubility of the gas and the $\dot{V}_A/\dot{Q}$ ratio of that unit.

mild intermittent asthma Least severe of the four classes of asthma severity, characterized by symptoms of coughing or wheezing less than 2 times per week with asymptomatic or normal peak expiratory flows (PEF) between brief exacerbations, nocturnal symptoms of coughing, wheezing, or breathlessness less than 2 times per month, and measured FEV$_1$ or PEF consistently more than 80% of predicted, while maintaining less than 20% variability in PEF routinely.

mild persistent asthma Category of asthma characterized by symptoms of coughing or wheezing more than 2 times per week but less than once per day with symptoms that affect normal daily activities of living or normal nighttime sleep patterns, nocturnal symptoms of coughing, wheezing, or breathlessness more than 2 times per month, and measured FEV$_1$ or PEF consistently more than 80% of predicted or personal best, while maintaining approximately 20% to 30% variability in PEF rates.

mitochondrial myopathy One of the manifestations of hereditary mitochondrial disorders, occurring as a result of a point mutation in mitochondrial DNA; can also affect other organ systems, particularly the brain.

mixed apnea Combination of central and obstructive apnea.

mode of ventilation Represents a combination of control, phase, and conditional variables that establish a set pattern of spontaneous and/or mandatory breaths.

moderate persistent asthma Category of asthma characterized by symptoms of coughing or wheezing on a near-daily basis, with exacerbations experienced more than 2 times per week, and often persisting for multiple days; manifests symptoms that routinely interfere with normal daily activities of living or normal nighttime sleep patterns and nocturnal symptoms of coughing, wheezing, or breathlessness more than 1 time per week, plus measured FEV$_1$ or PEF routinely 60% to 80% of predicted or personal best, while consistently maintaining more than 30% variability in PEF rates.

molar solution Solution containing 1 mole (mol) of solute per liter of solution.

mold Form of fungus that grows as long multicellular forms called *hyphae*, which associate to form structures called *mycelia*.

mole Quantity of a substance equal to its gram molecular weight, which contains 6.02×10^{23} atoms (Avogadro's number).

molecular diffusion Transport mechanism derived from random thermal oscillation of a molecule; so long as the molecules have a constant temperature, molecular diffusion always occurs and is responsible for gas exchange at the level of the alveolar-capillary membrane.

monitoring Continuous, or nearly continuous, evaluation of the physiologic function of a patient for the purpose of guiding management decisions, including when to make therapeutic interventions and assessment of those interventions.

monoplace chamber Hyperbaric chamber for one person with one lock and compressed with 100% oxygen.

monosaccharide Basic unit of the carbohydrate molecule; a simple sugar.

moral philosophy Individual's behavioral code, defining behavior in a given situation, based on personal principles the individual has previously adopted.

motivation Patient's interest in changing an undesirable behavior associated with his or her condition.

mouth occlusion pressure ($P_{0.1}$) Test of central respiratory drive that is independent of underlying respiratory mechanics; maximum negative mouth pressure generated during the first 100 milliseconds (0.1 seconds) of inspiration measured during complete airway occlusion.

mucociliary apparatus Mechanism that clears inhaled agents from the lower respiratory tract.

mucokinetic agent Drug, such as acetylcysteine, intended to reduce mucus viscosity and assist with the mobilization of airway secretions.

multiplace chamber A hyperbaric chamber compressed with air and designed for more than one person and with more than one lock (not including a medical lock).

multiple sclerosis (MS) Demyelinating disease of the central nervous system characterized clinically by repeated remissions and exacerbations of symptoms, including paresthesias, motor weakness, diplopia, blurred vision, bladder incontinence, and ataxia.

multiple sleep latency testing (MSLT) Test that determines a person's propensity to fall asleep. A mean MSLT of 15 minutes is normal for a well-rested adult; a mean MSLT of less than 5 minutes indicates severe hypersomnia.

Munchausen syndrome by proxy Psychiatric disorder in which a caretaking individual, usually a parent, stages and even induces serious illness in his or her child or charge, usually for the purpose of seeking attention and interaction with medical personnel.

murmur Extra cardiac sound heard in conjunction with S_1 and S_2.

muscarinic agent Substance that stimulates the postganglionic parasympathetic receptor.

muscular dystrophy Heterogeneous group of progressive, hereditary degenerative skeletal muscle diseases in which the respiratory muscles, like any skeletal muscle, become progressively weak, eventually culminating in respiratory failure and death (respiratory complications are the most common cause of death in these diseases).

mutuality Characteristic considered essential in nurturing a relationship by agreeing on the problems and the means to resolve them.

myasthenia gravis (MG) Autoimmune disorder characterized by impaired transmission of neural impulses across the neuromuscular junction resulting from the destruction of the postsynaptic acetylcholine receptors.

mycobacterial pneumonia Any of a group of pneumonias caused by tuberculous and non-tuberculous mycobacteria (NTM) and diagnosed by acid-fast bacilli (AFB) smears and mycobacterial cultures, using nucleic acid probes to detect *Mycobacterium tuberculosis*, *Mycobacterium avium complex*, *Mycobacterium gordonae*, and/or *Mycobacterium kansasii*.

mycosis Any fungal disease.

myocardial ischemia Condition of inadequate blood flow in the coronary arteries that supply the heart muscle; often results in angina.

myocardial perfusion imaging Imaging technique that involves intravenous injection of a radionuclide agent, which accumulates in the myocardium in proportion to regional myocardial perfusion.

nasal continuous positive airway pressure (nCPAP) Therapeutic support for potential low lung volumes and associated hypoxemia (particularly in infants). nCPAP is also commonly used in the treatment of obstructive sleep apnea (OSA).

nasopharyngeal airway Plastic or rubber airway device inserted into the nose and directed along the floor of the nose parallel to the hard palate; available as an alternative to the oropharyngeal airway.

nasopharynx Uppermost region of the throat or pharynx, behind the nasal cavity and extending from the posterior nares to the level of the soft palate.

nasotracheal intubation Intubation technique used for specific indications, such as when access to the mouth is to be avoided, in oral surgery or oral trauma, or when the mouth cannot be opened adequately as in trauma, temporomandibular joint (TMJ) dysfunction, or mandibular fixation.

nasotracheal suction Maneuver used to remove secretions from the lower respiratory tract.

National Association of Apnea Professionals (NAAP) Professional organization of physicians, respiratory therapists, and other medical personnel who provide care for infants with apnea and related disorders.

National Association of Medical Directors of Respiratory Care (NAMDRC) Official corporate sponsor of the AARC, as of 1997.

National Asthma Education and Prevention Program Expert panel of the National Institutes of Health focusing specifically on the needs of, and programs affecting, individuals with asthma.

National Board for Respiratory Care, Inc. (NBRC) Voluntary health certifying board founded in 1960 for the purpose of the evaluation of professional competence for respiratory therapists by providing high-quality voluntary credentialing examinations for respiratory care and pulmonary function technology.

nebulizer Device that produces an aerosol, or suspension, of particles in gas.

negative pressure ventilation Use of a ventilator that applies less than ambient pressure to the external chest wall.

neoadjuvant therapy Preliminary cancer treatment, such as chemotherapy or radiation, that usually precedes another phase of treatment.

neuromuscular blocker Chemical substance that interferes locally with the transmission or reception of impulses from motor nerves to skeletal muscles.

neuromuscular disease Any one of a diverse group of disorders ranging from primary muscle diseases that impair all skeletal muscle functions to selected involvement of the diaphragm.

neutral thermal environment Environment that provides adequate warmth and humidity to minimize insensible heat and water loss for premature and newborn infants; can be achieved with an incubator or Isolette for a premature, sick, or low–birth weight infant.

neutron Particle with no mass but net charge located inside the nucleus of an atom.

nicotinic receptor Cholinergic receptor that is sensitive to nicotine acetylcholine, responding to stimulation with electrical depolarization of the muscular cell membranes.

nitric oxide Colorless gas that is naturally synthesized in human tissue and plays an important role in vascular smooth muscle relaxation, inhibition of platelet aggregation, neurotransmission, and immune regulation.

nitrogen balance Study involving a 24-hour urine collection and calculation of the difference between nitrogen intake and excretion; helps determine protein requirements and assess changes in visceral protein store status over time.

nitrogen dioxide (NO_2) Irritating brownish gas that can be produced spontaneously from NO and O_2.

nitrous oxide Colorless, odorless, and tasteless gas that can be used with oxygen as an anesthetic; referred to as "laughing gas."

nocturnal asthma Marker for uncontrolled or more severe asthma; includes mechanisms that seem to revolve around circadian alterations of body temperature, vagal tone, mediators, inflammation, epinephrine and β_2-receptor function, and possible gastroesophageal reflux, aspiration, sinusitis, increased mucus production, sleep apnea, and the normal decrease in lung function of patients sleeping.

noncompetitive inhibition Form of inhibition in which a substance occupies a receptor and cannot be displaced from the receptor by increasing the number of other molecules through the principle of mass action.

noninvasive positive pressure ventilation (NPPV) Mechanical ventilation provided noninvasively (by mask or similar interface) rather than through an endotracheal tube or tracheostomy.

nonmaleficence Principle in which the health care practitioner refrains from harming the patient.

nonprotected bronchial brush Instrument used for cytologic sampling of proximal airways and central tumors under direct vision or of peripheral lesions under fluoroscopic guidance; a catheter with a brush (open or enclosed in a sheath) at its distal end is introduced through the working channel of the bronchoscope for sampling of proximal airways or central tumors.

nonrebreathing mask Oxygen mask with a one-way valve between the bag and the mask and another one-way valve over one or both mask ports, causing all of the patient's exhaled volume to be directed out of the mask through the mask ports. The valve positioned between the mask and bag prevents exhaled gases from entering the bag.

non–REM sleep stages Phases of sleep during which there is an absence of rapid eye movement. Non-REM sleep is subdivided into four stages based on EEG patterns: stages 1 and 2 are considered light sleep, and stages 3 and 4 are termed "deep sleep" or "slow-wave sleep."

non–small cell carcinoma Major category of histologic types of lung carcinomas, including adenocarcinoma of the lung, large-cell carcinoma, and squamous cell carcinoma.

nonsteroidal antiinflammatory Drug or agent with antipyretic, analgesic, and antiinflammatory effects to counteract or reduce inflammation by inhibiting prostaglandin synthesis.

normal flora Bacteria that normally exist in a particular area of the healthy body and which do not usually cause disease at that site.

nosocomial pneumonia Pneumonia that is acquired in the hospital or nursing home.

nucleic acid Organic molecule, principally occurring as either deoxyribonucleic acid (DNA) or ribonucleic acid (RNA), that is made from chains of nucleotide, each of which consists of a phosphate group, a 5-carbon sugar, and a nitrogenous base.

numeric integration formula One method for approximating a definite integral; also called the *Riemann Sum*.

obstructive apnea Reduction in airflow to less than 90% of baseline despite persistent respiratory effort.

Ohm's law Principle describing properties of electric systems, assuming linear relations between a pressure, resistance, and flow term, without loss of thermal energy, or turbulence, thus allowing application of easily measured quantities, such as electric resistance, to other circular systems of single or connected circuits in which measure-

ment may be more technically difficult; the most general expression of this law describes the relation of voltage, resistance, and impedance.

oncotic pressure Osmotic pressure of a colloid in solution, such as exists in a higher concentration of protein in the plasma on one side of a cell membrane than in the neighboring interstitial fluid.

open-loop control Means of mechanical system control in which change in the input causes a change in the output but without flow of information from the output to generate a new input to "close the loop."

opiate Natural or synthetic derivative of morphine, derived from the opium poppy, stimulating mu (μ), delta (δ), and kappa (κ) opiate receptors in the brain and spinal cord to decrease the sensation of pain; also acts as a potent sedative or cough suppressant.

optode Intraarterial sensor placed through an arterial cannula and into an artery.

oral appliance Dental device for clinical use; can be characterized primarily as either a tongue retaining device (TRD) or mandibular advancing device (MAD).

oropharyngeal airway Airway device with a relatively rigid structure designed to be inserted into the mouth between the lips and teeth and extend from the lips to the pharynx, following the natural curvature of the tongue, without entering the larynx or esophagus.

oropharynx One of three components of the throat or pharynx, extending behind the mouth from the soft palate to the hyoid bone; contains the palatine and lingual tonsils.

orthopnea Breathlessness, especially when recumbent.

ORYX Set of requirements established by the Joint Commission on Accreditation of Healthcare Organizations (JCAHO) for medical information management that places a greater emphasis on performance as measured against external norms.

osmosis Process of transferring water molecules through a semipermeable membrane; involves the movement of water from an area of high concentration of water to an area of low concentration in an attempt to make the concentrations equal.

osmotic pressure Externally applied hydrostatic pressure that stops the flow of a solvent through a membrane.

osteoporosis Decrease in the amount of bone mass, which can lead to fractures after minimal trauma.

osteoradionecrosis Radiation tissue damage.

outcomes indicators Factors used in clinical quality outcome measures, including cost, service, and tracking of the patient not only during an episode of care but also between episodes of care and throughout the lifetime, as well as the long-term health status of the community.

outcomes research Utilization of statistics methods for scientific validation of interventions as they impact similar patient types in addition to the outcomes measures focused at the person-specific and short-term period.

Ovid Online technology service with more than 90 databases including MEDLINE and CINAHL, a Cumulative Index to Nursing and Allied Health Literature, with direct full-text versions for articles in more than 300 leading medical journals and several ease-of-use features.

oxidative phosphorylation Joining of a phosphate group to adenosine diphosphate (ADP) to form ATP during catabolism.

oximeter   Spectrophotometer using specific wavelengths in the oxyhemoglobin spectrum to measure hemoglobin oxegen saturation in the blood.

oximetry   Determination of the hemoglobin oxygen saturation of arterial blood using an oximeter.

oxygen analyzer   Device used to measure the concentration of oxygen administered to patients.

oxygen cannula   Most widely used device for administering low-flow oxygen to infants, children, and adults in the hospital and in the home; consists of a delivery tube that ends in two short prongs, each about one-half inch in length, made of soft, pliable plastic.

oxygen catheter   Standard low-flow oxygen delivery system of choice until the late 1960s (rarely used today); consists of a soft, pliable plastic tube about 12 inches in length with a series of small holes at the distal end and a fitting at the other end to connect it to the oxygen supply tubing.

oxygen concentrator   Device designed to produce a low flow (0.5 to 5.0 L/min) of high-purity oxygen (90% to 95%) from room air by either molecular adsorption of nitrogen or filtration of air through a membrane; the most widely used source of oxygen in the home and extended care facilities.

oxygen conserver   Device that supplies a flow of oxygen only when it is needed, on demand at the initiation of inspiration. The conserver is placed between the oxygen supply and the delivery device, which can be a nasal catheter, nasal cannula, or transtracheal catheter.

oxygen consumption ($\dot{V}O_2$)   Rate of O_2 uptake by the body, measured by analyzing inspired and expired O_2 in a ventilator circuit (approximately 220 to 250 mL/min in the adult under resting conditions); equal to cardiac output multiplied by the arterial-venous content difference.

oxygen delivery   Rate of O_2 transport to the peripheral tissues, expressed as DO_2, and also referred to as O_2 *availability* or O_2 *transport*; determined by the cardiac output and arterial O_2 content.

oxygen extraction ratio   Derived parameter relating the amount of oxygen removed by the peripheral tissues to the amount contained in the arterial blood, or global oxygen consumption divided by oxygen delivery.

oxygen hood   Round or rectangular, bottomless, clear rigid plastic device with a half moon-shaped cutout that allows it to be placed over the infant's neck and encloses the entire head. Because only the infant's head is enclosed, the body is accessible for medical and nursing care procedures.

oxygen tent   Device used for both oxygen administration and for high humidity therapy. Adult tents were widely used through the 1960s; however, they have been replaced by nasal cannulae and masks.

oxygen toxicity   Pathologic response of the body and its tissues from long-term exposure to high partial pressures of oxygen.

oxyhemoglobin equilibrium curve (OEC)   Nonlinear in vivo relationship between PO_2 and O_2 saturation; first demonstrated by Paul Bert in 1878; commonly called the *oxyhemoglobin dissociation curve.*

pack years   Measure of patient's smoking exposure; one pack a day for 1 year equals 1 pack year.

pallor   Diminished skin color accompanying anemia or in severe peripheral vasoconstriction accompanying shock.

palpation   Examiner's use of his or her hands to feel for body movement, lumps, masses, and skin characteristics.

paradoxic respirations   Flail chest movement, characterized by chest wall movement outward on expiration and inward on inspiration.

paralinguistics   Factor affecting communication on either a conscious or unconscious level through the use of sounds such as giggling, laughing, belittling, *ah*'s and *um*'s, cracking knuckles, or silence.

parameter   Particular aspect of a variable such as the peak or mean value.

parenteral   Intravenous, intramuscular, and subcutaneous routes of drug administration, which all bypass the gastrointestinal system.

parenteral nutrition   Administration of nutrients by a route other than the alimentary canal.

parietal pleura   Serous membrane of mesothelial cells and connective tissue that lines the chest wall, covers the diaphragm, and extends over the structures of the mediastinum.

Parkinson's disease   See *parkinsonism.*

parkinsonism   Group of neurologic disorders characterized by hypokinesia, tremor, and muscular rigidity.

paroxysmal nocturnal dyspnea   Sudden shortness of breath that occurs several hours after a patient lies down; suggests cardiac dysfunction.

partial liquid ventilation (PLV)   Process in which the lungs are partially filled with perfluorocarbon and a conventional ventilator provides gas ventilation. The perfluorocarbon is administered by direct instillation into the endotracheal tube.

partial-rebreathing mask   Simple oxygen mask with the addition of a 300- to 600-mL reservoir bag. The oxygen supply tube is positioned between the mask and the reservoir bag, and the oxygen flow is set at a rate sufficient to keep the bag at least partially inflated throughout inspiration.

partial thromboplastin time (PTT)   Clotting time in anticoagulation therapy, best if 2 to 2.5 times the control.

Pascal   Under the SI system, the primary unit of pressure, that is, one Newton/meter^2; for ease of calculation, the kilopascal (kPa) is commonly used, so that one standard atmosphere (at sea level) is approximately 101 kPa.

Pascal's law   Observation that pressure is transmitted without reduction throughout any enclosed static fluid.

passive expiration   Expiration in which the respiratory system is responding to a sudden release of inspiratory pressure that requires no muscular effort.

passive humidification   System of humidification that uses exhaled heat and moisture to humidify the inspired gas; a heat and moisture exchanger (HME) is a passive humidifier.

passover humidifier   Humidifying device that directs gas over the surface of a body of water; example includes the passover wick humidifier.

pathologic apnea   Category or type of cessation of air flow that disrupts breathing for at least 20 seconds, accompanied by bradycardia with heart rate reduction of 20% below baseline or oxygen saturation below 80%.

Patient Bill of Rights   Professional code established by the American Hospital Association to outline the rights and responsibilities patients have regarding their medical care, including their right to refuse treatment to the extent permitted by law and to be informed of the medical consequences of their actions.

patient-controlled analgesia (PCA) Popular method of pain control in which the patient can self-administer portions of a preset amount of intravascular pain medication; the computerized device administers portions and includes a lockout interval to automatically inactivate the system if a patient tries to increase the amount of drug used within a predetermined time period.

patient-ventilator dyssynchrony A condition in which the patient is not breathing in sychrony with the ventilator.

PCO_2 One of three primary measurements made in arterial blood gas analysis; significant in assessing ventilation.

peak flow meter Monitoring device for the management of asthma.

pectus carinatum Condition in which the chest bows out at the sternum similar to that of a pigeon.

pectus excavatum Condition in which the sternum is depressed and deviated somewhat like a funnel.

pendeluft ventilation Result of gas mixing between lung regions that have different time constants; also called *out-of-phase ventilation;* motion of gas between two neighboring units during phasic ventilation.

penetrating trauma Chest trauma that results from knife and gun shot wounds and whose mechanism of injury depends on the velocity and size of the penetrating object.

peptide Compound created when amino acids are linked together, the OH from the carboxyl group of one amino acid and the H from the amine group of another amino acid splitting off.

peptide bond Bond between the amino acids is called a *peptide bond.*

percent cycle time Ratio of inspiratory time to total cycle time expressed as a percentage.

percent solution Concentration measure of a solute usually expressed with units of mass or volume in ratios such as weight/weight, weight/volume, and volume/volume; commonly used in clinical situations.

percussion Examination technique in which the examiner places a finger firmly against a body part and then strikes that finger with a fingertip from the other hand, producing sounds that may suggest normal or abnormal tissue.

percussion therapy Technique of rapidly clapping, cupping, or striking the external thorax directly over the lung segment being drained, with either cupped hands or a mechanical device.

pericardiocentesis Procedure that is commonly used in the treatment of cardiac tamponade and involves removing blood from the pericardial sac by placing a needle into the pericardium and withdrawing the accumulated blood.

pericardium Fibroserous sac around the heart and the roots of the great vessels.

periodic breathing Regular respiration of up to 20 seconds followed by apnea periods of no more than 10 seconds occurring three times or more in succession; may be a normal event for some patients.

periodic leg movements of sleep Condition characterized by pathologic repetitive myoclonic contractions, which can result in frequent arousals or awakenings and can cause daytime symptoms such as excessive daytime sleepiness.

permissive hypercapnia High PaCO_2 resulting from protective ventilation strategies.

pH Expression of the concentration or strength of an acid or base; indicates the hydrogen ion concentration [H+] in a solution; mathematically defined as the negative logarithm of the hydrogen ion concentration.

pharmacodynamics Drug's action in the body, both at a molecular level and in terms of overall clinical effect.

pharmacokinetics Drug's movement in the body through the processes of absorption, distribution, and elimination.

pharmacology Science describing the chemical entities of drugs and their interactions with the body, focusing in particular on these five aspects of each drug: (1) its chemical and physical properties, (2) the movement of drug into, through, and out of the body (pharmacokinetics), (3) the effect of the drug on the body (pharmacodynamics), (4) drug indications and dosages, and (5) side effects and toxicity.

phase variable One of four factors measured and used to start, sustain, and end any phase of the respiration cycle: pressure, volume, flow, and time.

phospholipid Lipid similar to triglyceride except that instead of three fatty acids attached to a glycerol, one of the fatty acid chains is replaced by a chemical structure containing phosphorus and nitrogen; its "head" is composed of the phosphorus and nitrogen group, and its two "tails" are composed of the two fatty acids so that the head attracts water (hydrophilic) while the tails repel it (hydrophobic), allowing it to bridge or join two different chemical environments; a primary component of cell membranes and of pulmonary surfactant.

photoplethysmography Noninvasive technology to measure blood pressure that uses a small finger cuff and a technique similar to pulse oximetry: a light source and detector built into the cuff measure the absorption of a specific wavelength of light passed across the arterial bed of the finger; as the cuff inflates, it eliminates the pulsatile component of absorption, and cuff pressure equals intraarterial pressure.

physician extender Newer role of the respiratory therapist to help physicians meet goals of decreasing ER visits and hospital admissions by providing services their patients need in the physician office setting and providing the respiratory therapist more opportunity for primary care, rather than acute or critical care and patient education about their disease, treatment techniques, and medications, in addition to other aspects of general daily medical care.

piezoelectric plethysmography Type of plethysmography apparatus that replaces the wire coils from the elastic belts with a piezoelectric buckle, which encloses a sensor to generate a voltage in response to stretch passed through the ends of the belts.

Pin Index Safety System One of three indexing safety systems for medical gases. This system uses a specific combination of two holes in the post valve just below the gas outlet for each gas or gas mixture; any regulator or devise intended to connect to the valve will have pins that correspond to the holes, allowing a proper connection.

plateau pressure End-inspiratory peak alveolar pressure attained during mechanical ventilation and which should, ideally, be kept below 30 cm H_2O, in conjunction with overall lung protective ventilation strategy.

platelets Blood cells critical to clot formation after vascular injury; produced in the bone marrow.

platypnea Difficulty breathing unless lying flat.

plethora Fullness of blood vessels at the skin surface, often occurring with vasodilation or hypercapnia.

plethysmography See *body plethysmography*.

pleura Serous membrane enclosing the lung and composed of a single layer of flat mesothelial cells on a delicate membrane of connective tissue.

pleural friction rub Continuous grating sound heard in auscultation of the lungs; resembles two pieces of leather or two hands being rubbed together; occurring when pleurae are inflamed or when fluid accumulates in the pleural cavity.

pleural space Space between the visceral and parietal layers of the pleurae.

pneumobelt Unconventional ventilation that consists of an inflatable rubber bladder held over the abdomen by an adjustable corset and assists diaphragmatic motion by causing piston-like motions of the abdominal viscera.

pneumogram 12- to 24-Hour recording of heart rate, respiratory impedance, oxygen saturation, nasal-oral airflow, and esophageal pH.

pneumonia Any of several subgroups of respiratory infections that are among the most frequent clinical problems respiratory therapists encounter and the sixth leading cause of death in the United States; characterized by the inflammation and consolidation of lung tissue caused by infectious agents.

pneumothorax Air in the pleural space that can cause collapse of the lung and shortness of breath; may result following blunt chest injury resulting from direct puncture of the lung by a fractured rib, with deceleration injuries causing a tear in the lung tissue, or as a result of a crush injury rupturing alveoli.

PO$_2$ One of three primary measurements made in arterial blood gas analysis, significant in assessing oxygenation.

point of service Type of health insurance plan that is a hybrid of the HMO and PPO plans. Point-of-service plans attempt to provide the tight utilization controls of the HMO coupled with the ability to choose a nonparticipating provider at the point (time) of receiving the service, thus the name "point of service."

polar Type of molecule that forms as the result of unequal charge distribution on a molecule, rather than the sharing or transfer of electrons.

poliomyelitis Acute viral disease now rare in the United States, characterized by fever, sore throat, headache, and vomiting, with stiffness of neck and back; possibly progressing to involvement of the CNS, pleocytosis in the spinal fluid, and perhaps paralysis.

polymerase chain reaction (PCR) See also *antigen detection*. Newer technique applied to sputum samples to help in the rapid identification of pathogens that may be difficult to culture or pathogens scarcely growing because of prior antibiotic treatment; application of PCR to BAL fluid increases the sensitivity and is rapid in detecting CMV, PCP, and mycobacterial pulmonary infection.

polynomial function Linear or quadratic function whose highest power is called its *degree*; a linear function is a first-degree function, whereas a quadratic function is a second-degree function.

polysaccharide Type of carbohydrate that is a complex sugar.

polysomnogram 8- to 24-Hour comprehensive recording made in a special diagnostics lab; includes all multichannel respiratory recording variables with the addition of EEG, EOG, and EMG electrodes to determine sleep states, leg and intercostal muscle movements; typically performed on children and adults (but not infants) to provide definitive diagnosis of obstructive sleep apnea or narcolepsy; to evaluate sleep state disturbances; to determine effectiveness of OSA treatment/or refine treatment (such as CPAP or mask ventilation); to evaluate the relationship of sleep disturbances to seizures or GER; to document presence or absence of OSA in patients with enlarged tonsils/adenoids; to document the absence of OSA following surgery.

Pores of Kohn Openings between alveoli that allow collateral ventilation between adjacent alveoli.

portable pressure ventilator Device designed to provide noninvasive positive-pressure ventilation (NPPV); examples are the BiPAP/ST series, Synchrony BiPAP, VPAP, and Knightstar 335. Features include the delivery of pressure support ventilation, small size and lightweight design, continuous flow, flows that vary according to patient demand, lack of sophisticated alarms (with a few exceptions), flow compensation for leaks, dependence on leak to clear CO_2, tidal volume monitoring, and responsive triggering.

portable volume ventilator Device designed to deliver alternate site mechanical ventilation. First- and second-generation models vary in terms of size, weight, cost, and reliability.

positive end-expiratory pressure (PEEP) Addition of positive airway pressure during the exhalation phase.

positive expiratory pressure (PEP) Airway clearance technique in which the patient exhales against a fixed-orifice flow resistor to aid in the movement of secretions into the larger airways.

positron emission tomography (PET) Imaging modality used for assessing thoracic pathology, in particular for tumor imaging, providing physiologic and metabolic information, focusing on the biochemical properties of cells.

postpoliomyelitis muscular dystrophy Progressive muscle weakness occurring, on average, 29 years after recovery from an acute episode of acute poliomyelitis.

postural drainage Use of positioning and gravity to drain secretions from areas of the bronchi and lungs into the trachea.

potency Amount of drug necessary to achieve a given level of effect; a more potent drug will produce the same effect at a lower concentration than a lower potency drug.

practice variation Gap in feasibility for clinicians using outcomes research, as imposed by the type of practice or care setting and possible limitations to conducting research, especially in terms of time, statistical relevant subject number, and financial resources.

PRECEDE-PROCEED model Model heavily used in the health promotion movement, focusing on factors external to the individual that shape health care behavior. In addition to issues of motivation and self-care, one's physical and psychological state can also have a major bearing on readiness to learn. The acronym PRECEDE stands for *p*redisposing, *r*einforcing, and *e*nabling constructs in *e*ducation/*e*nvironmental *d*iagnosis and *e*valuation; the acronym PROCEED stands for *p*olicy, *r*egulatory, and *o*rganizational *c*onstructs in *e*ducational and *e*nvironmental *d*evelopment.

precipitate Crystallization of a solute.

precordium Part of the front chest wall that overlays the heart and epigastrium.

preferred provider organization Organization in which member physicians, pharmacists, and hospitals offer their health services to subscriber patients on a discounted fee-for-service basis.

preload Distending pressure within the ventricle during diastole.

President's Council Ex-officio member group of the BOD consisting of past presidents of the AARC.

pressure amplitude Means for manipulating in P_{CO_2} level during HFOV; increasing the amplitude increases displacement of the bellows, thus increasing tidal volume delivery, which is measured as an increased pressure amplitude at the airway opening and results in a lower Pa_{CO_2}.

pressure-controlled ventilation (PCV) Mode of ventilation in which airway pressure is set and remains constant with changes in resistance and compliance; may prevent localized alveolar overdistention with changes in resistance and compliance.

pressure trigger Effort or force required to trigger the ventilator, representing an imposed load for the patient, occurring in response to a pressure drop in the system.

pressurized metered dose inhaler (pMDI) The most commonly prescribed method of aerosol delivery; used to administer bronchodilators, anticholinergics, antiinflammatory agents, and steroids. A pMDI consists of a pressurized canister containing a drug in the form of a micronized powder or solution that is suspended with a mixture of propellants, surfactant, preservatives, flavoring agents, and dispersal agents.

prevalence Rate of how many persons have a given disease or condition in a location at a given time.

prevention See *disease prevention*.

primary pulmonary hypertension (PPH) Uncommon disorder of the pulmonary vessels associated with severe elevation in pulmonary vascular resistance.

principle of double effects Situation in which the benefits or beneficence of a treatment is accompanied by undesired side effects that could cause harm.

problem-based learning Teaching-learning model designed to facilitate critical thinking and clinical decision-making abilities, using equal participation of students in small problem-solving groups to promote self-directed learning and enhance students' abilities to develop their reasoning and communication skills.

programmed instruction Learning method and materials that allow the patient to learn at his or her own pace and require little time on the part of the respiratory therapy patient educator.

prone position Position in which the patient is lying face downward. Changing patients with ARDS from a supine to a prone position may result in a significant improvement in oxygenation; prone positioning may also improve secretion clearance from the lungs.

prospective payment system (PPS) Managed care type of reimbursement in which the hospital or health care facility receives a set fee per diagnosis on each patient covered.

With PPS, health care professionals provide whatever care they feel is appropriate, and if the care costs less than the set fee that is paid, they make a profit. PPS is a popular replacement for the more traditional "fee-for-service" approach to paying for medical care.

prospective studies Studies that are proposed and then conducted to avoid bias.

prostacyclin (epoprostenol, PGI_2) Pulmonary vasodilator that has proven to be the most effective therapy available in the treatment of patients with primary pulmonary hypertension.

prostaglandin Lipid composed of a 20-carbon unsaturated fatty acid that contains a 5-carbon ring; often referred to as a tissue hormone.

protected specimen brush (PSB) Collection device used in the quantitative culture of bronchoscopic specimens in the diagnosis of ventilator-associated pneumonia.

protein Large molecule composed of carbon, hydrogen, oxygen, and nitrogen; formed when a long chain of peptides reaches about 100 amino acids or more in length.

protein-calorie malnutrition (PCM) Nutritional deficit affecting all muscle fiber types, impairing fast-twitch fibers most profoundly, resulting in decreased contractile strength; the primary component of the immune system adversely affected by protein-calorie malnutrition is cell-mediated immunity.

prothrombin time (PT) Test for coagulation defects, used to evaluate the extrinsic pathway, depending on the levels of factors V, VII, X, and eventually I and II.

protocols Written plans specifying the procedures to be followed in giving a particular examination, in conducting research, or in providing care for a certain condition.

proton Particle with a charge of positive one ($+1$) located inside the nucleus of an atom.

proto-oncogene Gene that can potentially be a primary inducer of cancer.

provider Health care professional offering diagnostic, assessment, treatment, guidance, educational, or evaluative services to patients and health care clientele.

proxemics Form of nonverbal cues that affect communication through interpretation of space.

prudent heart living Risk factor reduction approach to reducing cardiovascular disease that includes weight control, physical fitness, smart eating habits, and avoidance of stress and cigarette smoking.

psychomotor One of three learning domains, entailing "doing."

psychosocial assessment Important step prior to participation in a pulmonary rehabilitation program since the most common emotional consequences of COPD are depression and anxiety, both of which can further reinforce social isolation and inactivity.

PubMed Free search tool provided by the NLM to search MEDLINE, with a retrieval engine that links articles in more than 400 journals.

pulmonary alveolar proteinosis Interstitial lung disease characterized by filling of alveolar spaces with a lipoproteinaceous exudate and interstitial fibrosis; usually presents with dyspnea and cough.

pulmonary angiography Radiographic examination of the blood vessels of the lungs after injection of an opaque contrast medium into the pulmonary circulation.

pulmonary arteries Arteries supplying blood to the lungs.

pulmonary artery catheter (PAC) Swan-Ganz catheter, which is inserted into the pulmonary artery, providing pressure measurements, cardiac output determinations, and mixed venous blood analysis.

pulmonary artery wedge pressure (PAWP) Measure that provides an estimate of left atrial (LA) and left ventricular end-diastolic or filling pressure (LVDEP).

pulmonary cachexia Debilitating muscle and weight loss, often seen in patients with severe COPD, lung cancer, and other respiratory diseases, and which has a negative effect on survival.

pulmonary contusion Bruise in the lung that is usually the primary culprit in gas exchange abnormalities following chest trauma.

pulmonary edema Accumulation of excess fluid in the interstitial and alveolar spaces in the lung.

pulmonary embolism (PE) Blockage of a pulmonary artery by foreign matter, such as fat, air, tumor tissue, or a thrombus; characterized by dyspnea, sudden chest pain, shock, and cyanosis.

pulmonary hypertension Abnormally high pressure within the pulmonary circulation.

pulmonary hypoplasia Incomplete development or underdevelopment of lung tissue.

pulmonary rehabilitation Any of a variety of outpatient programs that provide opportunities to restore patients to the highest possible level of independence and functioning in the community; typically includes exercise training, education for patients and family, instruction in respiratory and chest physiotherapy, and psychologic support.

pulmonary vascular resistance (PVR) Resistance in the pulmonary vascular bed against which the right ventricle must eject blood.

pulse oximetry Technique that measures oxyhemoglobin saturation noninvasively in arterial blood; rapidly detects changes in arterial oxygen saturation.

pulsus paradoxus Abnormal decrease in systolic pressure and pulse wave amplitude during inspiration.

purified protein derivative (PPD) Dried form of tuberculin injected subcutaneously during a Mantoux test to detect past or present infections with tubercle bacilli by eliciting a delayed-type hypersensitivity response.

pursed-lip breathing Respiration characterized by prolonged expirations through pursed lips; done to help prevent airway closure.

quadratic function Type of second-degree polynomial function.

quadriplegia Paralysis of the arms, legs, and trunk of the body below the level of an associated injury to the spinal cord, usually caused by spinal cord injury.

qualitative outcomes Categorization of outcomes of respiratory care that includes respiratory therapist job satisfaction, patient satisfaction with a rehabilitation program, and recruitment success.

quality outcomes Categorization of outcomes of respiratory care that includes mortality, missed or delayed aerosol therapy treatments, and readmission rates from skilled nursing facilities for patients with pneumonia.

quantitative outcomes Categorization of outcomes of respiratory care that include length of stay (LOS) in acute care hospital, mortality rate, respiratory therapist turnover rates and recruitment costs, and number of missed or delayed aerosol therapy treatments.

quick reliever medication Any of a group of primarily short-acting agonists used to combat acute exacerbations of bronchoconstriction or provide quick, complete resolution of airflow obstruction and its accompanying symptoms of cough, wheezing, and chest tightness; includes short-acting β_2-agonist and anticholinergics.

racemic A mixture of two complementary stereoisomers, or racemates, that makes it optically inactive under polarized light.

radiation therapy Primary treatment of the intrathoracic tumor or for metastatic disease, involving the use of x-rays or gamma rays to slow or stop the proliferation of malignant cells.

radiographic opacity Property of an object in an x-ray image that proves it to be neither transparent nor translucent.

radionuclide angiocardiography Noninvasive technique for evaluating left ventricular function, using intravenous injection of a radioisotope (most commonly technetium-99m) and the use of a gamma-ray scintillation camera to detect the isotope's signal within the left ventricle.

Raman spectroscopy Method used to measure CO_2 in capnographs.

rate of change Amount of change in a function's dependent variable for a given change in the independent variable.

receptor Chemical structure on the surface of a cell that combines with an antigen to produce a discrete immunologic component; also, a sensory nerve ending that responds to various kinds of stimulation.

recruitment maneuver Sustained inflation at high airway pressure that has been advocated as an adjunct to mechanical ventilation in patients with ARDS; the result of a recruitment maneuver is decreased atelectasis.

reflecting Key skill used in critical thinking; involves the ability to "think about thinking" so as to explore assumptions, opinions, biases, and decisions; may be considered introspective or "inward think" or, if retrospective, "past think."

registered pulmonary function technologist (RPFT) Individual previously certified in pulmonary function technology, who has gained appropriate education and/or experience and who has successfully passed the pulmonary function registry examination of the NBRC.

registered respiratory therapist (RRT) Respiratory therapist who has successfully passed the advanced-level exam of the NBRC.

regulator High-pressure reducing valve that is attached to the outlet of a cylinder of gas to reduce the pressure in the cylinder to the standard and safe working pressure of 50 psig.

REM sleep Phase of the sleep cycle marked by the presence of rapid eye movements on electrooculography.

resistance Opposition to a force; ratio of pressure change to flow change; lung characteristic that, with compliance, serves as a determinant in the mechanics of air flow in and out of the lungs.

resistive load Pressure necessary to overcome the flow resistance of the airways (including endotracheal tube) along with lung and chest wall tissue resistance.

resonance Type of sound produced in percussion, which is loud, low, and long such as may be heard over normal lung tissue.

respiratory acidosis Abnormal increase in hydrogen ion concentration associated with an elevated $PaCO_2$.

respiratory alkalosis Abnormal decrease in $[H^+]$ associated with reductions in $PaCO_2$.

respiratory bronchiolitis Rare lung disorder that occurs exclusively in cigarette smokers; characterized by intracytoplasmic golden-brown, granular pigment within alveolar macrophages in respiratory and terminal bronchioles.

respiratory care protocol Patient care plans initiated and implemented by respiratory therapists, one purpose being the standardization of decision making. Respiratory care protocols provide flexibility because clinicians can modify them according to the needs of the patient; also referred to as *therapist-driven protocols (TDPs)*, *patient-driven protocols (PDPs)*, or simply *protocols*.

respiratory distress syndrome Condition of the newborn characterized by dyspnea with cyanosis; the most common cause for hypoxemic respiratory failure in premature neonates.

respiratory exchange ratio (RER) Ratio of $\dot{V}CO_2$ to $\dot{V}O_2$ ($\dot{V}CO_2/\dot{V}O_2$). During steady state exercise at moderate to low levels of exertion, the RER reflects the respiratory quotient (RQ), which is the ratio of $\dot{V}CO_2$ to $\dot{V}O_2$ in the mitochondria.

respiratory inductance plethysmography (RIP) Method for indirectly measuring tidal volume; sensors use a circuit of coiled wire woven into an elastic band and excited by an AC current. Inductance results from alternating electrical currents creating magnetic fields around themselves and those changing magnetic fields altering other electrical currents that they encounter.

respiratory quotient Ratio of carbon dioxide produced to oxygen consumed in the stoichiometric oxidation of a particular substrate.

retinopathy of prematurity Formation of fibrous tissue behind the lens of the eye caused by excessive oxygen administration to premature infants; produces blindness in its worst form; also called *retrolental fibroplasias*.

retrospective studies Studies that look back at records to study what has been done.

Reynolds' number Dimensionless number that describes factors associated with generation of laminar or turbulent flow such that units of measurement cancel each other when consistent units are used; the associated equation demonstrates that density and viscosity are independent factors affecting turbulence. On a qualitative basis, the Reynolds' number describes a ratio of inertial forces to viscous forces.

rhonchus Deep, rumbling respiratory sound that is more pronounced in auscultation on expiration and is usually continuous, caused by air passing through an airway partially obstructed by thick secretions, spasm of the airways, or presence of a tumor; higher-pitched or sibilant rhonchi arise in smaller bronchi, whereas lower-pitched, sonorous or snoring rhonchi are more common with thick secretions in larger airways.

ribonucleic acid (RNA) Nucleic acid in which the sugar component is ribose; acts as the machinery for this protein synthesis process by translating the genetic information stored in DNA into protein structures.

ribosome Tiny cellular particle that provides a surface for protein synthesis and provides enzymes to catalyze the process.

Riemann sum One method for approximating a definite integral; also called the *numerical integration formula*; often used to approximate exhaled volume.

rigid bronchoscopy Bronchoscopy using a nonflexible instrument, particularly useful in assessing patients with massive hemoptysis, removing aspirated foreign bodies (especially in children) and performing laser bronchoscopy or dilatation of tracheobronchial strictures or for retrieval of large volumes of tenacious secretions, necrotic debris, or large biopsy specimens.

rocking bed Unconventional ventilation device with action that has been compared to a piston in a cylinder. As the patient's head moves down, the piston-like viscera and diaphragm slide cephalad within the cylinder-like chest wall, assisting exhalation. In the foot-down position, the abdominal contents and diaphragm slide caudad, assisting inhalation.

roentgenography Radiography; the making of film records of internal structures of the body by passage of x-rays or gamma rays through the body to act on specially sensitized film.

role fidelity Principle dealing with one's faithfulness to duty.

Rule of nines Formula for estimating the amount of body surface covered by burns by assigning 9% to the head and each arm, twice 9% (18%) to each leg and the anterior and posterior trunk, and 1% to the perineum; modified in infants and children because of the different body proportions.

Sanz electrode Modern pH electrode, which has a small sampling chamber, allowing the use of aliquots of blood volume as small as 25 μL.

sarcoidosis Interstitial lung disease in which multiple organ systems usually have noncaseating granulomas; most prevalent ILD of unknown etiology.

saturated Strength of a solution indicating that it contains the maximum amount of a given dissolved solute for given conditions.

saturated fatty acid Naturally occurring fatty acid that has all available bonds of its hydrocarbon chain filled with hydrogen atoms so that the chain contains all single carbon-carbon bonds.

scientific notation Method of abbreviating small or large numbers by the use of exponents to express the number with a power of 10 (positive or negative) factor.

scoliosis Lateral curvature of the spine.

sedative Substance that decreases the level of consciousness.

sedimentation The deposition of insoluble material that settles to the bottom of a container of liquid; for example, gravitational sedimentation occurs when aerosol particles settle out of a suspension as a result of gravity.

segments Subdivisions within each lobe of the lungs; each segment corresponds to the distribution of a specific bronchus.

self-inflating bag Manual resuscitator that inflates automatically and does not require an external gas source to provide positive pressure.

semipermeable membrane Structure that separates the body's various compartments from one another and allows certain fluids and solutes to move freely between them.

serum electrolyte Substance found in the blood that dissociates into ions when melted or dissolved and is able to conduct an electric current; the most common serum electrolytes are the cations Na^+, K^+, Ca^{+2}, and Mg^{+2}; and the anions HCO_3^-, PO_4^-, and SO_4^-.

serum proteins Proteins found in the blood, including albumin, ferritin, and globulins.

service outcomes Categorization of outcomes of respiratory care that includes patient and family satisfaction with care provided by respiratory therapists, time interval from order until performance of sleep study, and respiratory therapist turnover rates.

severe persistent asthma Highest level of the four classes of asthma severity, manifesting symptoms of coughing or wheezing almost continually with frequent exacerbations often persisting for multiple days or sometimes weeks; involves symptoms that limit normal daily activities of living or normal nighttime sleep patterns, with nocturnal symptoms of coughing, wheezing, or breathlessness almost every night and measured FEV_1 or PEF routinely less than 60% of predicted or personal best, while consistently maintaining more than 30% variability in PEF rates.

Severinghaus electrode Modern PCO_2 electrode, a modification of the electrode developed by Stowe in the early 1950s.

sieve bed Columnar space in an oxygen concentrator that holds a porous crystalline aluminosilicate material called zeolite, synthetically produced to contain microscopically sized pores, through which oxygen can pass.

significant figures Measurement whose degree of error is less than one half the place following the figure; for example, the number 6453 ± 40 can be reported as 6400 or 6500 because 40 is less than one half of the hundredths place.

silhouette sign Radiological sign, usually an obliterated border, that helps to localize a radiographic opacity; for example, if the contiguous lung becomes opacified from any cause, the normal contrast between these structures is lost and the border between them is obliterated, producing the silhouette sign.

single blinding Research method in which only the data collectors know whether participants are part of the experimental group or the control group; participants are unaware of their treatment status.

skilled nursing facility (SNF) Institution or part of an institution that fulfills criteria for accreditation outlined by the sections of the Social Security Act that determine the basis for Medicaid and Medicare reimbursement for skilled nursing care.

sleep apnea Sleep disorder in which the person temporarily does not maintain airflow through the nose and mouth, resulting in periodic absence of breathing.

sleep efficiency Sleep study scoring category that measures the amount of time the patient is asleep per EEG criteria divided by the total recording time.

sleep latency Sleep study scoring category that measures the time from when lights are turned off to when the patient falls asleep.

sniff test Test performed under fluoroscopy to confirm the elevation of a hemidiaphragm resulting from paralysis by demonstrating paradoxical upward movement of the affected hemidiaphragm when the patient sniffs rapidly.

solitary pulmonary nodule (SPN) Lesion, seen on a chest radiograph, that is completely surrounded by lung parenchyma, without other radiographic abnormalities such as pleural effusion or adenopathy.

solute Solid, liquid, or gaseous material that is being dissolved.

solution Homogeneous mixture of two or more substances, meaning that the substances mix evenly and occupy the entire volume in equal proportions.

solvent Liquid material into which a solute is dissolved.

spacer Simple open-ended tube or bag that, with sufficiently large device volume, provides space for the pMDI plume to expand by allowing the CFC propellant to evaporate. A spacer can reduce oropharyngeal deposition of drug, ameliorate the bad taste of some medications, eliminate the cold Freon effect, and (in the case of a valved holding chamber) decrease the need for hand-breath coordination.

speaking valve Device designed to enable a patient with a tracheostomy to verbally communicate.

specialty sections Nine divisions within the AARC that support various major subsets of therapists, including the following: Management, Education, Perinatal/Pediatrics, Adult Acute Care, Home Care, Subacute Care, Transport, Diagnostics, and Continuing Care and Rehabilitation; members of the AARC belong to different specialty sections based on their work activities and their personal interests in the profession of respiratory care.

specific gravity Weight of a substance compared with the weight of an equal volume of water.

specific heat Ability of water to lose and gain large amounts of heat with little change in temperature.

spectrophotometry Method that identifies substances by their absorption (also called *extinction*) of specific wavelengths in the electromagnetic spectrum.

spike formation Penetration by a high-energy wave impulse of gas into the center of an airway, enhancing bulk flow of gas in the upper airway and providing a more expansive area of gas mixing the more distal lung.

spontaneous breath Inspiration that is patient-triggered and patient-cycled.

spontaneous breathing trial (SBT) Oldest ventilator weaning technique, in which, traditionally, the patient is removed from the ventilator and humidified supplemental oxygen is provided to the airway; also used to identify extubation readiness.

sputum induction Method of facilitating the coughing up of material from the lungs, often through the administration of bland aerosols. Induced sputum contains a higher proportion of viable cells than spontaneous sputum.

squamous cell carcinoma Slow-growing malignant tumor of scaly or platelike epithelium.

Starling's law of cardiac function Statement that the longer the initial sarcomere length, the greater the force generated with contraction.

statistical analysis Evaluating and attaching meaning to averages (means) and variability (standard deviations) obtained in a study's measurements to allow inference to other settings in a meaningful way.

status asthmaticus Severe attacks of asthma poorly responsive to adrenergic agents and associated with signs or symptoms of potential respiratory failure.

steatorrhea Greater than normal amounts of fat in the feces, characterized by frothy, floating fecal matter with a foul odor; seen in celiac disease, some malabsorption syndromes, and any condition in which fats are malabsorbed by the small intestine.

stereoisomer One of two or more chemical compounds that contain the same atoms linked in the same way but organized differently in space.

sterilization Equipment processing modality that involves the complete killing of all organisms; requires adequate heat and time.

steroid Important lipid group widely distributed throughout the body and involved in many important structural and functional roles.

strain gauge Sensor that changes its electrical resistance in response to an applied force.

stress test Functional study of the coronary circulation using a stressor to induce an imbalance between the coronary blood supply and myocardial demand and a means to detect the ischemic response.

stridor Crowing sound heard during auscultation of the lungs, commonly caused by inflammation and edema of the larynx and trachea heard during postextubation when tracheal damage results in edema formation; commonly associated with croup.

stroke volume Absolute volume of blood ejected during a single contraction of a ventricle.

stroke Cerebrovascular accident; sudden brain abnormality characterized by occlusion by an embolus, thrombus, or cerebrovascular hemorrhage, resulting in ischemia of the brain tissues normally perfused by the damaged vessels.

strong ion difference (SID) Net negative or positive charge exerted by strong ions; principle similar to that of the anion gap, but with the advantage of functioning as an independent variable in acid-base regulation. In physiologic fluids, the main strong electrolytes Na^+, K^+, and Cl^- influence $[H^+]$ by the law of electrical neutrality and the dissociation of water such that in any system at equilibrium the net charge must be zero; thus in a solution of Na^+, K^+, and Cl^- in water: $[Na^+] + [K^+] + [H^+] - [Cl^-] - [OH^-] = 0$.

subacute care Programs and facilities for patients who are sufficiently stabilized and no longer require acute care services, but whose care is too complex for treatments in a traditional nursing center and who present with rehabilitation and/or medically complex needs and require physiological monitoring, including respiratory care services.

subcutaneous Route of drug administration (SC or SQ) that involves the injection of drug into the dermal or subdermal layer of skin, where it is taken up by the capillary bed.

sudden infant death syndrome (SIDS) Unexpected and sudden death during sleep of an apparently normal and healthy infant, and in the absence of physical or autopsy evidence of disease.

surface tension Property of liquid tending to reduce the surface of a liquid to a minimum.

surfactant Surface-active agent, such as soap or detergent, dissolved in water to decrease its surface tension or the tension between the water and another liquid.

surrogate Individual appointed by a patient, in a legal document such as an advanced directive, living will, or medical power of attorney, to make decisions for that patient in the event that the patient cannot.

suspension Liquid mixture in which particles consist of large clumps of molecules; properties include the following: consisting of an insoluble substance dispersed in a liquid, being heterogeneous, not being clear, settling out over time, not passing through filter paper, not passing through membranes.

sweat test Method of assessing sodium and chloride excretion from the sweat glands; often the first test done in the diagnosis of cystic fibrosis; involves stimulating the sweat glands with a drug, such as pilocarpine, and then analyzing the perspiration produced.

synchronized intermittent mandatory ventilation (SIMV) Mode for breath delivery or ventilation in which a mandatory breath rate is set and the patient determines the V_T and rate of the spontaneous breaths between the mandatory breaths, which are synchronized with the patient's spontaneous efforts.

Systeme Internationale d'Unites Internationally agreed system of units in wide but not universal use; generally preferred system, particularly in scientific and health care settings.

systemic lupus erythematosus (SLE) Autoimmune disease that can affect almost all the organ systems; complications are classified as (1) pleuritis and pleural effusions, (2) acute lupus pneumonitis, (3) interstitial lung disease and, (4) respiratory muscle weakness.

systole Period of contraction in the cardiac cycle during which the heart pumps blood into the pulmonary and systemic circulation.

systolic dysfunction Impaired ventricular contractility.

tachypnea Persistent rate of respiration faster than 20 breaths per minute.

tactile fremitus Palpation of vibrations of the chest wall as a patient speaks.

Taylor dispersion Augmented diffusion of gas in situations of parabolic gas flow, resulting in high energy spikes; this augmented diffusion process is facilitated by the increased surface area between two gas streams during HFV.

teaching moment Any opportunity to impart critical and meaningful information to a captive audience.

telemedical record Recording and storage of interactive video technology or live, real-time teleconsultations.

telemetry Data transmission to a remote location; measurement at a distance.

teleologic theory Ethical theory that guides decision making regarding the right or wrong qualities of an action based on consequences of predicted outcomes.

tetralogy of Fallot Congenital cardiac anomaly, consisting of four defects: ventral septal defect, an overriding of the ascending aorta, obstruction of the right ventricular outflow tract, and right ventricular hypertrophy.

tetraplegia Paralysis of all four limbs; quadriplegia.

therapeutic window Range of drug concentration bounded on the low side by the minimum effective concentration and on the high side by the onset of dose-related side effects.

therapist-driven protocol See *respiratory care protocol.*

thermistor Thermometer that can measure extremely small changes in temperature.

thermocouple Apparatus that detects bidirectional airflow at the nose and mouth by sensing the temperature difference between inspired room air and exhaled air that has been warmed to body temperature; an active sensor used to measure temperature.

thermodilution Method of measuring cardiac output by injecting a cold or cool indicator and sampling with a thermistor.

third-party payer Another term for the insurer, when considered as one of the stakeholders in the provision and delivery of health care services. The five major stakeholders in the health care delivery system are the purchasers, the plans, the providers, the payers, and the patient. At times, the role and function of each will overlap and clear lines of distinction are not always apparent.

thorax Lungs, pleura, respiratory muscles, and skeletal elements, including the sternum, ribs, thoracic vertebrae, the clavicles, and the scapulae; within the thorax, the mediastinum contains major blood vessels, the esophagus, and the heart enveloped within the pericardial sac.

Thorpe tube Flow control device that provides an accurate display of flow, provided it is in a vertical position and the inlet pressure is constant. Unlike flow restrictors and Bourdon gauges, pressure-compensated Thorpe tube flow meters display the actual outlet flow in the face of downstream resistance.

thrombolytic therapy (TT) Use of drugs such as tissue plasminogen activator, urokinase, or streptokinase to dissolve an arterial clot.

thrombolytic Any of several drugs that help dissolve clots, such as streptokinase, urokinase, and TPA (tissue plasminogen activator).

time constant Measure of the time required for the passive respiratory system to respond to abrupt changes in ventilatory pressure; expressed in units of time (usually seconds) and calculated as resistance times compliance.

timed walk test Test focused on functional performance that generally involves having a patient walk over a measured course at a set duration of time (for example, 6 or 12 minutes). Patients are encouraged to go as far as they can, and supplemental oxygen is given as necessary.

tissue plasminogen activator Common thrombolytic agent used to help dissolve clots.

tolerance Drug property in which the dose required to achieve the same effect increases gradually over time.

tonometry Measurement of exact gas tensions in whole, fresh blood; because of the unique O_2-binding characteristics of hemoglobin and complex viscosity characteristics of normal fresh blood, whole blood must be carefully tonometered so that exact gas tensions can be prepared for analysis by a blood gas instrument.

total anomalous pulmonary venous return Rare congenital cardiac defect in which the pulmonary veins attach directly to the right atrium or to various veins draining into the right atrium rather than directing flow to the left atrium. Clinical manifestations include cyanosis, pulmonary congestion, and heart failure.

total parenteral nutrition (TPN) Administration of a nutritionally adequate hypertonic solution that can meet the needs of a patient who cannot eat by mouth.

tracheal gas insufflation Injection of fresh gas into the central airways for the purpose of improving the efficiency of alveolar ventilation and/or minimizing the ventilatory requirement.

tracheobronchial stent Bronchoscopically placed slender rod- or threadlike device used as an airway support and indicated as a temporizing or palliative measure in a variety of patients.

tracheostomy tube Hollow, curved tube of metal, rubber, or plastic that is surgically inserted in the trachea to relieve a breathing obstruction.

transactional Reciprocal or "give and take" relationship between two or more individuals in which each alternates between being a sender and a receiver, each engaging in constant sending and receiving in the form of both verbal and nonverbal feedback.

transbronchial biopsy Primary bronchoscopic technique for evaluating the alveolar compartment, particularly useful for sampling peripheral parenchymal masses, diagnosing a select number of specific interstitial lung diseases, and obtaining tissue specimens for culture or documentation of tissue invasion/microorganism pathogenicity.

transbronchial needle aspiration (TBNA) Innovative bronchoscopic diagnostic technique used for staging mediastinal lymph nodes in suspected bronchogenic lung cancer, diagnosing submucosally infiltrating or extrinsically compressing tumors, approaching endobronchial tumors with necrotic or friable outer layers, and increasingly, diagnosing peripheral nodules.

transcutaneous monitor Means of respiratory monitoring of blood gases through electrodes applied to the skin.

transdiaphragmatic pressure (P_{di}) Specific measure of diaphragm strength; made by measuring esophageal (P_{es}) and gastric (P_{ga}) pressures via balloon-tipped catheters placed in the midesophagus and in the stomach, respectively. P_{di} is then calculated as the algebraic subtraction of P_{es} from P_{ga} [$P_{di} = P_{ga} - P_{es}$].

transducer Type of passive or active sensor that converts one form of energy directly into another, particularly, but not exclusively, in most medical applications, converting mechanical into electrical energy, such as with pressure or ultrasound transducers.

transesophageal echocardiography (TEE) Diagnostic test in which a small ultrasound transducer is passed posterior to the heart via the esophagus, allowing close investigation of valvular heart disease because of the proximity of the transesophageal probe to the heart and the absence of intervening anatomic barriers such as the thoracic ribs; includes all aspects of transthoracic imaging, including two-dimensional, Doppler, and color Doppler techniques.

transrespiratory pressure Ventilator or muscle pressure generated to expand the thoracic cage and lungs during inspiration (that is, airway pressure minus body surface pressure).

transthoracic needle aspiration (TNA) Sensitive, specific tissue sampling and testing used in the diagnosis of pneumonia, especially anaerobic. However, TNA and TTA are rarely performed in clinical practice.

transtracheal aspiration (TTA) Technique for collecting sputum that was designed to bypass the upper airway, with its potential contaminants, by inserting a sterile needle directly into the trachea through the cricothyroid membrane and aspirating tracheal secretions.

transtracheal catheter Small-diameter Teflon catheter that is surgically inserted into the trachea between the second and third tracheal rings, connected to a small flange, and held in place by an adjustable chain. Oxygen supply tubing connects directly to the catheter and delivers oxygen into the midtrachea.

trigger Any variable used for initiation of the inspiratory phase (that is, pressure, volume, flow, or time).

triglyceride Most abundant lipid, which functions as the body's most concentrated source of energy; its basic building blocks are a glycerol molecule and three fatty acids.

troubleshooting Key skill used in critical thinking; involves the ability to locate, correct, and process technical problems; sometimes called "technical think."

tube thoracoscopy Placement of a thoracostomy tube (chest tube) into the pleural space to evacuate air or blood in the presence of pneumothorax or hemothorax.

tuberculosis Infection that arises by inhalation of organisms from infected, coughing individuals and manifesting with malaise, fever, or no symptoms.

tumor suppressor genes Genetic unit that is able to reverse the effect of a specific kind of mutation in certain tumors.

turbulent flow Mixture of fluid velocities in which friction has a particularly prominent effect (as opposed to laminar flow) and which varies directly with square of flow rate, and carries a term for friction, implying greater resistance at equivalent flows.

tympany Loud, drumlike, high-pitched sound typically heard over a gastric bubble during percussion examination.

Type I cells Alveolar epithelial cells that form part of the alveolar-capillary complex and cover a large portion (90%) of the alveolar surface, facilitating the movement of gases across this surface.

Type II cells Alveolar cells that produce surfactant and surfactant-associated proteins.

typical pneumonia Any of several pneumonias usually caused by pneumococcus, but also by *H. influenzae, Enterobacteriaceae,* and *S. aureus;* characterized by abrupt onset of chills, high fever, pleuritic chest pain, and cough productive of rusty or purulent sputum; physical signs of consolidation such as bronchial breath sounds and inspiratory crackles are present; lobar or segmental consolidation is seen on the chest radiograph, and leukocytosis is present.

ultrasonic nebulizer Device that uses a piezoelectric crystal, vibrating at a high frequency, to convert electricity to sound waves, creating standing waves in the liquid immediately above the transducer, disrupting the liquid surface, and forming a geyser of aerosolized droplets.

United States Pharmacopeia (USP) Not-for-profit private organization founded to develop officially recognized quality standards for drugs, including medical gases.

units of pulmonary dose toxic (UPDT) Factor used to determine when a patient may be in trouble from oxygen toxicity, and to calculate the dose of oxygen when treatment tables are intermixed while treating a large number of patients in a multiplace hyperbaric chamber.

unmeasured anions Anionic proteins and other substances in serum that are not measured in routine serum electrolyte determinations but whose presence can be suspected by calculating the anion gap.

unsaturated fatty acid Naturally occurring fatty acid that has one or more double carbon-carbon bonds in its hydrocarbon chain because not all of the chain carbon atoms are saturated with hydrogen atoms.

utilitarian theory Most common type of consequential theory; looks for the best outcome, the one that is most useful.

uvulopalatopharyngoplasty (UPPP) Oldest and most commonly performed surgery to treat obstructive sleep apnea.

valance electron The number of electrons in the outer shell of an atom.

valvular heart disease Any valvular lesion or abnormality that can be differentiated hemodynamically into two types, though a combination of both may exist: stenotic lesions due to a decreased valve orifice size/impaired valve opening or regurgitant lesions due to impairment of valve closure.

valvular regurgitation Condition in which a proportion of the ventricular stroke volume moves retrograde through the value.

valvular stenosis Narrowing of a heart valve.

vapor pressure A colligative property of a solution that depends on the number of solute particles dissolved and not on chemical properties; for example, a solute added to a solvent dilutes it, displacing solution surface solvent particles and allowing fewer solvent particles to escape in the form of gas, thereby reducing the vapor pressure.

variance tracking Difference between patient care and outcomes described in the pathway, protocol, or guideline and what actually happened. A method of assessing the difference between what you expect and what you actually find.

vascular resistance Value used to follow relative changes in afterload after cardiac interventions; calculated as $SVR = [(MAP - CVP)/CO] \times 80$.

vasodilator Nerve or agent that causes dilation of blood vessels; also pertaining to the relaxation of the smooth muscle of the vascular system.

vasopressor Agent used to increase blood pressure through a combination of vasoconstriction—causing higher flow resistance, therefore higher pressure—and increased cardiac output.

velocity Property of flow that determines diffusion and is inversely proportional to the square root of the molecular weight of a substance; equivalent to the kinetic energy of a fluid.

venostasis Abnormally slow blood flow through the veins, often seen in distended veins. Also called *phlebostasis.*

venous return Filling of the heart with blood from the venous circulation.

ventilation Process by which gases are moved into and out of the lungs; in respiratory therapy, use of any of several devices that provide assisted respiration and intensive positive-pressure breathing.

ventilation/perfusion ratio Measure of effective gas exchange in the lung, or $\dot{V}/\dot{Q}$ ratio; this ratio should be 1 for the most effective gas exchange to occur.

ventilation-perfusion scan Imaging technique used in the diagnosis of pulmonary embolism.

ventilator assisted individual (VAI)   Patient who requires the assistance of an artificial device for breathing.

ventilator-associated pneumonia   Pneumonia in a mechanically ventilated patient developing after at least 48 hours of mechanical ventilation.

ventilator-induced lung injury   Damage to the lungs sustained during mechanical ventilation and caused by any of several factors, including alveolar overdistention and derecruitment resulting from high peak inflation volume (volutrauma), alveolar collapse (atelectrauma), or cyclical opening of an alveolus during inhalation and closure during exhalation, or by release of inflammatory mediators (cytokines, chemokines), which may translocate into the pulmonary circulation, resulting in systemic inflammation.

ventilatory equivalent   The relationship between minute ventilation and oxygen consumption or carbon dioxide production.

ventilatory period   Cycle time (or total cycle time); the reciprocal of ventilatory frequency.

ventricles   Small cavities making up two of the four chambers of the heart; the right side of the heart receives blood, and the right ventricle pumps it into the pulmonary arteries; blood returning from the pulmonary veins drain into the left atrium, into the left ventricle, and finally into the aorta, which dispenses it into the systemic circulation.

ventricular assist device (VAD)   Mechanical pump that can completely assume the workload of the right or left ventricle and restore normal hemodynamics; allows long-term support of circulation in patients with refractory heart failure and is used primarily as a bridge to transplantation.

ventricular interdependence   Interaction between the left ventricle (LV) and the right ventricle (RV) both in systole and diastole through alterations in systemic and pulmonary venous return, LV and RV dimensional changes, and functional changes.

ventriculography   Radiographic examination of a ventricle of the heart after injection of a radiopaque contrast medium.

Venturi meter   Mechanism designed by Giovanni Venturi to avoid generation of turbulent flow in a region of reduced diameter; ignoring any gravitational forces (minimal in low density gases and constant in a horizontal tube), the pressure gradient across a change of diameter will describe the velocity of flow.

Venturi principle   Physical rule stating that pressure drop across an obstruction can be restored provided that the angle of divergence is less than 15 degrees.

veracity   Principle in which the health care practitioner tells the patient the truth.

verbal expressions   Set of communication tools that includes language, jargon, choice of words or questions, voice tone and quality, and feedback.

vesicular breath sounds   Low-pitched, low-intensity sounds heard over healthy lung issue.

vibration therapy   Maneuver used as part of conventional chest physiotherapy to assist patients in mobilizing secre-tions from the lower respiratory tract. Vibration is performed manually by pressing in the direction of the ribs and soft tissue of the chest during exhalation.

viral pneumonia   Uncommon but often severe pneumonia caused by any of the following viruses: influenza, parainfluenza, respiratory syncytial virus (RSV), cytomegalovirus (CMV), adenovirus, measles, varicella zoster, herpes simplex, Epstein-Barr, and hantavirus.

visceral pleura   Inner layer of pleura adjacent to the external lung tissue.

visceral pleural line   White line in a radiographic image of the pneumothorax that represents the visceral pleura visualized between air in the pleural space laterally and air in the aerated lung medially and that establishes the radiographic diagnosis of pneumothorax.

viscosity   Force applied to interaction between adjacent fluid molecules; also, the internal friction of a fluid, which is independent of the density of that fluid.

volume-controlled ventilation (VCV)   Mode of ventilation in which the ventilator controls the inspiratory flow and tidal volume is determined by the flow and the inspiratory time; in practice, the tidal volume in this mode is delivered regardless of resistance or compliance.

volume of distribution   Means used to convey drug distribution by calculating how much volume the drug would occupy if it were uniformly at its plasma concentration.

volumetric diffusive respiration   Pressure-controlled ventilation with a superimposed subtidal oscillation that facilitates clearance of endobronchial debris.

weaning   Removing a patient gradually from dependency on mechanical ventilation while maintaining an appropriate balance between the load placed on the respiratory muscles and the ability of the muscles to meet that load.

wedge pressure   See *pulmonary artery wedge pressure (PAWP)*.

wellness programs   Programs aimed at keeping people healthy through classes that educate consumers so that they can maintain, and possibly even improve their quality of life, covering such topics as the benefits of diet, good sleep habits, relaxation techniques, routine exercise, diagnostic screenings, and the psychosocial aspects of health, with an emphasis on preventing disease and establishing and maintaining healthy habits for life.

Wheatstone bridge   Circuit used to measure electrical resistance changes in strain gauges built into pressure transducers; solid-state bridge circuits have replaced the classic galvanometer and resistor array.

wheezes   Form of rhonchus characterized by either high- or low-pitched musical quality, caused by high-velocity air flow through a narrowed airway.

whispered pectoriloquy   Voice sound heard during auscultation of the lungs, typically heard with lung consolidation.

work of breathing   Pressure needed to move a volume of gas into the lungs.

yeast   Single-cell, nucleated fungus that reproduces by budding.

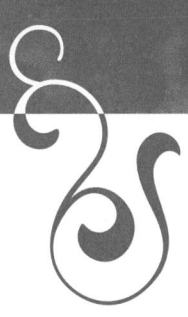

Index

b Indicates boxes; *f* indicates figures; *t* indicates tables.